PART IV
Analytes *299*

PART V
Pathophysiology *681*

Tietz Fundamentals of
Clinical Chemistry

Tietz Fundamentals of Clinical Chemistry

Fifth Edition

Carl A. Burtis, PhD

Chief, Clinical Chemistry
Health Division
Oak Ridge National Laboratory
Oak Ridge, Tennessee;
Clinical Professor of Pathology
University of Utah School of Medicine
Salt Lake City, Utah

Edward R. Ashwood, MD

Professor of Pathology
University of Utah School of Medicine
Director, Clinical Chemistry Laboratories
ARUP Laboratories, Inc.
Salt Lake City, Utah

Consulting Editor
Barbara G. Border, PhD, MT(ASCP)
Associate Professor of Clinical Laboratory Science
Texas Tech University Health Sciences Center
School of Allied Health
Department of Clinical Laboratory Sciences
Lubbock, Texas

W.B. SAUNDERS COMPANY
An Imprint of Elsevier Science
Philadelphia London New York St. Louis Sydney Toronto

W.B. SAUNDERS COMPANY
An Imprint of Elsevier Science

The Curtis Center
Independence Square West
Philadelphia, Pennsylvania 19106

Acquisitions Editor: Karen Fabiano
Developmental Editor: Sarahlynn Lester
Project Manager: Linda McKinley
Associate Production Editor: Kristin Hebberd
Book Design Manager: Judi Lang
Interior/Cover Design: Rokusek Design

Library of Congress Cataloging in Publication Data

Tietz fundamentals of clinical chemistry / [edited by] Carl A. Burtis, Edward R.
Ashwood; consulting editor, Barbara Border.—5th ed.

p.;cm.

Includes bibliographical references and index.

ISBN 0-7216-8634-6 (hard cover: alk. paper)

1. Clinical chemistry. I. Title: Fundamentals of clinical chemistry. II. Burtis, Carl A.
   III. Ashwood, Edward R., 1953- IV. Border, Barbara, PhD. V. Tietz, Norbert W., 1926-
   [DNLM: 1. Chemistry, Clinical. QY 90 T564 2000]

RB40 .F84 2000
616.07′56--dc21

00-061891

TIETZ FUNDAMENTALS OF CLINICAL CHEMISTRY   ISBN 0-7216-8634-6

Last digit is print number: 9 8 7 6 5 4 3 2

CONTRIBUTORS

John J. Albers, PhD
Research Professor of Medicine
Adjunct Research Professor, Pathology
University of Washington
Director, Northwest Lipid Research Laboratories
Seattle, Washington
Lipids, Lipoproteins, and Apolipoproteins

Fred S. Apple, PhD
Professor, Laboratory Medicine and Pathology
University of Minnesota School of Medicine
Medical Director of Clinical Laboratories
Hennepin County Medical Center
Minneapolis, Minnesota
Cardiac Function

K. Owen Ash, PhD
Professor of Pathology
University of Utah Health Science Center
Executive Vice President/Director of Business Development
ARUP Laboratories, Inc.
Salt Lake City, Utah
Laboratory Management

Hassan M.E. Azzazy, PhD, SC(ASCP), DABCC
Assistant Professor
Department of Medical and Research Technology
University of Maryland School of Medicine
Research Associate, Clinical Pathology
University of Maryland Medical Center
Baltimore, Maryland
Amino Acids

Paul S. Bachorik, PhD
Professor of Pediatrics and Associate Professor of Pathology
The Johns Hopkins University School of Medicine
Affiliate Staff Clinical Chemist
The Johns Hopkins Hospital
Baltimore, Maryland
Lipids, Lipoproteins, and Apolipoproteins

Edward W. Bermes, Jr., PhD
Professor Emeritus
Department of Pathology
Loyola University Medical Center
Maywood, Illinois
General Laboratory Techniques, Procedures, and Safety
Specimen Collection and Other Preanalytical Variables

Barbara G. Border, PhD, MT(ASCP)
Associate Professor of Clinical Laboratory Science
Texas Tech University Health Sciences Center
School of Allied Health
Department of Clinical Laboratory Sciences
Lubbock, Texas
Nucleic Acid Techniques
Inherited Disease

Larry D. Bowers, PhD, DABCC
Professor, Department of Pathology and Laboratory Medicine
Director, Athletic Drug Testing and Toxicology Laboratory
Indiana University School of Medicine
Indianapolis, Indiana
Chromatography/Mass Spectrometry

James C. Boyd, MD
Associate Professor of Pathology
University of Virginia Health Sciences Center
Director, Systems Engineering and Specimen Support Services
Associate Director, Clinical Chemistry and Toxicology
University of Virginia Health System
Charlottesville, Virginia
Automation in the Clinical Laboratory

Daniel W. Chan, PhD, DABCC, FACB
Professor of Pathology, Oncology, Radiology, and Urology
The Johns Hopkins University School of Medicine
Director, Clinical Chemistry Division
Department of Pathology
Johns Hopkins Medical Institutions
Baltimore, Maryland
Tumor Markers

Robert H. Christenson, PhD
Professor of Pathology
Professor of Medical and Research Technology
University of Maryland School of Medicine
Director, Clinical Chemistry and Rapid Response
Director, Point of Care Services
University of Maryland Medical Systems
Baltimore, Maryland
Amino Acids

June Y. Cope, MT(ASCP)SC
Send-out Area Supervisor
Dynacare Tennessee Laboratory
University of Tennessee Medical Center at Knoxville
Knoxville, Tennessee
Reference Information for the Clinical Laboratory

Laurence M. Demers, PhD, DABCC
Distinguished Professor of Pathology and Medicine
The Pennsylvania State University College of Medicine
The Milton S. Hershey Medical Center
Director, Clinical Chemistry and Automated Testing Laboratory
Director, Core Endocrine Laboratory
Hershey, Pennsylvania
Pituitary Function
Adrenocortical Function

Richard A. Durst, PhD
Professor of Chemistry and Chairman
Department of Food Science and Technology
Director, Cornell Analytical Chemistry Laboratories
Director, Cornell Institute of Food Science
Cornell University
Geneva, New York
Electrochemistry

Franklin R. Elevitch, MD
Associate Clinical Professor of Laboratory Medicine
University of California—San Francisco Medical Center
San Francisco, California;
President
Health Care Engineering
Palo Alto, California
Clinical Laboratory Informatics

David B. Endres, PhD
Professor of Clinical Pathology
School of Medicine
University of Southern California
Director, Chemistry
USC Pathology Reference Laboratory
Consultant, Chemistry
Los Angeles County—University of Southern California
Medical Center
Los Angeles, California
Mineral and Bone Metabolism

Merle A. Evenson, PhD
Professor of Medicine and Pathology
Laboratory Medicine
University of Wisconsin—Madison
Madison, Wisconsin
Spectrophotometric Techniques

Ann M. Gronowski, PhD
Assistant Professor of Medicine and Pathology
Washington University School of Medicine
Assistant Director, Clinical Chemistry
Barnes-Jewish Hospital
St. Louis, Missouri
Reproductive Endocrine Function

A. Ralph Henderson, MB, ChB, PhD, FRCPath
Professor and Chairman, Medical Biochemistry
College of Medicine and Medical Science
Arabian Gulf University
Consultant, Department of Pathology
Salmaniya Medical Complex
Manama, Bahrain, Arabian Gulf
Principles of Clinical Enzymology
Enzymes
Gastric, Pancreatic, and Intestinal Function

Jonathan W. Heusel, MD, PhD
Resident Physician in Clinical Pathology
Washington University School of Medicine
St. Louis, Missouri
Electrolytes and Blood Gases
Physiology and Disorders of Water, Electrolyte, and Acid-Base Metabolism

A. Myron Johnson, MD
Clinical Professor of Pediatrics and of Obstetrics and Gynecology
University of North Carolina
School of Medicine
Chapel Hill, North Carolina
Proteins

Raymond E. Karcher, PhD
Clinical Chemist
William Beaumont Hospital
Royal Oak, Michigan;
Adjunct Associate Professor
Oakland University
Rochester, Michigan
Electrophoresis

George G. Klee, MD, PhD
Professor of Laboratory Medicine
Mayo Medical School
Consultant, Department of Laboratory Medicine and Pathology
and Department of Health Sciences Research
Mayo Clinic and Mayo Foundation
Rochester, Minnesota
Quality Management
Vitamins
Analytes of Hemoglobin Metabolism—Porphyrins, Iron, and Bilirubin

David D. Koch, PhD, DABCC
Associate Professor
Department of Pathology and Laboratory Medicine
Medical School, University of Wisconsin
Director, Clinical Chemistry
University Hospital and Clinics
Madison, Wisconsin
Evaluation of Methods—with an Introduction to Statistical Techniques

Larry J. Kricka, DPhil, FRCPath
Professor of Pathology and Laboratory Medicine
University of Pennsylvania
Director, General Chemistry Laboratory
Hospital of the University of Pennsylvania
Philadelphia, Pennsylvania
Principles of Immunochemical Techniques

Mary E. Landau-Levine, MD
Scottsdale Pathology Associates
Scottsdale, Arizona
Reproductive Endocrine Function

Vicky A. LeGrys, DA, MT(ASCP), CLS(NCA)
Professor, School of Medicine
University of North Carolina
Chapel Hill, North Carolina
Electrolytes and Blood Gases

Donald B. McCormick, PhD
Fuller E. Callaway Professor Emeritus
Department of Biochemistry
School of Medicine, Emory University
Atlanta, Georgia
Vitamins

David B. Milne, PhD
Retired Research Chemist
USDA/ARS
Grand Forks Human Nutrition Research Center
Grand Forks, North Dakota
Trace Elements

Donald W. Moss, PhD, DSc
Emeritus Professor of Chemical Pathology
University of London
London, England
Principles of Clinical Enzymology
Enzymes

Thomas P. Moyer, PhD
Professor of Laboratory Medicine
Division of Clinical Biochemistry and Immunology
Mayo Clinic
Rochester, Minnesota
Therapeutic Drug Monitoring
Clinical Toxicology

David J. Newman, MSc, PhD, MCB, MRCPath
Honorary Senior Lecturer
Consultant Scientist and Scientific Director
South West Thames Institute for Renal Research
St. Helier Hospital
Surrey, United Kingdom
Nonprotein Nitrogen Metabolites
Renal Function

Kern L. Nuttall, MD, PhD
Consultant in Clinical Chemistry
Salt Lake City, Utah
Electrophoresis
Analytes of Hemoglobin Metabolism—Porphyrins, Iron, and Bilirubin

John F. O'Brien, PhD
Professor of Laboratory Medicine
Mayo Medical School
Consultant, Department of Laboratory Medicine and Pathology
Division of Laboratory Genetics
Mayo Clinic—Mayo Foundation
Rochester, Minnesota
Inherited Disease

Pennell C. Painter, PhD
Professor of Pathology
Department of Pathology
University of Tennessee Medical Center at Knoxville
Technical Director
Dynacare Tennessee Laboratory
Knoxville, Tennessee
Reference Information for the Clinical Laboratory

Theodore Peters, Jr., PhD
Adjunct Assistant Professor, College of Physicians and Surgeons
Columbia University
New York, New York;
Research Scientist Emeritus
Mary Imogene Bassett Hospital
Cooperstown, New York
Evaluation of Methods—with an Introduction to Statistical Techniques

Margaret A. Piper, PhD, MPH, SI(ASCP)
Senior Consultant
Technology Evaluation Center
BlueCross BlueShield Association
Chicago, Illinois
Nucleic Acid Techniques

William H. Porter, PhD
Professor, Pathology and Laboratory Medicine
Director, Clinical Chemistry, Toxicology, and Core Laboratories
University of Kentucky Medical Center
Lexington, Kentucky
Clinical Toxicology

Edward R. Powsner, MD
Formerly of Eastside Nuclear Medicine, P.C.
Grosse Pointe Farms, Michigan
Basic Principles of Radioactivity and Its Measurement

Christopher P. Price, PhD, FRSC, FRCPath
Professor of Clinical Biochemistry
St. Bartholomew's and Royal London School of Medicine and
Dentistry
Director of Pathology
Royal Hospital, NHS Trust
London, United Kingdom
Nonprotein Nitrogen Metabolites
Renal Function

Robert Rej, PhD
Associate Professor, Department of Biomedical Sciences
School of Public Health
State University of New York at Albany
Wadsworth Center for Laboratories and Research
New York State Department of Health
Albany, New York
Liver Function

Nader Rifai, PhD
Associate Professor, Department of Pathology
Harvard Medical School
Director of Clinical Chemistry
Children's Hospital
Boston, Massachusetts
Lipids, Lipoproteins, and Apolipoproteins

Elizabeth M. Rohlfs, PhD
Molecular Laboratory Director
Genzyme Genetics
Framingham, Massachusetts
Proteins

Thomas G. Rosano, PhD, DABCC, DABFT
Professor of Pathology and Laboratory Medicine
Albany Medical College
Director of Laboratory Medicine
Albany Medical Center Hospital
Albany, New York
Catecholamines and Serotonin

Robert K. Rude, MD
Professor of Medicine
University of Southern California
Director, Bone and Mineral Metabolism Laboratory
Orthopaedic Hospital
Los Angeles, California
Mineral and Bone Metabolism

David B. Sacks, MB, ChB, FACP, FRCPath
Associate Professor of Pathology
Harvard Medical School
Medical Director of Clinical Chemistry
Director, Clinical Pathology Training Program
Brigham & Women's Hospital
Boston, Massachusetts
Carbohydrates

Mitchell G. Scott, PhD
Associate Professor of Pathology
Washington University School of Medicine
Associate Director, Clinical Chemistry
Barnes-Jewish Hospital
St. Louis, Missouri
Electrolytes and Blood Gases
Physiology and Disorders of Water, Electrolyte, and Acid-Base
Metabolism

Stewart Sell, MD
Professor of Pathology and Laboratory Medicine
Albany Medical College
Attending Pathologist
Albany Medical Center
Albany, New York
Tumor Markers

Ole Siggaard-Andersen, MD, PhD
Professor of Clinical Biochemistry
University of Copenhagen
Copenhagen, Denmark;
Department of Clinical Biochemistry
Herlev Hospital
Herlev, Denmark
Electrochemistry
Electrolytes and Blood Gases
Physiology and Disorders of Water, Electrolyte, and Acid-Base
Metabolism

Lawrence M. Silverman, PhD
Professor of Pathology and Laboratory Medicine
University of North Carolina School of Medicine
Director, Molecular Pathology
University of North Carolina Hospitals
Chapel Hill, North Carolina
Proteins

Jane L. Smith, MS, MT(ASCP)SI, DLM
Supervisor, Immunology
Dynacare Tennessee Laboratory
University of Tennessee Medical Center at Knoxville
Knoxville, Tennessee
Reference Information for the Clinical Laboratory

Helge Erik Solberg, MD, PhD
Associate Director, Department of Clinical Chemistry
Rikshospitalet
Oslo, Norway
Establishment and Use of Reference Values

Kent A. Spackman, MD, PhD
Associate Professor of Pathology
Oregon Health Sciences University
Portland, Oregon
Clinical Laboratory Informatics

Thomas O. Tiffany, PhD
Chief Executive Officer
Pathology Associates Medical Laboratories
Spokane, Washington
Light Emission and Scattering Techniques

Keith G. Tolman, MD
Professor of Medicine
Director of Hepatology
University of Utah School of Medicine
Salt Lake City, Utah
Liver Function

M. David Ullman, PhD
Research Associate Professor
Department of Biochemistry and Molecular Biology
University of Massachusetts Medical Center
Worcester, Massachusetts;
Research Biochemist
ENRM Veterans Memorial Hospital
Bedford, Massachusetts
Chromatography/Mass Spectrometry

Elizabeth R. Unger, PhD, MD
Acting Chief, Human Papillomavirus Section
Centers for Disease Control and Prevention
Clinical Associate Professor
Department of Pathology and Laboratory Medicine
Emory University School of Medicine
Atlanta, Georgia
Nucleic Acid Techniques

Megan S. Veldee, MS, RD
University of Washington
Seattle, Washington
Nutritional Assessment, Therapy, and Monitoring

Ronald L. Weiss, MD
Professor of Pathology
University of Utah
Director of Laboratories
ARUP Laboratories, Inc.
Salt Lake City, Utah
Laboratory Management

James O. Westgard, PhD
Professor, Department of Pathology and Laboratory Medicine
University of Wisconsin Medical School
Director, Laboratory Quality Management Services
University of Wisconsin Hospital and Clinics
Madison, Wisconsin
Quality Management

Ronald J. Whitley, PhD
Professor, Department of Pathology and Laboratory Medicine
College of Medicine
University of Kentucky
Associate Director of Clinical Chemistry
University of Kentucky Medical Center
Lexington, Kentucky
Hormones
Catecholamines and Serotonin
Thyroid Function
Adrenocortical Function

John C. Widman, PhD
Certified Health Physicist
JCW Enterprises, Inc.
Southfield, Michigan
Basic Principles of Radioactivity and Its Measurement

Donald S. Young, MB, PhD
Professor and Vice-Chair for Laboratory Medicine
University of Pennsylvania
Director, William Pepper Laboratory
Hospital of the University of Pennsylvania
Philadelphia, Pennsylvania
General Laboratory Techniques, Procedures, and Safety
Specimen Collection and Other Preanalytical Variables
Automation in the Clinical Laboratory

NOTICE

Pharmacology is an ever-changing field. Standard safety precautions must be followed, but as new research and clinical experience broaden our knowledge, changes in treatment and drug therapy may become necessary or appropriate. Readers are advised to check the most current product information provided by the manufacturer of each drug to be administered to verify the recommended dose, the method and duration of administration, and contraindications. It is the responsibility of the treating physician, relying on experience and knowledge of the patient, to determine dosages and the best treatment for each individual patient. Neither the publisher nor the editor assumes any liability for any injury and/or damage to persons or property arising from this publication.

THE PUBLISHER

To my daughters:
Laura
Linda
Lisa

and granddaughters:
Kristen
Lindsey

For their love and support.
Life with them has never been dull.

CAB

To my nieces and nephews:
Teresa, Kenneth, and Rebecca
Veronica, Alexander, and Katherine
Michael and Melissa

ERA

FOREWORD

The fifth edition of Burtis and Ashwood's *Tietz Fundamentals of Clinical Chemistry* is a uniquely different book. Although pathologists will find this text useful, it is written primarily for students and instructors of laboratory science programs. With the recent upsurge in information related to laboratory analyses strongly fueled by the Human Genome Program, the proliferation of new methods for exploring human health has refined old concepts, provided new insights, and opened new areas of investigation. As scientists unravel the functions of many newly discovered proteins and the importance of polymorphisms, development of new laboratory tests is expected to continue at a faster pace. The challenge is to synthesize this new information with the established principles of clinical chemistry in a reasonable, understandable, and efficient fashion. The authors of this textbook have integrated the most pertinent new material with basic concepts. Explanations of complicated topics have been simplified, and material considered in depth in other disciplines (for example, hematology and microbiology) is not duplicated. This text, with its many illustrations and diagrams, provides complete coverage of the field of clinical chemistry.

There are as many goals in learning and instructing as there are students and teachers. As an instructor, my challenge is to make the enormous detail of clinical chemistry accessible and understandable while organizing the material to the students' advantage. Most students are interested in what their knowledge of clinical chemistry and laboratory practice will enable them to do, rather than in chemistry for its own sake. The fifth edition of *Tietz Fundamentals* addresses this issue, focusing on providing students with an in-depth yet practical understanding of the laboratory aspects of chemistry. For me, the *Tietz Fundamentals of Clinical Chemistry* books have always been the essential adjunct to my classroom lectures and laboratory instruction. Not only will this textbook continue to be a requirement for my laboratory science students, but it also will remain my primary source of information in the preparation and presentation of my lectures. When clinical training and practice take the place of classroom education, I recommend the textbook to students as an outstanding reference for all aspects of the chemistry laboratory.

I am particularly excited about the fifth edition of *Tietz Fundamentals,* not only because of my participation in its compilation and organization, but also because it presents a formidable amount of material in a user-friendly, accessible format. Although the chapters can be read independently of one another, they are organized into a logical sequence of five sections—Laboratory Principles, Analytical Techniques and Instrumentation, Laboratory Operation, Analytes, and Pathophysiology, and are supported by the Reference Information for the Clinical Laboratory. Cross-referencing among the chapters makes accessible a diversity of information on a similar topic, more straightforward than in previous editions. Other invaluable changes include the addition of a Key Words list at the beginning of each chapter. Not knowing what is considered important, my students often attempt the impossible—to learn everything! The list of Key Words will help students focus on the main points of the chapter, as well as provide them with an excellent quick reference for definitions. The objectives listed at the beginning of the chapters enumerate student learning goals for the material in each chapter. The addition of these objectives will assist me, as an educator, in the clarification of my instructional goals as well, and I intend to use the objectives to prepare study questions and examinations for my students. Another addition that I welcome in this edition is the inclusion of more intensive review of nucleic acid techniques and genetic disease. With predictive laboratory testing taking a more prominent place in the clinical laboratory, it is essential that students and educators become aware of the procedures involved in genetic assessment and how the results obtained from these procedures can be interpreted. The information in these chapters provides an excellent background and serves as a springboard for more detailed coursework.

Barbara G. Border, PhD, MT(ASCP)

PREFACE

As the discipline of clinical laboratory science and medicine has evolved and expanded, each new edition of *Tietz Fundamentals of Clinical Chemistry* has been revised to reflect these changes. The fifth edition of this series is no exception, as we have made significant revisions in its format and content. **First,** we added ten new chapters—four to the Analytes and six to the Pathophysiology sections. **Second,** several new authors joined our team of veterans from the fourth edition to revise and produce chapters that reflect the state of the art in their respective fields. Consequently, this new edition covers many new topics and updates information on older ones. With these changes, the fifth edition now contains 46 chapters that are grouped into five sections, entitled Laboratory Principles, Analytical Techniques and Instrumentation, Laboratory Operation, Analytes, and Pathophysiology and a final chapter that provides laboratory reference information. **Third,** to each chapter was added a list of Learning Objectives and a list of Key Words with definitions. Many of the definitions were obtained from the 28th edition of *Dorland's Illustrated Medical Dictionary*, with permission kindly granted by W.B. Saunders Company, Philadelphia, Pennsylvania. **Finally,** digital technology was used to produce this edition, with each chapter being electronically submitted, edited, and typeset. The Internet also was utilized in the preparation of this edition, as authors used it to find information and sources of products. In addition, the reader will note that references to electronic sources of information are found throughout the text. As editors, we found that the availability of Medline online (http://www.ncbi.nlm.nih.gov/PubMed/) was an invaluable resource, one that we used extensively to find and check references.

To assist us in preparing the fifth edition, we invited Barbara G. Border, PhD, MT(ASCP), to join our editorial team as an educational consultant. An educator from the School of Allied Health at Texas Tech University, Professor Border has used previous editions of *Tietz Fundamentals of Clinical Chemistry* in teaching Medical Technology and Medical Laboratory Assistant students. Because of her experience with using *Tietz Fundamentals* as a teaching text and her perspective as an educator, Professor Border's advice and assistance were invaluable to us as we revised and produced the fifth edition. Many of the significant changes that have been made are the results of her recommendations.

We greatly appreciate the opportunity provided to us to prepare the fifth edition of *Tietz Fundamentals of Clinical Chemistry*. It has been an exciting, challenging, and educational experience. We trust that this edition will live up to the reputation and success of its distinguished predecessors. We have enjoyed working with the team of dedicated authors that have spent many hours preparing comprehensive chapters that are authoritative and timely. We believe that they have produced a textbook that is reflective of the diverse, technical, and practical nature of the current practice of clinical laboratory science and medicine.

We also have benefited from and enjoyed working with the staff and consultants of Harcourt Health Sciences, especially Karen Fabiano, Acquisitions Editor; Sarahlynn Lester, Developmental Editor; Linda McKinley, Project Manager; and Kristin Hebberd, Associate Production Editor. Their cooperation, sound advice, and professional dedication are gratefully acknowledged.

Carl A. Burtis
Edward R. Ashwood

CONTENTS

Tietz Fundamentals of
Clinical Chemistry

PART I

Laboratory Principles

CHAPTER 1

General Laboratory Techniques, Procedures, and Safety

EDWARD W. BERMES, Jr., PhD, and DONALD S. YOUNG, MB, PhD

Objectives

1. Distinguish between the different types of water used in the laboratory based on preparation and use.
2. List the different available pipets, based on their use, type, and capability, and calibrate them using several methods.
3. Recognize, name, and state the use of common laboratory glass and plasticware.
4. Understand centrifugation and balances and the terminology related to each and calculate RCF and rpm when given the appropriate information.
5. State the properties of solutes, solvents, and solutions and express and calculate solution concentration using various methods.
6. Define units of measure and relate the differences among various units.
7. Recognize and interpret various laboratory hazard signage and state the appropriate course of action when an accident occurs.
8. Describe Universal Precautions and the OSHA Hazard Exposure Plan.

Key Words

Analyte A substance or constituent on which the laboratory conducts testing

Analysis The procedural steps performed to determine the kind or amount of analyte in a specimen

Balance An instrument used for weighing

Blood-Borne Pathogens Pathogenic microorganisms present in human blood, including but not limited to, hepatitis B virus (HBV) and human immunodeficiency virus (HIV)

Buffer A solution or reagent that resists a change in pH with the addition of either an acid or a base

Chemical Hygiene Plan (CHP) A set of written instructions describing the procedures required to protect employees from health hazards related to hazardous chemicals in the laboratory

Centrifugation The process of molecule separation by size or density through the use of centrifugal forces generated by a spinning rotor; G-forces of several hundred thousand times gravity being generated in ultracentrifugation

Certified Reference Material (CRM) A reference material in which one or more values are certified by a technically valid procedure and that is accompanied by or traceable to a certificate or other document by a certifying body

Desiccator A container filled with a hydrophilic compound (desiccant) and used to store substances in a water-free environment

Dilution The process (diluting) involving reduction of a solute's concentration through the addition of additional solvent

Exposure Control Plan   A set of written instructions describing the procedures necessary to protect laboratory employees against potential exposure to blood-borne pathogens

Gravimetry   The process used to measure the mass (weight) of a substance

Material Safety Data Sheet (MSDS)   A technical bulletin that contains information about a hazardous chemical, such as chemical composition, chemical and physical hazards, and precautions for safe handling and use

Metric System   A system of weights and measures based on the meter as a standard unit of length

Primary Reference Material   A thoroughly characterized, stable, homogeneous material of which one or more physical or chemical properties have been determined experimentally within stated measurement uncertainties; used in the calibration of definitive methods; the development, evaluation, and calibration of reference methods; and the assignation of values to secondary reference materials

Reagent Grade Water   Water purified and classified for specific analytical uses

Reference Material   A material or substance in which one or more physical or chemical properties are sufficiently well established to be used for the calibration of an apparatus, verification of a measurement method, or assignation of values to materials; types include *certified*, *primary*, and *secondary* materials

Relative Centrifugal Force (RCF)   The weight of a particle in a centrifuge relative to its normal weight

Secondary Reference Material   A reference material that contains one or more analytes in a matrix that reproduces or stimulates the expected matrix; used primarily for internal and external quality assurance purposes

Système International d'Unites (SI)   An internationally adopted system of measurement, the units of which are called *SI units*

Standard Reference Material (SRM)   A certified reference material (CRM) that is certified and distributed by the National Institute of Standards and Technology (NIST), an agency of the U.S. government formerly known as the *Bureau of Standards*

Test   In the clinical laboratory, a qualitative, semiqualitative, quantitative, or semiquantitative procedure for the detection of the presence or the measurement of the quantity of an analyte in a specimen

Universal Precautions   An approach to infection control based on the concept that all human blood and certain human body fluids should be treated as if known to be infectious for HIV, HBV, and other blood-borne pathogens

---

To reliably perform qualitative and quantitative analyses on body fluids and tissues, the clinical laboratorian must understand the following basic principles and procedures that affect the analytical process and operation of the clinical laboratory.

■ CHEMICALS AND RELATED SUBSTANCES

Laboratory chemicals are available in a variety of grades. The solutes and solvents used in analytical work are known as *reagent grade chemicals*, among which water is a solvent of primary importance. The International Union of Pure and Applied Chemistry (IUPAC) has established the criteria for primary standards. The National Institute of Standards and Technology (NIST) has a number of standard reference materials (SRMs) available for the clinical chemistry laboratory, and the College of American Pathologists also supplies some CRMs. The National Committee for Clinical Laboratory Standards (NCCLS) has established a standard for reagent grade water[14] and published several documents that describe and discuss the role of reference materials in the National Reference System for the Clinical Laboratory.[9-11]

CRMs of clinical relevance also are available from the World Health Organization and the Institute for Reference Materials and Measurements in Geel, Belgium.[18]

Reagent Grade Water

The preparation of most reagents and solutions used in the clinical laboratory requires "pure" water. Single-distilled water fails to meet the specifications for Type I Clinical Laboratory Reagent Water established by the NCCLS.[14]

NCCLS specifications for reagent grade water are given in Table 1-1. Although in many laboratories the term *deionized water* may have replaced *distilled water*, the use of both terms should be discouraged because they describe methods of preparation and do not in themselves reflect the quality of the final product. The term **reagent grade water,** followed by the designation of type (I through III), better defines the specifications of the water and is independent of the method of preparation.

In general, no single process of purification produces water that meets the rigid specifications for reagent grade water Type I set forth by the NCCLS (see Table 1-1). The processes or any combination thereof may be used in the preparation of reagent grade water as long as the final prod-

TABLE 1-1   NCCLS Specifications for Reagent Grade Water

Factor	Type I	Type II	Type III
Microbiological content:* cfu/mL (maximum)	10	10^3	NS
pH	NS	NS	5.0 to 8.0
Resistivity†: MΩ -cm, 25 °C	10 (in-line)	1.0	0.1
Silicate: mg SiO_2/L (maximum)	0.05	0.1	1.0
Particulate matter‡	Water passed through 0.22-μm filter	NA	NA
Organics§	Water passed through activated carbon or distillation or reverse osmosis	NA	NA

From National Committee for Clinical Laboratory Standards: Preparation and Testing of Reagent Water in the Clinical Laboratory. 2nd edition. Approved Standard. NCCLS Document C3-A3. Wayne, Pa, National Committee for Clinical Laboratory Standards, 1997.

NCCLS, National Committee for Clinical Laboratory Standards; *NS*, not specified; *NA*, not available; *cfu*, colony forming units; *MΩ/cm*, Mohm centimeter.

*The microbiological content of viable organisms, as determined by total colony count after incubation at 36 ± 1 °C for 14 hours, followed by 48 hours at 25 ± 1 °C, and reported as cfu/mL

†The electrical resistance in ohms measured between opposite faces of a 1.00-cm cube of an aqueous solution at a specified temperature; for these specifications, the resistivity is corrected for 25 °C and reported in MΩ/cm. The higher the amount of ionizable materials, the lower the resistivity and the higher the conductivity.

‡When water is passed through a membrane filter with a mean pore size of 0.2 μm, it is considered to be free of particulate matter.

§When water is passed through a bed of activated carbon, it is considered to contain minimal organic material.

uct meets the specifications. The combination selected usually is dictated in part by the quality of the source water and in part by the intended use of the water.

Preparation of reagent grade water

Distillation, ion exchange, and reverse osmosis are processes used to prepare reagent grade water. In practice, water often is filtered before any of the previously mentioned processes are used.

Distillation

Distillation is the process by which a liquid is vaporized and condensed to purify or concentrate a substance or separate a volatile substance from less volatile substances. It is the oldest method of water purification. Problems with distillation in the preparation of reagent water include the carryover of volatile impurities and entrapped water droplets that may contain impurities into the purified water. This carryover results in contamination of the distillate with volatiles, sodium, potassium, manganese, carbonates, and sulfates. As a result, water treated with distillation alone does not meet the specific conductivity requirement of Type I water.

Ion exchange

Ion exchange is a process that removes ions to produce mineral-free deionized water. Such water is prepared most conveniently with commercial deionizing equipment, which ranges in size from small, disposable cartridges to large, resin-containing tanks. Deionization is accomplished by the passing of feed water through columns containing insoluble resin polymers that exchange H^+ and OH^- ions for the impurities present in ionized form in the water. The columns may contain cation exchangers, anion exchangers, or a mixture of cation- and anion-exchange resins in the same container, known as a *mixed-bed resin exchanger*. A typical cation-exchange resin reacts as follows:

$$(RSO_3)H + Na^+ \rightarrow (RSO_3)Na + H^+$$

where R is the matrix on which the cation-exchange functional groups are attached.

The structure of an anion-exchange resin with a quaternary ammonium functional group is as follows:

$$(RNR'_3)OH + Cl^- \rightarrow (RNR'_3)Cl + OH^-$$

Depending on how they are configured, deionizers are capable of producing water that has specific resistance exceeding 1 to 10 Mohm/cm (MΩ/cm).

Reverse osmosis

Reverse osmosis is a process by which water is forced through a semipermeable membrane that acts as a molecular filter. The membrane removes 95% to 99% of organic compounds, bacteria, and other particulate matter and 90% to 97% of all ionized and dissolved minerals, but fewer of the gaseous impurities. Although the process is inadequate for the production of reagent grade water for the laboratory, it may be used as a preliminary purification method.

Quality, use, and storage of reagent grade water

Type III water may be used for glassware washing. (Final rinsing, however, should be done with the water grade suitable for the intended glassware use.) Type III water also may be used for certain qualitative procedures, such as those used in general urinalysis.

Type II water is used for general laboratory **tests** that do not require Type I water. Storage should be kept to a minimum, and storage and delivery systems should be constructed to ensure minimal chemical or bacterial contamination.

Type I water should be used in test methods requiring minimal interference and maximal precision and accuracy. Such procedures may include trace metal determination, enzyme measurements, electrolyte measurements, and preparation of all calibrators and solutions of reference materials. This water should be used immediately after production. No specifications for storage systems for Type I water are given because maintenance of the high resistivity during drawing off and storage of water is impossible.

Specific systems for the preparation of reagent grade water

Type I reagent water, with a neutral pH and 170 ppm of total dissolved solids, is produced from municipal feed water through the use of a primary dual filtration cartridge to remove particulate matter and organic compounds, followed by two tanks containing a mixed-bed ion-exchange resin. The water then passes through a $0.2-\mu m$ membrane filter. A conductivity light installed between the two ion-exchange tanks is turned off automatically when the resistance of the effluent from the first tank drops below 200,000 Ω/cm. The second tank then "polishes" the water to yield water with a resistance of up to 15 MΩ/cm. When the deionizers are exchanged, the first tank is removed for regeneration and replaced by the second tank, and the new tank takes over the second position. The spigot for water delivery should be within a few feet of the final filter.

Testing for water purity

At a minimum, water should be tested for microbiological content, pH, resistivity, and soluble silica.[1]

Reagent Grade or Analytical Reagent Grade Reagents

Chemicals that meet specifications of the American Chemical Society are described as reagent or analytical reagent grade. These chemicals are available in two forms—lot-analyzed reagents, in which each individual lot is analyzed and the actual amount of impurity reported, and maximum impurities reagents, for which maximum impurities are listed.

Ultra-pure reagents

Selected chemicals are available that have been especially purified to meet specific needs. No uniform designation exists for these chemicals and organic solvents. Terms such as *spectrograde, nanograde,* and *HPLC pure* have been used. Data of interest to the user are supplied with the reagent.

Other designations of chemical purity

Several other designations of chemical purity exist. In general, chemicals so designated often are not of sufficient purity for use as analytical reagents.

TABLE 1-2	Common Grades of Organic Solvents
Grade	Description
Practical	Contains some impurities; usually adequate for most organic preparations
USP and NF	Meet standards established by USP or NF; may contain impurities for which testing has not been performed
Chemically pure	Is almost as pure as reagent grade chemicals
Spectroscopic	Is spectrally pure in the visible, ultraviolet, and near- and mid-infrared ranges
Chromatographic	Contains a minimal purity of greater than 99% as determined by gas chromatography; no single impurity exceeding 0.2%
Reagent	Certifiably contains impurities below levels established by the Committee on Analytical Reagents of the American Chemical Society

USP, United States Pharmacopeia; *NF,* National Formulary.

Chemically pure is a designation that fails to reveal the tolerance limits of impurities, and the practices that different manufacturers follow in the use of this designation are not uniform. Manufacturers use the term *highest purity* for organic chemicals that they have purified to as great a degree as is practical. The purity usually is determined by measurement of melting or boiling points. However, highest-purity chemicals occasionally may have to be used in clinical chemical analyses when higher-purity biochemicals are not available.

USP and NF grade are chemicals produced to meet specifications set down in the United States Pharmacopeia (USP) or the National Formulary (NF). In many cases these compounds may be very pure and are used in chemical **analysis** and in the preparation of various reagents, but high purity cannot be assumed in all instances.

Purified, practical, technical, or commercial grade chemicals should not be used in clinical chemical analysis without prior purification.

Purity of organic reagents

The purity of commercially obtained organic reagents for clinical chemistry purposes is generally inferior to that of inorganic reagents. In addition, some organic compounds oxidize or decompose on standing, and the amount of impurities from this cause depends on how long a bottle of reagent has been opened or stored and under what conditions. Stability often is improved when the compounds are stored in amber bottles and refrigerated; however, phenols and amines oxidize on standing and tend to darken even when refrigerated.

Organic solvents are available in several grades of purity. The common grades are listed in Table 1-2. The degree of purity required for the solvent depends on the application.

TABLE 1-3	SRMs Used in the Clinical Laboratory (Revised)*	

Analyte	SRM Number
Antiepilepsy drug level assay (phenytoin, ethosuximide, phenobarbital, and primidone)	900
Human serum	909b
Sodium pyruvate	910
Cholesterol	911b
Urea	912a
Uric acid	913
Creatinine	914a
Calcium carbonate	915a
Bilirubin	916a
D-Glucose (dextrose)	917a
Potassium chloride	918a
Sodium chloride	919a
D-Mannitol	920
Cortisol (hydrocortisone)	921
Lithium carbonate	924a
VMA (4-hydroxy-3-methoxymandelic acid)	925
Bovine serum albumin	927c
Lead nitrate	928
Magnesium gluconate, clinical	929
Glass filters	930d
Thermometer, clinical laboratory	934
Iron metal	937
4-Nitrophenol	938
Lead in blood	955b
Electrolytes in frozen human serum	956a
Glucose in frozen human serum	965
Fat-soluble vitamins in human serum	968b
Angiotensin 1 (human)	998
Marijuana metabolite in urine	1507b
Benzoylecgonine (cocaine metabolite) in freeze-dried urine	1508a
Multidrugs of abuse in urine	1511
Tripalmitin	1595
Anticonvulsant drug level assay (valproic acid and carbamazepine)	1599
Ethanol-water solution	1828
Lipids in frozen human serum	1951a
Gallium	1968
Morphine-codeine in urine	2381
Morphine glucuronide in urine	2382
Amino acids/hydrochloric acid	2389
Toxic metals in urine	2670
Urine fluorine (freeze-dried)	2671a
Urine mercury (freeze-dried)	2672
Cotinine in human urine (freeze-dried)	8444
Drugs of abuse in powdered human hair	8449

SRM, Standard reference material.

*Additional SRMs and further information may be obtained via the National Institute of Standards and Technology Special Publication 260 (1997-1998) at the U.S. Department of Commerce, National Institute of Standards and Technology, Building 202, Room 2094, Gaithersburg, MD 20899. Alternatively, the National Institute of Standards and Technology may be accessed on the World Wide Web (www.nist.gov).

Because of the variety of grades available, the redistilling of reagents in the clinical laboratory is rarely necessary. Organic solvents in general should be considered potential health hazards, and thus inhalation of fumes should be avoided. Unless a solvent is known to be nonflammable, it should be considered a potential fire hazard. For example, diethyl ether has a particularly high flammability rating. The maximum quantities of solvents that should be stored in particular types and sizes of containers are described in the Occupational Safety and Health Administration (OSHA)[16] regulations and are detailed in this chapter's discussion on safety.

Reference Materials

Reference materials are materials or substances with physical or chemical properties that are established sufficiently for use as calibrators, the verification of a measurement method, or the assignation of values. Classes include primary, secondary, and certified (CRM).

Primary reference material

A **primary reference material**[9] is a highly purified chemical that is weighed out directly for the preparation of a solution of specified concentration or for the calibration of solutions of unknown strength. Each of these materials is supplied with a certificate of analysis for each lot. A primary reference material is a stable substance of definite composition that is dried, preferably at 104 to 110 °C, without a change in composition. It must not be hygroscopic. The IUPAC has proposed a degree of 99.98% purity for primary reference materials.

Secondary reference material

A **secondary reference material** is a material with values that have been assigned by a formal process of value transfer from a primary reference material and is used to assign values to tertiary reference materials.[9]

Certified reference material

A **certified reference material (CRM)** is a material that has had one or more of its values certified by a technically valid procedure. Each CRM is accompanied by or traceable to a certificate or other document by a certifying body. Each certified value is accompanied by an uncertainty at a stated level of statistical confidence. The term **standard reference material** is a CRM and a trademark name of the NIST. SRMs and CRMs for clinical laboratories are available from the NIST (Table 1-3) and the European Institute for Reference Materials and Methods.[18]

Desiccants and use of desiccators

Often in the clinical laboratory, drying a chemical before using it is necessary. Various techniques are used to dry chemicals, including placement into drying ovens, or

TABLE 1-4	Chemistry and Activity of Desiccants					
Drying Agent	Activity*	Capacity	Deliquescence	Easy Regeneration	Chemical Reaction
Phosphorus pentoxide	0.02	Very low	Yes	No	Acidic
Barium oxide	0.6 to 0.8	Moderate	No	No	Alkaline
Alumina	0.8 to 1.2	Low	No	Yes	Neutral
Magnesium perchlorate (anhydrous)	1.6 to 2.4	High	Yes	No	Neutral
Calcium sulfate (Drierite)	4 to 6	Moderate	No	Yes	Neutral
Silica gel	2 to 10	Low	No	Yes	Neutral
Potassium hydroxide (stick)	10 to 17	Moderate	Yes	No	Alkaline
Calcium chloride (anhydrous)	330 to 380	High	Yes	No	Neutral

*Micrograms of residual water per liter of air at 30 °C

desiccators, for a length of time. Various desiccants are used (Table 1-4), but compounds such as granular calcium chloride that produce dust in desiccators should be avoided. Drying agents that incorporate cobalt chloride or another moisture-sensitive salt to indicate exhaustion are preferable to those that do not contain such indicators. Silica gel and anhydrous calcium sulfate (Drierite) are sold with indicators included.

Desiccators should be opened carefully. Ordinary desiccators often contain air at less than atmospheric pressure as a result of the cooling of warm air formed from hot samples added before closure. If such a desiccator is not opened slowly, the inrush of air may create drafts sufficient to dislodge materials from open vessels or stir up dust particles from the drying agent that subsequently may settle in the vessels being stored.

■ LABORATORYWARE

Most laboratoryware used in the clinical laboratory, including beakers, bottles, burets, flasks, graduated cylinders, funnels, centrifuge tubes, tubing, and pipets, is manufactured of either glass or plastic, both of which may be made of one of several different types. Various types of tubing are used in the laboratory to connect pieces of equipment.

Glassware

Various types of glass are used in the manufacture of laboratory glassware, and various processes are used to clean the glass.

Types of glass

The thermal properties of glass are altered significantly by the addition of boron oxide (B_2O_3). Glassware containing boron oxide, known as *borosilicate glass,* is used extensively in clinical laboratories. Borosilicate glass is free from zinc-group elements and heavy metals (arsenic and antimony) and resists heat, corrosion, and thermal shock. Because its dimensions change very little with temperature, this type of glassware should be used whenever heating or sterilization by heat is to be performed.

Boron-free glassware has high resistance to alkali and was developed particularly for use with strongly alkaline solutions. Its thermal resistance is much less than that of borosilicate glass, and therefore it must be heated and cooled carefully. Its primary use should be with solutions or digestions involving strong alkali. This glass is often referred to as *soft glass.*

Corex (Corning) is a special alumina-silicate glass that has been strengthened chemically rather than thermally. It is at least six times stronger than borosilicate glass. Corex laboratory glassware is also harder than conventional borosilicates and more resistant to clouding due to alkali and scratching. This glass also is used for higher-temperature thermometers (>250 °C), graduated cylinders, and centrifuge tubes.

Vycor (Corning) brand laboratory glassware is recommended for use in applications involving high temperatures, drastic heat shock, and extreme chemical treatment with acids and dilute alkalis. This transparent glassware is resistant to attack by all acids except hydrofluoric. Even in the upper temperature range it is more resistant to alkali than is borosilicate glass. Vycor ware is used primarily in ashing and ignition techniques. It can be heated to 900 °C and withstand the shock of a temperature drop from 900 to 0 °C.

Low-actinic glassware contains materials that usually impart an amber or red color to the glass and thus reduce the exposure of the contents to light. This glass was developed to provide a highly protective laboratory glassware for the handling of materials such as bilirubin, carotene, and vitamin A that are sensitive to light in the 300- to 500-nm range.

Flint glass is a soda-lime glass composed of a mixture of silicon, calcium, and sodium oxides. This type of glass is the least expensive of all glasses and is fabricated readily in a wide variety of shapes. Such glass has poor resistance to high temperatures and sudden changes in temperature, and its resistance to chemical attack is only fair. Because this glass is relatively easy to melt and shape, it has been used to make bottles and some disposable laboratory glassware. Users of flint-glass pipets must rinse the pipets before use if the pipets have not been water-rinsed by the manufacturer.

Cleaning of glassware

In many institutions the glassware is washed in an automatic washer, rinsed in a special rinse cycle, and placed in an automatic dryer. The equipment manufacturer should be able to recommend a detergent that is compatible with the equipment and effective with the local water supply. Residual detergent may be detected through measurement of the pH of water added to the glassware or use of a dilute solution of an acid-base indicator that demonstrates an alkaline residue.

For general washing without an automatic washer, most laboratories prefer detergents that are nonionic, metal free, and not highly alkaline. Again, special care must be taken to ensure adequate rinsing. All clean laboratoryware should drain with a continuous thin film of water. Imperfect wetting, or the presence of discrete droplets of water, indicates that the vessel is not sufficiently clean.

Ultrasonic cleaners also may be used to supplement the action of detergent. In baths where extremely high-frequency vibrations cause the soil break free from the walls of the vessel, neutral detergents usually are preferred.

Air-drying or oven-drying at temperatures below 100 °C, with the laboratoryware placed bottom up, is the preferred drying method. Occasionally, rinsing the glassware with a water-miscible organic solvent and subsequently exposing it to a stream of air or nitrogen is desirable. To prevent contamination, the solvent must be of high quality, and the gas must be pure. Storage should be such that the laboratoryware is protected from dust.

Plasticware

Many types of laboratoryware are manufactured from plastic and possess unique qualities that make them ideal for use in situations that require high corrosion resistance and unusual impact and tensile strength. The physical and chemical properties of various resins used in the preparation of laboratory plasticware are listed in Table 1-5.

Whenever possible, plastics should be used in place of glass; plasticware, unlike glass, is unbreakable and does not release ions into solutions. However, plasticware does tend to bind various solutes and leach surface-bound constituents into solutions subsequently prepared in them.

Types of plasticware

Polyethylene and polypropylene are types of plastic used in most disposable plasticware. Polypropylene has a distinct advantage in that it withstands higher temperatures and can be sterilized; however, it absorbs pigments and tends to become discolored.

Polyethylene is permeable to water vapor, and even in tightly stoppered bottles evaporation may occur, resulting in an increased concentration of the reagents and calibrators. In practice, small volumes of reagent should never be stored in oversized plastic bottles for long periods. Polyethylene also is not completely inert and may bind or absorb proteins, dyes, stains, iodine, and picric acid. Slow reduction of ceric and cuprous ions has been observed in solutions stored in polyethylene bottles. Such solutions also may develop significant fluorescence after storage in plastic containers for extended periods.

The polyolefins are a unique group of resins that are chemically relatively inert (see Table 1-5). Although concentrated sulfuric acid slowly does attack polyethylene at room temperature, the polyolefins as a group are unaffected

---

TABLE 1-5	**Physical Properties of Plastics**						
Plastic	Maximum Usable Temperature (°C)	Brittleness Temperature (°C)	Transparency	Autoclavability	Specific Gravity	Flexibility	Microwavability*
Low-density polyethylene	80	−100	Translucent	No	0.92	Excellent	Yes
High-density polyethylene	120	−100	Translucent	No	0.95	Rigid	No
Polypropylene	135	0	Translucent	Yes	0.90	Rigid	Yes
Polymethylpentene ("TPX")	175	20	Clear	Yes	0.83	Rigid	Yes
Teflon FEP	205	−270	Translucent	Yes	2.15	Excellent	Marginal
Tefzel ETFE	150	−100	Translucent	Yes	1.70	Moderate	Yes
Polycarbonate	135	−135	Clear	Yes†	1.20	Rigid	Marginal
PVC	70†	−30	Clear	No‡	1.34	Rigid	Yes
Polystyrene	90	−20	Clear	No	1.05	Rigid	No
Polysulfone	165	−100	Clear	Yes	1.24	Rigid	Yes

Courtesy Nalgene Labware, Rochester, N.Y.

FEP, Fluorinated ethylene propylene; *ETFE,* ethylene-tetrafluoroethylene; *PVC,* polyvinyl chloride.

*Based on a 5-minute test at 600 watts of exposed, empty laboratoryware.

†Sterilizing reduces mechanical strength. Do not use PVC vessels for vacuum applications if they have been autoclaved.

‡Except for PVC tubing, which will withstand temperatures of 121 °C and can be autoclaved.

by acids, alkalis, salt solutions, and most aqueous solutions. Aromatic, aliphatic, and chlorinated hydrocarbons cause moderate swelling at room temperature; organic acids, essential oils, and halogens slowly penetrate these plastics. Strong oxidizing agents attack this group of resins at elevated temperatures only.

Polycarbonate is twice as strong as polypropylene and may be used at temperatures ranging from -100 to $+160$ °C. However, it lacks resistance to some chemicals and is unsuitable for use with strong acids, bases, or oxidizing agents. Polycarbonate also is dissolved by chlorinated aliphatic and aromatic hydrocarbons. Polycarbonate resin is insoluble in aliphatic hydrocarbons, some alcohols, and dilute aqueous acids and salts. Because laboratoryware molded from this resin is clear as glass and shatterproof, polycarbonate is used extensively in centrifuge tubes and graduated cylinders.

Fluorocarbon resins (Teflon) have unique qualities that make them almost chemically inert and therefore ideal when high corrosion resistance at extreme temperatures is essential. Because Teflon (fluorinated ethylene propylene [FEP]) resists extreme temperatures ranging from -270 to $+255$ °C, bottles and beakers made of this material are suitable for use in cryogenic experiments. Laboratoryware made of fluorocarbon resins (for example, Teflon) is pure, translucent, white, and inert to such corrosive reagents as boiling aqua regia, nitric and sulfuric acids, boiling hydrocarbons, ketones, esters, and alcohols. Because of its unique antiadhesive properties and nonwettable surface, Teflon is used in the manufacture of self-lubricating stopcocks, stirring bars, bottlecap liners, and tubing. It is also easy to clean and dries quickly, but it is easily scratched and warped.

Cleaning of plasticware

Linear polyethylene, polypropylene, Teflon, polymethylpentene, and polycarbonate plastics are cleaned in ordinary glassware washing machines. Ultrasonic cleaners also may be used, provided the plasticware does not rest directly on the transducer diaphragm. The use of abrasive cleaners and strong oxidizing agents should be avoided.

Polypropylene, Teflon, and polymethylpentene may be autoclaved repeatedly under normal conditions. Polycarbonate shows some loss of mechanical strength when autoclaved; thus the procedure should be limited to 20 minutes at 121 °C. Polystyrene, polyvinyl chloride (PVC), styrene acrylonitrile, and conventional polyethylene are not autoclavable, but they may be gas-sterilized with ethylene oxide or chemically sterilized via rinsing with benzalkonium chloride. With the exception of Teflon, none of the previously listed resins should be hot–air-sterilized because of the potential for accelerated oxidative degradation.

Some transparent plastics (for example, polycarbonate and polystyrene) may absorb minute quantities of water vapor and appear cloudy after autoclaving. This clouding effect is transient and disappears as the plastic dries; it may be accelerated by drying of the plasticware in an oven at 110 °C.

Synthetic and Rubber-Base Tubing

Tygon is a modified polyvinyl plastic substance that is clear and resistant to chemical attack and used extensively in the manufacture of tubing. It is inert to most chemicals and has been used to transfer liquids, gases, and colloidal suspensions. Tygon comes in a variety of sizes and is specified by inside diameter, outside diameter, and wall thickness. Because Tygon tubing is flexible, it curves around corners and avoids obstructions. It occupies a minimum of space and is used with a variety of positive-action (peristaltic) fluid pumping systems. Because it is available in continuous lengths, Tygon requires few joints or couplings. It is cut readily with a sharp blade and connected to other, larger-bore Tygon tubings with a small amount of solvent (cyclohexanone) to soften and bond the tubing ends.

A soapy solution or synthetic wetting agent is used to facilitate the slipping of Tygon tubing over metal or glass during connection. Simple collar clamps ensure the connection on glass or metal. Tygon is incompatible with polystyrene and acrylics and becomes discolored during contact at high temperatures with solutions containing zinc or copper.

Other available tubing types are made of Teflon, amber latex rubber, and neoprene. Teflon tubing is chemically inert to synthetic substances, organic solvents, acids, and alkalis and withstands continuous temperatures to 300 °C. It replaces Tygon in circumstances requiring its special properties. Amber latex rubber tubing is translucent and recommended for all kinds of glass connections in which a highly elastic tubing with a long life is required. Neoprene is a soft, pliable synthetic rubber with a smooth finish. Neoprene is not affected by oil, alkalis, hot water, and many corrosive substances. It is not recommended for use with chlorinated or aromatic hydrocarbons.

■ VOLUMETRIC EQUIPMENT AND ITS CALIBRATION

To ensure accurate volumetric measurements in the laboratory, only Class A glassware should be used. Class A glassware is certified to conform to the specifications outlined in the NIST circular NBSIR-74-461 (available from the National Technical Information Service, Springfield, VA 22161 as document Number PB246-623).

Pipets

A wide variety of pipets are used in the clinical laboratory, including manual transfer and measuring pipets, micropipets, and mechanical devices.

Transfer and measuring pipets

Transfer and measuring pipets are the two principal types of manual pipets used in the clinical laboratory (Figure 1-1).

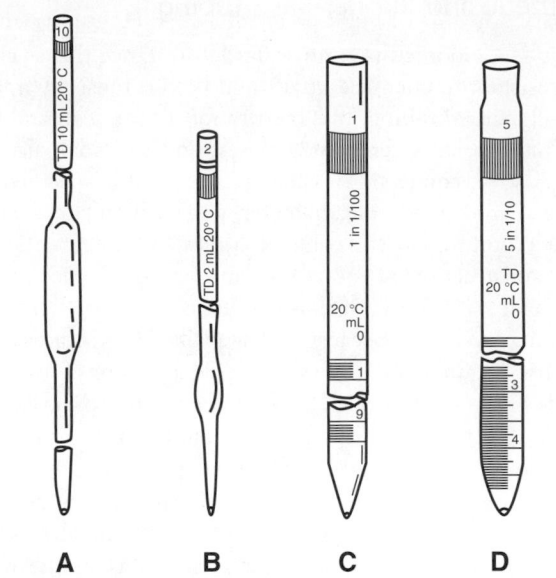

Figure 1-1 Pipets. **A,** Volumetric (transfer). **B,** Ostwald-Folin (transfer). **C,** Mohr (measuring). **D,** Serological (measuring). *TD,* To deliver as indicated.

Certain common techniques apply to the pipets described in this section. First, mouth pipetting is *never* allowed. Instead, pipetting bulbs should be used. Pipets must be held in a vertical position during adjustment of the liquid level to the calibration line and during delivery. The lowest part of the meniscus, when it appears at eye level, should be level with the calibration line on the pipet. The flow of liquid should be unrestricted during use with volumetric pipets, and the tips should touch the inclined surface of the receiving container until 2 seconds after the liquid has ceased to flow.

Transfer pipets

Transfer pipets, which include volumetric and Ostwald-Folin pipets, are designed to deliver (TD) a fixed volume of liquid. Each has a cylindrical bulb joined at both ends to narrower glass tubing. A calibration mark is etched around the upper suction tube, and the lower delivery tube is drawn out to a gradual taper. The bore of the delivery orifice should be sufficiently narrow so that rapid outflow of liquid and incomplete drainage does not create measurement errors beyond tolerances specified.

A volumetric transfer pipet (see Figure 1-1, *A*) is calibrated to deliver accurately a fixed volume of a dilute aqueous solution or nonviscous sample. The most commonly used sizes are 1, 2, 3, 4, 5, and 10 mL. Less frequently used sizes delivering 6, 8, 25, 50, and 100 mL also are available. The reliability of the volumetric pipet's calibration decreases as volume decreases; therefore special micropipets have been developed for microanalysis.

Ostwald-Folin pipets (see Figure 1-1, *B*) are similar to volumetric pipets, but the bulb is closer to the delivery tip, reducing the surface area in contact with the liquid. Com-

monly used sizes are 0.5, 1, 2, and 3 mL. These pipets are used for the accurate measurement of viscous fluids, such as blood or serum. In contrast to a volumetric pipet, an Ostwald-Folin pipet has an etched ring near the mouthpiece, indicating that it is a blowout pipet. With the use of a pipetting bulb, the liquid is blown from the pipet only after the blood or serum has drained to the last drop in the delivery tip. When the pipet is filled with opaque fluids such as blood, the top of the meniscus must be read. Controlled slow drainage is necessary with all viscous solutions so that no residual film remains on the pipet walls.

Measuring pipets

A graduated, or measuring, pipet is composed of a piece of glass tubing that is drawn out to a tip and graduated uniformly along its length. The Mohr and serological pipets are examples of this type. The Mohr pipet (see Figure 1-1, *C*) is calibrated between two marks on the stem, whereas the serological pipet has graduated marks down to the tip. The serological pipet (see Figure 1-1, *D*) has an etched ring (or pair of rings) near the bulb end that signifies its classification as a "blowout" pipet, which means that its contents must be blown out to deliver the entire volume. Mohr pipets require a controlled delivery of the solution between the calibration marks. Serological pipets have a larger orifice than do the Mohr pipets, and thus drain faster. Measuring pipets commonly are supplied in several sizes. In clinical laboratories measuring pipets are used principally for the measurement of reagents and generally are not considered sufficiently accurate for the measuring of samples and calibrators.

Measuring pipets are made of borosilicate glass. Any pipets with tips that are broken or have become badly etched must be discarded. Pipets made of special, chemically tempered glass also are available; although expensive, these pipets do not break as easily as the borosilicate types and are less susceptible to scratching and chipping.

Micropipets

A micropipet is used to handle quantities of liquids up to 1000 μL. In micro work the remaining volume that coats the inner wall of a pipet causes significant error. For this reason most micropipets are calibrated to contain (TC) the stated volume rather than deliver it. Proper use requires rinsing of the pipet with the final solution after contents are delivered into the diluent. Volumes are expressed in microliters (μL); the older term *lambda* no longer is recommended. (One lambda [λ] = 1 μL = 0.001 mL.) Micropipets generally are available in small sizes, ranging from 1 to 1000 μL.

Semiautomatic and automatic pipets and dispensers

Semiautomatic and automatics pipets and dispensers use either positive or air displacement. In positive displacement a piston displaces the volume of liquid dispensed. During air

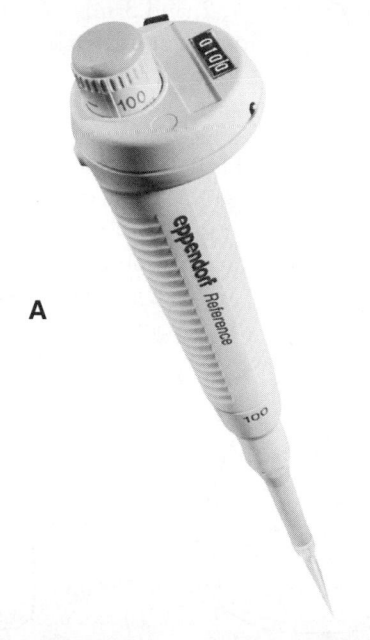

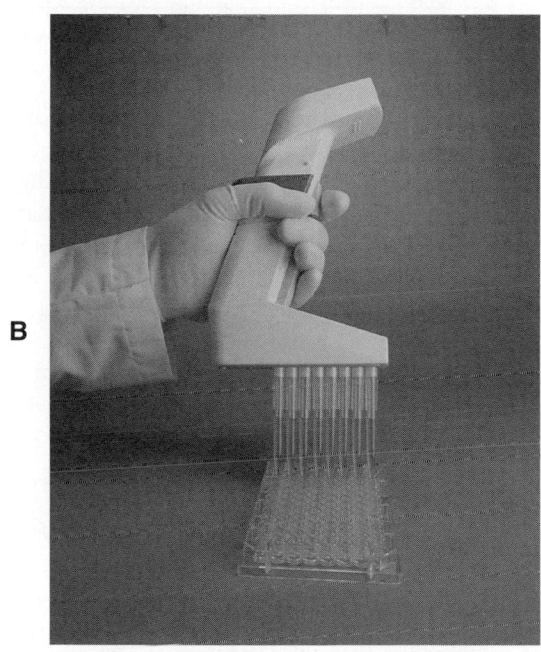

Figure 1-2 **A,** Adjustable volume micropipetting device. (Courtesy Brinkman Instruments, Inc., Westbury, N.Y.) **B,** Electronic programmable multichannel pipet. (Courtesy Matrix Technologies Corp., Hudson, N.H.)

displacement a piston displaces a quantity of air, which in turn displaces the volume of liquid dispensed.

Figure 1-2, *B,* illustrates a type of single or multirange micropipetting device. This electronic device is programmable and used to dispense aliquots of liquid into multiple wells simultaneously. In practice the use of disposable plastic tips allows simultaneous aspiration and delivery of solutions to as many as 12 microwells. Each channel is piston driven to allow the user to pipet with as few or as many tips as

needed. Aliquots of liquid as small as 0.5 μL are dispensed at three different aspiration or dispense rates.

Semiautomatic pipets and dispensers are available in sizes from 1 μL to 20 mL. Figure 1-2, *A,* illustrates a manually operated, positive-displacement device that draws up and dispenses its predefined volume (from 0.1 to 2500 μL) when its plunger is moved through a complete cycle. Its disposable fluid-containment tip is made of a plastic that tends to retain less inner surface film than does glass. Such pipets avoid the risk of cross-contamination among samples, eliminate the need for washing between samples, and improve the precision of measurements. Models also are available that allow for digital adjustment of the volume aspirated and dispensed.

Figure 1-3, *A,* shows a semiautomatic dispensing apparatus that aspirates and dispenses preset volumes of two different liquids via two motor-driven syringes, one for metering a volume of the sample and one for metering a volume of the diluent. This device can be adjusted to aspirate as little as 1 μL of one liquid and deliver it with as much as 25 mL of the other.

A more automatic and versatile piece of equipment is shown in Figure 1-3, *B.* This device is a complete liquid handling system that aspirates programmed volumes of samples and dispenses them with programmed volumes of diluent. The device is microprocessor controlled and easily programmable. Its accuracy is claimed to be better than ± 0.5% of the volume dispensed and its reproducibility to be better than ± 0.1% when at least 10% of syringe volume is dispensed. The minimum volume of a sample is 1 μL and of diluent, 25 mL. The device is capable of storing and retrieving 20 dispensing programs from its memory.

Automated pipetting stations for use with either reaction tubes or microtiter plates are available. Depending on the design of the system, either a single probe or multiple probes are used to transfer programmed volumes of solution from one container to microtiter plates rapidly so that the transfer to all 96 wells is complete in 1 minute. In some systems liquid sensing is incorporated into the sample probes to minimize contact with samples and reagents even though automatic washing of the probes is performed between specimens. Two-dimensional (X-Y) movement of probes and tubes or microtiter plates is built into the pipetting stations to minimize the need for operator intervention.

Volumetric flasks

Volumetric flasks (Figure 1-4) commonly are found in sizes ranging from 1 to 4000 mL. They are used primarily in the preparation of solutions of known concentrations and are available in various grades. The most accurate are certified to meet standards set forth by the NIST.

An important factor in the use of a volumetric apparatus is the need for an accurate adjustment of the meniscus. A card that is half black and half white is most useful. The card is placed 1 cm behind the apparatus, with the white half uppermost and the top of the black area about 1 mm below

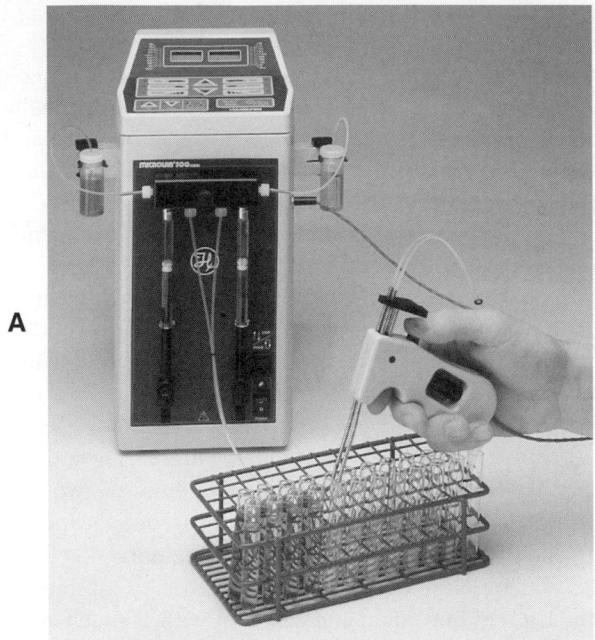

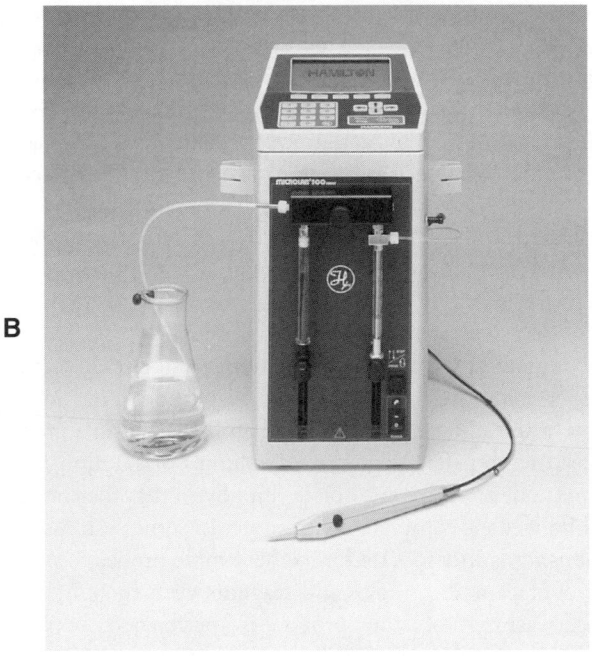

Figure 1-3 **A,** A semiautomatic dispensing apparatus that aspirates and dispenses preset volumes of two different liquids via two motor-driven syringes. **B,** An automatic programmable dilutor that aspirates and delivers diluent and sample. (**A** and **B** courtesy Hamilton Co., Reno, Nev.)

the meniscus. The meniscus then appears as a clearly defined, thin black line. Volumetric equipment should be used with solutions equilibrated to room temperature. Solutions diluted in volumetric flasks should be mixed repeatedly during the time in which dilution occurs so that the contents are homogeneous. The solution then is diluted to the indicated mark on the flask. This action also is known as *diluting to mark.*

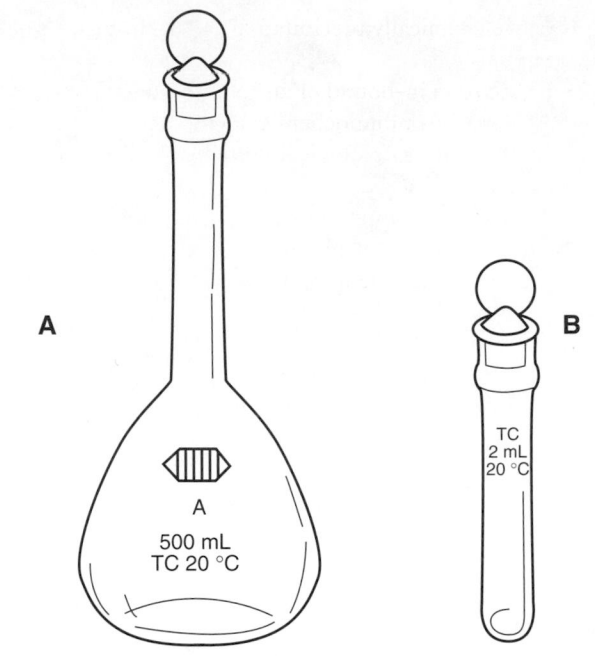

Figure 1-4 Volumetric flasks. **A,** Macro. **B,** Micro. *TC,* To contain.

Volumetric flasks should be cleaned and dried thoroughly before calibration. The flask should then be weighed and filled with carbon dioxide-free deionized water to slightly above the graduation mark. The neck of the flask just above the water level should be kept free of water. The meniscus mark is set at the graduation line by the removal of excess water, and the flask is reweighed. The final weight is corrected for the equilibrated water and air temperature to obtain the flask's volume. Flasks also may be calibrated with the gravimetrical and spectrophotometric techniques described in an expanded version of this chapter.[2]

■ LABORATORY OPERATIONS

A number of routine operations, including centrifugation, weighing, and thermometry, frequently take place inside a typical clinical laboratory.

Centrifugation

Centrifugation is the process by which centrifugal force is used to separate the lighter portions of a solution, mixture, or suspension from the heavier portions. A centrifuge is a device by which centrifugation is performed. In the clinical laboratory centrifugation is used to perform the following functions:

1. Remove cellular elements from blood to provide cell-free plasma or serum for analysis
2. Concentrate cellular elements and other components of biological fluids for microscopical examination or chemical analysis

3. Remove chemically precipitated protein from analytical specimens
4. Separate protein-bound or antibody-bound ligand from free ligand in immunochemical and other assays
5. Extract solutes in biological fluids from aqueous to organic solvents
6. Separate lipid components such as chylomicrons from other components of plasma or serum and separate lipoproteins from one another

Types of centrifuges

Horizontal-head, or swinging-bucket; fixed-angle, or angle-head; and ultracentrifuge are the three types of centrifuges used in the clinical laboratory.

Horizontal-head, or swinging-bucket, centrifuges

The horizontal-head, or swinging-bucket, centrifuge allows the tubes placed in the cups of the rotor to assume a horizontal position when the rotor is in motion and a vertical position when it is at rest. During centrifugation, particles travel constantly along the tube while the tube is positioned at a right angle to the shaft of the centrifuge; thus the sediment is distributed uniformly against the bottom of the tube. The surface of the sediment is flat (parallel to the shaft of the centrifuge) and remains so, with a column of liquid on top when the rotor stops and the tube assumes a vertical position. Supernatant liquid is removed with a pipet, negligibly disturbing the packed sediment. If the sediment is well packed, the supernatant is decanted.

The spinning rotor of a horizontal-head centrifuge offers considerable resistance to rotation and generates heat as a result of air friction. This resistance is lessened if the swinging buckets are enclosed in a windshield.

Fixed-angle, or angle-head, centrifuge

In the rotor of an angle-head centrifuge tubes are held in fixed positions at angles from 25 to 40 degrees to the vertical axis of rotation. On the start of centrifugation, particles are driven outward horizontally but strike the side of the tube so that the sediment packs against the side and bottom of the tube, with the surface of the sediment parallel to the shaft of the centrifuge. As the rotor slows down and stops, gravity causes the sediment to slide down the tube; usually, a poorly packed pellet is formed.

Ultracentrifuge

An ultracentrifuge is a high-speed centrifuge that typically uses a fixed-head rotor. The most common application of an ultracentrifuge in the clinical laboratory is the separation of lipoproteins (see Chapter 24). Because the separation may require hours or days and generate considerable heat as a result of high-speed friction, ultracentrifugation requires a refrigerated chamber. Ultracentrifuges are available in both analytical and preparative models. A tabletop model exists as a miniature air turbine with a small rotor capable of achieving a centrifugal force of 165,000 times gravity. This model is used in the clinical laboratory to clear the serum of chylomicrons so that accurate analyses may be performed on the infranatant.

Components of a centrifuge

Each centrifuge contains a rotor or centrifuge head, drive shaft, and motor. The rotor is enclosed in a chamber with a cover and latch. Most centrifuges also include a power switch, timer, speed control, tachometer, and brake. Some include a protective shield to minimize aerosol production in case a tube breaks or a refrigerator to reduce the temperature within the chamber. Most modern centrifuges contain programmable microprocessors that control the acceleration and deceleration of the rotor, as well as the overall running time. For a particular type of specimen the necessary program is recalled from memory to ensure reproducible separations. Centrifuges also may include audible or visible alarms to indicate malfunctions (for example, an imbalance of the rotor).

During operation, centrifuges generate heat; the temperature in the chamber in many centrifuge models may increase by as much as 5 °C after a single run. The change in temperature depends on the initial ambient temperature in the centrifuge chamber, rotor speed, duration of centrifugation, and rotor design. Consequently, when the material to be centrifuged is thermolabile, a refrigerated centrifuge should be used. In the simplest form a refrigerator unit is mounted beside the centrifuge, and cold air is blown into the rotor chamber. This approach usually is inadequate to stabilize the low temperature. In more sophisticated centrifuges, refrigeration coils around the chamber ensure maintenance of a preset temperature within ±1 °C. In addition, some centrifuge models are available with plastic covers over the rotor chambers or over each swinging bucket to reduce aerosol formation when a tube breaks during centrifugation.

Principles of centrifugation

The correct term to describe the force required to separate two phases in a centrifuge is **relative centrifugal force (RCF)**, also called *relative centrifugal field*. Units are expressed as the number of times greater than gravity (for example, $500 \times g$). (NOTE: One gravity is equal to the force of gravitational attraction at the surface of the Earth.) RCF is calculated as follows:

$$RCF = 1.118 \times 10^{-5} \times r \times rpm^2$$

where

1.118×10^{-5} = An empirical factor

r = Radius in centimeters from the center of rotation to the bottom of the tube in the rotor cavity or bucket during centrifugation

rpm = Speed of rotation of the rotor in revolutions per minute

The RCF of a centrifuge also may be determined from a nomogram distributed by manufacturers of centrifuges (see Chapter 46). RCF is derived from the distance from the rotor center to the bottom of the tube, whether the tube is horizontal or at an angle to the rotor center. The RCF as calculated above is the maximum RCF. However, not all the contents of a tube are subjected to the maximum RCF. The minimum RCF, calculated in the same way but from the center of rotation to the surface of the liquid, may be several hundred g less than the maximum value. Note also that RCF applied to a tube in a fixed-angle head is much less than that applied to the same tube in a horizontal-head rotor because the tube in the former is unable to swing outward.

The time required to separate particles depends on the rotor speed, radius of the rotor, and effective path length traveled by the sedimented particles (that is, the depth of the liquid in the tube). Duplication of conditions of centrifugation is often desirable. The following is a useful formula for the calculation of the speed required of a rotor with a radius that differs from the radius with which a prescribed RCF originally was defined:

$$\text{rpm (alternate rotor)} = 1000 \times \sqrt{\frac{\text{RCF, original rotor}}{11.18 \times r \text{ (cm), alternate rotor}}}$$

The length of time for centrifugation also can be calculated so that running with an alternate rotor of a different size is equivalent to running with the original rotor:

$$\text{Time (alternate rotor)} = \frac{\text{time} \times \text{RCF (original motor)}}{\text{RCF (alternate rotor)}}$$

Note, however, that the reproduction of exact conditions may not be possible when a different centrifuge is used. Descriptions of times of centrifugation include the time for the rotor to reach operating speed (which may vary from instrument to instrument) and do not include deceleration time, during which sedimentation still occurs, but less efficiently. Even with maximum braking, deceleration may take as long as 3 minutes in some centrifuges.

Operation of the centrifuge

For proper operation of a centrifuge only those tubes recommended by its manufacturer should be used. The material used for the tube must withstand the RCF to which the tube is likely to be subjected. Polypropylene tubes generally can withstand RCFs up to 5000 $\times$ g. The tube should have a tapered bottom, particularly if a supernatant is to be removed, and should be sized to fit securely into the rack to be centrifuged. The top of the tube should not protrude so far above the bucket that the rotor impedes the swing into a horizontal position.

For smooth operation of the centrifuge the rotor must be balanced properly. The weight of racks and tubes, as well as their contents on opposite sides of a rotor, should not differ by more than 1% or an acceptable limit established by the manufacturer. The smaller the difference, the smoother the centrifugation. Before centrifuging any laboratory specimens, pairs of adapters, and specimen tubes should be placed on opposite pans of a balance and the tubes rearranged so that the weights are equal and the placement of tubes is symmetrical. Tubes filled with water also may be used to equalize the weights. The total weight of each rack should not exceed the limits stated by the centrifuge manufacturer at a rated speed. In addition, centrifuges that automatically balance their rotors now are available.[3]

Tubes of collected blood should be centrifuged before their stoppers are removed to reduce the probability of the production of an aerosol when the tube is opened. Using a wooden applicator to release a clot stuck to the top of the tube or its stopper should be avoided; this practice may produce hemolysis. Centrifugation at an appropriate RCF usually ensures that the clot is released from the tube wall and drawn to the bottom of the tube.

Through years of experience with centrifuges a few specific recommendations for RCF or time for centrifugation of blood specimens have been developed. For example, NCCLS standard H18-A[5] proposes an RCF of 1000 to 1200 $\times$ g for 10 $\pm$ 5 minutes.

Operating practice

The cleanliness of a centrifuge is important; it minimizes the possible spread of infectious agents, such as hepatitis viruses. With proper operation, few tubes break, but when they do break, both the racks and the chamber of the centrifuge must be cleaned carefully. Any spillage should be treated as a possible blood-borne pathogen hazard. Gray dust arising from the sandblasting of the chamber by fragments of glass indicates tube breakage and possible contamination, necessitating chamber cleaning. Broken glass embedded in cushions of tube holders may cause continual breakage if cushions are not inspected and replaced in the cleanup procedure.

The speed of a centrifuge should be checked at least once every 3 months via a stroboscopical light or vibrating-reed external tachometer of known accuracy. The measured speed should not differ by more than $\pm 5\%$ from the rated speed under specified conditions. The centrifuge timer should be checked weekly against a reference timer (such as a stopwatch) and should not be more than $\pm 10\%$ in error. The temperature of a refrigerated centrifuge should be measured monthly under reproducible conditions and should be within ± 2 °C of the expected temperature. Commutators and brushes in the centrifuge motor should be checked at least every 3 months. Brushes (when used) should be replaced when they show considerable wear. However, in many modern induction-drive motors, brushes have been eliminated, removing a source of dust that causes motor failure.

Weighing

Mass is an invariant property of matter. **Gravimetry** is the process used to measure the mass of a substance. Weight is a function of mass under the influence of gravity, a relationship expressed by the following equation:

$$Weight = mass \times gravity$$

Two substances of equal weight that are subject to the same gravitational force have equal masses. Mass is determined through use of a **balance** to compare an unknown with a known mass. This comparison is called *weighing*, and the absolute standards with which masses are compared are called *weights*. In practice the terms *mass* and *weight* are used synonymously.

The classic form of a balance is a beam poised on an agate knife-edge fulcrum, with a pan hanging from each end of the beam and a rigid pointer hanging from the beam at the poise point. With the object to be weighed on one pan and weights of equal mass on the other, the pointer rests at an equilibrium point, or balance, between the extremes of the path of excursion. The weight required to achieve equilibrium therefore is equal to the weight of the substance being weighed.

Although the classic form of balance is antiquated, modern mechanical and electronic balances continue to apply the principle of equilibrium in a variety of ingenious ways. More than one type of balance is required for a clinical laboratory because of the need to weigh a variety of compounds and materials ranging from microgram to kilogram in weight. Coarse balances of large capacity (up to 5 kg) have detection limits of 0.1 g. The typical analytical balance has a capacity of 200 g and a detection limit of about 10 µg. Microbalances may have maximum capacities of as little as 5 g and detection limits of 0.1 µg.

All balances require a vibration-free location. The more sensitive a balance, the more protection it needs, not only from vibration but from air currents that disturb the equilibrium between the weighed object and the weights. The zero, or null, point of the balance (that is, the rest point in the absence of either weights or an object to be weighed) must be known or adjusted. Scrupulous attention to cleanliness is essential. Chemical substances being weighed should never be placed in direct contact with the pans. Disposable plastic weighing boats in various sizes provide convenient weighing of most chemicals. A good weighing technique for samples less than 1 g calls for the handling of weights with forceps and weighed objects with suitable utensils to avoid deposition of moisture, oils, or salts from the analyst's skin.

Principles of weighing

Two general principles of weighing exist—substitution and direct comparison. In weighing by substitution weights are removed from the side of a balance to which the object to be weighed has been added in order to restore equilibrium. In weighing by direct comparison weights are added to one side of the beam to counterbalance the weight of the object on the other side. The latter approach is more common.

In practice, two modes of weighing are used: (1) analytical weights are added to equal the weight of the object being weighed or (2) the material to be weighed is added to a balance pan to achieve equilibrium with a preset weight. Before a chemical is weighed, the weight of the container must be determined or allowed for via taring to reset the equilibrium point.

Types of balances

Double- and single-pan and electronic balances frequently are used in the clinical laboratory.

Double-pan balance

A double-pan balance conforms to the classic design, consisting of a single beam with arms of equal length. Standard weights usually are added by hand to the right-side pan to counterbalance the weight of the object on the left, but in some models a dial or vernier with chain is used to make fine adjustments to the mass associated with the right-side pan. In single-pan balances the arms are unequal in length, and the object to be weighed is placed on the pan attached to the shorter arm. A restoring force is applied mechanically or electronically to the other arm to return the beam to its null position. Double- and triple-beam balances are forms of the unequal-arm balance. A pan on a short arm is balanced about a fulcrum by a larger arm consisting of two or three parallel beams to which weights or poises of different weights are attached. In general, these balances are designed to weigh bulk reagents and have relatively low accuracy levels.

Single-pan balance

The single-pan balance commonly is used in the clinical laboratory. It most often operates electronically and self-balances. Such a balance may be interfaced directly to a computer or recording device. In the electronic single-pan balance a load on the pan causes the beam to tilt downward. A null detector senses the position of the beam and indicates when the beam has deviated from the equilibrium point.

Electronic balance

In an electronic balance an electromagnetic force is applied to return the balance beam to its null position. The electromagnetic force takes the place of weights in a two-pan balance. The restoring force is proportional to the weight on the pan and applied through a solenoid or torque motor. The current required to produce the force is displayed digitally by liquid crystals or light-emitting diodes in a form equivalent to the mass on the balance pan. The accuracy of an electronic balance depends on the linearity of both the digital voltmeter and the torque motor.

Almost all electronic balances have built-in provisions for taring so that the mass of the container is subtracted easily from the total mass measured. Thus operation of an electronic balance is simple—switching on the balance, placing a container to hold the material to be weighed on the balance pan, taring off the weight of the container, transferring the material to be weighed to the container, and recording the mass of the material as shown on the digital display. In many modern balances a built-in microprocessor compensates for changes in temperature and provides both automatic zero tracking and calibration.

Analytical weights

Analytical weights are used to counterbalance the weight of objects weighed on double-pan balances and verify the performance of both single- and double-pan balances. The NIST recognizes the following five classes of analytical weights:

1. Class M weights are of primary standard quality and are used only to calibrate other weights.
2. Class S weights are used for the calibration of balances. In the clinical laboratory balances should be calibrated at least monthly and before accurate analytical work.
3. Class S-1 weights have greater tolerance levels than class S weights and are used for routine analytical work.
4. Class P weights demonstrate even greater tolerance levels.
5. Class J weights are intended for microanalytical work and range from 0.05 to 50 mg, in contrast to the range of 1 mg to 100 g of the other classes.

The integral weights of a set of class S weights are made from brass or stainless steel and are lacquered or plated for protection. The fractional weights of a set of class S standards are usually made of platinum or aluminum. Tolerances of the different weights have been defined by the NIST. For class S weights from 1 to 5 g the tolerance is ± 0.054 mg; from 500 to 100 mg, ± 0.025 mg; and from 1 to 50 mg, ± 0.014 mg.

Thermometry

In the clinical chemistry laboratory measurements of temperature are made primarily to verify that devices measure within the prescribed temperature limits. Water baths or heated cells where reactions take place are examples of such devices, as are refrigerators, the temperatures of which must be measured and recorded daily.

The two most popular types of thermometers in the chemistry laboratory are liquid-in-glass (for example, mercury-in-glass) thermometers and thermistor probes. A thermistor is an electronic device that uses a semiconductor in which resistance varies as a function of temperature.

All thermometers must be verified against a NIST-certified thermometer. SRM 934 is a mercury-in-glass thermometer with calibration points at 0 °C, 25 °C, 30 °C, and 37 °C. Liquid-in-glass thermometers that have ranges greater than the SRM thermometer and are verified to have been calibrated against the NIST thermometers also are

available. Details of the verification of a thermometer's calibration are provide in an NCCLS document.[6]

The NIST also supplies several materials that melt at known temperatures. Gallium (SRM 1968) and rubidium (SRM 1969), which melt at 29.7723 °C and 39.3 °C, respectively, are particularly useful in the clinical laboratory (see Table 1-2).

■ SOLUTIONS

A solution is a homogeneous mixture of one or more substances (solutes) dispersed molecularly in a sufficient quantity of dissolving medium (solvent). The colligative properties of a solution depend on the number of molecules present in a given space and not on their size, molecular weight, or chemical constitution. Colligative properties of solutions include osmotic pressure, boiling point elevation, freezing point depression, and vapor pressure lowering. From an analytical perspective the quantity of the solute(s) in solution is important. The terms used to express quantity are also important, as are techniques used to process solutions.

Concept of Solute and Solvent

Many measurements in the clinical laboratory concern the determination of dissolved solutes in a solvent. In practice a clinical laboratorian is concerned primarily with the measurement of solids in liquids, in which a relatively large amount of solvent exists in comparison to the amount of solute.

When a solution holds as much of a dissolved solute as it can at a specific temperature, it is said to be *saturated*. The temperature of the solution, atmospheric pressure, and nature of the solute and solvent influence saturation. Solvents usually dissolve more solute at higher temperatures, whereas the solubility of gases usually decreases with increases in temperature. For those substances that dissolve when heat is added, previously dissolved solute may separate from the solution when it is cooled. An unsaturated solution is one that contains less solute than the solvent is capable of holding, and a supersaturated solution is one that contains more solute than it can hold when the solution is saturated. Adding undissolved substance, jarring, or stirring the supersaturated solution causes precipitation of the excess solute and produces a saturated solution.

Compounds of similar chemical composition usually are more soluble in one another than in compounds of very different structure (that is, "like dissolves like"). When two liquids dissolve in each other in any proportion, they are completely *miscible*. If the liquids do not dissolve at all in each other, they are completely *immiscible*. When each of two liquids is partially soluble in the other, they are said to be *partially miscible*. In practice a clinical laboratorian often has to dilute solutions and must express the concentration of analytes in a solution in a consistent and acceptable manner.

Expressing concentrations of solutions

In the United States laboratory data typically is reported in terms of mass of solute per unit volume of solution, usually the deciliter. Although considered incorrect by metrologists, mass concentration also is reported in terms of grams percent or percent. This is typically the way in which concentrations of ethanol in blood are expressed.[13] The terminology indicates an amount of solute per mass of solution (for example, grams per 100 g) and would be appropriate only if reference materials against which the unknowns were compared also were measured in the same terms. The following equations define the expressions of concentrations:

$$Mole = \frac{mass\ (g)}{gram\ molecular\ weight}$$

$$Molarity\ of\ a\ solution = \frac{number\ of\ moles\ of\ solute}{number\ of\ liters\ of\ solution}$$

$$Molality\ of\ a\ solution = \frac{number\ of\ moles\ of\ solute}{number\ of\ kilograms\ of\ solvent}$$

$$Normality\ of\ a\ solution = \frac{number\ of\ gram\ equivalents\ of\ solute}{number\ of\ liters\ of\ solution}$$

Normality (in oxidation-reduction reaction)
$$= molarity \times difference\ in\ oxidation\ state$$

Gram equivalent weight (as oxidatant or reductant)
$$= \frac{formula\ weight\ (g)}{difference\ in\ oxidation\ state}$$

For example, using these equations, a 1 molar solution of H_2SO_4 contains 98.08 g H_2SO_4 per liter of solution. Note that the symbol M, previously used to denote molarity, has been replaced by mol/L. A molal solution contains 1 mol of solute in 1 kg of solvent. Molality is expressed properly as mol/kg.

Likewise, a 1 normal solution contains 1 g equivalent weight of solute in 1 L of solution; that is, 1 mol HCl, 0.5 mol H_2SO_4, and 0.33 mol H_3PO_4, each in 1 L of solution, are 1 normal solutions. The use of normality is limited in that a given solution may have more than one normality, depending on the type of reaction for which the solution is used. The molarity of a solution, however, is a fixed number because only one molecular mass exists for any substance. *Normality* no longer is recommended in the expression of concentrations.

A milligram equivalent of a substance is its equivalent weight expressed in milligrams. The equivalent mass of H_2SO_4 is 49.04 g; therefore 1 mg equivalent of H_2SO_4 equals 49.04 mg H_2SO_4. Because substances may react on the basis of their valence, 1 mol calcium (atomic weight of 40), which is bivalent, has twice the combining power of 1 mol sodium (atomic weight of 23). Therefore 40 mg Ca is equivalent to 46 mg Na.

An older unit of measurement used to express the concentration of electrolytes in plasma is the milliequivalent (mEq), which is one-thousandth of an equivalent.

$$Milliequivalents\ (mEq) = \frac{weight\ (g)}{milliequivalent\ mass\ (g)}$$

Milligrams per 100 mL (deciliter) is converted to mEq per liter using the following formula:

$$mEq/L = \frac{mg/dL \times 10 \times valence}{mg\ atomic\ mass}$$

Example: If the serum sodium concentration is 322 mg/dL, then the serum contains 3220 mg/L. The equivalent mass of sodium is 23, and the valence is 1; therefore

$$mEq/L = \frac{322 \times 10 \times 1}{23} = 140$$

The recommended units for sodium concentration in plasma are millimoles per liter (mmol/L). In the previous example the concentration of sodium is

$$mmol/L = \frac{mg/L}{mg\ molecular\ mass} = \frac{322 \times 10 \times 1}{23} = 140$$

In chemical terms the titer of a solution is the mass of a substance equivalent to a unit volume of the solution.

$$Titer = \frac{grams\ of\ substance}{liters\ of\ solution} = \frac{mg\ substance}{mL\ solution}$$

However, a titer also is considered the lowest dilution at which a particular reaction takes place. Titer customarily is expressed as a ratio (for example, 1 to 10 or 1:10).

Procedures for processing of solutions

Several procedures routinely are used to process solutions in the clinical laboratory, including those for diluting, concentrating, mixing, and filtering.

Dilution

Dilution is the process by which the concentration or activity of a given solution is decreased by the addition of solvent. In the clinical laboratory most dilutions are made through the transfer of an exact volume of a concentrated solution into an appropriate flask and the subsequent addition of water or other diluent to the required volume, with appropriate mixing to ensure homogeneity. A serial dilution is a sequential set of dilutions in mathematical sequence. A given dilution is expressed as the amount, either volume or weight, of a solute (**analyte**) in a specified volume. For example, a 1:5 volume to volume (v/v) dilution contains 1 volume in a total of 5 volumes (1 volume plus 4 volumes).

Errors made in the performance of a dilution can be both random and determinate. Random errors vary nonreproducibly from one measurement to another and are minimized by careful technique. A determinate error affects each in a set of measurements, remaining fixed for all measurements.

Such errors are avoided through the use of properly calibrated equipment.

To avoid errors that arise when two liquids of very different compositions are mixed, the technique of dilution to volume is used. Instead of adding 90 mL water to 10 mL concentrated solution, the 10-mL concentrated solution should be pipetted into a 100-mL volumetric flask and water added to bring the volume to the 100-mL mark on the neck of the flask, also known as *diluting to mark*.

In the performance of a dilution, the following equation is used to determine the volume (V_2) needed to dilute a given volume (V_1) of solution of a known concentration (C_1) to the desired lesser concentration (C_2)

$$C_1 \times V_1 = C_2 \times V_2$$

Likewise, this equation also is used to calculate the concentration of the diluted solution when a given volume is added to the starting solution.

Procedures used to concentrate solutions

Evaporation.   This is a process used to convert a liquid or volatile solid into vapor. It is used in the clinical laboratory to remove liquid from a sample, which increases the concentrations of analyte(s) left behind. A procedure frequently used for the evaporation of volatile solvents involves the direction of a stream of air through a fine nozzle onto the surface of liquid in a tube to flush out vapors in equilibrium with the solution. With a suitable manifold, this procedure can be applied to many tubes simultaneously and the time required decreased by placement of the tubes in a heated water bath. The procedure should be carried out in a fume hood to prevent health hazards resulting from evaporating solvents. If compressed air is used, it should be passed through a filter and over a desiccating agent to prevent particulate matter and moisture from contaminating the solution.

Rapid removal of large volumes of solvent best is achieved through the combination of reduced pressure and heat. The solution is placed in a round-bottom flask no larger than 100 mL to avoid the danger of implosion. Vacuum is applied to the flask through a safety trap while the flask is swirled in a heated water bath. Swirling produces a large surface area, speeding evaporation and reducing bumping. Alternatively, a thick-walled Erlenmeyer flask may be used at ambient temperature. A water aspirator, an institution vacuum line, or a mechanical vacuum pump may be used to reduce the pressure. With any system a suitable trap is essential to collect the vapors. To concentrate a larger volume of solution, a rotary evaporator is used. To concentrate many specimens of small volume, vortex evaporators or multiple unit rotary evaporators are available.

Lyophilization.   This procedure, also known as *freeze-drying*, is used in laboratory medicine for the preparation of calibrators, control materials, reagents, and to a lesser extent, individual specimens for analysis. More than 99% of the water in a substance is removed in the typical lyophilization process. The composition of the lyophilized material usually remains unchanged except for the loss of water or some volatile organic matter. Lyophilization first entails freezing of a material at −40 °C or lower and subsequent subjection of the material to a high vacuum. Extremely low temperatures cause the ice to sublime; solid nonsublimable material, initially locked in an ice matrix, remains behind in a dried state.

Mixing and homogenizing

Efficient mixing of solutions of extremely different densities is facilitated via mechanical agitation. Depending on the application, a fixed- or variable-speed motor should be selected. For viscous solutions, high-torque, low-speed motors should be used, whereas in the presence of explosive vapors, an air-driven motor should replace an electrical version.

Laboratory mixers are rated according to the type of duty—continuous (8-hour uninterrupted) or intermittent. The design of the rotating device is dictated by its intended application, such as shearing, mixing, or homogenizing. Most stirrers are made of glass, stainless steel, or Teflon. Solutions in a flask also may be mixed by the insertion of a Teflon-coated stirring bar in the flask. The flask is placed above the stirring module that contains a rotating magnet.

A vortex mixer is a useful device for the mixing of solutions. These mixers come with cups or platform heads for test tubes and beakers, flasks, and other small containers, respectively. When a tube is pressed against the vibrating cup head, the liquid in the tube is mixed rapidly through the formation of a vortex. Variable speed control allows precise mixing, from a gentle shake to an aggressive vortexing action.

Measurements on cell contents require initial preparation of the tissues. Preparation may involve grinding of the tissue in a ground-glass tissue blender through manual force or a rotor driven by a simple electrical motor. For large quantities of material a tissue blender similar to the typical kitchen blender is used to emulsify and pulverize the tissue. Several different designs of blades are available and may be exchanged easily if a different application is required. The speed at which the blades rotate is usually more than 15,000 rpm.

Filtration

Filtration is defined as the passage of a liquid through a filter and is accomplished via gravity, pressure, or vacuum. Filtrate is the liquid that has passed through the filter. The purpose of filtration is to remove particulate matter from the liquid. Many filtrations in the clinical laboratory are performed with filter paper. Different types of filter paper include low-ash or ashless paper, as well as various grades related to thickness. Vacuum filtration requires paper known as *hardened-grade paper*, with high, wet tensile strength. Fiberglass papers have the greatest strength and combine the advantages of retention of fine particles with fast filtration. *Retention* refers to the particle size of precipitate that a given grade can retain; *speed* refers to relative mean flow rates.

Filtration also is performed with membranes of controlled pore size. These filters are made from homogeneous polymeric materials, such as polyvinylidene fluoride, cellulose esters, cellulose acetate, polytetrafluoroethylene, and PVC, depending on the intended application of the filter. The most widely used filter is composed of cellulose acetate and cellulose nitrate. The filters contain no loose fibers or particulate matter and are manufactured in a variety of sizes up to almost 30 cm in diameter and with pore sizes that vary from 10 to 0.025 μm, the latter being capable of sterilizing the filtrate by retaining microorganisms. In addition, 80% of the surface area of a typical membrane filter is occupied by pores; therefore high flow rates occur through a filter with pores of even the smallest diameter. The basic structure of a membrane filter is hydrophobic, although the surface of the membrane can be modified chemically to make it hydrophilic.

Filtration with filter paper often is conducted under gravity or pressure or in a vacuum. The latter method accelerates the filtration rate by combining the influences of gravity, suction, and capillary attraction. Filters have been incorporated into certain disposable tips for use with semiautomatic pipets. These filters minimize the exchange of aerosol droplets between the tips and the pipet, an action that is particularly important in DNA amplification and microbiological procedures. Other membrane filters are designed for ultrafiltration and available in a variety of pore sizes for selective filtration. *Ultrafiltration* is a term that describes a technique for the removal of dissolved particles through the use of an extremely fine filter. The technique concentrates macromolecules, such as proteins, because smaller dissolved molecules pass through the filter.

Many small specimens of biological fluids may be concentrated at the same time through the use of porous cellulose acetate filter cones and a centrifuge. The filter cones fit inside centrifuge tubes, and centrifugal force drives water and molecules with a molecular weight of less than 50,000 through the anisotropic membrane filter. This approach is used widely to concentrate proteins in urine or cerebrospinal fluid in preparation for electrophoretic analysis.

Surface filtration

Surface filtration, also known as *screen filtration*, is performed with filter papers, membranes, or sieves. Surface filtration retains the solid material on the filter medium, and the filtrate passes through the filter to be collected or discarded as required. The number and size of pores are controlled accurately in the manufacture of the separation medium so that determination of the appropriate filter for a given task is possible.

Depth filtration

With depth filtration a thick separation medium allows particles to remain in the body of the filter and on the surface. Depth filters usually are made of cotton, fiberglass, asbestos, or other materials, such as diatomaceous earth.

Combining depth and surface filters into a single filter is useful in the purification of solutions. The depth filter is a prefilter that traps large particles, thus lengthening the life of the secondary surface filter. Fiberglass or sintered glass often is used as a refilter for coarse materials.

■ BUFFER SOLUTIONS AND THEIR ACTIONS

A **buffer** is defined as a chemical system that prevents change in the concentration of another chemical substance. In the clinical laboratory, proton donor and acceptor systems are used as buffers to prevent changes in hydrogen ion concentration. All weak acids or bases, in the presence of their salts, form buffer systems. The action of buffers and their role in the maintenance of a solution's pH is explained with the aid of the Henderson-Hasselbalch equation.

The ionization of a weak acid, HA, and of a salt of that acid, BA, is represented as:

$$HA \leftrightharpoons H^+ + A^-$$

$$BA \leftrightharpoons B^+ + A^-$$

The dissociation constant (K_a) for a weak acid may be calculated from the following equation:

$$K_a = \frac{[H^+][A^-]}{[HA]}$$

Thus

$$[H^+] = K_a \times \frac{[HA]}{[A^-]}$$

or

$$\log[H^+] = \log K_a + \log \frac{[HA]}{[A^-]}$$

where brackets indicate the concentration of the compound contained within. Now multiplying throughout by -1

$$-\log[H^+] = -\log K_a - \log \frac{[HA]}{[A^-]}$$

Because by definition, pH equals -log [H$^+$], and pK_a equals -log K_a

$$pH = pK_a + \log \frac{[A^-]}{[HA]}$$

Because A$^-$ is derived principally from the salt, the equation may for practical purposes be written

$$pH = pK_a + \log \frac{[salt]}{[undissociated\ acid]}$$

or simply

$$pH = pK_a + \log \frac{[salt]}{[acid]}$$

where [salt] = [A$^-$] = concentration of dissociated salt, and [acid] = [HA] = concentration of undissociated acid.

Consequently, the pH of the system is determined by the pK_a of the acid and the ratio of [A$^-$] to [HA]. The buffer has its greatest buffer capacity at its pK_a, that is, that pH at which the [A$^-$] = [HA]. This factor, entered into the preceding equation, gives:

$$pH = pK_a + \log 1$$
$$pH = pK_a + 0$$

The capacity of the buffer decreases as the ratio deviates from 1. In general, a buffer should not be used at a pH greater than 1 from its pK_a. If the ratio is more than 50:1 or 1:50, the system is considered to have lost its buffering capacity. This point is approximately ±1.7 pH units of the pK_a of the acid.

The chemical mechanisms by which buffers exert their effect may be seen through consideration of the reactions involved when a base is added to a buffer solution containing acetate ions, CH_3COO^-, and acetic acid molecules, CH_3COOH. When NaOH is added:

$$
\begin{array}{lll}
CH_3COO^- \, H^+ & & CH_3COO^- \, NA^+ \\
& + \, Na^+ + OH^- \longrightarrow & \\
CH_3COO^- \, NA^+ & & CH_3COO^- \, NA^+
\end{array} \quad +HOH
$$

Base OH$^-$ is removed through combination with the hydrogen ion dissociated from acetic acid, thus minimizing pH changes.

The addition of alkali decreases the [CH_3COOH] in the buffer and increases the [CH_3COONa]. The pH of the solution increases in proportion to the change in ratio of salt to acid in the buffer solution. When HCl is added

$$
\begin{array}{lll}
CH_3COO^- \, H^+ & & CH_3COO^- \, H^+ \\
& + \, H^+ + Cl^- \longrightarrow & + \, Na^+ + Cl^- \\
CH_3COO^- \, NA^+ & & CH_3COO^- \, H^+
\end{array}
$$

H$^+$ is removed through combination with acetate to form poorly dissociated acetic acid. In this case the addition of HCl acts to decrease [CH_3COONa] and increase [CH_3COOH] in the buffer. The pH of the solution drops in proportion to the change in ratio of salt to acid in the solution; however, because the pH is related to the logarithm of the A$^-$/HA ratio, only a small change in pH occurs.

■ UNITS OF MEASUREMENT

A meaningful measurement is expressed with both a number and a unit. The unit identifies the dimension—mass, volume, or concentration—of a measured property. The number indicates the number of units contained in the property.

Traditionally, measurements in the clinical laboratory have been expressed in metric units. In the early develop-

TABLE 1-6	SI Base Units		
Quantity		Name	Symbol
Length		meter	m
Mass		kilogram	kg
Time		second	s
Electric current		ampere	A
Thermodynamic temperature		Kelvin	K
Amount of substance		mole	mol
Luminous intensity		candela	cd
Catalytic amount		katal	kat

SI, International System of Units.

ment of the **metric system,** units were referenced to length, mass, and time. The first absolute systems were based on the centimeter, gram, and second (CGS) and then the meter, kilogram, and second (MKS). The **Système International d'Unites (SI),** commonly referred to also as the *International System of Units,* is a different system that was accepted internationally in 1960. The units of the system are called *SI units.* Schemes also have been developed to report test results in a standard format.

International System of Units

Three classes of SI units exist—base, derived, and supplemental. The seven base units, plus the provisionally accepted katal, are listed in Table 1-6. A derived unit is derived mathematically from two or more base units (Table 1-7). A supplemental unit conforms to the SI but has not been classified as either base or derived. For example, the radian (for plane angles) and the steradian (for solid angles) are supplemental units. The minute, hour, and day have such longstanding use in everyday life that they have been retained for use with the SI.

Decimal multiples and submultiples of SI units

In practical application of SI units certain values are too large or too small to be expressed conveniently in base or derived units. A numerical value is expressed in a convenient size when the unit is modified appropriately by official SI prefixes. In general, the prefixes are such that the value of the unit changes a thousand-fold. However, certain common previously accepted multiples or submultiples, such as deci- and hecto-, still are accepted in the SI framework. The SI prefixes are listed in the Appendix.

Applications of SI in laboratory medicine

Many international organizations and nations have accepted the International System of Units for reporting results produced by the clinical laboratory. They also have accepted the liter as the preferred unit of volume. When SI units are used, the amounts of constituents of body fluids are reported as substance concentrations rather than mass

TABLE 1-7 Examples of SI-Derived Units Important in Clinical Medicine, Expressed in Terms of Base Units

Quantity	Name	SI Symbol	Expression in Terms of Other SI Units	Expression in Terms of SI Base Units
Volume	Cubic meter	m^3		m^3
Mass density	Kilogram per cubic meter	kg/m^3		kg/m^3
Concentration of amount of substance	Mole per cubic meter	mol/m^3		mol/m^3
Frequency	Hertz	Hz		s^{-1}
Force	Newton	N		$m \times kg \times s^{-2}$
Pressure	Pascal	Pa	N/m^2	$m^{-1} \times kg \times s^{-2}$
Energy, work, quantity of heat	Joule	J	$N \times m$	$m^2 \times kg \times s^{-2}$
Power	Watt	W	J/s	$m^2 \times kg \times s^{-3}$
Electric potential, potential difference, electromotive force	Volt	V	$W \times A^{-1}$	$m^2 \times kg \times s^{-3} \times A^{-1}$

SI, International System of Units.

TABLE 1-8 Typical Values for Analytes and Reporting Increments

Analyte	Conventional Units	Recommended Units	Rounded Recommended Units	Smallest Recommended Reporting Increment
Albumin	3.8 g/dL	550.6 µmol/L	550 µmol/L	10 µmol/L
Bilirubin	0.2 mg/dL	3.42 µmol/L	3 µmol/L	2 µmol/L
Calcium	9.8 mg/dL	2.45 mmol/L	2.45 mmol/L	0.02 mmol/L
Cholesterol	200 mg/dL	5.17 mmol/L	5.2 mmol/L	0.05 mmol/L
Creatinine	0.8 mg/dL	90.48 µmol/L	90 µmol/L	10 µmol/L
Glucose	90 mg/dl	5.00 mmol/L	5.0 mmol/L	0.1 mmol/L
Phosphorus	3.0 mg/dL	0.97 mmol/L	1.0 mmol/L	0.05 mmol/L
Thyroxine	7.0 µg/dL	90.09 nmol/L	90 nmol/L	10 nmol/L
Triglycerides	100 mg/dL	1.14 mmol/L	1.15 mmol/L	0.05 mmol/L
Urea nitrogen*	10 mg/dL	3.57 mmol/L	3.5 mmol/L	0.05 mmol/L
Uric acid	5.0 mg/dL	297 µmol/L	300 µmol/L	10 µmol/L

*Urea nitrogen is reported as urea (mmol/L) when SI units are used.

concentrations (for example, 2.5 mmol/L instead of 10.0 mg/dL for calcium and 3.9 mmol/L instead of 70 mg/dL for glucose). The rationale for this change is that compounds react on a molar basis, and expression of amounts of substances in such terms allows for a better understanding of the relative proportion of compounds. Although physicians initially have little comprehension of the meaning of results when expressed in units of substance concentration, experience in other countries has shown that they soon adjust to the units. Nevertheless, during and after the transition from one set of units to another, numbers must be associated unequivocally with units; therefore no cause exists for misinterpretation. A comparison of results of some of the most commonly measured serum constituents, at concentrations found in healthy individuals, is shown in Table 1-8.

Problem areas in the use of SI units

Problems in the implementation of SI units in the clinical laboratory have been encountered in the expression of:

(1) acidity, (2) enzyme units,* (3) protein concentration, (4) drug concentration, (5) osmolality, (6) units of energy, and (7) units of pressure. Details of these problems are found in an expanded version of this chapter.[2]

Standardized Reporting of Test Results

To describe test results properly, all necessary information must be included in the test description. Systems to express

---

*The proposed base unit katal (symbol *kat*), mol/s, is the catalytic amount of any catalyst, including enzymes, that catalyzes a reaction rate of one mole per second in an assay system. The kind of quantity measured is identified as *catalytic amount*. A constant relationship exists between the International Unit (1 µmol/min) and the katal (1 mol/s); to convert a value in International Units to nmol/s, the value is multiplied by 16.67. Note, however, that dependence on reaction conditions applies to SI units in the same way as it applies to International Units; therefore data reported in the same units but obtained under different conditions may not be comparable. See Chapter 20 for further details on the expression of enzyme activity.

the results produced in the clinical laboratory include the International Federation of Clinical Chemistry (IFCC)/IUPAC system and Logical Observation Identifier Names and Codes (LOINC) system.

IFCC/IUPAC system

The IFCC/IUPAC system recommends that the following items be included in any test description:

1. The name of the system or its abbreviation
2. A dash (two hyphens)
3. The name of the component (never abbreviated) with an initial capital letter
4. A comma
5. The quantity name, or its abbreviation
6. An equal sign
7. The numerical value and the unit or its abbreviation.

LOINC System

The LOINC system is an alternative set of codes developed to provide a set of universal names and identification codes for laboratory tests; the coding system facilitates the electronic transmission of laboratory data within and between institutions. This set of codes was developed by an ad-hoc group of clinical chemists, clinical pathologists, and representatives from the diagnostic industry. It was supported in part by grants and contracts from the John A. Hartford Foundation of New York, U.S. National Library of Medicine, Agency for Health Care Policy and Research, and Regenstrief Institute for Healthcare. A similar standard is being promulgated in Europe.

▦ SAFETY

Since 1970 OSHA and the Centers for Disease Control and Prevention (CDC) have published numerous safety standards that apply to clinical laboratories. Consideration for the health and safety of employees now is accepted as an obligation of all employers and laboratory directors. In May of 1988 OSHA expanded the Hazard Communication Standard to apply to hospital employees.

Safe operation of a clinical laboratory encompasses many aspects, including a formal safety program, various mandated plans (for example, chemical hygiene and blood-borne pathogens plans), and identification of various hazards, such as chemical, fire, electrical, and biological.

Safety Program

Every clinical laboratory should have a formal safety program. Although safety is each individual's responsibility, even in a small laboratory a specific individual should be assigned the title of *safety officer*. This individual should provide guidance to management officials and supervisors whose responsibility it is to provide a safe workplace for all

employees. OSHA[16] mandates that each laboratory have a chemical hygiene officer, designated based on training or experience, to provide technical guidance in the development of the chemical hygiene plan discussed later. Each new employee should receive a copy of the general laboratory safety manual as part of orientation. Each employee should know the location of available evacuation routes and firefighting equipment, as well as the manner in which the equipment is used. The laboratory's continuing education program should include periodic talks on safety. Several audiovisual aids are available from a variety of sources to support the educational part of the program.

Ensuring that the laboratory environment meets accepted safety standards is the second part of a safety program. This effort includes, but is not limited to, attention to proper labeling of chemicals, types and locations of fire extinguishers, maintenance of hoods in good working order, proper grounding of electrical equipment, and provision of means for proper handling and disposal of biohazardous materials, including all patient specimens. An NCCLS approved guideline details the management of clinical laboratory waste.[8]

A good laboratory practice is to organize a safety inspection team from the laboratory staff. This team then is responsible for conducting periodic and scheduled safety inspections.[12] In the United States OSHA inspectors have the authority to enter a clinical laboratory unannounced and, on presentation of credentials, inspect it. The inspection may be regular or the result of a complaint. Although the Joint Commission on Accreditation of Healthcare Organizations (JCAHO) accepts the College of American Pathologists accreditation of a laboratory, the JCAHO may still conduct a safety inspection of the laboratory when it inspects the hospital.

State or local health departments and local fire departments also may conduct regular inspections to determine conformance with their particular requirements. Currently, a laboratory that meets federal or state OSHA requirements is likely to satisfy the standards of any other inspecting agency.

Mandated Plans

In 1991 OSHA mandated that all clinical laboratories in the United States must implement a CHP[16] and an exposure control plan.[17]

Chemical hygiene plan

Topics that must be covered in a **chemical hygiene plan (CHP)** are listed in Table 1-9. Among them is the stipulation that each laboratory must have a complete chemical inventory updated annually. A copy of the **material safety data sheet (MSDS),** which defines each chemical as toxic, carcinogenic, or dangerous, must be on file and readily accessible and available to all employees 24 hours a day, 7 days a week. The chemical manufacturer's information as sup-

TABLE 1-9	Suggested Elements in a CHP

Glossary of terms
Standard operating procedures
Criteria used to determine and implement control measures
Chemical inventory/MSDS
Chemical labeling and storage
Environmental monitoring and maintenance of safety devices
Hazardous waste
Education and training of employees
Personal protective equipment
Responsibilities of chemical hygiene officer, supervisor, and employee
Circumstances under which particular procedures require prior approval
Medical consultation and examination
Record keeping

CHP, Chemical hygiene plan; *MSDS,* material safety data sheet.

plied on the MSDS is used to ascertain whether a certain chemical is hazardous. Each MSDS must provide the product's identity as it appears on the container label, as well as the chemical and common names of its hazardous components. The MSDS also provides physical data on the product, such as boiling point, vapor pressure, and specific gravity, and lists easily recognized characteristics, such as appearance and odor. Information about hazardous properties is given in detail on the MSDS; this data details fire and explosion hazards and health-related information, including the threshold limit value, exposure limits, and toxicity values. The threshold limit value is the allowable exposure for a given employee during an 8-hour day. The MSDS also notes the effects of overexposure and provides information on first-aid, spill, and disposal procedures and protective personal gear and equipment requirements.

Exposure control plan

OSHA regulations[17] require that each laboratory develop, implement, and adhere to a plan that ensures the protection of laboratory employees against potential exposure to **blood-borne pathogens,**[7,12,17] and ensures that the medical wastes the laboratory produces are managed and handled in a safe and effective manner.[8,12] The plan's organization should include sections on (1) purpose, (2) scope, (3) applicable references, (4) applicable definitions, (5) definitions of responsibilities, and (6) detailed procedural steps. In addition, each laboratory employee must be placed into one of three following groups:

- Group I: a job classification in which *all* employees have occupational exposure to blood or other potentially infectious materials
- Group II: a job classification in which *some* employees have occupational exposure to blood or other potentially infectious materials

Employees in this group should be those whose performance of duties defined by their job classifications or whose special assigned tasks put them at risk for *possible* exposure to human blood or other potentially infectious materials. An example of an employee who fits this classification is an instrument technician whose duties require routine maintenance or repair of an instrument in which blood or other potentially infectious materials have been stored. These individuals should receive the same training and orientation as employees in Group I.

- Group III: a job classification in which employees do *not* have *any* occupational exposure to blood or other potentially infectious materials

OSHA does not mandate that employees who qualify for this group receive training on the OSHA Bloodborne Standard. However, these employees must never be asked to perform any procedure that would subject them to occupational exposure. If in the future an employee in this group has any duties added to the job that would include exposure-prone tasks, the employee must be added to the Group II list. Training of this employee in all aspects of the OSHA Bloodborne Standard *must* be completed before the employee's actual performance of the new duties. In addition, the employee must be offered vaccination for hepatitis B within 10 working days of initial assignment to a position involving exposure.

Hazards in the Laboratory

Various types of hazards are encountered in the operation of a clinical laboratory. These hazards must be identified and labeled, and work practices must be developed to deal with them. Types of hazards may include, biological, chemical, electrical, and fire.

Identification of hazards

Clinical laboratories deal with each of the nine classes of hazardous materials, which are classified by the United Nations (UN) as (1) explosives, (2) compressed gases, (3) flammable liquids, (4) flammable solids, (5) oxidizer materials, (6) toxic materials, (7) radioactive materials, (8) corrosive materials, and (9) miscellaneous materials not otherwise classified.

Warning labels aid in the identification of chemical hazards during shipment. Under regulations of the U.S. Department of Transportation (DOT), chemicals transported within and into the United States must carry labels based on the UN classification.

DOT placards or labels are diamond-shaped, with a digit imprinted on the bottom corner that identifies the UN hazard class (1 to 9). The hazard is identified more specifically in printed words placed along the horizontal axis of the diamond. Color-coding and a pictorial art description of the hazard supplement the identification of hazardous material on the label; the artwork appears in the top half of the dia-

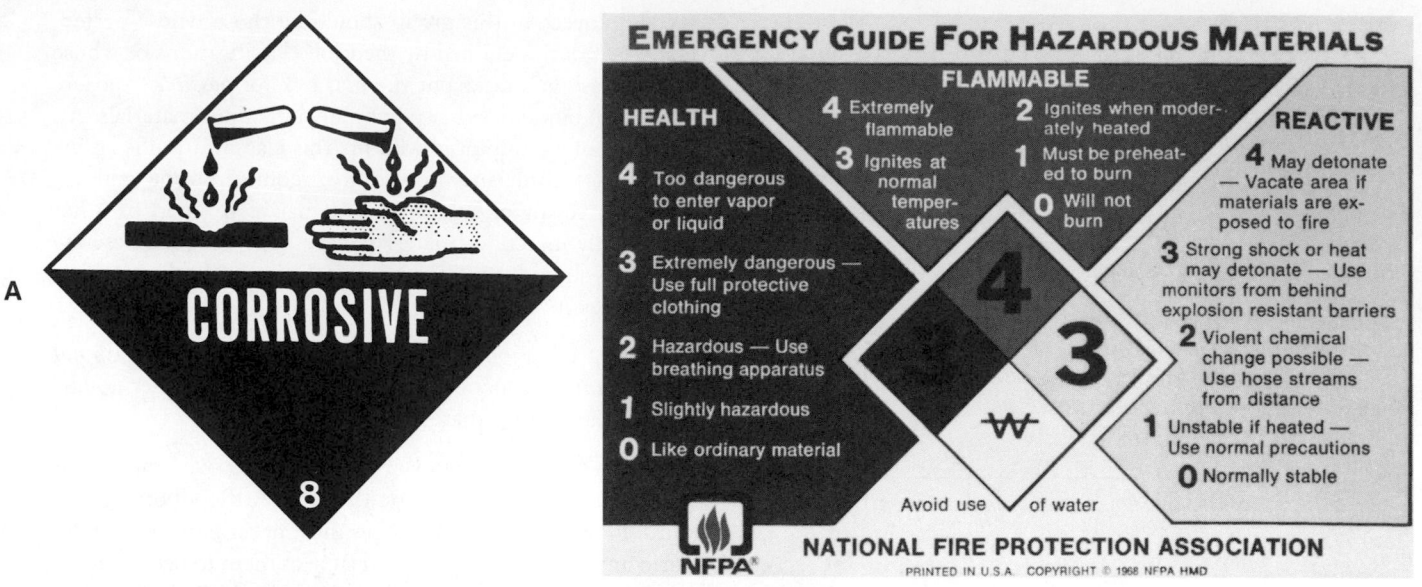

Figure 1-5   **A,** Department of Transportation label for corrosives. **B,** Labeling identification system of the National Fire Protection Association.

mond (Figure 1-5, *A*). The upper half of the label for corrosives shows a metallic bar and a hand, both of which are being eaten away by drops of fluid; the black bottom half of the label is in white with the word *corrosive*. The bottom corner shows the digit *8.*

The DOT uses the UN system to ship hazardous materials; however, when the hazardous material reaches its destination and is removed from the shipping container, the identification is lost. The laboratory then must label each individual container. Usually, the information necessary to classify a container's contents appropriately is listed on the shipping label and should be noted. Important first-aid information also usually is provided on this label.

Although OSHA prescribes the use of labels or other appropriate warnings, at present no single, uniform labeling system for hazardous chemicals exists for clinical laboratories. Appropriate hazard warnings include words, pictures, symbols, or combinations that convey the health or physical hazards of the container's contents and must specify the chemical's effect and the specific target organs involved.

The National Fire Protection Association (NFPA) has developed the 704-M Identification System, which classifies hazardous material by number from 0 to 4 (4 being most hazardous) according to flammability and reactivity (instability). This system uses diamond-shaped labels, available from most companies that sell laboratory safety equipment, that are color coded and divided into quadrants. Each of the three quadrants has a characteristic color that represents a type of hazard, and a number in the quadrant indicates the degree of the hazard. The fourth (lower) quadrant contains information of special interest to firefighters; for example, *W* indicates a water-ignitable material (see Figure 1-5, *B*).

Some chemicals require labels using two or three quadrants to convey the necessary information.

Descriptive labels, such as those labeled *corrosive, flammable, poison,* and *explosives,* also may be used. Obviously, some containers may require two or three labels because several types of hazards are involved. Kits containing assorted safety signs are available from most laboratory supply dealers. These contain most general labels needed in a clinical laboratory. An example kit may include labels that read *eye wash, use in hood, safety shower, empty cylinder,* and *wear eye protection in this area.*

Biological hazards

To operate a clinical laboratory safely, prevention of laboratory employee exposure to infectious agents, such as the hepatitis viruses and HIV, is essential. Exposure to infectious agents results from (1) accidental puncture with needles, (2) spraying of infectious materials by a syringe or spilling and splattering of these materials on benchtops or floors, (3) centrifuge accidents, and (4) cuts or scratches from contaminated vessels. Any unfixed tissue, including blood slides, also must be treated as potentially infectious material.

As discussed previously in this section, OSHA has mandated that all U.S. laboratories implement an **exposure control plan.**[17] In addition, the National Institute for Occupational Safety and Health, a functional unit of the CDC, has prepared and widely distributed a document entitled **"Universal Precautions"** that specifies how U.S. clinical laboratories should handle infectious agents.[15] In general, the document mandates that clinical laboratories treat all human blood and other potentially infectious materials as if they were known to contain infectious agents, such as HBV,

HIV, and other blood-borne pathogens. The precautions apply to all specimens of blood, serum, plasma, blood products, vaginal secretions, semen, cerebrospinal fluid, synovial fluid, and concentrated HBV or HIV viruses. In addition, any specimen that contains visible traces of blood should be handled through use of the Universal Precautions.

Universal Precautions also specifies that laboratory employees must use barrier protection to prevent skin and mucous membrane contamination. These barriers, also known as *personal protective equipment*, include gloves, gowns, laboratory coats, face shields or mask and eye protection, mouthpieces, resuscitation bags, pocket masks, and other ventilator devices. In practice, latex allergy has been a problem with some individuals when latex gloves are required. By September 1992, 1100 reactions and 15 fatalities related to latex allergy had been reported to the Federal Drug Administration.[4]

The NCCLS also has published a similar set of recommendations,[7,12] several of which are specified as requirements in the OSHA Exposure Control Plan. They include the following:

1. Never perform mouth pipetting and never blow out pipets that contain potentially infectious material.
2. Do not mix potentially infectious material by bubbling air through the liquid.
3. Use barrier protection, such as gloves, masks, and protective eyewear and gowns, when drawing blood from a patient and handling all patient specimens, including when removing stoppers from tubes. Disposable, non-sterile latex or vinyl gloves provide adequate barrier protection. Phlebotomists should change gloves and dispose of them between patients.
4. Wash hands whenever gloves are changed.
5. Use facial barrier protection if a significant potential exists for the spattering of blood or body fluids.
6. Avoid using syringes whenever possible and dispose of needles in rigid containers without handling them (Figure 1-6).
7. Dispose of all sharps appropriately.
8. Wear protective clothing, which is an effective barrier against potentially infective materials. When leaving the laboratory, remove the protective clothing.
9. Try to prevent accidental injuries.
10. Encourage frequent hand washing in the laboratory; employees must wash their hands whenever they leave the laboratory.
11. Make a habit of keeping your hands from your mouth, nose, eyes, and other mucous membranes to reduce the possibility of self-inoculation.
12. Minimize spills and spatters.
13. Decontaminate all surfaces and reusable devices after use with appropriate EPA-registered hospital disinfectants. Sterilization, disinfection, and decontamination are discussed in detail in NCCLS publication M29-A2.[7]

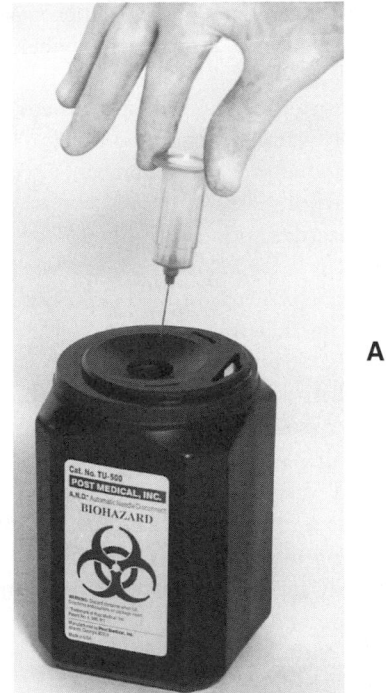

A

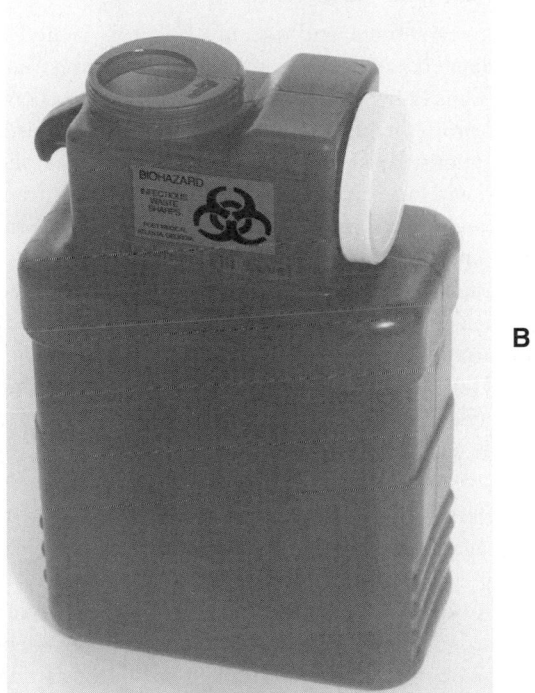

B

Figure 1-6 Convenient needle disposal system for sharps: **(A)** small (for blood-drawing tray) or **(B)** large. (Courtesy Post Medical, Inc., Atlanta.)

14. Do not use warning labels on patient specimens.

15. Use biosafety Level 2 procedures whenever appropriate.[12]

16. Before centrifuging tubes, inspect them for cracks. Inspect the inside of the trunnion cup for signs of erosion or adhering matter. Ensure that rubber cushions are free from all bits of glass.

17. Use biohazard disposal techniques (for example, "Red Bag").

18. Never leave a discarded tube or infected material unattended or unlabeled.

19. Periodically clean the freezer and dry-ice chests to remove broken ampules and tubes of biological specimens. Use rubber gloves and respiratory protection during cleaning.

20. Offer HBV vaccine to all employees at risk of potential exposure as a regular or occasional part of their duties; provision of the vaccine is an OSHA mandate. The CDC's Advisory Committee on Immunization Practices recommends that medical technologists, phlebotomists, and pathologists all be vaccinated with HBV vaccine.

Chemical hazards

The proper storage and use of chemicals is necessary to avoid dangers such as burns, explosions, fires, and toxic fumes. Thus knowledge of the properties of the chemicals in use and proper handling procedures greatly reduces dangerous situations. Bottles of chemicals and solutions should be handled carefully, and a cart should be used to transport a heavy container or multiple number of containers from one area to another. Glass containers with chemicals should be transported in rubber or plastic containers that protect them from breakage and contain the spill if breakage does occur. Appropriate spill kits should be available in strategical locations. General spill kits are available commercially and should contain specific materials to be used with spills of acid or caustic or organic materials. Directions for appropriate use of these materials are specified in these kits.

Spattering from acids, caustic materials, and strong oxidizing agents probably represents the greatest hazard to clothing and eyes and is a potential source of chemical burns. A bottle should never be held by its neck, but instead firmly around its body with one or both hands, depending on the size of the bottle. Acids must be diluted through slow addition to water; *water should never be added to concentrated acid.* During work with acid or alkali solutions, safety glasses should be worn. Acids, caustic materials, and strong oxidizing agents should be mixed in the sink, which provides water for cooling, as well as for confinement of the reagent in case the flask or bottle breaks.

All bottles containing reagents must be labeled properly. A good practice is to label the container before adding the reagent, thus avoiding the possibility of an unlabeled reagent. The label should bear the name and concentration of the reagent, the initials of the individual who made up the reagent, and the date on which the reagent was prepared. When appropriate the expiration date also should be included. The labels should be color-coded or an additional label added to designate specific storage instructions, such as the need for refrigeration or special storage related to a potential hazard. All reagents found in unlabeled bottles should be disposed of with the appropriate procedures and precautions. Strong acids, caustic materials, and strong oxidizing agents should be dispensed via any of a number of commercially available automatic dispensing devices. Under *no* circumstances is mouth pipetting permitted.

Perchloric acid, because it is potentially explosive in contact with organic materials, requires careful handling procedures. Perchloric acid should not be used on wooden bench tops, and bottles of the acid should be stored on a glass tray. Adding the acid dropwise (with a splatter shield) to at least 100 volumes of cold water and pouring the diluted acid down the drain with large amounts of additional cold water is an accepted method of disposal. Special perchloric acid hoods, with special wash-down facilities, should be installed if large amounts of this acid are used.

Special care is needed with mercury. Even small drops of mercury on benchtops and floors can poison the atmosphere in a poorly ventilated room. Mercury's ability to amalgamate with a number of metals is well known. After an accidental spillage of mercury, the spill area should be cleaned carefully until no droplets remain. All containers of mercury should be kept well stoppered.

The U.S. Environmental Protection Agency controls the disposal of nonradioactive hazardous wastes. The Resource Conservation and Recovery Act of 1976 (RCRA) states that disposal of materials classifiable within any of the nine UN hazardous materials classes is enforced in such a way that health and safety professionals involved in the disposal of such materials are liable personally for each individual violation. An NCCLS publication[8] also addresses hazardous waste disposal. However, many municipalities and states have their own regulations, and the laboratory should contact them for specifics.

Hazards from volatile chemicals

The use of organic solvents in a clinical laboratory represents a potential fire hazard and other health hazards from the inhalation of toxic vapors or from skin contact. These solvents should be used in a fume hood. Storage of organic solvents is regulated by rules set down by OSHA (Table 1-10). However, some local fire department rules are more stringent. Solvents should be stored in an OSHA-approved metal storage cabinet that is properly vented. The maximum working volume of flammable solvents allowed outside storage cabinets is 5 gallons per room. No more than 60 gallons of Type I and II solvents may be stored in a single cabinet. No more than three cabinets may be located in each 5000

TABLE 1-10 Maximum Allowable Size of Containers for Storage of Solvents Inside Buildings (OSHA)

| Container Type | Maximum Allowable Size of Containers | | | |
	Class IA	Class IB	Class IC	Classes II and III
Glass or approved plastic	1 pt	1 qt	1 gal	1 gal
Safety cans*	1 gal	2 gal	5 gal	5 gal
Metal drums (DOT)	60 gal	60 gal	60 gal	60 gal

Class	Definition
IA	Flash point below 22.8 °C; boiling point below 37.8 °C
IB	Flash point below 22.8 °C; boiling point above 37.8 °C
IC	Flash point between 22.8 °C and 37.8 °C
II	Flash point between 37.8 °C and 60 °C
III	Flash point above 60 °C

OSHA, Occupational Safety and Health Administration; *DOT*, Department of Transportation.
* A safety can is a metal or plastic container with a spring-closing spout cover designed to relieve internal pressure when the container is subjected to the heat of fire and prevent leakage if the container is tipped. A safety can also is equipped with a flame-arrester screen. Portable safety cans range in size from 1 pint to 5 gallons in numerous styles that feature faucets, pouring spouts, and dispensing hoses. Only safety cans tested and approved by the Factory Mutual Engineering Corporation of the Factory Mutual System or by Underwriters Laboratories, Inc. should be used.

square feet of laboratory space. Larger amounts than those shown in Table 1-10 must be stored in special refrigerated storage rooms or in outside storage buildings.

Vaporization is the major problem in the ignition and spread of fires. Vapors from flammable and combustible liquids and solids form a flammable mixture with air. These vapors are characterized by their flash point, the lowest temperature at which a solvent gives off flammable vapors in the close vicinity of its surface. The mixture at its flash point ignites when exposed to a source of ignition. At temperatures below the flash point the vapor is considered too dilute for ignition.

Disposal of flammable solvents in storm sewers or sanitary sewers generally is prohibited. Exceptions include small amounts of those materials miscible with water, but even disposal of these should be followed by large amounts of cold water. Other solvents should be collected in safety cans. Separate cans should be used for ether and chlorinated solvents; all other solvents may be combined in a third can. The cans should be stored, in keeping with storage quantity rules, in a safety cabinet until pickup by a waste-disposal firm. A more economical approach is to transfer the solvents to larger cans or drums in an outside storage facility so that pickup is less frequent. Some large institutions have their own in-house disposal facilities.

Hazards from compressed gases

DOT regulations cover the labeling of cylinders of compressed gases that are transported by interstate carriers. The diamond-shaped labels described previously are used on all large cylinders and any boxes containing small cylinders. Some general rules for handling large cylinders of compressed gas include the following:

1. Always transport cylinders with a hand truck to which the cylinder is secured.
2. Leave the valve cap on a cylinder until the cylinder is ready for use, before which time the cylinder should be secured by a support around the upper one third of its body. Disconnect the hose or regulator, shut off the valve, and replace the cap before the cylinder is completely empty to avoid the possibility of the development of a negative pressure. Place a sign or label that reads *empty* on the container.
3. Chain or secure cylinders at all times, even when they are empty.
4. Always check cylinders for the composition of their contents before connection to the regulator.
5. Never force threads; if a regulator does not thread readily onto the tank, something is wrong.

The precautions cited for large refillable gas cylinders also apply to small disposable cylinders, such as propane cylinders of the type frequently secured to flame photometers and cylinders of calibrating gases for blood gas equipment. Cylinders in floor-standing base supports require the additional security of a chain or strap attached to a wall or fixed piece of furniture. Local fire department regulations, which vary considerably, govern the disposal of exhausted cylinders.

Electrical hazards

Wherever electrical wires or connections exist, the potential for shock or fire hazard also exists. Worn wires on all electrical equipment should be replaced immediately; all equipment should be grounded through use of three-prong plugs. OSHA regulations stipulate that the requirements for grounding of electrical equipment stated in the National Electrical Code (published by the NFPA) be met. If grounded receptacles are unavailable, a licensed electrician should be consulted for proper alternative grounding techniques. Some local codes are more stringent than OSHA requirements and do not allow for two-pole mating receptacles for a three-pole plug.

Use of extension cords is prohibited. This standard is more stringent than any other existing regulation. However, in some instances an extension cord may be used temporarily, in which case the cord should be less than 12 feet long, have at least 16 AWG (American Wire Gauge) wire, be approved by the Underwriters Laboratory (UL), and have only one outlet at the end. If several outlets are needed in an area, a power strip with its own fuse or circuit breaker

TABLE 1-11	Classification of Fires and Fire Extinguisher Requirements		
Type of Hazard		**Class of Fire**	**Recommended Extinguisher Agents**
Ordinary Combustibles			
Wood, cloth, paper		A	Water, dry chemical foam, loaded steam
Flammable Liquids and Gases			
Solvents and greases, natural or manufactured gases		B	Dry chemical, carbon dioxide, loaded steam, Halon 1211 or 1301 foam
Electrical Equipment			
Any energized electrical equipment; if electricity is turned off at the source, equipment reverts to a Class A or B		C	Dry chemical, carbon dioxide, Halon 1211 or 1301 foam
Combinations of Hazards			
Ordinary combustibles and flammable liquids and gases		A and B	Dry chemical, loaded steam, foam
Ordinary combustibles and electrical equipment		A and C	Dry chemical
Flammable liquids and gases and electrical equipment		B and C	Dry chemical, carbon dioxide, Halon 1211 or 1301 foam
Ordinary combustibles, flammable liquids and gases, and electrical equipment		A, B, and C	Triplex dry chemical

may be installed at least 3 inches above benchtop level. Several manufacturers now sell devices that check for high resistance in neutral or ground wiring or excess voltage in the neutral wiring.

Electrical equipment and connections should not be handled with wet hands, nor should electrical equipment be used after liquid has been spilled on it. The equipment must be turned off immediately and dried thoroughly; a fan or hair dryer will speed this process. In case a wet or malfunctioning electrical instrument is used by several individuals, the plug should be pulled and a note cautioning all employees against its use should be placed prominently on the instrument.

Fire hazards

The ideal solution to the problem of fires and indeed to all laboratory accidents is prevention. However, all fires cannot be prevented, so provisions must be made for those that do occur. NFPA and OSHA publish standards covering subjects from emergency exits to safety and firefighting equipment. NFPA also publishes the National Fire Codes. Many state and local agencies have adopted these codes, some of which are more stringent than OSHA requirements, making them legally enforceable.

Every laboratory should have the necessary equipment to extinguish or confine a fire in the laboratory, as well as on the clothing of an individual. Easy access to safety showers is essential. A safety shower should have a pull chain either attached to the wall at a convenient height or hanging from the shower head; the chain should have a large ring attached to it so that an individual may activate the shower easily in an emergency, even with closed eyes. Fire blankets to smother flaming clothing should be available in an easily accessible, wall-mounted case. To use them the individual should unroll the blanket from its case and roll it around the body by taking hold of the rope attached to the blanket and turning the body around. The local fire marshal dictates the location of this equipment, as well as the locations of fire alarms and maps of evacuation routes.

Various types of fire extinguishers are available for use in various types of fires. Because every area practically cannot contain several types of fire extinguishers, dry chemical fire extinguishers are among the best all-purpose extinguishers. An extinguisher should be located near each laboratory door and also at the end of the room opposite the door in particularly large laboratories. Every individual in the laboratory should be instructed in the use of these extinguishers and other available firefighting equipment. All fire extinguishers should be tested by qualified personnel at intervals specified by the manufacturer. The three classes of fires and the type of fire extinguisher for each are listed in Table 1-11. Each fire extinguisher is labeled based on the type of fire it should be used to extinguish.

Two additional types of fires, designated D and E, should be handled only by trained personnel. Type D fires include those involving powdered metal materials, such as magnesium. A special powder is used to fight this hazard. A type E fire is one that cannot be extinguished or is liable to result in a detonation, such as an arsenal fire. A type "E" fire usually is allowed to burn out while nearby materials are protected.

To minimize fire damage many clinical laboratories now have computers housed in temperature- and humidity-controlled rooms. The most popular automatic fire control system used for these rooms is Halon 1301 (bromotrifluoromethane). Although it is the least toxic of the halons, NFPA regulations require a warning sign at the entrance to the room and the availability of self-contained breathing equipment.

References

1. American Society for Testing and Materials: ASTM Standards 11.01-Water 1 and 11.02-Water 2. Philadelphia, American Society for Testing and Materials, 1991.

2. Bermes EW Jr, Young DS: General laboratory techniques and procedures. In Burtis CA, Ashwood ER (eds): Tietz Textbook of Clinical Chemistry, 3rd edition, pp 3-41, Philadelphia, WB Saunders, 1999.

3. Dudley AW, Lin JJ, Leu NC: Automatic balancing centrifuge (ABC). Am J Clin Pathol 1994; 101:399.

4. Landwehr L, Boguniewicz M: Current perspectives on latex allergy. Pediatrics 1996; 128:305-312.

5. National Committee for Clinical Laboratory Standards: Procedures for the Handling and Processing of Blood Specimens: Approved Guideline. NCCLS Document H18-A2. Wayne, Pa, National Committee for Clinical Laboratory Standards, 2000.

6. National Committee for Clinical Laboratory Standards: Temperature Calibration of Water Baths, Instruments, and Temperature Sensors: Approved Standard. 2nd edition. NCCLS Document I2-A2. Wayne, Pa, National Committee for Clinical Laboratory Standards, 1990.

7. National Committee for Clinical Laboratory Standards: Protection of Laboratory Workers From Infectious Disease Transmitted by Blood, Body Fluids, and Tissue: Tentative Guideline. NCCLS Document M29-A2. Wayne, Pa, National Committee for Clinical Laboratory Standards, 1997.

8. National Committee for Clinical Laboratory Standards: Clinical Laboratory Waste Management: Approved Guideline. NCCLS Document GP5-A. Wayne, Pa, National Committee for Clinical Laboratory Standards, 1993.

9. National Committee for Clinical Laboratory Standards: Terminology and Definitions for Use in NCCLS Documents: Proposed Standard. 3rd edition. NCCLS Document NRSCL8-A. Wayne, Pa, National Committee for Clinical Laboratory Standards, 1998.

10. National Committee for Clinical Laboratory Standards: Source Book of Reference Methods, Materials, and Related Information for the Clinical Laboratory: Proposed Guideline. NCCLS Document NRSCL12-P. Wayne, Pa, National Committee for Clinical Laboratory Standards, 1994.

11. National Committee for Clinical Laboratory Standards: The Reference System for the Clinical Laboratory: Criteria for Development and Credentialing of Methods and Materials for Harmonization of Results: Proposed Guideline. NCCLS Document NRSCL13-P. Wayne, Pa, National Committee for Clinical Laboratory Standards, 1995.

12. National Committee for Clinical Laboratory Standards: Clinical Laboratory Safety: Approved Guideline. NCCLS Document GP17-A. Wayne, Pa, National Committee for Clinical Laboratory Standards, 1996.

13. National Committee for Clinical Laboratory Standards: Blood Alcohol Testing in the Clinical Laboratory: Approved Guideline. NCCLS Document T/DM6-A. Wayne, Pa, National Committee for Clinical Laboratory Standards, 1999.

14. National Committee for Clinical Laboratory Standards: Preparation and Testing of Reagent Water in the Clinical Laboratory. Approved Guideline. 3rd edition. NCCLS Document C3-A3. Wayne, Pa, National Committee for Clinical Laboratory Standards, 1997.

15. National Institute for Occupational Safety and Health: Guidelines for Prevention of Transmission of Human Immunodeficiency Virus and Hepatitis B Virus of Health-Care and Public Safety Workers. DHSS (NIOSH) Publication No. 89-107. Washington, DC, Department of Health and Social Services, February, 1989.

16. Occupational Exposure to Hazardous Chemicals in the Laboratory: Occupational Safety and Health Administration (OSHA). Document 29 CFR, Part 1910. Federal Register 1991; 55:3300-3335.

17. Occupational Exposure to Bloodborne Pathogens: Occupational Safety and Health Administration (OSHA) Final Rule. Federal Register 1991; 56:64,004-64,182.

18. Reference Samples/Reference Materials. Geel, Belgium, Institute for Reference Materials and Measurements, European Commission, Joint Research Center, 1996.

Additional Reading

American Society for Testing and Materials: ASTM Standard E542-94. Calibration of Laboratory Volumetric Apparatus. Philadelphia, American Society for Testing and Materials, 1996.

Committee on Hazardous Substances in the Laboratory: Prudent Practices for Handling Hazardous Chemicals in Laboratories: National Research Council. Washington, DC, National Academy Press, 1985.

Dean JA: Analytical Chemistry Handbook. New York, McGraw-Hill, 1995.

Laboratory Waste Management: A Guidebook, Washington, DC, American Chemical Society, 1994.

Montgomery, L: Health and Safety Guidelines for the Laboratory, Chicago, ASCP Press, 1995.

Young DS, Hirth EJ: SI Units for Clinical Measurements. Philadelphia, American College of Physicians, 1997.

CHAPTER 2

Specimen Collection and Other Preanalytical Variables

DONALD S. YOUNG, MB, PhD, and EDWARD W. BERMES, JR., PhD

Objectives

1. State the types of specimens that can be assayed in a clinical laboratory and determine the correct specimen type for the common laboratory tests.
2. Describe the proper method of specimen collection, handling, and transport for the most common specimen types tested in a clinical laboratory.
3. Determine the type of color-coded, evacuated tube that is appropriate for assessment of various analytes.
4. List anticoagulants and state both their action on whole blood and their appropriate uses in various laboratory tests.
5. State the effects of physiological, biological, and environmental factors on laboratory analyses.

Key Words

Additives   Compounds added to biological specimens to prevent them from clotting or preserve their constituents

Anticoagulant   Any substance that prevents blood from clotting

Hemoconcentration   A decrease in the fluid content of the blood that results in an increase in the concentration of the blood constituents

Hemodilution   An increase in the fluid content of the blood that results in a decrease in the concentration of the blood constituents

Hemolysis   Disruption of the red cell membrane, causing release of hemoglobin

Phlebotomist   An individual who practices phlebotomy; the individual who withdraws a specimen of blood

Phlebotomy   The puncture of a blood vessel to collect blood

Preanalytical Variables   Factors that affect specimens before tests are performed; classified as either *controllable* or *noncontrollable*

Preservative   A substance or preparation added to a specimen to prevent changes in the constituents of the specimen

Plasma   The fluid portion of the blood in which the cells are suspended; differs from serum in that it contains fibrinogen and related compounds removed from serum when blood clots

Serum   The clear liquid that separates from blood on clotting

Specimen   A sample or part of a body fluid or tissue collected for examination, study, or analysis

Tourniquet   A device applied around an extremity to control the circulation and prevent the flow of blood to or from the distal area

Venipuncture   The process by which a blood specimen is obtained from a patient's vein

---

Many factors besides disease affect the composition of body fluids, including preanalytical variables that occur before analysis and are classified as either *controllable* or *noncontrollable*. The effects of these variables on test values must be recognized and considered in the evaluation of laboratory data. Because many controllable, preanalytical variables are associated with specimen collection, this chapter begins with a discussion of proper specimen collection techniques. Other controllable and noncontrollable variables that affect test values and their interpretations are discussed in the latter part of the chapter.

■ SPECIMEN COLLECTION

Examples of biological **specimens** analyzed in clinical laboratories include whole blood; serum; plasma; urine; feces; sweat; saliva; cerebrospinal, synovial, amniotic, pleural, pericardial, and peritoneal fluids; and various types of solid tissues. The National Committee for Clinical Laboratory Standards (NCCLS) publishes a number of procedures for the collection of many such specimens under standardized conditions.[8-15] In addition, the National Institute for Occupational Safety and Health, a functional unit of the Centers for Disease Control and Prevention, has prepared for wide distribution a document entitled *Universal Precautions* that specifies how U.S. clinical laboratories should collect specimens safely.

Blood

Blood is the fluid that the heart circulates through the body's arteries, capillaries, and veins. It consists of **plasma** (a pale yellow liquid), erythrocytes (red blood corpuscles), leukocytes (white cells or corpuscles), and platelets (thrombocytes). **Serum** describes the normally clear liquid that separates from blood when it clots.

Blood for analysis may be obtained from veins, arteries, or capillaries. Venous blood is usually the specimen of choice, and venipuncture is the method used to obtain this specimen.[13] In young children skin puncture frequently is used to obtain what is predominantly capillary blood; arterial puncture is used mainly for blood gas analysis.

Venipuncture

In the clinical laboratory **venipuncture** is the process by which a blood specimen is obtained from a patient's vein.[13] The procedure is accomplished through insertion of a needle into the vein followed by withdrawal of a volume of blood into an evacuated tube* or syringe. The *draw* is defined as the quantity of blood withdrawn, whereas the removal of a blood sample from a vein is known as **phlebotomy.**

Preliminary steps

Before a specimen is collected, the **phlebotomist** should ask patients to verify their identities by asking them to state their names. If appropriate, the phlebotomist should verify that patients are fasting. Patients should be comfortably seated or in supine positions and should have been in the position for 20 minutes before the specimen is drawn. This standardization minimizes differences in concentrations of blood constituents due to variations in blood volume (**hemoconcentration** or **hemodilution**).

The patient's arm should be extended in a straight line from the shoulder to the wrist. An arm with an inserted intravenous line should not be used, nor should an arm with extensive scarring or a hematoma at the intended site. If a woman has had a mastectomy, arm veins on that side of the body should not be used because the surgery may have caused lymphostasis, which affects the blood composition.

Before performing a venipuncture, the phlebotomist should estimate the volume of blood to be drawn and select the appropriate number and types of tubes for the plasma or serum tests requested, as well as an appropriate needle. The most commonly used sizes are gauges 19 to 22. The larger the gauge size, the smaller the bore of the needle. The usual choice for an adult with normal veins is gauge 20; if veins tend to collapse easily, a size 21 is preferred. For volumes of blood from 30 to 50 mL, an 18-gauge needle may be required to ensure adequate blood flow and reduce the chance of hemolysis. All needles must be sterile, sharp, and free from barbs. If blood is drawn for trace-element measurements, the needle should be stainless steel and free from contamination. For trace element determinations all objects that come into contact with the specimen should be acid-washed or should be free of trace metal contamination (see Chapter 29).

Location

The median cubital vein in the antecubital fossa, or crook of the elbow, is the preferred site for collection of venous blood in adults because the vein is both large and close to the surface of the skin. Veins on the back of the hand or at the ankle may be used, but these are less preferable and should be avoided in diabetics and other patients with poor circulation. In severely ill patients or those requiring many intravenous injections, an alternative blood-drawing site should be selected.[1] Selection of a vein for puncture is facilitated by palpation. An arm containing a cannula or arteriovenous fistula should not be used without consent of the patient's physician. If fluid is being infused intravenously into

---

*Evacuated tubes are tubes that are sealed and maintained under vacuum. This vacuum is used to pull the blood specimen into the tube. The extent of the vacuum is such that a predetermined volume of blood is withdrawn into the tube. Evacuated tubes have expiration dates, beyond which time the vacuum may not be maintained or the anticoagulant may not be effective. The expiration date and tube type are printed clearly on each individual tube.

a limb, the fluid should be shut off for 3 minutes before a specimen is obtained, and a suitable note should be made in the patient's chart and on the result report form. Specimens obtained from the opposite arm or below the infusion site in the same arm may be satisfactory for most tests except for those analytes that are contained in the infused solutions (for example, glucose or electrolytes).

Preparation of the site

The area around the intended puncture site should be cleaned with a prepackaged alcohol swab or gauze pad saturated with 70% isopropanol. Cleaning of the puncture site should be performed in a circular motion and outward from the site. The skin should air-dry. No alcohol should remain on the skin because traces of it may cause hemolysis and invalidate test results. When specimens are to be collected for ethanol determinations, the skin should be cleaned with an alcohol-free, benzalkonium chloride solution (Zephiran chloride solution, 1:750). Povidone-iodine should be avoided as a cleaning agent because it may interfere with several analytical procedures. Once the skin has been cleaned, it should not be touched until after the venipuncture has been completed.

Timing

The time at which a specimen is obtained is important[3,6] for those blood constituents that undergo marked diurnal variation (for example, corticosteroids and iron) and those used to monitor drug therapy (for example, digoxin or prothrombin time) because the interval after drug administration affects the drug concentration. Furthermore, special precautions in the collection and handling of specimens are required for tests for alcohol and tests of medicolegal importance for which a chain of custody for the specimen must be established.

Venous occlusion

After the skin is cleaned, either a blood pressure cuff or **tourniquet** is applied 4 to 6 inches (10 to 15 cm) above the intended puncture site to obstruct the return of venous blood to the heart and distend the veins. When a blood pressure cuff is used as a tourniquet, it usually is inflated to approximately 60 mm Hg (8.0 kPa). Tourniquets typically are made from precut soft rubber strips or from Velcro-type bands. A tourniquet usually needs to be left in place no longer than 1 minute, but even within this short time the composition of blood changes. Although the changes that occur in 1 minute are slight, marked changes have been observed after 3 minutes (Table 2-1).

The composition of blood drawn first—that blood closest to the tourniquet—is most representative of the composition of circulating blood. The first-drawn specimen therefore should be used for those analytes such as calcium that are pertinent to critical medical decisions. Blood drawn later demonstrates a greater effect of venous stasis. The concen-

TABLE 2-1	Changes* in Composition of Serum When Venous Occlusion Is Prolonged from 1 to 3 Minutes			
Increase	Percent (%)	Decrease	Percent (%)
Total protein	4.9	Potassium	6.2
Iron	6.7		
Total lipids	4.7		
Cholesterol	5.1		
Aspartate aminotransferase	9.3		
Bilirubin	8.4		
Mean values obtained from 11 healthy individuals			

From Statland BE, Bokelund H, Winkel P: Factors contributing to intraindividual variation of serum constituents. 4. Effects of posture and tourniquet application on variation of serum constituents in healthy subjects. Clin Chem 1974; 20:1513-1519.
*To estimate the probable effect of a factor on results, relate the percent increase or decrease shown (or intimated) in the table to analytical variation (± % CV) routinely found for analytes. CV, Coefficient of variation.

tration of protein-bound constituents also is influenced by stasis and may be sufficient to increase the concentration of protein or protein-bound constituents by 15%. A uniform procedure for the order of draw for tests therefore should be established. In addition, the increase in activity of creatine kinase and aspartate aminotransferase in serum after venipuncture may be due to hemoconcentration, the slight trauma to tissue as the needle pierces the skin, or stasis of blood in the tissues.

Pumping of the fist before venipuncture should be avoided because it causes an increase in the plasma potassium, phosphate, and lactate concentrations. The lowering of the blood pH by accumulation of lactate causes the plasma ionized calcium concentration to increase. The ionized calcium concentration reverts to normal 10 minutes after the tourniquet is released.

Stress associated with blood collection can produce unwanted effects in patients of all ages. As a consequence, plasma concentrations of cortisol and growth hormone may increase. Stress occurs particularly in young children who are frightened, struggling, or held in physical restraint. Collection under these conditions may cause adrenal stimulation, leading to an increased plasma glucose concentration, or create increases in the serum activities of enzymes that originate in skeletal muscles.

Collection with an evacuated blood tube

Evacuated blood tubes usually are less expensive and considered more convenient and easier to use than syringes. Several types of evacuated tubes are available for venipuncture collection.[10] They differ by the additive used and volume of the tube. The different types are identified by the

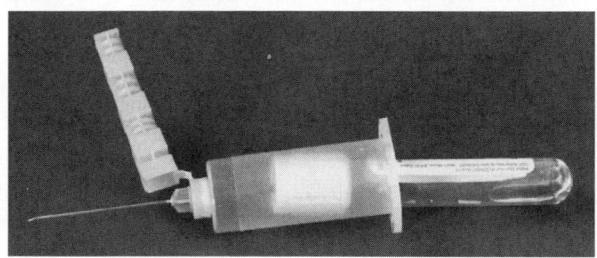

Figure 2-1   Assembled venipuncture set. (From Flynn JC: Procedures in Phlebotomy, 2nd edition, p 79, Philadelphia, WB Saunders, 1999.)

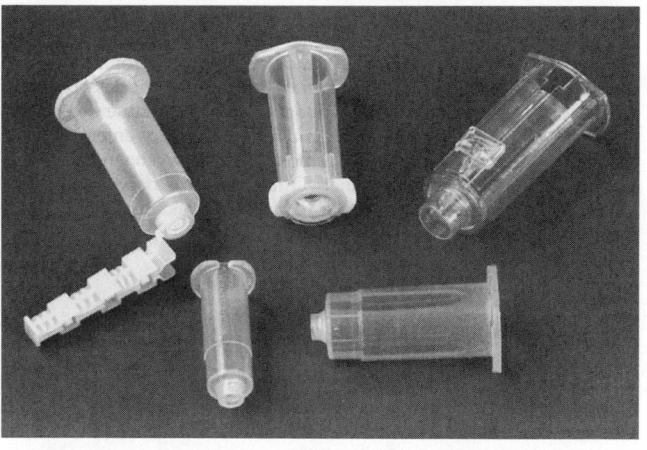

Figure 2-2   Various tube holders used in venipuncture. (From Flynn JC: Procedures in Phlebotomy, 2nd edition, p 79, Philadelphia, WB Saunders, 1999.)

TABLE 2-2   Coding of Stopper Color in Evacuated Blood Tubes

Tube Type	Additive	Stopper Color	Alternative
Gel separation tubes	Polymer gel/silica activator	Red/gray	Gold
	Polymer gel/silica activator/lithium heparin	Green/gray	Light gray
Serum tubes (nonadditive)	Silicone-coated interior	Red	Red
	Uncoated interior	Red	Pink
Serum tubes (with additives)	Thrombin (dry additive)	Yellow/gray; beige	Orange
	Particulate clot activator	Yellow/red	Red
	Thrombin (dry additive)	Light blue	Light blue
Whole blood/plasma tubes	K_2 EDTA (dry additive) K_3 EDTA (liquid additive) Na_2 EDTA (dry additive)	Lavender	Lavender
	Citrate, trisodium (coagulation)	Light blue	Light blue
	Citrate, trisodium (erythrocyte sedimentation rate)	Black	Black
	Sodium fluoride (antiglycolic agent)	Gray	Light gray
	Heparin, lithium (dry or liquid additive)	Green	Green
	Potassium oxalate	Light gray	Light gray
	Lithium iodoacetate	Light gray	Light gray
Special chemistry tubes			
Lead	Heparin, sodium (liquid additive)	Brown	Brown
	Heparin, sodium (dry additive)	Royal blue	Royal blue
Trace elements	Silicone-coated interior (serum tube)	Royal blue	Royal blue
Stat chemistry	Thrombin	Gray/yellow	Orange
Plasma preparation tube*	K_2 EDTA (dry additive)/polymer Gel/silica activator	Pearlescent white	Pearlescent white

Modified from the National Committee for Clinical Laboratory Standards: Evacuated Tubes and Additives for Blood Specimen Collection: Approved Standard H1-A4. 4th edition. Wayne, Pa, National Committee for Clinical Laboratory Standards, 1996; and information listed on the Becton Dickinson webpage (http://www.bd.com/).
EDTA, Ethylenediaminetetraacetic acid.
*The plasma preparation tube (Becton Dickinson, Franklin Lakes, N.J.) is a plastic evacuated tube used for the collection of venous blood that, on centrifugation, separates undiluted plasma for use in molecular diagnostic test methods. It has a pearlescent white hemogard closure and a purple band on the label.

color of the stopper (Table 2-2). Some tubes are siliconized to reduce adhesion of clots to walls or stoppers and decrease risk of hemolysis. The silicone–coated wall also may activate and accelerate the clotting mechanism. Blood collected into a tube containing one additive should never be transferred into another tube because the first additive may interfere with tests for which a different additive is specified. Thrombin is added to some tubes to accelerate clotting.

An assembled venipuncture set is shown in Figure 2-1. A needle is screwed into the collection tube holder (Figure 2-2), and the tube then is inserted gently into the holder. Before use, the tube should be tapped gently to dislodge any additive from the stopper before the needle is inserted into a vein; this action prevents aspiration of the additive into the patient's vein. Both single-draw and multidraw needles are available.

After the skin is cleaned, the needle should be aligned with the intended vein and pushed into the vein at an angle approximately 15 degrees to the skin (Figure 2-3). Once the needle is in place, the tube should be pressed forward into the holder to puncture the stopper and release the vacuum. When blood begins to flow into the tube, the tourniquet should be released without movement of the needle. The tube is filled until the vacuum is exhausted, and the tube then is withdrawn from the holder and replaced with another tube. Other tubes may be filled, if required, through use of the same technique and with the holder in place. However, when multiple tubes are drawn during a single venipuncture, tubes without **additives** should be drawn before tubes with additives to prevent contamination. When several tubes are required from a single blood collection, a shut-off valve, consisting of rubber tubing that slides over the needle opening inside the tube, often is used to prevent blood spillage during tube exchange.

Because metabolic changes occur when the clot or cells are in direct contact with the serum or plasma,[22] separator collection tubes are available to eliminate this problem. Each tube contains an inert, thixotropic, polymer gel material with a specific gravity of approximately 1.04 that is intermediate between plasma or serum and the cellular components of blood. On centrifugation of a filled tube, this gel rises from the bottom of the tube and becomes layered between the liquid and cellular components of the sample (Figure 2-4). Note that the gel serves as a mechanical barrier and eliminates the metabolic changes that occur when the clot or cells are in direct contact with the serum or plasma. In a few patients backflow from blood tubes into veins occurs because of a decrease in venous pressure. The dangerous consequences of this occurrence may be avoided when sterile tubes are used for blood collection. Backflow is minimized if the arm is held downward and blood is kept from contact with the stopper during the collection procedure.

Blood collection with a syringe

Syringes are used on patients with difficult veins. If a syringe is used, the needle is placed firmly over the nozzle of the syringe and the needle cover removed. If the syringe has an eccentric nozzle, the needle should be arranged with the nozzle downward but the bevel of the needle upward. The syringe and needle should be aligned with the intended vein and the needle pushed into the vein at an angle approximately 15 degrees to the skin. When the initial resistance of the vein wall is overcome as it is pierced, forward pressure on the syringe is eased and the blood is withdrawn through gentle pulling back of the syringe plunger. If a second syringe is needed, a gauze pad may be placed under the hub of the needle to absorb spill; the first syringe then quickly is disconnected and the second put in place to continue the draw. After removal of the needle from the syringe, drawn blood should be transferred quickly by gentle ejection into

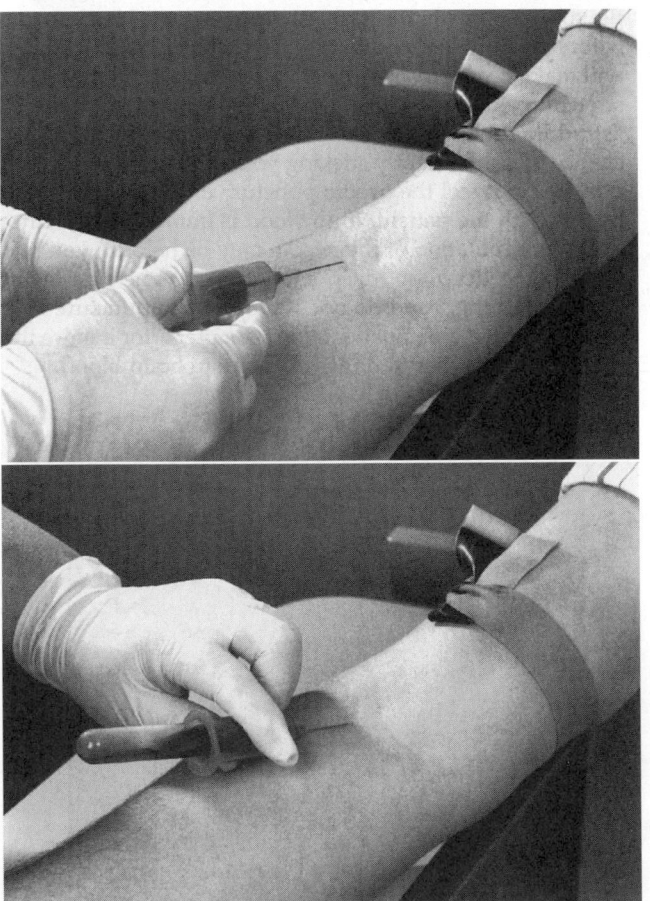

Figure 2-3   Venipuncture. (From Flynn JC: Procedures in Phlebotomy, 2nd edition, p 94, Philadelphia, WB Saunders, 1999.)

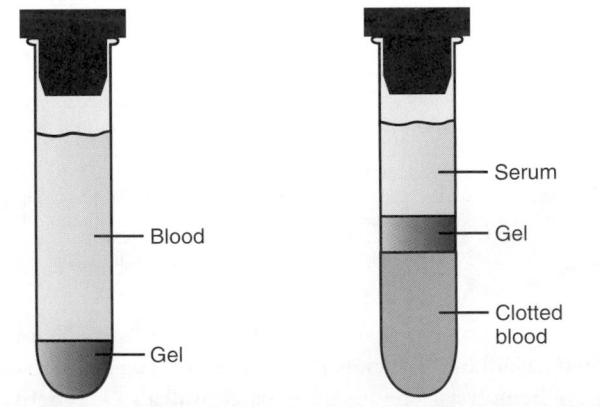

Figure 2-4   Blood collection tube with gel separator before *(left)* and after *(right)* centrifugation. (From Flynn JC: Procedures in Phlebotomy, 2nd edition, p 72, Philadelphia, WB Saunders, 1999.)

prepared tubes. The tubes then should be capped; if they contain additives or anticoagulants, they should be mixed-gently (5 to 10 inversions). Vigorous suction on a syringe during collection or forceful transfer from the syringe to the receiving vessel should be avoided because it may cause hemolysis.

Completion of collection

When blood collection is complete, the needle is with-drawn and the patient asked to hold a dry gauze pad over the puncture site, with the arm raised to lessen the likeli-hood of leakage. The pad subsequently is held in place by a bandage, which is removed after 15 minutes. The used needle from the syringe or collection tube should be dis-carded into a "sharps" container.

Venipuncture in children

The techniques for venipuncture in children and adults are similar. However, children are likely to make unexpected movements, and assistance in keeping them still is often de-sirable. Either a syringe or evacuated blood tube system may be used to collect specimens. A syringe should be either the tuberculin type or a 3–mL-capacity syringe, except when a large volume of blood is required for analysis. A 21- to 23-gauge needle or 20- to 23-gauge butterfly needle with at-tached tubing is appropriate to collect specimens.

Skin puncture

Skin puncture is an open collection technique in which the skin is punctured by a lancet[5,9] and a small volume of blood collected into a microdevice, such as a capillary tube. In practice it is used in situations in which (1) sample volume is limited (for example, pediatric applications), (2) repeated venipunctures have resulted in severe vein damage, (3) pa-tients have been burned or bandaged and veins therefore are unavailable for venipuncture, or (4) veins must be preserved for intravenous chemotherapy. Skin puncture most often is performed on the tip of a finger, an earlobe, or the heel or big toe of an infant. For example, in an infant younger than 1 year of age the lateral or medial plantar surface of the foot should be used for skin puncture; suitable areas are illus-trated in Figure 2-5. In older children the plantar surface of the big toe also may be used, but blood collection on ambu-latory patients from anywhere on the foot should be avoided. The proper procedure for the collection of blood from infants is described in NCCLS standard H4-A3.[12]

To collect a blood specimen by a skin puncture the phle-botomist first thoroughly cleans the skin with a gauze pad saturated with 70% isopropanol. All alcohol must evaporate from the skin so that hemolysis does not occur. When the skin is dry, it is punctured quickly by a sharp stab with a lan-cet. The depth of the incision should be less than 2.5 mm to avoid contact with bone. To minimize the possibility of in-fection a different site should be selected for each finger puncture. The finger should be held in such a way that grav-

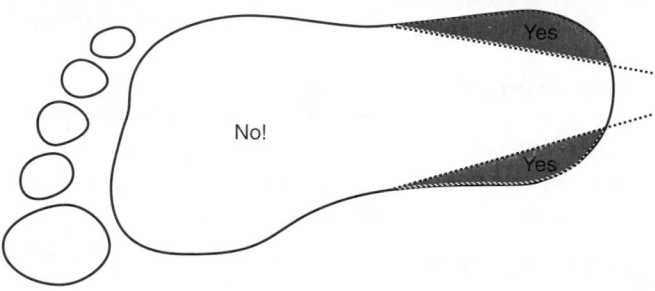

Figure 2-5 Acceptable sites for skin puncture to collect blood from an infant's foot. (Modified from Blumenfeld TA, Turi GK, Blanc WA: Rec-ommended site and depth of newborn heel punctures based on anatomi-cal measurements and histopathology. Lancet 1979; 1:230-233.)

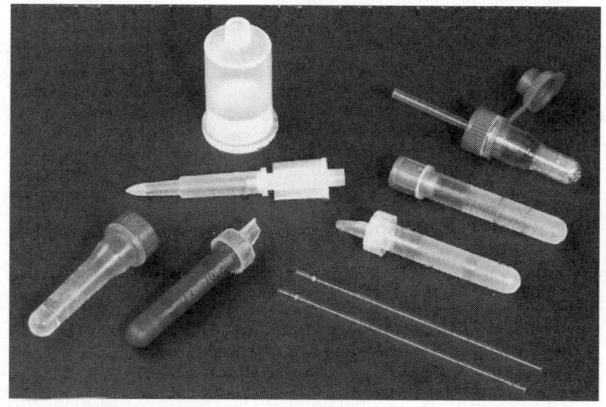

Figure 2-6 Microcollection tubes. (From Flynn JC: Procedures in Phlebotomy, 2nd edition, p 73, Philadelphia, WB Saunders, 1999.)

ity assists the collection of blood on the fingertip. Massag-ing the finger to stimulate blood flow should be avoided be-cause it causes the outflow of debris and tissue fluid, which does not have the same composition as plasma. To improve blood circulation the finger may be warmed by application of a warm, wet washcloth for 3 minutes before puncture. The first drop of blood is wiped off, and subsequent drops are transferred to the appropriate collection tube by gentle contact. Filling should be done rapidly to prevent clotting, and introduction of air bubbles should be avoided.

Blood also may be collected into capillary blood tubes by capillary action. A variety of collection tubes is commercially available (Figure 2-6). Such containers are available with different anticoagulants, such as sodium and ammonium heparin. Brown glass containers also are available for collec-tion of light-sensitive analytes, such as bilirubin.

In the collection of blood specimens on filter paper for neonatal screening,[8] the skin is cleaned and punctured as described previously. Then the filter paper is touched gently against a large drop of blood, which is allowed to soak into the paper to fill the marked circle; only a single application per circle should be made. The paper is examined to verify complete penetration, and the procedure is repeated to fill all the circles. Milking or squeezing of the foot should be avoided because it contributes tissue fluids. The filter papers should be air-dried. Blood should not be transferred onto filter paper after it has been collected in capillary tubes because partial clotting may have occurred.

Arterial puncture

Arterial puncture requires considerable skill and usually is performed only by physicians or specially trained technicians or nurses. The preferred sites of arterial puncture in order are as follows:

1. The radial artery at the wrist
2. The brachial artery in the elbow
3. The femoral artery in the groin

Because the femoral artery tends to leak a greater amount of blood, especially in elderly patients, sites in the arm are used most often. The proper technique for arterial puncture is described in NCCLS Standard H11-A3.[11]

In the neonate an indwelling catheter in the umbilical artery is best to obtain specimens for blood gas analysis. In the older child or adult in whom an arterial puncture is not possible, a capillary puncture may be performed to obtain arterial capillary blood. Such a specimen yields acceptable values for pH and PCO_2, but not always for PO_2. In the older child or adult the preferred puncture site is the earlobe; in the young child or infant it is the heel. Capillary blood specimens are particularly inappropriate when blood circulation is poor and thus should be avoided when a patient demonstrates reduced cardiac output, hypotension, or vasoconstriction. For each capillary puncture the skin should be warmed first with a hot, moist towel to improve circulation. The puncture itself should be performed as described previously; a free flow of blood is essential. Capillary tubes containing heparin and a small metal bar are used to collect the blood. Tubes should be sealed quickly and the contents mixed thoroughly through use of a magnet to move the metal bar up and down inside the tube.

Factors affecting blood collection

Factors affecting the collection of a blood sample include the use of anticoagulants and preservatives, site of collection, and hemolysis of a collected sample.

Anticoagulants and preservatives for blood

To prepare a whole blood or plasma sample, an **anticoagulant** must be added to the specimen during the collection procedure. A number of anticoagulants are used, including heparin, ethylenediaminetetraacetic acid (EDTA), sodium fluoride, citrate, oxalate, and sodium iodoacetate. The differences between plasma and serum concentrations of commonly ordered analytes are shown in Table 2-3. Triglyceride concentration is also higher in serum than in plasma.

TABLE 2-3	Differences in Composition Between Plasma and Serum	
Value Ratio	Analyte	Percent (%)
Plasma value greater than serum value	Calcium	0.9
	Chloride	0.2
	Lactate dehydrogenase	2.7
	Total protein	4
No difference between serum and plasma values	Bilirubin	
	Cholesterol	
	Creatinine	
Plasma value less than serum value	Albumin	1.3
	Alkaline phosphatase	1.6
	Aspartate aminotransferase	0.9
	Bicarbonate	1.8
	Creatine kinase	2.1
	Glucose	5.1
	Phosphate	7
	Potassium	8.4
	Sodium	0.1
	Urea	0.6
	Uric acid	0.2

From Ladenson JH, Tsa L-MB, Michael JM et al: Serum versus heparinized plasma for 18 common chemistry tests. Am J Clin Pathol 1974; 62:545-552; and copyright 1974 by the American Society of Clinical Pathologists. See footnote, Table 2-1.

Heparin. Heparin is the most widely used anticoagulant and causes the least interference with tests. It is a mucoitin polysulfuric acid and is available as sodium, potassium, lithium, and ammonium salts. This anticoagulant accelerates the action of antithrombin III, which neutralizes thrombin and thus prevents the formation of fibrin from fibrinogen. Most blood tubes are prepared with approximately 0.2 mg heparin for each milliliter of blood collected. The heparin usually is present as a hygroscopic, dry powder that dissolves rapidly.

However, downsides to heparin include expense, temporary action, and the production of a blue background in blood smears stained with Wright's stain. In addition, heparin is said to inhibit acid phosphatase activity and interfere with the binding of calcium to EDTA in calcium methods involving the formation of a complex with EDTA. Heparin also reportedly has affected the binding of triiodothyronine and thyroxine to their carrier proteins, producing higher free concentrations of these hormones.

Ethylenediaminetetraacetic acid. EDTA is a chelating agent that forms a complex with calcium necessary for coagulation. It is used as the disodium, dipotassium, or tripotassium salt, the latter two being more soluble. It is effective at a final concentration of 1 to 2 mg/mL of blood; higher concentrations hypertonically shrink the red cells. EDTA prevents coagulation by binding calcium, which is essential for the clotting mechanism. Blood collection tubes are prepared through the addition of a 0.1% solution of an EDTA salt, followed by evaporation of water at room temperature.

EDTA inhibits alkaline phosphatase, creatine kinase, and leucine aminopeptidase activities. Its chelation of calcium makes EDTA unsuitable for specimens of calcium and iron analyses using photometric or titrimetric techniques. As an anticoagulant it has little effect on other clinical tests.

Sodium fluoride. Sodium fluoride is a weak anticoagulant but often is added as an antiglycolytic agent to preserve blood glucose. As a preservative, together with another anticoagulant such as potassium oxalate, it is effective at a concentration of approximately 2 mg/mL of blood. It exerts its preservative action by inhibiting the enzyme systems involved in glycolysis. Most specimens are preserved at 25 °C for 24 hours or at 4 °C for 48 hours. Without an antiglycolytic agent the blood glucose concentration decreases approximately 10 mg/dL (0.56 mmol/L) per hour at 25 °C. The rate of decrease is faster in newborns because of the increased metabolic activity of their erythrocytes and in leukemic patients because of the high metabolic activity of the white cells.

Sodium fluoride is poorly soluble, and blood must be mixed thoroughly before effective antiglycolysis occurs. When sodium fluoride is used alone for anticoagulation, three to five times greater concentrations than the usual 2 mg/mL are required. This high concentration and the inhibition of the glycolytic cycle are likely to cause fluid shifts and change the concentration of some analytes. Fluoride is also a potent inhibitor of many serum enzymes and in high concentrations also affects urease, the enzyme used to measure urea nitrogen in many analytical systems.

Citrate. Sodium citrate solution, at a concentration of 3.4 to 3.8 g/dL in a ratio of 1 part to 9 parts of blood, is used widely for coagulation studies because the effect is reversible easily by the addition of Ca^{2+}. Because citrate chelates calcium, it is unsuitable as an anticoagulant for specimens used to measure this element. It also inhibits aminotransferase and alkaline phosphatase but stimulates acid phosphatase when phenylphosphate is used as substrate. Because citrate forms a complex with molybdate, it decreases the color yield in phosphate measurements that involve molybdate ions and produces low results.

Oxalates. The sodium, potassium, ammonium, and lithium salts of oxalic acid inhibit blood coagulation by forming rather insoluble complexes with calcium ions. Potassium oxalate ($K_2C_2O_4 \times H_2O$), at a concentration of approximately 1 to 2 mg/mL of blood, is the most widely used oxalate. At concentrations of greater than 3 mg oxalate/mL, hemolysis is likely to occur.

Combined ammonium/potassium oxalate does not cause shrinkage of erythrocytes. However, other oxalates cause shrinkage by drawing water into the plasma. Reduction in hematocrit may be as much as 10%, causing a reduction of 5% in the concentration of plasma constituents. As fluid is lost from the cells, an exchange of electrolytes and other

TABLE 2-4	Difference in Composition Between Capillary and Venous Serum		
Value Ratios		Analyte	Percent (%)
Capillary value greater than venous value		Glucose	1.4
		Potassium	0.9
No difference between capillary and venous values		Phosphate	
		Urea	
Capillary value less than venous value		Bilirubin	5
		Calcium	4.6
		Chloride	1.8
		Sodium	2.3
		Total protein	3.3

From Kupke IR, Kather B, Zeugner S: On the composition of capillary and venous blood serum. Clin Chim Acta 1981; 112:177-185. See footnote, Table 2-1.

constituents across the cell membrane occurs. Oxalate inhibits several enzymes, including acid and alkaline phosphatases, amylase, and lactate dehydrogenase, and may cause precipitation of calcium as the oxalate salt.

Sodium iodoacetate. At a concentration of 2 g/L, sodium iodoacetate is an effective antiglycolytic agent and substitute for sodium fluoride. Because it has no effect on urease, it has been used when glucose and urea tests are performed on a single specimen. Sodium iodoacetate inhibits creatine kinase but appears to have no significant effects on other clinical tests.

Influence of site of collection on blood composition

Blood obtained from different sites differs in composition. Skin puncture blood is more like arterial blood than venous blood, and no clinically significant differences exist between freely flowing capillary blood and arterial blood in pH, P_{CO_2}, P_{O_2}, and oxygen saturation. The P_{CO_2} of venous blood is up to 6 to 7 mm Hg (0.8 to 0.9 kPa) higher. Venous blood glucose is as much as 7 mg/dL (0.39 mmol/L) less than the capillary blood glucose as a result of tissue utilization. Blood obtained by skin puncture is contaminated to some extent with interstitial and intracellular fluids. The major differences between venous serum and capillary serum are illustrated in Table 2-4.

Hemolysis

Hemolysis is the disruption of the red cell membrane, which causes the release of hemoglobin. Serum shows visual evidence of hemolysis when the hemoglobin concentration exceeds 20 mg/dL. Slight hemolysis has little effect on most test values. Severe hemolysis causes an increase in the plasma activities of aldolase, aspartate aminotransferase, total acid phosphatase, lactate dehydrogenase, and isocitrate dehydrogenase. Hemolysis specifically increases the plasma concentrations of potassium, magnesium, and phosphate. The inorganic phosphate in serum increases rapidly as the organic esters in the cells are hydrolyzed. Hemolysis also may affect many tests when measured by unblanked or inadequately blanked analytical methods.[20]

Urine

Urine is the fluid excreted by the kidneys, passed through the ureters, stored in the bladder, and discharged through the urethra. Urine typically has an amber color and a peculiar odor and is slightly acidic. Under normal dietary conditions, 1000 to 2000 mL of urine is excreted every 24 hours. Its specific gravity varies from 1.005 to 1.030. Various types of urine specimens are collected, and a variety of techniques are used to preserve them.[15]

Types of urine specimens

The type of urine specimen to be collected is dictated by the tests to be performed. The various types of specimen collections are described in this section.

Random specimen

As its name implies, a *random urine specimen* is collected at an unspecified time, often when an analysis for drugs of abuse is to be performed (see Chapter 32).

First-morning or 8-hour specimen

This type of specimen typically is collected after an individual arises from a night's sleep. It is the specimen of choice for microscopic examinations, as well as for the detection of abnormal amounts of constituents of proteins or unusual compounds, such as chorionic gonadotropin, because it is likely the most concentrated specimen. Any urine voided during the night is collected and added to the first specimen collected in the morning. Other 8-hour periods may be used to accommodate unusual situations.

Timed specimen

A timed specimen is collected over a predetermined interval of time, such as 1, 4, or 24 hours. Before beginning a timed collection, a patient should be instructed about diet or drug ingestion, if appropriate, to avoid interference of ingested compounds with analytical procedures.

For timed collections the volume of the collection bottle is important. For example, with a 2-hour specimen a prelabeled 1-L bottle is adequate. For a 12-hour collection a 2-L bottle usually suffices; a 3- or 4-L bottle is appropriate for most 24-hour collections. Appropriate information, including warnings with respect to handling of the specimen, should appear on the bottle label.

24-Hour specimen

This strictly timed collection is required in situations in which the total amount of a given analyte must be measured

in a 24-hour period or in which an analyte may exhibit diurnal variation. For example, the lowest and highest concentrations of analytes such as catecholamines, 17-hydroxysteroids, and electrolytes occur in the early morning and around noon, respectively.

"Clean-catch" specimen

The "clean-catch" type of collection is used to obtain a urine specimen for bacterial culture only minimally contaminated with bacteria from the external genitalia or rectum. While the patient urinates, a midportion is collected into a sterile, inert plastic disposable urine container without contamination of the container (clean catch). Neither the urine stream nor the specimen container should touch the perineum. The container should have a capacity between 50 and 100 mL, with at least a 2-inch opening at the top and a spill-proof lid.

Catheter specimen

The catheter specimen is collected after a catheter is inserted into the bladder through the urethra. A urine specimen then is collected as a single specimen from the outflow end of the catheter. Catheter specimens are used for microbiological examination in critically ill patients or in patients with urinary tract obstruction. Such specimens normally should not be obtained merely for examination of chemical constituents.

Suprapubic specimen

A suprapubic urine specimen is collected to obtain a specimen directly from the bladder, which is uncontaminated by urethral bacteria. Used primarily to determine whether bacteria are present in the bladder, this type of collection is especially useful in infants. To obtain the specimen a needle is inserted through the thoroughly cleaned suprapubic skin and abdominal wall into the distended bladder. A specimen of urine is obtained via aspiration.

Urine collection from children

Collection of a timed specimen from an infant is difficult, but newborn and pediatric urine specimen collection bags with hypoallergenic skin adhesive are available for such specimens. The collection of specimens from older children is done as in adults, through the assistance of a parent when necessary.

Urine preservation

If a urine specimen cannot be transported and analyzed immediately, it should be refrigerated (at 2 to 8 °C) or frozen (at −24 to −16 °C) after collection. In addition, specimens not analyzed within 2 hours of collection should have a chemical preservative added to the collection container. **Preservatives** have different roles but usually are added to reduce bacterial action or chemical decomposition or solubilize constituents that might otherwise precipitate from the solution. Some specimens should not have *any* preservatives added because of the possibility of interference with analytical methods. Table 2-5 lists the preservatives commonly used in urine specimen collection and the analytes for which preservatives are required.

Feces

Small aliquots of feces frequently are analyzed to detect the presence of "hidden" blood, so-called occult blood, which is recognized as one of the most effective clues to the presence of a bleeding ulcer or malignant disease in the gastrointestinal tract. The utility of screening for occult blood is such that it is included as part of many periodical health examinations. Tests for occult blood should be performed on aliquots of excreted stools rather than on material obtained on the glove of a physician performing a rectal examination.

Feces from children may be screened for tryptic activity to detect cystic fibrosis. In infants fecal material for these tests usually is recovered from the diaper. In adults measurement of fecal nitrogen and fat in 72-hour specimens is used to assess the severity of malabsorption; measurement of fecal porphyrins occasionally is required to characterize the type of porphyria (see Chapter 30).

Sweat

The analysis of sweat for increased electrolyte concentration is used to confirm the diagnosis of cystic fibrosis. Chapter 25 details the manner in which sweat specimens are obtained.

Saliva

Saliva is the clear, alkaline, viscous fluid secreted from the parotid, submaxillary, sublingual, and smaller mucous glands of the mouth. Approximately 0.8 to 1.2 L of saliva is produced daily. Constituents such as viruses, bacteria, proteins, hormones, therapeutic drugs, and drugs of abuse have been measured in saliva.

Several techniques exist for the collection of saliva, and collection kits now are commercially available. In one such kit the patient must chew an absorption roll of dental cotton for several minutes. After being soaked with saliva, the roll is placed into a plastic tube and the saliva collected in the bottom of the tube via centrifugation. Another device uses a vacuum-type aspirator similar in concept to a dental aspirator. With this device, saliva automatically flows into a disposable cassette designed to hold up to 10 tests in a panel format.

Cerebrospinal Fluid

Cerebrospinal fluid (CSF) is that fluid contained within the four ventricles of the brain and the subarachnoid space. CSF normally is obtained through a puncture ("spinal tap") of the lumbar region by a physician. Occasionally a physician may request analysis of fluid obtained during surgery from the cervical region or from a cistern or ventricle of the brain. CSF is examined when a question exists as to the presence of a cerebrovascular accident, meningitis, demyelinating disease, or meningeal involvement in malignant disease.

Up to 20 mL of CSF can be removed safely from an adult, although this amount usually is not required. Antiglycolytic agents normally are not added to the tube for glucose measurement; the rapid processing of specimens, a clinical requirement for tests on CSF, ensures that little metabolism of glucose occurs even in the presence of many bacteria. To allow proper interpretation of CSF glucose values, a simultaneous blood specimen should be obtained.

Synovial Fluid

Synovial fluid is a fluid found in the joint cavities, bursae, and tendon sheaths. It is transparent, alkaline, viscous, and straw colored. Normally, only a very small amount of fluid is present in any joint, but this volume is increased substantially with inflammatory conditions. The technique used to obtain a specimen of synovial fluid is called *arthrocentesis*. It is performed by a physician, who uses sterile procedures, and must be modified from joint to joint depending on the anatomical location and size of the joint. Synovial fluid is withdrawn from joints to aid characterization of the type of arthritis and differentiate noninflammatory effusions from inflammatory fluids.

Amniotic Fluid

During pregnancy amniotic fluid lies within the amniotic cavity and is produced by the amnion during the early embryonic period and later by the kidney and lungs. The amount in a full-term patient normally varies from 500 to 1500 mL. The technique used to obtain a specimen of amniotic fluid is called *amniocentesis*. Details of this technique are discussed in Chapter 43.

Pleural, Pericardial, and Peritoneal Fluids

Serous fluids are found in the pleural, pericardial, and peritoneal cavities, where they lubricate the opposing parietal and visceral membrane surfaces. Inflammation or infection affecting the cavities causes fluid to accumulate. The process involving excessive accumulation of free fluid (ascitic fluid) in the abdomen is known as *ascites*. The fluid may be removed to determine whether it is an effusion or an exudate, a distinction possible by protein or enzyme analysis. Depending on the cavity sampled the collection procedure is called *thoracentesis* (chest), *pericardiocentesis* (heart), or *paracentesis* (abdomen). Only skilled and experienced physicians should perform these procedures.

The skin over the intended puncture site should be cleaned with 70% isopropanol and allowed to air-dry. A spinal needle then is inserted into the body cavity through a small bleb in the skin raised by injection of a local anes-

TABLE 2-5 Techniques and Chemical Additives Used to Preserve Urine Specimens (Revised)

Analyte	Refrigerate	Freeze	Add 6 mol/L HCl*	Add Boric Acid*	Add Acetic Acid*	Other Additives
Albumin	X	X		X		
Aldosterone	X	X	X	X		
Amino acids	X	X	X	X		Toluene
5-Aminolevulinic acid		X	X		X	Protection from sunlight Adjustment of pH to ≥7
Amylase	X					
Calcium			X			
Catecholamines		X	X		X	
Chloride	X			X		
Chorionic Gonadotropin				X		
Citrate	X	X	X	X		Toluene
Cortisol	X	X		X	X	
C-peptide		X				
Copper			X			
Creatine	X	X		X		
Creatinine	X	X	X	X		
Cystine		X	X			Toluene
Dehydroepiandrosterone				X		
Electrolytes (Na and K)	X			X		
Estradiol	X			X		
Estriol	X			X		
Estrogens, total	X			X	X	
Estrone	X			X		
Follicle Stimulating Hormone	X			X		
Glucose				X		
Histamine		X	X			
Homogentisic acid						None
Homovanillic acid			X		X	
17-Hydroxycorticosteroids				X	X	
Hydroxyproline		X	X	X		Toluene
5-Hydroxyindoleacetic acid	X		X	X		
Immunoelectrophoresis	X	X				
17-Ketosteroids			X	X	X	
Lead	X		X		X	
Lipase	X					
Magnesium	X		X			
Metanephrines			X		X	
Mercury						Nitric acid
Methoxyhydroxyphenolglycol (MHPG)	X	X				
N-Methylimidazoleacetic acid					X	
β2-Microglobulin	X	X				
Nitrogen	X		X			
Osmolality		X				
Oxalate	X		X			
p-Aminobenzoic acid (PABA)	X					
Phosphate	X	X	X	X		
Phosphoethanolamine			X			
Porphyrins	X	X				Sodium bicarbonate and EDTA; protection from sunlight
Pregnanetriol				X	X	
Protein, total	X			X		
Pyridinium collagen crosslinks			X	X		
Tetrahydro compound S				X	X	
Urea nitrogen	X			X		
Uric acid	X	X		X		Toluene or sodium bicarbonate
Urobilinogen						Addition of sodium bicarbonate to pH of 8 to 9; protection from sunlight
Vanillylmandelic acid			X	X	X	
Xanthine and hypoxanthine		X				
Zinc			X			

Modified from National Committee for Clinical Laboratory Standards: Routine Urinalysis and Collection, Transportation, and Preservation of Urine Specimens. Approved Guideline. GP16-A. Wayne, Pa, National Committee for Clinical Laboratory Standards, 1995.
EDTA, Ethylenediaminetetraacetic acid.
*Recommended concentration and pH varies.

thetic. A syringe is used to withdraw fluid, which is transferred to appropriate tubes for analysis.

Solid Tissue

Many types of solid tissue are sent to the laboratory for analysis. Malignant tissue from tumors and hair are examples.

Malignant tissue

A solid tissue sometimes analyzed in the clinical laboratory is malignant tissue (for example, breast tissue for estrogen and progesterone receptors).[4] During surgery at least 0.5 to 1 g of tissue should be removed and trimmed of fat and nontumor material. The tissue should be frozen rapidly, preferably in liquid nitrogen or a mixture of dry ice and alcohol. The time between collection and freezing should be less than 20 minutes. A histological section always should be examined at the time of specimen analysis to confirm that the specimen is indeed malignant tissue.

Hair

Hair is used as a sample for trace and heavy-metal analysis.[7] Recently the analysis of hair for the presence of drugs has increased (see Chapter 32) because more than 50 pharmaceuticals or drugs of abuse have been detected in hair after oral or parenteral administration. For these applications hair is advantageous as a biological specimen because it is obtained easily without loss of the individual's privacy or dignity. Snipping of a small amount of hair from the back of the head is sufficient for a specimen. However, hair analysis has been hindered by a lack of standardized procedures for collection, preparation, and analysis.

Handling of Specimens for Testing

Maintenance of specimen identification

Proper identification of the patient with the correct specimen begins wherever the specimen is collected. This identifying link must be maintained throughout the collection process, transport of the specimen to the laboratory, subsequent analysis, and preparation of a report. A variety of manual and automated techniques are used to establish and maintain specimen identification (see Chapter 12). Currently, bar coding is the identification technology of choice.

Preservation of specimens

The specimen must be treated properly from the time of its collection, during its transport to the laboratory, to the point at which it is analyzed. For some tests, such as ammonia and blood gas determinations, specimens must be preserved at ~4 °C from the time the blood is drawn until the specimen is analyzed or the serum or plasma is separated from the cells. Specimens for acid phosphatase, lactate and pyruvate, and certain hormone tests (for example, gastrin and renin

activity) also should be maintained at ~4 °C. For all test constituents that are thermolabile, serum and plasma should be separated from cells in a refrigerated centrifuge. Specimens for bilirubin or carotene must be protected from both daylight and fluorescent light to avoid photodegradation. Table 2-6 lists certain special handling requirements.

Separation and storage of specimens

Plasma or serum should be separated from cells as soon as possible, and certainly within 2 hours after collection.[22] Premature separation of serum, however, may permit continued formation of fibrin and lead to the obstruction of sample probes in testing equipment. Coagulation in plain or silicone-coated glass tubes usually is complete in 20 to 30 minutes but is prolonged in plastic containers. If centrifugation of a blood specimen within 2 hours is impossible, the specimen should be stored at room temperature rather than at 4 °C to decrease hemolysis and the risk thereof. If the specimen cannot be analyzed at once, the separated serum usually should be stored in a capped tube at 4 °C until the time of analysis. If a specimen for a particular test is unstable at 4 °C, the serum specimen should be maintained at −20 °C. Frost-free freezers should not be use because their temperature range between the freeze/thaw cycle swings too wide. Although 4 °C or −20 °C is the optimum storage temperature for many analytes, certain specimens, such as lactate dehydrogenase, are more stable at room temperature.

Specimen tubes should be centrifuged with stoppers in place. Closure reduces evaporation, which occurs rapidly in a warm centrifuge with the air currents set up via centrifugation. Stoppers also prevent aerosolization of infectious particles. Specimen tubes containing volatile analytes such as ethanol *must* be stoppered while they are spun. Centrifuging specimens with the stopper in place maintains anaerobic conditions that are important in the measurement of carbon dioxide and ionized calcium. Removal of the stopper before centrifugation allows the loss of carbon dioxide and an increase in blood pH. Control of pH is especially important in the enzymatic measurement of acid phosphatase, which is labile under the alkaline conditions resulting from carbon dioxide loss.

Specimen transport

The time required to transport a specimen from its time of collection until it reaches the laboratory varies from a few minutes to as long as 72 hours. The container or tube used to hold a specimen (primary container) should be constructed so that the contents do not escape if the container is exposed to extremes of heat, cold, or sunlight. Reduced pressure of 0.50 atmosphere (50 kPa) may be encountered during air transportation, together with vibration, and specimens should be protected inside a suitable container from these adverse conditions.

The shipping, or secondary, container used to hold one or more specimen tubes or bottles must be constructed to pre-

TABLE 2-6 Selected Blood Constituents Requiring Special Collection and Storage Conditions*†

Constituent	Anticoagulant	Handling Requirements
S-Acetone, acetoacetate†‡		Freeze; use stopper
S-Acid phosphatase		Add citrate (10 mg/mL); freeze
P-ACTH (corticotropin)	Heparin, 0.2 mg/mL	Freeze within 15 min of collection
S-Alcohol		Add NaF (10 mg/mL) to serum
S-Aldolase		Freeze
P,S-Aldosterone		Add boric acid (25 mg/mL) or freeze
P-Amino acids	Heparin, 0.2 mg/mL	Freeze
S-Androstenedione		Draw sample in morning (between 0000 and 1200 h)
S-Ascorbic acid		Freeze
S-Barbiturates		Do not use heparin
S-Bile acids		Freeze
S-C-peptide		Draw from fasting patient; freeze
S-Calcitonin		Freeze
P-Carcinoembryonic antigen (CEA)	EDTA, 2 mg/mL	
B-Cholinesterase	Heparin, 0.2 mg/mL	
S-Citric acid		Freeze
S-Complement		Freeze
P-Cortisol	Heparin, 0.2 mg/mL	Separate immediately
S-Creatine		Freeze
S-Creatine kinase isoenzymes		Freeze
S-Creatinine		Freeze
S-Cryoglobulins		Maintain above 20 °C
P-11-Deoxycortisol	Heparin, 0.2 mg/mL	Separate immediately
P,S-Digitoxin		Draw 6 to 12 h postadministration
S-Digoxin		Draw 8 h postadministration
P-Estradiol	Heparin, 0.2 mg/mL	Freeze
P-Fatty acids (free and esterified)	Heparin, 0.2 mg/mL	Freeze
P-Fibrinogen	Citrate, ~4 mg/mL	Do not use heparin
S,B-Fluoride		Do not collect in glass container
P-Folate (tetrahydrofolate)		Freeze
B-Galactose	Heparin, 0.2 mg/mL	Add NaF (10 mg/mL) with heparin
S-Gastrin		Collect from fasting patient; freeze
B-Glucose-6-phosphate dehydrogenase†	EDTA, 2 mg/mL	
P-HDL-cholesterol	EDTA, 2 mg/mL	Collect after 12- to 14-h fast; freeze
B-Hemoglobins (for quantitation and electrophoresis)	EDTA, 2 mg/mL	
S-Histidine		Freeze
S-17-Hydroxyprogesterone		Draw between 0900 and 1100 h
S-Insulin		Collect from fasting patient; freeze
S-Isocitrate dehydrogenase		Freeze
B-Lactate		Immediately dilute with an equal volume of 5% (50 g/L) perchloric acid; shake and mix
B-Lead	Heparin, 0.2 mg/mL	Collect in lead-free tube containing heparin
S-Lipoprotein phenotyping		Freeze
S-Lysozyme		Freeze
S-Magnesium		Separate immediately
S-Parathyroid hormone (PTH)		Freeze
S-Pepsinogen		Freeze
S-Placental lactogen		Freeze
S-Prolactin		Freeze
S-Prostaglandin $F_{2\alpha}$		Freeze
P-Pyridoxal phosphate (vitamin B_6)	EDTA, 2 mg/mL	Protect from light
B-Pyruvate		Immediately dilute with an equal volume of 5% (50 g/L) perchloric acid; shake and mix
P-Renin	EDTA, 2 mg/mL	Chill during collection and centrifugation
S-Vitamin A		Protect from light
S-Zinc		Use only acid-washed glass; avoid hemolysis

From Winsten S, Gordesky SE: Transportation of specimens. In Faulkner WR (ed): Selected Methods of Clinical Chemistry, vol 9, pp 11-15, Washington, DC, AACC, 1982.

P, Plasma; S, serum; B, whole blood; ACTH, adrenocorticotropin hormone; EDTA, ethylenediaminetetraacetic acid; HDL, high-density lipoprotein.

*All specimens listed, except those to be assayed for cryoglobulins, should be transported at temperatures below 15 °C, except as noted.

†A sealable Styrofoam container with "freezer packs" usually is sufficient to keep the specimen frozen for 12 hours. Solid carbon dioxide is necessary for longer periods.

‡Some question exists as to whether this constituent remains stable, even with this procedure.

vent breakage. Corrugated, fiberboard, or Styrofoam boxes designed to encircle a single specimen tube may be used. A padded shipping envelope provides adequate protection for shipping of single specimens. When specimens are shipped as drops of blood on filter paper (for example, for neonatal screening), the paper should be enclosed in a plastic bag and mailed in a regular envelope.

For transportation of frozen or refrigerated specimens an insulated container is used. It should be vented to prevent buildup of carbon dioxide under pressure and possible explosion. Ice packs commonly are used for refrigerated specimens. Solid carbon dioxide (dry ice) is a convenient refrigerant material that helps maintain frozen specimens, and temperatures as low as $-70\ °C$ are achievable. The amount of dry ice required depends on the size of the container and efficiency of its insulation, as well as the amount of time the specimen must be kept frozen.

Various laws and regulations apply to the shipment of biological specimens. Although they theoretically apply only to etiological agents (known infectious agents), all specimens should be transported as if the same regulations applied.[14] Airlines have rigid regulations covering the transport of specimens. Airlines deem dry ice a hazardous material; thus the transport of most clinical laboratory specimens is affected by such regulations.

■ PREANALYTICAL VARIABLES

Preanalytical variables that affect laboratory test values fall into two categories—those that are controllable and those that are not.

Controllable Variables

Many preanalytical variables related to specimen collection and discussed in the previous section are examples of controllable variables. Others include physiological variables and those associated with diet, lifestyle, stimulants, and drugs.

Physiological variables

Controllable personal variables that affect analytical results include posture, prolonged bed rest, exercise, physical training, and circadian variation.

Posture

In an adult a change from a supine to an upright position results in the reduction of an individual's blood volume about 10% (~ 600 to 700 mL). Because only protein-free fluid passes through the capillaries to the tissues, this change in posture results in the reduction of the plasma volume of the blood and an increase ($\sim 8\%$ to 10%) in the plasma protein concentration. Normally the decrease with the change from a supine position to standing is complete

within 10 minutes. However, 30 minutes is required for such a change when the individual goes from standing to the supine position.

The decrease in plasma volume that occurs with a postural change from the supine position to standing results in an increase in the concentration of all proteins, including enzymes and protein hormones and such compounds as drugs, calcium, and bilirubin that circulate partly bound to protein. In addition, the change in posture increases the secretion of catecholamines, aldosterone, angiotensin II, renin, and antidiuretic hormone. Epinephrine and norepinephrine concentrations in serum may double within 10 minutes, but their urinary excretion does not change. The increase of plasma aldosterone and plasma renin activity is slower, but their concentrations still may double within 1 hour. In general the concentrations of freely diffusible constituents with molecular weights of less than 5000 are unaffected by postural changes. However, a significant increase (~ 0.2 to 0.3 mmol/L) in potassium (K^+) occurs with 30 minutes of standing. This increase in K^+ has been attributed to the release of intracellular potassium from muscle. Although postural changes affect urinary sodium excretion, sodium concentration in plasma is affected only slightly. Table 2-7 lists the changes in the concentrations of some major serum constituents that accompany changes in posture.

Prolonged bed rest

With prolonged bed rest, fluid retention occurs and serum protein and albumin concentrations may be decreased by an average of 5 and 3 g/L, respectively. The concentrations of protein-bound constituents also are reduced, although mobilization of calcium from bones with an in-

TABLE 2-7	Changes in Concentration of Serum Constituents with Changes from Supine to Standing Positions
Constituent	Average Increase (%)
Alanine aminotransferase	7
Albumin	9
Alkaline phosphatase	7
Amylase	6
Aspartate aminotransferase	5
Calcium	3
Cholesterol	7
IgA	7
IgG	7
IgM	5
Thyroxine	11
Triglycerides	6

From Felding P, Tryding N, Hyltoft PP, et al: Effects of posture on concentrations of blood constituents in healthy adults: practical application of blood specimen collection procedures recommended by the Scandinavian Committee on Reference Values. Scand J Clin Lab Invest 1980; 40:615-621. *IgA*, Immunoglobulin A; *IgG*, Immunoglobulin G; *IgM*, Immunoglobulin M. See footnote, Table 2-1.

creased free ionized fraction compensates for the reduced protein-bound calcium, so serum total calcium is less affected. Prolonged bed rest also is associated with increased urinary nitrogen excretion. Calcium, sodium, potassium, phosphate, and sulfate excretions are increased; hydrogen ion excretion is reduced, presumably due to the decreased metabolism of skeletal muscle.

When an individual becomes active after a period of bed rest, more than 3 weeks are required before calcium excretion reverts to normal; another 3 weeks is necessary before positive calcium balance is achieved. Several weeks are required before positive nitrogen balance is restored.

Exercise

The influence of exercise on the composition of body fluids is related to the duration and intensity of the activity. Moderate exercise results in an increase in the concentration of blood glucose, which in turn stimulates insulin secretion. Plasma pyruvate and lactate also are increased with the increased metabolic activity of skeletal muscle. Even mild exercise may increase the plasma lactate twofold. Arterial pH and $P\text{CO}_2$ are reduced by exercise. Reduced renal blood flow due to exercise causes a slight increase in the serum creatinine concentration. Competition between uric acid and lactate and products of increased tissue catabolism for renal excretion cause the serum uric acid concentration to increase. Exercise causes a reduction in cellular adenosine triphosphate, which increases cellular permeability. The increased permeability causes slight increases in the serum activities of enzymes originating from skeletal muscles, such as aspartate aminotransferase, lactate dehydrogenase, creatine kinase, and aldolase. As little as 5 minutes of walking increases the activity of these enzymes in plasma. Mild exercise produces a slight decrease in the serum cholesterol and triglyceride concentrations that may persist for several days.

In general the effects of strenuous exercise are exaggerations of those occurring with mild exercise. Some representative changes in concentration or activity of serum constituents induced by strenuous exercise are listed in Table 2-8.

Physical training

Athletes generally have higher levels of serum activity for enzymes of skeletal muscular origin at rest than do nonathletes. However, the response of these enzymes to exercise is less in athletes than in other individuals. Serum concentrations of urea, uric acid, creatinine, and thyroxine are higher in athletes than in comparable untrained individuals, a situation probably related to the increased muscle mass and good turnover of muscle mass in athletes.

The total serum lipid concentration is reduced by physical conditioning, with serum cholesterol being lowered by as much as 25%. High-density lipoprotein (HDL) cholesterol, however, is increased. Thus the decrease is due mostly to a reduction in low-density lipoprotein (LDL) cholesterol. The concentration of serum apolipoprotein A-1 increases with training, whereas the concentration of apolipoprotein B decreases. The serum triglyceride concentration may be reduced by up to 20 mg/dL (0.23 mmol/L), but the free fatty acid concentration is higher in fit individuals than in others. Loss of body fat is associated with improvement in lipid concentrations. In general the same exercise produces a less-marked biochemical response in the fit than in the unfit individual.

Circadian variation

Many constituents of body fluids exhibit cyclical, or circadian, variations throughout the day. Factors contributing to such variations include posture, activity, food ingestion, stress, and daylight/darkness, and sleep/wakefulness. These

---

TABLE 2-8 **Effects of Strenuous Exercise on Selected Serum Constituents***

Constituent Value	Increase (%)	Constituent Value	Decrease (%)
Acid phosphatase	11	Albumin	4
Alanine aminotransferase	41	Bilirubin	4
Alkaline phosphatase	3	Iron	11
Aspartate aminotransferase	31	Lactate dehydrogenase	1
Calcium	1	Potassium	8
Chloride	1	Sodium	1
Cholesterol	3	Total lipids	12
Creatinine	17		
Phosphate	12		
Total protein	3		
Urea nitrogen	3		
Uric acid	4		

From Statland BE, Winkel P, Bokelund H: Factors contributing to variation of serum constituents in healthy subjects. In Siest G (ed): Organisation des Laboratoires: Biologie Perspective, pp 717-750, Paris, L'Expansion Scientifique Francaise, 1975.
See footnote, Table 2-1.
*Changes were determined 15 minutes after conclusion of 20 minutes of exercise.

cyclical variations may be large, and therefore the time of the specimen drawing must be controlled strictly. The concentration of serum iron, for example, may change by as much as 50% from 0800 to 1400 hours and that of cortisol by a similar amount between 0800 and 1600 hours. Serum potassium has been reported to decline from 5.4 mmol/L at 0800 hours to 4.3 mmol/L at 1400 hours. Table 2-9 illustrates the typical total variation of several commonly measured serum constituents over 6 hours. The total variation is listed along with analytical error.

Hormones are secreted in bursts, and this fact, coupled with the cyclical variation to which most hormones are subject, may make proper interpretation of their serum concentrations difficult. Corticotropin secretion is influenced by cortisol-like steroids, but it is also affected by posture, light/darkness, and stress. Its secretion is increased threefold to fivefold from its minimum between afternoon and midnight to its maximum around waking. Cortisol concentrations are greatest around 0600 to 0800 hours and may be twice as high as those observed at 2400 hours.

Maximum renin activity normally occurs early in the morning during sleep; the minimum occurs late in the afternoon. The plasma aldosterone concentration demonstrates a similar pattern. Glomerular filtration rate (GFR) varies inversely with the secretion of renin; GFR is least at the time of maximum renin secretion and ~20% greater in the afternoon, when renin activity is at its minimum. No circadian variation exists in the plasma concentrations of follicle-stimulating hormone (FSH) and luteinizing hormone in men, but a 20% to 40% increase of plasma testosterone occurs during the night. Serum thyroid-stimulating hormone is at its maximum between 0200 and 0400 hours and its minimum between 1800 and 2200 hours. The variation in amount is about 50%.

Growth hormone secretion is greatest shortly after the onset of sleep. Conversely, basal plasma insulin is higher in the morning than later in the day, and its response to glucose is also greatest in the morning and least about midnight. When a glucose tolerance test is administered in the afternoon, higher glucose values occur than when the test is given early in the day. The higher plasma glucose occurs in spite of a greater insulin response, which nevertheless is delayed and less effective.

Blindness

With blindness the normal stimulation of the hypothalamic-pituitary axis is reduced. Consequently, certain features of hypopituitarism and hypoadrenalism may be observed. In some blind individuals the normal diurnal variation of cortisol may persist; in others it does not. Urinary excretion of 17-ketosteroids and 17-hydroxycorticosteroids is reduced. Plasma sodium and chloride are often low in blind individuals, probably as a result of reduced aldosterone secretion. Plasma glucose may be reduced in the blind, and insulin tolerance is often less. The excretion of uric acid is reduced. Renal function may be slightly impaired, as evidenced by slight increases in serum creatinine and urea nitrogen.

Travel

Travel across several time zones affects the normal circadian rhythm. Five days are required to establish a new stable diurnal rhythm after travel across 10 time zones. The changes in laboratory test results are attributable to altered pituitary and adrenal function. Urinary excretion of catecholamines is usually increased for 2 days; serum cortisol is reduced. During a flight, serum glucose and triglyceride concentrations increase, while glucocorticoid secretion is stimulated. During a prolonged flight, fluid and sodium retention occur, but urinary excretion returns to normal after 2 days.

Diet

An individual's typical diet has considerable influence on the composition of plasma. Studies with synthetic diets have shown that day-to-day changes in the amount of protein are reflected within a few days in the composition of the plasma and in the excretion of end products of protein metabolism. In addition to the types of food and drink ingested, specific food-related situations also influence plasma composition,

TABLE 2-9	Total and Analytical Variation for Serum Tests on Specimens Obtained at 0800 and 1400 Hours*		
Constituent	Mean	Total Variation (%)	Analytical Variation (%)
Sodium (mmol/L)	141	1.9	1.8
Potassium (mmol/L)	4.4	7.1	2.8
Calcium (mg/dL)	10.8	3.2	2.7
Chloride (mmol/L)	102	3.8	3.4
Phosphate (mg/dL)	3.8	10.7	2.4
Urea nitrogen (mg/dL)	14	22.5	2.5
Creatinine (mg/dL)	1.0	14.5	6.3
Uric acid (mg/dL)	5.6	11.5	2.6
Iron (μg/dL)	116	36.6	3.4
Cholesterol (mg/dL)	193	14.8	5.7
Albumin (g/dL)	4.5	5.5	3.9
Total protein (g/dL)	7.3	4.8	1.7
Total lipids (g/L)	5.3	25.0	3.6
Aspartate aminotransferase (U/L)	9	25	6
Alanine aminotransferase (U/L)	6	56	17
Acid phosphatase (U/L)	3	15	8
Alkaline phosphatase (U/L)	63	20	3
Lactate dehydrogenase (U/L)	195	16	12

From Winkel P, Statland BE, Bokelund H.: The effects of time of venipuncture on variation of serum constituents. Am J Clin Pathol 1975; 64:433-447; and copyright 1975 by the American Society of Clinical Pathologists. See footnote, Table 2-1.

*Based on 11 male subjects, ages 21 to 27 years, studied at 0800, 1100, and 1400 hours.

including vegetarianism, obesity, malnutrition, and fasting and starvation.

Food ingestion

The concentration of certain plasma constituents is affected by the ingestion of a meal. The biggest increases in serum concentrations occur for glucose, iron, total lipids, and alkaline phosphatase. The increase in alkaline phosphatase (mainly intestinal isoenzyme) is greater when a fatty meal is ingested and is influenced by the blood group of the individual and the substrate used for the enzyme assay. Lipemia may affect some analytical methods used to measure serum constituents. Ultracentrifugation or the use of serum blanks reduces the analytical effects of lipemia.

The effects of a meal may be long lasting. Thus ingestion of a protein-rich meal in the evening may cause increases in the serum urea nitrogen, phosphate, and uric acid concentrations that are still apparent 12 hours later. Nevertheless, these changes may be less than the typical intraindividual variability. Large protein meals at lunch or in the evening also increase the serum cholesterol and growth hormone concentrations for at least 1 hour afterward. The effect of carbohydrate meals on blood composition is less than that of protein meals. No change in the cortisol concentration is noted when breakfast is ingested, probably because cortisol occupies completely all cortisol-binding sites on its binding protein in the early morning. Glucagon and insulin secretions are stimulated by a protein meal, and insulin also is stimulated by carbohydrate meals. The effects of ingestion of a 700-kcal (2.93 MJ) meal on some commonly measured blood constituents are illustrated in Table 2-10.

Ingestion of beverages and specific foods

Constituents in food and drink affect the composition of plasma. Bran, serotonin, and caffeine are common examples of such constituents.

Bran.   Habitual ingestion of bran impedes the absorption of certain compounds, including calcium, cholesterol, and triglycerides, from the gastrointestinal tract. The serum concentration of calcium may be reduced by as much as 0.3 mg/dL (0.08 mmol/L) and that of triglycerides by 20 mg/dL (0.23 mmol/L), especially if triglycerides were high initially. Pectin and dietary fibers reduce the serum apolipoprotein-B and cholesterol concentrations.

Serotonin.   Many fruits and vegetables that contain 5-hydroxytryptamine (serotonin), such as bananas, cause an increase in the excretion of 5-hydroxyindoleacetic acid. Avocados impair glucose tolerance by affecting insulin secretion. Onions reduce both the plasma glucose and insulin response to glucose.

Caffeine.   Caffeine, a common ingredient in many beverages, including coffee, tea, and colas, has a considerable effect on the concentration of blood constituents. It stimulates the adrenal medulla, causing an increased excretion of the catecholamines and their metabolites and a slight in-

TABLE 2-10	Influence of a Standard 700-kcal Meal on Serum Constituents*		
Constituent		Before Meal	After Meal (2 h)
Alanine aminotransferase (U/L)		31	33
Albumin (g/dL)		4.5	4.6
Alkaline phosphatase (U/L)		46	46
Aspartate aminotransferase (U/L)		22	28
Bilirubin (mg/dL)		0.7	0.8
Calcium (mg/dL)		9.9	10.0
Cholesterol (mg/dL)		220	220
Glucose (mg/dL)		71	82†
Lactate dehydrogenase (U/L)		198	198
Phosphate (mg/dL)		3.1	3.6†
Potassium (mmol/L)		3.8	4.0†
Sodium (mmol/L)		140	141
Total protein (g/dL)		7.8	7.9
Urea nitrogen (mg/dL)		16	16
Uric acid (mg/dL)		6.0	6.2

From Steinmetz J, Panek E, Sourieau F et al: Influence of food intake on biological parameters. In Siest G (ed): Reference values in human chemistry, pp 193-200, Basel, Karger, 1973.
See footnote, Table 2-1.
*Results are mean values in 200 healthy individuals.
†Note also that other studies have reported greater increases in glucose concentration and reductions in phosphate and potassium concentrations, depending on the type of meal.

crease in the plasma glucose concentration with impairment of glucose tolerance. The adrenal cortex also is affected; plasma cortisol is increased, accompanied by an increased excretion of free cortisol, 11-hydroxycorticoids, and 5-hydroxyindoleacetic acid. The effect of caffeine may be so marked that the normal diurnal variation of plasma cortisol may be eliminated.

Caffeine also has a marked effect on lipid metabolism. Ingestion of two cups of coffee may increase the plasma free fatty acid concentration by as much as 30% and glycerol, total lipids, and lipoproteins to a lesser extent. Prolonged ingestion of caffeine (for example, over several weeks) causes a slight reduction of the serum cholesterol concentration but an increase in the serum triglyceride concentration.

Caffeine is also a potent stimulant of gastric secretion of hydrochloric acid and pepsin. It increases the absolute amounts of sodium, potassium, calcium, and magnesium in urine—an effect not observed with decaffeinated coffee.

Vegetarianism

In longtime vegetarians the concentrations of LDL and very-low-density lipoproteins (VLDL) are low. The total lipid and phospholipid concentrations are reduced, and the concentrations of cholesterol and triglyceride may be only two thirds of those in individuals who ingest mixed diets. Both HDL and LDL cholesterol concentrations are affected. The effects are less marked in individuals who have been on vegetarian diets for only short periods of time. The lipid concentrations are also less in individuals who eat only vegetable diets (vegan) than in those who also consume eggs and milk. When individuals previously on mixed diets begin vegetarian diets, their serum albumin concentrations may drop by 10% and their urea concentrations by 50%. However, little difference exists in the concentration of protein or enzymes activities in the serum of longtime vegetarians and individuals on mixed diets.

Obesity

The serum concentrations of cholesterol, triglycerides, and β-lipoproteins are correlated positively with obesity.[18] Serum uric acid concentration also correlates with body weight, especially in individuals who weigh more than 80 kg. Serum lactate dehydrogenase activity and glucose concentration increase in both sexes as body weight increases.[18] In men, serum aspartate aminotransferase, creatinine, hemoglobin, and total protein increase as body weight increases, whereas serum calcium increases in women as their body weights increase. In both sexes, serum phosphate decreases as body mass increases; the fasting concentrations of pyruvate, lactate, citrate, nonesterified fatty acids, gastric juice volume, and acid output increase in obese individuals.

Cortisol production is increased in obese individuals. However, increased metabolism ensures that the serum concentration remains unchanged so that urinary excretion of 17-hydroxycorticosteroids and 17-ketosteroids is increased. Because growth hormone concentration is reduced in obese individuals, it responds poorly to the normal challenges, such as fasting or eating. Plasma insulin concentration is increased, but glucose tolerance is impaired in obese individuals (see Chapter 24). Although the serum thyroxine concentration is unaffected by obesity, the serum triiodothyronine correlates significantly with body weight and increases further with overeating. In obese men the serum testosterone concentration is reduced.

Malnutrition

In malnutrition the concentrations of total serum protein, albumin, and β-globulin and the activities of most commonly measured enzymes are reduced. The concentration of γ-globulin is increased, but this increase does not fully compensate for the decrease in other proteins. The concentrations of complement C3, retinol-binding globulin, transferrin, and transthyretin (prealbumin) decrease rapidly with the onset of malnutrition and are measured to define the severity of the condition. The plasma concentrations of lipoproteins are reduced, and serum cholesterol and triglycerides may be only 50% of such concentrations in well-nourished individuals. In spite of severe malnutrition, glucose concentration is maintained close to that in healthy individuals. However, the concentrations of serum urea and creatinine are reduced greatly as a result of decreased skeletal mass; creatinine clearance also is decreased.

Plasma cortisol concentration is increased because of decreased metabolic clearance. The plasma concentrations of

total triiodothyronine, thyroxine, thyroid-stimulating hormone, thyroxine-binding globulin and transthyretin (prealbumin) are reduced considerably. In addition, erythrocyte and plasma folate concentrations are reduced in protein-calorie malnutrition, but the serum vitamin B_{12} concentration is unaffected or may be increased only slightly. The plasma concentrations of vitamins A and E are reduced significantly. Although the blood hemoglobin concentration is reduced, the serum iron concentration initially is affected only minimally by malnutrition.

Fasting and starvation

Under a fasting or starvation regimen the body attempts to conserve protein at the expense of other sources of energy, such as fat. Consequently, the blood glucose concentration decreases by as much as 18 mg/dL (1 mmol/L) within the first 3 days of the start of a fast in spite of the body's attempts to maintain glucose production. Insulin secretion is reduced markedly, whereas glucagon secretion may double in an attempt to maintain normal glucose concentration. Lipolysis and hepatic ketogenesis are stimulated, and the concentrations of ketone bodies, fatty acids, and glycerol in serum increase considerably. Serum triglycerides increase by 20% after 48 hours of fasting but decline thereafter; the cholesterol concentration also decreases. Amino acids are released from skeletal muscle, and the plasma concentration of the branched-chain amino acids may increase by as much as 100% with just 1 day of fasting.

With the catabolism of tissue, induced by starvation, the concentration of serum protein eventually increases. However, the catabolism of nucleoproteins causes an immediate increase in the concentration of serum uric acid. This increase is exacerbated by the reduced GFR and competition for excretion between lactate and ketoacids. A metabolic acidosis is common, with associated reduction of the blood pH and P_{CO_2}; often the blood P_{O_2} also is reduced.

With the onset of starvation, aldosterone secretion increases, resulting in increased urinary excretion and decreased plasma concentration of potassium. Magnesium, calcium, and phosphate are affected similarly, although the urinary excretion of phosphate gradually declines. In addition, plasma growth hormone concentration may increase by as much as 15 times at the start of a fast but may return to normal after 3 days. Free and total triiodothyronine decrease by up to 50% within 3 days of the start of a fast. Free thyroxine concentration also is affected, but to a lesser extent; total thyroxine is changed very little. Urinary free cortisol is decreased by fasting, and the plasma cortisol concentration (free and total) shows a slight increase, along with loss of the normal diurnal variation.

Lifestyle

Lifestyle factors that affect the levels of commonly measured analytes include smoking and alcohol ingestion.

Smoking

Smoking, through the action of nicotine, affects several laboratory tests. The extent of the effect is related to the number of cigarettes smoked and the amount of smoke inhaled. Some effects of smoking on serum constituents are listed in Table 2-11. In addition, smoking increases the plasma concentrations of lactate, insulin, epinephrine, growth hormone, 11-hydroxycorticosteroids, and cortisol and the urinary excretion of 5-hydroxyindoleacetic acid and catecholamines and their metabolites. Nicotine is also a potent stimulant of the secretion of gastric juice. Both volume and acid secretion are increased within 1 hour of the smoking of several cigarettes. In contrast, the bicarbonate concentration and volume of pancreatic juice are reduced.

The blood erythrocyte count is increased in smokers. The amount of carboxyhemoglobin may exceed 10% of the total hemoglobin in heavy smokers, and the increased number of cells compensates for impaired ability of the red cells to transport oxygen. The blood Po_2 of the habitual smoker is usually about 5 mm Hg (0.7 kPa) less than that of the non-smoker, whereas the Pco_2 is unaffected. The blood leukocyte concentration is increased by as much as 30% in smokers, but the leukocyte concentration of ascorbic acid is reduced greatly. The lymphocyte count is increased in proportion to the total leukocyte count.

Smoking affects the body's immune response, and the serum concentrations of the immunoglobulins IgA, IgG, and IgM are in general lower in smokers than in nonsmokers, whereas the IgE concentration is higher. Smokers more often than nonsmokers may demonstrate the presence of antinuclear antibodies and weakly positive tests for carcinoembryonic antigen. Sperm counts in male smokers often are reduced, compared with those in nonsmokers, because the number of abnormal forms is greater and sperm motility is less. In addition, the serum vitamin B_{12} concentration often is markedly reduced in smokers, and the decrease is in inverse proportion to the serum concentration of thiocyanate.

Alcohol ingestion

A single moderate dose of alcohol has few effects on laboratory tests. Ingestion of enough alcohol to produce mild inebriation may increase the blood glucose concentration by 20% to 50%. The increase may be more marked in diabetics. More commonly, inhibition of gluconeogenesis occurs and becomes apparent as hypoglycemia and ketonemia. Lactate accumulates and competes with uric acid for excretion in the kidneys so that the concentration of serum uric acid also is increased. Marked hypertriglyceridemia also occurs after alcohol ingestion and is most noticeable when alcohol is ingested with a fatty meal; the effect may persist for longer than 12 hours. When moderate amounts of alcohol are ingested for 1 week, the serum triglyceride concentration is increased by more than 20 mg/dL (0.23 mmol/L).

Intoxicating amounts of alcohol stimulate the release of cortisol, although the effect is more related to the intoxi-

TABLE 2-11	Reported Changes in Serum Composition in Smokers

Constituent	Change (%)
Albumin	3
Cholesterol	4
Glucose	10
Phospholipids	5
Triglycerides	20
Urea nitrogen	10

From Siest G, Henny J, Schiele F (eds): Interpretation des Examens de Laboratoire, Basel, Karger, 1981.
See footnote, Table 2-1.

cation than to the alcohol per se. Sympatheticomedullary activity is increased by acute alcohol ingestion but without detectable effect on the plasma epinephrine concentration and with only a mild effect on norepinephrine. Plasma concentrations of catecholamines are increased markedly in intoxicated individuals. Acute ingestion of alcohol leads to a sharp reduction in the plasma testosterone in men, with an increase in the plasma luteinizing hormone concentration.

Chronic alcohol ingestion affects the activity of many serum enzymes, including isocitrate dehydrogenase, ornithine carbamoyl transferase, and especially γ-glutamyltransferase (GGT). In practice the increased activity of GGT commonly is used as a mark of persistent drinking. Chronic alcoholism is associated with many characteristic biochemical abnormalities, including abnormal pituitary, adrenocortical, and medullary function. Alcohol ingestion also has considerable influence on serum HDL cholesterol and total cholesterol concentration.

Drug administration

Drugs may have both in vivo and in vitro effects on laboratory tests. The in vivo effects arise from the therapeutic intent of drugs, their side effects, and patient idiosyncrasies. Effects on the composition of body fluids are likely to be more apparent when large doses of a drug are administered for long periods of time than when administration of a single dose occurs on an isolated occasion. Young[19,20] has published comprehensive listings of the effects of drugs on laboratory tests.

Noncontrollable Variables

Examples of noncontrollable preanalytical variables include those related to biological, environmental, and long-term cyclical influences and to underlying medical conditions.

Biological influences

The age and sex of the patient influence the results of individual laboratory tests.[16,17]

| TABLE 2-12 | Influence of Age on Mean Concentration of Serum Constituents in Males |

Constituent	Measured Value: <29 y	Change Compared With <29-y Value			
		30 to 39 y	40 to 49 y	50 to 59 y	60 to 69 y
Albumin (g/dL)	4.6	−0.2	−0.3	−0.4	−0.6
Alkaline phosphatase (U/L)	51	−3	−1	1	4
Aspartate aminotransferase (U/L)	41	3	3	1	1
Bilirubin (mg/dL)	0.4	0.1	0	0	0
Calcium (mg/dL)	9.8	−0.1	−0.2	−0.2	−0.3
Cholesterol (mg/dL)	211	29	43	48	36
Creatinine (mg/dL)	1.1	0	0.1	0.1	0
Glucose (mg/dL)	108	1	6	2	9
Phosphate (mg/dL)	4.0	−0.1	−0.3	−0.2	−0.2
Total protein (g/dL)	7.6	−0.1	−0.2	−0.2	−0.2
Urea nitrogen (mg/dL)	15	1	1	2	3
Uric acid (mg/dL)	5.9	0	0.2	−0.1	−0.2

From Leonard PJ: The effect of age and sex on biochemical parameters in blood of healthy human subjects. In Siest G (ed): Reference Values in Human Chemistry, pp 134-140, Basel, Karger, 1973.
See footnote, Table 2-1.

Age

Table 2-12 lists typical changes in serum composition occurring with age. In general, individuals are considered in four groups—newborn, childhood to puberty, adult, and elderly adults.

Newborn.   In the mature infant, most of the hemoglobin is the adult form, hemoglobin A, whereas in the immature infant, much of the hemoglobin may be the fetal form, hemoglobin F. In both mature and immature infants the arterial blood oxygen saturation is very low initially. A metabolic acidosis develops in newborns that results from the accumulation of organic acids, especially lactic acid. The acid-base status, however, reverts to normal within 24 hours.

The concentration of bilirubin rises after birth and peaks about the third to fifth day of life. However, this physiological jaundice of the newborn rarely produces serum bilirubin values greater than 5 mg/dL (85 μmol/L). Distinguishing this naturally occurring phenomenon from other conditions that produce neonatal hyperbilirubinemia may be difficult, and the chronological course of the hyperbilirubinemia is important.

A variety of other differences may be seen in the newborn. Because of their small glycogen reserves, the concentration of blood glucose is low in newborns, although low glucose may be due to adrenal immaturity. Blood lipid concentrations are low but reach ~80% of the adult values after 2 weeks. The plasma urea nitrogen concentration decreases after birth as the infant synthesizes new protein, and the concentration does not begin to rise until tissue catabolism becomes prominent. The serum thyroxine concentration of the healthy newborn, like that of the pregnant woman, is considerably higher than in the nonpregnant woman. After its birth, an infant secretes thyroid-stimulating hormone, which causes a further increase in the serum thyroxine concentration. The physiological hyperthyroidism gradually declines over the first year of life.

Childhood to puberty.   Many changes take place in the composition of body fluids between infancy and puberty. Most of the changes are gradual, and only rarely do abrupt changes occur in adult concentrations. Plasma protein concentrations increase after infancy, with adult concentration values being attained by 10 years of age. Serum IgG increases slightly out of proportion to the increase in concentration of α_2-globulin.

The serum activity of most enzymes decreases during childhood to adult values by puberty or earlier, although the activity of alanine aminotransferase may continue to rise, at least in men, until middle age. Serum alkaline phosphatase activity is high in infancy but decreases during childhood and rises again with growth before puberty. The activity of the enzyme is correlated better with skeletal growth and sexual maturity than with chronological age; it is greatest at the time of maximum osteoblastic activity occurring with bone growth. The activity decreases rapidly after puberty, especially in women. In addition, the serum creatinine concentration increases steadily from infancy to puberty, parallel with development of skeletal muscle; until puberty little difference exists in this concentration between sexes. The serum uric acid concentration decreases from its high at birth until 7 to 10 years of age, at which time it begins to increase, especially in boys, until about 16 years of age.

Adult.   The concentrations of most test constituents remain fairly constant between puberty and menopause in women and between puberty and middle age in men. During the midlife years, serum total protein and albumin concentrations decrease slightly. A slight decrease may occur in the serum calcium concentration in both sexes. In men the serum phosphate decreases markedly after 20 years of age; in women the phosphate also decreases until menopause, when a marked increase takes place. Serum alkaline phosphatase begins to rise in women at the time of menopause so that in elderly women, the activity of this enzyme actually may be higher than in men.

Serum uric acid concentrations peak in men in their 20s and in women during middle age. Urea concentration increases in both sexes in middle age. Age does not affect the serum creatinine concentration in men but does increase its concentration in women. The serum total cholesterol and triglyceride concentrations increase in both men and women at a rate of ~2 mg/dL (0.02 mmol/L) per year to a maximum between 50 and 60 years of age. The activity of most enzymes in serum is less during adult life than during adolescence. This increased enzyme activity presumably reflects the greater physical activity of adolescents. The concentration of glucose in plasma 1 hour after a loading dose of glucose rises ~8 mg/dL (0.44 mmol/L) per decade.

Elderly adults. Significant increases in the plasma concentrations of many constituents occur in women after the start of menopause (Table 2-13). For example, estrogen secretion in women begins to decrease before menopause and continues at a greater rate after menopause, whereas gonadotropins show a feedback-mediated reciprocal rise. Serum concentrations of estrogens decrease by 70% or more, and urinary excretion of estrogens is decreased comparably. The decreased estrogen secretion may be responsible for the increase of serum cholesterol that occurs up to 60 years of age in women. Estrogen secretion in men, although always less than in women, declines with age.

The secretions of triiodothyronine, parathyroid hormone, aldosterone, and cortisol also are reduced in the elderly. The reduced secretion of cortisol leads to a ~50% reduction in the urinary excretion of 17-hydroxycorticosteroids. Basal insulin concentration is unaffected by age, but its response to glucose is reduced. In men the secretion rate and concentration of testosterone are reduced after 50 years of age. In women the concentration of pituitary gonadotropins, especially FSH, is increased in the blood and urine.

Renal concentrating ability is reduced in the elderly adult, and creatinine clearance may decline by as much as 50% between the third and ninth decades of life. The tubular maximum capacity for glucose also is reduced. However, the plasma urea concentration rises with age, as does the urinary excretion of protein.

Sex

Until puberty few differences exist in laboratory data between boys and girls. After puberty the serum activities of alkaline phosphatase, aminotransferases, creatine kinase, and aldolase are greater in men than in women. The higher activity of enzymes originating from skeletal muscle in men is related to their greater muscle mass. After menopause the activity of alkaline phosphatase increases until it is higher in women than in men. Although total lactate dehydrogenase (LD) activity is similar in men and women, the LD-1 and

TABLE 2-13	Changes in Composition of Serum with Menopause

Constituent	Increase (%)
Alanine aminotransferase	12
Albumin	2
Alkaline phosphatase	25
Apolipoprotein A-1	4
Aspartate aminotransferase	11
Cholesterol	10
Glucose	2
Phospholipids	8
Phosphate	10
Sodium	1.5
Total protein	0.7
Uric acid	10

From Wilding P, Rollason JG, Robinson D: Pattern of change for various biochemical constituents detected in well-population screening. Clin Chim Acta 1972; 41:375-387.
See footnote, Table 2-1.

LD-3 activities are higher, whereas LD-2 is less in young women than in men. These differences disappear after menopause.

The concentrations of albumin, calcium, and magnesium are higher in men than in women, but the concentration of γ-globulin is lower. Blood hemoglobin concentrations are lower in women; thus the serum bilirubin concentrations also are slightly lower. Serum iron is low during a woman's fertile years, and the plasma ferritin may be only one-third that of men. The reduced iron concentration in women is attributable to menstrual blood loss. Cholesterol concentration is typically higher in men than in women, whereas the α-lipoprotein concentration is lower. The plasma amino acid concentrations and concentrations of creatinine, urea, and uric acid, are higher in men than in women. The effect of age on the difference in concentrations of serum constituents between males and females is illustrated in Table 2-14.

Race

Total serum protein concentration is known to be higher in blacks than in whites, a fact largely attributable to a much higher γ-globulin in blacks, although usually the concentrations of α_1- and β-globulins also are increased. The serum albumin is typically less in blacks than in whites. In black men, serum IgG is often 40% higher and serum IgA as much as 20% higher than in white men.

The activity of creatine kinase and lactate dehydrogenase is usually much higher in both black men and women than in whites. This occurrence is presumed to be related to the amount of skeletal muscle, which tends to be greater in blacks than in whites. Because of their greater skeletal development, black children usually demonstrate higher serum alkaline phosphatase levels at puberty than do white children.

Racial differences also exist in carbohydrate and lipid metabolism. For example, glucose tolerance is less in blacks,

TABLE 2-14 Influence of Sex on Composition of Serum at Different Ages

Constituent	Difference Between Sexes*				
	29 y	30 to 39 y	40 to 49 y	50 to 59 y	60 to 69 y
Albumin (g/dL)	0.1	0.1	0	0	−0.1
Alkaline phosphatase (U/L)	14	12	−8	2	−1
Aspartate aminotransferase (U/L)	5	8	8	1	−1
Bilirubin (mg/dL)	0.1	0.1	0.1	0.1	0.1
Calcium (mg/dL)	0.1	0.1	0.1	−0.1	−0.2
Cholesterol (mg/dL)	−14	2	6	−16	−34
Creatinine (mg/dL)	0.2	0.2	0.2	0.2	0.1
Glucose (mg/dL)	5	3	6	0	6
Phosphate (mg/dL)	0.1	0.1	0	−0.1	−0.2
Total protein (g/dL)	−0.1	−0.1	−0.1	−0.1	−0.2
Urea nitrogen (mg/dL)	3	3	3	2	0
Uric acid (mg/dL)	1.5	1.7	1.7	1.0	0.5

From Leonard PJ: The effect of age and sex on biochemical parameters in blood of healthy human subjects. In Siest G (ed): Reference Values in Human Chemistry, pp 134-140, Basel, Karger, 1973.
See footnote, Table 2-1.
*Male values are higher than female values, except where indicated by a minus (−) sign.

Polynesians, Native Americans, and Inuits than in comparable age- and sex-matched whites. After 40 years of age the serum cholesterol and triglyceride concentrations are consistently higher in whites than in blacks. These may be dietary rather than racial factors because the concentration of plasma lipids has been shown to differ for the same racial group in different parts of the world. The blood hemoglobin concentration is as much as 1 g/dL higher in whites than in blacks. Some groups indigenous of the Pacific region (for example, Maoris of New Zealand) have significantly higher mean serum uric acid concentrations than white populations.

Environmental factors

Environmental factors that affect laboratory results include altitude, ambient temperature, and place of residence.

Altitude

Individuals living at high altitudes demonstrate marked increases in blood hemoglobin because of reduced atmospheric PO_2. Erythrocyte 2,3-diphosphoglycerate also is increased, and the oxygen dissociation curve is shifted to the right. The increased erythrocyte concentration leads to an increased turnover of nucleoproteins and excretion of uric acid. The fasting, basal concentration of growth hormone concentration is high in individuals living at high elevations.

Ambient temperature

Environmental temperature affects the composition of body fluids. Acute exposure to heat causes the plasma volume to expand by an influx of interstitial fluid into the intravascular space and by reduction of glomerular filtration. The plasma protein concentration may decrease by up to 10%. Salt and water may be lost through sweat, but usually no changes in the plasma sodium and chloride concentrations occur. The plasma potassium concentration may de-

crease by as much as 10% as potassium is taken up by the cells. If sweating is extensive, hemoconcentration rather than hemodilution may occur.

Place of residence

The geographical location in which an individual lives may affect the composition of body fluids. For example, an increase in the serum concentrations of cholesterol, triglycerides, and magnesium has been observed in individuals living in areas with hard water. Trace element concentrations also are affected by locale; for example, in areas in which ore smelting is common, serum concentrations of the trace elements involved may be increased. Carboxyhemoglobin concentrations are higher in areas in which heavier automobile traffic is common than in rural areas (as was true for blood lead in the 1970s in the United States).

Long-term cyclical changes

Long-term cyclical changes also affect laboratory results. Seasonal influences and the menstrual cycle are examples of such changes.

Seasonal influences

Seasonal influences on the composition of body fluids are small and probably related to seasonal dietary changes and altered physical activity. Evaluations of seasonal variation are difficult because they depend on the definition of a season and the magnitude of temperature change from one season to another. Day-to-day variability in the composition of body fluids is greater in summer than in winter. Table 2-15 lists some seasonal effects on the composition of body fluids.

Menstrual cycle

The plasma concentrations of many female sex hormones, as well as other hormones, are affected by the men-

TABLE 2-15　Seasonal Effects on Composition of Serum

| | Concentration | | Difference between High |
Constituent	Highest	Lowest	and Low (%)
Alanine aminotransferase	Winter	Spring, summer	5
Albumin	Fall	Summer	1.2
Aspartate aminotransferase	Spring	Fall	11.7
Calcium	Fall	Winter	1
Creatinine	Summer	Winter	4.7
Glucose	Fall	Spring	1.5
Lactate dehydrogenase	Summer	Winter	1.8
Triglycerides	Spring	Fall	5.4
Urea nitrogen	Fall	Spring, summer	3.2
Uric acid	Summer	Winter	4.3

From Letellier G, Desjarlais F: Study of seasonal variations for eighteen biochemical parameters over a four-year period. Clin Biochem 1982; 15:206-211; and copyright 1982 by Canadian Society of Clinical Chemists.
See footnote, Table 2-1.

TABLE 2-16　Effect of Fever on Composition of Serum

| | | Concentration after Induction of Fever | | | |
Constituent	Baseline Value	18 h	48 h	72 h	96 h
Sodium (mmol/L)	141	130	130	132	135
Chloride (mmol/L)	99	91	89	92	94
Potassium (mmol/L)	3.6	3.5	3.0	3.4	3.6
Calcium (mg/dL)	9.7	8.4	8.5	9.0	9.1
Phosphate (mg/dL)	3.3	2.3	3.2	3.2	3.7
Magnesium (mg/dL)	1.85	1.62	1.73	1.78	1.70
Creatinine (mg/dL)	1.10	1.03	1.04	1.00	1.09
Urea nitrogen (mg/dL)	13.4	14.0	15.2	18.5	17.4
Uric acid (mg/dL)	5.0	5.5	5.7	6.2	6.2

From Beisel WR, Goldman RF, Joy RJT: Metabolic balance studies during induced hyperthermia in man. J Appl Physiol 1968; 24:1-10.
See footnote, Table 2-1.

strual cycle.[21] Thus the plasma corticosterone concentration is as much as 50% higher in the luteal phase than in the follicular phase. The urinary excretion of 17-hydroxycorticosteroids reaches a peak at midcycle. Plasma-androstenedione and plasma-aldosterone concentrations increase from the follicular phase to the luteal phase of the menstrual cycle. On the preovulatory day the aldosterone concentration actually may be twice that during the early part of the follicular phase. The change in renin activity is almost as great. These changes are usually more marked in women who retain fluid before menstruation. Urinary catecholamine excretion increases at midcycle and remains high throughout the luteal phase.

Underlying medical conditions

Fever, shock and trauma, and transfusion all affect laboratory results.

Fever

Fever provokes many hormone responses. Hyperglycemia occurs soon after the onset of fever and stimulates the secre-

tion of insulin, which improves glucose tolerance. However, growth hormone and glucagon also increase with fever, further influencing glucose homeostasis. Fever also appears to reduce the secretion of thyroxine, as do acute illnesses that do not involve fever. In response to increased corticotropin secretion, the plasma cortisol concentration is increased and its normal diurnal variation may be abolished. The urinary excretion of free cortisol, 17-hydroxycorticosteroids, and 17-ketosteroids is increased. As acute fever subsides, or as it lessens but persists for a prolonged period, the hormone responses diminish. Table 2-16 lists some representative changes in serum composition induced by fever.

Shock and trauma

Shock and trauma result in certain characteristic biochemical changes. For example, after shock or trauma, corticotropin secretion is stimulated to produce a threefold to fivefold increase in the serum cortisol concentration. The 17-hydroxycorticosteroid excretion is increased greatly, although the excretion of 17-ketosteroids and metabolites of adrenal androgens may be unaffected. Aldosterone secretion

TABLE 2-17 Incidence of Increased Activity of Serum Enzymes and Isoenzymes After Surgery

Enzyme	Increase (%)
Creatine kinase	76
CK-2 isoenzyme	6
Aspartate aminotransferase	50
α-Hydroxybutyrate dehydrogenase	28
LD-1 isoenzyme	18
LD-1 > LD-2	10
LD-5 isoenzyme	20

From Krafft J, Fink R, Rosalki SB: Serum enzymes and isoenzymes after surgery. Ann Clin Biochem 1977; 14:294-296.
CK, Creatine kinase; *LD,* lactate dehydrogenase.
See footnote, Table 2-1.

is stimulated, and plasma renin activity is increased, as are the secretions of growth hormone, glucagon, and insulin. Anxiety and stress increase the excretion of catecholamines. The stress of surgery has been shown to reduce the serum triiodothyronine concentration by 50% in individuals without thyroid disease.

The general metabolic response to shock includes the normal response to stress by mobilization of lipids, although the serum triglyceride concentration usually is not affected. Plasma glucose concentration is increased, and glucose tolerance is reduced.

Immediately after an injury, a loss of fluid to extravascular tissues occurs, with a resulting decreased plasma volume. If the decrease is enough to impair circulation, glomerular filtration is diminished. Diminished renal function leads to the accumulation of urea and other end products of protein

metabolism in the circulation.[2] In burned patients, serum total protein concentration drops by as much as 0.8 g/dL (8 g/L) because of both loss to extravascular spaces and loss to catabolism of protein. Serum α_1-, α_2-, and γ-globulin concentrations increase but not enough to compensate for the reduced albumin concentration. The plasma fibrinogen concentration responds dramatically to trauma and may double within 2 to 8 days after surgery.

With tissue destruction comes increased urinary excretion of the major components of skeletal muscle. The muscle damage associated with the trauma of surgery increases markedly the serum activity of enzymes originating in skeletal muscle, and this increased activity may persist for several days. Typical alterations in the activity of serum enzymes after surgery are illustrated in Table 2-17.

Transfusion

Transfusion of whole blood or plasma raises the plasma protein concentration; the amount of the increase depends on the amount of blood administered. Serum lactate dehydrogenase activity, primarily LD-1 and LD-2, is increased by the breakdown of transfused erythrocytes. Transfusions to replace blood lost because of injury reduce sodium, chloride, and water retention precipitated by the injury. Serum iron and transferrin concentrations are reduced immediately after an injury, but extensive blood transfusions can lead to siderosis and an increased serum iron concentration. Serum potassium may increase with the transfusion of stored blood.

Infusions of glucose solutions usually result in reductions of both the plasma phosphate and the potassium concentrations as these compounds are taken up by the erythrocytes. Infusions of solutions of albumin may increase plasma alkaline phosphatase activity if the albumin has been prepared from placentas.

References

1. Beto JA, Bansal VK, Ing TS et al: Variation in blood sample collection for determination of hemodialysis adequacy. Council on Renal Nutrition National Research Question Collaborative Study Group. Am J Kidney Dis 1998; 31:135-141.

2. Beto JA, Bansal VK, Kahn S: The effect of blood draw methodology on selected nutritional parameters in chronic renal failure. Adv Ren Replace Ther 1999; 6:85-92.

3. Dale JC, Steindel SJ, Walsh M: Early morning blood collections: a College of American Pathologists: Q-Probes study of 657 institutions. Arch Pathol Lab Med 1998; 122:865-870.

4. Kurman RJ, Amin MB: Protocol for the examination of specimens from patients with carcinomas of the cervix: a basis for checklists. Cancer Committee, College of American Pathologists. Arch Pathol Lab Med 1999; 123:55-61.

5. Larsson BA, Tannfeldt G, Lagercrantz H et al: Venipuncture is more effective and less painful than heel lancing for blood tests in neonates. Pediatrics 1998; 101:882-886.

6. Leppanen E, Dugue B: When to collect blood specimens: midmorning vs. fasting samples. Clin Chem 1998; 44:2537-2542.

7. McPhillips MA, Strang J, Barnes TR: Hair analysis: new laboratory ability to test for substance use. Br J Psychiatry 1998; 173:287-290.

8. National Committee for Clinical Laboratory Standards: Blood Collection on Filter Paper for Neonatal Screening Programs: Approved Standard LA4-A3. 3rd edition. Wayne, Pa, National Committee for Clinical Laboratory Standards, 1997.

9. National Committee for Clinical Laboratory Standards: Procedures for Collection of Skin Puncture Blood Specimens: Approved Standard H4-A4. 4th edition. Wayne, Pa, National Committee for Clinical Laboratory Standards, 2000.

10. National Committee for Clinical Laboratory Standards: Evacuated Tubes and Additives for Blood Specimen Collection: Approved Standard H1-A4. 4th edition. Wayne, Pa, National Committee for Clinical Laboratory Standards, 1996.

11. National Committee for Clinical Laboratory Standards: Procedures for the Collection of Arterial Blood Specimens: Approved Standard H11-A3. 3rd edition. Wayne, Pa, National Committee for Clinical Laboratory Standards, 1999.

12. National Committee for Clinical Laboratory Standards: Procedures for the Collection of Diagnostic Blood Specimens by Skin Puncture: Approved Standard H4-A3. 3rd edition. Wayne, Pa, National Committee for Clinical Laboratory Standards, 1991.

13. National Committee for Clinical Laboratory Standards: Procedures for the Collection of Diagnostic Blood Specimens by Venipuncture: Approved Standard H3-A4. 4th edition. Wayne, Pa, National Committee for Clinical Laboratory Standards, 1991.

14. National Committee for Clinical Laboratory Standards: Procedures for the Handling and Transport of Domestic Diagnostic Specimens and Etiologic Agents: Approved Standard H5-A3. 3rd edition. Wayne, Pa, National Committee for Clinical Laboratory Standards, 1994.

15. National Committee for Clinical Laboratory Standards: Routine Urinalysis and Collection, Transportation, and Preservation of Urine Specimens: Approved Guideline GP16-A. Wayne, Pa, National Committee for Clinical Laboratory Standards, 1995.

16. Pelsers MM, Chapelle JP, Knapen M et al: Influence of age and sex and day-to-day and within-day biological variation on plasma concentrations of fatty acid-binding protein and myoglobin in healthy subjects. Clin Chem 1999; 45:441-443.

17. Sebastian-Gambaro MA, Liron-Hernandez FJ, Fuentes-Arderiu X: Intra- and inter-individual biological variability data bank. Eur J Clin Chem Clin Biochem 1997; 35:845-852.

18. Siest G, Henny J, Schiele F (eds): Interpretation des Examens de Laboratoire. Basel, Karger, 1981.

19. Young DS: The effects of frequently prescribed drugs on common laboratory procedures. In Spittell JA Jr (ed): Practice of Medicine, pp 1-21, Philadelphia, JB Lippincott, 1984.

20. Young DS: Effects of Drugs on Clinical Laboratory Tests, 5th edition, Washington, DC, AACC Press, 1999.

21. Young DS: Effects of Preanalytical Variables on Clinical Laboratory Tests, 2nd edition, Washington, DC, AACC Press, 1997.

22. Zhang DJ, Elswick RK, Miller WG et al: Effect of serum-clot contact time on clinical chemistry laboratory results. Clin Chem 1998; 44:1325-33.

Additional Reading

Antonsen S: The estimation of biological and preanalytical variations of inflammation markers. Scand J Clin Lab Invest Suppl 1994; 219:55-60.

Dugue B, Leppanen E, Grasbeck R: Preanalytical factors and the measurement of cytokines in human subjects. Int J Clin Lab Res 1996; 26:99-105.

Faulkner WR, Meites S: Geriatric Clinical Chemistry, Reference Values, Washington, DC, AACC Press, 1993.

Flynn JC: Procedures in Phlebotomy, 2nd edition, Philadelphia, WB Saunders, 1999.

Irjala KM, Gronroos PE: Preanalytical and analytical factors affecting laboratory results. Ann Med 1998; 30:267-272.

Kallner A: Preanalytical procedures in the measurement of ionized calcium in serum and plasma. Eur J Clin Chem Clin Biochem 1996; 34:53-58.

Keffer JH: Preanalytical considerations in testing thyroid function. Clin Chem 1996; 42:125-134.

Narayanan S: Preanalytical aspects of coagulation testing. Haematologica 1995; 80(2 Suppl):1-6.

Narayanan S: The preanalytic phase: an important component of laboratory medicine. Am J Clin Pathol 2000; 113:429-452.

Petersen H, Larsen ML, Horder M et al: Influence of analytical quality and preanalytical variations on measurements of cholesterol in screening programmes. Scand J Clin Lab Invest 1990; 198(Suppl):66-72.

Soldin SJ, Hicks JM, Gunter KC et al (eds): Pediatric Reference Ranges, 2nd edition, Washington, DC, AACC Press, 1997.

Withold W: Monitoring of bone turnover biological, preanalytical and technical criteria in the assessment of biochemical markers. Eur J Clin Chem Clin Biochem 1996; 34:785-799.

PART II

Analytical Techniques and Instrumentation

CHAPTER 3

Spectrophotometric Techniques

MERLE A. EVENSON, PhD

Objectives

1. Provide two definitions for *electromagnetic radiation,* in terms of photon and wavelength, and state the wavelengths associated with the ultraviolet, infrared, and visible spectra.
2. State Beer's law and calculate the absorbance or concentration of a solution using the formula.
3. Define *photometry, absorbance, percent transmittance, bandwidth, stray light,* and *linearity.*
4. Determine absorbance from measured percent transmittance.
5. List the components of a spectrophotometer and provide examples of each component.
6. State the principles of flame emission spectrophotometry and atomic absorption spectrophotometry and list the substances analyzed by each technique.

Key Words

Absorbance (A) The capacity of a substance to absorb radiation; expressed as the logarithm (log) of the reciprocal of the transmittance (T) of the substance

$$A = \log(1/T) = -\log(T)$$

Absorption Spectrum The graphical plot of absorbance versus wavelength (the absorbance spectrum) for a specific compound

Absorptivity A measure of the absorption of radiant energy at a given wavelength and/or frequency as it passes through a solution of a substance at a concentration of 1 mol/L; expressed as the absorbance divided by the product of the concentration of a substance and the sample path length

Atomic Absorption Spectrophotometry An analytical method in which a sample is vaporized and the concentration of a metal is determined from the absorption of light by the neutral atom at one of the strong emission lines of the element

Bandpass The range of wavelengths passed by a filter or monochromator; also called *bandwidth;* expressed as the range of wavelengths transmitted at a point equal to one-half the peak intensity transmitted

Beer's Law A mathematical equation that stipulates that the absorbance of monochromatic light by a solution is proportional to the absorptivity *(a),* the length of the light-path *(b),* and the concentration *(c)*

$$A = abc$$

Blank A solution consisting of all the components of a reaction except the analyte

Flameless Atomic Absorption A type of atomic absorption spectrophotometry in which the element is converted to a vapor phase without the use of a flame

Infrared Radiation The 770- to 12,000-nm region of the electromagnetic spectrum

Line Spectrum The spectrum characteristic of an atom or ion, consisting of a series of discrete spectral lines that correspond to changes in energy levels of electrons

Molar Absorptivity (ε) A constant for a one molar solution of a given compound at a given wavelength and a 1-cm pathlength under prescribed conditions of solvent, temperature, pH, etc; expressed as L/mol × cm

Monochromatic Electromagnetic radiation of one wavelength or an extremely narrow range of wavelengths

Photodetector   A device used to measure or indicate the presence of light

Photodiode Array   A two-dimensional matrix of light-sensitive semiconductors that is used to record complete absorption spectrum in milliseconds

Photometer/spectrophotometer   Device used to measure intensity of light emitted by, passed through, or reflected by a substance

Photometry   The measurement of light

Photon   A quantum of radiant energy

Reflectance Photometry   A spectrophotometric technique in which light is reflected from the surface of a reaction and used to measure the amount of the analyte

Refraction   The oblique deflection from a straight path undergone by a light ray or wave as it passes from one medium to another

Refractive Index (Index of Refraction)   The ratio of the velocity of light in one media relative to its velocity in a second media

Spectrophotometry   The measurement of the intensity of light at selected wavelengths

Stray Light   Any light from outside a photometer or spectrophotometer or from scattering within the instrument that is detected and causes errors in the measured transmittance or absorbance

Ultraviolet Radiation   The 180- to 390-nm region of the electromagnetic spectrum

Visible Light   The 390- to 780-nm region of the electromagnetic spectrum that is visible to the human eye

Wavelength   A characteristic of electromagnetic radiation; the distance between two wave crests

Many determinations in the clinical laboratory are based on measurements of radiant energy emitted, transmitted, absorbed, or reflected under controlled conditions. The optical principles involved in photometry, spectrophotometry, flame photometry, and atomic absorption spectrophotometry are discussed in this chapter.

PHOTOMETRY AND SPECTROPHOTOMETRY

Photometry is the measurement of the luminous intensity of light or the amount of luminous light falling on a surface from such a source. **Spectrophotometry** is the measurement of the intensity of light at selected wavelengths. The term *photometric measurement* was defined originally as the process used to measure light intensity independent of wavelength. Modern instruments, however, isolate a narrow wavelength range of the spectrum for measurements. Those that use filters for this purpose are referred to as *filter* **photometers,** whereas those that use prisms or gratings are called *spectrophotometers*. The primary analytical utility of filter photometry or spectrophotometry is the isolation and use of discrete portions of the spectrum for purposes of measurement.

Basic Concepts

Energy is transmitted via electromagnetic waves that are characterized by their frequency and wavelength. The physical definition of *wavelength* is the distance that a periodic wave propagates in one period or the distance between wave crests. Analytically the term **wavelength** describes a posi-

tion within a spectrum. Electromagnetic radiation includes radiant energy that extends from cosmic rays with wavelengths as short as 10^{-9} nm up to radio waves longer than 1000 km. However, in this chapter the term *light* is used to describe radiant energy from the visible and ultraviolet portions of the spectrum (290 to 800 nm).

In addition to possessing wavelength characteristics, light also behaves as it is composed of discrete energy packets called **photons.** The relationship between the energy of photons and their frequency is illustrated in

$$E = h\nu \qquad (1)$$

where:

E = Energy in ergs
ν = Frequency of the light given in cycles per second
h = Planck's constant (6.62×10^{-27} erg seconds)

The frequency of light (ν) is related to the wavelength by

$$\nu = \frac{c}{\lambda} \qquad (2)$$

where:

ν = Frequency of light in cycles per second
c = Speed of light in a vacuum (3×10^{10} cm/sec)
λ = Wavelength in centimeters.

By combining equations (1) and (2), the product is

$$E = \frac{hc}{\lambda} \qquad (3)$$

This equation shows that the energy of light is inversely proportional to the wavelength. For example, **ultraviolet (UV) radiation** at 200 nm possesses greater energy than **infrared (IR) radiation** at 750 nm.

TABLE 3-1	UV, Visible, and Short IR Spectrum Characteristics	
Wavelength (nm)	Region	Color Observed*
<380	UV†	Not visible
380 to 440	Visible	Violet
440 to 500	Visible	Blue
500 to 580	Visible	Green
580 to 600	Visible	Yellow
600 to 620	Visible	Orange
620 to 750	Visible	Red
800 to 2500	Near-IR	Not visible
2500 to 15,000	Mid-IR	Not visible
15,000 to 1,000,000	Far-IR	Not visible

UV, Ultraviolet; *IR,* infrared.
*Because of the subjective nature of color, the wavelength intervals shown are only approximations.
†The UV portion of the spectrum sometimes is divided further into "near" UV (200 to 380 nm) and "far" UV (<220 nm). This arbitrary distinction has a practical basis because silica used to make cuvets transmits light effectively at wavelengths ≥220 nm.

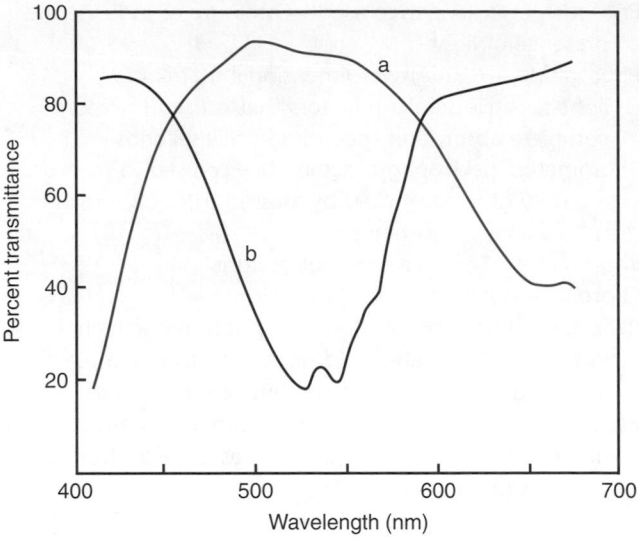

Figure 3-1   Spectral transmittance curves of nickel sulfate *(a)* and potassium permanganate *(b)*. Arbitrary concentrations read versus water as a blank (Beckman DB-G spectrophotometer).

The human eye responds to radiant energy with wavelengths between about 380 and 750 nm, but modern instrumentation permits measurements at both shorter-wavelenth (UV) and longer-wavelength (IR) portions of the spectrum. Sunlight, or light emitted from a tungsten filament, is a mixture, or spectrum, of radiant energy of different wavelengths that the eye recognizes as "white."

Table 3-1 shows the approximate relationships between wavelengths and color characteristics for the UV, visible, and short IR portions of the spectrum. A solution appears green when viewed against white light if it transmits light maximally between 500 and 580 nm but absorbs light at other wavelengths. Similarly, a solid object appears green if it reflects light in this region (500 to 580 nm) but absorbs light at other portions of the spectrum. In general, comparing the intensity of light transmitted by a colored solution with that of a **blank,** or reference, solution over the entire spectrum yields a typical spectral transmittance curve characteristic for that spectrum. Such curves are shown in Figure 3-1 for solutions of nickel sulfate *(a)* and potassium permanganate *(b)*. Inspection of the curves should lead to the prediction that the color of solution *a* is green inasmuch as light is transmitted maximally near the green portion of the spectrum. Curve *b,* on the other hand, illustrates the spectrum of a solution that transmits light maximally in the blue, violet, and red portions of the spectrum. The eye recognizes this mixture of colors as purple.

Relationship between transmittance and absorbance

Consider an incident light beam with intensity I_O passing through a square cell containing a solution of a compound that absorbs light of a certain wavelength, λ (Figure 3-2).

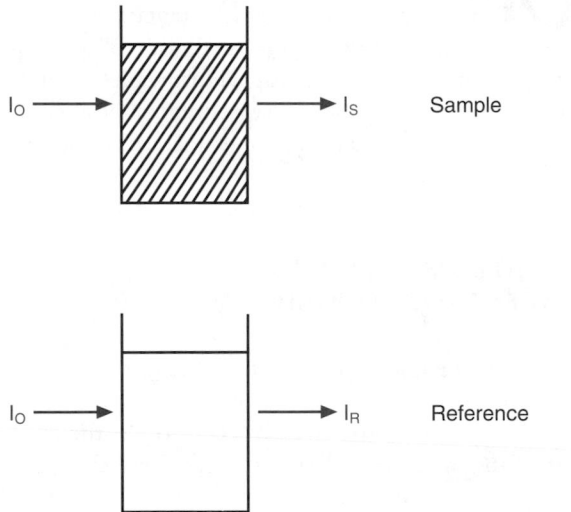

Figure 3-2   Transmittance of light through sample and reference cells. Transmittance of sample versus reference is I_S divided by I_R. I_O, Intensity of incident light; I_S, transmittance for compound in solution; I_R, transmittance through reference cell.

The intensity of the transmitted light beam I_S is less than I_O, and the transmittance (T) of light defined as

$$T = \frac{I_S}{I_O}$$

Some of the incident light, however, may be reflected by the surface of the cell or absorbed by the cell wall or solvent. To focus attention on the compound of interest, elimination of these factors is necessary. This action is done through use of a reference cell identical to the sample cell, except that the compound of interest is omitted from the solvent in the reference cell. The transmittance (T) through this reference

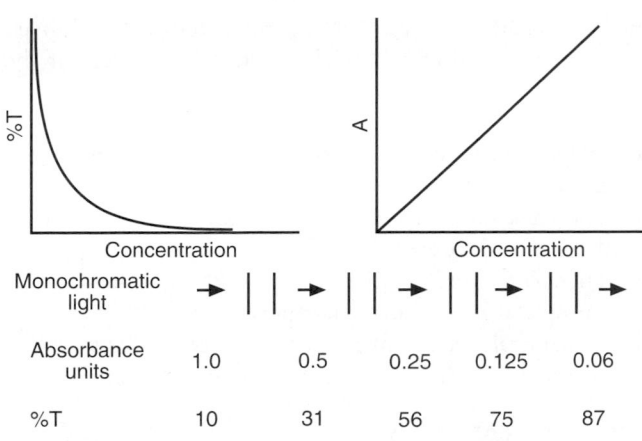

| Absorbance units | 1.0 | 0.5 | 0.25 | 0.125 | 0.06 |
| %T | 10 | 31 | 56 | 75 | 87 |

Figure 3-3　Absorbance and percent transmittance (%T) relationship. (From Tietz NW: Fundamentals of Clinical Chemistry, Philadelphia, WB Saunders, 1970.)

TABLE 3-2　Spectrophotometry Nomenclature

Name	Symbol	Definition
Absorbance	A	$-\log T$ or $\log I_0/I$
Absorptivity	a	A/bc (with c in g/L)
Molar absorptivity	ϵ	A/bc (with c in mol/L)
Path length	b	Internal cell or sample length, in cm
Transmittance	T	I/I_0
Wavelength unit	nm	10^{-9} m
Absorption maximum	λ_{max}	Wavelength at which a maximum absorption occurs

I/I_0, Ratio of the intensity of transmitted light to incident light.

cell is I_R divided by I_O; the transmittance for the compound in solution then is defined as I_S divided by I_R. In practice the reference cell is inserted and the instrument adjusted to an arbitrary scale reading of 100 (corresponding to 100% transmittance), after which the percent transmittance reading is made on the sample. The amount of light absorbed *(A)* as the incident light passes through the sample is equivalent to

$$A = -\log \frac{I_S}{I_R} = -\log T$$

Beer's law

Beer's law states that the concentration of a substance is directly proportional to the amount of light absorbed or inversely proportional to the logarithm of the transmitted light (Figure 3-3). Mathematically, Beer's law is expressed as

$$A = abc \tag{4}$$

where:

　A = Absorbance
　a = Proportionality constant defined as **absorptivity**
　b = Light path in centimeters
　c = Concentration of the absorbing compound, usually expressed in grams per liter

This equation forms the basis of quantitative analysis by absorption photometry. **Absorbance** values have no units; hence, the units for a are the reciprocal of those for b and c.

When b is 1 cm and c is expressed in moles per liter, the symbol ϵ (epsilon) is substituted for the constant a. The value for ϵ is a constant for a given compound at a given wavelength under prescribed conditions of solvent, temperature, pH, etc., and is called the **molar absorptivity.** The nomenclature of spectrophotometry is summarized in Table 3-2. Values for ϵ are useful to characterize compounds, establish their purity, and compare sensitivities of measurements obtained on derivatives. Pure bilirubin, for example,

when dissolved in chloroform at 25 °C, has a molar absorptivity of 60,700 ± 1600 at 453 nm. The molecular weight of bilirubin is 584. Hence a solution containing 5 mg/L (0.005 g/L) should have an absorbance of 0.520.

$$A = 60{,}700 \times 1 \times \frac{0.005}{584} = 0.520$$

Conversely, a solution of this concentration showing an absorbance of 0.490 could be assumed to have a purity of 0.490 divided by 0.520, or 94%.

The molar absorptivity of the complex between ferrous iron and *S*-tripyridyltriazine is 22,600, whereas that with 1,10-phenanthroline is 11,000. Thus for a given concentration of iron, *S*-tripyridyltriazine produces a complex with an absorbance about twice that of the complex with 1,10-phenanthroline. Thus *S*-tripyridyltriazine is a more sensitive reagent to use in the measurement of iron.

In toxicological work, listing of constants based on concentrations in grams per deciliter rather than in moles per liter is customary. This listing also may be necessary when the molecular weight of a substance is unknown. For $b = 1$ cm and $c = 1$ g/dL (1%), A is written as

$$A_{1cm}^{1\%}$$

This constant is called the *absorption coefficient.* An older symbol, now obsolete, was called the *extinction coefficient.*

Application of Beer's law

In practice the direct proportionality between absorbance and concentration must be established experimentally for a given instrument under specified conditions. Frequently a linear relationship exists up to a certain concentration or absorbance. When this relationship occurs, the solution is said to obey Beer's law up to this point. Within this limitation a calibration constant (K) may be derived and used to calculate the concentration of an unknown solution by comparison with a calibrating solution. From Equation (4)

$$a = \frac{A}{bc} \tag{5}$$

Therefore

$$\frac{A_1}{b_1 c_1} = \frac{A_2}{b_2 c_2} \qquad (6)$$

where subscripts 1 and 2 indicate the absorbance *(A)*, pathlength *(b)*, and concentration *(c)* of calibrating and unknown solutions, respectively.

Because the light path *(b)* remains constant in a given method of analysis with a fixed cuvet size, $b_1 = b_2$, and equation (6) then becomes

$$\frac{A_1}{c_1} = \frac{A_2}{c_2} \quad \text{or} \quad \frac{A_c}{c_c} = \frac{A_u}{c_u} \qquad (7)$$

where *c* and *u* represent calibrator and unknown, respectively. Solving for the concentration of unknown

$$c_u = \frac{A_u}{A_c} \times c_c \qquad (8)$$

or the equivalent expression

$$c_u = A_u \times \frac{c_c}{A_c} = A_u \times K \qquad (9)$$

where $K = c_c/A_c$. The value of the constant K is obtained through measurement of the absorbance (A_c) of a calibrator of known concentration (c_c).

Certain precautions must be observed with the use of such calibration constants. Under no circumstances should the constant be used when either the calibrator or unknown readings exceed the linear portion of the calibration curve (that is, when the curve no longer obeys Beer's law). At least two and preferably more calibrators should be included in each series of determinations to permit direct comparison of unknown with calibrator or to calculate the calibration constant because variations in reagents, working conditions, cell diameters, and deterioration or changes in instruments may result in day-to-day changes of the absorbance value for the calibrator. A nonlinear calibration curve may be used if a sufficient number of calibrators of varying concentrations is included to cover the entire range encountered for readings on unknowns.

In some cases a pure reference material may not be readily available, and constants may be provided that were obtained on pure materials and reported in the literature. In general, published constants should be used only if the method is followed in detail and readings are made on a spectrophotometer capable of providing light of high spectral purity at a verified wavelength. Use of broader-band light sources usually leads to some decrease in absorbance. The absorbance of NADH at 340 nm, for example, frequently is used as a reference for the determination of enzyme activity, based on a molar absorptivity of 6.22×10^3 (see Chapter 20). This value is acceptable only under the carefully controlled conditions previously described and should not be used unless these conditions are met. Published values for molar absorptivities and absorption coefficients should be used only as guidelines until they are veri-

fied by readings on pure reference materials for a given instrument. In addition, Beer's law is followed only if the following conditions are met:

- Incident radiation on the substance of interest is monochromatic.
- The solvent absorption is insignificant, compared with the solute absorbance.
- The solute concentration is within given limits.
- An optical interferant is not present.
- A chemical reaction does not occur between the molecule of interest and another solute or solvent molecule.

Measurement errors

Experience has shown that with most photometers the response of the detector to a signal of transmitted light is such that any uncertainty in %T is constant over the entire %T scale. The uncertainty derives from electrical and mechanical imperfections in the instrument and individual variations in the use of the instrument.

A fixed distance on the linear scale (for example, 1% T) represents a greater change in absorbance for low values of %T than for high values of %T. For this reason the absolute concentration error or uncertainty is greater when readings are taken at high absorbance. However, the relative concentration error is greater for readings at both low and high absorbances. Studies have shown that the relative error is minimal at an absorbance of 0.434 (36.8% T). Consequently, methods should be designed within an absorbance interval of approximately 0.1 and 0.7 (20% and 80% T).

Types of Spectrophotometers

Both single- and double-beam spectrophotometers are used in the clinical laboratory.

Single-beam spectrophotometer

The major components of a single-beam spectrophotometer are illustrated schematically in Figure 3-4. In practice a beam of light is passed through a monochromator that provides selection of the desired region of the spectrum to be used for measurements. Slits are used to isolate a narrow beam of the light and improve its chromatic purity. The light then passes through an absorption cell (cuvet), where a portion of the radiant energy is absorbed, depending on the nature and concentration of the solution. Any light not absorbed is transmitted to a detector (photocell or phototube), which converts light energy to electrical energy that is registered on a meter or recorder or displayed digitally.

In operation an opaque block is substituted for the cuvet to ensure that no light reaches the photocell, and the meter is adjusted to 0% T. Next, a cuvet containing a reagent blank is inserted, and the meter is adjusted to 100% T (that is, zero absorbance). The composition of the reagent blank should be identical to that of the calibrating or unknown solutions except for the substance to be measured. Calibrating solu-

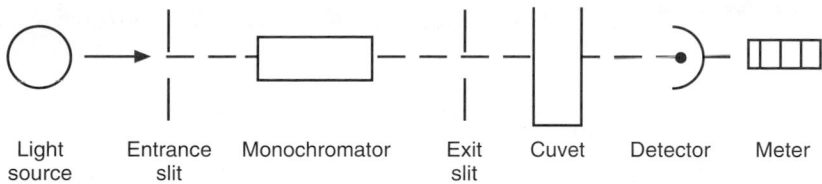

Figure 3-4   Major components of a single-beam spectrophotometer.

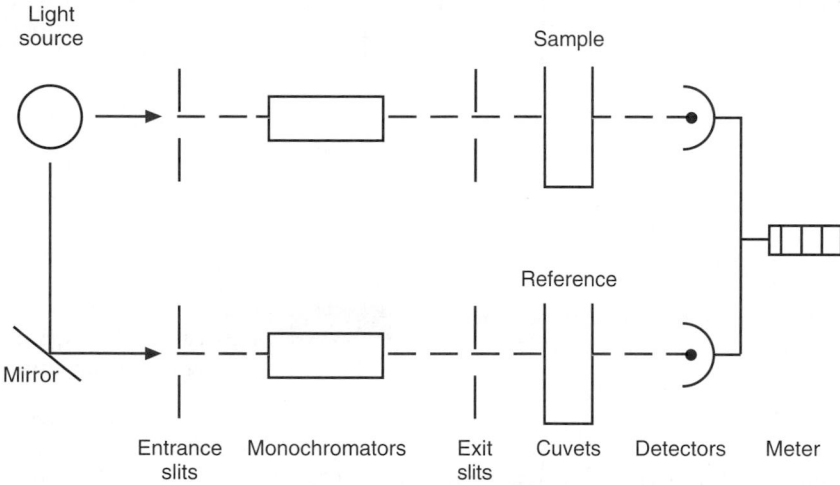

Figure 3-5   Double-beam-in-space spectrophotometer.

tions containing various known concentrations of the substance are inserted, and readings are recorded. Finally, a reading is made of the unknown solution, and its concentration is determined by comparison with the readings obtained on the calibrators. In most spectrophotometers digital hardware and software are integral components and perform these functions automatically.

Double-beam spectrophotometers

Figure 3-5 illustrates schematically a typical double-beam system. This system is referred to as a *double-beam-in-space spectrophotometer*. Another approach is to use a light-beam chopper (a rotating wheel with alternate silvered and cutout sections) inserted after the exit slit (Figure 3-6). A system of mirrors passes the portions of the light reflected off the chopper alternately through the sample and a reference cuvet onto a common detector. This system is referred to as a *double-beam-in-time spectrophotometer*. The chopped-beam approach, through use of one detector, compensates for light source variation and sensitivity changes of the detector.

Components of Spectrophotometers

The basic components of a spectrophotometer include the following:

1. Light source
2. Means to isolate light of a desired wavelength
3. Fiber optics

4. Cuvets
5. Photodetector
6. Readout device
7. Recorder
8. Microprocessor

Light sources

Types of light sources used in spectrophotometers include incandescent lamps and lasers.

Incandescent lamps

The light source for measurements in the **visible light** portion of the spectrum is usually a tungsten light bulb. The lifetime of a tungsten filament is increased greatly by the presence of low-pressure iodine or bromine vapor within the lamp. An example is the quartz-halogen lamp, which has a fused-silica envelope and provides high-intensity light over a wide spectrum. The quartz-halogen source has high intensity and longer lifetime than other lamps. Frequently these lamps operate for 2000 to 5000 hours before replacement is necessary.

The tungsten lamp is acceptable for measurements of moderately dilute solutions in which the change in absorbance varies significantly with small changes in concentration. A common disadvantage with older photometers is that a considerable amount of heat was generated by the light source; this heat caused problems in measurement either through changes in the geometry of the optical system or the sensitivity of the photocell. A tungsten light source does not supply sufficient radiant energy for measurements

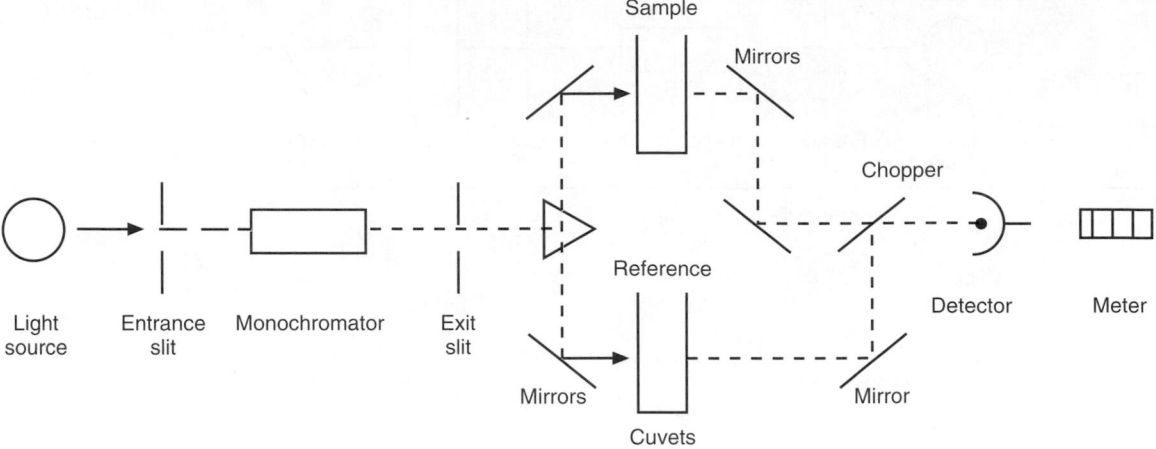

Figure 3-6 Double-beam-in-time spectrophotometer.

below 320 nm. In the UV region of the spectrum a low-pressure, mercury-vapor lamp, which emits a discontinuous, or **line spectrum,** is useful for calibration purposes but is not practical for absorbance measurements because it is used only at certain wavelengths. Hydrogen and deuterium lamps provide sources of continuous spectra in the UV region with some sharp emission lines, as do high-pressure mercury and xenon arc lamps; these sources are used more commonly in UV absorption measurements. A deuterium lamp is more stable and has a longer life than a hydrogen lamp.

Some photometers used as high-performance liquid chromatographic (HPLC) detectors employ miniature hollow-cathode lamps as narrow wavelength-intense sources (see Chapter 8). For example, a zinc hollow-cathode lamp gives a line at 214 nm that is adequately close to the maximum wavelength of peptide bond absorption (206 nm) and is used to measure peptides and proteins. The hollow-cathode lamp also has a long, useful lifetime if a lower-current, nonpulsed power supply is used.

Laser sources

Lasers (**L**ight **A**mplification by **S**timulated **E**mission of **R**adiation) also are used as light sources for spectrophotometers. These devices transform light of various frequencies into an extremely intense, focused, and nearly nondivergent beam of monochromatic light. Through selection of different materials, different wavelengths of light emitted by the laser are obtained (Table 3-3).

Inexpensive, near-IR lasers (0.8- to 2.5-μm wavelengths) are also available. They are solid-state devices constructed of a gallium-arsenic material, and energy is pumped into them at a low potential of ~1.5 V.

Spectral isolation

A system to isolate radiant energy of a desired wavelength (**monochromatic** light) and exclude that of other wavelengths is called a *monochromator.* Filters, prisms, and dif-

TABLE 3-3	Types of Lasers and the Wavelengths at Which They Operate
Laser	Wavelength(s) (nm)
Aluminum oxide doped with chromous oxide (ruby)	690
Argon	488 to 568
Carbon dioxide	337
Gallium-arsenic diode	325
Nitrogen	9200 to 10,800
Helium-cadmium	800 to 900
Helium-neon	633
Organic dye	400 to 800
Neodymium-YAG	1060

YAG, Yttrium aluminum garnet.

fraction gratings are used as monochromators. Combinations of lenses and slits also are inserted before or after the monochromator to render light rays parallel or isolate narrow portions of the light beam. Variable slits may be used to adjust total radiant energy reaching the photocell.

Filters

The simplest type of filter is a thin layer of colored glass. Certain metal complexes or salts, dissolved or suspended in glass, produce colors corresponding to the predominant wavelengths transmitted. Strictly speaking, a glass filter is not a true monochromator because it transmits light over a relatively wide range of wavelengths. The spectral purity of a filter or other monochromator usually is described in terms of its spectral **bandpass,** also known as *spectral bandwidth.* The bandpass is defined as the width, in nanometers, of the spectral transmittance curve at a point equal to one-half the peak transmittance (Figure 3-7). Commonly used glass filters have spectral bandwidths of approximately 50 nm and are referred to as *wide-bandpass filters.*

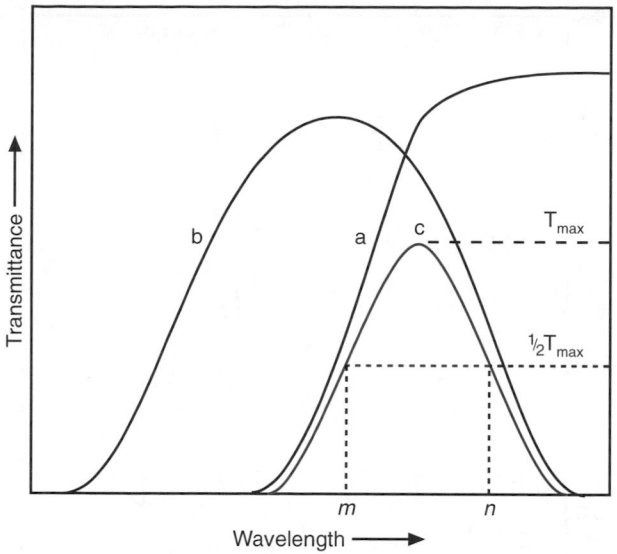

Figure 3-7   Spectral characteristics of a sharp-cutoff filter *(a)* and a wide-bandpass filter *(b)*. The narrow-bandpass filter *(c)* is obtained through combination of filters *a* and *b*. T_{max}, Maximum transmittance;

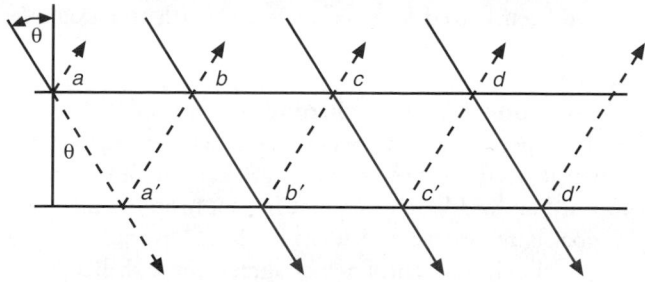

Figure 3-8   Passage of light through an interference filter. The heavier lines indicate reinforcement of entering light rays.

Other glass filters include the narrow-bandpass and sharp-cutoff types (see Figure 3-7). As implied, the latter filter typically shows a sharp rise in transmittance over a narrow portion of the spectrum and is used to eliminate light below a given wavelength. Narrow-bandpass filters may be constructed through the combination of two or more sharp-cutoff filters or regular filters; however, the availability of high-intensity light sources now favors the use of narrow-bandpass interference filters.

Another approach for construction of narrow-bandpass filters is to use a dielectric material of controlled thickness sandwiched between two thinly silvered pieces of glass. The thickness of the layer determines the wavelength of energy transmitted. Energies of wavelengths that are multiples of this thickness stay in phase as they reflect back and forth through the dielectric materials and finally emerge, whereas other wavelengths cancel one another because of their phase differences (Figure 3-8). These filters have narrow spectral bandwidths, usually from 5 to 15 nm, and are referred to as *interference filters*. Because they also transmit harmonics, or multiples, of the desired wavelength, accessory glass filters are required to eliminate these undesired wavelengths. Thus an interference filter designed for 620 nm also transmits some radiation at 310 and 1240 nm unless accessory cutoff filters are provided to absorb this undesired stray light.

Prisms and gratings

Prisms and diffraction gratings also are widely used as monochromators. A *prism* separates white light into a continuous spectrum through **refraction** with shorter wavelengths that are bent, or refracted, more than longer wavelengths as they pass through the prism. This action results in a nonlinear spectrum with the longer wavelengths closer to-

gether, but with suitable accessories, a narrow-bandwidth portion of the spectrum may be isolated. A diffraction grating is prepared through deposition of a thin layer of aluminum-copper alloy on the surface of a flat glass plate, with subsequent ruling of many small parallel grooves into the metal coating. Better gratings contain 1000 to 2000 lines/mm and are made with great care. These then are used as molds to prepare less expensive replicas for general use in instruments.

Modern holographic gratings are made through the use of a laser in a "high-precision machining" mode. The focused beam of the laser is scanned accurately over a photosensitive material termed a *photoresist*. After multiple lines have been etched on the photoresist, chemicals are used to dissolve and elute the laser-etched lines to create the channels that become the lines of the grating. A reflective layer of a highly reflective material then is sputtered onto the channels of the laser-etched, chemically eluted surface, and the grating is ready for use. Either a flat photoresistive surface or a concave surface is used to construct gratings of this nature, which are extremely accurate, demonstrate low light scatter, and are used widely in spectrophotometers in clinical chemistry instruments. For example, most UV-visible spectrophotometers and virtually all IR spectrophotometers use reflective gratings. In addition, HPLC detectors frequently use concave holographic reflective gratings in their optical systems.

Each line ruled on the grating, when illuminated, gives rise to a tiny spectrum. Wave fronts are formed that reinforce those wavelengths in phase and cancel those not in phase. The net result is a uniform linear spectrum. Some instruments contain diffraction gratings that produce spectral bandwidths of 20 nm or more; higher-priced instruments may have resolutions of 0.5 nm or less. The flat surface grating discussed previously is called a *plane transmission grating*. Lines are engraved on the surface of a mirror, which may be either a polished metal slab or a glass plate on which a thin, metallic film has been deposited. A grating also may be ruled at a specified angle so that a maximum fraction of the radiant energy is directed into wavelengths diffracted at a selected angle. This type of grating is called an *echelette* and is said to have been given a *blaze* at a particular angle or to have been blazed at a certain wavelength (for example, 250 nm).

Selection of a monochromator

The type of monochromator selected depends on the analytical needs of any given assay. For example, narrow spectral bandwidths are required in spectrophotometers if the goal is to resolve and identify sharp absorption peaks that are closely adjacent. Lack of agreement with Beer's law occurs when a part of the spectral energy transmitted by the monochromator is not absorbed at all by the substance being measured. This instance is observed more commonly with wide-bandpass instruments.

Some increase in absorbance, as well as improved linearity with concentration, usually is observed with instruments that operate at narrower bandwidths of light. This increase is especially true for substances that exhibit sharp peaks of absorption. Spectral absorbance curves for a solution of coproporphyrin I (Figure 3-9) demonstrate the marked decrease in maximum absorbance as the spectral bandwidth is increased from 1 to 20 nm. The *natural bandwidth* of an absorbing substance is defined as the bandwidth of the spectral absorbance curve at a point equal to one-half the maximum absorbance. Curve *a* in Figure 3-9, scanned at a spectral bandwidth of 1 nm, shows a natural bandwidth of approximately 10 nm. As a general rule the spectral bandwidth should not exceed 10% of the natural bandwidth for peak absorbance readings to be within 99.5% of true values. For example, many chemistry procedures used in the clinical laboratory produce absorbing species for which the natural bandwidth ranges from 40 to more than 200 nm.[4] The natural bandwidth of NADH is 58 nm (λ_{max} = 339 nm). Therefore for accurate measurements of this compound a spectral bandwidth of 6 nm or less should be used. Actual studies have shown that use of a 10-nm spectral bandwidth at 340 nm produces absorbance values approximately 98% of those obtained with a 1-nm spectral bandwidth.[8]

The wavelength selected is usually at the peak of maximum absorbance to achieve maximal sensitivity; however, choosing another wavelength to minimize interfering substances may be desirable. For example, turbidity readings on a spectrophotometer are greater in the blue region than in the red region of the spectrum, but the latter region is chosen for turbidity measurements to avoid absorption of light by bilirubin (460 nm) or hemoglobin (417 and 575 nm). The absorbing species developed in the alkaline picrate procedure for creatinine produces a relatively flat peak in the visible region of the spectrum at approximately 480 nm, but the reagent blank itself absorbs light strongly below 500 nm. A compromise is made through selection of a wavelength at 520 nm to minimize the contribution of the blank. Blank readings should of course be kept to a minimum. A small difference between two large numbers is subject to greater uncertainty; hence minimizing absorbance of the blank improves precision and accuracy. The linear working range of

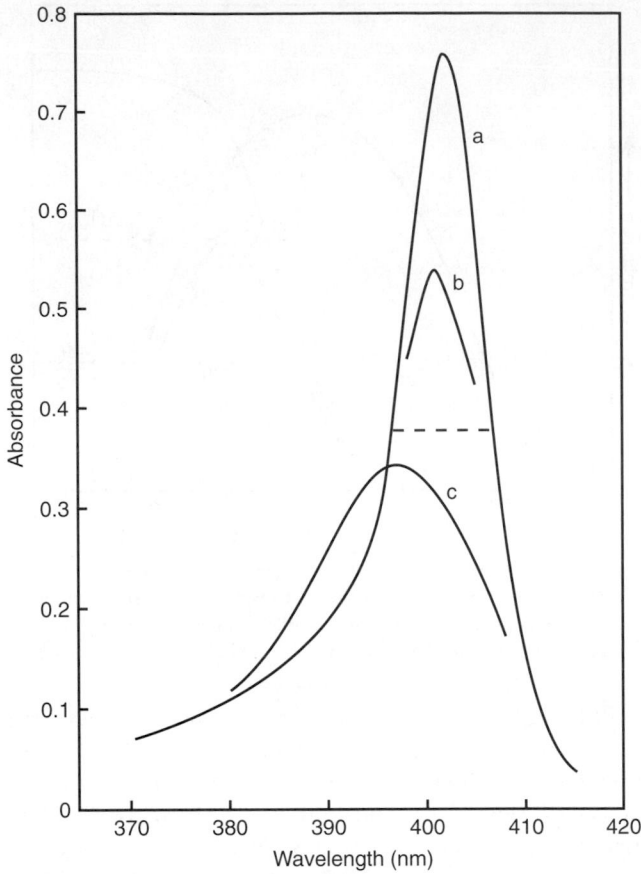

Figure 3-9 Effect of spectral bandwidth (SBW) on the absorption spectrum of coproporphyrin I at a nominal concentration of 1 μg/mL in HCl, 0.1 mol/L. SBW: Curve *a*, 1 nm, Beckman DB-G spectrophotometer; curve *b*, 10 nm; and curve *c*, 20 nm, Beckman DB spectrophotometer. The dotted horizontal line shows a natural bandwidth of 10 nm for coproporphyrin I when scanned at a spectral bandwidth of 1 nm. The shift of the absorbance maximum (A_{max}) to lower wavelengths as SBW is increased is related to skewness of the absorption spectrum to the left.

a method can be expanded also when measurements are not made at the peak absorbance. However, measurements should not be taken on the steep slope of an absorption curve because a slight error in wavelength adjustment can introduce a significant error in absorbance readings.

Fiber optics

In the single- and double-beam spectrophotometers shown diagrammatically in Figures 3-4, 3-5, and 3-6, the positioning of the individual components dictates the path that the light beam must follow as it travels from the source to the detector. This approach places certain restrictions on the design, size, and cost of such instruments. To overcome these restrictions, fiber optics now are integrated into the optical design of spectrophotometers. Fiber optics, also known as *light pipes*, are bundles of thin, transparent fibers of glass, quartz, or plastic that are enclosed in material of a lower refraction index and that transmit light throughout their lengths by internal reflections. The use of fiber optics in spectrophotometers offers the advantage of better directional control of the beam of light within the instrument; this control allows for the design and manufacture of miniature and inexpensive optical subsystems for use in automated instruments. For example, a single light source is multiplexed with multiple detectors by fiber optics for optimal positioning of the source and detectors in an automated system. Disadvantages of fiber optics include greater amounts of stray light; **refractive index** changes in the glass, quartz, or plastic rods; and loss of transmitted energy after continued use in the UV region of the spectrum. This loss of energy is known as *solarization* and results in a decrease in the optical sensitivity of an instrument.

Cuvets

Cuvets, also known as *absorption cells,* may be round, square, or rectangular and constructed from glass, silica (quartz), or plastic. Square or rectangular cuvets feature plane-parallel optical surfaces and constant light paths. The most popular have 1-cm light paths held to close tolerances. Ordinary borosilicate glass cuvets are suitable for measurements in the visible portion of the spectrum. For readings below 340 nm, however, quartz absorption cells usually are required. Some plastic cells have good clarity in both the visible and UV ranges but present problems relating to tolerances, cleaning, etching by solvents, and temperature deformations. Many plastic cuvets are designed for disposable, single-use applications.

Cuvets must be clean and optically clear; etching or deposits on the surface obviously affect absorbance values. Cuvets used in the visible range are cleaned by copious rinsing with tap and distilled water. Alkaline solutions should not be left standing in cuvets for prolonged periods because alkali slowly dissolves glass and produces etching. Cuvets may be cleaned in mild detergent or soaked in a mixture of concentrated HCl, water, and ethanol (ratio of 1:3:4). Cuvets should never be soaked in dichromate cleaning solution because the solution is hazardous and tends to adsorb onto and discolor the glass.

Cuvets used for measurements in the UV region should be handled with special care. Invisible scratches, fingerprints, or residual traces of previously measured substances may be present and demonstrate significant absorbance. A good practice is to fill all such cuvets with distilled water and measure the absorbance for each against a reference blank over the wavelengths to be used. This value should be essentially zero.

Photodetectors

Photodetectors are devices that convert light into an electric signal that is proportional to the number of photons striking its photosensitive surface. The photomultiplier (PM) tube is a commonly used photodetector for measurement of light intensity in the UV and visible regions of the

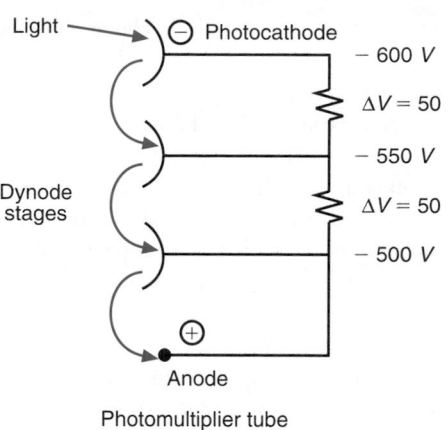

Figure 3-10   Schematic diagrams of a glass photomultiplier tube.

spectrum (Figure 3-10). Solid-state devices, such as photodiodes, photodiode arrays, and charge-coupled detectors, also are used in modern instruments. In older instruments barrier layer cells (also known as *photovoltaic cells*) were used as photodetectors because they were rugged and less expensive.[3]

Photomultiplier tubes

A PM tube is an electron tube that is capable of significantly amplifying a current (see Figure 3-10). The PM tube has as its cathode a light-sensitive metal that absorbs light and emits electrons in proportion to the radiant energy that strikes the surface of the light-sensitive material. The electrons produced by this first stage go to a secondary stage (surface), where each electron produces between four and six additional electrons. Each of these electrons goes on to another stage, again producing four to six electrons. Each electron cascades through the PM stages; thus the final current produced by such a tube may be 1 million times as much as the initial current. As many as 10 to 15 stages or dynodes are present in common PM tubes.

During operation of a PM tube, voltage is applied between the photocathode and each successive stage. The normal increment of voltage increase of each PM stage is from 50 to 100 V larger than that of the previous stage. A common PM tube may have approximately 1500 V applied to it.

PM tubes have extremely rapid response times, are very sensitive, and do not show as much fatigue as other detectors. Because these tubes have excellent sensitivity and rapid response, they must be shielded carefully from all stray light and daylight. A PM tube with the voltage applied should never be exposed to room light because the tube will burn out. Because of the fast response time of the PM tube, this detector is used readily with interrupted light beams such as those produced by choppers, and it therefore has significant advantages when used as a UV-visible detector in spectrophotometers. The rapid response times are needed when a spectrophotometer is being used to determine the absorption spectrum of a compound. The PM tube also has adequate sensitivity over a wide wavelength range.

When voltage is applied to PM tubes and all light has been blocked from them, some current usually is produced. This current is called *dark current*. Having the dark current of a PM tube at its lowest level is desirable because this current also is amplified and appears as background noise.

Solid-state detectors

Photodiodes and charge-coupled devices are solid-state devices used as detectors in spectrophotometers.

Photodiodes. A photodiode is a photosensitive semiconductor diode, the use of which as a detector in spectrophotometers has resulted in instruments capable of measuring light at a multitude of wavelengths. When a photodetector consists of two-dimensional arrays of diodes, each of which responds to a specific wavelength, it is known as a **photodiode array.** For example, photodiode arrays have been designed with 2-nm resolutions per diode from 200 to 340 nm, and 1-nm resolutions per diode from 340 to 800 nm.

In practice all diodes initially are charged to 5 V, and they discharge when they are struck by light. Each diode then is sequentially scanned and recharged to 5 V. The amount of energy required for recharging is proportional to the quantity of light striking that diode. Because scan time for all diodes are in the millisecond range, many scans are taken. The resultant data then are processed through use of a variety of algorithms, including signal averaging, background subtraction, and correction for scattered light. Consequently, an optical spectrum of an ongoing chemical reaction is monitored as a function of time with a high degree of resolution and accuracy.

Charge-coupled detectors. Charge-coupled detectors are multichannel devices with good dynamic ranges and signal-to-noise ratios that are superior to those of PM tubes.[9] These solid-state devices operate like a large number of photodetecting shift registers that are read horizontally and vertically. Because of their ability to detect very low levels of light, they have been used for molecular fluorescence measurement of very low concentrations of fluorescent molecules[10] (see Chapter 4).

Readout devices

Electrical energy from a detector is displayed on some type of meter or readout system—either direct-reading or null-point systems. In direct reading systems the output of the photocell is used to drive a sensitive meter directly, without further amplification. Other instruments use amplifiers to increase the output of the detector. In the null point system the output of the detector is balanced against the output of a reference circuit. The meter may be replaced by a servomotor activated by an imbalance of current, which stops when the two circuits are balanced. Direct digital readouts thus are obtained.

Also popular are digital readout devices that provide visual numerical displays of absorbance or converted values of concentrations. These operate on the principle of selective illumination of portions of a bank of light-emitting diodes (LEDs) or tubes controlled by the voltage signal generated. Typical examples include visible LEDs, which incorporate gallium as the major component. At present, gallium diodes that emit red light are used most widely. Compared with meters, digital readout devices have faster responses, are easier to read, and decrease operator fatigue.

Recorders

Spectrophotometers may be equipped with recorders in addition to or instead of the digital display of values. These devices are synchronized to provide line traces of transmittance or absorbance as a function of either time or wavelength. When a continuous tracing of absorbance versus wavelength is recorded, the resultant graphical representation is an **absorption spectrum.** If a substance absorbs light, distinct peaks are observed (Figure 3-11). Measuring the absorption spectra of an unknown sample and comparing it with spectra from known compounds is very useful for qualitative purposes. For example, this type of procedure is especially useful for identification of drugs that absorb in the UV region. Several criteria are used, including determination of those wavelengths showing maximum and minimum absorbance in both dilute acid and alkaline solutions, absorptivity at the wavelength of maximum absorbance, and ratios of absorbance at two wavelengths. Finally, the entire spectrum is compared with that of a known sample of the suspected drug.

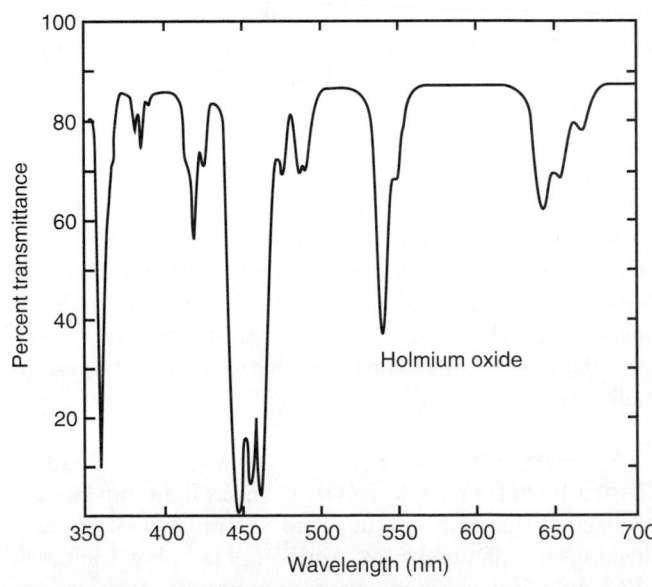

Figure 3-11   Spectral transmittance curve of holmium oxide filter.

Microprocessors

Microprocessors typically are incorporated in spectrophotometers. Operationally, signal output from calibrators is stored digitally, digital signals from blanks are subtracted from both the calibrators and unknowns, and the concentration of unknowns automatically is calculated. Data from multiple calibrators may be used to store a complete calibration curve, display or print out the curve for visible inspection, and calculate results of unknowns based on the curve or some mathematical transformation of it. A microprocessor and its resident software also is used to convert kinetic data into terms of enzyme activity. For example, change of absorbance with time is used widely to measure enzyme activity (see Chapter 20). Thus in the kinetic determination of lactate dehydrogenase, the rate of disappearance of NADH is monitored at 340 nm as pyruvate is converted to lactate. Multiple readings at short intervals also may be taken electronically and fed into a microprocessor to identify the linear portion of the curve, calculate the slope as the change in absorbance per minute (ΔA/min), and multiply by an appropriate constant to provide readout and printout of the final result.

Performance Parameters

With most analytical procedures based on a spectrophotometric measurement the absorbance of an unknown is compared directly with that of a calibrator or series of calibrators. Under these circumstances minor errors in wavelength calibration, variation in spectral bandwidths, presence of stray light, etc., do not usually contribute serious errors. Use of a series of calibrators covering a wide range of concentrations also provides a measure of linearity (that is, agreement with Beer's law) for a given procedure and instrument. When calculations are based on published or previously determined values for molar absorptivities or absorption coefficients, however, the spectrophotometer must be checked more rigorously. Performance verification of spectrophotometers on a periodic basis also improves reliability of routine comparative analyses.

To verify that a spectrophotometer is performing satisfactorily, the device must be shown to be able to operate within the specifications provided for it. Parameters to be tested include the following:

1. Wavelength accuracy
2. Spectral bandwidth
3. Stray light
4. Linearity
5. Photometric accuracy

The National Institute of Standards and Technology, formerly the National Bureau of Standards, provides several standard reference materials (SRMs) for spectrophotometry that are useful in the calibration or verification of the performance of photometers or spectrophotometers (Table 3-4).

Wavelength accuracy

For many analytical purposes the chosen wavelength is satisfactory if it is close to the λ_{max} of the chromogen being measured and the wavelength is reproducible. Most filters fall into this category and are quite satisfactory because unknowns are compared with calibrators at fixed wavelengths and spectral bandwidths. With prisms and diffraction gratings, however, a continuous choice of wavelengths is available, and verification of their accuracy and reproducibility becomes necessary. Knowledge of exact wavelength becomes critical when published molar absorptivities are used for identification of substances in toxicological studies and differential absorption techniques. Enzyme assays using the NAD-NADH reaction, for example, are based on a molar absorptivity constant for NADH of 6.22×10^3 at 340 nm. The wavelength settings therefore must be accurate and reproducible, and the instrument must show spectrophotometric accuracy if the constant is to be used in results calculation.

For the narrow-spectral-bandwidth instruments a holmium oxide glass may be scanned over the range of 280 to 650 nm. This material shows very sharp absorbance peaks at well-defined wavelengths (see Figure 3-11), and the wavelength scale readings that produce maximum absorbance may be compared with established values. If these readings do not coincide, a calibration curve then is constructed to relate scale readings to true wavelengths. Seven absorption peaks from holmium oxide glass that are suitable for calibration purposes are found at wavelengths (nm) of the following:

1. 279.3
2. 287.6
3. 333.8
4. 360.8
5. 418.5
6. 536.4
7. 637.5

Solutions of holmium oxide in dilute perchloric acid also have been recommended and may be used with any spectrophotometer.[2]

With broader-bandpass instruments a didymium* filter may be used to verify wavelength settings. This filter should show a minimum %T at 530 nm against an air blank (Figure 3-12). Because didymium has several absorption peaks, the setting should be verified grossly by visual examination of transmitted light, which should appear green at 530 nm.

Spectral bandpass/bandwidth

The spectral bandpass or bandwidth of a spectrophotometer customarily is stated by the manufacturer. It commonly is measured by use of a mercury-vapor lamp, which shows a

---

*Didymium is a rare metallic substance composed of neodymium and praseodymium.

TABLE 3-4   **SRMs Available from the NIST* for Calibration and Verification of Spectrophotometric and Spectrofluorometric Measurements**

SRM 930e

This SRM is for the verification and calibration of the transmittance and absorbance scales of visible absorption spectrometers. It consists of three Schott NG-type glass filters with nominal percent transmittances of 10%, 20%, and 30%. Each filter is certified individually for transmittance at wavelengths of 440.0, 465.0, 546.1, 590.0, and 635.0 nm.

SRM 931f

This SRM is for the verification and calibration of the absorbance scales of UV and visible absorption spectrometers having narrow spectral bandpasses. It consists of three sets of four solutions in sealed 10-mL ampules. The four solutions include a blank solution and three concentrations of an empirical inorganic solution prepared from high-purity cobalt and nickel metals dissolved in a mixture of nitric and perchloric acids. The net absorbances are certified for each concentration at wavelengths of 302, 395, and 512 nm, and a plateau in the region of 678 nm.

SRM 935a

This SRM is for the verification and calibration of the absorbance scales of UV absorption spectrometers having spectral band-passes not exceeding 2 nm. It consists of crystalline potassium chromate of established purity. Solutions made with this SRM are certified for apparent specific absorbances at wavelengths of 235, 257, 313, 345, and 350 nm. Acidic solutions of this SRM may be prepared to provide a standard with the desired absorbance at a specified wavelength.

SRM 936a

This SRM is for use in the evaluation of methods and the calibration of fluorescence spectrometers. Issued in 1-g units, it consists of solid quinine sulfate dihydrate. A solution made from it is certified for its relative molecular emission spectrum for a solution of 1.28×10^{-6} mol/L quinine sulfate dihydrate in 0.105 mol/L perchloric acid using an excitation wavelength of 347.5 nm. The values of the molecular emission spectrum are certified at 5-nm wavelength intervals from 375 to 675 nm.

SRM 1921a

This SRM is for use in the calibration of the wavelength scale of spectrometers in the IR spectral region from 3.2 to 18 μm (555 to 3125 cm^{-1}). Each unit consists of five cards made of a matte finish polystyrene film, approximately 38 μm thick, with a 25–mm-diameter clear aperture and centered 38 mm from the bottom of a cardboard holder 5 cm $\times$ 11 cm $\times$ 2 mm in size. The certified wavelength values, the corresponding peak wavelength values for 13 absorption peak positions in the 3.2- to 18-μm spectral region, and a spectrum marked with arrows identifying the certified peaks are provided with each unit.

SRM 1930

This SRM complements SRM 930e for the verification and calibration of the transmittance and absorbance scales of visible ab-sorption spectrometers. It consists of three Schott NG-type glassfilters with nominal percent transmittances at 1% T, 3% T, and 50% T. Each filter is certified individually for transmittance at wavelengths of 440.0, 465.0, 546.1, 590.0, and 635.0 nm.

SRM 1931

This SRM is for use in the evaluation and calibration of the relative spectral response of fluorescence spectrometers. It consists of four fluorescent standards and a "blank" specimen. The standards are composed of inorganic phosphors in a sintered poly-tetrafluoroethylene matrix and are certified for the relative corrected emission spectrum in energy/wavelength units. The values of the blue (400 to 550 nm), green (490 to 600 nm), yellow (490 to 740 nm), and orange (530 to 740 nm) emission spectra are certified at wavelength intervals of 2 nm.

SRM 2030a

This SRM is for use in the one-point verification of the transmittance and absorbance scales of spectrometers at the given wavelength and measured transmittance. It consists of one glass filter in its holder and one empty holder. The certified transmittance value at a wavelength of 465.0 nm and for a maximum spectral bandpass of 2.7 nm is provided for each unit.

SRM 2031a

This SRM is for use in the verification and calibration of the transmittance and absorbance scales of UV and visible absorption spectrometers. It consists of three individual filters mounted in separate holders and one empty holder. The nominal percent transmittance of the three filters are 10% T, 30% T, and 90% T. They are individually certified for transmittances at 10 wavelengths in the UV and visible spectral regions, including 250.0, 280.0, 340.0, 360.0, 400.0, 465.0, 500.0, 546.1, 590.0, and 635.0 nm.

SRM 2032

This SRM is for use in the assessment of heterochromatic stray radiation energy (stray light) in UV absorption spectrometers in the spectral region below 260 nm. Issued in 25-g units, this SRM consists of reagent-grade crystalline potassium iodide (KI). Aqueous solutions made with this SRM are certified for their specific absorbances under well-defined conditions at 240, 245, 250, 255, 260, 265, 270, and 275 nm.

SRM 2034

This SRM is for use in the verification and calibration of the wavelength scale of UV and visible spectrometers having nominal spectral bandwidths not exceeding 3 nm. It is a liquid consisting of 4% (w/v) holmium oxide in an aqueous solution of 10% (v/v) perchloric acid and is sealed in a nonfluorescent, fused-silica cuvet of optical quality. It is batch-certified for wavelength location of minimum transmittance of 14 bands in the spectral interval from 240 to 650 nm for six spectral bandwidths, ranging from 0.1 to 3 nm.

*From NIST Standard Reference Materials (SRM) Catalog: NIST special publication 260, Gaithersburg, Md, U.S. Department of Commerce, National Institute of Standards and Technology, 1998.
SRM, Standard reference material; *NIST,* National Institute of Standards and Technology; *IR,* infrared; *UV,* ultraviolet.

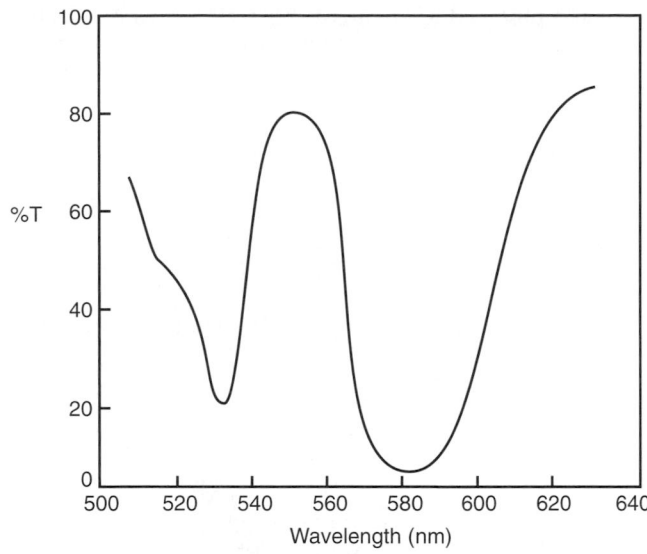

Figure 3-12 Spectral transmittance curve of a didymium filter (Perkin-Elmer Model 35 spectrophotometer, 8-nm nominal spectral bandwidth).

number of sharp, well-defined emission lines between 250 and 580 nm. The apparent width of an emission band at half-peak height is taken as the spectral bandpass of the instrument (see Figure 3-7). The width also may be calculated from the manufacturer's specifications.[6] Interference filters with spectral bandpasses of 1 to 2 nm are available and may be used to check those instruments with nominal spectral bandpasses of 8 nm or more.

Stray light

Stray light is the radiant energy reaching the detector that is outside the narrow band of wavelengths nominally transmitted by the monochromator. A perfect monochromator would transmit light only within its specified band of wavelengths. In practice, scattering and diffraction inside the monochromator introduce light of other wavelengths into the exit beam. This light is modified further by other components of the spectrophotometer and by the sample itself. Stray light usually is expressed as a ratio or percent of the stray light to the total detected light. Other sources of unwanted light include light leaks and fluorescence of the sample. Light leaks should be excluded by covering of the cell compartments. Light arising from fluorescence increases the signal to the detector and causes an apparent decrease in absorbance. These sources of light are not included in the usual definition of stray light.

The major effect of stray light on the performance of a spectrophotometer is an absorbance error, especially in the upper end of the absorbance range of the instrument. Most spectrophotometers are equipped with one or more stray-light filters. Thus a blue filter is used with a tungsten lamp for wavelength settings below about 400 nm. When the spectrophotometer is set to 350 nm, for example, most of

the stray light is of wavelengths in the visible range. The blue filter absorbs most visible light but transmits well in this UV portion of the spectrum. By analogy, a red filter is used for wavelengths in the range of 650 to 800 nm.

A cutoff filter is satisfactory for the detection of stray light. Such filters may be made of glass, similar to the stray-light filters discussed previously, and produce sharp cuts in the spectrum, with almost complete absorption on one side and high transmittance on the other. Liquid cutoff filters are satisfactory and convenient in the UV range, where stray light is usually more of a problem. A 50 g/L aqueous solution of sodium nitrite should show essentially 0% T when read against water over the range of 300 to 385 nm. Acetone, read against water, should show 0% T over the range of 250 to 320 nm.

Linearity

For a spectrophotometer to give accurate absorbance measurements throughout its absorbance range, its response to changes in light intensity must be linear. Under this condition a linear relationship exists between the light absorbed and the instrument readout.

Various liquid solutions have been used to check instrument linearity. Several sources of error may be encountered in this type of reference material, such as dilution errors and errors from lack of stability, shifts in pH, and temperature effects. An alternative procedure is to use a solid-glass filter that, at a given wavelength, has an absorbance that is a small fraction of the total linear range of the instrument.[5] The didymium filter shown in Figure 3-12 has an absorbance of approximately 0.09 at 550 nm and is satisfactory for the establishment of linearity. The procedure is as follows:

1. Set the wavelength at 550 nm, cover the empty cuvet compartment, and set the absorbance to zero.
2. Read the absorbance of the didymium filter and record the value.
3. Remove the filter and set the absorbance to 0.25.
4. Read the didymium filter and record the value.
5. Set the absorbance to 0.50, 0.75, 1.00, 1.25, etc., with the compartment empty, and read the absorbance as instructed in the previous steps.
6. Calculate ΔA for each increase in settings.

Linearity is satisfactory as long as the ΔA increments remain constant. The same general procedure may be used with a suitable filter on those spectrophotometers in which the blank reference settings are adjusted in steps up to approximately 1 unit of absorbance.

Photometric accuracy

Solutions of potassium dichromate ($K_2Cr_2O_7$) are recommended for overall checks on photometric accuracy.[2] These solutions also indicate wavelength calibration, linearity, cuvet light path, and freedom from stray light in the UV re-

TABLE 3-5	Recommended Absorbance Values for Acidic Potassium Dichromate Solutions	
	Absorbance	
Wavelength (nm)	Solution A	Solution B
235 (min)	0.626 ± 0.009	1.251 ± 0.019
257 (max)	0.727 ± 0.007	1.454 ± 0.015
313 (min)	0.244 ± 0.004	0.488 ± 0.007
350 (max)	0.536 ± 0.005	1.071 ± 0.011

gion. In practice, analytical reagent grade $K_2Cr_2O_7$ is dried at 110 °C for 1 hour. The following solutions in 0.005 mol/L sulfuric acid are prepared:

Solution A: 0.0500 g/L for the absorbance range from 0.2 to 0.7

Solution B: 0.1000 g/L for the absorbance range from 0.4 to 1.4

Measurements should be made in 10-mm cells, with the temperature controlled in the range of 15 to 25 °C and 0.005 mol/L sulfuric acid used as the reference. Table 3-5 provides the expected values for the two absorbance maxima and minima of the solutions based on literature values. Because the natural bandwidth of solution A at 350 nm is approximately 63 nm, the values shown apply strictly to spectrophotometers with spectral bandwidths of 6 nm or less.

Multiple-Wavelength Readings

Background interference typically is eliminated or minimized either by inclusion of blanks or by reading of absorbance at two or three wavelengths. In one approach, termed *bichromatic,* absorbance is measured at two wavelengths, one corresponding to peak absorbance and another at a point near the base of the peak as a baseline. The difference in absorbance at the two wavelengths is related to concentration. In effect this method provides a blank reference point for each individual sample. Another method to correct for background interference is to measure absorbance at the peak wavelength and at two other wavelengths equidistant from the peak. Values for the latter are averaged to obtain a baseline under the peak, which then is subtracted from the peak reading. The value thus obtained is known as a *corrected absorbance* and is related to the concentration, provided that the background absorbance is linear with the wavelength over the region in which readings are made. This correction also must be applied to absorbances obtained from calibrators.

Before the correction is used, knowledge of the shape of the absorption curve for the substance of interest and of the interference is required. The linearity of the baseline shift should be verified through measurement of the absorption spectrum of commonly encountered interferences. Care should be exercised in the use of the correction because if it is not properly used, it may introduce larger errors than

would be observed without correction. For example, such a situation may occur if the background reading is not linear over the region measured.

Other Photometric Techniques

In **reflectance photometry,** diffuse reflected light is measured.[1] The reflected light results from illumination, with diffused light, of a reaction mixture in a carrier or from the diffusion of light by a reaction mixture in an illuminated carrier. The intensity of the reflected light from the reagent carrier is compared with the intensity of light reflected from a reference surface. Because the intensity of reflected light is nonlinear in relation to the concentration of the analyte, either the Kubelka-Munk equation or the Clapper-Williams transformation commonly is used to convert the data into a linear format (see Chapter 12). The electro-optical components used in reflectance photometry are essentially the same as those required for absorbance photometry.

When a laser beam passes through a solution, the area where the beam passes through the cell is heated. The heating causes a refractive index change of the solution in the path of the laser beam, compared with the surrounding solution. When examined carefully, a change in the focal point of the scattered light on the outer surfaces of the laser beam can be measured. This process is called the *thermo-lens effect* and is extremely sensitive as an absorption detector.

In addition, Piezoelectric detectors have been developed for use in ultrasensitive mass measuring devices or other pressure-measuring detectors. This type of detector causes a small current to flow in a crystal when pressure is applied to that crystal. Hence, any process in which strain is produced or pressure is changed (for example, ultrasensitive balances) can be measured. In a similar fashion photoacoustic devices have been used as detectors when absorption of energy causes gas-volume changes or pressure changes in the detector. Such a device usually is attached to a membrane that senses slight pressure changes when radiant energy is absorbed. The membrane then is attached to a current- or potential-generating device that produces a measurable signal.

IR diode lasers are used in compact disc players and laser printers (see Chapter 15) and bar code readers (see Chapter 12) and are being applied for use in noninvasive glucose monitors. In the latter application the beam from a near-IR laser is focused on the skin of a patient. By measurement of the relative absorbance differences at several lines of the near-IR spectrum, computer subtraction of blank signals, and computer-mathematical enhancement of the signal-to-noise ratios (Fourier transform), measurement of the patient's glucose concentration is possible. Different companies select different approaches to their glucose monitoring instruments. Some do not use a near-IR lasers as a source, whereas others use transmission rather than reflection, and some do not use Fourier transform to process the data. However, various combinations of the aforementioned options make up the instrumental design principles used in this type of instrument. Several research groups actively are investigating improvements in the accuracy of such measurements.

FLAME-EMISSION SPECTROPHOTOMETRY

Flame-emission spectrophotometry is used for the quantitative measurement of sodium and potassium in body fluids. Lithium, although present in serum in very low concentrations, also may be measured in connection with the therapeutic use of lithium salts in the treatment of some psychiatric disorders.

Atoms of many metallic elements, when given sufficient energy such as that supplied by a hot flame, emit this energy at wavelengths characteristic for the element. A specific amount or quantum of thermal energy is absorbed by an orbital electron. The electrons, being unstable in this high-energy (excited) state, release their excess energy as photons of a particular wavelength as they change from the excited to their previous, or ground, state. If the energy is dissipated as light, the light may consist of one or more than one energy levels and therefore be different wavelengths. These line spectra are characteristic for each element. Sodium, for example, emits energy primarily at 589 nm. The wavelength to be used for the measurement of an element depends on the selection of a line of sufficient intensity to provide adequate sensitivity, as well as freedom from other interfering lines at or near the selected wavelength.

Alkali metals are comparatively easy to excite in the flame of an ordinary laboratory burner. Lithium produces a red, sodium a yellow, potassium a violet, rubidium a red, and magnesium a blue color in a flame. These colors are characteristic of the metal atoms that are present as cations in solution. Under constant and controlled conditions the light intensity of the characteristic wavelength produced by each atom is directly proportional to the number of atoms emitting energy, which in turn is directly proportional to the concentration of the substance of interest in the sample. Thus flame photometry lends itself well to direct concentration measurement of some metals.

Although this technique once was widely used for the analysis of sodium, potassium, and lithium in body fluids, it now has been replaced largely by electrochemical techniques. For readers who desire more information on this technique, additional details can be found in a previous version of this chapter.[3]

ATOMIC ABSORPTION SPECTROPHOTOMETRY

Atomic absorption (AA) spectrophotometry is a powerful optical technique that is used widely in clinical laboratories for elemental analysis.

Basic Concepts

AA spectrophotometry in some respects is the inverse of flame-emission photometry. In emission methods the sample is excited to measure the radiant energy emitted as the element returns to its lower energy level. In AA spectrophotometry, the element is not excited appreciably in the flame but merely is dissociated from its chemical bonds and placed in an unexcited, or ground, state (neutral atom). Thus the neutral atom is at a low-energy level in which it is capable of absorbing radiation at a very narrow bandwidth corresponding to its own line spectrum. A hollow-cathode lamp with a cathode made of the material to be analyzed is used to produce a wavelength of light specific for the material. Thus if the cathode is made of sodium, sodium light at predominantly 589 nm is emitted by the lamp. When the light from the hollow-cathode lamp enters the flame, part of it is absorbed by the ground-state atoms in the flame, resulting in a net decrease in the intensity of the beam from the lamp. This process is referred to as *atomic absorption.*

The process is analogous to absorption spectrophotometry. A specific hollow-cathode lamp serves as the light source, and the sample heated in the flame replaces the sample in the cuvet. The pathlength of the flame is analogous to the light path through the cuvet. As noted previously, only a small fraction of the sample in the flame contributes emission energy, and only a fraction of this is transmitted to the detector. Hence, most of the atoms are in the ground state and able to absorb light emitted by the cathode lamp. In general, AA methods are approximately 100 times more sensitive than flame-emission methods. In addition, due to the unique specificity of the wavelength from the hollow-cathode lamp, these methods are highly specific for the element being measured.

Components of Atomic Absorption Spectrophotometers

The basic components of an AA spectrophotometer are shown in Figure 3-13. The hollow-cathode lamp is the light source. The cathode of the lamp is made of the metal of the substance to be analyzed and is different for each metal analysis. In some cases an alloy is used to make the cathode, resulting in a multielement lamp. A nebulizer sprays the sample into the flame; the monochromator, slits, and detectors have similar functions to those in a spectrophotometer.

On most AA instruments an electric beam chopper and a tuned amplifier are incorporated. The power to the hollow-cathode lamp may be pulsed so that the light is emitted by the lamp at a certain number of pulses per second. On the other hand, all the light coming from the flame is continuous. When light leaves the flame, it is composed of pulsed, unabsorbed light from the lamp and a small amount of unpulsed flame spectrum and sample emission. The detector senses all light, but the amplifier is tuned electrically to accept only pulsed signals. In this way the electronics in

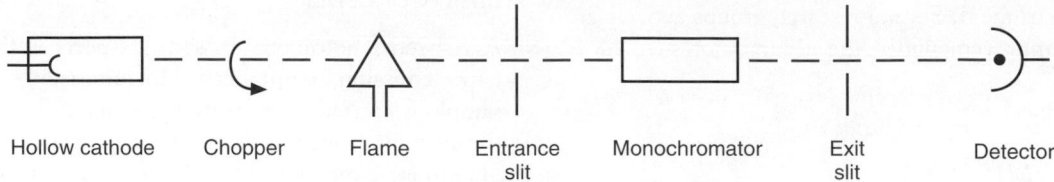

Figure 3-13   Components of an atomic-absorption spectrophotometer.

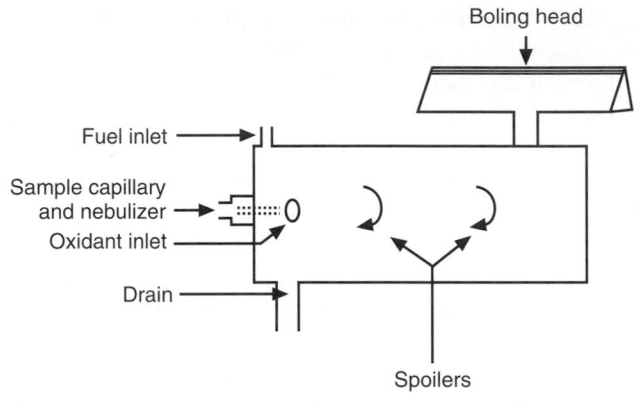

Figure 3-14   Laminar flow burner.

conjunction with the monochromator discriminate between the flame spectrum and sample emission.

The hollow-cathode lamp usually contains argon or neon gas at a pressure of a few millimeters of mercury. An argon-filled lamp produces a blue-to-purple glow during operation, and the neon produces a reddish-orange glow inside the hollow-cathode lamp. Quartz, or special glass that allows transmission of the proper wavelength, is used as a window. A current is applied between the two electrodes inside the hollow-cathode lamp, and metal is sputtered from the cathode into the gases inside the glass envelope. When the metal atoms collide with the neon or argon gases, they lose energy and emit their characteristic radiation. Calcium has a sharp, intense, analytical emission line at 422.7 nm, which is used most frequently for calcium analysis. In an interference-free system only calcium atoms absorb the calcium light from the hollow cathode as it passes through the flame.

Figure 3-14 shows a premix burner (laminar-flow burner) and illustrates the method in which the sample is aspirated, volatilized, and burned. Note that the gases are mixed and the sample is atomized before being burned. An advantage of this system is that the larger droplets go to waste while the fine mist enters the flame, thus producing a less noisy signal. In addition, the pathlength through the flame of the burner is longer than that of the total-consumption burner, which also is used in AA instruments.[2] This system produces a greater absorption and increases the sensitivity of the measurement. A disadvantage of the premix burner is that the flame usually is not as hot as that of the total-consumption burner,[3] and thus it cannot suffi-

ciently dissociate certain metal complexes in the flame (for example, calcium-phosphate complexes).

In **flameless atomic absorption (AA)** techniques (carbon rod, or "graphite furnace"), the sample is placed in a depression on a carbon rod in an enclosed chamber. Strips of tantalum or platinum metal also may be used as sample cups. In successive steps the temperature of the rod is raised to dry, char, and finally atomize the sample into the chamber. The atomized element then absorbs energy from the corresponding hollow-cathode lamp. This approach is more sensitive than the conventional flame methods and permits determination of trace metals in small samples of blood or tissue.

Zeeman Correction

With flameless AA, a novel approach called the *Zeeman correction* has been used to correct for background absorption.[7] In Zeeman background correction either the light source or the atomizer is placed in a strong magnetic field. In practice the analyte is placed in the magnetic field, and the intense magnetic field splits the atomic energy levels, which have equal energy, into two components that are polarized parallel and perpendicular to the magnetic field, respectively. The parallel component is at the resonance line of the source, whereas the two perpendicular components are shifted to different wavelengths. The two components interact differently with polarized light. A polarizer is placed between the source and the atomizer, and two absorption measurements are taken at different polarizer settings. One measures both analyte and background absorptions (A_t), whereas the other measures only the background absorption (A_{bc}). The difference between the two absorption readings is the corrected absorbance.

The major advantage of the Zeeman correction method is that the same light source at the same wavelength is used to measure the total and background absorptions. The implementation is complex and expensive and the strength of the magnetic field must be optimized for every element, but the method provides more accurate results at higher background levels than do the other correction techniques.

Interference in Atomic Absorption Spectrophotometry

Interferences in AA spectrophotometry are divided into spectral and nonspectral interferences.

Spectral interferences

Spectral interferences include the following:

1. Absorption by other closely absorbing atomic species
2. Absorption by molecular species
3. Scattering by nonvolatile salt particles or oxides
4. Background emission, which is electronically filtered

Absorption by other atomic species usually is not a problem because of the extremely narrow bandwidth (0.01 nm) used in the absorption measurements. Absorption and scattering by molecular species are particularly problematic at lower atomizing temperatures.

Nonspectral interferences

Nonspectral interferences encountered in AA spectrophotometry are either nonspecific or specific. Nonspecific interferences affect the nebulization by altering the viscosity, surface tension, or density of the analyte solution, and consequently the sample flow rate. Certain contaminants also decrease the desolvation and atomization efficiency by lowering the atomizer temperature. Specific interferences also are called *chemical interferences* because they are more analyte dependent. *Solute volatilization interference* refers to a situation in which the contaminant forms a nonvolatile species with the analyte. An example of this instance is the phosphate interference in the determination of calcium that is caused by the formation of calcium-phosphate complexes. The phosphate interference is overcome by the addition of a cation, usually lanthanum or strontium, that competes with calcium for the phosphate. Enhancement effects also are observed in which the addition of contaminants increases the volatilization efficiency. Such is the case with aluminum, which normally forms nonvolatile oxides but in the presence of hydrofluoric acid forms more volatile aluminum fluoride.

Dissociation interferences affect the degree of dissociation of the analyte. Analytes that form oxides or hydroxides are especially susceptible to dissociation interferences. Ionization interference occurs when the presence of an easily ionized element, such as K, affects the degree of ionization of the analyte, which leads to changes in the analyte signal. In case of excitation interference the analyte atoms are excited in the atomizer, with a subsequent emission at the absorption wavelength. This type of interference is more pronounced at higher temperatures.

References

1. Boyd JB, Young DS: Automation in the clinical laboratory. In Burtis CA, Ashwood ER (eds): Tietz Textbook of Clinical Chemistry, 3rd edition, pp 226-261, Philadelphia, WB Saunders, 1999.
2. Burgess C, Knowles A (eds): Standards in Absorption Spectrometry, New York, Chapman and Hall, 1981.
3. Evenson ME: Spectrophotometric techniques. In Burtis CA, Ashwood ER (eds): Tietz Textbook of Clinical Chemistry, 3rd edition, pp 75–93, Philadelphia, WB Saunders, 1999.
4. James GP, Djang MH: Evaluation of clinical laboratory instruments. Part III. Spectral bandwidth and wavelength accuracy. Am J Med Technol 1981; 47:477-483.
5. Lucas DH, Blank RE: Spectrophotometric standards in the clinical laboratory. Am Lab 1977; 9:77-83.
6. Passey RB, Gillum RL, Fuller JB: Measurement of spectral bandwidth, as exemplified with the Beckman "Enzyme Analyzer System TR Spectrophotometer." Clin Chem 1975; 21:1582-1584.
7. Slavin W: Atomic absorption spectroscopy: the present and future. Anal Chem 1982; 54:685A-694A.
8. Surles T, Erickson JO: Absorbance measurements at various spectral bandwidths. Clin Chem 1974; 20:1243-1244.
9. Sweedler JV, Billhorn RB, Epperson PM et al: High performance charge transfer devices. Anal Chem 1988; 60:282A-291A.
10. Tiffany TO: Fluorometry, nephelometry, and turbidimetry. In Burtis CA, Ashwood ER (eds): Tietz Textbook of Clinical Chemistry, 3rd edition, pp 94-112, Philadelphia, WB Saunders, 1999.

Additional Reading

Clark RJH, Hester RE (eds): Biomedical Applications of Spectroscopy, New York, John Wiley & Sons, 1996.

Dean JH: Analytical Chemistry Handbook, New York, McGraw-Hill, 1995.

Gore MG, Gore M: Spectrophotometry and Spectrofluorimetry: A Practical Approach, London, Oxford University Press, 2000.

Hargis LG, Howell JA, Sutton RE: Ultraviolet and light absorption spectrometry. Anal Chem 1996; 68:169R-183R.

Harris DC: Quantitative Chemical Analysis, 4th edition, New York, WH Freeman, 1995.

Ingle JD, Crouch SR: Spectrochemical Analysis, Englewood Cliffs, NJ, Prentice-Hall, Inc, 1988.

Jackson KW, Chen G: Atomic absorption, atomic emission, and flame emission spectrometry. Anal Chem 1996; 68:231R-256R.

Skoog DA, Holler FJ, Timothy A et al: Principles of Instrumental Analysis, 5th edition, Philadelphia, Saunders College Publishers, 1998.

Willard H, Merritt L, Dean J et al: Instrumental Methods of Analysis, 7th edition, Belmont, Calif, Wadsworth, 1988.

CHAPTER 4

Light Emission and Scattering Techniques

THOMAS O. TIFFANY, PhD

Objectives

1. Define *luminescence, fluorescence, fluorescence polarization, nephelometry,* and *turbidimetry.*
2. State the principle of fluorometry and the factors that interfere with fluorescence measurements.
3. List the components of a basic fluorometer.
4. State the principle of nephelometry and the principle of turbidimetry and the factors that interfere with light-scattering measurements.

Key Words

Bioluminescence   The emission of light as a consequence of the cellular oxidation of some substrate (luciferins) in the presence of an enzyme (luciferases); exists in bacteria, fungi, protozoa, and species belonging to 40 different orders of animals

Chemiluminescence   The emission of light by molecules in excited states produced by a chemical reaction, as in fireflies

Fluorescence   The emission of electromagnetic radiation by a substance after the absorption of energy in some form (for example, the emission of light of one color [wavelength] when a substance is excited by irradiation with light of a different wavelength); distinguished from phosphorescence in that its lifetime is less than 10 milliseconds after the excitation ceases

Fluorescence Microscopy   A highly sensitive microscopic technique for the demonstration of naturally fluorescent materials, such as nucleic acids, lipids, or steroid hormones; slide specimens stained with fluorescent dyes; or fluorescent-labeled antibodies

Luminescence   The emission of light due to a nonthermal process such as a chemical reaction or the absorption of ionizing radiation

Nephelometry   A technique that uses a nephelometer to measure the number and size of particles in a suspension; measures the intensity of light, scattered by the particles, with a detector at an angle to the incident light beam

Phosphorescence   Luminescence produced by certain substances after they absorb radiant or other types of energy; distinguished from fluorescence in that it continues even after the radiation causing it has ceased

Stokes Shift   The phenomenon by which luminescent or fluorescent substances emit light at longer wavelengths than the exciting wavelength at which the light is absorbed

Turbidimetry   The measurement of turbidity; generally performed through use of an instrument (spectrophotometer or photometer) that measures the ratio of the intensity of the light transmitted through dispersion to the intensity of the incident light

Turbidity   The cloudiness of a solution caused by suspended particles that scatter light; the amount of light scattered being related in a complex way to the concentration and sizes and shapes of the particles

---

Luminescence is the emission of light or radiant energy when an electron returns from an excited or higher energy level to a lower energy level. Light scattering occurs when radiant energy passing through a solution strikes a particle and is scattered in all directions.

■ LUMINESCENCE

Fluorescence, phosphorescence, chemiluminescence, and electrochemiluminescence are types of luminescence.

Basic Concepts

Figure 4-1 diagrammatically illustrates the relationship between absorption, fluorescence, and phosphorescence. Absorption of a quantum of light energy by a molecule causes the transition of an electron from its ground state to one of a number of possible excited vibrational levels. Once the molecule is in an excited state, several ways exist for it to return to its original energy state, including radiationless vibrational equilibration, fluorescence process, quenching of the excited state, radiationless crossover to a triplet state, quenching of the first triplet state, and phosphorescence process.

Fluorescence

Fluorescence is the emission of light by an atom or molecule after absorption of an exciting photon or x-ray. An atom or molecule that can fluoresce is termed a *fluorophor*. In theory fluorescence is a similar but competitive process to phosphorescence; however, three important differences exist between the two processes. First, as shown in Figure 4-1, vi-

brational equilibration before fluorescence results in some loss of the excitation energy. The emitted fluorescence light is therefore of less energy, or has a longer wavelength, than the excitation light. Second, the difference between the maximum wavelength of the excitation light and the maximum wavelength of the emitted fluorescence light is a constant referred to as the **Stokes shift.** This constant is a measure of the energy lost during the lifetime of the excited state before its return to the ground state (fluorescence emission). Third, the emission of fluorescence light is characterized by a rapid (10^{-8} second) decay time.

Fluorescence intensity measurements are more sensitive than absorbance measurements. The magnitude of absorbance of a chromophor in solution is determined by its concentration and the path length of the cuvet. The magnitude of fluorescence intensity of a fluorophor is determined by its concentration and the path length and intensity of the light source. Thus through the use of more intense light sources, digital signal filtering techniques, and sensitive emission photometers, fluorescence measurements are 100 to 1000 times more sensitive than absorbance measurements. All these factors are incorporated in conventional spectrofluorometric instrumentation, described later in this chapter.

Time relationships of fluorescence emission

The time relationship between fluorescence excitation and emission is shown in Figure 4-2. Phase I represents the time period between absorbance of light energy and radiationless loss of energy during vibrational rearrangement to the lowest excited energy state. This time period is represented by the up and down arrows in the diagram. Phase II shows the emission and decay of both a short-lived *(b)* and a longer-

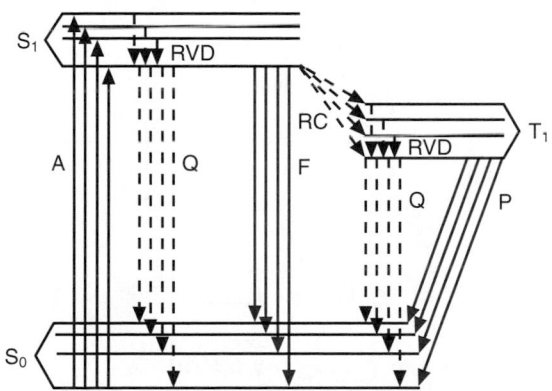

Figure 4-1   Luminescence energy-level diagram of a typical organic molecule. S_0, Ground level singlet state; S_1, first excited singlet state; *A*, absorption process; T_1, first excited triplet state; *RVD*, radiationless vibrational deactivation; *Q*, quenching of the excited singlet or triplet state; *F*, fluorescence process from the first excited singlet state; *P*, phosphorescence process from the first excited triplet state; *RC*, radiationless crossover from the first excited singlet state to the first excited triplet state.

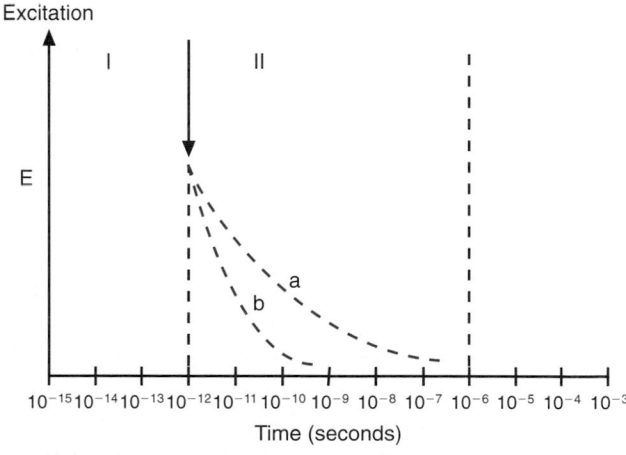

Figure 4-2   Fluorescence decay process. *E*, Absorption of energy; *I*, vibrational deactivation time phase; *II*, fluorescence emission time phase; *a*, long fluorescence decay time; *b*, short fluorescence decay time.

life *(a)* fluorophor. If the fluorescence emission is measured over time after a pulse of light from an excitation source, such as a xenon lamp or laser, the intensity of the emitted light decays as a first-order process. The time required for the emitted light to reach 1/e of its initial intensity, where *e* is the Naperian base 2.718, is the average lifetime of the excited state of the molecule, also known as the *fluorescence decay time.*

The time delay between absorption of quanta of energy and fluorescence can be used in fluorescence instruments called *time-resolved fluorometers.*[10] The advantage of a time-resolved fluorometer is the elimination of background short-lived fluorescence and light scattering, with the consequent dramatic increases in signal-to-noise and detection sensitivity.

Time-resolved fluorometry[2] is categorized as either (1) pulse fluorometry, in which the sample is illuminated with an intense brief pulse of light, and the intensity of the resulting fluorescence emission is measured as a function of time with a fast detector system, or (2) phase fluorometry, in which a continuous-wave laser illuminates the sample, and the fluorescence emission response is monitored for impulse and frequency response.[3]

Relationship of concentration and fluorescence intensity

The relationship between concentration and intensity of fluorescence emission is derived from the Beer-Lambert law. By rearrangement and expansion through a Taylor series, the following equation is obtained:

$$F = \phi\,[I_0\,(2.3\,abc)] \tag{1}$$

where

F = Relative intensity
ϕ = Fluorescence efficiency (that is, the ratio between quanta of light emitted and quanta of light absorbed)
I_0 = Initial excitation intensity
a = Molar absorptivity
b = Volume element defined by geometry of the excitation and emission slits
c = Concentration in mol/L

The previous equation indicates that fluorescence intensity is directly proportional to the concentration of the fluorophor and the excitation intensity. However, this relationship is true only for dilute solutions, in which absorbance is less than 2% of the exciting radiation. Above 2% the fluorescence intensity becomes nonlinear. This phenomenon is called the *inner-filter effect*, and it is discussed in more detail in a later section. Other factors influencing the measurement of fluorescence intensity are autofluorescence, the sensitivity of the detector, and the degree of background light scatter detected.

Fluorescence polarization

Light waves produced by standard excitation sources have their electrical vectors oriented randomly. However, when light waves are passed through a polarizer, their electrical vectors are oriented in a single plane and said to be *plane-polarized.* Fluorophors absorb light most efficiently in the planes of their electronic energy levels. If the rotational relaxation (Brownian movement) is slower than the fluorescence decay time, as is the case for large fluorescent-labeled molecules, the emitted fluorescence light is polarized. Because small molecules have rotational relaxation times much shorter than their fluorescence decay times, their emitted fluorescence light is depolarized. However, if the small fluorescent molecule is attached to a macromolecule or placed in a viscous solution, the small molecule emits polarized light. Fluorescence polarization, *P,* is defined by the following equation:

$$P = \frac{I_v - I_h}{I_v + I_h} \tag{2}$$

where I_v is the intensity of the emitted fluorescence light in the vertical plane, and I_h is the intensity of the emitted fluorescence light in the horizontal plane.

Fluorescence polarization is measured via placement of a mechanically or electrically driven polarizer between the sample cuvet and the detector. A diagram of a fluorescence polarization measurement system is shown in Figure 4-3. In the normal instrumentation mode the sample is excited with polarized light to obtain maximal sensitivity. The polarization analyzer first is positioned to measure the intensity of the emitted fluorescence light in the vertical plane *(I_v),* and then the polarization analyzer is rotated 90 degrees to measure the emitted fluorescence light intensity in the horizontal plane *(I_h).* Using equation (2), *P* then is calculated manually or automatically. In the laboratory fluorescence polarization is used to quantify analytes by use of the change in fluorescence depolarization after immunological reactions (see Chapter 10).

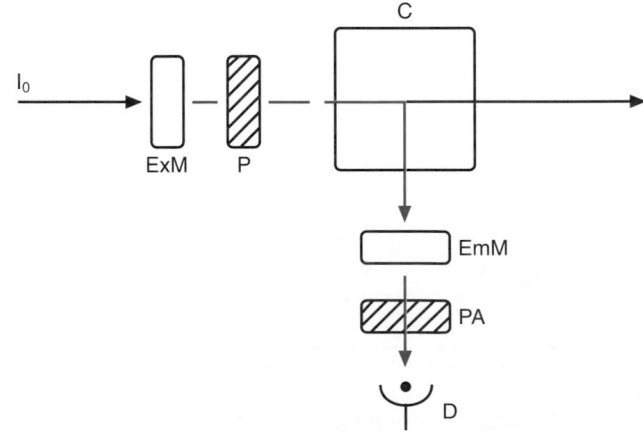

Figure 4-3   Schematic diagram of a fluorescence polarization analyzer. *P,* Polarizer to provide polarized excitation light; *PA,* polarizer analyzer, which is rotated to provide the measurement of parallel and perpendicular polarized fluorescence-emission intensity; *ExM,* excitation monochromator; *EmM,* emission monochromator; *D,* detector; *C,* reaction cell or cuvet; I_0, incident intensity.

Instrumentation for measurement of fluorescence

The instruments used to measure fluorescence are fluorometers and spectrofluorometers. The fluorometer uses interference or glass filters to produce monochromatic light for sample excitation and isolation of fluorescence emission, whereas the spectrofluorometer uses a grating or prism monochromator for the same purposes.

Basic instrumentation

The basic components of a spectrofluorometer are the following:

1. Excitation source
2. Excitation monochromator
3. Sample cell
4. Emission monochromator
5. Detector

Excitation source.   Many excitation sources are used in fluorometers and spectrophotometers, including xenon, quartz-halogen, and mercury arc lamps and lasers. These sources are capable of emitting radiant energy over a large spectral region, which is desirable. Some provide high-intensity spectra at one or more wavelengths, whereas others provide a continuum over the spectral range of interest (300 to 700 nm).

The xenon lamp provides a continuum of relatively high-intensity radiant energy over the spectral region of 250 to 800 nm. Arc wandering or flicker are limitations of xenon lamps in analytical use. However, the use of current-stabilized power supplies has improved the performance of xenon lamps used in fluorescence instrumentation.

Xenon flash lamps are used widely for certain fluorescence applications because of their high energy output, stability of lamp flashes, and higher ultraviolet and visible spectral output. These flash lamps can be pulsed at rates up to 2500 pulses per second. Light output is typically in the 0.01- to 0.1-J interval, with a spectral distribution ranging from 200 to 1100 nm. The life of a flash lamp varies from 10^6 to 10^9 flashes, with the spectral stability being maintained throughout the life of the flash lamp.

Laser sources also are used widely in fluorescence applications in which highly intense, well-focused, and essentially monochromatic light is required (see Chapter 3). Examples of these applications include time-resolved fluorometry, flow cytometry, pulsed-laser confocal microscopy, laser-induced fluorometry, and light-scattering measurements for particle size and shape.

Several types of lasers are available for fluorescence and light-scattering applications (see Chapter 3, Table 3-3). The argon ion laser is used widely in flow cytometry, where its monochromaticity (488 nm), spatial coherence, ease of optical alignment, and light intensity have made it the light source of choice over mercury and xenon arc lamp sources. Also available are air-cooled argon ion lasers that produce about 25 mW of energy output at 488 nm and have plasma tube lifetimes of 6000 hours or more. Continuous-wave dye lasers typically use argon ion lasers with outputs of 1 W or less as energy pumps and use different fluorescent dyes to achieve excitation wavelength ranges of 260 to 300 nm, 400 to 600 nm, and 540 to 900 nm. These lasers also have been used as modulated excitation sources for phase-resolved fluorescence measurements.

In addition, Helium-neon (He-Ne) and helium-cadmium (He-Cd) lasers are useful because of their low cost and ease of operation and because they emit a number of excitation wavelengths. He-Ne lasers, which operate at 633 nm, typically have been used for light-scattering applications. He-Ne lasers have been developed that emit excitation energy at 543 nm (green), 594 nm (yellow), and 611 nm (orange). However, power output has been limited to about 2 mW at 594 nm. One potential application is to provide excitation frequencies that are compatible with different fluorescent dye-labeled immunoassays. An He-Cd laser also is available that emits from 5 to 40 mW of power at 441 nm and from 1 to 10 mW of output power at 325 nm (that is, blue and ultraviolet excitation).

Excitation and emission monochromator.   A monochromator is a device used to isolate a narrow portion of the spectrum. Monochromators used in fluorescence instrumentation include interference filters, colored glass filters, gratings, and prisms (see Chapter 3).

Most modern analytical instruments using interference filters combine them with an appropriate sharp cutoff glass filter to form single filter packages. This type of combination filter removes undesired transmission of higher orders and provides narrow bandwidth, higher peak wavelength transmission, and increased band slope, the latter of which is important for the spectral separation of excitation and emission bands with small Stokes shifts.

Colored glass filters selectively absorb certain wavelengths of light. These filters have been used both for excitation and for emission wavelength selection, but they are more susceptible to transmitting stray light and exhibit unwanted fluorescence.

Grating monochromators are devices that isolate regions of the spectrum. Their function and construction are described in Chapter 3. The spectral resolution of the light at the slit is a function of the slit width and the resolution of the grating. Spectrofluorometers generally use larger slit widths than absorbance spectrophotometers to obtain higher excitation intensities. The advantage the grating monochromator provides is the selectivity of excitation and emission wavelengths required during work with new fluorophors with absorbance and emission maxima for which specially fabricated interference filters may not exist. The rotation of the grating can be computer controlled to automate spectral scans of fluorescence excitation and emission. In the conventional operation of a spectrofluorometer either the excitation wavelength or the emission wavelength is held constant while the other is scanned. Due to their high degree of monochromaticity, lasers are being used as both excitation light sources and monochromators. When a laser is

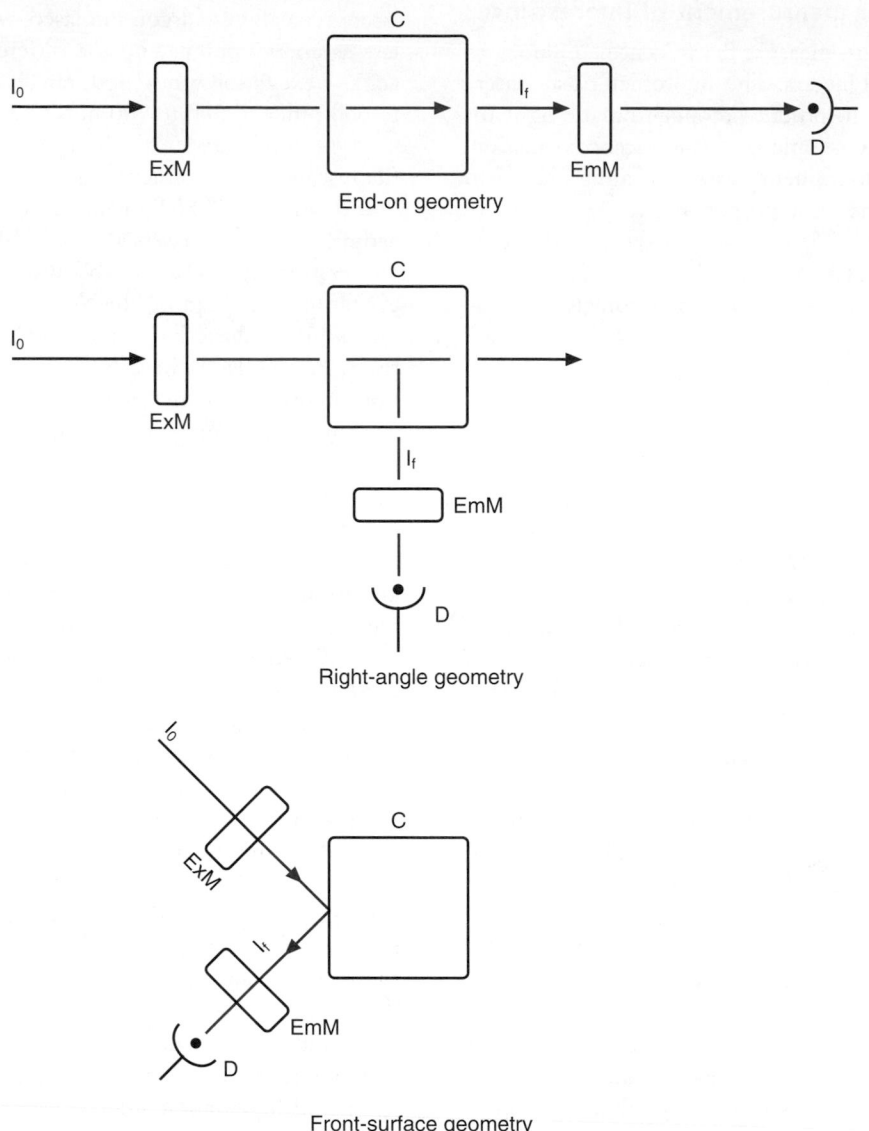

Figure 4-4   Fluorescence excitation-emission geometries. I_0, Initial excitation energy; *ExM*, excitation monochromator; *C*, sample cuvet; I_f, fluorescence intensity; *EmM*, emission monochromator; *D*, detector.

used as a combination excitation source and monochromator, a narrow-band interference filter usually is placed before the detector to eliminate additional orders of emission.

Sample cell compartment.   Because fluorescence light is emitted in all directions from a molecule, several excitation-emission configurations are used to measure fluorescence (Figure 4-4). The sample cell can be oriented at different angles in relation to the excitation source and detector to accommodate these different configurations. Most commercial spectrofluorometers and fluorometers use the right-angle-detector approach because it minimizes background signal that limits analytical sensitivity. The end-on approach allows the adaptation of a 180-degree fluorescence detector to existing spectrophotometers. Its sensitivity, however, is limited by the quality of the excitation-emission interference filter pair, excitation-emission spectral band over

lap, and inner-filter effect. The front-surface approach provides the greatest linearity over a broad range of concentrations because it minimizes the inner-filter effect. The front-surface approach is as sensitive as the right-angle detector but more susceptible to background light scatter. Front-surface fluorometry has been applied widely to heterogeneous, solid-phase fluorescence immunoassay systems.

The major concerns related to the geometry of the sample cell are light scattering, the inner-filter effect, and the sample volume element seen by the detector. Figure 4-5 shows the sample cell and slit arrangement for a conventional fluorescence spectrophotometer, with the excitation and emission slits oriented at a right angle. S_1 and S_2 designate the excitation and emission slits, respectively, within the figure. The position and width of the emission slit are important; if the emission slit is located near the front edge of the sample cell, as shown in Figure 4-5, *B*, the inner-filter effect is minimized. If the emission slit width is increased, sensitivity increases, but specificity may decrease.

The material of the sample cell generally is fused silica or quartz. Plastic cuvets can be used for certain applications, but certain ultraviolet absorbers in the plastics will fluoresce, causing unwanted background signal and loss of sensitivity.

Photodetectors.   For quantitative assays the most commonly used detector in fluorometers and spectrofluorometers is the photomultiplier (PM) tube, which is described in Chapter 3. The important features of the PM tube for fluorescence measurements include a wide choice of spectral responses, rapid photon response time (that is, nanosecond re-

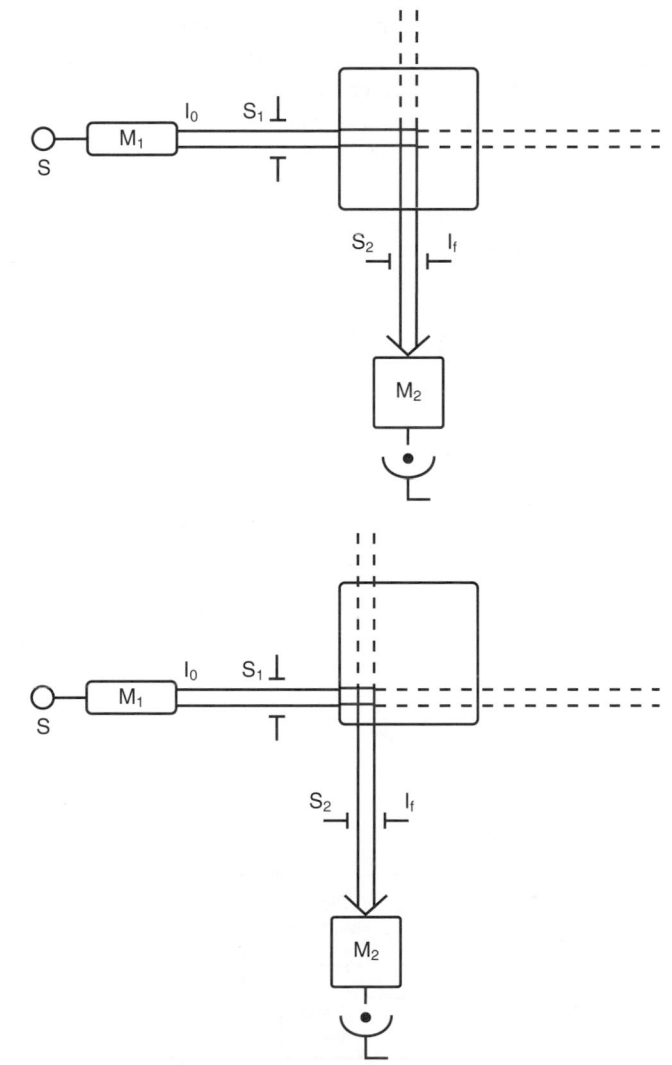

A

B

Figure 4-5   Two right-angle fluorescence sample cuvet positions. **A,** Standard 90-degree configuration. **B,** Offset positioning of the cuvet to minimize the inner-filter effect. *S,* Light source; M_1, excitation monochromator; I_0, initial excitation energy; S_1, excitation slit; I_f, fluorescence intensity; S_2, emission slit; M_2, emission monochromator.

sponse time), and sensitivity. Sensitivity is due to the possible gain of 10^6 electrons at the anode of the PM tube for each incident photon hitting the photo cathode.

Depending on the light level (photon flux) striking the PM cathode and the desired sensitivity, the measurement of electron flow at the PM tube anode is accomplished in different ways. At high light intensities, analog techniques for measurement of a PM tube current are used. The analog signal then is converted to a digital signal for computer use or panel digital display. At low light levels spikes or pulses are generated at the cathode of the PM tube and counted. The number of pulses that occur per unit time is directly proportional to the intensity of emitted fluorescence light striking the PM tube. This method is called *photon counting*. The use of photon counting increases the signal-to-noise ratio and sensitivity of the measurement of fluorophors at very low concentrations.

Charge-coupled detectors (CCD) are multichannel devices that also are used as photodetectors because they have good dynamic range and a signal-to-noise ratio that is superior to that of PM tubes.[7] This solid-state device can be thought of as a matrix containing a large number of photodetecting shift registers that can be read horizontally and vertically. CCDs have been used for molecular fluorescence measurements of very low concentrations of fluorescent molecules and as quantitative electronic imagers for quantitative confocal microscopy. A data-reading technique called *binning* has been developed that allows multielement devices to feature linked-together functional elements much like rectangular slit widths. In addition, use of a fluorometer constructed with a CCD and a 30-W mercury pen lamp as its light source has decreased detection limits by one order of magnitude.

Manual fluorometers and spectrofluorometers

Fluorometers and fluorescence spectrophotometers with many different features are available commercially, including both manual fluorometers and spectrofluorometers.

Manual fluorometers.   The simplest type of fluorometer consists of a light source (S), a sample compartment, excitation and emission filters or monochromators (M_1 and M_2), a detector, and a simple digital or meter display (see Figure 4-5, *A).* The operation of this device requires that the fluorometer display first be set to zero by use of a sample blank. A calibrating solution then is placed into the fluorometer and the range adjusted. This process usually is accomplished through adjustment of the high-voltage control of the PM tube, but it also may be controlled through adjustment of the emission slit (S_2). Once the zero and calibrator settings have been made, unknown solutions are read. If a number of unknown solutions are to be read, the zero and calibrator must be checked several times during the course of the analysis to compensate for electronic and light-source drift. This simple single-beam fluorometer, like the ratio-referencing fluorometers described in the text that follows, is capable of measuring concentrations over three or four orders of magnitude.

Spectrofluorometer. The block diagram and light path of a typical ratio-referencing spectrofluorometer are shown in Figures 4-6 and 4-7, respectively. The ratio-referencing spectrofluorometer is a basic simple right-angle instrument that uses two monochromators (M_1 and M_2), two PM detectors (D_1 and D_2, the reference and sample PM detectors), and a xenon lamp source. The light from the exciter monochromator (M_1) is split, and a small portion (10%) is directed to the reference PM detector (D_1) for ratio-referencing purposes. The remaining excitation light is focused into the sample cuvet (C). Emission optics are positioned at a right angle to the excitation optics. An emission monochromator (M_2) is used to select or scan the desired portion of the emission spectra, which is directed to the sample PM tube (D_2) for measurement of the emission intensity. The output signals from the reference and sample PM detectors are amplified (A_1 and A_2), and a ratio of the sample to the reference signal is provided by a digital display or chart recorder.

If excitation and emission interference filters are substituted for monochromators (M_1 and M_2), the instrument shown in Figure 4-6 becomes a simple ratio fluorometer. The operational mode of a ratio fluorometer is similar to that of the spectrofluorometer; however, only discrete excitation and emission wavelengths are available, and the use of this type of instrument is precluded from scanning of fluorophors to obtain emission and excitation spectra. The ratio-filter fluorometer is most useful for the obtaining of concentration measurements at defined excitation and emission wavelengths.

The ratio-referencing spectrofluorometer (see Figure 4-7) is operated at fixed excitation and emission wavelength settings for concentration measurements or used to measure the excitation or emission spectrum of a given compound. The measurement of concentration of unknowns is accomplished in a manner similar to that of the single-beam fluorometer. The fluorescence of each a blank and a calibrating solution first are measured, followed by measurement of unknown samples. The ratio-referencing spectrofluorometer provides two advantages over the single-beam spectrofluorometer. First, it eliminates short- and long-term xenon lamp energy fluctuations, such as arc flicker and lamp decay, and thus minimizes the need for frequent calibration of the instrument during analysis. Second, it provides "essentially" corrected excitation spectra by compensating for wavelength-dependent energy fluctuations.

Some spectrofluorometers can perform synchronous scanning of both the excitation and the emission monochromators, a process accomplished at a constant wavelength increment of 5 to 50 nm or more; intervals in the range of 15 to 30 nm, however, yield the most distinctive spectra. This technique has been valuable in the area of forensic chemistry as another approach to qualitative and quantitative

analyses of mixtures of fluorophors, such as drugs and their metabolites in solution. Other instrumental approaches to the measurement of mixtures of fluorophors exist, including the excitation-emission matrix approach and excitation scan with modulation of the emission signal.

Time-resolved and phase-resolved fluorometers

The time-resolved fluorometer is similar to the ratio-referencing fluorometer, with the exception that the light source is pulsed.[9] The detector then monitors, in a fast, photon-counting mode, decay of the fluorescence signal. Time-resolved fluorometry requires the use of long-lived fluorophors, such as the lanthanide or rare earth metal ions, such as europium (Eu^{3+}).[2] Whereas most fluorescence compounds have decay times of 5 to 100 ns, europium chelates decay in 0.6 to 100 μs. Thus time-resolved fluorescence assays take advantage of the difference in the lifetimes of fluorophor and background fluorescence by monitoring only its decaying fluorescence signal over a period of several lamp pulses. This action eliminates background interferences and at the same time averages the signal to improve the precision of measurement. Detection limits of approximately 10^{-13} mol/L are achievable with time-resolved fluorometry, an improvement of about four orders of magnitude over conventional fluorometric measurements.

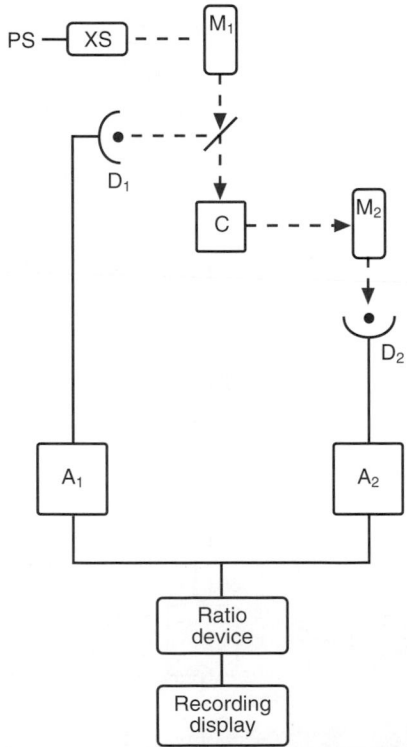

Figure 4-6 Block diagram of a typical spectrofluorometer. *XS*, Xenon source; *PS*, power supply; M_1, excitation monochromator; *C*, sample cell; M_2, emission monochromator; D_1, detector monitoring the variation in excitation intensity; D_2, detector measuring fluorescence emission intensity; A_1, excitation signal amplifier; A_2, emission signal amplifier.

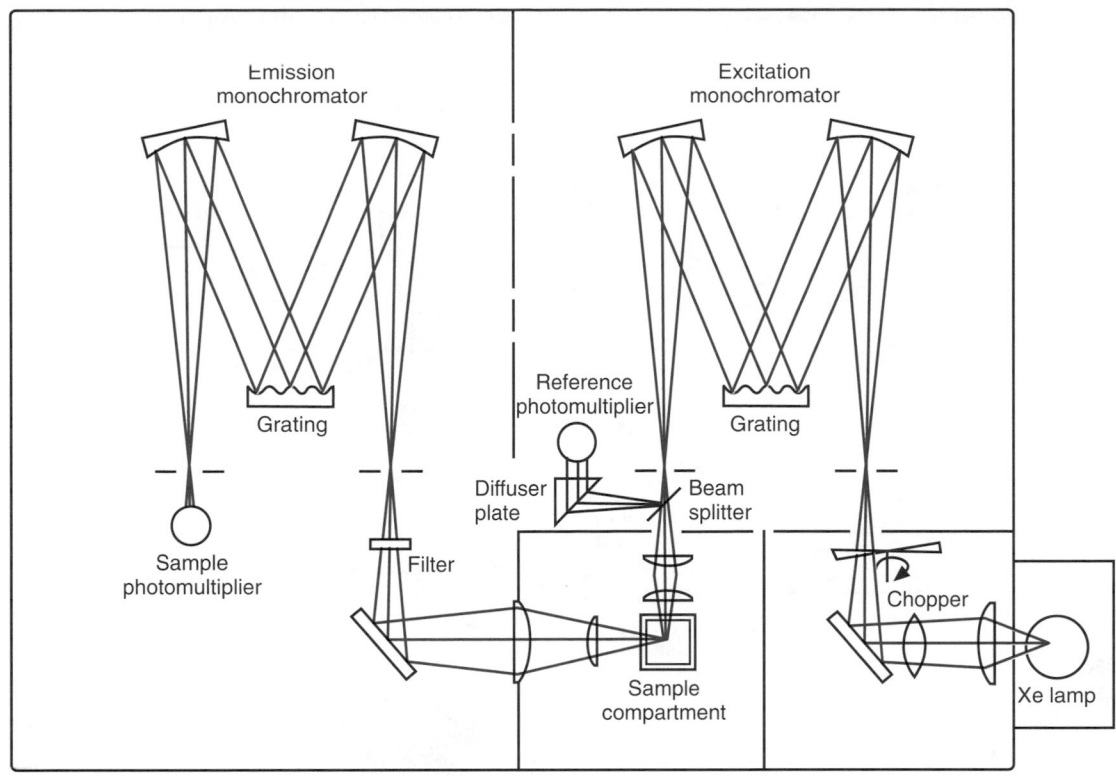

Figure 4-7   Diagram of the light path of a spectrofluorometer.

Transient-state polarized fluorescence is a time-resolved fluorescence technique used for the homogeneous detection of nucleic acids.[1] With this technique a pulsed laser diode operating in the near-infrared region is used to excite an appropriately labeled oligonucleotide probe. The fluorescence polarization of the excited probe then is measured through use of time-correlated, single-photon counting. The fluorescence emission is monitored in the perpendicular and horizontal modes for 10 seconds each. The difference in these two readings provides the transient-state fluorescence polarization measurement, which can result in the elimination of background Raman light scatter. The fluorescence polarization measurement of single-strand to double-strand DNA enables the measurement of probe formation without the need for strand separation, and the use of the near-infrared region reduces matrix fluorescence.

In a phase-resolved fluorometer a modulated excitation source, such as a flash lamp or continuous-wave laser, is used and the frequency response of fluorescence measured and used to determine fluorescence decay times.[3] A simple apparatus for measurement of luminescence lifetimes through use of the phase-resolved fluorescence approach is shown in Figure 4-8, *A*. The phase-resolved method allows for the measurement of nanosecond to picosecond fluorescence lifetimes and the use of shorter-lived fluorophors. The technique is used in homogeneous fluoroimmunoassays that are based on changes in decay time and charge transfer caused by the binding of labeled antigens and antibodies.

Fluorometers for special applications

Several automated fluorometric analyzers have been developed for special applications in clinical chemistry. These include the hematofluorometer, laser-induced fluorometer, flow cytometer, fluorescence and confocal fluorescence microscopes, and blood gas analyzer.

Hematofluorometer. The hematofluorometer is a single-channel front surface photofluorometer dedicated to the analysis of zinc protoporphyrin in whole blood (see Chapter 30). A typical hematofluorometer uses a quartz tungsten lamp, a narrow-bandpass excitation filter (420 nm), front surface optics, a narrow-bandpass filter (594 nm), and a PM tube. A drop of whole blood is placed on a small rectangular glass slide that serves as a cuvet.

Laser-induced fluorometers. A schematic diagram of a laser-induced fluorometer is shown in Figure 4-8, *B*. An argon ion laser is used for excitation energy and its beam focused tightly through a sheath-flow capillary flow cell. Fluorescence is collected through a microscope objective and a 580-nm bandpass filter before detection with a PM tube. An amplifier discriminator is used to adjust the signal counts to minimize background interference. The resulting sample counts are processed through a multichannel scaler and stored for data analysis by a computer. This type of fluorometer records the passage of individual fluorescent or fluorescent-labeled molecules, cells, or particles through a flow cell cuvet on which the laser beam is focused. The use of laser-induced fluorescence to detect a small number of

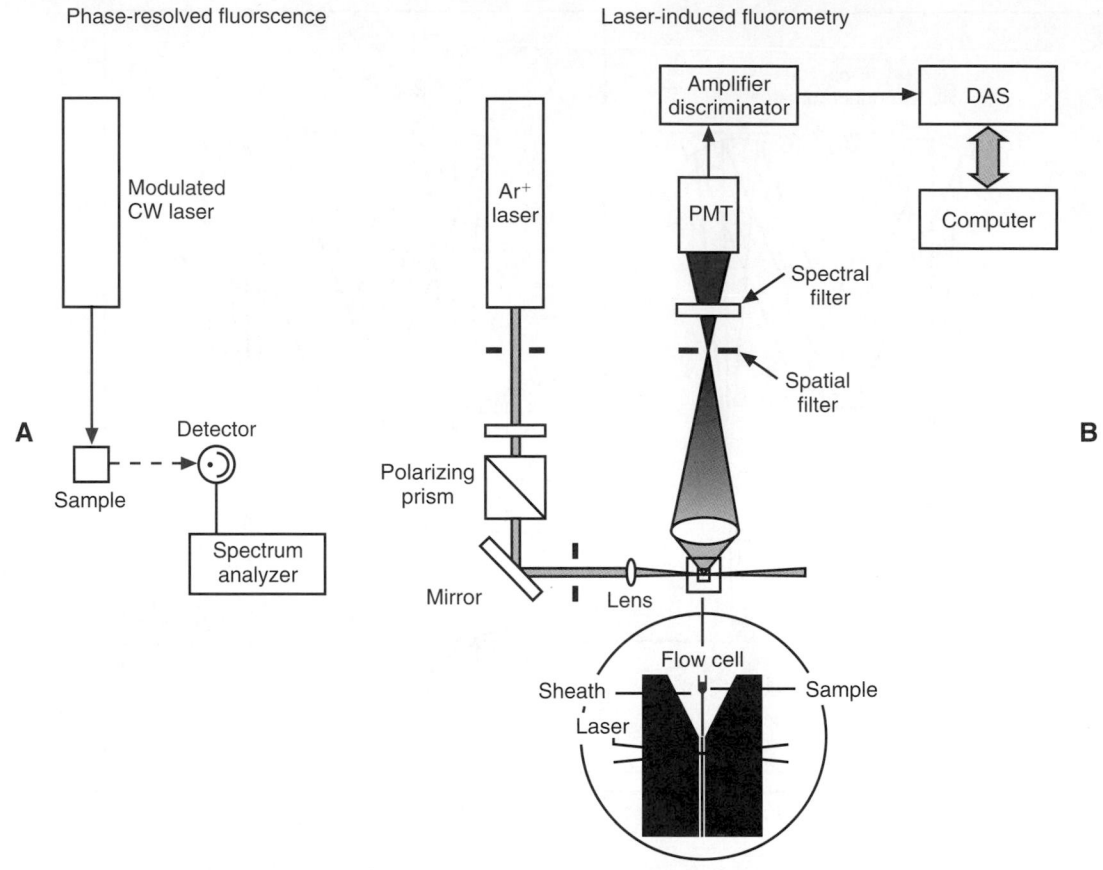

Figure 4-8   Special fluorometric instrumental applications. **A,** Phase-resolved fluorometry. **B,** Laser-induced fluorometry.

molecules in a flowing stream is important in the applications of flow cytometry, flow injection analysis, high-performance liquid chromatography, and capillary zone electrophoresis.

Flow cytometer. A flow cytometer combines laser-induced fluorometry and particle light-scattering analysis in a single instrument.[8] In such an instrument different populations of molecules, cells, or particles are differentiated by size and shape through the use of low- and right-angle light scattering. These cells, molecules, or particles can be labeled with different specific fluorescent labels, such as β-phycoerythrin, fluorescein isothiocyanate, and rhodamine-6G, as well as dye-labeled antibodies. As the cells, molecules, or particles flow through the flow cell, simultaneous fluorescence and light-scattering measurements automatically are performed by the flow cytometer. Most flow cytometers incorporate two or more fluorescence-emission detection systems so that multiple fluorescent labels can be used. In this manner molecules, cells, and particles are classified by size, shape, and type according to their light-scattering and fluorescent properties.

A schematic diagram of a flow cytometer is shown in Figure 4-9. An optical stop is placed in the 180-degree beam after the flow capillary to block the main laser beam and permit low-angle, forward light-scattering measure-

ments. The 90-degree emission signal is split and directed to two PM tubes to determine right-angle light scattering and detect at least two separate fluorescence emission signals. Two narrow-bandpass interference filters (530 and 596 nm) are placed in front of the two 90-degree fluorescence emission PM tubes. A computer with substantial resident software is used to reduce the acquired data to appropriate histograms for final result reporting. Cell-sorting electrodes are shown in the schematic drawing. Most commercial flow cytometers use a single argon ion laser (488 nm), which excites fluorescein isothiocyanate and phycoerythrin. When excited, fluorescein isothiocyanate-labeled cells emit green light (E_{max} = 530 nm), and phycoerythrin-labeled cells emit orange light (E_{max} = 596 nm).

Flow cytometers measure multiple parameters, including cell size (forward scatter), granularity (90-degree scatter), DNA content, RNA content, DNA nucleotide ratios ([A + T]/[G + C]), chromatin structure, antigens, total protein content, cell receptors, membrane potential, and calcium ion concentration as a function of pH. These parameters are used in hematology, immunology (T-cell subsets, tissue typing, lymphocyte stimulation, and antigen-antibody reactions), oncology (diagnosis, prognosis, and treatment monitoring), microbiology (bacterial identification and antibiotic sensitivity), virology, genetics (karyotyping and car-

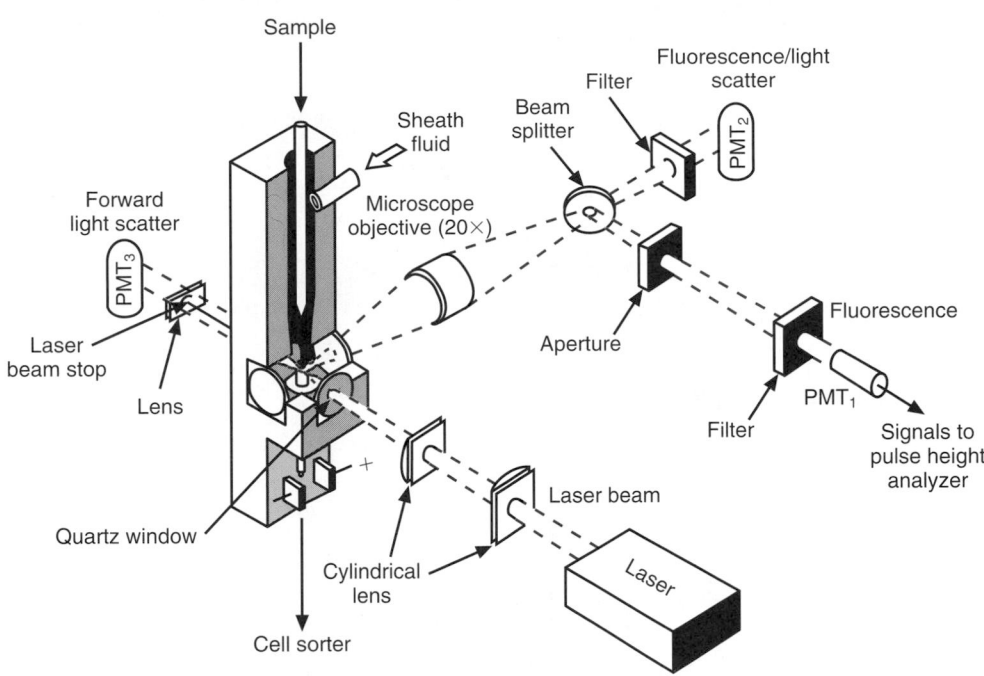

Figure 4-9   Schematic diagram of a flow cytometer. PMT_1, Photomultiplier tube for fluorescence; PMT_2, photomultiplier tube for fluorescence or 90 degrees light scatter; PMT_3, photomultiplier tube for low-angle light scatter.

rier state detection), parasitology, and reproduction and fertility studies; they also may have applications in cervical cytology.

Fluorescence microscope. A fluorescence microscope (Figure 4-10, *A*) is used to observe cellular components and properties. In practice, light from an excitation light source is focused through an appropriate narrow-bandpass interference filter to a chromatic beam splitter, which directs the excitation light through the objective lens to the specimen. The emission light from the specimen is focused by the objective lens through the chromatic beam splitter and passed through a barrier filter to the detector (eye, PM tube, or CCD).[7] **Fluorescence microscopy** is applied diagnostically to observation of antinuclear antibody patterns and urine microscopic examinations and to the use of highly specific fluorescent-labeled monoclonal antibodies for the identification of viral culture isolates for cytomegalovirus, herpes, varicella zoster, influenza A and B, respiratory syncytial virus, and immunofluorescence confirmation of human immunodeficiency virus antibodies.

A fluorescence microscope also is used in a technique called *fluorescence in situ hybridization (FISH)* that is becoming widely used as a means to study cellular genetics. In FISH, fluorochromes bound to DNA or antibodies are used as probes in biological systems. When a fluorescent-labeled probe binds to its DNA target sequence, the chromosome or chromosomal region can be identified through the use of the fluorescence microscope.

Confocal fluorescence microscope. A confocal fluorescence microscope provides three-dimensional images of fluorescence-labeled specimens. A schematic representation of a confocal fluorescence microscope is shown in Figure 4-10, *B*. Confocal microscopy uses a point source and point detector through the use of narrow slits or pinholes and provides a sharper image than conventional microscopy in that only a narrow point source of light excites the sample, and the reflected light is from the same point source. In confocal microscopy, either through the use of disks containing many specially drilled pinholes or by x-y scanning with laser light, high-resolution images are obtained. These scans of the image are recorded by a PM tube or CCD scanner. Confocal fluorescence microscopy is used for the measurement of redox potential in living cells and in conjunction with optical endoscopes to external redox confocal fluorometric microscopes to permit redox imaging of internal organs and tissues.[6]

Fluorescence blood gas analyzers. This type of analyzer uses fluorescence to determine pH, PO_2, and PCO_2 and does not require the removal of blood from the patient or transport of the sample. The sensor is added to the patient's existing arterial line. Arterial blood gas (ABG) measurements are made through the drawing of a small blood sample from the arterial line, which is injected into the ABG sensor module and returned to the patient.[11]

Limitations of fluorescence measurements

Factors that influence fluorescence measurements include concentration effects (for example, inner-filter effect and concentration quenching), background effects (due to Rayleigh and Raman light scattering), solvent and cuvet effects

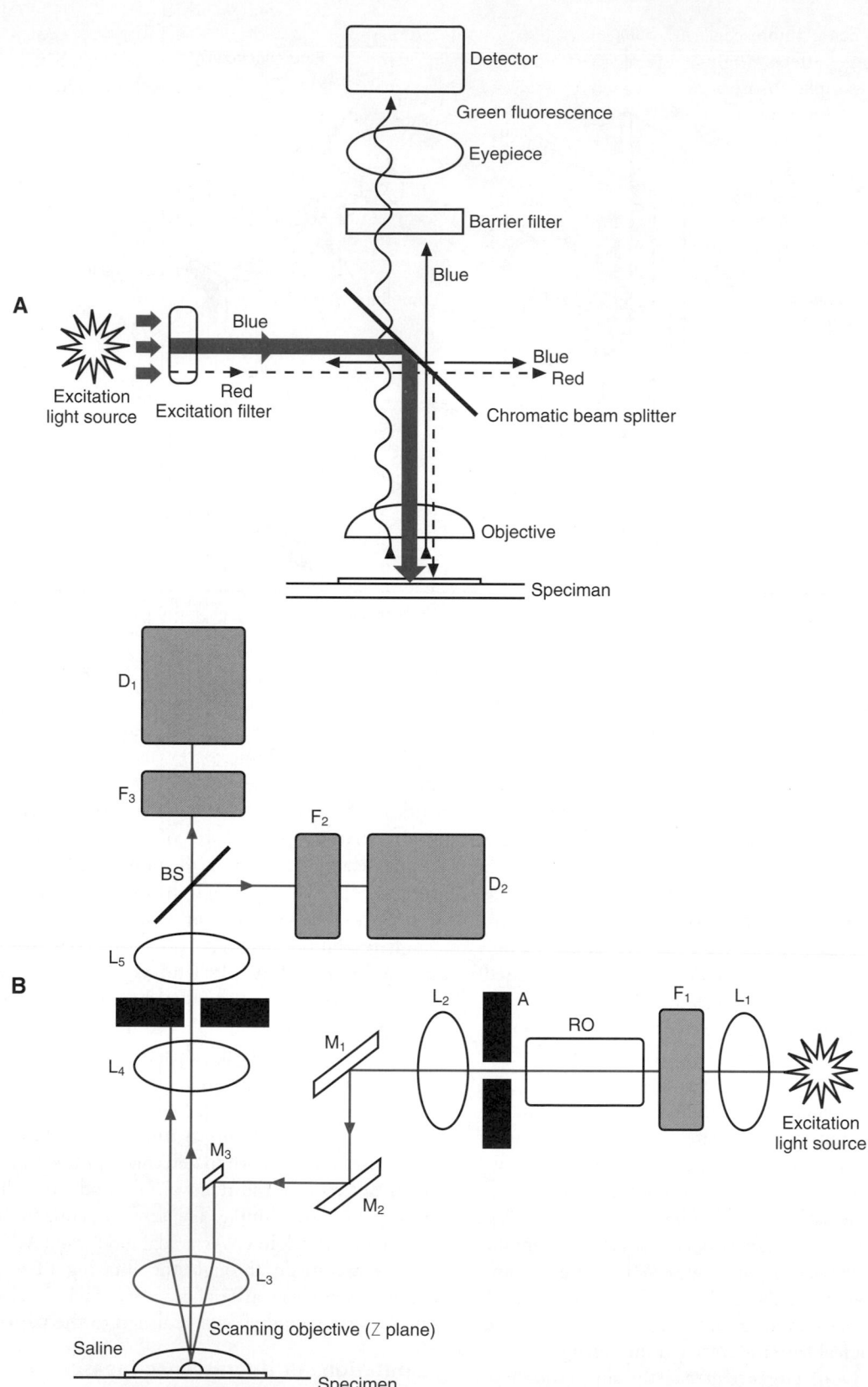

Figure 4-10   Schematic diagram of a fluorescence microscope **(A)** and a scanning confocal microscope **(B)**. *A*, Aperture; *BS*, beam splitter; D_1 and D_2, detectors; F_1, F_2, and F_3, filters; L_1, L_2, L_3, L_4, and L_5, lenses; M_1, M_2, and M_3, mirrors.

(interfering nonspecific fluorescence and quenching from the solvent), sample effects (light scattering, interfering fluorescence, and sample absorption), temperature effects, and photodecomposition (bleaching) of the sample.

Concentration effects

Inner-filter effect.   The inner-filter effect is caused by a loss of excitation intensity across the cuvet path length as the fluorophor absorbs the excitation light. As the fluorophor becomes more concentrated, the absorbance of the excitation intensity increases and the loss of the excitation light increases as it travels through the cuvet. This situation most often is encountered with a right-angle fluorescence instrument, in which the emission slits are set to monitor the center of the sample cell, where the absorbance of excitation light is greater than at the front surface of the cuvet. Using dilute solutions that absorb less than 2% of the exciting light or a front-surface fluorescence instrument minimizes the inner-filter effect.

Concentration quenching.   Another related phenomenon that results in a lower quantum yield than expected is called *concentration quenching*. This phenomenon can occur when a macromolecule, such as an antibody, is labeled heavily with a fluorophor, such as fluorescein isothiocyanate. When this compound is excited, the fluorescence labels are so spatially close that radiationless energy transfer occurs. Thus the resulting fluorescence is much lower than expected for the concentration of the label. This problem is common in flow cytometry and laser-induced fluorescence during attempts to enhance detection sensitivity through an increase in the density of the fluorescing label.

Light scattering

Light scattering, both Rayleigh and Raman types, limits the use of fluorescence measurements. Rayleigh scattering occurs with no change in wavelength. For fluorophors with small Stokes shifts, the excitation and emission spectra overlap and are particularly susceptible to loss of signal due to background light scatter. Rayleigh-type light scatter is controlled by the use of well-defined emission and excitation interference filters or by appropriate monochromator settings and the use of polarizers.

Raman-type scattering is independent of excitation wavelength and is a property of the solvent. Because Raman light scattering appears at longer wavelengths than the exciting radiation, it is a difficult interference to eliminate during work at very low fluorophor concentrations. In practice, setting the excitation and emission wavelengths far enough apart to avoid the Raman scatter or narrowing the slit width on the excitation monochromator is used to control Raman scattering. Both options tend to decrease sensitivity.

Solvent and cuvet effects

Quenching by the solvent should be investigated during the setup of a new fluorometric method. Quenching is related to the interaction of the fluorophor with the solvent or with a solute dissolved in the solvent. Such interaction results in a loss of fluorescence attributable to energy transfer or other mechanisms. An example of quenching is the loss of fluorescence when halides are added to quinine in dilute sulfuric acid. In addition, some solvents, such as ethanol, also cause appreciable fluorescence. During development of a fluorescence assay, checking of the background fluorescence of all components of the reaction mixture therefore is important. Fluorescence grade solvents with minimum fluorescence emissions that minimize these types of fluorescence background problems are available commercially.

Certain quartz glass and plastic materials used to manufacture cuvets contain ultraviolet absorbers that fluoresce and contribute to background florescence. Checking the background fluorescence of the cuvets is important for this purpose. Cuvets with minimal fluorescence emissions that minimize this type of fluorescence background are available commercially.

Sample matrix effects

A serum or urine sample contains many compounds that fluoresce and contribute to unwanted background fluorescence. The most serious contributors to this fluorescence are proteins and bilirubin. However, because protein excitation maxima are in the spectral region of 260 to 290 nm, their contribution to overall background fluorescence is minor when excitation occurs above 300 nm.

The light scattering of proteins and other macromolecules in the sample matrix also causes unwanted background fluorescence. Lipemic samples, for example, are noted for their intense light scattering, and the relative contribution of lipids to the background signal of a fluorescence measurement should be investigated during the setup of a new method.

Dilute solutions of fluorophors can exhibit additional problems besides unwanted background interference. Some fluorophors in the concentration range of $\leq 10^{-9}$ mol/L adsorb to the surface of glass and plastic cuvets and other reaction vessels. In addition, dilute solutions of fluorophors, when excited over long periods of time, are susceptible to photodecomposition by intense excitation light. Selecting proper reaction vessels, adding wetting agents, and minimizing the length of time a sample is exposed to the excitation light all help prevent these problems.

Temperature effects

The fluorescence quantum efficiency of many compounds is sensitive to temperature fluctuations. Therefore the temperature of the reaction must be regulated to within ± 0.1 °C. In general, fluorescence intensity decreases with increasing temperature by approximately 1% to 5% per degree Celsius. Temperature effects are minimized through control of reaction temperature and warming of samples or reagents, or both, if they have been refrigerated.

Photodecomposition

In conventional fluorometry, excitation of weakly fluorescing or dilute solutions with intense light sources may cause the photochemical decomposition of the analyte. Photodecomposition effects are minimized in the following ways:

1. Use of the longest feasible wavelength for excitation that does not introduce light-scattering effects
2. Decrease in the duration of excitation of the sample through measurement of the fluorescence intensity immediately after excitation
3. Protection of the unstable solutions from ambient light through storage in dark bottles
4. Removal of dissolved oxygen from the solution

Highly intense laser light sources with energy outputs greater than 5 to 10 mW that are used for flow cytometry, fluorescence microscopy, and laser-induced fluorescence measurements also rapidly photodecompose fluorescence analytes. This decomposition introduces nonlinear response curves and loss of the majority of the sample fluorescence. Fluorescence-based assays for analytes at ultra-low concentrations require optimization of laser intensity and the use of a sensitive detector.

Phosphorescence

Phosphorescence is the luminescence produced by certain substances after they absorb radiant or other types of energy. Phosphorescence is distinguished from fluorescence in that it continues to occur even after the radiation causing it has ceased. The decay time of emission of phosphorescence light is longer (10^{-4} to 10^2 seconds) than the decay time of fluorescence emission. Decay times are expressed in time ranges of several orders of magnitude and vary with the molecule and its solution environment. Phosphorescence shows a larger shift in emitted light wavelength than does fluorescence.

Chemiluminescence and Bioluminescence

Chemiluminescence and bioluminescence are types of luminescence in which the excitation event is caused by a chemical or electrochemical reaction, not by photolumination. The physical event of the light emission in chemiluminescence and bioluminescence is similar to fluorescence in that it occurs from an excited singlet state and the light is emitted when the electron returns to the ground state.

Chemiluminescence involves the oxidation of an organic compound, such as luminol, isoluminol, acridinium esters, or luciferin, by an oxidant (for example, hydrogen peroxide, hypochlorite, or oxygen); light is emitted from the excited product formed in the oxidation reaction. These reactions occur in the presence of catalysts, such as enzymes (for example, alkaline phosphatase, horseradish peroxidase, and microperoxidase), metal ions or metal complexes (for example, Cu^{2+} and Fe^{3+} phthalocyanine complex), and hemin.

Bioluminescence is a special form of chemiluminescence found in biological systems. In bioluminescence an enzyme or photoprotein increases the efficiency of the luminescence reaction. Luciferase and aequorin are two examples of these biological catalysts. The quantum yield (total photons emitted per total molecules reacting) is approximately 0.1% to 10% for chemiluminescence and 10% to 30% for bioluminescence.[4]

The reaction schemes for chemiluminescence and bioluminescence range from simple, single-step reactions, such as those involving 1,2-dioxetane substrates with alkaline phosphatase, to the more complex multiple-step reactions, such as those involving glucose-6-phosphate dehydrogenase and bacterial luciferase coupled with NADH:FMN (reduced nicotinamide adenine dinucleotide:flavine mononucleotide) oxidoreductase.

The applications of chemiluminescence and bioluminescence have increased greatly with the development of automated instrumentation and several new reagent systems. Because of their attomole to zeptomole detection limits, chemiluminescence and bioluminescence reactions have been used widely as direct and indicator labels in the development of immunoassays (see Chapter 10)[4] and nucleic acid assays.[5] Several such schemes have been used in new automated immunochemistry analyzers (see Chapter 12).

Electrochemiluminescence

Electrochemiluminescence differs from chemiluminescence and bioluminescence in that the reactive species that produce the chemiluminescent reaction are electrochemically generated from stable precursors at the surface of an electrode. Electrochemiluminescence processes have been demonstrated for many different molecules by several different mechanisms, including an oxidation-reduction-type reaction with tris (2,2′ bipyridyl) ruthenium and tripropylamine. The chemiluminescence precursors are stable and relatively small and can be used to label haptens or large molecules. Multiple labels can be coupled to proteins or oligonucleotides. The electrochemiluminescence process has been used in homogeneous immunoassays and nucleic acid assays. The advantages of this process include improved reagent stability, simple reagent preparation, and enhanced sensitivity. With its use, detection limits of 200 fmol/L and a dynamical range extending over six orders of magnitude can be obtained.

▮ LIGHT-SCATTERING TECHNIQUES

Light scattering is a physical phenomenon resulting from the interaction of light with particles in solution. Unlike fluorescence emission the scattered light is of the same frequency as the incident light. Turbidimetry and nephelometry are techniques used to measure scattered light. Light-scattering measurements are applied best to immunoassays of specific proteins and haptens. (See Chapters 10, 19, and 24 for discussions of specific applications.)

Basic Concepts

Factors important in the consideration of light scattering include the following:

1. Particle size
2. Wavelength dependence
3. Distance of observation
4. Polarization of incident light
5. Concentration of the particles
6. Molecular weight of the particles

Particle size

When the dimensions of the particles are considerably smaller than the wavelength of the incident light, each entire particle is subjected to the same electric field strength at the same time. The scattered light waves from the small particles are in phase and reinforce each other. As the particles become larger than the incident light wave, the radiated light waves are no longer all in phase. Reinforcement of radiation occurs in some directions, and destructive interference occurs in others. The scattering patterns from these large particles are characteristic of their size and shape.

Wavelength dependence of light scattering

Equation (3) illustrates the relationship of the intensity (i_s) of scattered light to the intensity (I_0) of incident light

$$\frac{i_s}{I_o} = \frac{16\pi^2 \, a \, \sin^2\theta}{\lambda^4 r^2} \qquad (3)$$

where:

i_s = Intensity of scattered light
I_0 = Intensity of excitation light
a = Polarizability of small particle
θ = Angle of observation
λ = Wavelength of incident light
r = Distance from light scattering to detector

As the equation indicates the intensity of light scatter increases by the fourth power of the wavelength as the wavelength of the incident light is decreased. The light intensity decreases by the square of the distance r from the light-scattering particles to the detector. A greater signal is obtained when the detector is located close to the analytical cuvet.

Concentration and molecular weight factors in light scattering

Equation (4) is derived from equation (3) to demonstrate the direct relationship of light scattering to the concentration and molecular weight of the particles

$$\frac{i_s}{I_o} = \frac{4\pi^2 (dn/dc)^2 Mc \sin^2\theta}{N_a \lambda^4 r^2} \qquad (4)$$

where:

i_s = Intensity of scattered light from small particles excited by polarized light
I_0 = Incident intensity
dn/dc = Change in refractive index of solvent with respect to change in solute concentration
M = Molecular weight (g/mol)
c = Concentration (g/mL) of particles
θ = Angle of observation
N_a = Avogadro's number
λ = Wavelength of incident light
r = Distance from light scattering to detector

Effect of polarized light on light scattering

Figure 4-11, *A*, illustrates the effect of polarized and nonpolarized light on light-scattering intensity from small particles as a function of scattering angle. Curve 2 shows a spherically symmetrical intensity diagram as predicted in equation (3). Curve 3 is the resultant intensity diagram when curves 1 and 2 are added and the scattering angular-intensity diagram obtained when light scatters from small particles excited with nonpolarized light. Curves 1 and 2 represent intensity diagrams from vertically and horizontally polarized light components that can be thought of as com-

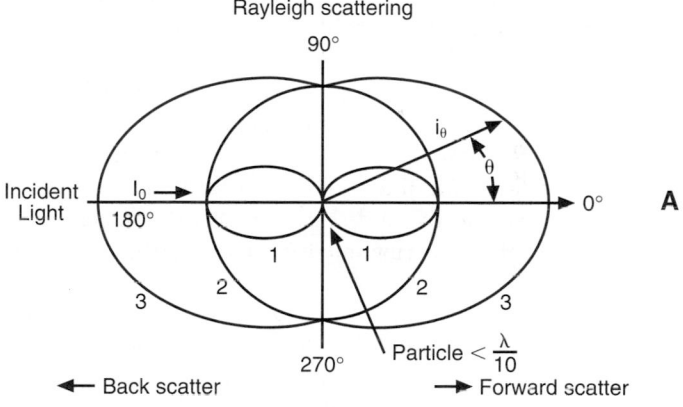

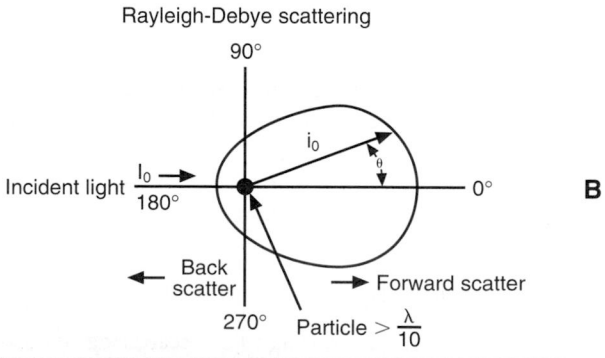

Figure 4-11   The angular dependence of light-scattering intensity with nonpolarized and polarized incident light for small particles **(A)** and the angular dependence of light scattering with nonpolarized light for larger particles **(B)**.

prising nonpolarized light. The light-scattering expression for small particles excited by nonpolarized light is provided in equation (5)

$$\frac{i_o}{I_o} = \frac{2\pi^2 (dn/dc)^2 Mc(1 + \cos\theta)}{N_a \lambda^4 r^2} \tag{5}$$

where i_0 is the intensity of scattered light by small particles excited with nonpolarized light, and I_0 is the incident intensity. Other terms are as indicated in the listing for equation (4).

Two important observations may be made from equation (5) and Figure 4-11, A. First, the total light scattered by small particles is less when particles are excited by polarized light than by nonpolarized light, and a reduction of background signal from light scattering in fluorescence measurements is achieved if an appropriately oriented polarizer is used in front of the emission detector. Second, the light-scattering intensity from small particles excited by nonpolarized light shows a symmetrical angular dependence of light scattering about the 90-degree axis (see Figure 4-11, A, curve 3).

Angular dependence of light scattering

The angular dependence of light scattering from small particles (less than $\lambda/10$) is represented in Figure 4-11, A. Careful examination of curve 3 shows that the light-scatter intensity for forward scatter (i_0 at 0 degrees) and back scatter (i_0 at 180 degrees) from small particles excited by nonpolarized light is equal. However, light-scatter intensity at 90 degrees is much less. As the particles become larger ($>\lambda/10$), the angular dependence of light scatter takes on the dissymmetrical relationship shown in Figure 4-11, B. In this case the light-scattering intensities at forward and back angles are unequal; the forward-scatter intensity is much larger. Also, the light-scattering intensity at 90 degrees is much less than the intensity at the forward (0-degree) angle.

As particles become even larger, dissymmetry increases further. This dissymmetry and the change of angular dependence of light scattering with change in the size of particles is useful in the characterization and differentiation of various classes of macromolecules and cells. As was mentioned previously, this property of light scattering is used in the design of flow cytometers. These instruments measure near-forward and right-angle light scattering from cellular particles flowing through an optical cell and excited by a high-intensity laser. These instruments use the ratio of the near-forward light scattering intensity to the right-angle light intensity to distinguish different cell sizes.

Light Scattering and Plasma Proteins

The expression for Rayleigh light scattering in equation (3) holds true in dilute solution for small particles with dimensions no larger than less than one-tenth the wavelength of the incident light. Thus the upper limit on size of particles

exhibiting Rayleigh scattering is about 40 nm when visible light at 400 nm is used. Many of the plasma proteins, such as immunoglobulins, β-lipoproteins, and albumin, are below this limit. As the particle becomes larger in size from ~ 40 to 400 nm, the angular dependence of the scattered light loses the symmetry around the 90-degree axis, as illustrated in Figure 4-11, A and B, and demonstrates an increase in forward scattering. Some plasma proteins of the immunoglobulin M class, chylomicrons, and aggregating immunoglobulin/antigen complexes fall into this size category. The scattering from particles in this size range is known as *Rayleigh-Debye* scattering, and the equation for this type of scattering becomes more complex. Particles such as red blood cells and bacteria are larger yet (that is, 7000 to 40,000 nm). These particles show a complex angular dependence of light scattering, and this type of scattering from very large particles is termed *Mie* scattering. The large particles produce a predominance of scattered light in a narrow angular region in the forward direction.

Measurement of Scattered Light

Turbidimetry and nephelometry are methods used to measure scattered light. Both are useful for measurement of serum proteins.

Turbidimetry

Turbidity causes the intensity of the incident beam of light to decrease as it passes through a solution of particles. The measurement of this decrease in intensity of the incident light beam that is caused by scattering, reflectance, and absorption of the light is **turbidimetry**. Analogous to absorption spectroscopy, turbidity can be defined as

$$I = I_o e^{-bt} \tag{6}$$

or

$$t = \frac{1}{b} \ln \frac{I_o}{I} \tag{7}$$

where:

t = Turbidity
b = Path length of the incident light through the solution of light-scattering particles
I = Intensity of transmitted light
I_0 = Incident intensity

Turbidity is measured at 180 degrees from the incident beam, or more simply in the same manner as absorbance and fluorescence (end-on geometry; see Figure 4-5) measurements are made in a spectrophotometer. Turbidity can be measured on most spectrophotometers and automated clinical chemistry analyzers. The stability and resolution of modern microprocessor-driven spectrophotometers and photometers have improved significantly the ability to measure turbidity with accuracy and precision.

Nephelometry

Nephelometry is the detection of light energy scattered or reflected toward a detector that is not in the direct path of the transmitted light. Common nephelometers measure scattered light at right angles to the incident light. The ideal nephelometric instrument would be free of stray light; neither light scatter nor another signal would be seen by the detector when no particles are present in the solution in front of the detector. However, due to stray light-generating components in the optical path and in the sample cuvet or sample itself, a truly dark field situation is difficult to obtain for nephelometric measurements. Some nephelometers are designed to measure scattered light at angles other than 90 degrees to take advantage of the increased forward-scatter intensity caused by light scattering from larger particles (for example, immune complexes). These instruments use the principal illustrated in Figure 4-11, *B*.

Selection of turbidimetry or nephelometry

The choice between turbidimetry and nephelometry depends on the application and available instrumentation. Until recently small changes in absorption due to turbidity were difficult to measure with precision, and nephelometry was the method of choice. However, with the advent of stable, high-resolution photometric systems, turbidimetric measurements have become competitive in sensitivity with nephelometric methods for immunological quantitation of serum proteins. Nephelometry, however, still offers an advantage in sensitivity when low-level antigen-antibody reactions are measured.

Light-Scattering Instrumentation

The intensity of light scattering is measured in the clinical laboratory with either a turbidimeter or a nephelometer.

Turbidimeter

Turbidimetric measurements are performed easily on photometers or spectrophotometers and require little optimization. The principal concern in turbidimetric measurements is signal-to-noise ratio. Photometric systems with electro-optical noise in the range of ± 0.0002 absorbance unit or less are useful for turbidity measurements.

Nephelometer

Although light scattering can be measured with standard analytical fluorometers or photometers, the angular dependence of light-scattering intensity has resulted in the design of special nephelometers. These devices place the PM detector at appropriate angles to the excitation light beam. The major operational difference between a fluorometer and a nephelometer is that the excitation and detection wavelengths are set to the same value in nephelometers.

The principle concerns of light-scatter instrumentation are excitation intensity, wavelength, distance of the detector from the sample cuvet, sample slits, and minimization of external stray light. Figure 4-12 shows a schematic diagram of the basic components of an instrument in the measurement of light scattering. It consists of a light source; collimating excitation optics; a sample cell; and the collection optics, which include light-scattering optics, a detector optical filter, and a detector. The schematic diagram also shows the

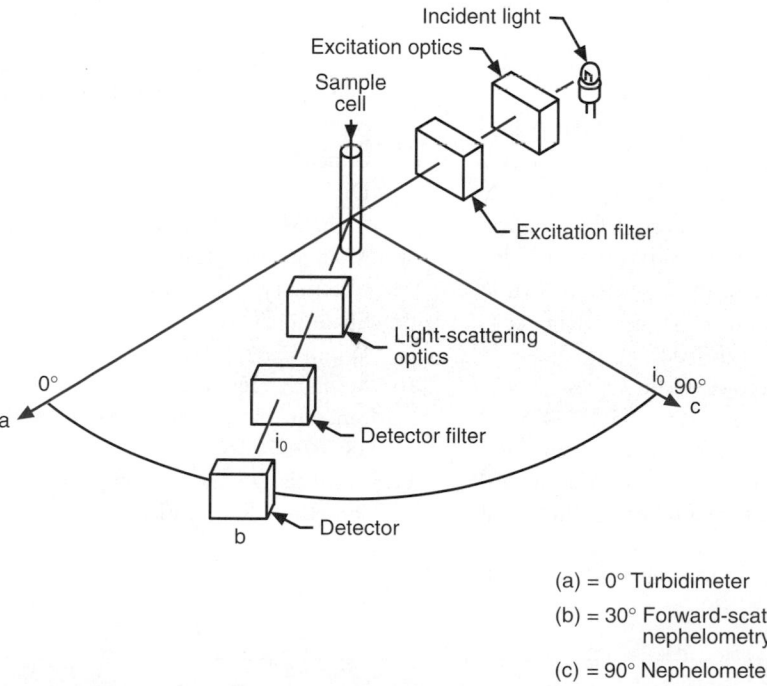

(a) = 0° Turbidimeter

(b) = 30° Forward-scatter nephelometry

(c) = 90° Nephelometer

Figure 4-12   Schematic diagram of light-scattering instrumentation showing the optics position for a turbidimeter *(a)*, forward-scattering nephelometer *(b)*, and right-angle nephelometer *(c)*.

different angles from the incident light beam where the detector, filter, and optics are placed to measure light scattering. In Figure 4-12, *a* is the straight-through arrangement for turbidimetry, whereas *b* and *c* illustrate arrangements frequently found in nephelometers. The detector arrangement shown in *b* is for measurement of forward scatter at 30 degrees. Some high-precision research instruments for light-scattering measurement provide detectors that move around the sample cell to take advantage of the angular dependence of light-scatter intensity. The movable detector is useful in determination of the molecular properties of the scattering particle. Most clinical instruments capable of measuring light scattering have fixed optical arrangements.

The optical components used for the nephelometer or turbidimeter are similar to those used in fluorometers or photometers. The light sources commonly used are quartz-halogen lamps, xenon lamps, and lasers. The laser beam is used specifically in some nephelometers because of its high intensity; in addition, the coherent nature of laser light makes it ideally suited for nephelometric applications. Ratio-referencing fluorometers and specifically designed nephelometers are well suited for nephelometric measurements.

Limitations of Light-Scattering Measurements

Antigen excess and matrix effects are problems encountered with light-scattering measurements.

Antigen excess

Antigen-antibody reactions are complex and appear to result in a mixture of aggregate sizes. As the turbidity increases during addition of antigen to antibody, the signal increases to a maximum value and then decreases. The point at which the decrease begins marks the beginning of the phase of antigen excess; this phenomenon will be explained in Chapter 10. Light-scattering methods for quantification of antigen-antibody reactions must provide a method for the detection of antigen excess. Most modern instruments have computer algorithms that flag antigen excess automatically.

Matrix effects

Particles, solvent, and all serum macromolecules scatter light. Lipoproteins and chylomicrons in lipemic serum provide the highest background turbidity or intensity. With appropriate dilutions the relative intensity of light scattering from a lipemic sample is less than that of the antiserum blank. However, as the concentration of the antigen in serum decreases and correspondingly less dilute samples are used, the background interference from lipemic samples becomes greater. An effective method for the minimization of this background interference is the use of rate measurements, where the initial sample blank is eliminated.

Large particles, such as suspended dust, also can cause significant background interference. This interference is controlled through filtering of all buffers and diluted antisera before analysis is attempted.

References

1. Diamandis E: Automation of molecular diagnostics. Clin Chem 1996; 42:7-8.
2. Diamandis E, Christopoulos TK: Europium chelate labels in time-resolved fluorescence immunoassays and DNA hybridization assays. Anal Chem 1990; 62:1149A-1157A.
3. Heiftje GM, Vogelstein EE: Time-resolved fluorometry: linear theory approach. In Wehry EL (ed): Modern Fluorescence Spectroscopy, New York, Plenum Press, 1981.
4. Kricka LJ: Chemiluminescent and bioluminescent techniques. Anal Chem 1995; 67:499R-502R.
5. Kricka LJ: Nucleic acid detection technologies—labels, strategies, and formats. Clin Chem 1999; 45:453-458.
6. Masters BR, Chance B: Redox confocal imaging: intrinsic fluorescent probes of cellular metabolism. In Mason WT (ed): Fluorescent and Luminescent Probes for Biological Activity: A Practical Guide to Technology for Quantitative Real-Time Analysis, London, Academic Press, 1993.
7. Masters BR, Kino GS: Charge coupled devices for quantitative Nipkow Disk real-time scanning confocal microscopy. In Shotton D (ed): Electron Light Microscopy: The Principles and Practice of Video-Enhanced Contrast, Digital Intensified Fluorescence, and Confocal Scanning Light Microscopy, New York, Wiley-Liss, 1993.
8. Melmed MR, Lindmo T, Mendelsohn ML (eds): Flow Cytometry and Sorting, New York, Wiley-Liss, 1990.
9. Shapiro HM: Practical Flow Cytometry, New York, Wiley-Liss, 1995.
10. Soini E, Hemmila I, Dahlen P: Time-resolved fluorescence in biospecific assays. Ann Biol Clin (Paris) 1990; 48:567-571.
11. Wolfbeis OS: Fiber Optic Chemical Sensors and Biosensors, Boca Raton, Fla, CRC Press, 1991.

Additional Reading

Henderson LO, Marti GE, Gaigalas A et al: Terminology and nomenclature for standardization in quantitative fluorescence cytometry. Cytometry 1998; 33:97-105.

Slavik S: Fluorescent Probes in Cellular & Molecular Biology, Boca Raton, Fla, CRC Press, 1994.

CHAPTER 5

Basic Principles of Radioactivity and Its Measurement

EDWARD R. POWSNER, MD, and JOHN C. WIDMAN, PhD

Objectives

1. Describe an atom and define *atomic number, mass number, isotope, half-life,* and *nuclide.*
2. Define *radioactive decay.*
3. List four types of radioactive decay, the type of particle produced by each, and the manner in which each type of particle interacts with matter.
4. Define excitation and ionization.
5. State the principles of autoradiography and scintillation counting.
6. List two types of scintillation counters and their uses in the laboratory.
7. Describe the hazards of radiation and the risks of radiation exposure.

Key Words

Autoradiography   Use of a photographic emulsion (x-ray film) to visualize radioactively labeled molecules

Beta (β-) Particle   High-energy electron emitted as a result of radioactive decay

Gamma (γ-) Ray   High-energy photon emitted as a result of radioactive decay

Half-Life   The time period required for a radionuclide to decay to one-half the amount originally present

Radioactivity   Spontaneous decay of atoms (radionuclides) that produces detectable radiation

Radiation Counter   Liquid or crystal scintillation counter or gas-filled (for example, Geiger) counter used to detect and measure radiation

Radiation Dose   The amount of radiation energy absorbed in matter, conventionally expressed in rads, defined as 100 ergs absorbed per gram of matter

Radiation Risk   Risk of cancer from radiation, used as the basis for regulations limiting radiation doses

Radiation Safety   Use of regulations and practices to ensure that radiation is used safely

Total Effective Dose Equivalent (TEDE)   Total radiation dose from both internal and external sources corrected for type of radiation; limits stated in governmental regulations

ATOMIC STRUCTURE, RADIATION, AND RADIOACTIVITY

The value of radionuclides for diagnosis, therapy, and medical research is fully established. Understanding both the risks and the benefits of these applications requires knowledge of the basic principles of **radioactivity** and its measurement and biological effects.

The Atom

An atom is the smallest unit of an element having the properties of that element.

Atomic theory

The ancient Greeks gave the word *atom* to hypothetical indivisible particles of matter. We now know that the atom is divisible, composed of even smaller particles, and that it has a definite structure. The modern model of the atom is mathematical and relies heavily on quantum theory. However, an earlier model proposed by Danish physicist Niels Bohr almost 100 years ago permits easy visualization of most major aspects of the atom. Bohr's atom consists of a tiny, positively charged nucleus, about 0.01 pm in diameter. Around this nucleus revolve negatively charged electrons in orbits that are roughly 100 pm in diameter, about 10,000 times larger than the diameter of the nucleus. The attractive electrical force between the negatively charged electrons and positively charged nucleus keeps the electrons in orbit, much as gravitational force keeps the planets in our solar system in orbit around the sun. The electrons occur in distinct orbits, or "shells;" the reactivity of the electrons in these shells determines the chemical properties of the atom.

The nucleus is composed of protons and neutrons tightly bound together. The forces and structure of the nucleus are more complicated than those of the electrons orbiting the nucleus. The masses of the proton and neutron are about (but not exactly) the same. As their names suggest the proton carries a positive charge, whereas the neutron has no charge. Both the neutron and the proton are referred to as *nucleons*.

Atomic species

The *atomic number (Z)* is the term given to the number of protons in the nucleus; the total number of nucleons—protons plus neutrons—is known as the *mass number (A)*. A *nuclide* is the name of an atomic species with a given atomic number and a given mass number. The generally accepted written representation of a nuclide is to place its mass number as a left superscript to its chemical symbol and its atomic number as a left subscript directly underneath the mass number (for example, $^{32}_{15}P$ and $^{14}_{6}C$). Because both atomic number and chemical symbol identify the element, the subscript often is omitted, for example, ^{32}P and ^{14}C.

Those nuclides with the same atomic number but·different mass numbers are known as *isotopes,* which represent various nuclear species of the same element. Most elements occurring in nature are mixtures of isotopes. For example, natural carbon is predominantly ^{12}C with about 1% ^{13}C and a trace of ^{14}C. The naturally occurring isotopes of the lighter elements, such as carbon and iron, are stable, but among the heavy elements, such as lead and bismuth, some or all of the naturally occurring isotopes are unstable. These unstable nuclides undergo spontaneous transitions to stable nuclides via a process referred to as *radioactive decay*. Decay typically is accompanied by the emission of energy in the form of radiation.

In the electrically neutral, nonionized atom the number of orbital electrons equals the number of protons. Because chemical properties depend on the number and arrangement of the orbital electrons and only slightly on the atomic mass, the chemical properties of all isotopes of an element are virtually identical. This identity of chemical properties is the basis for isotopic tracer methodology, the fundamental principle of which is that the living system does not differentiate among isotopes of the same element.

Masses of atoms and other particles are expressed in atomic mass units (amu). By definition, 1 amu is one-twelfth the mass of one atom of carbon-12. This is the isotope of carbon with a nucleus of 12 nucleons (6 protons and 6 neutrons). Also, 1 amu is about 1.6604×10^{-27} kg. The mass of one nucleon is slightly more than 1 amu.

Nuclear stability

In the neutron-proton model of the nucleus, protons contribute mass and positive charge, whereas neutrons contribute only mass; the combination of protons and neutrons provides stability. Binding energy and nuclear stability depend on the number of neutrons relative to the number of protons (n-p ratio). Only a small number of possible proton-neutron combinations are stable. A nucleus with an excess of either protons or neutrons is unstable; it emits radiation of a type that brings the daughter nucleus toward the region of stability. The unstable nucleus can adjust its n-p ratio by emitting particles of matter. This readjustment, known as *radioactive decay,* is the subject of the following discussion.

A solitary neutron is not stable but decays to a proton and an electron; in contrast, a solitary proton is stable. It is, in fact, the nucleus of an ordinary hydrogen atom ($^{1}_{1}H$). With this one exception, all atomic nuclei have both protons and neutrons. The simplest combination, one proton with one neutron, is the nucleus of the stable atom deuterium ($^{2}_{1}H$), sometimes referred to as "heavy" hydrogen. When combined with oxygen, heavy hydrogen is known as "heavy" water (H_2O). The next heavier member of this series of hydrogens, one proton with two neutrons, is unstable radioactive tritium ($^{3}_{1}H$). Beyond this, the one-proton, three-neutron combination, if it exists at all, would be an extremely unstable form of hydrogen. Combinations containing two protons are called *helium*. There is no stable nuclide of two protons alone; at least one neutron is required to stabilize a nucleus with two or more protons. The two-proton combination with one neutron is helium ($^{3}_{2}He$), with two neutrons it is still helium ($^4_2$He). Both heliums are stable, but helium isotopes with more than two neutrons are unstable.

In stable nuclides of low atomic number, hydrogen through neon (atomic number 10), the numbers of protons and neutrons are equal or approximately equal. Moderately massive nuclides have more neutrons than protons; for example, the stable isotopes of iron (atomic number 26) have between 28 and 32 neutrons for their 26 protons. The difference between the number of neutrons and the number of protons increases as the atomic number increases. Bismuth has an isotope with 126 neutrons for its 83 protons and decays so slowly that it long was believed to be stable. Its half-life is about 2×10^{17} years (10 million times the age of the universe!). No stable nuclides are found with more than 83 protons.

Radiation

Radiation from the atom and its nucleus may be classified as either particulate or electromagnetic. *Particulate radiation,* as the name suggests, consists of small bits of high-velocity matter, such as the electron, positron, proton, neutron, or the more complex particles composed of protons and neutrons. *Electromagnetic radiation* is characterized by its energy (or equivalently by its frequency or wavelength). Visible light is the most familiar example of electromagnetic radiation.

Electromagnetic radiation exists over a wide spectrum of energies. The parts of this spectrum are named by their features, just as parts of visible spectrum are named by their colors, from red at the low end to violet at the high end. Electromagnetic radiations with very low energy levels, low frequencies, and long wavelengths are called *radio waves,* whereas those of higher energy levels and frequencies and shorter wavelengths are called *light.* Those with the highest energy levels are called *x-rays* and *gamma rays* (Table 5-1). γ- and x-rays are distinguished by their origins; thus **gamma (γ-) ray** implies origin in the de-excitation of an atomic nucleus, whereas *x-ray* implies origin from the acceleration of orbital or other electrons. Nevertheless, both are electromagnetic radiation, and once emitted, a 35-keV γ-ray physically is indistinguishable from a 35-keV x-ray.

A major tenet of modern physics is that all types of radiation have properties resembling those of both particles and waves. For all electromagnetic radiation, including γ- and x-rays, *photon* is the name for the particle or quantum of radiation. The photon has no rest mass; indeed, it does not exist except while traveling at the speed of light. This fact is consistent with the photon's wavelike properties. The wavelength of the photon is inversely proportional to its energy. For the high-energy electromagnetic radiation classified as γ-rays or x-rays, the physical properties related to the particle-like aspects are more important than the wavelike aspects, and they are usually referred to as *x-ray photons* and *γ-ray photons.*

Radioactive Decay

Radioactive decay is a property of the atomic nucleus and is evidence of nuclear instability. Through radioactive decay the nucleus alters its composition or configuration to increase its stability. Decay is manifested by a spontaneous change within the nucleus that results in the loss of mass and emission of energetic radiations. Some radionuclides used in clinical pathology are listed in Table 5-2.

Alpha decay

To achieve stable configurations, a heavy element, particularly one with an atomic number above 70, may shed some of its nuclear mass by emitting a two-proton, two-neutron fragment identifiable after emission as a *helium nucleus.* Because nuclear radiations were observed before their identities were known, this fragment was called an *alpha* (α) *particle,* and its emission was termed α-*decay.* These names still are used. As an example, radium-226 decays by α-emission to produce radon and helium

$$^{226}_{88}\text{Ra} \rightarrow \,^{222}_{86}\text{Rn} + \,^4_2\text{He}$$

Most α-emitters are naturally occurring radioisotopes of the heavy elements. Although they continue to be evaluated (for example, in the treatment of bone neoplasms), they as yet have had very limited clinical applications.

Beta decay

For some heavy nuclides and almost all those with atomic numbers below 60, stability is achieved through a rearrangement of the nucleus in which the total number of nucleons are unchanged. In terms of the neutron-proton model of the nucleus, this rearrangement is the conversion of a neutron to a proton, or vice versa. During such conversions the nucleus emits either a negative electron or its positive equivalent, known as a *positron.* The emission of the negative electron, the **beta (β) particle,** is what is usually meant by the term β-*decay.*

The emission of a negative β-particle leaves the nucleus with one additional positive charge. Normally, a neutron is converted to a proton, and the nucleus assumes the next highest atomic number. Negative β-emission is characteristic of a nucleus that has more neutrons than are required by its protons for stability. Figure 5-1 *(lower detail)* shows the

TABLE 5-1	Classification of Electromagnetic Radiation	
	Name	Frequency (Hz)
	Radio waves	10^4 to 10^{11}
	Infrared light	10^{12} to 10^{14}
	Visible light	10^{14} to 10^{15}
	Ultraviolet light	10^{15} to 10^{17}
	Gamma (γ-) and x-rays	10^{17} to 10^{20}

TABLE 5-2   Radiation Properties of Some Radionuclides Used in the Clinical Laboratory

Nuclide	Half-Life	Decay Type*	Maximum Energy of Radiation (MeV)† Beta (β)	Maximum Energy of Radiation (MeV)† Gamma (γ)
^{3}H	12.3 y	β$^-$	0.186	None
^{14}C	5730 y	β$^-$	0.155	None
^{32}P	14.3 days	β$^-$	1.71	None
^{35}S	87 days	β$^-$	0.167	None
^{51}Cr	27.7 days	EC	None	0.320
^{57}Co	272 days	EC	None	0.122, 0.136, 0.014
^{58}Co	71 days	EC, β$^+$	0.474	0.811; annihilation photons only
^{59}Fe	45 days	β$^-$	0.475, 0.273	1.10, 1.29
^{99}Mo	66 h	β$^-$	1.21, 0.450	0.740, 0.181, 0.778
^{99m}Tc	6.0 h	IT	None	0.141
^{125}I	60 days	EC	None	0.035
^{131}I	8.04 days	β$^-$	0.607, 0.336	0.364, 0.637, 0.284

β$^-$, β-Decay; β$^+$, positron decay; EC, electron capture; IT, isomeric transition.
*Where a nuclide is known to have more than one mode of decay, each is listed in order of prevalence.
†Energies are given only for the more prevalent β- and γ-radiations and are in approximate order of prevalence. EC decay also yields the characteristic x-rays of the daughter; the energies of the x-rays are not included in this listing. As noted in the gamma column, positron decay (β$^+$) is accompanied by annihilation radiation, which consists principally of a pair of 0.511 MeV photons.

decay scheme for ^{131}I, which decays by β-emission. Other examples of nuclides that decay by negative β-emission are carbon-14, hydrogen-3 (tritium), and iron-59. Emission of a positive β-particle, referred to as *positron emission,* has the opposite effect; a proton becomes a neutron, and the atomic number decreases by one. This process is characteristic of a nucleus with more protons than neutrons. Positron emitters include carbon-11, fluorine-18, and iron-52.

Electron capture

In the type of radioactive decay known as *electron capture* an orbital electron is "absorbed" by the nucleus. After either electron capture or positron emission, the change in the nucleus is the same: the addition of one neutron and loss of one proton, an unchanged atomic mass, and a decrease in the atomic number by one. As an example, Figure 5-1 *(top)* shows the decay scheme for ^{125}I, which decays exclusively by electron capture. A simple explanation is that the orbits of the atomic electrons, particularly those of the innermost shells, have some probability of overlapping the nucleus and permitting the nucleus to capture the electron.

Although the n-p ratio is in the stable range after electron capture, the atom is left with a vacancy in one of its inner electron shells, or s orbital. This is an unstable or excited state for the atom. Atomic de-excitation is accomplished by rearrangement of the orbital electrons, usually a jump of an electron from a higher-energy orbital to the inner-orbital vacancy. As the electron falls to the inner orbit, energy is released either in the form of an x-ray or ejection of a more weakly bound orbital electron (Auger electron).

Gamma emission and internal conversion

The original observations of naturally occurring radioactive nuclides disclosed a third radiation, the γ-*ray.* Its ability to

penetrate materials that block α- and β-radiation distinguish this radiation. We now know that γ-radiation is high-energy electromagnetic radiation emitted during nuclear de-excitation. After either α- or β-decay or electron capture the nucleus may be left in an excited state, from which it returns to the ground state by shedding the excess energy either through the emission of a γ-photon or the ejection of an orbital electron (conversion electron). In either case the energy emitted equals the energy released in de-excitation, a process that may occur in one or more steps. Each step produces a photon of corresponding energy. For every radionuclide, the de-excitation steps and corresponding γ-ray energies provide a unique γ-ray spectrum that can be used to identify unknown nuclides. The γ-emissions following β-decay or electron capture are diagrammed in Figure 5-1.

Rate of Radioactive Decay

The rate of decay is characteristic of each individual radionuclide. The rate is unaffected by temperature, pressure, concentration, or any other chemical or physical condition. Ernest Rutherford (1871-1937) observed that the decay of a radionuclide is a random event. The decay of any single atom cannot be predicted, but in a group of millions of atoms the number that disintegrates during a given time interval can be predicted within statistical limits.

Activity and half-life

The rate of decay of a radioactive source is called its *activity* and is simply the rate at which radioactive parent atoms decay to form more stable daughter atoms (see Table 5-3). It is convenient to describe the rate of decay in terms of **half-life,** $t_{1/2}$, the time required for sample activity to decrease to half its initial value. The relationship between the initial ac-

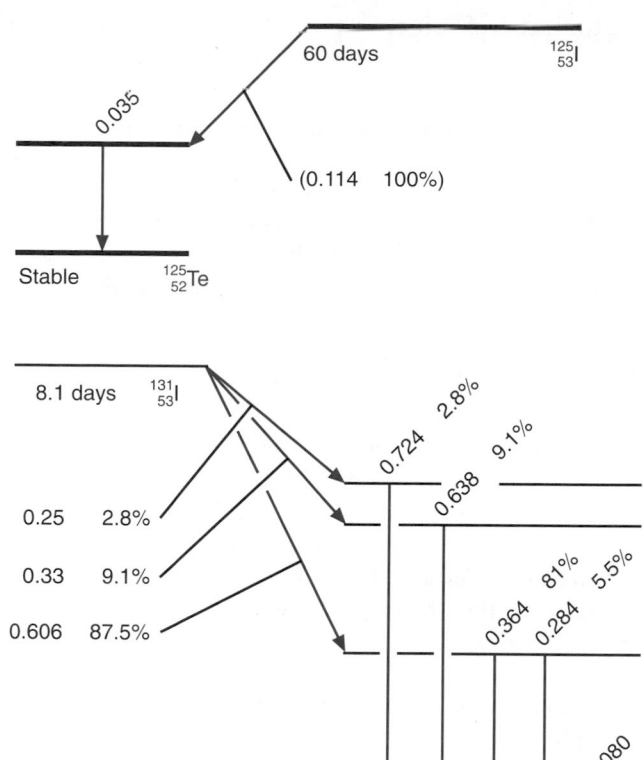

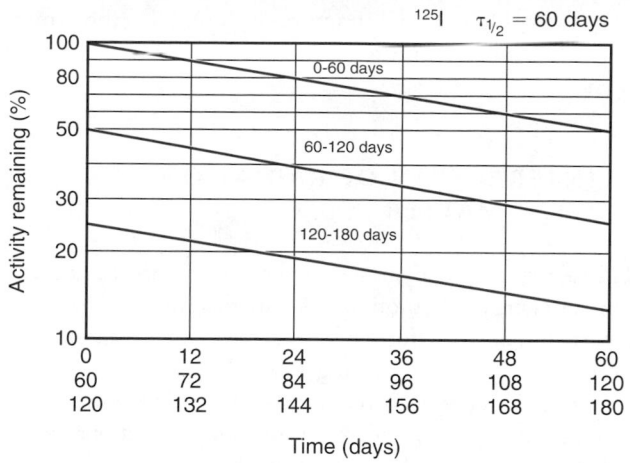

Figure 5-2 Radioactivity versus time for ^{125}I ($\tau_{1/2} = 60$ days). The logarithm of activity remaining is plotted against elapsed time over a period of three half-lives. $\tau_{1/2}$, Half-life.

Figure 5-1 Atomic mass-energy diagram for two iodine isotopes. *Top,* Electron capture decay of ^{125}I to ^{125}Te. *Bottom,* β-decay of ^{131}I to ^{131}Xe. In these diagrams the symbol for the nuclide is given just below the lowest or only horizontal line of each stack. The time to the left of the symbol for a radionuclide is its half-life; nonradioactive nuclides are simply labeled *stable*. The height of a horizontal line is proportional to its energy with respect to the ground state of the stable nuclide. The relative position of a line from right to left indicates relative atomic number. Arrows sloping down to the right indicate negative β-emission. Vertical arrows indicate γ-emission. Arrows sloping down to the left are used to indicate electron capture. The first number assigned to each arrow is the energy in MeV released during the transition; the second number, when given, is the frequency in percent. For example, 87.5% of the ^{131}I decays is 0.606 MeV β-particles, followed by a 0.364 MeV photon in 81% of the total number of decays. (Data from Powsner ER, Raeside DE: Diagnostic Nuclear Medicine, New York, Grune & Stratton, 1971; and Way K et al: Nuclear Data Sheets, New York, Academic Press, 1966.)

tivity (A_0) at time zero and the activity *(A)* after an elapsed time *(t)* is given by

$$A = A_0 \times 2^{-t/\tau_{1/2}}$$

This relationship is pictured conveniently with a plot of the logarithm of the percent activity remaining against time (Figure 5-2). Over each half-life the activity decreases by half; the effect is cumulative. In general,

$$A = A_0 \times 2^{-n}$$

where *n* is the number of half-lives. This equation is useful in the planning of experiments and disposal of radioactive

waste. For disposal a rule of thumb is that a decay time of seven half-lives reduces the activity to less than 1% of its original value ($2^{-7} = 1/128 = 0.78\%$), and that after 10 half-lives, to less than 0.1%.

Another formula, mathematically equivalent to the above formulas, is

$$A = A_0 \times e^{-(0.693/\tau_{1/2})t}$$

where *e* is the base of natural logarithms, and 0.693 is the natural logarithm of 2. This formula is used frequently because the exponential function (a built-in function of many small calculators) is tabulated, facilitating quick solutions to problems.

Units of radioactivity

The Becquerel (Bq) is the Système International d'Unites (SI) unit of radioactivity and is defined as one decay per second (dps). Because 1 Bq is a very small amount of activity, the activity of typical chemistry samples often is expressed in kiloBecquerels (kBq). The curie (Ci) is the older, conventional unit; it is defined as 3.7×10^{10} dps. This number originally was selected because it approximates the activity of 1 g of the prevalent isotope of radium. One curie equals 37 gigaBecquerels (GBq). (See Table 5-3 for a summary of units.)

Specific activity

The term *specific activity* has several meanings. It may refer to any one of the following: radioactivity per unit mass of an element, radioactivity per mass of labeled compound, or radioactivity per unit volume of a solution. The denominator of reference must be specified. In terms of radioactivity per unit mass, the maximum specific activity attainable for each radionuclide is that for the pure radionuclide. For example, pure ^{14}C has a specific activity of 62 Ci/mol or 4400 Ci/kg. As usually available ^{14}C is a tracer for compounds, in which it represents only a small fraction of the total carbon, most of which is the naturally occurring mixture of stable ^{12}C and stable ^{13}C.

INTERACTION OF RADIATION WITH MATTER

Radioactive emissions possess energy either in the form of kinetic energy of motion, as in the case of α- and β-particles, or in the form of electromagnetic radiation, as in the case of γ-rays. In passing through matter these radiations transfer energy to the atoms and molecules they encounter, chiefly through excitation and ionization. Alpha and β-particles transfer energy by the interaction of their electrical fields. Gamma rays, which are uncharged, interact by other processes and are discussed in subsequent sections. The ability of radiation to produce excitation and ionization is one of its most important properties. This property is the basis for the detection of radioactivity and is responsible for the biological effects of radiation.

Excitation and Ionization

Excitation describes the process whereby energy of the incident radiation is transferred to matter through raising of the electrons of the irradiated material to higher energy levels. If the energy absorbed from the radiation completely removes an electron from its atom or molecule, the process is called *ionization*. The resulting positive ion and negative electron are referred to as an *ion pair*. The ejected electron itself is called a *secondary electron*.

Particulate Radiation

The most important particle interactions are those of the charged particles, α and β. Both α- and β-particles cause ionization and excitation as a result of their velocities and charges. In mechanical terms, α- and β-particles are rapidly moving, charged bodies capable of forcing electrons from the atoms they pass. At each encounter the α- or β-particle loses energy, and after many encounters it finally comes to rest.

Electromagnetic Radiation

The nature of the initial interaction of photons, including γ-rays, is energy dependent. At the low end of the energy spectrum, particularly if the energy is insufficient to cause ionization, photons induce electronic and molecular motions that register as heat. This result is the predominant effect of the radio waves used in microwave or radar heaters. Photons higher on the energy spectrum can eject electrons from matter by several mechanisms, of which the most important are the photoelectrical and Compton interactions.

Photoelectrical effect

The ejection of an atomic electron (Figure 5-3) is the most likely action of a moderately energetic photon. The photoelectrical effect first was observed for photons of visible light and derives its name from this association. The photoelectrical effect occurs only if the energy of the incoming photon at least equals the binding energy of the electron. Photon energy in excess of the binding energy imparts kinetic energy to the ejected photoelectron, and the photon itself is absorbed.

Compton effect

The Compton effect (see Figure 5-3) predominates if the energy of the photon is greatly in excess of the binding energies of the atomic electrons. In a Compton interaction the incoming photon interacts with a free or weakly bound, outer-shell electron as though the photon and electron were billiard balls in collision. The electron is propelled in one direction while the photon is scattered in another direction, simultaneously losing some of its energy to the electron. The electron deposits its energy in the surrounding matter through ionization and excitation of other atoms. The scattered photon has a lower level of energy than the original photon.

DETECTION AND MEASUREMENT OF RADIOACTIVITY

Darkening of photographic emulsion, ionization of gas, or fluorescent scintillation are still the bases for most modern clinical detection techniques. The underlying physical process in all these methods is the detection of excitation or ionization caused by radiation. In radiology and autoradiog-

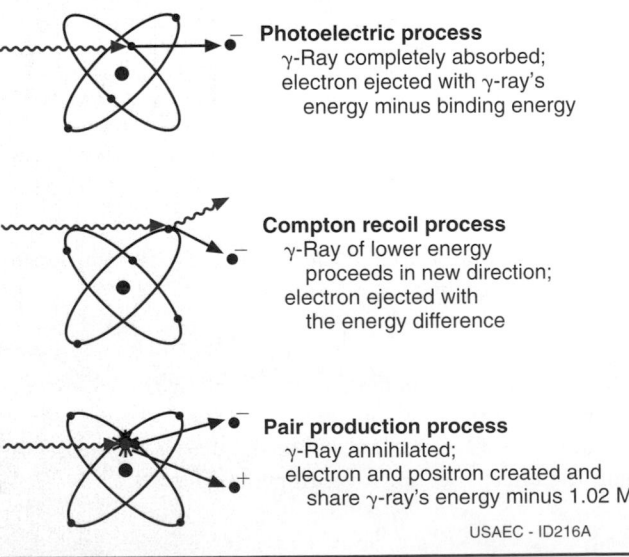

Photoelectric process
γ-Ray completely absorbed; electron ejected with γ-ray's energy minus binding energy

Compton recoil process
γ-Ray of lower energy proceeds in new direction; electron ejected with the energy difference

Pair production process
γ-Ray annihilated; electron and positron created and share γ-ray's energy minus 1.02 MeV

USAEC - ID216A

Figure 5-3   Interactions of γ-rays with matter (see text). (Courtesy U.S. Atomic Energy Commission, ID216A.)

raphy, exposure and observation of a photographic film are principal procedures. In the clinical chemistry laboratory almost all measurements use scintillation detectors.

Autoradiography

In **autoradiography** a photographic emulsion (x-ray film) is used to visualize radioactively labeled molecules. This technique has been used extensively in laboratories in which nucleic acid techniques are performed. Nucleic acid probes containing ^{32}P are readily available. The nucleic acid fragments are separated by gel electrophoresis. The gel is covered with a plastic film, and the photographic film is applied to the covered gel. Alternatively, the nucleic acid fragments can be transferred to a nylon membrane and the photographic film applied to the membrane. Exposure time varies from 30 minutes to 1 week, depending on the specific activity of the probe and its concentration. The film is developed, and the resulting image reflects the radioactivity of nucleic acid fragments.

In research applications the film is applied to a sample, typically a tissue slice, containing radioactive material. The emitted radiations expose the emulsion, forming an image of the points in the tissue from which radiations emanated. Thus cells or organelles can be identified specifically by their radioactivity.

Gas-Filled Detectors

Detectors filled with certain gases or gas mixtures are designed to capture and measure the ions produced by radiation within the detector. In ionization chambers a low-intensity electrical field moves the positive and negative ions through the gas in opposite directions; the resulting current is amplified and measured. If the applied field is moderately high (for example, several hundred volts over a few centimeters), the electrons move with enough velocity to ionize additional gas molecules. This process is referred to as *gas amplification* and is advantageous because the current it generates is easier to measure than the small current of the primary ions alone. The Geiger counter, which uses gas amplification, is a type of gas-filled counter commonly seen in the clinical chemistry laboratory, where it is used as a portable **radiation counter,** or monitor.

Scintillation Detectors

The operating principle for the scintillation detector is similar to that of the gas-filled detector, at least at the beginning. In both scintillation and gas detectors the absorption of radiation causes excitation and ionization, but in the scintillation detector the absorbed energy produces a flash of light rather than a pulse of current. The principal types of scintillation detectors found in the clinical chemistry laboratory are the sodium iodide crystal scintillation detector and or-

ganic liquid scintillation detector. Of these the crystal detector is the easier to use and the more economical. Consequently, most clinical laboratory procedures have been designed around radionuclides, such as ^{125}I, which can be counted efficiently in crystal scintillation detectors. Nevertheless, a few procedures still require compounds labeled with pure β-emitters, such as tritium or ^{14}C, nuclides that are assayed best within liquid scintillation detectors.

Crystal scintillation detector

Figure 5-4 presents a diagram of the crystal scintillation detector. The usual form of a crystal scintillation detector in the chemistry laboratory is the well detector, which has a hole drilled in the end or side of the cylindrical crystal to accept a test tube. Because it is hygroscopic, the crystal is sealed hermetically in an aluminum can with a transparent quartz window at one end, through which the blue-violet

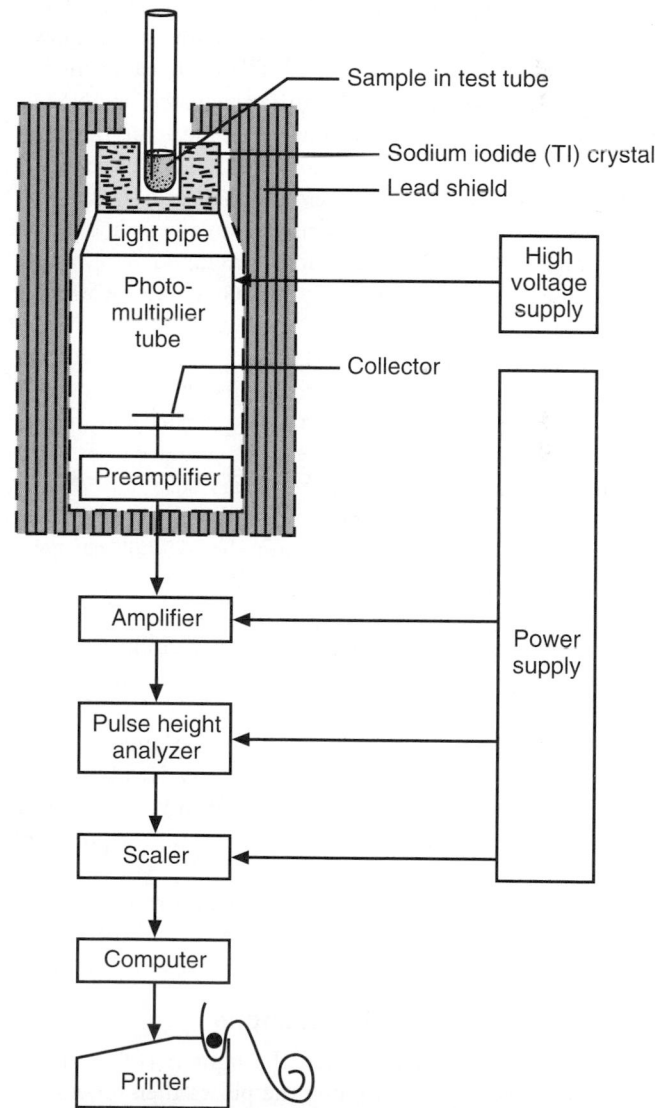

Figure 5-4   Crystal scintillation well detector.

(420 nm) scintillations can be seen. The aluminum can follow the contours of the well. Photons of ^{125}I in the sample easily penetrate the specimen tube and thin, low-density can and enter the crystal, where they are likely to be absorbed in the thick, high-density sodium iodide. Of course, only photon energy that is actually absorbed in the crystal produces scintillations and can be detected.

The well detector is the instrument of choice for γ– and x–ray-emitting nuclides, such as ^{51}Cr, ^{57}Co, ^{59}Fe, ^{125}I, and ^{131}I, and for this reason is often referred to as a *γ-counter*. It is not suitable for β-radiation, which usually cannot penetrate the sample container and aluminum lining of the well. For a typical well detector the counting efficiency for ^{125}I, expressed as the percentage of decay that produces counts, approximates 70%.

Liquid scintillation detector

As sketched in Figure 5-5, the liquid scintillation detector measures radioactivity by recording scintillations occurring within a transparent vial that contains both the unknown radioactive sample and a liquid scintillator. Because the radionuclide is mixed intimately with or actually dissolved in the liquid scintillator, the technique is ideal for the pure β-emitters of low energy and short range. Examples are tritium (maximum β-energy 19 keV and maximum range <10 μm in water) and ^{14}C (156 keV maximum energy and <300 μm range). Typical efficiencies for liquid-scintillation counting in the absence of significant quenching are 50% for tritium and 90% for ^{14}C.

The liquid scintillator, also known as the *scintillation cocktail*, contains at least two components—the primary solvent and the primary scintillator. The primary solvent absorbs the radiation energy, whereas the primary scintillator in turn absorbs energy from the primary solvent and converts that energy into light, typically in the ultraviolet range. In addition to the primary scintillator, the cocktail may contain the following:

1. A secondary solvent to improve the solubility of aqueous samples or a surfactant to stabilize or emulsify the sample
2. A secondary scintillator, sometimes referred to as a *wavelength shifter*, to absorb the ultraviolet photons of the primary scintillator and reemit the energy at a longer wavelength, which facilitates the response of some photomultiplier (PM) tubes
3. One or more adjuvants, such as suspension agents, solubilizers for biological tissues, and antifreezes, to prevent freezing and separation of water at low temperatures

Electronics of scintillation counting[3]

After each burst of scintillation the light is collected and converted to an electrical pulse; the pulses then are amplified, sorted by size, and counted. Because the amount of scintillation light produced is directly proportional to the

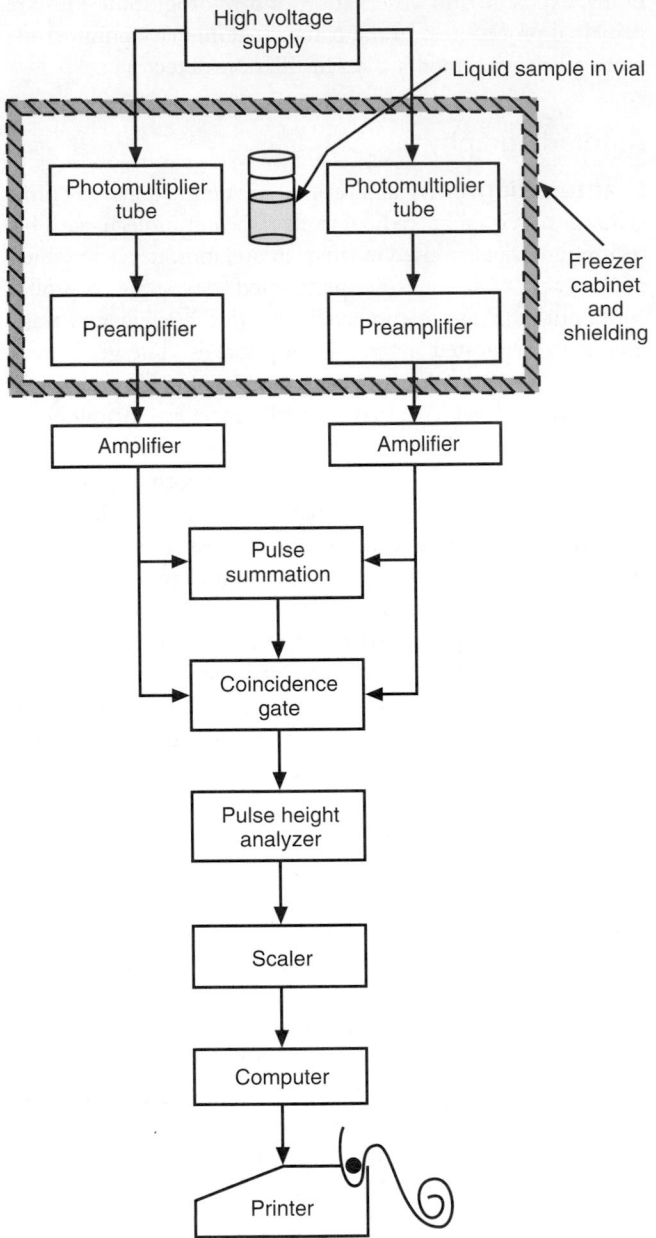

Figure 5-5   Liquid scintillation detector.

energy absorbed from each γ-ray or β-particle, measurement of the size of a pulse is really a measure of the incoming γ-ray or β-particle energy. These detected radiation events ("counts") often are sorted according to energy. The resulting energy spectrum permits, among other things, distinguishing of the counts of two nuclides in the same sample according to the energy of their characteristic emissions. Instruments that perform this function are called *spectrometers*.

The components that perform these functions in crystal and liquid scintillation detectors are shown in Figures 5-4 and 5-5, respectively. The more important of these components are discussed in the following sections.

Photomultiplier

The PM tube is a vacuum tube that converts the scintillations into electrical pulses (see Chapter 3). As used in a well detector the light of the scintillations in the crystal is transmitted to the PM through a short light pipe. For liquid scintillators the sample vial is placed in a lightproof opening between two PM tubes. Whether from a crystal or liquid scintillator, the photons of light enter the PM tube through its quartz window. Within the PM these photons strike the photosensitive layer (cathode), from which they eject outer-shell electrons. Sensitivity varies from tube to tube; on average, one electron is ejected for every 3 or 4 photons entering the tube. These electrons are accelerated toward the first of several intermediate electrodes, called *dynodes,* each of which is maintained at a progressively higher positive potential relative to the photosensitive cathode. As each electron strikes a dynode, it ejects several additional electrons from the dynode surface, thus effectively multiplying the number of electrons traveling down the tube. All these electrons are accelerated by their increasing potential differences into successive dynodes, where the multiplication is repeated.

Preamplifier

Despite the multiplication of electrons that occurs in the PM tube, the output of the tube still requires further amplification. A preamplifier, typically placed close to the PM tube, is used to boost the current before it is analyzed.

Pulse-height analyzer

Pulses are sized electronically by an analyzer, which ignores pulses outside an acceptable window or channel. Typically, the window is delimited by a pair of discriminators, one set to the bottom of the desired window, the other set to the top. Each responds only if the height of the pulse exceeds the value to which it has been set. A pulse is within the window if the lower discriminator responds and the upper discriminator does not. Conversely, the pulse is not in the window if both or neither of the discriminators respond.

The analyzer for a well detector usually is supplied with one or more windows, often factory set, each corresponding to the narrow, γ-energy peak of a specific nuclide. Generally, a window is centered around the peak; when multiple energy peaks are present in the nuclide's γ-ray spectrum, the window may be widened to include more than one peak, thereby increasing the counting efficiency. The windows in liquid scintillation counters must be wider than those in γ-counters. This size accommodates the wider spectrum of β-energies. When necessary, the window is adjustable to accommodate the effect of the sample itself on the apparent energy of the scintillation.

Efficiency of scintillation counting

The overall efficiency of a scintillation detector can be defined as the ratio of count rate to decay rate. The factors that affect the count rate and hence the efficiency include the following:

1. The fraction of all decays that yield useful radiation (that is, radiation capable of affecting the scintillator)
2. The fraction of potentially useful radiations that are directed into the scintillator
3. The fraction of photons entering the scintillator that deposit energy therein
4. The scintillation efficiency (that is, the ratio of energy emitted as light to the energy deposited as radiation)
5. The detector threshold (that is, the number of light photons, usually 10 to 20, required to trigger a count in the electronic circuits monitoring the scintillator)

Of these five factors, scintillation efficiency is the one most likely to require the attention of the clinical laboratorian. For solid crystal scintillation detectors a decrease in efficiency may indicate that the crystal has cracked or otherwise failed and should be replaced. For liquid scintillation detectors, changes in efficiency may be related to the sample or its preparation. Monitoring the efficiency of a scintillation detector is an important part of the quality control program.

Quenching

The term *quenching* implies a reduction in scintillation efficiency, usually in reference to liquid scintillation counters. A reduction in efficiency may occur whenever a portion of the energy of a photon emitted in the scintillator is absorbed before it is detected. Because quenching can cause batch-to-batch or sample-to-sample variations in efficiency, monitoring of and, when necessary, correcting for quenching are important in every assay. Some instruments perform these functions automatically; effective manual methods are available, but many are labor intensive.

Counting Statistics

The counting statistics of measuring radioactivity depend on the number of counts obtained from the radioactive sample and the superimposed background radioactivity.

Poisson distribution

Rutherford observed that the number of decays of a radioactive sample in successive, equal time intervals follows a Poisson distribution. For a typical assay in which thousands of decays are counted, the Poisson distribution closely resembles the bell-shaped Gaussian distribution—with one provision: the standard deviation *(s)* of the Poisson distribution is always equal to the square root of its mean

$$s = \sqrt{\bar{x}}$$

For example, if 10,000 counts are recorded from a specimen the standard deviation for this measurement is the square root of 10,000, or 100 counts. Of particular note is that this relationship refers to "counts;" the standard deviation is calculated from the number of counts, not from the count rate. The standard deviation is important because it allows the clinical laboratorian to estimate the uncertainty in the results. As in the Gaussian distribution the confidence limit for the Poisson distribution at $\pm 1s$ is 68%, and at $\pm 2s$ is 95.5%.

To illustrate the significance of this concept, notice that when 10,000 counts are collected, as in the above example, one s is 100 counts and the error at the 95.5% level is 2%.

$$\frac{2s \times 100 \text{ counts/s}}{10,000 \text{ counts}} = 0.02$$

If only 100 counts are collected, however, a similar calculation shows that the error can be as large as 20% at the same level of confidence. The square-root relationship between the standard deviation and the mean also dictates that quadrupling the number of counts cuts the counting error in half, at least to the extent that background is negligible. In the previous example counting to 40,000 reduces the error from 2% to 1%. Of course, doubling the count requires either doubling of the sample's activity or doubling of the time spent counting the sample. Either factor most likely will increase the cost of the assay.

Effect of background count rate

The *count* referred to in the previous section is the actual or gross count as read from the scintillation counter. In practice, samples always are counted in the presence of background radiation, which originates both from naturally occurring sources in the environment and from other samples in the laboratory. Electronic "noise" in the instrumentation also may contribute to this apparent activity. Unless the background is negligible, a clinical assay must include a correction for background. The corrected, or net, count is obtained by subtraction; thus if sample and background are counted for equal time

$$C_n = C_{n+b} - C_b$$

where:

C = Counts, specified in subscripts
n = Sample net
b = Background
$n + b$ = Sample with background (the gross count)

Consequently, the background count also must be considered during calculation of uncertainty, usually referred to as *counting error.*

The calculation of the counting error follows the rules for propagation of errors. In the case of a sum or difference the rule states that the square of the error in the result equals the sum of the squares of the individual errors. Following this rule

$$s_n^2 = s_{n+b}^2 + s_b^2$$

where the standard errors (sample standard deviations), s, are specified by the subscripts in the preceding equation.

For example, for a 10-minute measurement the background is 2500 counts, and the gross count of the sample is 10,000; the standard error of the net count is

$$s^2 = 2500 + 10,000 = 12,500$$

or

$$s = 111.8$$

In the calculation, s, the standard error of a count, is equal to the square root of the count, so s^2 equals the count. This equation illustrates that the standard error of the net count is higher than that of the gross count, even though the net count is lower.

■ RADIATION SAFETY

Users of radioactive materials regulated by the U.S. Nuclear Regulatory Commission (NRC) must comply with requirements for training in **radiation safety.** (The federal requirements referred to here and subsequently are found in the Code of Federal Regulations, Title 10, sections 19.12, 20.1003, 20.1201, 31.11, and Part 30). These regulations state the following:

All individuals who, in the course of employment, are likely to receive in a year an occupational dose of more than 1 mSv (100 millirem), shall be instructed in the health protection problems associated with exposure to ionizing radiation or radioactive material, precautions and procedures to minimize exposure, and the purposes and functions of protective devices.

This section is intended to meet this requirement.

Units of Radiation Exposure and Radiation Dose

The most important quantities, along with their units and definitions, used in radiation protection are provided in Table 5-3. The first of the quantities, radioactivity, more simply referred to as activity, and its units, Becquerel and curie, were defined in a previous portion of this chapter.

Absorbed dose

The effects of ionizing radiation are dependent largely on the amount of energy absorbed. The SI unit is the gray (Gy), equal to one joule (J) of energy per kilogram of absorber. The conventional unit is the rad (**r**adiation **a**bsorbed **d**ose), which equals 100 ergs per gram. One rad equals 0.01 Gy.

Exposure

Exposure is defined as the amount of charge liberated through the ionization of radiation per mass of air. The conventional unit is the roentgen (R). It is an older quantity that has certain limitations, but because it is easy to measure

TABLE 5-3	Quantities and Units Used in Radiation Protection		
Quantity	Conventional Unit	SI Unit	Meaning
Activity	curie (Ci) 1 Ci = 37GBq	becquerel (Bq)	Number of disintegrations of radioactive material per second
Absorbed dose	rad 1 rad = 10 mGy	gray (Gy)	Energy absorbed from ionization of radiation per unit mass of absorber
Exposure	roentgen (R) 1 R = 258 μC/kg	coulombs per kilogram (C/kg)	Amount of charge liberated by ionization of radiation per unit mass of air
Dose equivalent	rem 1 rem = 10 mSv	sievert (Sv)	Absorbed dose multiplied by quality factor (Dose × Q)

SI, International System of Units.

accurately, meters calibrated in mR/h are in widespread use. In SI units 1 R produces ionization, measured in coulombs (C), of 0.258 mC/kg. Additionally, exposure of dry air to 1 R results in the deposition of 0.87 rad in that air. During the exposure of soft tissue, because tissue is of different composition than air, 1 R deposits 0.93 to 0.97 rad, depending on photon energy. In other words, exposure to 1 R results in an absorbed dose of roughly 1 rad. This one-to-one relationship between roentgen and rad works only with conventional units; it does not apply in the SI system. The word *exposure* sometimes is used loosely, as in "exposure to radiation." This use should not be confused with the quantity defined in Table 5-3.

Dose equivalent

This quantity was introduced because the biological effect of radiation was found to depend on the type of radiation, as well as on the absorbed dose. This dependence is caused in part by differences in the density of ions produced. For example, ionization is very dense along the track of an α-ray but much less dense along the track of a γ-photon. The quality factor, a dimensionless factor that is determined by international agreement, takes this phenomenon into account. The dose equivalent is simply the absorbed dose multiplied by the quality factor. In a medical environment, β-particles and γ- and x-rays are used almost exclusively. For these types of radiations the quality factor equals one, which means that the absorbed dose and the dose equivalent are numerically equal.

Regulatory Requirements

Federal regulations govern licensing, radiation dose limits, and "reasonable" practices to limit doses of radiation.

Licensing

The NRC issues licenses permitting possession and use of byproduct material. *Byproduct* is an NRC term for radioactive material produced in a nuclear reactor. Many radioactive materials used in hospitals (^{99m}Tc, ^{131}I, some ^{125}I) are byproduct materials. A lesser number of materials are produced by cyclotrons and are not regulated by the NRC (for example, ^{123}I, ^{67}Ga, ^{57}Co, ^{201}Tl, some ^{125}I). These materials usually are regulated by the state; state regulations generally are similar to NRC regulations. Some states are known as *agreement states,* each of which has developed its state's radiation protection program so that it meets NRC standards and entered into an agreement with the NRC to enforce that agency's standards. In agreement states all radioactive materials, byproduct and other, are regulated by the state.

Radiation dose limits

The background **radiation dose** to all living things from natural sources (for example, cosmic rays and naturally occurring radioactive materials in the Earth and in living tissue) is, on average, about 0.3 rem per year. This natural background level varies considerably at different locations on the Earth's surface.

The NRC has published limits for the radiation dose equivalent for employees at all federally licensed facilities. Non-NRC activities of workers typically are covered by similar state government regulations. The radiation dose may come from external sources, such as laboratory radioactive sources or medical x-ray machines, or from radioactive material taken into the body. These two modes of exposure to radiation are called *external exposure* and *internal exposure,* respectively. The dose equivalent from external and internal exposures together constitute the **total effective dose equivalent (TEDE)** for the body. Federal regulations governing occupational exposure specify 5 rem per year as the limit for TEDE. For individual organs of the body, comparable limits are given in terms of *total organ dose equivalent.* The limit for an individual organ other than the eye is 50 rem per year. Because of the greater potential for radiation damage, lower limits apply to the lens of the eye (15 rem per year) and to an embryo or fetus (0.5 rem per year).

Regulations also require NRC licensees to ensure that their licensed activities do not cause the TEDE of members of the general public (that is, nonoccupationally exposed individuals) to exceed 0.1 rem per year.

The ALARA principle

The following text is paraphrased from NRC regulations cited in the previous section:

In addition, the licensee shall use, to the extent practicable, procedures and . . . controls . . . to achieve occupational doses and doses to members of the public that are as low as reasonably achievable (ALARA) . . . by making every reasonable effort to maintain exposures to radiation as far below dose limits . . . as practical . . . taking into account the state of technology, the economics of improvements . . . and other societal and socioeconomic factors . . .

This injunction should be regarded as a required part of the radiation safety program; however, just what is "reasonable" under ALARA is a matter of judgment by both the licensee and the regulators.

Health Risks of Radiation Exposure

Health effects from radiation may be classified in several ways; for example, according to the clinical outcomes: somatic, genetic, and teratogenic.

Somatic effects are those that occur to the exposed individual. These effects may manifest promptly after a large acute dose, (for example, 100 rem) or they may occur years after exposure to high or low doses. The somatic effect of concern from doses of radiation in the occupational range (that is, less than NRC limits) is the induction of cancer. Although it is known with a high degree of confidence that high doses of radiation cause cancer, it is not known with certainty that the same is true of low doses.

Genetic effects are abnormalities that may occur in future children of exposed individuals and in subsequent generations. The possibility of genetic effects in humans is of concern. However, genetic effects exceeding normal incidence have not been observed in any studies of irradiated human populations, even in the Japanese atomic bomb survivors. Continuing studies of the Chernobyl accident may change this observation. In any case genetic effects have been observed reliably in studies of exposed animal populations, including mammals. Radiation scientists are confident that such effects exist in humans and would be observed if the doses and sizes of irradiated populations were large enough.

Teratogenic effects are those that may be observed in children who were exposed during the fetal and embryonic stages of development. Teratogenic effects, such as cancer, congenital malformation, and reduced intelligence, have been observed in certain irradiated groups (for example, Japanese atomic bomb survivors) but only at relatively high doses (20 rem or more acute exposure).

Risks for cancer induction and loss of life expectancy

The **radiation risk** to an individual whose exposure history is known can be estimated when the absorbed dose is multiplied by the risk factor. The risk factor currently used by the NRC for cancer induction is 4×10^{-4} cases of cancer per rem.[4] A medical technologist who has received 250 millirem per year (0.25 rem) for 20 years has a lifetime dose of 5 rem. Thus the technologist's increased risk of cancer is $4 \times 10^{-4} \times 5 = 0.002$. The natural incidence of fatal cancer is about 20%, so this exposure to radiation has increased the total risk of cancer for this individual from 20% to 20.2%.[1,2]

An alternative method characterizing the risk from radiation is through assessment of the loss of life expectancy. The loss from receipt of 0.1 rem each year from 18 to 65 years of age is 5 days. This number may be compared to 60 days with occupational hazards in nonradiation industries, 205 days with motor vehicle accidents, and 158 days with all other accidents.[1]

Limiting external exposure

Three principal methods help reduce exposure from external sources:

Reduce time. Minimize the time spent in the vicinity of a source of radiation. Work efficiently, but do not rush.

Increase distance. Maintain as large a distance from the source as practical. The radiation intensity from a source diminishes rapidly as the distance from the source is increased. Tools such as tongs can effectively reduce exposure to hands and forearms.

Use shielding. When time and distance alone are insufficient, shielding provides another safeguard. Shields take many forms, including lead aprons, syringe shields, vial shields, countertop shields (often with leaded glass), fixed and portable (on casters) lead barriers, and thinner shields of plastic, which may be used for β-emitting and low-energy γ-emitting sources.

Limiting internal exposure

The protection techniques are designed to prevent radioactive material from entering the body. Entrance is most commonly via inhalation, but ingestion, absorption through intact skin, and intake through skin puncture also are possible.

Limiting inhalation is accomplished through proper laboratory design, including attention to adequate air-exchange and air-flow patterns, use of fume hoods, and following of other laboratory practices developed with the goal to minimize inhalation. For example, when working with a volatile radioactive source, an employee should be upwind of the source (that is, the source should be between the employee and an exhaust, such as a hood).

Limiting ingestion is accomplished through good laboratory hygiene, such as wearing of protective gloves and gowns; knowledge of proper glove removal; hand washing before eating; prohibition of pipetting by mouth, as well as food and cosmetics application in the laboratory; and effective recognition and cleanup of spills.

Absorption through intact skin is not significant for most compounds; nevertheless, when dealing with a material which may be absorbed, individuals should exercise extra care to properly cover the hands, forearms, and other parts that could become contaminated.

Employer and Employee Responsibilities in Control of Risk

The NRC requires licensees to post form NRC-3, which summarizes employee rights and responsibilities, as follows:

Employer If an employee is likely to receive more than 10% of any annual limit, the employer must perform monitoring. In the case of external exposure, this step usually is performed with a personal dosimeter, such as a film badge or other type of monitor. If the exposure is internal (for example, from vapors of ^{125}I), monitoring must as-sess the body's burden, either via direct measurement of body activity or measurement of excreta (for example, through urine counts). Determining the clearance rate from the body also may be necessary. Employers are required to notify each monitored employee of the employee's dose at least annually and notify the employee if any limit has been exceeded.

Employee If an employee decides that the risks associated with occupational radiation exposure are too high, the employee may request a reassignment from the employer; however, the employer is not required to provide such a reassignment. An employee should notify his or her supervisor(s) immediately on a suspicion that a work condition is unsafe or an NRC regulation or provision of the license has been violated.

References

1. Cohen BL: Catalog of risks extended and updated. Health Phys 1991; 61(3):317-335.
2. International Commission on Radiological Protection: Problems Involved in Developing an Index of Harm. Publication No. 27 (Annals of the ICRP vol 1, no 4), New York, Pergamon Press, 1977.
3. Krugers J: Instrumentation in Applied Nuclear Chemistry, New York, Plenum Publishing, 1973.
4. U.S. Nuclear Regulatory Commission: Regulatory Guide 8.29, Instruction Concerning Risks from Occupational Radiation Exposure. Revision 1, Washington, DC, NRC, February 1996.

Additional Reading

Bushong SC: Radiologic Science for Technologists, 6th edition, St Louis, Mosby-Year Book, 1997.

Early PJ, Sodee DB: Principles and Practice of Nuclear Medicine, 2nd edition, St Louis, Mosby-Year Book, 1994.

Hendee WR: Radioactive Isotopes in Biological Research, Malabar, Fla, Krieger, 1984.

Howard PL, Trainer TD: Radionuclides in Clinical Chemistry, Boston, Little, Brown, 1980.

Noz ME, Maguire GQ: Radiation Protection in the Health Sciences, River Edge, NJ, World Scientific, 1995.

Powsner ER, Raeside DE: Diagnostic Nuclear Medicine, New York, Grune & Stratton, 1971.

Powsner RA, Powsner ER: Essentials of Nuclear Medicine Physics, Malden, Mass, Blackwell Science, 1998.

Ross H, Noakes JE, Spaulding JD: Liquid Scintillation Counting and Organic Scintillators, Chelsea, Mich, Lewis, 1991.

Weber DA, Eckerman KF, Dillman LT et al: MIRD: Radionuclide Data and Decay Schemes, New York, Society of Nuclear Medicine, 1989.

CHAPTER 6

Electrochemistry

RICHARD A. DURST, PhD, and OLE SIGGAARD-ANDERSEN, MD, PhD

Objectives

1. Define *electrochemistry* and draw an electrochemical cell.
2. Define *potential* and state the principle of potentiometry and its use in the laboratory.
3. List four types of electrodes available for laboratory use.
4. State the principles of amperometry and coulometry and list the uses of each technique in a clinical laboratory.
5. Define *biosensor* and provide examples of biosensors as used in a clinical setting.

Key Words

Amperometry An electrochemical process in which current is measured at a fixed (controlled) potential difference between the working and reference electrodes in an electrochemical cell

Biosensor A special type of sensor in which a biological/biochemical component, capable of interacting with the analyte and producing a signal proportional to the analyte concentration, is immobilized at or in proximity to the electrode surface; the biocomponent interaction with the analyte being either a biochemical reaction (for example, enzymes) or a binding process (for example, antibodies) that is sensed by the electrochemical transducer

Conductometry An electrochemical process used to measure the ability of an electrolyte solution to carry an electric current by the migration of ions in a potential field gradient; an alternating potential being applied between two electrodes in a cell of defined dimensions

Coulometry An electrochemical process in which the total quantity of electricity (that is, charge = current × time) required to electrolyze a specific electroactive species is measured in stirred solutions under controlled-potential or constant-current conditions

Electrochemical Cell An electrochemical device that produces an electromotive force; classes including galvanic and electrolytic

Electrode A conductor through which an electrical current enters or leaves a nonmetallic portion of a circuit; indicator, working, and reference electrodes being examples of such devices used for electroanalytical purposes

Electrolytic Electrochemical Cell A type of electrochemical cell in which chemical reactions occur through the application of an external potential difference; forms the basis for amperometric, conductometric, coulometric, and voltammetric electroanalytical techniques

Galvanic Electrochemical Cell A type of electrochemical cell that operates spontaneously and produces a potential difference (electromotive force) through the conversion of chemical into electrical energy; forms the basis for potentiometric electroanalytical techniques

Ion-Selective Electrodes A type of special-purpose, potentiometric electrode consisting of a membrane selectively permeable to a single ionic species; the potential produced at the membrane-sample solution interface being proportional to the logarithm of the ionic activity or concentration; also known as *ion-selective membrane electrodes*

Polarography A special form of the voltammetric process that uses a dropping mercury electrode as the working electrode

Potentiometry   An electrochemical process in which the potential difference is measured between an indicator electrode and a reference electrode (or second indicator electrode) when no current is allowed to flow in the electrochemical cell

Voltammetry   An electrochemical process in which the cell current is measured as a function of the potential when the potential of the working electrode versus the reference electrode is varied as a function of time

---

Several types of analytical methods that are based on electrochemical measurements are applied to procedures used in the clinical laboratory.[3] These electrochemical techniques include potentiometry, voltammetry, coulometry, amperometry, and conductometry. They are coupled with biological systems to produce biosensors.

POTENTIOMETRY

Potentiometry is the measurement of the electrical potential difference between two electrodes in an **electrochemical cell.**[6] A **galvanic electrochemical cell** (Figure 6-1) consists of two electrodes (electron or metallic conductors) connected by an electrolyte solution (ion conductor). An **electrode,** or half-cell, consists of a single metallic conductor in contact with an electrolyte solution. The ion conductors may be composed of one or more phases that are either in direct contact with each other or separated by membranes permeable only to specific cations or anions. One electrolyte solution is the unknown, or test, solution, which may be replaced with an appropriate reference solution for calibration purposes. A salt solution or bridge may be interposed in the cell to reduce any liquid-liquid junction potential present. By convention the left electrode (M_L) is the reference electrode; the right electrode (M_R) is the indicator (measuring) electrode.

The electromotive force *(E or emf)* is defined as the maximum difference in potential between the two electrodes (right minus left) obtained when the cell current is zero. The cell potential is measured with a potentiometer, of which the common pH meter is a special type. The direct-reading potentiometer is a voltmeter that measures the potential across the cell (between the two electrodes); however, to obtain an accurate potential measurement, current must not flow through the cell. Incorporating a high resistance within the voltmeter (input impedance $>10^{12}$ ohms [Ω]) helps ensure the absence of current through the cell. Modern direct-reading potentiometers are as accurate as the classical compensation potentiometers and largely have replaced them. To facilitate the reading and recording of data, these instruments can be equipped with accessories that provide direct digital display, printouts, or computer interfacing.

Within any one conductive phase the potential is constant as long as the current flow is zero. However, a potential difference arises between two different phases. The overall potential of an electrochemical cell is the sum of all the potential gradients that exist between different phases of the cell (see Figure 6-1). The potential of a single electrode with respect to the surrounding electrolyte and absolute magni-

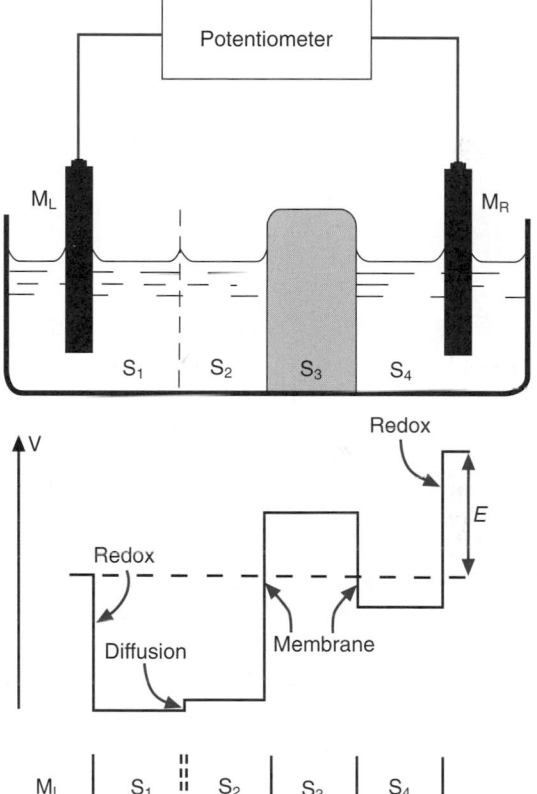

Figure 6-1   Schematic diagram of an electrochemical cell. The liquid junction between S_1 and S_2 may be an open contact between the two solutions, a porous membrane, or a fiber junction. The two electrodes (M_L and M_R) are connected externally via a high-impedance potentiometer. The electromotive force of the cell then is read directly. M_L and M_R, Two metallic conductors; S_1, S_2, S_3, and S_4, variable number of ion-conductive phases; S_1 may be a saturated KCl solution, S_2, a given test solution, S_3, an ion-selective membrane (not necessarily a thin membrane), and S_4, a given reference solution. The lower half of the figure illustrates the potential gradients at the phase boundaries produced by (1) redox potentials, (2) membrane potentials, and (3) diffusion potentials (liquid junction potentials). At the bottom the cell is described with symbols; vertical lines indicate phase boundaries, and the double dotted line indicates a liquid junction.

tude of the individual potential gradients between the phases actually cannot be measured; only the potential differences between two electrodes (half-cells) can be measured. The potential gradients can be classified as (1) redox potentials, (2) membrane potentials, or (3) diffusion potentials. Generally, devising a cell in such a manner that all the potential gradients except one are constant is possible. This potential then can be related to the activity of some specific ion of interest (for example, H^+ or Na^+).

Measurement of Ion Activity Versus Ion Concentration

Most analytical methods provide the total ionic concentration (also called the *stoichiometric concentration*) of the analyte in question. Direct potentiometric measurement on the undiluted sample provides a means through which the concentration of free unbound ion, or more exactly the activity of the ion, can be determined. This quantity is relevant for most purposes because chemical equilibria and biological phenomena are dependent on the activity of the ions rather than on the total ionic concentration.

The relationship between free ion activity and concentration of free ion and total ion is

$$aCa^{2+} = \gamma Ca^{2+} \times \frac{mCa^{2+}}{mol/kg} \tag{1}$$

where a is the relative activity of the ion in question, γ, the activity coefficient, which equals the molality, $m/[mol/kg]$, of free ion in question (for example, Ca^{2+}).

Notice that the symbol of a quantity (for example, mCa^{2+}) represents the numerical value multiplied by the unit (for example, $mCa^{2+} = 1.25 \times 10^{-3}$ mol/kg). Both the activity and the activity coefficient are dimensionless quantities.

The activity coefficient depends on the ionic strength (I) of the solution $(I = \frac{1}{2} \Sigma m \times z^2$, where z is the charge number of the ions) and generally decreases as ionic strength increases. For dilute aqueous solutions, calculation of the activity coefficients from the ionic strength is possible through use of the Debye-Hückel equation

$$-\log_{10} \gamma = \frac{z^2 \times A \times I^{1/2}}{1 + \mathring{a} \times B \times I^{1/2}} \tag{2}$$

where $\mathring{a}$ is the ion size parameter for the solution, (for example, H^+ [0.9], Na^+ [0.45], K^+ [0.3], Ca^{2+} [0.6], Cl^- [0.3], HCO_3^- [0.45]; unit: nm) and A and B are temperature-dependent constants (at 37 °C, $A = 0.5213$ $[mol \times kg^{-1}]^{-1/2}$ and $B = 3.305$ $nm^{-1} \times [mol \times kg^{-1}]^{-1/2}$). At higher ionic strengths $(I = >0.1$ mol/kg), the equation should be extended by two terms that take into account the hydration of the ions (according to the Stokes-Robinson hydration theory).

The previous equation shows that the decrease in the activity coefficient that occurs with an increase in ionic strength is more pronounced the higher the charge number (z) of the ion; thus activity coefficients are generally much lower for divalent than for monovalent ions. For most biological fluids, calculation of the activity coefficients accurately is difficult because the contribution of the protein ions to ionic strength is highly uncertain. Examples of estimated activity coefficients for normal human blood plasma are 0.75 for Na^+, 0.74 for K^+, and 0.31 for Ca^{2+}.

The amount-of-substance concentration *(c)*, often known as the *molarity*, equals the molality *(m)* times the mass concentration of water (ρH_2O); for example, for Ca^{2+}

$$cCa^{2+} = mCa^{2+} \times \rho H_2O \tag{3}$$

For normal human blood plasma the mass concentration of water is about 0.93 kg/L, but in pathological specimens from individuals with hyperlipidemia or severe hyperproteinemia the value may be as low as 0.8 kg/L; thus the substance concentration *(c)* may be 20% lower than the molality *(m)*.

The concentration of free ions equals the concentration of total ions *(ct)* multiplied by a factor (β), which may be called the *degree of dissociation;* for example, for Ca^{2+}

$$cCa^{2+} = \beta Ca^{2+} \times ctCa^{2+} \tag{4}$$

The degree of dissociation is different for different ions. For Ca^{2+} in normal blood plasma, its value is about 0.5 but varies with the albumin concentration (decreasing with increasing albumin concentration) and pH (decreasing with increasing pH). Na^+ and K^+ are dissociated almost completely in normal plasma (that is, only slightly bound), the values for β being about 0.99 for Na^+ and 0.96 for K^+.

Results of potentiometric measurements on undiluted whole blood, plasma, or serum usually are reported as the activity multiplied by an appropriate factor *(f)*. Thus the normal reference interval is the same as the conventional normal reference interval for substance concentration. For Na^+ the factor may be derived theoretically from the values for ρH_2O, γNa^+, and βNa^+ of normal plasma as follows:

$$fNa^+ = \frac{\rho H_2O}{\gamma Na^+ \times \beta Na^+} \times (mol/kg) = \frac{0.93 \times kg/L}{0.75 \times 0.99} \times (mol/kg)$$
$$= 1.25 \times 10^3 \text{ mmol/L}$$

Thus if the activity is measured as 112×10^{-3}, the result is reported as

$$112 \times 10^{-3} \times 1.25 \times 10^3 \text{ mmol/L} = 140 \text{ mmol/L}$$

For K^+ the factor is derived similarly; that is,

$$fK^+ = \frac{0.93}{0.74 \times 0.96} \times 10^3 \text{ mmol/L} = 1.31 \times 10^3 \text{ mmol/L}$$

For Ca^{2+} the factor is

$$fCa^{2+} = \frac{\rho H_2O}{\gamma Ca^{2+}} \times mol/kg = \frac{0.93}{0.31} \times 10^3 \text{ mmol/L}$$
$$= 3.0 \times 10^3 \text{ mmol/L}$$

That is, $f\text{Ca}^{2+}$ does not include βCa^{2+} because the activity is converted to the concentration of *free* Ca^{2+}, not the concentration of *total* calcium.

With such corrections major discrepancies between the results obtained through use of flame photometry and direct potentiometry for Na^+ and K^+ occur only when the mass concentration of water deviates significantly from the normal (because pathological variations in γ and β are insignificant in this respect). In severe hyperlipidemia, which the mass concentration of water may be as low as 0.80 kg/L, the result for Na^+ given by flame photometry might be 120 mmol/L, whereas that given by direct potentiometry might be 140 mmol/L. The flame photometric value may be misinterpreted to indicate Na^+ deficiency or water intoxication, or both. The potentiometric result shows that the Na^+ activity is normal. In actual practice, activity is converted to concentration through calibration directly in concentration units (by selection of suitable calibration solutions with compositions similar to normal plasma or serum).

In general, activity determinations are based on the comparison of the potential of the unknown solution with the potential of several calibration solutions with known activity. The best example is the pH determination

$$\text{pH(X)} = \text{pH(S}_1) + \frac{\text{pH(S}_2) - \text{pH(S}_1)}{E(\text{S}_2) - E(\text{S}_1)} \times [E(\text{X}) - E(\text{S}_1)] \qquad (5)$$

where:

$E(\text{S}_1)$ and $E(\text{S}_2)$ = Readings for two different calibration
    solutions
pH(X) = pH for the unknown
$E(\text{X})$ = Reading for the unknown

The precision of potentiometric measurements is limited by the standard deviation for the measured potentials (about 50 μV). This uncertainty is equivalent to a standard deviation of about 0.001 for log a for a monovalent ion, which corresponds to a coefficient of variation for the activity of a monovalent ion of about 0.2%. For divalent ions the coefficient of variation is about twice as great. The accuracy of direct potentiometric measurement is limited by the uncertain liquid junction potential, which can vary by about ± 0.5 mV as a function of the serum composition. The variation corresponds to a bias in the measured concentration of about $\pm 2\%$ for monovalent ions.

If potentiometric measurements are used for the determination of the concentration of total ions (free plus bound), the sample must be diluted with a suitable diluent that liberates the complex-bound ion from its binding agent (for example, by a pH adjustment). The dilution at the same time should establish a constant ionic strength so that a constant activity coefficient is obtained that is independent of variations in ionic strength of the original sample. This method is sometimes called *indirect potentiometry,* as opposed to *direct potentiometry,* which involves direct measurement in the undiluted sample. A different approach involves

titration with a potentiometric end-point detection. In this case the electrode is used only to sense the sudden change in activity as the end point is reached. Although more labor intensive, this technique generally is considered among the most accurate and precise analytical methods available.

Redox electrodes

Redox potentials are the result of chemical equilibria involving electron transfer reactions

$$\text{Oxidized form (Ox)} + z e^- \rightleftharpoons \text{Reduced form (Red)} \qquad (6)$$

where z represents the number of electrons involved in the reaction (the numerical stoichiometric number).
For example,

$$\text{Fe}^{3+} + \text{e}^- \rightleftharpoons \text{Fe}^{2+}$$

$$2\text{H}^+ + 2\text{e}^- \rightleftharpoons \text{H}_2$$

Any substance that accepts electrons is an oxidant (Ox), and any substance that donates electrons is a reductant (Red). The two forms, Ox and Red, represent a redox couple (conjugate redox pair). Usually, homogeneous redox processes take place only between two redox couples; in such cases the electrons are transferred from a reductant (Red_1) to an oxidant (Ox_2). In this process Red_1 is oxidized to its constant, whereas Ox_1 is reduced to Red_2.

$$\text{Red}_1 + \text{Ox}_2 \rightleftharpoons \text{Ox}_1 + \text{Red}_2 \qquad (7)$$

For example,

$$2\text{S}_2\text{O}_3^{2-} + \text{I}_2 \rightleftharpoons \text{S}_4\text{O}_6^{2-} + 2\text{I}^-$$

In an electrochemical cell, electrons may be accepted from or donated to an inert metallic conductor (for example, platinum). A reduction process tends to charge the electrode positively (remove electrons), and an oxidation process tends to charge the electrode negatively (add electrons). By convention a heterogeneous redox equilibrium (equation [7]) is represented by the cell

$$M_\text{L}|\text{Red}_1 - \text{Ox}_1 :: \text{Ox}_2 - \text{Red}_2|M_\text{R} \qquad (8)$$

where M_L and M_R are the left and right electrodes, respectively, and the cell potential is measured between these electrodes: $M_\text{R} - M_\text{L}$.

A positive potential ($E > 0$) for cell (8) signifies that the cell reaction (7) proceeds spontaneously from left to right; $E < 0$ signifies that the reaction proceeds from right to left, whereas $E = 0$ indicates that the two redox couples are at mutual equilibrium.

The electrode potential (reduction potential) for a redox couple is the couple's potential measured with respect to the standard hydrogen electrode, which is set equal to zero. (Hydrogen electrodes will be discussed in more detail in a later section of this chapter.) This potential, by convention, is the electromotive force of a cell, where the standard hydrogen electrode is the reference electrode (left electrode) and the given half-cell is the indicator electrode (right electrode). The reduction potential for a given redox couple is given by the Nernst equation. (For the derivation of this equation, the reader should consult a textbook of physical chemistry.)

$$E = E^\circ - \frac{N}{z} \times \log \frac{a\text{Red}}{a\text{Ox}} = E^\circ - \frac{0.0592 \text{ V}}{z} \times \log \frac{a\text{Red}}{a\text{Ox}} \quad (9)$$

where

E = Electrode potential of the half-cell
E° = Standard electrode potential when $a\text{Red}/a\text{Ox} = 1$
z = Number of electrons involved in the reduction reaction
F = Faraday constant ($= 96,487 \text{ C} \times \text{mol}^{-1}$), C = Coulomb
$N = \text{R} \times T \times \ln 10/\text{F}$ (the Nernst factor if $z = 1$),*
$N = 0.0592$ V if $T = 298.15$ K (25 °C)
$N = 0.0615$ V if $T = 310.15$ K (37 °C)
R = Gas constant ($= 8.31431 \text{ J} \times \text{K}^{-1} \text{ mol}^{-1}$)
T = Absolute temperature (unit: K [kelvin])
1n 10 = Natural logarithm of 10 = 2.303
$a\text{Red}/a\text{Ox}$ = Product of mass action for the reduction reaction
a = Activity

The redox electrodes presently in use can be divided into two major groups or classes—(1) inert metal electrodes immersed in solutions containing redox couples or (2) metal electrodes in which the metal functions as a member of the redox couple.

Inert metal electrodes

Platinum and gold are examples of inert metals used to record the redox potential of a redox couple dissolved in an electrolyte solution.†

The hydrogen electrode is a special redox electrode for pH measurement. It consists of a platinum or gold electrode that is electrolytically coated (platinized) with highly porous platinum (platinum black) to catalyze the electrode reaction.

$$\text{H}^+ + \text{e}^- \rightleftharpoons \frac{1}{2}\text{H}_2$$

The electrode potential is given by

$$E = E^\circ - N \times \log \frac{(f\text{H}_2)^{1/2}}{a\text{H}^+}$$

---

*N should not be mistaken for Avogadro's constant.
†Attempts have been made to measure the redox potential of blood and plasma. However, this potential is an undefined quantity as long as the redox couple is unspecified. The different redox couples of blood and plasma are not in thermodynamic equilibrium; in contrast, the different acid-base pairs are in equilibrium. If it were not for this disequilibrium, life would be impossible, because all organic substances would oxidize rapidly to carbon dioxide and water. The redox potential in blood measured with a gold electrode (with a calomel reference electrode) appears to be the redox potential of the ascorbic acid/dehydroascorbic acid couple, which is of much less clinical interest than that of redox couples such as NADH/NAD$^+$.

or

$$E = E^\circ - N \times [\log(f\text{H}_2)^{1/2} - \log a\text{H}^+]$$

where:

$E^\circ = 0$ at all temperatures (by convention)
$f\text{H}_2$ = Fugacity of hydrogen gas
$a\text{H}^+$ = Activity of hydrogen ions
$-\log a\text{H}^+$ = Negative log of the H$^+$ activity (paH$^+$ or pH)

When the partial pressure of hydrogen ($P\text{H}_2$) in the solution (and hence $f\text{H}_2$) is maintained constant through bubbling of hydrogen through the solution, the potential is a linear function of $\log a\text{H}^+$ ($= -$pH). In the standard hydrogen electrode, the electrolyte consists of an aqueous solution of hydrogen chloride with $a\text{HCl}$ equal to 1.000 (or $c\text{HCl} \sim 1.2$ mol/L, in which c is the amount-of-substance concentration) equilibrium with a gas phase and with $f\text{H}_2$ equal to 1.000 (or $P\text{H}_2 = 101.3$ kPa = 1 atm).

Metal electrodes participating in redox reactions

The silver electrode consists of a silver wire immersed in a solution containing silver ions. The electrode process consists of the reduction of Ag$^+$ to metallic silver

$$\text{Ag}^+ + \text{e}^- \rightleftharpoons \text{Ag}$$

The expression for the electrode potential reduces to

$$E = E^\circ + N \times \log a\text{Ag}^+$$

because the activity of pure silver is unity. According to this equation the electrode measures the Ag$^+$ activity in the solution. An application for this electrode is the determination of Cl$^-$ by titration with silver nitrate. In this method the silver electrode is coupled with a mercurous sulfate reference electrode for the end-point determination. When all Cl$^-$ ions are precipitated as silver chloride, the excess of Ag$^+$ causes a sudden change in the electrode potential, which indicates the end point of the reaction.

The silver/silver chloride electrode consists of a silver wire that has been coated thermally or electrolytically with silver chloride. The electrode dips into a solution containing Cl$^-$. The electrode process is as follows:

$$\text{AgCl (solid)} + \text{e}^- \rightleftharpoons \text{Ag (metal)} + \text{Cl}^-$$

Because $a\text{AgCl}$ and $a\text{Ag}$ are both unity (because both components are present as pure substances), the expression for the electrode potential reduces to

$$E = E^\circ - N \times \log a\text{Cl}^-$$

This equation shows that the electrode measures Cl$^-$ activity. This electrode has been used for direct measurement of the Cl$^-$ activity in serum. By placing it directly on the skin surface, the electrode also is used for the measurement of the Cl$^-$ activity of sweat in connection with the diagnosis of cystic fibrosis (see Chapter 25).

Similarly, a silver/silver bromide electrode, a silver/silver iodide electrode, and a silver/silver sulfide electrode measure Br^- activity, I^- activity, and S^{2-} activity, respectively. Unfortunately, because the porous silver halide coating allows the solution to come in contact with the silver metal substrate, these electrodes are quite sensitive to other redox couples in the test solution and thus often fail to function properly in biological solutions.

The calomel electrode consists of mercury covered by a layer of calomel (Hg_2Cl_2), which is in contact with an electrolyte solution containing Cl^-. The electrode process is as follows:

$$1/2\ Hg_2Cl_2\ (solid) + e^- \rightleftharpoons Hg\ (metal) + Cl^-$$

Because aHg and aHg_2Cl_2 are both unity (present as pure substances), the electrode potential reduces to

$$E = E^\circ - N \times \log aCl^-$$

This equation shows that the calomel electrode also functions as a chloride electrode and that its potential varies with the Cl^- activity. Cl^- activity generally is maintained constant, either as saturated potassium chloride or at a concentration of 3.5 (or 4.0) mol/L. Calomel electrodes frequently are used for pH measurement as reference electrodes together with glass electrodes.

Ion-selective membrane electrodes

Membrane potentials are caused by the permeability of certain types of membranes to selected anions or cations. Biological membranes often are permeable to small ions but impermeable to protein ions. This fact gives rise to the Donnan potential, which in turn leads to an uneven distribution of the diffusible ions on both sides of the membrane. For analytical applications, membranes that possess selective permeabilities for a single ion species are required.

The ion-selective membrane, which separates the solution on the left side (1) from the solution on the right side (2), can be illustrated as

$$1\,|\,Membrane\,|\,2 \qquad\qquad (10)$$

The membrane potential is defined conventionally as the right-side potential minus the left-side potential. The potentials of solutions 1 and 2 are measured with any suitable reference electrode. When a glass membrane is used, the potential of the reference solution (1) generally is measured by means of a silver/silver chloride electrode, whereas the potential of a test solution (2) is measured by means of a calomel (or silver/silver chloride) electrode via a salt-bridge junction between the saturated potassium chloride and test solutions.

If the activity of a diffusible cation is higher in solution 1 than in solution 2, a positive membrane potential develops. On the left side, where the cation activity is high, cations are bound to the membrane surface by specific binding groups; the membrane thus becomes positively charged. This charging of the membrane causes a dissociation of cations from the other side of the membrane into the solution on the right side, which thus becomes positively charged with respect to the solution on the left side. Therefore it appears as if the membrane were permeable to the cation only. This process proceeds until an equilibrium is established, which occurs when the electrical potential difference across the membrane matches the difference in activity of the diffusible ions on the two sides of the membrane. The membrane potential is given by the Nernst equation

$$E = -\frac{R \times T}{z \times F} \times \ln \frac{a(2)}{a(1)} \qquad\qquad (11)$$

where z is the ion charge number (positive for cations, negative for anions), and a is the activity of the diffusible ion (cation or anion). If solution 2 is a reference solution with constant activity of the diffusible ion (constant $a[2]$), the equation reduces to

$$E = E' + \frac{N}{z} \times \log a(1) \qquad\qquad (12)$$

where E' is constant and the membrane potential is proportional directly to the logarithm of the activity of the diffusible ion in the test solution (Figure 6-2).

Many different types of membrane electrodes have been designed. For example, electrodes may be flat or bulb shaped, inverted flat or bulb shaped, capillary type, needle type, or flow through. Miniaturize electrodes also have been designed for direct measurement in the blood stream (catheter-tip electrodes)[2,9] or for measurements in single cells (glass capillary microelectrodes).

Ion-selective membrane electrodes are classified arbitrarily as (1) glass electrodes, (2) solid-state electrodes, or (3) liquid ion-exchange electrodes. These electrodes may be modified further into gas electrodes or enzyme electrodes through the use of additional membranes.

Glass electrodes

Glass electrodes are constructed from specially formulated glasses consisting of a melt of silicon dioxide with added oxides of various metals. Membranes with varying compositions of the glass and with directed selectivities for H^+, Na^+, K^+, Li^+, Rb^+, Cs^+, Ag^+, Tl^+, and NH_4^+ have been prepared. The membranes generally have thicknesses of 10 to 100 μm. Depending on the type of glass, the electrical resistance is high (about 10 to 800 MΩ at room temperature) and increases considerably as the temperature decreases.

H^+-selective glass electrodes (pH electrodes) can be manufactured from a special type of glass (Corning 015) consisting of silicon dioxide, sodium oxide, and calcium oxide in the molar ratio of 72.2 : 21.4 : 6.4. An alternative glass that is more selective to H^+ consists of silicon dioxide, lithium oxide, and calcium oxide in the ratio 68 : 25 : 7. Other suitable compositions also exist.

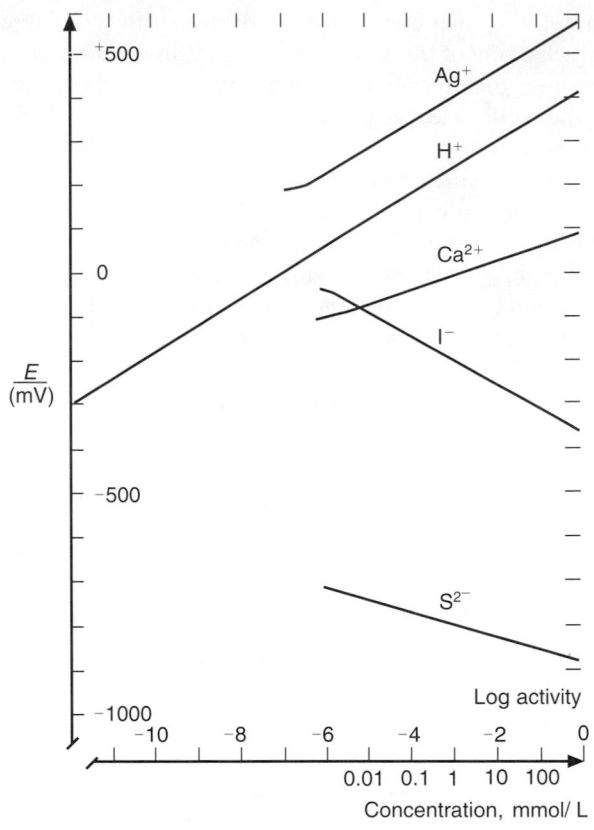

Figure 6-2   Illustration of the Nernst equation, that is, the relationship between the electromotive force of an ion-selective electrode chain (E) and the logarithm of the activity of the ion (log aI')

$$E = E' + \frac{R \times T \times \ln 10}{z \times F} \times \log aI'$$

where E' is constant at constant temperature (depending on the type of reference electrodes), and z is the charge number for the ion (positive for cations, negative for anions). The slope for the monovalent ions is ± 59.16 mV; for divalent ions, it is ± 29.58 mV ($T = 298.15$ K). The abscissa also indicates the concentration of free ions, provided the activity coefficient is taken to be 1.

The glass membrane of the electrode may be shaped according to the requirements of the application. It is bulblike for most titration purposes and flat for surface measurements, but it has an inverted bulb shape when used for microanalysis. For pH measurements in blood, thermal regulation of the capillary glass electrode has proved especially useful (Figure 6-3).

Na^+-selective glass electrodes are prepared from glass consisting of silicon dioxide, sodium oxide, and aluminum oxide in the ratio of 71:11:18. Lithium aluminum silicates also are suitable. Electrodes with flat surfaces have been used for the direct measurement of Na^+ activity on the skin surface for the diagnosis of cystic fibrosis. Capillary electrodes have been constructed for measurements of Na^+ in serum or serum dilutions.

Because of insufficient selectivity of K^+ over Na^+, K^+-selective glass electrodes are less satisfactory for serum measurements than are the Na^+-electrodes. Attempts have

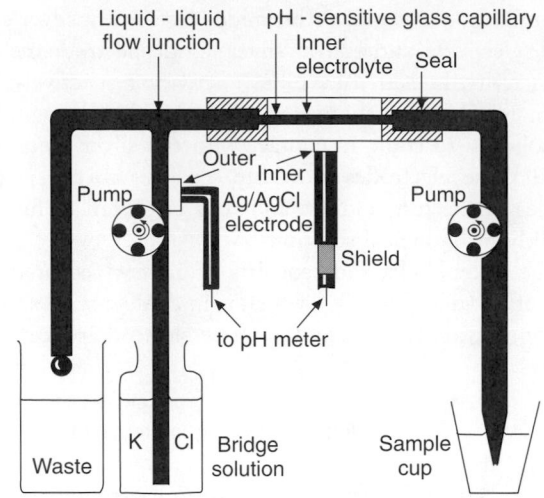

Figure 6-3   Schematic illustration of a capillary glass electrode for pH measurement in a flow system. The sample and salt bridge solution are pumped simultaneously through the tubing. An open liquid-liquid flow junction is established where they meet.

been made to measure H^+, Na^+, and K^+ in serum simultaneously with three different glass electrodes by use of a computer for calculation of the correction for the different electrodes based on their selectivity. Glass electrodes selective to Li^+ and NH_4^+ also are available.

Solid-state electrodes
A membrane used in a solid-state electrode is either a homogeneous membrane consisting of a "single" crystal or a heterogeneous membrane consisting of an active substance embedded in an inert matrix.

The homogeneous-membrane electrodes include those for F^- (europium-doped lanthanum fluoride crystal), Cl^- (silver chloride), Br^- (silver bromide), I^- (silver iodide), S^{2-} (silver sulfide), Cu^{2+} (cupric selenide), and others. The silver salt solid-state membrane electrodes are less susceptible to interference from redox systems than are the equivalent silver/silver salt redox electrodes. The silver chloride membrane electrode is used for measurement of the activity of Cl^- in sweat by direct measurement on the skin surface. The fluoride electrode has been used for measurements of the F^- concentration in blood, urine, and saliva, as well as in bone and tooth enamel after dissolution.

Ion-exchange electrodes
An ion-exchange electrode utilizes a liquid ion-exchange membrane consisting of an inert solvent in which ion-selective carrier substances are dissolved. The membrane solution can be separated from the test solution by means of a collodion membrane, or a porous matrix can be impregnated with the membrane solution. The inert solvent (plasticizer) and the ion-selective carrier often are embedded in a matrix of polyvinyl chloride (PVC) that is obtained when solutions of PVC in tetrahydrofuran are evaporated into thin semi-

solid membranes. Many different membranes with selectivities for specific cations or anions (for example, for K^+, NH_4^+, Ca^{2+}, and H^+) have been prepared.

K^+-selective membranes are made when the antibiotic valinomycin is dissolved in a suitable solvent. Valinomycin is a neutral carrier that binds K^+ in the center of a ring of oxygen atoms (Figure 6-4). This membrane is highly selective for K^+ and is used widely for the measurement of K^+ in blood and biological tissues.

The NH_4^+-selective membrane is based on a mixture of the neutral-carrier antibiotics nonactin and monactin. A Ca^{2+}-selective membrane is made when the calcium salt Ca^{2+}-bis(di-p-octylphenyl phosphate) is dissolved in PVC. Two di-p-octylphenyl phosphate ions bind to a calcium ion to act as the Ca^{2+} carrier. A neutral carrier also has been used that binds the Ca^{2+} in a neutral pocket in a manner similar to the binding of K^+ by valinomycin.

Operationally, the ion-selective membrane of an ion-exchange electrode often becomes coated with protein, causing a lack of reproducibility. This problem is avoided by covering of the ion-selective membrane with a dialysis membrane. The ion-selective membrane then measures the activity of the ion in a thin layer of protein-free dialysate under the dialysis membrane. The activity of the ion is not the same in this dialysate as in the original sample because the nondiffusible protein ions cause an uneven distribution of the diffusible ions (Donnan distribution). However, this apparent bias is balanced exactly by the Donnan potential across the dialysis membrane, and the Donnan potential is included in the total cell potential. A disadvantage of using a dialysis membrane is the significant prolongation of the response time of the electrode from less than 1 second to more than 20 seconds for a 98% response.

Gas electrodes

Gas electrodes are specially designed for the measurement of specific gases in gas mixtures or in solutions. Examples are the carbon dioxide and ammonia electrodes, both of which are based on potentiometric measurement through the use of a pH-glass electrode. The oxygen electrode is based on amperometric measurement with a polarized platinum cathode. (The latter will be discussed in a subsequent section of this chapter.) In one design the gas electrode is separated from the test solution by a thin, hydrophobic, gas-permeable membrane (for example, one made of polyethylene, polypropylene, microporous Teflon, or silicone rubber), but the separation may also simply be a small "air gap."

The carbon dioxide electrode (or more correctly termed, the *carbon dioxide cell*, because both electrodes are incorporated into a single sensor) represents a special application of a pH-glass electrode (Figure 6-5). The sample in this case is in contact with a membrane that is permeable to gas but not to solutions. This membrane is separated from the actual glass electrode by a thin film of bicarbonate solution (5 mmol/L). The carbon dioxide gas diffuses from the sample

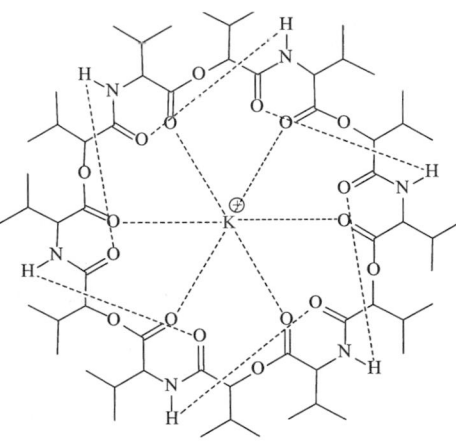

Figure 6-4 Valinomycin has a heterocyclical structure consisting of alternating peptide and ester linkages. The molecule is cylindrical, stabilized by six hydrogen bridges (from $-NH$ to $C=O$). The outer surface of the cylinder is strongly hydrophobic, and the interior is strongly hydrophilic. The size of the central cavity nearly equals the diameter of an unhydrated potassium ion.

(or test gas) through the membrane and rapidly equilibrates with the bicarbonate solution, thus altering its pH. The pH of the bicarbonate solution is a simple function of the partial pressure of carbon dioxide (P_{CO_2}) obtained by rearrangement of the Henderson-Hasselbalch equation

$$pH = -s \times \log P_{CO_2} - \log \alpha + pK' + \log cHCO_3^-$$

where:

s — Relative sensitivity of the electrode (normally 0.95 to 1.00)

α = Solubility coefficient of carbon dioxide in the bicarbonate solution

K' = Apparent, overall, first dissociation constant of carbonic acid

The carbon dioxide electrode has been used extensively for transcutaneous and arterial blood sample measurements.

The ammonia electrode is the same as the carbon dioxide electrode except that the bicarbonate solution is replaced with an ammonium chloride solution. Again, the measured pH of the ammonium chloride solution behind the gas-permeable membrane varies linearly with the logarithm of the partial pressure of ammonia (P_{NH_3}).

Combination ion/carbon dioxide sensors

Polymer membrane electrodes have been developed for the simultaneous measurement of an ionic constituent (for example, hydrogen or potassium ions) and the partial pressure of carbon dioxide in the sample. These devices, easily fabricated and mass produced by thick-film technology (that is, screen printing and automated solution dispensing equipment), have become the basis for some of the newer blood pH/gas measurement systems for point-of-care testing.[4,7,15]

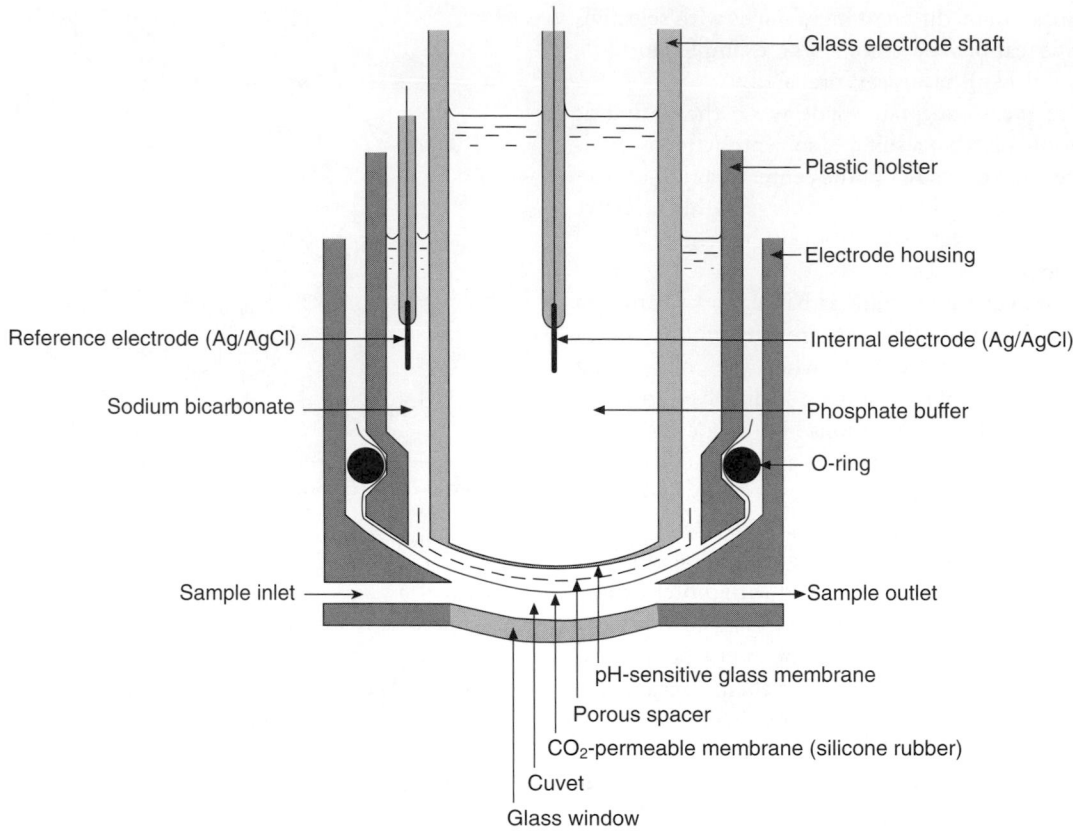

Reference electrode (Ag/AgCl)

Sodium bicarbonate

Sample inlet →

Glass electrode shaft

Plastic holster

Electrode housing

Internal electrode (Ag/AgCl)

Phosphate buffer

O-ring

→ Sample outlet

pH-sensitive glass membrane

Porous spacer

CO_2-permeable membrane (silicone rubber)

Cuvet

Glass window

Figure 6-5   Schematic illustration of a P_{CO_2} (partial pressure of carbon dioxide) electrode. (From Siggaard-Andersen O: The Acid-Base Status of the Blood, 4th edition, p 172, Baltimore, Williams & Wilkins, 1974.)

As illustrated in Figure 6-6, the sensor consists of an ionophore-containing polymeric membrane (for example, tridodecylamine for H^+ or valinomycin for K^+) sealed atop separate compartments containing the internal reference solutions in contact with internal Ag/AgCl reference electrodes. One reference solution contains a strong pH buffer plus KCl, whereas the second contains a solution of bicarbonate and KCl. For example, in the pH/CO_2 sensor, both membranes respond identically to pH because the hydrogen ion activity is sensed only by the outer surface of the membrane containing the lipophilic, tertiary amine ionophore. However, although the membrane is readily permeable to CO_2 (for example, silicone rubber, polyurethane, or PVC), the strong pH buffer in one compartment is not affected by changes in the P_{CO_2}. The bicarbonate solution in the second compartment, however, acts like a classical Severinghaus electrode (see Figure 6-5), whereby the pH of this inner solution reflects the P_{CO_2}, and this pH change is sensed by the inner surface of the pH membrane. Consequently, one half of the sensor responds to pH alone, whereas the other half responds to both pH and P_{CO_2}. By the use of an external reference electrode and differential amplifiers, separate outputs, corresponding to the two analytes, are monitored.

These sensors are mass-produced and consequently are inexpensive, disposable, and sufficiently reproducible for

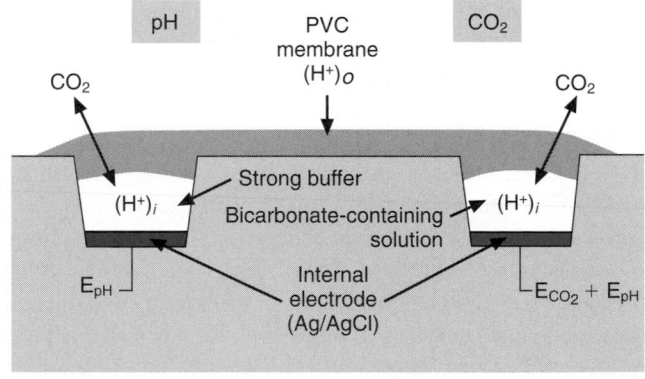

Figure 6-6   Schematic illustration of a combination pH-CO_2 sensor. Except for differences in the internal solutions the sensor components are identical and can be mass-produced easily for use in point-of-care blood gas analyzers.

multiple measurements. Also, because of their small size, they can be dried partially for long-term storage and rehydrated almost immediately on contact with the sample or calibrant solution.

Liquid junction potential

The liquid junction potential constitutes the most important source of bias in potentiometric measurements of ion activities. Diffusion potentials arise at a liquid junction (1∶∶2), where two solutions of different ionic compositions are in direct contact. If cations diffuse faster from left to right than do anions, a positive liquid junction potential develops at the interface. Diffusion potentials are due to irreversible processes and therefore are more difficult to calculate than true equilibrium potentials; however, such potentials often can be calculated with good approximation through use of the Henderson equation.

Operationally, a need exists for reduction of the liquid junction potential to a value as low and as reproducible as possible. This reduction is achieved through use of a concentrated potassium chloride solution as a bridge solution (3.5 mol/L, or saturated = 4.52 mol/L at 37 °C). The potential then is dominated by the large excess of K^+ and Cl^- diffusing at almost the same rates into the test solution, and the potential becomes largely independent of the composition of the test solution. As an example, the following values may be calculated for the liquid junction potential *(Ej)* at 37 °C:

$$KCl(4.32\ mol/kg) ∶∶ NIST\text{-}phosphate\ buffer\ (7.395),$$
$$E_j = -3.7\ mV$$
$$KCl\ (4.32\ mol/kg) ∶∶ normal\ plasma, \quad E_j = -2.5\ mV$$

The difference between the junction potential with the test solution (plasma) and calibration solution (phosphate buffer) is called the *residual liquid junction potential;* in the previous example this potential is +1.2 mV. Such a residual liquid junction potential gives a positive bias on the measured hydrogen ion activity of approximately 5%. To reduce the residual liquid junction potential, the composition of the calibration solution should match that of the test solution as closely as possible.

Erythrocytes present at the junction with concentrated potassium chloride as the bridge solution increase the liquid junction potential (about +0.6 mV when whole blood and plasma are compared). This action may be due to an osmotic effect of the concentrated bridge solution; water is drawn out of the red cells, changing the ionic concentrations at the liquid junction. This event occurs because precipitated proteins and cremated erythrocytes at the liquid junction act as ion exchangers, influencing the diffusion rate of the ions (slowing Cl^- more than K^+). When a flowing junction is used, the effect is reduced to about one third. Using a different bridge solution also is possible. For example, with 4 mol/kg sodium formate as a bridge solution, the effect of erythrocytes on the junction potential is negligible, and measurements on whole blood give the same result as measurements on the corresponding plasma. The potential of the junction: 1∶∶2, may be estimated by the Henderson equation

$$E_j = \frac{R \times T}{F} \times \frac{f(1) - f(2)}{g(1) - g(2)} \times \ln\frac{g(1)}{g(2)}$$

$$f = \Sigma m_i \times \frac{\lambda_i}{z_i}$$

$$g = \Sigma m_i \times \lambda_i \qquad (13)$$

where λ_i is the limiting molar conductance of the ions

$$unit,\ mS \times \frac{m_2}{mol}$$

For example, at 37 °C, for K^+ [9.1]; Na^+ [6.4]; Cl^- [9.6]; HCO_3^- [5.9]; $HCOO^-$ [6.8]; $H_2PO_4^-$ [4.8]; $HPO_4^=$ [15.1]; Ca^{2+} [14.0]. The liquid junction potential is, in principle, inaccessible for direct measurement, and the calculated value is only a rough estimate. Note that thermal diffusion potentials may arise at a liquid junction at which two identical solutions of different temperatures are in contact. Such thermal diffusion potentials should be avoided through maintenance of the whole cell at the same constant temperature.

■ VOLTAMMETRY

Voltammetry is an **electrolytic electrochemical cell** technique in which the electrolytic cell current is measured when the potential between the working electrode and reference electrode is varied as a function of time. Voltammetric techniques are used to study solution composition based on the current-potential relationships obtained when the potential of an electrochemical cell is varied under the control of a three-electrode potentiostat. In a three-electrode system the polarizable working electrode potential is measured potentiometrically at zero current between the working and reference electrodes, and the cell current is measured between the working and counter (or auxiliary) electrodes. Consequently, errors in the measurement of the cell potential, which are caused in a conventional two-electrode cell by the current flow through the resistive solution (known as the *IR drop*), are eliminated.

Because of the wide variety of excitation (potential-time) waveforms that can be used, a broad repertoire of voltammetric methods exists, including linear potential sweep (classical polarography and cyclical voltammetry), potential step (normal and differential pulse, and square-wave voltammetry), anodic and cathodic stripping voltammetry, and phase-sensitive AC voltammetry. **Polarography** describes the special case in which the working electrode is a dropping mercury electrode. This electrode is unique in that the electrode surface is renewed continuously, thus reducing the possibility of electrode fouling (contamination) by sample solution components, such as proteins and products of the electrochemical reaction.

Voltammetric methods are extremely sensitive and capable of multielement and speciation studies. For example, the pulse and stripping methods are among the most sensitive analytical techniques available, with detection limits as low as subparts-per-billion for certain electroactive analytes. Through judicious choice of experimental conditions and methods, several analytes often can be determined simultaneously in a single voltammetric experiment. In addition, voltammetric methods can distinguish between oxidation states, a factor that is often important in determination of the reactivity or toxicity of a substance.

In a voltammetric method the working electrode is placed in a solution of the particular electroactive substance or substances to be measured. As the potential of the working electrode is increased, a characteristic potential eventually is reached at which a current begins to flow; this potential signals the onset of an electrochemical reaction. If the test solution contains substances that are reduced more easily than H^+, the cathode is depolarized by these substances, and a current begins to flow through the cell. For example, if the test solution contains oxygen, the oxygen is reduced at the cathode according to the following reaction:

$$O_2 + 2H_2O + 4e^- \longrightarrow 4OH^-$$

When the characteristic potential for this reaction (~ -0.3 to -0.4 V) is reached, the current increases until it reaches a plateau (the so-called polarographic diffusion current). The height of the plateau is dependent on the rate at which oxygen can diffuse from the surrounding solution to the surface of the cathode (where partial pressure of oxygen [Po_2] is zero). The diffusion current therefore is directly proportional to the Po_2 of the test solution. Any substance that is reduced at the cathode is characterized by two parameters— (1) the polarographic half-wave potential (the potential at

which the current is equal to one-half the plateau current) that characterizes the substance being reduced and (2) the diffusion current, which is proportional to the concentration of the substance in the test solution (Figure 6-7).

In practice, polarography is used to identify and quantify analytes. For clinical applications, polarographic analysis is used for the determination of some metals, such as copper, lead, and zinc, and the characterization of proteins (for example, the Brdicka reaction between cobalt and the SH-groups of mucoproteins) in addition to the determination of oxygen. (The latter use will be discussed in subsequent sections.)

In the more sensitive technique of anodic stripping voltammetry a mercury-coated graphite rod frequently serves as a working electrode. When a negative potential is applied to the electrode, the trace metal ions in the sample are reduced and plate onto the electrode. The plating time is usually from 1 to 30 minutes, depending on the concentration of the metal ions. A voltammogram then is recorded, with the plated electrode as the anode and a nonpolarizable cathode. The metals are stripped off the anode via oxidation to the respective cations. The order in which they are stripped off is a function of the metal's unique redox potential. The current flow during the stripping of a given metal is a function of the amount of metal present. Thus trace metals in a biological fluid or tissue are both identified and quantified.

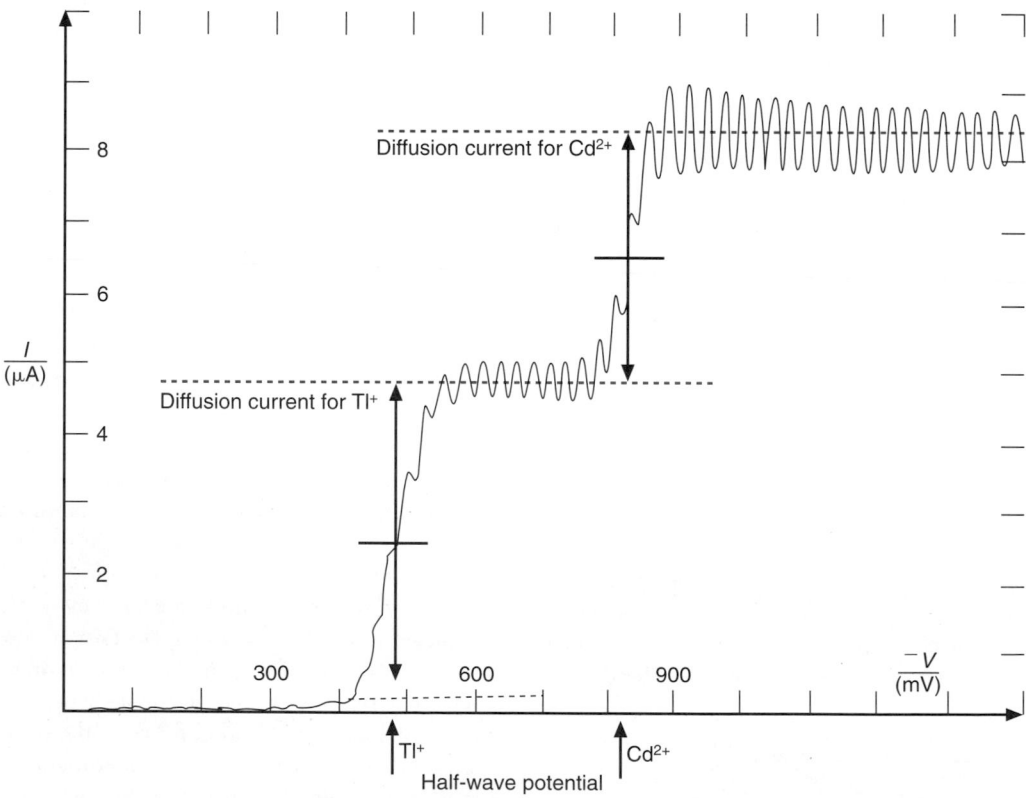

Figure 6-7   Voltammogram (polarogram) of a test solution containing TlCl (1.0 mmol/L) and CdCl$_2$ (0.5 mmol/L) in an ammonia/ammonium chloride buffer (1 mol/L). The abscissa shows the potential of the working electrode. The ordinate shows the current through the cell. The current oscillates because of the growth and detachment of the mercury drop at the dropping mercury electrode.

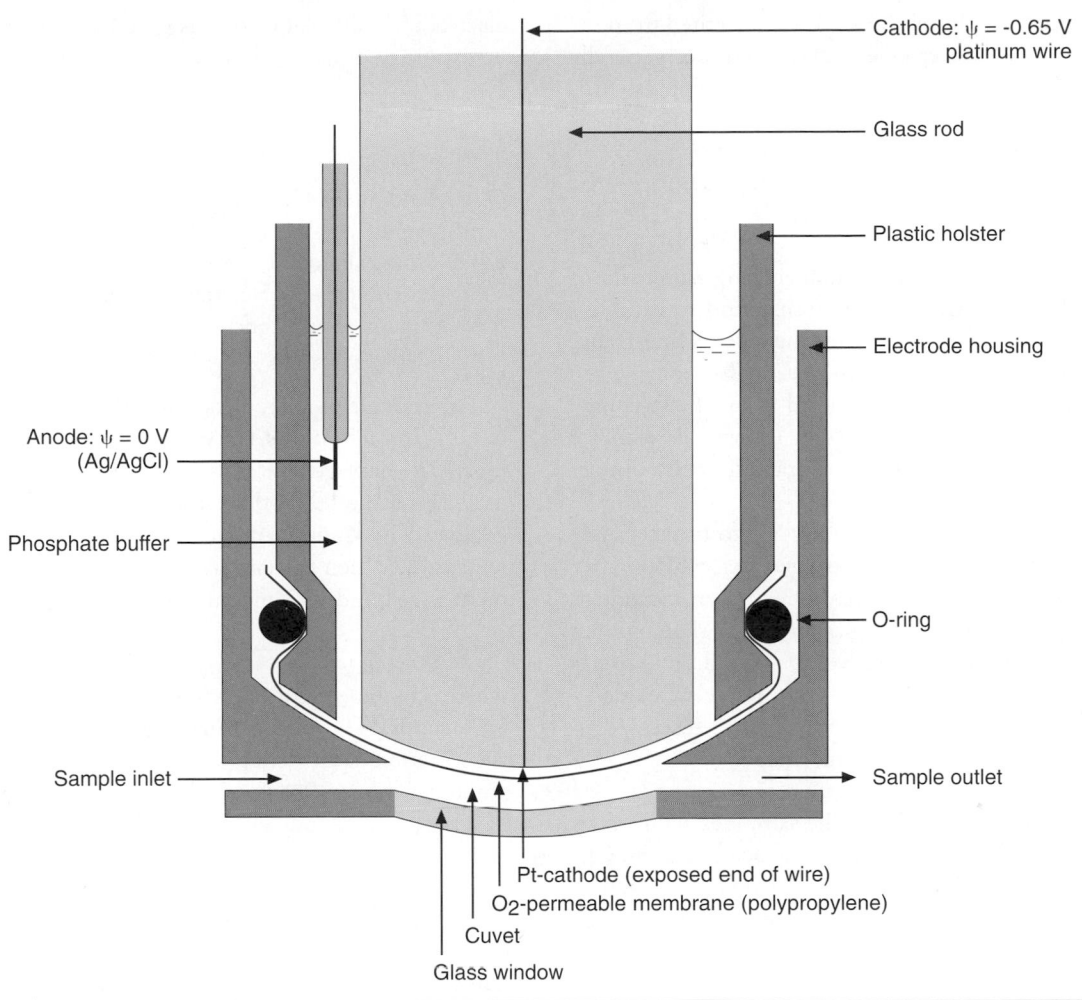

Figure 6-8   Schematic illustration of a PO_2 (partial pressure of oxygen) electrode. (From Siggaard-Andersen O: The Acid-Base Status of the Blood, 4th edition, p 178, Baltimore, Williams & Wilkins, 1974.)

In addition, the preconcentration (plating) step permits the analysis of extremely dilute samples.

A modification of the anodic stripping technique is known as *potentiometric stripping analysis.* After the initial plating step the electrode is left undisturbed, and the cell potential then measured as a function of time. The electrode reactions proceed in the reverse direction because of the presence of oxidizing species in the solution, such as Hg^{2+} or oxygen. During this process the potential remains almost constant, and the length of the plateau on the potential-time curve is proportional to the concentration of the first metal (chronopotentiometry). When the next metal begins to strip, a shift in potential is observed and the process is repeated.

■ AMPEROMETRY

Amperometry is an electrochemical technique based on the measurement of the current flowing through an electrochemical cell when a constant potential is applied to the electrodes.

The PO_2 Clark electrode, (Figure 6-8) is a complete electrochemical cell consisting of a small platinum cathode (with an area of about 300 μm^2) and a silver/silver chloride anode in a phosphate buffer with added potassium chloride. The platinum cathode, which is covered by a thin film of electrolyte, is separated from the test solution by a gas-permeable membrane such as polypropylene. The cathode potential is adjusted to -0.65 V. When oxygen is not present in the test solution, the current is nearly zero because the cathode is polarized. In the presence of oxygen a current is observed, caused by the the diffusion of oxygen from the test solution, through the membrane, and to the cathode, where it is reduced. The current is directly proportional to the PO_2 in the test solution. The sensitivity of commercial PO_2 electrodes is on the order of $\Delta I/\Delta PO_2 = 10^{-4}$ A/Pa, depending on the size of the cathode area and thickness of the gas-permeable membrane.

The purpose of the membrane is to (1) prevent proteins and other (dissolved) oxidants from gaining access to the cathode surface and (2) limit the diffusion zone to the membrane. Consequently, variations in the diffusion coefficient of oxygen in the test solution (or gas) are prevented from influencing the result. Nevertheless, PO_2 electrodes generally produce higher values in gases than in liquids; this gas-liquid ratio must be taken into account during calibration of the electrodes.

The PO_2 electrode has widespread application in the measurement of PO_2 in arterial and capillary blood. For example, special PO_2 electrodes with built-in heating coils have been developed for the transcutaneous measurement of arterial PO_2. Such electrodes have been found to exhibit a reasonably good correlation between the arterial and transcutaneous PO_2, especially in newborns. Unfortunately, the response is quite sensitive to the local blood flow; consequently, the correlation deteriorates in individuals who are in shock or whose conditions are characterized by diminished peripheral blood flow.

The PO_2 electrode also has been applied to the measurement of the concentration of total oxygen in the blood after liberation of hemoglobin-bound oxygen with ferricyanide or carbon monoxide (through formation of methemoglobin and carboxyhemoglobin, respectively). In addition, it has been used as the transducer in a broad range of oxidase-based enzyme electrodes. (These uses will be discussed in detail in a subsequent section of this chapter.)

Amperometric end-point determinations may be applied in the titration of Cl^- with Ag^+. The sample is acidified by means of nitric acid (or nitric plus acetic acid) and the Cl^- titrated with Ag^+. The Ag^+ may be added as a solution of silver nitrate (volumetric titration) or generated from a silver electrode by means of an electrical current (coulometric titration; see subsequent discussion). During titration the Ag^+ concentration remains low because of the reaction $Ag^+ + Cl^- \rightleftharpoons AgCl$, which causes the precipitation of silver chloride. At the end-point, Ag^+ appears in excess, and the increase in Ag^+ activity may be detected either potentiometrically (with a silver electrode and a mercury/mercurous sulfate reference electrode) or amperometrically. In the latter case two silver electrodes are used, and a negative potential of 0.15 to 0.25 V is applied to the cathode. During titration, the cathode is polarized, and the current is kept low. At the end of the titration the excess of Ag^+ depolarizes the cathode by the reaction $Ag^+ + e^- \rightleftharpoons Ag$, and a current flows; this current is proportional to the excess of Ag^+. When the current has reached a preset value the titration can be stopped automatically. This indicator principle is applied in the Cotlove chloride titrator, which also relies on the coulometric generation of Ag^+.

electrodes. This relationship is called *Faraday's law* and can be expressed as

$$Q = z \times n \times F \qquad (14)$$

where:

Q = Amount of electricity (unit: C [coulomb] = ampere $\times$ second) passing through the cell
z = Numerical stoichiometric number of electrons involved in the reduction (or oxidation) reaction (unit: 1)
n = Amount of substance reduced or oxidized (unit: mol)
F = Faraday constant (96,487 C $\times$ mol^{-1})

An example of an application is the coulometric titration of Cl^- (through use of the Cotlove titrator), in which silver ions (Ag^+) are generated by electrolysis from a silver wire used as the anode. At the cathode, H^+ is reduced to hydrogen gas. The amount of Ag^+ generated is measured coulometrically. When the current is kept constant, the measurement is reduced to a measurement of time according to

$$Q = I \times t \qquad (15)$$

where I is the electrical current (in amperes), and t is time (in seconds). The current also may be decreased gradually as the titration approaches the end point. In this case the amount of electricity is calculated as the integral

$$Q = \int_0^t I \times dt$$

This calculation is performed electronically by the coulometer. The end point of the titration may be detected either amperometrically or potentiometrically.

Acid-base titrations also can be performed coulometrically with a platinum generator electrode in the test solution separated from the other electrode by a sintered-glass filter. If the generator electrode is the cathode, H^+ is removed ($H^+ + e^- \rightleftharpoons 1/2H_2$), which is equivalent to the addition of base. If the generator electrode is the anode, H^+ is added ($H_2O \rightleftharpoons 1/2O_2 + 2H^+ + 2e^-$). In either case two sets of electrodes are necessary—the generator electrodes and the indicator electrodes. The latter may be used for direct potentiometric determination of the end point or in connection with an amperometric end-point determination. The position of the indicator electrode is adjusted in relation to the generator electrodes so that the current through the latter does not disturb the performance of the former. Coulometric titrations are among the most accurate analytical determinations available.

COULOMETRY

Coulometry is the electrochemical technique used to measure the amount of electricity (or charge) passing between two electrodes in an electrochemical cell. The amount of electricity is directly proportional to the amount of substance produced or consumed by the redox process at the

CONDUCTOMETRY

Conductance (G) is defined as the current (unit: A) divided by the potential difference (unit: V); its unit is the siemen (S). One siemen (S) is equal to one reciprocal ohm (Ω^{-1}). Electrolytic conductance is a measure of the ability of a solution of electrolytes to carry an electrical current by the migration of ions under the influence of a potential gradient. The rate of ionic migration (the current) is dependent on the ionic charge and size, solvent viscosity, and magnitude (and frequency) of the applied potential. Conductivity (κ) is defined as the current density (unit: $A \times m^{-2}$) divided by the electrical field strength (unit: $V \times m^{-1}$); the unit therefore is $\Omega^{-1} \times m^{-1} = S \times m^{-1}$.

Conductometry is the measurement of the current flow between two nonpolarized electrodes and between which a known electrical potential is established. To avoid polarization of the electrodes an alternating potential with a frequency between 100 and 3000 Hz usually is applied. As the conductivity of the solution increases, impedance (resistance) lessens and current flow in turn increases. (Because the applied potential is alternating, the resulting current also is alternating.) The current is directly proportional to the conductivity of the solution.

The conductivity of aqueous solutions is dependent on the concentration of electrolytes and closely related to their ionic strength. The conductivity of pure water is $\kappa = 4.9 \times 10^{-6}\ S \times m^{-1}$ at 18 °C. In ordinary distilled or deionized water the value is $\kappa < 2 \times 10^{-4}\ S \times m^{-1}$. A higher conductivity indicates the presence of electrolytes; thus conductivity measurements monitor the performance of water deionizers and indicate whether the ion exchange resin should be regenerated.

Some chemical reactions are associated with a change in conductivity of the reaction medium. For example, urea can be measured rapidly and accurately by the change or initial rate of change in conductivity that accompanies the urease-catalyzed formation of NH_4^+ and HCO_3^-. However, the high conductivity of biological fluids prevents the use of this technique for analytes of low concentrations in which the change in conductivity caused by the analyte is small, compared with a high-background conductivity. Conductivity measurement also is used for end-point detection in many kinds of titrations (for example, acid-base, precipitation, and compleximetric).

The Coulter principle for electronic counting of blood cells in suspension relies on the fact that the conductivity of blood cells is lower than that of the salt solution used as suspension medium. The cell suspension is forced through a tiny orifice. Two electrodes are placed on either side of the orifice, and a constant current is established between the electrodes. Each time a cell passes through the orifice, the resistance increases, causing a spike in the electrical potential difference between the electrodes. The pulses then are amplified and counted.

■ BIOSENSORS

For the purposes of this text a **biosensor** is a device or system in which an immobilized biological/biochemical component interacts with the analyte to produce, via an appropriate transducer, a signal proportional to the quantity or activity of analyte. The recognition interaction may entail either a binding process with antibodies, DNA probes, and natural cell receptors, or a biochemical reaction mediated by enzymes, organelles, intact cells, tissues, or entire organs.[5,16] Transduction can be achieved by any of the electrochemical measurement techniques discussed previously. However, many of the same biorecognition processes are used with other transduction mechanisms, such as optical, mass, and heat measurements.

Enzyme Biosensors

In an enzyme biosensor an enzyme-catalyzed reaction is coupled with either an amperometric or potentiometric electrode.

Amperometric biosensors

In 1962 Clark and Lyons developed an enzyme electrode for glucose that coupled a PO_2 electrode with a glucose oxidase catalyzed reaction. Under standardized conditions the electrode response to the decrease in PO_2 was a measure of the glucose concentration of the sample. In the original design the enzyme solution physically was trapped between a gas-permeable membrane and a dialysis membrane through which the glucose and oxygen, but not the enzyme, could pass. By reversing its polarity, the oxygen electrode becomes specific for hydrogen peroxide and can be coupled with any enzyme reaction that produces it. However, because hydrogen peroxide is produced and not consumed, as is oxygen, the electrode response to this quantity is related directly to analyte concentration and is independent of variations in the oxygen content of the sample. Analytes that have been analyzed through this amperometric technique include acetylcholine, lactate, uric acid, and ethanol. In these cases the membrane contains acetylcholinesterase, lactate oxidase, uricase, or alcohol oxidase, respectively. Sensors using multienzyme cascades (for example, a sucrose electrode using invertase, mutarotase, and glucose oxidase) also have been developed.[3]

Another development in the area of amperometric enzyme electrodes is the coupling of the electron-transfer (redox) process to the metal or carbon transducer electrode. However, direct coupling of an oxido-reductase enzyme and an electrode generally is not feasible because of slow electron-transfer kinetics. Alternative strategies have involved (1) "reengineering" of the enzyme itself, (2) modification of the electrode surface, or (3) use of electron-transfer mediators. In the modified enzymes, redox centers are incorporated into the structure of the enzyme to promote electron conduction to the surface, where electron transfer to an electrode can occur. Chemical modification of the electrode surface usually entails the immobilization of the enzyme through covalent binding via a prosthetic group, such as flavin adenine dinucleotide, or through the use of an electrically conducting polymer film, such as polypyrrole, or conducting organic salts, such as tetrathiafulvalene tetracyanoquinodimethane. The use of electron-transfer mediators, which shuttle electrons between the enzyme and the electrode surface, also has been successful in the coupling of the enzymatic redox process to the electrode. The mediators are reduced more easily than is the usual cofactor, oxygen; thus they provide independence from variations in the oxygen tension of the sample and either are solubilized in the ambient sample solution or immobilized onto the electrode surface. However, even the soluble mediators are usually of low solubility, and they tend to adsorb onto the electrode. Examples of electron-transfer mediators are benzoquinone, methylene blue, viologen, and ferrocene and its derivatives.

A successful application of a mediated enzyme electrode is the amperometric glucose electrode, which uses a ferrocene derivative as its mediator. In the original design, dimethyl ferrocene was incorporated into a graphite electrode, onto which glucose oxidase was immobilized. In operation the glucose oxidase that was reduced in the enzymatic reaction is reoxidized by electrochemically generated ferricinium ions. The current flowing in this regeneration process is proportional to the glucose concentration. Commercial devices based on this reaction are available to diabetic patients for home use. Additional membranes often are necessary to obtain the desired measurement range, which is the case with the glucose electrode for direct measurement in whole blood. Without a membrane the glucose electrode only measures glucose concentrations up to about 54.5 mg/dL (3 mmol/L), at which point the glucose oxidase becomes saturated. Covering the electrode with a polyurethane membrane reduces glucose diffusion to the enzyme layer, and the upper limit of the measurement range is increased to 550 to 900 mg/dL (30 to 50 mmol/L).

Potentiometric biosensors

The first potentiometric enzyme electrodes were based on glass-pH and cation- or anion-selective electrodes. An example of this type of biosensor was the urea-sensing electrode, in which urease is entrapped in a gel layer on the surface of a NH_4^+-sensitive electrode (Figure 6-9). The urease-catalyzed reaction produces ammonia that hydrolyzes to form NH_4^+ that is sensed by the electrode. This approach can be used with most deaminase enzymes. A variety of such potentiometric sensors also has been based on the pH electrode (for example, electrodes for penicillin, in which penicillinase hydrolyzes the β-lactam ring of penicillin, causing an increase in the H^+ activity; and for glucose, in which the enzymatic production of gluconic acid is measured). In addition, the I^--selective electrode has been used for the determination of glucose, cholesterol, and alcohols through use of a double-enzyme approach in which peroxidase is combined with various oxidase enzymes. In the resulting reaction the hydrogen peroxide produced by the oxidase enzyme is reduced to water by the peroxidase while it simultaneously oxidizes I^- to iodine. The resulting decrease in the iodide activity is sensed by the I^--selective electrode.

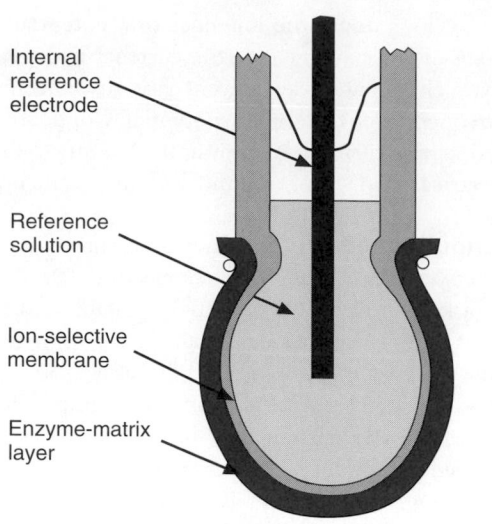

Figure 6-9 Schematic illustration of a potentiometric enzyme electrode. The cation-selective glass electrode surface is modified with an enzyme entrapped in a gel layer. (From Durst RA: Ion-selective electrodes in science, medicine, and technology. Am Sci 1971; 59:353.)

Potentiometric, gas-sensing electrodes that incorporate enzymes have been developed to measure ammonia and carbon dioxide. These sensors are used with deaminase and decarboxylase enzymes, which produce the respective gases that pass through the gas-permeable membrane of the gas-sensing electrode. These electrodes are basically the same as the conventional gas-sensing electrode (see Figure 6-5), with the addition of a thin layer of enzyme between the gas-permeable membrane and the solution and often with a dialysis membrane separating the enzyme layer from the actual biological fluid sample. One of the most important advantages of this sensor design, especially for complex biological media, is the freedom from ionic interferences that cannot pass through the gas-permeable membrane. However, variations in the natural levels of these gases in clinical samples produce errors, and consequently, differential measurements are required. Examples of successful ammonia-based enzyme electrodes are urea, aspartame, and creatinine, as well as amino acids, such as phenylalanine and adenosine. Enzyme sensors based on the carbon dioxide electrode include urea, oxalate, and amino acids.

Nonenzymatic Biosensors

In addition to purified enzymes and enzyme combinations used effectively in the development of biosensors, biological cells, tissues, and organs also have been used for such purposes.[12] In general, the design of these sensors is similar to enzyme biosensors with the biocomponent being isolated between the sensing transducer and a microporous retaining membrane. Examples of these types of electrodes include various alcohols and sugars (with bacterial cultures), amino acids and urea (with plant and animal tissue slices), and amino acids and hormones (with chemoreceptors and neuronal structures).

Because of its high specificity, immunological recognition is finding increasing application in the field of biosensors.[13] The antigen-antibody binding reaction occurs without product generation or significant measurable perturbations, so the coupling of this process to a transducer requires considerable ingenuity to obtain meaningful signals. In general, when the antibody is the component immobilized on the transducer, the complementary ligand is the measured analyte. When the ligand is immobilized, the receptor molecule concentration is detected. However, these schemes have been modified through the use of various competitive binding strategies.

Detection is achieved with immnosensors by direct or indirect approaches. In the direct sensing scheme a detectable physical or chemical signal accompanies the immulological reaction. This signal may involve a change in the spectral properties of the receptor or ligand, heat evolution or absorption, or a mass change produced by the binding interaction. Usually, such changes are small and difficult to measure and quantify, as evidenced by the relatively few reports of successful applications in the literature.

Most of the "immunobiosensors" use indirect sensing, in which a secondary process that is related to the immunological reaction is measured.[8] The secondary process usually entails the use of a label that is covalently attached to either the ligand or receptor and normally used in a competitive binding approach. In general, these sensors cannot be used for continuous monitoring because washing and regeneration steps are required between discrete sample measurements. The most commonly used electrochemical assay formats are those of competitive or sandwich enzyme immunoassays in which many of the same approaches used with conventional enzyme electrodes are incorporated into the biosensor. These approaches include amperometric immunoassays based on enzymes that produce peroxide (or remove oxygen) or that generate nongaseous electroactive products and nonenzymatic approaches that use electroactive labels conjugated to the receptors or ligands. Potentiometric immunosensors are based on the potential changes that occur when immobilized receptors or ligands undergo specific binding reactions or on more sensitive approaches that use enzymes to generate products detected by gas- or ion-selective electrodes.

Applications

Biosensors are useful for a variety of clinical applications and are incorporated into many point-of-care devices. For example, new or improved biosensors now are available to measure bacteria, bile acids, blood gases, cholesterol, choline, creatinine, DNA, ethanol, glucose in vivo, heparin, homocysteine, lactate, proteins, toxic metals, and urea.[1,3,8,10,11,14]

References

1. Billard P, DuBow MS: Bioluminescence-based assays for detection and characterization of bacteria and chemicals in clinical laboratories. Clin Biochem 1998; 31:1-14.

2. Csoregi E, Quinn CP, Schmidtke DW et al: Design, characterization, and one-point in vivo calibration of a subcutaneously implanted glucose electrode. Anal Chem 1994; 66:3131-3138.

3. Durst RA, Siggaard-Andersen O: Electrochemistry. In Burtis CA, Ashwood ER (eds): Tietz Textbook of Clinical Chemistry, 3rd edition, pp 133-149, Philadelphia, WB Saunders, 1999.

4. Erickson KA, Wilding P: Evaluation of a novel point-of-care system: the i-STAT portable clinical analyzer. Clin Chem 1993; 39:283-287.

5. Hill HA, Davis JJ: Biosensors: past, present and future. Biochem Soc Trans 1999; 27:331-335.

6. Inczedy J, Lengyel T, Ure AM: IUPAC Compendium of Analytical Nomenclature, 3rd edition, Oxford, Blackwell Science, 1998.

7. Jacobs E, Vadasdi E, Sarkozi L et al: Analytical evaluation of i-STAT portable clinical analyzer and use by nonlaboratory health-care professionals. Clin Chem 1993; 39:1069-1074.

8. Morgan CL, Newman DJ, Price CP: Immunosensors: technology and opportunities in laboratory medicine. Clin Chem 1996; 42:193-209.

9. Moussy F, Harrison DJ, O'Brien DW et al: Performance of subcutaneously implanted needle-type glucose sensors employing a novel trilayer coating. Anal Chem 1993; 65:2072-2077.

10. Pandey PC, Weetall HH: Application of photochemical reaction in electrochemical detection of DNA intercalation. Anal Chem 1994; 66:1236-1241.

11. Ramanathan S, Ensor M, Daunert S: Bacterial biosensors for monitoring toxic metals. Trends Biotechnol 1997; 15:500-506.

12. Rechnitz GA, Ho MY: Biosensors based on cell and tissue material. J Biotechnol 1990; 15:201-217.

13. Van Regenmortel MH, Altschuh D, Chatellier J et al: Measurement of antigen-antibody interactions with biosensors. J Mol Recognit 1998; 11:163-167.

14. Wang J: Electroanalysis and biosensors. Anal Chem 1995; 67:487-492R.

15. Wong RJ, Mahoney JJ, Harvey JA et al: StatPal II pH and blood gas analysis system evaluated. Clin Chem 1994; 40:124-129.

16. Ziegler C, Gopel W: Biosensor development. Curr Opin Chem Biol 1998; 2:585-591.

Additional Reading

Anderson JL, Bowden EM, Pickup PG: Dynamic electrochemistry: methodology and application. Anal Chem 1996; 68:379-492R.

Bard AJ, Faulkner L: Electroanalytical Chemistry, New York, Marcel Dekker, 1994.

Hamann CH, Vielstich W, Hamnett A: Electrochemistry, New York, John Wiley & Sons, 1998.

Henry C: Getting under the skin: implantable glucose sensors. Anal Chem 1998; 70:594A-598A.

Wang J: Analytical Electrochemistry, New York, VCH, 1994.

CHAPTER 7

Electrophoresis

RAYMOND E. KARCHER, PhD, and KERN L. NUTTALL, MD, PhD

Objectives

1. Define *electrophoresis* and provide a brief description of its theory.
2. State the uses of electrophoretic procedures in a laboratory setting.
3. State the purposes of the following in an electrophoretic procedure:
   Buffers
   Stains
   Support media
   Power supply
4. Discuss separation, detection, and quantification in an electrophoretic procedure.
5. List five different types of electrophoresis.
6. Define *blotting* and describe its use in a clinical laboratory.
7. Define *electroendosmosis*.
8. Identify the way in which each of the following affects electrophoresis:
   Inappropriate buffer pH
   Electroendosmosis
   Poor staining solution
   Sample overload
   High voltage
   Inappropriate support media
   Hemolyzed specimen

Key Words

Ampholyte   A molecule that is either positively or negatively charged (also called a *zwitterion*)

Capillary Electrophoresis (CE)   A separation method in which the classic techniques of zone electrophoresis, isotachophoresis, isoelectric focusing, and gel electrophoresis are carried out in a small-bore, fused silica capillary tube

Densitometry   An instrumental method for measurement of the absorbance, reflectance, or fluorescence of each separated fraction on an electrophoretic strip (or other medium) as it is moved past a measuring optical system

Electrophoresis   The migration of charged solutes or particles in a liquid medium under the influence of an electrical field

Electrophoretic Mobility   The rate of migration (cm/s) of a charged solute in an electric field per unit field strength (volts/cm); carries the symbol μ and units of $cm^2/(V \times s)$

Electrophoretogram   A display of protein zones on a support material after separation and staining

Endosmosis (Endosmotic, Electroendosmotic Flow)   Preferential movement of water in one direction through an electrophoresis medium due to selective binding of one type of charge on the surface of the medium

Isoelectric Focusing (IEF)   An electrophoretic method that separates amphoteric compounds in a medium that contains a stable pH gradient

Micellar Electrokinetic Chromatography (MEKC)   A hybrid of electrophoresis and chromatography involving the addition of chemical agents to the buffer to produce micelles, which help separate uncharged molecules

Proteomics   A type of analysis concerned with the global changes in protein expression as visualized most commonly by two-dimensional gel electrophoresis and analyzed by mass spectrometry

Wick Flow   Movement of water from the buffer reservoirs toward the center of an electrophoresis gel or strip to replace water lost by evaporation

Electrophoresis is a versatile and powerful analytical technique used to separate and analyze a diverse range of ionized analytes. Analytes of interest in the clinical laboratory that are separated by electrophoresis include proteins, peptides, amino acids, nucleic acids, oligonucleotides, nucleotides, nucleosides, organic acids, and small anions and cations in body fluid and tissues. This chapter includes discussions of the basic concepts and definitions, theory, description, and types of electrophoresis, including capillary electrophoresis.

■ BASIC CONCEPTS AND DEFINITONS

Electrophoresis is a comprehensive term that refers to the migration of all charged solutes or particles in a liquid medium under the influence of an electrical field. *Iontophoresis* is a similar term but applies only to the migration of small ions. *Zone electrophoresis* is the name of the technique most commonly used in clinical applications and refers to the migration of charged molecules as zones, usually in a porous supporting medium, such as cellulose acetate sheets or agarose gel film, after the sample is mixed with a buffer solution. It generates an **electrophoretogram,** a display of protein zones, each sharply separated from neighboring zones, on the support material. Protein zones are visualized when the support medium is stained with a protein-specific stain; the medium then is dried and quantified in a densitometer. The support medium also can be handled after drying and kept as a permanent record.

■ THEORY OF ELECTROPHORESIS

Chemical species carrying electrical charges because of ionization move toward either the cathode (negative electrode) or the anode (positive electrode) in an electrophoresis system, depending on the kind of charge they carry. For example, positive ions (cations) migrate toward the cathode, and negative ions (anions) migrate toward the anode (Figure 7-1). An **ampholyte,** which is a molecule that is either positively or negatively charged and formerly was called a *zwitterion,* takes on a positive charge (binds protons) in a

solution more acidic than its isoelectric point (pI)* and migrates toward the cathode. In a more alkaline solution the ampholyte takes on a negative charge (gives up protons) and migrates toward the anode. Because proteins contain many ionizable amino ($-NH_2$) and carboxyl ($-COOH$) groups, and the bases in nucleic acids also may be charged positively or negatively, proteins and nucleic acids behave as ampholytes in solution.

The rate of migration is dependent on factors such as the (1) net electrical charge of the molecule, (2) size and shape of the molecule, (3) electric field strength, (4) properties of the supporting medium, and (5) temperature of operation. **Electrophoretic mobility (μ)** is defined as the rate of migration (cm/s) per unit field strength (volts/cm). Equation (1) expresses electrophoretic mobility and is derived from two formulas, one expressing the driving force of the electric field on the ion and the other expressing the retarding force due to frictional resistance of the medium.[8]

$$\mu = \frac{Q}{6\pi\, r\eta} \tag{1}$$

where:

μ = Electrophoretic mobility in $cm^2/(V \times s)$
Q = Net charge on the ion
r = Ionic radius of the solute
η = Viscosity of the buffer solution in which migration is occurring

Thus electrophoretic mobility is directly proportional to net charge and inversely proportional to molecular size and viscosity of the electrophoresis medium.

Other factors that affect mobility include endosmotic flow (which will be discussed in a later section of this chapter) and wick flow. When electrophoresis is in progress, heat is generated, resulting in evaporation of solvent from the electrophoretic support. The drying effect causes the buffer to rise into the electrophoresis support from both buffer compartments. This flow of buffer from both directions is **wick flow,** and it affects protein migration and mobility.

---

*The isoelectric point of a molecule is the pH at which it has no net charge and will not move in an electric field.

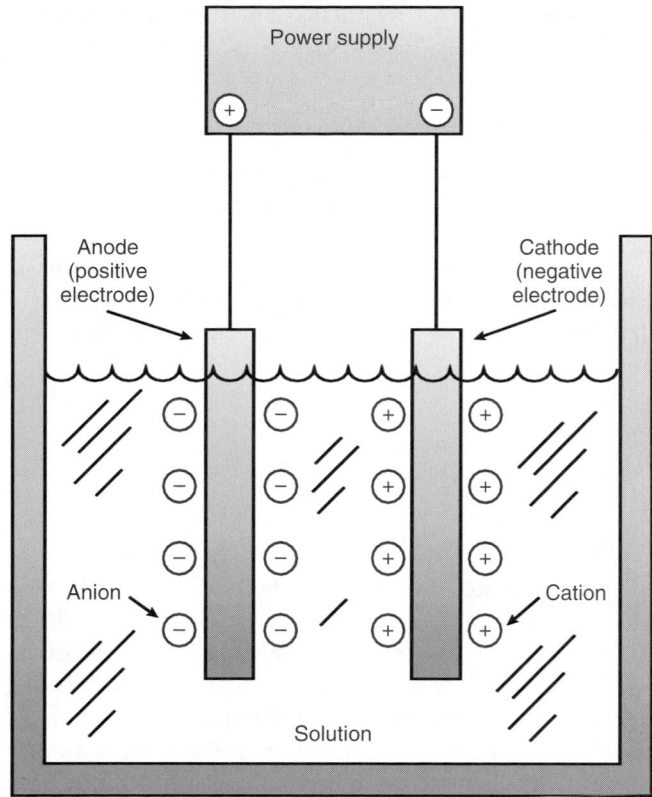

Figure 7-1   Movement of cations and anions in an electrical field.

■ DESCRIPTION OF TECHNIQUE

Electrophoretic instrumentation and reagents are discussed in this section, and a typical electrophorectic separation is described.

Instrumentation and Reagents

A schematic diagram of an electrophoresis system is shown in Figure 7-2. Two buffer boxes (1) with baffle plates contain the buffer used in the process. Each buffer box contains an electrode (2) of either platinum or carbon, the polarity of which is fixed by the mode of connection to the power supply. The electrophoresis support (3) on which separation takes place may contact the buffer directly, or by means of wicks (4). The entire apparatus is covered (5) to minimize evaporation and protect the system and is powered by a direct current power supply.

Support media

Starch gel was the first material to be used as a support medium for electrophoresis to separate macromolecules on the basis of both surface charge and molecular size. Because preparation of a reproducible starch gel is difficult, this medium is used rarely in the clinical laboratory. Currently, gels made of agarose, cellulose acetate, and polyacrylamide are the support media of choice for electrophoresis.

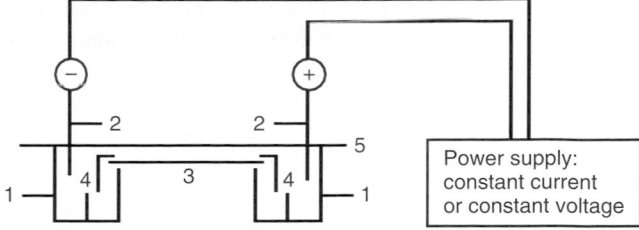

Figure 7-2   A schematic diagram of a typical electrophoresis apparatus showing two buffer boxes with baffle plates (1), electrodes (2), electrophoretic support (3), wicks (4), cover (5), and power supply.

Agarose

Agar is a complex acidic polysaccharide that contains monomers of sulfated galactose. Agarose is a sulfate-free fraction of agar. However, depending on its purity, agarose contains varying amounts of agaropectin. Agaropectin contains acid sulfate and carboxylic acid groups that account for the problems with unwanted liquid movement (which will be discussed in the later section on endosmosis) and background staining that are observed when unfractionated agar or impure agarose is used as an electrophoretic support. Agarose, which is essentially free of ionizable groups, exhibits few of these problems. Operationally, 0.5 to 1.0 g of agarose/dL of buffer provides a gel with suitable strength and good migration properties for proteins and DNA fragments in the range of 0.5 to 20.0 kbp (kilobase pairs; see also Chapter 11). Smaller DNA fragments (10 to 500 bp) may be resolved with special low-gelling-temperature grades of agarose.

The pore size produced in an agarose gel is independent of its concentration and large compared with the molecular size of proteins. This size causes proteins to be separated only on the basis of their charge-to-mass ratio; the resolved zones contain several proteins with the same electrophoretic mobility. The zones also tend to be broad because proteins diffuse during electrophoresis. These factors limit the resolving power of agarose and cellulose acetate (described below) when compared with higher-resolution gels, such as starch or polyacrylamide. Advantages of agarose, however, include lower affinity for proteins and clarity after drying, which permits excellent **densitometry.**

Because nucleic acids all have essentially the same charge to mass ratios, separation is based solely on molecular size, which determines how fast the molecule or fragment can migrate through the pores of the gel. This speed depends partly on whether the molecule is circular (form I), nicked-circular (form II) or linear (form III) DNA. Smaller DNA fragments have migration rates in agarose that are inversely proportional to the logs of their molecular weights, but this relationship decreases as their fragment size increases. Fragments larger than 50 to 100 kbp all migrate at the same rate through agarose and require an alternative technique, such as pulsed-field electrophoresis for separation. Alkaline agarose, which incorporates sodium hydroxide (NaOH) in its preparation, is used to analyze single-stranded DNA. One potential problem with the use of agarose for nucleic acids is that it may contain inhibitors, which could disrupt further enzymatic treatment of DNA eluted from the gel after separation.

Cellulose acetate

Treating cellulose with acetic anhydride acetylates the hydroxyl groups and forms the raw material for cellulose acetate membranes. Commercially available membranes contain about 80% air space within the interlocking cellulose acetate fibers and come as dry, opaque, brittle films that crack easily if not handled gently. When the film is soaked in buffer, the air spaces fill with liquid and the film becomes quite pliable. Characteristics of the membrane vary with the extent of acetylation, prewashing procedure used by the manufacturer, additives used, and pore size and thickness of the membrane. Serum samples (0.3 to 2.0 μL) generally are applied to cellulose acetate strips (presoaked with buffer) with a twin-wire applicator or the edge of a glass slide.

Cellulose acetate membranes become transparent after soaking in a solvent mixture containing 95 parts methanol and 5 parts glacial acetic acid. As they soak, the cellulose acetate fibers partially dissolve through the action of the solvent and coalesce to eliminate the original air spaces. Such transparent membranes are then suitable for analysis by densitometry.

Polyacrylamide

Polyacrylamide is a polymer formed when acrylamide is heated with a variety of catalysts, with or without cross-linking agents. Polyacrylamide gel is thermostable, transparent, strong, and relatively chemically inert. Furthermore, these gels are uncharged, thus eliminating electroendosmosis, and are prepared in a variety of pore sizes. Compared with agarose gel, the average pore size in a typical 7.5% polyacrylamide gel is about 5 nm (50 Å), large enough to allow most serum proteins to migrate unimpeded. However, proteins with molecular radii and/or lengths that exceed critical limits are more or less impeded in their migration; examples include fibrinogen, β_1-lipoprotein, α_2-macroglobulin, and γ-globulins. Proteins therefore are separated on the basis of both charge-to-mass ratio and molecular size, a phenomenon referred to as *molecular sieving*. Because of the potential carcinogenic character of acrylamide, appropriate caution must be exercised in handling of this material during gel preparation.

When used for the separation of nucleic acids, polyacrylamide can resolve DNA molecules that differ by as little as 0.2% in length (1 bp in 500 bp). It also can accommodate a larger amount of sample (up to 10 μg) in a single sample slot, and compared with DNA from agarose, the DNA recovered from a polyacrylamide gel, is extremely pure, containing no inhibitors. Polyacrylamide is most useful for mixtures of smaller DNA fragments and can resolve fragments smaller than 1 kbp; however, its small pore size prevents super-coiled DNA from entering the gel.

Power supplies

The function of a power supply in an electrophoretic process is to supply electric power. Commercially available power supplies allow operation at conditions of constant current, constant voltage, or constant power, all of which are adjustable. The flow of current through a medium that offers electrical resistance is associated with production of Joule heat

$$\text{Heat} = E \times I \times t \tag{2}$$

where:

E = EMF in volts (V)
I = Current in amperes (A)
t = Time in seconds (s)

Heat generated during electrophoresis increases the conductance of the system (decreases resistance). With constant-voltage power sources the resultant rise in current, because of the increase in thermal agitation of all dissolved ions, causes an increase in both the migration rate of the protein and the rate of evaporation of water from the stationary support medium. The water loss causes an increase in ion concentration and further decreases the resistance *(R)*. To minimize these effects on migration rate, a constant-current power supply is recommended. According to Ohm's law

$$E = I \times R \tag{3}$$

Therefore if R is decreased, the applied electromotive force also decreases (current remaining constant). This event in turn decreases the heat effect and keeps the migration rate relatively constant.

For isoelectric focusing (IEF), a power supply capable of constant power is recommended. If IEF is carried out with a constant-voltage power supply, frequent adjustments of the voltage may be necessary as the current drops because of lower conductivity of the carrier ampholytes when they reach their isoelectric points. Constant-current power supplies are not recommended for IEF.

Pulsed-power, or pulsed-field, techniques[1] periodically change the orientation of the applied field relative to the direction of migration by alternately applying power to different pairs of electrodes or electrode arrays. During each cycle, molecules must reorient themselves to the new field direction to fit through the pores in the gel before migration continues. Because reorientation time depends on molecular size, net migration becomes a function of the frequency of field alteration. This relationship permits separation of very large molecules, such as DNA fragments that are not resolved by the relatively small pores in agarose or polyacrylamide gels.[11]

Buffers

The buffer serves as a multifunctional component in the electrophoretic process as it (1) carries the applied current, (2) establishes the pH at which electrophoresis is performed, and (3) determines the electrical charge on the solute. The buffer's ionic strength influences the thickness of the ionic cloud (buffer and non-buffer ions) surrounding a charged molecule, its rate of migration, and the sharpness of the electrophoretic zones. As the concentration of ions increases, the ionic cloud increases in size and the molecule becomes more hindered in its movement. High ionic-strength buffers yield sharper band separations but also produce more Joule heat due to increased current levels, an effect that leads to denaturation of thermolabile proteins. Many buffer systems have been used in electrophoretic procedures; however, the barbital buffers and the Tris-boric acid-ethylenediaminetetraacetic acid (EDTA) buffers are those used most widely in protein separations. Buffers used for nucleic acid applications typically contain EDTA and either Tris-acetate, Tris-borate, or Tris-phosphate at about 50 millimole/L concentration and with a pH between 7.5 and 7.8.

Stains

Stains used to visualize and locate the separated protein and nucleic acid fractions are listed in Table 7-1 and differ according to type of application. The amount of dye taken up by the sample is affected by many factors, such as the type of protein and the degree of its denaturation by the fixing agents. Some stains are not suitable for polyacrylamide gel-isoelectric focusing (PAGE-IEF) because of their reactivity toward carrier ampholytes, but members of the Coomassie Brilliant Blue (CBB) series of dyes have been used successfully in PAGE-IEF. Silver nitrate, or silver diammine, has been used to stain proteins and polypeptides with sensitivities tenfold to 100-fold greater than dyes used for the same purpose.[15] Ethidium bromide is used most commonly for nucleic acids and has the additional effect of opening up the superhelical turns of the molecule. If ^{32}P has been incorporated into the DNA, autoradiography may be used to visualize bands.

Automated systems

Traditionally, electrophoresis has been a manual technique. However, the introduction of prepackaged gels and integration of computers with electrophoretic instrumentation has resulted in the availability of analytical systems that automatically perform electrophoretic separations and analyses. For example, the Helena REP automates much of the process, from sample application through electrophoresis, staining, scanning of gels, and computation of results. Other systems have automated the procedure partially or incorporated the ability to process multiple gels of different compositions sequentially. Most capillary electrophoresis (CE) systems have auto-sampling capabilities and some even feature multicolumn capabilities.[10] For example, the Beckman CZE system permits simultaneous processing of seven samples through the use of multiple capillaries. These advances have reduced the labor component associated with this technique significantly.

TABLE 7-1	Suggested Wavelengths for Quantitation of Protein and Nucleic Acid Zones by Direct Densitometry	
Separation Type		Nominal Wavelength (nm)
Serum Proteins in General		
Amido Black (Naphthol Blue Black)		640
Coomassie Brilliant Blue G-250 (Brilliant Blue G)		595
Coomassie Brilliant Blue R-250 (Brilliant Blue R)		560
Ponceau S		520
Isoenzymes NAD(P)H (NBTH→formazan)		
Nitrotetrazolium Blue (as the formazan)		570
Lipoprotein Zones		
Fat Red 7B (Sudan Red 7B)		540
Oil Red O		520
Sudan Black B		600
DNA Fragments		
Ethidium bromide (fluorescent)		254 (Ex)
		590 (Em)
[32]P Autoradiography		—
CSF Proteins		
Silver nitrate		—

DNA, Deoxyribonucleic acid; *CSF,* cerebrospinal fluid; *Ex,* excitation; *Em,* emission; *NAD(P)H,* reduced nicotinamide adenine dinucleotide; *NBTH,* reduced nitortetrazolium blue.

General Procedures

The separation is the primary step in an electrophoretic analysis. It then is followed by detection and quantification of the separated analytes.

Separation

To perform an electrophoretic separation, a hydrated support material, such as freshly prepared agarose gel or previously wetted cellulose acetate, is blotted to remove excess buffer and then placed into the electrophoresis chamber. Care should be taken to ensure that the gel has neither excess liquid nor bubbles on it. Next, the sample is added to the support, which is placed in contact with the buffer previously added to the electrode chambers. Electrophoresis is conducted for a determined length of time under conditions of either constant voltage or constant current. When electrophoresis is completed, the support is removed from the electrophoresis cell and rapidly dried or placed in a fixative to prevent diffusion of sample components. It is stained to locate and visualize the individual protein zones. After excess dye is washed out, the support is dried or placed in a clearing agent.

Detection and quantification

Once electrophoretic separation and staining are complete, direct densitometry is used to quantify the individual zones, either as a percentage of the total or as absolute concentration if the total quantity of protein is known. In this instrumental method the electrophoretic strip, also known as the *electrophoretogram,* (or other medium) is moved past a measuring optical system and the absorbance of each fraction displayed on a recorder chart or cathode ray tube (CRT). In most cases the area under each peak is integrated automatically. Reliable quantification of stained zones by densitometry requires light of an appropriate wavelength, a linear response from the instrument, and a transparent background in the strip being scanned. The response linearity may be tested with a neutral density filter designed with either separated or adjacent zones of linearly increasing density. Each zone has an expected value of absorbance. Recording the pattern of increasing density and subsequent return to baseline checks the optical, mechanical, and electrical functions of the densitometer.

Features generally considered essential in a densitometer include the following:

1. The ability to scan electrophoresis support lengths of 25 to 150 mm
2. Automatic gain control to prevent the most intense peak or zone of an electrophoretogram from going off scale
3. Automatic background zeroing for background correction, which allows the instrument to choose the lowest point in the electrophoretogram as baseline so that minor peaks are not lost or "cut off"
4. Variable wavelength control, either as a continuously variable monochromator or as selectable interference filters, to allow operation in the 400- to 700-nm range
5. Variable slits to allow for adjustment of the beam size
6. An integrating device
7. Automatic indexing, a feature that advances the electrophoresis strip from one sample channel to the next
8. The ability to measure ultraviolet fluorescence

Although not essential for routine laboratory use, the following features are desirable:

1. Computerized integration and printout
2. Built-in diagnostics (microcomputerized) for instrument trouble-shooting
3. Choice of one of several scanning speeds
4. The ability to measure in the reflectance mode

Most clinical applications use agarose gels and very small sample sizes to satisfy the requirement for a clear background and eliminate undesirable light-scattering effects associated with uncleared cellulose acetate strips. Nevertheless, problems associated with densitometry persist because of differences in the quantities of stain taken up by individual proteins and in protein zone sizes.

Modern DNA analysis techniques, which may produce several dozen bands of different-length DNA fragments, require the use of a new type of densitometer referred to as a *flat bed scanner,* or *digital image analyzer.*[6] These instruments use ultrasensitive charge-coupled device detectors or cameras (see Chapter 3), have resolutions of up to 1200 dots per inch, and are capable of scanning and storing digitized light intensity readings from large areas.

In addition to scanning by densitometry, electrophoresis gels now are being analyzed by mass spectrometers to determine the molecular weights of proteins and their cleavage products,[12] and for peptide sequencing.[7,14]

■ TYPES OF ELECTROPHORESIS

The first electrophoresis method used to study proteins was the free solution or moving boundary method devised by Tiselius in 1937. Tiselius' apparatus resolved the serum proteins into only four component mixtures, albumin/α_1, α_2, β, and γ-globulins, with the α-1 fraction incompletely separated from albumin. Results similar to those obtained with moving-boundary electrophoresis now can be achieved with the electrophoretic techniques described in this chapter.

Zone Electrophoresis

Zone electrophoresis techniques produce zones of proteins, which are heterogeneous and physically separated from one another. They usually are classified according to the type of support material used.

Agarose gel electrophoresis

Agarose gel electrophoresis (AGE) has been applied successfully to the analysis of serum proteins, nucleic acids, hemoglobin variants, lactate dehydrogenase and creatine kinase isoenzymes, lipoprotein fractions, and other substances. Most AGE procedures now are performed with commercially produced, prepackaged microzone gels. Aliquots of samples are applied by means of a thin plastic template with small slits corresponding to sample application points. The aliquots are allowed to diffuse into the agarose for 5 minutes, excess sample is removed by blotting, and the template is removed. Because the agarose surface remains undisturbed, this technique avoids any surface artifact. An AGE separation typically requires a sample volume of 0.6 to 3 μL and an electrophoresis time of 30 to 90 minutes. Figure 7-3

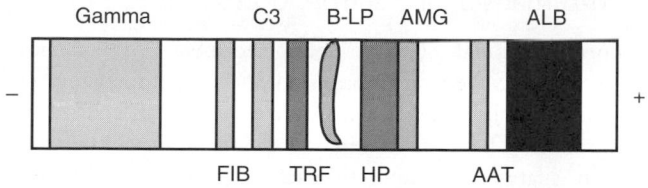

Figure 7-3 A simplified schematic diagram of plasma proteins separated on a high resolution agarose gel (Paragon, Beckman Instruments, Inc., Brea, Calif.) at pH 8.6. *AAT*, α_1-Antitrypsin; *ALB*, albumin; *AMG*, α_2-macroglobulin; *B-LP*, β-lipoprotein; *C3*, C3 complement; *FIB*, fibrinogen (not present if serum is used); *Gamma*, γ-globulins (immunoglobulins IgG, IgM, IgA); *HP*, haptoglobin; *TRF*, transferrin.

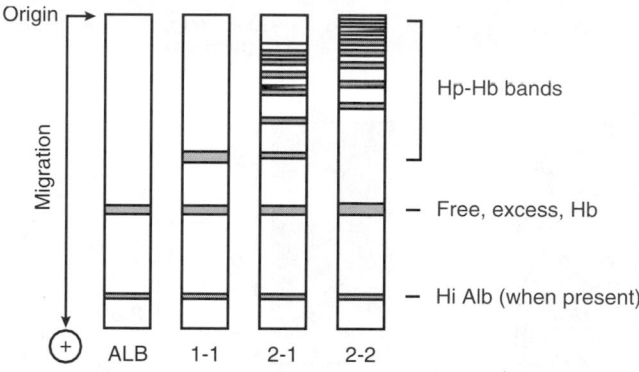

Figure 7-4 Electrophoretograms of the three main haptoglobin types, obtained with a PAGE procedure. Albumin is shown as a blank because it is used in the electrophoretic procedure. Excess control hemoglobin *(Hb)* as a hemolysate is added to the serum, and albumin is added to the control hemolysate to increase the viscosity of the solution. Staining is performed with *o*-dianisidine and hydrogen peroxide. Haptoglobin-hemoglobin complexes *(Hp-Hb)* are seen readily. At times an unstable Hb hemolysate causes the formation of the methamalbumin *(Hi Alb)*. *PAGE*, Polyacrylamide gel electrophoresis; *ALB*, albumin.

illustrates a separation of serum proteins and demonstrates the resolution possible on modern agarose gels.

Cellulose acetate electrophoresis

Cellulose acetate electrophoresis (CAE) uses cellulose acetate membranes as an electrophoretic support. An advantage of CAE is its speed of separation (20 minutes to 1 hour) and ability to store the transparent membranes for long periods of time. However, because of the need for presoaking before use and clearing of the strips prior to densitometry, cellulose acetate has been replaced by agarose in most clinical applications.

Polyacrylamide gel electrophoresis

Polyacrylamide gel electrophoresis (PAGE) uses gels cast in slabs or individual glass tubes (Rod or Tube PAGE). In the Rod PAGE technique a small-pore separation gel is poured into the tubular-shaped electrophoresis cell and allowed to gel for 30 minutes. Then a large-pore monomer solution containing a small amount of serum, about 3 µL, is polymerized above the separation gel so that the finished product is composed of two different layers of gel. When electrophoresis begins, all protein ions migrate through the large-pore gel (which does not impair movement of most proteins in serum) and stack up on the separation gel in a very thin zone. This process improves resolution and concentrates protein components at the border, or starting, zone. Separation then takes place in the bottom separation gel, with retardation of some proteins because of the molecular sieve phenomenon.

PAGE may yield 20 or more fractions and may be used to study individual proteins and nucleic acids in serum, especially genetic variants and isoenzymes. A schematic representation of haptoglobin typing by PAGE is shown in Figure 7-4. Often a detergent is added to PAGE and, when this detergent is sodium dodecyl sulfate (SDS), the combined procedure is termed SDS-PAGE. Functionally, the SDS coats protein molecules, giving all proteins an almost constant charge-mass ratio. This ratio overcomes any of the proteins' original differences in charge and improves their separation, which then is based on molecular size only.

Isotachophoresis

Isotachophoresis is a technique applicable specifically to small ions; the process separates them into adjacent zones all migrating at the same rate. Individual zones border one another but represent completely separated components without overlap. In isotachophoresis no background electrolyte (buffer) is mixed with the sample, so current flow is carried only by charged sample ions. Once a faster-moving component separates completely from a slower-moving one, it creates a region of depleted charge between the two that increases the resistance and therefore the local voltage in that region. This increased voltage causes the slower component to migrate faster and close the gap, thereby concentrating it and increasing the conductivity of its zone until it matches that of the faster ion. Ultimately, all ions migrate at the rate of the fastest ion in zones that differ in thickness, depending on their original concentrations.

Isoelectric Focusing

Isoelectric focusing (IEF) separates amphoteric compounds, such as proteins, in a medium possessing a stable pH gradient. The protein migrates to a zone in the medium where the pH is equal to its isoelectric point (pI), and at this pH its charge becomes zero and migration ceases. Figure 7-5 illustrates the procedure in a schematic diagram and shows the electrophoretic conditions before and after current is applied. In IEF the protein zones are very sharp because the pI of a protein is confined to a narrow pH range. Normal diffusion also is counteracted because the protein acquires charge if it diffuses from its pI position and subsequently is driven back due to electrophoretic forces (Figure 7-6). Proteins that differ in their pI values by only a 0.02 pH unit have been separated by IEF.

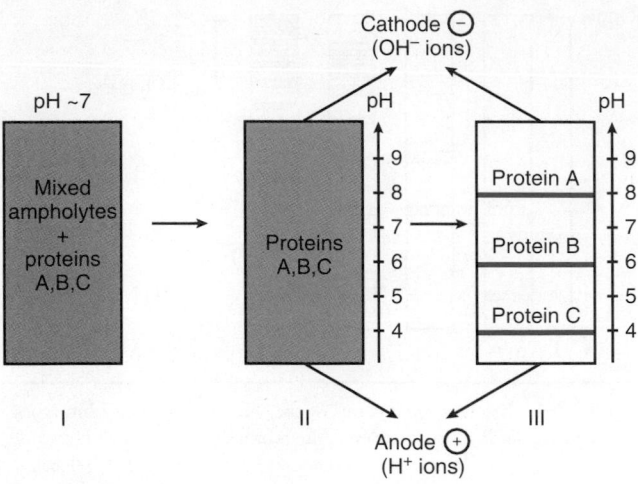

Figure 7-5 Schematic illustration of an IEF procedure. *I,* A homogeneous mixture of carrier ampholytes, pH range 3 to 10, to which proteins A, B, and C with pI 8, 6, and 4, respectively, were added. *II,* Current is applied, and the carrier ampholytes rapidly migrate to the pH zones, where net charge is zero (the pI value). *III,* The proteins A, B, and C migrate more slowly to their respective pI zones, where migration ceases. The high buffering capacity of the carrier ampholyte creates stable pH zones in which each protein may reach its pI. *IEF,* Isoelectric focusing; *pI,* isoelectric point.

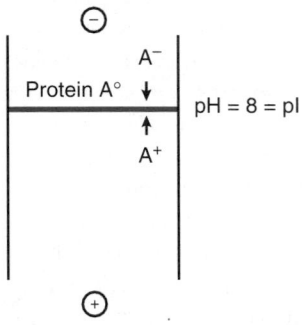

Figure 7-6 After the pH level at which protein A has a net charge of zero *(A°)* is obtained, diffusion toward the cathode bestows a negative charge on A *(A⁻)* and migration in the electric field forces A⁻ back to A°. Diffusion toward the anode causes A to take on the opposite charge *(A⁺),* and migration is toward the cathode and to the point where A° exists. IEF processes of this kind cause sharp zones to form (that is, the protein is focused).

The pH gradient is created through the use of amphoteric polyaminocarboxylic acids (carrier ampholytes), a group of compounds with molecular weights of 300 to 1000 and slightly differing pKa (acid dissociation constant) values. Mixtures of 50 to 100 different compounds quickly separate in an electric field to create a "stable pH gradient" when the individual ampholytes reach their pI values. As Figure 7-5 illustrates, the anode is surrounded by a dilute acid solution and the cathode by a dilute alkaline solution. Because carrier ampholytes generally are used in relatively high concentrations, a high-voltage power source (up to 2000 V) is necessary and power is in the vicinity of 2 to 50 W. As a result the electrophoretic matrix must be cooled.

Two-Dimensional Electrophoresis

Two-dimensional (2D) electrophoresis uses charge-dependent IEF electrophoresis in the first dimension and molecular weight-dependent electrophoresis in the second dimension. The first-dimension electrophoresis is carried out in a large-pore medium, such as agarose gel or large-pore polyacrylamide gel. Ampholytes are added to yield a pH gradient. The second dimension is often polyacrylamide in a linear or gradient format. This type of electrophoresis is used to achieve the highest resolving power for the separation of DNA fragments. In this application normal AGE is carried out in the first dimension and ethidium bromide is added to the gel for the second dimension to open the fragments and cause changes in their electrophoretic mobility.

The 2D electrophoresis method of O'Farrell uses rod PAGE-IEF for the first dimension and incorporates ampholytes that cover a pH range of 3 to 10 units. The gel is forced from the gel tube at the end of electrophoresis and placed in contact with a thin, polyacrylamide gradient gel slab that incorporates SDS. Separated proteins may be detected through use of Coomassie dyes, silver stain, radiography (exposure of photographic film to emissions of isotopically labeled polypeptides), or fluorographic analysis (x-ray film exposed to tritium-labeled polypeptides in the presence of a scintillator). The latter two methods provide the greatest analytical sensitivity because they are 100 to 1000 times more sensitive than the Coomassie dyes.

Analytical and preparative 2D electrophoresis is used to characterize the individual components of complex protein mixtures.[14] It remains the highest-resolution technique for protein separation and is the method of choice when complex samples must be arrayed for characterization, as in proteomics.[5] *Proteome* is the word used to describe the expressed protein complement of a genome, and *proteomics* is the term applied to functional genomics at the protein level.[3] **Proteomics** is the study of global changes in protein expression, as well as the systematic study of protein-protein interactions through the isolation of protein complexes. The goal of proteomics is a comprehensive, quantitative description of protein expression and its changes under the influence of biological perturbations, such as disease or drug treatment.[2]

Capillary Electrophoresis

In **capillary electrophoresis (CE),** the classic techniques of electrophoresis are carried out in a small-bore (10 to 100 μm), fused-silica capillary tube 20 to 200 cm long.[9] This capillary tube serves as a capillary electrophoretic chamber that is connected to a detector at its terminal end and, via buffer reservoirs, to a high-voltage power supply (Figure 7-7). The main advantage of CE comes from efficient heat dissipation, compared with traditional electrophoresis. Improved heat dissipation permits the application of voltages in the range of 25 to 30 kV, which enhance separation effi-

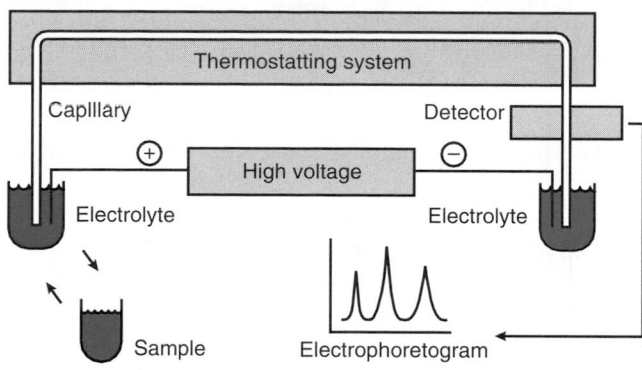

Figure 7-7   A schematic diagram of a typical capillary electrophoresis instrument. Power may be applied as either voltage or current. To introduce a sample, the inlet electrolyte vial is replaced briefly by a sample vial.

ciency and reduce separation time in some cases to less than 1 minute. Sample volumes are kept in the picoliter-to-nanoliter range to minimize distortions in the applied field caused by the presence of sample.

An additional advantage of the capillary format is its ease of automation. Commercial instruments resemble many high-performance liquid chromatography (HPLC) instruments in terms of automated sample loading and data analysis. Applications are also more extensive and include the separation of low-molecular-weight ions, proteins and other macromolecules. In addition, CE has proved useful in separations of inorganic ions, amino acids, organic acids, drugs, vitamins, porphyrins, carbohydrates, oligonucleotides, and DNA fragments.[4,9,13,16] Even uncharged molecules are separated with CE in the micellar electrokinetic chromatography mode.

Sample injection

In CE, sample volumes of 1 to 50 nL are loaded into the capillary chamber by either hydrodynamic or electrokinetic injection. With hydrodynamic injection an aliquot of sample is introduced by application of pressure at the inlet vial or reduction of pressure at the outlet vial. With electrokinetic injection an aliquot of a sample is introduced through the application of a voltage for a timed interval, typically at a field strength three to five times lower than that used for separation.

Detection

As in HPLC (see Chapter 8), ultraviolet-visible photometers are used widely as CE detectors and interface with a terminal section of the capillary tube that serves as an in-line cuvet. This configuration increases efficiency in that separation continues in the optical window of the cuvet, and no zone broadening occurs due to component mixing or dead volume. However, because the inner diameter of the capillary tube is also the pathlength of the cuvet, the detection limit of such a detector is limited. To improve the de-

tection limit, a capillary chamber with a "bubble" and Z geometry has been developed. Other in-capillary optical methods also have been used, including fluorescence, refractive index, chemiluminescence, Raman, and circular dichroism.[16] In general, the most sensitive optical detection method used in CE is laser-induced fluorescence.[13]

Modes of operation

Capillary zone electrophoresis (CZE) is the simplest form of CE and may be referred to also as *open-tube*, or *free-solution*, *CE*. The term *capillary ion electrophoresis* sometimes is used to refer to the analysis of inorganic ions by CZE. **Micellar electrokinetic chromatography (MEKC)**, sometimes called *capillary electrokinetic chromatography*, is a hybrid of electrophoresis and chromatography. It is an effective electrophoretic technique and is used for the separation of neutral and charged solutes. The separation of neutral species is accomplished through inclusion of micelles in the running buffer, formed by the addition of surfactants to the solution at concentrations above the critical micelle concentration. During migration the micelles interact with solutes in a chromatographic manner through both hydrophobic and electrostatic interactions. For neutral species, only partitioning in and out of the micelle affects the separation.

Capillary gel electrophoresis (CGE) is directly comparable to traditional slab or tube-gel electrophoresis because the separation is achieved by movement of solutes through a suitable polymer (for example, polyacrylamide), which acts as a molecular sieve or sizing mechanism. Macromolecules, such as DNA and SDS-saturated proteins, are not separated without a gel or some other mechanism because they contain mass-to-charge ratios that do not vary with size.

Blotting Techniques

In 1975 Edward Southern developed a widely used technique for the separation and detection of DNA fragments. This technique is known as *Southern blotting* and requires an electrophoretic separation. Subsequently, Northern and Western blotting techniques have been developed to separate and detect ribonucleic acids (RNAs) and proteins, respectively.

Southern blotting

In the Southern blotting technique, DNA or fragments of DNA first are separated by AGE. Next, a strip of nitrocellulose or a nylon membrane is laid over the agarose gel, and the DNAs or DNA fragments are transferred or "blotted" onto it by capillary blotting, electroblotting, or vacuum blotting. They are subsequently detected and identified by hybridization with a labeled, complementary nucleic acid probe. This technique is used widely in molecular biology for the identification of a particular DNA sequence; determination of the presence, position, and number of copies of a gene in a genome; and typing of DNA. (See Chapter 11 for a more detailed discussion.)

Northern blotting

The technique of Northern blotting was named by analogy to Southern blotting and is used to separate and detect RNAs and RNA fragments, as opposed to DNAs and DNA fragments. The RNAs or RNA fragments are separated and blotted according to the Southern technique and then detected and identified by hybridization to a labeled RNA probe. (See Chapter 11 for a more detailed discussion of this technique.)

Western blotting

Western blotting, also named by analogy to the Southern blotting technique, is a method used to separate, detect, and identify one or more proteins in a complex mixture. It involves initial separation of the individual proteins by SDS-PAGE into bands that subsequently are transferred or "blotted" onto an overlying strip of nitrocellulose or a nylon membrane via electroblotting. Then a reagent that contains a labeled antibody raised against the protein of interest is layered over the strip or membrane for detection.

■ TECHNICAL CONSIDERATIONS

Several technical aspects of the electrophoretic process have to be considered to obtain acceptable performance. They include electroendosmosis, handling of buffers and stain solutions, sampling considerations, and a number of problems commonly encountered in the performance of electrophoresis.

Electroendosmosis or Endosmosis

Certain electrophoretic support media in contact with water take on negative charges because of adsorption of hydroxyl ions. These ions become fixed to the surface and are rendered immobile relative to the other ions in the solution. Positive ions in the solution cluster about the fixed negative charge sites, forming an ionic cloud of mostly positive ions. The number of negative ions associated with this ionic cloud increases as the distance from the fixed negative charge sites increases until eventually, positive and negative ions are present in equal concentration (Figure 7-8). The potential that exists between the fixed ions and the associated cloud of ions is termed the *electrokinetic potential*, or the *zeta potential (ζ)*.

When current is applied to such a system, charges attached to the immobile support remain fixed but the cloud of ions in the solution is free to move to the electrode of opposite polarity. Because these ions are highly hydrated, their movement causes movement of the solvent as well. This

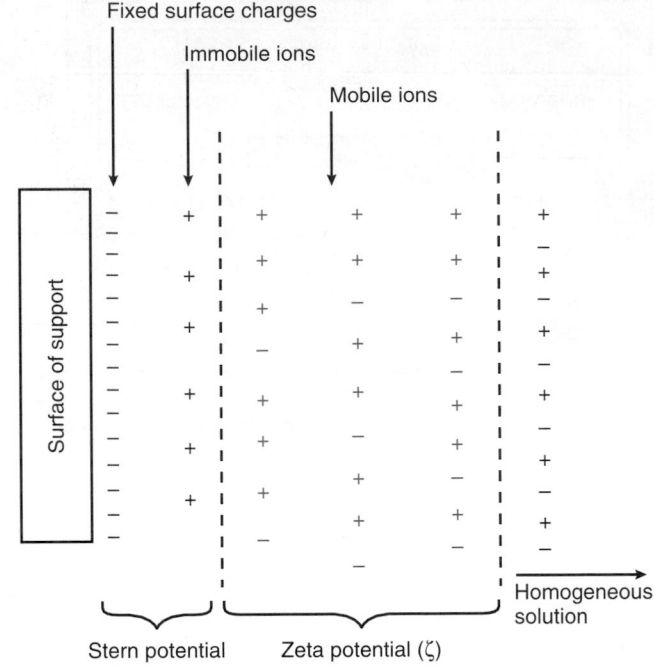

Figure 7-8 Distribution of positive (+) and negative (−) ions around the surface of an electrophoretic support. Fixed on the surface of the solid is a layer of − ions. (These may be + ions under suitable conditions.) A second layer of + ions is attracted to the surface. These two layers compose the Stern potential. The large, diffuse layer containing mostly + ions is the electrokinetic, or zeta (ζ), potential. Extending further from the surface of the solid is a homogeneous solution. The Stern potential plus the ζ-potential equals the electrochemical, or epsilon (ε), potential.

phenomenon, **endosmosis,** causes preferential movement of water in one direction. Macromolecules in solution that move in the direction opposite this flow may remain immobile or even be swept back toward the opposite pole if they are charged insufficiently. In media in which endosmosis is strong, such as conventional cellulose acetate and conventional agarose gel, γ-globulins are swept back from the application point. In electrophoretic media in which surface charges are minimal, such as starch or polyacrylamide gel, endosmosis also is minimal.

Buffers

Buffers are good culture media for the growth of microorganisms and should be refrigerated when not in use. Moreover, a cold buffer improves resolution and reduces evaporation from the electrophoretic support. The buffer used in a small-volume apparatus should be discarded after each run because of pH changes caused by the electrolysis of water that accompanies electrophoresis. If larger volumes (from 700 mL to 1 L) are used, buffer from both buffer boxes may be poured into a common container, stored at 4 °C, and reused for four subsequent electrophoretic runs.

Stain Solution

A typical stain solution may be used several times. A good rule of thumb is that 100 mL of stain solution may be used for a combined total of 387 cm^2 (60 in^2) of cellulose acetate or agarose film. With methods involving isoenzymes, the stain or substrate reagent may be considered faulty if stained protein zones are leached in the wash or clearing solution (cellulose acetate only) or whenever protein zones appear too lightly stained. Stain solution must be stored tightly covered to avoid evaporation.

Sampling

Because albumin in serum is about 10 times more concentrated than the α_1-globulins, the amount of serum applied should avoid overloading with albumin but be adequate to quantify α_1-globulin. Typical amounts of serum applied in agarose gel electrophoresis are 0.6 to 2.0 μL, depending on the test requirements, and 0.3 to 1.6 μL with cellulose acetate, depending on the size of the twin-wire applicator. When procedures call for multiple applications, such as in isoenzyme analysis, the concern about albumin overloading is no longer a factor because it is not detected.

Common Problems

Many of the following common problems are encountered frequently in the performance of electrophoresis:

1. Discontinuities in sample application may be due to dirty applicators. To clean applicators thoroughly, they should be agitated in water and gently pressed against absorbent paper. Caution must be used, and wires should not be cleaned with manual wiping.
2. Unequal migration of samples across the width of the gel may be because of either dirty electrodes causing uneven application of the electric field or uneven wetting of the gel.
3. Distorted protein zones may be due to bent applicators, incorporation of an air bubble during sample application, over-application of the sample, excessive drying of the electrophoretic support before or during electrophoresis, or improper tension on a cellulose acetate film resulting in zones that look "bent over."
4. Irregularities (other than broken zones) in sample application probably are due to excessively wet cellulose acetate films or agarose gels. Parts of the applied samples may appear washed out.
5. Unusual bands are normally artifacts that may be recognized easily. Hemolyzed samples are frequent causes of increases in β-globulin (where free hemoglobin migrates) or an unusual band between the α_2- and β-globulins, the result of a hemoglobin-haptoglobin complex. A band at the starting point may be fibrinogen and the sample should be verified as being serum before this band is reported as an abnormal protein. Split α_1-, α_2-, and β-globulin bands are not unusual and should not to be considered errors. Occasionally, a split albumin zone is observed in bis-albuminemia, but a grossly widened albumin zone may be due to certain medications that are albumin bound.
6. Atypical bands in an isoenzyme pattern may be the result of binding by an immunoglobulin. An irregular but sharp protein zone at the starting point that lacks the regular, somewhat diffuse appearance of proteins actually may be denatured protein resulting from a deteriorated serum or from damage done to the cellulose acetate by the twin-wire applicator. When faced with an unusual band anywhere in a serum protein pattern, the possibility that it is a true paraprotein (see Chapter 19) always must be considered. Finally, good laboratory practice dictates inclusion of a control serum with each electrophoretic run to aid in the evaluation of its quality.

References

1. Abbal P, Picou C: A general-purpose pulsed field controller. Electrophoresis 1990; 11:893-894.
2. Anderson NL, Anderson NG: Proteome and proteomics: new technologies, new concepts, and new words. Electrophoresis 1998; 19:1853-1861.
3. Blackstock WP, Weir MP: Proteomics: quantitative and physical mapping of cellular proteins. Trends Biotechnol 1999; 17:121-127.
4. Deyl Z , Tagliaro F , Miksik I : Biomedical applications of capillary electrophoresis. J Chromatog 1994; 656:3-27.
5. Herbert B: Advances in protein solubilisation for two-dimensional electrophoresis. Electrophoresis 1999; 20:660-663.
6. Horgan G, Glasbey CA: Uses of digital image analysis in electrophoresis. Electrophoresis 1995; 16:298-305.
7. Jensen ON, Wilm M, Shevchenko A et al: Peptide sequencing of 2-DE gel-isolated proteins by nanoelectrospray tandem mass spectrometry. Methods Mol Biol 1999; 112:571-588.
8. Karcher RE, Nuttall KL: Electrophoresis. In Burtis CA, Ashwood, ER (eds): Tietz Textbook of Clinical Chemistry, 3rd edition, pp 150-163, Philadelphia, WB Saunders, 1999.
9. Landers JP: Clinical capillary electrophoresis. Clin Chem 1995; 41:495-509.

10. Liu Z, Wang J, Luo J et al: Application of multichannel flow electrophoresis to separation of biomolecules: a survey. J Mol Recognit 1998; 11:149-150.
11. O'Reilly MJ, Kinnon C: The technique of pulsed field gel electrophoresis and its impact on molecular immunology. J Immunol Methods 1990; 131:1-31.
12. Ogorzalek Loo RR, Loo JA, Andrews PC: Obtaining molecular weights of proteins and their cleavage products by directly combining gel electrophoresis with mass spectrometry. Methods Mol Biol 1999; 112:473-485.
13. Paquette DM, Sing R, Banks PR et al: Capillary electrophoresis with laser-induced native fluorescence detection for profiling body fluids. J Chromatogr B Biomed Sci Appl 1998; 714:47 57.
14. Quadroni M, James P: Proteomics and automation. Electrophoresis 1999; 20:664-677.
15. Rabilloud T: A comparison between low background silver diammine and silver nitrate protein stains. Electrophoresis 1992; 13:429-439.
16. St Claire RL: Capillary electrophoresis. Anal Chem 1996; 68:569R-586R.

Additional Reading

Anderson NG, Anderson L: Twenty years of two-dimensional electrophoresis: past, present and future [review]. Electrophoresis 1996; 17:443-453.

Gersten D: Gel Electrophoresis of Proteins. Essential Techniques Series, New York, John Wiley & Sons, 1996.

Jones P, Rickwood D: Gel Electrophoresis: Nucleic Acids. Essential Techniques Series, New York, John Wiley & Sons, 1995.

Keren DF: High-Resolution Electrophoresis and Immunofixation. Techniques and Interpretation, Oxford, Butterworth-Heinemann, 1994.

Landers JP (ed): Handbook of Capillary Electrophoresis, 2nd edition, Boca Raton, Fla, CRC Press, 1996.

Righetti PG, Hancock W: Capillary Electrophoresis in Analytical Biochemistry, Boca Raton, Fla, CRC Press, 1995.

Westermeier R: Electrophoresis in Practice: A Guide to Theory and Practice, Basel, VCH Publishers, 1993.

CHAPTER 8

Chromatography/Mass Spectrometry

LARRY D. BOWERS, PhD, DABCC, M. DAVID ULLMAN, PhD, and CARL A. BURTIS, PhD

Objectives

1. Define *chromatography, stationary phase, mobile phase,* and *resolution.*
2. State the two basic forms of chromatography and the basic principle of each.
3. List five separation techniques used in chromatographic procedures and state the principle of each.
4. State the principle of thin-layer chromatography and its use in a clinical laboratory.
5. Define *retention factor,* calculate the retention factor, and discuss how the retention factor is used to identify compounds in a chromatographic procedure.
6. State the theory of gas chromatography and its use in a clinical laboratory.
7. State the principle of high-performance liquid chromatography and its use in a clinical laboratory.
8. List examples of detectors used in chromatographic procedures and how they quantify substance concentration.
9. Discuss the principle of mass spectrometry analysis and its uses in a laboratory.

Key Words

Chromatogram A graphical or other presentation of detector response, concentration of analyte in the effluent, or other quantity used as a measure of effluent concentration versus effluent volume or time

Chromatography A physical method of separation in which the components to be separated are distributed between two phases, one of which is stationary (stationary phase), whereas the other (mobile phase) moves in a definite direction

Column Chromatography A separation technique in which the stationary bed is within a tube

Gas Chromatography (GC) A separation technique in which the mobile phase is a gas

Gas Chromatography/Mass Spectrometry (GC/MS) An analytical process that utilizes a gas chromatograph coupled to a mass spectrometer

High-Performance Liquid Chromatography (HPLC) A type of liquid chromatography that uses an efficient column containing small particles of stationary phase

Ion-Exchange Chromatography A mode of chromatography in which separation is based mainly on differences in the ion-exchange affinities of the sample components

Liquid Chromatography (LC) A separation technique in which the mobile phase is a liquid

Liquid Chromatography/Mass Spectrometry (LC/MS) An analytical process that utilizes a liquid chromatograph coupled to a mass spectrometer

Mass Spectrometry (MS) An analytical technique that uses the mass spectrometer to identify and quantify substances in a sample by their mass-fragment spectrum

Mass Spectrometer An instrument in which beams of ions are separated (analyzed) according to their mass-to-charge ratios and measured electrically

Mobile Phase A gas or liquid that percolates through or along the stationary bed in a definite direction

Partition Chromatography A mode of chromatography in which separation is based mainly on differences between the solubilities of the sample components in the stationary phase (gas chromatography) or on differences between the solubilities of the components in the mobile and stationary phases (liquid chromatography)

Planar Chromatography   A separation technique in which the stationary phase is present as or on a plane, which is either a sheet of paper (paper chromatography [PC]) or a layer of solid particles spread on a support (thin-layer chromatography [TLC])

Resolution (R_s)   A measure of how completely two adjacent peaks are separated from each other

Reversed-Phase Chromatography   A type of liquid-partition chromatography in which the mobile phase is significantly more polar then the stationary phase

Stationary Phase   One of the two phases forming a chromatographic system; may be a solid (may or may not contribute to the separation process), gel or liquid (may be distributed on a solid)

Chromatography and chromatography/mass spectrometry are versatile and powerful analytical tools used in the clinical laboratory for the separation and quantification of a variety of clinically relevant analytes. This chapter begins with general discussions on basic concepts and definitions and covers the various separation mechanisms used in chromatography. Specific types of chromatography, including planar, gas, and high-performance liquid chromatography are discussed in detail. Because both gas and liquid chromatographs often are interfaced with mass spectrometers, the chapter concludes with a discussion on mass spectrometry and coupled techniques.

■ BASIC CONCEPTS AND DEFINITIONS

Chromatography is a physical method of separation in which the components (solutes) of a sample mixture are separated by their differential distribution between two phases—stationary and mobile. In the laboratory these solutes are the analytes to be measured. During the chromatographic process of separation the **mobile phase** carries the sample through a bed, layer, or column containing the **stationary phase.** As the mobile phase flows past the stationary phase, the solutes distribute between the two phases. Those solutes with lower affinities for the stationary phase reside more in the mobile phase than those with greater affinities for the stationary phase. Thus the lower affinity solutes travel faster and separate from solutes having greater affinities for the stationary phase. Strongly bound solutes subsequently are displaced from the stationary phase by changing the physical or chemical nature of the mobile phase. The term *chromatograph* is used as either a verb or a noun. As a verb, it means to separate by chromatography. As a noun, it refers to the assembly of components that are needed to carrying out a chromatographic separation.

The two basic forms of chromatography are planar and column (Figure 8-1). In **planar chromatography** the stationary phase is coated on a sheet of paper or bound to glass or plastic plate. For paper chromatography the stationary phase is a layer of water or a polar solvent coated onto the paper fibers. In thin-layer chromatography (TLC), a thin layer of particles of a material such as silica gel is spread uniformly on a glass plate or a plastic sheet. When the thin layer consists of particles with small diameters (4.5 μM), the technique is known as *high-performance thin-layer chromatography* (HPTLC).

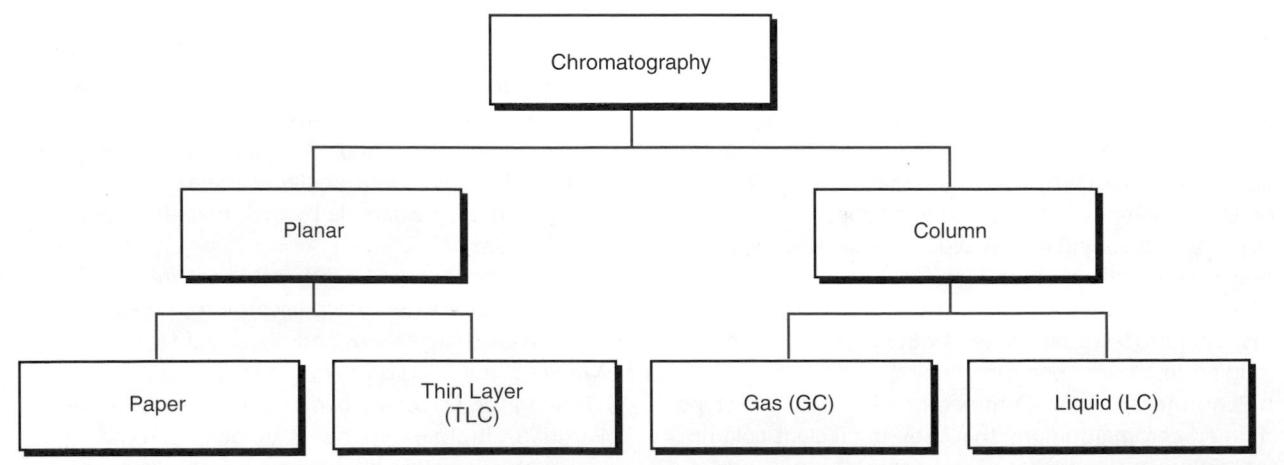

Figure 8-1   Forms of chromatography.

In **column chromatography** support particles, on which the stationary phase is coated or chemically bonded, are "packed" into a tube or the stationary phase is coated onto the inner surface of the tube. The technique is either **gas chromatography (GC)** or **liquid chromatography (LC)**, depending on whether the mobile phase is a gas or a liquid. In practice the instrument used to perform a GC or LC separation is known as either a *gas* or *liquid chromatograph*. When the stationary phase in LC consists of small-diameter particles, the technique is **high-performance liquid chromatography (HPLC).** When a gas or liquid chromatograph is connected to a mass spectrometer, the combined or "hyphenated" techniques are **gas chromatography/mass spectrometry (GC/MS)** and **liquid chromatography/mass spectrometry (LC/MS),** respectively.

In analytical GC and LC the mobile phase, or eluent, exits from the column and passes through a detector or series of detectors that produce a series of electronic signals

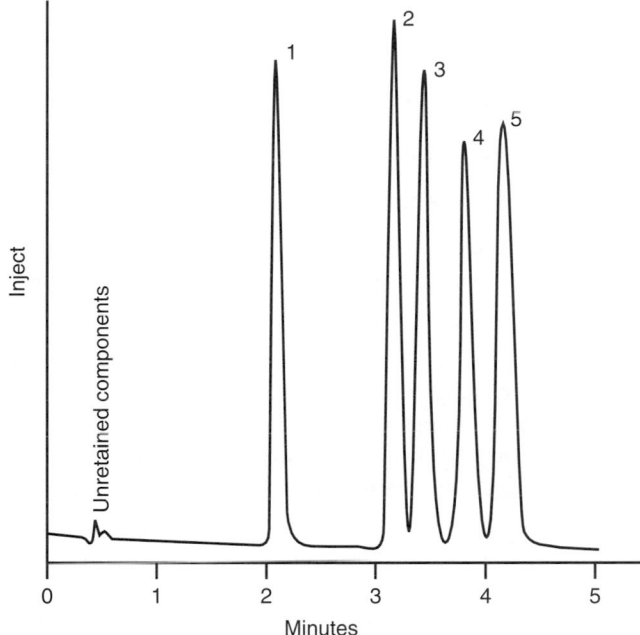

Column: C18, 3μ, 0.46 × 10 cm
Eluent: Isocratic, 0.025 M phosphate
Buffer: pH 3.0 in 25% acetonitrile
Flow rate: 2 mL/min
Detection: 215 nm, 0.1 aufs

Compounds: 1. Doxepin
              2. Desipramine
              3. Imipramine
              4. Nortriptyline
              5. Amitriptyline

Figure 8-2 Chromatogram from an HPLC reversed-phase separation of tricyclic antidepressants with the use of a UV photometer detector set at 215 nm. Signal is displayed at 0.1 aufs. *HPLC,* high-performance liquid chromatography; *UV,* ultraviolet; *aufs,* absorbance units full scale. (Courtesy Vydac/The Separations Group, Hesperia, Calif.)

that are plotted as a function of time, distance, or volume. The resulting graphical display is a **chromatogram** (Figure 8-2). The retention time or volume is the time or volume when a solute exits the column and passes through the detector. The data represented by the chromatogram are used to help identify and quantify the solute(s). Because eluting solutes are displayed graphically as a series of peaks, they are frequently referred to as *chromatographic peaks.* These peaks are described in terms of peak width, peak height, and peak area. In planar chromatography the separated zones are detected by their natural colors or visualized through chemical modification that produces colored "spots" or "bands."

■ SEPARATION MECHANISMS

Chromatographic separations are classified by the chemical or physical mechanisms used to separate the solutes. These include adsorption, affinity, ion-exchange, partition, and steric-exclusion mechanisms. For clinical applications chromatographic separations based on ion-exchange and partition mechanisms are used most widely.

Ion-Exchange Chromatography

As its name implies, **ion-exchange chromatography** is based on an exchange of ions between a charged stationary surface of one sign and solutes and mobile phase of the opposite sign (Figure 8-3). Operationally, solutes are separated by the differences in their signs and magnitudes of ionic charges. In this type of chromatography the surfaces of particles of a plastic resin or silica serve as the stationary phase. The stationary phase has functional groups with fixed cationic or anionic charges bound to it. To maintain electrochemical neutrality, an exchangeable ion termed the *counterion* is found in close proximity to the fixed charge. Solute ions in the mobile phase exchange with the counterions. The solute ions then are eluted selectively by variation of the mobile phase pH, ionic strength, or both.

Cation-exchange particles contain covalently bound, negatively charged functional groups. Both weak (CCOOH) and strong (CSO$_3$H) acidic functional groups are used to separate or "exchange" cationic solutes. Anion-exchange packings are used to separate anionic solutes. They have strongly basic quaternary amines with positive charges. Examples include triethylaminoethyl groups or weakly basic groups such as aminoethyl (AE), diethylaminoethyl (DEAE), guanidoethyl (GE), and epichlorohydrin-triethanolamine (EC-TEOLA) groups.

Ion-exchange chromatography has many clinical applications, including the separation of amino acids, peptides, proteins, nucleotides, oligonucleotides, and nucleic acids. Another important application of ion-exchange chromatography is the separation and removal of inorganic ions from aqueous mixtures. Thus most water-purification units

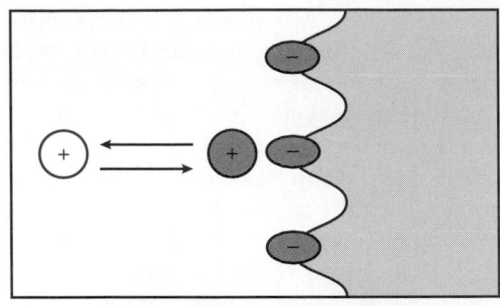

Ion-exchange chromatography

Separation is based on exchange of
ions between surface and eluents.

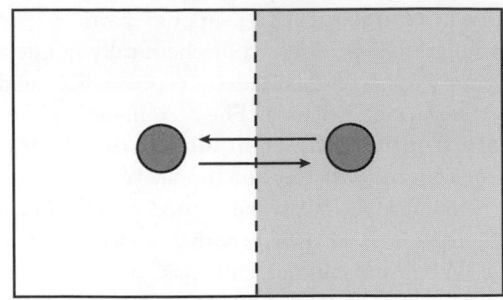

Partition chromatography

Separation is based on solute
partitioning between two liquid
phases.

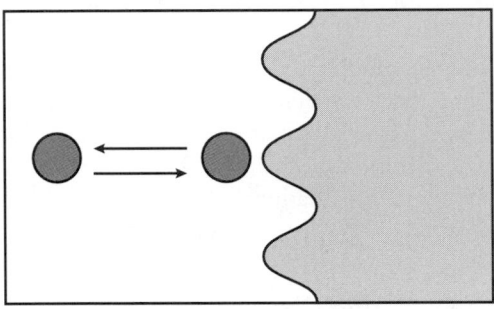

Adsorption chromatography

Separation is due to a series of
adsorption/desorption steps.

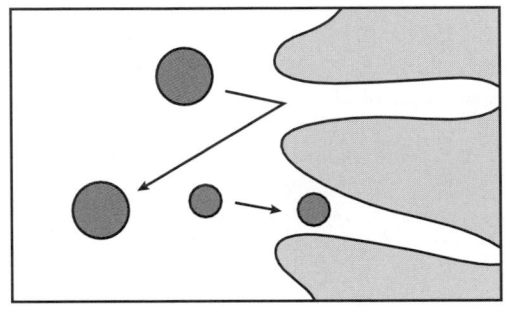

Size-exclusion chromatography

Separation is based on molecular size.

Figure 8-3   Examples of separation mechanisms used in chromatography. (Courtesy James K. Hardy, Akron, Ohio [http://ull.chemistry.uakron.edu/].)

used to prepare deionized water for the laboratory contain "mixed-bed" columns of cation and anion resins.

Partition Chromatography

The differential distribution of solutes between two immiscible liquids is the basis for separation by **partition chromatography** (see Figure 8-3). In practice, one of the immiscible liquids serves as the stationary phase. To prepare this phase a thin film of the liquid is adsorbed or chemically bonded onto the surface of support particles or onto the inner wall of a capillary column. Separation is based on differences in the relative solubility of solute molecules between the stationary and mobile phases.

Partition chromatography is categorized as either GLC or liquid-liquid chromatography (LLC). LLC further is categorized as either normal-phase or reversed-phase. For normal phase chromatography a polar liquid is used as the stationary phase, and a relatively nonpolar solvent or solvent mixture is used as the mobile phase. In reversed-phase partition chromatography the stationary phase is nonpolar, and the mobile phase is relatively polar.

Ion-suppression and ion-pair chromatography are two forms of **reversed-phase chromatography** used to

separate ionic solutes. With ion-suppression chromatography the ionic character of a weakly acidic or basic analyte is neutralized or suppressed through modification of the mobile phase pH. By neutralizing its ionic group, the solute then is less polar and better able to interact with the nonpolar stationary phase. The suppressed analyte thus has the properties of a neutral species and is separated by reversed-phase chromatography. In ion-pair chromatography a counter ion—opposite in charge to that of the analyte—is added to the mobile phase, where it forms ion pairs with ionic analytes, displaces the usual base pairs, and neutralizes the analyte ion(s). These ion pairs then are separated by reversed-phase chromatography. In practice, ion-pair chromatography is particularly useful for separations of therapeutic drugs and their metabolites.

Adsorption Chromatography

Differences between the adsorption and desorption of solutes at the surface of a solid particle are the basis of separation by adsorption chromatography (see Figure 8-3). Electrostatic, hydrogen-bonding, and dispersive interactions are the physical forces that control this type of chromatography. However, technical problems associated with the reproduc-

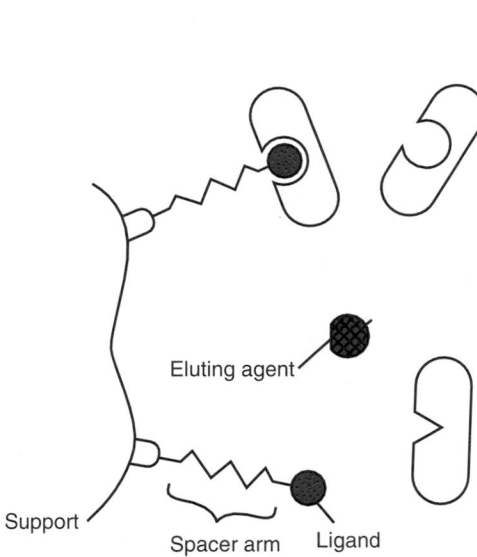

Figure 8-4   Principle of affinity chromatography. The analyte (enzyme, antibody, antigen, tissue receptor, etc.) binds to the support-bound ligand. It subsequently is eluted with a general eluent (such as a chaotropic agent), pH change, or biospecific eluent (such as an inhibitor or substrate).

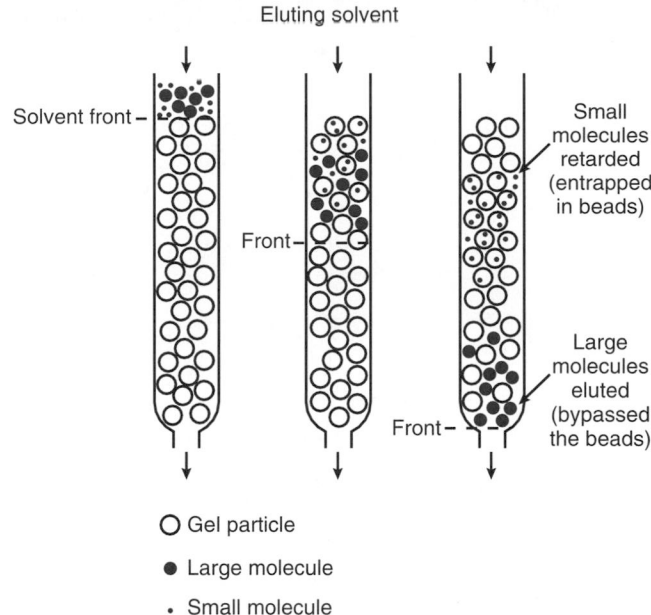

Figure 8-5   Schematic representation of gel-filtration column chromatography. (Modified from Bennett TP: Graphic Biochemistry, vol 1. Chemistry of Biological Molecules. New York, Macmillan, 1968.)

ibility of solute retention have reduced the popularity of this chromatography mode in the clinical laboratory.

Affinity Chromatography

In affinity chromatography the unique and specific biological interaction of the analyte and ligand is used for the separation (Figure 8-4). The specificity resulting from enzyme-substrate, hormone-receptor, or antigen-antibody interactions has been used in this type of chromatography.

The power of affinity chromatography lies in its selectivity. In the clinical laboratory affinity chromatography has been used to separate and prepare larger quantities of proteins and antibodies for study. Cells with different surface carbohydrate moieties are separated with lectin columns; low-density and very-low-density lipoproteins are separated with heparin columns; glycated hemoglobins are separated with phenyl boronate columns.

Steric-Exclusion Chromatography

Steric exclusion chromatography, also known as *gel-filtration, gel-permeation, size-exclusion, molecular-exclusion,* or *molecular-sieve chromatography,* separates solutes on the basis of their molecular sizes (Figure 8-5; see Figure 8-3). Molecular shape and hydration, however, are also factors in the process.

A variety of materials are used as stationary phases for steric-exclusion chromatography, including cross-linked dextran (Sephadex), polyacrylamide (Bio-Gel), agarose (Sepharose), polystyrene-divinylbenzene, porous glass, and

combinations of the above (Ultrogel, Synchrompak). The beads have tightly controlled pore sizes that allow small molecules to remain trapped temporarily inside them. Molecules too large or with shapes that prohibit them from entering the pores remain exclusively in the mobile phase and are eluted rapidly from the column. Molecules that are intermediate in size have access to various fractions of the pore volume and elute between the large and small molecules.

▓ RESOLUTION

Resolution (R₅) is a measure of a successful chromatographic separation (Figure 8-6). It is expressed mathematically as follows:

$$R_s = \frac{V_r(B) - V_r(A)}{\left[\dfrac{w(A) + w(B)}{2}\right]} \tag{1}$$

where

$V_r(A)$ = Retention volume for solute A
$V_r(B)$ = Retention volume for solute B
$w(A)$ = Bandwidth (units of volume) measured at base for solute A
$w(B)$ = Bandwidths (units of volume) measured at base for solute B

Resolution also is expressed in terms of time, with $V_r(A)$ and $V_r(B)$ being replaced with retention times $t_r(A)$ and $t_r(B)$ and $w(A)$ and $w(B)$ being expressed in units of time.

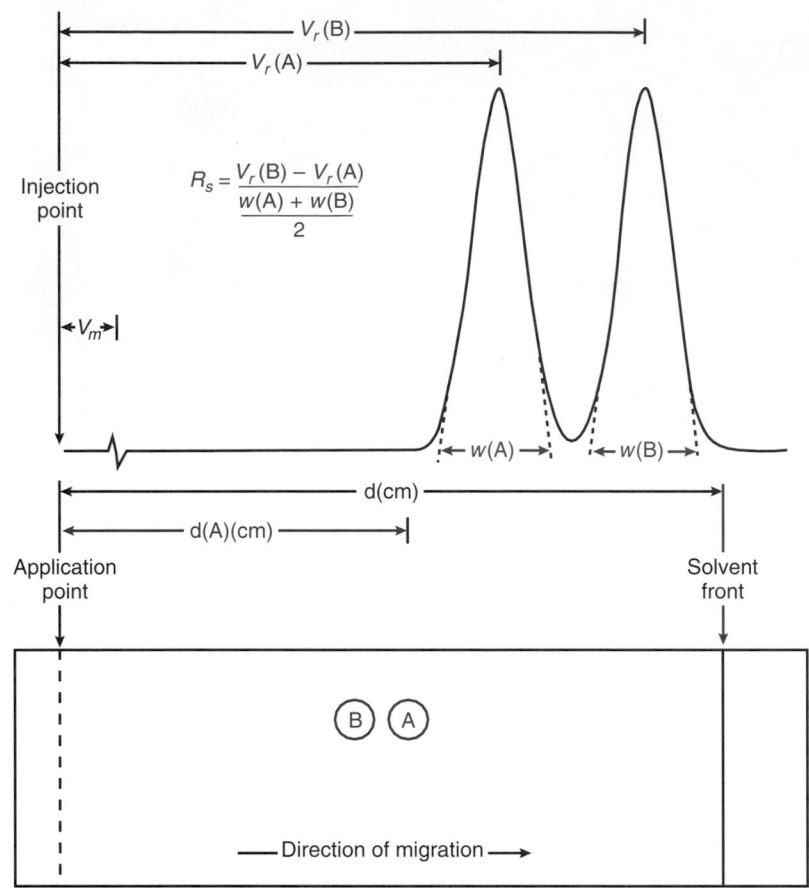

Figure 8-6 Schematic diagram of a chromatogram obtained from a column and open-bed chromatograph (planar). In open-bed chromatography *(bottom)*, strongly retained compounds (B) move more slowly than less strongly retained compounds. In column chromatography *(top)*, compound B is eluted later than compound A, again because of stronger retention. R_s, Resolution; $V_r(A)$, retention volume for solute A; $V_r(B)$, retention volume for solute B; $w(A)$, bandwidth (units of volume) measured at base for solute A; $w(B)$, bandwidth (units of volume) measured at base for solute B; Vm, volume between injector and detectors; $d(A)$, distance traveled by solute A; A, compound A; B, compound B.

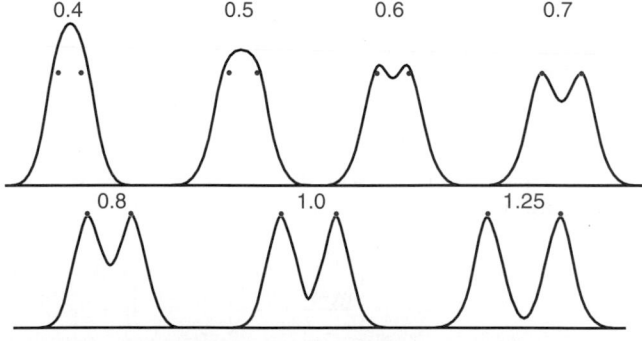

Figure 8-7 Separation of chromatographic peaks present in a 1:1 ratio as a function of resolution *(R_s)*. (From Snyder LR: A rapid approach to selecting the best experimental conditions for high-speed liquid column chromatography. Part I. Estimating initial sample resolution required by a given problem. J Chrom Sci 1972; 10:202.)

Incomplete separations occur when the calculated value for R_s is less than 0.8, whereas baseline separation is obtained when R_s is greater than 1.25 (Figure 8-7). As demonstrated in Figure 8-8, when R_s is unacceptable for a given separation, it is improved through a change in (1) the column retention factor *(k')*, (2) column efficiency *(N)*, or (3) column selectivity (α). The retention factor describes the distribution of solutes between stationary and mobile phases. Column efficiency accounts for the ease of physical interaction between solute molecules and column-packing material. Selectivity characterizes the specific chemical affinity between solute molecules and column packing. Thus by rearranging equation (1) and expressing the parameters in terms of retention, efficiency and selectivity, resolution also is expressed as follows:

$$R_s = \left(\frac{k'}{k' + 1}\right) \times \frac{\sqrt{N}}{4} \times \left(\frac{\alpha - 1}{\alpha}\right) \qquad (2)$$

A practical approach to improve resolution first is to adjust the retention factor to an acceptable value and then improve the efficiency. Finally, if required, the selectivity is changed.*

---

*For a more detailed description of these parameters and their impact on chromatographic resolution, the reader should consult Ullman MD, Bowers LD, Burtis CA: Chromatography/mass spectrometry. In Burtis CA, Ashwood ER (eds): Tietz Textbook of Clinical Chemistry, 3rd edition, Philadelphia, WB Saunders, 1999.

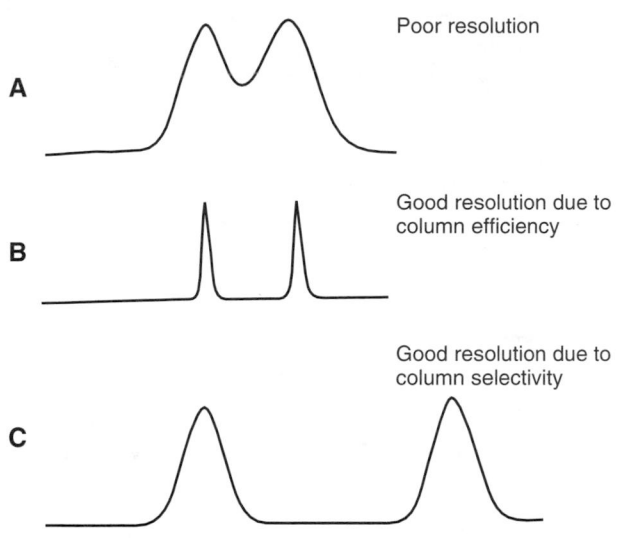

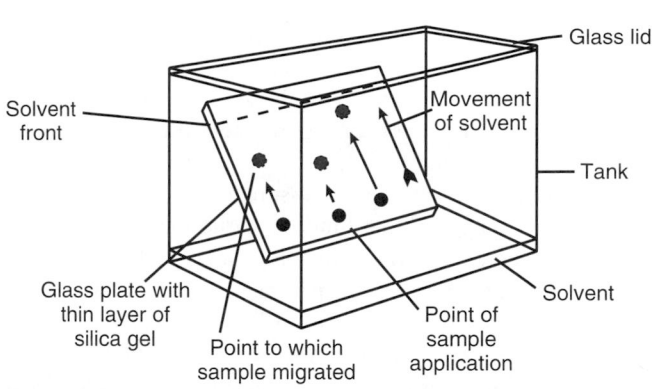

Figure 8-8   Effect of selectivity and efficiency on chromatographic resolution. **A,** Poor resolution. **B,** Good resolution due to column efficiency. **C,** Good resolution due to column selectivity. (From Johnson EL, Stevenson R: Basic Liquid Chromatography, Palo Alto, Calif, Varian Associates, 1978.)

Figure 8-9   Illustration of TLC. The solvent moves up the thin layer of absorbent by capillary action. In practice the TLC plate usually is developed as the solvent is allowed to move in an ascending direction. *TLC,* Thin-layer chromatography. (Modified from Bennett TP: Graphic Biochemistry, vol 1. Chemistry of Biological Molecules, New York, Macmillan, 1968.)

PLANAR CHROMATOGRAPHY

In planar chromatography solutes are separated on a planar surface of the stationary phase. Paper and thin-layer are subclassifications of planar chromatography. In paper chromatography the stationary phase is a layer of water or a polar solvent coated onto the paper fibers. Although once popular, this technique now is used seldomly in the clinical laboratory.

In TLC a thin layer of sorbent, such as silica gel (usually only 0.2-mm thick) is spread uniformly on a glass plate or plastic sheet. Prepared plates coated with a variety of sorbents (for example, silica gel, microcellulose, alumina, or Sephadex) are available commercially. The sample is added as a small spot or band near an edge of the plate. The plate then is placed in a closed glass container or tank with the lower edge in and the sample band just above the mobile phase (Figure 8-9). The mobile phase then migrates up the plate by capillary action. After the mobile phase travels a desired distance, the plate is removed from the tank and dried. Additional separation is achieved if the plate is developed in a second direction. In addition to this "ascending" technique, thin-layer plates also are developed in a radial mode. After the plate is dry, the separated components are located and identified by a variety of procedures, such as ultraviolet (UV) illumination; spraying with specific, color-generating reagents; or autoradiography. Provided the detection method was nondestructive, the appropriate sorbent region is scraped from the plate and extracted to recover the solute for further study or analysis.

The use of small-diameter, stationary-phase particles led to the development of HPTLC. The HPTLC separations are more efficient and reproducible because particles of

small diameters are used. Inadequate wetting and solvent evaporation must be controlled carefully. Laser-coded TLC plates are available in which each plate is identified individually to prevent recording and archiving errors.

To aid in compound identification, reference materials also are spotted on the plate and chromatographed along with the samples. Tentative identification is made by comparison of the migration distances and detection characteristics of the spots from the reference compounds with those arising from the samples. The relative migration distance of a compound is represented as its R_f value, which is defined as the spot migration distance divided by the mobile phase migration distance. However, more than one compound have the same R_f value in a particular chromatographic system, so further study often is necessary to determine the identity of an unknown compound.

When coupled with densitometry, TLC has been used successfully to quantify drugs, lipids from serum and amniotic fluid, and a number of other compounds of clinical interest. The advantages of TLC include the following:

1. Ease with which a compound is separated and visualized
2. Potential to chromatograph "dirty" samples without a cleanup step
3. Capacity to analyze multiple samples in a single run
4. Relative low cost

COLUMN CHROMATOGRAPHY

In column chromatography, support particles, on which the stationary phase is coated or chemically bonded, are "packed" into a tube, or the stationary phase is coated onto the inner surface of the tube.

Gas Chromatography

In GC a gaseous mobile phase is used to pass a mixture of volatile solutes through a column containing the stationary phase. The mobile phase is typically an inert gas, such as nitrogen, helium, hydrogen, or argon, referred to as the *carrier gas*. Solute separation is based on the relative differences in solutes' differences in vapor pressure and interactions with the stationary phase. Thus a more volatile solute elutes from the column before a less volatile one does. In addition, a solute that selectively interacts with the stationary phase elutes from the column after one with a lesser degree of interaction. The column effluent carries separated solutes to the detector in the order of their elution. Solutes are identified qualitatively by their similar retention times. Peak size (area or height) is proportional to the amount of the solute detected and is used to quantify it.

Gas-solid chromatography (GSC) and GLC are variations of GC. In GSC, separations occur primarily by differences in absorption at the solid phase surface. In GLC a nonvolatile liquid is coated onto particles of column packing or directly onto the wall of a capillary column. Separation occurs primarily by differences in solute partitioning between the gaseous mobile phase and the liquid stationary phase.

Instrumentation

A basic gas chromatograph (Figure 8-10) consists of the following features:

1. A chromatographic column to separate the solutes
2. A supply of carrier gas and flow-control apparatus to regulate the flow of carrier gas through the system
3. An injector to introduce an aliquot of sample or derivatized analyte into the column
4. A column oven to heat the column
5. An on-line detector to detect the separated analytes as they elute from the column
6. A computer to control the system and process data

Column technology

The chromatographic column is the heart of a gas chromatograph. The main types of columns are packed and capillary. Packed columns are filled with support particles that are used uncoated (GSC) or have been coated with the stationary phase (GLC). They vary from 1 to 4 mm in internal diameter (ID), from 1 meter or more in length, and are fabricated from tubes of glass or stainless steel. Although narrow columns are more efficient, wider columns have increased sample capacities. Longer columns also are more efficient but require increased carrier gas pressures.

Capillary columns, also known as *wall-coated open tubular columns*, are fabricated by coating of the inner wall of a

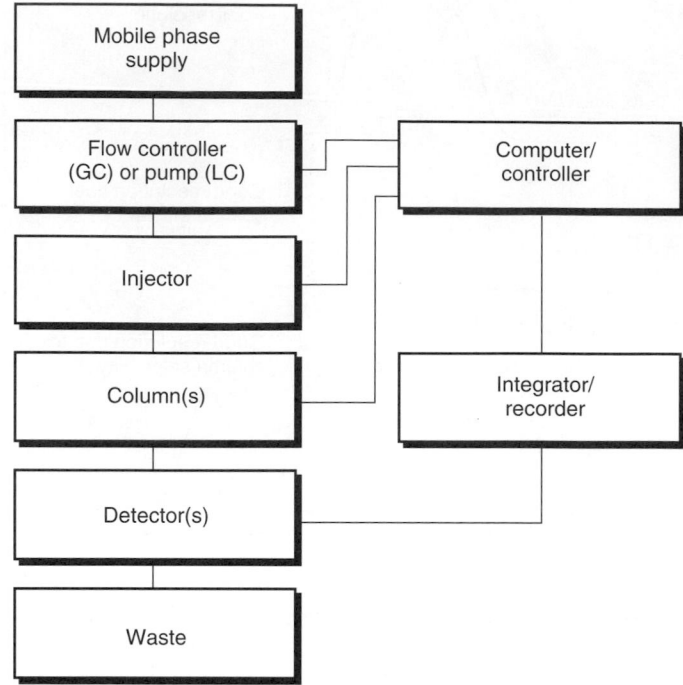

Figure 8-10 Schematic diagram of a gas or liquid chromatograph. *GC*, Gas chromatography; *LC*, liquid chromatography.

fused-silica tube with a thin film of liquid phase. They vary from 0.1 to 0.5 mm in ID and from 10 to 150 m in length. The ultrapure fused silica used to fabricate capillary tubing is very fragile. A thin outside coating of polyimide or aluminum improves column durability. These modified capillary columns have the structural strength and flexibility necessary to withstand coiling and placement in ovens. Capillary columns are very efficient but have a low sample capacities.

A variety of compounds have been used as the stationary phase in GLC. These include methyl silicone polymers, substituted silicone polymers, and silicone polyesters. These materials are coated or chemically bonded onto the surface of the support particles or onto the walls of the column. Although more expensive, bonded materials are preferable because of their stability.

Carrier gas supply and flow control

A constant flow of carrier gas is required for column efficiency and reproducible elution times. Systems that provide constant flow rates vary, from simple mechanical devices to sophisticated electronic ones. For example, a simple system consisting of a tank of compressed gas, a needle valve to adjust flow, a flow meter, and a pressure gauge is sufficient for many applications. More demanding temperature-programmed operation (which will be discussed in a subsequent section of this chapter) requires a more sophisticated differential-flow controller, such as an electronic pressure control system programmed to regulate the carrier gas flow rate and pressure during a chromatographic run. Such a controller is operated in either a constant-flow or a constant-

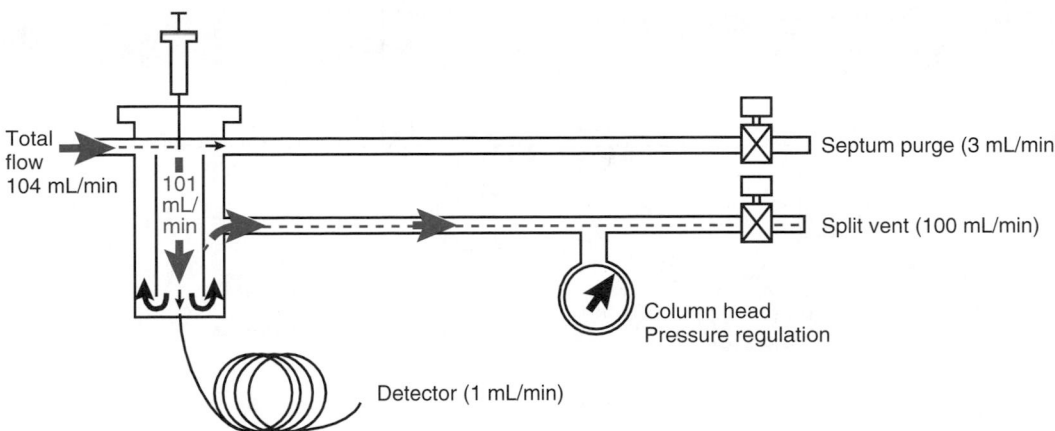

Figure 8-11   Flow diagram of a GC inlet system for split injection. The head pressure and total flow are adjusted to achieve a desired flow rate in the column and a fractional split between the column and the split vent. *GC*, gas chromatography.

pressure mode. In the constant-flow mode the pressure required to maintain a constant flow independent of carrier gas viscosity is calculated. A pressure transducer then measures and maintains the inlet pressure required for the constant flow.

Operationally, the flow rate depends on the type of column. For example, packed columns require a flow rate from 10 to 60 mL/minute. Flow rates for capillary columns are much lower (1 to 2 mL/minute), and the maintenance of a constant flow rate is even more critical for the efficient operation of these columns.

Carrier gases should be pure and dry. A number of gases are used as carrier gases, depending on the column and detector. Hydrogen and helium are the carrier gases of choice with capillary columns. Only high-purity hydrogen and helium should be used, however, because carrier-gas impurities harm the column, decrease the performance of some detectors, and adversely affect quantification in trace analysis. For packed columns the most frequently used carrier gas is nitrogen, which is used with flame-ionization (FID), electron-capture (ECD), or thermal-conductivity (TCD) detectors. Helium is used with FIDs and TCDs, and nitrogen-argon-methane mixtures are used with the ECD.

Injector

In most clinical GC methods samples are dissolved in nonaqueous liquids introduced into the column via an inline injector. With packed columns a glass microsyringe is used to inject a 1- to 10-μL aliquot of the dissolved sample through a septum that serves as the interface between the injector and the chromatographic system. In practice, the syringe needle is inserted through the injector septum and into a heating region. The volatile analytes and the solvent are then "flash-vaporized" and swept into the column by the carrier gas. To ensure rapid and complete solute volatilization the temperature of the injector is maintained at 30 to 50 °C higher than the column temperature.

Common problems with GC analysis include septum leaks and absorbance of components from the sample onto the septum during injection. In addition, because the septum is heated, decomposition products form and "bleed" into the column. This bleeding results in spurious peaks—termed "ghost" peaks—appearing in the chromatogram. Septum bleed is greater at higher injection-port temperatures. To minimize this problem a Teflon-coated, low-bleed septum is used. The inner surface of the septum is purged continuously with the carrier gas that is vented before it passes into the column. This approach is especially effective, and most commercial injectors are equipped with continuous-purge capabilities. The septum is a consumable component of the gas chromatograph and should be replaced at least once every 100 injections.

Because of the low sample capacities and carrier-gas flow rates used with capillary columns, split and splitless injection techniques are used to introduce samples into the columns. In the split mode (Figure 8-11), only a small portion of the vaporized sample enters the column, whereas in the splitless mode most of that sample enters the column (Figure 8-12). Operationally, the split flow mode is used for samples that contain relatively high concentrations of the target analyte(s); the splitless mode is used for samples containing low levels of the target analyte.

Temperature control

To operate properly, both packed and capillary columns require careful control of the column, injector, and detector temperatures. Control of the column temperature is achieved when the column is placed in an oven. Injector and detector temperatures usually are controlled by electrical resistance heating. Depending on the application, the column temperature is maintained at either a constant preset level (isothermal operation) during the chromatographic run or varied as a function of time (temperature-programmed operation).

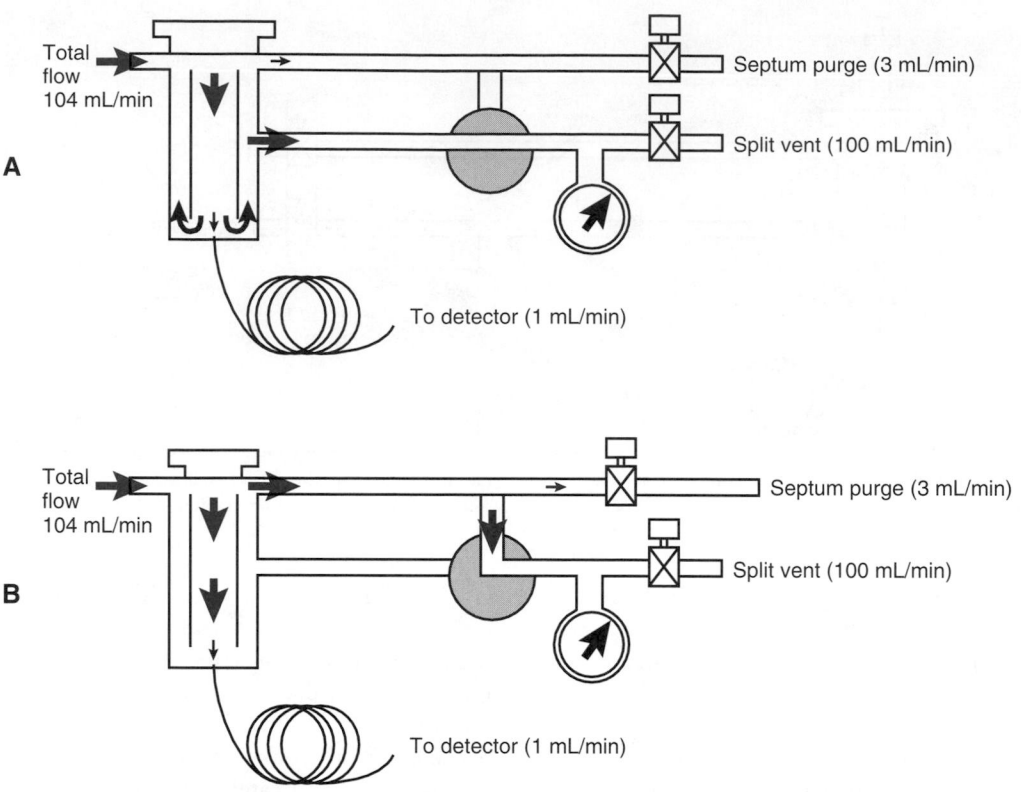

Figure 8-12   Flow diagram of a GC inlet system for splitless injection. Initially, the system has most of the flow through the injection liner, with the majority of it directed to the split vent **(A).** When an injection is made, flow is directed through the septum purge line, and all material in the injec- tion liner is transferred into the column **(B).** After 50 to 80 seconds, the flow again is directed through the liner **(A)** to purge any material remaining in the liner through the split vent; meanwhile, a constant flow is maintained through the column. *GC,* Gas chromatography.

Detectors

A variety of sensitive detectors are used with gas chromatographs, including universal units that detect most analytes to extremely selective devices that detect only specific ones (Table 8-1). Examples include FIDs, photoionization detectors (PIDs), TCDs, ECDs, thermionic-selective detecors (TSDs), and mass spectrometers.

The flame-ionization detector (FID) is the most commonly used detector for clinical analysis (Figure 8-13). Its advantages include simplicity, reliability, versatility, sensitivity, and ease of operation. During operation the column effluent is mixed with hydrogen and air, and the eluting compounds are burned by a flame. About one molecule in 10,000 produces an organic cation and releases an electron, which is detected by a collector electrode positioned above the flame. The current generated is related to the mass of carbon material delivered to the detector; after measurement, it is used for detection and quantification of the eluting solutes.

The photoionization detector (PID) is a variant of the FID. With the PID the energy for ionization is provided by an intense UV lamp rather than by a flame. The thermionic-selective detector (TSD), also known as the *nitrogen-phosphorus detector (NPD),* is a modification of the FID in which an alkali bead is heated electrically in the area above the jet. In the presence of alkali atoms in the flame,

nitrogen-containing compounds give a 15-times-greater, and phosphorous-containing compounds a 300-times-greater, response.

The thermal-conductivity detector (TCD) is based on the principle that addition of a compound to a gas alters the thermal conductance of the gas. It is used often with capillary GC. The operating principle of the electron-capture detector (ECD) is based on the reaction between electronegative compounds, such as fluorine, chlorine, bromine, and iodine, and thermal electrons. Because not all compounds contain these functional groups, derivatization with reagents containing polychlorinated or polyfluorinated moieties is a common practice used with an ECD.

Different types of mass spectrometers also are used as detectors for gas chromatographs. (These devices will be discussed in more detail in a subsequent section of this chapter.)

Computer/controller

The incorporation of computer technology into chromatographic instrumentation has resulted in cost effective, easy-to-operate automated systems with improved analytical performance. In these systems a computer provides both system-control and data-processing functions (Figure 8-14). As a process controller the computer regulates various pa-

TABLE 8-1	Examples of Detectors Used in Gas Chromatographs			
Type of Detector	Principle of Operation	Selectivity	Limit of Detection	Comments
Thermal conductance (TCD)	Measures thermal conductivity change in carrier gas on elution of compounds	Universal	<400 pg propane/mL He	
Flame ionization (FID)	$CHNO + heat \rightarrow CHNO^+ + e^-$; electrons collected for detection	Hydrocarbon	10 to 100 pg CHO	
Thermionic selective (TSD; NPD)	Alkali bead selectively ionizes N- or P-containing compounds	N, P	0.4 to 10 pg N 0.1 to 1.0 pg P	
Electron capture (ECD)	$e^- + R + N_2 \rightarrow Re^- + N_2 + e^-$; excess electrons collected; concentration inversely related	Electronegative groups	0.05 to 1.0 pg Cl-containing compounds	
Mass spectrometer (MS)	$e^- + ABC \rightarrow A^+ + BC$; monitor mass-to-charge ratio by either scanning or single-ion monitoring (SIM)	Universal (tunable)	1 ng scan 10 pg SIM	Provides structural confirmation; ion ratios constant in SIM
Photoionization (PID)	$CHNO + photon \rightarrow CHNO^+ + e^-$; detect electron	Hydrocarbon	1 to 10 pg CHO	May be improvement on FID
Electrolytic conductivity (Hall)	Postcolumn reaction detector for selective detection of halogen-, S-, or N-containing compounds	Halogen-, S-, and N-containing compounds	0.1 to 1.0 pg Cl 2.0 pg S 4.0 pg N	
Flame photometric (FPD)	P- and S-containing hydrocarbons emit light when burned in FID-type flame; emitted light detected	P- and S-containing compounds	0.9 pg CHP 20 pg CHS	
Fourier transform infrared (FTIR)	Infrared wavelength light absorbed by the compound of interest	Universal (tunable)	1 ng strong infrared absorber	Scanned for structural information or absorbance-measured for quantitation

NPD, Nitrogen-phosphorus detector.

rameters, such as mobile-phase composition and flow rate, column back-pressure, column and detector temperatures, sample injection, detector selection and operation, and the various timing steps that command the operation of the system. For data processing the computer monitors signals generated by the system's detectors and commands the acquisition and storage of data at specified time intervals. The area, or height, of each chromatographic peak is determined from the stored data and used to compute the analyte concentration represented by each peak. Available algorithms for this computation include those based on calibration curves or conversion factors from internal or external calibration. A complete report is prepared and printed for each chromatographic run. Computerized data systems also provide flexibility because stored data can be recalled and reprocessed with different integration parameters.

Practical considerations

Several techniques affect the practical application of GC in the clinical laboratory, including those used to prepare and derivatize samples for analysis and to identify and quantify analytes.

Sample extraction

For GC analysis, extraction of the analyte from the sample often is necessary. For example, to extract barbiturates from serum, the serum first is acidified to convert the barbiturates into a form soluble in an organic solvent such as dichloromethane. A volume of this solvent then is shaken vigorously with the acidified serum. When the aqueous and organic layers separate, most of the barbiturates are present in the organic phase, and many interferences, such as proteins, remain in the aqueous phase. Solvent extraction also is used frequently to increase the concentration of an analyte prior to chromatographic analysis.

Sample derivatization

Many clinically relevant compounds are nonvolatile and therefore difficult to separate by GC. However, chemical modification or derivatization of such compounds increases

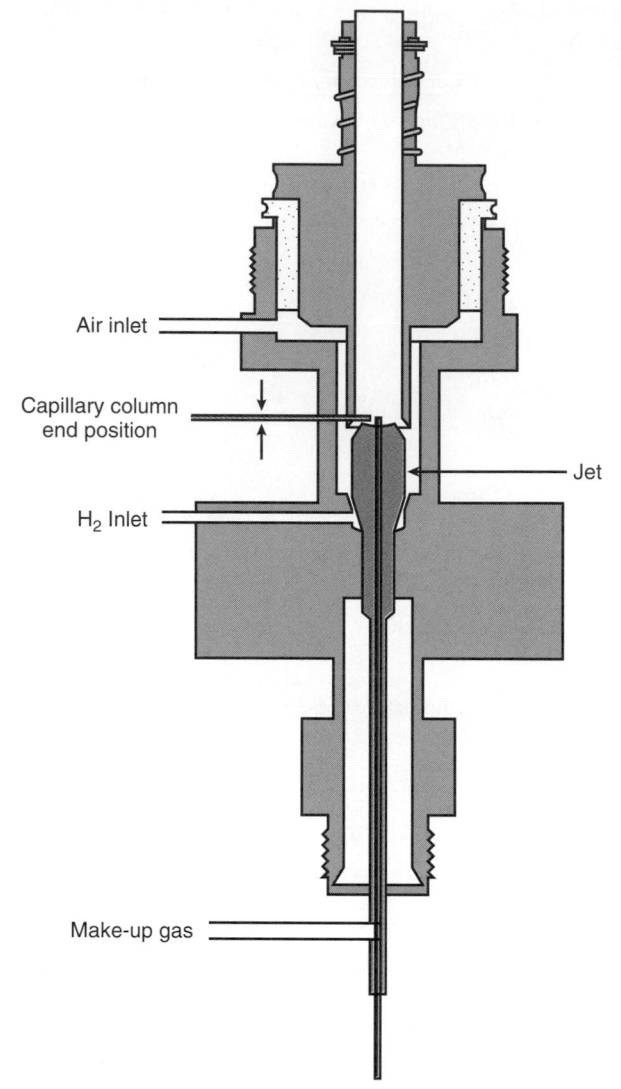

Air inlet

Capillary column
end position

Jet

H$_2$ Inlet

Make-up gas

Figure 8-13 Schematic diagram of a FID equipped with makeup gas. *FID,* Flame-ionization detector. (Modified from Hyver KJ: High Resolution Gas Chromatography, 3rd edition, Palo Alto, Calif, Hewlitt Packard, 1989.)

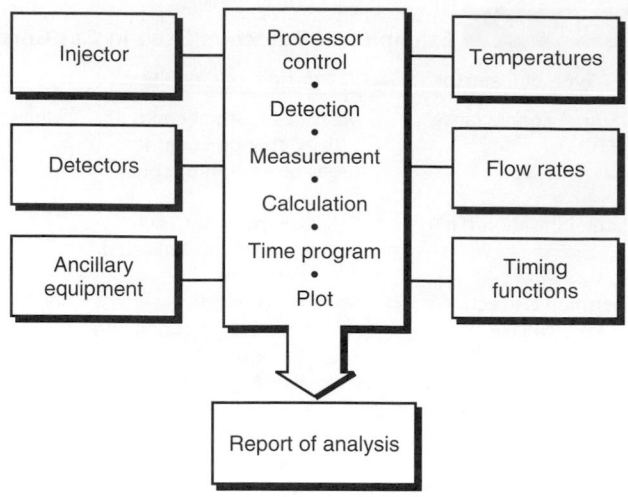

Injector	Processor control	Temperatures
Detectors	Detection · Measurement · Calculation	Flow rates
Ancillary equipment	Time program · Plot	Timing functions

Report of analysis

Figure 8-14 Functions of computers in gas and liquid chromatographs.

their volatility for GC analysis. Chemical reactions used to form these nonpolar derivatives include acylation, silylation, esterification, and oximation. In addition to enhancing solute volatility, derivatization also is used to enhance the specificity and sensitivity of particular separations. For example, the use of a chiral reagent to derivatize amphetamine improves specificity and allows the separation of the D- and L-isomers on a standard GC column. Enhanced detectability also is achieved via preparation of pentafluoropropyl derivatives for use with the ECD.

Analyte identification
The retention time, or volume, at which an unknown solute elutes from a column often is matched to that of a reference compound. The appearance of a solute peak at the

same time as that of a reference compound is consistent with the belief that the two compounds are the same. The simultaneous appearance does not prove identity, however, because other compounds may have the same retention time as the reference compound.

With capillary columns, introduction of the components of a single injection into two columns simultaneously is possible. The columns are connected to separate detectors of the same or a different type. Matching the retention properties of a single analyte with a reference compound on two columns of dissimilar phases enhances the chance for correct identification of the analyte. The most reliable analyte identification is provided by a detector that features structural information, such as a mass spectrometer.

Analyte quantification
The electronic signals from the detector(s) also are used to produce quantitative information. Both external or internal calibrating techniques are used. With external calibration, reference solutions containing known quantities of analytes are processed in a manner identical to the samples containing the analyte (Figure 8-15). A calibration curve of peak height or peak area versus calibrator concentration is constructed and used to calculate the concentration of the analyte in the samples. With internal calibration, also called *internal standardization,* reference solutions of known concentrations of analytes are prepared, and a constant amount of a different compound, the internal standard, is added to each reference solution and each sample (Figure 8-16). By plotting the ratio of the peak height (or area) of the analyte to the peak height (or area) of the internal standard versus the concentration of the analyte, a calibration curve that corrects for systematic losses is constructed. This curve then is used to compute the concentration of the analyte in the samples by interpolation.

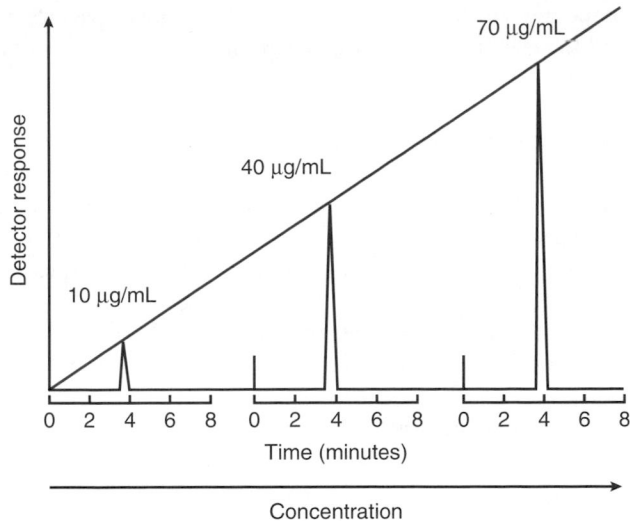

Figure 8-15   The use of external calibrators in the production of a calibration plot. (From Krull I, Swartz M: Quantitation in method validation. LC-GC 1998; 16:1084-1090.)

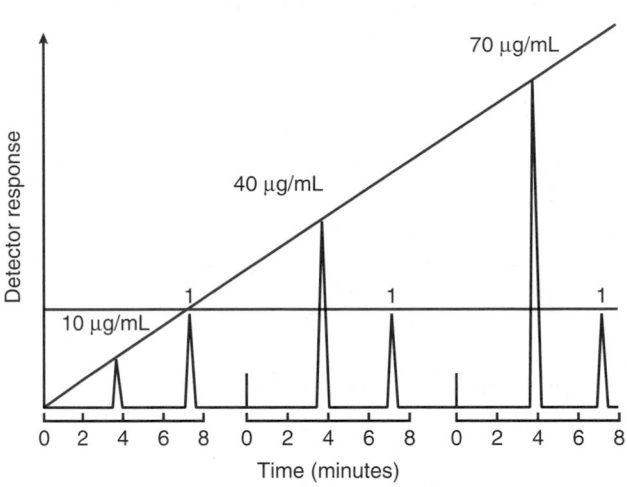

Figure 8-16   The use of internal calibrators in the production of a calibration plot (peak 1 being the internal standard). (From Krull I, Swartz M: Quantitation in method validation. LC-GC 1998; 16:1084-1090.)

Liquid Chromatography

Separation by LC is based on the distribution of the solutes between a liquid mobile phase and a stationary phase. When particles of small diameter are used as the stationary-phase support, the technique is high-performance liquid chromatography (HPLC). Because column efficiency is inversely related to the column-packing particle size and pressure drop is related to the square of the particle diameter, relatively high pressures are required to pump liquids through efficient HPLC columns. Consequently, the technique has also been referred to as *high-pressure liquid chromatography*. In the clinical laboratory HPLC is the most widely used form of LC. It has been used for assaying or monitoring many clinically relevant analytes, including amino acids, peptides, proteins, carbohydrates, lipids, nucleic acids and related compounds, vitamins, hormones, metabolites, and drugs, such as antiarrhythmics, antibiotics, antiepileptics, analgesics, bronchial smooth muscle relaxants, and tricyclic antidepressants.

Instrumentation

A basic liquid chromatograph (see Figure 8-10) consists of the following elements:

1. A chromatographic column to separate the solutes
2. A solvent reservoir to hold the mobile phase
3. One or more pumps to force the liquid mobile phase through the system
4. An injector to introduce an aliquot of sample into the column
5. An on-line detector to detect the separated analytes as they elute from the column
6. A computer that controls the system and processes data

TABLE 8-2   Types of Columns Used in HPLC

Column Terminology	Column ID (mm)	Optimum Flow Volume
Standard	4.6	1.25 mL/min
	4.0	1.0 mL/min
Narrow Bore	3.0	0.6 mL/min
	2.0	200 μL/min
Microbore/Capilllary	1.0	50 μL/min
	0.5	12 μL/min
	0.3	4 μL/min

HPLC, High-performance liquid chromatography; *ID*, internal diameter.

With these components various types of HPLC systems are assembled. These range from single-pump, single-solvent units to versatile, automated systems.

Column technology

Advances in column technology have improved the selectivity, stability, and reproducibility of LC analytical columns. This section describes (1) column dimensions, (2) the use of guard columns, and (3) the different types of column packings used in analytical columns.

Column dimensions.   Most analytical HPLC columns used in the clinical laboratory are fabricated from tubes made of 316 stainless steel. The IDs of these columns range from 0.3 mm to 5 mm (Table 8-2) and the lengths from 50 mm to 250 mm. Column end-fittings, which have zero dead volume and frits to retain the support particles, are used to connect the column to the injector on the inlet end and the detector on the outlet end. Generally, lower detection limits are achieved with columns having smaller IDs. Furthermore, the amount of mobile phase used with smaller ID columns is less than that with larger ID columns. For example, a 2-mm-ID column requires about fivefold less solvent than a 4.6-mm-ID column (see Table 8-2).

Columns of the dimensions described previously are packed with small, uniform, porous particles with surfaces covered by the stationary phase. Such particles have diameters ranging from 3 to 10 μm. The packings provide efficient columns with acceptable operating back pressures. Irregularly shaped or spherical packings that provide lower back pressures also are available. In addition, capillary columns are used in LC and are fabricated through coating of the inner wall of a fused-silica tube with a thin film of liquid phase. They vary from 0.1 to 0.5 mm in ID and from 10 cm to 50 cm in length.

Guard columns. To prevent an analytical column from irreversibly adsorbing proteins with a concurrent reduction in both resolution and column life, a guard column is placed between the injector and analytical column. A guard column is packed with the same or similar stationary phase as the analytical column. It collects particulate matter and any strongly retained components from the sample and thus conserves the life of the analytical column. After a predetermined number of separations, a guard column routinely is replaced.

Column packings. Analytical columns are packed with a variety of stationary phases, providing enormous versatility in the separation process. These materials include bonded, polymeric, chiral, and restricted access packings.

Bonded-phase packings—In bonded-phase packings the stationary phase is bonded chemically to the surface of silica particles through a silica ester or silicone polymeric linkage. Bonded-phase packings are mechanically and chemically stable, have long lifetimes, and provide excellent chromatographic performance. Bonded-phase packings are available for ion-exchange and both normal-phase and reversed-phase chromatography. In normal-phase HPLC the functional groups of the stationary phase are polar relative to those of the mobile phase, which usually consists of nonpolar solvents such as hexane. Examples of polar functional groups for normal-phase HPLC packings are silanol, amino, and nitrile groups. Reversed-phase HPLC requires a nonpolar stationary phase. The most popular reversed-phase packing is the C18 type, in which octadecylsilane molecules are bonded to silica particles. A column with octadecyl packing often is called an *ODS column* (ODS, octadecyl silica). Reversed-phase column retention and selectivity characteristics are altered via attachment of other groups, such as octyl, phenyl, or cyanopropyl, to the silica.

Polymeric packings—Graphitized carbon or mixed copolymers are used as polymeric packing (for example, polystyrene-divinyl benzene) or further derivatized with ion-exchange or C4, C8, or C18 functional groups. Columns filled with these packings feature levels of performance comparable to those of silica-based columns and are stable from pH 2 to 13.

Chiral packings—Chiral packings are used to separate enantiomers, which are mirror-image forms of the same compound. In the clinical laboratory this type of packing is used to separate and quantify drug enantiomers.

Restricted-access packings—With restricted access packings the outer surfaces of the support particles are protected by a hydrophilic network. Smaller solutes such as drugs pass through the network into the pores, which are coated with hydrophobic stationary phase. Large protein molecules are denied access to the inner core and pass through the column. Columns filled with restricted-access packing allow the direct injection of biological samples with high protein concentrations, which bypasses sample preparation and improves analytical accuracy.

Solvent reservoir

Solvents used as the mobile phase are contained in solvent reservoirs. In their simplest forms the reservoirs are glass bottles or flasks into which "feed lines" to the pump are inserted. To remove particles from solvents, in-line filters are placed on the inlets of the feed lines. Sophisticated mobile-phase handling systems available commercially contain specially designed bottles with internal, conically shaped bottoms that allow small solvent volumes to be utilized. These handling systems also feature three or four valve caps that permit the filtration, storage, and delivery of solvents and a stopcock for vacuum degassing.

Pump

Both constant-pressure and constant-displacement pumps are used in liquid chromatographs. However, constant displacement pumps are used more widely. During its operation the constant-displacement pump withdraws (aspirates) mobile phase from the solvent reservoir and delivers a reproducibly constant flow of it through the chromatographic system. Several different types of pumps are used for this purpose, including the syringe pump, single-piston rapid-refill reciprocating pump, diaphragm pump, and the most widely used dual-piston reciprocating pump.

A dual-piston reciprocating pump uses an asymmetrical cam to drive two pistons into and from two pumping chambers (Figure 8-17). The reciprocating action of the pump, however, creates "pump pulsations," or changes in the flow rate. The changes affect the output signals of some detectors, thereby increasing baseline noise that influences the detection limit of the system. Thus most reciprocating pumps utilize mechanical or electronic pulse dampers and/or multiple heads that operate out of phase to deliver mobile phase continuously. Another technique uses a significantly more rapid refill stroke than delivery stroke. Reciprocating pumps operate at up to 10,000 psi and generate flow rates from 0.01 mL/minute to 20 mL/minute or greater, depending on pump head size and configuration.

The HPLC pump is operated in either an isocratic or gradient mode (Figure 8-18). In the isocratic mode the mobile-phase composition remains constant throughout the chromatographic run. This mode is usually used for simpler separations and separations of those compounds with simi-

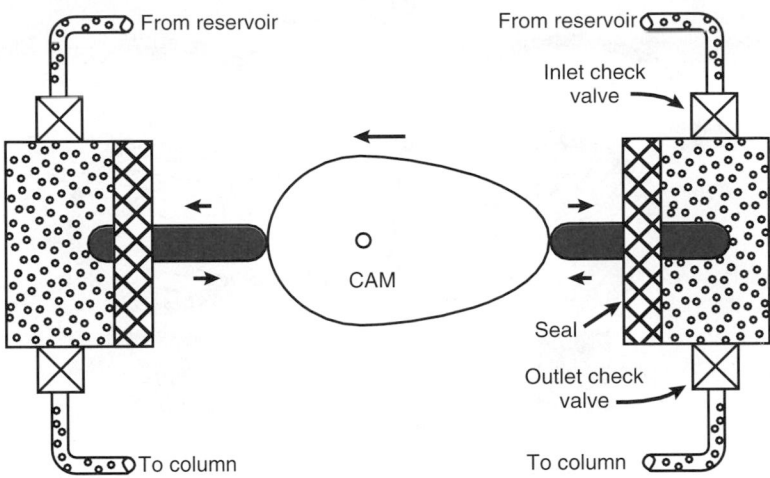

Figure 8-17   Cross-sectional view of a dual-piston reciprocating liquid pump. (From Walker JQ, Jackson MT Jr, Maynard JB: Chromatographic Systems: Maintenance and Troubleshooting, 2nd edition, New York, Academic Press, 1977.)

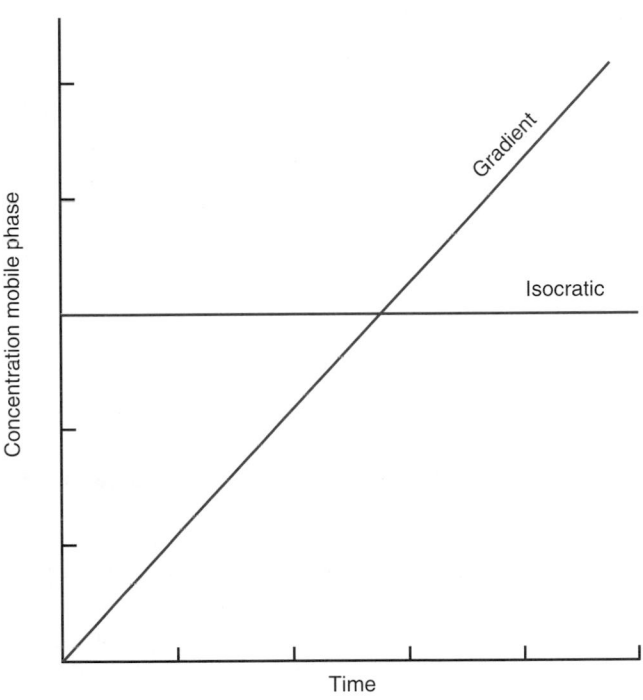

Figure 8-18   Examples of isocratic and gradient elution in LC. *LC,* Liquid chromatography.

lar structures and/or retention times. An isocratic mobile phase can be a single solvent (for example, methanol), or a prepared mixture of several solvents (for example, methanol, acetonitrile, and water) delivered from a single-solvent reservoir. Alternatively, a multisolvent mobile phase can be metered and proportioned from two or more reservoirs.

Most HPLC separations are performed under isocratic conditions. When a separation is more complex, gradient elution is used. In the gradient mode, mobile-phase composition is changed during the run in either a stepwise or continuous fashion. Many different techniques are used to generate gradient profiles. In one technique two or more pumps are used in parallel. A variety of gradient profiles are generated through programming of the output of each pump. Alternatively, the mobile phase is proportioned on the inlet side of a single pump. For example, up to four solvent reservoirs may be connected via proportioning valves to the inlet check valve of a single pump. The composition of the mobile phase then is varied through programming of the time during which solvent is delivered through each of the proportioning valves.

Injector

An aliquot of sample (for example, 0.2 to 50 μL) is introduced into a liquid chromatograph via an injector. The most widely used type is the fixed-loop injector (Figure 8-19). In the fill position an aliquot of sample is introduced at atmospheric pressure into a stainless-steel loop. In the inject mode the sample loop is rotated into the flowing stream of mobile phase, and the sample is swept into the chromatographic column. These injectors are precise, function at high pressures, and can be programmed for use in automated systems.

Digitally-controlled autosamplers that incorporate a loop injector are available commercially. These sophisticated devices are extremely precise and can be programmed for continuous and automated operation. In addition, the sample loop is flushed automatically with mobile phase between samples to avoid sample carry-over. The ability to inject multiple aliquots from a single sample vial is another feature of most autosamplers.

Detectors

Many detectors have been developed for use with liquid chromatographs (Table 8-3). Examples include photometric, spectrophotometric, fluorometric, and electrochemical detectors. A key and integral component of such detectors is the flow cell (Figure 8-20), through which the eluate from the chromatographic column passes. Dissolved analytes

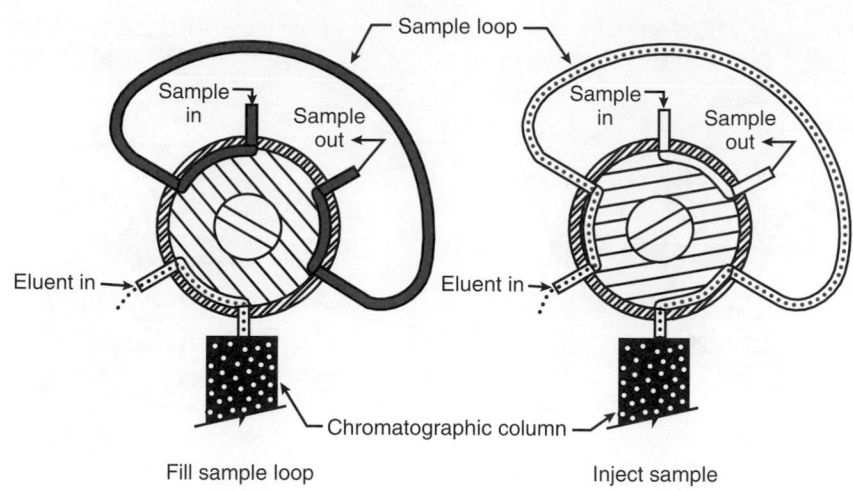

Figure 8-19 Cross-sectional view of a commonly used sample loop injector.

TABLE 8-3	Examples of Detectors Used in High-Performance Liquid Chromatographs

Type of Detector	Principle of Operation	Range of Application	Detection Limit	Comments
UV photometer (fixed wavelength)	Measures absorbance of UV light	Selective	<1 ng	Analyte must absorb UV light or be derivatized
UV photometer (variable wavelength)	Measures absorbance of UV light	Selective	<1 ng	Detector can be "tuned" to a specific wavelength
Diode array	Measures absorbance of light	Selective	<1 ng	Detector provides complete spectra
Fluorometer	Measures fluorescence	Very selective	pg to ng	Analyte must fluoresce or be derivatized
Refractometer	Measures change in refractive index	Universal	1 μg	
Electrochemical	Electrochemically measures oxidized/reduced analyte	Selective	pg to ng	Detector is useful for catecholamines

UV, Ultraviolet.

then are detected and an electronic signal generated. (Mass spectrometers, which also have been used as LC detectors, will be discussed in detail in a later section of this chapter.)

Photometers and spectrophotometers. UV and visible photometers measure the radiant energy absorbed by compounds as they elute from the chromatographic column (see Chapter 3). These detectors operate in the radiant energy regions of 190 to 400 nm and 400 to 700 nm, respectively. These devices are versatile and detect many solutes because most organic compounds absorb in the UV region, with a few in the visible region, of the electromagnetic spectrum.

Photometers operate as either fixed-wavelength or variable-wavelength detectors. Most fixed-wavelength UV photometers use the intense 254-nm resonance line produced by a mercury arc lamp (Figure 8-20). This type of detector is extremely sensitive and operates at 0.005 absorbance units full scale (aufs).* To provide the fixed-

wavelength detectors with greater flexibility, other less intense resonance lines of the mercury lamp are used. Alternatively, a phosphor is placed between the lamp and the flow cell, and the emitted fluorescence resulting from the 254-nm excitation is used as the light source. This latter approach is used in the dual-wavelength photometers that operate at two fixed wavelengths (for example, 254 nm and 280 nm). The intense 214-nm or 229-nm resonance lines of a zinc or cadmium arc lamp, respectively, also are used for detection at lower wavelengths, where more compounds absorb.

The second type of photometer is the variable-wavelength detector. It operates at a wavelength selected from a given wavelength range. Thus the detector is "tuned" to operate at the absorbance maximum for a given analyte or set of analytes, which enhances greatly the applicability and selectivity of the detector (see Figure 8-2). Another advantage of this detector is its ability to operate at lower wavelengths (for example, 190 nm). Because more compounds (for example, cholesterol) absorb at lower wavelengths, this capability enhances the versatility of the detector. At lower wavelengths, however, many solvents absorb UV light and

---

*An aufs is a unit of measure used to describe the full scale deflection on a recorder. For example, an aufs of 0.005 indicates that a full-scale deflection on a recorder corresponds to 0.005 absorbance units.

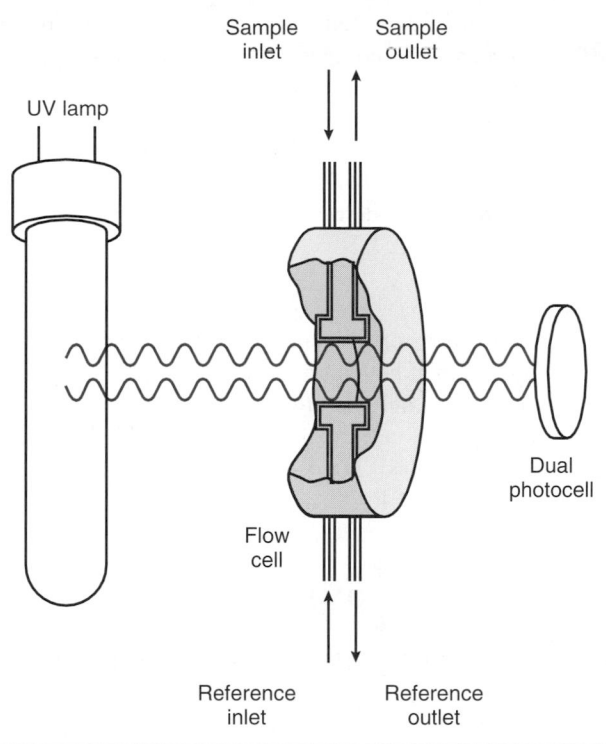

Figure 8-20 Optical schematic of a simple photometer and flow cell. *UV*, Ultraviolet.

cannot be used as mobile phases. Fortunately, acetonitrile and methanol, two widely used solvents in reversed-phase chromatography, have minimal UV absorptions at 200 nm.

In addition, diode arrays are used as HPLC detectors because they rapidly yield spectral data over the entire wavelength range of 190 to 600 nm in about 10 milliseconds. During operation the diode array detector passes polychromatic light through the detector flow cell. The transmitted light is dispersed by a diffraction grating and then directed to a photodiode array, where the intensity of light at multiple wavelengths in the spectrum is measured. Such detectors have been helpful in the identification of drugs in urine and serum.

Fluorometers.   As discussed in Chapter 4, fluorescence occurs when a molecule absorbs light at one wavelength and reemits light at a longer wavelength. On-line fluorometers are used in liquid chromatographs to detect fluorescing compounds as they elute from the column. In addition, either a precolumn or postcolumn reactor chemically tags a compound with a fluorescent label for subsequent detection. For example, amino acids or other primary amines often are labeled with either a dansyl or fluorescamine tag and followed with HPLC separation and fluorometric detection. Most fluorometers used with liquid chromatographs are relatively simple in design and extremely selective and sensitive for compounds fluorescing within the detector's operating wavelength range. Deuterium or xenon arc lamps or lasers have been used as light sources in such detectors.

Electrochemical detectors.   In amperometric electrochemical detectors an electroactive analyte enters the flow cell, where it is either oxidized or reduced at an electrode surface under a constant potential. Electroactive compounds of clinical interest conveniently analyzed by HPLC with electrochemical detection include the urinary catecholamines. In addition, electrochemically active tags (for example, bromine) are added to compounds such as unsaturated fatty acids or prostaglandins.

Coulometric detectors also are used. When placed in series such detectors are used to detect and quantify co-eluting compounds that differ in their half-wave potentials (the potential at half-signal maximum) by at least 60 mV. These detectors are extremely selective and sensitive, with reasonably wide linear response ranges. They are used in the clinical laboratory for the analysis of metanephrines, vanillymandelic acid, homovanillic acid, and 5-hydroxyidole acetic acid in human urine without extensive sample preparation.

Computer

As with gas chromatographs the incorporation of computer technology into HPLC instrumentation has resulted in cost effective, easy-to-operate automated systems with improved analytical performances (see Figure 8-14). In these systems a computer provides both system-control and data-processing functions. For details, the reader should consult the previous discussion on the use of computers in gas chromatographs.

Practical considerations

Several techniques affect the practical application of HPLC in the clinical laboratory, including those used to prepare samples and mobile phases and maintain the system.

Sample preparation

Sample preparation is an important step in chromatographic analysis by HPLC and includes procedures for sample concentration, purification, and derivatization.

Sample concentration/purification.   Concentrating or purifying an analyte in a sample often is necessary before separation and quantification by HPLC. Several liquid- and solid-phase extraction techniques are used for this purpose. The latter has become very popular because solid-phase extraction cartridges greatly simplify sample preparation. These cartridges are usually 1- or 3-mL syringe barrels made of polypropylene that contain stationary phase (for example, C18-reversed phase or silica). As an aliquot of urine or serum passes through the column, it retains the analytes. The column then is rinsed with solutions of different pH values or solvent compositions to selectively elute interfering substances. The analytes then are eluted with a different mobile phase. Alternatively, analytes are eluted directly, and unwanted solutes are retained on the cartridge. This sample preparation approach is popular in the preparation of samples for therapeutic drug monitoring, drugs of abuse testing, and catecholamine analysis.

Devices now are available for automated on-line extraction and sample preparation. These consist mainly of robotic arms and mechanisms for highly accurate and precise delivery of solvent volumes. Depending on the instrument, samples may be prepared and analyzed individually or in batches.

Sample derivatization. For HPLC analyses many analytes are derivatized before or after chromatographic separation to increase detectability. For example, in automated amino acid analyzers, eluted amino acids are reacted with ninhydrin in a postcolumn reactor. The resulting chromogenic species then are detected with a photometer. Other examples include labeling amino acids or other primary amines with dansyl or fluorescamine tags either before or after the chromatographic step.

Preparation of mobile phase

In preparing mobile phase, dissolved gases in the solvent must be removed or suppressed. The solvent also must be free of particulate matter. When the mobile phase comprises two or more solvents, they must be adequately mixed.

Solvent degassing. A common problem in LC is the evolution of dissolved gas bubbles generated as solvents pass from the solvent reservoirs into and through the chromatographic system. These bubbles should be removed or suppressed because they create an unstable electronic signal (noisy baseline) when they pass through a detector at ambient pressure. Operationally, vacuum degassing, helium purging, or postdetector back pressure are techniques used to prevent this problem.

With vacuum degassing the mobile phase is stirred in a side-armed flask or mobile-phase handling system under reduced pressure. Nonpolar mobile phases require less than 1 minute to degas, but polar mobile phases require several minutes. However, prolonged degassing under vacuum should be avoided because it alters the mobile phase composition, especially when volatile solvents are used.

Another degassing technique, helium "sparging," requires a constant, gentle stream of helium bubbled through the solvents in the solvent reservoirs. The relatively insoluble helium extracts the dissolved gases, which then are vented into the atmosphere. Placing a drying agent in the helium line (between the helium tank and solvent reservoir) is helpful because it removes any water in the gas. Finally, a back-pressure valve is attached to the outlet of the system's detector, forcing gases to remain in the solution until they have passed through the detector cell. Other degassing procedures include mild heating and ultrasonic vibration of the mobile phase.

Solvent clarity. Mobile phases should be prepared from HPLC-grade solvents free of particulate matter. Most commercial HPLC solvents are prefiltered. However, if the solvent has not been prefilterd, it should be filtered through a 0.5-μm screen.

Solvent mixing. During gradient operation the HPLC solvents that compose the mobile phase must be mixed adequately, most commonly with either a static or dynamic mixer. Static mixers rely on laminar-flow dynamics, whereas dynamic mixers use magnetic stirrers. Solvent viscosity affects mixing characteristics; inadequate mixing is detected by many UV detectors and may be expressed as an unstable baseline.

Safety

Normal laboratory precautions must be exercised during HPLC operation. The column effluent should be collected in a suitable container and stored appropriately before disposal. The explosive release of pressure in an HPLC system is not a major hazard; liquids compress only slightly, and therefore accumulate little energy.

■ MASS SPECTROMETRY

Mass spectrometry (MS) is a powerful qualitative and quantitative technique. In the clinical laboratory mass spectrometers are used to measure many clinically relevant analytes, especially when coupled with gas or liquid chromatographs.

Basic Concepts and Definitions

A **mass spectrometer** is an analytical instrument that first ionizes a target molecule into ions of a specific mass-to-charge (m/z) ratio and then separates and measures those ions. The instrument produces a mass spectrum, where the relative abundance of each ion is plotted as a function of its m/z ratio (Figure 8-21). The ion with the highest abundance in the mass spectrum is assigned a relative value of 100% and is called the *base peak*. For example, the base peaks of the mass spectra from the two derivatives of D-methamphetamine shown in Figure 8-21 are 204 and 308, respectively. The unfragmented ion of the original molecule is called the *molecular ion*. Data from a mass spectrometer is used to determine the structure and concentration of both inorganic and organic compounds.

All MS techniques require an ionization step that produces an ion from a neutral atom or molecule. A number of processes are used to ionize target molecules, many of which are discussed in the following section. If a low energy or "soft" ionization technique such as chemical ionization (CI) is used, the molecular mass of an analyte is determined (Figure 8-22, *B*). Advances in soft ionization techniques have extended the use of MS to the direct measurement of peptide and protein mass. Ionization at higher energy results in more extensive fragmentation of target molecules (see Figure 8-22, *A*).

The chemical nature of a molecule determines its fragmentation at specific bonds. The structure of an analyte

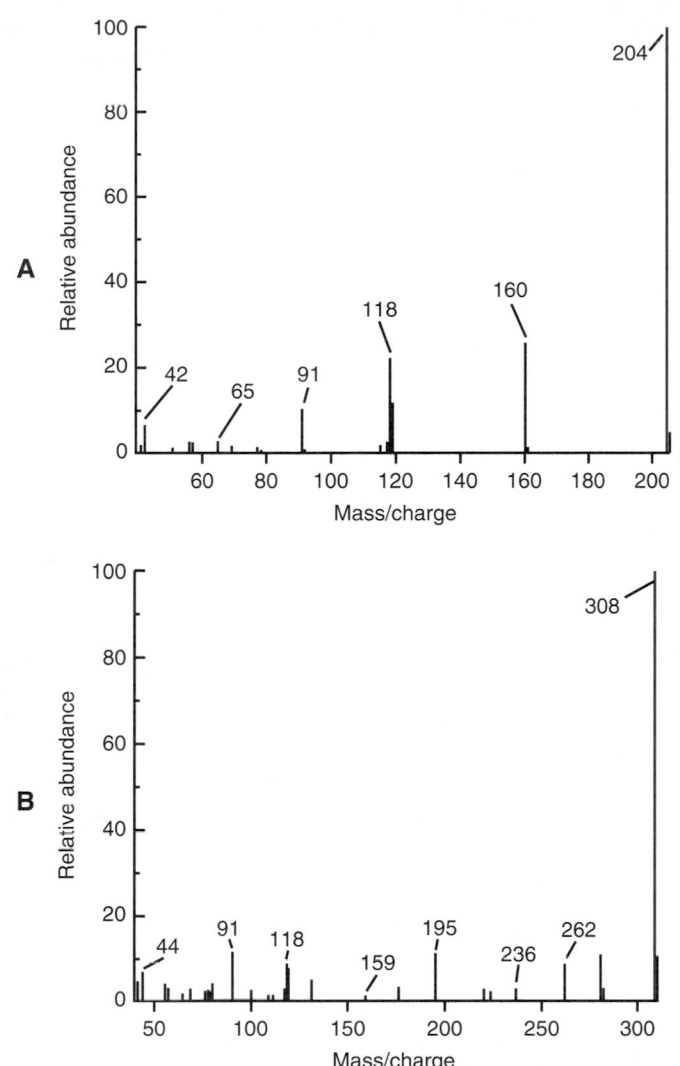

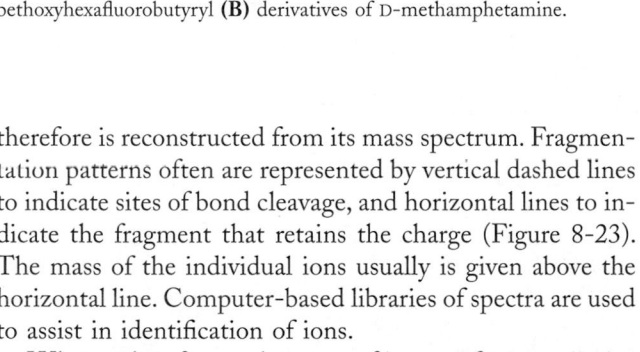

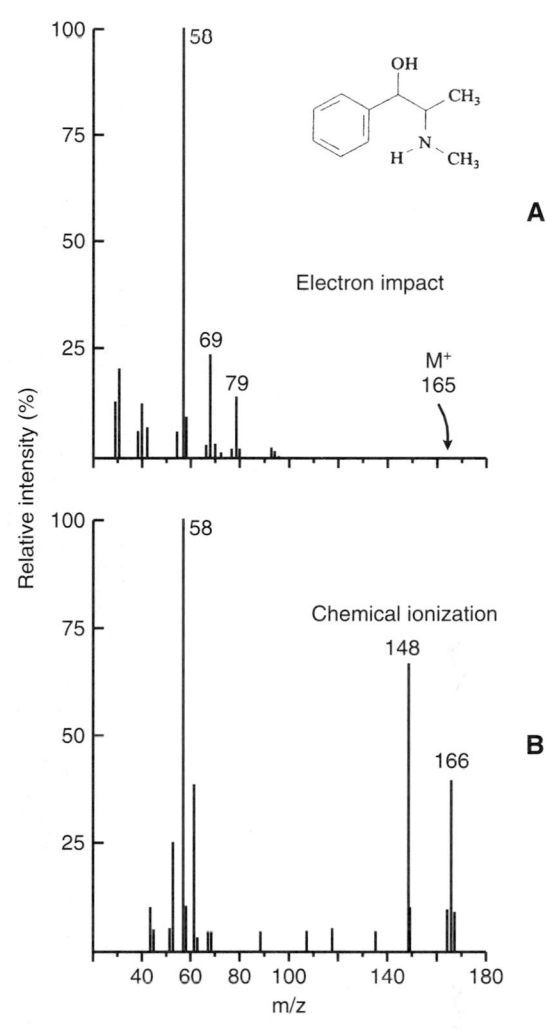

Figure 8-21   Mass spectrum of the pentafluoropropionyl **(A)** and carbethoxyhexafluorobutyryl **(B)** derivatives of D-methamphetamine.

Figure 8-22   Mass spectral comparisons of ephedrine utilizing electron impact **(A)**, and chemical ionization (methane) **(B)** techniques. *m/z*, Mass-to-charge ratio.

therefore is reconstructed from its mass spectrum. Fragmentation patterns often are represented by vertical dashed lines to indicate sites of bond cleavage, and horizontal lines to indicate the fragment that retains the charge (Figure 8-23). The mass of the individual ions usually is given above the horizontal line. Computer-based libraries of spectra are used to assist in identification of ions.

When only a few analytes are of interest for quantitative analysis and their mass spectra are known, the mass spectrometer is programmed to monitor only those ions of interest. This selective detection technique is known as *selected-ion monitoring (SIM)*. Because SIM focuses on a limited number of ions, more signal is collected for each selected mass, increasing the signal-to-noise ratio for the analyte.

A mass spectrometer also is used simultaneously to differentiate and quantify a compound with a normal

abundance of isotope from an analog enriched with a stable isotope. For example, a compound containing ^2H is measured relative to one containing ^1H; likewise ^{13}C relative to ^{12}C; ^{15}N relative to ^{14}N; and ^{18}O relative to ^{16}O. Thus a compound labeled with a stable isotope is used as an internal standard because it behaves nearly identically to the native compound during sample preparation and subsequent chromatographic analysis. This ability to quantify a compound relative to an isotopic species of known or fixed concentration is called *isotope dilution analysis*. The specific mass spectrometric technique is known as *isotope dilution mass spectrometry* (IDMS). The IDMS technique has been used to develop definitive methods to assign target values for a number of clinically relevant analytes in certified reference materials and proficiency testing samples.

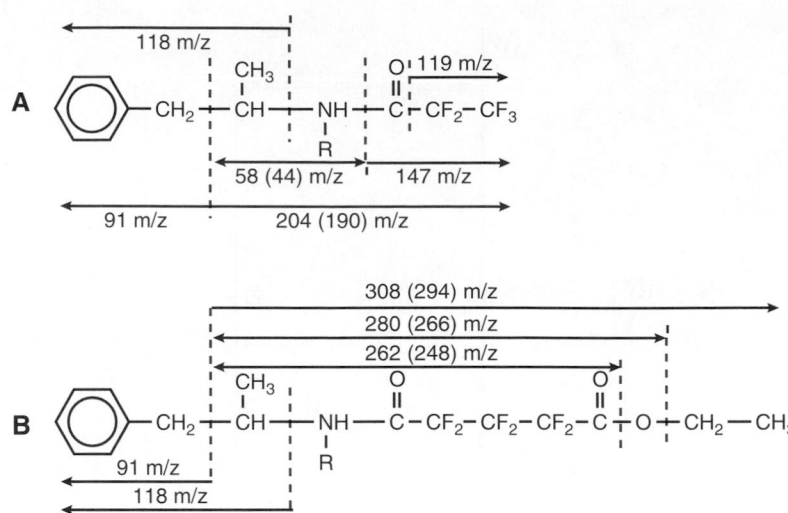

Figure 8-23   Fragmentation patterns for the pentafluoropropionyl **(A)** and carbethoxyhexafluorobutyryl **(B)** derivatives of methamphetamine (R=CH3) and amphetamine (R=H; masses in parentheses). Compare the predicted masses with the spectrum shown in Figure 8-21. Note that for the pentafluoropropionyl derivative, only one ion (204, 190 m/z) is characteristic of the aliphatic portion of each molecule. *m/z*, Mass-to-charge ratio.

Instrumentation

A mass spectrometer (Figure 8-24) consists of the following:

1.   Ion source
2.   Vacuum system
3.   Mass analyzer
4.   Detector
5.   Computer

Ion source

Many approaches have been used to form ions, both in high-vacuum and under near-atmospheric pressure conditions. For the majority of clinically relevant analytes the most important ionization techniques are electron ionization (EI) and chemical ionization (CI). Other ionization techniques include fast atom bombardment (FAB), and matrix-assisted laser desorption ionization (MALDI). In addition, the thermospray, atmospheric pressure chemical ionization (APCI), and electrospray (ES) interfaces used in HPLC/MS instruments also are used as ionization sources.

Vacuum system

Ion separation in a mass analyzer requires that the ions do not collide with any other molecules during interaction with the magnetic or electric fields. This requires the use of a vacuum from 10^{-5} to 10^{-9} torr, depending on mass analyzer type. To reach this level of vacuum, a mass spectrometer uses both a mechanical vacuum and an efficient high-vacuum pump. During operation the mechanical vacuum pump evacuates the system to a pressure at which the high-vacuum pump is then effective. A diffusion pump is the least expensive and most reliable high-vacuum pump. Turbomolecular pumps and cryopumps also are used.

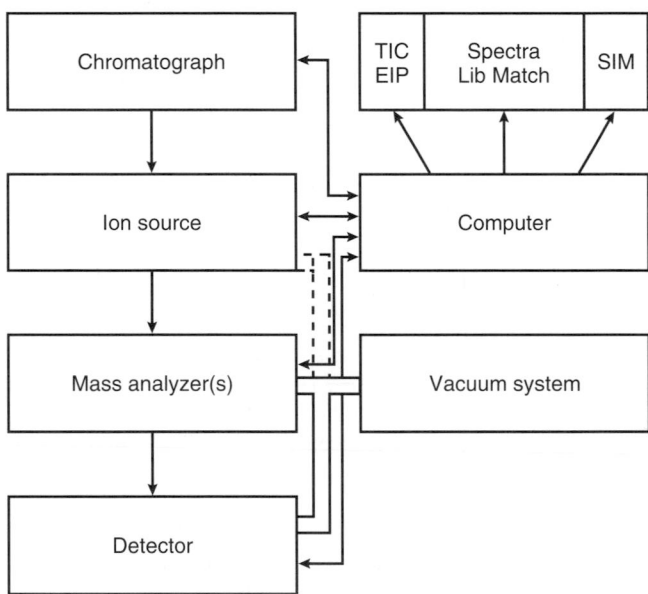

Figure 8-24   Block diagram of the essential components of a mass spectrometer. The ion source, inlet port, mass filter, and detector are all under high vacuum (10^{-7}). *TIC,* Total ion chromatogram; *EIP,* extracted ion profile; *Lib,* library; *SIM,* selective-ion monitoring.

Mass analyzers

The mass analyzer separates ions according to their m/z ratios and allows them to reach the detector. Several types of mass analyzers are available. These include the magnetic-sector, quadrupole mass filter, quadrupole ion trap, time-of-flight, and ion cyclotron resonance mass analyzers. Furthermore, with the development of soft ionization techniques, additional structural information is gained through use of tandem mass spectrometry (MS/MS).

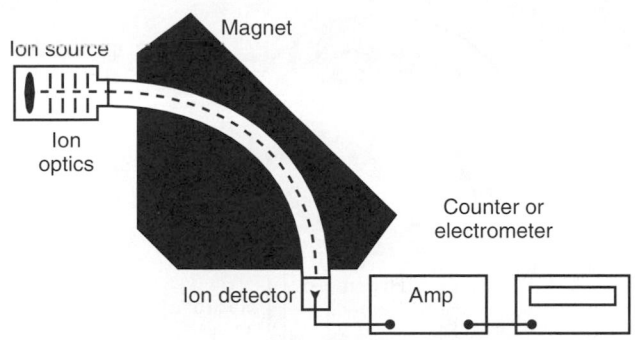

Figure 8-25 Ion path through a strong external magnetic field. Ion trajectories and radius of curvature (R) are related to the accelerating voltage (V), magnetic field strength (H), and m/z. Only when a specific V, H, and rm/z condition is met does an ion follow the unique path leading to the detector.

Magnetic sector

In a magnetic sector mass analyzer, ions first are accelerated and then directed into a magnet (Figure 8-25), imposing a magnetic field perpendicular to the flight path. Thus each ion follows a different arched path to the detector that is related to the ion's m/z ratio. Because the resolution of a magnetic sector mass analyzer is limited, an electronic sector is added to focus ions according to their kinetic energy. Like the magnetic sector the electric sector applies a force perpendicular to the direction of ion motion, and therefore has the form of an arc. An instrument that contains both magnetic and electric sectors is known as a *double focusing mass spectrometer*.

Quadrupole mass filter

The quadrupole mass filter (QMF) uses radio frequency (RF)- and direct current (DC)-induced electric fields to separate ions. QMFs first were described in the early 1950s, and they are the most commonly used mass analyzers. The QMF consists of four parallel rods in which the opposite pairs of rods are connected to the same DC and RF voltage (Figure 8-26). By rapidly changing the relative polarity and magnitude of the voltage applied to the pairs of rods, ions emanating from the ion source alternately are attracted to and repelled from pairs of rods. As a result the ions follow a corkscrew path as they move toward the detector. At a particular set of RF and DC voltages, ions with one specific m/z ratio have a stable trajectory, which allows them to enter the detector. All other ions collide with the rods or are pumped away by the vacuum system. Because of their lower cost and relative simplicity in comparison with magnetic sector analyzers, QMFs commonly are interfaced with both gas and liquid chromatographs.

Quadrupole ion trap

The operating principle of the quadrupole ion trap (QIT) is similar to the QMF in that ion stability in an oscillating electric field is used to manipulate ions. An impor-

tant distinction between the trap and the filter is that ions are stored in the QIT, whereas they only transiently pass through the QMF (see Figure 8-26). This capability is used to improve the resolution of the QIT and sensitivity for SIM. The QIT also has proven popular to interface with both gas and liquid chromatographs.

The ion storage capability of the QIT also is used when two or more mass analyzers are operated in tandem. The operation of MS/MS may be thought of as the taking of a mass spectrum of an ion. In MS/MS the targeted compound is ionized selectively and its characteristic ions separated from others in the mixture. The selected ions then collide with molecules of a neutral gas in an interconnecting collision chamber to produce fragments that are separated and identified in the second spectrometer. This permits the selective and specific analysis for many compounds of various structural classes. The need for a chromatographic step often is eliminated as separation and analysis are performed automatically by MS/MS.

Other mass analyzers

A time-of-flight (TOF) mass analyzer measures the time it takes ions of different masses to move from the ion source to the detector. A TOF instrument is well suited to ionization techniques that produce ions in well-defined pulses, such as MALDI. The major advantage of the TOF design is that all ions reach the detector, but at different times, so mass spectral "scan times" are extremely fast. This speed makes TOF the only MS technique at present that scans fast enough to be coupled to "fast GC" separations.* The TOF instrument also has a mass range sufficient to measure the mass of singly charged proteins.

The ion-cyclotron resonance (ICR) mass analyzer causes ions to move in a circular path by using a very high-strength magnetic field. The cyclotron frequency of the ion is dependent on its mass. Because the ions are stored in the analyzer and measured nondestructively, MS/MS analyses are performed easily with an ICR mass analyzer.

Detectors

A number of detectors are used to transform the intensity of the separated ions into an electronic signal. The continuous dynode is an example of such a detector. Basically, it is a glass trumpet with a tin oxide coating on the inner surface. When it is struck by an ion, the surface emits a number of electrons, each of which causes the emission of additional electrons in a cascade. The resulting signal is amplified by 10^5 to 10^6. The voltage applied across the dynode determines both the number of ions attracted into the horn and the magnitude of the amplification.

---

*Fast GC provides high-speed separations using short lengths of conventional columns of 0.25 mm ID.

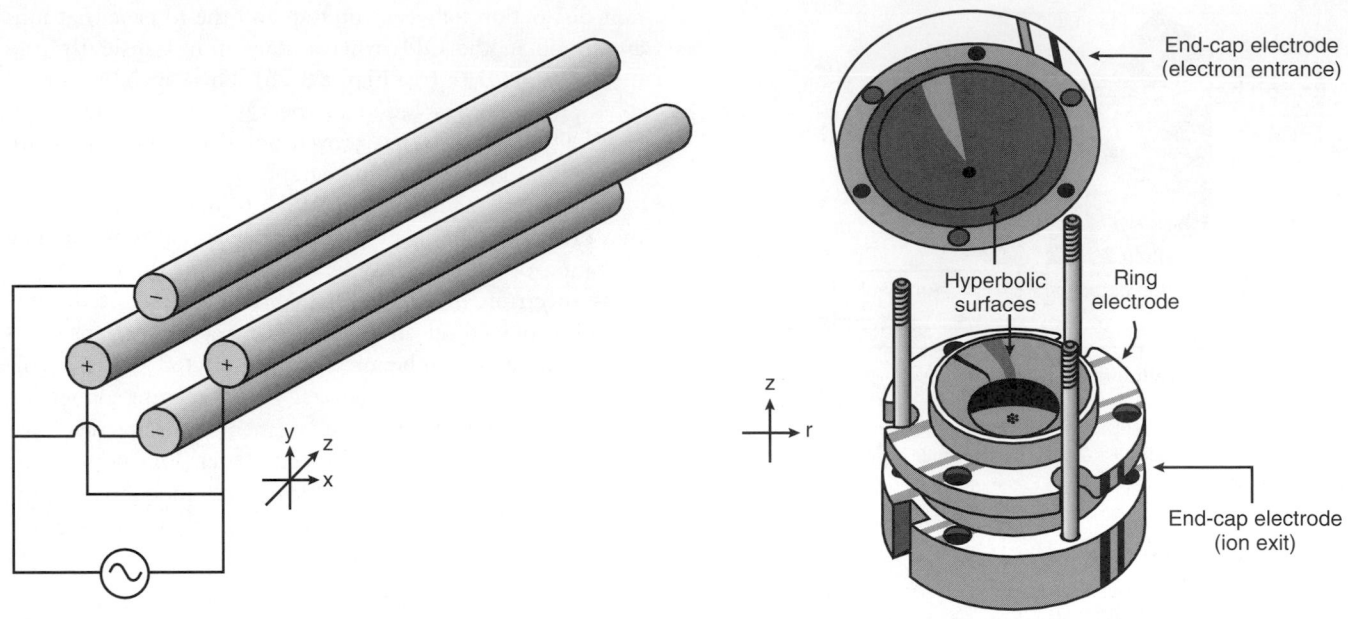

Figure 8-26   Diagram of QMF *(left)* and QIT *(right)*. *QMF,* Quadrupole mass filter; *QIT,* quadrupole ion trap.

Computer

The rapid rate of data generation in chromatographic/mass spectrometric systems requires a computer for data acquisition and display. One of the most important functions of a mass spectrometer computer is the ability to search libraries of chemical structures to assist in compound identification. Many laboratories generate their own libraries, whereas others are available commercially.

Coupled Techniques

Mass spectrometers coupled with gas and liquid chromatographs (GC/MS and LC/MS) result in versatile analytical instruments that combine the resolving power of the chromatographs with the exquisite specificity and sensitivity of a mass spectrometer. Such instruments are powerful analytical techniques that are used by clinical laboratories to identify and quantify organic analytes. They provide structural and quantitative information in real time on individual analytes as they elute from a chromatographic column. By acquiring several mass spectral scans across an eluting peak, the sum of all ions produced is displayed as a function of time to yield a total ion chromatogram. The resultant display has the appearance of a chromatogram with signal intensity plotted as a function of time. As in chromatographic analysis, retention times are measured and peak heights or peak areas integrated for use in quantitative analysis. These coupled techniques are extremely sensitive, and only nanogram or picogram quantities of an analyte are required for analysis. (Chapters 31 and 32 discuss their specific applications.)

Gas chromatography/mass spectrometry

GC/MS is used in the clinical laboratory primarily for the analysis of drugs. Such analyses are applicable particu-

larly in sports medicine, military, government, and private programs that test for drugs of abuse. For example, the U.S. Substance Abuse and Mental Health Services Administration (formerly the National Institute for Drug Abuse) and the U.S. Department of Transportation mandate that only GC/MS be used to confirm the presence of drugs in samples presumptively found to be positive by immunochemical analyses. In addition, GC/MS is used by the U.S. National Institute of Standards and Technology (NIST) as a definitive method to qualify standard reference materials and assign certified values to many clinical analytes, including cholesterol, glucose, creatinine, and urea nitrogen.

The gas chromatograph and mass spectrometer are coupled easily because both require the analyte to be in the gas phase. However, the mismatch in operating pressures between the gas chromatograph and mass spectrometer requires the use of an interface to couple the two (Figure 8-27). The interface requires either a large-capacity vacuum system or restriction on the volume of GC effluent. When packed GC columns are used with flow rates of 30 to 40 mL/minute at room temperature and pressure, much of the carrier gas must be removed before the analytes are introduced into the vacuum area of the interface. Jet or membrane separators have been used for this purpose. In capillary GC, with its lower flow rates, the column is connected to the mass spectrometer by direct coupling or through an open split interface. Generally, with most QMF and QIT instruments using small diffusion pumps (50 to 60 L/s), a capillary column of 0.2-mm ID or less is inserted directly into the ion source of the mass spectrometer. A 0.32-mm-ID capillary column can be coupled to a similar instrument when a larger diffusion pump (200 to 500 L/s) is used.

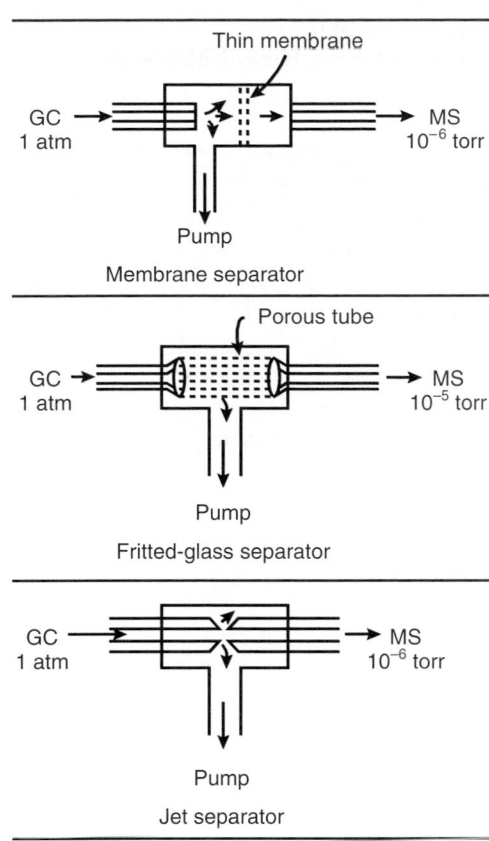

Figure 8-27 Techniques used to remove helium (carrier gas) and enrich the sample as it elutes from the end of the gas chromatographic column. The membrane, fritted glass, and jet separator all remove the helium through the use of an external vacuum pumping system, which draws the helium preferentially from the sample. *GC*, Gas chromatography; *MS*, mass spectrometry.

Liquid chromatography/mass spectrometry

Liquid chromatographs have been more difficult to interface with mass spectrometers than gas chromatographs because the analytes are dissolved in liquid. A number of interfaces have been developed that feature four key elements—(1) nebulization of the liquid phase, (2) removal of the bulk solvent, (3) dissociation of the solvent-analyte clusters, and (4) ionization of the analytes. Thus these interfaces are bifunctional in that they separate the solvent from the analyte and also ionize it. However, in contrast to GC/MS, ionization in these interfaces frequently takes place at near-atmospheric pressure, resulting in soft ionization and production of ions with minimal fragmentation. Thus MS/MS frequently is used in conjunction with LC/MS.

Specific interfaces developed to couple a liquid chromatograph to a mass spectrometer include the APCI, ES/ion-spray, particle-beam (PBI), and thermospray interfaces. All except the PBI are soft ionization techniques. They produce only a few ions, which are useful for quantification but not for structural identification. The PBI produces EI-like spectra that are searched in standard NIST libraries. Limits of detection are comparable to those achieved with GC/MS.

Atmospheric pressure chemical ionization

In an APCI interface the LC effluent is nebulized and desolvated and the resulting gas-phase compounds ionized by proton-transfer or charge-transfer reactions. Relatively little fragmentation occurs, and APCI has been used primarily for quantitative analysis or MS/MS. It is a robust interface that is useful for compounds of moderate-to-high polarity. Interface designs have accommodated liquid flow rates of up to 1 mL/minute.

Electrospray

The emergence of ES revolutionized the use of LC/MS, particularly in the analysis of biological macromolecules. The technique also is being used in clinical laboratories for small molecules. It is most effective for ionic or extremely polar compounds. The ES interfaces operate at flow rates up to 200 μL/minute. One unique feature of ES ionization is the production of multiply charged ions, particularly from peptides and proteins. This increases the sensitivity of their measurement and extends the mass range.

Particle-beam interface

The PBI interface is most efficient in the analysis of compounds of low-to-intermediate polarity. Because of this efficiency a PBI interface is used with HPLC columns of 4.6-mm ID. Both EI or CI techniques are used with a PBI interface. These techniques produce full-scan spectra that are searched with standard libraries.

Thermospray

In a thermospray interface the outlet from the liquid chromatograph enters a chamber, where it is heated and vaporized into small droplets. With the use of a high-throughput pump attached to the ion source, up to 2 mL/minute of aqueous solvents is introduced into the mass spectrometer vacuum system. The thermospray interface now is used rarely as an LC/MS interface, however, because of the development of the previously described techniques.

Additional Reading

GENERAL
Walker JQ, Minneci J (eds): Chromatography Fundamentals Applications & Troubleshooting, Niles, Ill, Preston Publications, 1996.

GAS CHROMATOGRAPHY
Grant DW: Capillary Gas Chromatography, New York, John Wiley & Sons, 1996.
Grob RL (ed): Modern Practice of Gas Chromatography, 3rd edition, New York, John Wiley & Sons, 1995.

GAS CHROMATOGRAPHY/MASS SPECTROMETRY

Gerhards P, Bons U, Sawazki J et al (eds): GC/MS in Clinical Chemistry, Weinheim, Germany, Wiley-VCH, 1999.

Kitson FG, Larsen BS, McEwen CN: Gas Chromatography & Mass Spectrometry: A Practical Guide, San Diego, Academic Press, 1996.

LIQUID CHROMATOGRAPHY/HIGH-PERFORMANCE LIQUID CHROMATOGRAPHY

Luogh WJ, Wainer IW (eds): High Performance Liquid Chromatography: Fundamental Principles and Practice, 1st edition, London, Chapman & Hall, 1995.

Hage DS: Affinity chromatography: a review of clinical applications. Clin Chem 1999; 45:593-615.

Snyder LR, Glajch JL, Kirkland JJ: Practical High Performance Liquid Chromatography—Method Development, 2nd edition, New York, John Wiley & Sons, 1997.

LIQUID CHROMATOGRAPHY/MASS SPECTROMETRY

Ardrey A: LC-MS: An Introduction, New York, VCH Publishers, 1996.

MASS SPECTROMETRY

Burlingame AL, Carr SA, Baldwin MA (eds): Mass Spectrometry in Biology and Medicine, Totowa, NJ, Humana, 1999.

McLafferty FW, Fridriksson EK, Horn DM et al: Biomolecule mass spectrometry. Science 1999; 284:1289-1290.

Russell DH, Edmondson RD: High-resolution mass spectrometry and accurate mass measurements with emphasis on the characterization of peptides and proteins by matrix-assisted laser desorption/ionization time-of-flight mass spectrometry. J Mass Spectrom 1997; 32:263-276.

PLANAR CHROMATOGRAPHY

Touchstone JC: Practice of Thin Layer Chromatography, 3rd edition, New York, John Wiley & Sons, 1992.

CHAPTER 9

Principles of Clinical Enzymology

DONALD W. MOSS, PhD, DSc, and A. RALPH HENDERSON, MB, ChB, PhD, FRCPath

---

Objectives

1. Define *enzyme* and describe how enzymes are classified based on their structures or their actions on substrates.
2. Define the following terms:
   Active site
   Apoenzyme
   Holoenzyme
   Cofactor
   Coenzyme
   Activator
   First-order and zero-order kinetics
   K_m, V_{max}, enzyme inhibition (competitive, noncompetitive, uncompetitive)
3. State the Michaelis-Menten and Lineweaver-Burk equations and relate them to enzyme kinetics by defining reaction velocity, V_{max} and K_m.
4. Draw and label a Michaelis-Menten curve and a Lineweaver-Burk plot.
5. List the factors that affect the velocity of an enzymatic reaction and how these factors affect enzyme kinetics.
6. State the way in which each type of inhibition affects enzyme kinetics and illustrate how each of the three types affects enzymatic reaction rate using a Lineweaver-Burk plot.
7. List the physiological factors that affect blood enzyme levels.
8. Compare the methods available for analysis of clinically significant enzymes and describe how the rate of an enzyme-catalyzed reaction relates to the amount of enzyme activity present in a system.

Key Words

Activation Energy In enzymology, the energy required for a molecule to form an activated complex; in an enzyme-catalyzed reaction, corresponds to the formation of the activated enzyme-substrate complex

Activator An effector molecule that increases the catalytic activity of an enzyme when it binds to a specific site

Active Center That part of the enzyme or other protein at which the initial binding of substrate and enzyme occurs to form the intermediate enzyme-substrate complex

Apoenzyme The protein part of an enzyme without the cofactor necessary for catalysis

Catalyst A substance that increases the rate of a chemical reaction but is not consumed or changed by it; an enzyme being a biocatalyst

Catalytic Activity The property of a catalyst that is measured by the catalyzed rate of conversion of a specific chemical reaction produced in a specific assay system

Coenzyme A diffusible, heat-stable substance of low molecular weight that, when combined with an inactive protein called an *apoenzyme,* forms an active compound or a complete enzyme called a *holoenzyme*

Continuous Monitoring   A reaction mode in which the reaction is monitored continuously and the data presented in either an analog or digital mode

Denaturation   The partial or total alteration of the structure of a protein without change in covalent structure by the action of certain physical procedures (heating, agitation) or chemical agents

Enzyme   A protein molecule that catalyzes chemical reactions without itself being destroyed or altered

First-Order Reaction   A reaction in which the rate of reaction is proportional to the concentration of reactant

Fixed-Time Reaction   A two-point reaction mode in which measurements are taken at specified (fixed) times; preferred mode for assays in which the reaction rate is first order in regard to the initial substrate concentration

Holoenzyme   The functional compound formed by the combination of an apoenzyme and its appropriate coenzyme

Immobilized Enzymes   Soluble enzymes bound to an insoluble organic or inorganic matrix or encapsulated within a membrane to increase their stability and ensure their repeated or continued use

Induction   In enzymology, a biological process that results in the increased biosynthesis of an enzyme, which increases its apparent activity; results from the presence of an inducer

Inhibitor   A substance that diminishes the rate of a chemical reaction; the process being called *inhibition*

Isoenzyme   One of a group of related enzymes catalyzing the same reaction but having different molecular structures and characterized by varying physical, biochemical, and immunological properties

International Unit (U)   The amount of enzyme activity that catalyzes the conversion of one micromole of substrate per minute under the specified conditions of the assay method

Katal   The amount of enzyme activity that converts one mole of substrate per second under specified reaction conditions

Lineweaver-Burk Plot   A plot of the reciprocal of velocity of an enzyme-catalyzed reaction (ordinate; y-axis) versus the reciprocal of substrate concentration (abscissa; x-axis)

Michaelis-Menten Constant   Operationally, the substrate concentration that allows an enzyme reaction to proceed at one-half its maximum velocity

Product   The substance produced by the enzyme-catalyzed conversion of a substrate

Substrate   A reactant in a catalyzed reaction

Zero-Order Reaction   A reaction in which the rate is independent of the concentration of reactant

---

Enzymes are proteins that have catalytic properties due to their powers of specific activation of their substrates. This definition indicates the characteristic properties of enzymes, which in turn govern the principles of methods of enzyme analysis. This chapter surveys the principles of basic and diagnostic enzymology.

■ BASIC ENZYMOLOGY

This section begins with a discussion of enzyme nomenclature and is followed with discussions of enzymes as proteins, antigens, and catalysts. The section ends with a discussion of enzyme kinetics.

Enzyme Nomenclature

Historically, individual enzymes were identified with the name of the **substrate** or group on which the enzyme acts and the addition of the suffix *-ase*. For example, the enzyme hydrolyzing urea was known as *urease*. Subsequent methods also identified the type of reaction, as in carbonic anhydrase, D-amino acid oxidase, and succinic dehydrogenase. In addition, some enzymes were given

empirical names such as trypsin, diastase, ptyalin, pepsin, and emulsin.

Because this combination of trivial common names and semisystematic names was imperfect, the International Union of Biochemistry (IUB) appointed an Enzyme Commission (EC) in 1955 to study the problem of enzyme nomenclature. Its proposals, with periodic updating, provide a rational and practical basis for the identification of all enzymes (http://www.chem.qmw.ac.uk/iubmb/enzyme/).

With the IUB system a systematic and trivial name is provided for each enzyme. The systematic name describes the nature of the reaction catalyzed, which is assigned a unique numerical code designation. The trivial or practical name, which may be identical to the systematic name but is often a simplification of it, is suitable for everyday use. The unique numerical designation for each enzyme consists of four numbers, each separated by a period (for example, 2.2.8.11). The number is preceded by the letters *EC*, denoting Enzyme Commission. The first number defines the class to which the enzyme belongs. All enzymes are assigned to one of six classes, characterized by the type of reaction they catalyze (1) oxidoreductases, (2) transferases, (3) hydrolases, (4) lyases, (5) isomerases, and (6) ligases. The next two numbers indicate the subclass and sub-subclass to which the enzyme is assigned. For example, these may differentiate the amino-transferring subclass from the phosphate-transferring category or the ethanol acceptor sub-subclass from that accepting acyl groups. The last number is the specific serial number given to each enzyme within its sub-subclass.

The systematic name of each enzyme consists of two parts—the first gives the name of the substrate or substrates acted on, and the second, a word ending in -ase, indicates the type of reaction catalyzed by all enzymes in the group. If two substrates are involved, both names are used and separated by a colon (for example, L-lactate:NAD oxidoreductase). An expression in parentheses, such as (decarboxylating), occasionally may be inserted to identify the reaction further. Because of the exact rules governing terminology, an enzyme is identified by both its code number and its systematic name. Table 9-1 lists some selected enzymes of clinical interest identified by trivial, abbreviated, and systematic names and by their code numbers (http://expasy.hcuge.ch/sprot/enzyme.html).

Although it is not recommended by the EC, a common and convenient practice is the use of capital-letter abbreviations for the names of certain enzymes, such as *ALT* (formerly *GPT*) for alanine aminotransferase (EC 2.6.1.2). Other examples are *AST* for aspartate aminotransferase, *LD* for lactate dehydrogenase, and *CK* for creatine kinase (see Table 9-1).

Enzymes As Proteins

Structure

All enzyme molecules possess the primary, secondary, and tertiary structures characteristic of proteins in general (see Chapter 19). Most enzymes also exhibit the quaternary level of structure (Figure 9-1). This structure consists of the association of small groups of subunits (also called *protomers*), each consisting of one polypeptide chain in its characteristic conformation, to make up an oligomeric protein molecule (for example, CK being a dimer, LD a tetramer). Biological activity, such as the catalytic activity of enzymes, often is a property of the oligomeric molecule so that activity is lost under conditions in which the subunits separate from one another. The protomers that compose a particular type of enzyme molecule frequently are identical (for example, as in the MM isoenzyme of CK, or the H_4 LD isoenzyme). However, association of unlike subunits occur and give rise, for example, to the heteropolymeric isoenzymes described later in this chapter.

The catalytic activity of an enzyme molecule depends generally on the integrity of its structure. Therefore any disruption of the structure is accompanied by a loss of activity, a process known as **denaturation.** If denaturation has not gone too far, it may be reversed with recovery of activity when the denaturing agent is removed. However, prolonged or severe denaturing conditions result in an irreversible loss of activity. Denaturing conditions include elevated tem-

---

TABLE 9-1	EC Numbers, Systematic and Trivial Names, Together with Frequently Adopted Abbreviations of Enzymes of Major Diagnostic Importance		
EC Number	Systematic Name	Trivial Name	Abbreviation
1.1.1.27	L-Lactate:NAD$^+$ oxidoreductase	Lactate dehydrogenase	LDH, LD
1.1.1.42	Threo-D$_s$-isocitrate:NAD(P)$^+$ oxidoreductase (decarboxylating)	Isocitrate dehydrogenase	ICD
1.4.1.3	L-Glutamate:NAD(P)$^+$ oxidoreductase (deaminating)	Glutamate dehydrogenase	GLDH, GLD
2.3.2.2	(5-Glutamyl)-peptide:amino-acid 5-glutamyltransferase	γ-Glutamyltransferase	GGT
2.6.1.1	L-Aspartate:2-oxoglutarate aminotransferase	Aspartate aminotransferase (transaminase)	AST
2.6.1.2	L-Alanine:2-oxoglutarate aminotransferase	Alanine aminotransferase (transaminase)	ALT
2.7.3.2	ATP:creatine N-phosphotransferase	Creatine kinase	CK
3.1.1.3	Triacylglycerol acylhydrolase	Lipase	Lip
3.1.1.7	Acetylcholine acetylhydrolase	Acetylcholinesterase, true cholinesterase, choline esterase I	—
3.1.1.8	Acylcholine acylhydrolase	Pseudocholinesterase, benzoyl cholinesterase, choline esterase II (serum cholinesterase)	ChE (SChE)
3.1.3.1	Orthophosphoric-monoester phosphohydrolase (alkaline optimum)	Alkaline phosphatase	ALP
3.1.3.2	Orthophosphoric-monoester phosphohydrolase (acid optimum)	Acid phosphatase	ACP
3.1.3.5	5′-Ribonucleotide phosphohydrolase	5′-Nucleotidase	5NT, NTP
3.2.1.1	1,4-α-D-Glucan glucanohydrolase	Amylase	Amy
3.4.21.4		Trypsin	—
4.1.2.13	D-Fructose-1,6-bisphosphate D-glyceraldehyde-3-phosphate-lyase	Aldolase	ALD

ATP, Adenosine triphosphate; *NAD,* nictinamide adenine dinucleotide.

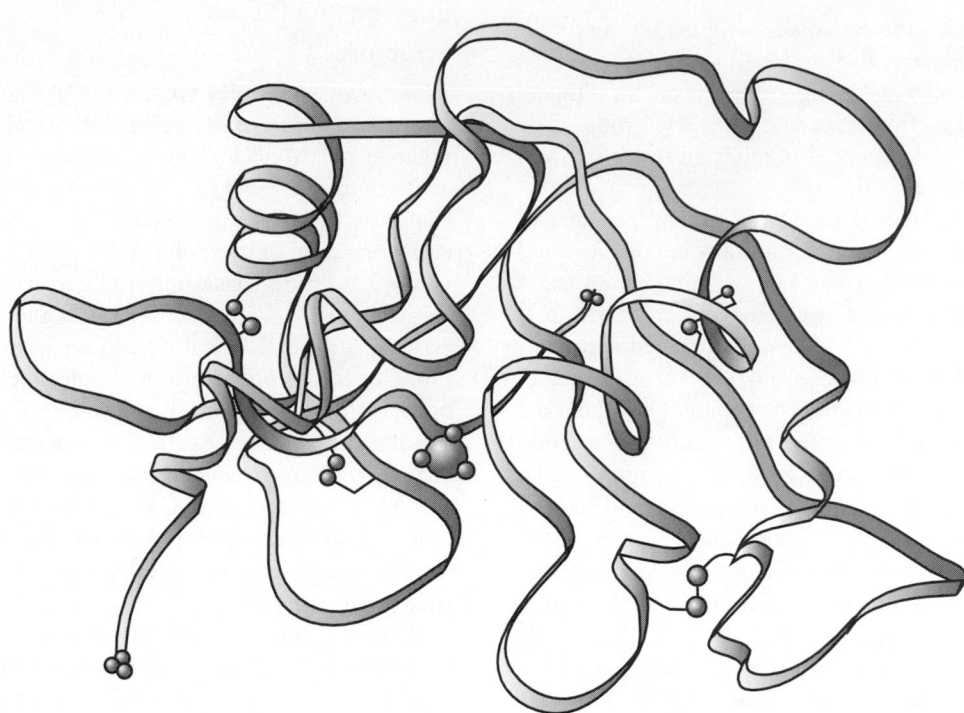

Figure 9-1   Plane projection of the three-dimensional structure of ribonuclease A. The phosphate group lies in the "active center" of the enzyme, situated in a cleft in the three-dimensional structure. (From Kartha G: Accounts Chem Res 1968; 1:374; and copyright 1968 American Chemical Society.)

peratures, extremes of pH, and chemical addition. Heat inactivation of most enzymes takes place at an appreciable rate at room temperature and becomes extremely rapid in most cases above about 60 °C. Low temperatures therefore are necessary to preserve enzyme activity, especially in aqueous solutions such as serum. Extremes of pH also cause unfolding of enzyme molecular structures and, except in a few cases, should be avoided during preservation of enzyme samples. Urea and related compounds disrupt hydrogen bonds and hydrophobic interactions so that exposure of enzymes to strong solutions of these reagents results in inactivation.

Isoenzymes and other multiple forms

Isoenzymes are multiple forms of an enzyme that possess the ability to catalyze the enzyme's characteristic reaction but differ in structure because they are encoded by distinct structural genes. The structural variations of isoenzymes are reflected to various degrees in their properties.

Genetic origins of enzyme variants

True isoenzymes may be due to the existence of more than one gene locus that codes for the structure of the enzyme protein. A substantial proportion of human enzymes (perhaps more than one-third) seems to be determined by more than one structural gene locus. The structural genes at the separate loci have undergone different modifications during the course of evolution, so the enzyme proteins coded by them no longer have identical structures.

Multiple gene loci have become disseminated throughout a whole species during the course of evolution so that these genes and their resultant isoenzymes typically are present in all individuals of that species. However, a large number of human enzymes exist in multiple molecular forms that differ in type from one individual to another. Family studies show that the various forms of a given enzyme are inherited according to Mendelian laws. In these cases the different enzyme forms originate from modified genes, or alleles. Allelic genes are alternative forms of the gene that occur at a particular locus and give rise to gene products with the same function. The isoenzymes that result from the existence of allelic genes are termed *allelozymes*. The proportion of human gene loci subject to allelic variation is considerable, and the probability that individuals will differ to some degree in their allelozyme patterns is correspondingly high.

In many cases the products of allelic genes are functionally adequate, and their inheritance causes no adverse effects. In other cases the individual who inherits particular allelozymes may experience illness when exposed to certain drugs or foods because of functional abnormalities of the allelozymes. In extreme cases the allele may produce no active isoenzyme at all, so metabolic disease of varying degrees of severity results.

Another category of multiple molecular forms arises in the case of enzymes that are oligomeric, consisting of molecules composed of subunits. The association of different types of subunits in various combinations gives rise to a

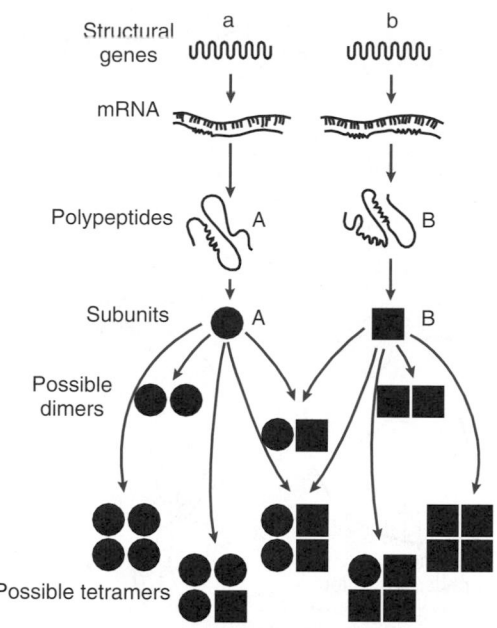

Figure 9-2   Diagram of the origin of isoenzymes, assuming the existence of two distinct gene loci. When the active enzymes are polymers containing more than one subunit, hybrid isoenzymes consisting of mixtures of different subunits may be formed. One such isoenzyme is formed in the case of a dimeric enzyme, such as CK, and three if the enzyme is a tetramer, such as LD. In both cases two homopolymeric isoenzymes also exist. *CK*, Creatine kinase; *LD*, lactate dehydrogenase. (From Moss DW: Isoenzyme Analysis, London, The Chemical Society, 1979.)

group of active enzyme molecules. When the different subunits are derived from distinct structural genes—either multiple loci or multiple alleles—the hybrid molecules so formed are included within the definition of isoenzymes and are called *hybrid isoenzymes*. The ability to form hybrid isoenzymes is evidence of considerable structural similarities among the different subunits. Hybrid isoenzymes are formed in vitro, but they also are formed in vivo in cells in which the different types of constituent subunits are present in the same subcellular compartment.

The number of different hybrid isoenzymes formed from two nonidentical protomers depends on the number of subunits in the complete enzyme molecule. For a dimeric enzyme one mixed dimer (hybrid isoenzyme) is formed in addition to two homopolymeric isoenzymes. If the enzyme is a tetramer, three heteropolymeric isoenzymes are formed (Figure 9-2).

Nongenetic causes of multiple forms

Many different types of posttranslational modifications of enzyme molecules give rise to multiple forms that are commonly known as *isoforms* (Figure 9-3). Several such processes have been shown to cause the heterogeneity of various enzymes, either in living matter or as a result of changes taking place during extraction or storage.

Modifications affecting nonprotein components of enzyme molecules also may lead to molecular heterogeneity.

Many enzymes are glycoproteins, and variations in carbohydrate side chains are a common cause of nonhomogeneity of these enzyme preparations. Some carbohydrate moieties, notably *N*-acetyl neuraminic acid (sialic acid), are ionized strongly and have profound effects on the properties of enzyme molecules.

Aggregation of enzyme molecules with one another or with nonenzymatic proteins may give rise to multiple forms separated by techniques that depend on differences in molecular size. A specific form of interaction between enzymatic and nonenzymatic proteins is the cause of unusual enzyme components seen when some samples of human plasma are fractionated by electrophoresis or chromatography. These components are due to the combination of apparently normal enzyme or isoenzyme molecules with plasma immunoglobulins. The enzyme-protein complexes thus formed may be heterogeneous themselves. Since the identification of "macroamylase," the first such enzyme-immunoglobulin complex to be identified, similar complexes involving LD, alkaline phosphatase (ALP), and CK have been observed.

Differences in properties among multiple forms

The structural differences between multiple forms of an enzyme give rise to differences in physicochemical properties, such as electrophoretic mobility, resistance to inactivation, and solubility, or in catalytic characteristics, such as ratio of reaction with substrate analogues or response to inhibitors. Methods of isoenzyme analysis therefore are designed to investigate a wide range of catalytic and structural properties of enzyme molecules. However, only limited deductions usually are possible about the nature of the underlying structural differences among isoenzymes responsible for the dissimilar properties.

Techniques of molecular biology, such as gene cloning and sequencing, have revolutionized the investigation of the primary structures of isoenzymes. The differences in primary structures between isoenzymes, whether derived from multiple gene loci or different alleles, now are known in a large number of cases.

Isoenzymes that are due to the existence of multiple-gene loci usually differ quantitatively in catalytic properties. These differences may be demonstrated in characteristics such as molecular activity, kinetic values for the substrate or substrates, sensitivity to various inhibitors, and relative rates of activity with substrate analogues (when the specificity of the isoenzymes allows the substrate to be varied); presumably, these differences are the basis of the biological importance of this type of isoenzymatic variation. In contrast, multiple enzyme forms that arise by such posttranslational modifications as aggregation usually have similar catalytic properties.

Enzymes as Antigens

As is the case with other proteins, enzymes usually elicit the production of antibodies when they are injected into animals

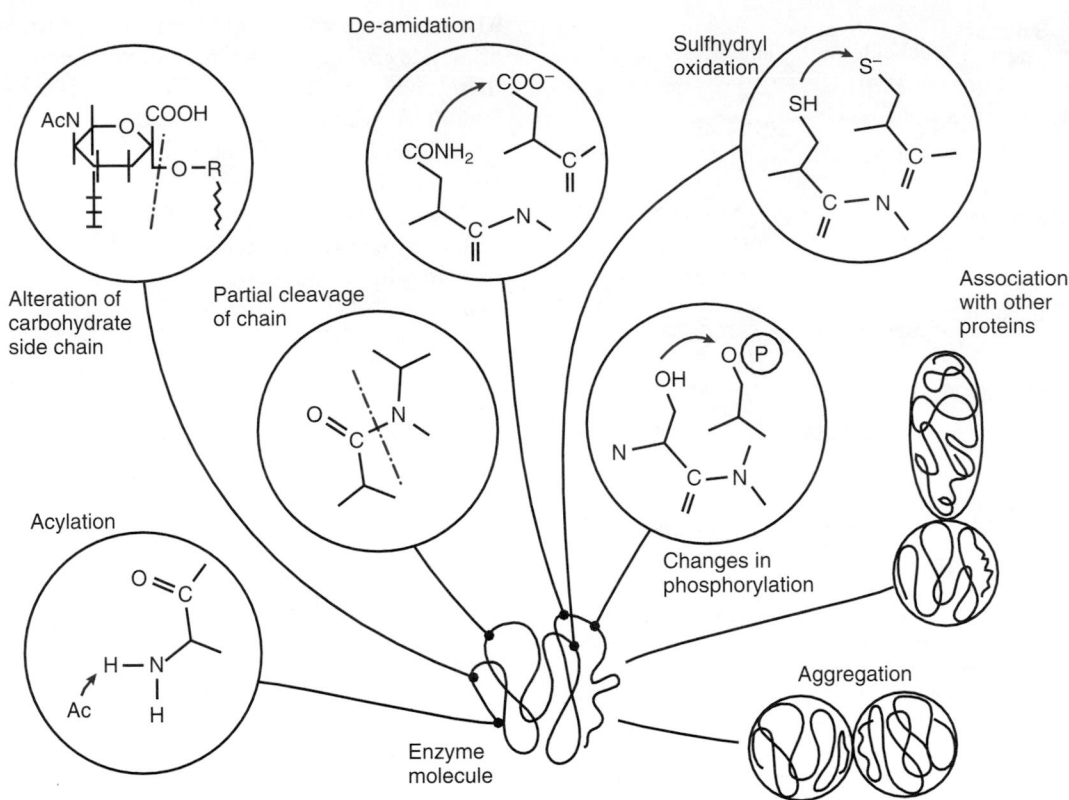

Figure 9-3 Nongenetic modifications that may give rise to multiple forms of enzymes. (From Moss DW: Isoenzymes, London, Chapman & Hall, 1982.)

of a species other than that in which they originated. The availability of enzyme-specific antisera opens a wide range of methods in enzyme analysis (see Chapter 10). The availability of immunochemical methods is particularly important in the analysis of isoenzyme mixtures.

The multilocus isoenzymes previously discussed usually differ in antigenic specificity, although these differences may not be great among isoenzymes that have presumably emerged relatively recently in evolutionary history and are related closely in structure. Immunological cross-reaction also is not uncommon among multilocus isoenzymes. Multiple enzyme forms due to postsynthetic modification frequently have common antigenic determinants. Isoenzymes derived from allelic genes (allelozymes) often are antigenically similar, even to the extent that substances that cross-react with antisera to the common isoenzyme may be detectable when mutation has abolished enzyme activity altogether. However, the greater specificity of monoclonal antibodies usually can reveal differences among otherwise antigenically similar isoenzyme molecules.

Enzymes As Catalysts

A **catalyst** is a substance that increases the rate of a particular chemical reaction without being consumed or permanently altered. Enzymes are protein catalysts of biological origin. Virtually all chemical reactions that take place in

living matter are catalyzed by specific enzymes. Thus life itself is regarded as an integrated series of enzymatic reactions and some diseases as a derangement of the normal pattern of metabolism. It is the **catalytic activity** of enzymes that makes them such sensitive indicators of pathological change.

Efficiency

Because of their remarkable catalytic activities, a given number of enzyme molecules convert an enormous number of substrate molecules to **products** within a short period of time. Therefore the appearance of increased amounts of enzymes in the bloodstream is detected easily, although the amount of enzyme protein released from damaged cells is small, compared with the total level of nonenzymatic proteins in blood. Thus a particular enzyme is recognized by its characteristic effect on a given chemical reaction, despite the presence of a vast excess of other proteins.

Like any other catalyst, an enzyme changes only the rate at which equilibrium is established between reactants and products; it does not alter the equilibrium constant of the reaction. In a reaction in which only one set of products is chemically possible, the catalyst does not produce any change in the nature of the products; however, when several different possible pathways exist, the enzyme directs the reaction along only one pathway.

Specificity and the active center

Interaction between the enzyme and its substrate involves the combination of one molecule of enzyme with one substrate molecule (or two, in the case of bisubstrate reactions). The reaction involves the attachment of the substrate molecule to a specialized region of the enzyme molecule, its **active center** (see Figure 9-1). The various groups that are important in substrate binding are brought together at the active center, and there the processes of activation and transformation of the substrate take place. The composition and spatial arrangement of the active center also form the basis for the specificity of an enzyme.

Each enzyme catalyzes only one reaction or, at most, a limited number of chemical reactions. The degree of specificity varies from one enzyme to another. Some enzymes show absolute specificity—catalyzing a unique reaction and no others. Pyruvate kinase, for example, catalyzes the transfer of a phosphate group between phosphoenolpyruvate and adenosine diphosphate (ADP) and functions in no other reaction. A somewhat lesser degree of substrate specificity is found in hexokinase, which transfers a phosphate group from adenosine triphosphate (ATP) to D-glucose but also phosphorylates D-fructose, D-mannose, and 2-deoxy-D-glucose at almost equivalent rates. Hexokinase does not act, however, on D-galactose or various other hexoses or pentoses, although some of these substances are bound to the enzyme and competitively inhibit enzyme activity. Disaccharides, methylated sugars, and sugar alcohols neither bind to the enzyme nor inhibit its activity.

The phosphatases are examples of enzymes with group specificity. These enzymes split phosphate from any of a large variety of organic phosphate esters, although at somewhat different rates. Substances as varied as glucose-6-phosphate (G-6-P), phenyl phosphate, and β-glycerophosphate serve as substrates. The esterases hydrolyze esters to alcohols and carboxylic acids and are enzymes of even lower specificity.

Stereoisomeric specificity is characteristic of many enzymes. The enzymes involved in glycolysis act only on the D-stereoisomers of glucose and its derivatives and never on the L-forms. The transaminases convert oxo-acids only to the L-isomers* of the amino acids, and the fumarase hydrates fumarate to the L-form of malate rather than to the D-glucose (related mirror image D-) form. Human α-amylase hydrolyzes only the linear segments of starches, in which the D-glucose residues are linked by α-1,4-linkages. It is inactive toward cellulose, in which the sugar residues are connected by β-1,4-linkages, and toward the branch points (α-1,6-linkages) in glycogen and amylopectin.

*Although the D and L designations are retained in this chapter, readers should be aware that in the Cahn-Ingold-Prelog system, a series of sequence rules determines configurations. In this system the symbols R and S are used instead of D and L to designate configurations. For further information readers are referred to March J: Advances in Organic Chemistry: Reactions, Mechanisms, and Structure, 4th edition, New York, John Wiley & Sons, 1992.

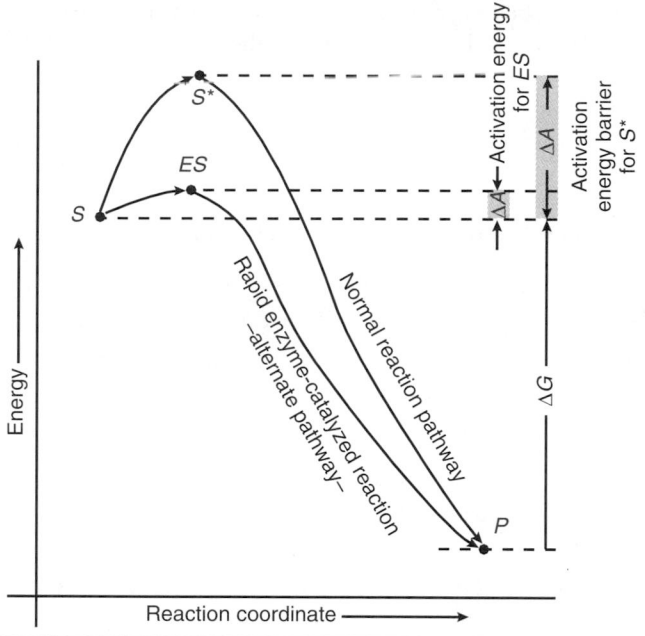

Figure 9-4   Activation energy barrier and reaction course, with and without enzyme catalysis. S, Substrate; ES, enzyme-substrate complex; S*, activated state; ΔG, free energy released by reaction; P, product.

Enzyme Kinetics

Enzymes act through the formation of an enzyme-substrate complex *(ES)* in which a molecule of substrate is bound to the active center of the enzyme molecule. The binding process transforms the substrate molecule to its activated state. The **activation energy** required for this transformation is provided by the free energy of binding of substrate *(S)* to enzyme *(E)*. Therefore activation takes place without the addition of external energy so that the energy barrier to the reaction is lowered and breakdown to products accelerated (Figure 9-4). The *ES* complex breaks down to give the reaction products *(P)* and free enzyme *(E)*.

$$E + S \leftrightarrow ES \leftrightharpoons P + E \qquad (1)$$

All reactions catalyzed by enzymes are in theory reversible, the enzymes catalyzing the forward and backward reactions equally. However, in practice the reaction usually is more rapid in one direction than in the other so that an equilibrium is reached in which the product of either the forward or the backward reaction predominates, sometimes so markedly that the reaction is virtually irreversible.

If the product of the reaction in one direction is removed as it is formed, for example, because it is the substrate of a second enzyme present in the reaction mixture, the equilibrium of the first enzymatic process is displaced so that the reaction proceeds to completion in that direction. Reaction sequences in which the product of one enzyme-catalyzed reaction becomes the substrate of the next enzyme and so on, often through many stages, are characteristic of biological processes. In the laboratory also several enzymatic reactions may be linked together to provide a means to measure the activity of the first enzyme or the concentration of the initial substrate in the chain. For example, the activity of CK usually is measured through a series of linked reactions, and the concentration of glucose is determined through consecutive reactions catalyzed by hexokinase and G-6-P dehydrogenase.

When a secondary enzyme-catalyzed reaction, known as an *indicator reaction,* is used to determine the activity of a different enzyme, the primary reaction catalyzed by the enzyme to be determined must be the rate-limiting step. Conditions are chosen to ensure that the rate of reaction catalyzed by the indicator enzyme is directly proportional to the rate of product formation in the first reaction.

Factors governing the rate of enzyme-catalyzed reactions

Many factors influence the rate of enzyme-catalyzed reactions, including enzyme and substrate concentrations, pH, and temperature.

Enzyme concentration

In the enzymatic reaction represented in equation (1), the equilibrium reaction between enzyme and substrate is assumed to be very rapid, compared with the breakdown of *ES* into free enzyme and products. The overall rate of the reaction under otherwise constant conditions therefore is considered proportional to the concentration of the *ES* complex. Provided that an excess of free substrate molecules is maintained, the addition of more enzyme molecules to the reaction system increases the concentration of the *ES* complex and the overall rate of reaction. This increase accounts for the rate of reaction being proportional to the concentration of enzyme present in the system and is the basis for the quantitative determination of enzymes by measurement of reaction rates. Reaction conditions are selected to ensure that the observed reaction rate is proportional to enzyme concentration over as wide a range as possible.

Substrate concentration

In addition to explaining the dependence of reaction rate on enzyme concentration under conditions in which excess substrate is present, the formation of an *ES* complex also accounts for the hyperbolic relationship between reaction velocity and substrate concentration (Figure 9-5). Such curves are referred to as *Michaelis-Menten plots.*

Single-substrate reactions. If the enzyme concentration is fixed and the substrate concentration is varied, the rate of reaction is almost directly proportional to the substrate concentration at low values of the latter. Under these conditions the rate of the reaction is proportional and dependent on the substrate concentration, a situation termed *first order.* At low concentrations of substrate only a fraction of the enzyme is associated with substrate, and the

rate observed reflects the low concentration of the *ES* complex. At high substrate concentrations the reaction rate is known as *zero order* and is independent of substrate concentration. With a **zero-order reaction** the entire enzyme is bound to substrate, and a much higher rate of reaction is obtained. Moreover, because the entire enzyme is present in the form of the complex, no further increase in complex concentration and no further increment in reaction rate are possible. The maximum possible velocity for the reaction has been reached.

A typical Michaelis-Menten curve is described by the equation

$$v = \frac{V_{max}[S]}{K_m + [S]} \qquad (2)$$

where V_{max} is the velocity that the observed value of v approaches at high values of $[S]$. It increases with increasing enzyme concentration. K_m, the **Michaelis-Menten constant,** is the substrate concentration at which $v = V_{max}/2$, and it is a constant for a given enzyme acting under given conditions. If an equilibrium is set up between enzyme and substrate, K_m is the equilibrium constant of this reaction. However, the symbol K_S (substrate constant) is used if this meaning is intended, and K_m is reserved for the experimentally determined value of $[S]$ at which $v = V_{max}/2$.

Although setting up an experiment to determine the variation of v with $[S]$ is relatively simple, the exact value of V_{max} is not evaluated easily from the hyperbolic curve. Furthermore, many enzymes deviate from their ideal behavior at high substrate concentrations and indeed may be inhibited by excess substrate; thus calculating the value of V_{max} can be difficult. Therefore when enzyme constants are measured ex-

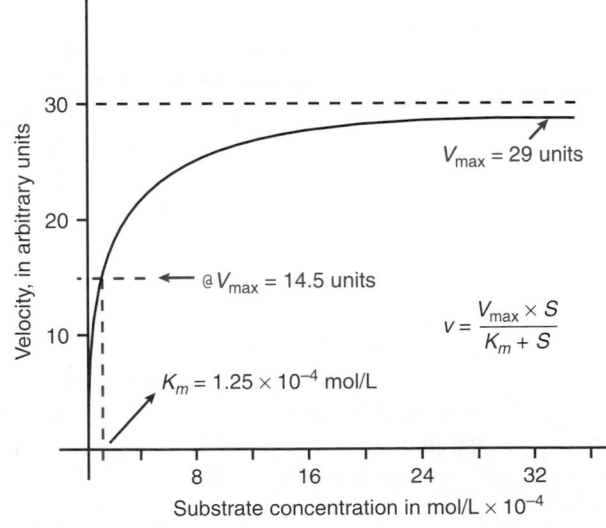

Figure 9-5   Michaelis-Menten curve relating velocity (rate) of an enzyme-catalyzed reaction to substrate concentration. The value of K_m is given by the substrate concentration at which one-half the maximum velocity is obtained. K_m, Michaelis-Menten constant; V_{max}, maximum velocity; S, substrate; v, velocity.

perimentally, the Michaelis-Menten equation (2) usually is transformed into one of several reciprocal forms, such as

$$\frac{1}{v} = \left(\frac{K_m}{V_{max}} \times \frac{1}{[S]}\right) + \frac{1}{V_{max}} \qquad (3)$$

This equation, when plotted, gives a straight line, with intercepts at $1/V_{max}$ on the ordinate and $-1/K_m$ on the abscissa. The graph on which the plots are made is the **Lineweaver-Burk plot** (Figure 9-6).

In practice, determining the reaction velocity over a wide range of substrate concentrations is necessary. Zero-order kinetics are maintained if the substrate is present at concentrations of at least 10 and preferably 100 times that of the value of K_m. When $[S] = 10 \times K_m$, v is approximately 91% of the theoretical V_{max}.

Two-substrate reactions.   Although the prior discussion has focused on the effect of changes in the concentration of only a single substrate on the rate of reaction, most enzymatic reactions are of the following type:

$$\begin{array}{cccccc} \text{Substrate 1} & + & \text{Substrate 2} & \overset{E}{\rightleftharpoons} & \text{Product 1} & + & \text{Product 2} \\ S_1 & & S_2 & & P_1 & & P_2 \end{array} \qquad (4)$$

Among the bisubstrate reactions important in clinical enzymology are the reactions catalyzed by dehydrogenases—in which the second substrate is a specific coenzyme, such as reduced nicotinamide-adenine dinucleotide (NADH) or reduced NAD phosphate (NADPH)—or by aminotransferases. The concentrations of both substrates affect the rates of two-substrate reactions. Values of K_m and V_{max} for each substrate are derived from experiments in which the concentration of the first substrate is held at saturating levels while the concentration of the second substrate is varied, and vice versa.

The selection of reaction conditions for the measurement of enzymatic activity involving two substrates is approached empirically; the concentration of the first substrate is varied, and that of the second substrate remains constant until maximum activity is reached. The process then is repeated, with the concentration of the first substrate held at the value thus determined, whereas the concentration of the second substrate is varied. However, this traditional empirical approach to optimization has been replaced by newer techniques of simplex co-optimization or response surface methods.

pH

The rate of enzyme-catalyzed reactions typically shows a marked dependence on pH (Figure 9-7). Many enzymes in blood plasma show maximum activity in vitro in the pH range from 7 to 8. However, activity has been observed at pH values as low as 1.5 (pepsin) and as high as 10.5 (alkaline phosphatase). The optimum pH for a given forward re-

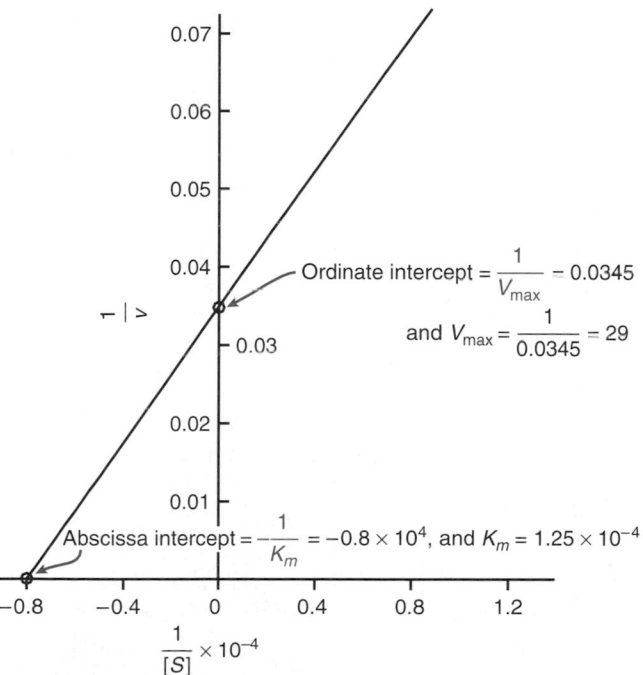

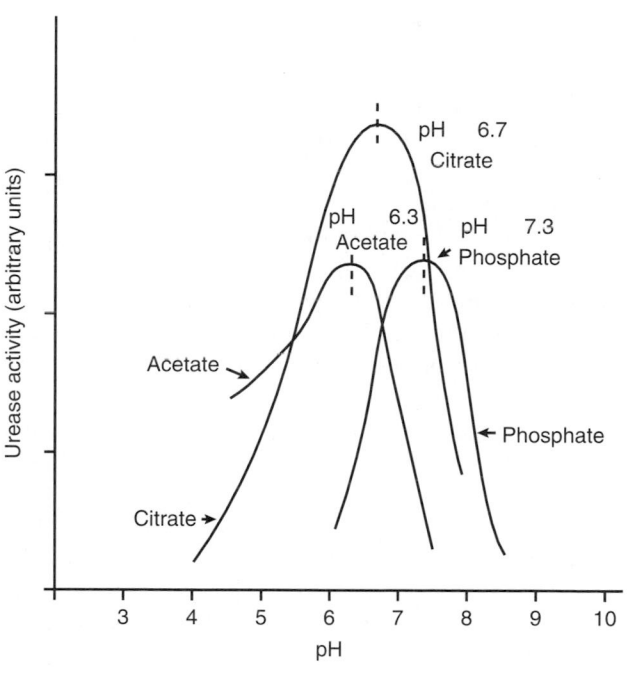

Figure 9-6   Lineweaver-Burk transformation of the curve in Figure 9-5, with $1/v$ plotted on the ordinate (y-axis), and $1/[S]$ on the abscissa (x-axis). The intercepts permit calculation of V_{max} and K_m. The units of v and $[S]$ are those given in Figure 9-5. *[S]*, Substrate concentration; V_{max}, maximum velocity; K_m, Michaelis-Menten constant; v, velocity.

Figure 9-7   The pH activity curves for urease demonstrate the effect of buffer species on optimum pH. (Modified from Howell SF, Sumner JB: The specific effects of buffers upon urease activity. J Biol Chem 1934; 104:619.)

action may be different from the optimum pH found for the corresponding reverse reaction. The form of the pH-dependence curve is a result of a number of separate effects, including the ionization of the substrate and extent of dissociation of certain key amino acid side chains in the protein molecule, both at the active center and elsewhere. Both pH and ionic environment also affect the three-dimensional conformation of the protein and therefore enzyme activity to such an extent that enzymes may be denatured irreversibly at extreme values of pH.

The pronounced effects of pH on enzyme reactions emphasize the need to control this variable by means of adequate buffer solutions. Enzyme assays should be carried out at the pH of optimal activity because the pH-activity curve has its minimum slope near this pH, and a small variation in pH causes a minimal change in enzyme activity. The buffer system must be capable of counteracting the effect of adding the specimen (for example, serum itself being a powerful buffer) to the assay system and the effects of acids or bases formed during the reaction (for example, formation of fatty acids by the action of lipase). Because buffers have maximal buffering capacities close to their pK_a values, whenever possible a buffer system should be chosen with a pK_a value within 1 pH unit of the desired pH of the assay. Interaction between buffer ions and other components of the assay system (for example, activating metal ions) may eliminate certain buffers from consideration.

Temperature

The rate of an enzymatic reaction is proportional to its reaction temperature. For most enzymatic reactions, values of Q_{10} (the relative reaction rates at two temperatures differing by 10 °C) vary from 1.7 to 2.5. However, an increase in the rate of the catalyzed reaction is not the only effect of an increase temperature on an enzymatic reaction. In theory the initial rate of reaction measured instantaneously should increase with as the temperature rises. In practice, however, a finite time is needed to allow the components of the reaction mixture, including the enzyme solution, to reach temperature equilibrium and permit the formation of a measurable amount of product. During this period the enzyme undergoes thermal inactivation and denaturation, a process that has a large temperature coefficient for most enzymes and thus becomes virtually instantaneous at temperatures of 60 to 70 °C.

The counteracting effects of the increased rate of the catalyzed reaction and more rapid enzyme inactivation as the temperature increases account for the existence of an apparent optimum temperature for enzyme activity (Figure 9-8). The apparent optimum temperature depends on the time taken to make the activity measurement. With previously used older assay methods that required lengthy periods of incubation of enzyme with substrate, enzyme inactivation took effect at lower temperatures and the phenomenon was more seen easily.

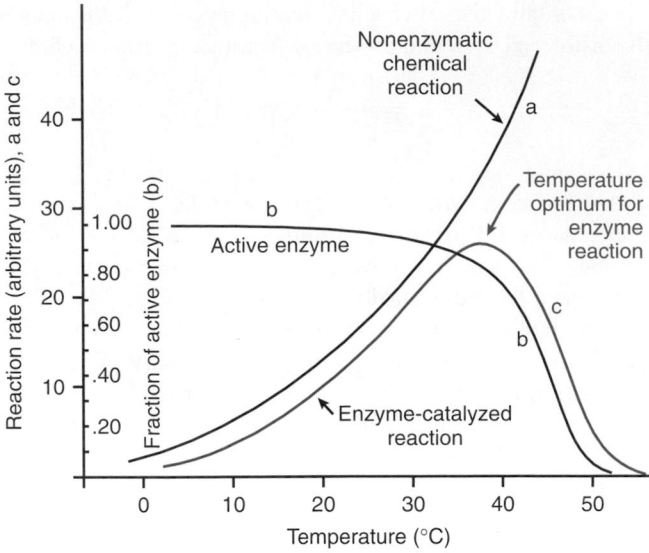

Figure 9-8 Schematic diagram illustrating the effect of temperature on the rate of nonenzyme-catalyzed and enzyme-catalyzed reactions.

The choice of temperature for the assay of enzymes of clinical importance still is under debate, but current opinion favors either 30 or 37 °C; each temperature has its advantages in particular circumstances. Whichever temperature is chosen, exact temperature control to within $\pm 0.1°$ C during the enzymatic reaction is essential.

Inhibition and activation of enzyme activity

Enzymatic rates often are affected by changes in the concentrations of substances other than the enzyme or substrate. These modifiers may be **activators,** which increase the rate of reaction, or **inhibitors,** the presence of which reduces the reaction rate. Activators and inhibitors are usually small molecules (compared with the enzyme itself) or even ions. They vary in specificity from modifiers that exert similar effects on a wide range of different enzymatic reactions to substances that affect only a single reaction.

Inhibition

Inhibition of an enzymatic reaction is either reversible or irreversible.

Reversible inhibition. Reversible inhibition implies that the activity of the enzyme is restored fully when the inhibitor physically is removed from the system. This type of inhibition is characterized by the existence of an equilibrium between enzyme *(E),* and inhibitor *(I)*

$$E + I \rightleftharpoons EI \qquad (5)$$

The equilibrium constant of the reaction, K_i (the inhibitor constant), is a measure of the affinity of the inhibitor for the enzyme, just as K_m generally reflects the affinity of the enzyme for its substrate.

A competitive inhibitor is usually a structural analogue of the substrate and binds to the enzyme at the substrate-binding site, but because it is not identical with the substrate, breakdown into products does not take place. When the process of inhibition is fully competitive, the enzyme combines with either the substrate or the inhibitor, but not with both simultaneously. At low substrate concentrations, the binding of substrate is reduced because some enzyme molecules are combined with inhibitor. Thus the concentration of ES and hence the overall reaction velocity are reduced, and K_m apparently is increased. At high $[S]$, however, all the enzyme molecules combine to form ES so that V_{max} is unaffected by the inhibitor. These characteristics of competitive inhibition are demonstrated in the Lineweaver-Burk plot (see Figure 9-9).

Competitive inhibition is responsible for the inhibition of some enzymes by excess substrate because of competition between substrate molecules for a single binding site. In two-substrate reactions, high concentrations of the second substrate may compete with the binding of the first substrate. Competitive inhibition also contributes to the reduction of the rate of an enzymatic reaction with time. For example, in a freely reversible reaction a rate reduction occurs because increasing concentrations of reaction products tend to drive the reaction backward. A product of a reaction itself may be an inhibitor of the forward reaction so that even if the reaction is not readily reversible, it proceeds against an increasing concentration of inhibitor. Product inhibition is thus one cause of nonlinearity of reaction progress curves.

A noncompetitive inhibitor is usually structurally different from the substrate. It is assumed to bind at a site on the enzyme molecule other than the substrate-binding site; thus no competition exists between inhibitor and substrate, and a ternary enzyme-substrate-inhibitor *(ESI)* complex forms. Attachment of the inhibitor to the enzyme does not alter the affinity of the enzyme for its substrate (that is, K_m is unaltered), but the *ESI* complex does not break down to provide products. Because the substrate does not compete with the inhibitor for binding sites on the enzyme molecule, an increase in the substrate concentration does not overcome the effect of a noncompetitive inhibitor. Thus V_{max} is reduced in the presence of such an inhibitor, whereas K_m is not altered, as the Lineweaver-Burk plot demonstrates (Figure 9-9).

In a rather unusual type of reversible inhibition, known as *uncompetitive inhibition*, parallel lines are obtained when plots of $1/v$ against $1/[S]$ with and without the inhibitor are compared (see Figure 9-9); that is, both K_m and V_{max} are decreased. Uncompetitive inhibition is due to combination of the inhibitor with the ES complex and is more common in two-substrate reactions, in which a ternary ESI complex forms after the first substrate combines with the enzyme.

Irreversible inhibition. An irreversible inhibitor combines covalently with the enzyme, with which it is not in equilibrium. The effect of an irreversible inhibitor is pro-

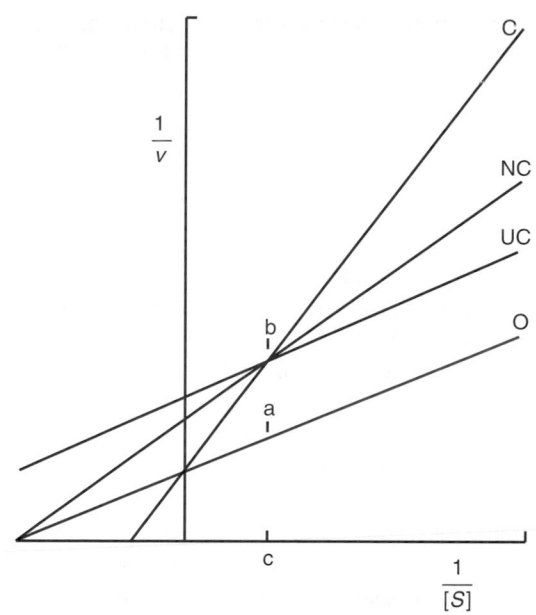

Figure 9-9   Effects of different types of inhibitors on the double-reciprocal plot of $1/v$ against $1/[S]$. Each inhibitor is assumed to reduce the activity of the enzyme by the same amount, represented by the change in $1/v$ from *a* to *b* at a substrate concentration of *c*. Line *O* is the plot for an enzyme without an inhibitor, *C* is that with a competitive inhibitor, *NC* is that with a noncompetitive inhibitor, and *UC* is that with an uncompetitive inhibitor. (From Moss DW: Measurement of enzymes. In Hearse DJ, de Leiris J (eds): Enzymes in Cardiology: Diagnosis and Research, New York, John Wiley & Sons, 1979.)

gressive with time, becoming complete if the amount of inhibitor present exceeds the total amount of enzyme. The rate of the reaction between enzyme and inhibitor is expressed as the fraction of the enzyme activity that is inhibited in a fixed time by a given concentration of inhibitor. When the inhibitor is added to the enzyme in the presence of its substrate, the reaction between the enzyme and inhibitor is delayed when some of the enzyme molecules are combined with the substrate and therefore are protected from reacting with the inhibitor. However, as the substrate molecules react chemically, the active centers become available for combination with the inhibitor. Thus inhibition eventually becomes complete even though an excess of substrate initially exists. Furthermore, addition of more substrate is ineffective in reversal of the inhibition, in contrast to its effect on reversible competitive inhibition, which was discussed previously.

Inhibition by antibodies. Combination of enzyme molecules with specific antibodies often has no effect on catalytic activity, which is retained by the enzyme-antibody complex. However, in some cases reaction of the enzyme and antibody reduces or even abolishes enzymatic activity. With this type of inhibition the antibody molecule is thought to restrict access of the substrate molecules to the active center by steric hindrance or by masking the substrate-binding site. However, some examples of enzyme inhibition by combination with antibodies appear to be due to a conformational change induced in the enzyme molecule.

Inhibition of the activity of an enzyme molecule as a result of combination with a specific antibody is the basis of homogeneous enzyme immunoassay. (See Chapter 10 for a more detailed discussion.)

Enzyme activation

Activators are considered to increase the rates of enzyme-catalyzed reactions by promoting formation of the most active state, either of the enzyme itself or of other reactants such as the substrate. This generalization covers a wide variety of mechanisms of activation.

Many enzymes contain metal ions as integral parts of their structures (for example, zinc in ALP and carboxy-peptidase A). The function of the metal may be to stabilize tertiary and quaternary protein structure. Removal of the divalent metal ions by treatment with an appropriate concentration of ethylenediaminetetraacetic acid (EDTA) solution is accompanied by conformational changes with inactivation of the enzyme. The enzyme is reactivated by dialysis against a solution of the appropriate metal ion or simply through the addition of the ion to the reaction mixture. Reactivation may take time because rearrangement of the polypeptide chains into the active conformation does not occur instantaneously.

The metal ion components of many enzymes appear to play a direct role in catalysis in addition to any possible structural role they may fulfill. A metal ion may function in catalysis, for example, by providing an electropositive center in the enzyme with which negatively charged groups in the substrate forms coordinate links.

When the activator ion is an essential part of the functional enzyme molecule, it is usually incorporated firmly into the enzyme molecule. Therefore adding the activator to reaction mixtures is not usually necessary, and excess amounts of the ion even may create an inhibitory effect. However, in many cases the activating ion is attached only weakly or transiently to the enzyme (or its substrate) during catalysis. Common activating cations are Mg^{2+}, Mn^{2+}, Fe^{2+}, Ca^{2+}, Zn^{2+}, and K^+. More rarely, anions may act as activators. For example, amylase functions at its maximum rate only if Cl^- or other monovalent anions, such as Br^- or NO_3^- are present. Some enzymes require the obligate presence of two activating ions. K^+ and Mg^{2+} are essential for the activity of pyruvate kinase, and both Mg^{2+} and Zn^{2+} are necessary for ALP activity.

The velocity of the reaction depends on the concentration of a reversible activator in a fashion similar to its dependence on substrate concentration. Activator-dependent enzyme reactions should be performed in the presence of both excess activator and excess substrate. In many cases, however, the addition of activator beyond a certain optimum concentration may result in a decrease in the reaction rate (inhibition by excess activator). In such cases the optimum concentration of activator must be used.

Coenzymes and prosthetic groups

Coenzymes are usually more complex molecules than are activators and are smaller molecules than the enzyme proteins themselves. Some compounds, such as the dinucleotides NAD and NADP, are classified as coenzymes and are specific substrates in two-substrate reactions. Their effect on the rate of reaction follows the Michaelis-Menten pattern of dependence on substrate concentration. The structures of these two coenzymes are identical except for the presence of an additional phosphate group in NADP; nevertheless, individual dehydrogenases, for which these coenzymes are substrates, are predominantly or even absolutely specific for one or the other form.

Coenzymes such as NAD and NADP are bound only momentarily to the enzyme during the course of reaction, as is the case for substrates in general. Therefore no reaction takes place unless the appropriate coenzyme is present in solution (for example, through its addition to the reaction mixture in the assay of dehydrogenase activity). In contrast to these entirely soluble coenzymes, some coenzymes are bound more or less permanently to the enzyme molecules, where they form part of the active center and undergo cycles of chemical change during the reaction.

The active **holoenzyme** results from the combination of the inactive **apoenzyme** with the *prosthetic group*, the term for a bound coenzyme. An example of a prosthetic group is pyridoxal phosphate (P-5′-P), a component of aspartate and alanine transaminases. The P-5′-P prosthetic group undergoes a cycle of conversion of the pyridoxal moiety to pyridoxamine and back again during the transfer of an amino group from an amino acid to an oxo-acid. Prosthetic groups, like activators with structural roles, usually do not have to be added to elicit full catalytic activity of the enzyme unless previous treatment has caused the prosthetic group to be lost from some enzyme molecules. However, both normal and pathological serum samples contain appreciable amounts of apo-aminotransferases, which are converted to the active holoenzymes by a suitable period of incubation with P-5′-P.

A study of the formulas of coenzyme and prosthetic groups shows that many contain structures derived from vitamins. Thus the nicotinamide portion of NAD and NADP derives from the vitamin niacin, whereas the P-5′-P prosthetic group of the aminotransferases is a derivative of pyridoxine, vitamin B_6. Other derivatives of the B-group vitamins participate in enzymatic reactions. (Chapter 28 will discuss this concept in more detail.)

■ DIAGNOSTIC ENZYMOLOGY

The clinical laboratorian is concerned principally with changes in the activity or mass in serum or plasma of enzymes that are predominantly intracellular and normally present in serum in low levels only (Table 9-2). By measur-

TABLE 9-2	Classification of Enzymes in Blood
Classification	Examples
Plasma-specific enzymes	Serine protease procoagulants: thrombin, factor XII (Hageman factor), factor X (Stuart-Prower factor), and others
	Fibrinolytic enzymes or precursors: plasminogen, plasminogen proactivator
Secreted enzymes	Lipase (from salivary glands, gastric oxyntic glands, and pancreas), α-amylase (from salivary glands and pancreas), trypsinogen, cholinesterase, prostatic acid phosphatase, prostate-specific antigen
Cellular enzymes	Lactate dehydrogenase, aminotransferases, alkaline phosphatases, and others

TABLE 9-3	Causes of Cell Damage or Death
Category	Examples
Hypoxia (an extremely common accompaniment of clinical disease)	Loss of blood supply due to narrowing (atheromatous plaques) or blocking (thrombosis) of artery or vein; ischemic-perfusion injury; inadequate oxygenation due to cardiorespiratory failure; loss of oxygen-carrying capacity; CO poisoning; and anemia
Chemicals and drugs (an important cause of cellular damage)	Environmental pollutants (lead, mercury); drugs, use and abuse; alcohol; tobacco
Physical agents	Trauma; extremes of heat and cold; radiation; electrical energy; toxic chemicals
Microbiological agents	Bacteria, viruses, fungi, protozoa, and helminths
Immune mechanisms	Immune disorders can cause tissue damage through a number of the following mechanisms: • Anaphylaxis (causing release of vasoactive amines) • Cytotoxicity (causing the target cell to be lysed) • Immune complex disease (leading to release of lysosomal enzymes) • Cell-mediated hypersensitivity (leading to cytotoxicity)
Genetic defects	Disorders with polygenic inheritance—diabetes mellitus, gout Mendelian disorders—X-linked disorders, autosomal dominant and recessive disorders, disorders with variable modes of transmission
Nutritional disorders	Protein-calorie malnutrition, vitamin deficiencies, mineral deficiencies, obesity and its consequences

Based on the classification by Robbins and colleagues. In Basic Pathology, 3rd edition, Philadelphia, WB Saunders, 1981.

ing changes in the levels of these enzymes in disease, inference of the location and nature of pathological changes in the tissues of the body is possible. Therefore understanding the factors that affect the rate of release of enzymes from their cells of origin and the rate at which they are cleared from the circulation is necessary so that changes in levels in disease are interpreted correctly.

Factors Affecting Enzyme Levels in Plasma or Serum

The measured level of an enzyme in blood is the result of the balance between the rate at which it enters the circulation from its cells of origin and the rate at which it is inactivated or removed.

Entry of enzymes into the blood

Leakage of enzymes from cells and altered productions are factors that influence the rate at which enzymes enter the circulation from the cells.

Leakage of enzymes from cells

Enzymes are retained within their cells of origin by the plasma membrane surrounding the cell. The plasma membrane is a metabolically active part of the cell, and its integrity depends on the cell's energy production. Any process that impairs energy production, either through deprivation of oxidizable substrates or restriction of access of oxygen necessary for energy production, promotes deterioration of the cell membrane. In such cases the membrane leaks its cellular components and, if cellular injury becomes irreversible, the cell dies. Small molecules are the first to leak from damaged or dying cells, followed by larger molecules, such as enzymes; ultimately the entire contents of the necrotic cell are discharged.

Direct attack on the cell membranes by such agents as viruses or organic chemicals also cause enzyme release, which is particularly significant in the case of the liver. A reduction in the supply of oxygenated blood perfusing any tissue also promotes enzyme release. An example of a clinical condition in which such a reduction occurs is that of myocardial infarction. The cells of the affected region begin to deteriorate rapidly and eventually die, releasing their enzyme contents to the systemic circulation; this release accounts for the rapid rise in serum enzyme activity characteristic of a myocardial infarction. The liver is particularly sensitive to hypoxia, which results from diminished cardiac output (heart failure). Increased activities of hepatocellular enzymes in the blood accompany a wide variety of conditions, such as congestive heart failure, shock, and hypoxemia.

Skeletal muscles also contribute enzymes to blood. Again the cause may be poor perfusion, hypothermia, or direct trauma to the muscles (crush injuries). Infection, inflammation (polymyositis), degenerative changes (dystrophies), drugs, and alcohol (alcoholic myopathy) all cause enzyme leakage from myocytes. Enzyme release from muscles and other tissues also occurs as a result of anesthesia. Table 9-3 summarizes a number of causes of cell damage or death.

Altered enzyme production

The small amounts of intracellular enzymes normally present in the plasma are thought to result from turnover of cells or leakage of enzymes from healthy cells. This contribution of enzymes to the circulating blood may decrease, either as the result of a genetic deficiency of enzyme production or the depression of enzyme production as a result of disease. However, cases in which enzyme production is increased are of more general interest in diagnostic enzymology. For example, an increase in the number and activity of the alkaline phosphatase-producing osteoblasts of bone is responsible for the increased level of alkaline phosphatase in the serum of normally growing children. Increased osteoblastic activity also accounts for the increased levels of the enzyme in serum in various types of bone disease. Toward the end of a normal pregnancy the placenta constitutes a new source of alkaline phosphatase and contributes its characteristic isoenzyme to the maternal circulation.

The process of enzyme **induction** also increases enzyme production. An example of such induction is the increased activity of γ-glutamyltransferase in serum, which results from the administration of drugs, such as barbiturates or phenytoin, and from the intake of ethanol. Biliary obstruction induces increased synthesis of alkaline phosphatase in the liver.

Clearance of enzymes

Because enzyme molecules are too large to pass through the healthy glomerulus of the kidney, urinary excretion is not a major route for elimination of enzymes from circulation. Amylase is an exception because increased levels of this enzyme are accompanied by increased excretion in the urine. The half-lives of enzymes in plasma vary from a few hours to several days, with an average half-life ($t_{1/2}$) of 6 to 48 hours. In addition, the existence of circulating inhibitors or activators of enzymes also has little effect on levels measured in the laboratory.

Measurement of Reaction Rates

The rate of an enzyme-catalyzed reaction is directly proportional to the amount of active enzyme present in the system. Consequently, the determination of the rate of reaction under defined and controlled conditions provides a very sensitive and specific method for the measurement of enzymes in samples such as serum.

Determination of reaction rate involves the kinetic measurement of the amount of change produced in a defined time interval. Both fixed-time and continuous-monitoring methods are used to measure reaction rates. In a **fixed-time reaction** the amount of change produced by the enzyme is measured after the reaction is stopped at the end of a

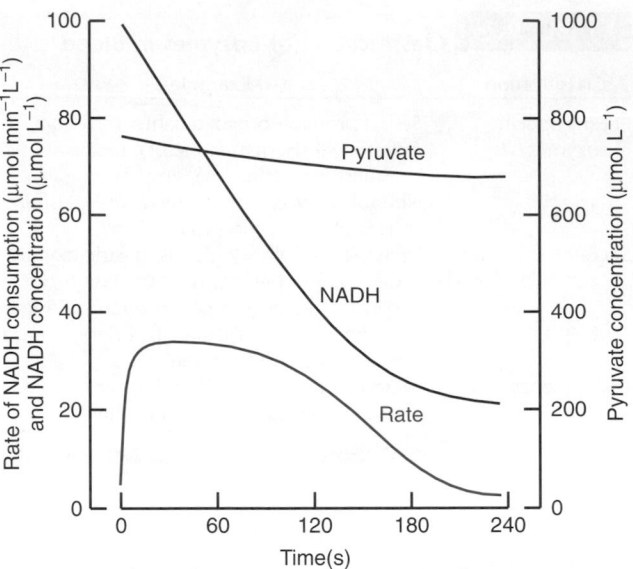

Figure 9-10 Changes in substrate concentrations and rates of reaction during an assay of LD activity at 37 °C in phosphate buffer, with pyruvate and NADH as substrates. The reaction is followed through observation of the fall in absorbance at 340 nm as NADH is oxidized to NAD^+. The rate of reaction rises rapidly to a maximum value, from which it declines only slightly until about half the NADH has been used. During this phase of the reaction the rate is essentially zero order with respect to substrate concentration. At the point at which the rate falls below about 90% of its maximum value, NADH concentration is approximately $10 \times K_m$. K_m for NADH is of the order of 5×10^{-6} mol/L, whereas for pyruvate it is 9×10^{-5} mol/L. Thus an initial pyruvate concentration approximately 10 times that of NADH is used. (Concentrations are per liter of reaction mixture.) *LD*, Lactate dehydrogenase. (From Moss DW: Measurement of enzymes. In Hearse DJ, de Leiris J (eds): Enzymes in Cardiology: Diagnosis and Research, New York, John Wiley & Sons, 1979.)

fixed-time interval. In the **continuous-monitoring** method the progress of the reaction is monitored continuously. These two methods have different advantages and limitations. To appreciate these, consideration of the way in which the rate of an enzymatic reaction varies with time is necessary.

The progress of conversion of the substrate into products in the presence of an enzyme is monitored through measurement of the decreasing concentration of the substrate or the increasing concentration of the products. Measurement of product formation is preferable because determination of the increase in concentration of a substance above an initially zero or low level analytically is more reliable than measurement of a decline from an initially high level.

The moment at which the enzyme and substrate are mixed, the rate of the reaction is zero. The rate then typically rises rapidly to a maximum value, which remains constant for a period of time (Figure 9-10). During the period of constant reaction rate, the rate depends only on enzyme concentration and is completely independent of substrate concentration. The reaction is said to follow zero-order ki-

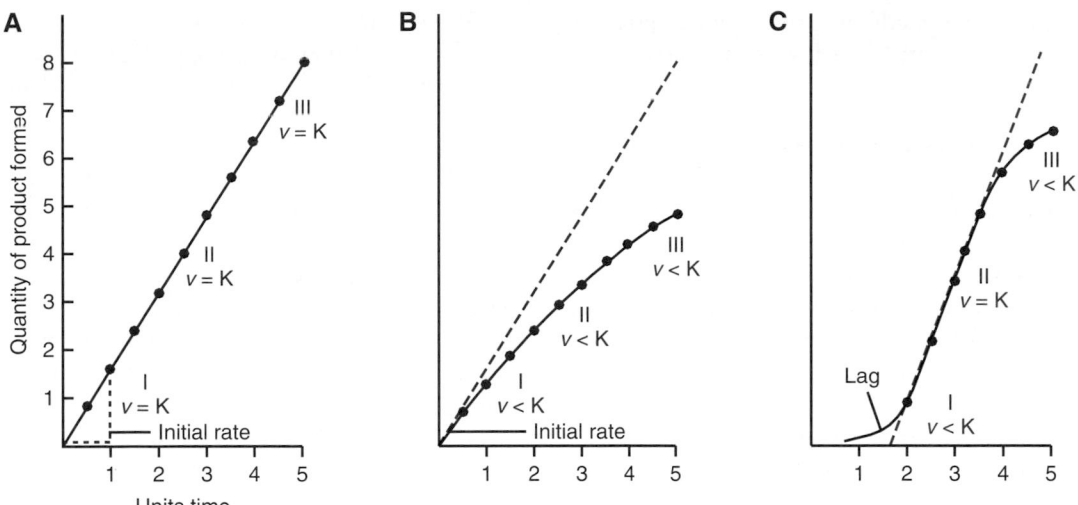

Figure 9-11   Forms of graphs demonstrating changes in enzyme reaction rates as a function of time. **A,** The rate is constant during the entire run, and rates *(v)* calculated as I, II, and III are identical to the initial rate (K). **B,** The rate falls off continuously; rates calculated at I, II, and III are different and less than the true initial rate (K). **C,** A measurement at II is representative of the maximum rate, but at I (lag period) and III (substrate depletion) it is less than at II.

netics because its rate is proportional to the zero power of the substrate concentration. Ultimately, however, as more substrate is consumed, the reaction rate declines and enters a phase of first-order dependence on substrate concentration. Other factors that contribute to the decline in reaction rate include accumulation of products that may be inhibitory, growing importance of the reverse reaction, and even enzyme denaturation.

In practice, enzyme assays are standardized, with enzyme concentration being the only variable that influences the reaction rate. Therefore enzyme assays are run under conditions that are initially saturating with respect to substrate concentration. The rate of reaction during the zero-order phase is determined via measurement of the product formed during a fixed period of incubation during which the rate remains constant (Figure 9-11). Measurement of reaction rates at any portion of the curve in Figure 9-11, *A,* provides results identical to the true "initial rate." However, the curve in Figure 9-11, *B,* deviates from linearity over its entire course, and rates fall off with time. From the curve in Figure 9-11, *C,* correct results are obtained only if the rate is measured along segment II. Incorrect results are obtained if the rate is measured during the lag phase (I) or during phase III.

Careful selection of reaction conditions, such as the concentrations of substrates and cofactors, improves the reaction progress curves, eliminating lag phases and prolonging the period of linearity so that fixed-time methods of analysis become feasible. Improvements in photometry, leading to more reliable and sensitive measurement of product formation, also have shortened the duration of incubation, compared with older assays, resulting in a corresponding increase in the interval over which enzyme activity is measured (Figure 9-12). Nevertheless, an upper limit of activity

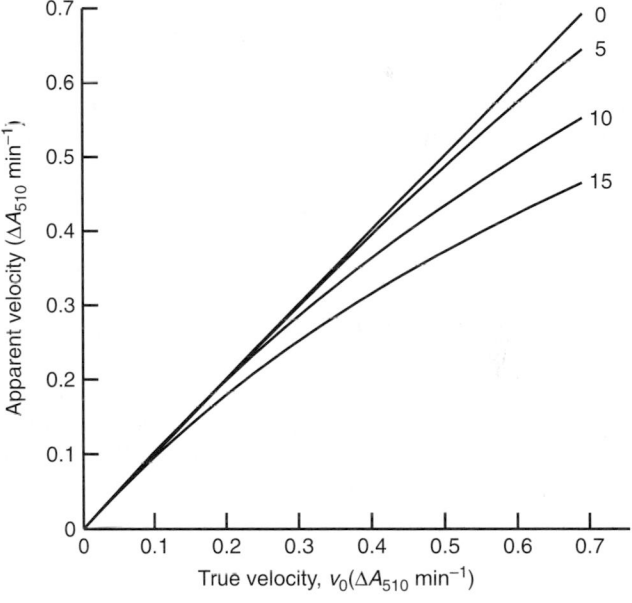

Figure 9-12   Apparent velocity of hydrolysis of phenyl phosphate by alkaline phosphatase measured over a fixed-time interval, as a function of the true initial velocity, v_0. The curves *5, 10,* and *15* correspond to incubation periods of 5, 10, and 15 minutes and illustrate the increasing deviation of the apparent velocity from the initial rate as the incubation period is lengthened. The initial substrate concentration is 4.75 mmol/L of reaction mixture in carbonate-bicarbonate buffer, pH 9.9 at 37 °C. (From Moss DW: Measurement of enzymes. In Hearse DJ, de Leiris J (eds): Enzymes in Cardiology: Diagnosis and Research, New York, John Wiley & Sons, 1979.)

exists in all fixed-time methods, above which progress curves no longer are linear; in such cases the amount of change measured over the fixed-time interval no longer represents true zero-order rate conditions.

The existence of an upper limit of enzyme activity implies that samples with activities above this limit must receive special attention. The upper limit of activity acceptable in the unmodified method must be chosen so that samples with activities below it are presumed, with a high degree of certainty, to give linear progress curves; on the other hand, if the limit is set too low, many samples are reanalyzed unnecessarily. Samples that are above the limit ideally should be reassayed through shortening of the incubation period until a constant reaction rate is obtained. However, this action is difficult or impossible in some automated methods, in which the duration of incubation is fixed by the configuration of the apparatus. In such cases dilution of the specimen becomes necessary; however, dilution may not always result in a proportionate change in activity.

The initial rate of reaction theoretically increases without limit as enzyme concentration increases, as long as no other factor, such as substrate concentration, becomes limiting. In practice, the reaction becomes so rapid at high enzyme activities that measurement of the initial rate of reaction is impossible, even with continuous-monitoring methods. Therefore an upper limit of activity that is accepted without modification of the assay procedure exists, even in continuous-monitoring methods, but this limit is usually much higher than that applicable in corresponding fixed-time methods. Fewer samples therefore require special treatment. Furthermore, continuous monitoring allows identification of the appropriate zero-order portion of the progress curve for each sample and identification of samples that require special treatment. Continuous-monitoring methods therefore possess a decisive advantage in enzyme assay and should be used whenever possible. Enzyme activity also can be measured by notation of the time required to consume all of a fixed amount of substrate, but methods of this type largely have been discontinued.

Units of enzyme activity

When enzymes are measured by their catalytic activities, the results of such determinations are expressed in terms of the concentration of the number of activity units present in a convenient volume or mass of specimen. The unit of activity is the measure of the rate at which the reaction proceeds (for example, the quantity of substrate consumed or product formed in a chosen unit of time). The quantity of substrate may be given in any convenient unit (milligrams, micromoles, change in absorbance, change in viscosity, or microliters of gas formed); time may be expressed in seconds, minutes, or hours. In clinical enzymology the activity of an enzyme generally is reported in terms of some convenient unit of volume, such as activity per 100 mL or per liter of serum or per 1.0 mL of packed erythrocytes. Because the

rate of the reaction depends on experimental parameters, such as pH, buffer type, temperature, nature of substrate, ionic strength, concentration of activators, and other variables, these parameters must be specified in the definition of the unit.

Historically, a multiplicity of units has been used to express enzyme activity. To standardize the way in which enzyme activities are expressed, the EC of the IUB proposed that the unit of enzyme activity be defined as the quantity of enzyme that catalyzes the reaction of 1 μmol of substrate per minute and that this unit be the **international unit (U).** Catalytic concentration is expressed in terms of U/L or mU/L, whichever gives the more convenient numerical value. In those instances in which some uncertainty exists as to the exact nature of the substrate or difficulty is present in calculations of the number of micromoles reacting (as with macromolecules, such as starch, protein, and complex lipids), the unit is expressed in terms of the chemical group or residue measured in the reaction (for example, glucose units or amino acid units formed).

Expectations are that the international unit itself eventually will be replaced by a new unit, the **katal**. Both the International Union of Pure and Applied Chemistry and IUB now recommend that enzyme activity be expressed in moles per second (mol/second) and that the enzyme concentration be expressed in terms of katals per liter (kat/L). This style is consistent with the SI (Systeme Internationale) scheme of units in that the mole is the measure of substrate transformed and the second is the unit of time (see Chapter 1). Thus 1 $U = 10^{-6}$ mol/60 seconds $= 16.7 \times 10^{-9}$ mol/second, or 1.0 nkat/L $= 0.06$ U/L.

Measurement of chemical changes

The amount of substrate transformed into products during an enzyme-catalyzed reaction is measured with any appropriate analytical method. For example, if an enzyme reaction is accompanied by a change in the absorbance characteristics of some component of the assay system (in either the visible or ultraviolet spectrum), it is observed spectrophotometrically during the process. "Self-indicating" reactions of this type are particularly valuable because they make possible continuous monitoring in a recording spectrophotometer. Important examples of self-indicating reactions are the determination of dehydrogenase activity through monitoring of the change in absorbance at 339 (340) nm of the coenzymes NADH or NADPH during oxidation or reduction and the measurement of ALP activity by the generation of the yellow *p*-nitrophenate ion from the substrate *p*-nitrophenyl phosphate (4-NPP) in alkaline solution. The advantages of continuous monitoring are so marked that coupled reactions frequently are used to provide an observable change in absorbance accompanying a primary reaction in which such a change is not present.

The spectrophotometric requirements of enzymatic analysis are no different from those of spectrophotometric quantitative analysis in general. However, the spectrophotometer used must be able to maintain the contents of the cuvet at a constant temperature during the reaction. In addition, because making use of the known molar absorptivity of reaction products has become customary, the absorbance and wavelength accuracy of the spectrophotometer should be checked regularly. (See Chapter 3 for details concerning the performance validation of a spectrophotometer.)

Optimization, standardization, and quality control

To measure enzyme activity reliably, all factors that affect the reaction rate, other than the concentration of active enzyme, must be optimized and controlled rigidly. Furthermore, because the reaction velocity is at or near its maximum under optimal conditions, a larger analytical signal is obtained that is more accurately and precisely measured than the smaller signal obtained under suboptimal conditions. Much effort therefore has been devoted to the determination of optimal conditions for the measurement of clinically important enzyme activities.

Optimization

Optimization of reaction conditions for enzyme assays traditionally has been performed through variation of a single factor and subsequent study of its effect on the reaction rate, followed by repeat of the experiment with a second factor until effects of all the variables have been tested. An optimal combination of variables is selected on the basis of these experiments, and the validity of the chosen conditions is verified. This single-variable approach is being replaced by techniques in which the effects of changes in more than one variable are studied simultaneously. Simplex cooptimization and response-surface methods are typical of these strategies.

Standardization

Two approaches to standardization of enzyme assays are possible. The first is to provide enzyme preparations of stated catalytic activity that are used as calibrators, in the way in which solutions of accurately known concentrations are used to calibrate determinations of other substances. However, this approach requires the availability of enzyme preparations of defined and reliable properties, particularly with regard to stability. A number of thoroughly characterized preparations of enzymes of diagnostic interest have the necessary stability during storage and currently are available.

The second approach is to standardize the conditions of assay, thus reducing the number of methods in use; this approach has been the objective of various national and international working parties and committees. Methods recommended by these groups range from methods intended for use in small groups of neighboring laboratories to rigorously specified reference methods intended to provide a criterion of analytical performance against which routine methods are judged.

In practice, reference methods set standards of precision and accuracy against which the relative performances of methods intended for routine use are judged. Sources of error identified in the development of reference methods then are taken into account in routine methods. Another approach is that as suitable enzyme calibrators become available, their activities may be assigned in terms of the reference method. These preparations then can be used to calibrate routine methods so that even if several routine methods are in use, the results obtained by all such methods are then expressed in a common set of units.

Quality control

Systematic application of quality control (QC) programs is essential in enzyme analysis to ensure that satisfactory analytical performance of enzyme assays is maintained on a day-to-day basis. Lyophilized and liquid preparations containing various enzymes are available from commercial sources and are used for QC purposes. In the past, serum pools prepared in the laboratory were used widely for QC purposes; their use has been discontinued largely for biosafety reasons. Typically, the reproducibility of results of enzyme assays on a day-to-day basis is usually less than ± 5 to 10% coefficient of variation.

Automation of enzyme activity measurements

As with other types of analysis, the increasing demand for enzyme estimation in diagnosis and treatment has been met by the introduction of automated methods of analysis (see Chapter 12). These systems are designed to mechanize the successive stages of sample and reagent volume measurement, preincubation and temperature control, initiation of the enzymatic reaction, monitoring of absorbance changes, and calculation of enzyme activity, which together constitute an enzyme measurement in the continuous-monitoring procedure. These automatic enzyme analyzers can provide satisfactory analytical data with greatly increased throughput of samples.

Measurement of enzyme mass

A considerable number of immunoassays for human enzymes have been developed that measure the mass of an enzyme rather than its activity. To develop such assays, purified enzyme must be prepared for use as a calibrator, to be labeled, and to be used to raise the enzyme-specific antibody. These methods determine all molecules with the antigenic determinants necessary for recognition by the antibody so that inactive enzyme molecules that are unaltered immunologically are measured along with active molecules. This fact is significant in the determination of some digestive enzymes, such as trypsin, when inactive precursors and inhibitors of catalytic activity are present in plasma. In some cases, such as serum cholinesterase, the amount of active enzyme is clinically the more significant quantity.

Enzymes as Analytical Reagents

Enzymes increasingly are being used as analytical reagents because they offer the advantage of enhanced specificity for the substance being determined. Uricase (urate oxidase), urease, and glucose oxidase are examples of highly specific enzymes used in clinically important assays. Coupled reactions often are used to construct an enzymatic analytical system for the determination of a particular compound. An example of this is the determination of glucose by the hexokinase reaction. Hexokinase converts sugars other than glucose to their 6-phosphate esters. However, the indicator reaction used to monitor this change is catalyzed by glucose-6-phosphate dehydrogenase (GPD), an enzyme that is highly specific for its substrate, so the overall process is highly specific for glucose.

In addition, both equilibrium and kinetic (rate) methods have been developed that use enzymes as reagents.

Equilibrium methods

The principle most widely used to determine the amount of a substance enzymatically is to allow the reaction to continue to completion so that all the substrate has been converted into a measurable product. These methods are called *end point* or, more correctly, *equilibrium methods*, because the reaction ceases when equilibrium is reached. Reactions in which the equilibrium point corresponds virtually to complete conversion of the substrate are preferable for this type of analysis. However, unfavorable equilibria often are displaced in the desired direction by additional enzymatic or nonenzymatic reactions that convert or "trap" products of the first reaction; for example, in measuring lactate with LD, the pyruvate formed then is trapped by the addition of hydrazine, with which it forms a hydrazone.

Theoretically, the time required to transform a fixed quantity, Q, of substrate into products is inversely proportional to the amount of enzyme, $[E]$, present.

$$Q = k_1 \times [E] \times t$$

and

$$[E] = \frac{Q}{k_1} + \frac{1}{t} \qquad (6)$$

where, k_1 is the rate constant, and t is the elapsed time. Therefore, $[E]$ is proportional to $1/t$.

Equilibrium methods may require the use of appreciable amounts of enzyme for each sample to avoid inconveniently long incubation periods. As the substrate concentration falls to low levels toward the end of the reaction, the K_m of the enzyme becomes important in the determination of the reaction rate. Enzymes with high affinities for their substrates (low K_m values) therefore are more suitable for equilibrium analysis. Equilibrium methods are largely insensitive to minor changes in reaction conditions. Having exactly the same amount of enzyme in each reaction mixture or maintaining the pH or temperature absolutely constant is not necessary,

provided that the variations are not so great that the reaction is not completed within the fixed time allowed.

Kinetic methods

In a kinetic method the amount of change produced in a fixed-time interval is measured, reducing the amount of reagent enzyme required for the time of reaction. As previously described, the rate of an enzyme-catalyzed reaction with initially high substrate concentration first follows zero-order kinetics and then, as the substrate concentration declines, passes into a first-order kinetic phase. For any **first-order reaction**, the substrate concentration $[S]$ at a given time t after the start of the reaction is given by the following:

$$[S] = [S_0] \times e^{-kt} \qquad (7)$$

where

$[S_0]$ = Initial substrate concentration
e = Base of the natural log
k = Rate constant

The change in substrate concentration $\Delta[S]$ over a fixed-time interval, t_1 to t_2, is related to $[S_0]$ by the following equation:

$$[S_0] = \frac{-\Delta[S]}{e^{-kt_1} - e^{-kt_2}} \qquad (8)$$

That is, the change in substrate concentration over a fixed-time interval is directly proportional to its initial concentration. This is a general property of first-order reactions.

For an enzymatic reaction, first-order kinetics are followed when $[S]$ is small, compared with K_m. Equation (2) then reduces to

$$v = \frac{V_{max}}{K_m} \times [S] \qquad \text{or} \qquad v = k[S]$$

Thus, the first-order rate constant, k, is equal to V_{max}/K_m.

Methods in which some property related to substrate concentration (for example, light absorbance) is measured at two fixed times during the course of the reaction are known as *two-point kinetic methods*. They are theoretically the most accurate for the enzymatic determination of substrates. However, these methods are more demanding technically than equilibrium methods. Because reaction rate is measured at two different points, all the factors that affect reaction rate, such as pH, temperature, and amount of enzyme, must be kept constant from one assay to the next, as must the timing of the two measurements. These conditions now are achieved readily in automatic analyzers (see Chapter 12). A reference solution of the analyte (substrate) must be used for calibration. To ensure first-order reaction conditions, the substrate concentration must be low, of the order of less than $0.2 \times K_m$. Enzymes with high K_m values therefore are preferable for kinetic analysis to provide a wider usable range of substrate concentration. Introduction of a competitive inhibitor has been suggested as a way to increase the apparent

K_m of a reagent enzyme. The low substrate concentrations necessary for kinetic analysis also require the measurement of small changes (for example, in absorbance).

Analytical Applications of Immobilized Enzymes

The consumption of relatively expensive enzymes, one of the disadvantages of enzymes used as analytical reagents, is reduced by the use of **immobilized enzymes** that have been bonded chemically to adsorbents and used as reusable reagents. Among enzymes available in such immobilized forms are urease, hexokinase, α-amylase, glucose oxidase, trypsin, and leucine aminopeptidase. Stability in heat and other forms of inactivation are increased considerably, compared with enzymes in solution. Immobilized proteolytic enzymes are not subject to autodigestion. However, some properties of the enzyme, such as its K_m or its optimum pH, may be altered.

Immobilized enzymes are useful mainly in analytical systems in which the reaction products are detected directly. Techniques such as potentiometry, polarography, and microcalorimetry therefore are chosen frequently to exploit the benefits of immobilized enzymes (see Chapter 6). Enzymes immobilized on the inner walls of plastic tubing and the inner surfaces of reaction vessels are used in a variety of analyzers. Enzymes incorporated into membranes form parts of enzyme electrodes. The surface of an ion-sensitive electrode is coated with a layer of porous gel in which an enzyme has been polymerized. When the electrode is immersed in a solution of the appropriate substrate, the action of the enzyme produces ions to which the electrode is sensitive. For example, an oxygen electrode coated with a layer containing glucose oxidase has been used to determine glucose by the amount of oxygen consumed in the reaction. In addition, urea has been estimated by the combination of a selective ammonium ion-sensitive electrode and a urease membrane.

Measurement of Isoenzymes and Isoforms

A number of analytical techniques are used to measure isoenzymes or isoforms. They include electrophoresis (see Chapter 7), chromatography (see Chapter 8), selective inactivation, and immunochemical methods, as well as those based on differences in catalytic properties.

Selective inactivation

Selective inactivation under controlled conditions has become an important technique in isoenzyme characterization. The method is based on differences in stability that result from small changes in the structure of protein molecules. Elevated temperatures or concentrated solutions of urea or other reagents frequently are chosen to denature the enzyme. Rates of enzyme inactivation by these agents are critically dependent on the conditions of the experiment, which therefore must be controlled strictly if reliable comparisons between samples are to be made. For example, temperature coefficients of inactivation by heat are of the order of 10 to 100 or more, so that variations in temperature of fractions of a degree markedly alter rates of inactivation. Therefore for heat inactivation studies, large, well-stirred water baths with high-performance thermostats are needed to minimize temperature fluctuations, and the duration of inactivation must be timed accurately. When urea is used as the inactivating agent, freshly prepared solutions must be used because cyanate is formed on storage of urea solutions and may itself act as an enzyme inhibitor.

Selective inactivation is a useful semiquantitative or quantitative method for the determination of the composition of isoenzyme mixtures in serum. However, the results are less easy to interpret when more than two isoenzymes are present, especially when hybrid isoenzymes form part of the mixtures, because these forms possess stability characteristics intermediate between those of their parent homopolymeric isoenzymes.

Immunochemical assays

Immunochemical methods of isoenzyme analysis are particularly applicable to isoenzymes derived from multiple gene loci because these are usually most clearly antigenically distinct. However, the greater discriminating power of monoclonal antibodies has brought potentially all multiple forms of an enzyme within the scope of immunochemical analysis. Some of these methods make use of catalytic activity of the isoenzymes. For example, residual activity may be measured after reaction with antiserum. Alternatively, enzymatic activity may be used to locate the enzyme-antigen precipitate in immunodiffusion or rocket electroimmunoassays if the reaction with antibody does not inhibit activity. Radioimmunoassays also have been applied to isoenzyme measurement, and these methods do not depend on the catalytic activity of the isoenzyme being determined.

Immunoassays of various kinds are the methods of choice for a variety of tumor markers, many of which are enzymes. Examples include the placental and germ-cell alkaline phosphatase isoenzymes that are overexpressed ectopically or eutopically in various cancers or the serine protease, prostate specific antigen. In some cases immunoassays and activity assays coexist in routine practice (for example, prostatic acid phosphatase). Immunoinhibition has become a popular method for the determination of MB-creatine kinase (CK-2) in serum, whereas activity-independent immunoassays are used increasingly to determine isoenzymes and isoforms of cardiac muscle proteins.

Differences in catalytic properties

Differences in catalytic properties, such as those in K_m, relative rates of reaction with substrate analogues (when the specificity of the enzyme allows for variation in the structure of the substrate), optimum pH, and response to inhibitors, typically exist between isoenzymes that are the products of multiple gene loci. These differences have formed the basis of methods of identification and measurement of particular isoenzymes. Under the most favorable circumstances, this approach to isoenzyme measurement has the advantage that only slight changes in the usual method of measuring en-zyme activity may be needed to provide information on the isoenzyme composition of a sample. Differences in catalytic properties have been used particularly in isoenzyme studies of LD and acid phosphatase.

Additional Reading

Cornish-Bowden A: Fundamentals of Enzyme Kinetics, Aldershot, United Kingdom, Ashgate Publishing Company, 1995.

Enzyme Nomenclature 1992: Recommendation of the Nomenclature Committee, San Diego, Academic Press, 1992.

Jung K, Mattenheimer H, Burchardt U: Urinary Enzymes in Clinical and Experimental Medicine, New York, Springer-Verlag, 1992.

Moss DW, Henderson AR: Enzymes. In Burtis CA, Ashwood ER (eds): Tietz Textbook of Clinical Chemistry, 3rd edition, pp 617-721, Philadelphia, WB Saunders, 1999.

Palmer T: Understanding Enzymes, Englewood Hall, NJ, Prentice Hall, 1995.

Passonneau JV, Lowry OH: Enzymatic Analysis: A Practical Guide, Clifton, NJ, Humana Press, 1993.

CHAPTER 10

Principles of Immunochemical Techniques*

LARRY J. KRICKA, DPhil, FRCPath

Objectives

1. Define the following terms:
   Antigen
   Antibody
   Hapten
   Immunogen
   Monoclonal
   Polyclonal
2. Diagram and label the components of an IgG antibody molecule.
3. Describe the type of interactions that occur between an antigen and an antibody.
4. Compare precipitin reactions with agglutination reactions.
5. Describe gel diffusion, immunoelectrophoresis, immunofixation, and Western blotting techniques and state the clinical utility of each.
6. Define *immunoassay*.
7. List the labels used in isotopic and nonisotopic immunoassays.
8. Compare competitive with noncompetitive immunoassays and heterogeneous with homogeneous immunoassays.
9. Describe enzyme immunoassay, enzyme-linked immunosorbent assay and enzyme-multiplied immunoassay.
10. Describe fluoroimmunoassay and fluorescence polarization immunoassay.
11. State the principle of immunocytochemistry.
12. State the clinical utility of immunoassays in a clinical laboratory.

Key Words

Antibody Immunoglobulin (Ig) class of molecule (for example, IgA, IgG, or IgM) that binds specifically to an antigen or hapten

Affinity Energy of interaction of a single antibody combining site and its corresponding epitope on the antigen

Antigen Any material capable of reacting with an antibody, without necessarily being capable of inducing antibody formation

Avidity Overall strength of binding of antibody and antigen; includes the sum of the binding affinities of all individual combining sites on the antibody

Bacteriophage Any virus that infects a bacterium

Enzyme-Linked Immunosorbent Assay (ELISA) A type of sandwich enzyme immunoassay in which one of the reaction components is attached to the surface of a solid phase to facilitate separation of bound- and free-labeled reactants

Enzyme-Multiplied Immunoassay Technique (EMIT) A nonseparation immunoassay based on an enzyme label

*The author gratefully acknowledges the original contributions of Dr. Gregory Buffone, on which portions of this chapter are based.

Hapten A chemically defined determinant that, when conjugated to an immunogenic carrier, stimulates the synthesis of antibody specific for the hapten

Immunoassay An assay based on the reaction of an antigen with an antibody specific for the antigen

Immunogen A substance capable of inducing an immune response

Label Any substance with a measurable property that can be attached to an antigen, antibody, or binding substance (such as avidin, biotin, or protein A)

Monoclonal Antiserum Product of a single clone or plasma cell line

Polyclonal Antiserum Antiserum raised in a normal animal host in response to immunogen administration

Western Blotting Membrane-based assay in which proteins are separated by electrophoresis, followed by transfer to a membrane and probing with a labeled antibody

---

Immunochemical reactions form the basis of a diverse range of sensitive and specific clinical assays known as *immunoassays*. In a typical **immunoassay** an antibody is used as a reagent to detect the analyte **(antigen)** of interest. The exquisite specificity and high affinity of antibodies for specific antigens, coupled with the unique ability of antibodies to cross-link antigens, allows for the identification and quantification of specific substances by a variety of methods, many of which are now automated. The principles of the methods most commonly used in the laboratory are discussed in this chapter.

■ BASIC CONCEPTS AND DEFINITIONS

Antibodies are immunoglobulins that can bind specifically to a wide array of natural and synthetic antigens, such as proteins, carbohydrates, nucleic acids, lipids, and other molecules. Immunoglobulin G (IgG) is the most prevalent immunochemical reagent in use. Currently, immunoglobulins A, M, D, and E do not play important roles in immunochemical analysis. IgG is a glycoprotein (molecular weight [MW] 158,000) composed of two duplex chains, each set composed of a heavy (γ) and light (λ or κ) chain joined by disulfide bonds (Figure 10-1). Interchain disulfide bonds hold the duplex chains together and create a symmetrical molecule. The variable amino acid sequence at the amino terminal end of each chain determines the antigenic specificity of the particular antibody. Each unique amino acid sequence is a product of a single plasma cell line or clone, and each plasma cell line produces antibodies with single specificities. A complex antigen elicits a multiplicity of antibodies with different specificities derived from different cell lines. An antibody derived in this manner is termed *polyclonal* and exhibits diverse specificities in its reactivity with the immunogen. Each unique region of the molecular antigen that binds a complementary antibody is termed an *epitope* (antigenic determinant).

An **immunogen** is either a protein or a substance coupled to a carrier, usually a protein. When an immunogen is introduced into a foreign host, it induces the formation of an antibody in the host. A **hapten** is a chemically defined determinant that by itself cannot stimulate an immune response. However, when conjugated to an immunogenic carrier, the conjugated molecule stimulates the synthesis of antibody specific for the hapten. Some general properties required for immunogenicity include the following:

1. Areas of structural stability within the molecule
2. Randomness of structure
3. Minimum MW of 4000 to 5000
4. Ability to be metabolized (a necessary but not sufficient criterion for some classes of antigens)
5. Accessibility of a particular immunogenic configuration to the antibody-forming mechanism
6. Structurally foreign quality

The strength or energy of interaction between the antibody and antigen is described in two terms. **Affinity** refers to the thermodynamic quantity defining the energy of interaction of a single antibody combining site and its corresponding epitope on the antigen. **Avidity** refers to the overall strength of the binding of antibody and antigen and includes the sum of the binding affinities of all the individual combining sites on the antibody. For example, IgG has two affinity-binding sites, whereas IgM has 10 affinity binding sites per antibody molecule. Thus affinity is a property of the substance bound (antigen), and avidity is a property of the binder (antibody).

Polyclonal antiserum is raised in a normal animal host in response to immunogen administration. In contrast, **monoclonal antiserum** is the product of a single clone or plasma cell line rather than a heterogeneous mixture of antibodies produced by many cell clones in response to immunization. Monoclonal antibodies now are used widely as reagents in immunoassay techniques.[5] The usual method of production of monoclonal antibodies involves fusing of sensitized lymphocytes from the spleens or lymph nodes of immunized mice with a murine myeloma cell line from tissue culture (an immortal B-cell line). The murine myeloma cell lines most commonly used are defi-

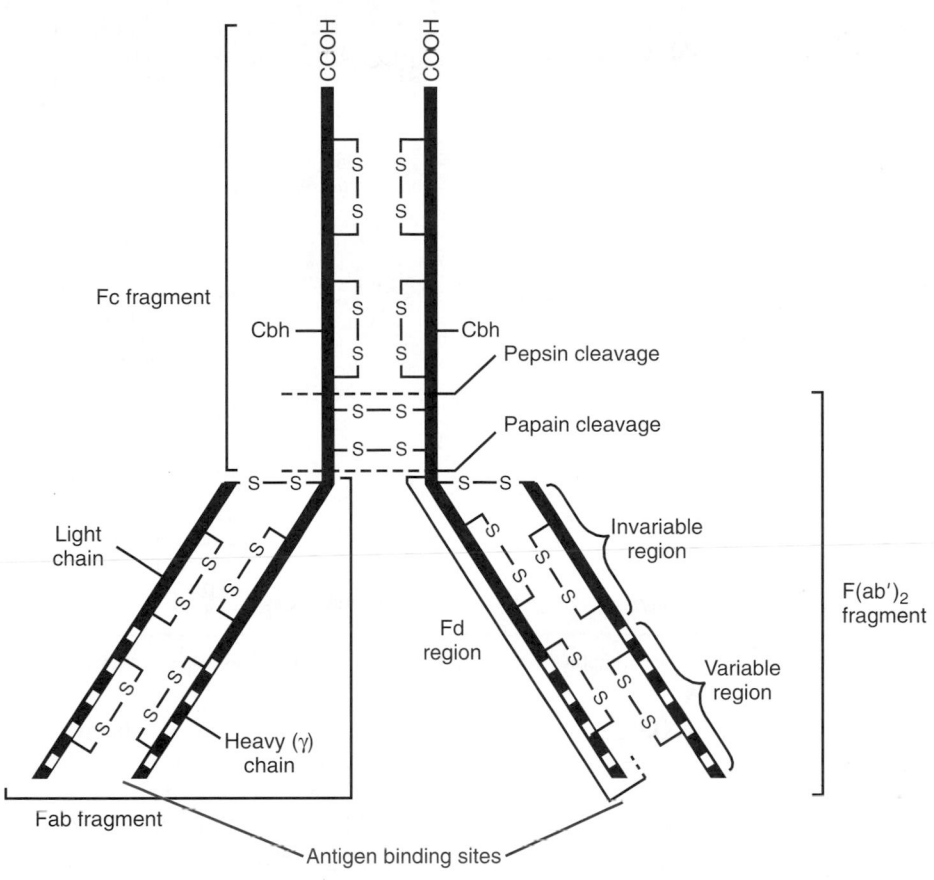

Figure 10-1   Schematic diagram of IgG (immunoglobulin G) antibody molecule showing carbohydrate (Cbh), disulfide bonds (—S—S—) and major fragments produced by proteolytic enzyme treatment (F(ab')$_2$, Fc, Fab, Fd).

cient in the enzyme hypoxanthine guanine phosphoribosyl transferase (HGPRT) and therefore cannot synthesize purine bases from thymidine and hypoxanthine in the presence of aminopterin. After the fusion the cells are placed into a selection medium containing hypoxanthine, aminopterin, and thymidine (HAT medium) to grow selectively fused hybrid cell lines. The fused hybrid cells can survive in a HAT medium because the cells combine the immortality of the myeloma cell with the genetic material of the spleen cell necessary for synthesis of HGPRT. Colonies arising from the fused cells then are screened for antibody production, and those cell lines secreting antibody of the desired specificity are cloned in subcultures. Thus a single clonal line can be isolated that produces an antibody with a specificity for a single antigen epitope and with a single binding energy or affinity.

Monoclonal antibodies have an analytical advantage in that two different antibody specificities can be used in a single assay. A solid-phase antibody specific for a unique epitope and another labeled antibody—specific for a different epitope—can be reacted with antigen in a single incubation step. This combination eliminates the two-step sequential addition of antigen and labeled antibody to the solid phase, as well as one incubation step and one wash-

ing step, which would be necessary when polyclonal antibodies binding to both sites are used. However, the unique ability of a monoclonal antibody to react with a single epitope on a multivalent antigen results in an inability of the majority of monoclonal antibodies to cross-link and precipitate macromolecular antigens. Thus monoclonal antibodies are not applicable for all immunoassays in the clinical laboratory, especially those that use traditional precipitin methods.

Phage-display technology is a new in vitro approach for the production of antibodies that mimic the immune system.[15,16] In this process, genes coding for the heavy and light chain variable domains of immunoglobulin isolated from lymphocytes are amplified by the polymerase chain reaction (see Chapter 11) and ligated into a filamentous bacteriophage vector to form combinatorial libraries of V_H and V_L genes. Individual **bacteriophages** display copies of a specific antibody on their surface, and the phage library can be screened for antibody of defined specificity through the use of immobilized antigen ("panning"). This technique mimics immune selection, and antibodies with many different binding specificities can be isolated. With this process large libraries displaying more than 10^{12} antibodies have been formed.

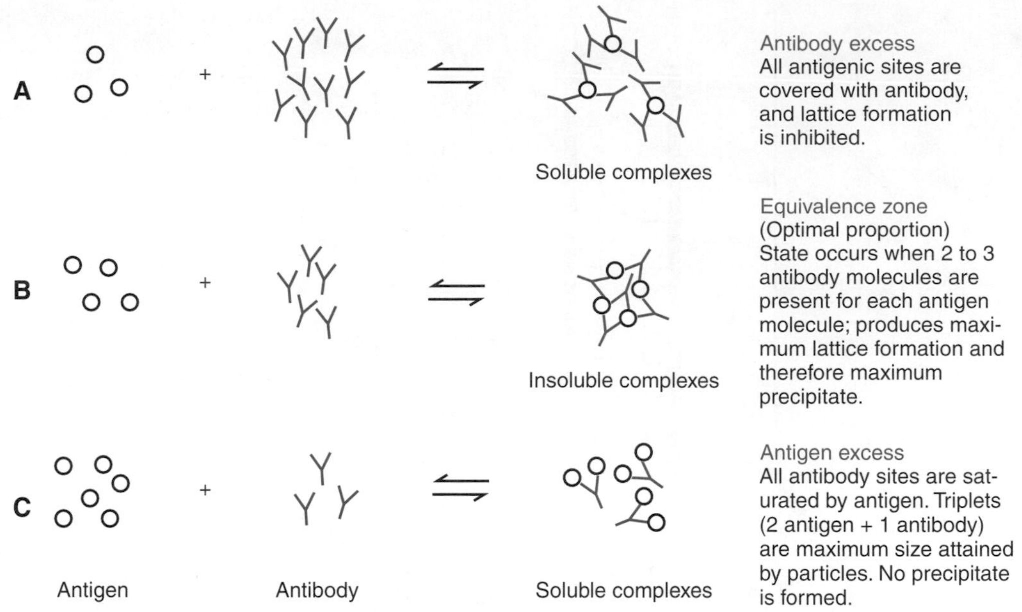

Figure 10-2   Schematic diagram for precipitin reaction. **A,** Antibody excess. **B,** Equivalence zone. **C,** Antigen excess.

ANTIGEN-ANTIBODY BINDING

Reaction Mechanism

Several forces act cooperatively to produce antigen-antibody binding. The three major contributing forces are (1) electrostatic Van der Waals-London dipole-dipole interactions, (2) hydrophobic interactions, and (3) ionic coulombic bonding (primarily between COO^- and NH_4^+ groups on the antigen and antibody).[4]

The binding of antigen to antibody is not static but is an equilibrium reaction that proceeds in three phases. The initial reaction (phase 1) of a multivalent antigen (Ag_n) and a bivalent antibody (Ab) occurs very rapidly in comparison to the subsequent growth of the complexes (phase 2) and is depicted by the following equation:

$$Ag_n + Ab \underset{k_{-1}}{\overset{k_1}{\rightleftharpoons}} Ag_nAb \underset{k_{-2}}{\overset{k_2}{\rightleftharpoons}} Ag_aAb_b \qquad (1)$$

where $k_1 >>> k_2$, n is the number of epitopes per molecule, and a and b are the number of antigen and antibody molecules per complex. Phase 3 of the reaction involves the precipitation of the complex after a critical size is reached. The speed of these reactions depends on electrolyte concentration, pH, and temperature, as well as on antigen and antibody types and the binding affinity of the antibody.

Precipitin Reaction

If the number of antibody combining sites, [Ab], is significantly greater than the antigen binding sites, [Ag], then antigen binding sites quickly are saturated by antibody before cross-linking can occur, and the formation of small antigen antibody complexes of the composition AgAb results (Figure 10-2, *A*). For the case in which antibody is in moderate excess (that is, [Ab]>[Ag]), the probability of cross-linking of Ag by Ab is more likely, and hence large complex formation is favored (Figure 10-2, *B*). In the case in which [Ag] is in great excess, large complexes are less probable, and the theoretical minimum size of complexes is Ag_2Ab (Figure 10-2, *C*).

This model describes the results observed when antigens and antibodies are mixed in various concentration ratios. The curve shown in Figure 10-3 is a schematic diagram of the classic precipitin curve. Although the concentration of total antibody is constant, the concentration of free antibody, $[Ab]_f$, and free antigen, $[Ag]_f$ varies throughout the range for any given Ag/Ab ratio. A low Ag/Ab ratio exists in section A of Figure 10-3 (zone of antibody excess). Under these conditions $[Ab]_f$ exists in solution, but $[Ag]_f$ does not. As total antigen increases, the size of the immune complexes increases up to equivalence (see Figure 10-3, section B,) where little or no $[Ab]_f$ or $[Ag]_f$ exists. This is the zone of equivalence and is the optimal combining ratio for cross-linking in the particular system under examination. As Ag/Ab increases (see Figure 10-3, section C), the immune complex size decreases and $[Ag]_f$ increases (zone of antigen excess).

Factors Influencing Binding

Factors that influence antibody/antigen binding include ionic species, ionic strength, and polymeric molecules.

Ion species and ionic strength effects

Cationic salts produce an inhibition of the binding of antibody with a cationic hapten. The order of inhibition by various cations is $Cs^+ > Rb^+ > NH_4^+ > K^+ > Na^+ > Li^+$. This order corresponds to the decreasing ionic radius and increasing radius of hydration. Similar results were found for

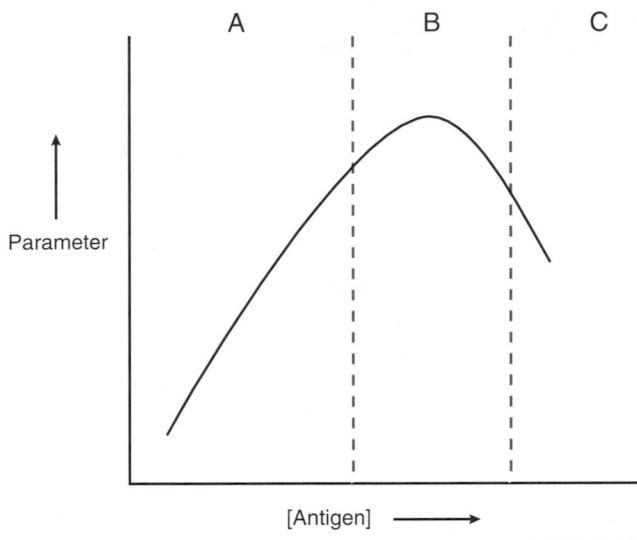

Figure 10-3   Schematic diagram of precipitin curve illustrating different antigen concentration zones. **A**, Antibody excess. **B**, Equivalence. **C**, Antigen excess. The parameter measured may be quantity of protein precipitated, light scattering, or another measurable parameter. Antibody concentration is held constant in this example.

anionic haptens and anionic salts. The order of inhibition of binding is $CNS^- > NO_3^- > I^- > Br^- > Cl^- > F^-$, again in the order of decreasing ionic radius and increasing radius of hydration.

Polymer effect

The addition of a linear polymer to a mixture of antigen and antibody causes a significant increase in the rate of immune complex growth and enhances the precipitation of immune complex, especially with low-avidity antibody. Numerous polymer species such as dextran (a high-molecular-weight polymer of D-glucose), polyvinyl alcohol, polyethylene glycol 6000 (PEG or Carbowax) have been used in immunochemical methods. The most desirable characteristics of the polymer are a high molecular weight, high degree of linearity (minimum branching), and high aqueous solubility. PEG 6000 has these characteristics and is particularly useful in immunochemical methods at concentrations of 3 to 5 g/dL.

■ QUALITATIVE METHODS

Various types of immunochemical techniques have been used for qualitative purposes, including passive gel diffusion, immunoelectrophoresis (IEP), and Western blotting.

Passive Gel Diffusion

Many qualitative and quantitative immunochemical methods are performed in semisolid mediums such as agar or agarose. This practice stabilizes the diffusion process with regard to mixing caused by vibration or convection and allows visualization of precipitin bands for qualitative and quantitative evaluation of the reaction. Antigen-antibody ratio, salt concentration, and polymer enhancement have the same influence on the antigen-antibody reaction in gels as they have on reactions in solution.

If the matrix does not interact with the molecular species under investigation, passive diffusion of reactants in a semisolid matrix can be described by Fick's equation

$$\frac{dQ}{dt} = -DA\frac{dC}{dx} \tag{2}$$

where:

dQ = Amount of diffusing substance that passes through the area A during time
t = Time
dC/dx = Concentration gradient
D = Diffusion coefficient.

The diffusion coefficient, D, is a direct function of temperature; it also is inversely proportional to the hydrated molecular volume of the diffusing species. The ratio dQ/dt is a function of dC/dx, the concentration gradient. The amount of diffusing species transferred from the origin to a distant point (over the migration distance) is dependent on the length of time diffusion is allowed to occur.

The initial concentration of antigen and antibody is critical. Each molecule in the system achieves a unique concentration gradient with time. When the leading fronts of antigen and antibody diffusion overlap, the reaction begins but formation of a precipitin line does not occur until moderate antibody excess is achieved. A precipitin band may form and be dissolved many times by incoming antigen before equilibrium is established and the position of the precipitin band is stabilized.

Two basic approaches to passive diffusion are in use today. One is simple diffusion in which a concentration gradient is established for only a single reactant. This approach is termed *single immunodiffusion* and usually depends on diffusion of an antigen into agar impregnated with antibody. A quantitative technique based on this principle is called *radial immunodiffusion* (RID). (RID will be discussed in more detail in subsequent sections of this chapter.)

The second approach is called *double diffusion*, in which a concentration gradient is established for both antigen and antibody (Figure 10-4). This approach is used widely and known as the *Ouchterlony technique*. In practice, it permits direct comparison of two or more test materials and provides a simple and direct method used to determine whether the antigens in the test specimens are identical, cross-reactive, or nonidentical.

Immunoelectrophoresis

IEP is an immunochemical technique that can be used to separate and identify the various protein species contained in a common solution, such as serum or spinal fluid (see Chapter 7). This technique has been used extensively for the study

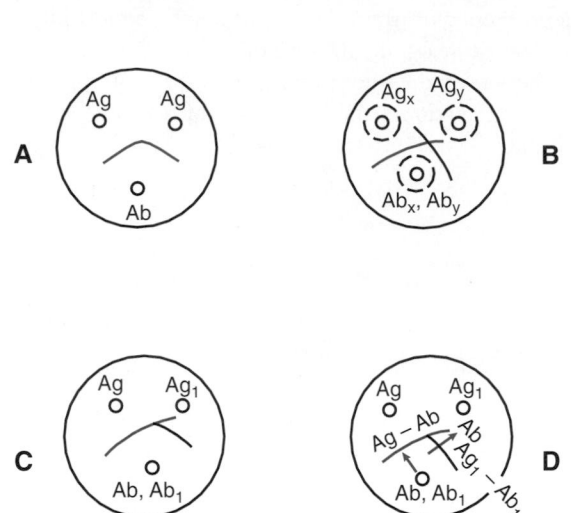

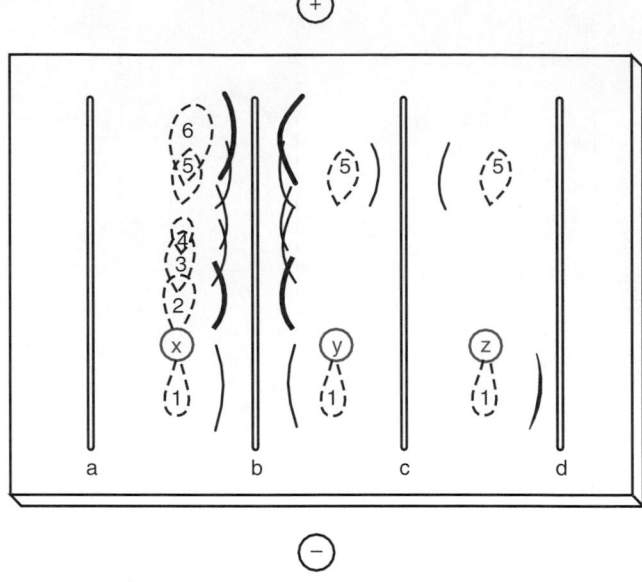

Figure 10-4   Double immunodiffusion in two dimensions by the Ouchterlony technique. **A,** Reaction of identity. **B,** Reaction of nonidentity. **C,** Reaction of partial identity. **D,** Scheme for spur formation. *Ag,* Antigen; *Ab,* antibody.

Figure 10-5   Configuration for immunoelectrophoresis. Sample wells are punched in the agar/agarose, sample is applied, and electrophoresis is carried out to separate the proteins in the sample. Antiserum is loaded into the troughs and the gel incubated in a moist chamber at 4 °C for 24 to 72 hours. Track *x* represents the shape of the protein zones after electrophoresis; tracks *y* and *z* show the reaction of proteins 5 and 1 with their specific antisera in troughs *c* and *d*. Antiserum against proteins 1 through 6 is present in trough *b*.

of antigen mixtures and the evaluation of human gammopathies. Proteins in the serum are separated according to their electrophoretic mobilities (Figure 10-5). After electrophoresis an antiserum against the protein of interest is placed in a trough parallel and adjacent to the electrophoresed sample. Simultaneous diffusion of the antigen from the separated sample and antibody from the trough results in the formation of precipitin arcs with shapes and positions characteristic of the individual separated proteins in the specimen.

In the clinical laboratory this procedure has been applied primarily to the evaluation of human myeloma proteins. However, the method gradually is being replaced by immunofixation electrophoresis, particularly in the study of protein antigens and their split products and the evaluation of myeloma.

Crossed immunoelectrophoresis (CRIE, also known as *two-dimensional immunoelectrophoresis*), is a variation of IEP wherein electrophoresis also is used in the second dimension to drive the antigen into a gel containing antibodies specific for the antigens of interest (Figure 10-6).[8] In practice, CRIE is more sensitive and produces higher resolution than that possible with IEP. An example of a clinical application of CRIE is shown in Figure 10-7.

In counter immunoelectrophoresis (CIE) two parallel lines of wells are punched in the agar. One row is filled with antigen solution, and the opposing row is filled with antibody solution (Figure 10-8). Voltage is applied across the gel to cause the antigen and antibody to move toward each other at a faster rate. A precipitin line is formed where they meet. This qualitative information can be used to identify the antigen and is provided within 1 to 2 hours. CIE has

found application in the detection of bacterial antigens in blood, urine, and cerebrospinal fluid.

Immunofixation (IF) has gained widespread acceptance as an immunochemical method used to identify proteins.[1] With this technique electrophoresis first is performed in agarose gel to separate the proteins in the mixture. Subsequently, antiserum spread directly on the gel causes the protein(s) of interest to precipitate. The immune precipitate is trapped within the gel matrix, and all other nonprecipitated proteins can be removed by washing of the gel. The gel then is stained for identification of the proteins. In practice, however, CRIE is more sensitive than IF in terms of detection limit and also demonstrates improved resolution. In addition, proteins of closely related or identical electrophoretic mobilities can be distinguished better by CRIE because in IF they appear as a single band. The utility of IF, which now is used widely for the evaluation of myeloma proteins, is illustrated in Figure 10-9.

Western Blotting

The previously discussed techniques use a direct examination of the immunoprecipitation of the protein(s) in the gel. However, certain media, such as polyacrylamide, do not lend themselves to direct immunoprecipitation, nor does sufficient antigen concentration always exist to produce an immunoprecipitate that is retained in the gel during subsequent processing. Under these circumstances the technique of

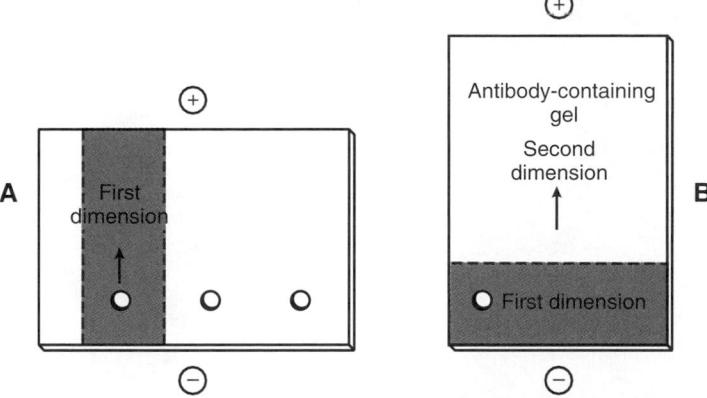

Figure 10-6   Two-dimensional crossed immunoelectrophoresis (CRIE). **A,** Configuration for the first dimension of CRIE. The segment of the gel denoted by the dashed lines is cut out and placed on a second plate. **B,** An upper gel containing antibody is added. Electrophoresis now is carried out at 90 degrees relative to the first dimension run.

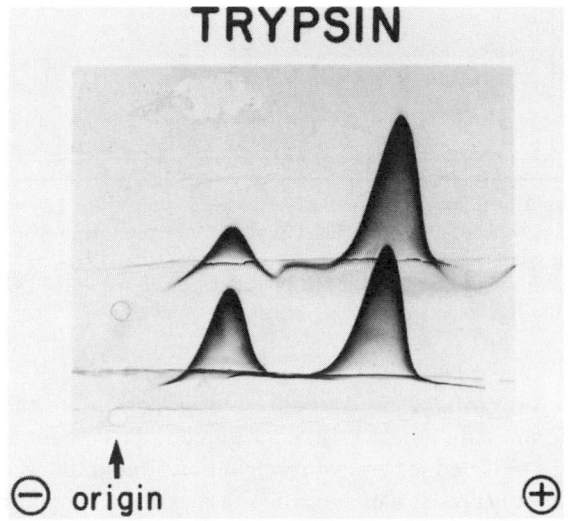

Figure 10-7   Crossed immunoelectrophoresis (CRIE) pattern obtained with two different concentrations of trypsin added to normal serum. The first dimension was carried out from left to right and the second dimension from bottom to top. Two separate gels are shown, with the highest trypsin concentration at the bottom. Antibody against α_1-antitrypsin was present in the second dimension gel. The resulting pattern shows two distinct α_1-antitrypsin species, the free protease inhibitor *(right)* and protease-antiprotease complex *(left)*. This example illustrates the ability of CRIE to evaluate changes in specific protein structure.

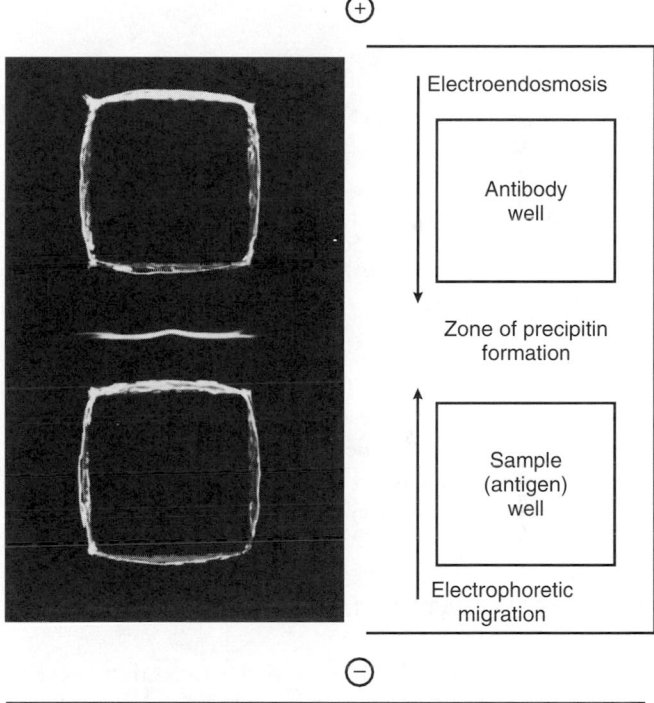

Figure 10-8   Counter immunoelectrophoresis showing positive reaction between anti-*Haemophilus influenzae B (upper well)* and a CSF sample containing *H. influenzae B (lower well).*

Western blotting can be used. This technique involves an electrophoresis step, followed by transfer of the separated proteins onto an overlying strip of nitrocellulose or a nylon membrane by a process called *electroblotting*. Once the proteins are fixed to the membrane, they can be detected with antibody probes labeled with either radioactive isotopes or enzymes. By using such probes, the limits of detection can be 10 to 100 times lower than those values obtained through direct immunoprecipitation and staining of proteins. This technique is analogous to Southern blotting (electrophoresed DNA blotted onto a membrane) and Northern blotting (electrophoresed RNA blotted onto a membrane).

An example of a Western blotting analysis for human immunodeficiency virus type 1 (HIV-1) antibodies is shown in Figure 10-10. When applied to antigen assays, concentrations of antigen as low as 500 ng/mL or 2.5 ng per band in the gel can be detected. The detection limit of the technique can be lowered even further to approximately 100 pg by chemiluminescent detection of the enzyme-labeled antibody and by detection of the light emission through the use of x-ray or photographic film.[7]

A simpler technique that bypasses the electrophoretic separation step is known as *dot blotting*. A protein sample to be analyzed is applied to a membrane surface as a small "dot" and dried. The membrane then is exposed to a labeled

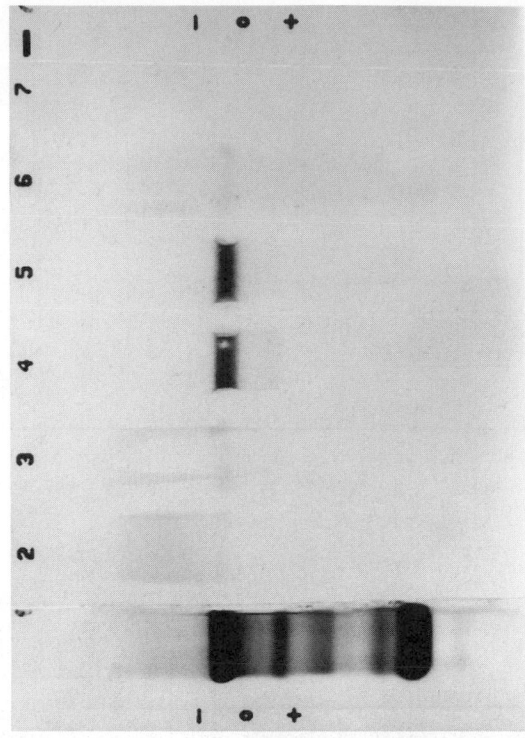

Figure 10-9   Immunofixation of a serum containing an IgM kappa paraprotein. Lane *1,* serum electrophoresis stained for protein; lane *2,* anti-IgG, Fc piece-specific; lane *3,* anti-IgA, α–chain-specific; lane *4,* anti-IgM, α–chain-specific; lane *5,* anti-κ light chain; lane *6,* anti-λ light chain. (Courtesy Katherine Bayer, Philadelphia.)

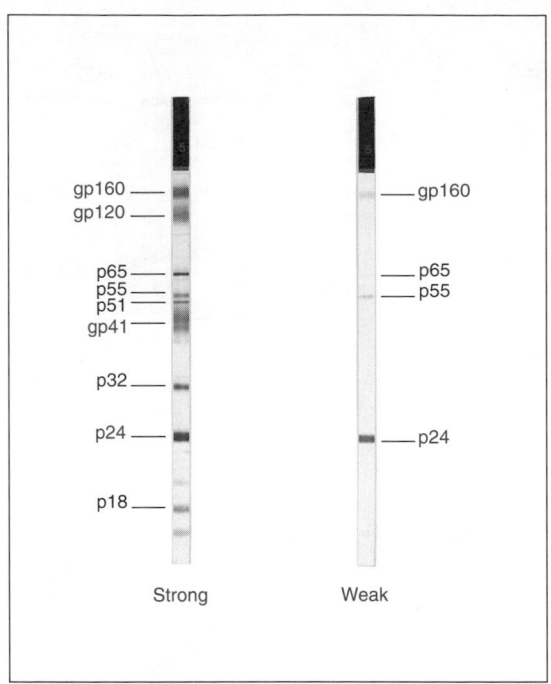

Figure 10-10   Western blot analysis of serum samples strongly positive and weakly positive for HIV-1 antibody. Core proteins (GAG, group-specific antigens) p18, p24, and p55; polymerase (POL) p32, p51, and p65; and envelope proteins (ENV) gp41, gp120, and gp160. (Courtesy Bio-Rad Laboratories Diagnostics Group, Hercules, Calif.)

antibody specific for the test antigen contained in the dotted protein mixture. After the membrane is washed, bound-labeled antibody is detected with a photometric or chemiluminescent detection system.

■ QUANTITATIVE METHODS

Immunochemical techniques have been used to develop quantitative methods that include radial diffusion and electroimmunoassays, turbidimetric and nephelometric assays, and labeled immunochemical assays. Many of these assays now have been automated.

Radial Immunodiffusion and Electroimmunoassay

RID and electroimmunoassay (known as the "rocket" technique) are two commonly used gel-based methods for quantitative immunochemical measurements.

Radial immunodiffusion immunoassay

RID is a passive diffusion method in which a concentration gradient is established for a single reactant, usually the antigen.[10] The antibody is dispersed uniformly in the gel ma-

trix. Antigen is allowed to diffuse from a well into the gel until antibody excess exists and immune precipitation occurs; a well-defined ring of precipitation around the well indicates the presence of antigen. The ring diameter continues to increase until equilibrium is reached. Calibrators are run simultaneous with the sample, and a calibration curve of ring area or diameter versus concentration is generated.

Electroimmunoassay

In electroimmunoassay a single concentration gradient is established for the antigen, and an applied voltage is used to drive the antigen from the application well into a homogeneous suspension of antibody in the gel (Figure 10-11).[9] This process produces a unidirectional migration of antigen and results in a decreased limit of detection. The height of the resulting rocket-shaped precipitin line is proportional to the antigen concentration. Quantification is achieved through the use of calibrators on the same plate along with the unknowns and subsequent estimation of the concentrations of unknowns from the heights of the rockets obtained. The calibration curve is linear only over a narrow concentration range, and consequently, samples may have to be diluted or concentrated as necessary.

In many clinical laboratories gel-based methods are restricted to qualitative studies or used as reference methods.

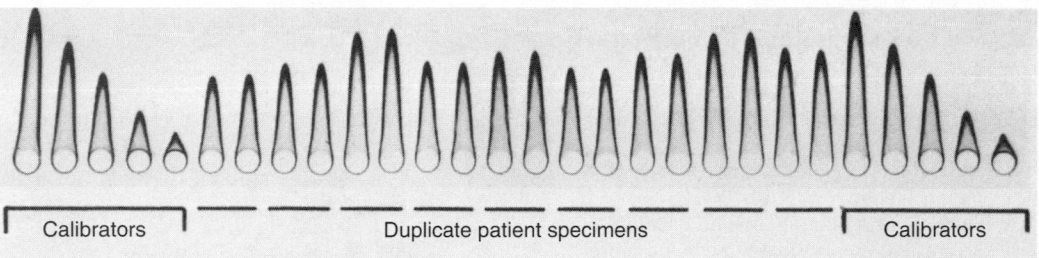

Calibrators   Duplicate patient specimens   Calibrators

Figure 10-11   Rocket immunoelectrophoresis of human serum albumin. Patient samples were applied in duplicate. Calibrators were placed at opposite ends of the plate.

Quantitative data are obtained more commonly by turbidimetric and nephelometric methods, radioimmunoassays, enzyme immunoassays, and fluorometric immunoassays.

Turbidimetric and Nephelometric Assays

Turbidimetry and nephelometry are convenient techniques used to measure the rate of formation of immune complexes in vitro. Instrumental principles for these methods are described in Chapter 4. Studies have shown that the reaction between antigen and antibody begins within milliseconds and continues for hours. The performance of both types of assays can be improved significantly through increases in the reaction rate by the addition of water-soluble linear polymers.

Both turbidimetric and nephelometric immunochemical methods using rate and pseudoequilibrium protocols have been described for proteins, antigens, and haptens. In rate assays measurements usually are made within the first few minutes of the reaction because the largest change (dI_s/dt) in intensity of scattered light (I_s) with respect to time is obtained during this time interval. For pseudoequilibrium assays, waiting 30 to 60 minutes is necessary so that the dI_s/dt is small, relative to the time required to make the necessary measurements. (NOTE: Such assays are termed *pseudoequilibrium* rather than *equilibrium* because true equilibrium is not reached within the time allowed for these assays.)

Nephelometric methods in general are more sensitive than turbidimetric assays and have an average lower limit of detection of approximately 1 to 10 mg/L for a serum protein. Lower limits of detection are obtained in fluids such as cerebrospinal fluid and urine because of their lower lipid and protein concentrations, which result in a better signal-to-noise ratio. In addition, for low-molecular-weight proteins such as myoglobin (MW 17,800), limits of detection can be lowered through the use of a latex-enhanced procedure based on antibody-coated latex beads.

Nephelometric and turbidimetric assays also have been applied to the measurement of drugs (haptens) with the use of inhibition techniques. To make the reagent, the drug of interest is attached to a carrier molecule, such as bovine serum albumin. The hapten-bound albumin then competes with free hapten (drug introduced in sample) for antihapten-

antibody. In the presence of free hapten, immune complex formation is decreased because more antibody sites are saturated; thus light scattering is decreased. The decrease in light scattering is related to the concentration of free hapten. Both kinetic and pseudoequilibrium methods have been described. In the absence of free hapten, bound hapten-albumin reacts with available antihapten-antibody sites to form cross-linked immune complexes with high light-scattering abilities.

Labeled Immunochemical Assays

The previously discussed methods rely on the examination of the immune complex formation as an index of antigen-antibody reaction. As demonstrated previously in equation (1), the overall reaction occurs in sequential phases, and only the final phase is the formation of the immune complex. However, the initial binding of the antibody and antigen also has been very useful analytically and thus used with antigens and antibodies that have **labels** to develop many sensitive and specific immunochemical assays. The reaction describing this initial binding and the kinetic constant for the overall reaction are shown in equations (3a) and (3b), respectively.

$$Ab + Ag \underset{k_{-1}}{\overset{k_1}{\rightleftharpoons}} AbAg \qquad (3a)$$

$$K = \frac{[AbAg]}{[Ab][Ag]} \qquad (3b)$$

where:

k_1 = Rate constant for the forward reaction
k_{-1} = Rate constant for the reverse reaction
K = Equilibrium constant for the overall reaction

As predicted from the law of mass action, the concentrations of Ab, Ag, and Ab:Ag are dependent on the magnitude of k_1 and k_{-1}. For polyclonal antiserum the average avidity of the antibody populations determines K, and the magnitude of k_1 in comparison to k_{-1} determines the ultimate limit of detection attainable with a given antibody population.

Types of labels

In the decade following the pioneering developments of Yalow and Berson,[17] all immunoassays used radioactive la-

TABLE 10-1	Labels for Nonisotopic Immunoassays
Label	**Example**
Chemiluminescent	Acridinium ester, acridinium sulfonamide, isoluminol
Cofactor	Adenosine triphosphate, flavin adenine dinucleotide
Enzyme	Alkaline phosphatase, marine bacterial luciferase, β-galactosidase, firefly luciferase, glucose oxidase, glucose-6-phosphate dehydrogenase, horseradish peroxidase, lysozyme, malate dehydrogenase, microperoxidase, urease, xanthine oxidase
Fluorophore	Europium chelate, fluorescein, phycoerythrin, terbium chelate
Free radical	Nitroxide
Inhibitor	Methotrexate
Metal	Gold sol, selenium sol, silver sol
Particle	Bacteriophage, erythrocyte, latex bead, liposome
Polynucleotide	DNA
Substrate	Galactosyl-umbelliferone

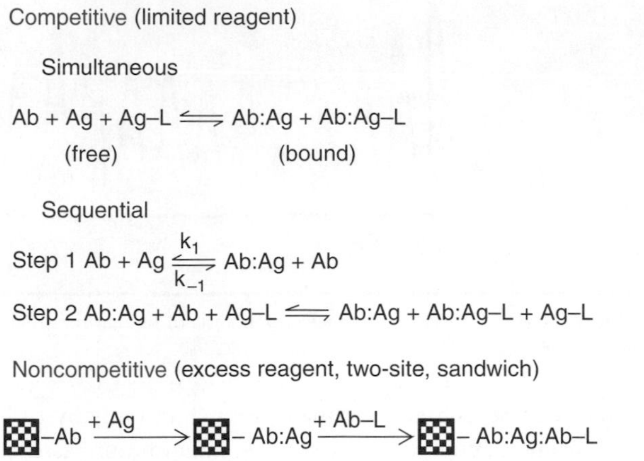

bels in competitive assays. Since the introduction of enzyme immunoassays in the 1970s, sophisticated assays with nonisotopic labels (Table 10-1)[6,13] have been developed.

Methodological principles

To capitalize on the exquisite specificity and enhanced sensitivity of immunochemical assays, various methodological principles have been applied in their development. These include competitive and noncompetitive reaction formats and different processing schemes to perform assays.

Competitive versus noncompetitive reaction formats

As shown in Figure 10-12, the two major types of reaction formats used in immunochemical assays are termed *competitive* (limited reagent assays) and *noncompetitive* (excess reagent, two-site, or sandwich assays).

Competitive immunoassays. In a competitive immunochemical assay all reactants are mixed together either simultaneously or sequentially. In the simultaneous approach the labeled antigen (Ag*) and unlabeled antigen (Ag) compete to bind with the antibody. In such a system the avidity of the antibody for both the labeled and the unlabeled antigen must be the same. Under these conditions the probability of the antibody binding the labeled antigen is inversely proportional to the concentration of unlabeled antigen; hence bound label is inversely proportional to unlabeled antigen concentration.

In a sequential competitive assay, unlabeled antigen first is mixed with excess antibody, and binding is allowed to reach equilibrium (see Figure10-12, step 1). Labeled antigen then is added sequentially (see Figure 10-12, step 2) and allowed to equilibrate. After separation the bound label is de-

Competitive (limited reagent)

Simultaneous

$$Ab + Ag + Ag–L \rightleftharpoons Ab{:}Ag + Ab{:}Ag–L$$

(free)   (bound)

Sequential

Step 1 $Ab + Ag \underset{k_{-1}}{\overset{k_1}{\rightleftharpoons}} Ab{:}Ag + Ab$

Step 2 $Ab{:}Ag + Ab + Ag–L \rightleftharpoons Ab{:}Ag + Ab{:}Ag–L + Ag–L$

Noncompetitive (excess reagent, two-site, sandwich)

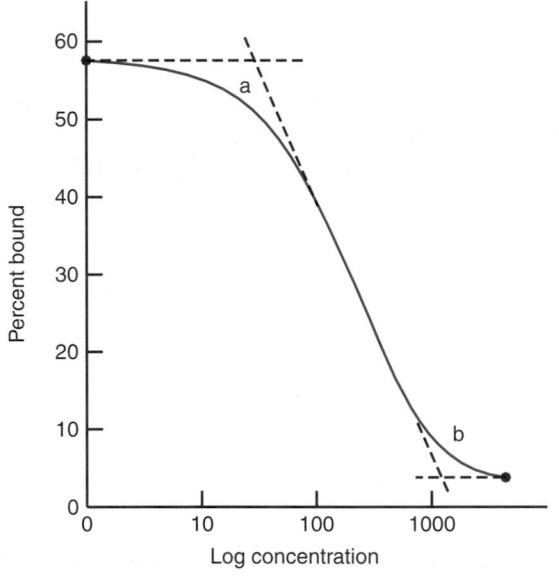

Figure 10-12   Immunoassay designs. *Ab,* Antibody; *Ag,* antigen; *L,* label, k_1, forward rate constant; k_{-1}, reverse rate constant.

Figure 10-13   Schematic diagram of the dose-response curve for a typical immunoassay. The analytically useful portion of the curve is bracketed by points *a* and *b.*

termined and used to calculate the unlabeled antigen concentration. Using this two-step method, a larger fraction of the unlabeled antigen can be bound by the antibody than that fraction in the simultaneous assay, especially at low antigen concentrations. Consequently, this strategy can provide a twofold to fourfold lowering of the detection limit of a sequential immunoassay, compared with that of a simultaneous assay, provided $k_1 \gg k_{-1}$. This improvement in detection limit results from an increase in AgAb binding (and thus in a decrease in Ag* binding), which is favored by the sequential addition of Ag and Ag*. If $k_1 \geq k_{-1}$, dissociation of AgAb becomes more probable, resulting in an increased competition between Ag* and Ag. A typical immunochemical binding curve is shown in Figure 10-13.

Noncompetitive immunoassays. In a typical noncompetitive assay, an antibody, called the "capture" antibody, first is passively adsorbed or covalently bound to the surface of a solid phase. In the second stage of the assay the antigen from the sample is allowed to react and is captured by the solid-phase antibody. Other proteins then are washed away, and a labeled antibody (conjugate) is added that reacts with the bound antigen through a second and distinct epitope. After additional washing to remove the excess unbound labeled antibody, the bound label is determined, and its concentration or activity is directly proportional to the concentration of antigen.

In noncompetitive assays the capture and labeled antibody can be either polyclonal or monoclonal. If monoclonal antibodies with specificity for distinct epitopes are used, simultaneous incubation of the sample and conjugate with the capture antibody are possible, thus simplifying the assay protocol.

Noncompetitive immunoassays can be performed in either simultaneous or sequential modes. However, in the simultaneous mode a situation can occur in which a high concentration of analyte can saturate both the capture and labeled antibodies. When this situation occurs, the calibration curve of the assay exhibits a "hook-effect," in which the assay response drops off at high analyte concentrations. Under these conditions the analyte is present in such high concentrations that it reacts simultaneously with the capture and labeled antibodies, reducing the number of complexes formed and producing a falsely low result. Assays for analytes for which the normal pathological concentration range is very wide (for example, CG, AFP) are particularly prone to this problem. Dilutions of a sample usually are reanalyzed to check for this type of analytical interference. The hook effect can be eliminated if a sequential assay format is adopted and the concentrations of capture and labeled antibody are sufficiently high to cover analyte concentrations over the entire analytical range of the assay.

Heterogeneous versus homogeneous immunochemical assays

Immunochemical assays that require a separation of the free from the bound label are termed *heterogeneous;* those that do not are called *homogeneous.*

Heterogeneous assays. Heterogeneous assays implicitly assume that $k_1 >> k_{-1}$. A variety of physical separation techniques (Table 10-2) are used to separate the free, labeled (Ag^*) from the bound, labeled antigen ($Ag^*{:}Ab$).

Precipitation of the bound, labeled antigen ($Ag^*{:}Ab$) from the reaction mixture can be achieved chemically by the addition of a protein-precipitating chemical, such as $(NH_4)_2SO_4$, or immunologically by the addition of a second, "precipitating" antibody. In liquid-phase adsorption the free antigen is adsorbed onto particles of activated charcoal or dextran-coated charcoal that are added directly to the reaction mixture. The particles of charcoal and the

TABLE 10-2 Separation Methods for Immunoassays
Adsorption
Charcoal, Florisil, talc
Precipitation
Polymer precipitation: polyethylene glycol
Solvent or salt precipitation: ethanol, dioxane, $(NH_4)_2SO_4$
Protein A or double (second) antibody precipitation
Solid-Phase Antibodies
Antibodies or other binding proteins (for example, protein A, biotin-avidin, and biotin streptavidin) adsorbed or covalently attached to an insoluble matrix (for example, plastic beads, inside surface of a plastic tube or microwell, and magnetic beads)
Miscellaneous
Electrophoresis
Gel filtration
Ion exchange
Radial partition

adsorbed antigen then are removed via particle settling or centrifugation.

Solid-phase adsorption is a widely used separation technique. With this method the binding and competition of the labeled and unlabeled antigens for the binding sites of the antibody occur on the surface of a solid support, onto which the capture antibody is attached either by physical adsorption or covalent bonding. Several different types of solid support are used, including the inner surface of plastic tubes or wells of microtiter plates and the outer surface of insoluble materials, such as cellulose or magnetic latex beads or particles.

Homogeneous assays. Homogeneous assays do not require a separation of the bound and free labeled antibody or antigen. In this type of assay the activity of the label attached to the antigen is modulated directly by antibody binding, with the magnitude of the modulation proportional to the concentration of the antigen or antibody being measured. Consequently, it is only necessary to incubate the sample containing the analyte antigen with the labeled antigen and antibody and then directly measure the activity of the label "in place," making these assays technically easier and faster. (See the descriptions of enzyme-multiplied, cloned enzyme donor, and fluorescence polarization immunoassays in subsequent sections of this chapter.)

Analytical detection limits

The analytical detection limits of competitive immunoassays are determined principally by the affinity of the antibody. Calculations have indicated that a lower limit of detection of 10 fmol/L (that is, 600,000 molecules of analyte in a typical sample volume of 100 μL) is possible in a competitive assay using an antibody with an affinity of 10^{12} L/mol.

TABLE 10-3	Detection Limits for Isotopic and Nonisotopic Immunoassay Labels	
Label	Detection Limit in Zeptomoles* $(10^{-21}$ mols)	Method
Alkaline phosphatase	50,000	Photometry
	300	Time-resolved fluorescence
	100	Fluorescence
	10	Enzyme cascade
	1	Chemiluminescence
β-D-galactosidase	5000	Chemiluminescence
	1000	Fluorescence
Europium chelate	10,000	Time-resolved fluorescence
Glucose-6-phosphate dehydrogenase	1000	Chemiluminescence
^{3}H	1,000,000	Scintillation
Horseradish peroxidase	2,000,000	Photometry
	25,000	Chemiluminescence
^{125}I	1000	Scintillation
Ruthenium (II) tris(bipyridyl)	20†	Electrochemiluminescence

*One zeptomole = 1000 attomoles, or 1,000,000 femtomoles.
†Obtained through personal communication.

For noncompetitive immunoassays the detector's ability to measure the label is the key factor that affects the detection limit of an assay.[3] Table 10-3 illustrates the detection limits for noncompetitive immunoassays using isotopic and nonisotopic labels. A radioactive label, such as ^{125}I, has low specific activity (7.5 million labels necessary for detection of 1 disintegration/second), compared with enzyme labels and chemiluminescent and fluorescent labels. Enzyme labels provide an amplification (each enzyme label producing many detectable product molecules), and the detection limit for an enzyme can be improved if the conventional photometric detection is replaced with chemiluminescent or bioluminescent detection. The combination of amplification and an ultrasensitive detection reaction makes noncompetitive chemiluminescent enzyme immunoassays among the most sensitive types of immunoassay. Fluorescent labels also have high specific activity; a single high–quantum-yield fluorophore can produce 100 million photon/second. In practice, several factors degrade the detection limit of an immunoassay; these include background signal from the detector, assay reagents, and nonspecific binding of the labeled reagent.

Secondary labels such as biotin also are used to introduce amplification into an immunoassay. The binding constant of the biotin-avidin complex is extremely high (10^{15} L/mol); capitalizing on this system allows for the creation of immunoassay systems that are even more sensitive than the simple antibody systems. A biotin-avidin system uses a biotin-labeled first antibody. Biotin can be attached to the antibody in relatively high proportion without loss of immunoreactivity by the antibody. When an avidin-conjugated label is added, a complex of Ag:Ab-biotin:avidin-label is formed. Further amplification can be achieved by a biotin:avidin:biotin linkage because the binding ratio of biotin:avidin is 4:1 (for example, Ag:Ab-biotin:avidin:[3 biotin labels]). If the label is an enzyme, large numbers of enzyme molecules in the complete complex provide a large increase in enzymatic activity, coupled with the small amount of antigen being determined, and the antigen assay is correspondingly more sensitive. Other strategies to lower the analytical detection limits of immunoassays include the use of streptavidin-thyroglobulin conjugates and macromolecular complexes of multiple-labeled thyroglobulin and streptavidin-thyroglobulin. In these reagents the thyroglobulin acts as a carrier for multiple labels (for example, Eu^{3+}), and amplification factors of several thousand are achieved.

Examples of labeled immunoassays

Specific examples of different types of labeled immunoassay are discussed in the following section. Others are described in Table 10-4.

Radioimmunoassay

Radioimmunoassay (RIA) is a sensitive and specific type of heterogeneous immunoassay that uses radiolabeled antigens or antibodies. Analytically, competition between radiolabeled and unlabeled antigen or antibody in an antigen-antibody reaction is used to determine the concentration of the unlabeled antigen or antibody. It takes advantage of the specificity of the antigen-antibody interaction and the sensitivity that derives from measurement of radioactively labeled materials. RIA can be used to determine the concentration of antibodies or any antigen against which a specific antibody can be produced. When used to measure the concentration of an antigen, RIA requires that the antigen is available in a pure form and can be labeled with a radioactive isotope. An alternative assay design uses labeled antibody (for example, immunoradiometric assay [IRMA]) and does not require purified antigen because the antigen need not be labeled. This also obviates potential problems that may be caused by iodination of labile antigens. Antibodies are more stable proteins and are easier to label without damage to the protein's function.

Nonseparation RIAs also have been developed based on the modulation of a tritium or a ^{125}I label by microparticles loaded with a scintillant.[12] These scintillation proximity assays have found routine application in high-throughput screening assays used for drug discovery.

RIAs were developed in the 1960s and used radioactive isotopes of iodine ^{125}I, ^{131}I and tritium (^{3}H) as labels.[17] Combinations of labels (for example, ^{57}Co and ^{125}I) also have been used for simultaneous assays (for example, vitamin B_{12} and folate). Although once popular, the use of RIAs in clinical laboratories has declined because of the (1) instability of the label and the radiolabeled antigens and antibodies, (2) concerns over the safe handling and disposal of

TABLE 10-4	Examples of Other Nonisotopic Immunoassays

Bioluminescent Immunoassays

Native or recombinant apoaequorin (from the bioluminescent jellyfish *Aequorea*) is used as the label. It is activated by reaction with coelenterazine, and light emission at 469 nm is triggered by reaction with calcium ions (calcium chloride).

Electrochemical-Differential Polarographic Immunoassay

Electroactive antigen is displaced from the antibody by the addition of unlabeled antigen. The unlabeled antigen concentration is proportional to the differential pulse measured at a dropping mercury electrode.

Enzyme Channeling Immunoassay

In this homogeneous assay a macromolecular antigen binds to two different antibodies labeled with different enzymes. The enzymes catalyze consecutive reactions; these reactions are more efficient when the enzymes are in close proximity in the immune complex.

Fluorescence Excitation Transfer Immunoassay

In this homogeneous competitive assay a fluorophore- (donor-) labeled antigen competes with antigen in the sample for binding sites on an antibody labeled with a fluorescent dye (acceptor). The fluorescence of the donor is quenched when it is bound to the acceptor-labeled antibody.

Immuno-PCR

In this heterogenous immunoassay a piece of single- or double-stranded DNA is used as a label for an antibody in a sandwich assay. Bound DNA label is amplified through use of the polymerase chain reaction (PCR). The amplified DNA product is separated by gel electrophoresis and quantitated by densitometric scanning of an ethidium-stained gel.

Luminescent Oxygen Channeling Immunoassay (LOCI)

In this homogeneous sandwich immunoassay an antigen links an antibody-coated sensitizer dye-loaded particle (250 nm in diameter) and an antibody-coated particle (250 nm in diameter) loaded with a mixture of a precursor of chemiluminescent compound and a fluorophore. Irradiation produces singlet oxygen at the surface of the sensitizer dye-loaded particle. This oxygen diffuses ("channels") to the other particle, held in close proximity by the immunochemical reaction between the antigen and antibodies on the particles. The singlet oxygen reacts with the chemiluminescent compound precursor in the particle to form a chemiluminescent dioxane, which then decomposes to emit light via a fluorophore-sensitized mechanism. No signal is obtained from precursor-fluorophore-loaded particles that are not linked via immunological reaction with an antigen.

Prosthetic-Group Immunoassay

In this competitive assay an enzyme cofactor is attached to hapten. Antihapten antibody blocks enzyme activity by restricting cofactor availability. Addition of free hapten results in an increase in both free cofactor and enzyme activity.

Solid-Phase Light-Scattering Immunoassay

Indium spheres are coated on glass to measure antibody binding to antigen. Binding of antibody to antigen increases dielectric layer thickness, which produces a greater degree of scatter than in areas where only antigen is bound. Quantitation is achieved by densitometry.

Solid-Phase Optical Diffraction Immunoassay

Periodic areas of antibody that are immobilized on a silicon surface react with antigen to form a grating that diffracts incident laser light. No grating is formed with a negative specimen, and hence no diffraction occurs.

Substrate-Labeled Fluorescent Immunoassay

In this competitive assay a free drug blocks binding of antibody to substrate drug complex, thus permitting enzymatic action that produces a fluorescent product.

Surface Effect Immunoassay

Antibody is immobilized on the surface of a waveguide (a quartz, glass, or plastic slide or a gold- or silver-coated prism), and binding of antigen is measured directly by total internal reflection fluorescence, surface plasmon resonance, or attenuated total reflection.

---

radioactive reagents and waste, and (3) lack of automated instrumentation.

Enzyme immunoassay

Enzyme immunoassay (EIA) utilizes the catalytic properties of enzymes to detect and quantify immunological reactions.[11,13] Alkaline phosphatase, horseradish peroxidase, glucose-6-dehydrogenase, and β-galactosidase are the enzymes most commonly used as labels in EIA.

Various detection systems have been used to monitor EIAs. Assays that produce compounds that can be monitored photometrically are very popular, because compact, high-performance photometers are now available that are versatile, reliable, simple to operate, and relatively inexpensive. However, EIAs that utilize fluorogenic or chemiluminogenic substrates are gaining popularity due to their inherent sensitivities. Enzyme cascade reactions also have been applied to the detection of enzyme labels in EIA; the principle of a cascade assay for alkaline phosphatase is illustrated in Figure 10-14. The advantage of such an assay is that it combines the amplification properties of two enzymes—the alkaline phosphatase label and the alcohol dehydrogenase in the assay reagent—producing an extremely sensitive assay (see Table 10-3).

Examples of EIA include **enzyme-linked immunoabsorbent assay (ELISA), enzyme-multiplied immunoassay technique (EMIT),** and cloned enzyme donor immunoassay (CEDIA).

Enzyme-linked immunosorbent assay. ELISA is a heterogeneous EIA technique that is used widely in clinical analyses. In this type of assay one of the reaction components is attached to the surface of a solid phase, such as that of a microtiter well. This attachment can be nonspecific adsorption or chemical or immunochemical bonding and facilitates separation of bound and free labeled reactants. Typically, during the use of the ELISA technique an aliquot of sample or

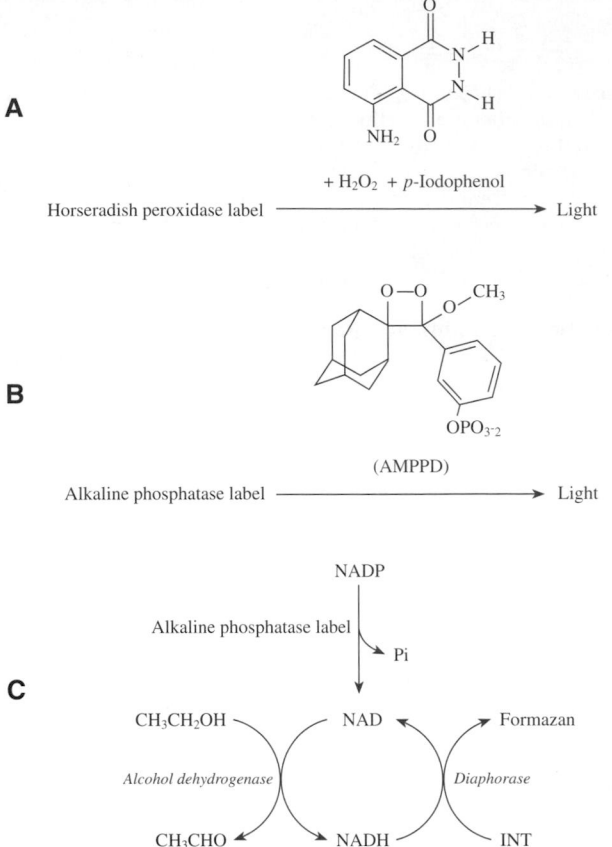

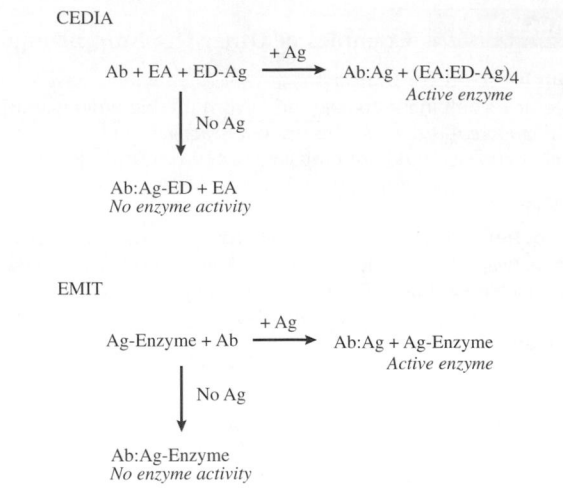

CEDIA

$$Ab + EA + ED\text{-}Ag \xrightarrow{+\ Ag} Ab\text{:}Ag + (EA\text{:}ED\text{-}Ag)_4$$

Active enzyme

No Ag

Ab:Ag-ED + EA
No enzyme activity

EMIT

$$Ag\text{-}Enzyme + Ab \xrightarrow{+\ Ag} Ab\text{:}Ag + Ag\text{-}Enzyme$$

Active enzyme

No Ag

Ab:Ag-Enzyme
No enzyme activity

Figure 10-15   Cloned enzyme donor immunoassay and enzyme-multiplied immunoassay technique homogeneous immunoassays. *EA,* enzyme acceptor; *ED,* enzyme donor; *SP,* scintillant-filled microparticle; *Ab,* antibody; *Ag,* antigen.

Figure 10-14   Ultrasensitive assays for horseradish peroxidase and alkaline phosphatase labels. **A,** Chemiluminescent assay for horseradish peroxidase label using luminol. **B,** Chemiluminescent assay for an alkaline phosphatase label using AMPPD (disodium 3-(4-methoxyspiro[1,2-dioxetane-3,2′-tricyclo[3.3.1.1]-decan]4-yl)phenyl phosphate). **C,** Photometric assay for an alkaline phosphatase label using a cascade detection reaction. *INT, p*-Iodonitrotetrazolium violet.

Enzyme-multiplied immunoassay technique.   EMIT is a homogeneous EIA (Figure 10-15). Because it does not require a separation step, an EMIT assay is simple to perform and has been used to develop a wide variety of drug, hormone, and metabolite assays.[14] EMIT-type assays are automated easily and included in the repertoire of most automated clinical and immunoassay analyzers (see Chapter 12).

In the EMIT technique, antibody against the analyte drug, hormone, or metabolite is added together with substrate to the patient's sample. Binding of the antibody and analyte then occurs. An aliquot of the enzyme conjugate of the analyte drug, hormone, or metabolite then is added as a second reagent; the enzyme-analyte conjugate then binds with the excess analyte antibody, forming an antigen-antibody complex. This binding of the analyte antibody with the enzyme-analyte conjugate affects the enzyme and alters its activity. The relative change in enzyme activity is proportional to the drug, hormone, or metabolite concentration in the patient's sample. Concentration of the analyte is calculated from a calibration curve prepared by analysis of calibrators that contain known quantities of analyte.

Cloned enzyme donor immunoassay.   CEDIA is a second type of homogeneous EIA (see Figure 10-15). It was the first EIA designed and developed through the use of genetic engineering techniques.[11,13] With this technique, inactive fragments (the enzyme donor and acceptor) of β-galactosidase are prepared by manipulation of the Z gene of the *lac* operon of *Escherichia coli*. These two fragments spontaneously reassemble to form active enzyme even if the enzyme donor is attached to an antigen. However, binding of antibody to the enzyme donor-antigen conjugate inhibits reassembly, and no active enzyme is formed. Thus competition between antigen and the enzyme donor-antigen conjugate for a fixed amount of antibody in the presence of the enzyme acceptor modulates the measured enzyme activity.

calibrator containing the antigen to be quantified is added to and allowed to bind with a solid-phase antibody. After the solid phase has been washed, an enzyme-labeled antibody different from the bound antibody is added and forms a "sandwich complex" of solid-phase-Ab:Ag:Ab-enzyme. Excess (unbound) antibody then is washed away, and enzyme substrate is added. The enzyme label then catalyzes the conversion of substrate to product(s), the amount of which is proportional to the quantity of antigen in the sample. Antibodies in a sample also can be quantified through the use of an ELISA procedure in which antigen instead of antibody is bound to a solid phase and the second reagent is an enzyme-labeled antibody specific for the analyte antibody. For example, in a microtiter plate format, ELISA assays have been used extensively for detection of antibodies to viruses and parasites in serum or whole blood. In addition, enzyme conjugates coupled with substrates that produce visible products have been used to develop ELISA-type assays with results that can be interpreted visually. Such assays have been very useful in screening, point-of-care, and home testing applications.

TABLE 10-5 Properties of Fluorescent Labels

Fluorophore	Excitation (nm)	Emission (nm)	Fluorescence Quantum Yield*	Lifetime (ns)
Fluorescein isothiocyanate	492	520	0.85	4.5
Europium (β-naphthoyl trifluoroacetone)	340	590, 613	—	500,000
Lucifer Yellow VS	430	540	—	—
Phycobiliprotein	550 to 620	580 to 660	0.5 to 0.98	—
Rhodamine B isothiocyanate	550	585	up to 0.7	3.0
Umbelliferone	380	450	—	—

*Fluorescence quantum yield refers to the fraction of molecules that emit a photon.

High concentrations of antigen produce the least inhibition of enzyme activity; low concentrations, the greatest.

Fluoroimmunoassay

Fluoroimmunoassay (FIA) utilizes a fluorescent molecule as an indicator label to detect and quantify immunological reactions. Examples of fluorophores used as labels in FIA and their properties are listed in Table 10-5. In the past, background fluorescence from drugs, drug metabolites, and protein-bound substances such as bilirubin limited the utility of this technique. However, this problem largely has been overcome by the use of time-resolved immunoassay techniques that use chelates of rare earth (lanthanide) elements as labels (see Chapter 4). These techniques are based on the fact that the fluorescent emissions from lanthanide chelates (for example, europium, terbium, and samarium) have long lives (>1 μs), compared with the typical background fluorescence encountered in biological specimens. In a time-resolved FIA a europium chelate label is excited by a pulse of excitation light (0.5 μs), and the long-lived fluorescence emission from the label is measured after a delay (400 to 800 μs); by this time any short-lived background signal has decayed.

Fluorescent polarization immunoassay is a type of homogeneous FIA that is used widely (Figure 10-16). With this technique the polarization of the fluorescence from a fluorescein-antigen conjugate is determined by its rate of rotation during the lifetime of the excited state in solution. A small, rapidly rotating fluorescein-antigen conjugate has a low degree of polarization; however, binding to a large antibody molecule slows the rate of rotation and increases the degree of polarization. Thus binding to antibody modulates polarization. The change in polarization then can be measured and related to antigen concentration.[11,13]

Another type of nonseparation FIA uses a multilayer device to eliminate the need for separation of bound and free fractions. The device consists of two agarose layers separated by an opaque layer of iron oxide. Sample is added to the upper (10-μm) layer and diffuses through the iron oxide (10-μm) layer to the thin (1-μm) signal layer that contains antibody:antigen-rhodamine complexes. Antigen-rhodamine conjugate is displaced from the signal layer by antigen in the sample and diffuses into the upper layer. Re-

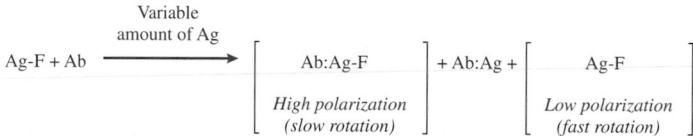

Figure 10-16 Homogeneous polarization fluoroimmunoassay. *F,* Fluorescein; *Ab,* antibody; *Ag,* antigen.

sidual bound antigen-rhodamine conjugate in the signal layer is measured by front-surface fluorometry. Displaced free conjugate does not contribute to the signal because it is shielded from the fluorescence excitation light by the iron oxide layer. As listed in Table 10-4, many other types of homogeneous FIAs have been developed.

Chemiluminescent immunoassay

Chemiluminescence is the light emission produced during a chemical reaction (see Chapter 4). In a chemiluminescent immunoassay a chemiluminescent molecule is used as an indicator label to detect and quantify immunological reactions. Isoluminol and acridinium esters are examples of chemiluminescent labels. Oxidation of isoluminol by hydrogen peroxide in the presence of a catalyst (for example, microperoxidase) produces a relatively long-lived light emission at 425 nm. Oxidation of an acridinium ester by alkaline hydrogen peroxide in the presence of a detergent (for example, Triton X-100) produces a rapid flash of light at 429 nm. Acridinium esters are high-specific activity labels (detection limit for the label being 800 zeptomoles) that can be used to label both antibodies and haptens (Figure 10-17, *A*).

Electrochemiluminescence immunoassay

Electrochemiluminescence immunoassay is a type of immunoassay in which an electrochemiluminescence molecule, such as ruthenium, is used as an indicator label in competitive and sandwich immunoassays. In such assays ruthenium (II) tris(bipyridyl) (see Figure 10-17, *B*) undergoes an electrochemiluminescent reaction (620 nm) with tripropylamine at an electrode surface. With this label, various assays have been developed in a flow cell, with magnetic beads as the solid phase. Beads are captured at the electrode surface, and unbound label is washed from the cell by a wash buffer. La-

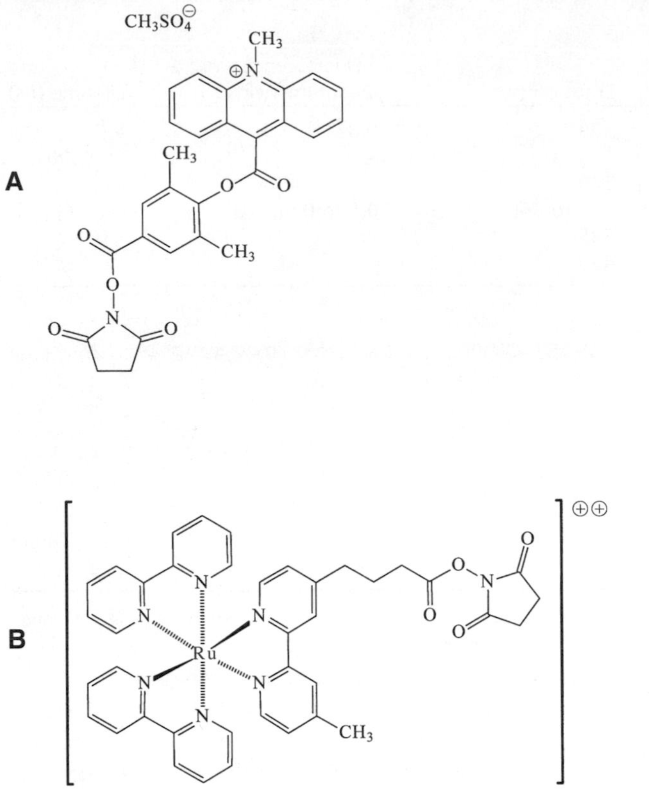

Figure 10-17 Luminescent labels. **A,** Chemiluminescent acridinium ester label. (From Law S-J, Miller T, Piran U et al: Novel poly-substituted aryl acridinium esters and their use in immunoassay. J Biolum Chemilum 1989; 4:88-98.) **B,** Electrochemiluminescent ruthenium (II) tris(bipyridyl) NHS (*N*-hydroxysuccinimide) ester label.

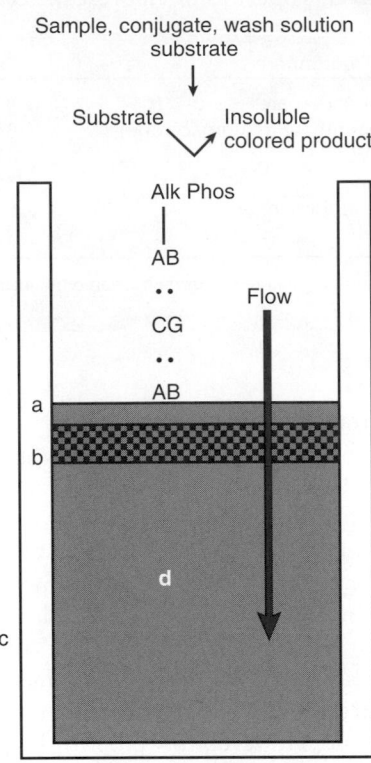

Figure 10-18 ICON immunoassay device illustrating immobilized antibody membrane *(a),* separating membrane *(b);* container *(c),* and adsorbent pad *(d). CG,* Human chorionic gonadotropin; *AB,* monoclonal antibody to CG; *Alk Phos,* Alkaline phosphatase.

bel bound to the bead undergoes an electrochemiluminescent reaction, and the light emission is measured by an adjacent photomultiplier tube.[2]

Simplified immunoassays

The integration of the technical advances made in molecular immunology with those made in the material and processing sciences has resulted in the development of a number of "simplified" immunoassays for use in physicians' offices or the home—the so-called point-of-care testing (POCT) market. The ICON pregnancy test (Hybritech, San Diego, Calif.) is an example of such a device. This device is built around a sandwich EIA. It is an operationally simple and sensitive assay for human chorionic gonadotropin (CG) and has a detection limit of 25 IU CG/L.[13] As shown in Figure 10-18, the ICON test uses a murine monoclonal antibody immobilized onto the surface of a microporous nylon membrane located on top of an adsorbent pad. The pad functions as a capillary pump to draw liquid through the membrane. To perform an analysis, an aliquot of urine is added to the surface of the membrane; CG is removed as liquid is drawn through it, resulting in the removal of CG in the sample through its binding to the capture antibody on the

membrane. Next, a matched murine monoclonal anti-CG antibody-alkaline phosphatase conjugate is added and allowed to drain into the adsorbent pad. Wash solution then is added, followed by an indoxyl phosphate substrate. Bound conjugate converts this substrate to an insoluble indigo dye, which appears as a discrete blue spot. The second generation of the ICON test includes two additional control zones. An immobilized anti-alkaline phosphatase zone acts as a procedural control; it binds the alkaline phosphatase conjugate and also appears as a blue spot. A further zone contains immobilized irrelevant murine monoclonal antibody; this zone detects the presence of heterophile antibodies in samples, particularly human antimouse antibodies (HAMA). These mimic antigen and bridge the capture and conjugated mouse antibodies, thus giving what appears to be a positive result.

Other POCT devices require only the addition of sample, simplifying the assay protocol and minimizing possible malfunction resulting from operator error. The TestPack Plus (Abbott Laboratories, Abbott Park, Ill.) is a one-step pregnancy test that illustrates the general principles of the new devices. It uses colloidal selenium particles (160-nm diameter) labeled with monoclonal anti-α-CG antibody, which is red in color and easily visible. Sample (urine) is applied to the sample well and soaks into a glass-fiber pad containing the conjugate. Any CG in the urine sample combines with the selenium-labeled antibody, and the mixture migrates along a nitrocellulose track to a region where a line of polyclonal anti-CG antibody and an orthogonal line of anti-β-CG:CG complex have been immobilized. The complex captures unreacted selenium-labeled anti-α-CG to form a minus sign visible in the viewing window. If CG was present in the urine sample, then the selenium-labeled anti-α-CG:CG complexes bind to the immobilized polyclonal anti-CG and a plus sign is formed, denoting a positive result. The remainder of the reaction mixture migrates to the end of the track and reacts with a Quinaldine red pH indicator in an "end-of-assay" window to signal that the flow in the device has functioned correctly. Variants of this type of device use antibody-coated beads loaded with blue dye and have separate windows for the positive, negative, and procedural controls (for example, Clearview; Unipath, Bedford, United Kingdom).

A quantitative dipstick test also is available that combines a competitive immunoassay assay for estrone-3-glucuronide and a sandwich immunoassay for luteinizing hormone. A small handheld portable reader also is included. The combined device is marketed as a personal contraception system that accurately predicts a woman's fertile phase (Persona, Unipath, Bedford, United Kingdom).

Simultaneous multianalyte immunoassays in which two or more analytes are detected in a single assay are becoming available widely. Two different strategies have been developed based on either discrete reaction zones or combinations of different labels. In the Triage panel for drugs of abuse POCT device (BioSite Diagnostics, San Diego, Calif.), seven drugs are analyzed simultaneously through the use of discrete test zones on a small piece of nylon membrane. Each test zone is composed of antibodies to a specific drug immobilized onto the membrane surface. This zone captures free gold sol-drug conjugate from the sample + anti-drug antibody + gold sol-drug conjugate reaction mixture and appears as a purple band. Combinations of distinguishable labels, such as europium (613 nm, emission lifetime of 730 μs) and samarium (643 nm, emission lifetime of 50 μs) chelates provide the basis of quantitative simultaneous immunoassays. These two chelates have different fluorescence emission maxima and different fluorescence decay times and thus can be distinguished easily from measurements at 613 nm, delay time 0.4 ms (europium), and 643 nm, delay time 0.05 ms (samarium). An assay for free and bound prostate-specific antigen and for myoglobin and carbonic anhydrase III are two examples of clinically useful tests combined in this simultaneous assay format.

Interferences

A particular problem that has been recognized for sandwich immunoassays is an interference caused by circulating human antibodies that react with animal immunoglobulins, particularly HAMA. This type of antibody can cause positive or negative interferences in two-site antibody-based sandwich assays that use mouse monoclonal capture antibody reagents. HAMA causes a false positive interference by bridging between a mouse immunoglobulin capture antibody and a mouse immunoglobulin conjugate and thus mimicking the specific analyte. A false-negative result is thought to be caused by HAMA reacting with one of the assay reagents (immobilized antibody or the conjugate) and preventing formation of the sandwich with specific analyte.

HAMA often are present in the blood of patients who have received mouse monoclonal antibody imaging or therapeutic agents. They also occur because of exposure to mouse antigens (for example, as a result of handling mice). Nonimmune mouse serum usually is included in mouse monoclonal antibody-based immunoassays to complex HAMA. However, despite this precaution, reactivity leading to false positive or negative results still is encountered. The presence of HAMA and other antianimal antibodies can be uncovered by dilution experiments because samples containing antianimal antibodies do not give proportional results. Reanalysis of a sample after incubation with an animal protein or serum (for example, mouse IgG or mouse serum for HAMA) also can confirm an interference.

◼ OTHER IMMUNOCHEMICAL TECHNIQUES

Immunocytochemistry

Labeled antibody reagents can be used as specific probes for protein and peptide antigens to examine single cells for synthetic capability and for specific markers for identification of various cell lines. Immunochemistry in recent years has been expanded rapidly by immunoenzymatic methods, such as horseradish peroxidase (HRP)-labeled (immunoperoxidase) assays. Using enzyme labels provides several advantages over fluorescent labels. First, they permit the use of fixed tissues (unembedded or embedded in paraffin), which provides excellent preservation of cell morphology and eliminates the problem of autofluorescence from tissue. Secondly, immunoperoxidase stains are permanent, and only a standard light microscope is needed to identify labeled features. The immunoperoxidase methods also are applicable in electron microscopy.

Immunochemical Agglutination Assays

Agglutination is the "clumping" together in suspension of antigen-bearing cells, microorganisms, or particles in the presence of specific antibodies, also known as *agglutinins*. Assays based on agglutination have been used for many years for the qualitative and quantitative measurement of antigens and antibodies. The visible clumping of particulates, such as cells and latex particles, is used to indicate the primary reaction of antigen and antibody. Agglutination methods require stable and uniform particulates, pure antigen, and specific antibody. IgM antibodies are more likely to produce complete agglutination than are IgG antibodies because of the size and valence of the IgM molecule. Therefore when only IgG antibodies are involved, the use of chemical enhancement or an antiglobulin-agglutination method may be necessary. As with all immunochemical reactions in which aggregation is the measured end point, the ratio of antigen to antibody is critical. Extremes in antigen or antibody concentration inhibit aggregation.

Hemagglutination describes an agglutination reaction in which the antigen is located on an erythrocyte. Erythrocytes are not only good passive carriers of antigen, but also are coated easily with foreign proteins and can be obtained and stored easily. Direct testing of erythrocytes for blood group, Rh, and other antigenic types is used widely in blood banks; specific antisera, such as anti-A, anti-C, and anti-Kell, are used to detect such antigens on the erythrocyte surface. In indirect or passive hemagglutination the erythrocytes are used as particulate carriers of foreign antigen (and in some tests, of antibody); this technique has wide applications. Other materials available in the form of fine particles, such as latex, also have been used as antigen carriers, but they are more difficult to coat, standardize, and store. In a related variation of this technique, known as *hemagglutination inhibition*, the ability of antigens, haptens, or other substances to inhibit specifically hemagglutination of sensitized (coated) cells by antibody is determined.

In general the agglutination methods are quite sensitive but not as quantitative as other immunochemical methods discussed previously. Nonisotopic immunoassays, especially EIAs, are as convenient as agglutination reactions and therefore are replacing agglutination methods in many laboratories.

References

1. Alper CA, Johnson AM: Immunofixation electrophoresis: a technique for the study of protein polymorphism. Vox Sang 1969; 17:445-452.
2. Blackburn GF, Shah HP, Kenten JH et al: Electrochemiluminescence detection for development of immunoassays and DNA probe assays for clinical diagnostics. Clin Chem 1991; 37:1534-1539.
3. Jackson TM, Ekins RP: Theoretical limitations on immunoassay. Methods Enzymol 1986; 74:28-60.
4. Kabat EA: Structural Concepts in Immunology and Immunochemistry, 2nd edition, New York, Holt, Rinehart & Winston, 1976.
5. Kohler G, Milstein C: Continuous cultures of fused cells secreting antibody of predefined specificity. Nature 1975; 256:495-497.
6. Kricka LJ: Ligand-Binder Assays, New York, Marcel Dekker, 1985.
7. Kricka LJ: Chemiluminescent and bioluminescent techniques. Clin Chem 1991; 37:1472-1481.
8. Laurell CB: Antigen-antibody crossed electrophoresis. Anal Biochem 1965; 10:358-361.
9. Laurell CB: Electroimmunoassay. Scand J Clin Lab Invest 1972; 29 Suppl 124:21-37.
10. Mancini G, Carbonara AO, Heremans JF: Immunochemical quantitation of antigens by single radial immunodiffusion. Immunochemistry 1965; 2:235-254.
11. Nakamura RM, Kasahara Y, Rechnitz GA (eds): Immunochemical Assays and Biosensor Technology for the 1990s. Washington, DC, American Association for Microbiology, 1992.
12. Picardo M , Hughes KT: Scintillation proximity assays. In Devlin JP: High Throughput Screening, pp 307-316, New York, Marcel Dekker, 1997.
13. Price CP, Newman DJ (eds): Principles and Practice of Immunoassay, 2nd edition, New York, Stockton Press, 1997.
14. Rubenstein KE, Schneider RS, Ullman EF: "Homogeneous" enzyme immunoassay: new immunochemical technique. Biochem Biophys Res Commun 1972; 47:846-851.
15. Winter G, Griffiths AD, Hawkins RE et al: Making antibodies by phage display technology. Ann Rev Immunol 1994; 12:433-455.
16. Winter G: Synthetic human antibodies and a strategy for protein engineering. FEBS Lett 1998; 430:92-94.
17. Yalow RS, Berson SA: Assay of plasma insulin in human subjects by immunological methods. Nature 1959; 184:1648-1669.

Additional Reading

Aller R: Automated immunoassay analyzers. CAP Today 1999; 13(4):49-82.
Chan DW (ed): Immunoassay Automation: An Updated Guide to Systems, San Diego, Academic Press, 1995.
Crowther JR: ELISA: Theory and Practice, Clifton, NJ, Humana Press, 1995.
Devlin JP (ed): High Throughput Drug Screening, New York, Marcel Dekker, 1997.
Diamandis EP, Christopoulos TK: Immunoassay, San Diego, Academic Press, 1996.
Wild D (ed): The Immunoassay Handbook, New York, Stockton Press, 1994.

CHAPTER 11

Nucleic Acid Techniques

ELIZABETH R. UNGER, PhD, MD, MARGARET A. PIPER, PhD, MPH, SI(ASCP),
and BARBARA G. BORDER, PhD, MT(ASCP)

Objectives

1. Describe a DNA molecule and compare its structure with that of an RNA molecule.
2. List the purines and pyrimidines and differentiate them.
3. Define the following terms:
   Nucleotide
   Base pair
   Complementarity
   Replication
   Transcription
   Translation
   Nuclease
   Polymerase
   Ligase
   Reverse transcriptase
   Restriction endonuclease
   Amplicon
4. List the steps involved in DNA replication, transcription, and translation.
5. Describe nucleic acid hybridization and give examples of hybridization assays used to answer diagnostic questions.
6. State the principles, advantages, and disadvantages of three amplification methods used for nucleic acid analysis.
7. Describe how restriction enzyme digestion produces reproducible nucleic acid fragment lengths and provide examples of methods that use this technique.

Key Words

Codon   A sequence of three nucleotides that specifies a specific amino acid during translation

DNA   Deoxyribonucleic acid; polymer of nucleotides containing a nitrogenous base, a deoxyribose sugar and phosphate; the most common genetic material of known organisms

Exon   The sequence of codons of a gene that are transcribed and retained during mRNA processing within the nucleus, exit the nucleus into the cytoplasm, and are translated into proteins

Gene   A segment of DNA involved in the production of a specific product; usually a protein or structural RNA; includes regions of the DNA involved in regulation of transcription and intervening noncoding sequences (introns)

Hybridization   The interaction between two single-stranded nucleic acid molecules to form a duplex (double-stranded) molecule based on the complementary base pairing of their respective sequences

Intron   Noncoding sequences present within a gene; present in the initial RNA transcript, but removed by splicing during processing to mature mRNA, after which the sequences remain in the nucleus

Ligase   An enzyme that joins two pieces of DNA

Mutation   Any change in the normal sequence of genomic DNA

Polymerase Chain Reaction (PCR)   A method for specific amplification of DNA segments that uses temperature cycling for synthesis and denaturation; DNA synthesis being directed by synthetic oligonucleotide primers through the use of a thermostable polymerase; number of copied segments doubling with each round of synthesis

Polymerase   Enzyme that uses mononucleotide molecular units and a parent nucleotide strand to produce a polynucleotide product that is complementary to the parent nucleotide strand

Primer   A short sequence of DNA or RNA that is paired with a single-stranded nucleic acid template providing a free 3'-OH end to "prime" the polymerase to initiate synthesis of a complementary strand

Restriction Fragment Length Polymorphism (RFLP)   Changes in the size of DNA fragments produced after digestion with a restriction enzyme; different fragment sizes resulting from changes in sequence that cause loss or introduction of a recognition site(s) for the restriction enzyme, or from the loss or gain of a significant amount of DNA between restriction enzyme recognition sites

Restriction Endonuclease (Restriction Enzyme)   One of more than 250 bacterial endonucleases that recognize specific short base sequences in the DNA (usually recurring sequences) and cleave the DNA in a specific location at or near this target (recognition) site

RNA   Ribonucleic acid; polymer of nucleotides containing a nitrogenous base, a ribose sugar and phosphate; the genetic material of some viruses and the template for protein production

Stringency   The extent of base pair mismatch tolerated in a stable duplex molecule; dictated by conditions of salt, formamide, and temperature during hybridization and washes; high stringency requiring the formation of nearly perfectly matched hybrids; low or relaxed stringency permitting related but not perfectly matched sequences to hybridize

Transcription   The process by which mRNA is produced from a DNA template

Translation   The process by which a polypeptide product is produced from an mRNA template

Variable Number of Tandem Repeats (VNTR)   Families of repetitive sequences in the human genome that are noncoding; their number of repeats being very polymorphic in the population; number of repeats also being inherited and relatively stable in family studies, which makes VNTRs useful sites in genetic identity testing

---

The fundamentals of nucleic acid biochemistry and basic principles of nucleic acid assays are discussed in this chapter. Continuing research in molecular biology, fueled recently by information from the Human Genome Project, changes our understanding of human disease pathology. Increasingly, genes responsible for inherited diseases as well as for susceptibility to infection, neoplasia, and chronic diseases (such as diabetes and atherosclerosis) are being identified. Molecular pathways of cell differentiation and proliferation that are altered during neoplasia are being discovered and characterized. Infectious agents increasingly are characterized and studied based on their nucleic sequences, as well as on their molecular interactions within the host. Diagnostic application of this new level of understanding is a logical consequence and requires that clinical laboratories implement assays based on nucleic acid techniques.

■ NUCLEIC ACID CHEMISTRY

Nucleic acids form the repository for hereditary information and provide the means to translate that information into the cellular machinery of life. **Deoxyribonucleic acid (DNA)** specifies the amino acid sequence of proteins and, with the exception of mutational and recombinational events, remains constant from generation to generation. DNA also specifies the sequence of a variety of **ribonucleic acid (RNA)** molecules that are used to translate DNA into protein or have specific functions within the cell. Detailing the structure and function of nucleic acids has been a central theme of molecular biology; a review of nucleic acid chemistry is fundamental to a description of nucleic acid diagnostic methods.

Molecular Structure and Chemical Properties

A single molecule of DNA is a polymer synthesized from monomers (nucleotides) composed of the sugar deoxyribose with a phosphate residue at the 5' carbon and a purine or pyrimidine base at the 1' carbon. The purines are adenine (A) and guanine (G), and the pyrimidines are cytosine (C) and thymine (T) (Figure 11-1). The nucleotides are joined by phosphodiester bonds that link the 5'-phosphate group of one sugar to the 3'-hydroxyl group of the adjacent sugar (see Figure 11-1, B). The repeating sugar-phosphate links con-

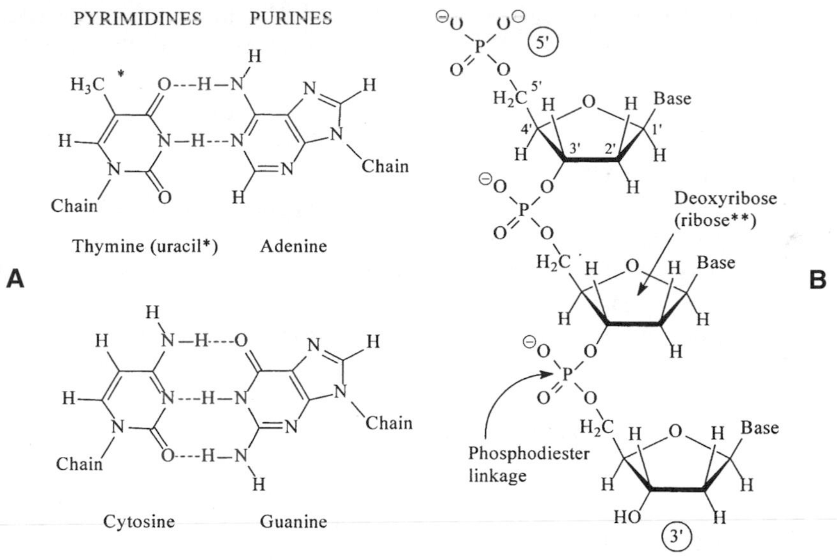

Figure 11-1 **A,** Purine and pyrimidine bases and the formation of complementary base pairs. Note the formation of hydrogen bonds *(dashed lines)*. (*In RNA thymine is replaced by uracil, which differs from thymine only in its lack of the methyl group.) **B,** A single-stranded DNA chain. Repeating nucleotide units are linked by phosphodiester bonds that join the 5′ carbon of one sugar to the 3′ carbon of the next. (**In RNA the sugar is ribose, which has a 2′-hydroxyl added to deoxyribose.) (Modified from Piper MA, Unger ER: Nucleic Acid Probes: A Primer for Pathologists, Chicago, ASCP Press, 1989.)

tribute an invariant highly charged backbone to the molecule. The sequence of the base side chains varies from molecule to molecule and uniquely identifies each DNA polymer.

Purines and pyrimidines differ in composition and size, but specific base pairing results in planar structures of similar dimensions (see Figure 11-1, *A*). Adenine (A) forms two hydrogen bonds with thymine (T), and guanine (G) forms three hydrogen bonds with cytosine (C). The hydrophobic nature of the bases combined with the A:T, G:C base pairing makes a right-handed, double-stranded helix the energetically favorable secondary structure of native DNA. The planar base pairs stack in the inside of the helix, whereas the hydrophilic sugar-phosphate backbone forms noncovalent bonds with surrounding water molecules. For the two DNA polymers to adopt the helical structure and form the proper base pairs, two requirements must be fulfilled: the polymers must run in opposite directions as defined by the free hydroxyl groups at each end (3′- 5′ versus 5′- 3′), and the sequence of the bases in each strand must be such that A:T and G:C hydrogen bonds always are formed. Two DNA strands that allow this appropriate hydrogen bonding are called *complementary*.

The phosphate esters of the nucleic acid backbone are strong acids that exist as anions at neutral pH. DNA is soluble in water up to about 1% weight of solute per volume of solution and is precipitated by the addition of alcohol. The bases are only weakly basic and uncharged over a pH range of approximately 4 to 9. Outside these limits the base pair hydrogen bonds are disrupted, and the helix unwinds.[3] Nucleic acid molecules absorb ultraviolet (UV) light maxi-

mally at 260 nm almost entirely because of the constituent bases. This property is used to quantitate the nucleic acid content of a solution.

Due to base pairing and the double-helical conformation, double-stranded DNA (dsDNA) is an exceptionally stable molecule. The helix conformation places each monomer in an identical orientation within the molecule and allows each to participate maximally in secondary bonding. The size similarity of the base pairs allows the helix to retain a constant angle of rotation. These features dictate that all dsDNA molecules, regardless of base sequence, have the same secondary structure within a physiological pH range and demonstrate nearly identical chemical properties. Thus DNA is extracted, precipitated, and manipulated in the laboratory through the use of the same chemical approach, regardless of its source.

RNA is chemically similar to DNA, but the sugar unit in RNA is ribose (containing an additional hydroxyl group at the 2′ position) and the demethylated pyrimidine uracil (U) replaces T. RNA exists in various functional forms, but it is always a single-stranded polymer of irregular three-dimensional structure that is much shorter than DNA. RNA conformations are not completely random; a portion of an RNA strand may fold and complementary portions anneal to form hairpin/loop structures with duplex sections. RNA is less stable than DNA because it lacks the double-stranded helical conformation and because the 2′-hydroxyl group of the ribose makes it subject to alkaline hydrolysis. In addition, although both DNA and RNA are degraded enzymatically by DNA- and RNA-specific nucleases (DNase and RNase, respectively), RNases are nearly ubiquitous, making work with native RNA molecules in the laboratory much more difficult. Special precautions must be taken to avoid RNase contamination.

◾ NUCLEIC ACID BIOCHEMISTRY

Whereas nucleic acid chemistry describes DNA and RNA molecules' composition and secondary structure, biochemistry describes the coordinated use and propagation of these molecules. Specific enzymes control the biochemical processes of nucleic acids. The processes of replication, transcription, translation, and hybridization, as well as the enzymes that interact with the nucleic acids, are described briefly in this chapter.

Replication, Transcription, and Translation

Every time a cell divides, the entire DNA content of that cell must be duplicated faithfully so that the total complement of hereditary information (the genome of the organism) is retained in each daughter cell. This process is called *replication*. Because of the laws of base pairing—that is, A pairs only with T and G only with C—the sequence of single-stranded DNA (ssDNA) dictates the sequence of its complementary strand. Replication proceeds in a semiconservative fashion, with the two parent strands of a dsDNA molecule each serving as the template for the synthesis of a daughter strand. The duplicated dsDNA molecules produced in this manner each are composed of one parent strand and one daughter strand. For replication to occur, the original double-stranded helix must be separated, an energetically unfavorable event. This event is accomplished with a combination of DNA-specific proteins and enzymes, and replication of both daughter strands proceeds as the parent strands separate. Replication is initiated at multiple sites during this process, but each origin of replication is used only once during a single cell cycle.

DNA specifies the amino acid sequence of proteins. However, the production of proteins is mediated by messenger RNA (mRNA) molecules that carry the information for specific proteins from the DNA in the nucleus to the cytoplasm, where the proteins are synthesized. An mRNA is synthesized directly from that part of the DNA that specifies the protein to be produced in a process termed **transcription**. The region of DNA that specifies or "codes" for the protein, along with regulatory sequences controlling transcription, is a **gene**. As in replication, transcription requires separation of the duplex DNA strands and use of the appropriate DNA strand as a template. An RNA polymerase recognizes and binds to specific DNA sequences, termed the *initiation site*, and starts joining the ribonucleotide units that pair with the template. The linkage of nucleotides continues as the polymerase moves across the gene template. Specific DNA sequences result in chain termination, and the newly synthesized mRNA quickly detaches from the template DNA because restoration of the

DNA-DNA duplex is more favorable energetically than retention of the DNA-RNA hybrid and section of ssDNA. The end product is a single-stranded poly-ribonucleotide that contains the information necessary for protein synthesis in its sequence of bases.

When mRNA first is synthesized, it is a faithful, complementary copy of the DNA gene sequence. Before export to the cytoplasm, however, mRNA molecules are modified further. Noncoding regions known as **introns** are excised from the mRNA by a molecular complex that enzymatically cleaves and ligates RNA at specific recognition sequences. After this step the mRNA contains only **exons,** or coding sequences. Further mRNA modification includes the addition of caps, or 7-methyl guanosine residues joined to the 5′ ends with triphosphate linkages, and tails, poly-A sequences added to the 3′ ends. After these modifications the mature mRNA is exported to the cytoplasm to direct protein synthesis.

Translation is the process whereby the mRNA sequence directs the amino acid sequence during protein synthesis. This direction is accomplished with the use of a code in which three nucleotides (a **codon**) specify one amino acid. The four bases may be combined into 64 possible codons, so most of the 22 amino acids are specified by more than one codon. In addition, several codons do not code for amino acids but signal termination of protein synthesis (stop codons). The genetic code is illustrated in Table 11-1. Translation takes place on ribosomes, which are ribonucleoprotein complexes that function as protein synthesis factories. During synthesis, codons are "read" by transfer RNA (tRNA), short RNA molecules with sequences complementary to amino acid codons (anticodons), and are bound to the amino acid molecule specified by the codon. As synthesis proceeds, the appropriate tRNA anticodon base-pairs with the next mRNA codon. An enzyme on the ribosome then catalyses the formation of a peptide bond between the amino acid bound to the tRNA and the growing protein chain. The previous tRNA is released, and the next tRNA is added. The ribosome moves along the mRNA until a stop codon is reached and synthesis is complete. The ribosome and the protein product then dissociate from the mRNA.

Nucleic Acid Enzymes: Tools for Molecular Biology

Many enzymes that function in replication and transcription have been purified and their biological activities used to direct specific reactions in vitro. Some enzymes are of particular use in cloning and amplification of nucleic acid sequences of interest, whereas others are used in the preparation of nucleic acid probes and modification of target samples in nucleic acid hybridization assays.

Nucleases are a category of nucleic acid-specific enzymes that hydrolyze the phosphodiester bonds of the nucleic acid polymer one nucleotide at a time. Nucleases may require free hydroxyl ends (exonucleases), with specificity for the 3′

TABLE 11-1	The Genetic Code (Translation of mRNA to Amino Acids during Protein Synthesis)			
		Third			
First	Second	U	C	A	G
U	U	Phenylalanine	Phenylalanine	Leucine	Leucine
	C	Serine	Serine	Serine	Serine
	A	Tyrosine	Tyrosine	Stop	Stop
	G	Cysteine	Cysteine	Selenocysteine*	Tryptophan
C	U	Leucine	Leucine	Leucine	Leucine
	C	Proline	Proline	Proline	Proline
	A	Histidine	Histidine	Glutamine	Glutamine
	G	Arginine	Arginine	Arginine	Arginine
A	U	Isoleucine	Isoleucine	Isoleucine	Methionine
	C	Threonine	Threonine	Threonine	Threonine
	A	Asparagine	Asparagine	Lysine	Lysine
	G	Serine	Serine	Arginine	Arginine
G	U	Valine	Valine	Valine	Valine
	C	Alanine	Alanine	Alanine	Alanine
	A	Aspartic acid	Aspartic acid	Glutamic acid	Glutamic acid
	G	Glycine	Glycine	Glycine	Glycine

U, Uracil; *C*, cytosine; *A*, adenine; *G*, guanine.
*The codon UGA can code for either selenocysteine or stop.

or 5′ end, or may act only on internal bonds (endonucleases). Nucleases can be DNA- or RNA-specific. DNase may be specific for single-stranded (for example, S1 nuclease) or double-stranded molecules (for example, DNase I). **Restriction endonucleases (restriction enzymes)** are enzymes found in bacteria that prevent replication of foreign DNA.[13] Each requires a different specific recognition sequence, usually 4 to 10 nucleotides, in a dsDNA molecule. At each location with this sequence the enzyme hydrolyzes both strands in a reproducible manner, forming either asymmetrical or blunt-end cuts. Restriction enzymes are useful for cutting large strands of DNA into sequence-specific reproducible fragments and for preparing DNA from different sources to be joined in cloning procedures.

Ligases catalyze the formation of phosphodiester linkages between two nucleic acid chains.[7] DNA ligases require the presence of a complementary template, whereas RNA ligases, used in mRNA processing, do not.

Polymerases catalyze the synthesis of complementary nucleic acid polymers using a parent strand as a template.[8] These enzymes are essential to nucleic acid cloning and amplification procedures.

Reverse transcriptase is found in retroviruses and catalyzes the synthesis of DNA from either an RNA or DNA template.[2] This enzyme activity is required as part of the life cycle of retroviruses. In vitro it is used to make complementary DNA copies of RNA in samples for use in cloning, probe preparation, and nucleic acid assays.

Nucleic Acid Hybridization

As described previously the thermodynamically favored structure of DNA under physiological conditions is an or-

dered, double-stranded helix formed of two separate DNA molecules held together by noncovalent interactions. The duplex structure is most stable when the rules of complementary base-pairing are followed, allowing for maximal hydrogen bonding and base stacking. The central binding between two DNA strands is both specific (that is, sequence dependent) and reversible (because of the noncovalent hydrogen bonds).

Denaturing agents (for example, high temperature [65 °C], formamide, or extremes of pH) favor dissociation of the double-stranded molecule into two separate random coils (Figure 11-2). When the denaturant is removed, single strands attempt to rejoin (anneal) to reform the duplex structure, strongly favoring interactions that maximize complementary base-pairing. Because temperature is the denaturant that is manipulated most easily, the helix-to-coil transformation is often referred to as *melting*, and the temperature at which one-half the DNA in solution is in the random coil configuration is referred to as the *melting point*, or T_m, of the DNA. The reverse process, in which two complementary strands of DNA recombine to form a stable duplex molecule, is referred to as *annealing* or **hybridization** (because the newly formed molecule may be a "hybrid" structure formed of complementary strands originating from different sources). Although the hybridization reaction thus far has been described in terms of DNA, RNA molecules also participate in the hybridization process. Base-pairing may occur between complementary strands of DNA, between DNA and RNA, and between complementary strands of RNA, resulting in DNA-DNA, DNA-RNA, and RNA-RNA duplex structures. A short, relatively well-characterized segment of nucleic acid used to search an unknown sample for the presence of complementary sequences

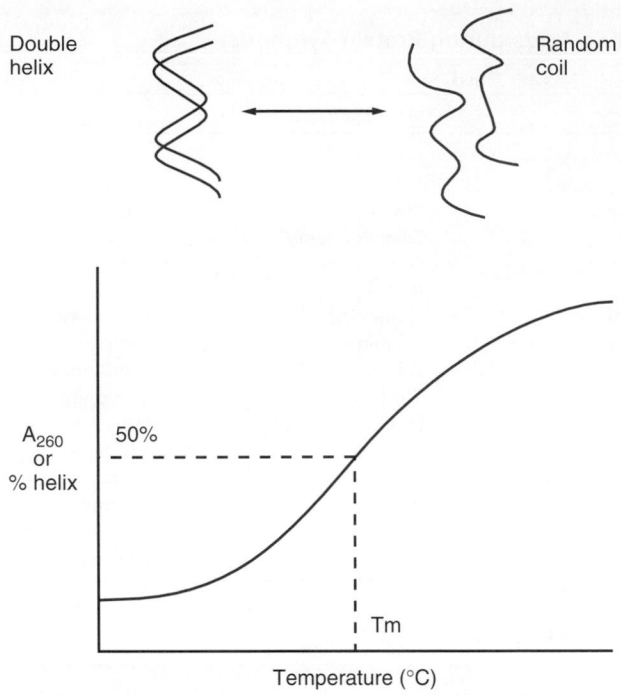

Figure 11-2 Dissociation curve of double-stranded helical nucleic acid. This reversible process is sequence dependent and forms the basis of the hybridization reaction. (Modified from Piper MA, Unger ER: Nucleic Acid Probes: A Primer for Pathologists, Chicago, ASCP Press, 1989.)

through the hybridization process is known as a *nucleic acid probe.*

Stringency

Although exact complementarity of base-pairing is favored, some degree of mismatch between the strands may be tolerated, depending on the conditions of the hybridization reaction. Duplex molecules with mismatched base pairs are less stable than those with a perfect sequence match and thus dissociate or melt at a lower temperature. The toleration (or lack thereof) for "mistakes" in base-pairing is referred to as the **stringency** of the hybridization reaction. Stringency is determined by the concentration of salt and formamide, as well as by temperature. Reduced salt, increased formamide, and increased temperature increase the stringency, requiring increasingly exact base-pairing for stable hybrids. Conversely, lowering the stringency increases the numbers of base-pair mismatches tolerated in a duplex structure. The stringency of the hybridization reaction is influenced by the environment during the hybridization reaction, as well as by subsequent washing steps designed for the removal of nonspecifically interacting nucleic acid.

Hybridization cocktail

The hybridization cocktail is the medium controlling the environment of the hybridization reaction. The composition of the cocktail and temperature of the hybridization determine the stringency of the hybridization reaction. The cock-

tail consists of empirically determined ingredients modulating stringency and favoring specific base-pair hydrogen bonding rather than charge interactions. The components vary widely but include buffers, salts, denaturants (for example, formamide, high-molecular-weight polymers, and carrier DNA or RNA), as well as various "magic" ingredients designed to reduce background (for example, detergents, bovine serum albumin, and ficoll). This complex mixture conveniently is referred to as a *cocktail.* Many commercially available formulations are ready for the addition of the specific probe. The ionic strength of both the hybridization cocktail and the subsequent washes can be modulated by the concentration of a saline-sodium citrate buffer (SSC), composed of 0.15 mol/L sodium chloride and 0.015 mol/L trisodium citrate (pH 7.0). The shorthand notation for these conditions refers to the strength of the SSC buffer (for example, 2 × SSC; 0.1 × SSC).

Hybridization kinetics

The kinetics of solution-phase hybridization are second order. The rate-limiting step is nucleation, the formation of a small number of base pairs in the correct orientation. Nucleation is followed by a rapid "zippering" of complementary sequences. An increase in probe concentration generally increases the hybridization rate, whereas temperature has a complex influence on the rate. Above the T_m, little tendency exists for hybrid formation. As the temperature is decreased below the T_m, the rate of hybridization increases and reaches a maximum at 20 to 25 °C below T_m. When the nucleic acid target or probe is immobilized to a solid support, such as nylon or nitrocellulose membrane, the kinetics of the hybridization are more complex. In practice, hybridization assays are designed empirically. Time and temperature of the hybridization reaction and probe concentration are the variables adjusted most frequently. Conditions that tend to maximize the extent of hybridization and minimize the background or nonspecific attachment of probe are selected.

Probes

In a hybridization assay the probe is analogous in its role and importance to the antibody molecule in an immunoassay. A probe is simply a known fragment of nucleic acid labeled with a reporter group for detection. Probes may be genomic, recombinant (cloned), or synthesized (oligonucleotide, or "oligos"). They may be DNA or RNA, single stranded or double stranded. The chemical nature of the probe influences the conditions of the assay and molecular stability; for example, dsDNA requires denaturation, and RNA probes must be kept under sterile RNase-free conditions. The label in many clinical applications is nonradioactive, although radioactive labels are still in use, particularly in research settings. Nonradioactive labels include directly detected fluorescent labels and indirectly detected affinity labels. A variety of detection formats are used for the same affinity label (Figure 11-3). For example, biotin may be detected by binding to avidin linked to an enzyme with sub-

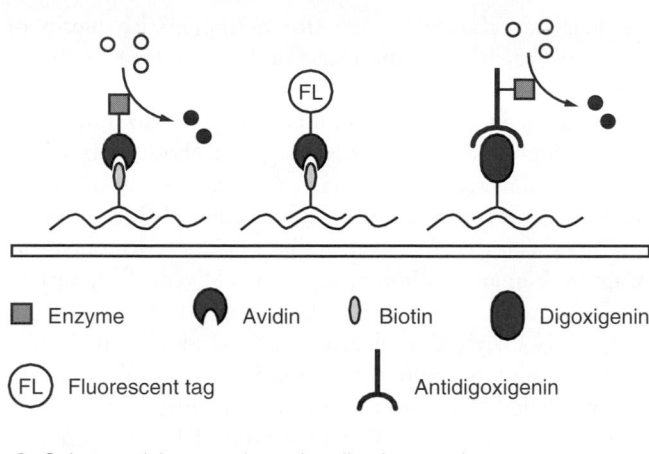

■ Enzyme   ◖◗ Avidin   ◗ Biotin   ⬮ Digoxigenin

(FL) Fluorescent tag   ⊥ Antidigoxigenin

○ Substrate (photometric or chemiluminescent)

Figure 11-3 Examples of affinity-labeled probe detection systems.

sequent photometric or chemiluminescent detection or avidin containing a fluorescent tag. For all nonradioactive methods the detection portion of the assay becomes identical to immunochemical assays (see Chapter 10) and is crucial in the obtaining of optimal sensitivity. Detection reagents with high background and suboptimal signal generation mar an effective hybridization reaction.

■ NUCLEIC ACID ANALYSES

The methods for manipulation of nucleic acids to yield clinical information are numerous and continuously evolving. The basic techniques involved in nucleic acid analysis include sample preparation, electrophoretic separation, hybridization assays, amplification methods, restriction fragment length polymorphisms, and sequencing. These techniques are interrelated and often combined; for example, some hybridization assays use electrophoretic separation, whereas some amplification methods utilize hybridization.

Sample Preparation

Key features of nucleic acid sample preparation include proper collection, storage, preservation, purification (that is, removal of substances that would prevent probe access to the target and inhibit action of polymerases), and concentration. In patient material, nucleic acids exist intimately mixed with a variety of proteins and lipids and are susceptible to enzymatic and chemical degradation. In some cases, as when the target of interest is of bacterial or yeast origin, strong lipopolysaccharide cell walls must be disrupted mechanically or with enzymes. Sample nucleic acids must be preserved adequately and made available for interaction with the probe and enzyme tools, such as restriction enzymes, ligases, and polymerases, used in assays.

The physical and chemical similarities among nucleic acids, regardless of source, allow for uniform methods of extraction and purification.[11] (This uniformity is unlike the situation with proteins, in which purification schemes must be tailored for the particular molecule.) Individual steps included in these uniform methods are cell lysis (mechanical and/or enzymatic), protein digestion, chloroform phenol extractions, and alcohol precipitation. A variety of new alternatives have been developed that minimize sample handling. One example is the use of chaotropic (denaturing) agents for lysis/extraction, followed by binding to various matrices in columns or microtitre plates and washing steps to remove impurities. The bound, purified nucleic acids then are released from the matrix. Automated methods of sample extraction also are being developed. For many assays complete purification is unnecessary, and shortened protocols are used.

Electrophoretic Separation

The sugar-phosphate backbone of both DNA and RNA imparts an evenly distributed net negative charge to these molecules. These highly charged molecules move in response to an electric field and separate according to molecular weight (see Chapter 7). Analysis of fragment size forms the basis for interpretation of some hybridization assays. The electrophoretic medium most frequently used is agarose, the percentage of which depends on the size of the fragments to be resolved. Most applications use a horizontal electrophoresis bed submerged in buffer. Detection may be achieved through staining of the gel with ethidium bromide, which intercalates adjacent bases in nucleic acid molecules and is visible with UV transillumination. Other formats in use include vertical polyacrylamide gel electrophoresis and capillary electrophoresis.

Genomic DNA is extremely long and complex. Before electrophoretic separation, the DNA must be cut with restriction enzymes to generate reproducible fragments of a size resolvable by electrophoresis. Restriction enzymes specific for a simple recognition sequence cut genomic DNA into smaller fragments than those specific for a complex recognition sequence because the simple sequence is represented more often within the molecule. Some restriction enzymes cut so infrequently that extremely large fragments, measured in megabase pairs (Mbp), result. Special electrophoretic systems that use pulsed electrical fields have been devised to separate these large molecules. RNA molecules, as transcripts of DNA, are "presized" and relatively small; thus no digestion is required before electrophoresis. Because of the high degree of secondary structure in the RNA molecule, the RNA gels generally are run under denaturing conditions.

Hybridization Assay

Conceptually, all hybridization assays are similar because they are based on the unique ability of nucleic acid molecules to hybridize. Complementary base-pairing allows fragments of known sequence (probe) to find matching sequences in an unknown sample. Hybridization assays require a probe and sample nucleic acid to be mixed under conditions that allow for specific complementary base-pairing. After probe and target have been allowed to interact, the assay must provide a way to detect the formation of probe-sample hybrids and interpret the results. Many different hybridization assay formats have been developed, and several of the more commonly used variations are described in the following text. Format selection depends on the clinical setting and the particular question to be answered. Each method has its strengths and weaknesses.

As with any assay, both positive and negative controls are necessary for validation. A positive sample control is one known to contain sequences complementary to the probe. It is used to establish that sample preparation is adequate to release target for the hybridization assay and to ensure that the probe hybridizes with the specific target under the assay conditions. The sample control also may be used to monitor the sensitivity of the assay if the positive control is chosen near the lower limit of detection. A negative sample control (that is, one known not to contain sequences complementary to the probe) is used to monitor specificity of the probe-target interactions. Controls for the probe include unrelated probes that are labeled, hybridized, and detected under identical assay conditions. These latter controls allow monitoring of the background signal generated by localization of probe through physical trapping or nonhybridized charge interactions.

Liquid or solution-phase hybridization

In liquid hybridization assays both the sample and the probe interact in solution. Because the hybridization takes place in a liquid phase, the reaction rates are maximal. The sample nucleic acids are generally purified from cell constituents by standard techniques and then randomly sheared and denatured before the assay is performed. The added probe must be single stranded and unable to self-hybridize.

Hybridization may be detected by the specific binding of hybrids to a solid matrix such as hydroxyapatite, which binds only duplex structures. Once hybrids are bound, nonhybridized probe may be removed efficiently by washing. Detection of the label on the bound probe permits quantitation of the hybridization reaction. An alternative analysis involves digestion of the hybridization reaction mixture with S1 nuclease, an enzyme active only on single-stranded nucleic acid. Duplex structures resist digestion and may be precipitated by addition of trichloroacetic acid. In a similar approach known as the *hybridization protection assay,* label on the probe is protected from chemical degradation only when the probe is involved in a duplex structure. Detection of label precipitated (in the S1 nuclease method) or resistant to degradation (the hybridization protection assay) allows for quantitation of the hybridization reaction.

Yet another variation of the solution-phase assay, termed *affinity-based hybrid collection assay,* uses two contiguous portions of the target nucleic acid as probes. One of the probe

sequences is affinity labeled (for example, with biotin or magnetic beads), and the other probe is labeled for signal generation. The only way for the two probes to interact with each other is through simultaneous hybridization with sample containing regions homologous to both probes. Hybrids are collected through the use of the affinity label, and signal is generated when the sample forms a bridge or sandwich between the two probes. The FDA approved Hybrid-Capture human papillomavirus assay (Digene Diagnostics, Inc., Beltsville, Md.) uses a bound antibody specific for RNA-DNA hybrid molecules to bind duplex molecules formed during solution phase hybridization of DNA sample and unlabeled RNA probe. The assay is being adapted to an enzyme-linked immunoabsorbent assay (ELISA) plate format, which is compatible with automatic detection.

Some sample degradation is tolerated by the assay, and many formats use minimally purified sample. Nonradioactive detection systems, both photometric and chemiluminescent, have been developed that are amenable to quantitation and automation. These features make solution phase assays attractive for clinical laboratories. However, this format does not permit identification of the size of the hybridizing product. In addition, low levels of specific target, high levels of weakly cross-reacting target, or a sample with high background each result in low positive readings that cannot be interpreted with certainty.

Solid-support hybridization

The discovery that nucleic acids could be bound simultaneously to a solid matrix and still be available for hybridization resulted in a dramatical increase in the use of hybridization as an analytical tool.[1] Many applications use some form of this assay because multiple samples can be processed simultaneously, facilitating control and simplifying some portions of the assay. Variations of the solid-support hybridization assays include dot blot hybridization, Southern and Northern hybridization, and in situ hybridization.

Dot blot or slot hybridization

In this assay format, multiple samples are immobilized in a geometric array on a nitrocellulose or nylon membrane. The name of the assay comes from the shape of each sample on the membrane. When samples are applied by hand, the shape is more random (blot). With the use of commercially available manifolds, samples usually are applied with suction, and the shape is very regular, either round (dot) or elongated (slot). Because all samples and controls are exposed to exactly the same reagents and conditions, the internal consistency of the assay is increased.

Depending on the application the extent of sample preparation varies between the extremes of direct application of crude patient material (blood, stool, sputum, cells, etc.) and full purification of nucleic acids. Purification increases the amount of sample that can be immobilized and minimizes nonspecific sticking of probe. However, purification requires individual handling of each sample and a relatively large amount of starting material. If patient material is applied directly to the matrix, a modified purification procedure can be performed on all samples simultaneously. This procedure usually involves a lysis and denaturation with strong base or chaotropic agent (for example, sodium iodide, protein removal with enzyme digestion, and sodium dodecyl sulfate treatment) and washing. The price for this convenience is lowered sensitivity, resulting from the limited amount of starting material that can be immobilized and the inefficiency of the extraction process. The unpurified starting material is also more subject to nonspecific binding of probe, which raises the background for the assay.

The sandwich hybridization assay is a modification of the dot blot hybridization assay and was designed to overcome some of the background problems encountered with the use of unpurified sample. This technique is analogous to the affinity-based hybrid collection assay in that two contiguous regions of the target are used as two separate probes. One probe is bound to the membrane and serves as the capture DNA. The second probe is labeled for signal generation. Signal molecules remain attached to the membrane only through sample-mediated hybridization; the sample nucleic acid forms a sandwich between the membrane, probe, and signal-generating probe.

Interpretation of the results of a dot blot hybridization assay is relatively straightforward. If hybridization has occurred, a signal is generated at the specified spot. Depending on the label used for signal generation, results may be quantitated; however, usually a simple yes or no interpretation is given (that is, the sample has more or less signal than adjacent samples and known positive and negative controls). Weak signals, resulting from a very small amount of specific target or from a large amount of weakly cross-reacting target, create problems in interpretation.

Similar assays have been developed substituting ELISA wells for membranes. This technique requires chemical modification of the plastic wells to bind short DNA probes at one end and allow the bound probe to hybridize to sample. As described for the solution phase assays, conversion to an ELISA plate format is conducive to automation of washing and detection.

Southern and Northern hybridizations

Both Southern and Northern hybridizations combine electrophoretic separation of test nucleic acid with transfer to a solid support and subsequent hybridization. Thus these assays not only provide information about the presence of hybridization, but they also permit determination of the molecular weight of the hybridizing species. The original procedure was termed *Southern blot hybridization,* or *Southern blotting,* after its inventor, E. M. Southern.[14] In this assay the test nucleic acid is DNA. Northern blotting was named not for its inventor but as a companion technique to Southern blotting that utilizes RNA as the test nucleic acid.

(Western blotting is a similar procedure in which proteins are subjected to electrophoresis and transfer.)

For optimal results the DNA sample must be purified with minimal shearing and other degradation. As indicated in the previous discussion of electrophoresis, the DNA sample must be digested with one or more restriction nucleases before electrophoretic separation occurs. Shearing introduces random breaks in the DNA, reducing the amount available to be cut specifically by recognition of restriction sites. Impurities in the sample also interfere with the ability of the restriction enzyme to digest the DNA completely. The particular restriction enzymes used must be determined for each probe. In some assays multiple aliquots of the sample are digested with a panel of restriction enzymes.

Because restriction enzyme digestion and electrophoresis are central to the results obtained, the inclusion of controls for these steps is important. A known sample, such as lambda phage DNA, is digested and subjected to electrophoresis. This procedure makes possible the monitoring of the activity of the restriction enzyme and provides molecular weight markers to evaluate electrophoretic separation. Before the large gel for Southern hybridization analysis is run, "test" gels often are run to evaluate digestion of the sample. A small aliquot of digested sample is subjected to agarose gel electrophoresis, stained with ethidium bromide, and visualized with UV transillumination. Appropriately digested genomic DNA appears as a smear down the electrophoresis lane.

The next step of the assay involves transfer of the DNA fragments in the agarose gel to a solid support. Details of the transfer process differ, but most variants utilize acid treatment to depurinate and fragment the DNA, making it smaller and easier to elute from the gel, followed by base denaturation (single strands binding to membranes much more efficiently) and neutralization. Original methods of transfer relied on capillary action, with the membrane in contact with the gel and absorbent paper stacked on top to blot the transfer buffer and DNA onto the membrane. The capillary transfer typically was allowed to proceed overnight. More recently, vacuum and pressure systems have been developed to speed the transfer. After transfer, DNA is immobilized permanently on the membrane by baking or UV cross-linking. At this point the membrane is ready for hybridization.

For Northern hybridizations, the starting material is RNA. Total RNA extracted from cells is primarily ribosomal RNA and tRNA, with mRNA accounting for 1% to 2% of total cellular RNA. Great care must be taken to avoid RNase degradation. As described earlier, RNA is composed of much shorter strands than is extracted DNA, so digestion prior to electrophoresis is not required. However, because of the secondary structure of RNA, electrophoresis under denaturing conditions is necessary. The use of good-quality RNA (that is, undegraded) is central to a successful Northern hybridization. After electrophoresis and ethidium bromide staining, undegraded RNA samples should demonstrate two clearly visible bands of ribosomal RNA with minimal low-molecular-weight material at the dye front. Transfer to solid support is similar to the technique used for Southern hybridizations. A control probe for a ubiquitously expressed mRNA (for example, actin) often is used to control for equal loading and transfer of RNA samples.

In both Southern and Northern blot tests, once transfer to the solid support membrane is complete, hybridization proceeds in a similar fashion to dot blot hybridization. Probes complementary to bound sequences hybridize at the location to which the fragments migrated in the gel. Detection of the probe results in autoradiographic, chemiluminescent, or photometric visualization of bands indicating the size and presence of the hybridizing species in the sample. An absence of bands in the sample lanes indicates an absence of complementary sequences. The presence of bands at molecular weights different from those of normal or germline (developmentally unaltered) samples can indicate a change in the genetic material. The Northern hybridization technique is used most often to evaluate the level of expression of a particular mRNA species so that quantitation or semiquantitation is necessary through reference to a control probe hybridization, such as actin. For specimens that have been subjected to sequence-specific polymerase chain reaction (PCR) amplification, gel electrophoresis, and ethidium bromide staining may be sufficient to visualize positive and negative results without the need for transfer and hybridization.

Amplification Methods

Achieving adequate sensitivity has been one of the difficulties in the clinical application of nucleic acid hybridization methods. Techniques that attempt to alleviate this difficulty by increasing either the sample or detection product may be grouped together as amplification methods. The PCR assay is the most well known and widely applied of these methods. Others include the ligase chain reaction, the self-sustained sequence replication assay, and the branched-chain DNA method.

Polymerase chain reaction

Kary Mullis[10] was awarded the Nobel Prize in Chemistry in 1993 for inventing the **polymerase chain reaction (PCR).** The method has been adopted widely and adapted for many research purposes, and commercial kits for clinical diagnosis are available. PCR uses the ability of an oligonucleotide probe to hybridize specifically to target and form an initiation site, or "primer," for DNA polymerase to synthesize a copy of the template. When oligonucleotides, referred to as **primers,** are selected to be complementary to opposite strands flanking the sequence to be detected, the action of the polymerase results in synthesis of two additional DNA strands containing the primers as the 5′ ends. After denaturation, four strands are available for the annealing of primers and subsequent polymerization or elongation.

The three steps of the reaction—denaturation, annealing, and elongation—are accomplished rapidly (within 20 to 30 seconds) and generally are performed at three different temperatures (denaturation at 94 °C, annealing at 55 °C, and elongation at 72 °C). Thus one "cycle" is executed through manipulation of temperature and accomplished in 60 to 90 seconds. The instrument that takes samples through the multiple steps of changing temperature is known as a *thermocycler.* Repetitive thermocycling eventually results in the geometric accumulation of the "short" product, which consists of primers and all intervening sequences. The process is shown schematically in Figure 11-4. With the addition of an initial reverse transcriptase (RT) step to form complementary DNA (cDNA) from RNA in the sample, RNA targets also can be amplified successfully. This modification of the reaction is known as *RT-PCR.*

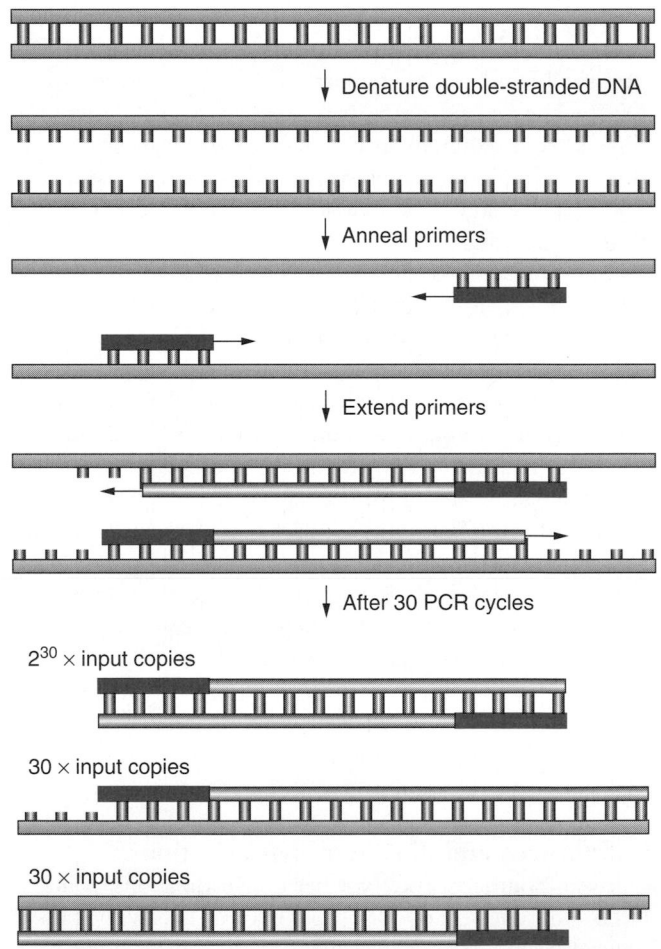

Figure 11-4 Schematic diagram of the PCR. One cycle of the reaction includes denaturation, annealing of primers, and primer-directed DNA polymerization or extension. With each cycle the number of the template in the reaction (input copies) doubles. Only the short product, bounded by primers, accumulates exponentially. A similar approach is used to amplify RNA targets by inclusion of an initial reaction with reverse transcriptase to produce a DNA copy of the RNA template. In this case the reaction is called *RT-PCR. PCR,* Polymerase chain reaction; *RT,* reverse transcriptase. (Courtesy David C. Swan, PhD, Atlanta.)

Reactants in a typical PCR reaction include the sample DNA, each deoxynucleotide (dATP, dCTP, dGTP, and dTTP, collectively known as *dNTPs*), primers, appropriate buffer, and thermostable polymerase in a volume of 50 or 100 μL. The exact conditions of the reaction and times for each phase of the cycle are dictated by the sample, length of the region to be amplified, and sequence of primers. Assuming perfect fidelity of the reaction, 20 cycles would result in a million-fold amplification of the target. Because practical levels of efficiency range from to 85% to 90%, actual amplification is "only" approximately 250,000-fold. Sources of inefficiency include the annealing of primers to nontarget regions of the sample DNA, gradual inactivation of the polymerase at elevated temperature, incomplete elongation of primed target, and presence of inhibitors.

Once the product has been amplified, detection of the DNA target is simplified greatly. Simple separation by gel electrophoresis with ethidium bromide staining may suffice, but often some form of hybridization is used to verify specificity of the amplified product and further increase sensitivity. Alternative methods of detection that are more amenable to automation and independent of hybridization are being developed. For example, one primer might be designed to include a nonannealing end with affinity label or magnetic bead. The other primer could include a signal-generating probe, such as an enzyme. Specific product would include both the affinity tag and the enzyme label and could be harvested and analyzed without hybridization.

Concerns about polymerase chain reaction in a clinical setting

The unprecedented sensitivity of PCR is both the method's greatest strength and its greatest weakness. Because PCR can detect a single molecule of target sequence, the potential for sample contamination is far greater than that normally encountered in the clinical laboratory. The greatest potential for contamination comes from the product of the amplification reaction referred to as the *amplicon*. After amplification each reaction mixture may contain as many as 10^{12} copies of the product. Thus aerosol droplets can contain sufficient targets for easy amplification. Amplicon can contaminate reagents, pipets, and glassware. Experience has dictated the use of laboratory procedures that minimize amplicon contamination.[9] These include the use of physically separated areas for preamplification and postamplification steps, barrier pipets tips and positive-displacement pipets to minimize aerosol contamination, UV light treatment of pipets, tips, tubes, and reaction mixes to inactivate DNA, and prealiquotted reagents. Clearly, the negative control or blank (all reactants minus target DNA) is one of the most important controls for the assay. Many laboratories use multiple blanks interspersed between samples to monitor the development of false-positive reactions.

The problem of amplicon carry-over has been addressed by two different chemical modifications of the amplicon that make it an unsuitable target for further amplification. The first method replaces dTTP in the PCR reaction with dUTP. A bacterial enzyme, uracil-*N*-glycosylase (UNG), degrades DNA that contains uracil. Because uracil normally is not found in DNA, only amplicons are susceptible to degradation by UNG treatment. All PCR reactants are mixed with UNG before the reaction begins to allow degradation of amplicon. UNG is inactivated during the first denaturation cycle, so newly formed amplicon can accumulate normally during the reaction. In the other approach a psoralen derivative is added at the start of the PCR reaction. This compound does not interfere significantly with the amplification reaction and is stable during the temperature cycles. After the amplification reaction the unopened tubes are exposed to UV light, resulting in the formation of psoralen-pyrimidine adducts. These adducts do not interfere with hybridization of the amplicon but do prevent subsequent copying by polymerase. Neither method prevents contamination from any source other than amplicon carry-over.

Introducing PCR testing into a clinical context presents challenges quite apart from the concern of false-positive reactions. The sensitivity of true-positive PCR reactions commonly is better than any other "gold standard" assay, and this fact presents difficulties in interpretation. The clinical relevance of small numbers of organisms or altered genetic sequences that are detectable by the assay requires careful work to correlate clinical outcome with results obtained by PCR testing.

PCR testing theoretically should be applicable to nucleic acids within minimally purified samples. In practice, clinical samples contain unpredictable amounts of impurities that inhibit polymerase activity. To ensure reliable amplification, some form of nucleic acid purification often is used. The idiosyncratic nature of PCR inhibitors within clinical samples requires demonstration that the sample lysate can support amplification. This important control often takes the form of amplification of an endogenous target, such as β-globin. Failure to amplify β-globin indicates that further purification of sample is required to remove inhibitors of the reaction or that the sample DNA is degraded or too dilute.

Ligase chain reaction

The ligase chain reaction (LCR; LCx Probe System, Abbott Laboratories, Abbott Park, Ill.), presented schematically in Figure 11-5, uses four complementary oligonucleotide sequences totally spanning the target and a thermostable ligase.[16] When the oligonucleotides are annealed specifically to the target, the break or space between the 5' and 3' ends of adjacent molecules is repaired by the ligase enzyme, resulting in chemical linkage of the oligonucleotides. After denaturation the newly ligated DNA strands form additional target. The ligation reaction is particularly sensitive to mismatches at the junction of the oligos; a single base-pair mismatch prevents ligation from occurring. If the oligonucleotides join at a known mutation site and are selected to

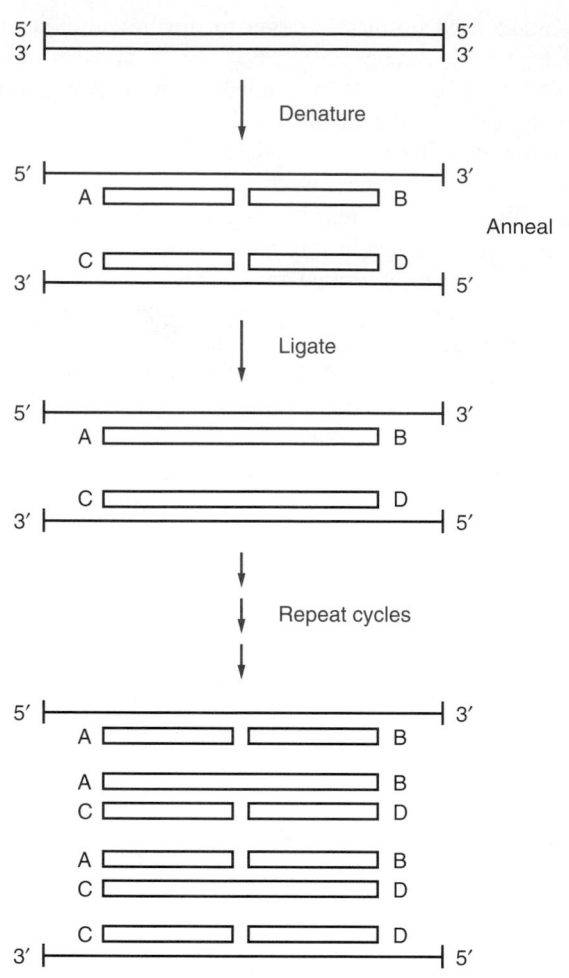

Figure 11-5 Schematic diagram of the LCR. *LCR,* Ligase chain reaction.

anneal with the mutated nucleotide, the LCR selectively enriches for the mutation. For example, the point mutation in an oncogene such as *ras* carried by a few malignant cells could be amplified selectively in a high background of normal *ras* genes carried by normal cells. Thus amplifications with the LCR detect point mutations easier than do PCR amplifications. The LCR is also more amenable to automation.

The disadvantages of LCR include the potential for blunt-end ligation—that is, target-independent ligation of oligos—which contributes to the background of the assay. LCR requires that the exact sequence of the region to be amplified is known. Synthesis of the annealing oligonucleotides, because of their length, is more expensive than synthesis of primers for PCR. Finally, the LCR does not permit detection of deletions.

Nucleic acid sequence-based amplification assays and transcription-mediated amplification

Nucleic acid sequence-based amplification[4] and transcription-mediated amplification[6] are commercial assay systems based on the self-sustained sequence replication

(3SR) assay.[5] Isothermal target amplification, through the use of the collective activities of reverse transcriptase—RNase H, and RNA polymerase—is common to these methods. The method may be applied to single-stranded RNA or dsDNA targets. With the exception of the initial denaturation for DNA targets, all the reactions proceed at the same temperature, so no temperature cycling is required. The reaction is adapted from the successful replication scheme of retroviruses. The single-stranded antisense RNA molecule is the amplicon that can accumulate to 10^9 copies. The RNA amplicon is hybridized readily, and carry-over contamination is less of a problem because of the labile nature of RNA.

Branched-chain DNA

Increased sensitivity can also be achieved by methods that amplify the detection or signal resulting from the hybridization assay. The branched-chain DNA (bDNA) approach developed by Chiron (Chiron Corporation, Emeryville, Calif.)[15] uses a sandwich hybridization assay, localizing the target nucleic acid with a capture probe affixed to a microtiter well and subsequently hybridizing with a target probe. After hybridization the target probe has free single-stranded portions that hybridize to the detection reagent, in this case a reporter probe that is a DNA molecule constructed of a recognition sequence and multiple side branches. Each branch has as many as three signal-generating enzymes, such as alkaline phosphatase, covalently bound. The result of this bottle-brush configuration is the very efficient localization of signal-producing enzymes to the target. Use of a chemiluminescent substrate allows the product to be quantitated with an ELISA-type format.

A significant strength of the signal amplification approach is that the danger of false-positive results from carry-over of target (amplified or native) is eliminated. The approach is well suited for quantitation. The limiting factor in these assays is that all initial hybridization steps before and including localization of the signal amplification reagent must be extremely specific. Any background or nonspecific localization of reagents results in background amplification (undesired), along with the desired signal amplification. The assay has been improved by the incorporation of artificial nucleotides (coined *iso-C* and *iso-G*). These nucleotides bind even tighter than the usual C and G, permitting extended washing and lower background signals.

Quantitation in amplification assays

Assays using amplification of target or signal to allow unprecedented sensitivity are highly complex and present significant challenges to quantitation of results. Variations in extraction efficiency and presence of enzyme inhibitors, lot to lot variation in enzyme and reagent performance, as well as day-to-day variation in reaction and detection conditions must be addressed in methods that attempt to yield a quantitative result. Despite these technical barriers, all the assays described previously have been adapted to quantify the original amount of target sequence in the sample analyzed. Several approaches are used. In the competitive assays a novel template is synthesized that is a different size from the expected amplicon. Each sample is assayed in multiple replicates, with a titered amount of competitive template added to each reaction. When target and competitor are present in equivalent amounts, the two different-sized products also are equivalent. The competitor is present in the same tube as the sample, so variations in enzyme activities affect both products identically. This approach is not used frequently in clinical applications because of the requirement for multiple aliquots of patient material and multiple assays for each patient.

Rather than relying on a competitive reaction, quantitation of sample nucleic acid may be determined by comparison to an added internal reference material or materials. The internal reference material may be added at the time of sample processing to control for efficiency of nucleic acid purification. Detection of target and standard in multiple dilutions of a single amplification reaction allows for quantitation. External calibrators, assayed as additional separate samples, also may be used to quantitate the results of these assays.

Restriction Fragment Length Polymorphisms

Hybridization assays are most specific when the probe utilized is unique for a disease-producing gene (for example, a marker gene for an infectious agent and a mutated sequence in a human gene that results in disease) so that the result directly discriminates between disease and nondisease in an individual. However, this approach requires a great deal of molecular information about the disease state before an appropriate probe and assay can be developed. In many situations this detailed information is not yet available. In other cases the goal is not disease detection but the establishment of identity or nonidentity between DNA samples, as in paternity or forensic testing. Analysis of **restriction fragment length polymorphisms** (**RFLP**, sometimes pronounced "rif-lip") provides an alternative method for characterization of a particular DNA sample.

As noted previously, restriction enzymes cut DNA into fragments of reproducible size; the same enzyme produces the same fragments in different samples if the samples contain the same DNA sequence. Southern blot analysis with a site-specific probe results in the detection of one or more fragments of a specified size. Changes in the sequence of the DNA may result in different fragment sizes when the changes result in loss or introduction of a recognition site for the restriction enzyme or when a significant amount of DNA is added or lost between restriction sites. The majority of such changes occur within noncoding DNA, so the RFLP pattern change may have no phenotypic expression. Sequence changes may be the result of mutation events or may occur because of differences in the lengths of repeat se-

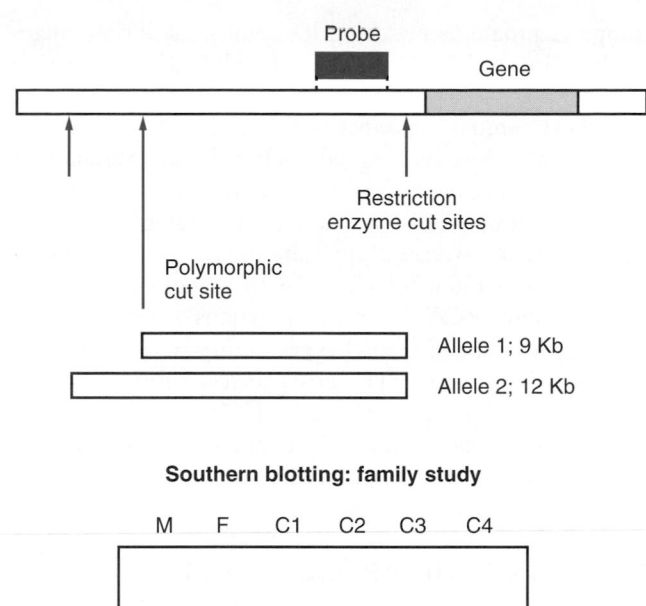

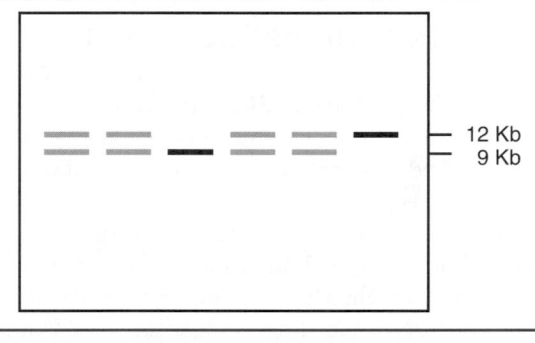

Southern blotting: family study

Figure 11-6   Example of RFLP analysis. For example, if the 12-kilobase (Kb) allele correlated with a recessive disease, child 4 would be affected, child 1 would be unaffected, and the rest of the family members would be unaffected heterozygotic carriers. *RFLP*, Restriction fragment length polymorphism; *M*, mother; *F*, father; *C*, child. (Modified from Piper MA, Unger ER: Nucleic Acid Probes: A Primer for Pathologists, Chicago, ASCP Press, 1989.)

quences. The human genome contains families of repetitive sequences, or **variable numbers of tandem repeats (VNTRs).** Particular fragment sizes or RFLPs at polymorphic sites, including VNTRs, tend to be inherited and are relatively stable in family studies, thus producing a genetic "fingerprint." They can be used for identity testing in paternity and forensic studies (see following discussion). Using combinations of restriction enzymes and probes, studies have linked particular RFLPs to genetic disease when the responsible gene is unknown. This technique can be used diagnostically in family studies (Figure 11-6).

Sequencing

Although DNA sequencing had only research applications in the past, a few clinical laboratories have begun to use this technique for clinical tests. The actual base sequence of the gene of interest can be determined and compared to the reference sequence. Usually the sequence is determined in each direction (sense and antisense) for accuracy. Any deviation from the reference sequence is identified through the use of computer programs matching the sequences. Base changes resulting in a stop codon or altered amino acid code, frame shift mutations, and deletions or insertions are identified. The most common automated sequencing procedures use four different florescent tagged nucleotides in a variation of the Sanger dideoxy sequencing method,[12] followed by agarose gel electrophoresis and automated reading of the dye-tagged products. Current applications include detection of germ-line mutations associated with malignancy, such as BRCA-1 and BRCA-2; somatic mutations occurring in malignancy, such as p53; and changes in infectious agents that may influence therapy or prognosis, such as human immunodeficiency virus (HIV) and hepatitis C virus (HCV). In each instance the number and size of possible genetic changes preclude an alternative, more rapid method of detection.

◼ DIAGNOSTIC APPLICATIONS

Clinical laboratory methods traditionally have provided information needed for accurate and specific diagnosis of disease. Nucleic acid analyses have the potential to expand the role of the laboratory beyond diagnosis to include assays guiding therapy and providing prognostic information. In most instances application of molecular techniques requires a well-founded clinical suspicion of a particular disease or condition. Open-ended screening assays based on this technology are not yet a reality. Thus rather than being replaced, standard laboratory methods are supplemented and enhanced by this technology. The following sections include examples of current types of diagnostic applications of nucleic acid analysis in the areas of infectious disease, hematological malignancies, solid tumors, genetic disease, and identity testing.

Infectious Disease

The traditional approach to detection and diagnosis of an infectious agent has been the use of appropriate stains and direct visualization, culture and isolation, or detection of host antibodies. However, many organisms are not identified easily by staining, culture is laborious and requires long periods of incubation, and some organisms require expensive media for culture or cannot be cultured at all. Measuring the host antibody response may not be informative during the acute phase of the infection or may not distinguish between past and present infection. Nucleic acid probes have the potential to detect directly genetic information of a pathogen in the specimen. Pathogen viability and specimen transport time and conditions no longer may be important issues because nucleic acid is a relatively stable target. Theoretically, probes also can be designed to detect antibiotic-resistance genes. Due to the cost of reagents, equipment, and trained personnel, molecular assays for infectious agents have tended to focus on those organisms that are otherwise difficult to identify within a clinically appropriate time frame.

Direct hybridization for the detection of microorganisms in patient samples is the simplest approach for pathogen diagnosis; however, the analytical sensitivity is limited. Direct probe hybridization methods require on the order of 10^4 copies of target sequence for detection. Selection of probes directed at naturally amplified targets, such as ribosomal sequences or repetitive genetic regions, improves sensitivity. Modifications of the hybridization format and detection systems to improve signal and reduce background also have been used. In some clinical settings the limit of detection in these assays is adequate, and further lowering of the limit of detection may result in detection of infections without clinical significance. Most commercially available tests utilize solution phase hybridization with chemiluminescent detection, and many have been adapted to microtitre plate format to facilitate automation.

In some instances combining in vitro culture with a hybridization assay may facilitate identification of infection. This approach relies on the ability of the hybridization assay to specifically detect very few organisms that could not be identified with conventional methods. The time of culture can be shortened significantly, a fact that is particularly important for slow-growing organisms.

Amplification methods first were introduced into the clinical laboratory for infectious disease applications. Amplification of target or signal significantly increases the analytical sensitivity of these assays. Commercial assays address concerns of false positive reactions through the use of chemical methods limiting amplicon carry-over. Quantitative amplification assays recently have been developed. Recent studies emphasize the importance of quantitative determination of HIV and HCV in the monitoring of the response of antiviral therapy.

Leukemias and Lymphomas

Leukemias and lymphomas are malignancies of the hematopoietic cells. They are diagnosed conventionally based on morphology and cell-surface proteins. Myeloid and lymphoid malignancies generally exhibit cell-surface markers that correspond to a normal developmental stage. Monoclonal antibodies and flow cytometry usually can characterize malignant populations according to the combination of markers present on the cell surface (immunophenotyping). This information is extremely useful for staging, prognosis, and treatment. In some cases, however, surface markers are not expressed or the abnormal population is too small to be detected. Nucleic acid hybridization assays complement conventional assays to provide additional information about cell lineage, clonality, molecular characterization of cytogenetic changes, and detection of minimal residual disease.

Cell lineage and clonality

Physical rearrangement of DNA is characteristic of the normal development of T- and B-lymphocytes. These rearrangements take place in the genes that code for immunoglobulins and other antigen-reactive cell-surface receptors. Using probes specific for particular coding regions of each of the receptor protein genes, together with a battery of restriction enzymes, visualization of DNA fragment sizes characteristic of the germline (nonlymphoid) and rearranged (lymphoid) receptor gene configuration is possible, through the use of Southern blot analysis of peripheral blood or bone marrow. In normal specimens only a germline band is visible because each lymphoid cell has a slightly different gene rearrangement and the individual different fragment sizes are below the limits of detection. However, if a clonal population is present, all the cells belonging to the clone have the same gene rearrangement and fragment size, and a new band is seen on the blot. This assay can detect a clonal population constituting 1% to 5% of the sample. By testing for both Ig and T cell receptor genes, the establishment of lymphoid cellular lineage in a clonal population is possible. PCR also can be used to amplify unique sequences that indicate gene rearrangement has occurred in various receptor genes. For this application a battery of probes or probes developed specifically for the patient's aberrant clone are used.

Molecular detection of characteristic cytogenetic changes

Translocations are the result of abnormal chromosomal breakage and exchange of large portions of chromosomes. Some translocations, as well as other extensive chromosomal abnormalities detectable by cytogenetic analysis, are associated nonrandomly with particular hematological malignancies. These cytogenetic changes can be used to classify disease and determine prognosis.

One well-known example is the reciprocal translocation between the c-*abl* gene on chromosome 9 and the breakpoint cluster region (bcr) on chromosome 22 that occurs in chronic myelogenous leukemia. This exchange results in an altered marker chromosome known as the *Philadelphia chromosome (Ph)*. Specific nucleic acid probes can detect DNA change from the c-*abl*-bcr gene rearrangement by Southern blot or interphase-fluorescence in situ hybridization (FISH). Alternatively, the production of the chimeric mRNA can be detected by Northern blot or RT-PCR. Translocations cannot be detected easily by direct DNA PCR because of the large fragments involved. Similar applications can detect a variety of chromosomal abnormalities in other kinds of leukemia and in lymphoma. These methods complement conventional cytogenetic analysis and may reduce the need for repeat analyses. However, because probes specific for each abnormality of interest must be chosen in advance, these assays are useful as screening assays only for the most common abnormalities.

Minimal residual disease

The same molecular methods that aid in diagnosis of leukemias and lymphomas can be used to monitor the response to therapy and detect disease that persists or recurs after therapy. Because of the high sensitivity of amplification methods the molecular signature of the malignant clone can be detected in samples that are normal by conventional morphological, immunochemical, or cytogenetic analysis. Clinical trials currently are being conducted to determine the clinical significance of these abnormal cells that otherwise would go undetected. The hope is that early detection of treatment failures can provide the opportunity for more effective salvage therapy.

Solid Tumors

Application of molecular biology to the study of cancer has led to the concept of cancer as a genetic disease of somatic cells. Characterization of the genes involved in the multistep process of malignant transformation has identified two broad categories of such genes—those that act to induce tumor formation (oncogenes) and those that act to inhibit tumor formation (tumor suppressor genes). The discovery of genes carried by retroviruses capable of conferring malignant properties to the infected cell gave rise to the concept of oncogenes, that is, genes capable of "causing cancer." This discovery proved to be an overly simplistic view, as further investigation into the nature of these genes demonstrated that very closely related genes (proto-oncogenes, or cellular oncogenes) are normal cell constituents involved in the normal physiology of cell growth, proliferation, and differentiation. Conversion of a proto-oncogene to an oncogene is referred to as *oncogene activation*. Oncogene activation may result from point mutations, altering stability or activity of the product; increased expression secondary to gene amplification; or a translocation that places the gene under the control of an abnormal promoter. Oncogenes act dominantly through the addition of abnormal product. Tumor suppressor genes are oncogenic through the loss of specific gene function. These genes apparently are involved in controlling or restraining cellular growth and division. Loss of the gene product thus could permit unregulated cell division. The prototypic example of this gene family is the retinoblastoma gene, *RB*. Other tumor suppressor genes include *p53* and *DCC* (deleted in colon cancer).

Hereditary cancer

Hereditary cancer and familial cancer syndromes are cancers associated with germ-line alterations in one or more genes. The mutations associated with several of these cancers have been identified and cloned, including hereditary retinoblastoma *(RB)*, medullary thyroid cancer *(RET)*, breast/ovarian cancer *(BRCA1* and *BRCA2)*, and colorectal cancer *(APC, MSH2,* and *MLH1)*. With the exception of BRCA mutations, the same genes often are found altered in sporadic cancers of the same sites, providing insight into the multiple steps involved in carcinogenesis. The identification of genes associated with inherited cancer syndromes raises the question of the appropriate role of genetic testing for these genes. In the hereditary colorectal cancer syndromes, presymptomatic genotyping of at-risk family members can alter clinical recommendations for surveillance. The situation for BRCA mutations is more difficult because of the large number of described alterations, the unproven predictive value of each mutation for lifetime risk of disease (variable penetrance and potential for polymorphisms), and the lack of effective methods for intervention. Further study is required to guide the appropriate clinical use of molecular testing in these hereditary cancer syndromes.

Molecular markers

Solid tumors have a myriad of somatic alterations, and much research is being directed toward the determination of which changes have diagnostic and prognostic importance. Although technology exists for the determination of oncogene translocations, mutations, deletions, amplifications, and message levels, this information is clinically useful only if it can be used to modify treatment (that is, predict outcome) or contribute to diagnosis. Morphological methods undoubtedly will remain central to solid tumor diagnosis, but molecular methods can be predicted increasingly to supply additional information to guide treatment. This trend is evidenced by the situation for breast cancer, in which Her-2/neu amplifications have prognostic significance and determine therapy. In addition, genetic alterations specifically associated with tumors can be used as molecular markers for the early detection of disease. These applications are still in development, but the principles are gaining acceptance.

Genetic Disease

Genetic mutations or DNA sequence changes that result in synthesis of a dysfunctional or nonfunctional protein or that alter the regulation or expression of a protein can cause disease. **Mutations** can be grouped into the following major categories:

1. Point mutations
2. Insertions or deletions with or without frameshift
3. Unstable expansion of trinucleotide repeats
4. Translocations

A point mutation is a single base pair substitution resulting in a missense or nonsense mutation. A missense mutation is caused by a base substitution that alters the translation of the affected codon triplet, resulting from an altered protein product. A nonsense mutation involves a base substitution that modifies a triplet codon to become a stop codon, resulting in a premature halt in translation. Insertion or deletion mutations can add or subtract amino acid codons. If the insertion or deletion base-pair length is not a multiple of three (that is, a codon length), the result is a shift in the reading frame and a subsequent amino acid sequence that may bear no relation to the normal sequence after the mutation point. In an exon region a mutation can change amino acid codons, result in a premature stop codon, or

change a stop codon to an amino acid codon. Any mutation in a regulatory sequence, such as a splice site, can have a profound effect on the protein product. Trinucleotide repeat expansions are due to an increase in the number of repeat sequences in genes. The affected gene normally contains a limited number of the short repeated sequence of three bases. Disease is associated with the expansion of the triplet repeat beyond the normal range. Some genetic diseases are the result of a single specific mutation that always characterizes that disease; others are characterized by a variety of mutations, resulting in variants of the same disease. In addition, not all mutations are inherited; some arise spontaneously (de novo mutations), adding to the difficulty of characterization of DNA changes associated with a genetic disease.

An essential requirement for the assay of genetic diseases is knowledge of the specific chromosome, gene, and mutation within the gene causing the disease. Direct analysis comprises those procedures that directly detect the mutation known to be responsible for a specific disease. Examples of these assays include dot or slot blot hybridization analysis (usually as a screening assay) of patient samples through the use of oligonucleotide probes to determine the presence of a subset of abnormal DNA molecules. Hybridization in these blot assays typically is assessed by autoradiography. Other direct mutation tests allow for the identification of the precise mutation of interest within a gene that might contain several possible mutations. This type of testing includes nuclease mapping assays that examine amplified DNA products through the use of digestion techniques with appropriate restriction enzymes and ensuing visualization of the generated restriction fragments.

If the genetic disease has a large component of unknown mutations or the disease-associated gene sequence or the disease-causing mutation is unknown, indirect analysis must be performed. Linkage analysis entails DNA sequence testing of affected and unaffected siblings and parents of the patient. This type of testing requires knowledge of closely linked or flanking polymorphic DNA sequences that reliably cosegregate with the normal or disease-causing genes. Linkage analysis depends on the idea that the polymorphic DNA marker and the gene are inherited together, and thus the gene need only be mapped to a specific location on a chromosome.

Applications of genetic testing fall into four basic classes. Carrier testing involves the detection of recessive mutations in healthy individuals who may be at risk for transmitting the mutations to offspring; it is characteristically performed for purposes of genetic counseling. Additionally, population-based carrier screening of large groups of individuals who have no family history of disease but may be at risk because of ethnicity can be performed. Diagnostic genetic testing is performed on a symptomatic individual with symptoms that are sufficiently suggestive of the disease in question. This type of testing is most advantageous for early or nonclassic clinical presentations but can be done postmortem, as in testing for sudden infant death syndrome genetic mutations. Detection of genetic disease in utero, prenatal genetic testing, is performed to identify an affected fetus with the possibility of termination of the pregnancy. The most controversial type of testing for genetic disease is referred to as *presymptomatic testing*. This form of testing may be used to help the offspring of individuals with late-onset dominant disorders determine his or her likelihood of inheriting the disease-associated mutations. Results obtained from these tests are used to make informed decisions regarding reproduction, initiation of preventive measures, or simple preparation for the future.

Identity Testing

Nucleic acid techniques can help determine relatedness between individuals or specimens and an individual. Common questions that arise include the following:

What is the chance that a kidney transplant will be rejected?
Is a specific man the father of a child?
Is this blood spot from a specific person?

Human leukocyte antigen typing for transplantation

In transplantation tissue typing the primary goal is to match donor and recipient human leukocyte antigen (HLA) phenotypes as closely as possible to diminish the likelihood of transplant rejection. The major histocompatibility complex on chromosome 6p in the human contains the HLA region, which is subdivided into three classes of highly polymorphic genes, two of which are important in tissue typing. Class I genes encode the classic transplantation antigens that function as targets in T-lymphocyte recognition sites and are found on the surface of all nucleated cells in association with β_2-microglobulin. Commercially available antibody panels using well-characterized antisera and patient leukocytes are used to type these antigens. The second set of genes, the class II genes, which are coded for in the HLA-D region, produces glycoproteins that are localized on the surface of B-lymphocytes, monocytes, macrophages, and activated T-cells. These protein antigens can stimulate the proliferation of T-cells from genetically dissimilar individuals in a mixed lymphocyte culture. Three distinct loci code for these antigens are referred to as *DR, DQ,* and *DP.* These regions, particularly DR and DQ, are the most useful clini-

cally when DNA probes are used to type polymorphisms in HLA phenotypes before organ transplantation. The DP locus appears to be related specifically to graft-versus-host reactivity, which can occur in bone marrow transplantation. The differences in nucleotide sequences of the D regions result in the presence or absence of recognition sites for specific restriction enzymes that give rise to DNA fragments. Nucleic acid techniques used in transplantation and tissue typing include amplification and nuclease mapping with allelic sequence-specific oligo probes. Some laboratories are beginning to use sequencing.

Paternity and forensic analysis

Class II antigen typing using DNA probes also has been applied to areas other than tissue transplantation. Because of the high degree of polymorphism discovered by molecular methods, molecular typing of DR and DQ alleles has been applied to forensic analysis and paternity testing, where polymorphic markers are useful in the establishment of identity or familial relationship.

Other types of polymorphic DNA markers are now in routine use for identity testing. For example, minisatellite or VNTR DNA (see previous RFLP discussion) can exhibit a high degree of polymorphism because of the variable number of repeat units. Minisatellite DNA from different individuals can result in different fragment sizes in a Southern blot analysis when an appropriate combination of probe and restriction enzyme is used. When minisatellite DNA probes are used at sufficient stringency to operate as single-locus probes, specific fragment sizes from this type of RFLP analysis behave as genetic markers and are inherited independently. Thus minisatellite DNA analysis can be used to establish paternity and identity among forensic specimens. Identity studies also have been performed with multilocus probes, probes that detect blocks of repeated DNA at more than one chromosomal location. RFLP analysis with these probes results in many more bands per probe and can be used in much the same way as a fingerprint. However, multilocus probes tend to be more difficult to use, less sensitive, and less useful in cases of mixed samples. As with most DNA hybridization assays, PCR can be added to the methodologies described previously to amplify the available DNA sample. This addition is extremely useful in forensic testing, in which the sample is often the limiting factor.

References

1. Anderson MLM, Young BD: Quantitative filter hybridisation. In Hames BD, Higgins SJ (eds): Nucleic Acid Hybridisation: A Practical Approach, pp 73-110, Oxford, IRL Press, 1985.
2. Baltimore D: Viral RNA-dependent DNA polymerase. Nature 1970; 226:1209-1211.
3. Blackburn GM, Gait MJ (eds): Nucleic Acids in Chemistry and Biology, pp 21-30, Oxford, IRL Press, 1990.
4. Compton J: Nucleic acid sequence-based amplification. Nature 1991; 350:91-92.

5. Guatelli JC, Whitfield KM, Kwoh DY et al: Isothermal, *in vitro* amplification of nucleic acids by a multienzyme reaction modeled after retroviral replication. Proc Natl Acad Sci USA 1990; 87:1874-1878.

6. Jonas V, Alden MJ, Curry JI et al: Detection and identification of *Mycobacterium tuberculosis* directly from sputum sediments by amplification of rRNA. J Clin Microbiol 1993; 31:2410-2416.

7. Kornberg A: Ligases and polynucleotide kinases. In Kornberg A, Baker T (eds): DNA Replication, 2nd edition, New York, WH Freeman, 1991.

8. Kornberg A: DNA polymerase I of *Escherichia coli.* In Kornberg A, Baker T (eds): DNA Replication, 2nd edition, New York, WH Freeman, 1991.

9. Kowk S, Higuchi R: Avoiding false positives with PCR. Nature 1989; 339:237-238.

10. Mullis KB, Faloona FA: Specific synthesis of DNA in vitro via a polymerase-catalyzed chain reaction. Methods Enzymol 1987; 155:335-350.

11. Sambrook J, Fritsch EF, Maniatis T (eds): Molecular Cloning: A Laboratory Manual, 2nd edition, p E.3, Cold Spring Harbor, NY, Cold Spring Harbor Laboratory, 1989.

12. Sanger F, Nicklen S, Coulson AR: DNA sequencing with chain-terminating inhibitors. Proc Natl Acad Sci USA 1970; 74:5463-5467.

13. Smith HO: Nucleotide sequence specificity of restriction endonucleases. Science 1979; 205:455-462.

14. Southern EM: Detection of specific sequences among DNA fragments separated by gel electrophoresis. J Mol Biol 1975; 98:503-517.

15. Ureda MS, Horn T, Fultz J et al: Branched DNA amplification multimers for the sensitive direct detection of human hepatitis viruses. Nucleic Acids Symp Ser 1991; 24:197-200.

16. Wu DY, Wallace RB: The ligation amplification reaction (LAR)-amplification of specific DNA sequences using sequential rounds of template-dependent ligation. Genomics 1989; 4:560-569.

Additional Reading

Alberts B, Bray D, Lewis J et al: Molecular Biology of the Cell, 3rd edition, New York, Garland Publishing, 1995.

Ausubel FM, Brent R, Kingston RE et al (eds): Current Protocols in Molecular Biology, New York, John Wiley & Sons, 1987 [looseleaf, three-volume manual with quarterly updates].

Bloomfield VA, Crothers DM, Ticoco I et al: Nucleic Acids: Structures, Properties, and Functions, Sausalito, Calif, University Science Books, 2000.

Coleman WD, Tsongalis GJ: Molecular Diagnostics for the Clinical Laboratory, Totowa, NJ, Humana Press, 1996.

Farkas DH (ed): Molecular Biology and Pathology: A Guidebook for Quality Control, San Diego, Academic Press, 1993.

Mitchell PS, Persing DH: Current trends in molecular microbiology. Lab Med 1999; 30:263-270.

Persing DH, Smith TF, Tenover FC et al (eds): Diagnostic Molecular Microbiology: Principles and Applications, Washington, DC, American Society for Microbiology, 1993.

CHAPTER 12

Automation in the Clinical Laboratory*

JAMES C. BOYD, MD, and DONALD S. YOUNG, MB, PhD

Objectives

1. Distinguish among the batch, random-access, discrete, sequential, single- and multiple-channel, centrifugal, and continuous-flow approaches to automation.
2. List the 11 most commonly automated operations of a chemical analysis and describe each operation individually.
3. Describe an integrated, automated laboratory workstation.
4. Define *point-of-care testing* and provide examples of point-of-care analyzers.

Key Words

Analyzer Configuration   The format in which analytical instruments are configured; available in both open and closed systems; in an open system the operator modifying the assay parameters and purchasing reagents from a variety of sources; in a closed system most assay parameters being set by the manufacturer, who also provides reagents in a unique container or format

Automation   The process whereby an analytical instrument performs many tests with only minimal involvement of an analyst; also defined as the controlled operation of an apparatus, process, or system by mechanical or electronic devices without human intervention

Batch Analysis   A type of analysis in which many specimens are processed in the same analytical session, or "run"

Carry-Over   The transport of a quantity of analyte or reagent from one specimen reaction into and contaminating a subsequent one

Centralized Testing   A mode of testing in which specimens are transported to a central, or "core," facility for analysis

Continuous-Flow Analysis   A type of analysis in which each specimen in a batch passes through the same continuous stream at the same rate and is subjected to the same analytical reactions

Core Laboratory   A type of centralized laboratory to which samples are transported for analysis

Discrete Analysis   A type of analysis in which each specimen in a batch has its own physical and chemical space separate from every other specimen

Multiple-Channel Analysis   A type of analysis in which each specimen is subjected to multiple analytical processes so that a set of test results is obtained on a single specimen; also known as *multitest analysis*

Parallel Analysis   A type of analysis in which all specimens are subjected to a series of analytical processes at the same time and in a parallel fashion

Point-of-Care Testing (POCT)   A mode of testing in which the analysis is performed at the site where health care is provided; also known as *bedside, near-patient, decentralized,* and *off-site testing*

Random-Access Analysis   A type of analysis in which any specimen, by a command to the processing system, is analyzed by any available process in or out of sequence with other specimens and without regard to their initial order

---

*The authors acknowledge the original contributions by Earnest Maclin, PE, on which portions of this chapter are based.

Sequential Analysis   A type of analysis in which each specimen in a batch enters the analytical process one after another, and each result or set of results emerges in the same order as the specimens are entered

Single-Channel Analysis   A type of analysis in which each specimen is subjected to a single process so that only results for a single analyte are produced; also known as *single-test analysis*

Specimen Throughput Rate   The rate at which an analytical system processes specimens

Unit-Dose Reagents   Reagents packaged such that only one package is used per assay

The term **automation** has been applied in clinical chemistry to describe the process whereby an analytical instrument performs many tests with only minimal involvement of an analyst. The availability of automated instruments enables laboratories to process much larger workloads without comparable increases in staff. The evolution of automation in the clinical laboratory has paralleled that in the manufacturing industry, progressing from fixed automation, whereby an instrument performs a repetitive task by itself, to programmable automation, which allows the instrument to perform a variety of different tasks. More recently, intelligent automation has been introduced into some individual instruments or systems to allow them to self-monitor and respond appropriately to changing conditions.

One benefit of automation is a reduction in the variability of results and errors of analysis through the elimination of tasks that are repetitive and monotonous for most individuals. The improved reproducibility gained by automation has led to a significant improvement in the quality of laboratory tests.

In recent years many small laboratories have consolidated into larger, more efficient entities in response to market trends involving cost reduction. The drive to automate these mega-laboratories has led to new avenues in laboratory automation. No longer is automation simply being used to assist the laboratory technologist in test performance, but it now includes (1) processing and transport of specimens, (2) loading of specimens into automated analyzers, and (3) assessment of the results of the performed tests. Automating these additional functions is key to the future prosperity of the clinical laboratory.[1,3]

This chapter discusses the principles that apply to automation of the individual steps of the analytical process—both in individual analyzers and in the integration of automation throughout the clinical laboratory.

■ BASIC CONCEPTS

Automated analyzers generally incorporate mechanized versions of basic manual laboratory techniques and procedures. However, modern instrumentation is packaged in a wide variety of configurations. The most common configuration is the random-access analyzer. In **random-access analysis** analyses are performed on a collection of specimens sequentially, with each specimen analyzed for a different selection of tests. The tests performed in the random-access analyzers are selected through the use of different vials of liquid reagents, different reagent packs, or different reagent tablets, depending on the analyzer. This approach permits measurement of a variable number and variety of analytes in each specimen. Profiles or groups of tests are defined for a specimen at the time the tests to be performed are entered into the analyzer via a keyboard (in most systems), by instruction from a laboratory information system in conjunction with bar coding on the specimen tube, or by operator selection of appropriate reagent packs.

Historically, other **analyzer configurations** used include centrifugal analyzers, continuous-flow analyzers, and modular analyzers. Centrifugal analyzers use discrete pipetting to load specimens and reagents sequentially into the discrete vessels in a rotor, and the specimens subsequently are analyzed by a **parallel analysis.** The rotor contains specimens for several different tests at the same time, each test being read at selected different optical wavelengths. All results for a single rotor typically are available in 2 to 6 minutes, determined by the length of time of the slowest reaction. Because the rotor has a fixed number of vessels, centrifugal analyzers are run in "batched" mode, performing **batch analysis** on the specimens loaded in each rotor.

Continuous-flow analyzers historically were the first automated analyzers used in clinical laboratories. Initially these analyzers were used in a **single-channel analysis** configuration and carried out a **sequential analysis** of each specimen. Subsequently, **multiple-channel analysis** versions were developed in which analysis of each specimen was performed on every channel in parallel. Results from nonrequested tests in the test profile were discarded as necessary after the analysis was complete. The inflexibility in the menu of tests that could be performed on these analyzers eventually led to their replacement in the marketplace by more versatile configurations.

Modular analyzers were developed by manufacturers to provide scaleability and increase operational efficiency. The addition of a module often is used to increase the analyzer's **specimen throughput rate** as measured in the number of test results produced per hour. Modules also may add functionality to an analyzer, such as with the addition of an ion-selective electrode module for measurement of electrolytes. In random-access analyzers additional modules may provide a wider menu of available tests.

AUTOMATION OF THE ANALYTICAL PROCESSES

The following individual steps required to complete an analysis often are referred to collectively as *unit operations:*

1. Specimen identification
2. Specimen preparation
3. Specimen delivery
4. Specimen handling and transport
5. Specimen processing
6. Sample introduction and internal transport
7. Reagent handling and storage
8. Reagent delivery
9. Chemical reaction phase
10. Measurement approaches
11. Signal processing, data handling, and process control

These operations are described individually in this section, with examples that demonstrate how they have been automated in terms of operational and analytical performance. In most automated systems these steps usually are performed sequentially, but in some instruments they may occur in parallel.

Specimen Identification

Typically the identifying link (identifier) between patient and specimen is made at the patient's bedside, and the maintenance of this connection throughout transport of the specimen to the laboratory, subsequent specimen analysis, and preparation of a report is essential. A variety of manual and automated techniques have been used to establish and maintain specimen identification. A wide variety of technologies are available for automatic identification and data collection purposes, including bar coding, optical character recognition, magnetic stripe and magnetic ink character recognition, voice identification, radiofrequency identification, touch screens, light pens, hand print tablets, optical mark readers, and smart cards. In practice, automatic identification includes only those technologies that electronically detect a unique characteristic or unique data string associated with a physical object. For example, identifiers, such as serial number, part number, color, manufacturer, patient number, and Social Security number, have been used to identify an object or patient through the use of electronic data processing. In the clinical laboratory bar coding has become the technology most widely used for purposes of automatic identification.

Identification by labeling

In many laboratory information systems electronic entry of a test order either in the laboratory or at a nursing station for a uniquely identified patient generates a specimen label bearing a unique laboratory accession number. A record is established that remains incomplete until a result (or set of results) is entered into the computer against the accession number. The unique label is affixed to the specimen collection tube when the blood is drawn. Proper alignment of the label on the collection tube is critical for subsequent specimen processing when bar-coded labels are used. Arrival of the specimen in the laboratory is recorded by a manual or computerized log-in procedure. In other systems the specimen is labeled at the patient's bedside, along with the patient identification and collection information, and enters the laboratory with a requisition form; there it is assigned an accession number as part of the log-in procedure, which may or may not be computer implemented.

After accessioning, specimens begin the technical handling processes. For those processes requiring physical removal of serum from the original tube, secondary labels bearing essential information from the original label must be affixed to any secondary tubes created. Some automated analyzers sample directly from the original collection tube while simultaneously reading the accession number from the bar-code label on the tube. Secondary bar-code labels, if necessary, may be generated at the time of accessioning or in some analyzers by a built-in printer that is activated when the analyzer is programmed.

Many methods are used to achieve secondary labeling when bar-coded labels are not available. A number may be handwritten on the specimen cup, or a coded label may be affixed to the original tube or to a specimen cup. The label numbers may require correlation with a manual or computer-generated work or load list. The load list usually records accession numbers in sequence with the physical positions of the cups or tubes in the loading zone of the analyzer. This loading zone may be a revolving tray or turntable, a mechanical belt, or a rack or set of racks by which specimens are delivered in a predetermined order to the sample aspiration station of the analyzer.

In those analyzers that do not link specimen identity and sample aspiration automatically, the sequence of results produced must be linked manually with the sequence of entry of specimens. Some analyzers print out or transmit to a host computer each result or set of results from a specimen, either through the position of the specimen in the loading zone or the accession number programmed to that position.

Bar coding

A major advance in the automation of specimen identification in the clinical laboratory is the incorporation of bar-coding technology into analytical systems. In practice a bar-coded label (often generated by the laboratory information system and bearing the sample accession number) is placed onto the specimen container and is subsequently "read" by one or more bar-code readers that have been strategically placed at key positions in the analytical sequence. The resultant identifying and ancillary information then is transferred to and processed by the system software.

Unequivocal positive identification of each specimen is achieved in analyzers with bar-code readers in less than 2 seconds. Advantages of the use of coded labels include the following:

1. Elimination of work lists for the system
2. Avoidance of mix-ups in the placement of tubes in the analyzer or during sampling
3. Analysis of specimens in a defined sequence
4. Avoidance of possible tube mix-up when serum must be transferred into a secondary container

Examples of bar codes that are used in chemistry analyzers are illustrated in Figure 12-1.

A bar-coding system consists of a bar code and a bar-code reader, or scanner. One- and two-dimensional bar-coding systems are available. Of the two, one-dimensional bar codes have been the most widely used in the clinical laboratory.

A one-dimensional bar code is an array of rectangular bars and spaces arranged in a predetermined pattern following unambiguous rules to represent elements of data referred to as *characters*. A bar code is transferred and affixed to an object by a "bar-code label" that carries the bar code and, optionally, other noncoded readable information. *Symbology* is the term used to describe the rules specifying the way the data are encoded into the bars and spaces. The width of the bars and spaces, as well as the number of each, is determined by a specification for that symbology. Different combinations of the bars and spaces represent different characters. When a bar-code scanner is passed over the bar code, the light beam from the scanner is absorbed by the dark bars and not re-flected; the beam is reflected by the light spaces. A photocell detector in the scanner receives the reflected light and converts that light into an electrical signal that then is digitized. A one-dimensional bar code is "vertically redundant" in that the same information is repeated vertically—the heights of the bars can be truncated without any loss of information. In practice, vertical redundancy allows a symbol with printing defects, such as spots or voids, to be read.

Identification errors

Many opportunities arise for the mismatch of specimens and results. The risks begin at the bedside and are compounded with each processing step a specimen undergoes between collection from the patient and analysis by the instrument. The risks are particularly great when hand transcription is invoked for accessioning, labeling and relabeling, and creation of load lists. An incorrect accession number, one in which the digits are transposed, or a load list with transposed accession numbers may cause test results to be attributed to the wrong patient. An additional hazard exists when specimens must be inserted into certain positions in the loading zone defined by a load list. Human misreading of either specimen label or loading list may cause misplacement of specimens, calibrators, or controls. Automatic reading of bar-coded labels reduces the error rate from 1 in 300 characters (for human entry) to about 1 in 1 million characters.

Specimen Preparation

The clotting of blood in specimen collection tubes, their subsequent centrifugation, and the transfer of serum to secondary tubes requires a finite time to complete. If performed manually, the process results in a delay in the preparation of a specimen for analysis. To eliminate the problems associated with specimen preparation, systems are being developed to automate this process. The following developments are noteworthy.

Use of whole blood for analysis

When whole blood is used in an assay system, specimen preparation time essentially is eliminated. Automated or semiautomated ion-selective electrodes, which measure ion activity in whole blood rather than ion concentration, have been incorporated into automated systems to provide certain test results within minutes of the drawing of a specimen. This approach now is used commonly for assays of electrolytes and some other common analytes. Another approach involves either manual or automated application of whole blood to dry reagent films and visual or instrumental observation of a quantitative change.

Automation of specimen preparation

Several manufacturers have developed fully automated specimen preparation systems. (These systems will be described in later sections of this chapter.)

Figure 12-1   Examples of bar codes used in chemistry analyzers; all examples contain the same information. **A,** Code 39. **B,** Code I 2/5. **C,** Code 128B. **D,** Codabar. (Courtesy Computer Transceiver Systems, Inc.)

Specimen Delivery

Several methods may be used to deliver specimens to the laboratory, including courier service, pneumatic tube systems, electric track vehicles, and mobile robots.

Courier service

Historically, couriers have been used to transport specimens from collection sites to the laboratory and between laboratories. Although in general reliable, courier service does create certain problems. Delivery is a batch process, and couriers usually only service a given pickup point at specified times. Arrangements for immediate pickup are possible, but they add costs to the analytical process and delay results reporting. In addition, specimen breakage or loss often occurs when specimens are handled manually.

Pneumatic tube systems

Pneumatic tube systems provide rapid specimen transportation and are reliable when installed as point-to-point services. However, when switching mechanisms are introduced to allow carriers (the bullet-shaped containers used to hold specimens) to be sent to various locations, additional mechanical problems arise and cause misrouting of carriers. Close attention to the design of the pneumatic tube system is necessary to prevent hemolysis of the specimen; avoidance of sudden accelerations and decelerations and the use of proper packing material inside the carriers are essential in this regard.

Electric track vehicles

Electric track vehicles have larger carrying capacities than do pneumatic tube systems and some automatically maintain the carrier in an upright position. Compared with pneumatic tube systems, electric track vehicles usually require larger stations for loading and unloading, and this fact often limits where a station may be placed. Electric track systems also promote batching of specimens, similar to courier services.

Mobile robots

Mobile robots have been used successfully to transport laboratory specimens both within[7] and outside the central laboratory.[15] Further studies are needed to establish the usefulness of mobile robots for specimen transport, but already apparent is that mobile robot transportation has many of the same limitations as courier services, including the need for batching of specimens and time delays in pickup notification.

Specimen Handling and Transport

In most situations the specimen for automatic analysis is serum. Many analyzers directly sample serum from primary collection tubes of various sizes. With such analyzers the collection tubes most frequently used contain separator material that forms a barrier between supernatant and cells (see Chapter 2).

Many analyzers also sample from cups or tubes filled with serum transferred from the original specimen tubes. Often the design of the sampling cup is unique for a particular analyzer. Each cup should be designed to minimize dead volume—that is, the excess serum that must be present in a cup to permit aspiration of the full volume required for testing. Cups must be made of inert material so that they do not interact with the analytes to be measured. Specimen cups also should be disposable to minimize cost, and their shape should be such that, even without a cap, minimal evaporation occurs.

Specimens may undergo other forms of degradation in addition to evaporation. Specimens that contain thermolabile constituents may undergo degradation of such analytes if held at ambient temperatures. Other constituents, such as bilirubin, are photolabile. Thermolability is minimized when both specimens and calibrators are held in a refrigerated loading zone. Photodegradation is reduced by the use of semiopaque cups and placement of smoke- or orange-colored plastic covers over the specimen cups.

The loading zone of an analyzer is the area in which specimens are held in the instrument before they are analyzed. The holding area may be a circular tray, a rack or series of racks built into a cassette, or a serpentine chain of containers into which individual tubes are inserted. When specimens are not identified automatically, they must be presented to the sampling device in the correct sequence, as specified by a loading list. The sampling mechanism determines the exact volume of sample removed from the specimen.

For most analyzers specimens for a second run may be prepared on a separate tray while one run is already in progress. This process permits machine operation and human actions to proceed in parallel for optimal efficiency. In some analyzers specimens may be added continuously by the operator as they become available. A desirable feature of any automated analyzer is the ability to insert new specimens ahead of specimens already in place in the loading zone. This feature allows for the timely analysis of a specimen with a high medical priority when it is received in the clinical laboratory. When specimen identification is machine-read, the operator easily can reposition specimens in the loading zone; however, when specimen identification is tied to a loading list, insertion or repositioning of specimens must be accompanied by revision of the loading list.

Transmission of infectious diseases by automated equipment is a concern in clinical laboratories. The method of transmission by equipment is primarily through splatter of serum or blood during the acquisition of samples from rapidly moving specimen probes. The use of level sensors, which restrict the penetration of sample probes into specimens and provide smoother motion control, greatly reduces splatter.

Because a potential for contamination exists when the stoppers of primary containers are opened or "popped" to decant serum into specimen cups, several firms have developed closed-container sampling systems for use in their automated hematology and chemistry analyzers. In these systems the specimen probe passes through a hollow needle that initially penetrates the primary container's rubber stopper. This configuration prevents damage or plugging of the specimen probe while allowing the level sensor (used to reduce carry-over and detect short sample) to remain active. After the specimen probe is withdrawn, the outer hollow needle also is withdrawn so that the stopper reseals and no specimen escapes (Figure 12-2). Closed-container sampling is used widely in hematology analyzers.

Specimen Processing

Automation of analytical procedures requires the capability to remove proteins and other interferents from some analytes and to separate free and bound fractions of heterogeneous immunoassays.

Removal of protein and other interferents

The removal of proteins and other interferents from analytes is sometimes necessary to assure specificity of an analytical method. Dialysis, column chromatography, and filtration have been used for this purpose.[2]

Separations in immunoassay systems

Automation of immunoassay procedures requires the separation of free and bound fractions of heterogeneous immunoassays. Several approaches have been used.

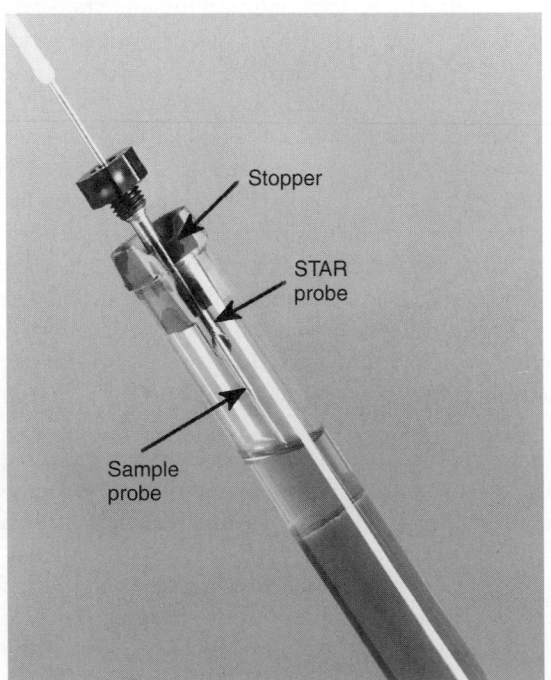

Figure 12-2 Major elements of the STAR probe used in the closed-container sampling system in Paramax 720 ZX. (Courtesy Dade-Behring International, Deerfield, Ill.)

To automate this separation step, several automated immunoassay analyzers use bound antibodies or proteins in a solid-phase format. In this approach the binding of antigens and antibodies occurs on a solid surface to which the antibodies or other reactive proteins have been adsorbed or chemically bonded. Different types of solid phases are used, including beads, coated tubes, microtiter plates, magnetic and nonmagnetic microparticles, and fiber matrices. Additional details on automated systems that use various solid phases are found in books by Chan[4] and Price and Newman.[16]

Sample Introduction and Internal Transport

The method used to introduce the sample into the analyzer and its subsequent transport within the analyzer is the major difference between continuous-flow and discrete systems. In continuous-flow systems the sample is aspirated through the sample probe into a stream of flowing liquid, whereby it is transported to analytical stations in the instrument. In **discrete analysis** the sample is aspirated into the sample probe and then delivered, often with reagent, through the same orifice into a reaction cup or other container. Carry-over is a potential problem with both types of systems.

Continuous-flow analyzers

Technicon Instruments Corporation pioneered the use of peristaltic pumps and plastic tubing to advance the sample and reagents in **continuous-flow analysis.** The peristaltic pump still is used in many analyzers with ion-selective electrodes. Peristaltic pumps trap a "slug" of fluid between two rollers that occlude the tubing. As the rollers travel over the tubing, the trapped fluid is pushed forward and, as the leading roller lifts from the tubing, is added to the fluid beyond the pump. To ensure proportionality between calibrators, controls, and specimens, the pump must act uniformly on the sample tube, and the roller speed must remain constant. Although polyvinyl tubing stretches with use, changes in flow rate over the duration of a typical run are minimal. On a short-term basis minor changes in proportionality between calibrators and unknowns are corrected by recalibration approximately every 20 minutes.

Discrete processing systems

Positive–liquid-displacement pipets are used for sampling in most discrete automated systems in which specimens, calibrators, and controls are delivered by a single pipet to the next stage in the analytical process.

A positive-displacement pipet may be designed for one of two operational modes: (1) to dispense only aspirated sample into the reaction receptacle or (2) to flush out sample together with diluent. Both systems use a plastic or glass syringe with a plunger, the tip of which usually is made of Teflon.

Pipets may be categorized as fixed-, variable-, or selectable-volume (see Chapter 1). Selectable-volume pipets allow the selection of a limited number of predetermined volumes. In general, pipets with selectable volumes are used in systems that allow many different applications, whereas fixed-volume pipets usually are used for samples and reagents in instruments dedicated to the performance of only a small variety of tests.

Carry-over

Carry-over is defined as the transport of a quantity of analyte or reagent from one specimen reaction into a subsequent one. As it erroneously affects the analytical results from the subsequent reaction, carry-over should be mimimized. Most manufacturers of discrete systems reduce the carry-over by setting an adequate flush-to-specimen ratio and incorporating wash stations for the sample probe. The ratio of flush to specimen may be as much as 4:1 to limit carry-over to less than 1%, although recent advances in materials and dispenser velocity control have permitted lower ratios. Appropriate choice of sample probe material, geometry, and surface conditions minimizes imprecision and inaccuracy.

Carry-over has been reduced in some systems through flushing of the internal and external surfaces of the sample probe with copious amounts of diluent. The outside of the sample probe is wiped in some instruments to prevent transfer of a portion of the previous specimen into the next specimen cup. In discrete systems with disposable reaction vessels and measuring cuvets, carry-over is caused by the pipetting system. In instruments with reusable cuvets or flow cells, carry-over may arise at each point through which samples pass sequentially. Disposable sample-probe tips eliminate both the contamination of one sample by another inside the probe and the carry-over of one specimen into the specimen in the next cup. Because a new pipet tip is used for each pipetting, carry-over is eliminated completely.

Compared with analyzers that perform nonimmunoassays, reduction of carry-over is a more stringent requirement for automated analyzers that perform immunoassays because for some analytes the concentration ranges in specimens are as high as six decades (for example, chorionic gonadotropin). Some systems use extra steps, such as additional washes, or an additional washing device to reduce carry-over to acceptable limits. Because extra steps reduce the overall throughput, additional rinsing functions are initiated (by computer operator selection) only for assays with large dynamical range.

Reagent Handling and Storage

Most automated systems use liquid reagents stored in plastic or glass containers. For those analyzers in which a working inventory is maintained in the system the volumes of reagents stored depend on the number of tests to be performed without operator intervention. Whenever possible, manufacturers use single reagents for test procedures, although two or more reagents may be required for some tests. Some analyzers use reagents in dry tablet form. Oth-

ers use reagent-impregnated slides or strips. Still others rely entirely on electrodes to react with specimens.

For many analyzers in which specimens are not processed continuously, reagents are stored in laboratory refrigerators and introduced into the instruments as required. In larger systems sections of the reagent storage compartments are maintained at 4 to 10 °C. Refrigerated storage for reagents also is provided in most immunoassay systems. Many of the reagents delivered in liquid form by the manufacturers of these systems are stable for 2 to 12 months.

Some systems use reagents or antibodies that have been immobilized in a reaction coil or chamber to allow for their repetitive use in a chemical reaction. Other systems use enzymes immobilized on membranes coupled to sensing electrodes. The reaction products then are measured by the sensing device. Only a buffer is required as a diluent and wash solution, and thus the membrane has an extended life of approximately several months. Some assemblies are recycled for as many as 7500 tests, which lowers the cost of each test.

Reagent identification

Labels on reagent containers include reagent identification, volume of the contents or number of tests for which the contents of the containers are to be used, expiration date, and lot number. Providing much of this information on labels is good laboratory practice and is required by law. Many reagent containers now carry bar codes that contain some or all of this information, and the manufacturer is able to retrieve any pertinent information when necessary.

Other advantages of using reagent bar codes include (1) facilitation of inventory management, (2) ability to insert reagent containers in random sequence, and (3) ability to automatically dispense a particular volume of liquid reagent. Furthermore, when a bar-code reader is coupled with a level-sensing system on the reagent probe, it alerts the operator as to whether a sufficient quantity of reagent exists to complete a workload.

In immunoassay systems a bar code on a reagent container contains key information about (multiple) calibrators, such as the definition of a calibration curve algorithm and values of curve constants defined at the time of reagent manufacture. Accompanying calibrator materials provided in their own bar-coded tubes at the time of manufacture ensure that calibration functions are integrated properly into the analysis.

Open versus closed systems

Automated analyzers also are classified as "open" or "closed." In an open analyzer the operator is able to change the parameters related to an analysis and to prepare "in-house" reagents or use reagents from a variety of suppliers. Such analyzers usually have considerable flexibility and adapt readily to new methods and analytes. A closed-system analyzer requires the reagent in a unique container or format provided by the manufacturer. In general, liquid reagents for open systems are less expensive than the proprietary components required for closed analyzers. Yet closed systems contain a hidden cost advantage because reconstitution or preparation of the reagents for use does not require a technologist's time. The variability arising from reconstitution of dry reagents has been overcome by the use of predispensed liquid reagents or through the provision of premeasured liquids. The stability of liquid reagents for some open systems now is approaching the longer stability that has characterized many closed systems. Most immunoassay systems are closed, as are most systems that have been developed for point-of-care applications.

Reagent Delivery

Liquid reagents are taken up and delivered to mixing and reaction chambers either by pumps (through tubes) or by positive-displacement syringe devices. In most high-throughput automated analyzers, reagents and diluent are drawn from bulk containers through tubes, and the sample from the specimen cup is drawn through the aspirating probe.

Syringe devices for both reagent and sample delivery are common to many automated systems. They are usually positive-displacement devices, and the volume of reagents they deliver is programmable. In those analyzers in which more than one reagent is acquired and dispensed by the same syringe, washing or flushing of the probe is essential to prevent reagent carry-over that may be deleterious to successive analytical steps in the same assay or to successive and different assays.

Chemical Reaction Phase

As its name implies the chemical reaction phase is where aliquots of sample and reagents are allowed to chemically react. Concerns related to this operation and the measurement of the reaction are addressed in the design of every automated analyzer. Design issues to be considered include the (1) vessel in which the reaction occurs and cuvet in which the reaction is monitored, (2) timing of the reaction(s), (3) mixing and transport of reactants, and (4) thermal conditioning of fluids. As discussed previously, separation of bound and unbound fractions is a fifth issue for some immunoassay systems.

Type of reaction vessel and cuvet

In a continuous-flow system, each specimen passes through the same continuous stream and is subjected to the same analytical reactions as every other specimen and at the same rate. In such systems the reaction occurs in the tube that serves as both a flow container and a cuvet.

In discrete systems each specimen in a batch has its own physical and chemical space, separate from every other specimen. Discrete analyzers use individual (disposable or reusable) reaction vessels transported through the system after sample and reagent have been dispensed or a stationary reaction chamber. In some discrete systems reaction vessels are reused; in others they are discarded after each use. The use of disposable cuvets has simplified automation and eliminated carry-over in the cuvets and the maintenance of flow cells. Disposable cuvets became possible through the development of improved plastics (notably acrylic and polyvinyl chloride) and manufacturing technology. Large-scale production of cuvets with excellent dimensional tolerances is an essential requirement. The cuvets must be transparent in the spectral range of interest. Disposable components are used increasingly in discrete automated systems.

Reaction vessels are reused in many instruments. The time before reusable cuvet/reaction vessels must be replaced depends on their composition (for example, 1 month for plastic and 2 years for standard glass vessels). Pyrex glass vessels usually are not replaced unless physically damaged.

The typical cleaning sequence of a reusable cuvet/reaction vessel involves aspiration of the reaction mixture from the cuvet at an *in situ* wash station. A detergent, alkaline, or acid wash solution then is dispensed repeatedly into and aspirated from the cuvet. The cuvet is rinsed several times with deionized water and dried by vacuum or pressurized air. Although the use of reusable cuvets reduces expenditure on consumables and extends walkaway time, it does contribute to instrument complexity and requires that a supply of cleaning liquids be maintained.

The dry reagent systems, which use slides of multilayer films or impregnated fiber strips, eliminate the need for dispensing and mixing of liquid reagents. Nevertheless, these instruments still require a mechanism to maintain a stable temperature and provide accurate positioning of the reaction unit for optical measurements.

Timing of reactions

The time allowed for a reaction to occur depends on a variety of factors. In some analyzers reaction time depends on the rate of transport of reaction mixture through the system to the measurement station, on timed events of reagent addition (or activation) relative to measurement, or on both. In discrete random access analyzers samples and reagents are added to a cuvet in a timed sequence, and absorbance readings are performed at intervals to follow the course of each reaction. Usually, the total read time for a reaction in these systems is constrained to a maximum value defined by the manufacturer but may be programmed to be shorter.

Mixing of reactants

Various techniques are used to mix reactants. In a discrete system, these include the following:

1. Forceful dispensing
2. Magnetic stirring
3. Vigorous lateral displacement
4. A rotating paddle
5. The use of ultrasonic energy

Continuous flow analyzers rely on the tumbling action of the stream in a mixing coil. Dry reagent systems obviate the need for mixing because the serum completely interacts with the dry chemicals as it flows through the matrix of the reaction unit. However, regardless of the technique used, mixing is a difficult process to automate.

Thermal regulation

Thermal regulation requires the establishment of a controlled-temperature environment in close contact with the reaction container and efficient heat transfer from the environment to the reaction mixture. Air baths, water baths, and contact with warm plates have been used for thermal regulation in commercial analyzers.

Measurement Approaches

Automated chemistry analyzers traditionally have relied on photometers and spectrophotometers for measurement of absorbance. Alternative approaches now being incorporated into analyzers include reflectance photometry and fluorometry. Immunoassay systems have used fluorescence, chemiluminescence, and electrochemiluminescence to enhance sensitivity. Ion-selective electrodes and other electrochemical techniques also are used widely. Principles of these measurement techniques have been discussed previously (see Chapter 6). This section reviews the special features and applications of the various approaches to automated analysis.

Photometry/spectrophotometry

The measurement of absorbance requires the following three basic components:

1. An optical source
2. A means of spectral isolation
3. A detector (see Chapter 3)

Optical source

The radiant energy sources used in automated systems include tungsten, quartz-halogen, deuterium, mercury, and xenon lamps, as well as lasers. In the quartz-halogen lamp, low-pressure halogen vapor (for example, iodine or bromine) is enclosed in a fused silica envelope in which a tungsten filament serves as an incandescent light source. The spectrum produced includes wavelengths from approximately 300 to 700 nm.

Spectral isolation

In automated systems spectral isolation commonly is achieved with interference filters. Such filters are quite inexpensive, and only a few are needed in any one instrument because only a limited number of wavelengths is required for analysis of a large number of absorbing species. Typical interference filters have peak transmissions of 30% to 80% and

bandwidths of 5 to 15 nm (see Chapter 3). In several multitest analyzers, filters are mounted in a filter wheel, and the appropriate filter is moved into place under command of the system's microprocessor or computer. Monochromators with moveable gratings and slits provide a continuous choice of wavelengths. They offer great flexibility and are suited especially for the development of new assays. However, because relatively few wavelengths are required for analyses in routine analyzers, many manufacturers use a stationary, holographically ruled grating, coupled with a stationary photodiode array, to isolate the spectrum. These two elements also are coupled with fiber-optic light guides to transfer the passage of light energy through cuvets at locations convenient for mechanization. Use of these passive elements enhances the reliability of a system because no moving parts are required for spectral isolation. Figure 12-3 illustrates a schematic arrangement of a grating/diode array.

Photometric detectors

Photodiodes are used as detectors in many automated systems, either as individual components or in multiples as an array. Photomultiplier tubes are required in many immunoassay systems to provide adequate sensitivity and fast detector response times for fluorescent and chemiluminescent measurements.

Analyzers that use time sharing of the optical system components tend to be less costly and still provide good performance and reliability. In general, an electrooptical package should offer an absorbance range up to 2.5 absorbance units *(A)* to permit the extended linearity desirable for some reactions.

Proper alignment of cuvets with the light path(s) is important in both automated and manual analyzers. In addition, stray energy and internal reflections must be kept to acceptable levels. If the light path is not perpendicular to the cuvet, inaccuracy and imprecision may occur, particularly in kinetic analyses.

Other forms of measurement

Several other optical techniques now are used widely as detectors in automated systems. Among these techniques are the following:

1. Reflectance photometry
2. Fluorometry
3. Fluorescence polarization
4. Turbidimetry and nephelometry
5. Chemiluminescence and bioluminescence

Reflectance photometry

In reflectance photometry diffuse reflected light is measured. The reflected light results from illumination, with diffused light, of a reaction mixture in a carrier or from the diffusion of light by a reaction mixture in an illuminated carrier. The intensity of the reflected light from the re-

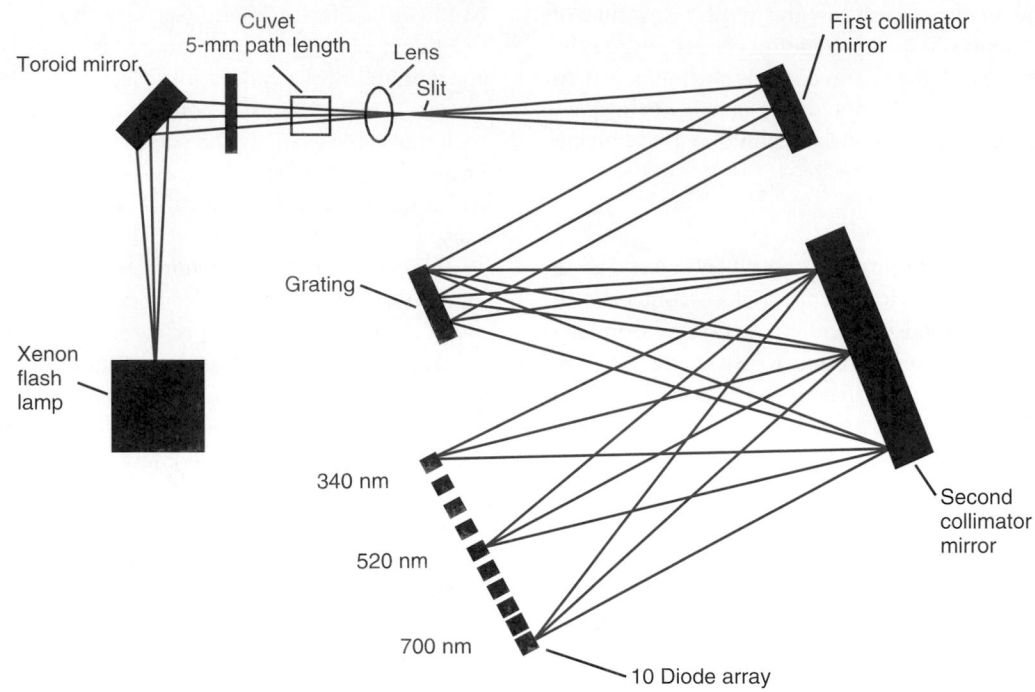

Figure 12-3   Using a diode array in a monochromator reduces requirements for moving parts. For simplicity, ray traces for three wavelengths only
are shown. (SYNCHRON CX7, Courtesy Beckman Coulter, Inc., Fullerton, Calif.)

agent carrier is compared with that reflected from a reference surface. Intensity of reflected light is not linear with
concentration of the analyte, and mathematical algorithms
commonly are used to linearize the relation of reflectance to
concentration.[2]

Fluorometry

Fluorescence is the emission of electromagnetic radiation
by a species that has absorbed exciting radiation from an
outside source. Intensity of emitted (fluorescent) light is directly proportional to concentration of the excited species
(see Chapter 4).

Fluorometry is used widely for automated immunoassay.
It is approximately 1000 times more sensitive than comparable absorbance spectrophotometry, but background interference due to fluorescence of native serum can create a major problem. This interference is minimized by careful
design of the filters used for spectral isolation, the selection
of a fluorophor with an emission spectrum distinct from
those of interfering compounds, or the use of time- or
phase-resolved fluorometry (see Chapter 4).

Different optical arrangements are represented in different manufacturers' equipment. Right-angle fluorescence
measurement is one of the common approaches, with emitted light passing through the emission interference filter to
a photomultiplier tube. In fluorescence polarization the light
source is in the form of polarized light. Measurement then
is made of the change in the degree of polarized light emitted by a fluorescent molecule (see Chapters 4 and 10).

Turbidimetry and nephelometry

These two optical techniques—turbidimetry and nephelometry—are applicable particularly to methods measuring
the precipitate formation in antigen-antibody reactions.
These techniques are used to measure plasma proteins and
for therapeutic drug monitoring. (See Chapter 4 for a more
detailed discussion of these techniques.)

Chemiluminescence and bioluminescence

Chemiluminescence and bioluminescence differ from fluorometry in that the excitation event is caused by a chemical
or electrochemical reaction and not by photolumination (see
Chapter 4). The applications of chemiluminescence and bioluminescence have increased significantly with the development of automated instrumentation and several new reagent
systems. Because of their attamole-to-zeptomole detection
limits, chemiluminescence and bioluminescence reactions
have been used widely as direct and indicator labels in the development of immunoassays (see Chapter 10).

Electrochemical methods

A variety of electrochemical methods have been incorporated into automated systems. The most widely used electrochemical approach involves ion-selective electrodes.
These electrodes have replaced flame photometry in the determination of sodium and potassium. Electrochemical detectors also have been used for the measurement of other
electrolytes and indirect application in the analysis of several
other serum constituents. The operating principle of ion-

selective electrodes is provided in some detail in Chapter 6. The relationship between ion activity and the concentration of ions in the specimens must be established with calibrating solutions, and such electrodes must be recalibrated frequently to compensate for alterations of electrode response.

Peristaltic pumps are used to move the sample into chambers containing fixed sample and reference electrodes. The electrodes must remain in contact with the specimen from 7 to 45 seconds to reach steady-state conditions. The most common arrangement is to provide electrodes to assay three analytes, typically sodium, potassium, and chloride. Because specimens and calibrators usually flow past a group of electrodes, results for all analytes are reported for most systems. Ion-selective electrode capability also has been incorporated into medium- and large-sized automated analyzers as integrated three- and four-parameter modules; this incorporation has increased significantly these systems throughputs because several results are produced in parallel.

Cell counters

Analyzers that perform a complete blood count have been automated through the use of the "Coulter principle," cell conductivity, light scatter, and flow cytometry. Individual blood cells are analyzed by application of one or more of these techniques. The Coulter principle is based on changes in electrical impedance produced by nonconductive particles suspended in an electrolyte as they pass through a small aperture between electrodes. In the sensing zone of the aperture the volume of electrolyte displaced by the particle (cell) is measured as a change in voltage that is proportional to the volume of the particle. By carefully controlling the quantity of electrolyte drawn through the aperture, several thousand particles per second are counted and sized individually. An electronic correction is applied if more than one cell passes through the aperture at the same time. Red blood cells, white blood cells, and platelets are identified by their sizes. Alternating current in the radiofrequency range short-circuits the bipolar lipid layer of the cell membrane, allowing energy to penetrate the cell. Information about intracellular structure, including chemical composition and nuclear volume, is collected with this technique.

Flow cytometry typically uses cells stained with a supravital or fluorescent dye that travel in suspension one by one past a laser light source. (Unstained cells also are measured.) Scattered light and emitted light are collected in front of the light source and at right angles, respectively (see Chapter 4). Information derived through measurement of light scatter when a cell is struck by the laser beam is then used to estimate cell shape, size, cellular granularity, nuclear lobularity, and cell surface structure. Some cell counters classify white cells using the Coulter principle, cell conductivity, and light scattering of unstained cells to differentiate cell types, whereas other cell counters use multiple flow cytometry channels or a combination of flow cytometry, cell conductivity, and light scattering.

TABLE 12-1 **Signal and Data Processing Functions Performed by Computers of Automated Analyzers**

Data Acquisition and Calculation

Acquisition of response signal and signal averaging

Subtraction of blank response

Correction of response of unknown for interferences (for example, Allen-type corrections)

First-order linear regression for slope determination ($[\Delta A/\Delta t]$ of rate reactions; $[\Delta A/\Delta C]$ of absorbance/concentration relation; $[\Delta R/\Delta C]$ of any response parameter to concentration)

Statistics (mean, SD, CV) on patient or control values

Mathematical transformation of nonlinear relations to linear counterpart

Monitoring

Test for fit of data to linearity criteria for calibration curves or rate reactions

Test of patient result against reference interval criteria

Test of control result against criteria of a quality control standard of performance

Display

Accumulation of sets of patient results

Collation of results for patient-oriented printout

Provision of warning messages to alert operator to instrument malfunction, need for maintenance, or unusual clinical situation

---

SD, Standard deviation; *CV*, coefficient of variation.

Signal Processing, Data Handling, and Process Control

The interfacing and integration of computers into automated analyzers and analytical systems has had a major impact on the acquisition and processing of analytical data. Analog signals from detectors routinely and rapidly (10^{-3} to 10^{-5} seconds) are converted to digital forms by analog-to-digital converters. The computer then processes the digital data into immediately useful and meaningful output. Data processing has allowed automation of such procedures as nonisotopic immunoassays and reflectance spectrometry because computer algorithms readily transform complex, nonlinear standard responses into linear calibration curves. Several functions performed by integrated computers in automated analyzers are listed in Table 12-1. Additional functions are the following:

1. Computers command and phase the electromechanical operation of the analyzer, thus ensuring that all functions are performed uniformly, in a repeatable manner, and in the correct sequence. Computer control of operational features of automated equipment, calculation of results, and monitoring of operation contribute to the increased reproducibility of results. These combined features allow less-skilled operators to operate such systems.

2. Computers acquire, assess, process, and store operational data from the analyzers. Built-in microprocessors monitor instrument functions for correct execution and react to improper function by recording the site and nature of the malfunction.

3. Computers enable communication interactions between the analyzer and operator. Computer messages to the user describing the site and type of problem enable quick identification of problems and prompt correction. Graphical displays provide detailed and interactive troubleshooting guidance to instrument operators and visual display of the status of each specimen and associated quality control data. Output data is flagged by comparison with preset criteria and displayed for the operator's evaluation and assessment. Such information may specify that linearity of a reaction has been exceeded, a reaction is nonlinear, substrate exhaustion has occurred, absorbance of a reagent is too high or too low, or baseline drift is excessive. Operators may reprogram certain functions of the analyzer (for example, the timing interval for a kinetic reaction and set point of the reaction temperature); enter certain values, such as calibrator concentrations; display stored information in raw or processed form; or define the format of printed output by simple interaction with the computer software.

4. Computers integrated into analytical systems provide communication with mainframe computers. Typical interfaces in the past have used serial RS-232 connections to permit interactive communication between computer systems in the modern laboratory analyzer and the Laboratory Information System (LIS). More recently, instrument manufacturers have been developing ethernet interfaces for networked connections with the TCP/IP (**T**ransmission **C**ontrol **P**rotocol/**I**nternet **P**rotocol) protocol.

■ INTEGRATED AUTOMATION FOR THE CLINICAL LABORATORY

Significant progress has been made in the integration of the individual steps of the analytical process into comprehensive analytical systems. Because of increased financial pressures to reduce costs, clinical laboratorians are integrating these analytical systems with "front-end" sample handling and transport systems to automate their laboratories "totally" and even are considering the automation of previously nonautomated areas.

Large commercial laboratories and a few academic medical centers have taken the lead in the development and implementation of large-scale automation. Such automation includes an automated specimen processing area, where specimen identification, labeling, scheduling, centrifugation, and sorting of samples are initiated. After specimen processing, automated specimen conveyor devices transport the sorted specimens to the appropriate workstations in the laboratory, where they are analyzed without human intervention. Rule-based expert system software assists with the review of laboratory results by automatically releasing results that have no associated problems and drawing any problematical results to the attention of trained laboratory professionals. After analysis, all specimens are stored in a central storage facility and their locations recorded to provide for automated retrieval.

Workstations

The task of integrating laboratory automation begins with the laboratory workstation. In general a clinical laboratory workstation is devoted to a defined task, such as the performance of chemistry profiles, complete blood counts, hormone testing, polymerase chain reaction testing, or urinalysis, and contains appropriate laboratory instrumentation to perform these tasks. Frequently the workstation in the modern laboratory is defined in terms of the automated analyzer that is used.

Current laboratory instruments and systems are highly developed for stand-alone operation and fit into the workstation concept. In most hospital and commercial laboratories workstations are run as isolated "islands of automation." Movement of specimens into and from the workstation is accomplished by manual transport, and the instrument operator's activities are largely independent of those at other workstations. If the analyzer has a bidirectional interface with an LIS (see Chapter 15) and bar-code reading capabilities, information regarding which assays to run on each sample is downloaded from the LIS and the instrument operator simply loads bar–code-labeled specimens into the sample input area. The built-in diagnostic software supplied in most modern analyzers (1) detects malfunctions during the assay process, (2) tracks use of reagents, and (3) notifies the operator of out-of-range results. In addition, this software provides sufficient "intelligence" to allow the operator the ability to walk away from the instrument for short periods, confident in its reliable operation. Nevertheless, the operator periodically needs to attend to instrument operation, replenish reagents, evaluate instrument diagnostic messages, and introduce new samples into the sample input tray.

Workcells

To reduce labor costs, instrument manufacturers are developing approaches to allow a single technologist to control and monitor the functions of several instruments simultaneously. Initially the designs have involved clusters of identical instruments called *workcells* (Figure 12-4). Each workcell has its own central control module (typically a personal computer) with software designed to help the technologist

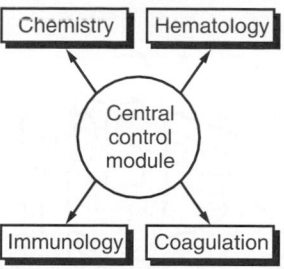

Figure 12-4 Workcell with clusters of like instruments enable one technologist to operate and monitor the functions of several analyzers simultaneously. The central control module usually is provided by the manufacturer of the analyzers in each cluster. (Modified from Boyd JC, Felder RA, Savory J: Robotics and the changing face of the clinical laboratory. Clin Chem 1996; 42:1901-1910.)

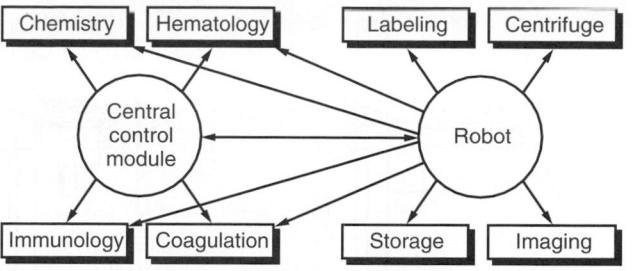

Figure 12-5 Although a workstation configured with a cluster of unlike instruments and robotic specimen processing is not yet commercially available, it could be useful in remote automated laboratories or in small outpatient laboratories. (Modified from Boyd JC, Felder RA, Savory J: Robotics and the changing face of the clinical laboratory. Clin Chem 1996; 42:1901-1910.)

monitor the functions of each analyzer and review laboratory results generated by the workcell. Access to the many front-panel functions of each analyzer is provided by the interface between the analyzer and central control module. The development of workcells is possible in large part because the manufacturers have designed sufficient diagnostic capacities into their instruments to enable the autonomous "walk-away" mode of operation discussed previously. Thus the technologist loads the samples onto each instrument in the workcell and then monitors subsequent instrument operation and reviews the results at the central control module. By incorporating the activities of what would be several workstations in most current laboratories into a single integrated workcell, this approach shows promise in saving laboratory manpower.

An extension of the workcell concept is to use several nonidentical analyzers and add robotic specimen handling and preparation (Figure 12-5).[13] The robot is used to perform all specimen preparation steps, including checks of sample adequacy, centrifugation, and labeling, and specimen storage after analysis. The robot then is responsible for introducing samples into the appropriate analyzer, allowing the technologist to assume a primarily monitoring role. An interface between the central control module and robot controller (or the combination of these functions on a single computer) allows the activities of the robotic cluster to be fully coordinated.

With sufficient monitoring capacity and intelligence built into the central control module, a robotic workstation is monitored electronically, not in the physical presence of the technologist. The remote automated laboratory system (which will be discussed in a subsequent section of this chapter) is an example of this concept.

Automated Specimen Transport

Different approaches have been developed to transport specimens within the laboratory, including mobile robots, conveyor belts, and robotic arms.

Mobile robots versus conveyor belts

Mobile robots and conveyor belts have been used in the laboratory to help transport specimens from one clinical laboratory workstation to another. Conveyor-belt technology has been applied successfully in the manufacturing industry for carefully defined transportation needs. However, the difficulty this technology demonstrates in handling the large variety of specimen containers in the clinical laboratory (ranging from microspecimen to large urine-collection containers) is a disadvantage. To increase the variety of types of specimen containers carried on a conveyor-belt system, specimens are placed into specially designed carriers that fit on the conveyor-belt line. Known as "pucks" or "racks" (depending on whether they carry individual samples or groups of samples, respectively), the carriers have receptacles for variously sized tubes. Although some conveyor-belt systems are custom manufactured for specific facilities, others are sold in modular forms, including straight and curved pieces of track of varying lengths, crossover modules, and gating modules assembled in various configurations to match a given laboratory's geometry. Others are configured uniquely for certain analyzers only.

Elevator modules are available for some systems that allow pucks or racks to be moved up to ceiling height or under the floor for transport. Elevator modules vary in the ability to maintain the specimen in an upright position, an important consideration if the tubes are being transported uncapped.

Transfer of samples from the conveyor belt to the laboratory workstation has been implemented in various ways. Many manufacturers are equipping their laboratory instruments with devices to obtain samples directly from conveyor-belt systems.

In contrast with the limited reconfigurability of conveyor belt systems and their limited ability to handle different-sized specimen containers, mobile robots are easily adapted to carry various sizes and shapes of specimen containers and have been reprogrammed to travel to new (and distant) locations with changes in laboratory geometry.

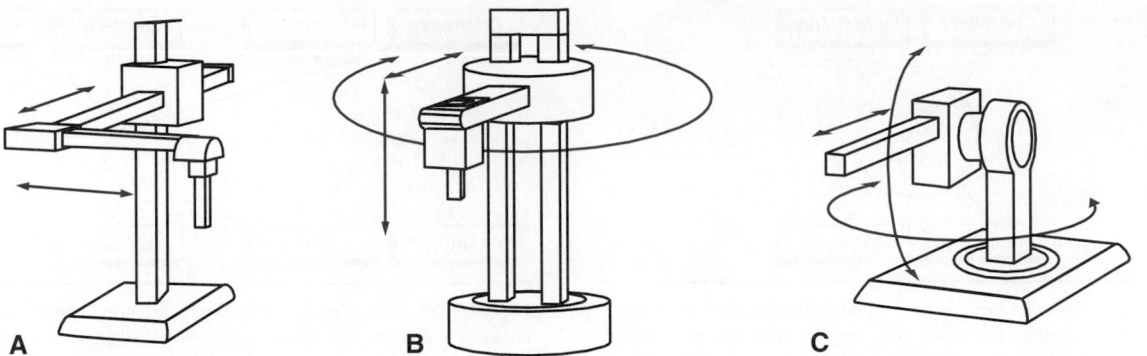

A **B** **C**

Figure 12-6 Three basic configurations of robotic devices that have applications in the clinical laboratory. **A,** Cartesian. **B,** Cylindrical. **C,** Articulating (polar) or jointed. (Modified from Journal of the International Federation of Clinical Chemistry, 1992; 4:175.)

Some limitations of mobile robots have been described previously, including their requirement to batch specimens and their difficulty in interfacing mechanically with laboratory analyzers so that specimens are introduced directly from the mobile robot onto the analyzer. In many situations laboratory personnel still are required to place samples onto or remove samples from the mobile robot at each stopping place. Mobile robots have been used to return conveyor-belt specimen carrier racks to the central dispatch area and transport specimens within and outside the laboratory.

Mobile robots have been equipped with simple or sophisticated guidance systems. A robot with a simple guidance system follows a predetermined route, such as a line on the floor, to reach its destination, whereas a robot with a more sophisticated guidance system is expected to navigate independently through a facility. The costs of the technology vary directly with the degree of sophistication. Sophisticated guidance systems require more built-in sensors to provide enough information about the robot's outside environment to enable independent navigation.

Robot arms

Robotic arms first were used by the pharmaceutical industry to conduct drug dosage studies and later by clinical laboratories to perform highly complex clinical assays. Three types of robotic devices are available commercially: Cartesian, cylindrical, and articulating (Figure 12-6). Robots, by virtue of their operational flexibility, enable the rapid reconfiguration of systems for new and varying protocols. This ability enhances versatility and safety, improves precision and productivity, and reduces errors due to human mismatch of specimen identity. However, misprogramming of the systems results in repetitive errors with potentially grave medical and legal consequences; thus great care is required to ensure that such errors do not occur.

Cartesian systems currently are the most common form of robotics in use in laboratories. These systems are built into programmable pipetting stations and provide flexible pipetting routines to suit varied protocols. They have been

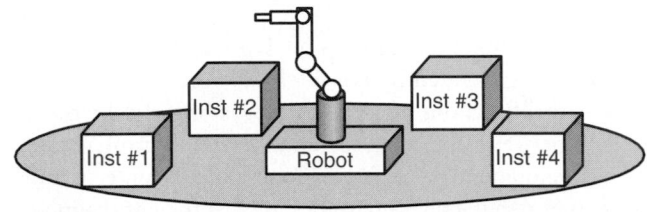

Figure 12-7 Radial arrangement of peripheral equipment around a centrally located robot. This type of workstation requires a circular work space in the laboratory with easy access from all sides. (Modified from Boyd JC, Felder RA, Savory J: Robotics and the changing face of the clinical laboratory. Clin Chem 1996; 42:1901-1910.)

applied most often to the automation of heterogeneous immunoassays.

Robot arms have varying configurations and degrees of freedom of movement. Two types of arms have been used in clinical laboratories: (1) cylindrical robot arms with interchangeable hands and (2) fully articulated robot arms with wrist and elbow joints. When the arm is attached to a stationary base, its range of motion is constrained (Figure 12-7) to a hemispherical or cylindrical space around the robot base (depending on the type of robot). This limit on the range of motion restricts the positions of devices with which the robot interacts to a radial pattern around the robot base. Some robot manufacturers have mounted their robot arms on mobile bases attached to a track (Figure 12-8). The track extends the range of motion of the robot so that instruments and devices with which the robot interacts are arrayed linearly along a table or bench.

Automated Specimen Processing

Although the manual operations carried out in a specimen processing area have the outward appearance of being simple, considerable complexity underlies these operations. Consequently, specimen processing has been one of the most difficult areas of the clinical laboratory to automate.

Automating the specimen processing area has been approached in various ways through the use of both integrated

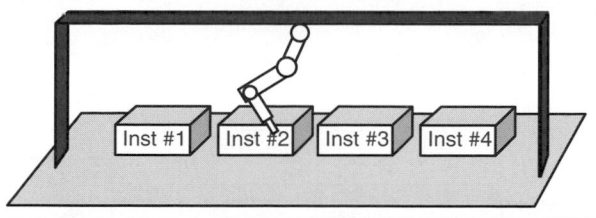

Figure 12-8   Using a robot on a linear track allows placement of peripheral equipment, with which the robot interacts, on a rectangular table. This workstation configuration uses a more conventional rectangular space that can be set along a wall. (Modified from Boyd JC, Felder RA, Savory J: Robotics and the changing face of the clinical laboratory. Clin Chem 1996; 42:1901-1910.)

approaches and modular approaches.[5] Each specimen passing through a specimen processing area has to undergo a series of operations, beginning with the following:

1. Receipt
2. Inspection appropriateness (labeling, container type, quantity of sample)
3. Logging into the LIS
4. Labeling with an accession number
5. Separation of urgent and stat samples from routine samples

In addition, samples must be sorted for centrifugation and aliquoting or otherwise prepared for the appropriate laboratory station. Centrifugation must be performed for the appropriate period of time, and each centrifuged sample must be inspected for appropriate quality, such as the presence of hemolysis, lipemia, and icterus, and according to its workstation destination. Adding to the difficulty of programming an automated system is the fact that clinical laboratories receive diverse specimens (ranging from blood to hair) in more than 50 types of specimen containers and often have repertoires exceeding 1000 tests.

Integrated specimen processing systems

Several manufacturers offer integrated automation systems for specimen processing. Although these systems are restricted to handling specific types of samples and specimen containers, they are capable of processing much of the daily workload of a laboratory and have been installed in hundreds of laboratories worldwide, mostly in Japan. Each system incorporates some or all of the following components:

1. *Sample inlet area* This holding area is where bar–code-labeled tubes are introduced into the system.
2. *Bar-code reading stations* Multiple bar-code readers are placed at critical locations in the processing system to track samples and direct their proper routing to various stations in the processing system.
3. *Sorter* This device separates tubes by type and passes them to the transport system.

4. *Transport system* The system is composed of segments of conveyor-belt line that move specimens to their appropriate locations.
5. *Automated centrifuge* In this area of the specimen processor, specimens that require centrifugation are removed from the conveyor belt, introduced into an automatically balanced centrifuge, centrifuged (either refrigerated or at room temperature), and removed from the centrifuge and placed back on the transport system.
6. *Level detection and evaluation of specimen adequacy* In this area sensors are used to evaluate the volume of sample in each tube and look for the presence of hemolysis, lipemia, or icterus.
7. *Decapping station* This area in the processing system is where tube caps are removed automatically.
8. *Aliquoter* This device aspirates appropriately sized aliquots from each mother tube and places them into bar-coded daughter tubes for sorting and transport to multiple analytical workstations.
9. *Take-out stations* These stations are temporary storage areas for samples before or after analysis.

Integrated specimen processing systems have been customized to optimize their use at individual facilities. Manufacturers of these systems emphasize the necessity of conducting a complete evaluation of each laboratory site to determine its specific needs before developing the specifications for an integrated specimen processing system.

Modular specimen processing systems

An alternative to integrated specimen processing involves a modular approach. Some manufacturers market several modules that either operate in stand-alone mode or are integrated into an overall specimen processing system. Modules include sorting, centrifugation, and aliquoting stations. Each module has its own on-board computer that is linked to a master controller computer system. Specimen transport systems also have been modularized with process-control software that provides a comprehensive solution for intralaboratory specimen transport.

Automated Specimen Sorting

The approach an automated specimen processing system takes to specimen sorting is an extremely important determinant of the overall scheme of automation in the laboratory. At least three approaches to specimen sorting have been taken. In the first and perhaps simplest approach the conveyor-belt system is configured as a continuous loop, and specimens are sampled either directly by the analytical instrument while on the conveyor or by a robot attached to the workstation, which removes selected specimens from the conveyor for analysis (Figure 12-9). This approach has the advantage that sample aliquoting is not required because samples pass all workstations at which tests are performed.

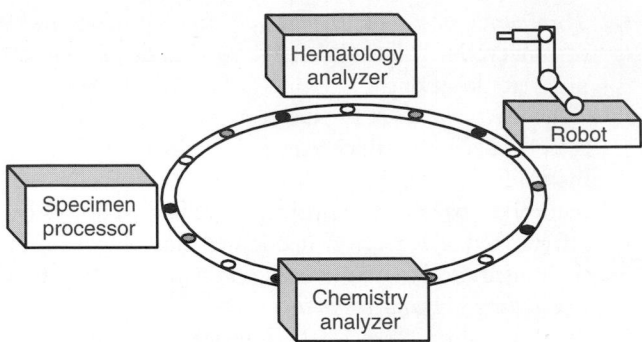

Figure 12-9   Direct sampling from a conveyor track in a loop configuration eliminates the need for separate equipment to sort specimens but also may limit the rate of sample movement on the track to the sampling speed of the slowest workstation. (Modified from Boyd JC, Felder RA, Savory J: Robotics and the changing face of the clinical laboratory. Clin Chem 1996; 42:1901-1910.)

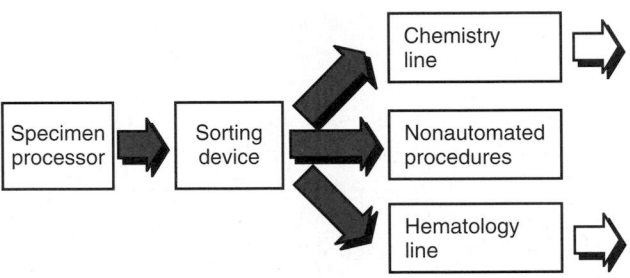

Figure 12-10   Sorting laboratory samples before introduction to an automated specimen conveyor system simplifies the design and construction of the conveyor. (Modified from Boyd JC, Felder RA, Savory J: Robotics and the changing face of the clinical laboratory. Clin Chem 1996; 42:1901-1910.)

However, the continuous loop also has some drawbacks in that sample throughput is limited by the slowest direct sampling analyzer on the loop, and finding an empty carrier into which to replace a sample removed from the line may be difficult. Some manufacturers have addressed both problems by creating multilane conveyors with a "through" lane and a local "holding" lane. In a continuous-loop system additional intelligence must be present at the workstation to detect samples that need to be analyzed at that workstation; a mechanical system also must exist to remove a sample tube from the loop. (This physical manipulation is known as "plucking," indicating that the tubes are pulled off or from the loop.)

In the second approach, specimens are separated by the automated specimen processing system into groups, according to their destination in the laboratory; afterward the separated specimens are routed down a dedicated conveyor line or carried batchwise on a mobile robot (Figure 12-10). This sorting method follows the approach used in most manual specimen processing areas and allows the implementation of an automated specimen processing system without the need to set up a transportation system simulta-

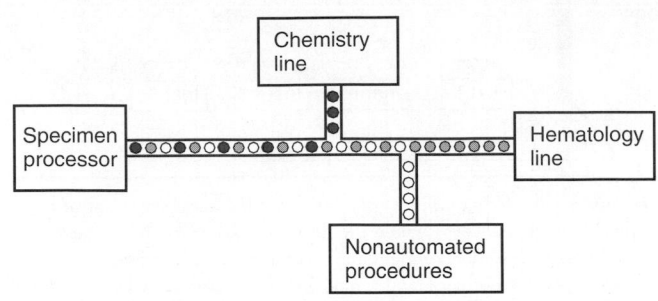

Figure 12-11   Using the conveyor system to sort samples dynamically during specimen transport eliminates the need for separate equipment to sort samples but requires a more sophisticated conveyor system with numerous bar-code reading stations and gates to direct the samples to the appropriate workstations. (Modified from Boyd JC, Felder RA, Savory J: Robotics and the changing face of the clinical laboratory. Clin Chem 1996; 42:1901-1910.)

neously. However, without a linked specimen transportation system the holding area for sorted specimens must be monitored to ensure that it does not overfill.

In the third approach the conveyor system sorts samples as they are transported (Figure 12-11). The advantages of this approach are that a dedicated specimen sorting device is not needed in the specimen processing system and with appropriate specimen rerouting the requirement for aliquoting of the specimen also is unnecessary. A disadvantage of this approach is the expense of multiple bar-code reading stations and specimen routing gates and the complexity of the process control software required.

Automated Specimen Storage and Retrieval

Automated capability to store and retrieve specimens on demand is an important aspect in automated specimen delivery systems. A few integrated systems offer specimen storage and retrieval modules that robotically store specimens refrigerated in specific locations and log them into a database maintained by the specimen delivery system. When a user requests a specific sample, the robot is given commands to retrieve the specimen from the appropriate archived location and route it to the requested station using the specimen transportation system.

Problems of Integration

Building a highly integrated laboratory generates many potential problems. Because a laboratory is not likely to use only the equipment of a single equipment manufacturer, integration of the instruments and robotic devices from different manufacturers is necessary. Decisions must be made concerning which device will be the master controller and which company will develop the software that provides overall control of the automation scheme. In addition, individuals or firms who will be responsible for configuration of the automation to the geometry and production schedule of the laboratory must be recruited and trained. Although industrial automation schemes have been developed to solve many of these problems, as yet insufficient experience exists with these approaches in the very different operating environment of a clinical laboratory.

Device integration

One objective in the development of an integrated laboratory is to link laboratory instruments and devices into an automated system so that the maximum number of instrument operator functions is automated. Automatic sample introduction requires the development of mechanical interfaces between each laboratory analyzer and devices such as conveyor belts, mobile robots, or robot arms. Enhancements to electronic interfaces for laboratory instruments are needed to allow remote computer control of front-panel functions, notification of instrument status information, and coordination of the distribution of specimens among instruments. Most existing LIS interfaces with laboratory analyzers provide only the abilities to download accession numbers and the tests requested on each sample and upload the results generated by the analyzer.

Process controllers and software

Process controllers provide computer integration of the many decision-making tasks that occur in the daily activity of a laboratory including the following:

1. Specimen tracking
2. Monitoring of specimen queues in the specimen distribution system
3. Monitoring of instrument function
4. Scheduling of analytical processes
5. Monitoring quality control

Process control software is needed to coordinate these activities in a large-scale automated laboratory. To integrate the various devices in the laboratory, communication with an overall master controller device must be established. In addition, communication is necessary among the LIS computer, specimen distribution controller, laboratory analyzers, and the specimen conveyor and specimen manipulation devices. The distribution of tasks must be specified carefully in the development of such a communications network.

■ AUTOMATION OF POINT-OF-CARE ANALYZERS

Point-of-care testing (POCT)[6,9,10] is a rapidly growing component of laboratory testing. Known by a variety of names, including *near-patient, decentralized,* and *off-site testing,* POCT offers the advantages of reduced turnaround time of test results and improved patient management in comparison with **centralized testing** in a **core laboratory.** Widespread POCT has become feasible through enhancements in the automation of instruments designed to serve satellite and near-patient care environments. The ease of use with these systems has improved dramatically with the incorporation of computers that provide automated diagnosis of analytical problems, automated calibration, and consistent application of quality control processes. In most cases manipulation of liquid reagents has been eliminated through the use of solid-phase reagents and ion-selective electrodes. Many systems can analyze whole blood, thus eliminating the need for centrifugation.

The attributes desirable for POCT instruments include the following:

1. First results in a minute or less
2. Portable instruments with consumable reagent cartridges
3. A one- or two-step operating protocol
4. Ability to perform direct specimen analysis on whole blood
5. Simple operating procedures that do not require a laboratory-trained operator
6. Flexible test menus
7. Quantitative results with accuracy and precision (in comparison to those of the central laboratory)
8. Built-in calibration and quality control
9. Ambient temperature storage for reagents
10. Results provided as hard copy and stored form and available for transmission
11. Low instrument cost
12. Service by exchange
13. Built-in regulatory record keeping[12]

The technical advances that have catalyzed the evolution of POCT instruments are the development of microchips and electrodes to measure electrolytes, blood gases, nucleic acids, and other analytes and solid-state stable reagents in disposable unit-dose devices. By offering individually packed test units, manufacturers provide convenience and assume the burden of quality assurance of the reagents.[14] Although the throughput of tests for these systems is low, the time required to produce the results is usually short. These systems are often small enough to be portable, further enhancing the possibility of bringing tests to the patient. Recent progress in miniaturization of laboratory instrumentation promises even more exciting developments for POCT.[11]

The initial cost of these systems is typically lower than the considerable cost for the more comprehensive routine analytical systems. However, the cost of the **unit-dose reagents** these systems require is often higher than that of bulk liquid reagents. This extra cost is offset partially by operational simplicity, which reduces labor expenditures.

Point-of-Care Testing Options

The need for rapid analytical results for the management of critically ill patients is well documented,[17] but many institutions that perform critical analytical tests in their central laboratories have turnaround times that exceed 20 minutes. POCT is viewed by some as the best means for the reduction of test turnaround times.[8] Various approaches in the provision of POCT have been considered, including operation of an off-site laboratory through the use of either laboratory or nonlaboratory personnel to perform the testing, mobile laboratories, handheld instruments at the bedside, and remote automated laboratories. A variety of analyzers and approaches have been developed for POCT, including handheld, desktop, portable, and mobile and remote laboratories.

Handheld analyzers

Whole-blood glucose analyzers were the first handheld instruments to receive widespread clinical application, and their use has become an accepted component of patient care in most hospitals. Many different glucose meters that have varying degrees of ease of use are available. Some require wiping, blotting, washing, or timing steps, but more recent models are simpler to use. Although the cost of bedside glucose testing is comparable to that of central laboratory testing, much of the cost of bedside testing is attributable to the high costs of quality control and quality assurance, training, and documentation.

Recently, portable analyzers that perform analyses of electrolytes (Na^+, K^+, Cl^-, Ca^{2+}), hematocrit, blood gases (pH, P_{CO_2}, P_{O_2}), urea, and glucose have been introduced into clinical use. Several calculated parameters based on the measured analytes also are provided. Disposable cartridges containing the microfabricated thin-film electrodes and immobilized enzymes are introduced into the handheld unit that houses the electronics. The user chooses a cartridge (with appropriate test repertoire), places several drops of whole blood on the cartridge receiving area, and places the cartridge into the handheld unit. Calibration fluid and subsequently the whole blood are flooded automatically over the electrodes. After the analysis is complete, the data are displayed on a liquid crystal display and stored in the unit for transfer to the LIS by infrared or wire connections. Quality control is performed on several cartridges in each box; otherwise, no other quality control is performed on the units because they feature built in self-diagnosis.

Maintaining adequate quality control of POCT instruments is a major concern because the Joint Commission for Accreditation of Healthcare Organizations (JCAHO) holds the hospital clinical laboratory accountable for the quality of these results, even though no laboratory staff members may have been involved in providing them. Most instrument manufacturers provide a means to record quality control data, and some provide a means to prevent the use of an instrument with out-of-range quality control results by a lockout mechanism. Nevertheless, the nonlaboratory user may not detect an instrument problem that might be detected by a trained technologist and is not always necessarily as diligent in performing quality control checks and instrument maintenance.

Desktop and portable analyzers

A few manufacturers market small desktop and portable analyzers that incorporate on-board centrifugation of the sample before it is analyzed. One approach incorporates a molded test pack specific for each analyte that ensures precise transfer of serum and metering of reagents. Optical measurements are made, as in other centrifugal analyzers. Another small centrifugal analyzer performs a panel of up to 12 tests on a single specimen. This analyzer includes a check system to inhibit the release of results from hemolyzed, lipemic, or icteric specimens, enabling unskilled operators to use the same criteria as medical technologists in a central laboratory to accept or reject test results.

Various whole-blood analyzers have been engineered for simplicity, accuracy, and robustness in the hands of nonlaboratory personnel. On-board quality control and totally replaceable fluid and electrode packs virtually eliminate maintenance problems. Some of these devices are battery-powered and easily transported to a patient's bedside to perform analyses.

Other POCT analyzers measure prothrombin and activated partial thromboplastin times, therapeutic drugs (such as digoxin, theophylline, and carbamazepine) or markers of myocardial damage (total creatine kinase, CK-2, myoglobin, and troponin T). Measuring thyroxine and cholesterol at a patient's bedside is even possible, although the clinical rationale for such measurements is questionable.

Mobile laboratories

Another approach to POCT is the use of laboratory instruments on a movable cart. One such device incorporates instruments on a rolling table to perform blood gas, coagulation, and complete blood count determinations. A computer is used to gather all the instrument data and provide the modem link with which to transmit analytical results and quality control data to the central laboratory. A mobile laboratory is dispatched to any location in which laboratory services are needed, including outpatient clinics, critical care units, and the emergency room.

Remote automated laboratory system

Unmanned satellite laboratories are possible alternatives to central laboratory facilities.[6] In concept these laboratories incorporate small laboratory analyzers (usually whole-blood analyzers) that have been interfaced to a computer that controls the instrument and provides a touchscreen interface for the walk-up user of the system. Once the instrument has generated results on a user-introduced specimen, these results are forwarded to a central monitoring facility, where they are reviewed by a trained medical technologist.

The remote automated laboratory system (RALS) approach allows testing to be performed at the point of care while central laboratory control is maintained over the process. The advantages of reduced labor costs for sample transportation and laboratory staff and reduced sample turnaround time outweigh the increased costs of equipment.

When used with a whole-blood analyzer a RALS requires no sample preparation steps. The RALS concept has obvious extensions to the outpatient clinic, but such extension requires a much more complex robotic instrument cluster with robotic sample preparation, chemistry, hematology, and coagulation instruments.

References

1. Boyd JC, Felder RA, Savory J: Robotics and the changing face of the clinical laboratory. Clin Chem 1996; 42:1901-1910.
2. Boyd JC, Young DS: Automation in the clinical laboratory. In Burtis CA, Ashwood ER (eds): Tietz Textbook of Clinical Chemistry, 3rd edition, pp 226-264, Philadelphia, WB Saunders, 1999.
3. Burtis CA: Converging technologies and their impact on the clinical laboratory. Clin Chem 1996; 42:1735-1749.
4. Chan DW: Immunoassay Automation: An Updated Guide to Systems, San Diego, Academic Press, 1995.
5. Felder RA: Automation of preanalyticalal processing and mobile robotics. In Kost CJ (ed): Handbook of Clinical Automation, Robotics, and Optimization, pp 252-282, New York, John Wiley & Sons, 1996.
6. Felder RA: Robotic automation of near-patient testing. In Kost CJ (ed): Handbook of Clinical Automation, Robotics, and Optimization, pp 596-619, New York, John Wiley & Sons, 1996.
7. Howanitz PJ, Sunseri DA, Love LA et al: Adapting mobile robotic technology to intralaboratory specimen transport. Arch Pathol Lab Med 1996; 120:944-950.
8. Kost GJ: New stat laboratory instrumentation: we can and should satisfy clinicians' demands for rapid response. Am J Clin Pathol 1990; 94:522-523.
9. Kost GJ: New whole blood analyzers and their impact on cardiac and critical care. Crit Rev Clin Lab Sci 1993; 30:153-202.
10. Kost G (ed): Point-of-care testing: pathology patterns. Am J Clin Pathol 1995; 104(Suppl):S1-S127.
11. Kricka LJ, Wilding P: Micromechanics and nanotechnology. In Kost CJ (ed): Handbook of Clinical Automation, Robotics, and Optimization, pp 45-77, New York, John Wiley & Sons, 1996.
12. Maclin E, Mahoney WC: Point-of-care testing technology. J Clin Lig Assay 1995; 18:21-33.
13. Markin SJ: Robotics, interfaces, and the docking device. In Kost CJ (ed): Handbook of Clinical Automation, Robotics, and Optimization, pp 235-251, New York, John Wiley & Sons, 1996.
14. Phillips DL: Quality systems for unit-use testing devices. Clin Chem 1997; 43:893-896.
15. Prasad P: Effective use of robots as mechanized couriers at Stanford University Hospital. Biomed Instrum Technol 1995; 29:398-404.
16. Price CP, Newman DJ (eds): Principles and Practice of Immunoassay, 2nd edition, New York, Stockton Press, 1997.
17. Zaloga GP, Hill TR, Strickland RA et al: Bedside blood gas and electrolyte monitoring in critically ill patients. Crit Care Med 1989; 17:920–925.

Additional Reading

Felder RA: Modular workcells: modern methods for laboratory automation. Clin Chim Acta 1998; 278:257-267.
Gochman N, Quint J: The new millennium in laboratory automation. Ann Clin Lab Sci 1999; 29:104-105.
Hicks JM, Price CP (eds): Point-of-Care Testing, Washington, DC, AACC Press, 1999.
Hoffmann GE: Concepts for the third generation of laboratory systems. Clin Chim Acta 1998; 278:203-216.
Hurst WJ: Automation in the Laboratory, New York, VCH Publishers, 1995.
Kost GJ (ed): Handbook of Clinical Automation, Robotics, and Optimization, New York, John Wiley & Sons, 1996.
Sasaki M, Kageoka T, Ogura K et al: Total laboratory automation in Japan: past, present, and the future. Clin Chim Acta 1998; 278:217-227.
Ward KM, Lehmann CA, Leiken AM: Clinical Laboratory Instrumentation and Automation, Philadelphia, WB Saunders, 1994.

PART III

Laboratory Operation

CHAPTER 13

Evaluation of Methods—with an Introduction to Statistical Techniques

DAVID D. KOCH, PhD, DABCC, and THEODORE PETERS, JR., PhD

Objectives

1. Discuss the need for method selection and evaluation in the context of a clinical laboratory.
2. Define and state the formulas for the following:
   Mean
   Median
   Standard deviation
   Correlation coefficient
   t-Test
   Regression analysis
   F-test
   Gaussian distribution
3. State the considerations that must be examined in the selection of a new analytical method.
4. Define *performance standards.*
5. Define the following:
   Accuracy
   Random and systematic error
   Total error
   Analytical range
   Analytical sensitivity
   Analytical specificity
   Interference
   Recovery
6. Outline the tasks involved in a methods evaluation, including statistical measures that must be performed.

Key Words

Accuracy   Closeness of the agreement between the measured value of an analyte and its "true" value

Analysis of Variance (ANOVA)   A technique that tests differences among two or more groups of observations; compares variation among groups with variation within them (one-way ANOVA)

Bias   The systematic deviation of the test results from the accepted reference value

Candidate Method   A method being considered for use in the laboratory; often referred to as "new" or "test" method

CLIA '88   An acronym for the Clinical Laboratory Improvements Amendments of 1988

Coefficient of Variation (CV)   A measure of relative precision (the ratio of the standard deviation to the mean, multiplied by 100 to convert it to percentage)

Degrees of Freedom (DOF)   An integer value equal to the number of linearly independent observations in a set of n observations; the DOF being equal to n minus the number of restrictions placed on the entire data set

F-Test   A statistical calculation to determine whether the variances of two groups of independent measurements differ from one another; the statistic being the ratio of the larger to the smaller variance

Gaussian Distribution   A normal distribution of observations characterized as being symmetrical and bell shaped; has a mean at the center of the distribution, with tail widths proportional to the standard deviation of the data about the mean; also known as a *normal distribution*

Least-Squares Analysis   A method by which unknown parameters for method comparison data or paired measurements are estimated through minimization of the sum of squared residuals

Linear Regression   A regression model in which the dependent variable (Y) is related linearly to each independent variable; simple linear regression being the case where only a single explanatory variable (X) exists

Mean   The arithmetical average of a set of numbers

Precision   The closeness of agreement between independent test results obtained under specified conditions; not typically represented as a numerical value but expressed quantitatively in terms of imprecision—the standard deviation (SD) or coefficient of variation (CV)

Standard Deviation (SD)   A measure of variability/dispersion that is the square root of the population variance

t-Test   A test used to compare the means of one or more normal distributions with variations that are unknown but must be estimated from the data

---

The introduction of new or revised methods into the clinical laboratory is a recurring task for clinical laboratorians who desire to ensure high-quality laboratory services. Method selection and evaluation are key steps in the implementation of new methods (Figure 13-1). Good laboratory practice requires that a new or revised method be selected with care and its performance evaluated rigorously and impartially under laboratory conditions before it is adopted for routine use. Because both a method and an instrument typically are involved in the production of an analytical result, this chapter's use of the term *method* implies both a methodological and an instrumental component. The term *method evaluation* very well may mean "instrument evaluation," although the question being asked in an evaluation experiment is not whether the instrument is acceptable for use but whether the methods furnished by the instrument are acceptable. If all or most of the methods perform favorably, then the instrument presumably is acceptable.

Abundant method performance data now are found in the open and commercial literature. With the availability of such information, accepting only these data to guide decisions about accepting a **candidate method** is tempting. Although this information is useful and probably should be consulted as a beginning point of reference, individual laboratories should have the confidence and capability to generate and apply such data themselves.

The purpose of this chapter is to outline techniques that allow clinical laboratorians to select and evaluate analytical methods objectively. Included in this chapter are the following components:

1. A brief summary of statistical terms used in this and other chapters
2. A list of definitions pertinent to the method selection and evaluation process
3. Various performance standards used to assess method performance objectively

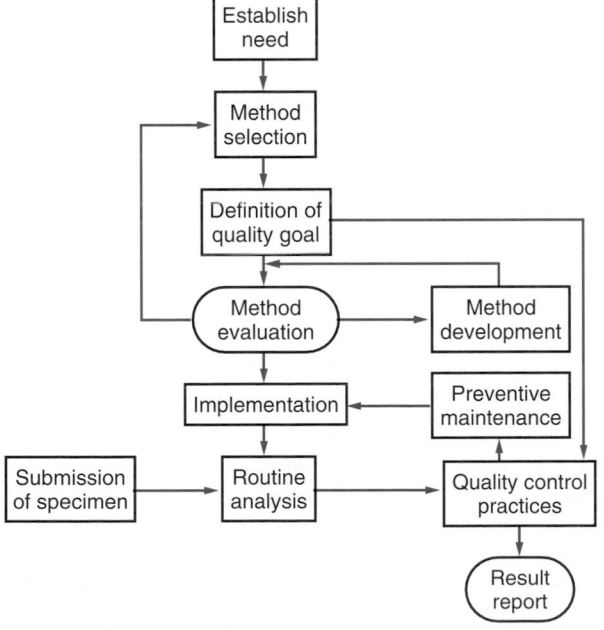

New method introduction approach

Figure 13-1   A flow diagram that illustrates the process by which a new method is introduced into routine use. The diagram highlights the key steps of method selection, method evaluation, and quality control.

4. Procedures for the selection and evaluation of a candidate method

■ BASIC STATISTICS

In method evaluation studies a large number of data points accumulates fairly quickly. Various statistics provide useful tools to help analyze these data points by reducing them to a manageable few numbers. The following is a brief review of the essential statistical techniques.

Mean, Standard Deviation, and Coefficient of Variation

The statistical terms *mean, standard deviation,* and *coefficient of variation* assume a **Gaussian distribution** of data that is symmetrical and bell-shaped (see Chapter 14) and focus on the distribution of errors from the analytical method, not the distribution of values from a healthy or patient population. Three key statistical terms often used by clinical laboratorians are the mean ($\bar{x}$), standard deviation, and the coefficient of variation. The **mean** is the arithmetical average of a set of numbers; the **standard deviation (SD)** is a measure of the variability/dispersion of a population of numbers; and the **coefficient of variation (CV)** is the ratio of the SD to the mean multiplied by 100 to convert it to percentage. The equations used to calculate $\bar{x}$, SD, and CV, respectively, are as follows:

$$\bar{x} = \frac{\Sigma x_i}{n}$$

$$SD = \sqrt{\frac{\Sigma x_i^2 - \frac{(\Sigma x_i)^2}{n}}{n - 1}}$$

$$CV = \frac{SD}{\bar{x}} \times 100\%$$

where x_i is an individual measurement, and n is the number of measurements. These statistical tests are used in comparison-of-methods studies and elsewhere.

Standard Deviation of Duplicates

When samples are analyzed in duplicate, the differences between duplicate analyses are used to estimate the SD, as follows:

$$SD_{dup} = \sqrt{\frac{\Sigma d^2}{2n}}$$

where d is the difference between the two results obtained from analysis of duplicate aliquots of a patient specimen, and n is the number of different patient samples analyzed. If the duplicates are performed in one run, SD_{dup} estimates within-run precision or random error; if the duplicates are analyzed in different runs, between-run variation is included in the estimate.

Paired *t*-Test

For comparison-of-methods studies a "paired" ***t*-test** is used to test the average difference of the pairs of values obtained by the candidate and reference methods. Note that a *t*-test is applied to means or average differences and provides a test for accuracy or the presence of systematic errors of a method.

Three statistics are calculated. The average difference, or bias, is calculated by the following equation:

$$\text{Bias} = \bar{y} - \bar{x}$$

where $\bar{y}$ is the mean of the test method values, and $\bar{x}$ is the mean of the reference method values. Next, the SD of the differences (SD_d) is calculated

$$SD_d = \sqrt{\frac{\Sigma[(y_i - x_i) - \text{bias}]^2}{n - 1}}$$

where y_i and x_i are the values for individual patient samples, as measured by the candidate and reference methods, respectively; bias is from the previous equation; and n is the number of patient samples tested. The *t*-value is obtained as follows:

$$t = \frac{[\text{bias}]\sqrt{n}}{SD_d}$$

To interpret the *t*-test the calculated *t*-value is compared with a "critical" *t*-value obtained from the appropriate table in a statistical handbook or textbook. The critical values are given for different probabilities (P) and **degrees of freedom (DOF)**. A probability of 0.05 usually is selected, which allows a 5% chance that the calculated *t*-value will exceed the critical *t*-value because of chance alone. In this example, DOF is equal to n-1.

If the calculated *t*-value is greater than the critical *t*-value, the difference **(bias)** is interpreted as statistically significant, meaning that a real difference has been observed between the two methods. If the calculated *t*-value is less than the critical *t*-value, then the bias is interpreted as not statistically significant; the data do not support a conclusion that a difference exists between the two methods.

For example, if a calculated *t*-value of 1.80 was obtained based on a comparison study that included 41 different specimens, the critical *t*-value would be found in a table of critical *t*-values in the row for 40 DOF (DOF = n − 1) and the column for $P = 0.025$. (This column should be used because the statistical analysis does not seek a difference in a specific direction but rather a simple "yes" or "no" answer.) For the example given here, the critical *t*-value is 2.02. Thus the calculated value is less than the critical value (1.80 < 2.02), meaning that the experimental data do not support a conclusion that bias exists between the two analytical methods.

Interpretation of the *t*-test is more difficult when the question is to determine whether a method's accuracy or systematic error is acceptable. For example, although the *t* increases directly as the bias increases, it also increases as the number of specimens increases and as SD_d decreases. Thus a very small bias may be statistically significant when a large comparison study (large n) has been performed between two methods, both with very good precision (small SD_d). On the other hand, a large bias may not be statistically significant when few specimens have been compared between two imprecise methods.

To judge acceptability, interpretation of the bias as an estimate of systematic error and comparison of its size to the previously defined allowable bias (B_A) or allowable total error (TE_A) is better than reliance on the *t*-test. When bias is smaller than either B_A or TE_A, the observed systematic error is less than the defined allowable error, and performance is judged acceptable. When bias is larger than either B_A or TE_A, the observed systematic error is larger than the allowable error, and performance is unacceptable.

F-Test

To compare the precision of two analytical methods the SDs of the methods are compared by use of the **F-test.** The F-value is calculated in the following equation:

$$F = \frac{(SD_1)^2}{(SD_2)^2}$$

where SD_1 is the larger SD and SD_2 the smaller one.

For example, consider a test method with an SD of 2 mg/dL (n = 31) and a reference method with an SD of 1 mg/dL (n = 21). The calculated F-value is 4.00 ($F = 2^2/1^2$).

To interpret the F-test the calculated F-value is compared with a critical F-value. When the calculated value is greater than the critical value, a statistically significant difference is observed, meaning that the SD of one method is larger than that of the other. When the calculated value is less than the critical value, no statistically significant difference is observed. Therefore based on the study data used, no evidence allows the conclusion that any difference exists between the two SDs.

Tables of critical F-values are found in most statistical handbooks or textbooks. For the values given in such tables, only a 5% chance ($P = 0.05$) exists that the critical F-value is exceeded due to chance alone. To look up a critical value the DOF of the numerator and denominator are necessary, which are both equal to n − 1. In the previous example, if 31 samples are analyzed by the test method and 21 samples analyzed by the reference method, the critical F-value is found in the appropriate table at the intersection of the column (numerator) with 30 DOF and the row (denominator) with 20 DOF (that is, a value of 2.04). If the observed F-value is greater than the critical F-value, a statistically sig-

nificant difference (at p = 0.05) exists between the SDs of the two methods. Therefore the reference method in this example is more precise than the test method.

Whether the precision of the test method is acceptable is a different question not answered by the F-test. To judge acceptability the observed SD (SD_{obs}) must be compared with the defined allowable SD (SD_A) or with the defined TE_A. If $SD_{obs} < SD_A$, or if $4SD_{obs} < TE_A$, precision is acceptable. If $SD_{obs} > SD_A$, or if $4SD_{obs} > TE_A$, the observed precision is unacceptable.

Linear Regression or Least-Squares Analysis

To describe the graphical plot of test values versus reference values from a comparison-of-methods experiment the best-fit straight line through the data is determined by **linear regression** or **least-squares analysis.** A straight line is given by an equation of the following form:

$$y = a + bx$$

where *a* is the y-intercept, and *b* is the slope of the regression line describing the way in which estimates of the test method values (*y*) are related to reference method values (*x*).

The slope (b) is calculated from the following equation:

$$b = \frac{n\Sigma xy - \Sigma x\Sigma y}{n\Sigma x^2 - (\Sigma x)^2}$$

The y-intercept (a) is calculated from the following equation:

$$a = \bar{y} - b\bar{x}$$

where

$\bar{y}$ = Mean value from test method sample
$\bar{x}$ = Mean value from the reference method sample
b = Slope calculated from the previous equation.

The SD about the regression line ($SD_{y/x}$) is calculated from the equation

$$SD_{y/x} = \sqrt{\frac{\Sigma(y_i - Y_i)^2}{n - 2}}$$

where y_i is the value observed for a sample by the test method, and Y_i is the value calculated from the regression equation, given the value by the reference method (x_i). The denominator gives the number of DOF, which is equal to n − 2 because the slope and intercept already have been calculated, thereby imposing two restrictions on the data set (leaving n − 2 independent comparisons or DOF).

Ideally the slope is 1.00; the y-intercept, 0.0; and $SD_{y/x}$, 0.0. Deviations from these ideal values are caused by different kinds of analytical errors. Proportional errors cause changes in the slope, constant errors cause changes in the y-intercept, and random errors cause increases in $SD_{y/x}$.

In applying linear regression to data from a comparison-of-methods experiment, graphing of the data for visual inspection is important. The response between the two methods must be linear (the numbers fitting a straight line), a wide analytical range must have been studied, and no widely discrepant values (outliers) should exist. Estimates of slope and intercept are unreliable if nonlinearity, a narrow range of concentrations, or outliers exist. When nonlinearity is present, the comparison data should be restricted to the linear range. If the range of data is narrow (also indicated by a correlation coefficient <0.95), an alternative statistical technique, such as Deming's regression, may be necessary. If outliers are present, those samples should be remeasured if possible. Otherwise, determination of whether the outliers affect the decision on acceptability should be done through analysis with and without the outlying values; if the decision changes, the presence of the outliers is critical and the study should be extended to obtain more reliable data.

Correlation Coefficient

Although it is not a necessary calculation, the correlation coefficient (r) commonly is used in comparison-of-methods studies. It is calculated from the following equation:

$$r = \frac{n\Sigma xy - \Sigma x \Sigma y}{\sqrt{[n\Sigma x^2 - (\Sigma x)^2][n\Sigma y^2 - (\Sigma y)^2]}}$$

where

x = The individual x values
y = The individual y values
n = The number of pairs of x, y data

Ideally, the value for r should be 1.00. Values less than 1.00 are due to random error within or between the methods. Systematic errors have no effect on r, which can have a value of 1.0 even when a method is inaccurate. Therefore the accuracy of a method should not be judged based on the value of r. The only use of r in comparison-of-methods experiments is to help assess the reliability of the linear regression estimates of slope and y-intercept. When $r > 0.95$ the estimates of slope and y-intercept are affected only slightly by variability in the comparative method.

■ BASIC CONCEPTS

Successful method evaluation occurs when five key points are followed (Table 13-1). In essence the process should seek to learn whether the candidate method exhibits sufficient analytical quality to produce results applicable clinically as intended. Statistical and economic considerations are also important but often compete with the clinical perspective. For example, statistical techniques are required for method evaluation, but statistical significance does *not* provide the sole basis with which to judge a method's acceptability. Instead a decision to accept or reject a method should be based on data, which lead to estimates of error that are

TABLE 13-1	The Keys to Successful Evaluation of a New Method

1. Apply a clinical perspective to the whole task.
2. Set analytical goals before you begin.
3. Conduct the correct experiments to collect the necessary data.
4. Use statistical tools properly so that you estimate the errors correctly.
5. Make objective conclusions about the method.

examined for clinical significance. Pressures to contain laboratory costs also have become exceedingly important and must be considered in the selection of a candidate method. However, selecting a method solely on the basis of cost is short-sighted reasoning that ultimately may increase costs and result in loss of physician trust, missed opportunities, or other negative consequences.

Confirming the need for the assay is the first step in the selection of a candidate method (see Figure 13-1). Carefully delineating the requirements for a candidate method at the outset helps ensure that the process of selection and evaluation is conducted in a straightforward and efficient manner. Consequently, these requirements guide the entire process of selection and evaluation of analytical methods. This process is part of the quality planning component that begins the continuous loop of quality management (see Chapter 17).

Practical Requirements

Certain practical factors first are considered in the decision of whether a method or instrument is implemented in a given laboratory. They include type of specimen, sample size, throughput, turnaround time, test repertoire, specimen handling, run size, personnel skill requirements, cost per test, method of calibration, calibration frequency, capability of random access, quality control approach, space needs (including reagent storage), waste disposal requirements, and chemical hazard and safety considerations. Most practical requirements are defined by laboratory personnel in discussion among analysts, supervisors, and directors. Candidate methods with practical characteristics not consistent with the requirements of the laboratory are not given further consideration.

Parameters of Analytical Performance

Properties relating to the performance of the method include its accuracy; analytical range, recovery, sensitivity, and specificity; blank reading; detection limit; interferences; precision; reagent stability; "ruggedness"; and sample interaction. A rugged method provides consistently reliable performance when used by different operators and with different batches of reagents over a long period of time. The assessment of these parameters requires experimental studies to estimate a method's performance; findings from these studies then are used as the basis for an informed decision as to whether the observed performance is acceptable for the medical use of the test results.

Accuracy

Accuracy is defined by the International Federation of Clinical Chemistry as the closeness of the agreement between the measured value of an analyte and its "true" value. The concepts of systematic error and total error are used to assess this closeness of agreement.

Systematic error

Systematic error is a measure of the agreement between the measured quantity and the true value. This aspect of accuracy usually is estimated by a comparison-of-methods experiment in which the clinical specimens are assayed by the method under evaluation and by a method with previously established and validated accuracy.[17] The terms *inaccuracy* and *bias* often are used to emphasize the lack of agreement among methods being compared. Systematic error is detected as either positive or negative bias for a given analytical method, in contrast to random error, which is both positive and negative. Systematic errors are subdivided into two types, constant and proportional. Constant systematic error is of the same magnitude even as the concentration of the analyte changes; in contrast, the magnitude of proportional systematic error is a percentage of the concentration of the analyte. Constant and proportional systematic errors are detected and clearly demonstrated through plotting of the results of a test method versus the "true values" for a group of samples (Figure 13-2). In Figure 13-2, *A*, random error appears as scatter in the data about the line of best fit. In Figure 13-2, *B*, constant error causes a shift of the line in one direction and is quantified best by the point at which the line intersects the ordinate (the y-intercept). Proportional error causes the slope of the line to vary from the ideal 45-degree angle. Thus careful inspection of such a plot provides meaningful information about these components of analytical error.

Total error

Information on the various components of error is valuable in any attempt to identify the source of errors and reduce their magnitude. On the other hand, what must be considered in judgment of a new method is the overall effect of the components of error, or the total error. The total error is that which determines the analytical quality achievable and the ultimate acceptability of the method for its intended clinical applications. Total error and its relationship to the random and systematic components are illustrated in Figure 13-3.

The distribution of values around a central value represents random error, whereas the shift of the central value of the distribution from the true value represents systematic error. The total error demonstrates how large the errors are

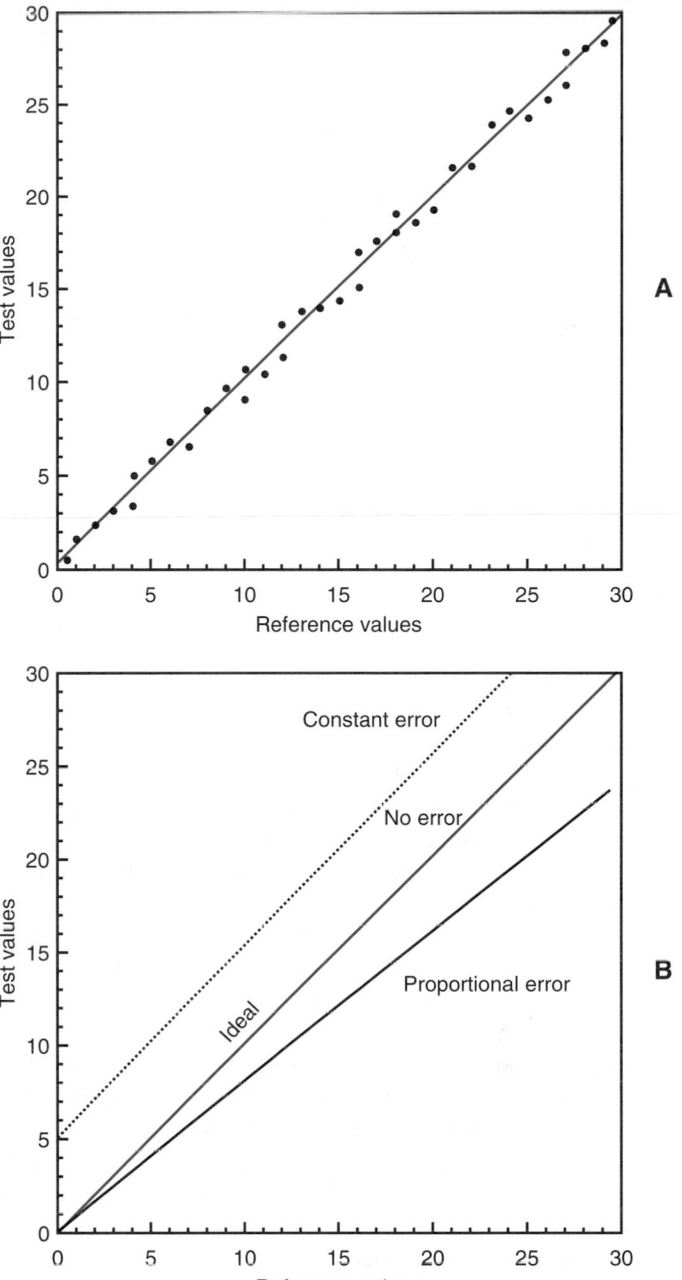

Figure 13-2 **A,** An indication of random error about the line. **B,** Appearance of constant and proportional types of systematic error.

when the random and systematic components occur in the same direction. This worst-case estimate of error appears larger than that for either component alone and therefore is a more judicious estimate in a decision of whether the quality of the analytical method is acceptable. Total error is a more comprehensive concept of accuracy than is traditional systematic error and is particularly applicable to clinical laboratory science, where often only a single measurement is performed. Test results are affected by both random and systematic errors.

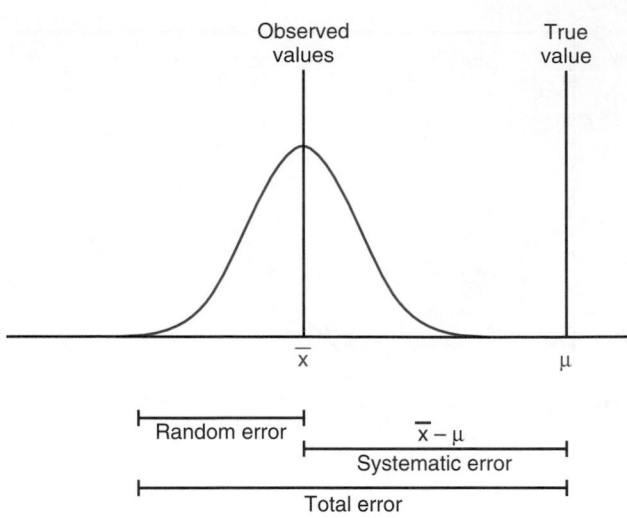

Figure 13-3   The total error concept of accuracy. (Modified from Westgard JO, de Vos DJ, Hunt MR et al: Method Evaluation, Houston, American Society for Medical Technology, 1978.)

Analytical range

The analytical range is the "range of concentration or other quantity in the sample over which the method is applicable without modification."[4] It is tested by a linearity experiment[13] in which reference solutions containing a wide range of specific quantities of an analyte are analyzed by the candidate method. Ideally the calibration curve (the plot of response versus analyte concentration) should be linear and pass through the origin. If the curve is linear, the range tested is termed the *linear range* of the method. If a linear response is not obtained, calibration procedures should use more calibrating solutions to define the response curve adequately and these solutions should bracket the unknowns. The analytical range of a method should be wide enough to include 95% to 99% of the expected samples without predilution. As defined by the Clinical Laboratory Improvements Amendments of 1988 **(CLIA '88),** Final Rule,[5] once the analytical range of a method is validated, it is termed the *reportable range* of that method.

Analytical sensitivity

The analytical sensitivity of a method is defined by the International Union of Pure and Applied Chemistry (IUPAC) as the slope of the calibration curve and the ability of an analytical procedure to produce a change in the signal for a defined change of the quantity. Basically, this term quantifies the change in signal relative to a change in the quantity, concentration, or property of the analyte. Commonly the terms *analytical sensitivity* and *detection limit* are confused and even misused. This confusion exists because the terms are interrelated; both are considered attributes of a "sensitive" method. In practice an ideal method would be characterized as having a high level of analytical sensitivity and a low detection limit.

Analytical specificity

The term *analytical specificity* is related to accuracy and refers to the ability of an analytical method to determine exclusively the analyte it claims to measure without reacting with other related substances.[4] For example, a glucose method is specific if it measures glucose accurately in the presence of similar hexose sugars (for example, mannose and galactose). Likewise, immunochemical methods are said to be specific for the analyte of interest when the antibody does not appreciably cross-react with like molecules. Analytical specificity also may be affected by substances commonly encountered in serum or plasma, such as bilirubin, hemoglobin, and lipids. These compounds may influence methods by virtue of their color, turbidity, or other physical or chemical properties.

Blank measurements

Responses observed during the measurement procedure that are due to reagent and sample constituents (rather than the studied analyte) are referred to as *blank measurements*. The analyst must be aware of the magnitude of blank measurements because they contribute to the total error of the measurement process. Blank values are obtained experimentally by measurement of (1) a solution of reagents without sample present (that is, a reagent blank) or (2) a solution of sample and reagents missing a key reagent that initiates the reaction or causes formation of the final reaction product (that is, a sample blank). The solutions used to obtain blank measurements should have essentially the same compositions as the solutions used in the measurement of unknown samples. Low blank measurements are preferable and provide optimal opportunity to obtain accurate and precise estimates of the analyte in question. If a method produces high blank measurements, its performance still may be satisfactory if the blank measurements are stable and precise; this precision permits small differences between analytical signals to be meaningful.

Detection limit

IUPAC defines detection limit (also called the *limit of detection*) as the smallest concentration or quantity of an analyte that is detected with reasonable certainty for a given analytical procedure. The detection limit depends on the amplitude of the blank readings and also is related to the precision of these measurements. The detection limit, (x_L), defines that point at which any smaller result should not be reported, except as "less than x_L."

Interferences

The term *interference* describes the effect that a compound (or group of compounds) other than the analyte in question has on the accuracy of measurement of an analyte. An example is the measurement of glucose by a glucose oxidase reaction, in which the intermediate product, hydrogen peroxide, may react with uric acid rather than the intended chromogen. Interferences may be subtle (for example, the presence of a drug that reacts with some of a diazo reagent intended for the analyte). Obviously, testing for all possible interferences for a given analytical method is difficult, if not impossible. To assist in this process the National Committee for Clinical Laboratory Standards has published a document that describes how to conduct interference testing of methods.[14] In addition, a listing of drugs and the ways in which they interfere with many clinical laboratory tests is available.[21]

Precision

The ability of an analytical method to produce the same value for replicate measurements of the same sample is known as its **precision,** also termed *random analytical error.* Precision usually is estimated by a replication experiment in which the same sample material is analyzed a minimum of 20 times and the SD calculated.

Different components of precision may be estimated, depending on how the experiment is performed. Within-run precision is the variability found when the same material is analyzed repetitively in the same analytical run or when duplicate analyses are made within a run on a series of clinical specimens and the SD of the duplicates calculated. Within-run precision usually underestimates total precision because minimal opportunity exists for conditions to change during the time between replicate analyses. Within-day precision or between-run precision is estimated when the same material is assayed repeatedly in several different runs on the same day. This variability is usually somewhat higher than that observed for within-run duplicates. Day-to-day precision or between-day precision is the variability found when the same material is analyzed repeatedly on different days. This last estimate is the most realistic assessment of the performance that a clinician observes in the applications of the test because it includes variations that arise from method performance by different operators, instrument changes from day to day, the use of different pipets, and variations in temperature or other laboratory conditions. All three components of precision are estimated through **analysis of variance (ANOVA)** calculations.[15] In practice the term *imprecision* is used frequently instead of *precision* because it quantifies the variability that occurs in replicate measurements.

Recovery

Recovery refers to the ability of an analytical method to measure an analyte correctly when a known amount of the analyte is added to authentic samples. Measurement of recovery is an effective means to obtain information about accuracy because it tests whether the method measures the analyte in the presence of all the other compounds contained in the matrices of authentic samples. Recovery experiments also test for competitive interferences (for example, the competition from protein for calcium in certain dye-binding methods for assaying of serum calcium). Unfortunately, recovery experiments often have been per-

formed poorly and their data improperly calculated. Also worth noting is that the addition of pure analyte in vitro is obviously an artificial approach; one cannot be sure that the physical or chemical state of the analyte (for example, its solubility and its binding to serum proteins) or metabolic circumstances (for example, conjugation in the liver) are the same as that occurring in vivo. However, when analytical reference methods and reference materials are limited or unavailable, a recovery experiment may be the only practical way to assess accuracy.

■ PERFORMANCE STANDARDS

To select and evaluate a candidate method objectively, performance standards must be established *before* analytical experiments are begun and a conclusion about the suitability of the method is made. Performing evaluation experiments to estimate errors and attempting to reach conclusions about the acceptability of a method without first defining the performance criteria diminishes the legitimacy of the study and results in the making of subjective statements, such as "shows good quality," "compares well," and "demonstrates acceptable performance," statements which have appeared in academic and commercial literature. Astute laboratorians must question whether such conclusions are valid. The laboratorian can avoid such doubt by establishing performance goals before conducting experiments and obtaining evaluation data. Actual performance then is compared with the goals to determine acceptability.

Performance goals should specify the total error allowed (TE_A) at a specific concentration (or concentrations) or activities of the analyte. These concentrations are selected at medical decision levels (X_C) at which test results are interpreted most critically by clinicians for diagnosis, monitoring, or therapeutic decisions. Several sources of information have been used to establish limits for total allowable error. These include professional judgment based on experience with the medical use of laboratory tests, surveys of clinicians, the intraindividual biological variation[7,8] of the analyte, limits based on state-of-the-art performance, and limits calculated from fractions of the reference interval of the analyte. No specifications are universally applicable. What is appropriate depends on the medical mission of the healthcare facility, patient population being served, particular application of the test, and manner in which the physician interprets the test result.[19] Thus performance goals may differ from laboratory to laboratory or even from application to application within a laboratory. For example, a creatinine method used to monitor kidney transplant recipients might have more stringent requirements than a method used as part of a health screening profile.

Several guidelines for the setting of analytical goals have been published.[1,9,18] For example, the CLIA regulations have established fixed limits for the assessment of method and laboratory performance for specific regulated analytes.[5] Given the legal and punitive ramifications of the CLIA regulations, these limits now have become, de facto, the maximum limits for allowable error in the United States. Consequently, in practice the total allowable error for a given analytical method must be less than the respective CLIA fixed limit for the analyte in question. For example, to produce acceptable performance on proficiency testing challenges, Ehrmeyer and colleagues[6] recommend that laboratories minimize bias and reduce internal coefficients of variation to one-third the CLIA fixed-limit goals. Their recommendation assumes a stable measurement process. Burnett and Westgard[3] further suggest that coefficients of variation for a method should not exceed one-fourth CLIA limits so as to include the possibility of unstable method performance and the utilization of cost-effective quality control procedures. On this basis the comparison of CLIA '88 limits with SD specifications is possible through division of the former by four. The authors of this text believe the use of CLIA limits is a practical and reasonable approach for method evaluation.

Maximum SD error goals from several sources are listed in Table 13-2. Wherever possible, the error recommendations are calculated in concentration units through the use of decision levels or critical concentrations (X_C). The source of these decision levels is either Barnett's[1] work or the limits of the reference or therapeutic intervals for the analyte in question.

SELECTING AN ANALYTICAL METHOD

Selecting a candidate method is the second step in the introduction of a new method into the laboratory (see Figure 13-1). Various approaches have been taken to identify candidate methods, including review of scientific literature, consultation with colleagues, review of commercial literature, or discussion of methods with manufacturers' representatives at professional meetings. Types of candidate methods include those discussed in the scientific literature, those available as commercial kits, those in a "closed" analytical system, and those requiring development by a laboratory (that is, an "in-house" method).

In the review of prospective methods, attention should be given to the following:

1. Principle of the assay, with original references
2. Composition of reagents and reference materials, as well as the quantities of such provided and storage requirements (for example, space, temperature, light, and humidity restrictions) applicable both before and after the opening of the original containers
3. Stability of reagents and reference materials (for example, shelf life)
4. Possible hazards, appropriate safety precautions, and Occupational Safety and Health Administration guidelines

5. Type, quantity, and disposal of waste generated
6. Specimen requirements (that is, conditions for collection, specimen volume requirements, the need for anticoagulants and preservatives, and necessary storage conditions)
7. Anticipated analytical performance (for example, accuracy, precision, sensitivity, and specificity)
8. Reference interval of the analyte, including information on how it was derived, typical values obtained in health and disease, and the need to determine a reference interval for the specific institution (see Chapter 14)
9. Detailed protocol for test performance
10. Instrumental requirements and limitations.
11. Availability of technical support, supplies, and service

In addition, the following questions should be asked regarding the situation in the laboratory:

1. Is the requisite measuring equipment available? If not, is sufficient space available for new equipment?
2. How much of a technologist's time is required, and what skill level is needed?
3. If training the entire staff in a new technique is required, is such training worth the possible benefit?
4. What is the estimated cost to perform an assay with the proposed method, including the cost of calibrators, quality control specimens, and the technologist's time?
5. Are the data generated compatible with the data processing equipment already available?

A qualitative assessment often is made from a review of a method's characteristics, but the use of a value scale to assign points to the various features of a method based on their relative importance also is possible; this latter approach results in a more quantitative selection process. Decisions then are made regarding the analytical methods that best fit the laboratory's requirements and that have the potential to achieve the necessary analytical quality.

EVALUATING AN ANALYTICAL METHOD

After the needs have been defined, the quality goals established, and a candidate method or methods selected, experiments are conducted to collect the necessary data that allow evaluation of the performance characteristics of the method(s).

Preliminary Evaluation

In general a preliminary period should be allowed for familiarization with the analytical method, its equipment, and its procedural steps; this familiarization period may involve trial runs to determine within-run precision and analytical range. Once the analyst is satisfied that the method is performing properly, precision should be measured by at least

TABLE 13-2   Allowable Error Recommendations

Analyte	Decision Level, X_C	Acceptable Performance, CLIA '88*	Precision Goals (Maximum SD) $X_C \times$ CLIA/4	Barnett†	Fraser‡	Fixed Limit Goals (Maximum Total Error), CLI A '88
Routine Chemistry						
Alanine aminotransferase§	50 U/L	20%	2.5		5.8[c]	10
Albumin	3.5 g/dL	10%	0.09	0.25	0.05[d]	0.35
Alkaline phosphatase	150 U/L	30%	11		5.1[d]	45
Amylase	100 U/L	30%	7.5		3.7[d]	30
Aspartate aminotransferase§	30 U/L	20%	1.5		1.2[c]	6.0
Bicarbonate	20 mmol/L			5.0	0.46[c]	
	30 mmol/L			5.0	0.69[c]	
Bilirubin, total§	1.0 mg/dL	0.4	0.10	0.2	0.08[c]	0.40
	20 mg/dL	20%	1.0	1.5	1.6[c]	4.0
Blood gas, P_{CO_2}	35 mm Hg	5 mm Hg	1.3	3.0	0.84[b]	5.0
	50 mm Hg	5 mm Hg	1.3	3.0	1.2[b]	5.0
Blood gas, P_{O_2}	30 mm Hg	3 SD‖	0.75 SD‖			3 SD‖
	80 mm Hg	3 SD	0.75 SD	5.0		3 SD
	195 mm Hg	3 SD	0.75 SD			3 SD
Blood gas, pH	7.35	0.04	0.01	0.004	0.01[b]	0.04
	7.45	0.04	0.01	0.006	0.01[b]	0.04
Calcium, total§	7.0 mg/dL	1.0	0.25	0.16	0.06[d]	1.0
	10.8 mg/dL	1.0	0.25	0.24	0.10[d]	1.0
	13.0 mg/dL	1.0	0.25	0.30	0.12[d]	1.0
Chloride§	90 mmol/L	5.0%	1.1	2.0	0.63[d]	4.5
	110 mmol/L	5.0%	1.4	2.0	0.77[d]	5.5
Cholesterol, total§	200 mg/dL	10%	5.0		5.4[d]	20
Cholesterol, high-density lipoprotein	35 mg/dL	30%	2.6		1.9[c]	10.5
	65 mg/dL	30%	4.9		3.6[c]	19.5
Creatine kinase§	200 U/L	30%	15		32[c]	60
Creatine kinase, MB isoenzyme	13 μg/L	3 SD	0.75 SD			3 SD
Creatinine	1.0 mg/dL	0.30	0.08	0.15	0.02[d]	0.30
	3.0 mg/dL	15%	0.11		0.07[d]	0.45
Glucose§	50 mg/dL	6.0	1.5	5.0	1.1[d]	6.0
	126 mg/dL	10%	3.15	5.0	3.1[d]	12.6
	200 mg/dL	10%	5.0		4.4[d]	20
Iron	150 μg/dL	20%	7.5		24[d]	30
Lactate dehydrogenase	300 U/L	20%	15		12[d]	60
Lactate dehydrogenase isoenzymes	100 U/L	30%	7.5			30
Magnesium	2.0 mg/dL	25%	0.13		0.02[d]	0.50
Phosphate, inorganic	4.5 mg/dL				0.11[c]	
Potassium§	3.0 mmol/L	0.50	0.13	0.25	0.04[c]	0.50
	6.0 mmol/L	0.50	0.13	0.25	0.07[c]	0.50
Protein, total§	7.0 g/dL	10%	0.18	0.30	0.10[d]	0.70
Sodium§	130 mmol/L	4.0	1.0	2.0	0.39[d]	4.0
	150 mmol/L	4.0	1.0	2.0	0.45[d]	4.0
Triglycerides	160 mg/dL	25%	10	15	18[d]	40
Urea nitrogen§	27.0 mg/dL	9%	0.6	2.0	1.7[d]	2.4
Uric acid	6.0 mg/dL	17%	0.25	0.5	0.25[d]	1.02

CLIA, Clinical Laboratory Improvements Amendments; *SD*, standard deviation.

*Clinical Laboratory Improvements Amendments of 1988. Final Rule. Laboratory Requirements. Federal Register February 28, 1992; 57:7002-7288.

†Barnett RN: Medical significance of laboratory results. Am J Clin Pathol 1968; 50:671-676.

‡Goal calculated from one-half the intraindividual biological variation data given by Fraser et al in:

  [b]Fraser CG: Generation and application of analytical goals in laboratory medicine. Annali dell' Instituto Superiore di Sanita 1991; 27:369-376.

  [c]Fraser CG: Biological variation in clinical chemistry—an update: collated data, 1988-1991. Arch Pathol Lab Med 1992; 116:916-923.

  [d]Fraser CG, Peterson PH, Ricos C et al: Quality specifications. In Haeckel R (ed): Evaluation Methods in Laboratory Medicine, pp 87-99, New York, VCH Publishers, 1993.

§Reference method/material credentialed by the National Reference System for Clinical Laboratories.

‖SD limits are based on peer group data from the Proficiency Testing program used.

Continued

TABLE 13-2 Allowable Error Recommendations—cont'd

Analyte	Decision Level, X_C	Acceptable Performance, CLIA '88*	Precision Goals (Maximum SD)			Fixed Limit Goals (Maximum Total Error), CLI A '88
			$X_C \times$ CLIA/4	Barnett†	Fraser‡	
Endocrinology and Related Markers						
11-Deoxycortisol	8.0 μg/L				0.86[d]	
17-OH Progesterone	0.5 μg/L				0.073[c]	
Aldosterone	15 ng/dL				2.2[c]	
	30 ng/dL				4.4[c]	
Androstenedione	260 ng/dL				15[c]	
CA 15-3	25 U/mL				0.65[d]	
CA 125	35 U/mL				2.4[d]	
CA 549	11 U/mL				0.5[d]	
Carcinoembryonic antigen	5 ng/mL				0.23[d]	
Chorionic gonadotropin	25 IU/L	3 SD	0.75 SD			
	10,000 IU/L	3 SD	0.75 SD			
Cortisol	5 μg/dL	25%	0.31		0.38[d]	1.25
	30 μg/dL	25%	1.88		2.3[d]	7.5
C-peptide	37 μg/L				1.7[d]	
Dehydroepiandrosterone sulfate	2000 μg/L				12[d]	
	4500 μg/L				27[d]	
Estradiol	60 ng/L				6.5[d]	
	450 ng/L				49[d]	
Follicle-stimulating hormone	10 U/L				0.15[d]	
	95 U/L				1.5[d]	
Luteinizing hormone	6 U/L				0.37[c]	
	55 U/L				3.4[c]	
Prolactin	15 μg/L				0.53[c]	
	200 μg/L				7.0[c]	
Prostate-specific antigen	2 μg/L				0.18[c]	
T₃ uptake	25%	3 SD	0.75 SD			3 SD
Testosterone	90 ng/dL				3.7[c]	
	1000 ng/dL				42[c]	
Thyroid-stimulating hormone	0.3 mIU/L	3 SD	0.75 SD		0.030[c]	3 SD
	5.0 mIU/L	3 SD	0.75 SD		0.50[c]	3 SD
Thyroxine, free	0.8 ng/dL	3 SD	0.75 SD		0.023[c]	3 SD
	4.0 ng/dL	3 SD	0.75 SD		0.11[c]	3 SD
Thyroxine, total	3.0 μg/dL	1.0	0.25		0.09[c]	1.0
	13 μg/dL	20%	0.65		0.39[c]	2.6
Transferrin	375 mg/dL				9.0[d]	
Triiodothyronine	80 ng/dL	3 SD	0.75 SD		3.4[c]	3 SD
	200 ng/dL	3 SD	0.75 SD		8.5[c]	3 SD
Toxicology and Therapeutic Drug Monitoring						
Alcohol, blood	0.10 g/dL	25%	0.006			0.025
Carbamazepine	8 mg/L	25%	0.50		0.51[d]	2.0
	12 mg/L	25%	0.75		0.77[d]	3.0
Digoxin	0.8 μg/L	0.20	0.05		0.03[d]	0.20
	2.0 μg/L	20%	0.10		0.08[d]	0.40
Ethosuximide	40 mg/L	20%	2.0		2.0[a]	8.0
	100 mg/L	20%	5.0		4.9[a]	20.0
Gentamicin	10 mg/L	25%	0.6			2.5
Lead, blood	10 μg/dL	4.0	1.0			4.0
	40 μg/dL	4.0	1.0			4.0
Lithium	0.5 mmol/L	0.3	0.08		0.02[d]	0.3
	1.5 mmol/L	20%	0.08		0.06[d]	0.3

[a] Fraser CG: Desirable standards of performance for therapeutic drug monitoring. Clin Chem 1987; 33:387-389.

TABLE 13-2   Allowable Error Recommendations—cont'd

Analyte	Decision Level, X_C	Acceptable Performance, CLIA '88*	Precision Goals (Maximum SD)			Fixed Limit Goals (Maximum Total Error), CLIA '88
			$X_C \times$ CLIA/4	Barnett†	Fraser‡	
Toxicology and Therapeutic Drug Monitoring—cont'd						
Phenobarbital	15 mg/L	20%	0.75		0.33[d]	3.0
	40 mg/L	20%	2.0		0.88[d]	8.0
Phenytoin	10 mg/L	25%	0.6		0.36[d]	2.5
	20 mg/L	25%	1.2		0.72[d]	5.0
Primidone	5 mg/L	25%	0.3		0.56[a]	1.3
	12 mg/L	25%	0.75		1.36[a]	3.0
Procainamide	4 mg/L	25%	0.25			1.0
	20 mg/L	25%	1.25			5.0
Quinidine	7 mg/L	25%	0.45			1.8
Theophylline	10 mg/L	25%	0.63		1.1[d]	2.5
	20 mg/L	25%	1.2		2.2[d]	5.0
Valproate	50 mg/L	25%	3.1		3.2[d]	12.5
	100 mg/L	25%	6.2		6.4[d]	25
Hematology						
Cell identification		90% consensus				
Erythrocyte count	4.5 M/µL	6%	0.07		0.09[d]	0.27
	5.9 M/µL	6%	0.09		0.12[d]	0.35
Fibrinogen	150 mg/dL	20%	7.5			30
Hematocrit	35%	6%	0.53%		0.46%[d]	2.1%
	50%	6%	0.75%		0.65%[d]	3.0%
Hemoglobin	12 g/dL	7%	0.21		0.14[d]	0.84
	17 g/dL	7%	0.30		0.20[d]	1.19
Leukocyte count	3.5 K/µL	15%	0.13		0.23[d]	0.52
	11 K/µL	15%	0.41		0.74[d]	1.65
Partial thromboplastin time	40 seconds	15%	1.5			6.0
Platelet count	50 K/µL	25%	3.12		2.0[d]	12.5
	500 K/µL	25%	31.2		20[d]	125
Prothrombin time	INR 3.6	15%	INR 0.14			INR 0.54
White cell differentiation		3 SD				3 SD
Immunology						
Alpha₁-antitrypsin	80 mg/dL	3 SD	0.75 SD			3 SD
Alpha-fetoprotein	10 µg/L	3 SD	0.75 SD			3 SD
Antinuclear antibody		2 Titers or ±	1 Titer			
Antistreptolysin O		2 Titers or ±	1 Titer			
Antihuman immunodeficiency virus		R/N	R/N			
Complement C3	100 mg/dL	3 SD	0.75 SD			3 SD
Complement C4	20 mg/dL	3 SD	0.75 SD			3 SD
Hepatitis (HBsAg, anti-HBc, HBeAg)		R/N	R/N			
IgA	400 mg/dL	3 SD	0.75 SD		17[c]	3 SD
IgE	200 IU/mL	3 SD	0.75 SD			3 SD
IgG	500 mg/dL	25%	31		13[c]	125
	2000 mg/dL	25%	125		52[c]	500
IgM	300 mg/dL	3 SD	0.75 SD		8.8[c]	3 SD
Infectious mononucleosis		2 Titers or ±	1 Titer			
Rheumatoid factor		2 Titers or ±	1 Titer			
Rubella		2 Titers or ±	1 Titer			

INR, International normalized ratio; *R/N*, reactive/nonreactive; *IgA*, immunoglobulin A; *IgE*, immunoglobulin E; *IgG*, immunoglobulin G.

TABLE 13-3	Criteria to Judge the Acceptability of Errors as Estimated from Different Evaluation Experiments	

Type of Error	Experiment	Criteria
Random error	Replication	$S_{obs} < S_A$, or $4 \times S_{obs} < TE_A$
Proportional error	Recovery	$\left|\dfrac{(\bar{B} - 100)}{100}\right| x_c < B_A$
Constant error	Interference	$|Bias| < B_A$
Systematic error	Comparison of methods	$|(a + bx_c) - x_c| < B_A$
Total error	Replication and comparison	$4 \times S_{obs} + |(a + bx_c) - x_c| < TE_A$

S_{obs}, SD determined in a replication experiment; $\bar{B}$, average recovery (in percent) determined in a recovery experiment; *bias*, average difference determined in an interference experiment; *a* and *b*, *y*-intercept and slope, respectively, determined by regression analysis with the comparison-of-methods data; x_c, decision level concentration at which medical interpretation is most critical; S_A, allowable SD; B_A, allowable bias; TE_A, allowable total error.

20 replicates with the use of material having concentrations at each decision level. Studies on recovery and interference then are performed. If the requisite comparative method with traceable or established accuracy and precision is available, accuracy should be tested in a comparison-of-methods experiment.

Quantitative values are obtainable for each type of error; these values are compared with the limits of error allowed by the specifications. In practice, estimates of these error quantities are obtained through the use of various statistical techniques. For example, the SD is used to estimate precision; thus one criterion to judge precision is that the experimental SD fall within the specified SD_A. Alternatively, when a random error goal has been specified, the experimental SD is multiplied by four (according to the recommendation of Burnett and Westgard[3]) to provide an estimate of random error; this estimate then is compared with the TE_A. Similar criteria subsequently are developed for interference, recovery, and comparison-of-methods experiments (Table 13-3).

Step-by-Step Outline of a Method Evaluation Experiment

To conduct a method evaluation the analyst should complete certain tasks. The following list incorporates pertinent stipulations from the CLIA '88 regulations:

1. Write a protocol for the evaluation, one for the procedure, and then maintain the latter for 2 years or the duration of application of the procedure, whichever is longer. A National Committee for Clinical Laboratory Standards document providing details used to describe a technical procedure is available.[16]

2. Document the validity of the method by recording all the information collected during evaluation to authenticate decisions.

3. Determine the reportable range by analyzing a set of reference solutions or a series of dilutions either of control materials or a specimen pool containing an elevated quantity of the analyte in question.[13] Choose the appropriate diluent; in some instances the only suitable diluent may be serum known to be free of the analyte of interest. Plot the observed value against the relative dilutions for the series of samples. Estimate the analytical range by visual inspection of the graph. Compare the observed range with the necessary analytical range or the range provided by the manufacturer.

4. Determine the components of precision of the assay. First, determine within-run precision by analyzing serum pools or control materials 20 times or more. Select materials with values that are near each decision level. Calculate mean and SD and assess acceptability by comparing the SD_{obs} with the SD_A or calculating random error appropriately for the test and comparing it with the TE_A (see Table 13-1). In the processing of data, results that appear questionable should be excluded only (1) if they are related to documented errors (for example, if they were obtained when an automated instrument indicated an "error" status), (2) if arbitrary exclusion of the results as undocumented mistakes is possible (for example, decimal point or transcription errors), or (3) if they are statistical outliers.[11]

   After excluding any outliers, calculate the mean and SD for each data set. If the within-run precision does not meet the requirement, attempt to locate the source of imprecision or abandon this procedure in favor of another. Steps at which imprecision is commonly a problem include the dispensing of specimens or reagents, mixing operations, and measurement of signal. If the within-run precision meets the requirement, proceed with further testing. Determine day-to-day precision by analyzing the pools or control materials each working day for at least 20 days.

5. Determine the accuracy of the method by comparing the performance of the candidate method with that of a definitive or reference method, performing a recovery experiment, or comparing the performance of the candidate method with that of the method being replaced.

   a. A scientifically valid technique to establish the accuracy of a candidate method is the comparison of its performance with that of a definitive or reference method with established accuracy (Figure 13-4). In actual practice, however, reference methods often are not readily accessible to routine clinical laboratories. In this situation use of the candidate method to analyze a reference material that has certified values for a number of clinically relevant analytes is a method of assessment. Values have been assigned for these materials through the use of either

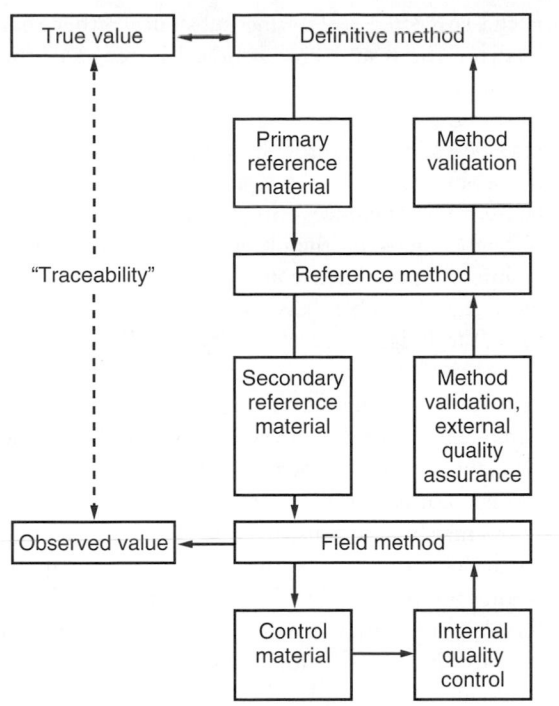

Figure 13-4   Structure of an accuracy-based measurement system illustrating relationships among reference methods and materials.

definitive or reference methodology. An example of such a material is standard reference material (SRM) 909, which is available from the National Institute of Standards and Technology. Values obtained from the candidate method then are compared with the target values listed in the documentation provided with the SRM.

b. For the recovery experiment, a set of samples that consists of authentic specimens (that is, baseline samples) to which specific quantities of the analyte in question (that is, test samples) have been added should be analyzed; next, the differences between the test and baseline concentrations or activities should be calculated to determine the amount recovered. Then the ratio of the amount recovered divided by the amount added is calculated. (This value should *not* be calculated as the total amount found divided by the total amount added because the true total amount added is unknown). Finally, this value should be multiplied by 100 to obtain the recovery in percent. The difference between the average recovery and the ideal 100% recovery provides an estimate of proportional error, which then is multiplied by a decision level of interest to determine the magnitude of the error at that critical concentration. This estimate of proportional error then is compared with the allowable error to judge acceptability.

c. If the candidate method is replacing an existing method, the performance of the two methods should be compared with a split-sample study. In such a study, 40 to 100 clinical specimens are collected, split into aliquots, and analyzed with both methods. In this situation the number of specimens is less important than the concentration range the specimens cover[12] and the variety of diseases and medical conditions they represent. If possible, specimens should be fresh. If stored specimens must be used, they should be preserved under conditions that prevent analyte degradation. The samples should be assayed by the two methods within a 4-hour period to minimize any change because of instability of the specimens themselves (for example, evaporation). They should be assayed in small groups over several days to provide data representative of the performance of both analytical methods.

d. Data analysis should begin as the method comparison studies progress. The results should be plotted on a timely basis, with the test method results on the *y*-axis and the comparative method results on the *x*-axis. Some data points ("outliers") almost inevitably fall outside the line of ideality; investigation of these outliers often reveals valuable information. If an outlier is identified, the sample should be reanalyzed by both methods, inspected for unique characteristics, and facts gathered about the patient's condition at the time the specimen was obtained. Obviously these steps are taken only if the outlier was observed in real time, underscoring the importance of data daily plotting.

Comparison data may be processed with a variety of statistical techniques. Although *r* and statistical tests for assessment of the significance of the difference in the means have been popular, they are of little value for in assessment of performance relative to the medically based analytical goals. In fact, depending on these statistics for method acceptability decisions is misleading and is a crucial mistake commonly made by those conducting method evaluation studies. In particular, the *r* should *never* be used to assess whether a test method is accurate relative to a comparative method.[2] Grossly inaccurate *x* and *y* data still produce high ("good") values for *r*. The *r* may be used to reveal whether the two methods are associated and—of greater value in method evaluation—it helps to justify the application of least-squares linear regression statistics to comparison-of-methods data by determining whether the range of data is suitably wide. An *r* greater than or equal to 0.975 indicates that the sample data are of an adequate range for the application of simple linear regression techniques.[17] No other use of the *r* is appropriate in method comparison studies.

The *t* value is used to determine whether a bias is statistically significant. This fact may be interesting, but it does not help in the making of decisions on acceptability of the method being tested, which, as has been discussed previously, should be based on clinical significance. Decisions to accept or reject a method should not be based on t values, or r, or any such statistic. Statistics are tools that help us estimate the observed errors.

Regression analysis determines the slope (b), y-intercept (a), and SD about the regression line ($SD_{y/x}$). The slope provides an estimate of proportional analytical error, the intercept gives an estimate of constant error, and $SD_{y/x}$ is an estimate of random error between the methods. The regression equation ($Y = a + bX$) is used to estimate the systematic error at the decision level concentrations. The Y-value (Y_C) corresponding to the X-value of interest (X_C) is calculated ($Y_C = a + bX_C$); systematic error (SE) is calculated as the difference between X_C and Y_C (SE = $|Y_C - X_C|$; see Table 13-3). Comparing SE with the specification for allowable bias or TE_A to judge acceptability then is possible. Using a total error criterion through addition of the observed systematic error to four times the SD_{obs} (TE = SE + 4 x SD_{obs}) also is possible; then this estimate is compared with the TE_A. Points that seem aberrant should be examined carefully on a timely basis. Outliers are excluded from the data set if an error is identified or on the basis of statistical grounds.[11] Often outliers provide some of the most informative data concerning the specificity (or lack thereof) exhibited by the new method.

6. Estimate the sensitivity of the new method by determining the slope of the calibration curve. This information is obtained from the analytical range experiment if the dilutions of the samples are adequately large. In addition, make sample and reagent blank measurements and note the magnitude of these signals in comparison with the signal for a low concentration of the analyte.

7. Estimate the detection limit (x_L) of the method with the following equation:

$$x_L = x_{bl} + ks_{bl}$$

where

x_{bl} = Mean of the blank measurements
s_{bl} = SD of the blank measurements
k = Numerical factor chosen based on the confidence level desired

In practice, k is assigned a value of either 2 or 3 to obtain a detection limit that has a probability of either 95% or 99%, respectively.

8. Test the specificity of the new method by assessing the interference caused by substances regularly found in blood samples, such as bilirubin, hemoglobin, lipids, anticoagulants, and common drugs.[14] To test interference, conduct an experiment that is analogous to the recovery experiment, with the exception that the material added

is the suspected interfering substance rather than the analyte. The results are expressed in terms of the difference in concentration between the sample containing the interferent and the baseline sample. Interference also may be estimated through comparison of results with those obtained by use of an analytical method known to be free of interference; using this method, again take the difference between the observed values as the estimate of interference. Then compare this difference, or bias, with the allowable bias or the allowable total error (TE_A) to judge its acceptability (see Table 13-2).

9. Establish the reference interval of the analyte. If the results from both the candidate and old methods are comparable, the reference interval used with the old method also is used with the new one. If the new method performs according to the manufacturer's claims, the laboratory may be able to use the reference interval published by the manufacturer. However, CLIA '88 requires the laboratory to verify that the manufacturer's reference interval is appropriate for the laboratory's patient population.[5] The reference interval must be determined if (1) the values produced by the new method do not agree with those from the old one, but the new method is an improvement, (2) the new method is accepted relative to the old method for other reasons, or (3) the new method is to be used to measure an analyte not previously assayed by the laboratory. (Protocols for determination of reference intervals will be discussed in Chapter 14.)

In addition to assessing the performance of the candidate method, the laboratory should also perform the following:

a. Determine the stability and uniformity of reagents and reference materials by comparing the results obtained when using different lots and using lots that have been stored for varying periods of time. The variation of results should be much less than that given in the defined error specifications.

b. Prepare a section for the laboratory's procedure manual that provides step-by-step performance instructions for the test, along with other required or desirable features.[16]

c. Prepare in-service training materials and instruct personnel on how to perform the test; all staff personnel who perform the test should study the test description and demonstrate competency in its performance after individualized instruction.

d. Implement quality control procedures (see Chapter 17) and establish control limits and procedures.

e. Prepare documentation for clinical staff members, including instructions on specimen collection, hours of test availability, expected turnaround time, reference intervals, potential interfering substances, and a short description of the test's clinical utility.

f. Inform clinical staff members of the test's availability and encourage feedback during the introductory phase of the new test's application. Monitor performance carefully during the first several months by using statistical control procedures.

An example of a method evaluation study has been published in an expanded version of this chapter.[10]

ASSESSING METHOD ACCEPTABILITY

When the previous steps of a method evaluation have been completed successfully, objective conclusions about the acceptability of method performance are reached through the following steps:

1. Comparison of the experimentally determined estimates of the errors with the limits defined by the specifications established for the analytical goals
2. Consideration of the performance of the candidate method as acceptable when the value obtained for the total error is less than the total error allowed for the method
3. Consideration of the performance of the candidate method as unacceptable when one or more of its analytical parameters is greater than the allowable error for the method

When this latter event occurs, the performance of the method must be improved; if it cannot be improved, the method is rejected.

This approach to method evaluation decision making is logical and rigorous, but graphical techniques also are available for the formation of objective decisions about method performance. For example, Westgard[20] has developed and introduced a graphical approach that he has called the *method evaluation decision chart (MEDx chart)*. The MEDx chart is based on the total error of the method being tested but plots the operating point in terms of the observed inaccuracy and imprecision. This operating point defines the performance of the method on the basis of where it appears with respect to allowable error criteria fixed on the chart. The allowable error lines depend on the total error quality goal defined by the laboratory for its projected use of the test. The charts actually allow three or four criteria and thus help classify a method one or two steps beyond simply "acceptable" or "unacceptable." Example MEDx charts may be found at the Westgard QC website (www.westgard.com).

References

1. Barnett RN: Medical significance of laboratory results. Am J Clin Pathol 1968; 50:671-676.
2. Bland JM, Altman DG: Statistical methods for assessing agreement between two methods of clinical measurement. Lancet 1986; 1:307-310.
3. Burnett RW, Westgard JO: Selection of measurement and control procedures to satisfy the Health Care Financing Administration requirements and provide cost-effective operation. Arch Pathol Lab Med 1992; 116:777-780.
4. Buttner J, Borth R, Boutwell JH et al (IFCC Committee on Standards): Provisional recommendations on quality control in clinical chemistry: general principles and terminology. Clin Chem 1976; 22:532-539.
5. Clinical Laboratory Improvements Amendments of 1988. Final Rule. Laboratory Requirements. Federal Register February 28, 1992; 57:7002-7288.
6. Ehrmeyer SS, Laessig RH, Leinweber JE et al: 1990 Medicare/CLIA final rules for proficiency testing: minimum intralaboratory performance characteristics (CV and bias) needed to pass. Clin Chem 1990, 36:1736-1740.
7. Fraser CG: Biological variation in clinical chemistry—an update: collated data, 1988-1991. Arch Pathol Lab Med 1992; 116:916-923.
8. Fraser CG, Petersen PH: Desirable standards for laboratory tests if they are to fulfill medical needs. Clin Chem 1993; 39:1447-1453.
9. Fraser CG, Petersen PH, Libeer J-C et al: Proposals for setting generally applicable quality goals solely based on biology. Ann Clin Biochem 1997; 34:8-12.
10. Koch DD, Peters T Jr: Selection and evaluation of methods. In Burtis CA, Ashwood ER (eds): Tietz Textbook of Clinical Chemistry, 3rd edition, pp 320-335, Philadelphia, WB Saunders, 1999.
11. Kringle RO, Bogovich M: Statistical procedures. In Burtis CA, Ashwood ER (eds): Tietz Textbook of Clinical Chemistry, 3rd edition, pp 265-309, Philadelphia, WB Saunders, 1999.
12. Linnet K: Necessary sample size for method comparison studies based on regression analysis. Clin Chem 1999; 45:882-894.
13. National Committee for Clinical Laboratory Standards: Evaluation of the Linearity of Quantitative Analytical Methods: Proposed Guideline. Document EP6-P. Wayne, Pa, NCCLS, 1986.
14. National Committee for Clinical Laboratory Standards: Interference Testing in Clinical Chemistry: Proposed Guideline. Document EP7-P. Wayne, Pa, NCCLS, 1986.
15. National Committee for Clinical Laboratory Standards: Evaluation of Precision Performance of Clinical Chemistry Devices: Tentative Guideline. 2nd edition. Document EP5-A. Wayne, Pa, NCCLS, 1999.

16. National Committee for Clinical Laboratory Standards: Clinical Laboratory Technical Procedure Manual: Approved Guideline. 3rd edition. Document GP2-A3. Wayne, Pa, NCCLS, 1996.

17. National Committee for Clinical Laboratory Standards: Method Comparison and Bias Estimation Using Patient Samples: Approved Guideline. Document EP9-A. Wayne, Pa, NCCLS, 1995.

18. Skendzel LP, Barnett RN, Platt R: Medically useful criteria for analytical performance of laboratory tests. Am J Clin Pathol 1985; 83:200-205.

19. Stockl D: European specifications for imprecision and inaccuracy compared with US CLIA proficiency-testing criteria. Clin Chem 1995; 41:120-121.

20. Westgard JO: A method evaluation decision chart (MEDx chart) for judging method performance. Clin Lab Sci 1995; 8:277-283.

21. Young DS: Effects of Drugs on Clinical Laboratory Tests, 5th edition, Washington, DC, AACC Press, 2000.

Additional Reading

Kristiansen J, Christensen JM: Traceability and uncertainty in analytical measurements. Ann Clin Biochem 1998; 35:371-379.

Shahangian S, Cohn RD: Variability of laboratory test results. Am J Clin Pathol 2000; 113:521-527.

CHAPTER 14

Establishment and Use of Reference Values

HELGE ERIK SOLBERG, MD, PhD

Objectives

1. Define the following terms:

Reference value	Selection criteria
Subject-based reference value	Random sample
Population-based reference value	Prevalence

2. Compare selection criteria and exclusion criteria and provide examples of each.
3. Determine reference intervals using parametric and nonparametric measures.
4. Define *sensitivity, specificity,* and *predictive value* of laboratory tests and calculate each.
5. Demonstrate, using a formula, how the predictive value of a laboratory procedure is affected by prevalence.

Key Words

Multivariate Analysis Consideration of more than one test simultaneously

Parametric A statistical approach to reference value analysis that requires specific distributional assumptions; nonparametric approaches, on the other hand, making no assumptions about a distribution

Partitioning The process by which a reference group is subdivided to reduce the biological variation in each group

Reference Value A value obtained by observation or measurement of a particular type of quantity on a reference individual

Reference Individual An individual selected, as basis for comparison with individuals under clinical investigation, through the use of defined criteria

Sensitivity (Clinical) The proportion of subjects with disease who have positive test results

Specificity (Clinical) The proportion of subjects without disease who have negative test results

---

■ ESTABLISHMENT OF REFERENCE VALUES

Data collected during medical interviews, clinical examinations, and supplementary investigations must be interpreted by comparison with reference data. If the condition of the patient resembles that typical of a particular disease, the physician may base the diagnosis on the observation (positive diagnosis). This diagnosis is made more likely if observed symptoms and signs do not fit the patterns characterizing a set of alternative diseases (diagnosis by exclusion).

The interpretation of medical laboratory data is just a special case of decision making by comparison. To follow this decision process, **reference values** are required for all tests performed in the clinical laboratory, not only from healthy individuals but also from patients with relevant diseases.[2,5,11,13] Ideally, observed values should be related to several collections of reference values—values from healthy individuals, the undifferentiated hospital population, individuals with typical diseases, and ambulatory individuals; in addition, previous values from the subjects under investigation are necessary.

Certain conditions are mandatory to make the comparison of a patient's laboratory results with reference values possible and valid:

1. All groups of reference individuals should be clearly defined.
2. The patient examined should resemble sufficiently the reference individuals (in all groups selected for comparison) in all respects other than those under investigation.
3. The conditions under which the samples were obtained and processed for analysis should be known.
4. All quantities compared should be of the same type.
5. All laboratory results should be produced with the use of adequately standardized methods under sufficient analytical quality control (see Chapter 17).
6. The stages in the pathogenesis of the diseases that are the objectives for diagnosis should be demarcated.
7. The diagnostic sensitivity and specificity, prevalence, and clinical costs of misclassification should be known for all laboratory tests used.

Reference Values

The term *normal values* has been used frequently in the past. Confusion arose because the word *normal* has several very different connotations. This term is obsolete and should not be used. The International Federation of Clinical Chemistry (IFCC)[5] recommends use of the term *reference values* and related terms, such as *reference individual, reference limit, reference interval,* and *observed values.* Reference values are results of a certain type of quantity obtained from a single individual or group of individuals corresponding to a stated description, which must be spelled out and made available for use by others.

A short description of qualifiers associated with the term reference values, such as *health-associated reference values* (close to what was understood by the obsolete term *normal values*) is convenient. Other examples of such qualifying words are *diabetic patient, hospitalized diabetic patient,* and *ambulatory diabetic patient.* These short descriptions prevent the common misunderstanding that reference values are associated only with health.

A further distinction exists between subject-based and population-based reference values. *Subject-based reference values* are previous values from the same individual, obtained when the individual was in a defined state of health. *Population-based reference values* are those obtained from a group of well-defined reference individuals and are usually

the type of values referred to when the term *reference values* is used without any qualifying words. This chapter deals predominantly with population-based values.

Selection of Reference Individuals

A set of selection criteria determines which individuals should be included in the group of **reference individuals.** Such selection criteria include statements describing the source population, specifications of criteria for health, or the disease of interest.[2,5,13] The selection of reference individuals is based essentially on the application of defined criteria to a group of examined candidates. The required characteristics of the reference values determine which criteria should be used in the selection process. Table 14-1 provides a list of important criteria to use in the production of health-associated reference values.

Ideally the group of reference individuals should be a random sample of all the individuals in the parent population who fulfill the selection criteria. However, a strictly random sampling scheme is impossible to obtain in most situations for a variety of practical reasons. It would imply the examination of and application of selection criteria to the entire population (thousands or millions of individuals) and the random selection (for example, by raffling) of a subset of individuals among those accepted. Therefore using the best reference sample that can possibly be obtained after all practical considerations have been taken into account is necessary. Data then should be used and interpreted with due caution because of the possible bias introduced by the non-randomness of the sample selection process.

Often separate reference values for sex, age group, and other criteria are necessary. Thus defining the partition crite-

TABLE 14-1	Examples of Exclusion Criteria for Health-Associated Reference Values*

Disease
Risk Factors
   Obesity
   Hypertension
   Risks from occupation or environment
   Genetically determined risks
Intake of pharmacologically active agents
   Drug treatment for disease or suffering
   Oral contraceptives
   Drug abuse
   Alcohol
   Tobacco
Specific physiological states
   Pregnancy
   Stress
   Excessive exercise

*The table lists only some major classes of criteria. This list should be supplemented with other relevant criteria based on known sources of biological variation (see Chapter 2).

ria for the subclassification of the set of selected reference individuals into more homogeneous groups also may be necessary (Table 14-2).[5,13] The number of partition criteria usually should be kept as small as possible to obtain sufficient sample sizes for the derivation of valid statistical estimates.

Age and sex are the most frequently used criteria for subgrouping because several analytes vary significantly among different age and gender groups (see Chapter 2). Age may be categorized by equal intervals (for example, by decades) or intervals that are narrower in the periods of life where greater variation is observed. In addition, the use of qualitative age groups (for example, postnatal, infancy, childhood, prepubertal, pubertal, adult, premenopausal, menopausal, or geriatric) often is convenient. Height and weight also can be used as criteria for the categorization of children.

Specimen Collection

Preanalytical standardization of the preparation of individuals before sample collection, sample collection itself, and handling of the sample before analysis may eliminate or minimize bias or variation from these factors. These steps may reduce biological "noise" that otherwise may conceal important biological "signals" of disease, risk, or treatment effect (see Chapter 2).

The magnitudes of preanalytical sources of variation clearly are not equal for different analytes. Therefore one may argue that only those factors causing unwanted variation for the biological quantity for which reference value production is intended should be considered. Body posture during sample collection is, for instance, highly relevant for the establishment of reference values for nondiffusible analytes, such as albumin in serum, but irrelevant for diffusible ones, such as serum sodium.

TABLE 14-2   Examples of Partition Criteria to be Used for Possible Subgrouping of the Reference Group

Age (not necessarily categorized by equal intervals)
Sex
Genetic factors
    Race (ethnic origin)
    Blood groups (ABO)
    Histocompatibility antigens (HLA)
Physiological factors
    Stage in menstrual cycle
    Stage in pregnancy
    Physical condition
Other factors
    Socioeconomic
    Environmental
    Chronobiological

HLA, Human leukocyte antigen.

On the other hand, several constituents usually are analyzed in the same clinical specimens. Therefore devising special systems for each type of quantity is impractical. For that reason standardized procedures for blood sample collection by venipuncture and skin puncture have been recommended.[7]

A special problem is caused by drug ingestion before sample collection. A distinction may be made between indispensable and dispensable medications. The latter category of drugs always should be avoided for at least 2 days before specimen collection. The use of indispensable drugs, such as contraceptive pills or essential medication, may be a criterion for exclusion or partition.

Analytical Procedures and Quality Control

Essential components of the required definition of a set of reference values are specifications concerning (1) analysis method, including information on equipment, reagents, calibrators, type of raw data, and calculation method, (2) quality control (see Chapter 17), and (3) reliability criteria (see Chapter 13). Specifications should be described so carefully that another investigator can reproduce the study and evaluate comparability of the reference values with values obtained by the methods used for production of the patient's values in a routine laboratory. To ensure comparability between reference and observed values, the same analytical method should be used.

Statistical Treatment of Reference Values

After the analysis of the reference specimens is performed, the reference values are subjected to a statistical treatment. This treatment includes partitioning of the reference values into appropriate groups, inspection of the distribution of each group, identification of outliers, and determination of reference limits.

Partitioning of reference values

The subset of reference individuals and the corresponding reference values may be partitioned according to sex, age, and other characteristics (see Table 14-2). **Partitioning** also is known as *stratification, categorization,* or *subgrouping,* and its results are called *partitions, strata, categories, classes,* or *subgroups.* The aim of partitioning is to reduce, if possible and necessary, variation among subjects to minimize biological "noise." Less intraclass variation gives narrower and more sensitive reference intervals. In general, reference values may be partitioned when the differences between the classes are statistically significant (rejection of the "null" hypothesis of equal distributions).[8,10]

In the following sections a homogeneous reference distribution is assumed to exist—either the complete subset distribution (if partitioning is unnecessary) or a subclass distribution after partitioning.

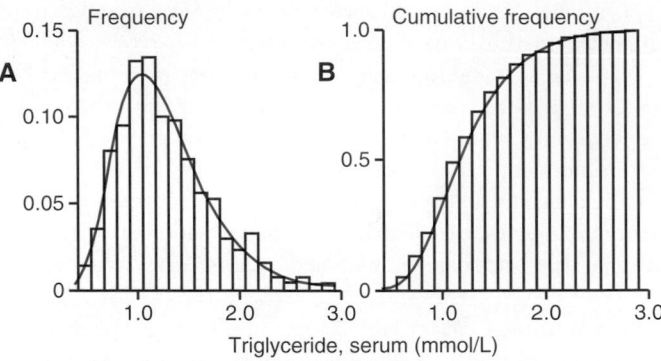

Figure 14-1   Observed and hypothetical distributions of 500 triglycerides values in serum (in mmol/L). **A,** The vertical bars of the histogram show the number of observations in the interval divided by the total number of observations. The curve is the estimated probability distribution of the population, assuming random sampling and a log-Gaussian distribution. **B,** The cumulated ratios (*bars*) and estimated cumulative probability distribution (*curve*). The data were computer generated for the purpose of this illustration.

Inspection of distribution

Displaying the reference distribution graphically and subsequently inspecting it always is advisable. A histogram, as shown in Figure 14-1, *A,* is prepared easily by hand or use of a computer program; it is the data display best suited for visual inspection. The examination of the histogram is a safeguard against the misapplication or misinterpretation of statistical methods, and it may provide valuable information about the data. The following characteristics should be sought in an examination of the distribution:

1. Highly deviating values (outliers) may represent erroneous values. (This subject will be discussed in more detail in a subsequent section in this chapter.)
2. Bimodal or polymodal distributions have more than one peak and may indicate that the distribution is nonhomogeneous because of the mixing of two or more distributions. If nonhomogeneity is the case, the criteria used to select reference individuals should be reevaluated or partitioning of the values according to age, sex, or other relevant factors attempted.
3. The shape of the distribution may be asymmetrical (skewed) or more or less peaked than the symmetrical and bell-shaped Gaussian distribution (non-Gaussian kurtosis).[8,10,11,13]
4. The visual inspection also may provide initial estimates of the location of reference limits that are useful as checks on the validity of computations.

Identification and handling of outliers

An erroneous value can be traced to a gross deviation from the prescribed procedure for establishment of reference values. Such values either may deviate significantly from the proper reference values (outliers) or be hidden in the refer-

ence distribution. Only a strict experimental protocol, with adequate controls at each step, can eliminate the latter type of erroneous values.

Visual inspection of a histogram is a reliable method for identification of possible outliers. However, the inspector must keep in mind that values near the furthest point on the long tail of a skewed distribution easily may be misinterpreted as outliers. If the distribution is positively skewed, inspection of a histogram displaying the logarithms of the values may aid in the identification of outliers. Some outliers also may be identified by statistical tests,[5,13] but no single method can detect outliers in every situation that may occur. The following are two main problems often encountered:

1. Many tests assume that the type of the true distribution is known before the tests are used. Some tests specifically require that the distribution be Gaussian. However, biological distributions are very often non-Gaussian, and their types seldom are known in advance. The range test is relatively robust[5] and involves identification of the extreme value as an outlier if the difference between the two highest (or lowest) values in the distribution exceeds one-third the range of all values.
2. Several tests for outliers assume that the data contain only a single outlier. Thus the range test usually fails in the presence of several outliers.

Deviating values identified as possible outliers should not be discarded automatically. Values should be included or excluded on a rational basis. The records of the dubious values should be checked and any errors corrected. In some cases deviating values should be rejected because noncorrectable causes have been found, such as previously unrecognized conditions that qualify individuals for exclusion from the group of reference individuals.

Determination of reference limits

In clinical practice an observed patient's value usually is compared with the corresponding reference interval, which is bounded by a pair of reference limits. This interval, which may be defined in different ways, is a useful condensation of the information carried by the total set of reference values.

The terms *reference limits* and *clinical decision limits* should not be confused. Reference limits describe the reference distribution; they provide information about the observed variation of values in the selected set of reference individuals. Thus comparison of new values with these limits only conveys information about similarity with the given set of reference values. In contrast, clinical decision limits provide optimal separation among clinical categories. The latter limits usually are based on analysis of reference values from several groups of individuals (healthy individuals and patients with relevant diseases) and thus are used for the purpose of differential diagnosis.

The term *reference range* sometimes is used for the term *reference interval,* but this use should be discouraged because

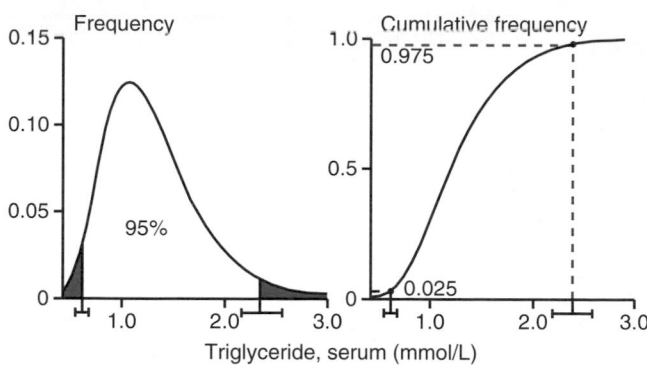

Figure 14-2   Central 95% reference interval with the 2.5 and 97.5 percentiles and their 0.90 confidence intervals of the 500 serum triglycerides concentrations (see Figure 14-1), as determined by the parametric method (see related text). The curves are the estimated probability distributions.

the statistical term *range* denotes the difference (a single value!) between the maximum and minimum values in a distribution.

Three kinds of reference intervals have been suggested—tolerance interval, prediction interval, and interpercentile interval.[5] The choice from among these types of intervals may be important for certain well-defined statistical problems, but their numerical differences are negligible when based on at least 100 reference values.

The interpercentile interval is simple to estimate, more commonly used, and recommended by the IFCC.[5] It is defined as an interval bounded by two percentiles of the reference distribution. A percentile denotes a value that divides the reference distribution such that a specified percentage of its values has magnitudes less than or equal to the limiting value. For example, if 2.32 mmol/L is the 97.5 percentile of serum triglycerides, 97.5% of the concentration values are equal to or below this value.

The definition of the reference interval as the central 95% interval bounded by the 2.5 and 97.5 percentiles is an arbitrary but common convention (Figure 14-2); that is, 2.5% of the values are cut off in both tails of the reference distribution.[5] Another size or an asymmetrical location of the reference interval may be more appropriate in particular cases.

The precision of a percentile as an estimate of a population value depends on the size of the subset; it is less precise when few observations are present. If the assumption of random sampling is fulfilled, determination of the confidence interval of the percentile (that is, the limits within which the true percentile is located with a specified degree of confidence) is possible (see Figure 14-2). The 0.90 confidence interval of the 97.5 percentile (upper reference limit) for serum triglycerides may, for example, be 2.22 to 2.62 mmol/L. The true percentile would be expected in this interval with a confidence of 0.90 if all serum triglycerides concentrations in the total reference population were measured. The theoretical minimum sample size required for the estimation of

the 2.5 and 97.5 percentiles is 40 values, but at least 120 reference values are required to obtain reliable estimates.

The interpercentile interval can be determined by both parametric and nonparametric statistical techniques. The **parametric** method for the determination of percentiles and their confidence intervals assumes a certain type of distribution, and it is based on estimates of population parameters, such as the mean and standard deviation (SD). For example, a parametric method is used if the true distribution is believed to be Gaussian and reference limits (percentiles) are determined as the values located two SDs below and above the mean. The majority of the parametric methods are in fact based on the Gaussian distribution. If the reference distribution has another shape, mathematical functions that transform data to approximately Gaussian shape may be used. The nonparametric method makes no assumptions concerning the type of distribution and does not use estimates of distribution parameters. The percentiles are determined simply by cutting off of the required percentage of values in each tail of the subset reference distribution.

When the results obtained by these two methods are compared, the estimates of the percentiles usually are very similar; the only difference is that the parametric estimates of percentiles are theoretically more precise (with narrower confidence intervals) than those obtained by the nonparametric method, especially with smaller sample sizes. The simple and reliable nonparametric method, especially in its bootstrap version (see following section), generally is preferable to the parametric method.

Nonparametric method

Several nonparametric methods are available,[13] but those based on ranked data are simple and reliable and allow nonparametric estimation of the confidence intervals of the percentiles.[3,5,12,13] The procedure is as follows:

1.   The *n* reference values are sorted in ascending order of magnitude and ranked. The minimum value has rank number 1, the next value number 2, and so on until the maximum value, rank *n*, is reached. Consecutive rank numbers should be given to two or more values that are equal ("ties"). The sorting and ranking may be done easily with spreadsheet software.
2.   The rank numbers of the 2.5 and 97.5 percentiles is computed as $0.025(n + 1)$ and $0.975(n + 1)$, respectively.
3.   One determines the percentiles by finding the original reference values that correspond to the computed rank numbers, provided that the rank numbers are integers. Otherwise, interpolation between the two limiting values is necessary.
4.   Finally, the confidence interval of each percentile is determined through use of the binomial distribution. Table 14-3 facilitates this step for the 0.90 confidence

---

TABLE 14-3 Nonparametric Confidence Intervals of Reference Limits*

| Sample Size | Rank Numbers | | Sample Size | Rank Numbers | |
	Lower	Upper		Lower	Upper
119 to 132	1	7	556 to 574	8	22
133 to 160	1	8	575 to 598	9	22
161 to 187	1	9	599 to 624	9	23
188 to 189	2	9	625 to 631	10	23
190 to 218	2	10	632 to 665	10	24
219 to 248	2	11	666 to 674	10	25
249 to 249	2	12	675 to 698	11	25
250 to 279	3	12	699 to 724	11	26
280 to 307	3	13	725 to 732	12	26
308 to 309	4	13	733 to 765	12	27
310 to 340	4	14	766 to 773	12	28
341 to 363	4	15	774 to 799	13	28
364 to 372	5	15	800 to 822	13	29
373 to 403	5	16	823 to 833	14	29
404 to 417	5	17	834 to 867	14	30
418 to 435	6	17	868 to 871	14	31
436 to 468	6	18	872 to 901	15	31
469 to 470	6	19	902 to 919	15	32
471 to 500	7	19	920 to 935	16	32
501 to 522	7	20	936 to 967	16	33
523 to 533	8	20	968 to 970	17	33
534 to 565	8	21	971 to 1000	17	34

Modified from International Federation of Clinical Chemistry: Approved recommendation on the theory of reference values: Part 5. Statistical treatment of reference values. J Clin Chem Clin Biochem 1987; 25:650.
*The table shows the rank numbers of the 0.90 confidence interval of the 2.5 percentile for samples with 119 to 1000 values. To obtain the corresponding rank numbers of the 97.5 percentile, subtract the rank numbers in the table from ($n + 1$), where n is the sample size.

---

interval of 2.5 and 97.5 percentiles. The bounding rank numbers for each percentile may be located in the table.

5. Table 14-4 shows an example of the nonparametric determination of percentiles using the serum triglycerides values shown in Figure 14-1.

Bootstrap estimation. The bootstrap method[3,9] is an extension of the nonparametric method. The method consists of the following steps:

1. Random samples of size n from the set of n reference values should be drawn, with replacement. Drawing "with replacement" is performed if each value randomly selected from the set is kept in the set so that it may participate in the random selection of the next value. The number of resamples should be high (500 being a reasonable default number).

2. For each resample, the upper and lower reference limits (percentiles) should be estimated by the rank-based nonparametric procedure described previously, with omission of the last step (estimation of the confidence interval).

3. The mean of the resample estimates of the two reference limits should be computed and the two mean values used as the final estimates.

4. The 0.90 confidence interval of each reference limit may be computed as $m \pm 1.645 \times s$, where m is the mean value of the lower or upper reference limit and s the corresponding SD.

Among available methods for estimation of reference limits and their confidence intervals, the bootstrap method probably is the most reliable. Because of the intense resampling a computer is necessary.[12]

Parametric method

The parametric method[3,5,11,13] is much more complicated than the nonparametric method and usually requires the use of a computer statistics program when large samples are to be processed.[12] The parametric method to estimate percentiles assumes that the true distribution is Gaussian. A critical phase in the parametric method therefore is to test the goodness-of-fit level of the reference distribution to a hypothetical Gaussian distribution. A simple test is the examination of a plot of the cumulative distribution (see Figure 14-1, *B*) on Gaussian probability paper, which features a nonlinear vertical axis based on the Gaussian distribution. The plot should be close to a straight line if the distribution is Gaussian. However, visual evaluation of the deviations from the straight line is very difficult because of the nonlinearity of the

TABLE 14-4   **Nonparametric Determination of Reference Interval***

Sorted and Ranked Serum Triglycerides Values in the Left Tail of the Distribution

Values:	0.41	0.43	0.45	0.46	0.47	0.49	0.51	0.55	0.55	0.55
Ranks:	1	2	3	4	5	6	7	8	9	10
Values:	0.56	0.58	0.58	0.61	0.62	0.62	0.64	0.64	0.65	0.65
Ranks:	11	12	13	14	15	16	17	18	19	20

Sorted and Ranked Triglycerides Values in the Right Tail of the Distribution

Values:	2.21	2.22	2.26	2.27	2.27	2.28	2.30	2.31	2.34	2.35
Ranks:	481	482	483	484	485	486	487	488	489	490
Values:	2.48	2.50	2.55	2.62	2.63	2.65	2.72	2.78	2.90	2.91
Ranks:	491	492	493	494	495	496	497	498	499	500

Calculation of Rank Numbers of the Percentiles
Lower: 0.025(500 + 1) = 12.5
Upper: 0.975(500 + 1) = 488.5

Finding the Original Values Corresponding to These Rank Numbers
Lower reference limit (2.5 percentile): 0.58
Upper reference limit (97.5 percentile): 2.32 (by interpolation)

Rank Numbers (See Table 14-3) and Values of the 0.90 Confidence Limit of the Lower Reference Limit
Rank numbers: 7 and 19
Confidence limits: 0.51 and 0.65

Rank Numbers (See Table 14-3) and Values of the 0.90 Confidence Limit of the Upper Reference Limit
Rank numbers: 500 + 1 – 19 = 482
500 + 1 – 7 = 494
Confidence limits: 2.22 and 2.62

Summary
Lower reference limit: 0.58 (0.51 – 0.65) mmol/L
Upper reference limit: 2.32 (2.22 – 2.62) mmol/L

*The table shows a worked-out example through use of the 500 serum triglycerides concentrations displayed in Figure 14-1. (See the text for a description of the nonparametric method.) The unit of all concentrations in the table is mmol/L.

vertical distances in the graph. Many statistical computer-programs have goodness-of-fit tests (for example, tests based on coefficients of skewness and kurtosis, the Kolmogorov-Smirnov test, or the Anderson-Darling test).[5,12,13]

If the reference distribution does not differ significantly from the Gaussian distribution, the 2.5 and 97.5 percentiles can be estimated by the values approximately two SDs on each side of the mean, or more accurately

$$2.5 \text{ percentiles} = \bar{x} - 1.96 \times SD$$

$$97.5 \text{ percentile} = \bar{x} + 1.96 \times SD$$

The 0.90 confidence interval of each percentile is estimated by the following two limits:

$$\text{Lower confidence limit} = \text{percentile limit} - 2.81 \times \frac{SD}{\sqrt{n}}$$

$$\text{Upper confidence limit} = \text{Percentile limit} + 2.81 \times \frac{SD}{\sqrt{n}}$$

If the reference distribution is non-Gaussian, mathematical transformation of data may provide a distribution similar to a Gaussian version. One frequent observation of interest is that logarithmically transformed values of a distribution with a long right tail (positively skewed) fit the Gaussian distribution rather closely. In other cases square roots of the values better approximate the Gaussian distribution. This information is the basis for the common use of the logarithmic and square root transformations when reference limits are estimated as described in the following section. If these two functions fail to transform data to fit a Gaussian distribution, more general transformations can be used. Such functions are described in other relevant literature.[2,5,11-13] To apply the parametric procedure the following steps must be observed:

1. The data is transformed by the logarithmic function $y = \log(x)$ through use of either natural logarithms, $\ln(x)$, or common Briggsian logarithms, $\log_{10}(x)$. Then the fit is tested to the Gaussian distribution through use of the methods described previously. If both transformations fail, either more general functions, which are usually more complicated, or the simple nonparametric method previously described should be used.

2. The mean ($\bar{y}$) and the standard deviation (SD_y) of the transformed data then are computed. Next, the percentiles and their confidence intervals are estimated in the transformed scale with the formulas discussed previously, with $\bar{y}$ for $\bar{x}$ and SD_y for SD.

3. The final step is reconversion of the percentiles and their confidence intervals to the original data scale through use of the inverse functions—antilogarithms or squares, respectively.

4. For example, the mean and SD of the serum triglycerides values of Figure 14-1 after logarithmic transformation (natural logarithms) are $\bar{y} = 0.172$ and $SD_y = 0.357$. The 2.5 percentile is

$$0.172 - 1.96 \times 0.357 = -0.528$$

$$2.5 \text{ percentile} = e^{-0.528} = 0.59$$

The lower reference limit of serum triglycerides thus is 0.59 mmol/L. The 0.90 confidence interval of this percentile is

$$-0.528 - 2.81 \times \frac{0.357}{\sqrt{500}} = -0.573$$

$$\text{Lower confidence limit} = e^{-0.573} = 0.56$$

$$-0.528 + 2.81 \times \frac{0.357}{\sqrt{500}} = -0.483$$

$$\text{Upper confidence limit} = e^{-0.483} = 0.62$$

That is, 0.56 − 0.62 mmol/L. The 97.5 percentile (and its 0.90 confidence interval) is by the same method found to be 2.39 (2.29 − 2.50) mmol/L. Readers may verify the latter results as a learning exercise.

Comparison with Table 14-4 demonstrates that the nonparametric and parametric methods both result in very similar estimates of reference limits (percentiles). The parametric confidence intervals, however, are somewhat narrower than the nonparametric ones.

■ USE OF REFERENCE VALUES

Interpreting medical laboratory data requires comparison of the patient's values with the reference values. This section of the chapter includes five aspects of this comparison: presentation of an observed value, use of multivariate reference regions, use of subject-based reference values, determination of the transferability of reference values, and use of sensitivity and specificity.

Presentation of an Observed Value in Relation to Reference Values

An observed value (patient's value) may be compared with reference values. This comparison is often similar to hypothesis testing, but it is seldom statistical testing in the strict sense. Thus consideration of the reference values as the yardstick for a less formal assessment than hypothesis testing is advisable.

The clinician should be supplied with as much information about the reference values as necessary for the interpretation.[2,5] Reference intervals for all laboratory tests may be presented to the physicians in a booklet, together with information about the analysis methods and their imprecision and descriptions of the reference values. A convenient presentation of the observed value and the reference interval on the same report sheet may be helpful for the busy clinician. For example, the reference intervals may be preprinted on report forms, or the computer system may select the appropriate age- and sex-specific reference interval from a file and print it next to the test result or in graphical form.

An observed value may be classified as low, usual, or high (three classes), depending on its location in relation to the reference interval. On reports a convenient practice is to flag unusual results (for example, through use of the letters *L* and *H* for low and high, respectively). A more detailed division of the value scale also has been advocated. The regions outside the reference interval may be subdivided to indicate the observed value's degree of unusualness. The reference interval also may be subclassified, but the advantages of this practice are doubtful because the shape of the reference distribution is not taken into account.

Another popular method of classification is to express the observed value by a mathematical distance measure. For example, the well-known SD-unit, or normal equivalent deviate, is such a measure. It is calculated as the difference between the observed value and the mean of the reference values divided by their SD.[2]

Multivariate, Population-Based Reference Regions

The previous sections of this chapter have discussed univariate population-based reference values and quantities derived from them. However, such values do not fit the common clinical situation, in which the observed values of several different laboratory tests are available for interpretation and decision making. For example, on average 8.4 individual laboratory tests are requested on each sample received in this author's laboratory. Two models exist for interpretation by comparison in this situation. Each observed value can be compared with the corresponding reference values or interval (that is, performance of multiple, univariate comparisons), or the set of observed values can be considered as a single multivariate observation and interpreted as such by a multivariate comparison. Only the latter method, which is known as **multivariate analysis**, can prevent the development of false-positive results (see following section).

The multivariate concept

A univariate observation, such as a single laboratory result, may be represented graphically as a point on a line, the

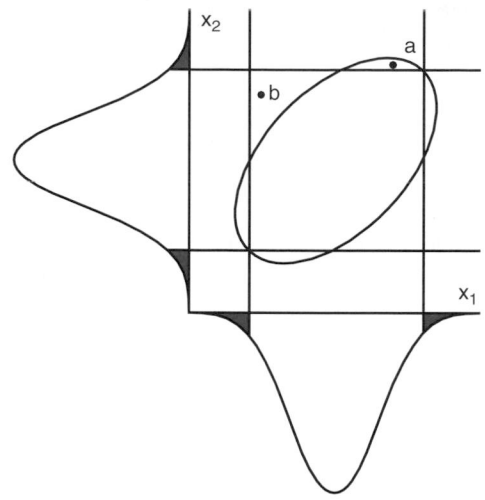

Figure 14-3   Bivariate reference region *(ellipse),* compared with the region defined by the two univariate reference intervals *(box).* The correct interpretation of the two patterns, *a* and *b,* is possible only by comparison with the bivariate reference region *(ellipse).* x_1, Values from test 1; x_2, values from test 2.

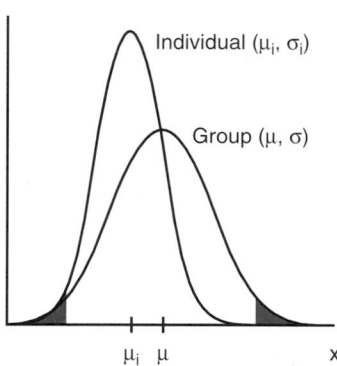

Figure 14-4   The relationship between population-based and subject-based reference distributions and reference intervals. The example is hypothetical, and the two distributions are, for simplicity, Gaussian. μ, True mean; μ_i, hypothetical mean; Φ, true standard deviation; Φ_i, hypothetical standard deviation; x, analysis result. (Modified from Harris EK: Effects of intra- and interindividual variation on the appropriate use of normal ranges. Clin Chem 1974; 20:1536.)

axis, or a scale of values. The results obtained by two different laboratory tests performed on the same sample (a bivariate observation) may be displayed as a point in a plane defined by two perpendicular axes. Three results yield a trivariate observation and a point in a space defined by three perpendicular axes, and so on. The possibility for visualization of a multivariate observation is lost when more than three dimensions exist. Still, the multivariate observation can be considered as a point in a multidimensional hyperspace with as many mutually perpendicular axes as are results of different tests. In this context the prefix *hyper-* signifies "more than three dimensions." Such multivariate observations also are known as *patterns* or *profiles.* A multivariate distribution thus is represented by a cluster of points on a plane, in a space, or in a hyperspace, depending on the dimensionality of the observation. Several statistical methods are based on multivariate methods, and some of them are straightforward extensions of well-known univariate methods.[6]

The multivariate reference region

Defining a common multivariate reference region based on the joint distribution of the reference values for two or more laboratory tests is possible. This multivariate region is not a right-angled area or (hyper-)box, but more like an ellipse in the plane (Figure 14-3) or an ellipsoid body or hyperbody. This region may be a straightforward extension of the univariate 95% interval to the multivariate situation; it may be set to enclose 95% of the central multivariate reference data points.[1,2] In that case only 5% false-positive results would be expected.

The use of multivariate reference regions usually requires the assistance of a computer program. The computer pro-

gram takes a set of results obtained by several laboratory tests on the same clinical sample and calculates an index. The interpretation of a multivariate observation in relation to reference values then involves comparison of the index with a critical value estimated from a corresponding set of reference values.[1,2]

Subject-Based Reference Values

Figure 14-4 illustrates the inherent problem associated with population-based reference values. It shows two hypothetical reference distributions. One represents the common reference distribution based on single samples obtained from a group of several different reference individuals. It has a true (hypothetical) mean μ and an SD of σ. The other distribution is based on several samples collected over time in a single individual, the *i*th individual. Its hypothetical mean is μ_i and the SD, σ_i.

If an observed value is located outside the subject's 2.5 and 97.5 percentiles, the personal or subject-based reference interval, the cause may be a change in the biochemical status, suggesting the presence of disease. Figure 14-4 demonstrates that such an observed value still may be within the population-based reference interval. The sensitivity of the latter interval to changes in a subject's biochemical status depends accordingly on the location of the individual's mean μ_i relative to the common mean μ and to the relative magnitudes of the corresponding SDs σ_i and σ. A mean μ_i close to μ and a small σ_i relative to σ may conceal the individual's changes entirely within the population-based reference interval.

TABLE 14-5　**Predictive Value of a Test Applied to Healthy and Diseased Populations**

Population	Number of Patients with Positive Test Result	Number of Patients with Negative Test Result	Totals
Number of patients with disease	TP	FN	TP + FN
Number of patients without disease	FP	TN	FP + TN
TOTALS	TP + FP	FN + TN	TP + FP + TN + FN

TP, True positives (number of diseased patients correctly classified by the test); *FP,* false positives (number of nondiseased patients misclassified by the test); *FN,* false negatives (number of diseased patients misclassified by the test); *TN,* true negatives (number of nondiseased patients correctly classified by the test).

Sensitivity = positivity in disease, expressed as percent = $\dfrac{TP}{TP + FN} \times 100$

Specificity = absence of a particular disease, expressed as percent = $\dfrac{TN}{FP + TN} \times 100$

Predictive value of positive test (PV^+) = percent of patients with positive results who are diseased

$$= \frac{TP}{TP + FP} \times 100 = \frac{\text{prevalence} \times \text{sensitivity}}{(\text{prevalence} \times \text{sensitivity}) + (1 - \text{prevalence})(1 - \text{specificity})}$$

Predictive value of negative test (PV^-) = percent of patients with negative test results who are nondiseased = $\dfrac{TN}{TN + FN} \times 100$

The following two possible solutions exist to the problem of the clinical insensitivity of population-based reference intervals:

1. Attempts may be made to reduce the variation in the reference values by partitioning of them into more homogeneous subclasses, as discussed previously.
2. The subject's previous values, obtained in a well-defined state of health, may be used as the reference for any future value.[2-4,13] The application of subject-based reference values becomes more feasible as "health-screening" by laboratory tests and computer storage of results become available to large sections of the general population.

Transferability of Reference Values

The determination of reliable reference values for each test in the laboratory's repertoire is a major task that is often far beyond the capabilities of the individual laboratory. Therefore the use of reference values in one facility that are generated in another laboratory would be convenient. This task is possible if the following conditions are fulfilled:

1. The populations should be described and matched adequately.
2. Subsets of data from both laboratories should be compared with one another to check for bias arising from analytical factors.
3. Analytical performance in both laboratories should agree.
4. Preparation of individuals before specimen collection and specimen collection itself should follow a standardized scheme in both laboratories.

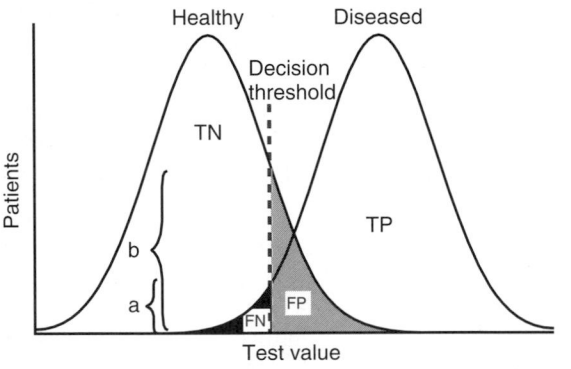

Figure 14-5　Simulated distributions of healthy and diseased populations. Note that at the decision threshold, the probability of a subject with disease, *a*, is much less than the probability of a healthy subject, *b*. *TP,* True positives; *TN,* true negatives; *FP,* false positives; *FN,* false negatives.

Sensitivity and Specificity

When a clinician uses a laboratory test to help establish a diagnosis (as opposed to following a trend or evaluating the effectiveness of treatment), knowing the test's sensitivity and specificity can assist with proper interpretation. The **sensitivity** of an assay is the fraction of those subjects with a specific disease that the assay correctly predicts. The **specificity** is the fraction of those individuals without the disease that the assay correctly predicts. Table 14-5 lists pertinent definitions and formulas.

Changing the decision limit of an assay affects both sensitivity and specificity. Consider the case when the disease group has higher values than the nondisease group (Figure 14-5). Values above the decision limit are classified as positive; those at or below are negative. Moving the upper decision limit to a lower value increases the sensitivity—but at the cost of a decrease in the specificity. Thus increased true-positive detection was traded for an increase in the number of false-positive results. This trade-off occurs in every test performed in medicine. Although it is not often appreciated, the trade-off affects the opinions of surgical pathologists and radiologists, as well as the care provider who performs a physical examination, as much as it affects the interpretation of quantitative laboratory test results.

Given a positive result, in how many cases does a patient actually have the disease? The predictive value positive of a test answers this question. The predictive value of a test combines disease prevalence with test sensitivity and specificity. Prevalence is the proportion of the population (or those being tested) with the disease. The predictive value positive of a test is the number of true-positive results divided by the number of positive results (true-positive and false-positive results combined). The number of true-positive and false-positive results is a function of the prevalence in the population and sensitivity and specificity of the test in question. The predictive value negative follows in a similar way but is used less often. It answers the question, "Given a negative result, how likely is it that a patient does not actually have the disease?" The formulas can be used for the predictive value positive and the predictive value negative found in Table 14-5 to combine the sensitivity and specificity of a test with the prevalence.

References

1. Boyd JC, Lacher DA: The multivariate reference range: an alternative interpretation of multi-test profiles. Clin Chem 1982; 28:259-265.
2. Gräsbeck R, Alström T (eds): Reference Values in Laboratory Medicine: The Current State of the Art, Chichester, England, John Wiley & Sons, 1981.
3. Harris EK, Boyd JC: Statistical Bases of Reference Values in Laboratory Medicine, New York, Marcel Dekker, 1995.
4. Harris EK, Cooil BK, Shakarji G et al: On the use of statistical models of within-person variation in long-term studies of healthy individuals. Clin Chem 1980; 26:383-391.
5. International Federation of Clinical Chemistry, Expert Panel on Theory of Reference Values: Approved recommendation on the theory of reverence values. Part 1. The concept of reference values. J Clin Chem Clin Biochem 1987; 25:337-342. Part 2. Selection of individuals for the production of reference values. J Clin Chem Clin Biochem 1987; 25:639-644. Part 3. Preparation of individuals and collection of specimens for the production of reference values. J Clin Chem Clin Biochem 1988; 26:593-598. Part 4. Control of analytical variation in the production, transfer, and application of reference values. Eur J Clin Chem Clin Biochem 1991; 29:531-535. Part 5. Statistical treatment of collected reference values: determination of reference limits. J Clin Chem Clin Biochem 1987; 25:645-656. Part 6. Presentation of observed values related to reference values. J Clin Chem Clin Biochem 1987; 25:657-662.
6. Morrison DF: Multivariate Statistical Methods, 3rd edition, New York, McGraw-Hill, 1990.
7. National Committee for Clinical Laboratory Standards: Procedures for the Collection of Diagnostic Blood Specimens by Venipuncture. Approved Standard. 4th edition. NCCLS Document H3-A4, 1998, and Procedures and Devices for the Collection of Diagnostic Blood Specimens by Skin Puncture. Approved Standard. 4th edition. NCCLS Document H4-A4, 1999, Wayne, Pa, National Committee for Clinical Laboratory Standards.
8. Sachs L: Applied Statistics: A Handbook of Techniques, New York, Springer-Verlag, 1984.
9. Shultz EK, Willard KE, Rich SS et al: Improved reference-interval estimation. Clin Chem 1985; 31:1974-1978.
10. Snedecor GW, Cochran WG: Statistical Methods, 8th edition, Ames, Iowa, Iowa State University Press, 1989.
11. Solberg HE: Establishment and use of reference values. In Burtis CA, Ashwood ER (eds): Tietz Textbook of Clinical Chemistry, 3rd edition, pp 336-356, Philadelphia, WB Saunders, 1999.
12. Solberg HE: RefVal: a program implementing the recommendations of the International Federation of Clinical Chemistry on the statistical treatment of reference values. Comput Meth Progr Biomed 1995; 48:247-256.
13. Solberg HE, Gräsbeck R: Reference values. Adv Clin Chem 1989; 27:1-79.

CHAPTER 15

Clinical Laboratory Informatics

FRANKLIN R. ELEVITCH, MD, and KENT A. SPACKMAN, MD, PhD

Objectives

1. Describe a basic computer system, including hardware and software.
2. Explain the need for computerized laboratory information systems in hospital laboratories, satellite laboratories, and clinician office laboratories.
3. List the types of information and demographics necessary to maintain a laboratory information database.
4. Describe the various ways in which a laboratory information system can communicate with laboratory instruments.
5. Illustrate the ways in which a laboratory information system interacts with a hospital information system.
6. Design a basic laboratory information system from data input to result output.

Key Words

Hospital Information System (HIS)   A system of computerized functions for the management of patient care within a hospital

Hypertext   A database feature that links displayed information to additional related information in the database

Internet   A worldwide network of computers available for public use.

Laboratory Information System (LIS)   A system of computerized functions for the management of laboratory operations and communication of laboratory test results

Operating System (OS)   A master computer program that controls the basic functions of the computer, including display terminal images, keyboard and mouse response, file management, and program control

Worldwide Web   A process on the Internet that allows computer users to navigate the network using graphical user interfaces and hypertext links between different Internet addresses

---

The term *informatics* refers to the management and processing of information, ordinarily involving computing. It encompasses the scientific and practical aspects of collection, indexing, storage, and retrieval of information. Also related to informatics are human factors, information needs assessment, and technology implementation and adoption. The scientific basis of informatics is not simply computer science but also psychology, engineering, anthropology, sociology, and business.

However, one could argue that the field of scientific endeavor that has had the greatest impact on informatics is computer hardware engineering. The size and expense of computers are diminishing rapidly while their capacity and speed are increasing nearly as rapidly. This dramatic and far-reaching change has been driven primarily by the industry leaders' ever-increasing ability to place large numbers of integrated circuits onto silicon chips. Gordon Moore, one of the founders of the Intel Corporation, observed in 1965 that the number of circuits that could be manufactured on a single chip seemed to be doubling approximately each year.[4,13] This observation has come to be known as "Moore's law" and has been restated in many ways. Some authors now quote Moore's law as an implication that computer power doubles every 18 months at half the price.

Microcomputers are currently in use within the laboratory in many areas, including process control, quality control, online monitoring, data interpretation, communications, and inventory control. Integrated through a common database and various communications networks, the modern microcomputer is capable of supporting the entire laboratory information system (LIS). In the 1990s the scope of computer applications in the laboratory broadened to include management of preanalytical and postanalytical tasks. Bar-code technology enables the automation of processes from patient and specimen identification to test tube handling within chemistry analyzers (see Chapter 12). Improved computer programs use laboratory data to produce additional information helpful in the improvement of patient care. Such information can be available as lists of possible diagnoses, suggestions for further tests, and reports of the identification of drug and test interactions.

This chapter provides only an introduction to basic informatics concepts and an overview of the application of the computer in the laboratory, especially the LIS. The material presented is supplemented with references to more detailed sources of information.[1,2]

■ THE COMPUTER SYSTEM

A computer system is composed of two components—hardware and software. Software is the set of logical instructions and information that determines how the computer behaves. Hardware is the physical computer itself, including monitors, keyboards, power supply, disk drives, and internal boards on which the silicon chips reside. Different chips may have different functions, such as memory or communications. The main chip that does the computing in today's small computers is called the *microprocessor*. A system designed as a general-purpose computer that uses this chip is called a *microcomputer*.

Computer Hardware

Computer hardware can be divided into three categories—the central processing unit (CPU), which is the computer itself; random access memory (RAM); and peripheral devices, or "peripherals," which are external to the CPU. Peripheral devices transfer information into and from the CPU (input/output [I/O] devices), store data and programs for use in the CPU (storage devices), and communicate with other computers (communication and network devices).

Central processing unit and memory

The CPU is the component of the hardware responsible for executing the instructions of the software. Software instructions are stored on magnetic media, such as floppy disks or hard disks, in files called binaries or executables. When a program or application is begun, its executable file is read from the disk into main memory (RAM), from which the CPU obtains the instructions to be executed.

Each CPU has a "pacemaker" called a *clock* that determines its speed; CPU clock speeds usually are measured in millions of cycles per second, or megahertz. A software instruction may take a minimum of one clock cycle to execute; thus clock speed is a rough way to compare the relative power of different CPUs. However, the internal design of the CPU is even more important in the determination of its power, so standard computer tasks called *benchmarks* are used to measure and compare the performance of different makes of processors.

Input and output devices

Devices that communicate with the user or instruments are I/O devices. One of the most common peripheral I/O devices is the video display device (monitor), which is very similar to a television set. The monitor is used to display information for the user. Monitors may be limited to displaying characters (often limited to 24 lines and 80 columns), or they may be able to display graphical images. A keyboard, mouse, or light pen may be used as an input device. A graphical user interface is achieved through the combination of a graphical output display with a point-and-click-input device such as a mouse, trackball, or touchpad.

The computer determines the number of pixels (picture elements, or discrete display points) displayed by a graphical monitor, as well as the number of different colors or grey levels that can be displayed. A common basic configuration is known as the *video graphics adapter standard*, which displays 640 pixels wide and 480 pixels high in 16 colors. More advanced video hardware and software often are installed to provide higher levels of resolution (more pixels) and more colors. Some monitors also double as input devices by providing touch-sensitive screens.

For interaction with users, LISs may use dumb terminals, microcomputers, or both. A dumb terminal is a combination keyboard input device and text-only video monitor. These terminals also may have bar-code readers or light pens attached as input devices. Most often, such terminals are connected directly (hardwired) to the central computer and depend on the central computer to process each character. On the other hand, a microcomputer can be connected directly to the main computer and mimic a dumb terminal. Other options include connection of microcomputers and main computers through a local area network (LAN) or in a client-server configuration.

For some situations, input with a voice recognition system is an ideal way to convert speech into text. Trainable systems for individual word recognition are available, and some speaker-independent systems require only brief pauses between spoken words.

Printers are important output devices. They generally are differentiated by speed (pages per minute), resolution (dots per inch), and color capacity. Higher speed, higher resolution, and color generally imply higher cost, although printing technology also seems to have been following Moore's law. One other aspect of printers is their capacity, or the total number of pages they are designed to print before replacement or extensive servicing. For high-speed, high-capacity printing jobs, such as daily cumulative reports, many LISs use a lineprinter, a device designed to print an entire line of text (generally 80 or 130 characters) at once. However, lineprinters do not produce graphics or print in color.

Storage devices

Storage is measured in bits and bytes. A bit is a binary digit (that is, a 0 or a 1). A byte is a sequence of eight bits and is the number of bits necessary to represent one character in ASCII (American Standard Code for Information Interchange). Because the size of electronic documents (often called *files*) can be measured conveniently by the number of characters (letters and numbers), measurement of storage in terms of bytes is customary. Computers store and retrieve data according to addresses represented in binary arithmetic. The maximum storage size that can be referenced by a binary address grows as a power of two of the number of bits in the address. Consequently, computer-addressable storage sizes are also generally some power of two. A kilobyte (KB) thus is not exactly 1000 bytes, but rather 1024 bytes (2^{10} bytes), and a megabyte (MB) is not exactly a million bytes but rather 1,048,576 bytes (2^{20} bytes).

Digital data, represented as 0s and 1s, are stored on magnetic media, such as magnetic disks or tapes. Data are written as magnetized spots that can be read easily by a magnetic sensing device, or read head. Hard disks are made of one or more spinning aluminum platters with magnetized surfaces, and may have either fixed or movable read/write heads. Among the magnetic storage media the hard disk has the fastest access time and highest total cost. Floppy disks and some hard disks may be removed from the disk drive for storage. Most floppy disks are 3½ inches in diameter and not actually floppy but enclosed in a rigid plastic shell. Older technology included 5¼- and 8-inch diameter disks with flexible plastic shells that actually were floppy. Magnetic tape, configured as either reels or cartridges, is the storage medium with the slowest access time but is useful because of its high storage capacity and low cost.

Optical media also may be used to store digital data. The CD-ROM (compact disk-read only memory) is, as its name suggests, a type of optical storage that, once manufactured, can be read but not changed. It is a convenient mechanism for widespread distribution of a fixed set of data, such as a publication or digitized audio recording. In addition, optical storage technologies also exist that allow data to be written to the optical disk only once (WORM [write once, read many]), and magneto-optical devices that allow multiple writes.

Computer communications and networks

Connecting an LIS to a hospital computer or connecting any two computers together may be accomplished through a direct connection or a networked connection. Direct connection requires special attention to a number of details to make the communication possible. Networked connection is becoming more commonplace because many of the communication issues are handled at the chip level through standard communication protocols.

Networked interconnections

Most institutions connect microcomputers together on a LAN that often also permits access to the central computers that run the LIS or the hospital information system. Each computer has its own set of chips (usually on a separate board) that provides a plug into which the network can connect. These technologies specify the way that signals are handled by each computer on the network so that they can share a common transmission medium (usually copper wire or fiber-optic cable) for communication among all connected computers and devices. LAN data transmission capacity is specified in millions of bits per second (Mbps). Transmission rates vary from 4 to 100 Mbps.

Many LANs have devices called *routers*, which allow the interconnection of LANs across a wide area, through use of telephone connections or dedicated fiber-optic cables; this creates wide area networks (WANs). The widespread adoption of the Internet Protocol (IP) for the transmission of data across LANs and WANs has resulted in the interconnection of a worldwide internetwork, known simply as the **Internet.** Each computer on the Internet must have its own IP address, a sequence of 8 bytes that uniquely identifies that computer. Each computer also may have a domain address, a series of alphanumeric names joined by periods, such as "main.ohsu.edu." Each domain address is linked to an IP address, and translation tables are maintained in various computers and routers on the network. The domain address is the computer destination for messages sent across the Internet.

New and faster communication technologies are being used to transmit internetwork traffic. For example, when optical carriers (fiber-optic cables) are used, a standard developed by Bellcore (Telemedia Technologies, Morristown, N.J.) for point-to-point links, known as *SONET (synchronous optical network),* supports transmission capacities from about 50 Mbps up to nearly 2500 Mbps.[15] This capacity represents as much as a 250-fold increase over today's capacity. Such vast increases in bandwidth are likely to be needed as graphics, sound, images, and video are shared across the Internet. (See the discussion on the Worldwide Web in a subsequent section of this chapter.)

Software

Software consists of the encoded instructions that determine the computer's behavior. Software programs are divided conveniently into those that supply basic functioning of the computer (**operating system [OS]** programs) and those that supply special functions for the user (application programs). A third category of programs is programming languages, that is, programs that facilitate the creation, debugging, and testing of OSs and applications. Microsoft Windows is an OS program; it provides facilities for formatting of storage media, copying of files, listing of the contents of storage devices, and other basic functions. Other OSs in widespread use include the Macintosh OS, UNIX, and Linux.* The most common microcomputer configuration, with an Intel or compatible microprocessor running a version of Microsoft's Windows as the OS, sometimes is referred to as the "Wintel" platform. Because of the large market share of this type of platform, a version of virtually every type of application program has been designed to run on it. Economies of scale in their production tend to make these programs relatively inexpensive.

■ MICROCOMPUTER APPLICATIONS

The personal computer is an essential tool for laboratorians because of the increased productivity potential it offers when used appropriately.

Types of Applications

Basic office applications often are sold together as a suite (word processor, spreadsheet, database, and presentation program). Special purpose programs are available for time management and scheduling. Software packages facilitate use of the Internet, including electronic mail systems, communications software, and Worldwide Web browsers. Numerous CD-ROM products provide online textbooks, encyclopedias, dictionaries, reference works, educational packages, and other useful information. Selecting and organizing these microcomputer capabilities requires some knowledge of the benefits they can provide and a willingness to learn how to use them.

Word processor applications do more than simply provide an electronic typewriter. They can check and correct spelling. Mailing lists can be merged with form letters to

appear personalized and save time. They provide tools for the outline and modification of articles, chapters, and books, and allow integration of tables, charts, graphs, and figures into documents.

Spreadsheet applications are useful for manipulation of numbers or names in tabular form; they are most useful for encoding of sums, averages, and other relationships among tables of data. Many individuals who learn to use a spreadsheet never go on to learn to use a database-management program because the spreadsheet meets their needs. When is a database-management system needed? The following are some criteria that can be used to determine whether a spreadsheet program alone is sufficient or a database-management program should be considered:

1. The information consists of more than one table of data, with inter-relationships between the tables (for example, one table listing patients' demographic data and another listing their laboratory test results).
2. Multiple different views of the data are required (for example, one view that sorts patient names alphabetically and another that sorts them by visit date).
3. Reports are required periodically, with abstracts of various aspects of the data (for example, the number of complete blood counts ordered from each hospital service each month).
4. Multiple individuals need to access the data for different purposes.
5. Several different individuals, who would benefit from a data entry form, enter new rows or elements of data.
6. Security, implemented through user accounts and passwords, is necessary.

Database-management systems are no longer too arcane and inaccessible for the average user. Learning how to use one of the newer microcomputer relational database-management systems generally does not take long and can be very useful for information management.

In addition, presentation programs provide many useful functions that enhance the creation of visual aids for teaching and expository speaking. They help convert outlines into full presentations, guide the creation of readable and attractive slides, and facilitate the automatic creation of handouts and lecture notes.

Information Literacy and the Worldwide Web

"Computer literacy" has come to mean the knowledge of a computer's workings and some level of skill in its operation. Laboratorians need some level of computer literacy because the appropriate use of information technology seems to be a major factor in increased employee productivity in the United States.[10] More useful is the broader set of skills that might be called "information literacy," the ability to effectively retrieve, evaluate, manage, and apply information to solve a problem or complete a task. Information literacy im-

---

*UNIX is an interactive time-sharing operating system invented in 1969 by Ken Thompson. Linux is a free operating system originally written from scratch with no proprietary code by Linus Torvalds and team of programmers over the Internet.

plies an individual's ability to know what sources of information exist, which are fastest and most reliable, and the best way in which to access them. Traditionally, important sources of information have included consultants, colleagues, librarians, textbooks, and published literature. Today an increasing trend exists for computer-based tools to include and subsume these other sources, placing a greater importance on skills involving electronic information tools.

The most interesting informatics development in the 1990s was the **Worldwide Web** (the Web). The technology of the Web consists of existing Internet technology, combined with a few new protocols (notably HTTP [**hypertext** transfer protocol]) that can be accessed with a freely available type of software, called a *browser*, that runs on all common computer systems (Macintosh, Wintel, and UNIX). The phenomenon of the Worldwide Web consists of a worldwide adoption of this technology by virtually all major organizations as a mechanism for electronic communication. Web pages, electronic publications accessed over the Internet through browsers, are published by governments, universities, corporations of all sizes, organizations of all types and sizes, and individuals. The amount of information on the Web and its growth rate are staggering. In 1996 more than 500,000 Web sites existed, mostly commercial domains, and the number of commercial domains had doubled in less than 6 months.[6] Automated searches of the Web retrieve information about virtually any concept imaginable—sometimes from authoritative or reputable sources,[12] sometimes not.

Many organizations separate their Web materials into those accessible publicly on the global Internet and those accessible only within the organization on its own local network, often called an *intranet*. An intranet permits an organization to exploit the broad capabilities of Web technology for communication and education, while maintaining better privacy, security, and consistency of network speeds and capacities.

LABORATORY INFORMATION SYSTEMS

A **laboratory information system (LIS)** integrates the clinical laboratory with the medical staff and most departments of a health-care organization.[1,2,7] The initial installation or upgrade of an LIS always should begin with a systematic study of the existing LIS. Because an LIS commits an organization to formal policies and procedures, a harmonious relationship among all parties is essential. Only then can a long-term institutional commitment to planning, implementation, operation, and maintenance of an LIS begin.

The study may show that improvements in the existing system are sufficient to correct problems and achieve enhanced service. If the decision is to purchase a new LIS, the next step is to write specifications for the new system. These

TABLE 15-1	Clinical Laboratory Information Data Transactions	
Transaction	Data Provider	Data Receiver
Patient identification	Patient	Admission clerk
Admission	Patient	Emergency room clerk
Transfer	Nurse	Nurse Laboratory clerk
Test ordering	Clinician	Phlebotomist Nurse
Specimen collection	Phlebotomist Nurse	Laboratorian Nurse Clinician
Test analysis	Laboratory instrument	Laboratorian
Test result reporting/ interpretation	Laboratorian Laboratory director	Clinician Nurse
Patient discharge	Clinician	Admission clerk Business clerk Laboratory clerk Medical records Nurse
Patient/guarantor billing	Laboratory clerk	Business clerk

specifications must be detailed and specific and address the needs of both the laboratory personnel and the health-care organization and medical staff members. If a **hospital information system (HIS)** exists (or is imminent), an LIS-HIS interface specification is included. The health-care organization may choose to develop its own LIS or purchase one from an LIS vendor through competitive bidding. In either case a lifelong relationship (at least for the life of the LIS) is established. The mutual obligations of this relationship are described clearly in a legal contract.

Patient identification, admission, transfer, and discharge information; test requests; and some specimen collections often are entered into the facility's system by nonlaboratory personnel. With an HIS this information is transmitted automatically to the LIS through either a shared database or an interface. Test results are returned from the LIS to the HIS for inquiry and reporting at nursing stations. Billing information is transferred to the hospital financial management system (FMS) electronically or by magnetic tape.

The flow of clinical laboratory information can be divided into seven steps (Table 15-1). Each step is characterized by a data transaction in which exists a unidirectional transfer of data from a data provider to a data receiver. Although laboratory personnel are involved at each step, the patient, medical staff members, and five other services participate in the overall process.

One major advantage of an LIS is that it establishes standard laboratory nomenclature and standardized information processing procedures. The basic unit of information in an LIS file is called a *data element*. All aspects of clinical laboratory testing are described by the appropriate combinations

TABLE 15-2   Data Elements of an LIS

Patient	Test
1. Number	1. Number
2. Name	2. Name(s)
3. Birthdate	3. Mnemonic identification
4. Sex	4. Source
5. Admission date	5. Turnaround time
6. Admission status	6. Container volume
7. Location	7. Special requirements
8. Room and bed	8. Department
9. Clinician(s)	9. Work list
10. Diagnosis/diagnoses	10. Method
11. Discharge date	11. Units of measurement
12. Financial status	12. Numeric?
13. Guarantor(s)	13. Required?
14. Billing number	14. Delta check
15. Addresses	15. Controls/calibrators
	16. Reference intervals
Specimen	17. Critical value(s)
1. Number	18. Charge code
2. Status	19. Charge
a. Ordered	20. Workunits
b. Collected	
c. Received	
d. Reported	
3. Date (year, month, day)	
4. Time (on a 24-hour clock)	
5. Employee identification	

LIS, Laboratory information system.

TABLE 15-3   LIS Interactions

Transaction	Inquiry/Reports
Patient identification, admission/ discharge/transfer	Daily listings
Test ordering	Clinicians' orders
	Uncollected specimens
Specimen collection	Collection lists
	Labels
	Master log
	Outstanding specimens
	Tests pending
	Work lists
	QNS report
	ND report
Specimen analysis	Quality control listings/graphs
Result reporting/interpretation	Stat
	Interim
	Cumulative
	Exception reports
	Abnormal values
	Critical values
	Delta check
Patient/guarantor billing	Billing listing
	Productivity/workload

LIS, Laboratory information system; *QNS,* quality not sufficient; *ND,* not done.

of fewer than 50 data elements grouped to define a patient, specimen, or test (Table 15-2). As LISs become more complex and sophisticated, additional data elements are added to this basic list. Actually, all the transactions shown in Table 15-1 translate into data-element processing in the LIS (that is, adding, deleting, and editing). The LIS facilitates not only data entry, but also storage, collation, and formatting of data for retrieval, inquiry, and reporting (Table 15-3).

Data elements are organized in an LIS into two functional types of files—definitional and descriptive. Definitional files, tables, or dictionaries are intended for long-term repetitive use. They include data elements that constitute the basic services of the laboratory. Definitional files include (1) test lists; (2) work list formats; (3) calibrators and controls; (4) coded comments; (5) laboratory sections; (6) hospital, emergency room, and clinic locations; (7) clinicians' names, addresses, and phone numbers; (8) diagnostic classifications; and (9) automated instrument interface specifications. Descriptive files retain the historic events in the LIS, such as (1) patient identification, admission, discharge, and transfer information; (2) test requests; (3) specimen data; and (4) test results. Relevant definitional data elements (see Table 15-2) are included in descriptive files that constitute each patient's record.

For each transaction in the LIS the appropriate data elements are incorporated into a descriptive file. With each new transaction, data elements are added. Because of the

cumulative process, repeated storage of data elements that are already filed with each new test request is necessary. All transactions relate specific test numbers to specific specimen numbers for a specific patient number.

Patient Identification

All hospital services for each patient are related to that individual's unique patient number. At the time of admission an admission clerk records the patient's name, birthdate, and sex. If an HIS is used, the HIS computer assigns a unique patient number and the four data elements—patient number, name, birthdate, and sex—are transmitted to the LIS. In a multiprocessor network the patient number is recognized by each processor so that a way to relate a specimen to the patient from whom it was obtained always is available.

Once a patient is identified properly, that individual's identification information is linked with all subsequent laboratory transactions. Although LIS-printed labels eliminate the illegibility problem sometimes associated with the use of embossed plates, introduction of an error still is possible if the wrong label is placed on a specimen. The use of bar-code readers reduces transcription and identification errors in specimen processing (see Chapter 12).

Data are retrieved in the LIS by either patient name or patient number. When a patient name is used for retrieval, a Soundex (that is "sounds like") code or partial lookup based on the patient's initials is helpful, in case the name is misspelled or illegible.

Admission, Transfer, and Discharge

A patient's demographic data elements may differ from one health-care encounter to another. Such elements include (1) admission date, (2) admission status, (3) location (ward, service, or outpatient site), (4) room or bed, (5) clinician(s) treating the patient, (6) diagnosis or diagnoses, (7) discharge date, (8) financial status, (9) guarantor(s), and (10) billing number.

Admission statuses include outpatient, inpatient, preadmission, ambulatory, surgery, and so on. In an LIS these classifications initiate report routing, define the length of time data are retained in the LIS, and organize pricing schedules. Charges for laboratory testing are based on admission status when cost differences exist between inpatient and outpatient services. Location (hospital room and bed) is used to track inpatient specimen collection rounds and report delivery. Outpatient reports are routed to the emergency room, clinics, or clinicians' offices.

Responsibility for documenting patient diagnoses is shared among health organization staff members and clinicians. Although clinicians make diagnoses, staff members enter the diagnostic codes (for example, ICD-9-CM [International Classification of Diseases, Clinical Modification]) into the medical record. These codes are used for billing non-Medicare services and are clustered into Diagnostic Related Groups (DRGs) for billing inpatient Medicare services.

In an LIS, patient identification, admission, transfer, and discharge data elements must be entered before tests can be ordered and processed. If an HIS also is present, these data elements are transmitted automatically to the LIS. The billing process is initiated at the time of admission by acquisition of the patient's financial status and guarantor information (see subsequent section on patient and guarantor billing). (The guarantor is the specific insurance company or government agency to which the statement of charges is sent.) Health-care accounting systems are becoming increasingly complex as health-care organizations integrate outpatient and inpatient services. The number of health insurance plans, including managed care, Medicare, Medicaid, and workers' compensation, is multiplying (see Chapter 16).

Test Order

Nursing service is the communications hub for patient care. All inpatient orders, including those for laboratory testing, pass through nursing service. When a clinician places an order directly into an HIS interfaced to an LIS, the order is recorded in the patient's chart as a printed report. Nursing service must ensure that all specimens are collected and all results recorded properly. Nonblood specimens (for example, urine and sputum) are collected by the nursing service. When tests are ordered in an HIS, a specimen number is assigned by the computer. This number is the unique identifier that both the HIS and the LIS use for inquiry and reporting. Entering the specimen number, test identification, date canceled, reason for cancellation, and user identification into the LIS maintains a record of cancellations. Duplicate test orders for a single specimen are rejected automatically.

Specimen Collection

The LIS records the receipt of a collected specimen in the laboratory by changing the specimen status from "ordered" or "collected" to "received." This specimen status change automatically completes the order in the HIS. An accession number is assigned in the HIS, and this number can be used in the LIS. Accession numbers also can be assigned by the LIS.

If additional tests are requested for a specimen that has been received by the laboratory, they should be added to the previous specimen accession number. Quality-control specimens should have separate accession numbers. Phlebotomist and nursing service identification also should be stored in the LIS.

Specimen Analysis

For specimen processing the LIS sorts tests with the appropriate calibrators and controls by work station or reference laboratory. These groupings are called *work lists* and may be reviewed either on a video terminal or in a printed report. The format for work lists is designed specifically for each work area. A work list may be a loading list for an automated instrument, or it may provide a format for recording of data if tests are performed manually. When a work list is completed partially, it is advanced automatically to the next work list. In this way work lists serve as "conveyor belts" for work in progress in the laboratory. To keep track of uncompleted work, the LIS produces operational reports on request throughout the day. This type of report includes a cumulative list of specimens received in the laboratory but not completed, a list of received specimens that were not processed because of insufficient quantity (or any other reason), a list of tests ordered but canceled, daily master logs of all specimens collected, and a cumulative summary of all tests ordered for each patient at the time of admission.

A variety of laboratory instruments are used to produce test results. Many instruments have built-in microprocessors with capability to display preformatted results, together with limit checks and the results of control samples. Once a laboratorian matches them with the proper patient identifiers, these values are transmitted directly to the LIS and HIS. Many instruments have sufficient memory to retain large numbers of patient and control values if the LIS becomes nonoperational. Supplemental memory storage devices (buffers) are available commercially as backups for those instruments that do not possess such capabilities.

Interfaces are electronic connections between analytical systems and LISs. Although test results may be transmitted automatically one-way from an analytical system to an LIS (that is, an unidirectional interface), two-way exchanges so that test orders, specimen identifiers, and patient identifiers and demographics can be sent to analytical systems by an LIS or HIS (that is, a bidirectional interface) may be advantageous. By replacing redundant data entry steps, interfaces can improve laboratory efficiency and productivity. However, care must be taken to design an interface network so that neither specimen processing in the analytical system nor the response times (the time intervals from entering a command into a computer to completion of the task) of the LIS or HIS are slowed. Standards for information exchange through interfaces have been developed and are maintained perpetually to accommodate advancements in analytical and network technologies.[18]

Interfaces facilitate result reporting. In general, on-line results should not be released until a laboratorian verifies them. Certain analytical systems allow release of tests without human intervention, provided quality control, format, and critical value checks are satisfied. Identification of the laboratorian running the instrument is reported, together with a flag indicating automatic verification. An example is in microbiology, in which organism identification can be released as a preliminary report if the analytical system meets extremely stringent criteria. Similarly, in chemistry all but the abnormal results may be reported automatically. Manual redundancies of reference laboratory ordering and reporting are facilitated greatly by interfaces linked by telephone to client LISs. In such cases a laboratorian in the client laboratory verifies the reference laboratory results before reporting to the ordering clinicians.

The LIS reports quality control results in several formats—the multirule Shewhart chart, a daily listing of observed raw and expected values, and a calculated running mean and standard deviation. A cumulative summary of observed control values is displayed monthly in a standard graphical format (see Chapter 17), together with a display of the expected mean and standard deviation and a list of observed means and their standard deviations for at least the 5 previous months.

Test Results

A laboratorian reviews and verifies all results before such results are available for inquiry or reporting. The LIS retains identification of the laboratorian who performed a test and verified the results. Free text and coded comment entries also are included with results. The LIS test list definitions (see Table 15-2) provide on-line editing capabilities for numerical and nonnumerical results, required results, and results outside of reference or critical limits (see Chapter 14). Coded comments are edited by user-definable tables of eligible responses. The LIS may record the time at which re-

sults were verified and use this time as a test completion time. The system also may record the start, stop, and elapsed times of automated instrument runs.

In addition to patient stat, interim, or cumulative reports, the LIS provides lists throughout the day of all patients with results that are abnormal or critical for review by the laboratory director.

Test Interpretation

Ideally, computer-generated interpretive reports should assist clinicians in evaluating patient problems and arriving at medical decisions with accuracy and efficiency. The first step in report design is to format data in such a way that abnormal results and pathophysiological relationships are highlighted. This format can be accomplished by grouping of physiologically related analytes in the print collation sequence of the cumulative report and flagging of abnormal and critical values with distinctive symbols.

The next step in interpretive reporting is the explanatory comment. The laboratory director may add this comment to emphasize an abnormal finding or caution against false-positive results. An elaboration of the comment is the categorical listing of disease entities that might be associated with abnormalities.

Computer-assisted interpretive reports have taken several different forms. The reports may list possible causes of a single abnormal result, differential possibilities offered by multiple abnormal results, and suggestions for further laboratory testing. They have been useful for analytes such as calcium, thyroid hormones, and serum proteins, for which the pathophysiology is defined.

The application of statistical protocols to interpretive reports is in its infancy. Such protocols require thoughtful design. Not only must study and reference populations be selected appropriately (see Chapter 14), but the ratio of patients to test variables must be adequate. This statement means that the laboratory must be able to monitor the prevalence of properly coded patient diagnoses while maintaining consistent test coding and calibration (accuracy) over extended periods of time.

Developing interpretive laboratory reports requires a professional team of clinicians, computer scientists, biostatisticians, and laboratorians. The underlying database must apply to the lifelong history of individual patients. Database elements should use standard descriptors and codes so that data can be shared within an institution and across multiple sources of data. Existing coding systems for diagnoses, such as ICD-9-CM, and for procedures, such as the Current Procedural Terminology, are incomplete. The College of American Pathologists has developed an extensive coding system called *SNOMED (Systematized Nomenclature of Human and Veterinary Medicine),* which has been recognized widely as the most complete standard nomenclature system for medicine.[5,19]

Patient and Guarantor Billing

The business office is responsible for processing laboratory charges. Together with the laboratory, administrators develop a charge list that includes the name, charge code, and charge for each test from the hospital's chart of accounts. The laboratory then must maintain both the LIS and FMS price lists when charges are revised or tests added to the laboratory's repertoire.

Outpatient laboratory services demand more accounting time than do inpatient services. Patient identification and admission information must be gathered efficiently so that patients are registered promptly. Missed diagnostic codes, addresses, guarantor names, or ZIP codes result in wasted time and inefficiency. When a large outpatient population exists, registration of patients at the outpatient laboratory service center, where the patient information must be edited, is helpful. In addition, keeping patients' accounts online with current postings is helpful because patients are as interested in their bills as they are in laboratory results. If the HIS, FMS, and LIS are not interfaced, a terminal from each system may be required. An interim solution is to have microfiche available for HIS and FMS information, although the accounting information in such cases may be several days old.

If a laboratory test cannot be performed once it is requested, proper credit can be given to the patient, or the charge can be deleted automatically if the billing report has not yet been issued. When the computer is inoperative for long periods of time, the laboratory must have a "downtime" procedure in place, one that ordinarily uses paper requisitions, logs, workbooks, and reports.

■ FUTURE USE OF COMPUTERS

Since the early 1980s the computer has had a profound impact on the structure, function, and management of the clinical laboratory. The microcomputer has revolutionized specimen tracking through bar coding and improved specimen analysis through the application of process control, automation, and applied mathematics. Computer engineers and programmers have become indispensable members of instrument design and development teams. Patient demographics and orders can be received automatically by instruments and the results returned to an LIS. The LIS has enabled clinical laboratories to manage ever-growing amounts of information.[9] To meet the challenge of cost reduction through economies of scale, LISs must find better ways to link dispersed geographical sites and instrumentation. Given the high cost of software development, an LIS vendor even may become closely associated with specific health-care organizations.

Computer technology also is addressing the challenge of interpretive reporting and data utilization. However, clinical laboratory data are only a portion of the total database required for making of accurate patient-specific diagnostic, therapeutic, and prognostic decisions. Facing this challenge requires computer access to clinical information and the development of rational models of medical decision-making processes. Another "layer" of software, the decision support system, is emerging; this software uses data from all computers in an organization to provide cost and resource utilization information for management planning. Decision support systems also can assist laboratory directors in managing organizational compliance with health plan accreditation requirements and clinical pathways for patient care.[8]

The stage is set for extraordinary advances in computerized information processing.[4] Health-care organizations, medical groups, and computer vendors will develop enterprise-wide information systems, enhanced by color graphics and sound, that connect a central data repository with multiple sites over broad geographical areas. The LIS will be a module within this system that is essential for quality control and the cost of patient care.

Generally accepted standards for data exchange among computer systems are required for these developments to happen.[15,20] Standards in this area are coordinated by the Health Informatics Standards Board of the American National Standards Institute. These standards are being developed in a coordinated effort by several standards development organizations, including the American Society for Testing and Materials,[3,16] the Institute for Electronics and Electrical Engineering,[17] Health Level Seven,[18] working groups of the American College of Radiology and the National Electrical Manufacturers Association, the Insurance Subcommittee of the Accredited Standards Committee X12, and the National Council for Prescription Drug Programs.

As Moore's law demonstrates, the price and size limitations of computer hardware will decrease steadily into the beginning of the 21st century. Thus the limiting and costly aspect of a computer system is its software. To reduce the high cost of programming, new approaches can be expected.[11,14]

References

1. Aller RD, Elevitch FR (eds): Laboratory and Hospital Information Systems, p 270, Philadelphia, WB Saunders, 1991.

2. Aller RD, Elevitch FR (eds): Symposium on Computers in the Clinical Laboratory, p 254, Philadelphia, WB Saunders, 1983.

3. American Society for Testing and Materials Subcommittee E31.07: Standard Guide for Computer Automation in the Clinical Laboratory, E792-86, Philadelphia, American Society for Testing and Materials, 1986.

4. Burtis CA: Converging technologies and their impact on the clinical laboratory. Clin Chem 1996; 42:1735-1749.

5. Campbell JR, Carpenter P, Sneiderman C et al: Phase II evaluation of clinical coding schemes: completeness, taxonomy, mapping, definitions, and clarity (CPRI work group on codes and structures). J Am Med Informatics Assn 1997; 4:238-251.

6. Chou D: Internet: road to heaven or hell for the clinical laboratory? Clin Chem 1996; 42:827-830.

7. Elevitch FR, Aller RD: The ABCs of LIS: Computerizing Your Laboratory Information System, p 291, Chicago, ASCP Press, 1989.

8. Elevitch FR, Silvers A, Sahl JD: Projecting corporate health plan utilization and costs from annual ICD-9-CM diagnostic rates: a value added opportunity for pathologists. Arch Pathol Lab Med 1997; 121:1187-1191.

9. Elevitch FR, Treling C, Spackman KA et al: A clinical laboratory information systems survey: challenge for the decade. Arch Pathol Lab Med 1993; 117:12-21.

10. Farrell C, Manel M, Weber J: Riding high: corporate America now has an edge over its global rivals. Business Week October 9, 1995; 134-146.

11. Kona proposal to create, exchange, and process electronic health-care records using SGML (Standard Generalized Markup Language), ISO8879: 1986. Available from URL: http://www.iso.ch/cate/d16387.html
(See also http://www.mcis.duke.edu/standards/h17/sigs/sgml/WhitePapers/KONA)

12. Lancet guide to the Internet. Lancet 13 July 1996; 348:9020. (See also http://www.thelancet.com)

13. Lenzner R: The reluctant entrepreneur. Forbes Sept. 11, 1995, 162. (See also http://otto.cmr.fsu.edu/[<]lakanen/digmus/student/people/moore.htm)

14. Lincoln TL, Essin DJ, Anderson R et al: The introduction of a new document processing paradigm into health care computing—a CAIT white paper. 1995. Available from URL: http://www.mcis.duke.edu/standards/SGML/proposals/CAIT-white-paper.txt

15. Malamud C: Stacks: Interoperability in Today's Computer Networks, p 80, Englewood Cliffs, NJ, Prentice-Hall, 1992.

16. McDonald CJ: A Standard Specification for Transferring Clinical Laboratory Data Messages Between Independent Computer Systems: ASTM E-31.11 Draft Standard, Philadelphia, American Society for Testing and Materials, 1987.

17. Simborg DW: Network Application Architecture: Proceedings of the 12th Annual Symposium on Computer Applications in Medical Care, pp 648-650, Washington, DC, IEEE Press, 1988.

18. Simborg DW: The case for the HL7 standard. Comput Healthcare, January 1988; 8:39-41.

19. Spackman KA, Campbell KE, Cote RA: SNOMED RT: a reference terminology for health care. Proc AMIA Annu Fall Symp 1997; 640-644.

20. Standards for medical identifiers, codes and messages needed to create an efficient computer stored medical record. J Am Med Informatics Assn 1994; 1:1-7.

Additional Reading

WORLDWIDE WEB SITES

www.aacc.org (American Association for Clinical Chemistry)
www.ama-assn.org (American Medical Association)
www.amia.org (American Medical Informatics Association)
www.ascp.org (American Society of Clinical Pathologists)
www.cap.org (College of American Pathologists)
www.cdc.gov (Centers for Disease Control and Prevention)

www.ifcc.org (International Federation of Clinical Chemistry)
www.hl7.org (Health Level Seven)
www.nccls.org (National Committee for Clinical Laboratory Standards)
www.nih.gov (National Institutes of Health, United States)
www.nlm.nih.gov (The U.S. National Library of Medicine)

CHAPTER 16

Laboratory Management

RONALD L. WEISS, MD, and K. OWEN ASH, PhD

Objectives

1. Define the following terms in regard to a clinical laboratory:
   Managed care   Reengineering
   Consolidation   Budget
   Downsizing   Network
2. State five cost-reduction strategies that clinical laboratory management can perform.
3. List five categories of financial management that laboratory managers can consider.
4. Compare and provide examples of direct and indirect costs.
5. List seven things a laboratory manager must do to provide an employee a positive culture or work environment.

Key Words

Billed Unit A unit of production or service actually delivered and billed to a customer; in the laboratory, a patient test result or group of tests billed as a unit

Capitation A method of reimbursement wherein the provider agrees to accept a fixed rate of payment for a particular range of services

Cost Center An organizational component to which a set of costs are allocated

Cost Shifting An activity that reallocates a cost from one cost center to another

Depreciation An accounting principle in which the decline in value of a capital asset is recorded over time, usually as a monthly expense; considered a noncash expense because no cash actually is used

Direct Cost A cost directly related to production of an individual product or service; examples including technologist labor, reagents, consumable supplies, quality control materials, and equipment depreciation

Fee-for-Service A form of reimbursement in which each unit of service (for example, a laboratory test) is billed to a patient, physician, or insurer based on a predetermined fee

Fixed Cost A cost that is fixed; does not change significantly with the volume of a product produced or service provided; technologist labor being considered a fixed cost provided that staffing coverage is independent of the actual volume of tests performed during a shift

Full-Time Equivalent A unit of labor representing the equivalent of one individual working 40 hours per week and 2080 hours per year

Indemnity Contract In business contracts, a commitment in which one individual or entity agrees to protect another against financial loss or cost; in health insurance, the traditional fee-for-service coverage in which each unit of service delivered is reimbursed at a predetermined amount

Indirect Cost A cost not attributable directly to a product or service provided but one necessary to create the required "environment" for production; examples including utilities, supervisor labor, administration, clerical support, marketing activities, building maintenance, and rent

Make-Versus-Buy Decisions A process used to determine whether a particular product or service should be produced by an organization or purchased from an outside supplier

Prospective Payment   A form of reimbursement that pays for defined services in advance; the basis for Medicare reimbursement under the Diagnosis Related Groups (DRG) formula used to pay hospitals for a defined in-patient care visit (for example, an appendectomy); pays a reasonable, average, predetermined cost and not the actual costs for a given patient

Revenue Center   In contrast to a cost center, a department or activity center that predictably generates revenue; used to be viewed as the laboratory before prospective payment and managed-care capitation

Variable Costs   In contrast to fixed costs, costs that vary over time or parallel the change in volume of a particular product or service activity; examples including reagents and consumable supplies

---

Social, political, economic, and technological changes are making impacts on the delivery of health care (Table 16-1) and on clinical laboratories.[1,2,7] Consequently, the need for effective and efficient management of the laboratory has never been greater.

This chapter begins with discussions on health-care delivery, financial strategies, and laboratory strategies for managed care. It concludes with discussions on ways in which clinical laboratorians may manage the financial, staff, and facility resources of the laboratory. Further information on these topics is found in the management publications listed in the section on additional reading.

HEALTH-CARE DELIVERY AND FINANCIAL STRATEGIES

In the past, patients in the United States customarily received their health-care insurance from their employers and generally had the freedom to choose their health-care providers. However, because health-care expenditures have increased dramatically, new delivery and financial strategies that have evolved to manage care and costs are replacing this traditional approach.

Managed Care

Managed care is a health-care delivery model with a defined network of providers who have agreed to provide a defined set of services to a population of beneficiaries in a cost-effective and quality-conscious manner. In practice, it attempts to integrate the delivery of health care with its financing, usually through a managed care organization (MCO), which acts as a third-party administrator. Examples of MCOs include health maintenance organizations (HMOs) and preferred provider organizations (PPOs). Providers (physicians, hospitals, and laboratories) contract with the MCOs to deliver high-quality, comprehensive care at cost-effective rates to a contracted source of patients (employers, Medicare). A primary focus of managed care is to optimize the utilization of health-care resources. Ideally, both overutilization and underutilization are discouraged through the use of financial-incentive and risk-sharing strategies. Successful managed-care contracting for laboratory services is a complex process that requires thorough preparation and understanding.[8,12,18] Table 16-2 describes the critical success factors associated with successful laboratory management.

Health maintenance organization

The oldest and most common MCO structure is the HMO. HMOs are prepaid health-care delivery organizations highly regulated through the federal HMO Act of 1973. Each plan enrollee pays a single premium to the HMO for defined care benefits. This premium is allocated to the providers on either a fixed-rate or discounted **fee-for-service** basis. To the extent that the costs of their services do not exceed their share of the premium, the providers financially benefit. The HMO takes a portion of the premium to cover its management costs and profit. Resource utilization is controlled by limits on the enrollee's choice of physicians and emphasis on the role of primary-care physicians as "gate-keepers" of utilization. These individuals deliver as much

---

TABLE 16-1	Current and Emerging Trends in Health-Care Delivery

Changes in the number of managed-care participants

Intense pressures to reduce costs

Reduction in hospital excess capacity through downsizing, consolidation, acquisition, and closure

Focus on ambulatory care delivery and reduced in-patient hospitalization

Focus on wellness and disease prevention

Aging population

Development of outcomes management

Provider consolidations and the development of integrated delivery systems

Development of health information networks and patient care data repositories

Systems designed to focus on patient-oriented care

Rapid technological advances, with particular focus on human genetics

TABLE 16-2	Factors to Consider in Competition for Managed-Care Contracts

Understand laboratory costs.
Review prevailing reimbursement rates.
Identify key contractual elements.
   Expected services and allowed exclusions
   Offered payment
   Payment schedule
   Criteria used to determine eligible plan members
   Existing utilization controls
   Stop-loss provision
   Conditions that trigger renegotiation
   "Standard-of-care" provisions
   Insurance and indemnification procedures
   Existence of exclusivity provisions
Review the MCO itself.
   Reputation in the community
   Member demographics (age, sex, etc.)
   Physician specialty mix
   Number of current enrollees and rate of growth
   Number of current and prospective employers
   Geographical coverage of the plan
   Current financial statements and the plan's credit history
   Nature of the quality-assurance program
Interview current plan providers, if possible.

MCO, Managed care organization.

care as they are able to deliver, while judiciously using specialist care and ancillary services, such as the laboratory, radiology, and pharmacy.

Preferred Provider Organization

The next most common MCO model is the PPO, which establishes contractual arrangements between providers and either insurance carriers, third-party administrators, or self-insured employers. The "preferred providers" agree to deliver care on a discounted fee-for-service basis. In return for access to a potential patient population these providers agree to accept certain controls, such as utilization review and pre-procedural or preadmission authorization. Patients have a wider choice of physicians than they do in an HMO and have financial incentives to use the preferred providers (for example, with deductibles and copayments). Unlike most HMO patients, however, they have the freedom, at a higher cost to them, to seek care outside the PPO. The point of service (POS), the most rapidly growing form of MCO, combines features of both an HMO and a PPO, allowing greater freedom of physician choice.

Managed Costs

Although the goal of managed care is to deliver high-quality, cost-effective care, emphasis has been placed increasingly on cost management. As a result, service components, such as laboratories, are isolated as **cost centers** (as opposed to **revenue centers**) and targeted for cost reduc-

tion. Thus laboratory services often are viewed as a commodity, and MCOs often seek out laboratory providers based solely on the lowest price.

The cornerstone of managed-care reimbursement is to spread the financial risk of the cost of patient care to the physician and hospital providers. This goal typically is accomplished through fixed-rate, **prospective payment** arrangements. Not unlike the Diagnosis Related Groups (DRG) system of in-patient Medicare reimbursement, MCOs establish arrangements that limit payment on the basis of a care encounter (for example, per diem and per discharge) or the number of beneficiaries enrolled at any one time in the MCO plan. This latter approach is known as **capitation,** a system in which providers receive a fixed amount per member per month, regardless of whether care is provided.

In the past, some laboratories have been successful at bidding managed-care contracts. Prices below cost have been sustainable because of the phenomenon of "pull-through," **cost shifting.** As long as managed-care patients with low reimbursement rates are outnumbered by Medicare and private insurance patients with higher reimbursement rates, a profitable patient mix exists. Based on service convenience, physicians caring for managed-care patients usually can be convinced to send their more profitable testing to the same laboratory. As managed-care patients grow in numbers and Medicare reimbursement fees decline, this revenue shifting is eliminated and shrinking profit margins make managed-care contracts less desirable. Bidding managed-care laboratory services at extremely low prices erodes profitability.

Despite the success of large commercial laboratories in obtaining managed-care contracts, smaller laboratories, with proper preparation and attention to detail, also can compete. In fact, independent local and regional laboratories may be in a better position to support the full spectrum of both in-patient and out-patient care than is a national laboratory.

Protecting (or improving) laboratory profitability with an **indemnity contract** or under capitation arrangements requires a focus on one or more of the following:

1. Reduction in cost per test (especially labor and supplies)
2. Reduction in referral testing costs
3. Reduction in laboratory utilization by plan physicians
4. Setting of contractual limitations on significant changes in laboratory utilization (for example, "stop-loss" clauses)

◾ LABORATORY STRATEGIES FOR MANAGED CARE

As hospitals move to reduce the cost of laboratory services, utilization controls and practice guidelines will decrease the ordering frequencies for many routine laboratory tests (for example, chemistry profiles, complete blood counts). As hospital laboratories are forced to reduce costs, test menus should be reviewed critically to identify tests that are performed more efficiently in a consolidated core laboratory or sent to a reference laboratory. Manual processes should be reviewed to determine opportunities for automation. Many hospital laboratories are seeking outreach opportunities to bring in additional test volumes and thereby increase efficiencies. The pressure to reduce costs has resulted in rapid consolidations affecting commercial, private, independent, and hospital-based laboratories.

To reduce costs, clinical laboratories have instituted a number of strategies, including process automation, utilization and outcomes management, restructuring and reengineering, management contracts, networking, and consolidation.

Process Automation

Automation improves the quality and efficiency of laboratory service (see Chapter 12). Technologies for automation of the analytical processes within the laboratory are well established and continue to expand to accommodate an increasing variety of tests.[6,7] To operate efficiently, many laboratories are automating the error-prone, labor-demanding logistical processes, such as order entry, labeling, report delivery, as well as specimen triage, storage, and retrieval. A growing segment of the laboratory diagnostics industry is developing products and systems with which to automate these logistical processes.[11] The same approach used in the selection of automated analyzers[5] is applicable in the selection of other products of automation. Steps in this approach include the following:

1. *Evaluation of existing processes* A team of capable, experienced, detail-oriented individuals should analyze the processes carefully to determine how each step contributes to the overall workflow.
2. *Simplification of the processes* The team should not assume that existing processes are optimal or even required but should simplify complex manual systems before attempting costly automation.
3. *Identification of the alternatives* An increasing number of vendors offer automation products and systems. The team should choose vendors that assist them in the automation planning and implementation, not just in the purchase.
4. *Performance of a cost-benefit analysis* The team should determine the criteria on which to make the decision and compare the financial analyses of the most viable alternatives. Each step of the overall process must be coordinated and integrated to achieve maximal efficiency. New instruments need to fit into the overall automation plan. Costs associated with the facilities renovations required to accommodate the automation or the cost of a necessary integration with the labora-

tory information system (LIS) should not be overlooked.

Utilization and Outcomes Management

Laboratories long have made an important contribution to improved patient outcome. Laboratory information is often a sizable component of the patient record. Laboratorians should participate in a process that prospectively determines the true value of laboratory information and the way in which constructive changes and constraints improve its overall effectiveness.

Optimal care should be accessible, improve the quality of life, increase longevity, improve functional status, and reduce morbidity, complications, and the cost of care. Patient satisfaction should not be overlooked and is influenced by convenience, provider courtesy and professionalism, and facility amenities ("the hospital-as-a-hotel" concept).

In practice the laboratory often is overutilized, underutilized, or poorly utilized, each of which contributes to an increase in costs. Overutilization is expensive because it consumes costly laboratory resources and may initiate expensive, inappropriate medical investigation of nonexistent disease. Underutilization results in a delayed or incorrect diagnosis or inadequate patient management. Poor utilization is costly because inappropriate testing leads to delays in necessary care or expensive unnecessary follow-up testing, including the use of obsolete tests. From the laboratory's standpoint the use of inadequately controlled or insensitive and nonspecific methods similarly contributes to mismanagement.

Physicians control laboratory utilization and use the information to influence patient outcome. Modifying laboratory utilization often requires multifaceted intervention strategies. Education on "proper" utilization and feedback on "improper" activities commonly is used. More enduring approaches include the provision of information on laboratory costs, especially those paid by the patient; the provision of financial incentives to physicians encourage cost-effective behavior; and the imposition of administrative changes. A rational mix of these measures, however, may be both effective and reasonably well received.

Outcome management employs a variety of tools. Professional societies and academies have developed practice guidelines for management of a number of diseases and conditions. Such disease management guidelines may be adapted to local patterns of practice and become institutionally formulated "care maps" that outline in detail how the typical patient with a particular disease or condition should be managed through all aspects of care, including laboratory services. Pathway-specific testing algorithms or diagnostic laboratory modules should be incorporated (for example, rapid diagnosis of acute chest pain).

Reengineering

Reengineering involves rethinking and radical redesign of processes to achieve dramatic improvements. In relation to the laboratory, reengineering is an effort to redesign the entire laboratory process from within to improve efficiency, productivity, and quality.[14] In 1995 Steiner, Root, and Michel[15] stated:

> During the next four to five years, not one single laboratory site will avoid major restructuring and reengineering of its existing facilities and operation . . . Our prediction is absolute: every single laboratory site will be restructured, probably more than once, over the next few years . . . change will be institutionalized and be an inevitable factor . . . for years to come.

In hospitals that have experienced declining in-patient occupancy rates and reduced lengths of stay, in-patient laboratory testing has decreased, leaving the hospital laboratory with significant excess in staff members and equipment. Consequently, many laboratories have reengineered their operations to reduce capacity ("downsize") or better fill unused capabilities. To reduce capacity, some laboratories have chosen to perform only a small number of tests. The rest are outsourced to another laboratory. As an alternative, excess capacity could be used to support new sources of patient specimens, such as testing from physicians' offices, clinics, long-term care facilities, other hospitals, and MCOs.

Laboratories that choose to expand must be competitive in both price and service. This goal is particularly formidable for laboratories that lack experience and the requisite infrastructure to do business outside the closed environment of the hospital. Detailed requirements are listed in Table 16-3.

The resources required to meet expanded service requirements have led some hospitals to consider alternative approaches, such as laboratory management contracts with large commercial laboratories and network alliances with other hospital laboratories to form stand-alone (core) laboratories.[15]

Management Contracts

In the past, management contracts with independent hospitals and commercial laboratories were relatively common. In such contracts an external contractor assumes partial or complete management of the laboratory operation, including employees, equipment, and supplies. Minimal services may be left within the hospital, whereas the more routine, high-volume and esoteric testing is sent to larger facilities owned by the managing contractor. This approach may be particularly attractive for laboratories looking to downsize. In practice, the cost savings depends on the relative costs for services remaining in the hospital. Organizational culture clashes often become a serious threat to management contracts.

TABLE 16-3   Attributes of a Laboratory Outreach Program

Technical Operations
Responsive testing schedules (rapid turnaround times)
Broad test menu (routine and reference)
Competent and knowledgeable personnel
Appropriate levels of quality

Marketing
Business and strategical planning capabilities and resources
Sales experience
Appropriate promotional materials
Competitive pricing models (fee-for-service and fixed-rate reimbursement)

Client Services
Market-oriented, customer-support mentality
Knowledgeable staff members
Easy access for information, inquiry, and problem solving (telecommunications)
Responsiveness and professionalism

Couriers
Flexible scheduling to meet client needs (routine pickups, stats, "will calls")
Adequacy of transport container to maintain specimen integrity

Financial Operations
Accurate test-cost accounting
Timely and accurate invoicing
Third-party billing capability (for example, Medicare, private insurers, managed care)

LIS
Well-formatted test reports
Facsimile reporting, where appropriate
Report printers, where needed
Remote electronic reporting and inquiry
Electronic mail capability

LIS, Laboratory information system.

Networking

A laboratory network is a group of laboratories that exchange information and laboratory services. The motivation is for the laboratory to become a regionally integrated laboratory provider, with participants maintaining their operational status quo as much as possible. With a "shared-services" or "centers-of-excellence" design, each facility becomes a referral site to the network members for certain specialty services. For example, one hospital may have a highly respected virology laboratory; another may have a large immunology laboratory. Efficient courier systems to transport specimens are required.

In addition, a complex specimen triage and logistics infrastructure managed by a supportive LIS is required. Test orders and results must be communicated promptly to and from these testing sites. Most current LISs do not support these complex needs. When member hospitals have different commercial LISs, getting them to "talk" to one another effectively and support interfacility specimen sharing may be difficult or prohibitively expensive. A stand-alone, computer-based system may tie facilities sharing testing together but usually does not tie their LISs together. Network hospitals most often do not have the same LISs. In such cases the development of an "interface engine" may be the best approach. This system becomes the "hub" through which each of the network LISs communicate.

Network success is tied closely to price competitiveness and a unified approach to managed-care contract negotiation. The costly and complicated logistics, inadequate LIS solutions, excess capacity, instrumentation redundancy, and inherent overstaffing may create economical disadvantages sufficient to inhibit necessary competitiveness.

Consolidation

Consolidation is defined here as the merger of several independent laboratories into a core laboratory. Partners in the formation of a consolidated core laboratory may include hospitals, pathology groups, or independent laboratories (local or regional). This laboratory partnering may be the first step for hospitals intent on consolidating all their services into integrated health systems spanning communities, regions, or entire states. Their ultimate goal is to expand patient access to the full continuum of care, consolidate unnecessary redundancies, and reduce the overall cost of care.

In practice, consolidation leads to improvements in efficiency, productivity, service, and quality, which eliminates unnecessary resource duplication and excess capacity. When a group of hospital laboratories agree to form a core laboratory in which the majority of the high-volume routine testing is performed, significant downsizing of individual hospital sites to "rapid response" laboratories follows. Overall staff size is reduced unless significant growth in outreach activities of the core laboratory necessitates increased capacity. Equipment usually is consolidated and standardized to deliver consistency in results and economies in purchasing.

When networked or consolidated laboratories attempt to expand their outreach activities, they must pay close attention to a number of critical strategic and operational considerations (see Table 16-3). Careful planning and capable management are necessary to ensure the success of these enterprises.

■ FINANCIAL MANAGEMENT

Effective management requires a systematic approach to management of financial resources. Such a system provides three main functions. First, effective financial management gives managers accurate, timely, and useful financial information necessary for ongoing control of operational expenses. Second, financial management provides information necessary for strategical decision making. Third, it provides summary information for owners and other interested parties that communicates the financial health of the organization. In addition, state and federal governments require financial information to assess appropriate taxation.

Categories of financial management that require consideration include (1) budgeting, (2) test-cost accounting, (3) capital expenditures, (4) expense reports, and (5) make-versus-buy decisions.

Budgeting

A laboratory budget is a financial plan that predicts expenditures for the upcoming fiscal year. Ownership of budget responsibilities and accountability is accomplished best through the direct involvement of all parties concerned. In this type of "bottom-up" budget, line managers are asked to predict the resources necessary to accomplish the workload projected by senior management for the new fiscal year. The line managers then may be provided a monetary incentive to maintain their expenses within the established budget. However, because external forces, such as market demands, generally control volume fluctuations, incentives should be adjusted for changes in volume. Such an incentive program brings ownership to those managers who control labor and material costs.

Budgets also may be incremental or zero based. The incremental budget begins with the actual expenses incurred during the current year. These expenses are corrected to reflect the anticipated growth rate and any increased efficiency resulting from increased testing volumes and/or process improvements. In contrast, the zero-based approach builds each new year's budget from zero.

Test-Cost Accounting

Any laboratory planning to compete successfully must determine how much its tests cost. Accurate costs allow managers to determine profitable pricing and assess how overall profitability is affected by operational interventions. Decisions about the introduction of new tests or instruments also are facilitated. Choosing among instrument alternatives is a combination of technical performance characteristics (for example, accuracy, throughput, and reliability) and cost accounting information.

Cost accounting begins with identification of the basic cost components. Costs are divided broadly into categories—direct or indirect and fixed or variable. **Direct costs** are attributable directly to production of the billable test or patient result. The most common direct costs are technical labor, reagents, disposable supplies, and quality control materials. All such costs are consumed on a per-test or incremental basis and vary with run frequencies, run failures, waste, and the number of specimens in each run. Examples of **indirect costs** include office supplies, supervision and administration, inspection fees, proficiency testing, rent, utilities, equipment and other capital **depreciation,** taxes, sales and marketing expenses, telephone, and information systems costs. In practice, indirect costs are more difficult to measure and assign on a per-test basis and generally are allocated as average costs spread over the total volume of billable tests.

Whether a cost is fixed or variable refers to the way in which it behaves with changes in the volume of billable tests. A **fixed cost** is one that does not vary as volume varies (for example, capital expenditures). **Variable costs** increase with each additional test increment and include reagents, disposable supplies, and technical labor.

Once laboratory expenses are segregated into cost categories, they are allocated to individual tests. Numerous techniques for laboratory cost accounting have been published.[13,16,17] Because it focuses on single billable tests, "job-order costing" is the most accurate, but also the most demanding, method of test-cost accounting.[17] "Process costing" results in an average cost per billable test and is both less time consuming and less accurate.

The direct cost for labor and reagents also provides the basis to determine the incremental cost-per-patient result (that is, the cost to add one additional test to a batch). Competitive pricing, particularly for high-volume outreach business, is facilitated greatly by knowledge of incremental costs.

Capital Expenditures

The cost-effective laboratory also must make wise investment decisions for capital expenditures. Most laboratories utilize both batch and random-access instrumentation systems, each having differing labor and supply costs. Even when automated systems provide random-access capabilities without significant increases in supply costs, increased staffing may be required to provide "on-demand/stat" testing. In addition, the per-test cost for reagents is generally higher with the random-access systems. Economies of scale often are substantial for batch analyses. However, this advantage decreases as run frequencies increase, and fewer patient specimens are analyzed per run. If less than four patient specimens are analyzed in a batch, the laboratory most likely is losing money on each run. Maintaining technical competency and performance proficiency is also more problematical for low-volume assays.

When differences in technological capability and analytical quality are deemed medically comparable, decisions among analytical systems should be made on a cost-per-billable-test basis. This step further emphasizes the importance of an accurate test-cost accounting system. Decisions on whether to purchase or lease instruments are facilitated

by an analysis of how soon investment costs are recovered. In the "payback" model the "break-even point" is the volume of billable test revenue required to offset all acquisition costs.

Net present value (NPV) and internal rate of return (IRR) are other common financial tools used for present value determinations. In present value determinations the devaluing effect of factors such as inflation and the value to forego other investment opportunities make a current dollar worth more than a dollar a year from now. Expressed mathematically

$$PV = \frac{future \ \$s}{(1 + r)^t}$$

where r is the discount rate (for example, inflation), and t is years. This adjusted value then is used in equations to compare investment alternatives.

The NPV is the present value of the discounted sum of all anticipated future revenues resulting from the new investment (that is, the net price per test multiplied by the anticipated annual volumes) less the costs of acquisition (that is, the purchase price or lease costs) and ongoing operation. Any investment with an NPV greater than 0 is considered an attractive investment. The IRR is the discount rate, r, at which the NPV equals 0. The derived r is compared with the rate predetermined by an organization as its minimum return on investment ("hurdle" rate). Any investment that produces an IRR greater than this minimum return is considered attractive.

Expense Reports

To effectively manage laboratory finances, expenses must be tracked closely. Detailed line-item expense reports that show actual performance against budgeted expenses should be provided to each manager monthly. Significant

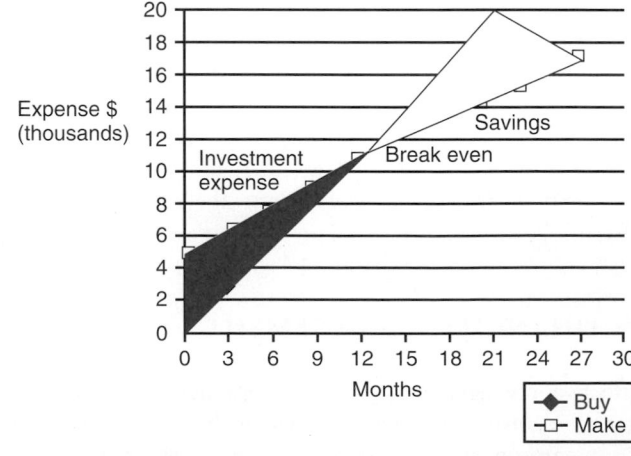

Figure 16-1   Example of the make-versus-buy decision process.

variances then are regularly addressed and communicated to management.

Make-Versus-Buy Decisions

Savings may be achieved through a variety of **make-versus-buy decisions.** Examples include (1) reference laboratory services, (2) other support services (for example, instrument maintenance, information systems, billing and finance, etc.), and (3) reagent preparation.

The manager is responsible for evaluating alternatives and making decisions that earn the greatest benefit for the organization. Financial considerations are not the only factors to consider. Periodic review of make-versus-buy decisions identifies ways to improve productivity. A time plot of expenses for the make-versus-buy alternatives (Figure 16-1) demonstrates the potential savings after the break-even point.

Several of the following parameters contribute to make-versus-buy decisions, and the relative importance of each depends on the circumstances of the individual laboratory:

1. Test volume and run frequency
2. Turnaround time required for optimal patient care
3. Reagent and supply costs, stability, and availability
4. Labor requirements, both costs and required expertise
5. Equipment
6. Space

Table 16-4 illustrates an example, which considers the make decision to bring a specific test in-house or the buy decision to continue sending it to a reference laboratory. In this simplified example, overhead costs (for example, building, space, computer, and administration) are not added to the in-house costs.

The total cost per test is determined through consideration of both the make and the buy alternatives. The cost per test for the buy alternative is obtained from current or potential vendors. Because volume estimates are critically important, two and four requests per week have been selected. For the buy alternative, start-up costs are spread over a 2-year period. A guideline is that the payback period should be 2 years or less, with the ratio of total savings being equal to or greater than the total investment expense over the 2-year period.

Laboratories should examine critically all low-volume tests—most of which are not cost effective to perform in house. To determine the cost of these low-volume tests, instrument maintenance, instrument capital costs, labor, controls, calibration, wastage, and space all must be included. Overall laboratory efficiency often dramatically improves with elimination of low-volume, inefficient tests and con-

---

TABLE 16-4 **Example of Make-Versus-Buy Decision Process**

Pertinent Facts

Test volume	Current	Two requests/week	= 104/y
	Projected after 2 y	Four requests/week	= 208/y
Vendor price	Current		= $35/test
	After 2 y		= $32/test

"Make" Costs

Start-up (development and training)	Labor: 106 h × $14.50/h	= $2320
	Reagents and controls	= $400
	Equipment	= $5000
	Supplies	= $70
		= $7790
Development costs per test	Two tests/week	= $37.45/test
	Four tests/week	= $18.73/test
Operation direct costs per patient assay (labor, controls, reagents)	Two tests/week	= $8.80/test
	Four tests/week	= $6.50/test
Two-year cost of "make" decision	Two tests/week = 208(37.45 + 8.80)	= $9620
	Four tests/week = 416(18.73 + 6.50)	= $10,496
Two-year cost of "buy" decision	Two tests/week = 208 × $35/test	= $7280
	Four tests/week = 416 × $32/test	= $13,312

Decision

At two tests/week	Buy decision saves $2340 over 2 y.
At four tests/week	Make decision saves $2816 over 2 y.*

*After development costs are recouped at the end of the second year, savings increase substantially. The make-buy decision is critically dependent on test volumes.

centration on more productive and efficient higher-volume tests.

The primary reason to consider make-versus-buy decisions is to improve overall laboratory productivity and expand laboratory services in a cost-effective manner.

■ HUMAN RESOURCE MANAGEMENT

Individuals are the most valuable assets of any organization. Successful organizations provide environments that challenges employees to assume increasing responsibilities consistent with their training, experience, and personal aspirations. In practice this environment includes building a positive culture and providing the employees with essential management tools. In such an environment, continuous improvement becomes a foundation of the corporate culture.

Building a Positive Culture

A positive culture is an environment that cultivates capable, dedicated, and informed employees. Components in the building of a positive culture include the following:

1. Development of a clear mission and vision statements
2. Leadership by example
3. Recognition of the employee contributions
4. A team approach to problem solving
5. An environment of open communication
6. Employee empowerment
7. Development of a system for performance measurement
8. Recruiting and nurturing of dedicated and enthusiastic employees

Mission and vision statements

Good managers realize that individuals want and need to contribute to the success of the organizations to which they belong. The key is a common understanding of the purpose of the organization and where it is headed. The mission statement should declare the purpose simply and concisely. The vision statement describes what the organization plans to become to accomplish its mission. Employees at all levels must understand both statements easily.

Leadership by example and attitude

Mutual respect is a key to successful management; each individual brings a unique set of talents, abilities, expectations, experiences, and weaknesses to the job. Leaders must be sensitive to the powerful effects of their own examples and attitudes on the culture of their organization.[4] Staff members closely monitor their supervisors, noting items such as dress, speech, attitudes, work habits, ethics, the cars they drive, and especially when they arrive and leave work. The attitudes supervisors have toward management responsibilities are reflected clearly through their interactions, communications, and work activities.

Recognition

Managers should build upon the strengths of their employees and provide positive recognition for their accomplishments. A manager contributes to a positive culture through recognition.[4] Effective techniques for a manager include the following:

- Personally greeting an employee, especially in front of peers
- Sending personal handwritten notes
- Inviting subordinates to report accomplishments
- Telling peers of individuals' accomplishments
- Issuing an award for outstanding accomplishments
- Starting an employee-of-the-month award
- Telling his or her supervisor of an employee's accomplishments
- Ensuring that an employee is recognized formally before colleagues and managers
- Privately informing employees that accomplishments are recognized and appreciated

Problem solving

Every problem represents an improvement opportunity, but problem resolution should be handled in a manner that preserves personal dignity for all concerned. Given the opportunity, properly trained and appropriately recognized employees take personal ownership for their job responsibilities, including problem resolution. Capable leaders are able to recognize others for successes and take the blame when things go wrong. In such an environment, problems are defined, owned, and resolved.

Open communications

Effective and timely communication regarding all aspects of the organization, helps employees take personal ownership in their areas of responsibility. Organizations that follow the following four mechanisms can improve communication:

1. Hold regular operational meeting for managers.
2. Report quarterly organizational progress measures.
3. Hold regular open meetings without agendas between employees and senior management.
4. Periodically publish an "executive briefing" that highlights important issues for managers to discuss with employees during regular staff meetings.

Empowerment

Empowering employees to act greatly expands a manager's influence. Once the limits of empowerment have been defined clearly, the manager must allow empowered employees to make decisions within the defined boundaries. Managers should seek employee input to identify areas in which they may be empowered. For example, employees may be empowered to make decisions regarding (1) hiring of co-workers, (2) establishment of work schedules, (3) ordering of supplies, and (4) improvements in system processes.

Performance measures

Progress measures direct, unify, focus, and motivate an organization. Both organizational and supportive departmental measures should be identified in the following four areas:[3]

1. *Activity* How much does the employee do (for example, number of tests per month)?
2. *Productivity* How efficient is the employee (for example, **billed units** per full-time equivalent staff member)?
3. *Quality* How good are the employee and organization (for example, turnaround time, percent of error-free performance)?
4. *Finance* Are the employee and organization fiscally responsible (for example, variance from budget, cost per test)?

Once established, organizational performance measures are tracked over time and communicated as a means to focus employee contribution to improvement.

Staffing

A positive corporate culture depends on recruiting and retention of good employees. Key features of successful staffing include selection of qualified new employees, promotion and transfer of employees within the organization, and steps to deal with problem employees.

Selecting new employees

The long-term success of any organization is determined by hiring decisions. Effective managers are familiar with the needs of their organization and hire individuals whose strengths compensate for existing weaknesses. The temptation to hire employees who duplicate existing strengths and weaknesses should be avoided.

Transferring and promoting employees

Transfer and promotion within allows trained employees who have proven their skills to further their career goals within the organization. Transferred employees generally require shorter training periods than newly hired employees and often promote increased cooperation within the organization. Internal transfers are a means to advance good and productive employees. Managers must, however, resolve problem employee situations and avoid transferring their problems to other managers.

Dealing with problem employees

When an employee is unhappy and unproductive in a job assignment, the manager's responsibility is to help solve the problem. Effective performance appraisals are very important. In these one-on-one sessions an employee's performance must be compared openly with clearly understood requirements. Corrective measures must be communicated and documented clearly, up to and including termination.

Management Tools

Successful management requires the effective use of meetings, memoranda, letters, reports, and time-management techniques.[4] These tools are great assets to both the manager and the employees and facilitate accomplishment, the real goal of all managers.

Meetings

Meetings are management tools only and must be kept in perspective. Properly planned, conducted, and controlled meetings are invaluable management tools with which to make decisions, train, motivate, encourage, recognize, clarify, inform, and communicate vital information to all levels of the organization. The following six guidelines are recommended for managers to improve meeting productivity:

1. Determine the primary purpose for the meeting and the goals to be accomplished.
2. Identify those who need to attend to accomplish the purposes; for decision making and planning, the number of attendees should be small. Informational and motivational meetings are effective with larger groups.
3. Schedule the day, time, and location for the convenience of the attendees.
4. Prepare and prioritize an agenda. The number of agenda items depends on the purpose and type of meeting, as well as the nature of the items.
5. Distribute the agenda and necessary materials in advance.
6. Document meeting proceedings. Always prepare and distribute minutes, which summarize the proceedings; highlight the assignments, including a date for completion; document decisions; and specify the time and place for the next meeting, if required.

Letters, memoranda, and reports

A variety of acceptable formats for letters, memoranda, and reports commonly are used. The purpose and any action to be taken should be stated clearly and concisely at the beginning of the document. When follow-up is requested, the document author always should specify a deadline for receipt of the requested information. The distribution list is also important and should be used to inform those who need

Department name_____ Department head _____
Contact person   _____ Phone number   _____
Date _____

Please fill in the boxes with your existing head count and projected head count. In addition, project your support area square footage and bulk storage cubic feet.

	Existing	Year 1	Year 2	Year 3	Year 4	Year 5
Area head count #						
Support area in square footage *equipment, file/storage/work area*						
Bulk storage in cubic feet						

Please list the departments with which you work closely and rate them according to the following "closeness rating" and "reason code" criteria.

VALUE	CLOSENESS
A	Absolutely necessary
E	Especially important
I	Important
O	Ordinary closeness

CODE	REASON
1	Work flow
2	Close working arrangement
3	Personnel tie-in
4	Convenience

DEPARTMENT NAME	CLOSENESS	REASON

Special Considerations:

Figure 16-2   Space-planning worksheet.

to know the document's contents but are not expected to take action.

Time management

In practice, time is the most important and critical resource to manage.[9,10] A time-management system is a required tool for managers and employees and should accommodate hourly, daily, weekly, monthly, and even yearly advance scheduling. The following tips are intended to help managers use their schedule to increase personal productivity:

1. Schedule in advance but retain flexibility to accommodate unplanned events.
2. Specify open times for appointments.
3. Block out sufficient focus time for special priority projects.

4. Schedule time for routine tasks, such as mail, telephone, and electronic correspondence.

■ SPACE AND FACILITY MANAGEMENT

The mission, visions, and strategic plans for the organization are also the foundation for effective facilities planning. Because alteration of an organization's physical facilities is time consuming, disruptive, and costly, an accurate long-range plan provides significant financial benefit.

Project Definition

The first task in facilities planning is to determine the scope of the project. The laboratory may need to build new space, expand existing space, or reorganize or remodel existing space. Careful preconstruction planning reduces costs. Important design limitations to consider are financial limits, size, location, and political constraints. Within limits, flexibility also should be built into the project.

Macro-Planning

Macro-planning is the process used to determine the future space needs of laboratory sections and how the sections interrelate. The plan should address relationships among laboratory sections, such as those concerning analytical laboratories, specimen processing, administration, information services, customer services, finance, and human resources. Employee input needs to be gathered to size and configure appropriately the proposed laboratory space. A simple space-planning worksheet is recommended to organize the coordination of functional and proximity relationships that optimize workflow (Figure 16-2). Laboratory space requires utilities and furnishings different from those found in a normal office space and therefore must be specified accurately and thoroughly before the start of construction to minimize expense.

Micro-Planning

The micro-planning process defines the architectural details and finalizes the relationships within, as well as among, each work group or department. This process begins with a summary of the existing space allocation for each function and **full-time equivalent.** The space requirements for each individual function depend not only on the growth or downsizing projections, but also on the (1) existing space capacity, (2) technological advances, (3) automation requirements, and (4) other specific factors the managers deem necessary. The information gathered with the space-planning worksheet provides objective data from each department. Fairness, open communication, and objectivity all help minimize emotional and territorial issues. After the individual functions have been sized and working relationships identified, specific locations then are assigned and approved provisionally.

At this point a small group should be assigned to work closely with the architect to complete the design details. Detailed architectural drawings are prepared for each area of the laboratory. After the floor plan and the design choices are specified clearly, the managers must work with the employees to optimize the design detail. Finally, the flexibility offered by modular laboratory and office furniture saves money during future reorganization projects.

Coordination During Construction

Detailed preconstruction planning expedites construction, but continual coordination is required throughout the bidding and building processes. Because neither the builder nor the architect is likely to be familiar with how a laboratory functions, a senior-level building coordinator should be assigned from the organization to become a member of the construction management team. No matter how well planned, construction adjustments sometimes may be required. The building coordinator's job is to ensure that the carefully developed plans become the reality within the scheduled time and budget parameters.

References

1. American Association for Clinical Chemistry: The changing environment for the practice of clinical chemistry. Report from the AACC Delta Group on the changing practice environment. Clin Chem 1996; 42:91-95.
2. Athena Society: The future of clinical chemistry and its role in healthcare. Clin Chem 1996; 42:96-101.
3. Ash KO: Laboratory adaptations to healthcare initiatives: part II. Clin Chem 1995; 41:128-130.
4. Ash KO, Weiss RL: Laboratory Management, Washington, DC, AACC Press, 1995.
5. Ash KO, Smith A, Ng RH et al: Selecting instrumentation. ASCP Check Sample. Clin Chem 1985; CC85-1 (CC-159), Chicago, American Society for Clinical Pathology, 1985.
6. Boyd JC, Felder RA, Savory J: Robotics and the changing face of the clinical laboratory. Clin Chem 1996; 42:1901-1910.
7. Burtis CA: Converging technologies and their impact on the clinical laboratory. Clin Chem 1996; 42:1735-1749.
8. Cooper RS: The Laboratory Guide to Negotiating Managed Care Contracts, Washington, DC, Washington G-2 Reports, 1995.
9. Frings CS: The Hitchhiker's Guide to Effective Time Management, Washington, DC, AACC Press, 1997.
10. Frings CS: Self-Management & Leadership Strategies for Success, Washington, DC, AACC Press, 1998.
11. Boyd JC, Young DS: Automation in the clinical laboratory. In Burtis CA, Ashwood ER (eds): Tietz Textbook of Clinical Chemistry, 3rd edition, pp 226-261, Philadelphia, WB Saunders, 1999.
12. Markel SF, Venner AM: A market analysis approach to bidding for capitated clinical laboratory and pathology services contracts. Arch Pathol Lab Med 1995; 119:627-634.
13. Patterson PP: Cost accounting in hospitals and clinical laboratories. Part I. Clin Lab Manag Rev 1988; 2:343-346; Part II. Clin Lab Manag Rev 1989; 3:26-33; Part III. Clin Lab Manag Rev 1989; 3:151-156.

14. Pomerantz P: The laboratory restructuring challenge: the reengineering imperative. Clin Lab Manag Rev 1995; 9:357-362.

15. Steiner JW, Root JM, Michel RL: The transformation of hospital laboratories: why regionalization, consolidation, and reengineering will lead laboratories into the 21st century. Hosp Technol Serv 1995; 14:1-33.

16. Travers EM: Managing Costs in Clinical Laboratories: A Manager's Fiscal Guide to Laboratory Cost Effectiveness and Productivity, New York, McGraw-Hill, 1989.

17. Travers EM: Laboratory manager's financial handbook. Cost accounting: the road map to financial success. Clin Lab Manag Rev 1996; 10:265-285.

18. Yablonsky T: How to stay competitive in a managed care environment. Lab Med 1996; 27:246-254.

Additional Reading

Johns M: Information Management for Health Professions, Albany, Delmar Publishers, 1996.

McLean R: Financial Management in Health Care Organizations, Albany, Delmar Publishers, 1997.

National Committee for Clinical Laboratory Standards: Cost accounting in the clinical laboratory; Tentative Guideline GP11-A. Wayne, Pa, National Committee for Clinical Laboratory Standards, 1998.

National Committee for Clinical Laboratory Standards: Laboratory design; Approved Guideline GP18-A. Wayne, Pa, National Committee for Clinical Laboratory Standards, 1998.

National Committee for Clinical Laboratory Standards: Training verification for laboratory personnel; Approved Guideline GP21-A. Wayne, Pa, National Committee for Clinical Laboratory Standards, 1995.

Richardson T: Total Quality Management Basics: A Primer for Technicians, Albany, Delmar Publishers, 1997.

Umiker WO: Coping with Difficult People in the Health Care Setting, Chicago, ASCP Press, 1994.

Varnadoe L: Medical Laboratory Management and Supervision: Operations, Review, and Study Guide, Philadelphia, FA Davis, 1996.

CHAPTER 17

Quality Management

JAMES O. WESTGARD, PhD, and GEORGE G. KLEE, MD, PhD

Objectives

1. Define *quality* and *total quality management.*
2. List examples of preanalytical, analytical, and postanalytical variables that affect laboratory test results and state how each is controlled.
3. Compare internal quality control with external quality assessment.
4. Define *control materials* and state their use in the clinical laboratory; define *quality control.*
5. Explain the need for control charts in the clinical laboratory and describe how to enter data on a control chart.
6. List and explain the Westgard rules for interpretation of laboratory control data.
7. Apply the Westgard rules to actual control data and determine what actions must be taken to correct out-of-limit control values.
8. Define *proficiency testing.*

Key Words

Control Limits Lines on a control chart that are used to assess the control status of a method; commonly calculated as the mean of the control material plus and minus a certain multiple of the standard deviation observed for that control material

Control Procedure (QC Procedure) The protocol and materials necessary for an analyst to assess whether a method is working properly and patient test results can be reported; can be described by the number of control measurements and the decision criteria (control rules) used to judge the acceptability of the results

Control Rules A decision criterion used to interpret quality control (QC) control data and make a judgment on the control status (for example, 1_{3s} representing a control rule where a run is judged out of control if a measurement exceeds the mean plus or minus 3 standard deviations)

External Quality Assessment A quality program in which specimens are submitted to laboratories for analysis and the results of an individual laboratory are compared

with the results for the group of participating laboratories

Error Detection A performance characteristic of a QC procedure that describes how often an analytical run is rejected when results contain errors in addition to the inherent imprecision of the method

False Rejections A performance characteristic of a QC procedure that describes how often an analytical run is rejected when no errors occur, except for the inherent imprecision of the method

ISO 9000 A series of international standards for quality management produced by the International Organization for Standardization

Levey-Jennings Control Chart A simple graphical display in which the observed values are plotted versus an acceptable range of values, as indicated on the chart by lines for upper and lower **control limits**, which commonly are drawn as the mean plus or minus 3 standard deviations

Proficiency Testing (PT) The process whereby simulated patient specimens made from a common pool are analyzed by laboratories; the results of this procedure being evaluated to determine the "quality" of the laboratories' performance

Quality　Conformance to the requirements of users or customers and the satisfaction of their needs and expectations

Statistical QC　Those aspects of quality control in which statistics are applied, in contrast to the broader scope of quality assurance that includes many other procedures, such as preventive maintenance, instrument function checks, and performance validation tests

Total Quality Management (TQM)　A management philosophy and approach that focuses on processes and their improvement as the means to satisfy customer needs and requirements

Total Testing Process　A broad definition of the laboratory testing process that includes the preanalytical, analytical, and postanalytical steps

Westgard Multirule　A control procedure that uses a series of control rules to test the control measurements; a 1_{2s} rule being used as a warning, followed by use of 1_{3s}, 2_{2s}, R_{4s}, 4_{1s}, and 10_x as rejection rules

---

The principles of quality management, assurance, and control have become the foundation by which clinical laboratories are managed and operated. This chapter begins with a discussion of the fundamentals of total quality management and follows with descriptions of total quality management of the clinical laboratory, control of preanalytical variables, control of analytical variables (with emphasis on statistical quality control and identification of sources of analytical errors), and **external quality assessment** and proficiency testing programs. The chapter concludes with a discussion of new quality initiatives, including the ISO 9000 certification process.

FUNDAMENTALS OF TOTAL QUALITY MANAGEMENT

Quality systems in health-care organizations are evolving.[13] Public and private pressures to contain costs now are accompanied by pressures to improve quality. The seemingly contradictory pressures for both cost reduction and quality improvement (QI) require that health-care organizations adopt new systems to manage quality. When faced with these same pressures, other industries have implemented a process termed **total quality management (TQM).** This process also is referred to as *total quality control (QC), total quality leadership, continuous quality improvement, quality management science,* or more generally as *industrial quality management.* It provides both a management philosophy for organizational development and a management process for improvement of quality in all aspects of work. Many health-care organizations,[4,17,30] including clinical laboratories,[11,12,18,26] have adopted the concepts and principles of TQM.

Concepts

In this chapter, **quality** is defined as conformance to the requirements of users or customers. The universal principles of total quality management are (1) customer focus, (2) management commitment, (3) training, (4) process capability and control, and (5) measurement through quality-improvement tools.[30] The focus on users and customers is important, particularly in service industries such as health care. The users of health-care laboratories are often the nurses and doctors; their customers are the patients and other parties who pay the bills.

Costs must be understood in the context of quality. If quality means conformance to requirements, then "quality costs" must be understood in terms of "costs of conformance" and "costs of nonconformance," as illustrated in Figure 17-1. In industrial terms, costs of conformance are divided into prevention costs and appraisal costs. Costs of nonconformance consist of internal and external failure costs. For a laboratory testing process, calibration is a good example of a cost incurred to prevent problems. Likewise, quality control is a cost for performance appraisal, a repeat run is an internal failure cost for poor analytical performance, and repeat

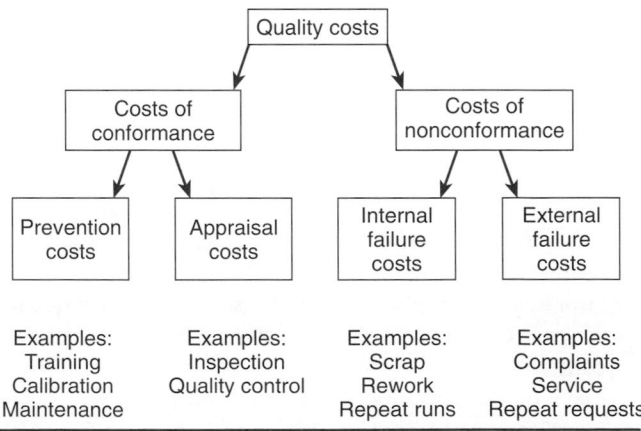

Figure 17-1　The cost of quality in terms of the costs of conformance and the costs of nonconformance to customer requirements. (From Westgard JO, Barry PL: Cost-Effective Quality Control: Managing the Quality and Productivity of Analytical Processes, Washington, DC, AACC Press, 1997.)

requests for tests—because of poor analytical quality—constitute an external failure cost.

This understanding of quality and cost leads to a new perspective of the relationship between these two concepts. Improvements in quality lead to reductions in cost. For example, with better analytical quality a laboratory eliminates repeat runs and repeat requests for tests. This repeat work is waste. If quality improves, waste is reduced, which in turn reduces cost. The father of this fundamental concept was the late W. Edwards Deming, who developed and internationally promulgated the idea that quality improvement reduces waste and leads to improved productivity, which in turn reduces costs and provides a competitive advantage.[3]

Methodology

Quality improvement occurs when problems are eliminated permanently. Problems arise primarily from imperfect processes, not from imperfect individuals. Industrial experience has shown that 85% of all problems are process problems, whereas the remaining 15% are problems requiring the action and performance improvement of individual employees. Thus quality problems are primarily management problems because only management has the power to change work processes.

This emphasis on processes leads to a new view of the organization as a system of processes (Figure 17-2). For example, physicians might view a health-care organization as a provider of processes for patient examination (A), patient testing (B), patient diagnosis (C), and patient treatment (D). Health-care administrators might view the same health-care organization in terms of processes for admission of patients (A), tracking of patient services (B), discharge of patients (C), and billing for costs of service (D). Laboratory

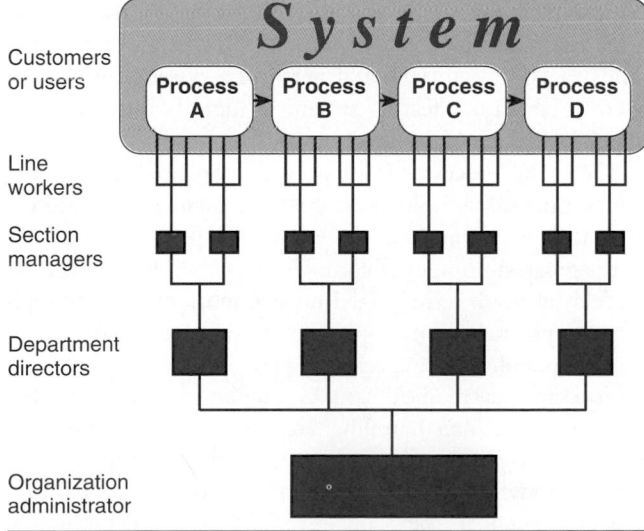

Figure 17-2 The total quality management view of an organization as a system of processes.

directors might understand their responsibilities in terms of processes for acquiring specimens (A), processing specimens (B), analyzing samples (C), and reporting test results (D). Laboratory analysts might view their work as processes for acquiring samples (A), analyzing samples (B), performing quality control (C), and releasing patient test results (D). The total system for a health-care organization involves the interaction of all of these processes and others.[13]

Given the primary importance of these processes for the organization, TQM views the organization as a support structure rather than a command structure. The most immediate processes required for the delivery of services are those of the frontline employees. Senior management's role is to support the frontline employees and empower them to identify and solve problems in their own work processes.

The importance of empowerment is understood easily if a problem involves processes from two different departments. For example, if a problem involves the link between process A and process B (see Figure 17-2), the traditional management structure requires that a problem be passed up from the line workers to a section manager or supervisor, a department director, and an organization administrator. The administrator then works back through an equal number of intermediaries in the other department. Direct involvement of line workers and their managers should provide more immediate resolution of the problem.

However, such problem solving requires a carefully structured process to ensure that root causes are identified and proposed solutions are verified. Juran's "project–by–project" quality improvement process[7] provides detailed guidelines that have been adopted widely and integrated into current team problem-solving methodology. The methodology outlines distinct steps for the following:

1. Careful definition of the problem
2. Establishment of baseline measures of process performance
3. Identification of root causes of the problem
4. Identification of a remedy for the problem
5. Verification that the remedy actually works
6. "Standardization" or generalization of the solution for routine implementation of an improved process
7. Establishment of ongoing measures for monitoring and control of the process

▮ TOTAL QUALITY MANAGEMENT OF THE CLINICAL LABORATORY

The principles and concepts of TQM have been formalized into a quality-management process (Figure 17-3). The traditional framework for quality management in a health-care laboratory emphasizes the establishment of quality laboratory processes (QLPs), QC, and more recently, quality assurance (QA). QLP includes analytical processes, as well as

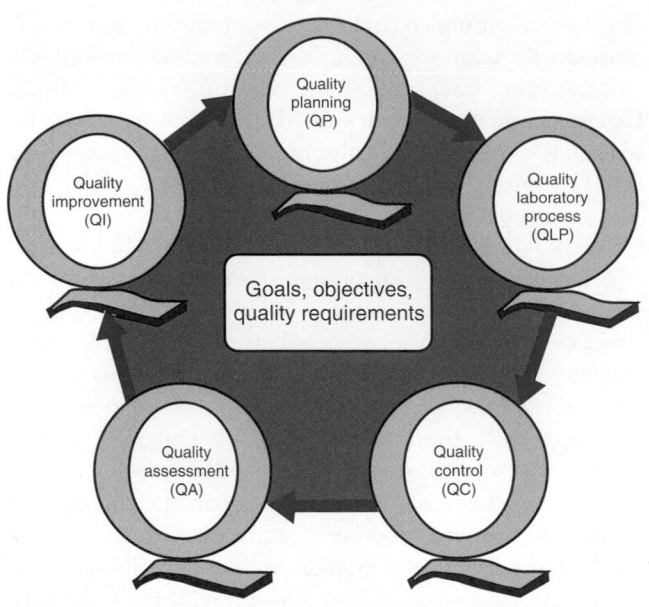

Figure 17-3 Total quality management framework for management of quality in a health-care laboratory. (From Westgard JO, Burnett RW, Bowers GN: Quality management science in clinical chemistry: a dynamic framework for continuous improvement of quality. Clin Chem 1990; 36:1712-1716.)

the general policies, practices, and procedures that define how all aspects of the work are done. QC emphasizes statistical **control procedures** but also includes nonstatistical check procedures, such as linearity checks, reagent and standard checks, and temperature monitors. QA, as currently applied, is concerned primarily with broader measures and monitors of laboratory performance, such as turnaround time, specimen identification, patient identification, and test utility. *Quality assessment* is the proper term for these activities, as opposed to *quality assurance*. Measuring performance does not by itself improve performance and often does not detect problems in time to prevent harmful effects. Quality assurance requires either that causes of problems be identified through QI and eliminated through quality planning (QP) or that QC detect the problems early enough to prevent their consequences.

To provide a fully developed framework for quality management, the QI and QP components must be established.[25] QI provides a structured problem-solving process to help identify the root cause of a problem and a remedy for that problem. QP is necessary to standardize the remedy, establish measures for performance monitoring, ensure that the performance achieved satisfies quality requirements, and document the new QLP. The new process then is implemented through QLP, measured and monitored through QC and QA, improved through QI, and replanned through QP. These five components, which work together in a feedback loop, illustrate how continuous QI is accomplished and quality assurance is built into laboratory processes.

The "five-Q" framework (see Figure 17-3) also defines how quality is managed objectively with the "scientific method," or the PDCA cycle (**p**lan, **d**o, **c**heck, **a**ct). QP provides the planning step, QLP establishes standard processes for the way things are done, QC and QA provide measures for checks on how well things are done, and QI provides a mechanism through which to act on those measures. The methodology naturally applied in scientific experiments also should be the basis for objective management decisions.

Objectivity, however, depends on the existence of quantitative quality requirements for evaluation of the performance of existing processes and planning of the performance of new processes.[28] Laboratories must define their service goals and objectives and establish clinical and analytical quality requirements for process testing. Without such quality goals, no objective way exists to determine whether acceptable quality is being achieved, identify processes that need improvement, or plan or design new processes that ensure the attainment of a specified level of quality.

THE TOTAL TESTING PROCESS

Accurate and timely test reports are the responsibility of the laboratory. However, many problems arise before and after submitted specimens are analyzed (see Chapter 2). Therefore the **total testing process** must be managed properly in the preanalytical, analytical, and postanalytical phases.

The many steps or subprocesses that take place from the time of the physician's initial request for a test to the time of the final interpretation of the test result are obtained through performance of a "systems analysis." Table 17-1 lists the steps or subprocesses for a typical clinical laboratory. Although such an analysis identifies the critical processes for a typical laboratory, each laboratory situation is different, and additional processes and sources of error may be present. Thus each laboratory should perform a systems analysis of its own laboratory testing system to identify those areas in which errors are likely to occur.

Once the processes have been documented, those processes most susceptible to error should be identified and receive the most attention. Many times the processes that lead to the greatest number of complaints, such as lost specimens or delayed results, are judged most important, even though other steps, such as the appropriateness of test selection and the acceptability of a specimen, may be more important to achieve optimal medical care. Guidelines describing procedures for specimen handling are available from organizations such as the National Committee for Clinical Laboratory Standards (NCCLS). Documents by accrediting agencies, such as the College of American Pathologists, Centers for Disease Control and Prevention, and state regulatory agencies, are also helpful.

TABLE 17-1 Laboratory Testing Processes and Potential Errors

Process	Potential Errors
Test ordering	Inappropriate test
	Illegible handwriting
	Incorrect patient identification
	Special requirements not specified
	Cost or delayed order
Specimen acquisition	Incorrect tube or container
	Incorrect patient identification
	Inadequate volume
	Invalid specimen (for example, hemolyzed or too dilute)
	Incorrect collection time
	Improper transport conditions
Analytical measurement	Incorrect instrument calibration
	Specimen mix-up
	Incorrect volume of specimen
	Presence of interfering substance
	Instrument precision problem
Test reporting	Incorrect patient identification
	Report not posted in chart
	Illegible report
	Delayed report
	Transcription error
Test interpretation	Interfering substances not recognized
	Specificity of test not understood
	Precision limitations not recognized
	Inappropriate analytical sensitivity
	Previous values unavailable for comparison

■ CONTROL OF PREANALYTICAL VARIABLES

Establishing effective methods for the monitoring and control of preanalytical variables is difficult because many of the variables are outside the traditional laboratory areas. Monitoring preanalytical variables requires the coordinated effort of many individuals and hospital departments, each of which must recognize the importance of these efforts in the maintenance of high-quality service. Accomplishing such monitoring may require support from outside the laboratory, particularly from the institution's clinical practice committee or some similar authority. A list of important variables to consider include the following:

- *Test utilization and practice guidelines* Traditionally, laboratory test utilization always has been monitored or controlled to some degree, but current emphasis on the cost of medical care and government regulation of medical care may increase the importance of this factor.
- *Patient identification* Correct identification of patients and specimens is a major concern for laboratories. The highest frequency of errors occurs with the use of handwritten labels and request forms. The use of bar-coding technology for patient identification has minimized this potential source of error (see Chapter 12).

- *Turnaround time* Delayed and lost test requisitions, specimens, and reports are major problems for laboratories. An essential feature for monitoring of the cause of delays is to record the actual times of specimen collection, receipt in the laboratory, and reporting of test results.
- *Laboratory logs* When the serum aliquot tubes arrive in the laboratory, a request/report form generally accompanies the specimens. The patient name and identification number and the tests requested on the form should be checked so that they match the information on the label of the specimen tube. The specimen should be inspected to confirm adequacy of volume and freedom from problems that may interfere with the assay, such as lipemia or hemolysis. The specimens then should be stored appropriately, and the identification information and arrival time recorded in a master log.
- *Transcription errors* In laboratories where electronic identification and tracking have not been implemented, a substantial risk of transcription error exists from manual entry of data, even when results are double-checked. Computerization reduces this type of transcription error because computerized systems have error-detection routines programmed into the terminal entry functions. These routines may include check digits, limit checks, test-correlation checks, and verification checks with master hospital files.
- *Patient preparation* Laboratory tests are affected by many patient factors, such as recent intake of food, alcohol, or drugs, as well as smoking, exercise, stress, sleep, posture during specimen collection, and other variables (see Chapter 2). Proper patient preparation is essential to obtain meaningful test results. The laboratory must define the instructions and procedures for patient preparation and specimen acquisition.
- *Specimen collection* The techniques used to acquire a specimen have affected many laboratory tests (see Chapter 2). Improper containers and incorrect preservatives also affect test results and make them inappropriate. One way to monitor and control this aspect of laboratory processing is to assign a specially trained laboratory team to specimen collection.
- *Specimen transport* The stability of specimens during transport from the patient to the laboratory may be critical for some tests performed locally and for most tests sent to regional centers and commercial laboratories.[14] To control specimen transport, the essential feature is the authority to reject specimens that arrive in the laboratory in an obviously unsatisfactory condition (such as a thawed specimen that should have remained frozen).
- *Specimen separation and aliquoting* Separating and aliquoting blood specimens are functions usually performed under the direct control of the laboratory. The main variables are the centrifuges, containers, and personnel. Centrifuges should be monitored through checks in the speed, timer, and temperature. Collection tubes, pipets,

stoppers, and aliquot tubes are sources of calcium and trace metal contamination; each lot number of materials used should be tested for contamination by calcium and possibly other elements.

CONTROL OF ANALYTICAL VARIABLES

Many analytical variables must be controlled carefully to ensure accurate measurements by analytical methods. Reliable analytical methods are obtained through a careful process of selection, evaluation, implementation, maintenance, and control (see Chapter 13). Smooth and uninterrupted laboratory service requires many procedures aimed to prevent the occurrence of problems. Different laboratories have experienced different problems with the same analytical methods because different amounts of effort were allocated to the care, maintenance, and support of those methods.

Certain variables—water quality; calibration of analytical balances; calibration of volumetric glassware and pipets; stability of electrical power; and the temperature of heating baths, refrigerators, freezers, and centrifuges— should be monitored on a laboratory-wide basis because they affect many laboratory methods (see Chapter 1). In addition, certain variables specifically affect individual analytical methods, and these require the development of procedures to deal specifically with the characteristics of the methods.

Documentation of Analytical Protocols

Step-by-step procedures for performance of analytical determinations are critical if the methods are to provide the same results when used by different analysts over a long period of time. Maintaining such consistency requires the development of written protocols or method and procedure manuals. Table 17-2 outlines the information that should be contained in such documents. More detailed guidelines are provided by the NCCLS.[15] Method manuals should be reviewed annually and revised whenever changes occur. In addition, retaining outdated procedures in an archival file is a good practice.

Monitoring Technical Competency

The personal characteristics and techniques of individual analysts may affect certain analytical methods significantly, particularly manual methods. Proper training of laboratory personnel to establish uniformity in technique is important, as is scheduling of sufficient routine service to maintain proper techniques. A written list of objectives that outline the critical tasks and knowledge is a helpful tool in training of personnel on new analytical methods. The objectives ensure systematic instruction that covers the critical points. Before analyses for clinical use are performed, the technical

---

TABLE 17-2   **Outline for a Procedure Manual**

A. Procedure Name
List the principal name of the procedure first and alternatives names next. List commonly used abbreviations.

B. Clinical Significance
Provide a brief explanation of how the test is used in clinical medicine. Include reference intervals for specific diseases and recommended diagnostic and therapeutic action limits.

C. Principle of Method
Briefly state the principles on which the method is based.

D. Specimen
List the type of specimens that can be used and recommended volume, as well as minimum volume. Indicate conditions that render the specimen unacceptable, such as hemolysis or lipemia. List patient preparation procedures. Provide instruction for specimen handling before testing.

E. Reagents and Equipment
Provide a list of reagents in order of their use, including standards. Indicate the names and addresses of suppliers and outline detailed instructions for preparation, including checks that should be performed before use. List equipment used and special promotions required.

F. Procedure
Describe the procedure step by step, including calibration and QC procedures. Provide enough detail so that the assay can be performed by an individual unfamiliar with the test. Include all necessary calculations.

G. Reference Values
List the reference intervals for healthy subjects. Indicate parameters, such as age, sex, or race, that affect reference values. Include the nature of the population studied, number of subjects, and date or reference for the original work.

H. Comments
Include any special analytical variables affecting the test, such as pH or temperature. Include the effects of commonly used drugs, any dangers or personal hazards in the procedure, and any special safety precautions and procedures.

I. References
Provide the primary literature references that describe the method or the references on which the method is based.

QC, Quality control.

---

competence of the personnel should be checked and practice runs performed. Periodic monitoring of competency may be difficult, but incident reports and results from internal and external QC checks can identify specific problems; these problems should be discussed directly with the personnel involved. Inservice and continuing-education programs help maintain and improve competence. Employee conferences also help uncover nontechnical problems that may affect work quality (see Chapter 16).

Statistical Control of Analytical Methods

The performance of analytical methods typically is monitored through analysis of specimens with known concentrations and subsequent comparison of the observed values with the known values.[2,19] The known values usually are represented by an interval of acceptable values, or upper and lower limits for control (control limits). When the observed values fall within the control limits, the analyst is assured that the analytical method is performing properly. When the observed values fall outside the control limits, the analyst is alerted to the possibility of problems in the analytical determination. A variety of sources of information on the application of **statistical QC** in the clinical laboratory are available.[1,6,10,22,24]

Control materials

Specimens that are analyzed for QC purposes are known as *control materials.* They need to be available (1) in a stable form, (2) in aliquots or vials, and (3) for analysis over an extended period of time. In addition, only minimal vial-to-vial variation should exist so that differences between repeated measurements are attributed to the analytical method alone. The control material should have preferably the same matrix as the test specimens of interest; for example, a protein matrix may be best when serum is the test material to be analyzed by the analytical method. Materials from human sources generally are preferred, but because of limited availability and biohazard considerations, bovine materials offer a certain advantage in safety and are more readily available. The concentration of analyte should be in the normal and abnormal reference intervals, corresponding to concentrations that are critical in the medical interpretation of the test results.

Most laboratories purchase control materials from one of several companies that manufacture control sera or "control products." These products generally are supplied in lyophilized or freeze-dried forms that are reconstituted by the addition of water or a specific diluent solution. Also available are materials with matrices representing urine, spinal fluid, and whole blood. Liquid control materials also are available and have the advantage of eliminating errors caused by reconstitution. However, the matrices of these liquid materials contain other materials that constitute a potential source of error with some analytical methods and instruments.

In addition to the product's matrix, several other factors must be considered in the selection of commercial control materials. Stability is critical because the laboratory often purchases a year's supply of one manufacturing lot or batch. Different batches (or lot numbers) of the same material have different concentrations, which require new estimates of the mean and standard deviation (SD). The size of the aliquots or vials should be convenient for the analytical methods to be monitored. Larger-sized vials are generally less expensive (on a per-milliliter basis), but unused materials may eliminate potential savings. Two or three different materials

should be selected to provide concentrations that monitor performance at different medical decision levels.

Control products are purchased as assayed or unassayed materials. Assayed materials come with a list of values for the concentrations that are expected for that material. This list often includes both the mean and SD for several common analytical methods and preferably for a reference method used to measure a particular analyte. Because of the work required to determine these values, the assayed materials are more expensive. Although the stated assay values are useful in selection of the desired materials, determination of the mean and SD in the user's laboratory is advisable because this process improves the performance characteristics of statistical control procedures.

General principles of control charts

A common method used to compare the values observed for control materials with their known values is the use of control charts.* Control charts are simple graphical displays in which the observed values are plotted versus the time when the observations are made. The known values are represented by an acceptable range of values, as indicated on the chart by lines for upper and lower control limits. When the plotted points fall within the control limits, this occurrence generally is interpreted to mean that the method is performing properly. When points fall outside the control limits, problems may be developing.

The control limits usually are calculated from the mean ($\bar{x}$) and SD (s) obtained from repeated measurements on the known specimens by the particular analytical method that is to be controlled. The mean and SD are calculated from the following equations:

$$\bar{x} = \frac{\sum x_i}{n}$$

$$s = \sqrt{\frac{n \sum_{i=1}^{n} x_i^2 - \sum_{i=1}^{n} (x_i)^2}{n(n-1)}}$$

where x_i is an individual control observation, and n is the number of observations in the time period being monitored.

The initial estimate should be based on measurements obtained over a period of at least 1 month when the method is working properly. In practice this initial estimate may not be entirely reliable because of the low number of data points and possible outliers in the data. The estimates are revised when more data have been accumulated by recording of n and the summations of x_i and (x_i^2) and subsequent use of the

---

*Control charts first were introduced into the clinical chemistry laboratory by Levey and Jennings in 1950. They demonstrated how the industrial control procedures could be used with the mean and range of duplicate measurements from clinical chemical methods.

cumulative totals in the previous equations to provide cumulative means and SDs. The effects of outliers are minimized by elimination of values exceeding the mean by more than $\pm$ 3.1 to 3.8 s's (where the exact factor depends on the total number of data points: 3.14 for $n = 30$; 3.22, $n = 40$; 3.33, $n = 60$; 3.41, $n = 80$; 3.47, $n = 100$; 3.66, $n = 200$; 3.83, $n = 400$).

Error distribution of the analytical method is assumed to be Gaussian (that is, symmetrical and bell-shaped; see Chapter 14). The control limits are set to include most of the control values, usually 95% to 99.7%, which correspond to the mean $\pm$ 2 or 3 SDs (s). Because observance of a value in the tails of the distribution should be a relatively rare occurrence (only 1 out of 20 times for 2 s limits, 3 out of 1000 for 3 s limits), such an observation is suspect and suggests that something may have happened to the analytical method. Such an occurrence could have caused a shift in the mean (an accuracy problem), which would result in a higher probability of exceeding the limits, or it could have caused an increase in the SD (a precision problem), which would widen the distribution and also result in a higher probability of exceeding the control limits of acceptability.

Figure 17-4, A, illustrates how the distributions of control values appear for three different situations: (1) stable performance in which only an occasional observation exceeds the control limits, (2) occurrence of a systematic error that shifts the mean of the distribution and causes a much higher expectation or probability that control values are may be observed outside one of the control limits; and (3) occurrence of an increase in random error or imprecision, which widens the distribution and causes a much higher probability that a control value may be observed outside either of the control limits.

Control charts are used to compare the observed control values with the control limits and provide a visual display that is inspected and reviewed quickly. On these charts the concentration or observed value is plotted on the y-axis versus time of observation on the x-axis. Commonly, one month's data is plotted on a chart, usually only one or two points a day, but the time axis should be appropriate for the method being monitored. An example of a **Levey-Jennings control chart** is shown in Figure 17-4, B, where the control values represent the three situations in Figure 17-4, A, with 10 values per situation (for a total of 30 values). If the analytical method is operating properly, the control values fall predominantly within the control limits. When an accuracy problem exists, the control values are shifted to one side and several values in a row may fall outside one of the limits. When a precision problem exists, the control values fluctuate much more widely and may exceed both the upper and lower control limits.

Interpretation of the control data is guided by certain decision criteria or **control rules,** which define when an analytical run is judged "in control" (acceptable) or "out of con-

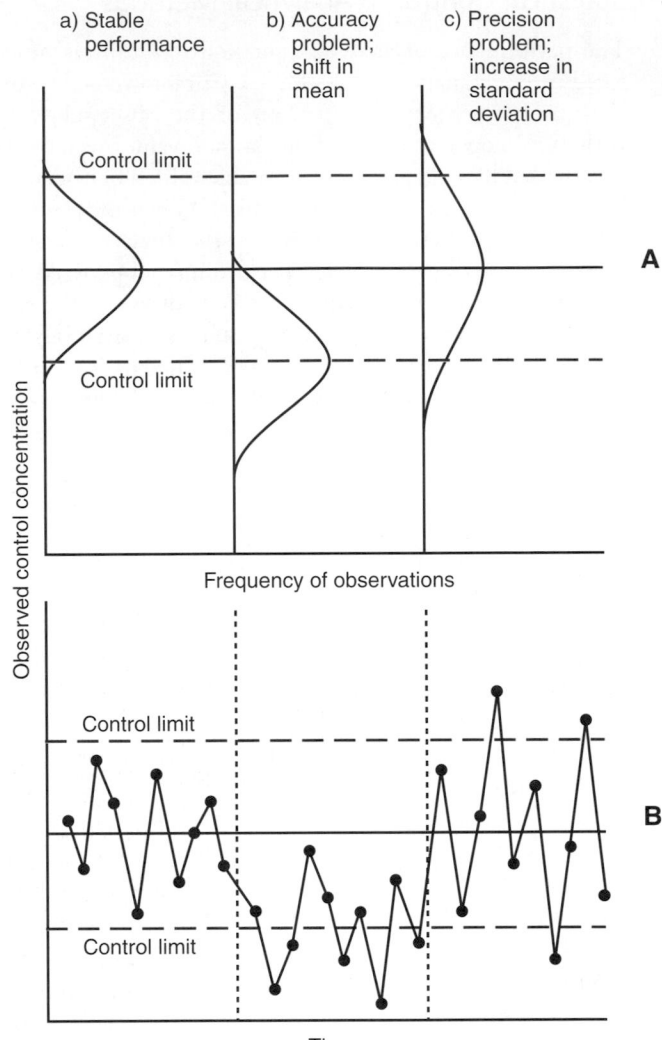

Figure 17-4 Conceptual basis of control charts. **A,** Frequency distributions of control observations for different error conditions. **B,** Display of control values representing those distributions when concentration is plotted versus time on a control chart.

trol" (unacceptable). *Analytical run* is used in this discussion to refer to that segment of data for which a decision on acceptability is to be made. This is the group of patient results that is to be reported, based on the control results available for inspection at that time. The total number of control observations available for inspection when a decision is to be made on the acceptability of an analytical run is designated as N. For example, when one control observation precedes and one follows a group of 10 patient samples whose results are to be reported, two control observations exist in that analytical run. The control rules are given symbols as A_L, or n_L, where A is the abbreviation for a statistic, n is the number of control observations, and L refers to the control limits. For example, 1_{3s} refers to a control rule in which 1 observation exceeding the mean $\pm$ 3 s control limits is the criterion for rejection of the analytical run. Similarly, 1_{2s} refers to a control rules in which 1 observation exceeds the mean $\pm\ 2\ s$.

Performance characteristics of a control procedure

The different control procedures discussed previously have different performance capabilities, depending on the control rules and the number of control observations chosen. For example, a Levey-Jennings control chart with control limits set as the mean $\pm\ 2\ s$ has a high rate of "false alarms" (that is, rejections when the method is actually performing satisfactorily), approximately 5% when n = 1, 9% when n = 2, and 14% when n = 3. Use of 3 s control limits, such as a 1_{3s} control rule, reduces the false alarms to 1% or less; however, the true alarms or **error detection** also experiences a reduction.

The selection of control rules and numbers of control measurements should be related to the quality goals set by the laboratory.[16] Many of the procedures in use today have not been chosen for best performance, but rather for ease of use in manual implementation or rule availability in the QC software of instruments and laboratory information systems. In addition, control rules vary from method to method. Knowledge of the performance characteristics of control procedures is necessary to select the control rules and n's that detect relevant laboratory problems without causing too many false alarms. Experienced analysts often use a series of informal rules or judgments to reduce the number of false alarms, without knowing their effects on the detection of real problems or true alarms. Some quantitative assessment of these two characteristics—false alarms and true alarms—should exist whenever capabilities of new control procedures are assessed, or established control procedures are reviewed.[23]

Recognizing the seriousness of the false-rejection problem and its relationship to the control limits chosen for the Levey–Jennings chart is important. These **false rejections** are in effect an inherent property of the control procedure. They occur because of the control limits that have been selected, not because of any problems with the analytical method. Therefore the use of 2 s control limits generally is not recommended. With the use of 3 s control limits the false-rejection problem is eliminated, but error detection unfortunately also is reduced.

Westgard multirule chart

The "multirule" procedure developed by Westgard and associates[27] uses a series of control rules to interpret control data. The probability for false rejections is kept low through selection of only those rules with low individual probabilities for false rejection (0.01 or less). The probability for error detection is improved through selection of those rules that are particularly sensitive to random and systematic errors. The **Westgard Multirule** procedure requires a chart with lines for control limits drawn at the mean $\pm\ 1\ s$, 2 s, and 3 s (that is, adapted to existing Levey-Jennings charts by the addition of one or two sets of control limits).

The following control rules are used:

- 1_{2s} One control observation exceeding the mean $\pm\ 2\ s$; used only as a "warning" rule that initiates testing of the control data by the other control rules
- 1_{3s} One control observation exceeding the mean $\pm\ 3\ s$; primarily sensitive to random error
- 2_{2s} Two consecutive control observations exceeding the same mean plus 2 s or mean minus 2 s limit; sensitive to systematic error
- R_{4s} One observation exceeding the mean plus 2 s and another exceeding the mean minus 2 s; sensitive to random error
- 4_{1s} Four consecutive observations exceeding the mean plus 1 s or the mean minus 1 s; sensitive to systematic error
- $10_{\bar{x}}$ 10 consecutive control observations falling on one side of the mean (above or below, with no other requirement on size of the deviations); sensitive to systematic error

The use of the multirule procedure is similar to the use of a Levey-Jennings chart, but the data interpretation is more structured. To use the multirule procedure, use the following steps:

1. Analyze samples of the control material by the analytical method to be controlled on at least 20 different days. Two different materials with appropriate concentrations are recommended. Calculate the mean and SD for the results for each control material being used.
2. Construct a control chart for each of the control materials being used. The observed concentration or control value should be plotted on the y–axis, setting the range of concentrations to include the mean $\pm\ 4\ s$. Draw horizontal lines for the mean, the mean $\pm\ 1\ s$, the mean $\pm\ 2\ s$, and the mean $\pm\ 3\ s$. In practice, use of different colors for these lines, perhaps green, yellow, and red for the 1 s, 2 s, and 3 s limits, respectively, is useful. The x–axis should be scaled for time, day, or run number and labeled accordingly.
3. Introduce two control specimens into each analytical run, one for each of the two concentrations (when two different materials have been selected). Record the control values and plot each on its respective control chart.
4. When both control observations fall within the 2 s limits, accept the analytical run and report the patient results. When one of the control observations exceeds a 2 s limit, hold the patient results. Inspect the control data using the 1_{3s}, 2_{2s}, R_{4s}, and $10_{\bar{x}}$ rules. When any of the rules indicates the run is out of control, reject the analytical run and do not report the patient results. When all the rules indicate that the run is in control, accept the analytical run and report the patient results.
5. When a run is out of control, determine the type of error based on the control rule that has been violated.

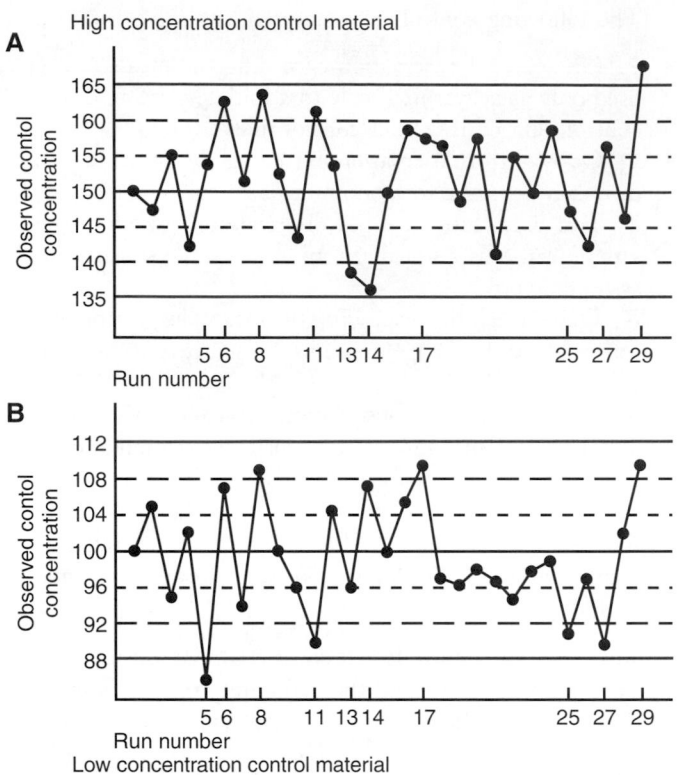

A, High concentration control material

B, Low concentration control material

Figure 17-5 Westgard multirule control chart with control limits drawn at the mean ± 1 *s*, 2 *s*, and 3 *s*. Concentration is plotted on the *y*-axis versus time (run number) on the *x*-axis. **A,** Chart for high-concentration control material. **B,** Chart for low-concentration control material. *s,* Standard deviation. (From Westgard JO, Barry PL, Hunt MR et al: A multi-rule Shewhart chart for quality control in clinical chemistry. Clin Chem 1981; 27:493-501.)

Look for sources of that type of error. Correct the problem, and then reanalyze the entire run, including both control and patient samples.

An example application of the multirule procedure is shown in Figure 17-5, where the top chart illustrates a high-concentration control material and the bottom chart a low-concentration material. Of note is that the R_{4s} rule is applied only within a run so that between-run systematic errors are not wrongly interpreted as random errors. However, the rule may be applied "across" materials, meaning that one of the observations is on the low material and the other on the high material, as long as they are within the same run. On the other hand, note that the 2_{2s}, 4_{1s}, and $10_{\bar{x}}$ rules are applied across runs and materials. This application effectively increases *n* and improves the error-detection capabilities of the procedure.

Identifying sources of analytical errors

Statistical control procedures provide a way to alert the analyst to analytical problems that cause the quality of analytical performance to fall short of the goals set for the laboratory. However, these control procedures do not identify the

sources of the analytical errors and solve the control problems. The analyst must respond to the out-of-control signal to correct the problem and prevent future occurrences.

QC guidelines from the NCCLS[16] emphasize the importance of problem correction, as opposed to routine repeat of controls, followed by trying of new control bottles; the latter process in effect repeats tests until the controls happen to fall within the acceptable range. When control procedures are selected properly on the basis of the quality required for the test and the imprecision and inaccuracy observed for the method, false rejections should be minimized; therefore routine repetition wastes time and effort. Practical tools for selection of appropriate QC procedures have been described in the literature.[23]

When alerted to a control problem, the analyst first should inspect carefully the analytical method, equipment, reagents, and specimens to ensure that everything looks, feels, smells, and sounds correct. An inspection may appear to be a qualitative and sensory technique, but it is a very powerful tool when performed with checklists developed for specific analytical methods. This inspection should include a review of records documenting changes that occur with the instrument and reagents. Brief instrument function checks often are performed to verify proper system performance and separate chemical and instrumental sources of errors. An experienced analyst often spots the problem by performing this kind of inspection, whereas inexperienced analysts are aided by formal checklists.

The type of error itself provides a clue about the source of the error. For example, systematic errors often are related to calibration problems, such as (1) impure calibration materials, (2) improper preparation of calibrating solutions, (3) erroneous set point and assigned values, (4) unstable calibrating solutions, (5) contaminated solutions, (6) inadequate calibration techniques, (7) nonlinear or unstable calibration functions, (8) unstable reagent blanks, and (9) inadequate sample blanks. Random errors more likely are due to (1) lack of reproducibility in the pipetting of samples and reagents, (2) dissolving of reagent tablets and mixing of sample and reagents, and (3) lack of stability of temperature baths, timing regulation, and photometric and other sensors. Individual analytical methods may not be subject to all these possible sources of error; rather, only a few plausible sources may exist for a particular type of error. Experienced analysts often know what these common sources are for their particular analytical methods and quickly identify the sources once the type of error is known.

A clue to the type of error is the control rule that is violated. Different control rules have different sensitivities to detect random and systematic errors, as illustrated by the multirule control procedure, in which the 1_{3s} and R_{4s} rules tend to respond to random error and the 2_{2s}, 4_{1s}, and $10_{\bar{x}}$ rules to systematic errors. Control procedures that use patient samples rather than stable control materials help identify preanalytical sources of error, such as sample handling and processing. External quality assessment procedures may provide more extensive information about systematic errors than what is available from internal procedures. The information from all these procedures is complementary and, when used in combination, provides a more complete assessment of the types of errors and their possible sources.

Limitations of internal quality-control programs

Internal QC procedures only detect changes in performance between the present operation and the "stable" operation that was characteristic during the baseline period, when the analytical method was thought to operate properly. Although the procedures detect systematic and random errors, the only systematic errors detected are those changes from the original baseline. If the method actually had some undetected systematic errors during the baseline period, those systematic errors would be included in the mean that was used to calculate the control limits for the procedure. Thus only systematic changes from this original mean are detected by internal QC procedures.

Initial method evaluation studies are essential to ensure that systematic errors are not present before the baseline period and the determination of the mean and control limits. The accuracy of the method should be established initially by comparison with other analytical methods (as well as recovery and interference studies). The method should continue to be monitored by comparison with other analytical methods. Ongoing comparison-of-methods studies are desirable to ensure that systematic errors do not increase slowly and go undetected by internal QC procedures. These ongoing comparison studies are provided by the external QA programs.

■ EXTERNAL QUALITY-ASSESSMENT AND PROFICIENCY TESTING PROGRAMS

All the control procedures described previously have focused on monitoring of a single laboratory. These procedures constitute what is often called *internal QC* to distinguish them from procedures used to compare the performances of different laboratories, the latter being known as *external QA*. The two procedures are complementary, internal QC being necessary for the daily monitoring of the precision and accuracy of the analytical method, and external quality assessment being important in the maintenance of long-term accuracy of the analytical methods.

Participation in an external proficiency testing program is required for all U.S. laboratories that perform tests classified as *moderate* and *high-complexity tests*. Many point-of-care testing sites perform some of these tests and also must enroll in proficiency testing programs. Current approved providers of proficiency testing programs deliver sets of up to five specimens for analysis by the laboratory 3 times per year. The laboratory reports its results to the provider, who then makes them available to the regulatory agencies.

Features of External Quality-Assessment Programs

Several external QA programs available to the clinical laboratory are sponsored by professional societies and manufacturers of control materials. The basic operation of these programs involves all the participating laboratories analyzing the same lot of control material, usually daily as part of the internal QC activities. The results are tabulated monthly and sent to the sponsoring group for data analysis. Summary reports are prepared by the program sponsor and distributed to all participating laboratories. This type of reporting is not available in real time and is useful only for monthly reviews and periodic problem-solving activities. However, with advances in telecommunications and the arrival of the World Wide Web, real-time external QC is anticipated.

The reports often include extensive data analysis, statistical summaries, and plots. The overall mean of all laboratories in the program or the mean of values of all laboratories is taken as the "true" or correct value and is used for comparison with the individual laboratory's mean. Different programs do this in different ways. For example, the *t*–test is used to test the statistical significance of any difference between an individual laboratory's observed mean and the group mean. When the difference is significant, the laboratory is alerted that its results are biased in comparison with the results of most of the other laboratories. Another approach is to divide the difference by the overall SD of the group and then express the difference in terms of the number of SDs

$$SDI = \frac{\text{lab mean} - \text{group mean}}{\text{group } s}$$

where *SDI* is the abbreviation for SD interval or index, and *group s* is the SD for the group or a selected subset of the group. Differences greater than 2 indicate that a laboratory is not in agreement with the rest of the laboratories in the program. These calculations reduce all the test results to the same values, which makes possible interpretation of the data from different analytes without reference to the exact mean and *s* for each analytical method. For example, a value of +2.0 has the same meaning for any test, indicating that the value is 2 *s* above its established mean.

Some additional information about the nature of the systematic error is obtained when two different control materials are analyzed by each laboratory. The laboratory's observed mean for material A is plotted on the *y*-axis, versus its observed mean for material B on the *x*-axis. These graphs are called *Youden plots*. Ideally, the point for a laboratory should fall at the center of the plot. Points falling from the center but on the 45-degree line suggest a proportional analytical error. Points falling from the center but not on the 45-degree line suggest either an error that is constant for both materials or one that occurs with just one material.

The report also may include Levey-Jennings plots of the data, but because this information is not available in real time, it does not effectively serve the purposes of internal QC. Blank control charts set up for each analyte and each control material save the laboratory the time required to prepare these charts manually.

The operation of external QA programs is improved significantly by the incorporation of a computer. The external comparisons are performed more quickly with the computer as a terminal for electronic transmission of data to the central computer. The results from the many different laboratories then are compared and processed, and the reports are returned electronically. When the individual control observations are entered into the computer, the control data is tested immediately by internal control procedures to determine control status. Thus, when used in this way, the computer integrates the internal and external procedures into a more efficient program for QA.

Role of Proficiency Testing in Accreditation

Proficiency testing (PT) is the process in which simulated patient specimens made from a common pool are analyzed by laboratories; the results of this procedure are evaluated to determine the "quality" of the laboratories' performance. Controversy exists over the validity of this laboratory evaluation process, but government and licensing agencies increasingly are using it as an objective method for laboratory accreditation. Media stories highlighting laboratory quality problems have aroused the U.S. government's concern for protecting patients' interests and the public welfare. Subsequently, Congress passed revisions to the Clinical Laboratory Improvement Act of 1967 (CLIA '67) and the Clinical Laboratory Improvement Amendments of 1988 (CLIA '88) that mandate PT as a major part of the laboratory accreditation process.[21]

The CLIA '88 proposed criteria that group laboratory tests into "specialty" and "subspecialty" categories and specify representative tests to be monitored in each category. To succeed in a given category, a laboratory must produce correct results on four of five specimens for each of the analytes in that category and score overall at least 80% for three consecutive challenges. If more than two incorrect results are produced for any analyte, the laboratory is considered "on probation." If a laboratory has two or more incorrect results for any analyte or an overall score less than 80% on two of three consecutive surveys, it is classified as "suspended" and must cease testing all analytes in that specialty category until it is reinstated.

The CLIA '88 regulations have established fixed limits (either percentages or absolute values from target) for PT

performance evaluation (see Chapter 13). The target values for these analytes are established by the agencies implementing the PT programs under the federal guideline[21] that states:

Target value means either the mean of all responses after removal of outliers (those responses greater than 3 SDs from the original mean) or the mean established by definitive or reference methods acceptable for use in the National Reference System for the Clinical Laboratory by the National Committee for Clinical Laboratory Standards. In instances where definitive or reference methods are not available, a comparative method may be used. If the method group is less than 20 participants, "target value" means the overall mean after outlier removal (as defined above) unless acceptable scientific reasons are available to indicate that such an evaluation is not appropriate.

Accepted reference methods do not exist for many of these "controlled analytes," and even when they do exist, the values obtained for PT specimens with some analytical systems may not match those obtained with the reference method; these mismatches may be caused by differences in matrices and analyte forms. The College of American Pathologists uses peer group mean values as the targets or groups of methods that agree with the definitive method. This target value is termed the *definitive method correlated target value (DMCTV)*. Alternatively, the all-method mean (or median) is used as the target value, but this use might cause problems if one manufacturer dominates the market, especially if the method used is calibrated in a manner different from the others. A listing of the CLIA fixed limits for PT performance evaluation is included in Chapter 13 and in an expanded version of this chapter.[29]

The CLIA '88 regulations specify that the PT specimens should be treated in the same manner as patient specimens and require that the individuals performing the tests sign a statement attesting that they have complied with the regulations. In reality, PT specimens must be treated differently than those from patients because many are lyophilized or sealed in containers; reporting of their results requires different forms and generally is not computerized. This "special handling" does not necessarily provide better test results. In a study of PT problems at a large reference laboratory,[5] error rates were higher if PT specimens were given special handling procedures than if they were submitted as blind patient specimens. Moreover, most problems with the specimens were caused by systematic errors, which were not corrected by the average of replicates.

PT programs are far from ideal monitors of laboratory performance. In a study of PT survey problems at the Mayo Clinic, over one-half the errors on surveys were related directly to deficiencies in the surveys (for example, invalid specimens and inappropriate evaluation criteria), and only 28% could be linked to specific analytical problems.[9]

■ NEW QUALITY INITIATIVES

Several organizations have begun quality initiatives to ensure that organizations incorporate the principles of quality management and QA in their daily operations. For example, the International Organization for Standardization (ISO), in Geneva, Switzerland, (http://www.iso.ch) has developed and promulgated the **ISO 9000** standards.

ISO is a worldwide federation of national standards bodies from some 100 countries. The mission of ISO is to promote the development of standardization and related activities in the world with a view toward facilitating the international exchange of goods and services and developing cooperation in the spheres of intellectual, scientific, technological, and economic activity. ISO's work results in international agreements, which are published as International Standards. The ISO 9000 standards are examples of such standards, and they have been applied worldwide. ISO also has organized several Technical Advisory Groups that address quality issues of interest to clinical laboratorians.

ISO 9000

ISO 9000 is a set of four standards enacted to ensure quality management and QA in manufacturing and service industries.[20] They first were published in 1987 and are used worldwide, with more than 80 countries adopting them.

ISO 9000 Standards

ISO 9001	Quality systems—model for QA in design, development, production, installation, and servicing
ISO 9002	Quality systems—model for QA in production, installation, and servicing
ISO 9003	Quality systems—model for QA in final inspection and test
ISO 9004	Quality management and quality system elements; guidelines

The ISO 9000 standards represent an international consensus on the essential features of a quality system to ensure the effective operation of any business, whether a manufacturer or service provider or other type of organization, in the public or private sector. ISO certification is performed by accredited organizations known as *registrars*. Registrars review the organization's quality manual and audit the process to ensure that the system documented in the manual is in place and effective. Many major diagnostic companies have received ISO 9000 certification, and in 1996 the Excel Bestview Medical Laboratories of Mississauga, Ontario, Canada became the world's first clinical laboratory to receive ISO 9002 certification. U.S. transfusion laboratories also have begun to adopt the ISO 9000 approach to quality management.[8]

ISO Technical Advisory Groups

ISO also has a number of other activities that relate to quality activities in the laboratory. In 1995, ISO organized a Technical Advisory Group (TC 212—Clinical Laboratory Testing and In Vitro Diagnostic Testing Systems), which is managed by NCCLS. This Technical Committee coordinates international standardization efforts in laboratory medicine and in vitro diagnostic test systems.

References

1. Cembrowski GS, Carey RN: Laboratory Quality Management, Chicago, ASCP Press, 1989.
2. Dechert J, Case KE: Multivariate approach to quality control in clinical chemistry. Clin Chem 1998; 44:1959-1963.
3. Deming WE: Out of the Crisis, Cambridge, Mass, Massachusetts Institute of Technology Center for Advanced Study, 1987.
4. Earnest MP, Grimm SM, Malmgren MA et al: Quality improvement in an integrated urban healthcare system: a necessary journey. Clin Perform Qual Health Care 1998; 6:193-200.
5. Gambino R, Mallon P, Woodrow G: Managing for total quality in a large laboratory: some examples. Arch Pathol Lab Med 1990; 114:1145-1148.
6. Harris EK, Boyd JC: Statistical Bases of Reference Values in Laboratory Medicine, New York, Marcel Dekker, 1995.
7. Juran JM, Endres A: Quality Improvement for Services, Wilton, Conn, Juran Institute, 1986.
8. Kalmin ND, Myers LK, Fisk MB: ISO 9000 model ideally suited for quality plan at blood centers. Transfusion 1998; 38:79-85.
9. Klee GG, Forsman RW: A user's classification of problems identified by Proficiency Testing Surveys. Arch Pathol Lab Med 1988; 112:371-373.
10. Kringle RO, Bogovich M: Statistical procedures. In Burtis CA, Ashwood, ER (eds): Tietz Textbook of Clinical Chemistry, 3rd edition, pp 265-309, Philadelphia, WB Saunders, 1999.
11. Le Neel T, Truchaud A, Cazaubiel M et al: Technologies for implementation of quality assurance in the clinical laboratory. Clin Chim Acta 1998; 278:103-110.

12. McQueen MJ: Laboratory quality assurance at the international level: the role of nongovernmental organizations. J Int Fed Clin Chem 1997; 9:144-146,148,150.

13. National Committee for Clinical Laboratory Standards: A Quality System Model for Health Care: Proposed Guideline GP26-A, Wayne, Pa, National Committee for Clinical Laboratory Standards, 1999.

14. National Committee for Clinical Laboratory Standards: Procedures for the handling and transport of diagnostic specimens and etiologic agents: Approved Standard H5-A3. 3rd edition. Wayne, Pa, National Committee for Clinical Laboratory Standards, 1994.

15. National Committee for Clinical Laboratory Standards: Clinical Laboratory Technical Procedure Manuals: Approved Guideline GP2-A3. 3rd edition. Wayne, Pa, National Committee for Clinical Laboratory Standards, 1996.

16. National Committee for Clinical Laboratory Standards: Statistical Quality Control for Quantitative Measurements: Principles and Definitions: Approved Guideline C24-A2. 2nd edition. Wayne, Pa, National Committee for Clinical Laboratory Standards, 1999.

17. O'Sullivan KE : How one British National Health Service Trust follows the path to continuous quality improvement. J Health Qual 1999; 21:16-22.

18. Ogram D, Lailey J, Rondeau K et al: Quality systems for the clinical laboratory. Canadian Society of Laboratory Technologists Working Group. Can J Med Technol 1995; 57:(Suppl)1-14.

19. Ohman S: Quality control for the clinical chemistry laboratory. Qual Assur 1997; 5:79-93.

20. Rabbitt JT, Bergh PA: The Miniguide to ISO 9000, New York, Quality Resources Press, 1995.

21. U.S. Department of Health and Human Services: Clinical Laboratory Improvement Amendments of 1988; Final Rules and Notice 42 CFR Part 493. The Federal Register 1992; 57:7188-7288.

22. Westgard JO: Basic QC Practices, Madison, Wis, Westgard QC, 1998.

23. Westgard JO: Error budgets for quality management: practical tools for planning and assuring analytical quality of laboratory testing processes. Clin Lab Manag Rev 1996; 10:377-403.

24. Westgard JO, Barry PL: Cost-Effective Quality Control: Managing the Quality and Productivity of Analytical Processes, Washington, DC, AACC Press, 1997.

25. Westgard JO, Barry PL: Total quality control: evolution of quality management systems. Lab Med 1989; 20:377-384.

26. Westgard JO, Barry PL, Tomar RH: Implementing total quality management in health care laboratories. Clin Lab Manage Rev 1991; 5:353-370.

27. Westgard JO, Barry PL, Hunt MR et al: A multi-rule Shewhart chart for quality control in clinical chemistry. Clin Chem 1981; 27:493-501.

28. Westgard JO, Burnett RW, Bowers GN: Quality management science in clinical chemistry: a dynamic framework for continuous improvement of quality. Clin Chem 1990; 36:1712-1716.

29. Westgard JO, Klee GG: Quality management. In Burtis CA, Ashwood, ER (eds): Tietz Textbook of Clinical Chemistry, 3rd edition, pp 369-383, Philadelphia, WB Saunders, 1999.

30. Widtfeldt AK, Widtfeldt JR: Total quality management in American industry. AAOHN J 1992; 40:311-318.

PART IV

Analytes

CHAPTER 18

Amino Acids

ROBERT H. CHRISTENSON, PhD, and HASSAN M. E. AZZAZY, PhD, SC (ASCP), DABCC

Objectives

1. Diagram the basic chemical structure of an amino acid.
2. Explain the formation (polymerization) of a peptide from amino acids.
3. State the primary source of amino acids.
4. State the metabolic cycle of amino acids.
5. Define *aminoaciduria* and compare primary and secondary aminoacidurias.
6. Describe the symptoms and deficient enzymes in phenylketonuria, tyrosinemia, alkaptonuria, homocystinuria, maple syrup urine disease, and cystinuria.
7. State the principle of the Guthrie test.
8. List the clinical laboratory procedures used to assess amino acid concentration.

Key Words

Alkaptonuria   An autosomal recessive aminoacidopathy caused by a deficiency of homogentisic acid oxidase and characterized by an accumulation of homogentisic acid (HGA) in the urine

Amino Acid   An organic compound containing both amino ($-NH_2$) and carboxyl ($-COOH$) functional groups.

Aminoaciduria   High blood levels of amino acids that result in significant renal excretion

Cystinuria   Massive urinary excretion of cystine, lysine, arginine, and ornithine, because of a defect of carriers in the proximal renal tubules

Essential Amino Acids   Amino acids that cannot be synthesized by most mammals and therefore are considered essential constituents of the diet for maintenance of health or growth

Guthrie Test   A semiquantitative microbiological assay for the determination of amino acids

Homocystinurias   A group of disorders characterized by excessive excretion of homocystine into the urine

Inborn Error of Metabolism   Primary disease caused by an inherited enzyme defect

Maple Syrup Urine Disease (MSUD)   Accumulation of the branched amino acids and their corresponding 2-keto acids in blood, urine, and cerebrospinal fluid

Oligopeptide   A relatively short chain of amino acids (3 to 5 residues)

Peptide Bond   The amide bond formed between the carboxyl group of one amino acid and the amino group of another

Phenylketonuria (PKU)   An autosomal recessive disorder characterized by accumulation and excretion of phenylalanine, phenylpyruvic acid, and related compounds

Polypeptide   A chain of amino acids containing approximately 6 to 30 residues

A mino acids are the basic structural units of proteins. Their measurement in physiological fluids provides important information for the diagnosis of many pathological and inherited conditions.

■ BASIC BIOCHEMISTRY

Amino acids are organic compounds containing both an amino group ($-NH_2$) and a carboxyl group ($-COOH$). Those occurring in proteins are called α-amino acids and have the empirical formula $RCH(NH_2)COOH$. The core of an α-amino acid is the α-carbon atom next to the carboxylic acid group, as follows:

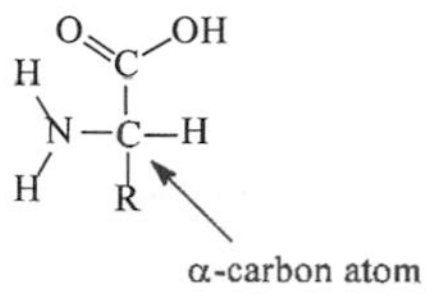

α-carbon atom

With the exception of glycine, all α-amino acids are asymmetrical, with a covalent bond between the α-carbon and hydrogen atom, a carboxyl group, an amino group, and a distinctive R group of a specific chemical structure.

Table 18-1 lists the amino acids that are of importance in protein chemistry. The 22 amino acids listed in section I are used to build the large number of biologically active peptides and proteins that exist in nature. Biochemically, the characteristic acid-base properties of individual amino acids, as well as the diverse nature of their R groups and their interactions, give peptides and proteins their versatility in structure and function.

Acid-Base Properties

The acid-base properties of amino acids depend on the amino and carboxyl groups attached to the α-carbon and on the basic, acidic, or other functional groups represented by R. In the physiological pH range of 7.37 to 7.47, the carboxyl group of an amino acid is dissociated and the amino group protonated, as follows:

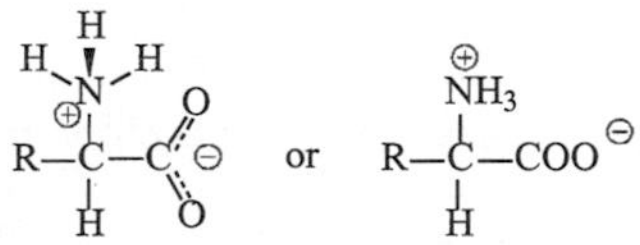

This kind of ionized molecule, with coexistent negative and positive charges, is called a *dipolar ion* or *ampholyte*. At low pH an amino acid is in its cationic form with both its amino and carboxyl groups protonated ($-N^+H_3$ and $-COOH$). As the pH rises, the carboxyl group loses its proton and the ampholyte form appears at about pH 6. With a further increase in pH the amino $-N^+H_3$ also is deproto-

nated, resulting in the anionic form of the molecule. This process for a monoamino and monocarboxylic amino acid is as follows:

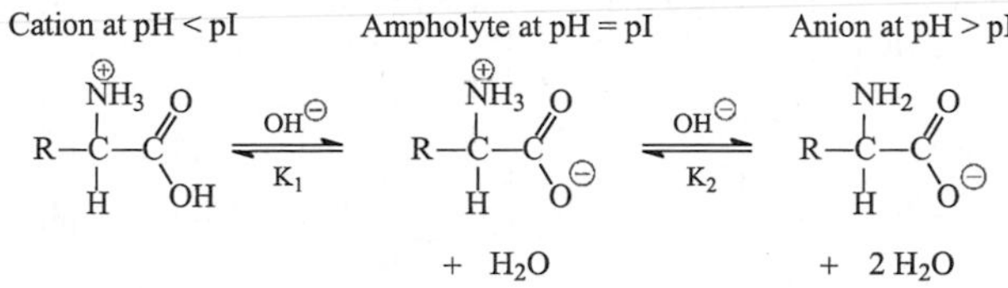

Cation at pH < pI   Ampholyte at pH = pI   Anion at pH > pI

The dissociation constants, K_1 (ratio of ampholyte to cation) and K_2 (ratio of ampholyte to anion) usually are expressed logarithmically as pK_1 and pK_2, where $pK = -\log K$, in a manner analogous to the notation for pH. A pK is the pH at which equal quantities of the protonated (associated) and unprotonated (dissociated) forms are present. The isoelectric point, pI, is the pH at which the molecules exist in the ampholyte form and have a net charge of 0. The isoelectric point of a neutral amino acid can be calculated from the pKs of its amino and carboxyl groups ($pI = 1/2 [pK_1 + pK_2]$). The concept of an ampholyte and its dissociation characteristics is also applicable to proteins because most proteins are negatively charged at physiological pH.

Influence of R Groups

The R groups of individual amino acids are responsible for their special properties. For example, some R groups are nonpolar and therefore hydrophobic; others are polar and hydrophilic (see Table 18-1). Still others can become charged, either negatively (the acidic amino acids) or positively (the basic amino acids). R groups may be linear (for example, valine) or cyclical (for example, proline), small (for example, glycine) or bulky (for example, tryptophan). Electron density may be low, as in aliphatic chains, or high, as in aromatic rings. This diversity in R-group structure and chemistry makes possible several kinds of interaction between R groups, a fact of significant importance in protein structure determination.

Some amino acids have R groups that contain charged or ionizable substituents. These substituents have their own pKs. At a pH of approximately 7 the second carboxyl groups of glutamic acid (Glu) and aspartic acid (Asp) are fully ionized and negatively charged. At this physiological pH, most basic amino acids are positively charged; however, less than 10% of histidine is positively charged. At pH ~6, glycine, with a pK_1 of 2.34 and pK_2 of 9.60, has a net charge near 0, illustrating the acid-base behavior of that group of amino acids with R groups that have no ionizable substituents. The differing solubilities and acid-base properties of amino acids provide the basis for their separation by electrophoresis, partition chromatography, or ion-exchange chromatography (see Chapters 7 and 8). Differences in the chemical nature of R groups permit, in some cases, the iden-

TABLE 18-1 Amino Acids

Name and Abbreviation	MW	Structure at pH 6 to 7	Comments
I. Amino Acids Found in Most Proteins			
HYDROPHOBIC AMINO ACIDS; NONPOLAR R GROUPS			
Alanine (Ala)	89.09		Substrate for ALT; least hydrophobic of the group
Leucine (Leu)	131.17		Branched-chain R group; essential; ketogenic; metabolism faulty in MSUD
Isoleucine (Ile)	131.17		Essential; partly ketogenic; see Leucine
Valine (Val)	117.17		Essential; partly ketogenic; see Leucine
Proline (Pro)	115.13		Important constituent of connective tissue proteins (for example, collagen and elastin); some hydroxylated to Hyp during collagen synthesis; destabilizes α-helical and β-structures; contains an α-imido group
Methionine (Met)	149.21		Essential; important in transfer of methyl groups; provides sulfur for other sulfur-containing compounds
Phenylalanine (Phe)	165.19		Essential; elevated levels in PKU
Tryptophan (Trp)	204.22		Essential; metabolites found in carcinoid disease; contains indole ring system; precursor of serotonin and melatonin
HYDROPHILIC AMINO ACIDS; UNCHARGED POLAR GROUPS			
Glycine (Gly)	75.07		Simplest amino acid; optically inactive; placed in this group because its R group (single H) is unable to affect polarity of the rest of the molecule; used in biosynthesis of purines and porphyrins; used in vitro as a buffer
Serine (Ser)	105.09		Constituent in active center of many enzymes; hydroxyl group able to be phosphorylated
Threonine (Thr)	119.12		Essential

ALT, Alanine transaminase; *AST,* aspartate transaminase; *MW,* molecular weight; *MSUD,* maple syrup urine disease; *PKU,* phenylketonuria.

TABLE 18-1   Amino Acids—cont'd

Name and Abbreviation	MW	Structure at pH 6 to 7	Comments

I. Amino Acids Found in Most Proteins—cont'd
HYDROPHILIC AMINO ACIDS; UNCHARGED POLAR GROUPS—CONT'D

Name and Abbreviation	MW	Comments
Cysteine (Cys)	121.16	Sulfhydryl group functional in the activity of many enzymes; is responsible for disulfide bridges in peptides and proteins; cystine being dicysteine, Cys–S–S–Cys; homocysteine having one carbon more than cysteine and forming homocystine (dihomocysteine)
Selenocysteine (Secys)	168.05	Active form of selenium; found in many enzymes involved in oxidation-reduction reactions
Tyrosine (Tyr)	181.19	Usually nonessential; intermediate in synthesis of catecholamines, thyroxine, and melanin; functional phenolic group; reacts with Folin's reagent in quantitative protein assay
Glutamine (Gln)	146.15	Storage form of ammonia in tissue; supplies the amido nitrogen used in purine and pyrimidine biosynthesis
Asparagine (Asn)	132.12	Storage form of ammonia in tissues
Hydroxyproline (Hyp)	131.13	Constituent of collagen—the only human protein to contain appreciable amounts; urinary output used to indicate bone matrix metabolism; contains an α-imino group

DICARBOXYLIC AMINO ACIDS; ACIDIC R GROUPS

Name and Abbreviation	MW	Comments
Aspartic acid (Asp)	133.10	Cosubstrate with Glu for AST; used in pyrimidine biosynthesis
Glutamic acid (Glu)	147.13	Cosubstrate with Ala for ALT and with Asp for AST

BASIC AMINO ACIDS; BASIC R GROUPS

Name and Abbreviation	MW	Comments
Lysine (Lys)	146.19	Essential; terminal NH_2 called ε-amino
Arginine (Arg)	174.20	Involved in urea synthesis; the basic group being a guanidinium group
Histidine (His)	155.16	Imidazole group of histidine being the most important buffer group in the physiological pH range

Continued

TABLE 18-1	Amino Acids—cont'd		
Name and Abbreviation	MW	Structure at pH 6 to 7	Comments
II. Miscellaneous Amino Acids			
Thyroxine (T_4)	776.93		Thyroid hormone
Triiodothyronine (T_3)	651.01		Thyroid hormone; more active than T_4
β-Alanine (β-Ala)	89.09		Constituent of the vitamin pantothenic acid
Dihydroxyphenylalanine (DOPA*)	197.18		Intermediate in catecholamine synthesis
γ-Aminobutyric acid (GABA*)	103.12		Metabolite of Glu; a neurotransmitter
Ornithine (Orn*)	132.16		Intermediate in urea synthesis
Citrulline (Citr*)	175.19		Intermediate in urea synthesis
Phosphoserine	185.08		In casein and other phosphoproteins
Pyrrolidine carboxylic acid	129.12		Cyclized form of Glu; rare; used to terminate peptide chains, as at N-terminal end of L-chains of γ-globulins
Taurine	125.14		Forms conjugates with bile acids; inhibits nerve impulse transmission
β-Aminoisobutyric acid (β-AIB*)	103.12		Present in urine; a metabolite of pyrimidines

ALT, Alanine transaminase; AST, aspartate transaminase; MW, molecular weight; MSUD, maple syrup urine disease; PKU, phenylketonuria.
*Abbreviation useful but not official.

tification or measurement of specific amino acids by photometric reactions.

Peptide Bond

A **peptide bond** is formed when the α-amino group of one amino acid is linked covalently with the α-carboxyl of a second amino acid, as follows:

First amino acid   Second amino acid   Dipeptide

The peptide bond is described by the structure in the enclosed area. For example, glycine and alanine can react to form two different dipeptides, either glycyl-alanine or alanyl-glycine.

In glycyl-alanine, alanine is called the *C-terminal residue* of the peptide; glycine is the *N-terminal residue* because its amino group is free. In alanyl-glycine the designations are reversed. The *C-* and *N*-terminal designations apply also to polypeptides and proteins. Very short chains often are designated *tripeptides, tetrapeptides,* or *pentapeptides,* and so on. Chains of up to five residues are called **oligopeptides.** Longer chains (6 to 30 residues) are referred to as **polypeptides.** When the number of amino acids linked together exceeds 40, the chain takes on the physical properties associated with proteins.

Other interactions among the R groups of amino acids include disulfide bond formation, hydrogen bond formation, hydrophobic interaction, association between charged R groups, and steric effects. The covalent disulfide bond contributes to polypeptide structure, as follows:

$$R-SH + HS-R \longrightarrow R-S-S-R$$

The other types of interactions are weaker but are often so numerous that their collective strength is large. Hydrogen bonds result from the sharing of a hydrogen atom between two electronegative atoms, such as N (nitrogen) or O (oxygen), that have unbonded electrons. In proteins, groups with a hydrogen atom that can be shared include $=N-H$ (peptide nitrogen, imidazole, and indole); $-OH$ (serine, threonine, tyrosine, and hydroxyproline); $-NH_2$ and $-N^+H_3$ (arginine, lysine, and α-amino); and $-CONH$ (carbamino). Groups that can accept the sharing of a hydrogen atom include $-COO^-$ (aspartate, glutamate, and α-carboxylate); $-S-S-$ (disulfide); and $>C=O$ (in peptides and ester linkages).

Hydrophobic interactions result because the association of nonpolar groups, such as methyl or phenyl, is favored energetically in aqueous or other polar solutions. In proteins this association serves to bend and fold a molecule in a way that brings nonpolar R groups inside to the less-polar interior; polar R groups are oriented outside toward the more polar aqueous environment.

Metabolism

In a healthy individual the primary supply of amino acids for endogenous protein synthesis is provided by intake of dietary proteins. Although most amino acids can be synthesized in vivo, 8 to 10 of the 22 common amino acids cannot be synthesized by most mammals. These are considered "essential" constituents (**essential amino acids**) of the diet for maintenance of health or growth, or both. Proteolytic enzymes in the gastrointestinal tract act on ingested proteins, releasing amino acids that then are absorbed from the jejunum into the blood and subsequently become part of the body's pool of amino acids. The liver and other tissues draw on this pool for synthesis of plasma and intracellular proteins. The liver and kidneys also are involved actively in interconverting amino acids by transamination and degrading them by deamination (Figure 18-1). Deamination produces ammonium ions, which are consumed rapidly in the synthesis of urea. Urea, in turn, is excreted by the kidneys.

Amino acids in blood are filtered through the glomerular membranes but normally are reabsorbed in the renal tubules by saturable transport systems. The mechanism of reabsorption is an active transport system dependent on membrane-bound carriers and intraluminal Na^+ concentration.

When the transport mechanisms become saturated or are defective, amino acids spill into urine, resulting in a condition known as **aminoaciduria.** Three types of aminoaciduria have been identified:

1. Overflow aminoaciduria occurs when the plasma level of one or more amino acids exceeds the renal threshold (capacity for reabsorption).
2. Renal aminoaciduria occurs when plasma levels are normal but the renal transport system has a congenital or acquired defect.
3. No-threshold aminoaciduria occurs when excessive amounts of an amino acid, arising from an inherited metabolic block, are present in urine, but plasma levels are essentially normal because all the amino acid is excreted. Note that no-threshold aminoacidurias, such as homocystinuria, are not due to congenital or acquired kidney defects but are due solely to saturation of the reabsorption by normal renal tubular mechanisms.

Plasma amino acid concentrations vary during the day by about 30%; values are highest in midafternoon and lowest in early morning. This diurnal variation is particularly important when specimens are analyzed for detection of heterozygous states of defective metabolism.

Plasma amino acid concentrations are high during the first days of life, especially in premature neonates, but they

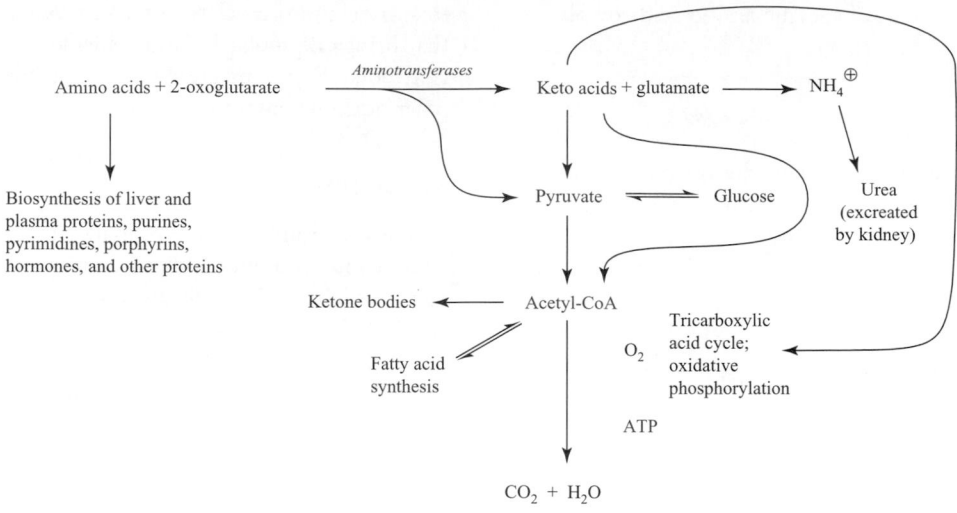

Figure 18-1   A generalized scheme of amino acid metabolism in the liver. *CoA,* Coenzyme A; *ATP,* adenosine triphosphate.

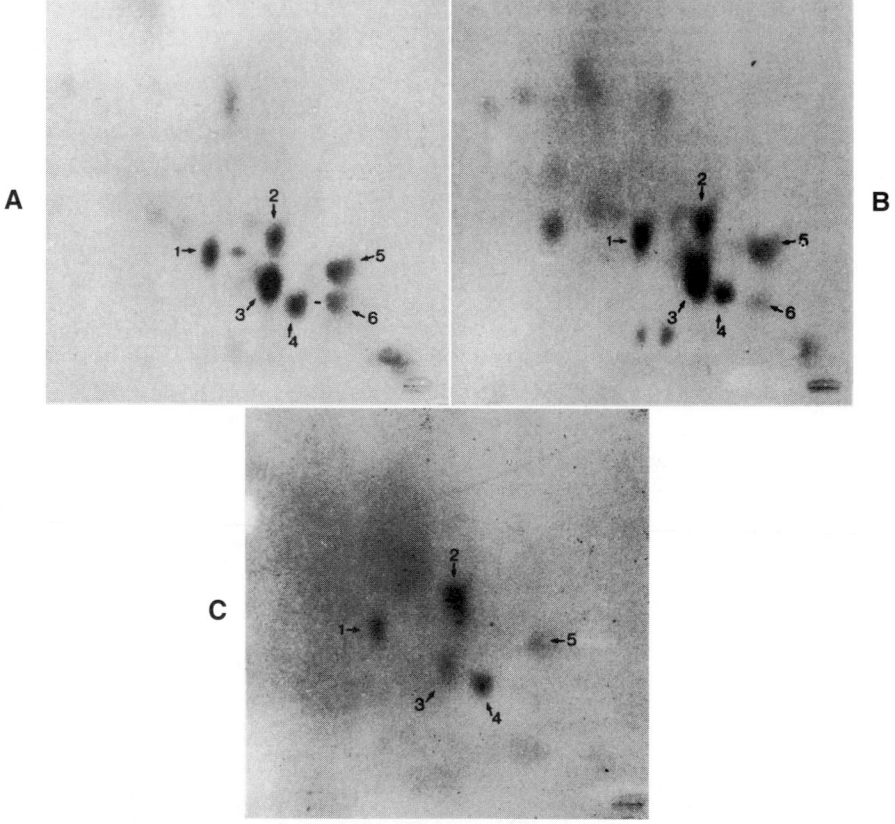

Figure 18-2   Two-dimensional chromatograms of urine showing the variability of amino acid excretion with age. **A,** Neonate. **B,** Infant. **C,** Adult. *1,* Alanine; *2,* serine; *3,* glycine; *4,* glutamine; *5,* histidine; *6,* lysine/ornithine.

tend to be low in infants with birth weights low for their gestational ages; malnutrition due to placental insufficiency is the cause. Maternal values are low in the first half of pregnancy.

Amino acid excretion in urine varies with age (Figure 18-2). Premature infants, especially during the first week of life, demonstrate a physiological generalized renal aminoaciduria; even in full-term infants aminoaciduria is more

marked than in normal adults. In the urine of normal adults, glycine usually is the dominant fraction. The renal threshold for many substances is lowered during pregnancy, and amino acids, such as histidine, phenylalanine, lysine, and tyrosine, commonly are present in urine.

An amino acid of particular note is selenocysteine. Structurally, selenocysteine is a selenium-containing analog of cysteine that is recognized as the 21st amino acid encoded by DNA.[18] It is the biologically active form of selenium, is tightly regulated, and is found in the prokaryotic and eukaryotic kingdoms in active sites of enzymes involved in oxidation-reduction reactions. Many experimental studies have shown that selenocysteine is an amino acid that is used in ribosome-mediated protein synthesis. The mRNA triplet codon for Secys is UGA, originally believed to be a "stop" codon but now is recognized to have two functions, depending on the adjacent DNA sequences.[6] Twelve mammalian selenoproteins, including glutathione peroxidase, iodothyronine deiodinases, selenoprotein P, selenoprotein W, and thioredoxin reductase, have been characterized, and each contains selenocysteine that is incorporated in response to the specific UGA codon.[6]

THE AMINOACIDURIAS

Aminoacidurias may be primary or secondary. Primary disease is due to an inherited enzyme defect, also called an **inborn error of metabolism.** The defect is located either in the pathway by which a specific amino acid is metabolized or in the specific renal tubular transport system by which the amino acid is reabsorbed. Secondary aminoaciduria is due to disease of an organ such as the liver, which is an active site of amino acid metabolism, to generalized renal tubular dysfunction, or to protein-energy malnutrition.

Primary Aminoacidurias

Primary aminoacidurias result from mutations in the DNA that codes for the specific amino acid sequence of a particular enzyme. The defect in the enzyme derived from the altered gene is reflected as diminished or absent biological activity, which blocks the metabolic path of that enzyme's substrate. The substrate accumulates or is diverted into alternative paths; products of the normal path are not formed at all or are formed in smaller amounts, or products of the alternative path are present in much-larger-than-normal amounts. Theoretically, diagnosis of primary aminoacidurias should be possible on three levels: (1) the DNA abnormality, (2) the enzyme defect, and (3) the metabolic abnormalities caused by the defect. Diagnosis depends heavily on recognition of clinical signs and symptoms and characterization of the chemical nature of primary aminoacidurias. Demonstration of an enzyme defect is confined to prenatal diagnosis or confirmation of a postnatal diagnosis by testing of cultured cells. Approaches for demonstration of DNA abnormalities are still under active development.

More than 70 inherited disorders of amino acid and organic acid metabolism are known, and most are encountered in the neonatal stage.[1] Most such inherited diseases are rare. Collectively, these diseases present an increasingly important diagnostic opportunity because some are treatable if diagnosed sufficiently early.

The symptoms and prognoses of the primary aminoacidurias that cause disease may vary from nearly benign, as in alkaptonuria, to lethal, as in maple syrup urine disease (MSUD). They usually are caused by a block in a major catabolic pathway, and their expression often indicates the diversion of substrate to an alternative, metabolically ineffective minor path. As a result, substrates and precursor substrates behind the block accumulate in the blood. When renal transport mechanisms for these substances are saturated, the products spill into the urine. Accumulation of keto acids in MSUD and of phenylalanine in individuals with phenylketonuria (PKU) are examples of precursors and substrates with toxic effects. If an alternative path is used, as it is for phenylalanine in cases of PKU, the quantities of products and intermediates of the alternative path are increased in blood and urine; in PKU these substances include phenylpyruvate and phenyllactate. An enzyme block occasionally occurs in an anabolic pathway, as in the synthesis of melanin, when the consequence is albinism. In some cases substrates do not accumulate in the blood because of a lack of reabsorption in the kidneys (no-threshold aminoaciduria); blood levels are low, and urine levels increase.

The renal types of primary aminoacidurias such as cystinuria do not demonstrate high levels of amino acids in blood because the defective protein coded by the abnormal gene is an element of the renal reabsorption mechanism for that amino acid. The transport defect may affect a single amino acid or a group of amino acids; in cystinuria, for instance, the dibasic amino acid transport system is impaired.

The primary aminoacidurias listed in Table 18-2 are inherited as autosomal recessive disorders. The overflow types (Table 18-2, *A*) probably involve a change in only one amino acid residue of the enzyme concerned. For an autosomally recessive disease to occur in an offspring, the gene defect must be present on the chromosomes of both parents and the offspring's genome then must be homozygous for the defect. A homozygote therefore fails to produce the critical protein with a correct amino acid sequence. In a heterozygote, enzyme activity typically is decreased, and the block in the metabolic path is only partial.

Secondary Aminoacidurias

The secondary aminoacidurias affect many amino acids simultaneously; as in primary aminoacidurias, these defects may be overflow or renal types. Examples of disorders that result in secondary overflow aminoaciduria are acute viral hepatitis and acetaminophen poisoning.

Generalized secondary renal aminoaciduria is caused by progressive damage to the kidney and has various causes, acquired or inherited, all of which cause proximal renal tubular dysfunction. If rickets (see Chapter 38) also is present, the condition is called *Fanconi's syndrome.* In childhood, secondary renal aminoaciduria is often secondary to cystinosis, an autosomal recessive disorder causing widespread intracellular deposits of cystine but without cystinuria. Generalized

TABLE 18-2 Primary Aminoacidurias

A Primary Overflow Aminoacidurias (Autosomal Recessive Disorders*)

Disorder	Prevalence	Abnormal Enzyme(s) (or Other Defects)	Excesses in Blood	Excesses in Urine	Clinical Features	Treatment
Hyperphenylalaninemia						
Classic PKU (type I)	1:10,000	Phenylalanine hydroxylase (absent)	Phenylalanine	Phenylalanine and its metabolites (phenylpyruvate, phenyllactate, o-hydroxyphenylacetate)	Mental retardation; seizures; eczema	Dietary restriction of phenylalanine
Variant PKU (type II)	1:14,000	Phenylalanine hydroxylase (deficient)	Phenylalanine	Variable	Mild mental retardation	Dietary restriction of phenylalanine
Transient neonatal (type III)	1:30,000	Phenylalanine hydroxylase (deficient)	Phenylalanine	Phenylalanine	Normal	None required
Type IV	Rare	Dihydropteridine reductase (absent)	Phenylalanine	Variable	Neurological disorders	DOPA, 5-OH-tryptophan
Type V	1:30,000	Defect in biopterin synthesis	Phenylalanine	Variable	Neurological disorders	DOPA, 5-OH-tryptophan
Tyrosinemia						
Type I (tyrosinosis)	1:100,000	Fumarylacetoacetate? (absent)	Tyrosine; methionine	Tyrosine and its metabolites (PHPPA, PHPLA, PHPAA); DOPA; generalized aminoacid uria (for example, Fanconi's syndrome)	Hepatic cirrhosis; renal damage	Dietary restriction of phenylalanine, tyrosine, methionine (treatment not a cure for liver disease)
Type II	Rare	Tyrosine aminotransferase (absent)	Tyrosine	Tyrosine and its metabolites; tyramine	Eye and skin lesions; mental retardation	Dietary restrictions of tyrosine, phenylalanine
Transient neonatal	Full term, 1:10; premature, 1:3	Liver immaturity	Tyrosine; phenylalanine	Tyrosine and its metabolites; tyramine	None; long term	Vitamin C; reduced protein intake
Alkaptonuria	1:250,000	HGA oxidase (absent)	HGA (slight)	HGA	Degenerative arthritis; cartilage pigmentation	None available
Homocystinuria	1:200,000	Cystathionine β-synthase (absent or deficient)	Homocystine; methionine	Homocystine; methionine and its sulfoxide	Ocular, skeletal, vascular effects	Pyridoxine; low-methionine diet supplemented with cystine
	Rare	Methylenetetrahydrofolate reductase (absent or deficient)	Homocystine with normal methionine	As in blood	Mental retardation	Folate
	Rare	Methyltransferase	Homocystine with normal methionine	Homocystine; methylmalonic acid	Failure to thrive; mental retardation	Vitamin B$_{12}$

CNS, Central nervous system; CSF, cerebrospinal fluid; DOPA, dihydroxyphenylalanine; PHPLA, p-hydroxyphenyllactic acid; PHPPA, p-hydroxyphenyl pyruvic acid; PHPAA, p-hydroxyphenyl acetic acid; MSUD, maple syrup urine disease; PKU, phenylketonuria; HGA, homogentisic acid.
*In some, probable rather than proven.

TABLE 18-2 Primary Aminoacidurias—cont'd

A PRIMARY OVERFLOW AMINOACIDURIAS (AUTOSOMAL RECESSIVE DISORDERS*)

Disorder	Prevalence	Abnormal Enzyme(s) (or Other Defects)	Excesses in Blood	Excesses in Urine	Clinical Features	Treatment
Histidinemia	1:20,000	Histidase (absent)	Histidine; alanine	Imidazole; pyruvic acid and other histidine metabolites	Sometimes normal; sometimes neurological symptoms, such as mental retardation or speech defects	Dietary restriction of histidine
Branched-chain ketoaciduria (MSUD)	1:250,000	Branched-chain keto acid decarboxylase (deficient)	During acute attacks: leucine, isoleucine, alloisoleucine, valine, and corresponding ketoacids	During acute attacks: as in blood; also odor	Overwhelming acidosis; vomiting and CNS symptoms; sometimes mental retardation; respiratory failure; may be fatal	Dietary restriction of leucine, isoleucine, valine
Nonketotic hyperglycemia	1:150,000	Block in glycine cleavage enzyme system	Glycine	Glycine (also in CSF)	Seizures, hypotonia, no ketosis; if severe, mental retardation; fatal within 2 y	None available
Propionic acidemia	Rare	Propionyl CoA carboxylase (deficient)	Glycine	Glycine; propionate; hydroxypropionate; methylcitrate	Metabolic ketoacidosis; developmental retardation	Low-protein diet
Methylmalonic acidemia	1:20,000	Methylmalonyl CoA mutase (absent or deficient)	Glycine; methylmalonic acid	Glycine; methylmalonic acid (also in CSF); ketonuria	Metabolic ketoacidosis; developmental retardation	Vitamin B_{12}
Cystathioninuria	1:70,000	γ-Cystathionase (absent or deficient)	Cystathionine	Cystathionine (also in CSF) and cystathionine metabolites	Benign	None required
Carnosinemia	1:500,000	Carnosinase (deficient)	Carnosine	Carnosine (carnosine and homocarnosine also in CSF)	Severe neurological disease	None available
Hyperprolinemia I and II	1:300,000	Type I: proline oxidase (deficient)	Proline	Proline; hydroxyproline; glycine	Probably benign	None required
		Type II: Δ^5-pyrroline-5-carboxylic acid dehydrogenase (deficient)	Proline	Proline; hydroxyproline; glycine	Probably benign	None required

Urea Cycle Disorders

Disorder	Prevalence	Abnormal Enzyme(s) (or Other Defects)	Excesses in Blood	Excesses in Urine	Clinical Features	Treatment
Citrullinemia	Rare	Argininosuccinate synthetase (deficient)	Citrulline; ammonia; alanine	Citrulline; glutamine	Vomiting; seizures; coma; mental retardation; hepatomegaly	Low-protein diet; arginine supplements

Continued

TABLE 18-2 | Primary Aminoacidurias—cont'd

A PRIMARY OVERFLOW AMINOACIDURIAS (AUTOSOMAL RECESSIVE DISORDERS*)

Disorder	Prevalence	Abnormal Enzyme(s) (or Other Defects)	Excesses in Blood	Excesses in Urine	Clinical Features	Treatment
Urea Cycle Disorders—cont'd						
Argininosuccinic aciduria	1:75,000	Argininosuccinate lyase (deficient)	Argininosuccinic acid; citrulline; ammonia after meals	Argininosuccinic acid and its anhydride; citrulline; increase argininosuccinic acid in CSF	Vomiting; growth failure; neurological dysfunction; trichorrhexis nodosa	Low-protein diet; arginine supplements
Argininemia	Rare	Arginase (deficient)	Arginine; ammonia after meals	Normal or excess arginine; cystine; ornithine	Vomiting; comas; spastic diplegia	Low-protein diet
Hyperornithinemia	Rare	Ornithine decarboxylase (deficient)	Ornithine; glutamine; alanine; ammonia after meals	Ornithine; homocitrulline	Vomiting; lethargy; coma; retardation	Low-protein diet
Ornithine transcarbamylase deficiency	Rare	Ornithine transcarbamylase (deficient, X-linked dominant)	Ammonia; glutamine	Orotic acid; uridine; uracil	Lethargy; irritability; vomiting; convulsions; coma; apnea; death	Low-protein diet
Carbamoylphosphate synthetase deficiency	Rare	Carbamoylphosphate synthetase (absent or deficient)	Ammonia; glycine; glutamine	Glycine; glutamine	Vomiting; lethargy; hypotonia; coma; pulmonary and gastrointestinal hemorrhages; developmental retardation	Low-protein diet

B PRIMARY RENAL AMINOACIDURIAS (AUTOSOMAL RECESSIVE DISORDERS*)

Disorder	Prevalence	Excess Amino Acids in Urine	Clinical Features†	Treatment
Cystinuria, classic	1:13,000	Lysine; ornithine; arginine; cystine	Cystine renal calculi	High fluid intake; urine kept alkaline; D-penicillamine; captopril
Hypercystinuria	Rare	Cystine	Cystine renal calculi	High fluid intake; urine kept alkaline; D-penicillamine; captopril
Dibasic aminoaciduria and lysinuric protein intolerance	Rare	Ornithine; lysine; arginine	Vomiting; hepatomegaly; growth failure; protein intolerance; mental retardation	Low-protein diet
Hartnup's disease	1:18,000	All neutral amino acids	Possibly no symptoms; usually pellagra-like dermatitis; neurological and psychiatric symptoms	Adequate-protein diet; nicotinamide
Iminoglycinuria	1:12,000	Glycine; proline; hydroxyproline	Benign	
Dicarboxylic aminoaciduria	Rare	Glutamic acid; aspartic acid	Probably benign	
Methionine malabsorption	Rare	Methionine; also tyrosine, phenylalanine, and branched-chain amino acids; α-hydroxybutyric acid; urinary odor	White hair; seizures; mental retardation	Low-methionine diet

CNS, Central nervous system; CSF, cerebrospinal fluid; DOPA, dihydroxyphenylalanine; PHPLA, p-hydroxyphenyllactic acid; PHPPA, p-hydroxyphenyl pyruvic acid; PHPAA, p-hydroxyphenyl acetic acid; MSUD, maple syrup urine disease; PKU, phenylketonuria; HGA, homogentisic acid.
*In some, probable rather than proven.
†Affected individuals usually have a transport defect in the jejunal mucosa and in the proximal renal tubules.

renal aminoacidurias may be caused by poisons (especially heavy metals), wasting from starvation or disease, acute tubular necrosis, or congenital conditions such as galactosemia and Wilson's disease.

Diagnosis of the Inherited Aminoacidurias

Inherited aminoacidurias are diagnosed by (1) examination of a sick infant or child, (2) routine neonatal screening, or (3) prenatal diagnosis.

Sick infant or child

An inherited aminoaciduria must be diagnosed rapidly before permanent damage is done; however, the diseases are uncommon and their symptoms are often nonspecific. An inborn error should be suspected when (1) a previous neonatal death is unexplained, (2) the parents are biologically related, (3) symptoms appear when feedings are changed, or (4) the condition improves when food is withheld and the infant or young child maintained on a glucose-saline drip. An inherited aminoaciduria also is suspected when an infant or young child demonstrates clinical symptoms of persistent vomiting, failure to thrive, or neurological or liver abnormalities.

Clinically, the determination of individual amino acids in plasma or urine is much more useful than the determination of total amino acids. Thin-layer chromatography (TLC) is used frequently for this purpose because it is a relatively simple and inexpensive technique and a large number of specimens can be processed as a batch (see Chapter 8). However, TLC is only semiquantitative and is difficult to automate. Simple chemical or microbiological tests for individual amino acids and metabolites often are used to supplement TLC. Alternatively, tandem mass spectrometry (MS/MS)[4] and capillary electrophoresis (CE)[8,10] increasingly are used to quantify numerous amino acids, organic acids, and other analytes of interest in the assessment of inborn errors of metabolism.

An attempt should be made as soon as possible to reach a provisional diagnosis that can be confirmed later if necessary. Failure to act carries the risk that the child may die or develop irreversible problems before any information is obtained from the laboratory. Ideally, the laboratory should perform a battery of tests to rule out inherited metabolic diseases in general, not only the aminoacidurias.

Neonatal screening

Genetic screening of newborns is practiced commonly to facilitate the earliest possible diagnosis of a potentially treatable inherited aminoaciduria. Most screening programs have been directed at early detection of PKU. One of the most widely used tests for PKU screening is the Guthrie test, a semiquantitative microbiological assay discussed later in the chapter.

To prevent false-negative results on the Guthrie test, the specimen must be free of drugs, such as antibiotics or endo-genous substances that inhibit bacterial growth. To minimize the occurrence of a false-negative result due to antibiotic therapy, a specimen can be autoclaved; this process degrades the antibiotic but not the amino acid of interest. False-positive results also may occur; therefore every positive result should be confirmed with a quantitative chemical or chromatographic test. Positive results obtained for premature infants must be interpreted in conjunction with additional tests because immaturity of the liver may cause increased amino acid levels. Specimens should not be obtained until 48 hours after birth because 2 days of protein intake is required to accumulate an abnormal concentration of an amino acid. Individuals should follow a normal diet for at least 24 hours before a specimen is collected. However, managed-care practices that require discharge of the mother and infant less than 24 hours after birth affect the sampling process.

Gas chromatography/mass spectrometry (GC/MS) and MS/MS (see Chapter 8) also have been used to screen for amino acids.[2,19] These analytical techniques permit rapid and simultaneous screening of more than 30 constituents.

Prenatal diagnosis

Prenatal diagnosis of an inherited aminoaciduria is particularly important when a mother previously has given birth to a child with a severe inherited defect. Preliminary study of parents, affected relatives, or the affected child—preferably by skin fibroblast cultures—is essential to define the defect to be excluded. The usual chemical tests for metabolites are not applicable to prenatal diagnosis. Although amniotic fluid is obtained easily, it may not reflect a metabolic defect in the fetus. Fetal blood, on the other hand, reliably can reflect the metabolic defect, but few physicians are willing to perform the high-risk procedures used to obtain the specimen.

Therefore prenatal diagnosis must be based on identification either of primary enzyme deficiency or a genetic mutation in fetal cells. A common approach is to collect amniotic fluid by amniocentesis at 12 to 18 weeks of gestation, culture the fetal cells, and then examine the cells for enzyme activity. Unfortunately, 3 to 6 weeks may be required to grow enough cells for the enzyme assays. The ideal prenatal test would lead to a diagnosis during the first 3 months of pregnancy. An example of such a test is chorionic villi sampling (CVS), which permits direct gene analysis of tissue obtained by biopsy (see Chapter 43). If amniotic fluid is used, fetal cells often are cultured to supply enough DNA for analysis.

■ DISORDERS OF AMINO ACID METABOLISM

Several inherited disorders result from errors in amino acid metabolism. Most such disorders involve a block or deficiency of a key enzyme involved in their normal metabolism. Amino acids of particular importance include pheny-

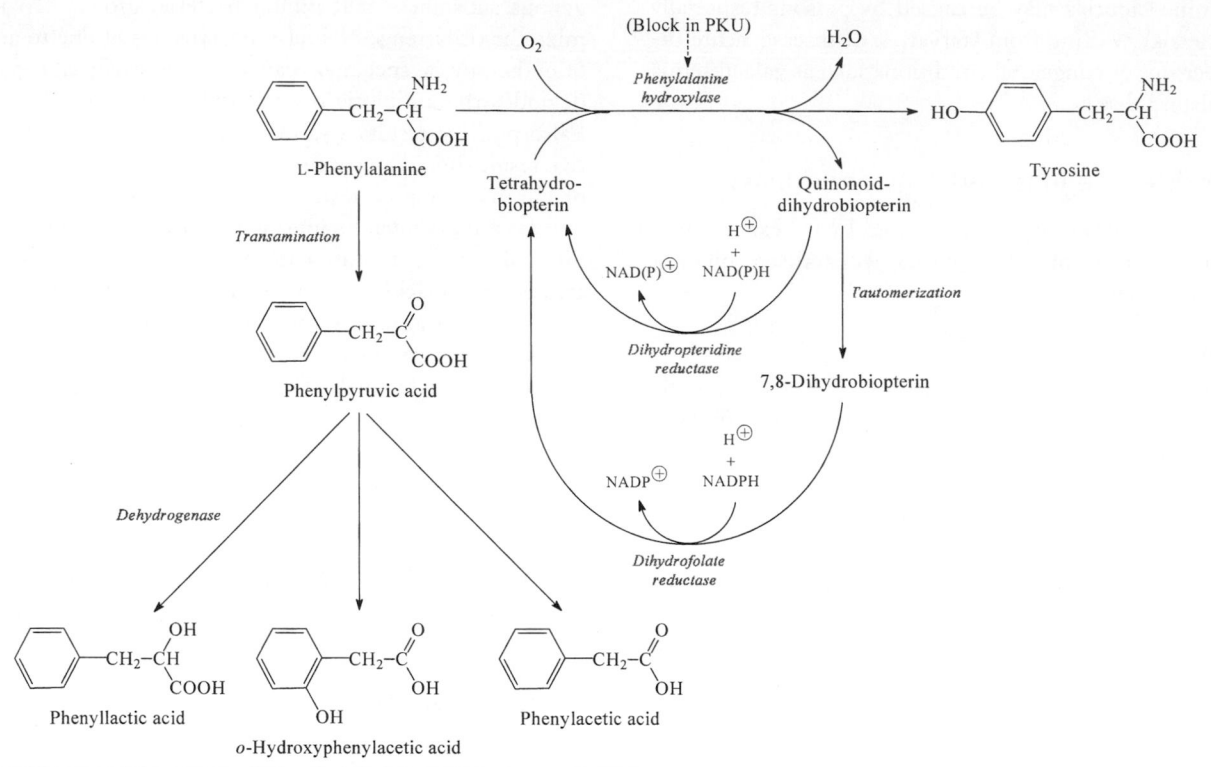

Figure 18-3   Metabolic pathway of phenylalanine. *PKU,* Phenylketonuria.

lalanine, tyrosine, cystine, homocysteine, histidine, and other simple and branched-chain amino acids.

Disorders of Phenylalanine Metabolism

The hyperphenylalaninemias are disorders of phenylalanine hydroxylation in which an afflicted individuals' phenylalanine levels are greater than 2 mg/dL (120 μmol/L).[16] In normal individuals phenylalanine hydroxylase hydroxylates phenylalanine to tyrosine (Figure 18-3). The hyperphenylalaninemias are due primarily to deficiencies of this enzyme. However, approximately 1% to 3% of cases are due to a defect in either dihydropteridine reductase or one of the enzymatic steps involved in biopterin synthesis.

Types of hyperphenylalaninemias

Types of hyperphenylalaninemias include classic PKU, maternal hyperphenylalaninemia, and other types of hyperphenylalaninemia.

Classic phenylketonuria

In classic **phenylketonuria (PKU),** which accounts for approximately 50% of all cases, phenylalanine hydroxylase activity is almost totally absent. As a direct consequence of impaired hydroxylation at the para position, phenylalanine accumulates in blood, urine, and cerebrospinal fluid (CSF).

In individuals with classic PKU, blood phenylalanine levels exceed 20 mg/dL (physiological blood levels of phenylalanine being less than 2 mg/dL). As a result of these high concentrations in blood, normally minor pathways of phenylalanine metabolism are activated, leading to increased production of metabolites such as phenylpyruvate, phenyllactic acid, *o*-hydroxyphenylacetic acid, and phenylacetic acid (see Figure 18-3). These metabolites are cleared rapidly by the kidneys and excreted into the urine. Approximately 2% of the Caucasian population in the United States are heterozygote carriers of the defective gene.

Maternal hyperphenylalaninemia

Maternal hyperphenylalaninemia is a condition that occasionally occurs in adult phenylketonuric pregnant women who have been treated successfully by dietary control since infancy. More cases of this disorder are arising as children treated for PKU become adults. High maternal levels of phenylalanine cross the placenta and can result in cardiac defects, intrauterine growth retardation, anencephaly, and mental retardation in the fetus. To reduce or prevent some or all of these adverse effects, the individual must follow a restricted diet before conception and throughout pregnancy. This restriction also applies to the consumption of the synthetic sweetener aspartame, which is a dipeptide of phenylalanine and aspartic acid.

Other types of hyperphenlyalaninemia

Hyperphenylalaninemia resulting from tetrahydrobiopterin deficiency is caused by a defect in dihydropteridine reductase or one of the enzymatic steps involved in biopterin synthesis. The disorder results in severe progressive neurological disease, probably arising from failure to synthesize the neurotransmitters serotonin, dopamine, and norepinephrine. Dietary control of phenylalanine blood levels usually has no beneficial effect, but replacement therapy with precursors of the neurotransmitters that appear after the block in the pathway, namely 5-hydroxytryptophan and dihydroxyphenylalanine (DOPA), has some benefits.

Another form of hyperphenylalaninemia is referred to as *transient neonatal hyperphenylalaninemia*. This disorder is caused by delayed hepatic maturation of the phenylalanine hydroxylase enzyme system. This condition is not an inherited defect, and blood phenylalanine levels may exceed 12 mg/dL initially but progressively decline toward normal as the neonate matures.

Less severe forms of hyperphenylalaninemia, often referred to as *PKU variants,* result from partial deficiencies of phenylalanine hydroxylase. In the atypical variant, phenylalanine hydroxylase activities typically are less than 6% of normal, and ketonuria may or may not be present.

Symptoms

Untreated PKU causes severe mental retardation. Affected children appear normal at birth, and the earliest symptoms are usually nonspecific—delayed development, feeding difficulties, and vomiting. In some children, an unusual but characteristic musty odor may be noted in urine or sweat, caused by the increased production of phenylpyruvate. Without treatment, irreversible retardation progresses. Older children frequently demonstrate hyperactivity, seizures, eczema, and hypopigmentation.

Actual injury to brain tissue begins within the second or third week of life and reaches maximum levels at about 8 or 9 months of age. Without therapy, the child may develop with a low IQ of less than 20.

Treatment

PKU is both a genetic (inborn error of metabolism) and a nutritional disease (phenylalanine being an essential amino acid but toxic in PKU). A lifetime low-phenylalanine diet is the current treatment of choice for afflicted individuals.[16] Once an individual is diagnosed, dietary restriction is initiated before the onset of brain damage so that the serum phenylalanine concentration does not exceed 8 mg/dL. Even when diagnosis is made as late as 4 to 6 months of age, institution of diet therapy decreases the rate of further mental deterioration.

Diagnosis of phenylketonuria in the neonate

Early diagnosis of PKU is essential to stop the occurrence of its severe effects. Consequently, neonatal screening has become widespread in the United States, Australia, Great Britain, and other European countries. Because up to 3% of cases are caused not by phenylalanine hydroxylase deficiency, but by deficiencies of enzymes necessary for biopterin synthesis, every newly diagnosed case of PKU should be evaluated for cofactor variants. Phenylalanine restriction alone is ineffective in these cofactor-variant cases, and thus the correct diagnosis is necessary to guide treatment. Evaluation should include measurement of biopterin and neopterin in urine and occasionally in serum.

Tests used to diagnose PKU in the neonate include chromatography, fluorometry, and a ferric chloride ($FeCl_3$) test for phenylpyruvic acid (PPA) in urine. These tests are discussed later in the chapter.

Diagnosis of the heterozygote or carrier state

To diagnose the heterozygote or carrier state, the suspected individual is given an oral dose of phenylalanine, 100 mg/kg body weight. Blood specimens then are obtained at baseline and hourly intervals for 4 hours and assayed for phenylalanine. In a noncarrier, phenylalanine concentrations rise from a fasting value of about 1.4 mg/dL to a value of 9 mg/dL at 1 and 2 hours and then drop to 5 mg/dL at 4 hours. In a heterozygote the phenylalanine concentration rises from normal to a value of about 19 mg/dL at the first hour and falls much more slowly than in a normal individual. In individuals with PKU (homozygotes) the rise in serum level is higher and more prolonged, reaching 30 mg/dL at 1 hour and 40 to 59 mg/dL at 2 to 5 hours. A phenylalanine tolerance index is calculated through summation of the 1-, 3-, and 4-hour values. The values of the index for normal individuals and carriers are sufficiently disparate to distinguish clearly between the two.

Alternatively, the elimination rate of phenylalanine is observed after an intravenous loading dose of 300 μmol/kg body weight. Distinction of normal from homozygotes and heterozygotes has been achieved with only a 2% overlap when an elimination rate of 4.34 mmol/h/m^2 was used as a discriminatory level.

Tyrosinemia and Related Disorders

Tyrosinemia, of which several forms exist, is accompanied by tyrosinuria and phenolic aciduria.[13] Tyrosine is essential for protein synthesis and serves as a precursor for thyroxine, melanin, and catecholamines. A number of different pathways exist for the metabolism of tyrosine (Figure 18-4). The major pathway leads to *p*-hydroxyphenylpyruvic acid (PHPPA) and then to homogentisic acid (HGA). The phenyl ring then is opened by HGA oxidase to form maleylacetoacetic acid, which then is isomerized and hydrolyzed to fumarate and acetoacetate.

In an alternate pathway, tyrosine is converted to DOPA and then to the pressor hormones norepinephrine and epinephrine. The skin pigments, melanins, also are derived

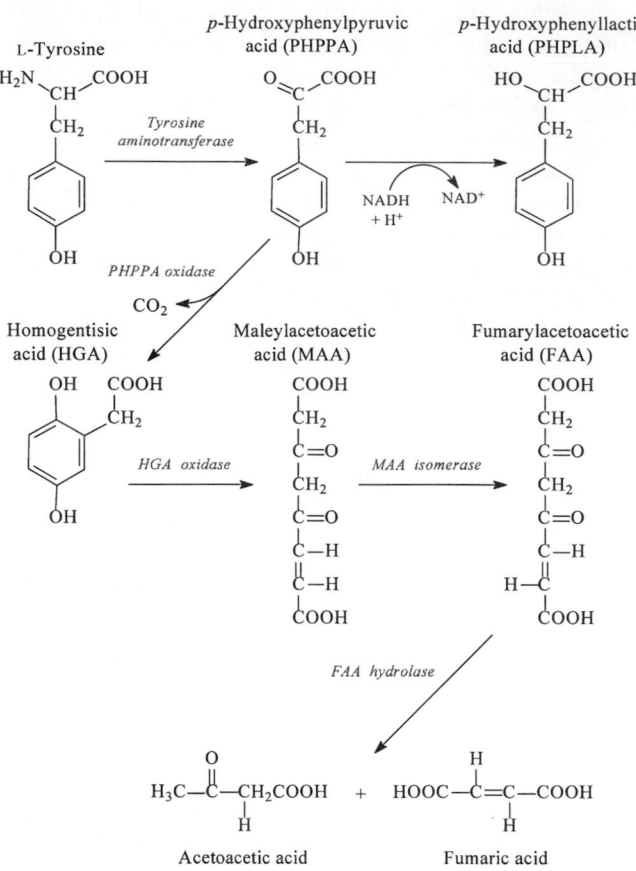

Figure 18-4   Metabolic pathway of tyrosine.

from tyrosine. Clinical syndromes resulting from inherited defects in melanin synthesis are collectively known as *albinism;* tyrosinase activity is frequently absent or deficient in many such disorders.

Types of tyrosinemia

Types of tyrosinemia include I, II, and transient neonatal tyrosinemia.

Tyrosinemia I (tyrosinosis, hepatorenal tyrosinemia)

In type I tyrosinemia, reduced activity of fumarylacetoacetate hydrolase is believed to be the primary defect in tyrosinosis. This defect results in (1) increased tyrosine levels in blood and urine, (2) increased methionine levels in blood, and (3) excretion of large amounts of DOPA and other tyrosine metabolites in urine. Other distinctive biochemical findings include increased serum α-fetoprotein, sometimes to very high levels, and increased urinary excretion of 5-aminolevulinic acid.

The disease primarily affects the liver and kidneys. Liver damage varies from acute hepatic failure and death in infancy to a chronic condition with cirrhosis later in life. A generalized transport failure (Fanconi's syndrome) develops in the proximal tubules of the kidneys with resulting vitamin D-resistant rickets (sometimes the presenting symptom),

hyperphosphaturia, glucosuria, and aminoaciduria. Most cases of type I tyrosinemia have been found in an isolated French-Canadian population in Quebec. Elsewhere, the disease has an incidence of about 1:100,000.[13]

Tyrosinemia II

Tyrosinemia II is a deficiency of the hepatic enzyme tyrosine aminotransferase. Distinctive clinical features of type II tyrosinemia include eye lesions, such as corneal erosions, and skin lesions of the palms and soles. Mental retardation also is an occasional feature. Elevated levels of tyrosine are found in blood and urine, as well as increased concentrations of phenolic acids and tyramine in urine. Unlike type I tyrosinemia, however, plasma methionine is not elevated.

Transient neonatal tyrosinemia

In this disorder, serum tyrosine levels are high in premature infants and in full-term infants of low birth weight resulting from an immature liver and its limited ability to synthesize the appropriate enzymes. As the liver matures, the accumulated tyrosine is metabolized and serum levels decrease to adult levels within 4 to 8 weeks of age.

Diagnosis of tyrosinemia

Ion-exchange column chromatography detects a substantial increase in the serum level of tyrosine and is regarded as a reference method. A number of chromatographic, photometric, and enzymatic methods also are used to diagnose tyrosinemia; these methods are discussed later in the chapter.

Alkaptonuria

Alkaptonuria is a rare hereditary metabolic disease resulting from deficient activity of HGA oxidase in the major catabolic pathway that converts tyrosine to fumarate and acetoacetate.[9] Reduced activity of this oxidase causes accumulation of HGA in cells and body fluids. Polymers of HGA, as well as monomeric HGA, bind to collagen in cartilage, intervertebral discs, and other connective tissue, eventually causing degenerative arthritis and pigmentation of cartilage. Pigment is often first apparent in the ears (ochronosis). A urine specimen from an affected individual darkens with time, on exposure to air, or on addition of alkali. Alkaptonuria usually is not diagnosed until middle age, when ochronosis and arthritis lead to suspicion, but it can be diagnosed in neonates if the dark stain in an unwashed diaper is noticed and investigated.

No satisfactory treatment exists for alkaptonuria. If the diagnosis is made early, dietary restriction of tyrosine or its precursor, phenylalanine, may be beneficial. The reduction tests for HGA is used to diagnose this disorder.

Cystinuria

Classic **cystinuria** is the most common inborn error of amino acid transport. This disease is characterized by massive urinary excretion of cystine, lysine, arginine, and ornithine.[15] Normally these amino acids are filtered by the glomerulus and reabsorbed in the proximal renal tubule, the latter by specific carrier molecules that are most likely membrane-fixed enzymes. Probably three specific classes of carriers exist—one for cystine; another for lysine, arginine, and ornithine; and a third that transports all four amino acids. Cystinuria is a transport defect of the third carrier system.

Because cystine is the least soluble of the naturally occurring amino acids, its overexcretion often leads to the formation of cystine calculi in the renal pelves, ureters, and bladder; obstruction, infection, and renal insufficiency occasionally result. Approximately 1% to 2% of all urinary tract stones are composed of cystine. Treatment involves reduction of the concentration of cystine in urine by ingestion of large amounts of water, which increases cystine solubility through maintenance of alkaline urine, and, if necessary, reduction of cystine excretion through use of D-penicillamine or administration of captopril.

Homocystinuria/Homocysteinemia

Homocysteine lies at an important metabolic branch point in the pathway from methionine to cysteine, where an alternative sulfur-conserving pathway exists back to methionine (Figure 18-5). Homocysteine normally does not accumulate in plasma because it is unstable and, when present in excess, undergoes oxidation to homocystine,[17] as follows:

Circulating levels of homocysteine in blood are less than 15 μmol/L. Concentrations of homocystine in normal urine are too low for detection, but decreased rates of homocysteine conversion to cystathionine (by cystathionine β-synthase) or back to methionine (by N^5-methyltetrahydrofolate transferase) may cause homocystinuria. Homocysteinemia has been linked to cardiovascular disease, and increased blood levels may be an important risk factor.[12,14]

Homocystinuria

The **homocystinurias** (incidence 1:200,000) are a group of disorders characterized by increased concentrations of homocysteine in body tissues. Examples are disorders linked to deficiency of cystathionine β-synthase and defects in the N^5-methyltetrahydrofolate-dependent methylation of homocysteine.[15]

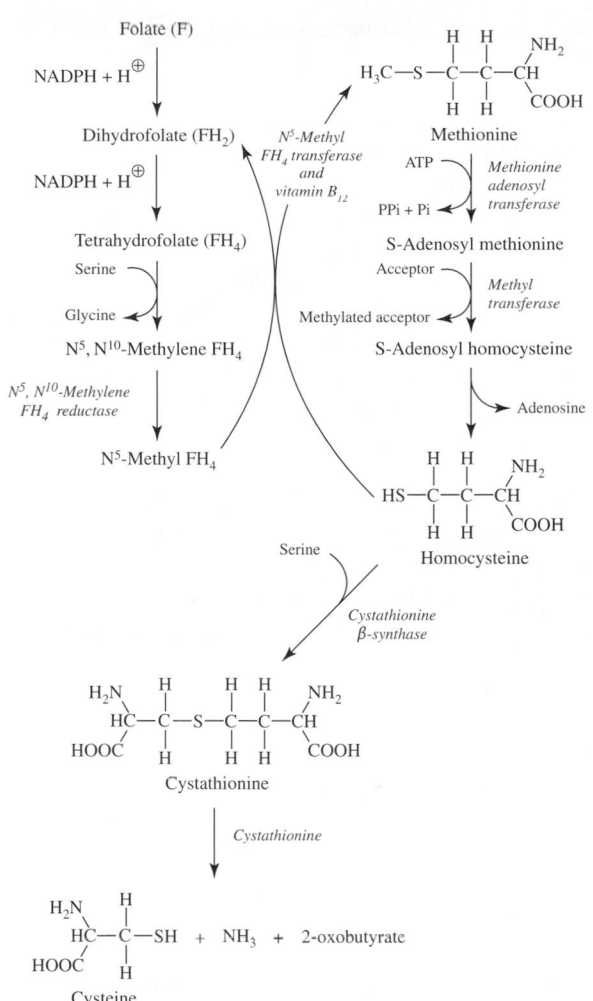

Figure 18-5 Biochemical pathways of the conversion of methionine to homocysteine and cysteine. *ATP,* Adenosine triphosphate; *Pi,* phosphate; *PPi,* pyrophosphate.

Cystathionine β-synthase deficiency

Cystathionine β-synthase deficiency is the most common cause of homocystinuria.[15] Deficient activity of this enzyme places a block between homocysteine and cystathionine; as a result, homocysteine and its precursor accumulate, and cysteine and cystine decrease in body fluids. Biochemical abnormalities include detectable plasma levels of homocystine, the oxidized from of homocysteine, and increased plasma methionine levels; the latter are normally approximately 0.45 mg/dL and may increase up to 30 mg/dL. The urine contains homocystine and other sulfur-containing amino acids, such as methionine, methionine sulfoxide, and the mixed disulfide of cysteine and homocysteine.

No symptoms are noticeable in neonates, but ocular, skeletal, and vascular symptoms gradually develop with age. Dislocation of the ocular lenses appears in the first few years, often followed by myopia, glaucoma, and retinal detachment. Skeletal abnormalities include osteoporosis, thinning and lengthening of the long bones, genu valgum (knock knee), and frequent chest, vertebral, and foot deformities. The most serious symptoms are caused by arterial or venous thromboses, which may be lethal even at an early age. The mental retardation that occurs in less than half the cases is probably a consequence of thrombotic complications.

Homocystinuria due to cystathionine β-synthase deficiency is genetically heterogeneous; enzyme activities measured in fibroblasts or lymphocytes vary from 0% to 10% of normal levels. Individuals in whom the enzyme defect is incomplete respond biochemically and clinically to large doses of pyridoxine, the cofactor needed to activate the enzyme. Those with complete enzyme deficiency should be treated with a diet low in methionine and supplemented with cystine.

Defects in the N^5-methyltetrahydrofolate-dependent methylation of homocysteine

Deficiencies of N^5-methyltetrahydrofolate or its transferase produce a block in the normal conversion of homocysteine back to methionine and cause rare forms of homocystinuria, distinguished by the absence of increased levels of plasma methionine.

Diagnosis of homocystinuria

Neonatal screening is practical only for cystathionine β-synthase deficiency. A Guthrie test for increased plasma methionine is performed. A positive result should be interpreted with care, however, because it may be transient or due to liver damage, tyrosinosis, or a deficiency of hepatic S-adenosylmethionine synthetase. The incidence of transient hypermethioninemia has decreased, probably because infant milk preparations now have lower protein content. In the absence of neonatal screening, homocystinuria is unlikely to be diagnosed until symptoms appear and the urine is tested.

Homocystine and cystine can be measured with the cyanide-nitroprusside test. To differentiate between homocystine and cystine, the silver-nitroprusside modification of this test may be used.

Organic Acidurias

The organic acidurias are characterized by excessive urinary excretion of aliphatic and aromatic organic acids and may be either congenital or acquired. Clinically, individuals with organic acidurias typically have unexplained, severe ketoacidosis; presenting symptoms of the various types are similar— vomiting, lethargy, seizures, coma, and, in survivors, mental retardation. Because most of the acids cannot be visualized by TLC, diagnosis within this group of aminoacidurias depends chiefly (with the exception of MSUD) on analysis by high-performance liquid chromatography (HPLC), GC/MS, or MS/MS.

Maple syrup urine disease
Maple syrup urine disease (MSUD) takes its name from the characteristic odor of the urine of affected individuals;

the maple syrup, or burnt sugar, odor is due to the high concentration of aliphatic keto acids. Amino acid analyses of blood and urine demonstrate high levels of leucine, isoleucine, and valine. These branched-chain amino acids normally are converted by transamination to their corresponding α-keto acids, which then are converted to acetylcoenzyme A (CoA) derivatives. An inherited defect of the decarboxylase step results in accumulation of the branched-chain amino acids and their corresponding α-keto acids in blood, urine, and CSF.

Several types of MSUD have been identified clinically and biochemically. In the classic type, affected infants appear normal at birth but then develop frequent vomiting and failure to thrive. Acute ketoacidotic episodes, often triggered by recurring infections, result from increased production of organic keto acids. Severe neurological dysfunction leads to seizures, coma, respiratory failure, and death in many individuals. Survivors usually are mentally retarded.

Antenatal diagnosis may be made by assay of decarboxylase activity in cultured cells from amniotic fluid. Treatment includes dietary restriction of branched-chain amino acids. Daily analysis of urine with dinitrophenylhydrazine (DNPH) and monthly measurement of plasma amino acid levels are important to monitor the effectiveness of the dietary therapy.

Disorders of propionate and methylmalonate metabolism

Individuals affected with disorders of propionic acid and methylmalonic acid metabolism usually have overwhelming illness early in life.[5] Intolerance of dietary protein, particularly amino acids such as leucine, isoleucine, valine, threonine, and methionine, is characteristic. These disorders involve deficiencies of propionyl CoA carboxylase and methylmalonyl CoA mutase. Chemically, massive ketonuria and elevated levels of glycine in body fluids are present. High concentrations of methylmalonic acid also can be demonstrated in methylmalonic aciduria, but not in propionic aciduria. Definitive diagnosis of propionic aciduria can be made by demonstration of the presence of methylcitrate in urine or analysis of organic acids in urine by GC/MS or MS/MS.

■ ANALYSIS OF AMINO ACIDS

Many procedures are available to measure amino acids in biological samples.[21] To diagnose pathological disorders, the following three groups of tests for amino acid analysis are important:

1. Screening tests, including TLC, urine color tests, and the Guthrie microbiological test
2. Quantitative tests to monitor treatment or confirm an initial diagnosis
3. Specific tests that identify an unknown amino acid or metabolite

TABLE 18-3	Drugs that Interfere with Urinary Amino Acid Assessment	
Methodological Interferences (Drugs Causing Ninhydrin-Positive Spots)	Physiological Interferences (Drugs Interfering with Amino Acid Metabolism)
Penicillins	Valproic acid
Cephalosporins	(hyperglycinuria)
α-Methyldopa	(hyperglycinemia)
Levodopa	Antimetabolites
Polythiazide	(secondary aminoaciduria)
X-ray contrast media	(β-alanine)
	(β-aminoisobutyric acid)
	6-Azouridine
	(homocystinuria)

Specimen Requirements

To diagnose accurately an inherited aminoaciduria, care must be taken to obtain valid and representative samples. For example, individuals should follow a normal diet for 2 to 3 days before collection. Blood and urine specimens should be collected simultaneously. Use of heparinized plasma is preferable to serum and other anticoagulants. The plasma must be deproteinized if analysis includes the sulfur-containing amino acids. Because some drugs administered either to the mother before she gives birth or to the infant interfere with specimens (Table 18-3), all medications should be noted.

Screening Tests

A variety of methods are used to screen for amino acids in body fluids. They include TLC, photometric assay, and the Guthrie test.

Thin-layer chromatography

TLC analysis of amino acids is conducted in three stages: (1) preparation of the sample, (2) chromatographic separation, and (3) identification of the separated amino acids. For analysis of amino acids in body fluids and tissues, often pretreatment of the sample is necessary to remove proteins, lipids, inorganic salts, or other substances that interfere with chromatographic resolution.

The amount of amino acids visible in a chromatogram is influenced not only by the disease process but also by the volume of fluid applied to the chromatogram. Therefore the sample volume is calibrated by reference to its total nitrogen content or the amount of creatinine in a specified volume of the specimen.

In practice, cellulose continues to be the stationary phase of choice because procedures using it provide superior chromatographic resolution and reduce the time required for solvent development (see Chapter 8). Procedures using paper, however, are very useful when blood or urine samples are collected on filter paper discs.

A large number of solvent systems have been proposed for separation of amino acid mixtures. One-dimensional TLC is favored by some laboratories because of its simplicity; multiple reference compounds and samples can be run easily on a single plate. In two-dimensional TLC after the first migration, the chromatogram is rotated 90 degrees and then transferred to another solvent system for a second migration. When selective staining reagents are used in conjunction with two-dimensional solvent systems, identification of more than 75 compounds of biochemical interest is possible.

Many staining reagents can be used to visualize amino acids separated by TLC. The most widely used reagent for both qualitative and quantitative assessment of amino acids is ninhydrin. A number of colored products are formed, but the major one presumably results from deamination and condensation as follows:

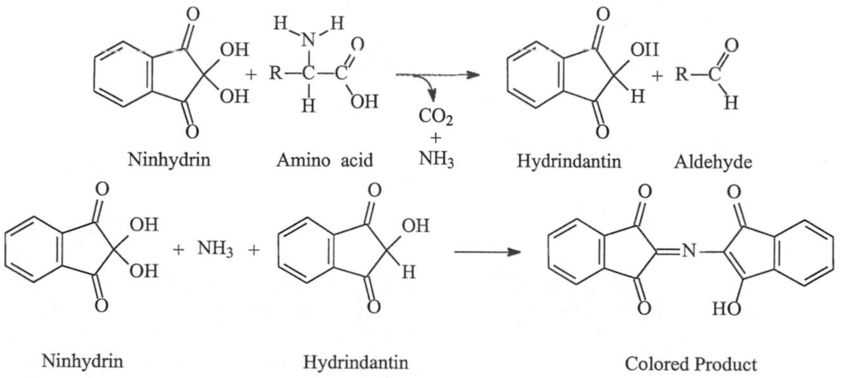

Most amino acids react with ninhydrin at ambient temperatures to form a blue color that turns purple on heating. However, proline and hydroxyproline yield yellow compounds that are less satisfactory for visual observation; consequently, additional stains such as isatin (indole-2,3-dione) often are used. Isatin converts proline and hydroxyproline to blue compounds that are detectable against a yellow background. The addition of organic bases, such as collidine, to ninhydrin solutions also produces polychromatic staining, which facilitates identification of individual amino

TABLE 18-4 Reagent Systems for Staining of Chromatographic Plates

Staining Method	Use	Reagent Composition	Procedures and Comments
Ninhydrin-isatin reagent	Large number of amino acids commonly encountered in biological fluids	a. Ninhydrin, 0.25 g/dL in acetone b. Isatin, 10 mg/dL in acetone c. Lutidine	1. Mix 50 mL of reagent (a) and 50 mL of reagent (b); then add 1 mL of lutidine. 2. Dip or spray chromatograms; dry at 40 °C for 20 to 30 min.
Ninhydrin-collidine reagent	Polychromatic reagent; facilitation of identification of individual amino acids	a. Ninhydrin, 0.2 g/dL in isopropanol b. Collidine (2,4,6-trimethylpyridine)	1. Mix 2.5 mL of reagent (b) with 100 mL of reagent (a). 2. Dip or spray chromatograms and heat for 10 min in a 70 °C-humidified oven.
Chlorine-o-toluidine	General reagent for amino acids; higher concentrations required for detection	a. Saturated solution of o-toluidine in 2% acetic acid b. Potassium iodide, 0.85 g/dL in H_2O c. Sodium hypochloride, 2 g/dL in H_2O	1. Mix equal volumes of reagents (a) and (b) just before use (solution 1). 2. Spray chromatograms lightly with solution (c) and dry for 1 to 1.5 h; overspray the chromatograms with solution 1.
Pauly's reagent	Histidine and other imidazoles; tyrosine and other phenolic compounds forming red, brown, and yellow azo dyes	a. Sodium nitrate, 5 g/dL in H_2O b. Sulfanilic acid, 9 g in 90 mL concentrated hydrochloric acid and 900 mL H_2O c. Sodium carbonate, anhydrous, 10 g/dL in H_2O	1. Mix 1 volume of solution (a) and 1 volume of solution (b). After 5 min, add 2 volumes sodium carbonate. *Caution:* Carbon dioxide is liberated vigorously. 2. May dip or spray chromatograms. Dry chromatograms at 100 °C for 4 to 5 min.
Ehrlich's reagent	Indoles: purple; hydroxyindoles: blue; aromatic amines: yellow	a. p-Dimethylaminobenzaldehyde, 10 g in 100 mL concentrated hydrochloric acid b. Acetone	1. Mix 1 volume of reagent (a) with 4 volumes of reagent (b) before use.
Fluorescamine	Very sensitive general reagent for amines, amino acids, peptides	a. Triethylamine, 10 g/dL in methylene chloride b. Fluorescamine, 20 mg/dL in anhydrous acetone	1. Dry chromatograms at 100 °C; then spray with reagent (a) and allow to dry for a few seconds. 2. Spray reagent (b) and allow to dry. Apply reagent (a) again; amino acid spots are visible at 360 nm. Sensitivity is very good at 250 to 300 pmol/L.
Iodoplatinate	Unoxidized sulfur amino acids form white spots on purple background	a. Chloroplatinic acid ($H_2PtCl_6 \cdot 6\ H_2O$), 1.0 g/L, in hydrochloric acid, 0.2 mol/L b. Potassium iodide, 16.7 g/L in H_2O	1. Just before use, combine 0.6 volume of reagent (a) with 10 volumes of reagent (b) and mix; subsequently add 40 volumes of acetone. 2. Watch for color development, which may take 24 h; plastic or glass plates *must* be used; chromatograms must be stored in a plastic bag in the dark.
Sakaguchi reaction	Arginine and other substituted guanidines form deep-red or orange spots (fades)	a. 8-Hydroxyquinoline, 0.1 g/dL in acetone b. Bromine liquid, 0.3 mL in 100 mL sodium hydroxide, 0.5 mol/L	1. Prepare fresh. 2. Dip chromatograms into solution (a) and evaporate acetone. 3. Dip into reagent (b).

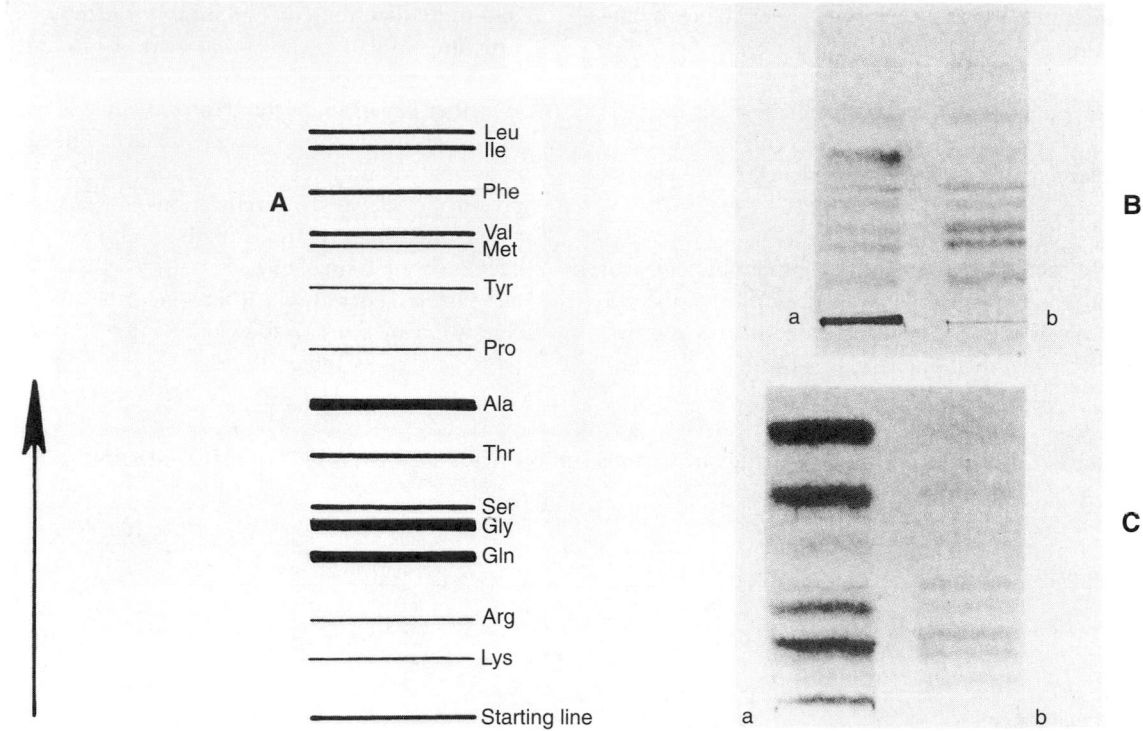

Figure 18-6   One-dimensional chromatography of amino acids in a solvent system consisting of n-butanol:acetone:acetic acid:water (35:35:10:20, v/v). **A,** Positions of several amino acids after their separation from a standard mixture. **B,** Separation of plasma amino acids in transient neonatal tyrosinemia. Note tyrosine band *a; b* is the amino acid standard. **C,** Separation of plasma amino acids in untreated maple syrup urine disease; the most prominent bands are those of isoleucine, leucine,

and valine (*a*); *b* is the amino acid standard. *Leu,* Leucine; *Ile,* isoleucine; *Phe,* phenylalanine; *Val,* valine; *Met,* methionine; *Tyr,* tyrosine; *Pro,* proline; *Ala,* alanine; *Thr,* threonine; *Ser,* serine; *Gly,* glycine; *Gln,* glutamine; *Arg,* arginine; *Lys,* lysine. (From Bremer HJ, Duran M, Kamerling JP et al: Disturbances of Amino Acid Metabolism: Clinical Chemistry and Diagnosis, Baltimore, Urban and Schwartzenberg, 1980.)

acids. Table 18-4 provides a brief summary of some useful stains.

One-dimensional thin-layer chromatography

The principle of one-dimensional TLC is described in Chapter 8. Although two-dimensional TLC is preferred for urine, one-dimensional TLC of plasma or urine can detect most aminoacidopathies and generally is adequate for screening. With this technique, specimens, reference solutions, and controls are applied to precoated cellulose thin-layer plates. Development is performed in an appropriate solvent-vapor system, followed by drying and staining of the chromatogram. The reference solution is a mixture of amino acids of known concentration. Examples of one-dimensional chromatograms are shown in Figure 18-6. When several samples of the same specimen are run on a single plate and each then stained with different specific stains, identification of many individual amino acids is often possible.

Two-dimensional thin-layer chromatography

Two-dimensional TLC can be used to identify free amino acids in blood, urine, CSF, and other biological fluids and tissues. With this technique, protein first is precipitated with absolute ethanol, followed by extraction with chloro-

form to remove urea and other organic and inorganic substances. Amino acids in the aqueous layer then are separated by TLC on precoated cellulose plates. Two developing solvents are used; the first contains ammonia to increase the mobility of amino acids with basic side chains, and the second contains formic acid to increase the mobility of amino acids with acidic side chains. A representative two-dimensional chromatogram is shown in Figure 18-7. Representative colors and R_f values obtained from amino acids with such a system are listed in Table 18-5.

In practice, an aliquot of sample is applied at one corner of a cellulose thin-layer plate, and after separation of amino acids in one direction, the plate is turned at a right angle and the amino acids further separated by a second solvent. After development, individual amino acids are visualized with ninhydrin-collidine. Then the distance migrated by each individual amino acid and the solvent front are measured from the point of application. The distances are used to calculate an R_f with the following equation:

$$R = \frac{\text{distance from application point to spot center}}{\text{distance from application point to solvent front}}$$

Presumptive identification is made by comparison of the R_f values and characteristic colors of unknowns with those of reference mixtures of authentic amino acids chromatographed at the same time.

Photometric screening tests for urine

Various qualitative tests are used for screening, spot checking, or supplemental information (Table 18-6).

Guthrie test

The **Guthrie test** is a semiquantitative microbiological assay. Bacterial spores, usually *Bacillus subtilis,* are incorporated into an agar medium to which a competitive growth inhibitor has been added, one that is specific for the amino acid to be determined. The inhibitor often has a molecular structure similar to the amino acid of interest. Technically, blood or urine from the individual is spotted onto a piece of soft filter paper, and a standardized circle is "punched" from the paper and laid on the agar surface. The agar plate then is incubated and later observed for bacterial growth. In the presence of elevated concentrations of the amino acid of interest, the effect of the growth inhibitor is diminished or overcome and zones of bacterial growth are observed. The test system is designed to show growth only when the concentration of the amino acid of interest exceeds its upper reference limit (Table 18-7).

TABLE 18-5 Color Reaction and R_f Values of Various Amino Acids on Cellulose TLC Plates Stained With Ninhydrin-Collidine

Amino Acid	Color	$R_f \times 100$ First Dimension	$R_f \times 100$ Second Dimension
1. Cystine	Gray	15	10
2. Cysteine	Gray	15	10
3. Cystathionine	Violet	8	13
4. Cysteic acid	Violet	15	14
5. Phosphoethanolamine	Violet	4	21
6. Argininosuccinic acid	Violet	7	27 to 40
7. Ornithine	Violet	23 to 28	23
8. Asparagine	Beige	21	24
9. Homocystine	Violet	18	33
10. Arginine	Violet	11	23 to 37
11. Lysine	Violet	30	23 to 35
12. 1-Methylhistidine	Gray	29	26 to 39
13. Histidine	Gray	36	19
14. Carnosine	Tan	34	20 to 30
15. Taurine	Violet	46 to 60	23
16. Glutamine	Violet	21	34
17. Aspartic acid	Aquamarine	8	37
18. Citrulline	Violet	22	41
19. Methionine sulfoxide	Violet	26	39
20. Methionine sulfone	Violet	40	40
21. Serine	Violet	40	40
22. Glycine	Rose	24	43
23. Hydroxyproline	Orange	28	43
24. Glutamic acid	Violet	9	47
25. Sarcosine	Gray-pink	31	51
26. Threonine	Violet	65	44
27. β-Alanine	Aquamarine	33	54
28. Alanine	Violet	31	57
29. Proline	Yellow	36	57
30. Tyrosine	Gray-brown	53	55
31. Tryptophan	Yellow-gray	53	55
32. Ethanolamine	Violet	80	47
33. γ-Aminobutyric acid	Violet	35	65
34. α-Aminobutyric acid	Violet	38	58
35. β-Aminoisobutyric acid	Violet	37	66
36. Methionine	Violet	49	65
37. Phenylalanine	Gray	59	69
38. Valine	Violet	44	72
39. Leucine	Violet	54	78
40. Isoleucine	Violet	54	78

TLC, Thin-layer chromatography. NOTE: Numbers that precede amino acids correspond to the numbers indicated in Figure 18-7.

Quantitative Tests

Amino acids can be measured quantitatively in body fluids with a variety of techniques, including CE,[8] GC,[22] HPLC,[20] ion-exchange liquid chromatography,[7,11] and MS/MS.[4] In addition, molecular genetic testing is beginning to be used for this purpose.

Capillary electrophoresis

In CE the classic techniques of electrophoresis are performed in small-bore (10 to 100 μm), fused-silica capillary tubes 20 to 200 cm in length (see Chapter 7). It is a very efficient, rapid, sensitive, and versatile analytical technique that is used to analyze a diverse spectrum of analytes, ranging from small ions to macromolecular proteins or nucleic acids.[8,10] When coupled with sensitive detectors, CE is capable of measuring femtomolar quantities of amino acids.

Gas chromatography

Advantages of GC include small sample size, sensitivity, and speed, but a major limitation is the relatively low volatility of amino acids at temperatures conventionally used in this technique. However, these compounds can be reacted with derivatizing agents to increase volatility and enhance their chromatographic and detection characteristics.

Because of the necessity for an initial cleanup step followed by derivatization, GC is not used routinely in the clinical laboratory. However, it is still used for investigation of organic acidurias.

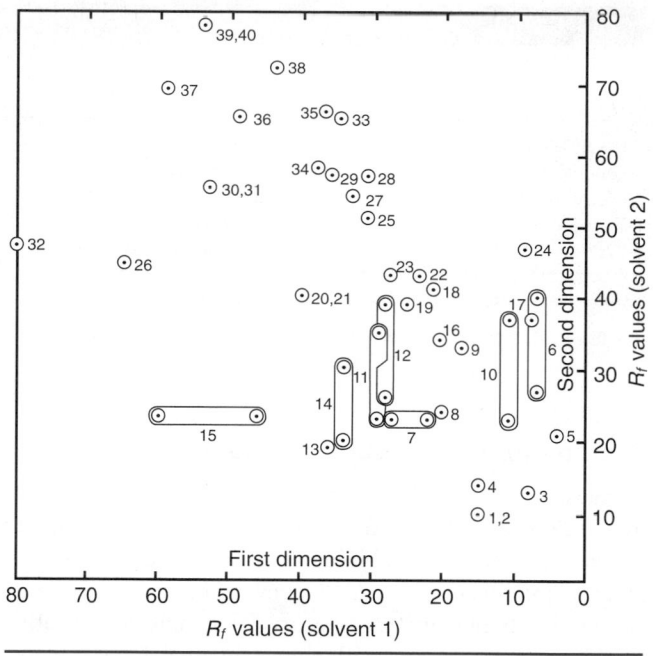

Figure 18-7   Composite map of R_f values ($\times$ 100) of amino acids obtained with two-dimensional chromatography on cellulose. First-dimension solvent—pyridine:acetone:concentrated ammonium hydroxide:water (40:30:5:20 by volume). Second-dimension solvent—2-propanol:concentrated formic acid:water (66:15:15 by volume). The origin is 0. The numbers correspond to the amino acids listed in Table 18-5.

TABLE 18-6	Color Tests on Urine	
Test and Color	Metabolites	Disorder
Ferric Chloride*		
Dark blue-green (persistent)	Phenylpyruvate	PKU
Green (transient)	p-Hydroxyphenylpyruvate	Tyrosinuria
Blue (transient)	HGA	Alkaptonuria
Gray-green	Imidazolepyruvate	Histidinemia
Gray-blue	Branched-chain keto acids	MSUD
Blue-green	5-Hydroxyindoleacetic acid	Carcinoid
Purple	Salicylates	(Interferent)
Purple-brown	Phenothiazines	(Interferent)
Cyanide/Nitroprusside		
Cherry-red	Cystine	Cystinuria; generalized aminoacidurias
	Homocystine	Homocystinuria
	Cysteine-homocysteine disulfide	Homocystinuria
	Penicillamine-cysteine disulfide	(Treatment)
2,4-Dinitrophenylhydrazine		
Yellow-white (ppt)	Branched-chain keto acids; phenylpyruvate; p-hydroxyphenylpyruvate	MSUD; PKU; tyrosinosis
Nitrosonaphthol		
Orange-red	Tyrosine and its metabolites (for example, p-Hydroxyphenylpyruvate, -lactate, -acetate)	Tyrosinosis; tyrosinemia

HGA, Homogentisic acid; *MSUD,* maple syrup urine disease; *PKU,* phenylketonuria.
*Phenistix (Bayer Corp., Elkhart, Ind.) is a commercial version of the ferric chloride test.

TABLE 18-7 Guthrie Test Systems

L-Amino Acid	Inhibitor	Disease	Upper Reference Limit (mg/dL)
L-Phenylalanine	β-2-Thienylalanine	PKU	4
L-Leucine	4-Azaleucine	MSUD	4
L-Methionine	Methionine sulfoximine	Homocystinuria	2
L-Tyrosine	L,D-Tyrosine	Tyrosinemia	8
L-Lysine	S(β-Aminoethyl) cysteine	Hyperlysinemia	4

MSUD, Maple syrup urine disease; *PKU,* phenylketonuria.

High-performance liquid chromatography

Because of its excellent sensitivity, high resolution, and relatively short analysis time, HPLC is used extensively to measure amino acids in biological samples (see Chapter 8). The major advantage of HPLC over GC is that the relatively high temperatures necessary for sample volatilization by GC are unnecessary with this technique. Thus the possibility of amino acid decomposition at high temperatures is averted.

Only a few amino acids are detected by the ultraviolet (UV) or visible spectrophotometers, fluorometers, or electrochemical detectors that are routinely used with HPLC analyzers. Consequently, amino acids typically are derivatized for analysis by HPLC. Postcolumn derivatizations with ninhydrin or fluorogenic reagents, such as *o*-phthaldialdehyde or fluorescamine, have been used successfully for detection purposes. Precolumn derivatization techniques using *o*-phthaldialdehyde, dansyl, phenyl isothiocyanate, or 9-fluorenylmethyl chloroformate derivatives have been used with reversed-phase HPLC. Electrochemical detection also has been coupled with derivatization methods to enhance analytical sensitivity.

Ion-exchange liquid chromatography

Ion-exchange liquid chromatography has been used widely to separate and quantify amino acids in a variety of specimens (see Chapter 8). After separation, the eluted amino acids are mixed with ninhydrin or some other indicator in a postcolumn reactor. The resultant colored species then are detected with an online spectrophotometer, fluorometer, or other detection device. The amino acids are identified by the comparison of the retention times of the components in the specimen to those of reference compounds. Quantitation is made by comparison of specimen peak areas or heights with those from sets of calibrators, or, alternatively, by use of an internal standardization technique. Fluorometric detection with fluorescamine and *o*-phthaldialdehyde has decreased the limits of detection, and shorter, narrower columns packed with smaller particles operating at higher flow rates have decreased the time required for analysis.

Tandem mass spectrometry

MS/MS is applicable to the rapid assay of specific analytes in complex biological fluids (see Chapter 8). MS/MS has been used to screen neonates for such amino acid metabolic disorders as PKU,[3] MSUD,[2] tyrosinemia,[3] hypermethioninemias,[4] and homocystinuria.[4,19] Although the initial cost for equipment is high and derivatization is required, MS/MS can be cost effective because it is an automated technique and can be used to screen for several diseases simultaneously.

Compared with older methods, MS/MS is a more sensitive technique, offers greater accuracy and precision, and has higher clinical specificity and sensitivity. Consequently, it produces fewer false-negative and false-positive results.

Molecular genetic testing

Many genes coding for enzymes involved in amino acid metabolism have been isolated, and some mutations have been identified. As knowledge regarding characterization of mutations and the chromosomal location of specific genes evolves, the identification of highly linked polymorphisms will allow carrier detection in affected families by linkage analysis or direct mutation analysis.

Tests for Specific Amino Acids

In addition to the general analytical techniques discussed previously, a variety of simple tests exist that are specific for individual amino acids. These tests are used in the diagnosis of specific disorders.

Methods for the determination of serum phenylalanine and related compounds

Tests used to assay for serum phenylalanine and related compounds include chromatography, fluorometry, and an FeCl₃ test for PPA in urine.

Chromatography

Automated ion-exchange column chromatography, GC, GC/MS, and one-dimensional paper chromatography are used both to confirm specimens yielding positive phenylalanine screening results or to monitor dietary treatment of individuals with PKU.

Fluorometry

In the fluorometric determination of serum phenylalanine, phenylalanine is reacted with ninhydrin in the presence of the dipeptide L-leucyl-L-alanine to form a fluorescent product that is proportional to the phenylalanine concentrations. The reaction is carried out at pH 5.88. An alkaline copper tartrate reagent is added to stabilize the fluorescent product.

In practice, blood specimens are drawn from infants into microcapillary tubes. If the assay must be delayed, the plasma is separated and frozen until it is analyzed. Before analysis, samples are treated with trichloroacetic acid to precipitate proteins. Next, ninhydrin-peptide reagent is added to an aliquot of the protein-free supernatant and mixed. After a 2-hour incubation, the fluorometer is read at excitation and emission wavelengths of 365 nm and 515 nm, respectively. The concentration of phenylalanine is determined with a calibration curve.

Ferric chloride test for phenylpyruvic acid in urine

The $FeCl_3$ test is used to detect PPA in urine for monitoring of the effectiveness of dietary therapy for individuals with PKU. However, the test is only qualitative, lacks specificity, and should not be used for screening purposes. In practice, PPA cannot be detected in an infant's urine until the serum phenylalanine concentration reaches levels between 12 and 15 mg/dL (usually 10 to 14 days after birth). Infants affected with PKU excrete up to 2 g/day of PPA. PPA is unstable.

Methods for determination of tyrosine in serum

A convenient method to measure tyrosine in plasma involves reaction of a trichloroacetic acid (TCA) filtrate with a mixture of α-nitroso-β-naphthol (ANBN) and nitrite in the presence of nitric acid. This fluorometric method is unsuitable for urine, in which interfering compounds are present in greater concentration.

Enzymatic methods have been developed to measure tyrosine in plasma by use of the enzymes tyrosinase (from mushrooms), L-amino acid oxidase (from snake venom), or ammonia lyase (from yeast). Tyrosinase catalyzes the oxidation of tyrosine to dopaquinone, and consumption of oxygen is measured amperometrically.

Detection of p-hydroxyphenylpyruvic acid in urine

Tyrosinemia can be diagnosed by chromatographic isolation and identification of PHPPA from urine. Urinary excretion of PHPPA in affected individuals may reach 1.6 g/d,

about twenty-fivefold greater than the amount excreted by normal subjects. More conveniently, Millon's reagent (a solution of mercuric sulfate and sulfuric acid) or the ANBN test can be used to detect a wide variety of substituted phenolic compounds in urine. These tests, however, are not specific for PHPPA; positive reactions also are given by tyrosine and tyrosine metabolites, such as p-hydroxyphenyllactate (PHPLA) and p-hydroxyphenylacetate (PHPA), which accompany increased urinary output of PHPPA.

Reduction tests for homogentisic acid

HGA reduces ammoniacal silver nitrate $(AgNO_3)$ very rapidly. In this procedure, aqueous $AgNO_3$ solution is added to urine, followed by a few drops of dilute ammonia hydroxide, (NH_4OH). If HGA is present, a brown-black to black precipitate of reduced elemental silver is formed immediately.

Cyanide-nitroprusside test for cystine and homocystine

The cyanide-nitroprusside test is based on the reaction of sodium nitroprusside with sulfhydryl compounds, such as cysteine and homocysteine, to produce a red-purple product. Oxidized disulfides (for example, cystine and homocystine) do not react but first must be reduced to their free thiol forms with alkaline sodium cyanide before they develop the red-purple color.

Silver-nitroprusside test for homocystine

A modification of the cyanide-nitroprusside test is used to differentiate between cystine and homocystine. Through substitution of $AgNO_3$ for sodium cyanide as the reducing agent, homocystine can be reduced to its thiol form (homocysteine), whereas cystine remains in the nonreactive oxidized form. Homocysteine then reacts with sodium nitroprusside and becomes pink-purple.

Dinitrophenylhydrazine test for keto acids

The basis for this test is the chemical reaction between DNPH and the keto group of an amino acid. For example, the DNPH reagent reacts with various aliphatic, cyclic, and aromatic carbonyl compounds to form relatively insoluble crystalline hydrazones. To perform the test, equal quantities of filtered urine are mixed with the DNPH solution. A yellow to yellow-white precipitate that forms within 5 minutes indicates a large quantity of keto acids. A slight precipitate or turbidity that forms after 1 minute may be normal. Interference contributed by acetone can be eliminated if the urine is heated briefly before testing.

References

1. Burlina AB, Bonafe L, Zacchello F: Clinical and biochemical approach to the neonate with a suspected inborn error of amino acid and organic acid metabolism. Semin Perinatol 1999; 23:162-173.

2. Chace DH, Hillman SL, Milllington DS et al: Rapid diagnosis of maple syrup urine disease in blood spots from newborns by tandem mass spectrometry. Clin Chem 1995; 41:62-68.

3. Chace DH, Milllington DS, Terada N et al: Rapid diagnosis of phenylketonuria by quantitative analysis for phenylalanine and tyrosine in neonatal blood spots by tandem mass spectrometry. Clin Chem 1993; 39:66-71.

4. Chace DH, Hillman SL, Milllington DS et al: Rapid diagnosis of homocystinuria and other hypermethioninemias by tandem mass spectrometry. Clin Chem 1996; 42:349-355.

5. Fenton WA, Rosenberg LE: Disorders of propionate and methylmalonate metabolism. In Scriver CR, Beaudet AL, Sly WS et al (eds): The Metabolic and Molecular Bases of Inherited Disease, 7th edition, pp 1423-1450, New York, McGraw-Hill, 1995.

6. Gladyshev VN, Hatfield DL: Selenocysteine-containing proteins in mammals. J Biomed Sci 1999; 6:151-160.

7. Hara K, Hijikata Y, Hiraoka E et al: Measurement of urinary amino acids using high performance liquid chromatography equipped with a strong cation exchange resin pre-column. Ann Clin Biochem 1999; 36:202-206.

8. Issaq HJ, Chan KC: Separation and detection of amino acids and their enantiomers by capillary electrophoresis: a review. Electrophoresis 1995; 16:467-480.

9. La Du BN: Alkaptonuria. In Scriver CR, Beaudet AL, Sly WS et al (eds): The Metabolic and Molecular Bases of Inherited Disease, 7th edition, pp 1371-1386, New York, McGraw-Hill, 1995.

10. Landers JP: Clinical capillary electrophoresis. Clin Chem 1995; 41:495-509.

11. Le Boucher J, Charret C, Coudray-Lucas C et al: Amino acid determination in biological fluids by automated ion-exchange chromatography: performance of Hitachi L-8500A. Clin Chem 1997; 43:1421-1428.

12. Miner SES, Evrovski J, Cole DEC: The clinical chemistry and molecular biology of homocysteine metabolism: an update. Clin Biochem 1997; 30:189-201.

13. Mitchell GA, Lambert M, Tanguay RM: Hypertyrosinemia. In Scriver CR, Beaudet AL, Sly WS et al (eds): The Metabolic and Molecular Bases of Inherited Disease, 7th edition, pp 1077-1108, New York, McGraw-Hill, 1995.

14. Molgaard J, Malinow MR, Lassvik C et al: Hyperhomocyst(e)inaemia: an independent risk factor for intermittent claudication. J Intern Med 1992; 231:273-279.

15. Mudd SH, Levy HL, Skovby F: Disorders of transsulfuration. In Scriver CR, Beaudet AL, Sly WS et al (eds): The Metabolic and Molecular Bases of Inherited Disease, 7th edition, pp 1279-1328, New York, McGraw-Hill, 1995.

16. Scriver CR, Kaufman S, Eisensmith RC et al: The hyperphenylalaninemias. In Scriver CR, Beaudet AL, Sly WS et al (eds): The Metabolic and Molecular Bases of Inherited Disease, 7th edition, pp 1015-1075, New York, McGraw-Hill, 1995.

17. Segal S, Thier SO: Cystinuria. In Scriver CR, Beaudet AL, Sly WS et al (eds): The Metabolic and Molecular Bases of Inherited Disease, 7th edition, pp 3581-3602, New York, McGraw-Hill, 1995.

18. Stadtman TC: Selenium biochemistry. Ann Rev Biochem 1996; 65:83-100.

19. Sweetman L: Newborn screening by tandem mass spectrometry (MS/MS). Clin Chem 1996; 42:345-346.

20. Teerlink T, van Leeuwen PAM, Houdijk A: Plasma amino acids determined by liquid chromatography within 17 minutes. Clin Chem 1994; 40:245-249.

21. Walker V, Mills GA: Quantitative methods for amino acid analysis in biological fluids. Ann Clin Biochem 1995; 32:28-57.

22. Zumwalt RW: Amino Acid Analysis by Gas Chromatography, Boca Raton, Fla, CRC Press, 1987.

Additional Reading

Bamforth FJ: Laboratory screening for genetic disorders and birth defects. Clin Biochem 1994; 27:332-342.

Cynober LA (ed): Amino Acid Metabolism in Health and Nutritional Disease, Boca Raton, Fla, CRC Press, 1995.

Massey KA, Blakeslee CH, Pitkow HS: A review of physiological and metabolic effects of essential amino acids. Amino Acids 1998; 14:271-300.

Scriver CR, Beaudet AL, Sly WS et al (eds): The Metabolic and Molecular Bases of Inherited Disease, 7th edition, pp 1015-1460, New York, McGraw-Hill, 1995.

CHAPTER 19

Proteins

A. MYRON JOHNSON, MD, ELIZABETH M. ROHLFS, PhD,
and LAWRENCE M. SILVERMAN, PhD

Objectives

1. Define the following terms:
Protein	Acute-phase reaction
Globulin	Paraprotein
Immunoglobulin	Complement protein
2. State and describe the four stages of protein structure.
3. Compare "fibrous" proteins with "globular" proteins and provide examples of each.
4. Describe the physiological functions of proteins.
5. List the properties that are unique to each protein.
6. List the principal plasma proteins and the clinical significance of each.
7. List the immunoglobulin classes and their clinical significance.
8. State the clinical laboratory analytical methods for determination of total protein concentration, albumin concentration, and globulin concentration, as well as the principle of each reaction.
9. State the principle of immunofixation electrophoresis and describe the migration patterns of the plasma proteins.

Key Words

Acute-Phase Reaction   The body's response to injury or inflammation, including fever, leukocytosis, and protein changes

Apoprotein   The protein moiety of a conjugated protein or protein complex

Bence-Jones Protein   An abnormal plasma or urinary protein, consisting of monoclonal immunoglobulin light chains, excreted in some neoplastic diseases and characterized by its unusual solubility properties as it precipitates on heating at 50 to 60 °C and redissolves at 90 to 100 °C

Complement   A functionally related system comprising at least 20 distinct serum proteins that help destroy foreign cells identified by the immune system

Conjugated Protein   A protein that contains one or more prosthetic groups

Globular Protein   A protein with a compact morphology that is soluble in water or salt solutions

Immunodeficiency   A deficiency or inability of certain parts of the immune system to function, which makes an individual susceptible to certain diseases that he or she ordinarily would not develop

Immunoglobulins   A class of proteins also known as *antibodies* made by the B cells of the immune system in response to a specific antigen and containing a region that binds to this antigen (antigen-binding site); five classes of immunoglobulins (IgA, IgD, IgE, IgG, and IgM)

Paraprotein   An abnormal plasma protein appearing in large quantities as a result of a pathological condition; also known as *myeloma components (MCs)*

Peptide Bond   The amide bond formed between the

carboxyl group of one amino acid and the amino group of another

Plasma Proteins   Proteins present in blood, including carrier proteins, fibrinogen and other coagulation factors, complement components, immunoglobulins, enzyme inhibitors, and many others; most being found in other body fluids, but in lower concentrations

Prosthetic Group   A nonpolypeptide structure that is

bound tightly to a protein and required for the activity of an enzyme or other protein

Protein   Any of a group of complex organic compounds that contain carbon, hydrogen, oxygen, nitrogen, and usually sulfur (the characteristic element being nitrogen) and are distributed widely in plants and animals

Proteinuria   The presence of an excess of serum proteins in the urine

The human body contains thousands of different **proteins.** Many are structural elements of cells or organized tissues; others are soluble in intracellular or extracellular fluids. The proteins most amenable to routine laboratory evaluation are those in blood, urine, cerebrospinal fluid (CSF), amniotic fluid, saliva, feces, and peritoneal or pleural fluids.

■ BASIC BIOCHEMISTRY

Proteins are polymers of amino acids that are linked covalently through **peptide bonds** (see Chapter 18). Very short chains of linked amino acids are designated as dipeptides, tripeptides, tetrapeptides, or pentapeptides. Chains more than five residues in length are called *oligopeptides.* Longer chains (6 to 30 residues) are referred to as *polypeptides.* When the number of amino acids linked together exceeds 40 (molecular mass = 5000 or 5 kD), the chain takes on the physical properties associated with proteins. The different R groups found in amino acids provide peptides and proteins with their versatility in structure and function.

Structure

Proteins are classified as fibrous (mainly structural) or globular. Although fibrous proteins, such as fibrinogen, troponin, collagen, and myosin, are of clinical interest, most proteins of clinical interest are soluble globular proteins, such as hemoglobin, enzymes, peptide hormones, and plasma proteins. The complex bending and folding of polypeptide chains are a result of the numerous interactions of their R groups. **Globular proteins** are compact and have little or no space for water in the interior of the molecule, where most of the hydrophobic R groups are located. Most polar R groups are located on the surface of the protein, where they exert a substantial influence on protein solubility, acid-base behavior, and electrophoretic mobility.

Most globular proteins retain their biological activities within narrow ranges of temperature and pH. Periods of exposure to high temperatures or extremes of pH cause the molecules of proteins to "denature" and lose their solubilities and biological activities. For example, many enzymes

lose their catalytic function after denaturation occurs (see Chapter 9).

Globular proteins have the following four levels of structure:

1. Primary structure refers to the identity and specific order of amino acid residues in the polypeptide chain. This sequence, which depends exclusively on covalent (peptide) bonds, is predetermined by the DNA coding. The three-dimensional structure and any special biological properties of the protein follow automatically from this amino acid sequence.

2. Secondary structure is a regularly recurring arrangement in space of the primary structure extending along one dimension. The secondary structures of many globular proteins have stretches of α-helix, β-pleated sheet, and random coils, all dependent on numerous hydrogen bonds and occasional disulfide covalent bonds.

3. Tertiary structure involves the intramolecular folding of the polypeptide chain into a compact three-dimensional structure with a specific shape. This structure is maintained by electrovalent linkages, hydrogen bonds, disulfide bridges, van der Waals forces, and hydrophobic interactions. Hydrophobic interactions are considered a major force in maintenance of the unique tertiary structure of proteins.

4. Quaternary structure refers to the association of several polypeptide chains or subunits into a larger "oligomeric" aggregate unit. This structure depends on the close fit of the polypeptide subunits through interactions at their contact surfaces and with any prosthetic groups.

Many proteins contain nonamino acid components known as **prosthetic groups.** Such proteins often are referred to as **conjugated proteins** and are classified according to the nature of their prosthetic groups as metalloproteins, lipoproteins, glycoproteins, mucoproteins, and phosphoproteins. Both glycoproteins and mucoproteins have covalently linked carbohydrate prosthetic groups, but the amount of carbohydrate varies between the two. In glycoproteins this amount may be approximately 5% to 15%, whereas in mucoproteins, it may be approximately 15% to 75%. Conjugated proteins freed of their prosthetic groups are known as **apoproteins.**

Properties

Many properties of proteins are used for their separation, identification, and assay. The following five properties are among them:

1. *Molecular size* Most proteins are macromolecules of high molecular mass. Because of their sizes and differing molecular masses, proteins are separated from smaller molecules by dialysis, ultrafiltration, molecular exclusion gel filtration chromatography, and density-gradient ultracentrifugation.
2. *Differential solubility* Protein solubility is affected by the pH, ionic strength, temperature, and dielectric constant of the solvent. When these parameters are varied, proteins become either more or less soluble. For example, through variations in the ionic strength of a solution, proteins become either more soluble ("salting-in") or less soluble ("salting-out").
3. *Electrical charge* The effect of pH to introduce, enhance, or change the surface charges on a protein creates various species of different charges that migrate at different rates in an electrical field; separation by electrophoresis and isoelectric focusing are based on this behavior (see Chapter 7). Ion-exchange chromatography is based on electrostatic interactions of charged proteins with oppositely charged solid media (see Chapter 8).
4. *Adsorption on finely divided inert materials* These materials offer large surface areas for interactions with proteins. These interactions are either hydrophobic, absorptive, ionic, or molecular (hydrogen bonding).
5. *Specific binding to antibodies, coenzymes, or hormone receptors* The unique property of a protein to recognize and bind to a complementary compound with high specificity is the basis for immunochemical assays (see Chapter 10). Proteins also are separated by affinity chromatography, in which a ligand attached to a solid medium provides high selectivity (see Chapter 8).

Function

Proteins demonstrate numerous biological functions. For example, enzymes catalyze biochemical reactions essential to metabolism; protein, polypeptides, and oligopeptide hormones regulate metabolism; and antibodies and components of the complement system protect against infection. In addition, plasma proteins maintain the osmotic pressure of plasma. They transport hormones, vitamins, metals, and drugs, often serving as reservoirs for their release and use; apolipoproteins solubilize lipids; hemoglobin carries oxygen; and protein coagulation factors affect hemostasis.

Hundreds of different proteins are present in blood plasma; they are known collectively as **plasma proteins.** They include acute-phase reaction proteins, carrier proteins, fibrinogen and other coagulation factors, complement components, immunoglobulins, enzyme inhibitors, precursors of substances such as angiotensin and bradykinin, and many others.

Most plasma proteins are synthesized in the liver and move into the bloodstream through the hepatic sinusoids and central veins of the liver (see Chapter 36). Plasma proteins circulate in the blood and between the blood and extracellular tissue spaces. Their extravascular movement occurs not only by passive diffusion but also by active transport mechanisms and pinocytosis and exocytosis through and from cells. Most plasma proteins are catabolized in the liver; for some plasma proteins the signal that marks them for degradation appears to be the loss of part or all of the sialic acid content.

Of relevance to the clinical laboratory, the most common changes in protein concentrations in disease result from the so-called **acute-phase reaction** or response (APR), a nonspecific response to inflammation (infections, autoimmune diseases, etc.) or tissue damage (trauma, surgery, myocardial infarction, or tumors). The proteins affected are known as acute-phase proteins (APPs). The concentrations of some APPs (α_1-antitrypsin, α_1-acid glycoprotein, haptoglobin, ceruloplasmin, C4, C3, and C-reactive protein) increase in response to an APR and are known as *positive APPs*. Others (transthyretin, albumin, and transferrin) decrease and are known as *negative APPs*. The protein APR is nonspecific and comparable to fever or increased leukocyte count. The changes in plasma protein levels are triggered by cytokines released at the site of injury. Plasma levels of the individual APP proteins change at different rates after the initial insult (Figure 19-1). In practice these changes are helpful in detection of inflammation, and sequential

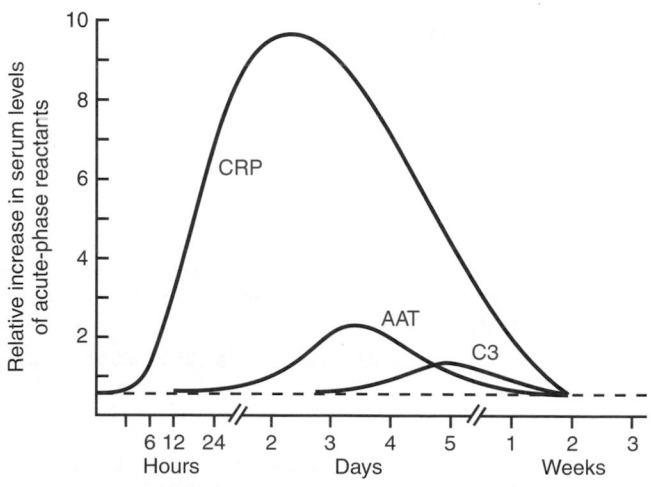

Figure 19-1 Relative increases of acute-phase reactants after an acute, short-lived insult. Concentrations are expressed as multiples of the upper limit of the reference interval. The dashed line represents the upper reference limit. *CRP,* C-reactive protein; *AAT,* α_1-antitrypsin; *C3,* complement factor 3.

TABLE 19-1 Properties of Selected Plasma Proteins

Electrophoretic Region	Protein	Half-Life	pI	Molecular Mass (daltons)	Preferred Analysis Method	Comments
	Retinol-binding protein (RBP)	12 h		21,000	Nephelometry, turbidimetry	
	Transthyretin (TTR)	48 h	4.7	54,980	Nephelometry, turbidimetry	Indicator of nutrition; transport protein
	Albumin	15 to 19 days	4 to 5.8	66,200	Nephelometry, turbidimetry, dye-binding	Reduced levels in many diseases; general transport protein; maintenance of plasma osmotic pressure
α_1	α_1-Antitrypsin (AAT)	4 days	4.8	51,800	Nephelometry, turbidimetry	Congenital deficiency possibly associated with emphysema or cirrhosis
	α_1-Acid glycoprotein (AAG, orosomucoid)	5 days	2.7 to 4	40,000	Nephelometry, turbidimetry	Function obscure; binds cationic drugs and hormones
	α_1-Fetoprotein (AFP)			69,000	RIA, fluorescence polarization	Principal fetal protein; albumin analogue
α_2	Haptoglobin (Hp, HAP)	2 days	4.1*	85,000 to 1 million	Nephelometry	Binding of hemoglobin; reduced by hemolysis
	α_2-Macroglobulin (AMG)	5 days	5.4	720,000	Nephelometry, turbidimetry	Increased levels in nephrotic syndrome; proteolytic enzyme inhibitor
	Ceruloplasmin (Cp)	4.5 days	4.4	132,000	Nephelometry, RID, turbidimetry	Decreased levels in Wilson's disease; contains copper; antioxidant
β_1	Transferrin (TRF, siderophilin)	7 days	5.7	79,600	Nephelometry, turbidimetry	Transport of iron; increased levels in hypochromic anemia and pregnancy/ estrogen effects
	C4			206,000	Nephelometry, turbidimetry	Complement factor
β_2	C3			185,000	Nephelometry, turbidimetry	Complement factor
	β_2-Microglobulin (BMG)			11,800	RIA	Useful in testing of renal tubular function; elevated levels in lymphocytosis or lymphocyte breakdown
γ	IgG	24 days	6 to 7.3	144,000 to 150,000	Nephelometry, IF, turbidimetry	Antibodies increased in immune reactions; monoclonal
	IgA	6 days		~160,000	Nephelometry, IF, turbidimetry	Increased levels in B-cell tumors
	IgM	5 days		970,000	Nephelometry, IF, turbidimetry	
	C-reactive protein (CRP)		6.2	~115,000	RID, RIA, nephelometry, homogeneous enzyme immunoassay, turbidimetry	Nonspecific defense against infectious agents

pI, Isoelectric point; *RID,* radial immunodiffusion; *RIA,* radioimmunoassay; *IF,* immunofixation.
*For Hp 1-1 phenotype.

measurements of proteins such as CRP are useful in monitoring of the progress of the inflammation or its response to treatment.

Table 19-1 lists the properties of the principal plasma proteins. The individual proteins are listed in the order of their electrophoretic mobilities in agarose gels at pH 8.6. Their interim reference intervals for adults, based on the international standard RPPHS/CRM 470, (Reference Preparation for Proteins in Human Serum/Certified Reference Material 470) are listed in Table 19-2.

TABLE 19-2 Interim Consensus Reference Intervals for 14 Plasma Proteins in Human Serum Referenced to CRM 470/RPPHS

Protein	g/L	mg/dL
α_1-Acid glycoprotein	0.5 to 1.2	50 to 120
Albumin	35 to 52	3500 to 5200
α_1-Antitrypsin	0.9 to 2.0	90 to 200
C3*	0.9 to 1.8*	90 to 180*
C4	0.1 to 0.4	10 to 40
Ceruloplasmin	0.2 to 0.6	20 to 60
C-reactive protein	<5	<0.5
Haptoglobin	0.3 to 2.0	30 to 200
IgA	0.7 to 4.0	70 to 400
IgG	7 to 16	700 to 1600
IgM	0.4 to 2.3	40 to 230
Transthyretin (prealbumin)	0.2 to 0.4	20 to 40
α_2-Macroglobulin	1.3 to 3.0	130 to 300
Transferrin	2.0 to 3.6	200 to 360

From Dati F, Schumann G, Thomas L et al: Consensus of a group of professional societies and diagnostic companies on guidelines for interim reference ranges for 14 proteins in serum based on the standardization against the IFCC/BCR/CAP reference material (CRM 470). Eur J Clin Chem Clin Biochem 1996; 34:517-520.
CRM 470/RPPHS, Certified Reference Material 470/Reference Preparation for Proteins in Human Serum.
*Values are slightly lower in fresh samples (assayed < 8 hours after draw). These values are applicable only to adults between 20 and 60 years of age.

■ INDIVIDUAL PLASMA PROTEINS

The following discussion is limited to several of the more important individual plasma proteins.

Albumin

Albumin is a small globular protein with a molecular mass of 66.3 kD. Normally, it is the most abundant protein found in plasma from midgestation until death, accounting for approximately one-half the plasma protein mass. Because of its high plasma concentration and relatively small size, albumin is also the major protein component of most extravascular body fluids, including CSF, interstitial fluid, urine, and amniotic fluid. Approximately 60% of the total body albumin is in the extravascular space. It has no carbohydrate side chains but is highly soluble in water due to its high net negative charge at physiological pH.

Biochemistry and function

Albumin is synthesized primarily by the hepatic parenchymal cells. The synthetic reserve of the liver is enormous. For example, in the nephrotic syndrome the synthetic rate may be 300% or more of its normal rate. The synthetic rate of albumin is controlled primarily by colloidal osmotic pressure (COP) and secondarily by protein intake; in addition, synthesis is decreased by inflammatory cytokines. Catabolism occurs primarily by pinocytosis in all tissues, with reutiliza-

tion of the resulting free amino acids for synthesis of cellular proteins. The normal plasma half-life of albumin is 15 to 19 days.

Albumin's primary function is the maintenance of COP in both the vascular and extravascular spaces, with continuous equilibration between. Albumin also binds and transports a large number of compounds, including free fatty acids, phospholipids, metallic ions, amino acids, drugs, hormones, and bilirubin.

Albumin is coded by a gene on the long arm of chromosome 4, closely linked to the genes for α-fetoprotein and vitamin D-binding globulin, both of which share extensive sequence homology with albumin. More than 80 genetic variants have been reported. All are inherited in autosomal codominant fashion, with expression of both gene products in heterozygotes. Many isotypes have altered electrophoretic migration, resulting in so-called bisalbuminemia. However, bound drugs and metabolites also may change albumin's electrophoretic migration. A few variants have abnormal binding affinities for thyroxine (T_4); affected individuals are euthyroid but have abnormal serum total and free T_4 levels.

Clinical significance

Increased levels of albumin are present only in acute dehydration and have no clinical significance. Decreased levels are seen in a multitude of clinical conditions, some of which are discussed in the following text.

Analbuminemia

Individuals with this rare genetic deficiency have plasma albumin levels less than 0.5 g/L but mild if any edema. Major clinical manifestations are related to abnormal lipid transport.

Inflammation

Acute and chronic inflammation are the most common causes of hypoalbuminemia, resulting from hemodilution, loss into the extravascular space, increased consumption by cells, and decreased synthesis.

Hepatic disease

The decreased levels of albumin present in most cases of hepatocellular disease result from increased immunoglobulin levels, loss into the extravascular space, and direct inhibition of synthesis by toxins and alcohol. However, the liver can synthesize increased amounts of albumin until hepatic parenchymal damage or loss is severe, with the loss of approximately 95% of function.

Urinary loss

The renal glomerulus acts as a molecular sieve, excreting any substance inversely proportional to its molecular radius. Because albumin is relatively small and globular, significant amounts filter into the glomerular urine. However, most of it is reabsorbed by the proximal tubular cells. Normal ex-

TABLE 19-3　Other Protease Inhibitors

Inhibitor	Molecular Mass (kD)	Physiological Proteases Inhibited	Diseases Associated with Deficiency
α_1-Antichymotrypsin	68	Cathepsin G; mast cell chymase; prostate-specific antigen*	Hepatic cirrhosis; asthma; ? emphysema
α_2-Antiplasmin	70	Plasmin	Hemorrhage (increases clot lysis)
Antithrombin III†	65	Thrombin	Thromboembolism
C1 inhibitor†	104	C1r, C1s	Hereditary angioedema
Inter-α-trypsin inhibitor	160	Unknown	None known

*Several inhibitors bind and inactivate prostate-specific antigen (PSA), including α_1-antitrypsin, α_2-macroglobulin, and α_2-antiplasmin. α_1-Antichymotrypsin complexes are usually the predominant ones in serum or plasma, probably because of rapid clearance of the others. Levels of complexed PSA are increased in most individuals with prostatic cancer, compared with normal individuals or those with benign prostatic hypertrophy.
†Quantitative and qualitative (functional) deficiencies reported.

creted urine contains up to 20 mg albumin per gram of creatinine. Excretion above this amount suggests either increased glomerular filtration, tubular damage, hematuria, or combinations of these.

Increased filtration also occurs with physical exercise and fever; therefore urinary albumin should be assayed under controlled conditions and repeated if a clinical question exists as to the cause of increased levels. Mildly increased excretion (20 to 300 mg/L), or microalbuminuria, appears to predict future development of clinical renal disease in individuals with hypertension or diabetes mellitus. Except for hereditary analbuminemia, the lowest levels of plasma albumin are present in individuals with active nephrotic syndrome, associated with marked albuminemia.

Gastrointestinal loss

Inflammatory disease of the intestinal tract is associated with increased gastrointestinal (GI) loss of albumin. This increase usually is of little concern unless the loss is excessive or persists. Chronic protein-losing enteropathy may result in loss similar to that present in the nephrotic syndrome.

Protein energy malnutrition

Albumin levels have been used to help detect and monitor protein nutritional status (see Chapter 45). However, low levels generally do not correlate with the degree of malnutrition and most often are due to APR.

Edema and ascites

Plasma levels of albumin are decreased in the presence of edema and ascites. However, edema and ascites are usually secondary to increased vascular permeability, rather than to hypoalbuminemia per se. The albumin levels in these fluids vary from very low to higher than those in plasma.

Alpha$_1$-Acid Glycoprotein

α_1-Acid glycoprotein (AAG), also known as *orosomucoid*, contains a high percentage of carbohydrate with a large number of sialic acid residues. Thus it has a very high net negative charge and is very soluble in water. AAG is the major constituent of the seromucoid fraction of plasma, a group of proteins precipitated by $HClO_4$ and other strong acids.

Biochemistry and function

AAG has a polypeptide chain with 181 amino acids and a total molecular mass of 40 kD, of which approximately 45% is carbohydrate, including 11% to 12% sialic acid. It is synthesized primarily by the hepatic parenchymal cells, and catabolism results in the removal of desialylated protein by the hepatic asialoglycoprotein receptors.

Although its true physiological role is unknown, AAG binds and inactivates basic and lipophilic hormones, including progesterone and the progesterone antagonist RU 486. AAG also binds and reduces the bioavailability of many drugs, including propranolol, quinidine, chlorpromazine, cocaine, and benzodiazepines. If AAG levels are elevated, drug dosage may be increased to compensate for this increased binding. AAG is classified as one of the lipocalins—proteins that bind lipophilic substances.

Clinical significance

AAG levels increase in the APR, especially in GI inflammatory disease and malignant neoplasms. Levels are increased by corticosteroids and some nonsteroid antiinflammatory drugs (NSAIDs). Estrogens (for example, from pregnancy or oral contraception) decrease synthesis of AAG. Levels also are low in protein-losing syndromes, such as nephrotic syndrome. Several known variants of AAG exist; however, they are not clinically significant.

Alpha$_1$-Antitrypsin

α_1-Antitrypsin (AAT; α_1-proteinase inhibitor) is one of the so-called serpins (*ser*ine *p*roteinase *in*hibitors) that inactivate serine proteases, especially those structurally related to trypsin. Other serpins include α_1-antichymotrypsin, α_2-antiplasmin, antithrombin III, and C1 inhibitor (Table 19-3).

Biochemistry and function

AAT is synthesized primarily by hepatic parenchymal cells. Catabolism occurs in hepatic parenchymal cells by two routes. AAT-protease complexes are removed by the serpin-enzyme complex receptors. In the second route, desialylated AAT is removed by asialoglycoprotein receptors.

AAT is the highest-concentration proteinase inhibitor in plasma on a molar basis. Physiologically, it is the most important inhibitor of leukocyte elastase, released in the process of phagocytosis by polymorphonuclear leukocytes. This enzyme reacts with elastin in the tracheobronchial tree and vascular endothelium. AAT's relatively small size and diffusion into these tissues are important in the prevention of loss of elastic recoil. Uninhibited elastase in the bronchial tree, because of either excess elastase or a deficiency in AAT, results in the development of emphysema.

At least 75 known genetic variants of AAT exist, several of which are associated with low concentrations of AAT. The common wild phenotype is Pi MM; the most common deficiency phenotypes of clinical importance are Pi ZZ and SZ. If the mean normal concentration is taken as 100%, levels in Pi MZ, Pi SS, Pi ZZ, and Pi SZ individuals average about 60%, 60%, 15%, and 35%, respectively. Rare null individuals do not have AAT. The Pi ZZ, and to a lesser extent Pi SZ, phenotypes are those most commonly associated with the clinical conditions in the discussion that follows.

Clinical significance

AAT levels are elevated by the APR and by estrogens (pregnancy, oral contraception). AAT levels are secondarily low in individuals with neonatal respiratory distress syndrome, severe pancreatitis, and protein-losing disorders. Decreased AAT levels due to primary, or genetic, deficiency are associated with a very high risk for development of basilar pulmonary emphysema (in contrast to the apical disease present in other forms of emphysema). Onset of disease is usually much earlier than it is for most other forms of emphysema, with changes beginning in the late second to fourth decades of life in 90% of Pi ZZ individuals. The process is increased by air pollution and cigarette smoking.

AAT deficiency also is associated with diseases of the liver, including neonatal cholestasis, cirrhosis, and hepatocellular carcinoma. Neonatal cholestasis, or "hepatitis," is present most commonly at 3 to 8 weeks of age and usually regresses after a few weeks. Intrahepatic and extrahepatic bile ducts may be small, probably because of decreased bile flow. Differentiating this fact from biliary atresia is important because mortality is high in Pi ZZ infants subjected to major surgery. In addition, a strong correlation exists between AAT deficiency and primary liver cancer.

One variant, Pi $M_{pittsburgh}$, has a met → arg amino acid substitution, which results in increased activity against clotting enzymes, including thrombin and kallikrein. Heterozygotes for this variant have a bleeding disorder because of its anticoagulant effects.

Alpha$_1$-Fetoprotein

α_1-Fetoprotein (AFP) is one of the first α-globulins to appear in mammalian sera during development of the embryo and is the dominant serum protein in early embryonic life. AFP reappears in the adult serum during certain pathological states.

Biochemistry and function

AFP is an albumin analog containing approximately 4% carbohydrate, with a molecular mass of approximately 70 kD. It is a major protein in fetal serum, synthesized primarily by the fetal yolk sac and liver. AFP is visible between albumin and AAT on electrophoresis of fetal or newborn serum.

Clinical significance

Elevated maternal serum or amniotic fluid AFP indicates the possibility of an open neural tube or abdominal wall defect in the fetus. Multiple fetuses, fetal demise, fetomaternal bleeds, and incorrect estimation of gestational age also may elevate maternal serum levels (see Chapter 43). In addition, serum AFP is increased in the presence of many forms of hepatocellular and germ cell carcinomas in children and adults (see Chapter 21).

Maternal serum levels are decreased in pregnant women with fetal trisomy 18 or 21 (see Chapter 43). Rare genetic deficiency of AFP does not appear to carry any clinical consequences.

Alpha$_2$-Macroglobulin

α_2-Macroglobulin (AMG) is a major plasma proteinase inhibitor. Unlike AAT and most other proteinase inhibitors, it is a very large molecule (molecular mass ~725 kD) and does not diffuse from the plasma space into extracellular fluids in significant amounts.

Biochemistry and function

AMG inhibits many different classes of proteinases, including those with serine, cysteine, and metal ions in their proteolytic sites. It is not an APP in human beings. It is synthesized primarily by the hepatic parenchymal cells.

Clinical significance

Increased levels of AMG occur with the effects of estrogen. For example, women of child-bearing age demonstrate higher levels than men of the same age. Levels in infants and children are two to three times adult levels, perhaps as a protective mechanism against increased exposure to intestinal proteases in infancy and bacterial or leukocytic proteases during childhood. Markedly increased levels may be present in individuals with nephrotic syndrome because of plasma volume loss and increased synthesis of all proteins to compensate for protein loss by the kidneys.

Decreased levels of AMG are present in individuals with severe acute pancreatitis and before treatment in individuals with advanced carcinoma of the prostate. Although genetic variants of AMG exist, they have no known clinical significance.

Beta₂-Microglobulin

β_2-Microglobulin (BMG) is a low-molecular-mass (11.8 kD) protein found on the cell surfaces of all nucleated cells.

Biochemistry and function

BMG is the light or β-chain of the human leukocyte antigens (HLAs) and consists of a single polypeptide chain with one intrachain disulfide bridge and no carbohydrate. Some BMG is shed into the plasma, particularly by lymphocytes and tumor cells. The small size of the molecule allows BMG to pass through the glomerular membrane, but normally less than 1% of the filtered BMG is excreted in the urine; the remainder is reabsorbed and catabolized in the proximal tubules of the kidneys.

Clinical significance

High plasma levels of BMG occur in individuals with renal failure, inflammation, and neoplasms, especially those associated with B lymphocytes. The principal clinical value of the BMG assay is to test renal tubular function, particularly in kidney transplant recipients, in whom rejection of the allograft manifests as diminished tubular function, and in cases of questionable heavy metal exposure. Because of the sensitivity of BMG to acid pH, other proteins, such as α_1-microglobulin (A1M) and cystatin C, may be more useful in urine. (Alternatively, urine specimens may be alkalinized.) Serial assays of BMG also are useful to monitor B-cell tumors.

Ceruloplasmin

Ceruloplasmin (Cp) is an α_2-globulin that contains approximately 95% of the total serum copper, giving it a blue color. When Cp levels are significantly elevated (for example, during pregnancy) or the normal yellow pigments of plasma are decreased, such as in active rheumatoid arthritis, plasma may have a greenish tint.

Biochemistry and function

Cp is synthesized primarily by the hepatic parenchymal cells. Copper is added to the peptide chain by an intracellular ATPase that is absent in Wilson's disease. Copper is essential for the normal folding of the polypeptide chain; apoCp is synthesized even in the absence of copper or the ATPase, but most is degraded intracellularly, with only moderate amounts released into circulation.

The primary physiological role of Cp involves plasma reduction and oxidation (redox) reactions. It functions as either an oxidant or antioxidant, depending on factors such as the presence of free ferric ions and ferritin binding sites (see Fig-

ure 19-2). Cp is vitally important in regulating the ionic state of iron in particular, oxidizing Fe^{2+} to Fe^{3+} and thus permitting incorporation of the iron into transferrin without the formation of toxic iron products. Albumin and transcuprein are probably the most important copper transport proteins.

Clinical significance

Cp levels increase as a result of a APR; however, Cp is a weak, late-reacting APP. Levels are increased significantly by estrogens, as in cases of pregnancy and oral contraception.

Individuals with primary genetic deficiency of Cp demonstrate a clinical picture similar to that present in those with hereditary hemochromatosis because of the inability to incorporate iron into transferrin. Deficient individuals have normal tissue copper but increased tissue iron stores and decreased serum iron.

Low plasma Cp levels secondary to a lack of incorporation of Cu^{2+} into the molecule during synthesis are much more common than primary deficiency. Secondary deficiency may be due to (1) dietary copper insufficiency (including malabsorption), (2) inability to release Cu^{2+} from the GI epithelium into the circulation (as in Menkes' disease), or (3) inability to insert Cu^{2+} into the developing Cp molecule (as in Wilson's disease). Levels also may be low in blood loss or GI or renal protein-losing syndromes.

Dietary deficiency, secondary to nutritional copper deficiency, is associated with neutropenia, thrombocytopenia, low serum iron, and hypochromic, normocytic, or microcytic anemia that does not respond to iron therapy.

Wilson's disease, or hepatolenticular degeneration, differs from dietary deficiency in that total body copper is increased markedly and deposited in tissues, including the hepatic parenchymal cells, the brain, and the periphery of the iris (resulting in the characteristic Kayser-Fleischer rings). Symptoms in individuals with Wilson's disease usually begin in the second or third decade of life, but may manifest earlier or later. Mutations that completely destroy gene function may be associated with the onset of liver disease as early as 3 years of age.

In addition to the rare genetic deficiency of Cp mentioned previously, several known variants exist, none of which has known clinical significance.

C-Reactive Protein

A substance present in the sera of acutely ill individuals that is able to bind the C-polysaccharide on the cell wall of *Streptococcus pneumoniae* first was described in 1930. In 1941, it was shown to be a protein and given the name *C-reactive protein (CRP)*. It is one of the first APPs to become elevated in inflammatory disease and also the one exhibiting the most dramatic increases in concentration. It consists of five identical subunits and is synthesized primarily by the liver.

Biochemistry and function

In the presence of Ca^{2+}, CRP protein binds not only the polysaccharides present in many bacteria, fungi, and protozoal parasites but also phosphorylcholine; phosphatidylcholines, such as lecithin; and polyanions, such as nucleic acids. In the absence of Ca^{2+}, CRP binds polycations, such as histones. Once complexed, CRP activates the classic complement pathway starting at C1q. Similar to antibodies, CRP thus initiates opsonization, phagocytosis, and lysis of invading organisms, such as bacteria and viruses. CRP also can recognize potentially toxic autogenous substances released from damaged tissue, bind them, and then detoxify them or clear them from the blood. CRP itself is catabolized after opsonization.

Clinical significance

CRP long has been recognized as one of the most sensitive APPs; levels in plasma usually rise dramatically after myocardial infarction, stress, trauma, infection, inflammation, surgery, or neoplastic proliferation. The increase begins within 6 to 12 hours of the infarction, and the level may reach 2000 times normal. Determination of CRP is clinically useful for (1) screening for organic disease; (2) assessment of the activity of inflammatory disease; (3) detection of intercurrent infections in systemic lupus erythematosus (SLE), in leukemia, or after surgery (secondary rise in plasma level); and (4) management of neonatal septicemia and meningitis, when specimen collections for bacteriological investigations may be difficult. Circulating levels of CRP may constitute an independent risk factor for cardiovascular disease. However, the manner in which CRP is involved in cardiovascular disease is still unclear.

Cord blood normally has low CRP concentrations (1 to 35 μg/dL), but in intrauterine infection, levels may be as high as 26,000 μg/dL. Levels in infancy normally rise for a few days after vaginal delivery, fall to very low levels, and then gradually rise over several weeks to adult levels.

Haptoglobin

Haptoglobin (Hp) is an α_2-glycoprotein that binds hemoglobin (Hb) irreversibly. Hp is synthesized by the liver and composed of four peptide chains linked by disulfide bonds into two pairs, an $(\alpha\beta)_2$ configuration similar to that of Hb. Each Hp 1 monomer binds up to two Hb $\alpha\beta$ dimers, or the equivalent of one intact Hb molecule; the Hp β-chain binds to Hb α-chains.

Biochemistry and function

During extracellular hemolysis, Hb is released from the erythrocytes and the free Hb dimers bind almost immediately to Hp. Hp-Hb complexes are large enough to prevent or greatly reduce renal loss of Hb and its iron. The complexes are removed very rapidly by the hepatic Kuppfer cells, where the proteins are degraded and the iron and amino acids reutilized. In addition, Hp-Hb complexes may be important for the control of local inflammatory processes; the Hp-Hb complex is a potent peroxidase capable of hydrolyzing peroxides released during phagocytosis and killing, by polymorphonuclear leukocytes, at sites of inflammation. Hp is also a natural bacteriostatic agent for iron-requiring bacteria, such as *Escherichia coli*, preventing the utilization of Hb iron by these organisms.

Genetic variants of both the α- and β-chains exist; the commonly recognized polymorphism involves the former. The α^2 chain is almost twice the size of the α^1 chain (142 versus 83 amino acids) and results in the formation of molecules of Hp polymers with high molecular mass.

Clinical significance

Hp levels are increased by corticosteroid hormones and many NSAIDs. Hp, like Cp, is a weak and late-reacting APP. Hp levels are elevated in selective protein-losing syndromes, such as nephrotic syndrome, in individuals with the Hp 2-1 or 2-1 phenotypes. Biliary obstruction in the absence of severe hepatocellular disease is associated with significant lipid alterations and increased Hp levels.

Hp depletion usually is the most sensitive laboratory indicator of hemolysis, followed by hemopexin depletion (or the presence of hemopexin-heme complexes) and by the presence of methemalbuminemia, hemoglobinuria, or both. Under normal circumstances, approximately 1% of circulating red blood cells are removed from the circulation or destroyed intravascularly each day. An increase to only 2% destruction per day will deplete plasma Hp completely in the absence of a stimulus to production, such as acute inflammation or corticosteroid therapy.

Estrogens decrease synthesis of Hp. Most forms of acute or chronic hepatocellular disease, including acute viral hepatitis and cirrhosis with jaundice, are associated with decreased levels of Hp due to altered estrogen metabolism in addition to increased red cell breakdown secondary to erythrocyte membrane lipid alterations. Genetic absence (ahaptoglobinemia) and hypohaptoglobinemia have been reported in many populations, especially in individuals of African descent. However, most reports have originated in populations with high rates of hemolytic disease. True *Hp0* (total deficiency) is rare in most if not all populations. More commonly, genetic hypohaptoglobinemia is associated with very low levels of Hp. In Hp 1-1 individuals, selective protein-losing syndromes (for example, nephrotic syndrome) usually are associated with low levels.

Hp always should be assayed in association with AAG because the other factors—with the exception of protein-losing syndromes—influence the levels of both proteins in parallel. Thus if an individual has a normal Hp level but high AAG level, the possibility of hemolysis plus either corticosteroid therapy or an APR must be considered.

Retinol-Binding Protein

As its name implies, retinol-binding protein (RBP) is a monomeric transport protein for all-*trans* retinol, a form of vitamin A (see Chapter 28).

Biochemistry and function

RBP circulates in plasma as a 1:1 complex with transthyretin (TTR) that migrates anodal to albumin on electrophoresis. The formation of the complex with TTR prevents RBP from being filtered by the renal glomeruli and stabilizes the interaction between retinol and RBP to reduce its release to nontarget cells. At the target cell, uptake of retinol is followed by dissociation of the TTR-RBP complex; apo-RBP (RBP without retinol) then is cleared from the circulation by the kidney. The half-life of RBP is 12 hours. It is synthesized by the liver.

Clinical significance

Serum RBP levels are increased in individuals with proximal tubular damage because of chronic renal disease, diabetic nephropathy, or heavy metal poisoning.

Decreased levels of RBP are associated primarily with APR, liver disease, and protein malnutrition (see Chapters 28 and 45). Zinc deficiency states are characterized by low serum levels of RBP and total vitamin A.

Transferrin

Transferrin (TRF, siderophilin) is the principal plasma transport protein for iron. Although it reversibly binds and transports a number of divalent cations, only iron and copper binding have known clinical significance. TRF accounts for most of the total iron binding capacity (TIBC; see Chapter 30) of plasma; one molecule binds two ferric ions if Cp is present to act as a ferroxidase (Figure 19-2). The

Ferroxidase activity of Cp

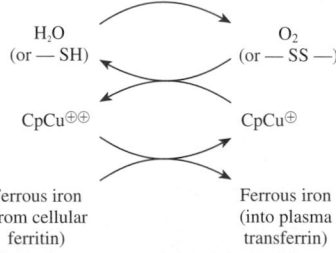

H_2O
(or — SH) O_2
                 (or — SS —)

$CpCu^{\oplus\oplus}$ $CpCu^{\oplus}$

Ferrous iron   Ferrous iron
(from cellular   (into plasma
ferritin)   transferrin)

Figure 19-2 Proposed function of $CpCu^{2+}$ as a proton (hydrogen ion) recipient from cellular ferrous iron. The resulting oxidation of Fe^{2+} to the ferric state permits its binding and transport by plasma TRF. $CpCu^{+}$ is oxidized (regenerated to $CpCu^{2+}$) by reaction with oxygen, oxidized thiol groups, or other oxidizing substances. *CpCu²⁺*, Ceruloplasmin copper. (Modified from Ritchie RF, Navolotskaia O (eds): Serum Proteins in Clinical Medicine. Vol. I. Laboratory Section, pp 13.01-13.03, Scarborough, Maine, Foundation for Blood Research, 1996.)

$TRF-Fe^{3+}$ complex then transports iron to cells for incorporation into cytochromes, Hb, and myoglobin, and to storage sites, such as the liver and reticuloendothelial system. Virtually every cell type has surface receptors for TRF.

Biochemistry and function

TRF is synthesized primarily in the liver and migrates in the area of the β-region on routine clinical electrophoresis of serum. At least 22 genetic variants of TRF have been identified, but only genetic atransferrinemia is biologically significant. Plasma levels are regulated primarily by availability of iron, with plasma levels rising with iron deficiency and falling on successful treatment. As with albumin, about one-half the TRF exists outside the vascular compartment in extracellular fluids, including lymph and CSF.

Clinical significance

Evaluation of plasma TRF levels is useful for the differential diagnosis of anemia and monitoring of treatment of iron deficiency anemia. In cases of iron deficiency the TRF level is increased, but the protein is less saturated with iron. If anemia is due to a failure to incorporate iron into erythrocytes instead of a deficiency of iron, the TRF level may be normal or low but the protein is highly saturated with iron. In iron-overload states, such as hereditary hemochromatosis, TRF concentration is normal, but saturation (normally 30% to 38%) is increased. High levels of TRF are present in pregnancy and during estrogen administration.

TRF is a negative APP, and low levels are present in inflammation or malignancy. Protein energy malnutrition (PEM) is associated with low levels, but PEM is less frequent than inflammatory disease in developed countries. Protein loss, such as in the nephrotic syndrome or protein-losing enteropathies, also causes low levels. In congenital atransferrinemia a very low level of TRF is accompanied by iron overload and severe hypochromic anemia that is resistant to iron therapy.

Many genetic variants of TRF exist; several are associated with altered electrophoretic mobility, which may be confused with a paraprotein (see immunoglobulins). Congenital atransferrinemia, discussed previously, is very rare.

Transthyretin (Prealbumin)

TTR previously was known as *prealbumin* because it electrophoretically migrates ahead of albumin. As discussed previously, TTR circulates in plasma as a 1:1 complex with RBP.

Biochemistry and function

The half-life of TTR is about 48 hours. It is a tetrameric protein that is synthesized by the liver. TTR also is a transport protein; it transports both T_4 and triiodothyronine. Normally, TTR binds about 10% of the thyroid hormones present in plasma.

Clinical significance

Levels of TTR are increased in the presence of a TTR-producing tumor or Hodgkin's disease and by glucocorticosteroid therapy, as well as some nonsteroidal NSAIDs.

Decreased levels of TTR are associated primarily with the APR, liver disease, and protein malnutrition (see Chapters 36 and 45). Low levels of TTR often are used to indicate protein nutritional status; however, levels must be interpreted carefully because the APR is much more common than PEM in developed countries.

A number of genetic variants of TTR have been described, some of which are associated with increased (familial euthyroid hyperthyroxinemia) or decreased T_3 and T_4 binding. Several variants are associated with extracellular deposition of amyloid fibrils in various tissues. These autosomal dominant hereditary amyloidoses include amyloidotic cardiomyopathy, familial amyloidotic polyneuropathy, and senile systemic amyloidosis.

■ COMPLEMENT PROTEINS

The **complement** system consists of at least 20 proteins in blood and tissue fluids. They interact sequentially with antigen-antibody (Ag-Ab) complexes, with one another, and with cell membranes in a complex but adaptable way to destroy viruses and bacteria and, pathologically, even the host's own cells. Complement proteins are divided into the following five groups by function:

1. The classic pathway, which includes C1, C4, C2, and C3 (in order of activation)
2. The alternative pathway, which includes C3, factors B and D, and properdin
3. The membrane attack complex, which includes C5 through C9
4. Inhibitors and inactivators of the previously mentioned pathways, including C1 inhibitor, factors H and I, and C4 binding protein, or C4bp
5. Cellular receptors for activated or cell-bound components

The classic pathway is activated primarily by Ab-Ag complexes or complexing of bacteria or other ligands with CRP, whereas the alternative pathway is activated by bacterial lipopolysaccharides, cellular proteases, and cobra venom. Activation of the classic pathway through C3 also activates the alternative pathway, which then amplifies the production of effector molecules. Other mechanisms also may activate the complement system, including the action of proteases released by leukocytes and other inflammatory cells. The common step involved is the activation of C3 to C3b.

During activation, many complement components are cleaved enzymatically into two fragments—in general one larger fragment that binds to various surfaces, such as bacterial membranes, plus a smaller fragment that may become active in chemotaxis and vascular permeability. The larger fragments are designated by a lowercase *b* and the smaller ones by a lowercase *a*. The larger fragments usually contain a binding site for cell membranes and immune complexes, plus in many cases an enzymatic site that then activates the next component(s). Thus the active, cell-bound fragment of C3 is C3b, whereas the anaphylotoxic peptide C3a is released into the surrounding fluid. Inactivated fragments are designated by the letter *i* (for example, C3bi).

The sequential activation of either the classic or the alternative pathway, with or without complete activation of the membrane attack complex, produces biological effector molecules that initiate inflammation and facilitate the elimination of antigens either by lysis (for example, bacteria) or phagocytosis (for example, immune complexes). Thus the complement system is one of the major mediators of inflammation. Secondary edema and stasis permit the passage of further antibody, complement, and phagocytes into the extravascular space, which helps kill and remove infectious agents and immune complexes.

Biochemistry and Function

The complement components are synthesized primarily by the liver, although small amounts probably are synthesized by monocytes and other cell types. The clinical importance of the complement system is demonstrated by the disease associations present in inherited or secondary deficiencies of the various components. Most complement components also demonstrate genetic polymorphism. C1, C1 inhibitor, C3, C3 proactivator (factor B), and C4 are the components most often measured for clinical purposes because their levels are important in relatively common disease states, and assays are available readily.

Clinical Significance

Several complement proteins, notably C3 and C4, are increased in number after an APR; however, they are weak and late-reacting APPs. Levels of C3 and C4 also are elevated in biliary obstruction.

Both genetic variants and deficiencies of nearly all complement components have been described. For example, genetic deficiency of C2 and C4 typically is associated with autoimmune, immune-complex diseases such as SLE, polymyositis, and glomerulonephritis. In contrast, deficiency of C3 (or its inhibitors) is associated with infection, often severe, particularly with encapsulated bacteria. Deficiency of any of the membrane-complex components (C5 through C9) may be associated with recurrent, persistent, and/or severe neisserial infections. Deficiency of C1 inhibitor results in hereditary angioedema (HAE), with continuous activity of C1 and thus of C2 and C4. HAE is characterized by recurrent attacks of subcutaneous, laryngeal, bronchial, and GI edema, which may be life-threatening. Decreased C4 levels have been used to screen for the disorder; if C1 inhibitor levels are normal in individuals with clinical symptoms and decreased C4, functional assays should be performed.

Secondarily decreased levels of any component may occur as a result of consumption. The classic examples of this are depletion of C4 in HAE and of C3 and C4 in acute poststreptococcal glomerulonephritis.

In diseases such as SLE and other disorders associated with formation of immune complexes, differentiation of genetic and secondary deficiency may require family studies, phenotyping, DNA analysis, or combinations of these.

■ IMMUNOGLOBULINS

Immunoglobulins, or humoral antibodies, recognize foreign antigens, such as those from bacteria or viruses, and initiate mechanisms to destroy them. The ability to recognize the enormous variety of antigens is accomplished by an unusual degree of structural heterogeneity based on gene rearrangement (see Chapter 11). The heterogeneity is illustrated by the diffuse bands seen on electrophoresis, particularly for IgG. Immunoglobulins are synthesized and secreted by plasma cells, which are derived from B-lymphocytes (Table 19-4).

All immunoglobulin molecules consist of basic units built of two identical heavy (H) chains and two identical light (L)

chains (see Chapter 10). Each of the four chains has a variable and constant region, with the variable region involved in antigen recognition and binding. The amino acid sequences of the variable regions (Fab "fragment") determine the antigenic specificity of the particular antibody molecules. The remainder of the molecule, the constant part, is the same for every immunoglobulin molecule of a given subclass and carries the effector sites.

Immunoglobulin Classes

The constant portions of the heavy chains (Fc) contain the sites that interact with cells and with complement. Variations in the Fc fragment are responsible for the classes and subclasses into which immunoglobulins are grouped: IgM, IgG with four subclasses, IgA with two subclasses, IgD, and IgE. (Their respective heavy chains are called μ, γ, α, δ, and ε.)

Immunoglobulin G

The major immunoglobulin produced by plasma cells is immunoglobulin G (IgG), which accounts for 70% to 75% of the total immunoglobulins. Its major functions are neutralization of toxins and destruction or removal of infectious agents, which it accomplishes by initiating either phagocytosis or the complement cascade. IgG antibodies are produced in response to most bacteria and viruses.

IgG has a molecular mass of 160 kD and less than 3% carbohydrate. On cellulose acetate or agarose gel electro-

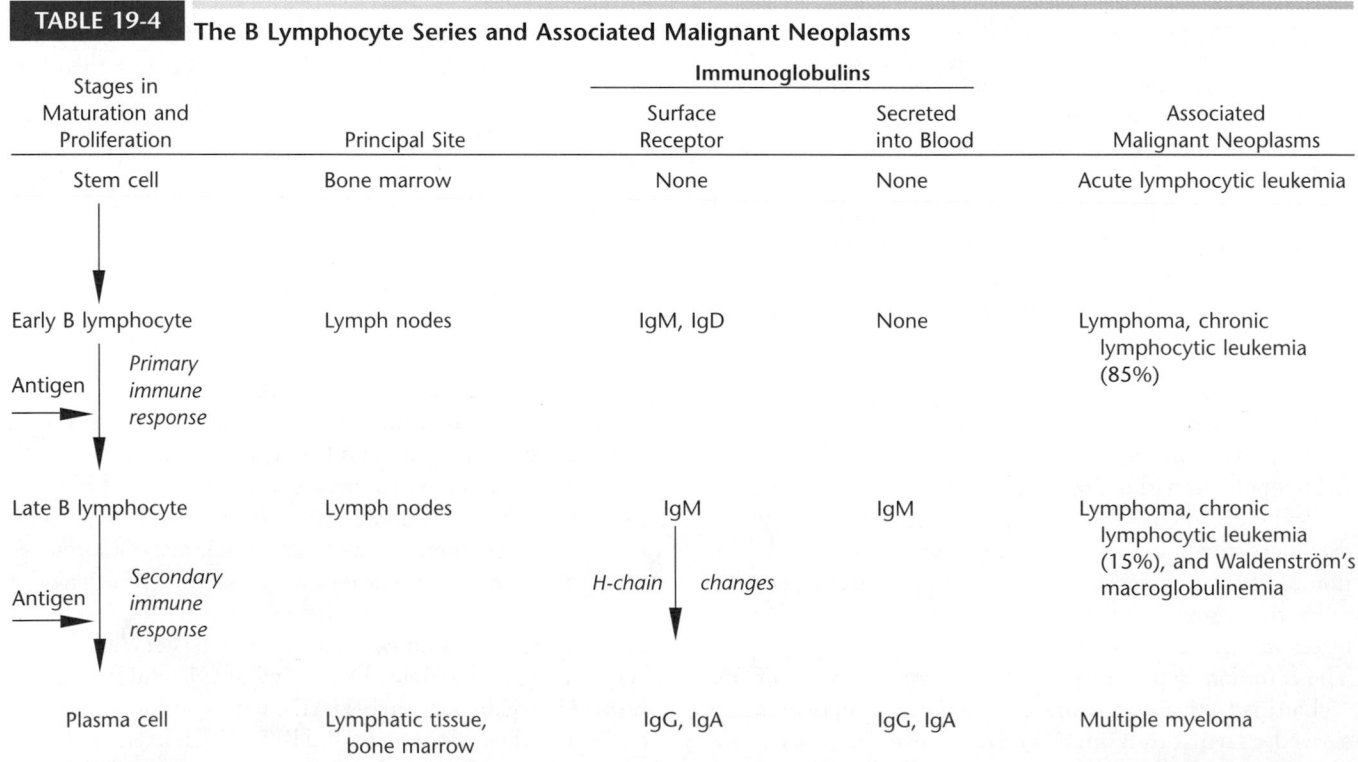

TABLE 19-4 **The B Lymphocyte Series and Associated Malignant Neoplasms**

Stages in Maturation and Proliferation	Principal Site	Immunoglobulins		Associated Malignant Neoplasms
		Surface Receptor	Secreted into Blood	
Stem cell	Bone marrow	None	None	Acute lymphocytic leukemia
Early B lymphocyte	Lymph nodes	IgM, IgD	None	Lymphoma, chronic lymphocytic leukemia (85%)
Late B lymphocyte	Lymph nodes	IgM	IgM	Lymphoma, chronic lymphocytic leukemia (15%), and Waldenström's macroglobulinemia
Plasma cell	Lymphatic tissue, bone marrow	IgG, IgA	IgG, IgA	Multiple myeloma

IgM, IgD, IgG, IgA, Immunoglobulins M, D, G, and A.

phoresis, most IgG migrates in the γ- and slow-β-regions; the heterogeneity of the IgG antibody molecules synthesized by different plasma cells causes the region to stain diffusely. The broad response to various antigens is called a *polyclonal response.*

IgG has four subclasses (IgG$_1$, IgG$_2$, IgG$_3$, and IgG$_4$) that differ primarily in the hinge region. IgG$_1$ and IgG$_3$ bind firmly to the Fc receptors of phagocytic cells, activate killer monocytes (K cells), and cross the placenta by an active transport process dependent on Fc binding. IgG$_1$ is the principal IgG to cross the placenta and protect neonates for the first 3 months of postnatal life (Figure 19-3). The half-lives of IgG$_1$, IgG$_2$, and IgG$_4$ are about 22 days. The half-life of IgG$_3$ is 7 days.

Immunoglobulin M

Immunoglobulin M (IgM) is the most primitive and least specialized immunoglobulin and the only one that a neonate normally synthesizes. In adult serum, it is the third most abundant immunoglobulin, accounting for 5% to 10% of the total circulating immunoglobulins. IgM as a membrane receptor molecule is monomeric, but most of the serum IgM is a pentamer (five monomers joined by J chains); each monomer is similar to the IgG molecule. Its large size (900 kD) prevents IgM's passage into extravascular spaces. B lymphocytes have IgM surface receptors and secrete IgM in the first, or primary, response to an antigen. The lymphocytes later switch heavy chain types, but the variable regions remain unchanged. As the cells change into plasma cells, a second dose of the same antigen causes a larger, or secondary, response primarily of IgG. IgM continues to be synthesized against antigens confined to the blood, such as erythrocyte surface antigens (for example, the naturally-occurring anti-A and -B hemagglutinins and tropical parasites). IgM is an efficient complement activator, the Fc chains being spaced at the correct distance to match the C1q binding sites.

IgM is not transported across the placenta and therefore is not involved in hemolytic disease of neonates. IgM present in umbilical cord serum and in neonates is synthesized by the newborn; levels of more than 25 mg/dL suggest the possibility of intrauterine infection but are not diagnostic of that condition.

Immunoglobulin A

Immunoglobulin A (IgA) contains 10% carbohydrate and has a molecular mass of 160 kD and a half-life of 6 days. Approximately 10% to 15% of serum immunoglobulin is IgA. In its monomeric form the structure of IgA is similar to that of IgG, but 10% to 15% of IgA in serum is polymeric, particularly IgA$_2$, which is more resistant to destruction by some pathogenic bacteria than IgA$_1$. On electrophoresis, IgA migrates in the β-γ region, anodal to most of the IgG.

Another and possibly more important form of IgA is called *secretory IgA,* found in tears, sweat, saliva, milk, colostrum, and GI and bronchial secretions. Secretory IgA has a molecular mass of 380 kD and consists of two molecules of IgA, a secretory component with a molecular mass of 70 kD and a J chain of 15.6 kD. It is synthesized mainly by plasma cells in the mucous membranes of the gut and bronchi and in the ductules of the lactating breast. The secretory component makes IgA more resistant to proteolytic enzymes, allowing it to protect the mucosa from bacteria and viruses. Its presence in colostrum and milk probably protects neonates from intestinal infections. IgA activates complement by the alternative pathway, but the exact role of IgA in serum is unclear.

Immunoglobulin D

Immunoglobulin D (IgD) accounts for less than 1% of serum immunoglobulins. It is monomeric, contains about 12% carbohydrate, and has a molecular mass of 184 kD. Its structure is similar to that of IgG. Like IgM, IgD is a surface re-

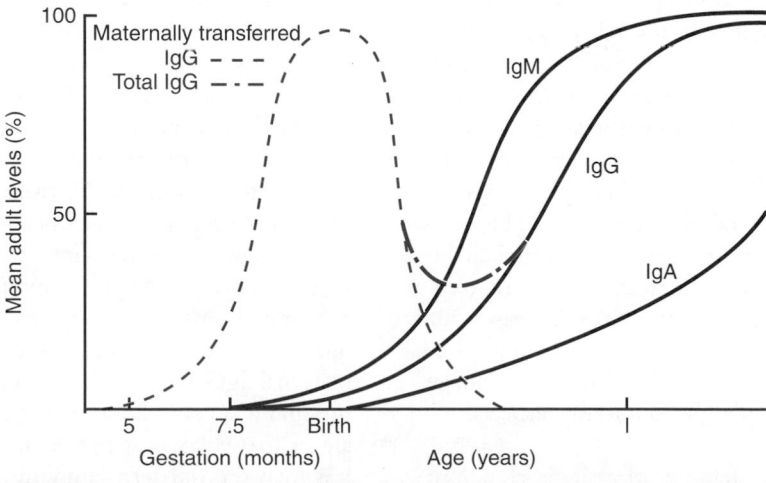

Figure 19-3   Serum immunoglobulin levels as percent of adult levels before birth and for the first year of life. *IgM, IgG, IgA,* Immunoglobulins M, G, and A.

ceptor for antigen on B lymphocytes, but its primary function is unknown.

Immunoglobulin E

Immunoglobulin E (IgE) is bound so rapidly and firmly to mast cells that only trace amounts of it normally are present in serum. IgE contains 15% carbohydrate and has a molecular mass of 188 kD; its structure is similar to that of IgG. IgE is attached to mast cells through binding sites on its Fc regions. When antigen (allergen) cross-links two of the attached IgE molecules, the mast cell is stimulated to release histamine and other vasoactive amines. These vasoactive amines are responsible for the vascular permeability and smooth muscle contraction that accompany such allergic reactions as hay fever, asthma, urticaria, and eczema.

Clinical Significance

A change in immunoglobulins levels in disease states may be a decrease or an increase in the normal polyclonal mixture of serum immunoglobulins or an increase in one or more monoclonal idiotypes (in multiple myeloma usually one, rarely two).

Increased levels

Elevated levels of immunoglobulins may be (1) polyclonal (a diffuse mixture of antibodies), (2) monoclonal (a single class, subclass, and idiotype, produced by a single clone of plasma cells or B lymphocytes), or (3) oligoclonal (a few to several "monoclonal" proteins of different specificities). Typically, clinical samples contain a polyclonal mixture of antibodies. Polyclonal increases are present in recurrent or chronic infection, autoimmune disease (for example, rheumatoid arthritis or SLE), hepatocellular disease, or parasitic infestations. In these cases a diffuse band is present on serum electrophoresis. IgG tends to predominate in autoimmune responses; IgA in skin, gut, respiratory, and renal infections; and IgM in primary viral infections and bloodstream infections, such as malaria. Chronic bacterial infections cause an increase in serum levels of all immunoglobulins. In such cases, estimations of the individual immunoglobulins seldom provide more information than protein electrophoresis. These estimations are valuable, however, in the differential diagnosis of liver disease and intrauterine infections. In primary biliary cirrhosis the IgM level is markedly increased; in chronic active hepatitis, IgG and sometimes IgM are increased; and in portal cirrhosis, IgA and sometimes IgG are increased. In intrauterine infections, production of IgM by the fetus increases, and at birth the IgM level in umbilical cord blood is increased. Estimations of IgE are used in the diagnosis and management of asthma and other allergic conditions, especially in children.

Benign or malignant proliferation of a single clone produces a high concentration of a single idiotype (a monoclonal antibody) that may appear as a single, sharp, narrow band on protein electrophoresis. Less commonly, malignant proliferation may occur in two or more clones, giving rise to additional bands.

If a few clones proliferate in response to infection, autoimmune disease, or bone marrow transplantation, oligoclonal banding is present; this banding is also the case on electrophoresis of CSF in demyelinating diseases, such as multiple sclerosis (see discussion of CSF proteins in this chapter).

Immunodeficiency

Immune defense depends on the following four complex, interactive systems:

1. Humoral antibodies (immunoglobulins)
2. Cell-mediated immunity of the T lymphocytes
3. The phagocytic system
4. The complement system

The latter two systems are nonspecific in that they have no immunological memory for antigen. Only the first and fourth systems are composed of plasma proteins. **Immunodeficiency** states characterized by recurrent infections may be the result of a defect in any one of these systems, or combinations thereof. Table 19-5 summarizes some causes and effects of immunoglobulin deficiency.

Marked reduction or absence of the γ-band on electrophoresis indicates deficiency of IgG antibodies. IgG deficiency may be secondary to protein loss or transient failure of synthesis; it also may be due to a primary congenital disorder. The diagnosis of a deficiency state is important because it dictates the need for replacement therapy with IgG. However, the presence of a normal-appearing γ-band on protein electrophoresis—and even a normal level of IgG—does not rule out immunoglobulin deficiency. Some deficiencies involve only one or two immunoglobulin classes or subclasses; if the total immunoglobulin level is not affected significantly, these deficiencies may not be obvious. Furthermore, some clinically immunodeficient individuals have normal IgG levels, but active antibodies are not synthesized in response to some or all antigens.

Physiological immunodeficiency, normally present in infants at 2 to 5 months of age, is a risk factor for infection. Figure 19-3 indicates how levels of maternal IgG, transferred across the placenta, rise in a fetus during the last 3 months of pregnancy, then begin to fall after birth. Contact of the infant with environmental antigens after birth causes B lymphocytes to begin to multiply, IgM levels to start to rise, and plasma cells producing IgG and IgA to increase in number. These developments are paralleled by a decrease of maternal IgG so that in the infant's blood, IgG falls to a minimum at about 3 months of age. Two groups of neonates are at particular risk: premature newborns, who start with less than the full-term amount of maternal IgG, and newborns in whom initiation of IgG synthesis is delayed tran-

TABLE 19-5   Causes of Immunoglobulin Deficiency

Secondary Causes (Common)

DEFECTIVE SYNTHESIS (IgM FALLING FIRST, THEN IgA, FINALLY IgG)

Lymphoid malignancy, multiple myeloma, lymphoma, chronic lymphocytic leukemia

Toxic reaction (for example, renal failure, diabetes mellitus)

Drugs (for example, phenytoin, penicillamine)

In neonates only: prematurity, transient delay in initiation of synthesis

ABNORMAL LOSS OF PROTEINS

Nephrotic syndrome, burns, protein-losing enteropathy

Primary or Inherited Causes (Rare)

FAILURE OF ANTIBODY PRODUCTION

GENERALIZED (SEVERE PYOGENIC INFECTIONS)

Infantile X-linked Bruton's type

Acquired, variable, unclassifiable, occurring at any age

SELECTIVE IMMUNOGLOBULIN DEFICIENCY

IgA: most common (1:700); symptomless but often present in individuals with allergic or autoimmune disease

IgG and IgA (IgM increased): recurrent pyogenic infections

IgA and IgM: giardiasis common

IgG: Recurrent pyogenic infections

IgM: Susceptibility to autoimmune disease and to septicemia after splenectomy

COMBINED FAILURE OF ANTIBODY- AND CELL-MEDIATED IMMUNITY

Severe combined immunodeficiency; Swiss and sex-linked types; death in infancy from fungal or viral infections

Associated with thymoma, achondroplasia, or thrombocytopenia and eczema (Wiskott-Aldrich syndrome)

IgA, IgG, IgM, Immunoglobulins A, G, and M.

---

siently. IgG determinations are invaluable in these cases because levels may become dangerously low if the newborn is not treated. Rising IgM and normal salivary IgA concentrations at 6 weeks of age suggest a favorable prognosis.

Monoclonal immunoglobulins (paraproteins)

A single clone of plasma cells produces immunoglobulin molecules with identical structures because of gene rearrangement. If the clone multiplies malignantly, as it does in cases of multiple myeloma or Waldenström's macroglobulinemia, the serum concentration of its particular protein may become so great that it produces a narrow, sharply discrete spike on electrophoresis. These monoclonal immunoglobulins, which are also called **paraproteins** or myeloma components (MCs), may be polymers, monomers, or fragments of immunoglobulin molecules; if they are fragments, they are usually light chains (**Bence-Jones proteins,** in urine) or, rarely, heavy chains or half-molecules; either intact immunoglobulins, chains, or fragments may be polymerized. About 60% of MCs result from multiple myeloma or to a solitary plasmacytoma; about 15% result from

overproduction of B lymphocytes (hematopoietic neoplasms), mainly in lymph nodes, lymphomas, chronic lymphocytic leukemia, Waldenström's macroglobulinemia, or (rarely) heavy-chain disease. Up to 25% of MCs are benign, and many never are discovered. However, such individuals must be monitored because of the possible later development of malignancy.

Multiple myeloma

Multiple myeloma is a malignant neoplasm of a single clone of plasma cells producing any MC other than IgM. The plasma cells most often proliferate diffusely throughout the marrow, but occasionally they form a solitary tumor called a *plasmacytoma.* Osteolytic bone lesions are produced, and the other bone marrow cells are reduced so that thrombocytopenia, anemia, and leukopenia develop. At the same time, development of normal clones of plasma cells is inhibited; consequently, synthesis of the other immunoglobulins is reduced, and recurrent infections may be seen. The incidence of multiple myeloma is low in individuals younger than 60 years of age but rises rapidly with age. Individuals may demonstrate local symptoms of a bone lesion but more often nonspecific symptoms, such as weight loss, obscure anemia, hemorrhage, repeated infections, or renal failure. A highly suggestive laboratory finding is a normal serum alkaline phosphatase level in an individual with destructive bone lesions. Cardinal diagnostic features of the disease include neoplastic plasma cells in bone marrow aspirate, radiological demonstration of osteolytic lesions, and identification of an MC in serum or in concentrated urine. All individuals who conceivably could have the disease should be screened for MCs because less than 1% of those with the disease fail to have detectable MCs. Table 19-6 lists the MCs that may be associated with multiple myeloma and some characteristic findings for them.

Lymphoid tumors

Lymphoid tumors, presenting as lymphomas or chronic lymphocytic leukemias, arise from less mature stages in B–lymphocyte development; about one in five produces an MC, usually of the IgM class.

Waldenström's macroglobulinemia

Waldenström's macroglobulinemia arises from mature B lymphocytes producing an IgM MC. It is the presence of this very-high-molecular-mass protein that produces the most salient symptom of the disease—an increase in viscosity of the blood. Bence-Jones proteinuria occurs in 80% of these cases, but the condition is much less malignant than multiple myeloma. The lymph nodes and spleen are enlarged, but the lymphoid infiltration is slow growing and symptoms are treatable by exchange transfusion. In rare cases, unusual forms of IgG, IgA, or light chains polymerize and cause a similar syndrome of high blood viscosity.

TABLE 19-6	Monoclonal Immunoglobulins (Paraproteins or MCs) in Multiple Myeloma			
Plasma Paraprotein or MC	Incidence* (%)	Age of Occurrence* (Mean) in Years	Incidence of Bence-Jones Proteinuria (%)	Comments
IgG	50	65	60	Are more susceptible to immunodeficiency; reach their highest levels
IgA	25	65	70	Tend to have hypercalcemia and amyloidosis
Bence-Jones (free light chains) only	20	56	100	Often experience renal failure; bone lesions; amyloidosis; poor prognosis
IgD	2	57	100	90% λ-type; often have extraosseous lesion, amyloidosis, renal failure; 50% with enlarged lymph nodes, liver, spleen; poor prognosis
IgM	1	—	100	May or may not have hyperviscosity syndrome
IgE	0.1	—	Most	—
Biclonal	1	—	—	—
None detected	<1	—	0	Usually experience a reduction of normal immunoglobulins

IgG, IgA, IgD, IgM, IgE, Immunoglobulins G, A, D, M, and E; *MC,* myeloma component.
*Approximate; incidence is the percentage of all MCs or paraproteins.

Heavy-chain diseases

Heavy-chain diseases are rare conditions, also associated with lymphoid infiltration, in which the MC consists only of a heavy chain, usually incomplete. The most common is α-chain disease, in which the intestine is infiltrated and a severe malabsorption syndrome produced. In addition, γ-chain disease and μ-chain disease also occur.

Cryoglobulinemia and amyloid disease

Cryoglobulinemia and amyloid disease sometimes are characterized by MCs. A cryoglobulin is a serum protein that precipitates at temperatures lower than body temperature. Individuals may develop peripheral thrombosis in cold weather. Most cryoglobulins are polyclonal immunoglobulin complexes, but many are monoclonal, usually IgM. For cryoglobulin examination a temperature of 37 °C must be maintained for blood collection and serum separation and storage to keep the cryoglobulin from precipitating from the serum. Amyloid disease is characterized by deposits of insoluble fibrillar protein complexes in various tissues; with special staining the deposits are visible easily in biopsy sections. Some deposits contain fragments of light chains, especially from the variable region. Amyloid deposits also may occur in multiple myeloma.

■ PROTEINS IN OTHER BODY FLUIDS

In addition to plasma, proteins are found in several other body fluids and tissue including urine, CSF, amniotic fluid, saliva, and feces.

Urinary Proteins
Biochemistry and function

The glomerular basement membrane (GBM) acts as an ultrafilter for plasma proteins. The degree to which individual proteins pass through the membrane is a function of (1) molecular size, (2) net ionic charge, (3) plasma concentration, and (4) reabsorption by the renal tubules. In general, transport of protein molecules through the glomerular membrane is inversely related to size and net negative charge. Normally, high-molecular-mass proteins such as IgM (molecular mass = 900 kD) are present in glomerular filtrate in trace amounts only. Relatively small yet significant amounts of albumin (molecular mass = 66 kD) are passed into the filtrate as a result of its high plasma concentration and relatively low molecular mass. Proteins with molecular masses of 15 to 40 kD filter more readily but in lesser quantities because of their low plasma concentrations.

The amount of a given protein in excreted urine depends on the extent of its reabsorption by the renal tubules, which also is inversely related to molecular size. Small proteins, such as BMG and A1M are reabsorbed almost completely if tubular function is normal.

Only a small amount of protein is present in normal excreted urine (20 to 150 mg/day), and most of it is albumin. The remainder is almost entirely the Tamm-Horsfall protein uromucoid, probably secreted by the distal tubules. Increased permeability of the GBM is signaled first by increased amounts of albumin in the urine. Loss of normal selectivity, or sieving, is demonstrated by the appearance in urine of proteins with increasingly greater molecular mass. Diminished or diminishing tubular reabsorption is suggested by increasing concentrations of low-molecular-mass proteins in urine (see Chapter 34).

Clinical significance

Proteinuria is defined as an increase in the amounts of protein in urine. Types include glomerular, tubular, overload, and postrenal proteinuria. (See Chapter 34 for a detailed discussion of each type of proteinuria.)

Glomerular proteinuria

Glomerular proteinuria is the most common and serious type of abnormal proteinuria. Because most of the excreted protein is albumin, glomerular proteinuria often is labeled *albuminuria*. Individuals routinely are screened for this disorder with a simple dipstick test for albumin. If the dipstick test result is negative, clinically significant glomerular proteinuria is precluded. If the test result is positive, further investigation, such as a quantitative evaluation of protein excretion, is indicated.

Tubular proteinuria

Tubular proteinuria is characterized by the appearance of low-molecular-mass proteins in the urine because of their defective reabsorption by the proximal renal tubules. It may occur alone (for example, in heavy metal poisoning) but is associated more commonly with glomerular proteinuria. When tubular proteinuria occurs alone, albumin excretion is increased only slightly, not enough to give a positive dipstick reaction. More specific tests are required to detect simple tubular proteinuria or identify it in the presence of glomerular proteinuria.

Overload proteinuria

Overload proteinuria includes hemoglobinuria, myoglobinuria, and Bence-Jones proteinuria, which is caused by high plasma concentrations of immunoglobulin light-chains (for example, in multiple myeloma). None of these proteins are detected by most urine dipsticks, which are designed to detect albumin. Detection of light chains depends on electrophoretic and immunochemical testing. Hb or myoglobin is detected by immunochemical or functional tests.

Postrenal proteinuria

Postrenal proteinuria refers to protein arising from the urinary tract below the kidneys and usually is caused by inflammation, bleeding, or malignancy. It is diagnosed by microscopic examination of the urinary sediment for inflammatory, blood, or malignant cells.

Proteins in Cerebrospinal Fluid

CSF is a clear, colorless fluid that contains small quantities of glucose and protein. As described in Chapter 2, CSF for laboratory testing normally is obtained from the lumbar region.

Biochemistry and function

CSF is the fluid synthesized and contained within the four ventricles of the brain and the subarachnoid space. More than 80% of CSF protein originates from plasma by ultrafiltration through the walls of capillaries in the meninges and choroid plexuses; the remainder results from intrathecal synthesis. The lowest concentration of total protein and the smallest proportion of the larger protein molecules are in the ventricular fluid. As the CSF passes down to the lumbar spine, the protein concentration increases.

Because CSF is mainly an ultrafiltrate of plasma, relatively low-molecular-mass plasma proteins, such as albumin, TRF, and TTR are the proteins normally found in it. No protein with a molecular mass greater than that of IgG is present in sufficient concentration to be visible on electrophoresis. The electrophoretic pattern of normal CSF after concentration of the fluid has a prominent TTR band and two TRF bands. The second (more cathodal) of the TRF bands is called the τ (tau) band; it is produced or transformed intrathecally and is deficient in sialic acid content.

Clinical significance

The total protein and specific protein content of CSF is measured to detect either increased permeability of the blood-CSF barrier to plasma proteins or increased intrathecal synthesis of immunoglobulins. Total CSF protein levels are increased in many diseases (Table 19-7).

Proteins in Amniotic Fluid, Saliva, and Feces

Amniotic fluid is analyzed for AFP and other analytes in antenatal screening for fetal defects (see Chapter 43). Saliva is tested for secretory IgA in evaluation of possible immunological deficiency and for BMG in Sjogren's syndrome. Assay of feces for AAT is used sometimes in the diagnosis of exudative enteropathy; unlike other plasma proteins, AAT is resistant to proteolytic hydrolysis in the gut. Stool AAT values exceeding 54 mg/L indicate abnormal intestinal absorption.

Pathological accumulations of fluid in the peritoneal and pleural cavities or elsewhere vary greatly in protein content; they may be ultrafiltrates with low protein concentrations and very low amounts of high-molecular-mass proteins or serous fluids with high protein concentrations and significant amounts of large proteins, such as immunoglobulins. These fluids are divided arbitrarily according to their protein concentrations into transudates, with total protein less than 3 g/dL, and exudates, with total protein concentrations more than 3 g/dL. Transudates ordinarily reflect changes in permeability of filtering membranes, whereas exudates usually result from infection or malignancy; the latter may contain large numbers of leukocytes or malignant cells.

TABLE 19-7 CSF Protein in Various Diseases		
Clinical Condition	Appearance and Cells $\times 10^6$/L	Total Protein (mg/dL)
Normal	Clear, colorless; 0 to 5 lymphocytes	15 to 45*
Increased Admixture of Proteins from Blood		
INCREASED CAPILLARY PERMEABILITY		
Bacterial meningitis	Turbid, opalescent, purulent; usually >500 polymorphs	80 to 500
Cryptococcal meningitis	Clear or turbid; 50 to 150 polymorphs or lymphocytes	25 to 200
Leptospiral meningitis	Clear to slight haze; polymorphs early, then 5 to 100 lymphocytes	50 to 100
Viral meningitis	Clear or slight haze, colorless; usually up to 500 lymphocytes	30 to 100
Encephalitis	Clear or slight haze, colorless; usually up to 500 lymphocytes	15 to 100
Poliomyelitis	Clear, colorless; up to 500 lymphocytes	10 to 300
Brain tumor	Usually clear; 0 to 80 lymphocytes	15 to 200 (usually normal)
MECHANICAL OBSTRUCTION		
Spinal cord tumor†	Clear, colorless, or yellow	100 to 2000
HEMORRHAGE		
Cerebral hemorrhage	Colorless, yellow, or bloody; blood cells	30 to 150
Local Immunoglobulin Production		
Neurosyphilis	Clear, colorless; 10 to 100 lymphocytes	50 to 150
Multiple sclerosis‡	Clear, colorless; 0 to 10 lymphocytes	25 to 50
Both Increased Capillary Permeability and Local Immunoglobulin Production		
Tuberculous meningitis	Colorless, fibrin clot, or slightly turbid; 50 to 500 lymphocytes	50 to 300 (occasionally up to 1000)
Brain abscess	Clear or slightly turbid	20 to 120
After Myelography (Inflammatory Reaction)		Slight increase

CSF, Cerebrospinal fluid.
*Premature infant: up to 400 mg/dL; children: 30 to 100 mg/dL; old age: up to 60 mg/dL.
†Froin's syndrome: lumbar fluid values are much higher than cisternal fluid values.
‡Similar values may occur in certain other chronic inflammatory conditions of the nervous system.

■ MISCELLANEOUS PROTEINS

In addition to the proteins discussed previously, other proteins, such as amyloid and heat-shock proteins, are found in body tissues and fluids.

Amyloid

Amyloid (Greek for "resembling starch") is a pathological extracellular deposit associated with a group of disorders collectively called *amyloidosis*. The deposits exert pressure on vital organs and eventually cause death. All types of amyloid bind Congo red, which emits an apple-green fluorescence under polarized light.

Clinically, amyloidosis is classified into the following five main groups:

1. Primary amyloidosis
2. Amyloidosis associated with multiple myeloma
3. Secondary amyloidosis associated with inflammatory or infectious diseases
4. Amyloidosis associated with aging
5. Familial amyloidosis

The first two types are characterized by bone marrow plasmacytosis and excess plasma cell production of antigenically identical monoclonal light chains and are collectively known as *AL amyloidosis*.

Secondary amyloidosis is associated with amyloid A (AA) deposits and is called *AA amyloidosis*. AA proteins are amino-terminal fragments of serum amyloid A protein (SAA), which circulates as a molecule of 220 to 235 kD, complexed mostly to high-density lipoprotein. SAA is an acute phase protein, increasing rapidly in infections or noninfectious inflammation. AA amyloidosis often is associated with chronic noninfectious inflammatory diseases, such as rheumatoid arthritis (incidence up to 20%) and other inflammatory joint diseases, as well as chronic suppurative and granulomatous infections, such as tuberculosis and osteomyelitis, and nonlymphoid tumors, such as renal and gastric carcinomas and Hodgkin's lymphoma. Deposits of AA protein are found most often in the kidneys, liver, and spleen and usually cause a nephrotic syndrome and hepatosplenomegaly.

Senile amyloid protein is found most often in the heart (senile cardiac amyloid) but also in the pancreas and brain (referred to as *amyloid plaque*). Nodular or infiltrative amyloid deposits also may be present in the skin, lungs, trachea, and endocrine organs, such as the pancreas (in long-standing diabetes) or thyroid (in medullary carcinoma). These forms usually are asymptomatic, except for the cardiac form.

Heat-Shock Proteins

When exposed to heat shock or other types of stress, a large number of prokaryotic and eukaryotic cells synthesize a family of proteins called *heat-shock proteins*. These proteins form complexes with many other proteins, and a wide variety of physiological and molecular functions have been postulated for them. For example, heat-shock proteins function as "molecular chaperones" in the synthesis and release of other proteins.

■ ANALYSIS OF PROTEINS

Methods used to analyze proteins in body fluids include the following:

1. Specific quantitative assays of particular proteins by immunochemical methods (see Chapter 10) with the use of specific antisera and measurement of the Ag-Ab complexes by nephelometry, turbidimetry, radial immunodiffusion (RID), or electroimmunoassay; or, if present in very low concentrations, by radioimmunoassay (RIA) or enzyme immunoassay (EIA)
2. Detection and identification of proteins by electrophoresis (see Chapter 7)
3. Quantitative measurements of total protein in serum, urine, and CSF
4. Analysis by mass spectrometry, which provides structural and quantitative information (see Chapter 8)

Quantitative Immunochemical Methods

Immunochemical methods generally are applicable for the measurement of any protein discussed in this chapter (see Chapter 10). Because of their speed and ease, nephelometric and turbidimetric methods are used most widely. These techniques are performed by measurement of the amount of Ag-Ab complex formation at either the endpoint (equilibrium methods) or at a timed interval, or by measurement of the rate of complex formation (kinetic methods). Turbidimetry and nephelometry at timed intervals are also efficient methods for assaying of large numbers of samples and are performed in many routine chemis-

try analyzers (see Chapter 4). Lipemic sera should not be assayed by these methods because of the extreme light scattering by the lipid particles in the samples. These sera must be centrifuged in a high-speed centrifuge to separate liquids and obtain clear sera before assay. Test tubes containing samples, controls, and calibrator must remain covered during assay to prevent dust and dirt particle contamination. The reaction cells also must remain covered during the assay and when they are stored. Dust particles and other particulate matter in the reaction mixture result in extraneous light-scattering signals and lead to erroneous results.

Specimen collection and storage

Test specimens for immunochemical methods must be non-hemolyzed, cell-free serum, urine, or CSF. CSF specimens are collected by a physician and need no additional processing except for centrifugation if cells are present. Serum and CSF samples may be stored at 2 to 8 °C for up to 3 days or at −20 °C for longer periods. Repeated freezing and thawing of specimens, which may cause many proteins to deteriorate, should be avoided. The minimum amount of specimen required is 100 μL.

Assay characteristics

A number of assay characteristics discussed in the following text must be considered in the selection of an appropriate immunochemical method to measure proteins in body fluids.

Limit of detection

Detection limits of approximately 1 to 2 mg/dL are attainable with many nephelometric and turbidimetric methods, especially with particle enhancement. Nephelometry, turbidimetry, and RID are sufficiently sensitive for quantification of most plasma proteins of clinical interest. RIA, EIA, and chemiluminescence methods are more sensitive and measure levels as low as nanograms per milliliter.

Precision

With nephelometry and turbidimetry, within-run coefficients of variation (CVs) of less than 5% are common. RID and EIA systems have higher within-run and run-to-run CVs, usually in the range of 5% to 15%. RIA, which measures much smaller amounts of protein, generally has within-run CVs of 5% to 10%.

Turnaround time

Kinetic or timed nephelometric and turbidimetric methods provide results within minutes, compared with equilibrium methods, which take up to 1 hour to complete. RID usually requires 24 to 48 hours of incubation. Depending on the procedure, turnaround time for RIA is usually several hours.

Instrumentation and equipment

Nephelometers and spectrophotometers equipped with microprocessors that generate calibration curves and calculate test results are required for the light-scattering and light-absorbing methods. Nephelometric and turbidimetric methods are included with many automated analytical systems (see Chapter 12). RID requires no instrumentation other than pipets, although some type of illuminated plate reader is advantageous. RIA requires radiation scintillation counters and an automated pipetting station.

Calibration of immunochemical methods

In 1993 and 1994 the Bureau Communitaire de Référence (BCR) of the European Economic Community, the International Federation of Clinical Chemistry (IFCC), and College of American Pathologists (CAP) jointly introduced a new reference preparation for serum proteins, with values assigned in International Units (IU) against World Health Organization (WHO) materials and in mass units against the U.S. National Reference Preparation (USNRP) for albumin, AMG, complement factors C3 and C4, Cp, Hp, and IgA, IgG, and IgM. Mass values were assigned for AAT, α_1-antichymotrypsin, AAG, and TRF against highly purified and thoroughly characterized purified proteins, and for CRP against WHO 85/506, through use of the factor 1 IU = 1 mg/dL. The new material is available from BCR as Certified Reference Material 470 (CRM 470) and from CAP as the Reference Preparation for Proteins in Human Serum (RPPHS). All manufacturers of immunochemical assays now have referenced their calibrators and controls against the new material, and both national and international studies have shown a significant decrease in interlaboratory variance since its introduction.

Special considerations for analysis of selected proteins

Special consideration must be taken in immunochemical measurement of some proteins, including the immunoglobulins, complement proteins, albumin, and Hp.

Immunoglobulins

Only immunochemical methods are sensitive enough to detect or quantify individual immunoglobulins at physiological levels. Because RID and electroimmunoassay gel techniques are considered obsolete, nephelometry or turbidimetry is preferred because of their ease, speed, and precision of analysis. Nephelometry and turbidimetry are applicable for serum and CSF IgG, IgA, and IgM assays, but for IgD and IgE, RIA or EIA is required.

Special genetic tests are used to determine the clonality of a T- or B-cell population in various myeloid or lymphoid leukemias (see Chapter 11).

Complement proteins

Serum usually is preferable for most protein assays; however, plasma from ethylenediaminetetraacetic acid (EDTA)-anticoagulated blood may be more suitable for assay of most complement factors. The most important requirements are prompt separation of plasma or serum from cells and prompt analysis or storage at -70 °C to preserve labile components.

Nephelometry, turbidimetry, or RID may be used for assays of C3, C4, and factor B, although C3 and C4 may be overestimated by RID when breakdown products are present. Breakdown products are detected and estimated readily by immunofixation. C1q and C1 esterase inhibitor also are assayed immunochemically, although reference materials have not been standardized.

Albumin

Immunochemical methods, such as RID and nephelometry, are highly specific and sensitive for albumin. Either pure protein or reference materials based on RPPHS/CRM 470 are used for calibration.

Haptoglobin

Immunochemical methods are preferred for quantification of Hp with either nephelometry or turbidimetry more satisfactory than RID. Typing of Hp is performed by gel electrophoresis (starch or polyacrylamide gel).

Electrophoretic Techniques

Electrophoresis is widely used in clinical laboratories to study and measure the protein content of biological fluids. Electrophoretic techniques used include cellulose acetate, gel and capillary electrophoretic techniques, and specialized electrophoretic techniques termed *Western blotting, immunofixation,* and *two dimensional (2D) electrophoresis.* Electrophoretic methods also are used to measure urinary and CSF proteins.

Serum protein electrophoresis

The principles of serum protein electrophoresis (SPE) are described in Chapter 7. It is used commonly as a screening tool for protein abnormalities, especially for MCs. Figure 19-4 illustrates SPE separations typical of normal and pathological conditions. In an electrophoretogram obtained from normal serum, usually only five bands (albumin, α_1, α_2, β, and γ) are visible, although a sixth band (β_2, C3 complement component) may be visible if the serum is fresh and a buffer containing Ca^{2+} ions is used. Densitometry may be used for approximate quantification of individual bands and for graphical displays of stained electrophoresis patterns. Many individual proteins have concentrations too low to manifest as distinct stained bands or are overshadowed by proteins of higher concentrations that migrate near them (for example, Cp masked by Hp and AMG).

Various stains may be used to visualize bands. However, some proteins stain poorly because they contain high proportions of lipid (lipoproteins) or carbohydrate (AAG). Amido Black and Ponceau S have been popular in the past; however, Coomassie Brilliant Blue (CBB) is more sensitive

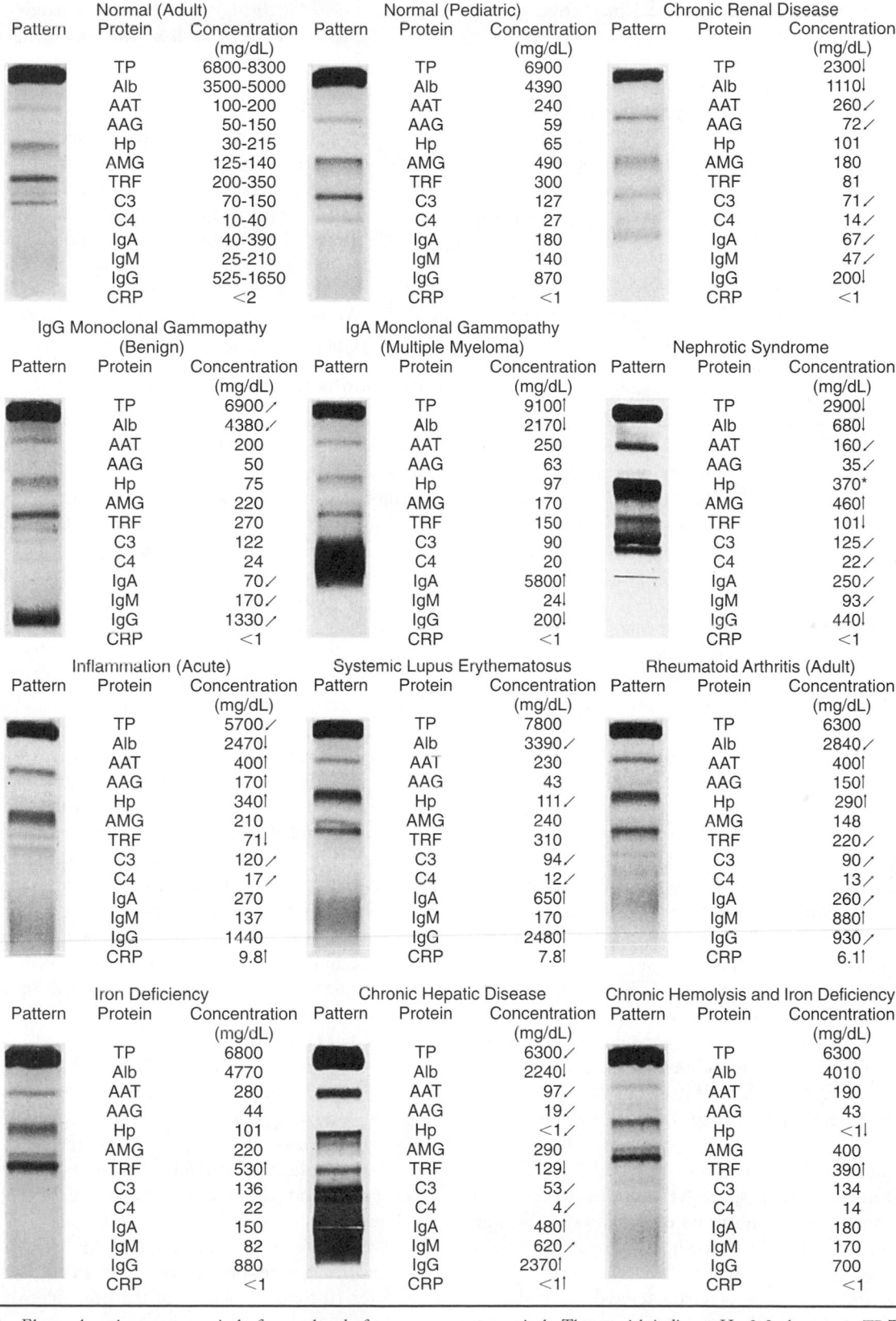

Figure 19-4 Electrophoretic patterns typical of normal and of some pathological conditions (agarose gel). Upward- and downward-pointing arrows indicate increases and decreases from the reference interval, respectively. Right- or left-slanting arrows indicate variations from normal to an increase or from normal to a decrease from the reference interval, respectively. The asterisk indicates Hp 2-2 phenotype. *TP,* Total protein; *Alb,* albumin; *AAT,* α_1-antitrypsin; *AAG,* α_1-acid glycoprotein; *Hp,* haptoglobin; *AMG,* α_2-macroglobulin; *TRF,* transferrin; *C3, C4,* complement factors 3 and 4; *IgA, IgM, IgG,* immunoglobulins A, M, and G; *CRP,* C-reactive protein.

and now used more widely. After visual inspection of the separated bands, the electrophoresis strips are cleared to allow semiquantitative evaluation of the bands by densitometry and then dried for preservation in a permanent record. Most laboratories provide a chart report bearing an image of the densitometric scan, of the stained strip, or both. Special fat stains are necessary to visualize lipoproteins. A patient's serum always should be run in parallel with a normal control serum; the two patterns are then compared and the following changes noted:

1. Intensely stained bands in the α- to the γ-regions in areas not containing normal proteins or free Hb suggest monoclonal immunoglobulins (MCs).

2. Multiple bands, absent bands, or different mobility of normal bands may appear. These may be due to genetic variants, such as Hp in the α_2-region, AAT in the α_1-region, and TRF or C3 in the β-region.

3. Other causes of altered mobility may be present. Increased mobility of albumin occurs when it is bound to penicillin or salicylates or to greater-than-normal amounts of bilirubin or fatty acids. Decreased mobility of AAT occurs when it binds thiol groups, enzymes, or Bence-Jones protein.

4. A band not normally seen may appear. The concentration of a normal protein may increase to such a level that it becomes visible as a line. For instance, a faint, sharp band may appear between albumin and the α_1-region as a result of a 100-fold increase of AFP from certain tumors. Similarly, a large increase of CRP in a severe APR may generate a faint band in the γ-region, or an increase of lysozyme in monocytic leukemia may produce a band in the post-γ-region.

5. Changes in relative concentrations may occur. The stained pattern also should be observed for changes in relative concentrations of the major plasma proteins. Such changes suggest the presence of certain pathological conditions:

   a. Decreased albumin and γ-bands in conjunction with an increased α_2-band suggest selective protein loss, such as that displayed in the nephrotic syndrome. Note, however, that the albumin concentration must fall by at least one third of its normal level before its decrease becomes evident on the electrophoretic strip.

   b. An increase in the α_1-band (AAT and AAG) and α_2-band (Hp) suggests an APR. An increase in only α_1-components may be noted in cases of chronic hepatitis and in APRs accompanied by hemolysis, as well as in individuals during estrogen therapy or pregnancy. In diseases characterized by vasculitis (such as rheumatoid arthritis) or in immune complex diseases, a predominant increase in the α_2-band may be observed.

   c. An increase in the β_1-band suggests iron deficiency anemia (TRF increase) or high levels of estrogen.

   d. Fusion or bridging of β- and γ-bands suggests an increase in IgA, such as that occurring in cases of cirrhosis, respiratory tract or skin infections, and rheumatoid arthritis.

   e. A diffuse increase in the γ-band suggests a polyclonal γ-globulin increase associated with an immune reaction, chronic inflammatory disease, liver disease, or disseminated neoplasms. Oligoclonal bands are present occasionally in cases of chronic aggressive hepatitis and chronic viral infections, as well as in some bacterial infections (for example, pneumococcal pneumonia).

   f. An absence or decrease of the γ-band suggests immune deficiency, either congenital or acquired.

Immunofixation electrophoresis

Immunofixation electrophoresis (IFE), or simply immunofixation, largely has replaced immunoelectrophoresis (IEP) for evaluation of MCs because of its rapidity and ease of interpretation. In IFE, aliquots of a patient's specimen are placed on separate tracks in an agarose gel or on a cellulose acetate strip, and the major protein groups are separated by electrophoresis. One of the tracks then is treated with a chemical fixative solution to fix all proteins and create an electrophoresis reference pattern for the specimen. The other tracks are treated with specific heavy- and light-chain antisera that immunoprecipitates relevant proteins in the agarose gel or cellulose acetate membrane. All unreacted proteins then are washed out, and the remaining proteins are stained. Through comparison of the locations of the stained immunofixed bands with a band of the same location in the reference pattern, a specific protein may be identified.

In monoclonal gammopathies, IFE usually yields a distinct, sharply defined precipitin band with one heavy-chain and one light-chain antiserum. These bands match the location of the particular immunoglobulin in the reference pattern (Figure 19-5). In polyclonal gammopathies a diffuse precipitin band occurs with the specific antiserum, in contrast to the sharp band observed in monoclonal gammopathies.

IFE patterns always should be confirmed by quantification of the immunoglobulins (IgG, IgA, and IgM) in the specimen with nephelometry or turbidimetry. Elevations of specific immunoglobulins should correspond to more intensely stained bands on the IFE pattern. To avoid antigen excess, quantification of the immunoglobulins before IFE is performed and dilution of the sample accordingly are helpful.

A comparison of IFE and IEP for two patients with monoclonal gammopathies is shown in Figure 19-5. (See Chapter 10 for a discussion of the principles of IEP.)

Capillary electrophoresis

In capillary electrophoresis (CE) the classic techniques of zone electrophoresis, isotachophoresis, isoelectric focusing, and gel electrophoresis are carried out in small-bore (10 to

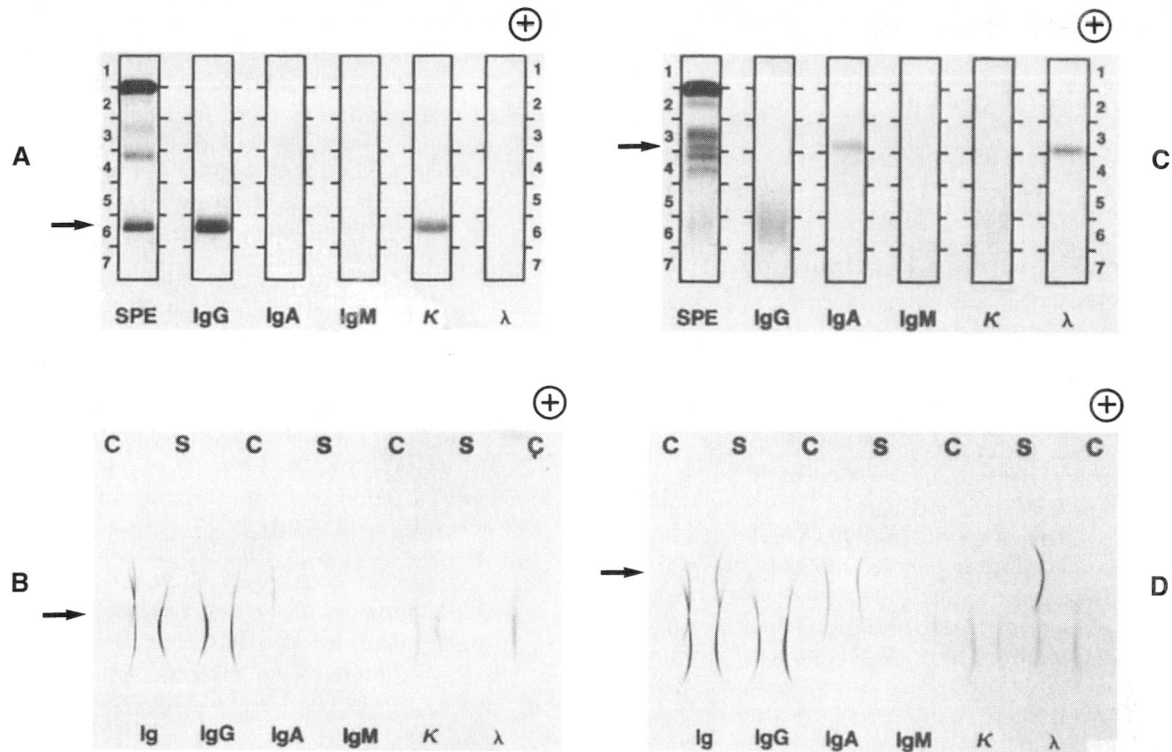

Figure 19-5   Comparison of immunofixation electrophoresis (IFE) and immunoelectrophoresis (IEP) for two patients with monoclonal gammopathies. **A,** Patient specimen with an IgG (kappa, κ) monoclonal protein as identified by IFE. Note the position of monoclonal protein *(arrow)*. After electrophoresis, each track except SPE is reacted with its respective antiserum; then all tracks are stained to visualize the respective protein bands. (IgG, IgA, IgM, κ and λ indicate antiserum used on each track.) **B,** Same specimen as in **A,** with proteins identified by IEP. Note the position of monoclonal protein *(arrow)*. Control C and patient sera S are alternated. After electrophoresis, antiserum is added to each trough, as indicated by the labels Ig, IgG, IgA, IgM, κ and λ. The antisera react with separated proteins in the specimens to form precipitates in the shape of arcs. The IgG and κ arcs are shorter and thicker than those in the normal control, showing the presence of the IgG (κ) monoclonal protein. The concentrations of IgA, IgM, and λ-light chains also are reduced. **C,** Patient specimen with an IgA (lambda, λ) monoclonal protein identified by the IFE procedure, as described in **A. D,** Same specimen as in **C,** with proteins identified by IEP, as described in **B.** The abnormal IgA and λ-arcs for the patient specimen indicate an elevated concentration of a monoclonal IgA (λ) protein. All separations were performed with the Beckman Paragon system. *SPE,* serum protein electrophoresis; *IgG, IgA, IgM,* immunoglobulins G, A, and M; *C,* normal control; *S,* patient sera.

100 μm), fused-silica capillary tubes 20 to 200 cm in length (see Chapter 7). It is a very efficient, rapid, sensitive, and versatile analytical technique that is used to analyze a diverse spectrum of analytes, ranging from small ions to macromolecular proteins or nucleic acids. CE has been used for both micropreparative and analytical purposes.

Western blotting

Western blotting (immunoblotting) is a method used to separate, detect, and identify one or more proteins in a complex mixture. It involves initial separation of the individual proteins by electrophoresis and subsequent transfer or "blotting" of them onto an overlaying nitrocellulose or nylon membrane by either passive diffusion or electroblotting. The membrane then is reacted with a labeled antibody specific for the protein of interest. (See Chapter 7 for a more detailed discussion of this technique.)

Two-dimensional electrophoresis

Analytical and preparative 2D-dimensional electrophoresis is used to characterize the individual components of com-

plex protein mixtures. It remains the highest resolution technique for protein separation and is the method of choice when complex samples must be arrayed for characterization, as in proteomics. The proteome is the expressed protein complement of a genome, and proteomics is functional genomics at the protein level. Proteomics is the study of (1) global changes in protein expression and (2) the systematic study of protein-protein interactions through the isolation of protein complexes. The goal of proteomics is a comprehensive, quantitative description of protein expression and its changes under the influence of biological perturbations, such as disease or drug treatment.

Electrophoretic separation of urinary proteins

The procedure for electrophoresis of urine on agarose gel or cellulose acetate is identical to that for serum, with the exception that urine must be concentrated before application unless more sensitive staining methods are used (for example, gold and/or silver stains). Simple electrophoresis of urine concentrated to a protein concentration of approximately 3 g/dL identifies the presence of immunoglobulin light chains (Bence-Jones protein) or other low-molecular-mass proteins typical of tubular proteinuria. Comparison of a urine separation with a corresponding serum separation also may indicate the degree of selectivity in glomerular proteinuria. An important point to remember is that normal urine may contain light-chain "ladders," which may be confused with Bence-Jones protein.

Electrophoretic separation of cerebrospinal fluid proteins

With sufficient concentration of CSF, use of the same electrophoretic procedures as those used for serum is possible but high-resolution techniques are recommended strongly. The use of silver staining and IFE enhances sensitivity and allows unconcentrated CSF to be electrophoresed. In addition, with this enhanced sensitivity, IgG bands are identified with certainty. Figure 19-6 illustrates an electrophoresis pattern and subsequent IFE, demonstrating the presence of oligoclonal bands.

The definition of oligoclonal banding is the presence in CSF of two or more IgG bands that stain with greater in-

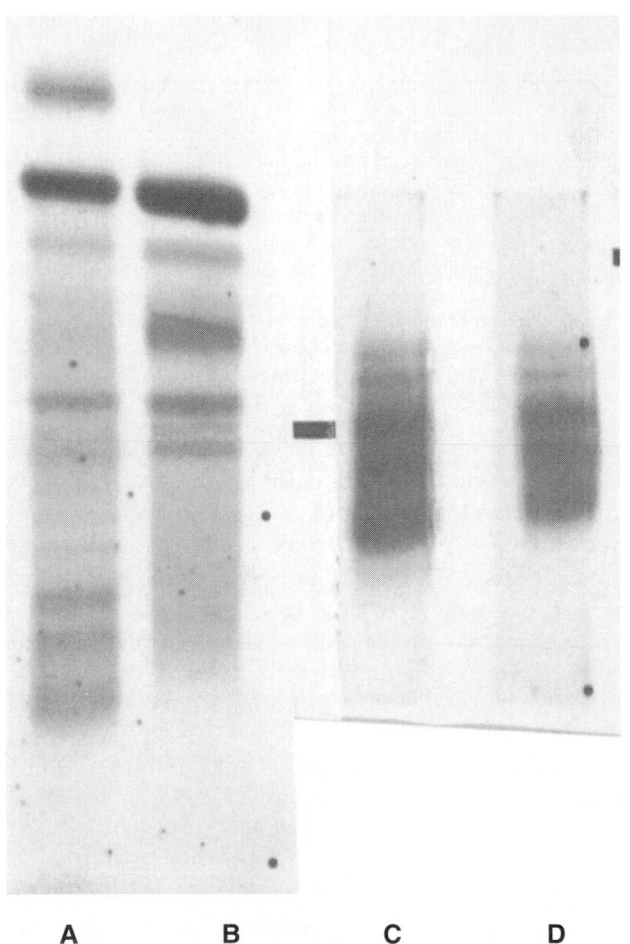

A　　　B　　　C　　　D

Figure 19-6　Cerebrospinal fluid (CSF) electrophoresis patterns stained with Paragon violet after preconcentration with a centrifugal device. **A,** CSF, concentrated fortyfold. **B,** Serum collected within 6 hours of CSF collection. **C,** Immunoglobulin G (IgG) immunofixation of the neat CSF concentrate. **D,** IgG immunofixation of a 1:3 dilution of the CSF concentrate.

tensity than in the concurrent serum sample. Reporting of oligoclonal banding is either "present" or "absent." Oligoclonal banding is often subtle, and densitometric scans seldom add information to visual inspection.

In general, use of CBB or Paragon violet stain is favored for methods using preconcentrated CSF samples; silver staining is necessary when analysis is performed with neat samples. Although some 20 to 50 times more sensitive than CBB, silver staining is a more complex procedure and less suited than CBB or Paragon violet for serum and other body fluids.

Quantitative Measurements of Total Protein in Body Fluids

When the total protein concentration of biological fluids such as serum, urine, and CSF is measured, the following two arbitrary assumptions are made:

1. All protein molecules are pure polypeptide chains, containing on the average 16% by weight of nitrogen.
2. Each of the several hundred individual proteins reacts chemically like every other protein.

Clearly the first assumption is not true, and the second is not always true. Nevertheless, these simplifying assumptions make measurement of total protein a practical, although empirical, procedure.

Specific methods

Many methods have been developed to measure the total protein content of biological fluids. A number of them are reviewed in the section that follows.

Biuret method

The biuret method depends on the presence of peptide bonds in all proteins. These peptide bonds react with Cu^{2+} ions in alkaline solutions to form a colored product, the absorbance of which is measured spectrophotometrically at 540 nm. The biuret reagent contains sodium potassium tartrate to form a complex with cupric ions and maintain their solubility in alkaline solution. Iodide is included as an antioxidant. In the biuret reaction a colored chelate is formed between the Cu^{2+} ion and the carbonyl oxygen and amide nitrogen atoms of the peptide bond. The reaction occurs with any compound containing at least two H_2N-C-, H_2N-CH_2-, CH_2-, H_2N-CS-, or similar groups joined together directly or through a carbon or nitrogen atom. One copper ion probably is linked to six nearby peptide linkages by coordinate bonds. Amino acids and dipeptides do not react, but tripeptides, oligopeptides, and polypeptides react to yield pink to reddish-violet products.

The intensity of the color produced is proportional to the number of peptide bonds that are reacting and therefore to the amount of protein present in the reaction system. Thus the biuret reaction with protein is suitable for quantitative determination of total protein by spectrophotometry.

Although small peptides present in serum also react, their concentration in serum is so low that they contribute little to the biuret color. Ammonium ions interfere but not at concentrations that occur in serum. Most biuret methods detect between 1 and 15 mg of protein in the aliquot measured, an amount present in 15 to 200 µL of a serum containing protein at 7 g/dL. Numerous versions of the biuret method have been developed and applied.

Either serum or plasma may be used for a biuret assay, but serum is preferred. A fasting specimen is not required but may be desirable to decrease the risk of lipemia. Hemolysis should be avoided. Tightly stoppered samples of serum are stable for 1 week or more at room temperature and for 1 month at 2 to 4 °C. Specimens that have been frozen and thawed should be mixed thoroughly before assay.

Direct photometric methods

Absorption of ultraviolet (UV) light at 200 to 225 nm and 270 to 290 nm has been used to measure the protein content of biological samples. Absorption of UV light at 280 nm depends chiefly on the aromatic rings of tyrosine and tryptophan at pH 8. Accuracy and specificity suffer from an uneven distribution of these amino acids among individual proteins in a mixture, as well as from the presence in body fluids of free tyrosine and tryptophan, uric acid, and bilirubin, which also absorb light near 280 nm. Peptide bonds are responsible chiefly for UV absorption (70% at A_{205}); specific absorption by proteins at 200 to 225 nm is 10 to 30 times greater than at 280 nm. Interference from free tyrosine and tryptophan is significant at these short wavelengths. However, a 1:1000 or 1:2000 dilution of serum with NaCl, 0.15 mol/L, circumvents this interference. The method has been used for CSF after removal of small interfering molecules by gel filtration. This approach is sensitive and simple but requires an appropriate spectrophotometer and high-quality cuvets with high transmission of light at 220 nm.

Dye-binding methods

Dye-binding methods are based on the ability of proteins to bind dyes such as Amido black 10B and CBB. The unequal affinities and binding capacities of individual proteins for dyes are a limitation in all these applications, which are complicated further by the inability to define a consistent material for use as a calibrator. The dye-binding method of greatest contemporary interest, particularly for assay of total protein in CSF and urine, uses CBB G-250. CBB binds to protonated amine groups of amino acid residues in the polypeptide chain, and the absorbance maximum for the bound species of the dye decreases at 465 nm and increases at 595 nm. The method is simple, fast, and linear up to 150 mg/dL.

Folin-Ciocalteu (Lowry) method

Most proteins contain tyrosine or tryptophan or both, but each protein contains a unique proportion of them. Albumin, for instance, has only 0.2% tryptophan by weight, whereas the tryptophan content of individual globulins varies between 2% and 3%. These amino acids, either free or in an unfolded polypeptide chain, reduce phosphotungstic-phosphomolybdic acid (Folin-Ciocalteu reagent) and produces a blue color. This property is more useful for assay of a pure protein with composition and relative reactivity that are known (for example, fibrinogen) than it is for a mixture of individual proteins with different concentrations and reactivities.

Kjeldahl method

In the Kjeldahl method, acid digestion is used first to convert nitrogen in the protein to ammonium ion. The concentration of ammonia nitrogen then is evaluated by titration or nesslerization, a correction is made for nitrogen contributed by nonprotein compounds also present in serum, and the ammonia nitrogen value is multiplied by a factor of 6.25 (100%/16%) to express protein nitrogen as total protein. The method is characterized and reproducible but time consuming, inconvenient, and impractical for routine use. Kjeldahl determination, however, still remains a means by which to characterize and validate reference materials for use with the biuret method.

Refractometry

Refractometry is a quick alternative to chemical analysis for serum total protein when a rapid estimate is required. Some laboratories find it a convenient way to determine total protein content before SPE is performed. At protein concentrations less than 3.5 g/dL, refractometric results are likely to be inaccurate. At a level greater than 11.0 g/dL, a valid result is obtained by dilution of the serum with equal parts of water, followed by reading of the diluted sample. A day-to-day CV of less than 2.0% is acceptable precision.

Turbidimetric and nephelometric methods

Precipitation of protein for turbidimetric or nephelometric assays is achieved with sulfosalicylic acid alone, with sulfosalicylic acid in combination with sodium sulfate or trichloroacetic acid (TCA), or with TCA alone. Precipitation methods for total protein assay depend on formation of a fine precipitate of uniform, insoluble protein particles, which scatter incident light in suspension.

Calibration of total protein methods

Bovine or human albumin is used routinely to calibrate biuret methods. Albumin is available in high purity, it contains only amino acids, its nitrogen content is a constant fraction of its molecular mass, and the number of peptide bonds per molecule is known.

For the calibration of precipitation and dye-binding methods the recommendation usually is to use a suitable dilution of a serum, or serum pool, with a normal albumin/globulin ratio. This calibrator is obtained from a healthy subject and analyzed for total protein with a correctly calibrated biuret or Kjeldahl method. For precipitation methods, bovine or human serum albumin should not be used as calibrators with sulfosalicylic acid because these pure proteins provide about 2.5 times the turbidity that serum globulins do; however, use of pure albumin is possible as a calibrator with TCA precipitation.

Reference intervals

The total protein concentration of serum obtained from a healthy ambulatory adult is 6.3 to 8.3 g/dL and from an adult at rest, 6.0 to 7.8 g/dL. The reference intervals for neonates and young children varies from 4.6 to 7.0, to 6.0 to 8.0 g/dL. The two general causes of a change in the concentration of serum total protein are a change in the volume of plasma water and a change in the concentration of one or more specific proteins in the plasma. Decrease in the volume of plasma water (hemoconcentration) is reflected as relative hyperproteinemia; concentrations of all the individual plasma proteins are increased to the same degree if the process is acute. Hyperproteinemia is noted in cases of dehydration due to inadequate water intake or excessive water loss, such as in cases of severe vomiting, diarrhea, Addison's disease, or diabetic acidosis. Hemodilution (increase in plasma water volume) is reflected as relative hypoproteinemia; again, concentrations of all the individual plasma proteins are decreased to the same degree if the loss is acute. Hemodilution occurs with water intoxication or salt-retention syndromes, during massive intravenous infusions, and physiologically when an individual assumes a recumbent position.

Determination of Albumin in Plasma

Most clinical laboratories assay albumin by automated dye-binding methods, using bromcresol green (BCG) or purple (BCP) dyes. These dyes have great affinity for albumin; therefore the initial rate of binding usually is measured and related to the concentration of albumin in the sample. The use of serum is recommended because these assays overestimate albumin in the presence of fibrinogen and heparin. In addition, they tend to be erroneous if the overall serum protein pattern is abnormal. Other ligands, including drugs and metabolites, bind to albumin but usually do not affect dye-binding assays of serum or plasma significantly unless their concentrations are extremely high.

Determination of Total Protein in Urine

Many methods have been used to measure urinary proteins. The biuret method applied to acid-precipitated protein or a concentrate obtained by membrane filtration has the advantage of equal sensitivity to each individual protein in the mixture. Many laboratories, however, find this approach too time consuming for routine use and prefer turbidimetric and dye-binding methods because they are fast and simple. Of the dye-binding methods, pyrogallol red, Ponceau S, and CBB are the most popular. The turbidimetric and dye-binding methods have nonlinear calibration curves and unequal sensitivities for individual proteins. Most underestimate low-molecular-mass proteins in tubular proteinuria and immunoglobulin light chains in overload proteinuria.

To quantify urinary proteins, a timed collection usually is used. Collection periods of 4, 8, and 12 hours have been used to monitor renal transplant recipients or a patient whose acute renal losses of albumin are being compensated with closely regulated replacement therapy. In most cases, however, a 24-hour collection time is chosen, both for quantitative total or specific protein assay and for electrophoretic separation. An alternative approach is to measure the protein/creatinine ratios of random specimens.

Dipstick tests often are used to measure excess protein in urine semiquanitatively. With these tests the reactive portion of the stick is coated with a buffered indicator that develops color in the presence of protein. Detection limits are approximately 7 mg/dL. Like all dye-binding techniques, the dipstick methods are more sensitive to albumin than to other plasma proteins. They are therefore excellent screening tests for glomerular proteinuria but unsatisfactory for detection of tubular or overload proteinuria. Although most tests measure protein in excess of 10 mg/dL, they are only semiquantitative and their use should be limited to screening and to approximate estimates required before the specimen is concentrated for electrophoresis or diluted for quantitative assay. A first-morning urine specimen is preferable because it tends to be concentrated and unaffected by postural factors.

The reference interval for urinary total protein is 1 to 14 mg/dL. The excretion rate at rest is 50 to 80 mg/day, but many laboratories indicate the reference value as less than 100 mg/day (<150 mg/day in pregnancy). The concentration may reach 300 mg/dL in urine of healthy subjects after exercise.

Determination of Total Protein in Cerebrospinal Fluid

The low levels of protein in CSF limit the methods that are used to measure its total protein content. Turbidimetric methods and versions of the CBB dye-binding method are used commonly for this purpose. The most serious disadvantage of turbidimetric methods is the requirement for 0.2 to 0.5 mL of sample. CBB methods are sensitive enough for use with samples as small as 25 μL, but they underestimate globulins. Because albumin is the predominant protein of CSF, this underestimation may not be serious enough to preclude the use of a CBB method.

Determination of specific proteins in cerebrospinal fluid

Nephelometry, immunoturbidimetry, electroimmunodiffusion, and RID are used most often to measure albumin and IgG. Apparent absence of IgG may be due to its degradation by proteinases in the specimen. RIA is required to determine specific proteins present in very low concentrations (for example, IgM). The reference interval for albumin levels in lumbar CSF by RID is 17.7 to 25.1 mg/dL. IgA, IgD, and IgM, measured by RIA, each are normally less than 0.2 mg/dL. Reference intervals for IgG are age related; their means increase from 3.5 mg/dL in the 15- to 20-year age group to 5.8 in adults 60 years of age and older. The usual reference interval for CSF IgG in adults is 0.8 to 4.2 mg/dL; for total protein, it is 15 to 45 mg/dL. Total protein levels are considerably higher in neonates, and in healthy elderly adults, concentrations up to 60 mg/dL are considered normal.

Mass Spectrometry

Mass spectrometry (MS) is a powerful qualitative and quantitative analytical tool that is used to assess the molecular mass and primary amino acid sequence of peptides and proteins. Technical advancements in MS have resulted in the development of matrix-assisted laser desorption ionization (MALDI) and electrospray (ES) ionization techniques that allow sequencing and mass determination of picomole quantities of proteins with masses larger than 100 kD (see Chapter 8). A time-of-flight mass spectrometer is used to detect the small quantities of ions that are produced by MALDI. In this type of spectrometer, ions are accelerated in an electrical field and allowed to drift to a detector. The mass of the ion is calculated from the time it takes to reach the detector. To measure the masses of proteins in a mixture or produce a peptide map of a proteolytic digest, a small quantity of sample (0.5 to 2.0 μL) is dried on the tip of the sample probe, which then is introduced into the spectrometer for analysis. With this technique, proteins located on the surfaces of cells are ionized and analyzed selectively.

With ES ionization a fine mist of highly charged particles is produced when a liquid flows from a capillary tube into a strong electrical field (3 to 6 kV). In practice, ES ionization sources often are coupled directly with reversed-phase high-performance liquid chromatography (HPLC) or capillary columns. The ability to couple a liquid chromatograph with an ES ionization source and a mass spectrometer allows the on-line removal of salts and contaminants and the analysis of complex mixtures. Although different from MALDI, ES provides similar sensitivity and application to the analysis of large proteins.

Tandem mass spectrometry (MS/MS) is a type of MS that is applicable to the rapid sequencing of peptides contained in a complex biological mixture. In a tandem mass spectrometer, two or more mass analyzers are connected in tandem. In the first analyzer the targeted compound is ionized selectively and its characteristic ions separated from others in the mixture. The selected primary ions then collide with molecules of a neutral gas to produce fragments that are separated and identified in the second spectrometer. Using two mass spectrometers in tandem permits the selective and specific analysis of many compounds of various structural classes. The need for a chromatographic step is eliminated because separation and analysis take place simultaneously in the tandem mass spectrometer. Compared with older methods, MS/MS offers greater analytical sensitivity, accuracy, and speed, as well as the ability to analyze peptides that contain a blocked N-terminus.

Additional Reading

Baudner S, Haupt H, Hubner R: Manufacture and characterization of a new reference preparation for 14 plasma proteins/CRM 470 = RPPHS lot 5. J Clin Lab Anal 1994; 8:177-190.

Copeland RA: Methods for Protein Analysis: A Practical Guide in Laboratory Protocols, London, Chapman & Hall, 1994.

Dati F, Schumnann G, Thomas L et al: Consensus of a group of professional societies and diagnostic companies on guidelines for interim reference ranges for 14 proteins in serum based on the standardization against the IFCC/BCR/CAP reference material (CRM 470). Eur J Clin Chem Clin Biochem 1996; 34:517-520.

Davies JS: Amino Acids, Peptides, and Proteins, vol 25, Boca Raton, Fla, CRC Press, 1994.

Johnson AM, Rohlfs EM, Silverman LM: Proteins. In Burtis CA, Ashwood ER (eds): Tietz Textbook of Clinical Chemistry, 3rd edition, pp 617-721, Philadelphia, WB Saunders, 1999.

Keren DF: High-Resolution Electrophoresis and Immunofixation: Techniques and Interpretation, 2nd edition, Newton, Mass, Butterworth-Heinemann, 1994.

Lagrand WK, Visser CA, Hermens WT et al: C-reactive protein as a cardiovascular risk factor: more than an epiphenomenon? Circulation 1999; 100:96-102.

Morgan BP: Complement: Methods and Protocols, Totowa, NJ, Humana Press, 2000.

Ritchie R (ed): Serum Proteins in Clinical Medicine. Vol I. Laboratory Section, Scarborough, Maine, Foundation for Blood Research, 1996.

Ritchie R (ed): Serum Proteins in Clinical Medicine. Vol II. Clinical Section, Scarborough, Maine, Foundation for Blood Research, 1999.

Whicher J, Ritchie RF, Johnson AM et al: New International Reference Preparation for Proteins in Human Serum (RPPHS). Clin Chem 1994; 40:934-938.

CHAPTER 20

Enzymes

A. RALPH HENDERSON, MB, ChB, PhD, FRCPath, and DONALD W. MOSS, PHD, DSC

Objectives

1. List the factors that affect enzyme levels in blood.
2. State the physiological actions, tissue distribution, clinical significance, and methods of analysis of the transaminases, creatine kinase, lactate dehydrogenase, the phosphatases, γ-glutamyltransferase, 5'-nucleotidase, the cholinesterases, amylase, lipase, and trypsin.
3. List the isoenzymes methods of analysis, and discuss the migration of creatine kinase and lactate dehydrogenase isoenzymes after electrophoresis.
4. List five additional important enzymes and state their clinical significance.

Key Words

Acid Phosphatase   An enzyme of the hydrolase class that catalyzes the cleavage of orthophosphate from orthophosphoric monoesters under acidic conditions

Angiotensin-Converting Enzyme (ACE)   An enzyme that cleaves the decapeptide angiotensin I to form active angiotensin II

Aldolase   A glycolytic enzyme that cleaves fructose 1,6-bisphosphate into dihydroxyacetone phosphate and glyceraldehyde 3-phosphate

Alkaline Phosphatase   An enzyme of the hydrolase class that catalyzes the cleavage of orthophosphate from orthophosphoric monoesters under alkaline conditions

Alpha Amylase   An enzyme that catalyzes the endohydrolysis of 1,4-α-glycosidic linkages in starch, glycogen, and related polysaccharides and oligosaccharides containing 3 or more 1,4-α-linked D-glucose units

Cholinesterase   An enzyme of the hydrolase class that catalyzes the cleavage of the acyl group from various esters of choline, including acetylcholine, and some related compounds

Chymotrypsin   A serine protease from pancreas that preferentially hydrolyses phenylalanine, tyrosine, or tryptophan peptide and ester bonds

Creatine Kinase (CK)   A dimeric enzyme that catalyzes the formation of adenosine triphosphate (ATP) from adenosine diphosphate (ADP) and creatine phosphate (CrP) in muscle; has three forms—CK-1, CK-2, and CK-3

Gamma Glutamyltransferase   An enzyme that catalyzes reversibly the transfer of a glutamyl group from a glutamyl-peptide and an amino acid to a peptide and a glutamyl-amino acid

Isoform   An enzyme molecule that has been modified after translation

Lactate Dehydrogenase (LD)   An enzyme of the oxidoreductase class that catalyzes the reduction of pyruvate to (L)-lactate, using NADH as an electron donor

Lipase   Any enzyme that cleaves a fatty acid anion hydrolytically from a triglyceride or phospholipid

Pancreatitis   Acute or chronic inflammation of the pancreas, which may be asymptomatic or symptomatic and is due to autodigestion of pancreatic tissue by its own enzymes; caused most often by alcoholism or biliary tract disease

Prostate-Specific Antigen (PSA)   A kallikrein-like serine proteinase produced by epithelial cells of both benign and malignant prostate tissue

Transaminases   A subclass of enzymes of the transferase class that catalyze the transfer of an amino group from a donor (generally an amino acid) to an acceptor

(generally a 2-keto acid); alanine and aspartate aminotransaminase being examples that are of significant clinical utility

Trypsin   A serine endopeptidase that catalyzes the cleavage of peptide bonds on the carboxyl side of either arginine or lysine

Enzymes are known as markers of cellular damage, and their measurement is an important function of clinical laboratories. The basic principles of clinical enzymology are discussed in Chapter 9, whereas this chapter deals with individual enzymes. For organizational purposes the individual enzymes are discussed relative to the organ function in which they are important. Thus enzymes used in the investigation of diseases of liver parenchyma, cardiac and skeletal muscle, the biliary tract, and the pancreas are discussed together. However, a considerable overlap exists in this classification because many enzymes are used to investigate disease in several organs.

BASIC CONCEPTS

The selection of which enzyme to measure in serum for diagnostic or prognostic purposes depends on a number of factors. An important factor is the distribution of enzymes among the various tissues, as shown for selected enzymes in Figure 20-1. The main enzymes of established clinical value, together with their tissues of origin and clinical applications, are listed in Table 20-1.

Not all intracellular enzymes are equally valuable as indicators of cellular damage. For example, isocitrate dehydrogenase (ICD) activity is high in heart muscle, but after a myocardial infarction, it is inactivated rapidly on entering the vascular compartment. Ornithine carbamoyltransferase is an enzyme of the urea cycle, and it is therefore almost totally liver specific, with a liver/blood ratio of about 1,000,000:1; thus even minor degrees of hepatocyte damage should create a readily detectable elevation in blood levels. However, this enzyme has not found particular favor in clinical enzymology, possibly because of the inconvenience of the assay and a consequent lack of wide clinical experience with the results of the assay.

The mass of the damaged or malfunctioning organ, together with the enzyme cell/blood gradient, also has a profound influence on the resulting elevation of enzyme activity in blood. Thus the gradient of activity of prostatic acid phosphatase (ACP) between prostate and blood is about 10,000:1, and the mass of that organ is 20 g. By contrast, the cell/blood gradient of alanine aminotransferase (ALT) in the liver cell is 100,000:1, and the mass

of the liver can exceed 1000 g. Fewer cells must be damaged in the liver than in the prostate for the abnormality to be detected by an enzyme elevation in blood. However, if a total organ involvement exists, then the vast number of affected liver cells markedly elevate blood levels of any liver enzyme. By estimation, if only one liver cell in every 750 is damaged, elevation in the blood level of ALT is detectable.

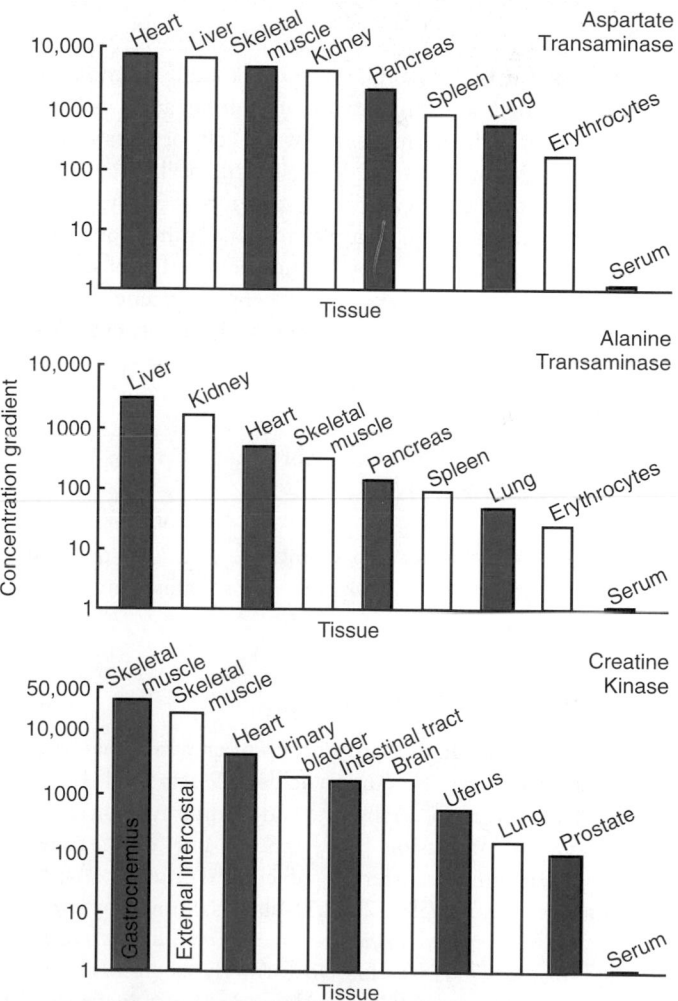

Figure 20-1   The concentration gradients among some human tissues and serum for aspartate transaminase, alanine transaminase, and creatine kinase. The concentration gradient axis is logarithmic.

TABLE 20-1   **Distribution of Diagnostically Important Enzymes**

Enzyme	Principal Sources	Principal Clinical Applications
Acid phosphatase	Prostate, erythrocytes	Carcinoma of prostate
Alanine aminotransferase	Liver, skeletal muscle, heart	Hepatic parenchymal disease
Aldolase	Skeletal muscle, heart	Muscle diseases
Alkaline phosphatase	Liver, bone, intestinal mucosa, placenta, kidney	Bone diseases, hepatobiliary diseases
Amylase	Salivary glands, pancreas, ovaries	Pancreatic diseases
Aspartate aminotransferase	Liver, skeletal muscle, heart, kidney, erythrocytes	Myocardial infarction, hepatic parenchymal disease, muscle disease
Cholinesterase	Liver	Organophosphorus insecticide poisoning, suxamethonium sensitivity, hepatic parenchymal diseases
Creatine kinase	Skeletal muscle, brain, heart, smooth muscle	Myocardial infarction, muscle diseases
Glutamate dehydrogenase	Liver	Hepatic parenchymal diseases
γ-Glutamyltransferase	Liver, kidney	Hepatobiliary disease, alcoholism
Lactate dehydrogenase	Heart, liver, skeletal muscle, erythrocytes, platelets, lymph nodes	Myocardial infarction, hemolysis, hepatic parenchymal diseases
5′-Nucleotidase	Hepatobiliary tract	Hepatobiliary disease
Prostate-specific antigen	Prostate	Carcinoma of prostate
Sorbitol dehydrogenase	Liver	Parenchymal hepatic diseases
Trypsin(ogen)	Pancreas	Pancreatic diseases

Pathological damage to a tissue embraces a wide spectrum of effects; thus a mild, reversible viral inflammation of the liver, such as a mild attack of viral hepatitis, is likely to increase only the permeability of the cell membrane and allow cytoplasmic enzymes to leak into the blood. A severe attack causing cell necrosis also disrupts the mitochondrial membrane, and both cytoplasmic and mitochondrial enzymes are detected in blood. Thus knowledge of the intracellular location of enzymes can help determine the nature and severity of a pathological process if suitable enzymes are assayed in the blood.

■ LIVER, CARDIAC, AND SKELETAL ENZYMES

Enymes in this category include the aminotransferases, creatine kinase, alkaline phosphatase, and lactate dehydrogenase.

Aminotransferases

The aminotransferases are a group of enzymes that catalyze the interconversion of amino acids to 2-oxo-acids by transfer of amino groups. Aspartate and alanine aminotransferase (Enzyme Commission [EC] 2.6.1.1 and 2.6.1.2) are examples of aminotransferases of clinical interest. Aspartate aminotransferase (EC 2.6.1.1) also is known as *aspartate transaminase, L-aspartate:2-oxoglutarate aminotransferase, AST,* or *AspAT.* It was known formerly as *glutamate oxaloacetate transaminase (GOT).* Alanine aminotransferase (EC 2.6.1.2) also is known as *alanine transaminase, L-alanine:2-oxoglutarate aminotransferase, ALT* or *AlaAT.* It was known formerly as *glutamate pyruvate transaminase (GPT).*

Biochemistry

The 2-oxoglutarate/L-glutamate couple serves as one amino group acceptor and donor pair in all amino-transfer reactions; the specificity of the individual enzymes derives from the particular amino acid that serves as the other donor of an amino group. Thus AST catalyzes the following reaction:

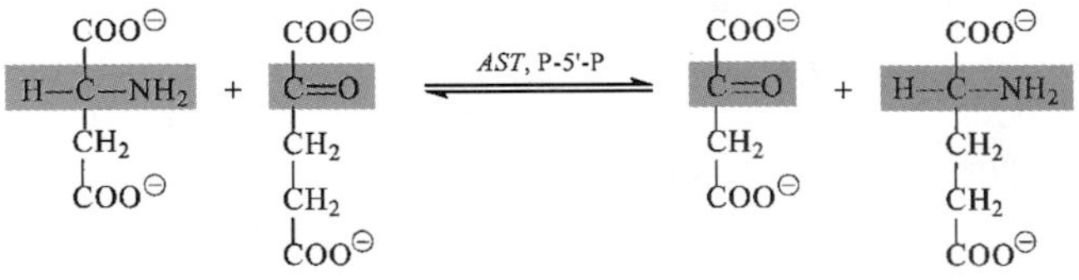

L-Aspartate   2-Oxoglutarate   Oxaloacetate   L-Glutamate

ALT catalyzes the analogous reaction, as follows:

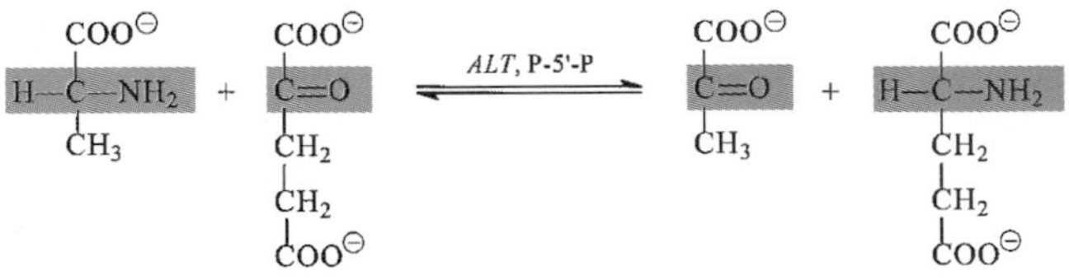

L-Alanine   2-Oxoglutarate   Pyruvate   L-Glutamate

The reactions are reversible, but the equilibria of the AST and ALT reactions favor the formation of aspartate and alanine, respectively.

Pyridoxal-5′-phosphate (P-5′-P) and its amino analogue, pyridoxamine-5′-phosphate, function as coenzymes in the amino-transfer reactions. The P-5′-P is bound to the apoenzyme and serves as a true prosthetic group. The P-5′-P bound to the apoenzyme accepts the amino group from the first substrate, aspartate or alanine, to form enzyme-bound pyridoxamine-5′-phosphate and the first reaction product, oxaloacetate or pyruvate, respectively. The

TABLE 20-2	Transaminase Activities in Human Tissues, Relative to Serum as Unity		
Tissue		AST	ALT
Heart		7800	450
Liver		7100	2850
Skeletal muscle		5000	300
Kidneys		4500	1200
Pancreas		1400	130
Spleen		700	80
Lungs		500	45
Erythrocytes		15	7
Serum		1	1

From King J: Practical Clinical Enzymology, London, D Van Nostrand, 1965.
AST, Aspartate aminotransferase; *ALT,* alanine aminotransferase.

coenzyme in amino form then transfers its amino group to the second substrate, 2-oxoglutarate, to form the second product, glutamate. P-5′-P thus is regenerated.

Both holoaminotransferases and the coenzyme-deficient apoenzymes may be present in serum. Therefore addition of P-5′-P under conditions that allow recombination with the enzymes usually produces a marked increase in aminotransferase activity. This increase ranges from zero to threefold or fourfold and averages approximately 50% for AST in normal serum and 20% for ALT. Adding P-5′-P during assays of aminotransferase activity for routine diagnostic purposes has not been customary, but the International Federation of Clinical Chemistry (IFCC) reference method specifies this addition.

Clinical significance

Transaminases are distributed widely in animal tissues. Both AST and ALT normally are present in human plasma, bile, cerebrospinal fluid (CSF), and saliva, but none is found in urine unless a kidney lesion is present. Transaminase activities in various tissues, relative to those in serum, are shown in Table 20-2.

With viral hepatitis and other forms of liver disease associated with hepatic necrosis (see Chapter 36), serum AST and ALT levels are elevated even before the clinical signs and symptoms of disease (such as jaundice) appear. Levels for both enzymes may reach values as high as 100 times the upper limit of the reference interval, although twentyfold to fiftyfold elevations are encountered most frequently. Peak values of transaminase activity occur between days 7 and 12; activities then gradually decrease, reaching normal levels by the third to fifth week if recovery is uneventful. Alcoholic hepatitis has more modest elevations.

In cases of infectious hepatitis and other inflammatory conditions affecting the liver, ALT is characteristically as high as or higher than AST, and the ALT/AST (De Ritis) ratio, which normally is less than 1, becomes greater than unity. The relatively similar elevations of AST and ALT in hepatitis cases have been attributed to the release of only the

cytoplasmic isoenzyme of AST into the circulation from reversibly damaged parenchymal cells. When necrosis of cells occurs, considerable amounts of mitochondrial AST also are released, depressing the ALT/AST ratio.

Extremely high ALT and AST activities are seen in severe cases of toxic hepatitis. Elevations up to 20 times the upper limit of the reference interval have been encountered in cases of infectious mononucleosis with liver involvement and somewhat lower values in those of intrahepatic cholestasis. Increased levels also have been observed in cases of extrahepatic cholestasis, with levels tending to be higher the more chronic the obstruction. The aminotransferase levels observed in cirrhosis vary with the status of the cirrhotic process and range from upper normal to four to five times normal. (The level of AST activity is higher than that of ALT activity.)

Fivefold to tenfold elevations of both enzymes occur in individuals with primary or metastatic carcinoma of the liver, with AST usually being higher than ALT, but levels are often normal in the early stages of malignant infiltration of the liver. Slight or moderate elevations of both AST and ALT activities have been observed after intake of alcohol, in delirium tremens, and after administration of various drugs, such as opiates, salicylates, or ampicillin.

Although serum levels of both AST and ALT become elevated whenever disease processes affect liver cell integrity, ALT is the more liver-specific enzyme.[2] Serum elevations of ALT activity are observed rarely in conditions other than parenchymal liver disease. Moreover, elevations of ALT activity persist longer than do those of AST activity. Measurement of both AST and ALT has some value in distinguishing of hepatitis from other parenchymal lesions.

After a myocardial infarction, increased AST activity appears in serum, as might be expected from the relatively high AST concentration in heart muscle (see Table 20-2). On average, serum levels do not become abnormal, however, until 6 to 8 hours after the onset of chest pain. Abnormal AST levels are observed in more than 97% of cases of myocardial infarction when correctly timed blood specimens are analyzed. Peak values of AST activity are reached after 18 to 24 hours, and the activity values fall to within the reference interval by the fourth or fifth day, provided no new infarct has occurred. The peak values of AST activity are roughly proportional to the extent of cardiac damage. Average increases are four to five times the upper limit of normal; levels of 10 to 15 times normal frequently are associated with fatal infarcts.

ALT levels are within normal limits or only marginally increased in cases of uncomplicated myocardial infarction because the concentration of ALT activity in heart muscle is only a fraction of that of AST activity.

AST (and occasionally ALT) activity levels are increased in progressive muscular dystrophy and dermatomyositis, reaching levels up to eight times normal; they are usually normal in other types of muscle diseases, especially those of neurogenic origin. Pulmonary emboli can raise AST levels to two to three times normal, and slight to moderate elevations (two to five times normal) are noted in cases of acute pancreatitis, crushed muscle injuries, gangrene, and hemolytic disease.

Methods for the measurement of transaminase activity

The assay system used to measure transaminase activity contains two amino acids and two oxo-acids. As no convenient method exists to assay either of the amino acids, formation or consumption of the oxo-acids is measured. Historically, various photometric substrates (2,4-dinitrophenylhydrazine and various dyes) were coupled to the transaminase reactions. Methods based on these reactions once were used widely but are now considered obsolete. Today, continuous-monitoring methods are used to measure transaminase activity.

Reaction principle

Transaminase reactions are monitored continuously by coupling of the transaminase reactions to specific dehydrogenase reactions. The oxo-acids formed in the transaminase reaction are measured indirectly by enzymatic reduction to the corresponding hydroxyacids, the accompanying change in NADH concentration being monitored spectrophotometrically. Thus oxaloacetate, formed in the AST reaction, is reduced to malate in the presence of malate dehydrogenase (MD), as follows:

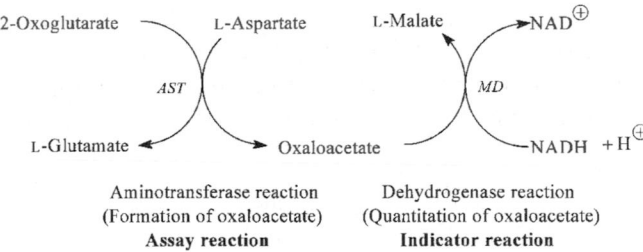

Aminotransferase reaction
(Formation of oxaloacetate)
Assay reaction

Dehydrogenase reaction
(Quantitation of oxaloacetate)
Indicator reaction

Pyruvate formed in the ALT reaction is reduced to lactate by the action of lactate dehydrogenase (LD). The substrate, reduced nicotinamide-adenine dinucleotide (NADH), and the auxiliary enzymes, MD and LD, must be present in sufficient quantity so that the reaction rate is limited only by the amounts of AST and ALT, respectively. As the reactions proceed, NADH is oxidized to NAD^+. The disappearance of NADH per unit time is followed by measurement of the decrease in absorbance at 339 (340) nm for several minutes, either continuously or at frequent intervals. The change in absorbance per minute (ΔA/min) is proportional to the micromoles of NADH oxidized and to the micromoles of substrate transformed per minute (international units).

Measurements should be made in a spectrophotometer with established spectrophotometric and wavelength accuracy and good resolution at 339 (340) nm. The temperature

of the reaction mixture in the cuvet must be controlled at a constant, known level with a thermostatically controlled cuvet compartment. A preliminary incubation period is necessary to ensure that NADH-dependent reduction of endogenous oxo-acids in the sample is completed before 2-oxoglutarate is added to start the transaminase reaction. After a brief lag phase, noted with most coupled reactions, the change in absorbance (ΔA) is monitored; alternatively, several readings (five to eight at 1-minute intervals) are taken to establish the linear portion of the curve.

Standardization

Because of the large numbers of AST and ALT activity measurements performed daily in many laboratories throughout the world, the development of standard or reference methods for these two enzymes was given priority by national and international groups. All such groups have chosen the coupled-reaction approach with MD or LD as the indicator enzyme. However, the methods proposed differ in several details, such as substrate concentrations, nature of buffer (for example, tris[hydroxymethyl]aminomethane [TRIS] or phosphate), and assay temperature. The technique of response-surface methodology has been used in the development of the most recent of these methods to select values for the many variables that affect the rate of reaction. As previously mentioned, supplementation with P-5'-P ensures that all the transaminase activity of the sample is measured.

Reference intervals

The AST reference interval for adults is 8 to 20 U/L at 30 °C (without P-5'-P) and 10 to 30 U/L at 30 °C (with P-5'-P). The ALT reference interval for adults is 10 to 40 U/L at 37 °C (with P-5'-P). Values in men are slightly higher than those in women.

Creatine Kinase

Creatine kinase (EC 2.7.3.2; also known as *adenosine triphosphate:creatine N-phosphotransferase; CK*) is a dimeric enzyme (82 kD) that catalyses the reversible phosphorylation of creatine (Cr) by ATP as follows:

Physiologically, when muscle contracts, ATP is consumed (to form ADP), and CK catalyzes the rephosphorylation of ADP (to form ATP), using creatine phosphate (CrP) as the phosphorylation reservoir.

The optimum pH values for the forward (Cr + ATP → ADP + CrP) and reverse (CrP + ADP → ATP + Cr) reactions are 9.0 and 6.7, respectively. The equilibrium position for the reaction depends on pH. At neutral pH, CrP has a much higher phosphorylating potential than does ATP; this higher potential favors the reverse reaction, with ATP being formed from CrP. The reverse reaction proceeds two to six times faster than the forward reaction, depending on the reaction conditions.

As is true for all kinases, Mg^{+2} is an obligate activating ion to form the ATP- and ADP-Mg^{+2} complexes. The optimal concentration range for Mg^{+2} is quite narrow, and excess Mg^{+2} is inhibitory. Many metal ions, such as Mn^{+2}, Ca^{+2}, Zn^{+2}, and Cu^{+2}, inhibit enzyme activity, as do iodoacetate and other sulfhydryl-binding reagents. Activity is inhibited by excess ADP and by citrate, fluoride, nitrate, acetate, iodide, bromide, malonate, and L-thyroxine. Urate and cystine are potent inhibitors of the enzyme in serum. Even chloride and sulfate ions inhibit activity, and the concentrations of these ions should be kept low in any enzyme assay system based on the CrP + ADP (reverse) reaction. The enzyme in serum is relatively unstable, activity being lost as a result of sulfhydryl group oxidation at the active site of the enzyme. Activity can be restored partially through incubation of the enzyme preparation with sulfhydryl compounds, such as N-acetylcysteine, monothioglycerol, dithioerythritol, dithiothreitol (Cleland's reagent), and glutathione. N-acetylcysteine and monothioglycerol, both being used at a final concentration of 20 mmol/L, are the current agents of choice.

Biochemistry

CK activity is greatest in striated muscle, brain, and heart tissue, which contain some 2500, 550, and 470 U/g of protein, respectively. Other tissues, such as the kidneys and the diaphragm, contain significantly less activity (<30 U/g protein), and the liver and erythrocytes are essentially devoid of activity.

CK is a dimer composed of two subunits, each with a molecular weight (MW) of about 40,000. These subunits (B, or brain; and M, or muscle) are the products of loci on chromosomes 14 and 19, respectively. Because the active form of the enzyme is a dimer, only three different pairs of subunits can exist: BB (or CK-1), MB (or CK-2), and MM (or CK-3). The Commission on Biochemical Nomenclature has recommended that isoenzymes be numbered on the basis of their electrophoretic mobility, with the most anodal form receiving the lowest number. Accordingly, the CK isoenzymes are numbered CK-1, CK-2, and CK-3. The distribution of these isoenzymes in the various tissues of humans is shown in Table 20-3.

TABLE 20-3   Creatine Kinase Isoenzyme Patterns of Human Tissues

Tissue	CK Activity (U/g Wet Weight)	CK-3 (%)	CK-2 (%)	CK-1 (%)
Skeletal muscle	2500	98.9	1.1	0.06
Rectus abdominis		98	2	
Pectoralis major		100	0	
Gastrocnemius		100	0	
Brain	555	0	2.7	97.3
Heart	473	78.7	20.0	1.3
Left ventricle		54 ± 6	41 ± 7	
Papillary muscle		52 ± 4	46 ± 5	
Stomach	190	4.3	0	95.7
		10	0	90
Small intestine	112	1.2	0	98.8
		11 to 13	7 to 9	78 to 80
Colon	138	2.1	0	97.8
		3 to 4	0 to 1	96
Rectum	267	1.2	0	98.8
Kidney	32	2.8	0	97.2
		8 to 12	0	88 to 92
Bladder	145	6.6	0	93.4
		2	6	92
Prostate	114	6	0	94
		34 to 39	2 to 6	59 to 60
Lung		27 to 72	0 to 4	18 to 69
Liver	~1	0	0	100
Uterus	115	2.3	0	97.4
		5 to 16	2 to 20	64 to 93
Placenta		0	0	100
Thyroid		4 to 26	0 to 1	73 to 96

From Lang H: Creatine Kinase Isoenzymes: Pathophysiology and Clinical Application, Berlin, Springer-Verlag, 1981.
CK, Creatine kinase.

All three of these isoenzyme species are found in the cell in the cytosol or associated with myofibrillar structures. However, a fourth form exists that differs from the others both immunologically and in electrophoretic mobility. This isoenzyme, CK-Mt, is located between the inner and outer membranes of mitochondria, and it constitutes in the heart, for example, up to 15% of the total CK activity. Its structure is determined by a locus on chromosome 15. CK activity also may be found in macromolecular form—the so-called macro CK. Macro CK is found, often transiently, in up to 6% of hospitalized patients, but only a small proportion of these patients have abnormal CK activities. It exists in two forms, types 1 and 2. Type 1 is usually a complex of CK-1 and immunoglobulin G (IgG), but other complexes have been described, such as CK-3 with immunoglobulin A (IgA). Prevalence has been estimated between 0.8% and 2.3%, but this fact depends on methodology and the population studied. Type 1 is associated with gastrointestinal diseases, adenoma or carcinoma, myocardial and vascular diseases, and other life-threatening conditions; it is associated with a higher mortality. Type 1 often occurs in women older than 50 years of age. Type 2 is found predominantly in adults who are severely ill with malignancies or liver disease or in children with myocardial disease. Type 2 can interfere with the assay of CK-2 by ion-exchange or immunoinhibition methods. Both macro CK types are heat stable and distinguishable from the CK isoenzymes. Type 2 can be differentiated from type 1 by its higher activation energy.

Both M and B subunits have a C-terminal lysine residue, but only the former can be hydrolyzed by the action of carboxypeptidases normally present in blood. Carboxypeptidases B (EC 3.4.17.2) or N (arginine carboxypeptidase; EC 3.4.17.3) sequentially hydrolyze the lysine residues from CK-3 (CK-MM) to produce two CK-3 **isoforms**—CK-3_2 (one lysine residue removed) and CK-3_1 (both lysine residues removed). The loss of the positively charged lysine produces a more negatively charged CK molecule with greater anodic mobility. Because the magnitude of mobility toward the anode is the basis for naming of isoforms, it follows that the gene product is named CK-3_3. Many alternative nomenclatures are in use, such as CK 3a, 3b, and 3c or MM_1, MM_2, and MM_3 for CK-3_1, CK-3_2, and CK-3_3, respectively. Because CK-2 (CK-MB) has only one M subunit, the gene product is named CK-2_2 and the lysine-hydrolyzed molecule is named CK-2_1. Alternative names are thus CK 2a and CK 2b or MB_1 and MB_2. Other CK-3 and CK-2 isoforms have been observed, but these are less well characterized than those described previously. The assay of the CK isoforms requires special techniques, such as high-voltage electrophoresis with gel cooling, high-performance liquid chromatography (HPLC), chromatofocusing, or immunoassay.[4]

Serum CK activity is subject to a number of physiological variations. Sex, age, muscle mass, physical activity, and race all interact to affect serum activities.

Clinical significance

CK activity is elevated in many diseases, including those involving skeletal muscle, the heart, the central nervous system, and the thyroid.

Diseases of skeletal muscle

Serum CK activity is elevated significantly in all types of muscular dystrophy, especially in Duchenne's type, in which the upper limit of normal may be encountered. In cases of progressive muscular dystrophy (particularly Duchenne's sex-linked muscular dystrophy), enzyme activity in serum is highest in infancy and childhood (7 to 10 years of age) and may be elevated long before the disease is clinically apparent. Serum CK activity characteristically falls as individuals get older and the mass of functioning muscle diminishes with the progression of the disease. About 50% to 80% of the asymptomatic female carriers of Duchenne's dystrophy show threefold to sixfold elevations in CK activity, but values may be normal if specimens are obtained after individuals have experienced a period of physical inactivity. Quite

high values of CK are noted in individuals with viral myositis, polymyositis, and similar muscle diseases (see also this chapter's discussion on necrotizing polymyopathy). However, with neurogenic muscle diseases, such as myasthenia gravis, multiple sclerosis, poliomyelitis, and parkinsonism, serum enzyme activity is normal. Very high activity also is encountered in cases of malignant hyperthermia, a familial disease characterized by high fever and brought on by administration of inhalation anesthesia (usually halothane) to the affected individual. Apparently, CK-2 replaces part of the CK-3 form in the muscles, resulting in impaired storage of CrP in muscle.

Usually, only CK-3 is present in serum in dystrophies and myopathies. However, diseased or damaged skeletal muscle (such as that following extreme exercise) may contain significant proportions of CK-2 because of the phenomenon of "fetal reversion," in which fetal patterns of protein synthesis reappear. Thus serum CK-2 fractions >5% may be detected in such circumstances. This explanation may account for the elevated CK-2 values sometimes observed in individuals with chronic renal failure (uremic myopathy).

Diseases of the heart

The serum enzyme changes after a myocardial infarction are detailed in Chapter 33. However, a number of other cardiac conditions and diagnostic or therapeutic procedures have been reported to cause serum CK-3 and CK-2 enzyme changes.[3] These conditions include cardioversion; cardiopulmonary resuscitation; cardiac catheterization; percutaneous transluminal coronary angioplasty; general effects of anesthesia and noncardiac surgery; cardiopulmonary bypass and coronary artery bypass surgery; perioperative myocardial infarction and cardiac transplantation; myocarditis; pericarditis; and polymyositis, pulmonary embolism, cardiac contusion, and acute cocaine abuse.

Diseases of the central nervous system

Serum CK activity may increase in individuals with acute cerebrovascular disease or neurosurgical intervention and those with cerebral ischemia. Isoenzyme studies show that the increase is entirely in the CK-3 isoenzyme; no CK-1 isoenzyme increase is demonstrable. By contrast, after head injury, serum CK-1 activity is detected readily in many of these individuals, and the extent of elevation may correlate with the severity of the injury and the prognosis. In addition, serum CK-2 often is detected in those individuals with head injuries and in cases of subarachnoid hemorrhage. This appearance of CK-2 suggests myocardial damage after the cerebral accident and indicates the need to monitor such individuals through determination of the serum CK isoenzyme levels. In cases of Reye's syndrome, a childhood disorder characterized by acute brain swelling with fatty infiltration and nonicteric dysfunction of the liver (see Chapter 36), total serum CK activity is increased as much as seventyfold, with CK-1 just detectable. The extent of the total CK elevation appears to indicate the severity of the encephalopathy.

Elevations of total CK activity in CSF have been found in some specimens from epileptic individuals and those with brain tumors, cerebral infarcts, cerebral hemorrhage, or cerebral damage caused by cerebral trauma; however, the elevations are not consistent with the degree of pathological change. Similarly, CSF specimens from a majority of individuals with either bacterial or nonbacterial meningitis and those with autism demonstrate increased levels of CK. After certain types of neurological injury, CK-1 levels in CSF increase. For example, after head injuries, the activity (or mass) of CK-1 in CSF inversely correlates with the Glasgow Coma Scale score. Clinically, individuals with activities more than 200 U/L always die, those between 100 and 200 U/L usually survive but have various degrees of neurological deficit, and those with less than 100 U/L have a chance of good recovery.

Diseases of the thyroid

Serum CK activity demonstrates an inverse relationship with thyroid activity. About 60% of hypothyroid subjects show an average elevation of CK activity fivefold more than the upper limit of the reference interval; elevations of as high as fiftyfold also have been found. The major isoenzyme present is CK-3, although up to 13% of CK activity may be present as CK-2, suggesting possible myocardial involvement. In hyperthyroidism the serum CK activity tends to be at the low end of the reference interval.

CK-1 in serum

During normal childbirth, maternal total serum CK activity elevates sixfold. The uterus and possibly the placenta are the probable sources of the CK-1. Surgical intervention during labor further increases the serum activity of CK-1. CK-1 may be elevated in neonates, particularly in brain-damaged or very low-birth-weight newborns. The presence of CK-1, usually at low levels, also has been reported in a wide variety of instances, such as in multisystem insult and many critical-care patients, as well as after aortocoronary bypass operations or cardiopulmonary resuscitation and in hypothermia. Certain gastrointestinal disorders, such as infarction or adenocarcinoma, and various lung tumors may cause elevated serum CK-1 activities. Tumors of the prostate, bladder, testes, kidneys, breasts, ovaries, and uterus, central nervous system neoplasms, and leukemias, lymphomas, and sarcomas have been associated to various degrees with elevations of serum CK-1.

Methods for the determination of creatine kinase activity

Numerous photometric, fluorometric, and coupled enzyme methods have been developed for the assay of CK activity, through use of either the forward (Cr → CrP) or reverse

(Cr ← CrP) reaction. Analytically, the reverse reaction is preferable because it proceeds faster than the forward reaction, although the cost of the starting chemicals, CrP and ADP, is greater than the cost of Cr and ATP.

Reaction principles

CK catalyzes the conversion of CrP to Cr with a concomitant phosphorylation of ADP to ATP as follows:

$$\text{Creatine phosphate} + \text{ADP} \xrightarrow[\text{pH 6.7}]{CK} \text{creatine} + \text{ATP}$$

$$\text{ATP} + \text{glucose} \xrightarrow{HK} \text{glucose-6-phosphate} + \text{ADP}$$

$$\text{Glucose-6-phosphate} + \text{NADP}^{\oplus} \xrightarrow{G6PD} \text{6-phosphogluconate} + \text{NADPH} + \text{H}^{\oplus}$$

The ATP produced is measured by hexokinase (HK)/ glucose-6-phosphate dehydrogenase (G6PD) coupled reactions that ultimately convert nicotinamide-adenine dinucleotide phosphate (NADP) to reduced NADP (NADPH), which is monitored spectrophotometrically. Oliver initially developed this method that Rosalki subsequently modified and improved by adding adenosine-5-monophosphate (AMP) to inhibit adenylate kinase (AK) and cysteine to activate CK. Subsequently, Szasz and his colleagues optimized the assay by incorporating N-acetylcysteine to activate CK, ethylenediaminetetraacetic acid (EDTA) to bind Ca^{+2} and increase the stability of the reaction mixture, and diadenosine pentaphosphate (Ap_5A) and AMP to inhibit AK.[6]

CK assays demonstrate a lag phase with a slow increase in reaction rate after the addition of substrate or serum to the assay mixture. Typical lag phases in an optimized assay system are 110 seconds at 25 °C, 90 seconds at 30 °C, and 60 seconds at 37 °C. This phenomenon has important practical implications because inappropriate timing of the measurement period causes incorrect and low estimations of the reaction rate.

Bioluminescent methods that are more sensitive than spectrophotometric methods have been developed to measure CK activity. In these methods the reverse reaction is linked to the luciferin/luciferase reaction as follows:

$$\text{Creatine phosphate} + \text{ADP} \xrightarrow{CK} \text{creatine} + \text{ATP}$$

$$\text{ATP} + \text{luciferin} + O_2 \xrightarrow{Luciferase} \text{AMP} + \text{oxiluciferin} + \text{PPi} + CO_2 + \text{light}$$

The light produced in this reaction is a measure of enzyme activity.

Specimen requirements

Serum is the preferred specimen for CK assay. Plasma containing heparin, EDTA, citrate, or fluoride may produce unpredictable reaction rates. CK activity in serum is unstable and is lost rapidly during storage. Stability decreases in the following order: macro forms of CK, CK-3, CK-2, and CK-1. The degree of stability varies with the individual specimen and with the activating efficiency of the assay mixture. CK is inactivated by bright daylight and increasing specimen pH because of the loss of carbon dioxide; accordingly, specimens should be stored in the dark in tightly closed tubes. CK is susceptible to thermal denaturation; the degree of inactivation corresponds to the degree of temperature increase and is not reversed by the addition of sulfhydryl (thiol) reagents. CK also is inactivated by oxidation of sulfhydryl groups at the active site; this inactivation is reversible by the addition of thiol agents. Therefore the serum specimen should be chilled to 4 °C as rapidly as possible after collection. The addition of a thiol agent for storage is probably unnecessary because an optimized assay formulation, containing EDTA, 2 mmol/L, and N-acetylcysteine, 20 mmol/L, reactivates CK in serum to 99% after it has been stored for 1 week at 4 °C.

A slight degree of hemolysis is tolerated because erythrocytes contain no CK activity. However, moderately or severely hemolyzed specimens are unsatisfactory because enzymes and intermediates (AK, ATP, and glucose-6-phosphate [G-6-P]) liberated from the erythrocytes may affect the lag phase and side reactions occurring in the assay system.

Reference intervals

In healthy individuals, the magnitude of serum CK activity is affected by age, sex, race, lean body mass, and physical activity, as well as other less defined genetic differences. These factors presumably explain the distributions for CK activity from reference populations that are skewed markedly toward higher values. However, children have higher CK values than adults, men have higher values than women, and blacks have higher values than nonblacks. North American experience derived from a population of blacks, Hispanics, Asians, and Caucasians suggests three broad race/gender CK subgroups for the 2.5th to 97.5th percentiles (at 37 °C): high CK activities of 50 to 520 U/L for black men, intermediate CK activities of 35 to 345 U/L for black women and all nonblack men, and low CK activities of 25 to 145 U/L for all nonblack women.

The CK levels in the sera of normal newborns are elevated during the first 24 hours after birth to about three times adult values, and a slight elevation remains throughout the first year of life.

In men, serum CK activity remains constant after the first year until 12 years of age; it then increases at about 15 years of age, a reflection of the increase in muscle mass during puberty. CK activity thereafter decreases slightly with age. In women, activity is stable from the first year until 12 years of age and then rises to the time of menstruation. Thereafter, activity falls, particularly during pregnancy; the mean level during pregnancy is less than half that of premenarchal girls. After menopause the serum CK level rises. For both sexes a distinct seasonal variation is present, with CK activities being higher in the summer months.

Exercise and muscle trauma (for example, contact sports, traffic accidents, intramuscular injections, surgery, convulsions, wasp or bee stings, and burns) elevate serum CK values. Mild exercise, such as a 3-mile jog, has no effect, but more strenuous or prolonged exercise produces CK elevations. Sustained exercise, such that practiced by well-trained long-distance runners, produces an increase in the CK-2 content of skeletal muscle, which may produce abnormal serum CK-2 activities. The CK-3 isoform pattern is altered by exercise, even mild forms of exercise. Many drugs elevate serum CK activity because they release enzyme from cells or exert direct toxic effects on cell membranes.

Examples of reference intervals (U/L) for Caucasian adults for serum CK are as follows:

Reaction Temperature	Man	Woman
25 °C	10 to 65	7 to 55
30 °C	15 to 105	10 to 80
37 °C	38 to 174	26 to 140

Methods for the separation and quantitation of creatine kinase isoenzymes

The three techniques most commonly used to separate and quantitate CK isoenzymes are electrophoresis, ion-exchange chromatography, and various immunological methods.

Electrophoresis

The CK isoenzymes are separated with agar, agarose, or cellulose acetate electrophoresis. The isoenzyme bands then are visualized by incubation of the support with a concentrated CK assay mixture with the reverse reaction. The NADPH formed in this reaction then is detected by observation of the bluish-white fluorescence after excitation by long-wave (360-nm) ultraviolet light. NADPH may be quantitated by fluorescent densitometry, which can detect 2 to 10 U/L. Typical examples of results obtained by this technique on the serum sample of a healthy adult and for an individual who has suffered a myocardial infarction 24 hours previously are shown in Figure 20-2, *A*. Alternatively, the NADPH can reduce a tetrazolium salt to form a colored formazan. The discriminating power of electrophoresis allows the detection of abnormal bands, many of which are shown in Figure 20-2, *B*. In individuals receiving maintenance hemodialysis for end-stage renal disease, albumin becomes endogenously fluorescent and may simulate the CK-1 band. This possibility is excluded readily through examination of the electrophoretic strip under fluorescent light before and after staining.

Ion-exchange chromatography

Ion-exchange techniques are used to separate the CK isoenzymes either by batch adsorption or by column (or minicolumn) chromatography. Various media have been

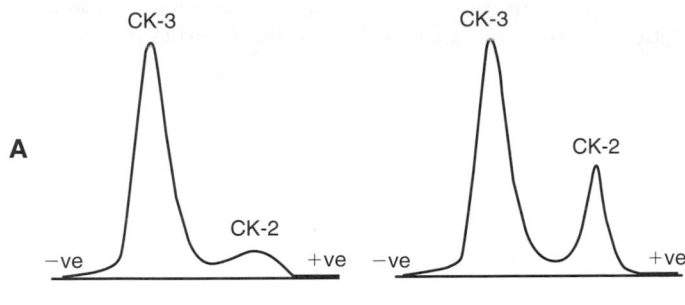

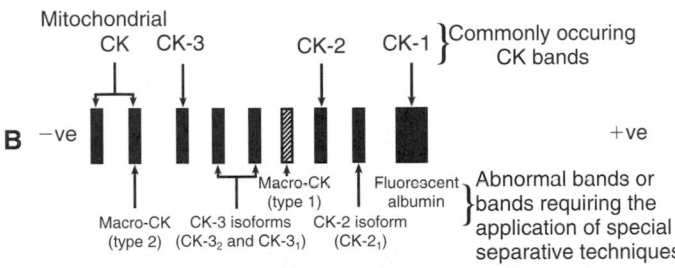

Figure 20-2   **A,** The electrophoretic separation of serum CK isoenzymes from a healthy adult *(left)* and an individual *(right)* who had a myocardial infarction 24 hours previously. **B,** A diagram representing the CK isoenzymes (some of which are only seen in disease states) and some of the reported anomalous isoenzymes. CK-3 and CK-2 isoenzymes are derived from the gene products CK-3 and CK-2. *CK,* Creatine kinase; CK-1, CK-2, CK-3, isoenzymes of CK.

used (DEAE-Sephadex A50, DEAE-cellulose, DEAE-Glycophase, DEAE-Biogel A), but DEAE-Sephadex A50, usually in the form of a minicolumn (0.5 by 6.0 cm) holding about 60 mg of gel, is the most popular. The CK isoenzymes and other proteins are adsorbed onto the gel; the gel then is washed, and the CK-3 is eluted with TRIS buffer, 50 mmol/L, pH 8.0, containing NaCl, 100 mmol/L. CK-2 is eluted next with the same TRIS buffer containing NaCl, 200 mmol/L. Finally, CK-1 is eluted with TRIS buffer, 50 mmol/L, pH 7.0, containing NaCl, 500 mmol/L. The lower limit of detection is about 1 to 5 U/L. The elution process considerably dilutes the CK isoenzymes. Therefore this dilutional effect needs to be reduced by (1) use of small volumes of eluting buffer, (2) concentration of each fraction after collection, or (3) use of the eluate as part solvent for the CK reagents.

Immunological methods

Immunological methods used to measure the CK isoenzymes require specific antisera against the M and B subunits. The antisera are used to precipitate specific isoenzymes (immunoprecipitation), or competitively bind specific isoenzymes (immunoassay). Goat antisera appear to inhibit subunit activity (immunoinhibition) more effectively, although they can be used together with donkey antigoat IgG to precipitate CK molecules previously inhibited with goat antisera.

In the procedure based on immunoprecipitation, anti-CK-B sera is used to precipitate (after centrifugation) all CK-1 (BB) and CK-2 (MB) from a serum sample, leaving only the CK-3 (MM) activity to be detected. Similarly, anti-CK-M sera precipitate all CK-3 and CK-2, leaving only CK-1 (if present) to be detected. The serum content of CK-2 then is measured by calculation of the difference between the total serum CK activity and the sum of CK-1 and CK-3 activities. The detection limit of this assay is about 4 U/L; the coefficient of variation of the CK-1 and CK-3 determinations is 4%, and that of CK-2 is between 10 and 20%. The greater coefficient of variation for CK-2 is due to the summation of errors in the separate determinations of total CK, CK-1, and CK-3 activities.

The technique of immunoinhibition is simpler and faster than immunoprecipitation and is used more widely. The inhibiting anti-CK-M sera inhibit both M subunits of CK-3 and the single M subunit of CK-2 and thus allow determination of the enzyme activity of the B subunit of CK-2, the B subunits of CK-1, any macro or mitochondrial CKs, and AK. To determine CK-2 effectively, this technique therefore assumes the absence of CK-1 (or the other sources of interference previously mentioned) from the tested serum, a circumstance that does not always occur. However, when CK-1 is present in a specimen, it usually has an activity of less than 5 U/L, which is below the detection limit of the immunoinhibition technique. Therefore CK-1 interference in this assay is generally negligible.

In contrast with immunoprecipitation and immunoinhibition, which measure the isoenzymes by determinations of enzyme activity, immunoassays measure enzyme mass. Although mass assays of CK-1 and CK-3 are achieved readily with less than 2% cross-reactivity, one of the CK-2 units is included in any determination of either the M or B subunits. Therefore specific measurements of CK-2 require the application of the "sandwich" technique, in which two antibodies with affinity for different parts of the CK-2 molecule are used sequentially. The first antibody, which is usually monoclonal, is rendered immobile on a matrix, and the second antibody is conjugated with a label, such as an enzyme or a marker molecule. The sandwich technique ensures that only CK-2 is estimated, because neither CK-3 nor CK-1 reacts with both antibodies. Mass assays are more sensitive than activity-based methods and detect serum abnormalities earlier. A number of mass assays, using various labels (see also Chapter 10), now are available commercially and used increasingly for routine and emergency assay of CK-2.

The lower limit of detection of these systems for CK-2 is usually less than 0.5 µg/L. Reference intervals for men are usually less than 5.0 µg/L, with values for women being less than those for men, although many laboratories use a single reference interval (male). Precision at physiological levels is usually between ± 5% and 10% (coefficient of variation). In addition to reporting the CK-2 mass, some laboratories also calculate a relative index (CK-2 mass [µg/L] ÷ total CK

TABLE 20-4 Creatine Kinase Isoenzyme Results in Sera of Patients with Various Clinical Conditions and Obtained by Several Different Techniques

| | CK Activity, U/L | | | | |
Clinical Condition	Total	CK-3	CK-2	CK-2 Activity (%)	Technique
Hospitalized noncardiac patients	131*	124.1	5.9	2.3	E
Myocardial infarctions	1556*	1338	178	11.3	E
Patients receiving morphine intramuscularly	347 ± 89	345 ± 89	3 ± 2	0.3 to 0.9	E
Dermatomyositis	1599	1419	89	5	E
Polymyositis	1725	1052	673	39	E
Normal	36-277	—	0 to 2.6	0 to 1	C
Myocardial infarctions	84-236	—	4.6 to 28	6 to 11	C
			CK Mass, μg/L: CK-2	RI[2]	Technique
Normal			0 to 5	up to 4	I
Myocardial infarction (24 hours after infarction)			262	30	I

CK, Creatine kinase; E, electrophoresis; C, column chromatography; I, immunoassay; RI, relative index = [total CK (U/L)/CK-2 (μg/L)] × 100.
*Average values; Scandinavian assay at 37 °C.

activity [U/L] × 100) or, in International System of Units (SI) units, as a decimal fraction, which does not require multiplication by 100. These values are usually about 5% (SI < 0.05). For mass assays of CK-3, men have values of 102 to 1688 μg/L and women 36 to 487 μg/L, whereas for mass assays of CK-1, values are less than 6 μg/L.

Table 20-4 provides representative CK isoenzyme results for various clinical conditions and techniques.

Lactate Dehydrogenase

Lactate dehydrogenase (EC 1.1.1.27; L-lactate:NAD$^+$ oxidoreductase; LD) is a hydrogen transfer enzyme that catalyzes the oxidation of L-lactate to pyruvate with the mediation of NAD$^+$ as hydrogen acceptor as follows:

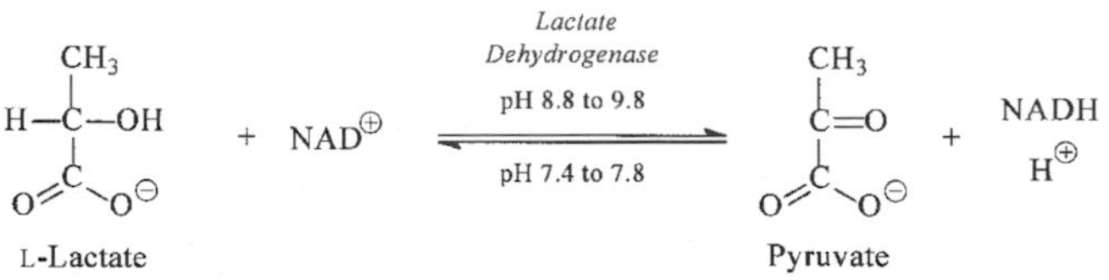

As indicated, the reaction is reversible, and the reaction equilibrium strongly favors the reduction of pyruvate to lactate (P → L), the "reverse reaction."

Biochemistry

The pH optimum for the lactate-to-pyruvate (L → P) reaction is 8.8 to 9.8, and an assay mixture, optimized for LD-1 at 37 °C, contains NAD$^+$, 9 mmol/L, and L-lactate, 80 mmol/L; for the P → L assay, at 37 °C, the pH optimum is 7.4 to 7.8, NADH 300 μmol/L, and pyruvate 0.85 mmol/L. The optimal pH varies with the predominant isoenzymes in

the sample and depends on the temperature and substrate and buffer concentrations. The specificity of the enzyme extends from L-lactate to various related 2-hydroxyacids and 2-oxo-acids. The catalytic oxidation of 2-hydroxybutyrate, the next higher homologue of lactate, to 2-oxobutyrate is referred to as *2-hydroxybutyrate dehydrogenase* (HBD) *activity*. LD does not act on D-lactate, and only NAD$^+$ serves as coenzyme. The enzyme has an MW of 134,000 and is composed of four peptide chains of two types: M (or A) and H (or B), each under separate genetic control. The structures of LD-M and LD-H are determined by loci on human chromosomes 11 and 12, respectively. The subunit compositions of the five isoenzymes, in order of decreasing anodal mobility in an alkaline medium, are LD-1 (HHHH; H$_4$); LD-2 (HHHM; H$_3$M); LD-3 (HHMM; H$_2$M$_2$); LD-4 (HMMM; HM$_3$); and LD-5 (MMMM; M$_4$). A different, sixth LD isoenzyme, LD-X (also called *LD$_c$*), composed of four X (or C) subunits, is present in postpubertal human testes. A seventh LD, called *LD-6*, has been identified in the sera of severely ill individuals.

LD is inhibited by reagents with reactivity against thiol groups, such as mercuric ions and *p*-chloromercuribenzoate, the inhibition being reversed by the addition of cysteine or glutathione. Borate and oxalate both inhibit LD by competing with lactate for its binding site on the enzyme; similarly, oxamate competes with pyruvate for its binding site. Both pyruvate and lactate in excess inhibit enzyme activity, although the effect of pyruvate is greater. Inhibition by either substrate is greater for the H form than for the M form, and substrate inhibition decreases with increases in pH. EDTA inhibits the enzyme, perhaps by binding Zn^{+2}; however, the postulated activator role for zinc ions is not fully established.

LD activity is present in all the body's cells and invariably is found only in the cytoplasm of the cell. Enzyme levels in various tissues (in U/g) are high, compared with those in serum—liver, 145; heart, 124; kidney, 106; skeletal muscle, 147; and erythrocytes (U/g hemoglobin), 36. Thus tissue levels are about 500 times greater than those normally found in serum, and therefore leakage of the enzyme from even a small mass of damaged tissue increases the observed serum level of LD significantly.

In addition to their higher enzyme concentrations, many of these tissues show different isoenzyme compositions. In cardiac muscle, kidneys, and erythrocytes, the electrophoretically faster moving isoenzymes LD-1 and LD-2 predominate, whereas in liver and skeletal muscle the more cathodal LD-4 and LD-5 isoenzymes predominate; however, skeletal muscle damage may also result in midzone or even anodic LD patterns. Isoenzymes of intermediate mobility account for the LD activity of many tissues (for example, endocrine glands, spleen, lungs, lymph nodes, platelets, and nongravid uterine muscle).

Clinical significance

Lactate dehydrogenase in serum

Changes in serum LD activity after a myocardial infarction are described in Chapter 33. Values may be elevated moderately in cases of myocarditis and cardiac failure with hepatic congestion (Figure 20-3) but are normal in cases of angina and pericarditis. Enzyme levels may be elevated moderately in cases of severe shock and anoxia.

Hemolysis, if sufficiently severe, produces an LD isoenzyme pattern similar to that present in myocardial infarction; however, research now suggests that this effect of hemolysis depends on a markedly increased percentage (for example, >10%) of reticulocytes. Megaloblastic anemias, usually resulting from the deficiency of folate or vitamin B_{12}, cause the erythrocyte precursor cell to break down in the bone marrow (ineffective erythropoiesis), resulting in the release of large quantities of LD-1 and LD-2 isoenzymes. Marked elevations of the total serum LD activity—up to 50 times the upper limit of the reference interval—have been observed in individuals with the megaloblastic anemias. These elevations rapidly return to normal after appropriate treatment is instituted.

Elevations of LD activity are present in the serum of individuals with liver disease, but these elevations are not as great as are the increases in aminotransferase activity. Elevations are especially high (10 times normal) in cases of toxic hepatitis with jaundice; slightly lower values are observed in cases of viral hepatitis and infectious mononucleosis, the latter often associated with elevations of LD-3. LD activity is normal or at most twice the upper limit of normal in individuals with cirrhosis and obstructive jaundice. Serum LD-5 often is elevated markedly in individuals with either primary liver disease or liver anoxia secondary to decreased oxygen perfusion.

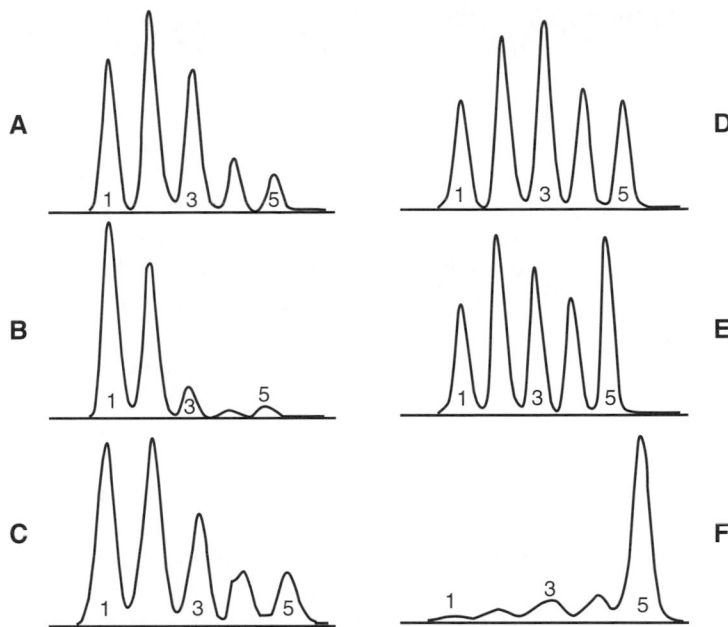

Figure 20-3   Serum lactate dehydrogenase (LD) isoenzyme patterns obtained with a thin-layer agarose gel electrophoresis system. The gel was incubated with a liquid overlay of NAD^+ and L-lactate to detect isoenzymes. The generated NADH was detected by fluorescent scanning. **A,** Normal serum. **B,** Acute myocardial infarction (common pattern showing "flipped" LD-1). **C,** Acute myocardial infarction (showing elevated LD-1 that has not "flipped"). **D,** Involvement of platelets or lymphatic tissue (obtained from an individual with infectious mononucleosis). **E,** Congestive cardiac failure showing elevated LD-5 as a result of hepatic anoxia. **F,** Acute circulatory shock showing the result of very severe hepatic anoxia.

Increased levels of the enzyme in serum also are found in about one third of individuals with renal disease, especially those with tubular necrosis or pyelonephritis. However, these elevations do not correlate well with proteinuria and other parameters of renal disease. The LD isoenzyme pattern in renal disease is very similar to a normal serum pattern, except for the higher absolute values. In renal infarction cases the serum LD pattern can mimic that in individuals with myocardial infarction.

Individuals with malignant disease demonstrate increased LD activity in serum; up to 70% of those with liver metastases and 20% to 60% of those who do not have hepatic metastases have elevated total LD activity. Especially high values are associated with Hodgkin's disease and abdominal and lung cancers. The isoenzyme pattern of the elevated LD occasionally reflects the organ affected by the malignancy, but it most often shows only a nonspecific increase in the slow-moving forms (LD-4 and LD-5), suggesting that the tissue has regressed into synthesizing the more embryonic, anaerobic LD types. One unusual exception to this observation is the markedly elevated LD-1 in germ cell tumors, such as teratoma, seminoma of the testis, and dysgerminoma of the ovary. As a rule the elevations of LD in individuals with cancer are too erratic to be useful in clinical diagnosis, although serum levels have been assayed to monitor changes in tumor burden after chemotherapy. More helpful in diagnosis are measurements of LD activity in exudative effusions obtained from areas near or adjacent to malignancies. In these fluids, LD levels are often higher than they are in serum, whereas the opposite is true for fluids bathing healthy tissues. In exudates caused by malignancies, LD-2 is unusually high in 33% of cases, and in 50% of cases, LD-2 exceeded 35% or LD-5 was less than 12% of the total LD activity. Leukemias are associated with only moderate elevations of serum LD.

Moderately increased LD activity is found in the sera of all individuals affected by progressive muscular dystrophy, especially those in the early and middle stages of the disease. The observed increase is confined to LD-5, the isoenzyme form characteristic of striated muscle. In the later stages of the disease, after a large mass of the tissue containing the LD-5 has been lost, the observed LD levels in serum even may decline to normal levels, with the predominant isoenzyme forms then being LD-1 and LD-2. Only occasionally is an elevated serum LD level found in individuals with other forms of neuromuscular disorders.

Elevated values of the enzyme in serum also are encountered in cases of pulmonary embolism; occasionally a raised LD level may be the only evidence to suggest the presence of a hidden embolus. The serum LD-3 level probably is elevated because of the massive destruction of platelets after the formation of an embolus.

Lactate dehydrogenase in urine

Elevations of LD activity in urine three to six times normal are associated with chronic glomerulonephritis, systemic lupus erythematosus, diabetic nephrosclerosis, and bladder and kidney malignances. Determination of LD activity in urine is affected by uncertainties arising from the presence of inhibitors, such as urea and small peptides, and from the possible inactivation of LD under adverse pH conditions in the urine.

Lactate dehydrogenase in cerebrospinal fluid

In healthy individuals, CSF-LD activity is normally much lower than is the serum activity, and LD-4 and LD-5 frequently are undetectable. The use of these analytes also is complicated by the possibility of contamination by hemorrhage or disruption of the blood-brain barrier by disease, which adds LD of systemic origin to the CSF. Additionally, LD isoenzymes may be released from cells that have infiltrated into the CSF. For example, in bacterial meningitis cases the resulting granulocytosis produces an elevation of LD-4 and LD-5, whereas viral meningitis produces lymphocytosis, which may create an elevation of LD-1 through LD-3.

For the previously mentioned reasons the correlation between CSF and LD activity, especially CSF-LD-1 activity, and the Glasgow Coma Scale score is not as close in individuals with head injuries as in those with CSF-CK, suggesting a preference for the latter assay. In many individuals, CSF-LD-5 is elevated in the presence of metastatic tumors, whereas primary brain tumors show an increase in all isoenzyme fractions (that is, an isomorphic LD isoenzyme pattern). In neonates, elevation of CSF-LD is observed in cases of intracranial hemorrhage and associated significantly with subsequent seizures and hydrocephalus.

Methods for the determination of lactate dehydrogenase activity

A multiplicity of forward (L → P) and reverse (P → L) reactions have been introduced in the past 30 years. Advantages of the L → P assay include the following:

1. Substrate inhibition by lactate is less than that produced by pyruvate.
2. NAD preparations used in the L → P reaction appear to contain fewer endogenous LD inhibitors than NADH preparations used in the L → P reaction. However, the problem with endogenous LD inhibitors is becoming a nonissue as commercial preparations of NADH now are substantially free of LD inhibitors.
3. The reaction linearity of the L → P assay is more prolonged than that of the P → L assay.[8]

Advantages of the P → L assay include the following:

1. A less expensive assay formulation (because of the much lower concentration of reactants)
2. A greater change in absorbance with time, allowing more precise measurements
3. Greater stability of the working reagents

Within the last decade, a significant move has shifted from the P → L to the L → P reaction and toward 37 °C as the assay temperature. For example, an L → P continuous-monitoring reference method has been developed by the IFCC Committee on Enzymes of the IFCC.[1] It is optimized for LD-1 at both 30 and 37 °C.

Reaction principle

LD catalyzes the conversion of L-lactate to pyruvate with the simultaneous reduction of oxidation of NAD to NADH. The change in absorbance with time because of the conversion of NAD to NADH is directly proportional to LD activity.

Specimen requirements

Serum is the preferred specimen to measure LD activity. Plasma samples should not be used because they may be contaminated with platelets, which contain high concentrations of LD. Serum should be separated from the clot as soon as possible after the specimen has been obtained. Hemolyzed serum must not be used because erythrocytes contain 150 times more LD activity (particularly LD-1 and LD-2) than does serum.

The different isoenzymes vary in their reactions to cold, LD-4 and LD-5 being especially labile. In tissue extracts, all activity of LD-4 and LD-5 is lost if the extracts are stored at $-20\,°C$ overnight. Loss of activity may be prevented by addition of NAD^+ or glutathione. Both types of monomers bind a molecule of NAD^+, but the binding of NAD to the M form is weaker and some dissociation occurs, with concomitant exposure of sulfhydryl groups to oxidation. In serum the sulfhydryl in albumin and other proteins retards inactivation of the M-rich isoenzymes (LD-4 and LD-5). Serum specimens should be stored at room temperature, at which no loss of activity occurs for 2 to 3 days. If specimens of sera must be stored for longer periods, they should be kept at 4 °C, with NAD^+ (10 mg/mL) or glutathione (3.1 mg/mL) added to decrease the rate of inactivation of LD-4 and LD-5.

Reference intervals

Values for LD activity in serum vary considerably, depending on the direction of the enzyme reaction, type of method used, and experimental parameters. The reference interval for the $L \rightarrow P$ reaction at pH 8.8 to 9.0 and at 30 °C is 35 to 88 U/L; at 37 °C, it is 125 to 225 U/L, with the female upper limit being 214 U/L. The reference interval for the $P \rightarrow L$ reaction at 30 °C and at pH 7.4 is 95 to 200 U/L. The reference values for CSF-LD are 7 to 30 U/L for the $P \rightarrow L$ reaction at 30 °C. In urine a reference interval of 42 to 98 U/L has been reported for the $L \rightarrow P$ reaction at 25 °C.

Methods for the separation and quantitation of lactate dehydrogenase isoenzymes

Techniques used to separate and measure the isoenzymes of LD include electrophoresis, chemical inhibition, ion-exchange chromatography, and immunoprecipitation. In addition, a photometric assay has been developed in which 2-oxobutyrate is used as a substrate to allow measurement of LD-1 and LD-2.

Electrophoresis

Electrophoretic separation on agarose gels or cellulose acetate membranes is the procedure most commonly used to demonstrate LD isoenzymes. With this technique the serum sample first is inserted into a well in the gel surface or touched onto the surface of the membrane. After the isoenzymes have been separated by electrophoresis, a reaction mixture is layered over the separation medium. The mixture (typically D,L-lactate, 500 mmol/L, and NAD^+, 13 mmol/L, often dissolved in a suitable pH 8.0 buffer) is applied as a liquid or in a gel. The overlay and medium are incubated at 37 °C. The NADH generated over the LD zones is detected either by its fluorescence, when it is excited by long-wave ultraviolet light (365 nm), or its reduction of a tetrazolium salt to form a colored formazan.

Through use of an agarose gel technique with fluorometric quantitation of the generated NADH, the following reference intervals for isoenzymes were obtained for a healthy population (n = 250), expressed as percent of total LD:

- LD-1, 14% to 26%
- LD-2, 29% to 39%
- LD-3, 20% to 26%
- LD-4, 8% to 16%
- LD-5, 6% to 16%.

The LD-1/LD-2 ratio was 0.45 to 0.74. A cellulose acetate method using tetrazolium staining produced the following reference intervals, expressed as percent of total LD:

- LD-1, 18% to 33%
- LD-2, 28% to 40%
- LD-3, 18% to 30%
- LD-4, 6% to 16%
- LD-5, 2% to 13%.

Selective chemical inhibition methods

Several selective chemical inhibition methods have been described to inhibit serum LD-2 through LD-5, thus permitting the assay of LD-1 alone. Chemicals used as inhibitors include 1,6-hexanediol (700 mmol/L), sodium perchlorate (825 mmol/L), and guanidine thiocyanate (190 mmol/L). Results from these assays correlate well ($r > 0.99$) with electrophoretic and immunoinhibition assays.

Ion-exchange chromatography

LD isoenzymes also have been separated with minicolumns packed with ion-exchange resin. This method allows the discrete estimation of serum LD-1 and LD-2 activities and the determination of the LD-1/LD-2 ratio. The separation is carried out in three steps. The first step elutes LD-3, -4, and -5; the second, LD-2; and the third, LD-1. The LD-1/LD-2 ratio then is calculated.

Immunoprecipitation

An immunoprecipitation method using a goat antiserum to purified rhesus monkey LD-5 has been used to measure LD-1. This antiserum binds LD isoenzymes LD-2 through LD-5. The bound isoenzymes are precipitated by the addition of a second antibody. Because this second antibody is conjugated to polyvinylidene fluoride particles, the particles with the immune complex are centrifuged readily from solution, leaving only LD-1 in the supernatant. The LD-1 activity is assayed by reaction rate methods. LD-1 results correlate well with those obtained with the electrophoretic assay.

Selected substrate to measure 2-hydroxybutyrate dehydrogenase activity

When 2-oxobutyrate is used as enzyme in place of pyruvate, the reduction of substrate proceeds at an appreciable rate only when LD-1 and LD-2 are present; the other LD isoenzymes are much less active. HBD, present in serum, represents the LD activity of (mostly) the LD-1 and LD-2 isoenzymes. HBD measurement thus indicates the activity of the cardiac LD isoenzymes.

Alkaline Phosphatase

Alkaline phosphatase (EC 3.1.3.1; orthophosphoric-monoester phosphohydrolase [alkaline optimum]; ALP) catalyzes the alkaline hydrolysis of a large variety of naturally occurring and synthetic substrates, but the natural substrates on which they act in the body are not known.

Biochemistry

ALP is present in practically all tissues of the body, especially at or in the cell membranes, and it occurs at particularly high levels in intestinal epithelium, kidney tubules, bone (osteoblasts), liver, and placenta. Several isoenzymes are known to exhibit optimal activity at a pH of about 10 in vitro, but the optimum pH and the activity observed vary with the nature and concentration of the substrate on which the action takes place, the type of buffer or phosphate acceptor present, and to some extent the nature of the isoenzymes. Although the exact metabolic function of the enzyme is not yet understood, the enzyme appears to be associated with lipid transport in the intestine and the calcification process in bone. Some divalent ions, such as Mg^{2+}, Co^{2+}, and Mn^{2+}, are activators of the enzyme, and Zn^{2+} is a constituent metal ion. The correct ratio of Mg^{2+}/Zn^{2+} ions is necessary to avoid displacement of Mg^{2+} and obtain optimal activity. Phosphate, borate, oxalate, and cyanide ions are inhibitors of all forms of the enzyme. The individual multiple forms are inhibited to different extents by L-phenylalanine, urea, excess Zn^{2+}, or AsO_4^{3-}. Variations in Mg^{2+} and substrate concentrations change the pH optimum. The type of buffer present (except at low concentrations) affects the rate of enzyme activity. Buffers can be classified as inert (carbonate, barbital), inhibiting (glycine, propylamine), or activating (2-amino-2-methyl-1-propanol [2A2M1P], TRIS, and diethanolamine [DEA]). Glycine apparently inhibits by complexing the activating Mg^{2+} ion.

The form present in the sera of normal adults probably originates mainly in the liver, with up to half the total activity coming from the skeleton. The respective contributions of these two forms to the total activity are markedly age dependent. In addition, a significant difference exists between the sexes in serum ALP activity at some ages, although this fact is less important for interpretation of values than the dependence on age. A small amount of intestinal ALP also may be present, particularly in the sera of individuals of blood group B or O who secrete blood-group substances. The enzyme found in urine probably is derived from renal tissue and does not represent serum enzyme cleared by the kidneys. ALP in serum is denatured rapidly at 56 °C but is relatively stable at lower temperatures. (The placental isoenzyme is most stable.) Sera kept at room temperature usually show a slight increase in activity, which varies from 1% over 6 hours to 3% to 6% over 1 to 4 days. Even sera stored at refrigerator temperature demonstrates a slow increase (2% per day) in activity. In frozen sera, activity decreases but slowly recovers after the sera thaws.

Similar enhanced activity occurs with reconstituted lyophilized preparations, such as those available as commercial "control sera" or "reference materials." In reconstituted material stored at 37 °C the increase in activity of some materials has been found to be as high as 50% to 100% over 24 hours, and the increases with storage at 4 and 20 °C are about 10% and 30%, respectively. Enhancement of activity continues for several days but at a decreasing rate.

Clinical significance

Serum ALP measurements are of particular interest in the investigation of two groups of conditions: hepatobiliary disease (see Chapter 36) and bone disease associated with increased osteoblastic activity (see Chapter 38).

Hepatobiliary disease

The response of the liver to any form of biliary tree obstruction is to induce the synthesis of ALP. The main site of new enzyme synthesis is the hepatocytes adjacent to the biliary canaliculi. Some of the newly formed enzyme enters the circulation to raise the enzyme level in serum. The elevation tends to be more marked (greater than threefold) in cases of extrahepatic obstruction (for example, by stone or by cancer of the head of the pancreas) than in those of intrahepatic obstruction and is greater the more complete the obstruction. Serum enzyme activities may reach 10 to 12 times the upper limit of normal and usually return to normal on surgical removal of the obstruction. Intrahepatic obstruction of the bile flow (for example by invasion of cancer tissue or by drugs, such as chlorpromazine, that affect the biliary tree) also raises serum ALP levels, but usually to a lesser extent than extrahepatic obstruction. Liver diseases that affect principally parenchymal cells, such as infectious hepatitis, typically also show only moderately (less than threefold) elevated or even normal serum ALP levels.

Bone diseases

Among the bone diseases the highest levels of serum ALP activity are encountered in individuals with Paget's disease (osteitis deformans) as a result of the action of the osteoblastic cells as they try to rebuild bone that is being resorbed by the uncontrolled activity of osteoclasts. Values from 10 to 25 times the upper limit of the reference interval are not unusual. Only moderate rises are observed in osteomalacia, the levels slowly declining in response to vitamin D therapy. Levels generally are normal in osteoporosis. In rickets cases, levels two to four times normal may be observed, and these fall slowly to normal on treatment with vitamin D. Slight to moderate elevations occur in individuals with Fanconi's syndrome. Primary and secondary hyperparathyroidism are associated with slight to moderate elevations of ALP activity in serum, the existence and degree of elevation reflecting the presence and extent of skeletal involvement. Very high enzyme levels are present in individuals with osteogenic bone cancer. Transient elevations may be found during healing of bone fractures. Physiological bone growth elevates ALP in serum, and this increase accounts for the fact that in the sera of growing children, enzyme activity is 1.5 to 2.5 times that in normal adult serum.

An increase of up to two to three times normal has been observed in women in the third trimester of pregnancy, with the additional enzyme originating in the placenta. Upward or downward trends in placental ALP may presage complications of pregnancy, such as hypertension or preeclampsia. However, because of the wide range of placental ALP activity in serum in normal pregnancy, single estimations are of little diagnostic value.

An unexpected result of the application of the techniques of isoenzyme analysis to the characterization of ALP in serum was the discovery that forms of the enzyme that are essentially identical to the normal placental isoenzyme appear in the sera of some individuals with malignant diseases. These carcinoplacental, or "Regan," isoenzymes appear to result from the derepression of the placental phosphatase gene. In some cases, modification of the gene or its product may cause the appearance of isoenzymes that differ in some respects from the normal placental isoenzyme while still retaining the latter's general characteristics. Tumors also have produced ALPs that appear to be modified forms of nonplacental isoenzymes.

Methods for the determination of alkaline phosphatase activity

Numerous methods have been developed to determine ALP activity. In general, methodological developments have been directed at increasing the speed and sensitivity of the assay by selecting readily hydrolyzed substrates and phosphate-accepting buffers and toward the use of continuous-monitoring methods based on "self-indicating" substrates.

The most popular of the chromogenic or self-indicating substrates for ALP is 4-nitrophenyl phosphate (usually abbreviated 4-NPP or PNPP from the older name, p-nitrophenyl phosphate). ALP catalyzes the hydrolysis of 4-NPP, forming phosphate and free 4-nitrophenol (4-NP, PNP), which in dilute acid solutions is colorless, as follows:

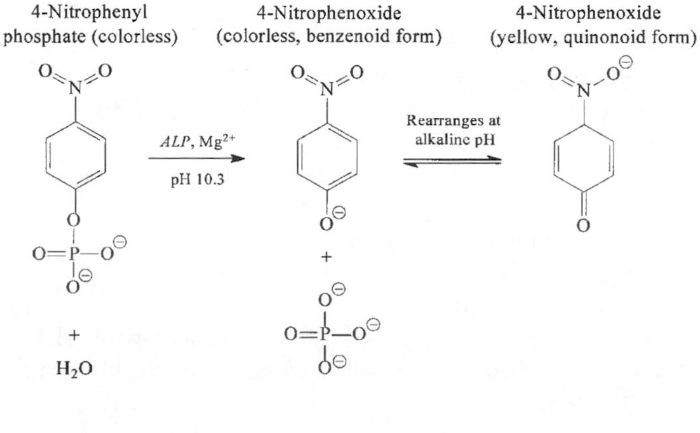

Under alkaline conditions 4-NP is converted to the 4-nitrophenoxide ion, which is an intense yellow color. The rate of formation of 4-NP by the action of the enzyme on 4-NPP at 37 °C then is monitored with a recording spectrophotometer. Other self-indicating substrates include phenolphthalein monophosphate, thymolphthalein phosphate, and α-naphthyl phosphate.

In these ALP methods the liberated phosphate group is transferred to water. The rate of phosphatase action is enhanced, however, if certain amino alcohols are used as buffers. Among these activators are compounds such as 2A2M1P, DEA, TRIS, ethylaminoethanol (EAE), and N-methyl-D-glucamine. Enzyme activity in the presence of optimal concentrations of these buffers is twofold to sixfold greater than activity in the presence of a nonactivating buffer, such as carbonate.

The IFCC recommended method uses 4-NPP as substrate and 2A2M1P as phosphate-acceptor buffer. It includes Mg^{2+} and Zn^{2+}, the concentrations of which are controlled at optimal levels by addition of Mg^{2+} and Zn^{2+}, as well as the chelating agent N-hydroxyethylethylenediaminetriacetic acid (HEDTA). Although Zn^{2+} ions are present in a total concentration of 1 mmol/L, most are bound to HEDTA, leaving only a small, experimentally determined optimal concentration of free ions. A similar situation exists for Mg^{2+} ions. Thus HEDTA acts as a metal ion buffer, maintaining optimal concentrations of the two ions. The temperature range of measurement is 30 ± 0.1 °C or 37 ± 0.1 °C, and the acceptable wavelength range is 405 ± 2 nm.

Specimen requirements

Serum or heparinized plasma, free of hemolysis, should be used. Complexing anticoagulants, such as citrate, oxalate, and EDTA, must be avoided. Freshly collected serum samples should be kept at room temperature and assayed as soon as possible but preferably not later than 4 hours after collection. Frozen specimens should be thawed and kept at room temperature (20 to 26 °C) for 18 to 24 hours before measurement to achieve full enzyme reactivation.

Reference intervals

With the IFCC method the following reference intervals have been established for adults in the fasting state:

Men 20 to 50 years of age: 38 to 94 U/L
Men ≥ 60 years of age: 43 to 88 U/L
Women 20 to 50 years of age: 28 to 78 U/L
Women ≥ 60 years of age: 40 to 111 U/L

Methods for the separation and quantification of alkaline phosphatase isoenzymes

ALP exists in multiple forms, some of which are true isoenzymes encoded at separate genetic loci (Figure 20-4). Criteria that have been used to differentiate the isoenzymes and other multiple forms of ALP include (1) differences in elec-

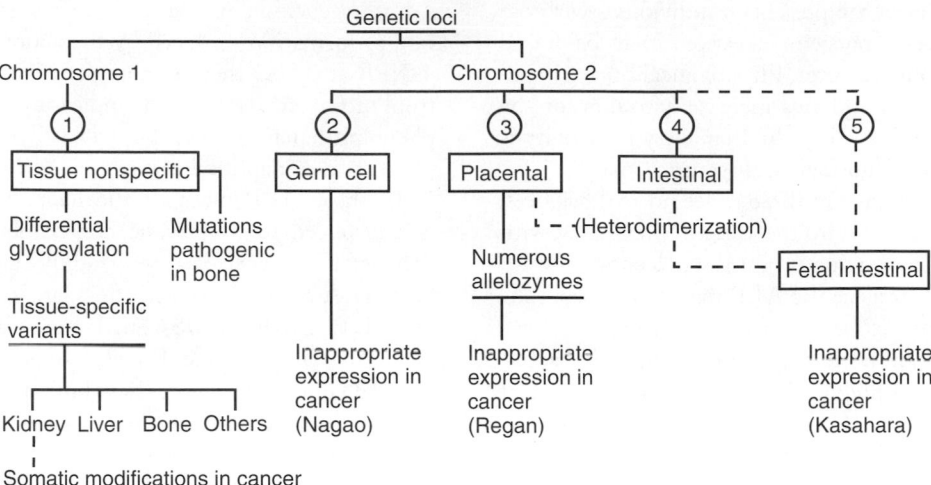

Origins of Alkaline Phosphate Isoforms

Figure 20-4 Identities, chromosomal assignments, and main physiological and pathological expression of genes encoding human alkaline phosphatases. Two alternative proposed origins of the fetal intestinal alkaline phosphatase are shown *(broken lines);* the existence of a fifth locus encoding this isoform is still debatable. All the isoenzymes and isoforms are glycoproteins, imposing a further level of microheterogeneity. Additional isoforms can be generated by different processes of cleavage or preservation of the membrane-anchoring domain. (Modified from Moss DW: Perspectives in alkaline phosphatase research. Clin Chem 1992; 38:2486-2492.)

trophoretic mobility, (2) variations in stability to denaturation by heat or urea, (3) differences in response to the presence of selected inhibitors, (4) differences in relative rates of reaction with various substrates, and (5) differences in immunochemical characteristics.

Electrophoretic separation

The same electrophoretic techniques are used for the separation of ALP isoenzymes in serum as for separations of serum proteins. Upon electrophoresis at an alkaline pH, the liver phosphatase typically moves most rapidly toward the anode. Bone phosphatase, which typically gives a more diffuse zone than the liver isoenzyme, has a slightly lower anodal mobility, although the two zones usually overlap to some extent. Intestinal phosphatase also migrates diffusely but more slowly than bone enzyme, and kidney phosphatase, which is present very rarely in serum, migrates even more slowly. The placental isoenzymes have mobilities of the same order as those of liver and bone, depending on the phenotype.

Additional minor phosphatase zones also are present in extracts of tissues and occasionally in serum. One such zone contains a high-MW form of ALP but also is strongly negatively charged. Therefore it moves slowly in starch gel or may even fail to enter polyacrylamide gel, but it migrates more anodally than the main liver zone on nonsieving media, such as cellulose acetate. This zone has been named the *fast liver fraction* because of the latter property and because it has been observed more frequently in serum in hepatobiliary disease of various types.

Two methodological approaches have improved the electrophoretic separation between bone and liver ALPs. In the first, electrophoresis is carried out in the presence of wheat germ lectin, which retards bone ALP to a greater extent than the liver enzyme. In the other, serum is treated briefly with neuraminidase to remove terminal sialic acid residues. After such treatment, the mobility of bone phosphatase is reduced more than that of liver phosphatase (Figure 20-5).

Incubation of the sample with neuraminidase also is used to confirm the presence of intestinal phosphatase. This treatment reduces the anodal mobility of all phosphatase isoenzymes except that of adult intestinal origin, which is neuraminidase resistant because terminal sialic acid residues are not present in the molecule.

Heat-inactivation analysis

Because placental ALP is heat stable, incubation of the enzyme at a temperature as high as 65 °C for 30 minutes provides a convenient and specific test for the presence of this isoenzyme. Pronounced heat stability also is shown by the Regan isoenzyme, a placenta-like fetal form of ALP that occurs in 5% to 15% of specimens from individuals with cancers of various types. Thus heating the sample at 65 °C also is used to detect this abnormal isoenzyme

Other isoenzymes of ALP are differentiated on the basis of their stability at temperatures lower than 65 °C. At 56 °C, for example, liver ALP is more stable than the bone isoenzyme. Thus if after 10 minutes at 56 °C less than 20% of the serum ALP activity remains, the enzyme present is probably largely bone type; residual activities of between 25% and 55% support electrophoretic evidence that liver phosphatase is the predominant isoenzyme.

Urea inhibition

Urea at high concentrations inhibits the activity of ALP, the inhibition being irreversible and varying with the tissue

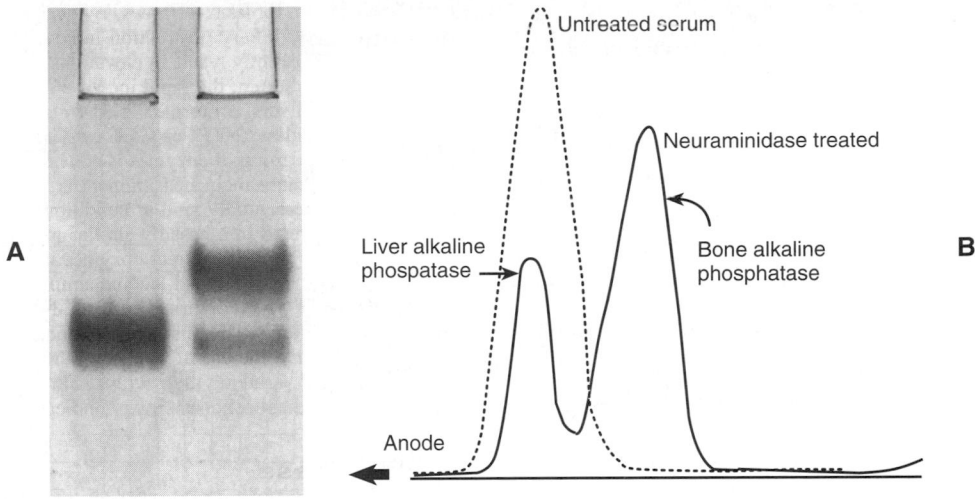

Figure 20-5 **A,** Polyacrylamide-gel electrophoresis of bone and liver alkaline phosphatases in human serum. Mixture of two sera containing entirely bone and entirely liver phosphatases *(left)*. Mixture of the same two sera after each has been treated with neuraminidase for 10 minutes at 37 °C *(right)*. The anodal direction is downward. The more anodal zone is liver phosphatase. **B,** Densitometric scans of electrophoretic pat-

terns shown in **A.** Scan of mixture of untreated sera *(broken line).* Scan of mixture of sera treated briefly with neuraminidase *(solid line).* The anode is to the left. (Modified from Moss DW, Edwards RK: Improved electrophoretic resolution of bone and liver alkaline phosphatases resulting from partial digestion with neuraminidase. Clin Chem Acta 1984; 143:177-182.)

TABLE 20-5   **Comparison of Results of ALP, NTP, and GGT in 174 Sera from Patients with Hepatobiliary Disease**

| | Average Activities (Multiples of Upper Reference Limits) | | | Incidence of Abnormal Results (%) in All Specimens | | |
Patient Condition	ALP	NTP	GGT	ALT	NTP	GGT
Biliary tract disease (primary biliary cirrhosis, carcinoma of the pancreas, biliary stricture, cholangitis)	4.0	6.2	11.9	57	43	74
Parenchymal cell disease (various forms of acute and chronic hepatitis)	1.5	1.1	2.3			

ALP, Alkaline phosphatase; *NTP,* 5'-nucleotidase; *GGT,* γ-glutamyltransferase.

origin of the enzyme. This urea inhibition provides an alternative to heat inactivation in isoenzyme analysis. Bone isoenzyme is most susceptible to urea denaturation (16% residual activity after treatment at 37 °C for 18 minutes in urea, 3 mol/L). The liver enzyme has intermediate resistance (44% residual activity), whereas the intestinal and placental enzymes are most resistant to urea denaturation (69% activity left).

Chemical inhibition

Specific chemical inhibitors also have been applied to the characterization of ALP isoenzymes in serum. For example, L-phenylalanine markedly inhibits intestinal, placental, and Regan isoenzymes when present at a concentration of 5 mmol/L but has less effect on the isoenzymes of bone or liver. In addition, Levamisole preferentially inhibits bone and liver phosphatases and is effective at much lower concentrations.

Immunological techniques

Antisera or antibodies also are used to discriminate between the ALP isoenzymes in serum. Polyclonal antisera

have been shown to distinguish between placental and intestinal ALPs and ALPs from other sources, although placental and intestinal ALPs cross-react with some antisera. Immunological methods with polyclonal antisera or monoclonal antibodies provide the best measurements of intestinal or placental ALPs. However, polyclonal antisera are incapable of distinguishing among the products of the tissue-nonspecific ALP gene, including the liver and bone-derived isoforms. Monoclonal antibodies have been developed that discriminate between liver and bone ALPs. Considerable cross-reaction remains, but the most discriminatory antibodies form the basis of useful methods to determine bone ALP in serum.

■ BILIARY TRACT ENZYMES

The activities of several enzymes in serum change in a manner similar to that of ALP in cases of hepatobiliary disease (Table 20-5). Because these changes are most pronounced in such diseases as intrahepatic and extrahepatic cholestasis, which focus principally on the biliary tract, these enzymes often are referred to collectively as *biliary tract enzymes*. 5′-Nucleotidase and γ-glutamyl transferase are examples of biliary tract enzymes. Although not discussed here, arylamidase (often erroneously called *leucine aminopeptidase*) also is considered a biliary tract enzyme.

5′-Nucleotidase

5′-Nucleotidase (EC 3.1.3.5; 5′-ribonucleotide phosphohydrolase; NTP) is a phosphatase that acts only on nucleoside-5′-phosphates, such as AMP and adenylic acid, releasing inorganic phosphate, as follows:

Adenosine-5′-monophosphate
(AMP)

Adenosine

Biochemistry

NTP is distributed widely throughout the tissues of the body and is localized principally in the cytoplasmic membrane of the cells in which it occurs. Its pH optimum is between 6.6 and 7.0.

Clinical significance

The activity of NTP in serum is increased twofold to sixfold in cases of those hepatobiliary diseases in which interference occurs with the secretion of the bile. This interference may be due to extrahepatic causes (a stone or tumor occluding the bile duct) or may arise from intrahepatic conditions, such as cholestasis caused by chlorpromazine, malignant infiltration of the liver, or biliary cirrhosis. When parenchymal cell damage is predominant, as it is in early infectious hepatitis, the serum NTP level is normal or elevated only moderately. Thus both NTP and ALP behave similarly in cases of hepatobiliary disease. Because an increase in NTP activity is minimal in individuals with skeletal disease, any significant rise in NTP activity is virtually specific for hepatobiliary disease.

Method for the determination of 5′-nucleotidase activity

The substrate most generally used to measure the activity of NTP is AMP. However, this substrate is an organic phosphate ester and thus also can be hydrolyzed to an appreciable degree by other nonspecific (alkaline) phosphatases, even at a pH as low as 7.5 (the pH previously assumed to be optimal for NTP activity). Methods used to estimate NTP in serum therefore must incorporate some means for correcting for the hydrolysis of the substrate by the nonspecific phosphatases. For example, NTP is inhibited by nickel ions, and this property is used to distinguish it from ALP.

Reaction principle

NTP catalyzes the hydrolysis of AMP to adenosine and phosphate. In this method, serum is incubated with AMP at pH 7.5 and 37 °C, with and without added nickel ions. After 30 minutes the amount of inorganic phosphate liberated is determined. Phosphate produced in the absence of nickel represents the combined activities of ALP and NTP, whereas that produced in the presence of nickel is due to the activity of ALP alone. Thus the difference between these two values for liberated phosphate corresponds to the activity of NTP in the serum sample. Manganese ions activate NTP.

Specimen requirements

Serum should be used for analysis. Plasma may cause turbidity, and although EDTA is said to be without effect, this and other metal-binding anticoagulants could interfere with activation by manganese.

Reference intervals

The reference interval for NTP activity in sera from normal men and normal nonpregnant and pregnant women is from 2 to 17 U/L. Lower values have been reported in children.

Gamma Glutamyltransferase

Peptidases are enzymes that catalyze the hydrolytic cleavage of peptides to form amino acids or smaller peptides. They constitute a broad group of enzymes of varied specificity, and some individual enzymes act as amino acid transferases and catalyze the transfer of amino acids from one peptide to another amino acid or peptide. **Gamma glutamyltransferase** (EC 2.3.2.2; γ-glutamyl-peptide:amino acid γ-glutamyltransferase; GGT) catalyzes the transfer of the γ-glutamyl group from peptides and compounds that contain this group to some acceptor. The γ-glutamyl acceptor is the substrate itself, some amino acid or peptide, or even water, in which case simple hydrolysis takes place. The enzyme acts only on peptides or peptidelike compounds containing a terminal glutamate residue joined to the remainder of the compound through the terminal (γ) carboxyl, as follows:

γ-Glutamyl-*p*-nitroanilide
Substrate (donor)

Glycylglycine
Acceptor

p-Nitroaniline
Donor residue

γ-Glutamylglycylglycine
Transfer product

Glycylglycine is five times more effective as an acceptor than is either glycine or the tripeptide (gly-gly-gly), but little is known about the optimal properties of the acceptor cosubstrate. The rate of the peptidase transfer reaction is considerably faster than that of the simple hydrolysis reaction.

Biochemistry

GGT is present in serum and in all cells except those in muscle. Some enzyme is present in cytosol, but the larger fraction is located in the cell membrane and may transport amino acids and peptides into the cell across the cell membrane in the form of γ-glutamyl peptides. GGT also may be involved in some aspects of glutathione metabolism.

Clinical significance

GGT present in serum appears to originate primarily from the hepatobiliary system, and GGT activity is elevated in all forms of liver disease. It is highest in cases of intrahepatic or posthepatic biliary obstruction, reaching levels some 5 to 30 times normal. It is more sensitive than ALP, NTP, (see Table 20-5) arylamidase, and the transaminases in detection of obstructive jaundice, cholangitis, and cholecystitis. The rise in GGT activity occurs earlier in these diseases than do these other enzymes and persists longer. Only moderate elevations (two to five times normal) occur in infectious hepatitis cases, and in this condition, GGT determinations are less useful diagnostically than are measurements of the transaminases.

High elevations of GGT also are observed in individuals with either primary or secondary (metastatic) neoplasms; again, changes occur earlier and are more pronounced than those of the other liver enzymes. Small increases (two to five times normal) of GGT activity are observed in individuals with fatty livers, and similar but transient increases are noted in cases of drug intoxication. In cases of acute and chronic pancreatitis and in some pancreatic malignancies (especially those associated with hepatobiliary obstruction), enzyme activity may be 5 to 15 times the upper limit of normal.

Normal levels of the enzyme are found in cases of skeletal disease (Paget's disease, bone neoplasms), children older than 1 year, and healthy pregnant women, all conditions in which ALP is elevated. Thus measurement of GGT levels in serum helps ascertain whether observed elevations of ALP are caused by skeletal disease or reflect the presence of hepatobiliary disease. NTP determinations provide the same information, but GGT has the advantage of becoming elevated earlier than NTP in liver disease cases and rising to greater levels than NTP. However, elevations of NTP sometimes have been more useful clinically because they are encountered only in hepatobiliary disease states.

Normal levels of GGT are observed in individuals with various muscle diseases and renal failure, but mild elevations may be noted in those individuals with untreated lipoid nephrosis. In individuals with myocardial infarctions, GGT levels usually are normal. If the level does rise, it occurs at about the 4th day and reaches a maximum value in another 4 days, the implication being liver damage secondary to cardiac insufficiency.

Elevated levels of GGT are noted in the sera of individuals with alcoholic cirrhosis and in the majority of sera from those who drink heavily. Individuals receiving drugs, such as phenytoin (Dilantin) and phenobarbital, demonstrate raised levels of the enzyme in serum specimens but not in specimens of CSF. Such an increase of activity may reflect induction of new enzyme activity by the action of the anticonvulsant drugs. The release of GGT into serum reflects the toxic effects of alcohol and other drugs on microsomal structures in liver cells. The enzyme level present correlates well with the duration of the drug action. Hepatic complications occurring in cases of cystic fibrosis (mucoviscidosis) also lead to elevations of GGT.

High levels of GGT are present in the prostate, which may account for the higher activity of GGT in sera of men, which is approximately 50% higher than in sera from women. Prostatic malignancy at times may be the source of elevated GGT activity in serum. Irradiation of tumors in patients with cancer may be accompanied by a rise in GGT activity, although LD activity in the course of such treatment remains unchanged.

GGT in urine probably originates in the kidneys and genitourinary tract. Elevated enzyme activity is present in the urine of individuals with acute urorenal infections and diseases involving renal tissue destruction. However, in cases of chronic renal disease and in older individuals, urine enzyme levels may be depressed.

Methods for the determination of gamma glutamyltransferase activity

Many of the early GGT assays used L-γ-glutamyl-*p*-nitroanilide (GGPNA) as the substrate, with glycylglycine serving as the γ-glutamyl residue acceptor. However, GGPNA has limited solubility in the reaction mixture, and saturating substrate concentrations therefore are difficult to reach with this substrate. The *p*-nitroaniline produced in the reaction is determined by its yellow color, which is monitored at 405 nm. Both two-point and continuous-monitoring methods have been described in the literature.

Derivatives of GGPNA also are available and have been used in other methods. In these derivatives, various groups have been introduced into the benzene ring to increase solubility in water. The most useful of these substrates is L-γ-glutamyl-3-carboxy-4-nitroanilide, which is soluble readily in water and split by GGT at a rate comparable to that observed with L-GGPNA. Activities in serum are higher with the carboxyl derivative than with the noncarboxylated substrate, partly because of the higher substrate concentrations attainable with the former.

Reaction principle

In the IFCC reference method for GGT, L-γ-glutamyl-3-carboxy-4-nitroanilide serves as the substrate, with glycylglycine serving as an acceptor. Buffering is provided by TRIS and glycylglycine ($pK_2 = 8.25$). Serum may be added to the buffer-acceptor solution, and the reaction is initiated by addition of substrate in HCl solution. Alternatively, the reaction is initiated by addition of serum. The wavelength of measurement is 410 nm, at which the product, 5-amino-2-nitrobenzoate, has an absorption coefficient of 7.908 $L \times mmol^{-1} \times cm^{-1}$.

Specimen requirements

Serum free from hemolysis is the preferred specimen, but EDTA-plasma (up to 1 mg/mL of blood) also has been used. Heparin produces turbidity in the reaction mixture; citrate, oxalate, and fluoride depress activity by 10% to 15%.

Reference intervals

The reference interval for GGT activity in the serum of women is 1 to 24 U/L at 37 °C. For men, it is 2 to 30 U/L at 37 °C.

■ DIGESTIVE ENZYMES OF PANCREATIC ORIGIN

Assays of serum amylase, lipase, trypsin, and chymotrypsin are applied almost exclusively to investigation of pancreatic disease. (Pancreatic function and pathology will be discussed in detail in Chapter 37.)

Amylase

Amylase (EC 3.2.1.1; 1,4-α-D glucan glucanohydrolase) is an enzyme of the hydrolase class that catalyzes the hydrolysis of 1,4-α-glucosidic linkages in polysaccharides. Both straight-chain (linear) polyglucans (such as amylose) and branched polyglucans (such as amylopectin and glycogen) are hydrolyzed—but at different rates. In the case of amylose the enzyme splits the chains at alternate α-1,4-hemiacetal (−C−O−C−) links, forming maltose and some residual glucose; maltose, glucose, and a residue of limit dextrins are formed if branched-chain polyglucans are used as substrate. The α-1,6-linkages at the branch points are not attacked by the enzyme.

Biochemistry

Animal amylases, including those present in human tissues, are **α-amylases.** They also are called *endoamylases* because they attack α-1,4-linkages randomly anywhere along the polyglucan chain. Large polysaccharide molecules thus are broken down rapidly into small units (for example, dextrins, maltose, and some glucose units). Beta-amylase is an exoamylase found in plants and bacteria. It acts only at the terminal-reducing end of a polyglucan chain splitting off two glucose units (maltose) at a time. Because both maltose and glucose are reducing sugars, the course of the hydrolytic reaction of amylase is paralleled by an increase in soluble reducing materials.

Amylase in human serum has a moderately sharp pH optimum at 6.9 to 7.0. The enzyme customarily is assayed at 37 °C, although it is active at 50 °C, and some automated procedures have used this higher temperature. The temperature coefficient is +6% increase in activity per degree Celsius increase in temperature ($Q_{10} = 1.6$). Alpha-amylases are calcium metalloenzymes, with the calcium being absolutely necessary for functional integrity; saturation with Ca^{2+} is obtained at approximately 1.0 mmol/L. However, full activity is displayed only in the presence of various anions, such as chloride, bromide, nitrate, cholate, or monohydrogen phosphate, with chloride and bromide being the most effective activators. The amylases normally occurring in human plasma are small molecules with MWs varying from 55,000 to 60,000. The enzyme thus is small enough to pass through the glomeruli of the kidneys, and amylase is the only plasma enzyme normally found in urine. Serum and urine amylases migrate electrophoretically with the β- and γ-globulins.

Amylase is present in a number of organs and tissues. The greatest concentration is present in the pancreas (P-type), where the enzyme is synthesized by the acinar cells and then secreted into the intestinal tract via the pancreatic duct system. The salivary glands also secrete a potent amylase (S-type) to initiate hydrolysis of starches while the food is still in the mouth and esophagus. The action of the salivary enzyme, once referred to as *ptyalin,* is terminated by acid in the stomach. In the intestinal tract the mildly alkaline conditions of the duodenum favor the effective action of pancreatic and intestinal amylase. Intestinal maltase then further hydrolyzes maltose to glucose.

Most pancreatic amylase in the lower portions of the intestinal tract is destroyed by trypsin activity, although some amylase activity is present in feces. Amylase activity also is found in semen, testes, ovaries, fallopian tubes, striated muscle, lungs, adipose tissue, colostrum, tears, and milk. Some tumors of the lung and ovary may contain considerable amylase activity. Little or no amylase activity exists in the liver. The enzyme found in urine is derived from the plasma. Ascitic and pleural fluids may contain amylase as a result of the presence of a tumor or **pancreatitis.**

The enzyme present in normal serum and urine is predominantly of pancreatic and salivary-gland origin. These isoenzymes are products of two closely linked loci on chromosome 1. Each gene is allelic; thus 12 distinct phenotypes exist for the salivary isoenzyme and 6 for the pancreatic isoenzyme. Amylase isoenzymes also undergo posttranslational modification of deamidation, glycosylation, and deglycosylation to form a number of isoforms. Indeed, nonenzymic deamidation appears to be the mechanism for "aging" that occurs when amylase is sequestered (for example, pancreatic pseudocysts) or subjected to prolonged in-vitro storage. Aged amylase possesses a different isoelectric point from the parent amylase and is detected by electrophoresis.

Although the pancreatic isoenzyme is not glycosylated, the salivary isoenzyme may exist in both glycosylated and deglycosylated forms; these isoforms can be separated because their MWs differ by as much as 3000. Multiple amylase isoenzymes have been found in both serum and urine through gel filtration, ion-exchange chromatography, isoelectric focusing, and electrophoresis techniques. Macroamylases sometimes are present in sera; these rare forms are probably complexes between ordinary amylase (usually S-type) and IgA, IgG, or other normal or abnormal high-MW plasma proteins.

Clinical significance

Assays of amylase activity in serum and urine are used primarily in the diagnosis of diseases of the pancreas and the investigation of pancreatic function (see also Chapter 37). In cases of acute pancreatitis, a transient rise in serum amylase activity occurs within 2 to 12 hours of the onset; levels return to normal by day 3 or 4. A fourfold to sixfold elevation in amylase activity above the reference limit is usual, with maximum levels attained in 12 to 72 hours. The magnitude of the elevation of serum enzyme activity is not related to the severity of pancreatic involvement; however, the greater the rise, the greater is the probability of acute pancreatitis. Studies suggest that up to 20% of all proven cases of acute pancreatitis are normoamylasemic, although the parallel assay of lipase improves the detection rate. In cases of acute pancreatitis associated with hyperlipemia, serum amylase activity may be normal; the spuriously normal amylase activity may be unmasked either by serial dilution of the serum or ultracentrifugation. A significant amount of the serum

amylase is excreted in the urine, and therefore elevation of serum activity is reflected in the rise of urinary amylase activity. Urine amylase, compared with serum amylase, appears to be *more* frequently elevated, reaches *higher* levels, and persists for *longer* periods of time. The urinary clearance of amylase is increased markedly in acute pancreatitis cases. In individuals with quiescent chronic pancreatitis, both serum and urine activities usually are subnormal.

Acute pancreatitis sometimes is difficult to diagnose because it must be differentiated from other acute intraabdominal disorders; in addition, an increase in serum amylase activity may not be due necessarily to pancreatitis. Table 20-6 lists some of the many causes of hyperamylasemia and

---

TABLE 20-6   Causes of Hyperamylasemia and Hyperamylasuria

Pancreatic Disease (P type↑)*
Pancreatitis
  Acute
  Chronic
  Complications
    Pseudocyst
    Ascites and pleural effusion
    Abscess
Pancreatic trauma, including investigative maneuvers
Pancreatic carcinoma

Disorders of Nonpancreatic Origin (Mechanism Unknown)
Renal insufficiency (mixed↑)
Neoplastic hyperamylasemia—usually bronchogenic or ovarian
  (usually S type↑)
Salivary gland lesions—for example, mumps, calculus disease
  (S type↑)
Macroamylasemia (predominantly S type)

Disorders of Complex Origin (Mechanism Unknown or Uncertain)
Biliary tract disease
Intraabdominal disease (other than pancreatic diseases; see above)
  Perforated peptic ulcer (P type↑)
  Intestinal obstruction (P type↑)
  Mesenteric infarction (P type↑)
  Peritonitis (mixed↑; dependent on cause)
  Acute appendicitis
  Ruptured ectopic pregnancy (S type↑)
  Aortic aneurysm with dissection
Cerebral trauma (type dependent on other organ damage)
Burns and traumatic shock
Postoperative hyperamylasemia (usually S type↑)
Diabetic ketoacidosis (mixed↑)
Renal transplantation (S type↑)
Acute alcoholism (mixed↑)
Drugs
  Medicinal opiates (P type↑)
  Heroin addiction →? Heroin lung (S type↑)

From Salt WB, Schenker S: Amylase—its clinical significance: a review of the literature. Medicine 1976; 155:269-289.
*Predominant isoenzyme type is shown in parentheses: P type (pancreatic); S type (salivary); mixed (either or both isoenzymes possibly present).

hyperamylasuria. Whether the major isoenzyme is type P or type S identifies the organ source.

Amylase assays also are valuable in detection of the development of complications, such as pseudocyst, ascites, and pleural effusion, after the onset of acute pancreatitis. Examining the pleural fluid for amylase activity is recommended; activities can be 100 times the serum reference interval after an attack. In cases of pancreatic abscess, serum amylase is elevated occasionally. In addition, traumatic lesions of the pancreas, including surgical trauma and radiological investigations, may cause transient hyperamylasemia; serious injury often leads to persisting elevations of the enzyme. If the pancreatic duct is obstructed by carcinoma of the pancreas, then elevation of serum amylase activity is likely. If an acute relapse of chronic pancreatitis occurs, serum amylase levels may be elevated; more often, however, the activity remains low within the reference interval.

Hyperamylasemia also is present with some nonpancreatic disorders. For example, in individuals with renal insufficiency the serum amylase activity is increased up to twofold of the upper limit of the reference interval and in proportion to the extent of renal impairment. Hyperamylasemia also is present with neoplastic diseases. Additionally, tumors of the lung and serous tumors of the ovary can produce hyperamylasemia (with an S-type isoenzyme mobility), with elevations as high as 50 times the upper limit of the reference interval. Both kinds of tumor produce pleural effusion; in the case of ovarian tumors, the result has been called *pseudo-Meigs' syndrome* (Meigs' syndrome being association of ascites and pleural effusion with fibroma of the ovary). The amylase activities in these effusions have been more than 200 times the upper limit of the reference interval for serum. Salivary gland lesions caused by infection, irradiation, obstruction, surgery, and tumor all have been reported to produce a significant S-type hyperamylasemia. Mumps (infective parotitis) and maxillofacial surgery have caused a twofold elevation, and salivary gland irradiation has produced a transient ninefold to eighteenfold elevation of serum amylase activity.

Biliary tract diseases such as cholecystitis have caused up to fourfold elevations of the serum amylase activity as a result of either primary or secondary pancreatic involvement. Various intraabdominal events (see Table 20-6) have led to a significant increase in serum amylase activities up to a fourfold elevation and sometimes beyond. Such increases may be due to leakage of the P-type amylase from the intestine into the peritoneal cavity and then into the circulation. Peritonitis and acute appendicitis have been reported to produce a slight elevation (up to twofold and threefold) of serum amylase activity. In cases involving ruptured ectopic pregnancy, serum amylase activities can be elevated as high as eight times the upper limit of the reference interval; the amylase isoenzyme is the S type. Dissecting aortic aneurysms can produce elevated serum amylase activities, but the mechanism is uncertain.

Cerebral trauma has also been associated with hyperamylasemia. Postoperative hyperamylasemia occurs in about 20% of all patients subjected to a wide variety of surgical interventions, including extraabdominal procedures. Fourfold elevations have been observed, with the principal isoenzyme being the S type. In individuals with diabetic ketoacidosis, elevations of approximately four times the upper limit of the reference interval are found in as many as 80% of these individuals. These abnormalities are more frequent when the blood glucose exceeds 500 mg/dL (28 mmol/L), and the onset of ketoacidosis is relatively acute. The source of the amylase is uncertain. After renal transplantation, about one fifth of the patients develop hyperamylasemia; only a small proportion of these instances are due to the occurrence of pancreatitis, whereas the remainder are asymptomatic. In cases of pneumonia and other nonneoplastic diseases of the lung, hyperamylasemia increasingly has been observed; although its exact incidence is uncertain, the isoenzyme likely is the S type. About 10% of individuals with acute alcoholic intoxication demonstrate a threefold elevation; the isoenzyme type is divided equally between the P and S types. Finally, a wide variety of drugs always must be considered as possible causes of hyperamylasemia.

Renal clearance of amylase, as related to the reasonably constant clearance of creatinine, is a useful diagnostic tool. The amylase/creatinine clearance ratio (ACCR) is defined and expressed as a percentage, as follows:

$$ACCR = \frac{\text{urine amylase (U/L)} \times \text{serum creatinine (mg/L)}}{\text{serum amylase (U/L)} \times \text{urine creatinine (mg/L)}} \times 100$$

The ACCR is calculated readily from amylase activity and creatinine concentration determined on the same urine and on a single serum sample obtained at the time of urine collection. A timed urine collection is unnecessary, and the only constraint is an adequate volume of specimen. Therefore random or short (2- to 4-hour) collections are adequate. The reference interval for ACCR is approximately 2% to 5%. Note, however, that the ACCR is affected by the type of amylase assay used. Thus establishment of a reference interval for the assay method currently in use is imperative.

In acute pancreatitis cases, tubular reabsorption of amylase and other proteins is reduced (probably secondary to competition from other low-MW proteins), and ACCR is increased; values exceeding 8% are not uncommon. Caution must be exercised in interpretations of increased ACCR values because elevations also have been observed in burns, ketoacidosis, renal insufficiency, myeloma, light-chain proteinuria, and march hemoglobinuria, as well as after extracorporeal circulation, large intravenous doses of corticosteroids, duodenal perforations, and extraperitoneal surgical procedures. In individuals with macroamylasemia, ACCR is usually less than 2%.

Methods for the determination of amylase activity

Based on different principles and various substrates, more than 200 methods have been developed for the assay of amylase activity. They include both starch-based and defined substrate methods.

Starch-based methods

Until a decade ago, saccharogenic, amyloclastic, and chromolytic starch methods were the assays of choice to determine amylase activity. These assays are used rarely today.

Saccharogenic assays. In saccharogenic assays the course of the enzyme reaction is followed by measurement of the quantity of reducing materials (sugars, dextrins) formed.

Amyloclastic assays. Amylase activity also has been measured by following of the decrease in starch substrate concentration rather than measurement of the product formed. Methods based on this approach are called *amyloclastic methods.*

Chromogenic assays. Chromogenic assays use dye-labeled amylase substrates. These substrates are synthesized as amylose, amylopectin, or a defined oligosaccharide is linked to various dyes or indicator groups. The dye-labeled substrates are suspended in buffer, and the added serum amylase attacks the α-1,4 bonds to produce small dye-containing fragments. These fragments then are measured photometrically after being separated from the unreacted substrate by centrifugation or filtration.

Defined substrate methods

The use of defined amylase substrates and auxiliary and indicator enzymes in the amylase assay has improved the reaction stoichiometry and led to more controlled and consistent hydrolysis conditions. Substrates used include small oligosaccharides and 4-nitrophenyl-glycoside substrates.

Oligosaccharide substrates. When hydrolyzed by α-amylase, small oligosaccharides substrates can provide better-defined products than can starches. For example, both maltopentaose and maltotetraose are excellent α-amylase substrates with good stability, consistent hydrolysis products, and unambiguous reaction stoichiometry. Other useful substrates include small oligosaccharides (of four to seven glucose units), with the 4-NP group covalently bound to the reducing end of the oligosaccharide. In one such assay, α-glucosidase (EC 3.2.1.20; maltase) is used to hydrolyze the disaccharides and trisaccharides produced by the action of amylase to glucose, as follows:[5]

$$\text{Starch} \xrightarrow{\alpha\text{-amylase}} \text{maltose} + \text{maltotriose} + \text{dextrins}$$

$$\text{Maltose} + \text{maltotriose} \xrightarrow{\alpha\text{-glucosidase}} \text{glucose}$$

$$\text{Glucose} + \tfrac{1}{2}\,O_2 \xrightarrow{\text{Glucose oxidase}} H_2O_2 + \delta\text{-gluconolactone}$$

The rate of glucose production then is determined with glucose oxidase (EC 1.1.3.4) and an oxygen electrode. For each mole of glucose oxidized, 0.5 mol of oxygen is consumed. Thus the rate of oxygen removal is related directly to the amylase activity in the sample.

An alternative method involves the same principle but requires the addition of peroxidase (EC 1.11.1.7) in an indicator reaction using the diammonium salt of 2,2'-azine-di-(3-ethylbenzthiazoline)-6-sulfonic acid (ABTS), as follows:

$$H_2O_2 + \text{ABTS (reduced)} \xrightarrow{\text{Peroxidase}} H_2O + \text{ABTS (oxidized)}$$
$$\text{(colorless)} \qquad\qquad\qquad \text{(colored)}$$

ABTS has an absorbance maximum of 410 nm when oxidized. Hydrogen peroxide formed from endogenous glucose during preincubation is decomposed by catalase (EC 1.11.1.6); at the end of the preincubation period, catalase activity then is blocked and the increase in absorbance at 410 nm is proportional to the amylase activity of the specimen.

Both these methods require a 10-minute preincubation period to consume the endogenous glucose and overcome the lag phase of the total reaction sequence.

Several variations of this reaction rate formulation have been devised. For example, the detection of glucose can be achieved by the hexokinase (EC 2.7.1.1) reaction, as follows:

$$\text{Maltopentaose} \xrightarrow{\alpha\text{-amylase}} \text{maltotriose} + \text{maltose}$$

$$\text{Maltotriose} + \text{maltose} \xrightarrow{\alpha\text{-glucosidase}} 5\ \text{glucose}$$

$$\text{Glucose} + \text{ATP} \xrightarrow{\text{Hexokinase}} \text{G-6-P} + \text{ADP}$$

$$\text{G-6-P} + \text{NAD}^{\oplus} \xrightarrow{\text{G-6-P dehydrogenase}} \text{6-P-gluconolactone} + \text{NADH} + H^{\oplus}$$

Maltotetraose also has been used as a substrate in the following reaction scheme:

$$\text{Maltotetraose} \xrightarrow{\alpha\text{-amylase}} 2\ \text{maltose}$$

$$\text{Maltose} + P_i \xrightarrow{\text{Maltose phosphorylase}} \text{glucose} + \text{glucose-1-P}$$

$$\text{Glucose-1-P} \xrightarrow{\beta\text{-Phosphoglucomutase}} \text{Glucose-6-P}$$

$$\text{G-6-P} + \text{NAD}^{\oplus} \xrightarrow{\text{G-6-P dehydrogenase}} \text{6-P-gluconolactone} + \text{NADH} + H^{\oplus}$$

Maltose generation is detected by the maltose phosphorylase (EC 2.4.1.8) reaction that avoids interference by the endogenous glucose of the sample.

With this method, two molecules of NADH are produced for each bond hydrolyzed by amylase. This fact holds true only if neither glucose nor maltotriose is produced by the action of amylase. However, subsequent studies have shown that these products are present in the reaction mixture in significant quantities. Thus the assay underestimates amylase activity. Note that endogenous glucose does not interfere with the estimation of amylase activity. However, LD contamination—both from the specimen and the assay reagents—and the presence of pyruvate cause negative interference because LD activity, in the presence of pyruvate (from the specimen) and NADH (generated by G-6-PD activity), produces lactate and NAD^+. The degree of this interference therefore depends on the LD activity, pyruvate concentration, and amylase activity of the individual specimen.

4-Nitrophenyl-glycoside substrates. Substrates for this assay are prepared by bonding of 4-NP to the reducing end of a defined oligosaccharide. If the oligosaccharide is maltoheptaose (G7), the substrate is then 4-NP-G7. Amylase splits this substrate to produce free oligosaccharides (G5, G4, G3) and 4-NP-G2 (9%), 4-NP-G3 (31%), and 4-NP-G4 (60%), as follows:

$$4\text{-NP-(glucose)}_7 \xrightarrow{\alpha\text{-}amylase} 4\text{-NP-(glucose)}_{4,3,2} + \text{(glucose)}_{5,4,3}$$

$$4\text{-NP-(glucose)}_{4,3,2} \xrightarrow{\alpha\text{-}glucosidase} 4\text{-NP-(glucose)}_4$$
$$+ \text{x-glucose} + \text{NP}$$

Note that G6, G1, 4-NP-G6, and 4-NP-G5 are not produced in appreciable quantities. If α-glucosidase is added, some of the 4-NP-G4 is hydrolyzed to free NP and free oligosaccharides; 4-NP-G3 and 4-NP-G2 are hydrolyzed to free NP and glucose. The pancreatic isoenzyme hydrolyzes the substrate at a greater rate than does the salivary isoenzyme in the ratio 1.8:1. The result of the combined hydrolysis by amylase in the specimen and by the reagent α-glucosidase is that more than 30% of the product is free NP. The free NP is detected by its absorbance at 405 nm. Alpha-glucosidase does not react with any oligosaccharide containing more than four glucose molecules in the chain; G4 is hydrolyzed only very slowly.

An alternative method based on the β-2-chloro-4-NP (CNP) indicator uses 2-chloro-*p*-nitrophenyl-α-D-maltotrioside (CNP-G3) as a substrate, as follows:

$$10\text{ CNP-G3} \xrightarrow{\alpha\text{-}amylase} 9\text{ CNP} + 1\text{ CNP-G2}$$
$$+ 9\text{ maltotriose} + 1\text{ glucose}$$

This assay does not require α- or β-glucosidases and is considered a "direct" assay. The optimum pH for the salivary and pancreatic isoenzymes is slightly different, but at an assay pH of 6.0, more than 95% of the activities of both isoenzymes is measured. Ninety percent of the CNP-G3 is converted to CNP in this reaction. Color development is rapid, reaction kinetics are linear for more than 5 minutes, and its measuring range is up to twentyfold the upper limit of the reference interval; the reagent also has proven very stable in liquid form. Its disadvantages include its low substrate conversion rate, compared with G4, G5, and G7 assays; the variation in molar absorptivity of CNP due to changes in pH, temperature, and protein content; and the presence of the activator, potassium thiocyanate (KSCN).

Specimen requirements

With the exception of heparin, all common anticoagulants inhibit amylase activity because they chelate Ca^{2+}; citrate, EDTA, and oxalate inhibit it by as much as 15%. As a consequence, amylase assays should be performed only on serum or heparinized plasma. Serum amylase is quite stable; activity loss is negligible at room temperature in the course of 1 week or at refrigerator temperatures over a 2-month period. In urine an acid pH may make the enzyme less stable; therefore the pH of urine specimens should be adjusted to approximately 7.0 before storage.

Reference interval

Reference intervals for amylase are very method dependent. Rather than list the reference intervals for the many amylase methods described previously, the reader is directed to the expanded version of this chapter[6] and to Chapter 46.

Methods for the determination of amylase isoenzymes

Analytical methods for human amylase isoenzymes (isoamylases) include electrophoresis, ion-exchange chromatography, isoelectric focusing, selective inhibition of the S-type isoamylase by a wheat germ inhibitor, and immunoinhibition. Up to three pancreatic and three salivary isoenzymes have been demonstrated after separation on agarose or cellulose acetate media. A minicolumn ion-exchange technique has been described that separates P-type from S-type isoamylases. Isoelectric focusing using thin-layer polyacrylamide gels separate both the S- and P-types. S-type amylase is inhibited preferentially by a protein isolated from wheat. In a method based on this principle the amylase activity of the serum specimen is determined in the presence and absence of the inhibitor. The extent of inhibition is proportional to the S-type isoenzyme content of the specimen.

A double monoclonal antibody assay is available commercially that uses the synergistic action of two immunoinhibitory monoclonal antibodies to the salivary isoenzyme. After the salivary amylase is inhibited by the addition of the antibodies, the uninhibited pancreatic amylase is measured with 4-NP-G7 as a substrate. A number of other immunoassays also have been developed.[6]

After birth, serum S-type amylase activity increases steadily with age and reaches normal adult levels of 83 U/L (interval, 35 to 155 U/L) or 48% of total activity at 5 years of age. Serum P-type amylase activity is not demonstrable in most children younger than 1 year, but activity rises slowly thereafter to reach adult levels (52% of total activity) at 10 to 15 years of age. With isoelectric focusing, values of 68% and 32%, respectively, for the S- and P-type isoamylases in serum have been reported.

Lipase

Human **lipase** (EC 3.1.1.3; triacylglycerol acylhydrolase) is a glycoprotein with an MW of about 54,000 and an isoelectric point of about 5.8. The lipase gene resides on chromosome 10. The lipase concentration in pancreas is about 100-fold greater than in other tissues, and the concentration gradient between pancreas and serum is ~20,000 fold. For full catalytic activity and greatest specificity, bile salts and a cofactor called *colipase* are required. The colipase gene resides on chromosome 6. Human lipase also can be activated fully in vitro by colipases from other species (for example, porcine colipase); this property is used in analytical formulations of the lipase assay.

Biochemistry

Lipases are defined as enzymes that hydrolyze glycerol esters of long-chain fatty acids. Only the ester bonds at carbons 1 and 3 (α-positions) are attacked, and the products of the reaction are 2 mol of fatty acids and 1 mol of 2-acylglycerol (β-monoglyceride) per mole of substrate. The latter is resistant to hydrolysis, probably because of steric hindrance, but it can isomerize spontaneously to the α-form (3-acylglycerol). This isomerization permits the third fatty acid to split off, but at a much slower rate. A scheme for the steps in the complete hydrolysis of a molecule of triglyceride to glycerol and three fatty acids is as follows:

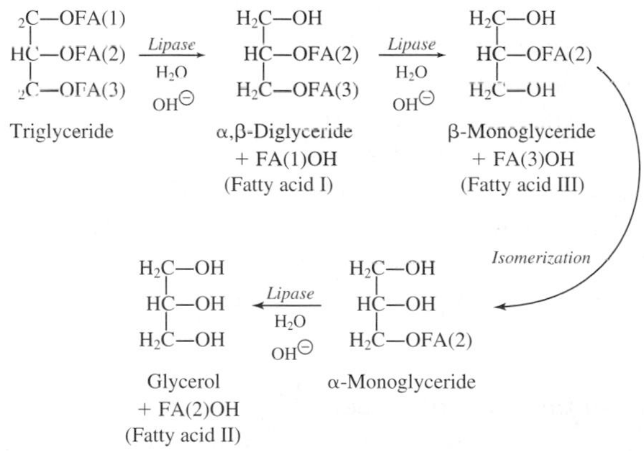

Lipase acts only when the substrate is present in an emulsified form at the interface between water and the substrate. The rate of lipase action depends on the surface area of the dispersed substrate. Bile acids ensure that the surface of the dispersed substrate remains free of other proteins, including lipolytic enzymes, by lining the surface of the insoluble substrate and the aqueous medium. Lipase seems to gain access to the substrate surface in the following manner: Colipase attaches to a micelle of bile salts, thus forming a colipase-bile salt complex that reconfigures the structure of colipase with the exposure of a site with high affinity and high specificity for lipase. This site therefore attracts lipase and anchors it to the substrate surface, allowing lipase action to proceed.

Most lipase found in serum is produced in the pancreas, but some also is secreted by the lingual salivary glands and gastric, pulmonary, and intestinal mucosa. Lipase activity also has been found in leukocytes, adipose tissue cells, and milk.

Clinical significance

Lipase measurements on serum, plasma, and ascitic and pleural fluid are used to investigate pancreatic disorders, usually pancreatitis. The complete absence of lipase or colipase has been reported. Such congenital absence results in severe steatorrhea.

After an attack of acute pancreatitis, serum lipase activity increases within 4 to 8 hours, peaks at about 24 hours, and decreases within 8 to 14 days; levels remain elevated longer than those of amylase. The serum half-life of lipase is between 7 and 14 hours. Elevations between 2 and 50 times the upper limit of the reference interval have been reported. Lipase elevations usually parallel those of amylase, but increases in lipase activity may occur sooner or later than increases in amylase activity and lipase may rise to a greater extent. Normoamylasemia may occur in up to 20% of individuals with acute pancreatitis. Likewise, the existence of hyperlipemia may cause a spurious normoamylasemia. Thus the two assays should complement and not exclude each other, and both enzymes should be assayed. The increase in serum lipase activity is not necessarily proportional to the severity of the attack.

Acute pancreatitis may produce ascitic fluid, pleural fluid (usually on the left side), or both. These fluids may contain lipase activity. Up to 50% of individuals with severe acute pancreatitis develop a pseudocyst; its presence usually is suspected when no clinical improvement is visible within a week of the acute attack. About 50% of individuals with pseudocyst formation show persistent serum amylase elevations, and lipase assays also may be useful under these circumstances.

Acute pancreatitis sometimes is difficult to diagnose because it has to be differentiated from other acute intraabdominal disorders with similar clinical findings, such as perforated gastric or duodenal ulcer, intestinal obstruction, mesenteric vascular obstruction, and many others. Elevation of serum lipase activity is probably a more specific diagnostic finding in these cases than serum amylase activity because many of these conditions are less likely to cause increases in lipase activity than in amylase activity.

Serum lipase assays also may be valuable in the diagnosis of chronic pancreatitis, but severe destruction of the acinar tissue in the later stages of the disease results in a reduction of the amount of enzyme that can enter the circulation and in subnormal serum activities. Marginal or no increase of serum lipase activity therefore is not unusual with this disease. Obstruction of the pancreatic duct by a calculus or carcinoma of the pancreas may cause an increase in serum lipase activity, depending on the location of the obstruction and the amount of remaining functioning tissue. Serum lipase activity is increased in individuals with acute and chronic renal disease, although this elevation is neither as frequent nor as pronounced as that of serum amylase activity.

In cases involving mumps (acute parotitis) without pancreatic involvement, serum lipase activity usually is not elevated but serum amylase activity is. Finally, investigation of the biliary tract by endoscopic retrograde pancreatography or treatment with opiates (which causes the sphincter of Oddi to contract) may cause elevation of serum lipase activity.

Methods used to measure lipase activity

Many lipase methods have been described; they have used both triglyceride and nontriglyceride substrates in titrimetric, turbidimetric, spectrophotometric, fluorometric, and immunological techniques.

Titrimetric methods

Lipase catalyzes the hydrolysis of fatty acids from an emulsion of olive oil or oleic acid. The liberated fatty acids are titrated with dilute alkali. In practice, a 100-μL aliquot of serum is incubated with a hydroxypropyl methylcellulose-stabilized olive oil (or triolein) emulsion at a reaction pH of 9.0 for up to 10 minutes at 30 °C. The liberated fatty acids are titrated continuously, potentiometrically, to maintain a pH of 9.0 with 15 mmol/L NaOH.

The relatively long incubation times of the earlier titrimetric methods posed a risk of enzyme denaturation because of lengthy exposure of enzyme to the relatively high reaction temperature. However, kinetic methods that use an automated potentiometric titrator (an instrument commonly referred to as a *pH-stat*) makes possible shorter incubation periods, and inactivation of the enzyme during the incubation period is reduced significantly. In one such method,[9] the pH is maintained constant at 9.0 at 30 °C by addition of dilute alkali. The amount of alkali used is recorded as a function of time and serves as a measure of fatty acid produced during the reaction. Good precision is obtained with a serum sample of 100 μL and a reaction time of 3 to 8 minutes. When olive oil is used as an substrate, the reported reference interval at 37 °C is less than 160 U/L ($<$ 2.72 μKat/L); with triolein as a substrate, slightly higher activities are obtained, with the upper limit of the reference interval increasing to 200 U/L ($<$ 3.4 μKat/L).

Turbidimetric methods

Lipase catalyzes the hydrolysis of fatty acids from an emulsion of oleic acid, with a simultaneous increase in the turbidity of the reaction mixture. In practice, a 100-μL aliquot of serum is added to a preincubated stabilized triolein emulsion-containing sodium deoxycholate, $CaCl_2$, and porcine colipase at pH 9.2 with TRIS buffer and triolein. Assay temperature is 30 °C. Absorbance at 340 nm is read after 4 minutes and again after an additional 5 minutes. The $\Delta A/$minute is taken as a measure of lipase activity. This method requires the use of a lipase calibrator. The reference interval for a turbidimetric lipase assay at 30 °C for an adult reportedly is 13 to 141 U/L (0.22 to 2.40 μKat/L).

Spectrophotometric and fluorometric methods

Some spectrophotometric methods used to measure lipase are based on extraction of free fatty acids released by lipolysis from the reaction mixture, followed by conversion of the acids to their cupric salts and reextraction into an organic phase containing diethyldithiocarbamate (DTC). The copper-DTC complex is colored brown and suitable for spectrophotometric quantification. Versions of this approach concentrate on minimization of the number of extractions and facilitation of phase separations.

A number of substrates and complex auxiliary and indicator systems are used in spectrophotometric and fluorometric methods.[6] Reference intervals are method dependent. However, a fluorometric method using 1-pyrenedecanoyl-2,3-dioleyl glycerol as a substrate produce a reference interval of 0-120 mU/L.

Methods that use short-chain triglyceride substrates

Short-chain triglycerides have the analytical advantage of greater solubility in aqueous media. Tributyrin emulsions have been suggested as substrates for assays of lipase activity. One study demonstrated that tributyrin was hydrolyzed 12 times faster than triolein by human pancreatic juice or duodenal fluid. A tributyrin derivative, 2,3-dimercaptopropan-1-ol tributyrate (BALB), also has been used in a spectrophotometric method. Hydrolysis of BALB by lipase in the presence of the surfactant sodium dodecyl sulfate produces 2,3-dimercaptopropan-1-ol. This product reacts with 5,5′-dithiobis-(2-nitrobenzoic acid) (DTNB) to form 5-thio-2-nitrobenzoate ions, which absorb strongly at 412 nm. Both serum arylesterase and carboxylic esterase hydrolyze BALB, but their effects are eliminated by pretreatment of serum with the potent esterase inhibitor phenylmethylsulfonylfluoride.

Immunoassay of lipase

A number of lipase immunoassays have been described, but few are available commercially. One such method is a sandwich technique that uses a specific antilipase antibody that is conjugated to horseradish peroxidase. This antibody binds pancreatic lipase in serum, with the subsequently measured peroxidase activity being proportional to the amount of lipase bound. The detection limit of the assay is 300 ng/L; the reference interval in a healthy adult population is 7.7 to 56 μg/L. The assay possesses a broad dynamic range of 20 times the upper limit of the reference interval. A particular advantage of the assay is its ability to determine low lipase concentrations characteristic of cystic fibrosis, chronic pancreatitis, and some cases involving carcinoma of the pancreas.

Trypsin

Trypsin (EC 3.4.21.4; no systematic name) is a serine proteinase characterized by the presence at the active site of serine and histidine, both of which participate in the catalytic process.

Biochemistry

Trypsin hydrolyzes the peptide bonds formed by the carboxyl groups of lysine or arginine with other amino acids, although esters and amides involving these amino acids actually are split more rapidly than peptide bonds. This specificity is illustrated in Figure 20-6, which presents the structures of three synthetic substrates, benzoyl-L-lysineamide (BLA), 2-toluenesulfonyl-L-arginine methyl ester (TAME), and benzoyl-L-arginine-4-nitroanilide (BAPNA); all are hydrolyzed rapidly by trypsin.

The acinar cells of the human pancreas synthesize two different trypsins (1 and 2) in the form of the inactive proenzymes (or zymogens), trypsinogens-1 and -2. These zymogens are stored in zymogen granules and secreted into the duodenum under the stimulus of either the vagus nerve or the intestinal hormone cholecystokinin-pancreozymin. The two trypsinogens represent approximately 19% of the total protein in pancreatic juice; trypsinogen-1 is present at about twice the concentration of trypsinogen-2. In the intestinal tract the trypsinogens are converted to the active enzyme trypsin by the intestinal enzyme enterokinase or by preformed trypsin (autocatalysis).

Trypsin-1 also is described as cationic and trypsin-2 as anionic because of their differing electrophoretic mobilities; the cationic form predominates and is the better documented enzyme. Trypsin-1 and trypsin-2 have MWs of 25,800 and 22,900 and pI values of 4.6 to 6.5 and greater than 6.5, respectively. The pH optimum for trypsin-1 for natural substrates is in the range of 8.0 to 9.0, but for synthetic substrates such as TAME or BAPNA, it is 7.8; the pH optimum for trypsin-2 is 8.0 to 10.0. Trypsin-2 differs from trypsin-1 in that it rapidly undergoes autolysis at neutral or alkaline pH values and is not stabilized against autolysis by

Ca^{2+}. Because the two trypsins show little immunological cross-reactivity, specific immunoassay of each is possible.

When trypsinogens are converted to active trypsin, a tetrapeptide (tetra-L-aspartyl-L-lysine) is cleaved from trypsinogen (trypsinogen activation peptide, or TAP). Measuring TAP by radioimmunoassay is possible, determinations of urinary TAP may provide useful early predictive information on the severity of acute pancreatitis (see Chapter 37).

Trypsin activity is stimulated by calcium and magnesium ions and to a lesser extent by cobalt and manganese ions and aliphatic alcohols. Cyanide, sulfide, citrate, fluoride, and heavy metals inhibit activity, as do those organic phosphorus compounds that combine with serine at the active site.

Materials such as soybeans, lima beans, and egg whites contain natural trypsin inhibitors—small polypeptides such as α_1-antitrypsin (α-1-protease inhibitor) and α_2-macroglobulin—that combine irreversibly with trypsin and inactivate it by blocking the active center. Similar nondialyzable trypsin inhibitors are present in pancreatic juice, serum, and urine. These inhibitors protect plasma and other proteins against hydrolysis by trypsin and other proteases if for some reason any appreciable quantity of the enzyme enters the vascular system. The absence of α_1-antitrypsin is associated with an increased tendency toward panlobular emphysema in early life; this example illustrates the effects of uninhibited proteases on organ function.

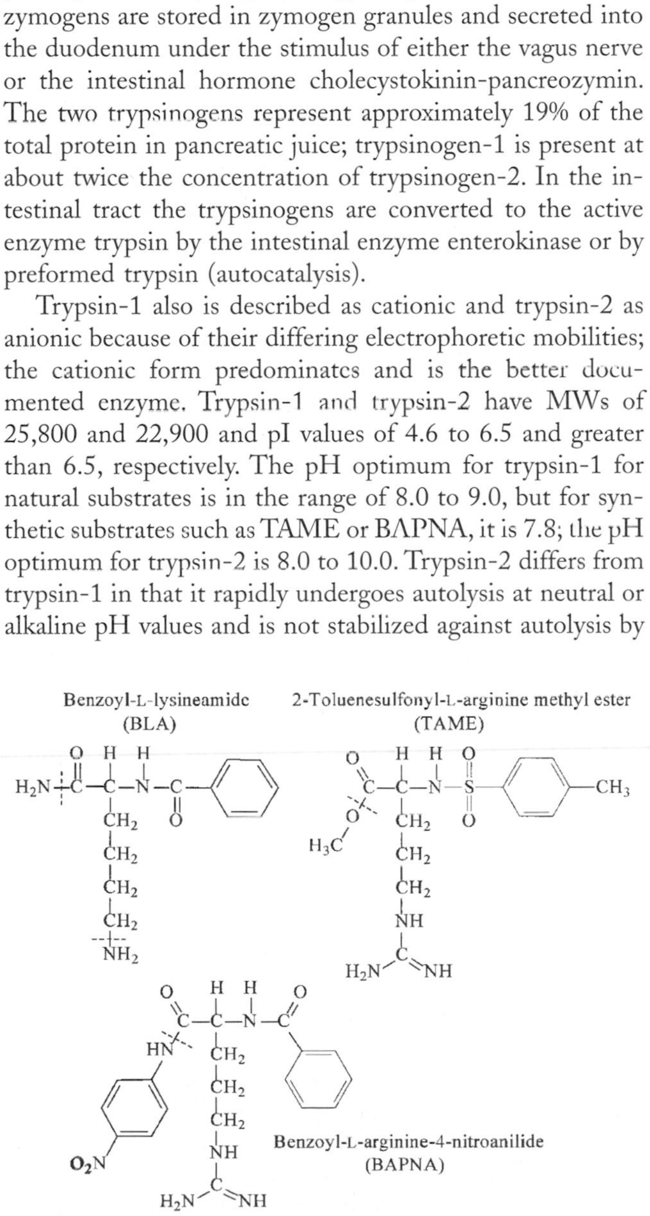

Clinical significance

Trypsin in duodenal content and feces

Determinations of trypsin in gastrointestinal secretions are used to help evaluate pancreatic function and diagnose chronic pancreatitis and fibrocystic disease (see Chapter 37). Trypsin assays are performed either on aspirated specimens of duodenal content or fresh feces. In current practice, determination of trypsin in feces is thought to be of limited value because much of the pancreatic trypsin may be destroyed by proteases as the intestinal contents pass through the tract; in addition, the remainder of those contents is not differentiated easily from proteases associated with intestinal bacteria.

Fibrocystic disease (cystic fibrosis, mucoviscidosis) in children is accompanied by deficient secretion of trypsin by the pancreas. The disease is diagnosed on clinical grounds and by the measurement of sweat electrolytes. Either at the time of presentation or at the stage when pancreatic insufficiency develops, little or no tryptic activity in duodenal contents usually is evident. Decrease in activity is demonstrated conveniently with the x-ray film test (described in a subsequent section of this chapter) or with one of the previously mentioned quantitative methods that use synthetic substrates.

Immunoreactive trypsin in serum

In serum, radioimmunoassay (RIA) detects trypsinogen-1, trypsin-1, and the trypsin-1:α_1-antitrypsin

Figure 20-6 Formulas for three synthetic substrates for trypsin, illustrating the bond specificity of the enzyme, which attacks bonds involving the −COOH of lysine and arginine. Note the bond that is hydrolyzed *(dashed line)*. Hydrolysis of TAME is an example of esterase activity; hydrolyses of BLA and BAPNA are examples of amidase activity.

complex, although only to the extent of less than 40% for the latter. It does not detect the trypsin-1:α_2-macroglobulin complex, for which special techniques are necessary. Free trypsin-1 usually is not found in serum; it is always complexed. Trypsin-2 exists in healthy individuals as trypsinogen-2, and it also is found in disease states complexed to α_1-antitrypsin and α_2-macroglobulin.

Trypsin-1 (cationic trypsin). In healthy individuals, free trypsinogen-1 is the major form found in serum. After an attack of acute pancreatitis, serum immunoreactive trypsin rises in parallel with serum amylase activity to peak values, ranging from 2 to 400 times the upper limit of the reference interval. The distribution of the different forms of trypsin appears to be related to the type and severity of the acute pancreatitis. Thus in the mildest form of acute pancreatitis, 80% to 99% of the immunoreactive trypsin exists as free trypsinogen-1, with smaller proportions existing as bound trypsin-1. In the more severe forms, in which mortality ranges from 20% to more than 50%, the proportion of free trypsinogen-1 may be as low as 30% of the total, with appreciable proportions existing as the α_1-antitrypsin- and α_2-macroglobulin-bound trypsin-1.

Immunoreactive trypsin-1 in serum is elevated in cases of chronic renal failure, as with serum amylase. Thus renal failure must be ruled out during interpretation of elevated levels. In cases of chronic pancreatitis without steatorrhea, plasma levels of immunoreactive trypsin-1 do not differ from those found in healthy individuals; when steatorrhea is present, however, fasting levels are extremely low. In the relapsing phase of chronic pancreatitis, plasma immunoreactive trypsin may be elevated considerably. In individuals with carcinoma of the pancreas, immunoreactive trypsin levels may be high, normal, or even low, thus limiting the usefulness of its measurement in this condition.

In fibrocystic disease cases, plasma immunoreactive trypsin levels reportedly have been high in neonates; as the disease progresses, the levels fall. Dried blood specimens have been suggested for use in screening tests. In both types 1 and 2 diabetic individuals, significantly lower than normal plasma immunoreactive trypsin levels have been reported, with a graded reduction in levels related to the degree of insulin failure.

Increased plasma levels have been reported in virologically confirmed cases of mumps and coxsackievirus B infections and in children with clinical diagnoses of mumps, pyrexia of unknown origin, and meningitis, as well as in adults with Bornholm's disease or cardiac and respiratory infections.

Trypsin-2 (anionic trypsin). Serum trypsin-2 determinations have demonstrated diagnostic utility in both acute and chronic pancreatitis cases. They also are useful in diagnosis of pancreatic cancer, in which a nonparallel rise of trypsin-1 and trypsin-2 occurs; this fact suggests that a specific rise in trypsin-2 signals pancreatic disease. Trypsinogen-2 also is useful as a biochemical marker of rejection of pancreatic grafts, and serum levels are used to establish the proper timing of graft biopsies and the use of immunosuppressive agents.

Methods for the determination of trypsin in duodenal fluid and stool

Semiquantitative determination by the x-ray film test

The test specimen may be either duodenal fluid or a fresh stool specimen. Serial twofold dilutions of the specimen in barbital buffer, 100 mmol/L (pH 8.0), are prepared. For a duodenal fluid specimen, the dilution may range from 1/2 to 1/256 and for a stool specimen, from 1/5 to 1/320. A drop of each dilution is spotted onto a small piece of unexposed x-ray film, along with a drop of barbital buffer to act as a control. The x-ray film with the series of specimen and control drops then is incubated for 30 minutes at 37 °C, cooled in a refrigerator to harden the gelatin, and washed with a slight stream of water to remove any loose or hydrolyzed gelatin. The piece of film then is examined for the presence of clear (digested) areas, indicating hydrolysis of the gelatin layer by the action of the enzyme; the control spot should show no evidence of digestion. The greatest dilution of the specimen that provides a cleared area is taken as the measure of the trypsin activity present. The test is not recommended for stool specimens from adults because of the high rate of false-negative results.

The stool of a normal infant younger than 1 year of age shows tryptic activity through a dilution of 1/80 or higher. With older children, activity may be evident only through a dilution of 1/20 or 1/40. Infants with fibrocystic disease rarely give positive results beyond the 1/10 dilution. In the case of duodenal contents, normal infants demonstrate positive results through a dilution of 1/32 or 1/64, fibrocystic children usually in dilutions of 1/4 or less.

Determination of trypsin in stool or duodenal fluid with TAME as substrate

Synthetic peptide substrates, such as benzoyl-L-arginine ethyl ester (BAEE), BLA, BAPNA, and TAME are the substrates of choice for trypsin assays. They are more specific for trypsin than chymotrypsin and are not attacked by other proteases found in duodenal contents and stool specimens. In addition, these synthetic substrates have only one bond that can be split, so expression of activity in international units is possible.

Procedures using these substrates are simple and convenient, although specimen color may on occasion be a source of interference. When possible, the change in absorbance at some fixed wavelength is observed during the course of the reaction. For example, because benzoyl arginine, a reaction product, has a greater absorbance at 253 nm than does the substrate BAEE, the reaction is monitored by measurement of the rate of increase in absorbance at 253 nm. If amides are used, the ammonia formed is measured by Berthelot's method (see Chapter 22). With the use of any synthetic substrate, monitoring of the reaction through measurement of the carboxyl H^+ produced is possible with a pH-stat. With BAPNA as a substrate, the yellow color of the p-nitroaniline split off in the reaction permits the measurement of trypsin activity by a continuous-monitoring photometric procedure.

A procedure using TAME in TRIS buffer has been developed and is based on measurement of tryptic activity by titration of the carboxyl hydrogen ion released on hydrolysis of the methyl ester. Tryptic activity is recorded as millimoles of NaOH required to maintain a constant pH and converted to micrograms of crystalline trypsin by comparison with a calibration curve. With this method, normal children and adults have trypsin values of 40 to 760 µg/g stool, adults with (alcoholic) pancreatic insufficiency provide values of 0 to 33 µg/g stool, and fibrocystic children demonstrate concentrations less than 20 µg/g stool.

Determination of immunoreactive trypsin in blood, serum, or plasma by immunoassay

Antibodies to purified human pancreatic trypsin-1 and trypsin-2 (and the precursor trypsinogens) have been developed. Immunoassays with these antibodies can detect the mass quantities of trypsin, trypsinogen, and trypsin bound to α_1-antitrypsin. The trypsin-1 bound to α_2-macroglobulin cannot be detected by immunoassay unless the complex is isolated and dissociated. The trypsin-1:α_2-macroglobulin complex is isolated from serum by gel filtration, and trypsin-1 is dissociated by treatment of the complex with acid, after which the freed trypsin-1 may be assayed. Trypsin-1 bound to α_2-macroglobulin can consist of more than 30% of the total serum trypsin in disease states, but many assays do not measure this particular trypsin fraction. Alternatively, the trypsin-1 bound to α_2-macroglobulin may be estimated photometrically by use of a synthetic substrate. Several commercial immunoassays also are available for measurement of trypsin-1.[6] In one such assay the reference interval for immunoreactive trypsin is 185 to 272 µg/L for individuals between 18 and 36 years of age. For adults the reference interval is 135 to 400 µg/L. Serum trypsin-1 levels increase with age, values are 50% higher in women than in men, and serum concentrations increase as renal function decreases.

Chymotrypsin

Chymotrypsin (EC 3.4.21.1; no systematic name) is also a serine proteinase. It hydrolyzes peptide bonds involving carboxyl groups of tryptophan, leucine, tyrosine, or phenylalanine, with preference for the aromatic residues. Specificity of chymotrypsin therefore is in contrast to that of pepsin, which splits bonds involving amino groups of the aromatic amino acids. Chymotrypsin also demonstrates hydrolytic activity for other types of bonds in the fol-

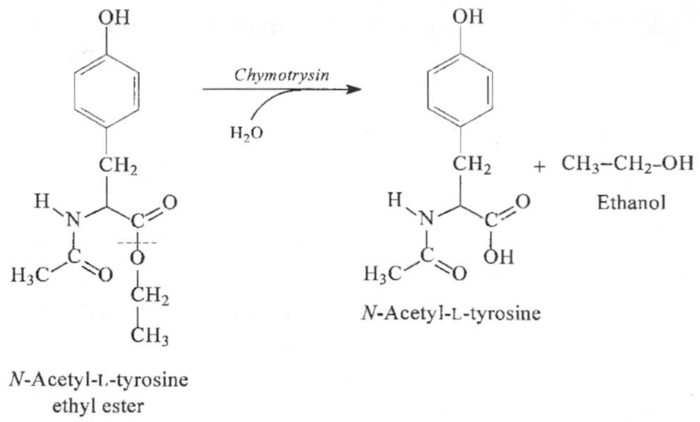

Figure 20-7   N-acetyl-L-tyrosine ethyl ester, a synthetic substrate for chymotrypsin.

lowing order: esters (especially N-substituted tyrosine esters) > amide > peptides. N-acetyl-L-tyrosine ethyl ester is an example of a synthetic substrate, used for chymotrypsin assays in duodenal aspirates and feces, that contains an ester bond and is not hydrolyzed significantly by trypsin (Figure 20-7).

Biochemistry

The acinar cells of the human pancreas synthesize two different chymotrypsins (1 and 2, with chymotrypsin-2 being the major species) in the form of the inactive proenzymes (or zymogens), chymotrypsinogens-1 and -2. These zymogens are stored in granules and are secreted as is trypsinogen into the pancreatic duct. In the intestinal tract the chymotrypsinogens are converted to chymotrypsin by the action of trypsin. Chymotrypsin is more resistant than trypsin to degradation in the intestine; it is therefore the enzyme of choice for assay in feces.

Chymotrypsin-1 also is described as anionic and chymotrypsin-2 as cationic because of their differing electrophoretic mobilities; the cationic form predominates. The MW of both forms is approximately 25,000. Close immunological identity exists among the chymotrypsins and chymotrypsinogens; immunoassay for chymotrypsin-2 reacts totally with chymotrypsinogen-2 and strongly with both chymotrypsin-1 and chymotrypsinogen-1. Chymotrypsin, like trypsin, is bound in blood plasma by α_1-antitrypsin and α_2-macroglobulin. The complex of chymotrypsin-1 (or -2):α_1-antitrypsin can be detected by the chymotrypsin-2 immunoassay; however, the chymotrypsin-1 (or -2):α_2-macroglobulin complex is not detected with this assay.

Clinical significance

The major application of chymotrypsin assays is in the investigation of pancreatic disease. In neonates, chymotrypsin-2 in umbilical cord blood is 2.2 to 7.5 times higher in infants with fibrocystic disease than in healthy infants. In adults, acute pancreatitis can elevate immunoreactive chymotrypsin-2 to 35 times the levels found in healthy adults. In those with pancreatic carcinoma, levels may be normal or slightly (2.5-fold) elevated. After total pancreatectomy, no chymotrypsin-2 is detectable in serum.

In gastric carcinoma cases, levels may be elevated slightly (up to 2.5-fold) but are usually within the reference interval. In hepatobiliary disease states, elevations up to twice the upper limit of the reference interval are found. As with trypsin and amylase, elevation of serum chymotrypsin-2 reaches eight times the reference interval in individuals with renal failure.

In duodenal aspirates (or pancreatic juice) and in feces, chymotrypsin levels are reduced variably in pancreatic dysfunction.

Methods for the determination of chymotrypsin in blood

Methods used to determine chymotrypsin with synthetic substrates or peptides no longer are preferred for use in the clinical laboratory and have been replaced by immunoassays. Several investigators have purified chymotrypsin-2 and prepared antichymotrypsin sera for immunoassay of chymotrypsin. These assays detect, by mass, chymotrypsinogen-2, chymotrypsin-2, and, to a lesser extent, chymotrypsin-2 bound to α_1-antitrypsin. A significant cross-reaction exists with chymotrypsinogen-1 (55% to 85%), chymotrypsin-1 (25% to 50%), and chymotrypsin-1:α_1-antitrypsin (20% to 32%) in these assays; however, the complex chymotrypsin-1 (or -2):α_2-macroglobulin is not detected.

In neonates (umbilical cord blood), total chymotrypsin is less than 24 μg/L. In adults, total chymotrypsin intervals from 15 to 78 μg/L (mean of 37.5 μg/L) have been reported, although an earlier report suggested a mean level of approximately 10 μg/L.

Methods for the determination of chymotrypsin in duodenal or pancreatic aspirates and feces

Synthetic substrates commonly are used for these applications. A sensitive kinetic assay has been developed that uses N-Succinyl-Ala-Ala-Pro-Phe-2-nitroanilide as a substrate. Duodenal or pancreatic aspirates are obtained after stimulation with test meals or by administration of secretin or secretin and cholecystokinin-pancreozymin (see Chapter 37). Stool specimens are collected either randomly or in a 24-hour period. When chymotrypsin is measured in stool specimens, prior treatment of the specimen with detergent to release particle-bound chymotrypsin is necessary. Reference intervals are method dependent, but one such method reported a reference interval for chymotrypsin of 120 to 1265 mg/kg of stool (120 to 1265 μg/g stool).

An indirect estimate of chymotryptic activity in the gut is made by oral administration of N-benzoyl-L-tryosyl-PABA (Bz-Tyr-PABA), usually with a standardized meal (see Chapter 37). Bz-Tyr-PABA is hydrolyzed specifically by chymotrypsin; in the gut the hydrolysis releases free p-aminobenzoic acid (PABA), which is absorbed, conju-

gated in the liver, and excreted in the urine, where it can be measured readily.

Because of the many and varied techniques used for these assays, reference intervals should be established in the laboratory performing the test.

■ OTHER ENZYMES OF CLINICAL UTILITY

Acid Phosphatase

Under the name **acid phosphatase** (ACP) are included all phosphatases with optimal activity below a pH of 7.0. Thus the name refers to a group of similar or related enzymes rather than to one particular enzyme species. However, the ACP of greatest clinical importance (EC 3.1.3.2; orthophosphoric-monoester phosphohydrolase [acid optimum]; ACP) is the one derived from the prostate that has a pH optimum in the range of 5 to 6.

Biochemistry

ACP is present in lysosomes, which are organelles in all cells, with the possible exception of erythrocytes. Extralysosomal ACPs also are present in many cells. The greatest concentrations of ACP activity occur in the liver, spleen, milk, erythrocytes, platelets, bone marrow, and the prostate gland. The prostate gland is the richest source, and it contributes a small proportion of the enzyme present in sera from healthy men. The majority of the normally low ACP activity of serum is of a tartrate-resistant type and probably originates mainly in osteoclasts.

The optimum pH for the individual ACPs varies, depending on the tissues from which they are obtained. The observed pH optimum also varies with the substrate on which the enzyme acts; the more acidic the substrate, the lower the pH at which maximum activity is obtained.

The ACPs are unstable, especially at temperatures above 37 °C and at pH levels above 7.0. Some of the enzyme forms in serum (especially the prostatic enzyme) are particularly labile, and more than 50% of the ACP activity may be lost in 1 hour at room temperature. Acidification of the serum specimen to a pH below 6.5 helps stabilize the enzymes.

In practice, differentiation specifically between increases in the concentrations of the prostatic and nonprostatic forms is necessary. Certain inhibitors enhance the discrimination between prostatic and nonprostatic ACPs. For example, the prostatic enzyme is inhibited strongly by dextrorotatory tartrate ions, whereas the erythrocyte isoenzyme is not. Erythrocyte ACP is inhibited by formaldehyde and cupric ions, to which prostatic ACP is resistant. Thus these inhibitors, particularly tartrate, allow a distinction to be made between prostatic and erythrocyte ACPs. However, interference by the erythrocyte isoenzyme in the measurement of prostatic ACP in serum is not a significant problem in blood specimens taken with precautions against hemolysis and from which serum has been separated without delay.

An alternative approach to increase the specificity of the assay is the use of substrates hydrolyzed rapidly by the prostatic enzyme but at a significantly slower rate by the other forms of the enzyme. For example, α-naphthyl phosphate and thymolphthalein monophosphate are less sensitive relatively to the action of nonprostatic ACPs than are such substrates as phenylphosphate and 4-NPP.

Clinical significance

Although once widely used to detect or monitor carcinoma of the prostate, determination of ACP activity in serum now is used rarely for this purpose. It has been replaced by digital rectal examination, transrectal ultrasonic imaging, histological examination of the biopsy specimen, total-body bone scan, and **prostate-specific antigen (PSA)** assay.

Slight or moderate elevations in total ACP activity often occur in individuals with Paget's disease, in those with hyperparathyroidism with skeletal involvement, and in the presence of malignant invasion of the bones by cancers, such as breast cancer in women. The serum ACP activity in these cases is not inhibited by tartrate and has the immunological and electrophoretic properties of the ACP from osteoclasts. The osteoclasts also are the source of the higher serum ACP in growing children, compared with adults. Raised levels of the osteoclast-derived ACP also are present in serum in osteoclastoma (giant-cell tumor), osteoclastic neoplasm, and osteopetrosis (marble bone disease), in which the osteoclasts fail to resorb bone. Thus raised levels of osteoclastic ACP in serum indicate increased osteoclastic activity—whether effective, as in normal bone growth, or ineffective, as in osteopetrosis.

This isoenzyme is therefore a potentially useful marker of conditions with a marked osteolytic component, such as osteoporosis. However, methods currently available lack the sensitivity and specificity necessary to measure reliably the small and often insidious changes in osteoclastic ACP levels in serum. The only nonbone condition is which elevated activities of tartrate-resistant, osteoclast-type ACP are found in serum is Gaucher's disease of spleen, a lysosomal storage disorder. Its source in this disease is the abnormal macrophages in spleen and other tissues, which overexpress this normal macrophage constituent. The hairy cells of hairy-cell leukemia (leukemic reticuloendotheliosis) also express the osteoclast-type ACP, providing a useful histological marker. However, in this condition the isoenzyme does not enter the plasma in increased amounts.

Because ACP is present in very high concentrations in semen, its measurement has become important in investigations of rape and similar offenses. In practice, swabs taken from alleged rape victims should be preserved by immersion in 2.5 mL of a protective broth (containing, per liter, 50 g of bovine albumin, 0.2 g sodium azide [NaN_3], 10 mmol phosphate buffer at pH 7.4, 9 g NaCl) and stored at either 4 °C or room temperature. Specimens stored in this fashion retain ACP activity for at least 1 month. When this technique and a thymolphthalein monophosphate substrate are used, vaginal ACP in noncoital women is less than 10 U/L of broth, whereas in recently postcoital women it exceeds 50 U/L. In vivo degradation of vaginal postcoital ACP activity follows a logarithmic course so that it reaches noncoital levels 4 days after intercourse.

An alternative preservative procedure involving placement of swabs in 1 mL of isotonic saline has been proposed. Samples then are frozen and allowed to thaw at 2 to 4 °C for 24 hours before assay. However, PSA has been advocated as a more sensitive and specific marker for semen detection in rape investigations because it is detected only in body fluids from women at very low levels. A comparison of immunoassay results of both analytes suggested that ACP probably is the better test.[7] In addition, because male sexual dysfunction is common in rape cases, ACP activity or PSA may not be detected in samples from alleged rape victims.

Methods for the determination of acid phosphatase

Methods used to measure ACP activity essentially are adaptations of those developed for ALP. Phenyl phosphate and 4-NPP, for example, have been used frequently in an acid pH medium for ACP estimation. However, the spectral differences between the phosphate ester and its parent phenol that are exploited in continuous-monitoring procedures for the assay of ALP are distinctive only at alkaline pH. Therefore the reaction mixture first must be made alkaline to stop the ACP reaction before the amount of product formed can be measured.

Continuous-monitoring methods for assay of ACP activity can be based on the principle introduced by Hillmann, in which α-naphthol released from its phosphate ester forms a colored product with the stabilized diazonium salt of 2-amino-5-chlorotoluene-1,5-naphthalene disulfonate (Fast Red TR). Fast Red TR does not react significantly with bilirubin, and coupling with α-naphthol takes place at the pH of enzyme action. Practical difficulties of the method include a pronounced lag phase and instability of the color produced. Nevertheless, the method has been used successfully in manual and automated procedures. The introduction of alcohols, such as 1,5-pentanediol, accelerates the reaction and increases sensitivity; the alcohols react as phosphate acceptors in transfer reactions.

As mentioned previously, nonprostatic ACPs hydrolyze certain substrates less readily than does the prostatic enzyme. Because the object of diagnostic assays is almost always to determine the prostatic phosphatase, the substrates preferred by the enzyme now usually are chosen for the assay systems. The two most popular of these are thymolphthalein monophosphate and α-naphthyl phosphate, the latter being favored for continuous-monitoring procedures. Although neither substrate is completely specific, tartrate inhibition to enhance specificity seldom is considered advantageous for methods using the mentioned substrates.

Immunological methods, such as RIA, counter immuno-electrophoresis (CIE), immunoprecipitation, and immunoenzymetric techniques derive their specificity from the specificity of the antiserum. The potential increase in sensitivity offered by RIA methods relates to the ability of antiserum to recognize all molecules of the enzyme, whether or not they are active catalytically. The specific antiserum may be combined with a photometric assay of activity; if the antiserum is used to "capture" or precipitate prostatic ACP activity, determination of total and residual activity again provides measurement, by difference, of the prostatic enzyme's activity.

Specimen requirements

Serum should be separated immediately from erythrocytes and stabilized by the addition of disodium citrate monohydrate at a level of 10 mg/mL of serum. Alternatively, 50 μL of acetic acid (5 mol/L) per milliliter of serum is added to lower the pH to 5.4, at which the enzyme is stable. Under these conditions, activity is maintained at room temperature for several hours and for up to a week if the serum is refrigerated. Although the substrate is relatively insensitive to erythrocyte ACP, hemolyzed serum specimens are contaminated with considerable amounts of this isoenzyme and should be rejected. Lipemic sera should not be used because of possible interference with measurement because of turbidity.

Reference intervals

In the sera of healthy adult men, the reference interval for prostatic ACP is 0 to 0.6 U/L. Results of RIA or other immunological methods for the determination of prostatic ACP usually are expressed in mass concentrations. Reference intervals are method dependent; representative values are less than 3 μg/L for RIA or immunoenzymetric assays or less than 20 μg/L for CIE.

Aldolase

Aldolase (EC 4.1.2.13; D-fructose-1,6-bisdiphosphate D-glyceraldehyde-3-phosphate-lyase; ALD) catalyzes the splitting of D-fructose-1,6-diphosphate (FDP) to D-glyceraldehyde-3-phosphate (GLAP) and dihydroxyacetone-phosphate (DAP), an important reaction in the glycolytic breakdown of glucose to lactate, as follows:

D-Fructose-1,6-diphosphate (FDP)   Dihydroxyacetone phosphate (DAP)   D-Glyceraldehyde-3-phosphate (GLAP)

The reaction equilibrium favors the formation of fructose diphosphate.

Biochemistry

ALD is a tetrameric enzyme with subunits determined by three separate gene loci. Only two of these loci, those producing A and B subunits, appear to be active simultaneously in most tissues; therefore the most common isoenzyme pattern consists of various proportions of the components of a five-membered set of isoenzymes, of which two members correspond to the A and B homopolymers. The locus that determines the structure of the C subunit is active in brain tissue, as is the A locus, so this tissue contains ALD A and C together with the three corresponding heteropolymers.

Clinical significance

Serum ALD determinations have been of greatest clinical interest in primary diseases of skeletal muscle. In general, however, measurement of ALD activity in serum does not provide information that is not available more readily by measurement of other, more easily assayed enzymes, such as AST, LD, and especially CK. Because of its greater diagnostic sensitivity and ease of measurement, CK generally is regarded as the enzyme of choice in the investigation of disorders of skeletal muscle.

Methods for the measurement of aldolase activity

All assay methods are based on the forward reaction. Both photometric fixed-time and continuous-monitoring procedures have been developed.

The ALD activity in serum is quite stable. Activity is unchanged at ambient temperatures for up to 48 hours and at 4 °C for several weeks. Hemolyzed specimens should not be used, and plasma is preferred over serum because of the possible release of platelet enzyme during the clotting process.

Reference interval

The accepted reference interval for the activity of ALD in serum in adults is 1.0 to 7.5 U/L, measured at 30 °C. However, a definite sex difference is present, with men having higher values.

Angiotensin-Converting Enzyme

Angiotensin-converting enzyme (EC 3.4.15-1; **ACE**) is a peptidyl-dipeptidase that catalyzes the conversion of inactive angiotensin I to the biologically active angiotensin II. Thus ACE is an important enzyme in the renin-angiotensin-aldosterone cycle. Potent ACE inhibitors commonly are used to control hypertension.

Biochemistry

Renin is released from the kidney when the sodium concentration is low. Renin enzymatically cleaves a decapeptide, angiotensin I, from the C-terminal end of angiotensinogen.

ACE then enzymatically cleaves the C-terminyl histidine (His)-leucine (Leu) dipeptide from angiotensin I, resulting in the octapeptide angiotensin II. Angiotensinase then converts angiotensin II to angiotensin III and eventually into inactive products. The lung and testes are major sources of ACE.

Angiotensin II is responsible for a variety of physiological effects on a number of target tissues. For example, it causes contraction of vascular smooth muscle and thus is a potent vasoconstrictor that raises blood pressure directly. Angiotensin II also stimulates aldosterone release from the adrenal glands. Aldosterone in turn causes sodium retention and an increase in plasma volume and elevated blood pressure and potassium loss (see Chapter 41).

Clinical significance

An elevated serum ACE supports the diagnosis of sarcoidosis. ACE activity is elevated in other conditions, including histoplasmosis, alcoholic cirrhosis, asbestosis, berylliosis, diabetes, Hodgkin's disease, hyperthyroidism, amyloidosis, primary biliary cirrhosis, idiopathic pulmonary fibrosis, pulmonary embolism, scleroderma, silicosis, tuberculosis, Gaucher's disease, and leprosy.

Methods for the measurement of angiotensin-converting enzyme activity

A manual assay is available for ACE measurement that uses benzoyl-glycyl-histidyl-leucine as substrate. The reaction is monitored spectrophotometrically by measurement of the rate of release of benzoylglycine (hippuric acid). Automated procedures have been developed that use either furoylacroyl-Phe-Gly-Gly or hippuryl-His-Leu as substrates. With the latter the His-Leu formed then is cleaved by leucine amino peptidase to yield free histidine. Histidase then converts histidine to ammonia and urocanic acid. The ammonia generated then is reacted with 2-oxoglutarate to yield glutamate in the presence of glutamate dehydrogenase, a reaction in which NADH is converted to NAD (see Chapter 22). The decrease in absorbance at 340 nm then is measured.

Reference intervals

Reference intervals for ACE are method dependent. For example, the reference interval for ACE with the furoylacroyl-Phe-Gly-Gly substrate has been reported to be 8 to 52 U/L (0.14 to 0.88 µKat/L) for individuals older than 14 years. For the hippuryl-His-Leu substrate, a reference interval of 7.2 to 26.6 U/L (0.12-0.45 µKat/L) has been reported for individuals between 17 and 19 years of age. In general, ACE levels increase with age.

Cholinesterases

Two related enzymes have the ability to hydrolyze acetylcholine. One is acetylcholinesterase (EC 3.1.1.7; acetylcholine acetylhydrolase), which is called *true cholinesterase,*

or *choline esterase I.* True cholinesterase is found in erythrocytes, the lungs and spleen, nerve endings, and the gray matter of the brain. It is responsible for the prompt hydrolysis of acetylcholine released at the nerve endings to mediate transmission of the neural impulse across the synapse. The degradation of acetylcholine is necessary for the depolarization of the nerve so that it is repolarized in the next conduction event. The assay of this enzyme is clinically useful.

The other **cholinesterase** is acylcholine acylhydrolase (EC 3.1.1.8; SChE); it is usually called *pseudocholinesterase, benzoyl cholinesterase,* or *choline esterase II.* Although it is found in the liver, pancreas, heart, white matter of the brain, and serum, its biological role is unknown. The type of reaction catalyzed by both cholinesterases is as follows:

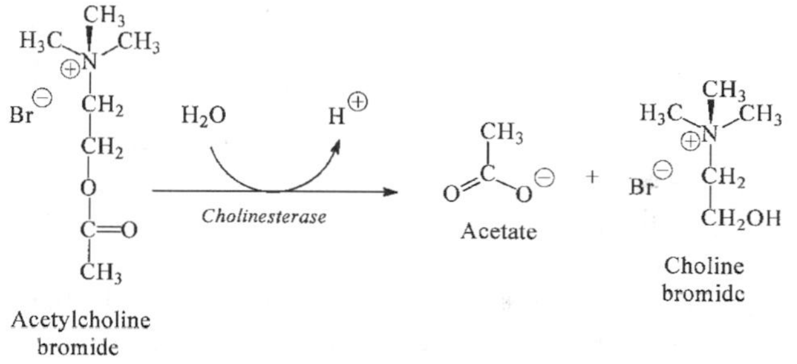

Biochemistry

The two enzymes differ in specificity toward some substrates while behaving similarly toward others. For example, the serum enzyme acts on benzoylcholine but cannot hydrolyze acetyl-β-methylcholine; the red cell enzyme acts on the latter but not on the former. Only choline esters are split by the red cell enzyme; aryl or alkyl esters are not attacked. The red cell enzyme is inhibited by its substrate, acetylcholine, if present at concentrations of approximately 10^{-2} mol/L; the serum enzyme is not inhibited by this substrate.

Both enzymes are inhibited by the alkaloids prostigmine and physostigmine, both of which contain quaternary nitrogen (also present in choline) in their structures. These two compounds are typical competitive inhibitors, competing with the choline residue of acetylcholine for its binding site on the enzyme surface. Both enzymes are inhibited irreversibly by some organic phosphorus compounds, such as diisopropylfluorophosphate. The phosphoryl group binds very tightly to the enzyme site, at which binding of the acyl group normally occurs, thus preventing attachment of the acetylcholine. Both enzymes also are inhibited by a large variety of other compounds, among which are morphine, quinine, tertiary amines, phenothiazines, pyrophosphate, bile salts, citrate, fluoride, and borate.

The cholinesterase present in normal sera is separated by electrophoresis into 7 to 12 bands, the number of which depends on the experimental technique used. The isoenzymes of SChE differ in molecular size and appear to be aggregates of different numbers of the same basic unit. Of more interest are the atypical (genetic) variants of the enzyme, characterized by diminished activity against acetylcholine and other substrates, which are found in the sera of a small fraction of apparently healthy individuals.

The gene controlling the synthesis of SChE can exist in many allelic forms. Four of the most common forms are designated as E_1^u, E_1^a, E_1^f, and E_1^s. At least 25 other forms exist, and another gene locus is recognized (E_2). The normal, most common phenotype is designated as $E_1^u E_1^u$, or UU. The gene E_1^a is referred to as the *atypical gene;* the sera of individuals homozygous for this gene ($E_1^a E_1^a$ = AA) are active only weakly toward most substrates for cholinesterase and possess increased resistance to inhibition of enzyme activity by dibucaine. The E_1^f gene also gives rise to a weakly active enzyme but with increased resistance to fluoride inhibition. The E_1^s gene (*s* for *silent*) is associated with absence of enzyme or the presence of a protein with minimal or no catalytic activity. The mutations that give rise to the atypical and fluoride-resistant SChE variants involve a change in the structure of the active center. The variant isoenzymes (allelozymes) are less effective catalysts than the usual form; the affinity of the enzymes for the substrates is reduced (that is, K_m is increased), and affinity for competitive inhibitors, such as dibucaine or fluoride, similarly is decreased. This occurrence gives rise to the characteristic dibucaine- or fluoride-resistant properties of the genetic variants that are exploited in their characterization.

The homozygous forms, AA or FF ($E_1^f E_1^f$), are found in only 0.3% to 0.5% of the Caucasian population; their incidence among blacks is even lower. Inheritance of increased SChE activity also has been reported in a few families. This fact apparently is due to increased production of the usual allelozyme.

Clinical significance

Cholinesterase levels in serum are useful for (1) an indication of possible insecticide poisoning (see Chapter 32), (2) the detection of individuals with atypical forms of the enzyme, or (3) a test of liver function. Among the organic phosphorus compounds that inhibit cholinesterase activity are many insecticides, such as parathion, sarin, and tetraethyl pyrophosphate. Individuals who work in agriculture and in organic chemical industries are subject to poisoning by inhalation of these materials or contact with them. If enough material is absorbed to inactivate all the acetylcholinesterase of nervous tissue, the individual dies. Both cholinesterases are inhibited, but the activity of the serum enzyme falls more rapidly than does that of the erythrocyte enzyme. A 40% drop in serum enzyme activity occurs before the first symptoms are felt, and a drop of 80% is required before neuromuscular effects become apparent.

Near-zero levels of enzyme activity require emergency treatment of the patient with such enzyme reactivators as pyridine-2-aldoxime.

Succinyldicholine (suxamethonium), a drug used in surgery as a muscle relaxant, also is hydrolyzed by cholinesterase, and its pharmacological effect persists only long enough to meet the needs of the surgical procedure. In individuals with low levels of enzyme activity or those with weakly active variants, the drug is not destroyed rapidly enough and the individual may enter a period of prolonged apnea requiring mechanical ventilation until the drug is eliminated by other routes. Preoperative screening has been advocated to identify individuals in whom suxamethonium administration may lead to complications.

The degree of sensitivity varies with the phenotype of the individual. Total activity declines—from individuals who are homozygous for the usual allele, through those who are heterozygous for the usual and a variant allele, and those who are homozygous or heterozygous for variant alleles—to zero in individuals in whom two "silent" alleles are paired. Those who possess one normal allele (that is, who are heterozygous for the normal and a variant allele) usually produce enough enzyme to protect them against suxamethonium sensitivity, whereas those with paired variant alleles (either as homozygotes or heterozygotes) show various degrees of sensitivity.

Measurements of total serum cholinesterase activity and determination of the "dibucaine number" and "fluoride number" are necessary to characterize cholinesterase variants fully. The latter values indicate the percentage inhibition of enzyme activity toward specified substrates in the presence of standard concentrations of dibucaine or fluoride. Measurement of serum cholinesterase activity also can serve as a sensitive measure of the synthetic capacity of the liver if the individual's normal (baseline) level is known. In the absence of genetic causes or known inhibitors, any decrease in activity in serum reflects impaired synthesis of the enzyme by the liver. A 30% to 50% decrease is observed in individuals with acute hepatitis and chronic hepatitis of long duration. Decreases of 50% to 76% occur in those with advanced cirrhosis and carcinoma with metastases to the liver. Essentially normal levels are seen in individuals with chronic hepatitis, mild cirrhosis, and obstructive jaundice.

Methods for the determination of cholinesterase activity

Contemporary methods to determine cholinesterase activity use acylthiocholine esters as substrates. These substrates are hydrolyzed at approximately the same rate as choline esters, and the thiocholine formed can be measured by reaction with chromogenic disulfide agents, such as DTNB (Ellman's reagent) or 4,4'-dithiodipyridine. The iodide salts of acetyl-, propionyl-, and butyrylthiocholine all have been used as substrates. The reactions for butyrylthiocholine, with DTNB as the chromogen, are as follows:

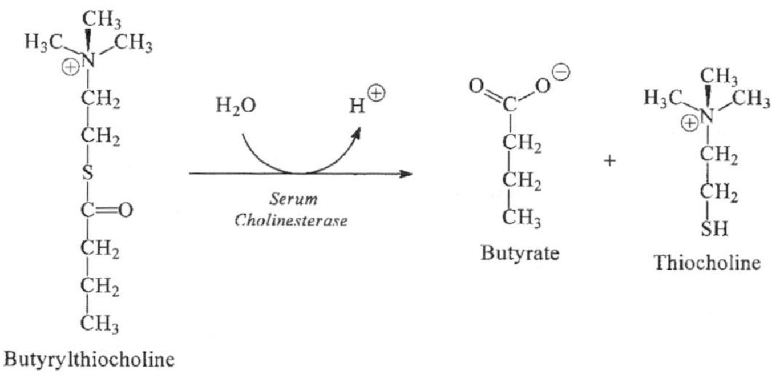

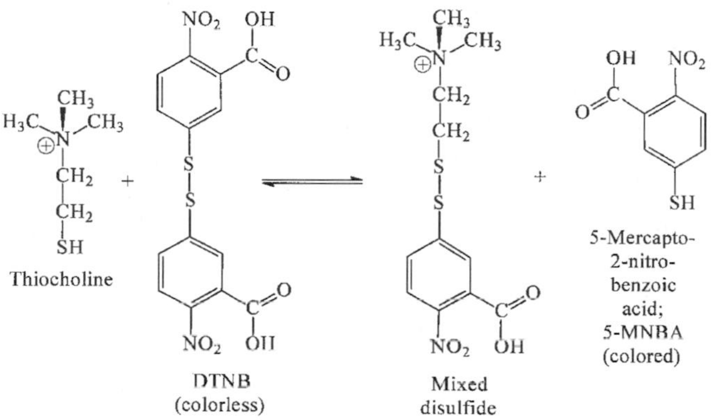

Butyrylthiocholine

Thiocholine

DTNB (colorless)

Mixed disulfide

5-Mercapto-2-nitro-benzoic acid; 5-MNBA (colored)

With this method, activity of SChE is determined from the rate of hydrolysis of propionylthiocholine in the presence of DTNB. The reaction of the thiocholine product with colorless DTNB forms colored 5-mercapto-2-nitro-benzoic acid (5-MNBA), which is measured spectrophotometrically at 410 nm. Dibucaine or fluoride inhibition is estimated by performance of concurrent assays in which dibucaine or fluoride is present in the substrate mixture. Percent inhibition is evaluated by comparison of activity in the inhibited system with that in the uninhibited system.

Specimen requirements

Serum is the sample of choice. Enzyme activity in serum is stable for several weeks, whether the specimen is stored at room temperature or under refrigeration. Moderate hemolysis does not interfere if separated serum has been centrifuged to remove red blood cell ghosts. Specimens from patients who have displayed apnea after succinylcholine treatment should not be obtained until after paralysis has passed; metabolites of the drug appear to interfere with the assay.

Reference interval

For the genotype UU, the mean $\pm$ SD for the foregoing method is 8440 ± 1780 U/L.

Glutamate Dehydrogenase

Glutamate dehydrogenase (EC 1.4.1.3; L-glutamate: NAD(P) oxidoreductase, deaminating; GLD) is a mitochondrial enzyme located mainly in the liver, heart muscle, and kidneys, but small amounts occur in other tissues, including the brain, skeletal muscle, and leukocytes.

Biochemistry

GLD is a zinc-containing enzyme consisting of six polypeptide chains. The smallest active molecule has an MW of approximately 350,000, but larger polymers are also found. The enzyme catalyzes the removal of hydrogen from L-glutamate to form the corresponding ketimino-acid that undergoes spontaneous hydrolysis to 2-oxoglutarate, as follows:

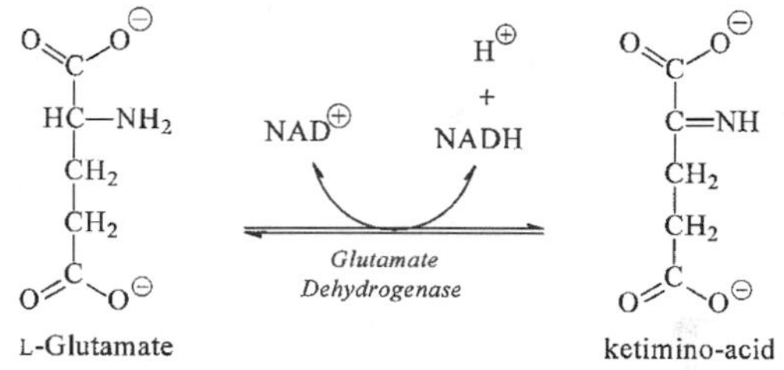

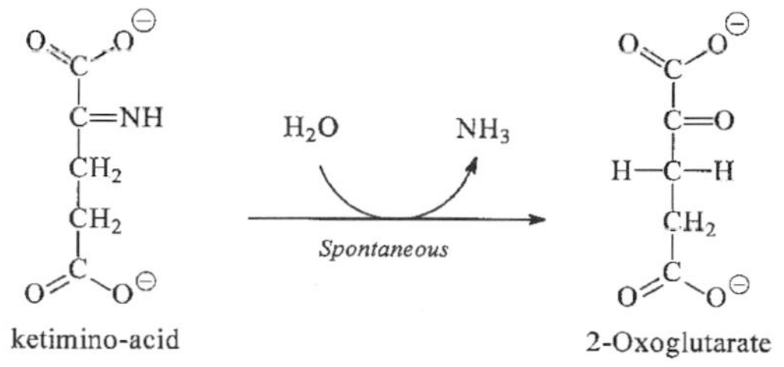

L-Glutamate

ketimino-acid

ketimino-acid

2-Oxoglutarate

Although NAD is the preferred coenzyme, NADP also acts as the hydrogen acceptor. Similarly, specificity for L-glutamate also is not absolute; a number of other amino acids, including L-norvaline and L-2-aminobutyrate, act as substrates. GLD is inhibited by metal ions, such as Ag^+ and Hg^+, by several chelating agents, and by L-thyroxine. ADP activates GLD above pH 7 and also reverses the inhibition caused by thyroxine and diethylstilbestrol.

The GLDs of human tissues may be separated by electrophoresis into several forms, most likely resulting from different polymeric states.

Clinical significance

GLD is present in normal serum in trace amounts only, but increased activities are observed in cases of liver disease in which hepatocellular damage is present. However, the degree of elevation is relatively much less than that of the transaminases. Fourfold or fivefold elevations are listed in cases of chronic hepatitis (similar to those for the transaminases); in cases of cirrhosis, increases are only up to twofold. Very large rises in serum GLD occur in individuals with halothane toxicity, and marked increases also occur in response to some other hepatotoxic agents. Compared with other hepatocellular enzymes, such as the transaminases, increases in the activity of GLD in serum are disproportionately large and may reach 10 to 20 times normal.

GLD potentially offers differential diagnostic utility in the investigation of liver disease, particularly when it is interpreted in conjunction with other enzyme test results. This interpretation often is done by calculation of the transaminase/GLD ratio.

The difficulties in the use of the additional diagnostic information potentially offered by GLD are similar to those discussed in the following section on ICD. Absolute levels of activity in serum are low; precision of assay, particularly the precision of ratios, is difficult to achieve and maintain.

Methods for the determination of glutamate dehydrogenase activity

Continuous-monitoring methods have been developed for the determination of GLD with both the forward and reverse reactions. The equilibrium favors the formation of glutamate, and higher reaction rates are observed when 2-oxoglutarate is used as substrate.

Reference intervals

Reference values up to 3 U/L (women) and 4 U/L (men) have been reported for optimized methods at 25 °C. The upper level is increased to 7.5 U/L when a method optimized at 37 °C is used.

Isocitrate Dehydrogenase

Isocitrate dehydrogenase (EC 1.1.1.42; threo-D_s-isocitrate: NADP oxidoreductase, decarboxylating; ICD) catalyzes the oxidative decarboxylation of isocitrate to 2-oxoglutarate, as follows:

D$_s$-Isocitrate   Oxalosuccinate

Hydrogen Transfer Reaction

Oxalosuccinate   2-Oxoglutarate

Decarboxylation Reaction

The enzyme is substrate specific because only D-isocitrate is acted on by the enzyme. It does not act on L-isocitrate. In addition, it is specific for NADP.

Biochemistry

ICD found in serum originates primarily in the liver, although it is found to some extent in all cells. Genetically distinct cytoplasmic (soluble) and mitochondrial isoenzymes exist. As with other isoenzymes determined by separate gene loci, the isoenzymes of NADP-dependent ICD differ in quantitative catalytic properties and physical properties.

The ICD discussed in this section must be distinguished from the NAD-dependent ICD (EC 1.1.1.41) that participates in the Krebs tricarboxylic acid cycle, a distinct enzyme with quite different properties. NAD-dependent ICD also is located in the mitochondria.

The NADP-dependent enzyme is found in high concentrations not only in the liver but also in heart, skeletal muscle, kidney, and adrenal tissue; platelets; and red blood cells. It has an MW of 64,000 and requires Mn^{2+} as an activator, the ion being essential for the decarboxylation reaction. The concentration that provides optimal activation is in the range of 0.5 to 1.5 mmol/L. Mg^{2+} or Co^{2+} also can activate ICD; however, only 60% to 80% of the activity possible with Mn^{2+} is obtained. The pH range for optimal activity is broad (pH 7.0 to 7.8).

Clinical significance

The main diagnostic use of ICD measurements is in the investigation of hepatobiliary disease, in which ICD is placed in the same category as other enzymes, such as the transaminases, which indicate the leakage of enzymes from damaged or dying cells. In this respect, ICD is perceived to have the advantage of sensitivity in that levels in individuals with hepatocellular disease are increased significantly in relation to the very low levels normally present in serum. However, this large relative increase is offset by the low absolute levels of the enzyme, which are difficult to measure. The high degree of organ specificity of ICD also is considered an advantage, but equivalent specificity can be obtained by combinations of other enzyme tests when an equivocal clinical presentation makes combination necessary.

Methods for the determination of isocitrate dehydrogenase activity

ICD activity has been determined spectrophotometrically through measurement of the increase in NADPH concentration (ΔA_{340}) during the course of the ICD-catalyzed reaction. Various ICD methods differ in the choice of buffer, temperature, and NADP and Mn^{2+} concentration; no "optimized" procedure yet has been developed.

Reference interval

The reference interval for ICD activity in the sera of normal adults is 1.2 to 7.0 U/L at 37 °C. No significant age- or sex-related variations exist, except that levels in newborns may be up to four times adult levels, falling to normal within 2 weeks after birth.

Prostate-Specific Antigen

Prostate-specific antigen (EC 3.4.21.77; semenogelase; PSA) is a 34,000-MW monomeric glycoprotein, a product of a locus on chromosome 19, related to the kallikrein family of proteases. It is a serine protease produced mostly by the epithelial cells lining the acini and ducts of the prostate gland. (The biochemical details, clinical significance, and analytical methodology used to measure PSA will be discussed in detail in Chapter 21.)

References

1. Bais R, Philcox M: Approved recommendation on IFCC methods for the measurement of catalytic concentration of enzymes. Part 8. IFCC method for lactate dehydrogenase (L-lactate: NAD+oxidoreductase, EC 1.1.1.27). International Federation of Clinical Chemistry (IFCC). Eur J Clin Chem Clin Biochem 1994; 32:639-655.

2. Ellis G, Goldberg DM, Spooner RJ et al: Serum enzyme tests in diseases of the liver and biliary tree. Am J Clin Pathol 1978; 70:248-258.

3. Henderson AR: Enzyme tests in cardiovascular disease. In Moss DW, Rosalki SB (eds): Enzyme Tests in Diagnosis, pp 90-135, London, Edward Arnold, 1995.

4. Kanemitsu F, Okigaki T: Characterization of human creatine kinase BB and MB isoforms by means of isoelectric focusing. Clin Chim Acta 1994; 231:1-9.

5. Kaufman RA, Tietz NW: Recent advances in measurement of amylase activity—a comparative study. Clin Chem 1980; 26:846-853.

6. Moss DW, Henderson AR: Clinical enzymology. In Burtis CA, Ashwood ER (eds): Tietz Textbook of Clinical Chemistry, 3rd edition, pp 617-721, Philadelphia, WB Saunders, 1999.

7. Roach BA, Vladutiu AO: Prostatic specific antigen and prostatic acid phosphatase measured by radioimmunoassay in vaginal washings from cases of suspected sexual assault. Clin Chim Acta 1993; 216:199-201.

8. Scandinavian Society for Clinical Chemistry and Clinical Physiology: Recommended methods for the determination of four enzymes in blood. Scand J Clin Lab Invest 1974; 33:291 306.

9. Tietz NW, Astles JR, Shuey DF: Lipase activity measured in serum by a continuous monitoring pH-stat technique—an update. Clin Chem 1989; 35:1688-1693.

Additional Reading

Colowick SP, Kaplan NO: Methods in Enzymology, San Diego, Academic Press [multivolume, multiyear series].

Cornish-Bowden A: Fundamentals of Enzyme Kinetics, Aldershot, United Kingdom, Ashgate Publishing Company, 1995.

CHAPTER 21

Tumor Markers

DANIEL W. CHAN, PhD, DABCC, FACB, and STEWART SELL, MD

Objectives

1. Define the following terms:
Cancer	Proto-oncogene
Tumor marker	Oncogene
Oncofetal antigen	Tumor-suppressor gene
Carbohydrate marker	
2. List and discuss the stages of cancer.
3. State the clinical application of tumor marker analysis and list potential uses of tumor markers.
4. Discuss the clinical relevance of prostate-specific antigen and its use in the detection of prostate cancer.
5. List the hormones and enzymes that are considered tumor markers and the type of cancer each detects.
6. List at least two oncofetal antigens that are considered tumor markers and the type of cancer each detects.
7. List the carbohydrate markers that are considered tumor markers and the type of cancer each detects.
8. Compare and contrast oncogenes and tumor-suppressor genes; list two oncogene markers and two suppressor gene markers.

Key Words

Cancer   A relatively autonomous growth of tissue

Cancer Staging   The process by which cancer is divided into groups of early and late disease; useful for prognosis and helps guide therapy selection

Carbohydrate-Related Tumor Markers   Antigens containing carbohydrate found on the tumor cell surface or secreted by the tumor cells (for example, high-molecular-weight mucins or blood group antigens)

DNA Chip   A thumb-nail-sized chip containing an array of up to 30,000 short DNA sequences; used mostly in research to discover new tumor markers

Ectopic Syndrome   Production of a hormone at a distant site by a nonendocrine cancerous tissue that normally does not produce the hormone (for example, small-cell carcinoma of the lung producing antidiuretic hormone)

Oncofetal Antigens   Proteins produced during fetal life; present in high concentrations in the sera of fetuses; decrease to low levels or disappear after birth; reappear in some cancer patients because certain genes are reactivated in the transformed malignant cells

Oncogene   A gene with a protein product that has the potential to cause a normal cell to become cancerous

Prognosis   The prospect of recovery as anticipated from the usual course of the cancer

Prostate-Specific Antigen (PSA)   A kallikrein-like serine proteinase produced by epithelial cells of both benign and malignant prostate tissue

Tumor Marker   A substance found in an increased amount in the blood, other body fluids, or tissues that may suggest the presence of a type of cancer

Tumor-Suppressor Gene   A gene with a protein product that constrains growth; loss of a tumor-suppressor gene, such as p53, possibly leading to cancer

INTRODUCTION TO TUMOR MARKERS

This chapter begins with an introduction to cancer, followed by a discussion on the definition of tumor markers, classification of these markers, their clinical applications, and methods for their evaluation. The biochemistry, methodology, and clinical applications of specific tumor markers of clinical interest are discussed in detail.

Cancer

In 2000 the estimated number of new U.S. cancer cases was 1.22 million. Breast cancer is the leader, followed by cancer of the prostate, lung, colon-rectum, and bladder.[14]

A simple definition of **cancer** is "a relatively autonomous growth of tissue." Understanding the cause of autonomous growth clearly would facilitate the search for a cure. Advances in molecular genetics have provided a better understanding of the genesis of human cancer. The proliferation of normal cells is thought to be regulated by growth-promoting **oncogenes** and counterbalanced by growth-constraining **tumor-suppressor genes.** The development of cancer appears to involve the activation or altered expression of oncogenes or the loss or inactivation of a tumor-suppressor gene.

Early detection of cancer offers the best chance for cure. The goal is to diagnose cancer when a tumor is still small enough to be removed completely through surgery. Unfortunately, most cancers do not produce symptoms until the tumors are either too large to be removed surgically or cancerous cells already have spread to other tissues (metastasized).

Although other modes of therapy, such as administration of chemical toxins or irradiation, often are effective in the destruction of most tumor cells, they usually are not curative. The few residual viable tumor cells are able to proliferate, develop resistance to further therapy, and eventually kill the individual.

Cancer Staging

Cancer staging is the process by which cancer is divided into groups of early and late cancer. Classification is useful for **prognosis** and helps guide clinicians in selecting therapy and evaluating clinical outcomes. "TNM" is currently the most widely used system to classify cancer, replacing the historical system of I to IV or A to D. This system describes the anatomical extent of disease in the following three components:

T—The extent of the primary tumor
N—The presence or absence and extent of regional lymph node metastasis
M—The presence or absence of distant metastasis

The addition of numbers to these components indicates the extent of the disease (for example, $T_0, T_1, T_2, T_3, T_4; N_0, N_1, N_2, N_3; M_0, M_1$). In general, two classifications—clinical and pathological—are described for each site. For a detailed description of the classification of malignant tumors, readers are referred to additional sources.[23]

Definition of a Tumor Marker

A **tumor marker** is a substance sometimes found in an increased amount in the blood, other body fluids, or tissues that may suggest the presence of a type of cancer. Tumor markers are found in cells, tissues, or body fluids. They are measured qualitatively or quantitatively by chemical, immunological, or molecular biological methods to identify the presence of a cancer.

Morphologically, cancer tissue is recognized as resembling fetal tissue more than normal adult differentiated tissue. Tumors are graded according to their degree of differentiation as being (1) well differentiated, (2) poorly differentiated, or (3) anaplastic (without form). Tumor markers are the biochemical or immunological counterparts of the differentiation state of the tumor. In general, tumor markers represent the reexpression of substances produced normally by embryogenically related tissues (Table 21-1).

An ideal tumor marker should be both specific for a given type of cancer and sensitive enough to detect small tumors for early diagnosis or during screening. Unfortunately, most known tumor markers are neither specific for a single, individual tumor nor sensitive enough for screening. Most are found with different tumors of the same tissue type (tumor-associated markers). They are present in higher quantities in cancer tissue or blood from cancer patients than in benign tumors or in the blood of normal individuals. Tumor markers are most useful in the determination of the progression of disease status after the initial therapy is complete and monitoring of subsequent treatment modalities.

Production of Tumor Markers by Various Tissues

Marker	Normal Producing	Embryogenically Closely Related	Distantly Related	Unrelated
CEA	Colon	Stomach, liver, pancreas	Lung, breast	Lymphoma
AFP	Liver, yolk sac	Colon, stomach, pancreas	Lung	
CG	Placenta	Germinal tumors	Liver	Epidermal lung
Serotonin	Enteroendocrine carcinoid	Adrenal	Oat cell, lung	Epidermal lung

Modified from Sell S: Cancer markers. In Moossa AR, Schempff SC, Robson MC (eds): Comprehensive Textbook of Oncology, 2nd edition, vol 1, pp 225-238, Baltimore, Williams & Wilkins, 1991.
CEA, Carcinoembryonic antigen; *AFP,* α-fetoprotein; *CG,* chorionic gonadotropin.

Historical Development

The first tumor marker was the Bence-Jones protein, which usually indicates the presence of multiple myeloma, a plasma cell malignancy. From 1928 to 1963, hormones, enzymes, isoenzymes, and proteins were demonstrated to be tumor markers. Occasionally, such markers were useful in the diagnosis of individual tumors, but the general application of tumor markers for monitoring of cancer patients did not begin until the discovery of α-fetoprotein (AFP) in 1963 and carcinoembryonic antigen (CEA) in 1965.

The production of such markers during fetal development, as well as in tumors, led to the use of the terms *oncodevelopmental markers* and oncofetal antigens. In 1975 the development of monoclonal antibodies for immunoassay led to the discovery of many oncofetal antigens and antigens derived from tumor cell lines. Examples include the carbohydrate antigens, such as CA 125, CA 15-3, and CA 27.29.

Finally, advances in molecular genetics (by use of nucleic acid probes and monoclonal antibodies) have led to the discovery of oncogenes and suppressor genes. Some of these have proven to be useful tumor markers. Examples include *ras* oncogene, c-*erb* B-2, and p53.

Clinical Applications of Tumor Markers

The potential uses of tumor markers are summarized in Table 21-2. In general, tumor markers are used for diagnosis, prognosis, and monitoring of effects of therapy and as targets for localization and therapy. Ideally a tumor marker should be produced by the tumor cells and detectable in body fluids. It should not be present in healthy individuals or benign conditions. Therefore a tumor marker can be used for cancer screening to find asymptomatic individuals within a general population. Most tumor markers are present in normal, benign, and cancer tissues and are not specific enough for cancer screening. However, if the incidence of cancer is high among certain populations, screening is feasible. An example is the use of AFP in the screening of hepatocellular carcinoma in China and Alaska. **Prostate-specific antigen (PSA)** has been used in conjunction with

Potential Uses of Tumor Markers

Screening in general populations
Differential diagnosis in symptomatic individuals
Clinical staging of cancer
Estimation of tumor value
Prognostic indicator of disease progression
Evaluation of success of treatment
Detection of recurrence of cancer
Monitoring of responses to therapy
Radioimmunolocalization of tumor masses
Determination of direction for immunotherapy

digital rectal examination for early detection of prostate cancer.

The clinical staging of cancer is aided by quantitation of the marker; that is, the serum level of the marker reflects the number of cancer cells present in the body (also known as the *tumor burden*). The marker value at the time of diagnosis is used as a prognostic indicator for disease progression and patient survival. This indication is possible for an individual patient, but different levels of markers produced by different tumors usually do not allow the clinician to determine the prognosis of a tumor from the initial level. However, after successful initial treatment, such as surgery, the marker value should decrease. The rate of the decrease is predicted by the half-life of the marker. For example, the half-life of PSA is 2 to 3 days; that of chorionic gonadotropin (CG), 12 to 20 hours; and that of AFP, 5 days. If the half-life after treatment is longer than the expected half-life, then the treatment has not been successful in removing the tumor. The magnitude of marker reduction may, however, reflect the degree of success of the treatment or the extent of disease involvement.

Detecting cancer recurrence permits early treatment or a change in therapy. Ultrasensitive PSA assays allow earlier detection of prostate cancer after a patient undergoes radical prostatectomy. The breast cancer marker CA 27.29 has been shown to detect recurrent disease before any clinical evidence exists in breast cancer patients receiving adjuvant chemotherapy.

Most tumor marker values correlate with the effectiveness of treatment and responses to therapy. In breast cancer cases the concentration of markers such as CA 549 changes with the treatment and clinical outcome of the patient. Marker values usually increase as the disease progresses, decrease with the onset of remission, and do not change significantly when the disease remains stable. The tumor marker kinetics in the monitoring of cancer may be more complicated. The marker values in response to treatment may show an initial delay before demonstrating the expected pattern of change.

Methods for Evaluation of Tumor Markers

To evaluate the usefulness of a tumor marker, reference values must be established, predictive values calculated, distribution of marker values evaluated, and the role of the values in disease management determined. In addition, new technologies, such as DNA chips, are being developed to enhance testing for tumor markers.

Reference values

Reference values of a tumor marker are obtained from a healthy population, preferably with age- and sex-matched individuals. The determination of reference values is time consuming and requires a large healthy population ($n \geq 120$ subjects). Statistical analysis using the mean ± 2 standard deviation (SD) for a population with a Gaussian (normal) distribution is the most frequently used method. For a non-Gaussian distribution the percentile method is probably the simplest approach (see Chapter 14).

The reference values determined in this fashion that use healthy individuals are applicable to analytes with physiologically well-defined concentrations. For testing with relatively specific applications, such as the use of tumor markers in the diagnosis and management of cancer, a decision level is more appropriate than the upper limit of the healthy population. In most cases, use of benign individuals as the nondisease group is more appropriate than healthy individuals. The decision level can be determined by use of a predictive value model.

Predictive value model

The predictive value model uses sensitivity, specificity, and the prevalence of disease. By varying the decision level, sensitivity and specificity change in opposite directions. An optimal decision level is selected based on the importance of disease detection, the ability to treat it, and the cost and pain associated with the testing and treatment.

A useful approach in the evaluation of multiple tests for the same analyte or multiple markers for the same type of cancer is the receiver operating characteristic (ROC) curve. The ROC curve is constructed through a plot of sensitivity versus 1 − specificity. The advantage of the ROC curve is the display of performance over the entire range of decision

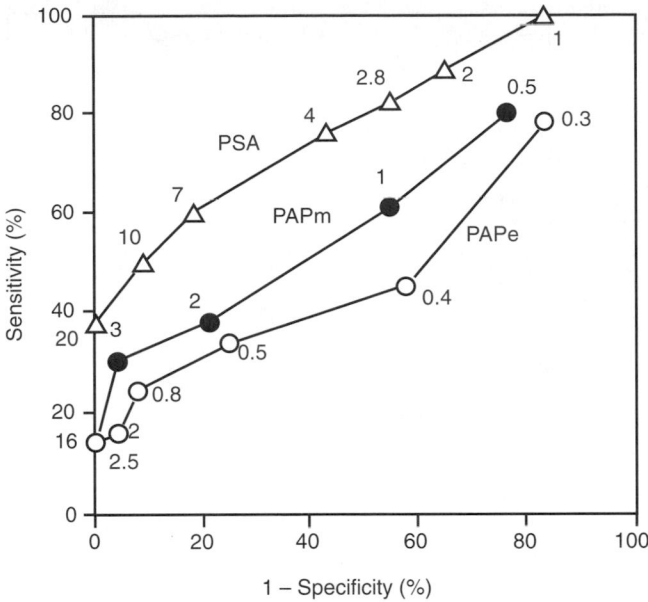

Figure 21-1   Receiver operating characteristic (ROC) curves for PSA, PAPm, PAPe. The data for all 128 subjects with prostate disease are plotted, with several quantitative decision levels (as indicated on the curve) for each assay. Units are in μg/L for PAPm and PSA, and in U/L for PAPe. *PSA,* Prostate-specific antigen; *PAPm,* prostatic acid phosphatase by monoclonal immunoassay; *PAPe,* enzymatic prostatic phosphatase. (Modified from Rock RC, Chan DW, Bruzek DJ et al: Evaluation of a monoclonal immunoradiometric assay for prostate-specific antigen. Clin Chem 1987; 33:2257-2261.)

levels. The decision level can be pinpointed where the optimal sensitivity and specificity are achieved. By superimposing of the ROC curves of several markers, the most predictive marker can be selected. Figures 21-1 and 21-2 both are examples.

Distribution of marker values

Application of the predictive value model is difficult for analytes that are not diagnostic for a single disease. Levels of most, if not all, tumor markers are elevated in more than one disease condition. When the predictive value model is used, selection of a population that includes groups with and without disease is necessary. Which individuals should be included in these two groups? The decision should be based on the specific clinical questions asked. If the question concerns the predictive value of CEA for active colorectal carcinoma, the disease group should include only those individuals with active colorectal carcinoma. Selection of the nondisease group is more challenging. Should healthy individuals and those with benign conditions be included? If so, how many benign condition groups should be included? Should those in remission be included as well because they do not have active diseases? The values calculated for sensitivity and specificity greatly depend on the types of groups included and the number of individuals in each group.

The distribution of tumor marker values usually is shown as the percentage of individuals with elevated values as de-

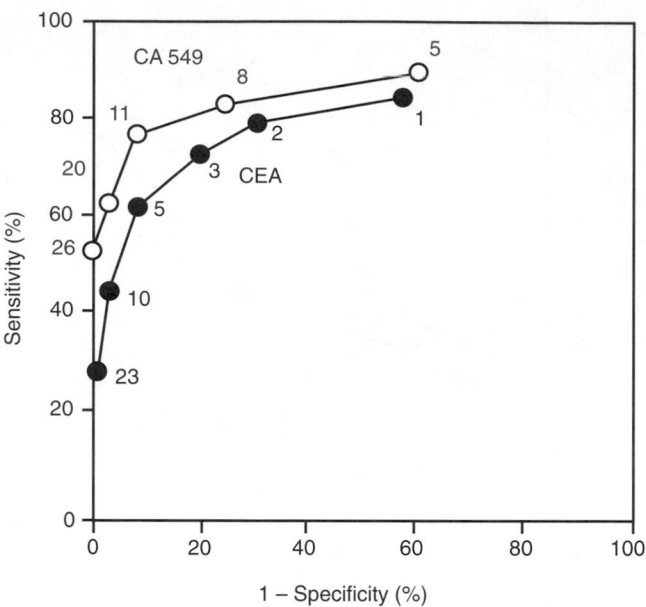

Figure 21-2   Receiver operating characteristic (ROC) curve for CA 549 (kU/L) and CEA (μg/L). The sensitivity and specificity at the decision level of CA 549 = 11 kU/L are 76.6% and 91.9%. The sensitivity and specificity at the decision level of CEA = 5 μg/L are 61.4% and 91.5%. The data include patients with breast cancer and benign breast diseases (331 for CA 549, and 322 for CEA). The decision values for CA 549 *(white circles)* and CEA *(black circles)* are indicated on the curve. *CA 549,* Carbohydrate antigen 549; *CEA,* carcinoembryonic antigen. (Modified from Chan DW, Beveridge RA, Bruzek DJ et al: Monitoring breast cancer with CA 549. Clin Chem 1988; 34:2000-2004.)

termined with various cutoff values in the healthy, benign, and cancerous groups. International staging criteria should be used to classify cancer patients. Diagnosis should be based on pathological findings. The groups are selected from past experiences of similar markers. With breast cancer, for example (Table 21-3), normal women are used as the healthy population for comparison. The nonmalignant or benign groups are selected to include those women with the most likely causes of marker elevation—benign liver and breast diseases and pregnancy. The nonbreast metastatic cancer groups are selected to show the specificity of the marker in endometrial, colon, lung, prostate, and ovarian carcinoma.

Grouping all breast cancer patients into a single category is not satisfactory because most markers are elevated in those with active breast cancer. The adjuvant group consists of women who presented with metastasis, underwent mastectomy and treatment with adjuvant chemotherapy, and have no evidence of disease. The adjuvant group should not have elevated marker values. The metastasis group includes women in complete remission, partial remission, or with progressive breast cancer accompanied by local or distant metastases. The progressive breast cancer group should have the highest percentage of elevated marker values; the partial remission group should have an intermediate per-

centage of elevated marker values. The complete remission group should have the lowest percentage of elevated marker values.

Disease management

Most tumor markers are used to monitor treatment and progression of cancer. The selection of subject groups is important to illustrate the usefulness of the marker in various clinical settings. Markers are used to determine the success of the initial treatment (for example, surgery or radiation), detect the recurrence of cancer, and monitor the effectiveness of the treatment modality. To determine the success of surgery, an elevated marker level before surgery should fall after a successful operation. The extent of the decrease in the marker value depends on the pretreatment tumor involvement.

If the cancer recurs after a successful initial treatment, the marker value may not fall within the normal half-life. It may fall to a steady level that is higher than normal, or it may fall within the reference interval of healthy individuals. A subsequent rise in the marker value suggests recurrence of the cancer. An example of monitoring in breast cancer is shown in Figure 21-3.

To monitor the effectiveness of cancer therapy, the marker value should increase as the cancer progresses, decrease as the cancer regresses, and remain unchanged if the disease remains stable. In the evaluation of candidate markers, all the events related to the progression, stability, and regression of disease are grouped; whether the marker value changes in the predicted direction in all these situations is evaluated next.[11]

The Working Group on Tumor Marker Criteria of the International Society for Oncodevelopmental Biology and Medicine has published the following criteria for the interpretation of changes in tumor marker values[1]:

If no therapy is given, at least a linear increase in three consecutive samples (i.e., two time intervals) on a log scale should be registered to establish a recurrence. Usual intervals could be three months but are clinically determined. After a first increase, next samples should be taken after 2-4 weeks, irrespective of the absolute level.

If therapy is initiated, the changes in marker values should reflect the clinical progression of the disease:

Progressive disease is defined by an increase in the marker level of at least 25%. Sampling should be repeated within 2-4 weeks for additional evidence . . . The sampling interval during therapy may depend on the type of tumor and should be related to clinical follow-up.

A decrease in marker value of at least 50% is indicative of partial remission:

. . . with the concept that tumor load is related to the changes in serum tumor marker levels.

TABLE 21-3 Distribution of CA 549 Values

Diagnosis	Number of Patients	Number (and %) of Individuals with CA 549 Values (kU/L)					
		0 to 8	>8	>11	>15	>20	>25
Normal Women	100	85 (85)	15 (15)	5 (5)	0 (0)	0 (0)	0 (0)
Nonmalignant							
Benign liver	42	19 (45)	23 (55)	11 (26)	3 (7)	0 (0)	0 (0)
Benign breast	69	63 (91)	6 (9)	1 (1)	1 (1)	0 (0)	0 (0)
Pregnancy	30	26 (87)	4 (13)	0 (0)	0 (0)	0 (0)	0 (0)
Nonbreast Metastatic Cancer							
Endometrial	8	7 (88)	1 (12)	1 (12)	1 (12)	1 (12)	0 (0)
Colon	41	25 (61)	16 (39)	7 (17)	3 (7)	1 (2)	1 (2)
Lung	40	22 (55)	18 (45)	13 (33)	11 (28)	6 (15)	6 (15)
Prostate	30	13 (43)	17 (57)	12 (40)	5 (17)	5 (17)	3 (10)
Ovarian	60	22 (37)	38 (63)	30 (50)	21 (35)	15 (25)	10 (17)
Breast Cancer							
Adjuvant	88	61 (69)	27 (31)	10 (11)	6 (9)	4 (5)	0 (0)
Metastatic							
Complete remission	16	11 (69)	5 (31)	3 (19)	1 (6)	1 (6)	1 (6)
Partial remission	52	12 (23)	40 (77)	33 (63)	27 (52)	22 (42)	16 (31)
No response (progressive)							
Local	12	5 (42)	7 (58)	5 (42)	3 (25)	2 (17)	2 (17)
Metastasis	94	7 (7)	87 (93)	83 (88)	79 (84)	73 (78)	69 (73)

From Chan DW, Beveridge RA, Bruzek DJ et al: Monitoring breast cancer with CA 549. Clin Chem 1988; 34:2000-2004.

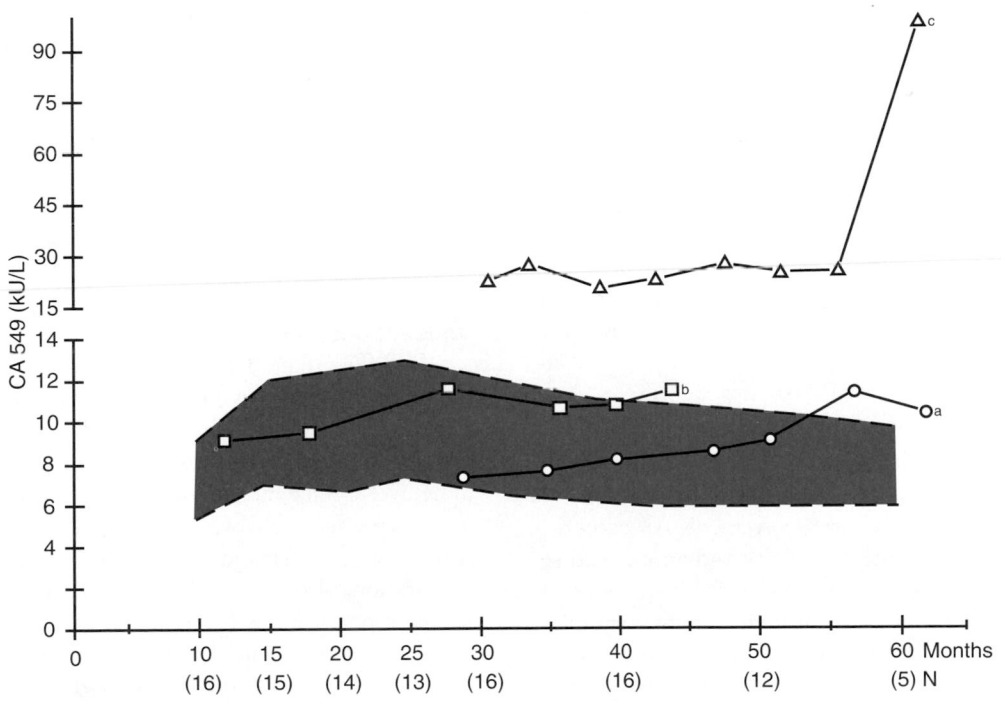

Figure 21-3   Example of use of a tumor marker to monitor disease progression. The blue area is the mean ±2 standard deviation of CA 549 values from 16 patients with breast cancer in the adjuvant group. Thus they demonstrated no metastasis, underwent mastectomy and treatment with adjuvant chemotherapy, and showed no evidence of disease during the 60 months of testing. Patient *a (circles)* may have cancer recurrence. Patient *b (squares)* is stable without recurrence. Patient *c*, however, *(triangles)* shows clear evidence of recurrence at 63 months. (Modified from Chan DW, Beveridge RA, Bruzek DJ et al: Monitoring breast cancer with CA 549. Clin Chem 1988; 34:2000-2004.)

The Working Group also provided a general opinion that:

> . . . a complete remission cannot be determined by marker levels, but if tumor marker levels are elevated, the clinical decision of complete remission based on conventional methods should be considered incorrect unless an explanation for the presence of the elevated level is given.

DNA chips

New methods are being developed that permit screening of a large number of genetic differences between cancer and normal tissue, or among types of cancer. One method compares the expression of messenger RNA (mRNA) from cancer tissue with other cancers or to germline cells.[13] DNA sequences from both ends of expressed gene fragments (that is, expressed sequence tags, or ESTs) are spotted mechanically onto a glass slide. More than 30,000 ESTs can be arrayed on a thumbnail-sized glass chip. These **DNA chips** thus allow the determination of different expressed mRNAs. For example, a red-labeled complementary DNA (cDNA) can be produced from mRNA extracted from cancer tissue. Likewise, a green-labeled cDNA can be produced from mRNA extracted from normal tissue. The labeled cDNAs are mixed and incubated on a DNA chip. The degree of different mRNA expression is determined by color comparison. Red indicates mRNA specific for tumor, green indicates mRNA specific for normal tissue, and yellow indicates mRNA produced by both tumor and normal tissue. When fully developed, DNA chips will allow for the discovery of many new tumor markers.

■ SPECIFIC TUMOR MARKERS

As discussed previously, tumor markers include enzymes, hormones, oncofetal antigens, carbohydrate markers, blood group antigens, proteins, receptors, or genes. Specific tumor markers from each of these groups are described in the following section.

Enzymes

With few exceptions an increase in an enzyme or isoenzyme is not specific or sensitive enough to be used to identify a type of cancer or specific organ involvement. An exception is PSA. PSA has mild protease activity and amino acid sequence homology with serine protease of the kallikrein family. It is expressed exclusively by normal, benign, hyperplastic, and cancerous prostate glands but not by other tissues. Until the application of PSA as a marker for prostate cancer, tumor enzymes had lost most of their popularity for use as cancer markers. Enzymes were used historically as tumor markers before the discovery of oncofetal antigens and the advent of monoclonal antibodies. The abnormalities of enzymes as markers for cancer are either the expression of the fetal form of the enzyme (isozyme) or the ectopic production of enzymes.

Enzymes are present in much higher concentrations inside cells and are released into the systemic circulation as the result of tumor necrosis or a change in the membrane permeability of the cancer cells. Increased enzyme levels also are observed in the blockage of pancreatic or biliary ducts and in renal insufficiency cases. The intracellular location of the enzyme affects the rate of the release. By the time enzymes are released into the systemic circulation, the metastasis of tumors may have occurred. Most enzymes are not unique for a specific organ; therefore enzymes are most suitable as nonspecific tumor markers. Elevated enzyme levels may signal the presence of malignancy.

Isoenzymes and multiple forms of enzymes sometimes provide additional organ specificity. Table 21-4 summarizes various enzymes, their associated types of malignancy, and the assays used to measure their activity or mass concentrations (radioimmunoassay [RIA] or immunometric assay). Enzymes traditionally are measured by their activities. With the introduction of antibody techniques, some enzymes, such as PSA, are measured as protein antigens rather than by their enzyme activity (see Chapter 20).

Alkaline phosphatase

Alkaline phosphatase (ALP) is present in practically all tissues of the body, with the liver, bone, and placenta being especially rich in this enzyme. The ALP in the sera of normal adults comes primarily from the liver or biliary tract. Elevated levels of ALP are present in individuals with primary or secondary liver cancer. Its level may be helpful in the evaluation of metastatic cancer with bone or liver involvement. Greatest elevations are seen in individuals with osteoblastic lesions, such as in cases of prostate cancer with bone metastases. Minimal elevations are seen in individuals with osteolytic lesions, such as breast cancer with bone metastases. In liver metastases the serum ALP level shows a better correlation with the extent of liver involvement than do those of other liver tests.

To differentiate the origin of elevated ALP levels, tests of other liver enzymes are performed, such as that for 5′-nucleotidase or γ-glutamyltransferase. Determination of ALP isoenzymes sometimes provides additional specificity. The liver isoenzyme is more stable thermally than the bone isoenzyme (see Chapter 20). Other malignancies, such as leukemia, sarcoma, and lymphoma complicated with hepatic infiltration, also may show elevated ALP levels. Placental alkaline phosphatase (PALP) is synthesized by the trophoblast and elevated in the sera of pregnant women. PALP first was identified as the Regan isoenzyme in 1968 by Fishman and recognized as one of the first oncodevelopmental markers, along with AFP and CEA. It is elevated in individuals with a variety of malignancies, including ovarian, lung, trophoblastic, and gastrointestinal cancers; seminoma; and Hodgkin's disease.

TABLE 21-4 Enzymes as Tumor Markers

Enzyme	Assay	Type of Cancer
Alcohol dehydrogenase	Activity	Liver
Aldolase	Activity	Liver
Alkaline phosphatase	Activity	Bone, liver, leukemia, sarcoma
Alkaline phosphatase, placental	Activity	Ovarian, lung, trophoblastic, gastrointestinal, seminoma, Hodgkin's disease
Amylase	Activity	Pancreatic, various
Aryl sulfatase B	Activity	Colon, breast
Creatine kinase-BB	Activity	Prostate, lung (small cell), breast, colon, ovarian
Esterase	Activity	Breast
Galactosyltransferase	Activity	Colon, bladder, gastrointestinal, various
γ-Glutamyltransferase	Activity	Liver
Hexokinase	Activity	Liver
Lactate dehydrogenase	Activity	Liver, lymphomas, leukemia, various
Leucine aminopeptidase	Activity	Pancreatic, liver
Neuron-specific enolase	RIA	Lung (small cell), neuroblastoma, carcinoid, melanoma, pheochromocytoma, pancreatic
5'-Nucleotidase	Activity	Liver
Prostate-specific antigen	IA	Prostate
Prostatic acid phosphatase	Activity/IA	Prostate
Pyruvate kinase	Activity	Liver, various
Ribonuclease	Activity	Various (ovarian, lung, large bowel)
Sialyltransferase	Activity	Breast, colon, lung
Terminal deoxytransferase	Activity	Leukemia
Thymidine kinase	RIA/Activity	Various, leukemia, lymphomas, lung (small cell)

IA, Immunoassay; *RIA,* radioimmunoassay.

Creatine kinase

Creatine kinase (CK) catalyzes the phosphorylation of creatine by adenosine triphosphate (ATP). CK is a dimer consisting of two subunits—M (muscle) and B (brain). Three isoenzymes—CK-1 (BB), CK-2 (MB), and CK-3 (MM)—exist. CK-1 is present in the brain, prostate gland, gastrointestinal tract, lung, bladder, uterus, and placenta. Cardiac muscle has the highest concentration of CK-2 (~20%). CK-3 is present in skeletal and cardiac muscles. Elevated levels of CK-1 have been demonstrated in individuals with prostate cancer and small-cell carcinoma of the lung. Although it is also elevated in other malignancies, such as those of the breast, colon, ovary, and stomach, the clinical usefulness of CK-1 as a tumor marker requires further investigation.

Lactate dehydrogenase

Lactate dehydrogenase (LD), an enzyme in the glycolytic pathway, is released as the result of cell damage. The elevation of LD in cases of malignancy is rather nonspecific. It has been demonstrated in a variety of cancers, including liver; non-Hodgkin's lymphoma; acute leukemia; nonseminomatous germ-cell testicular cancer; seminoma, neuroblastoma; and other carcinomas, such as breast, colon, stomach, and lung cancer. The serum LD level has been shown to correlate with tumor mass in solid tumors and provides a prognostic indicator for disease progression. Its value in the monitoring of therapy is rather limited. The isoenzymes provide only marginal specificity for organ involvement. For example, the elevation of the LD-5 isoenzyme is associated with liver metastases. The elevation of LD-5 in the spinal fluid may be an early indication of central nervous system metastases.

Neuron-specific enolase

Enolase is a glycolytic enzyme also known as *phosphopyruvate hydratase.* Neuron-specific enolase (NSE) is the form of enolase found in neuronal tissue and in the cells of the diffuse neuroendocrine system, the amine precursor uptake and decarboxylation (APUD) tissues. NSE is found in tumors associated with a neuroendocrine origin, including small-cell lung cancer (SCLC), neuroblastoma, pheochromocytoma, carcinoid, medullary carcinoma of the thyroid, melanoma, and pancreatic endocrine tumors. Serum NSE level is measured by RIA. The upper reference limit is 12.5 μg/L. In individuals with SCLC the sensitivity is reportedly 80%. The specificity is at least 80% to 90%. The NSE level appears to correlate with stages and provides a useful prognosis for disease progression. The value of NSE in detection of disease relapse has not been proven. Although the findings are mixed, NSE also appears to be useful in monitoring of chemotherapy, with increasing levels correlating with disease states. The immunostaining of NSE also may provide differential diagnosis among SCLC and other histological carcinoma types. Among children with advanced neuroblastoma, more than 90% have been reported to have elevated serum levels of NSE. High levels of NSE are associated with poor prognosis. The levels seem to correlate with the stage of the disease. Monitoring therapy with serum NSE is controversial, particularly with respect to the issue of specificity. However, elevated levels of NSE in children with stage IV neuroblastoma were associated with a poorer outcome.

Prostatic acid phosphatase

Acid phosphatases are a group of enzymes that hydrolyze phosphate esters with optimum pH of less than 7.0. They are present in the lysozymes of the secretory epithelial cells. Although acid phosphatase is produced primarily by the prostate gland (prostatic acid phosphatase, or PAP), it is also found in erythrocytes, platelets, leukocytes, bone marrow, bone, liver, spleen, kidney, and intestine (see Chapter 20). PAP was measured initially by its enzymatic activity and later by RIA. Elevated serum PAP is present in several malignant conditions, such as osteogenic sarcoma, multiple myeloma, and bone metastases of other cancers. It also may be elevated in some benign conditions, such as benign prostatic hyperplasia (BPH), osteoporosis, and hyperparathyroidism. The clinical use of PAP has been replaced by PSA.

Prostate-specific antigen

PSA has proven to be an extremely useful tumor marker. Prostate cancer is the leading cancer in older men. When detected early (organ confined), prostate cancer potentially is curable by radical prostatectomy. Therefore early detection is important. The role of PSA in prostate cancer has been reviewed by Chan and Sokoll.[3]

Biochemistry

PSA is a single-chain glycoprotein that is 7% carbohydrate. It has 237 amino acid residues and four carbohydrate side chains with linkages at amino acid 45 (asparagine), 69 (serine), 70 (threonine), and 71 (serine). The N-terminal amino acid is isoleucine, and the C-terminal residue is proline. Its molecular mass is 28.43 kD, and it has isoelectric points from 6.8 to 7.2 because of its various isoforms. The three-dimensional structure and antigenic domain of PSA have been characterized. The complete gene encoding PSA has been sequenced and located on chromosome 19. It is similar to the kallikrein-1 gene with 82% homology. Functionally, PSA is a serine protease of the kallikrein family. It is produced exclusively by the epithelial cells of the acini and ducts of the prostate gland. PSA is secreted into the lumina of the prostatic duct. In the seminal fluid, PSA cleaves a seminal vesicle-specific protein into several low–molecular-weight (MW) proteins. This action is part of the process of liquefaction of the seminal coagulum. Therefore PSA possesses chymotrypsin-like and trypsin-like activity.

Molecular forms of prostate-specific antigen

PSA exists in two major forms in blood circulation. The majority of PSA is complexed with protease inhibitor α_1-antichymotrypsin (ACT) (100 kD) or with α_2-macroglobulin (A2M) and a minor component of free PSA (28.43 kD). Most immunoassays measure both free and ACT-complexed PSA but not A2M-PSA.[15] In human seminal fluid, PSA can be fractionated into five isoforms. PSA-A and PSA-B are active, intact enzymes capable of forming a complex with ACT. PSA-C, PSA-D, and PSA-E are nicked forms with disulfide bonds cleaved; they possess low or no enzyme activity.[22]

The metabolic clearance rate of PSA follows a two-compartment model, with initial half-lives of 1.2 and 0.75 hours for free PSA and total PSA and subsequent half-lives of 22 and 33 hours.[16] Because of this relatively long half-life, 2 to 3 weeks may be necessary for the serum PSA to return to baseline levels after certain procedures, including transrectal biopsy, transrectal ultrasonography, transurethral resection of the prostate, and radical prostatectomy. Prostatitis and acute urinary retention also can elevate PSA concentration. Although the digital rectal examination has no clinically important effects on serum PSA levels in most individuals, in some it may lead to a twofold elevation. Serum PSA levels appear to possess significant physiological variation (up to 30%). Serum PSA has been reported to decrease by 18% after the patient has been hospitalized for 24 hours. Collecting serum samples from ambulatory individuals is a good practice.

Methods

Immunoassays, available commercially, are used to measure PSA. Most of them use nonisotopic labels, such as enzyme, fluorescence, or chemiluminescence. The majority of these assays are automated on an immunoassay system. Different assays and even the same assay with different lots of reagent may produce different results. The reasons for such differences are due to changes in assay calibration, production lot variation, assay reaction time, reagent matrices, assay sensitivity, and imprecision. Antibodies react with different PSA epitopes; therefore some antibodies react dissimilarly with the various molecular forms of PSA. Assays are classified as *equimolar* if they bind to free and complexed PSA equally and *nonequimolar* if they bind to free or complexed differently. The World Health Organization and the International Federation of Clinical Chemistry have developed two international preparations to facilitate the effort to standardize PSA assays—100% free PSA (code 96/686) and 90% PSA-ACT complex and 10% free PSA (code 96/700).

Clinical applications

PSA is an extremely useful tumor marker for prostate cancer. It is used to detect, stage, and monitor treatment of prostate cancer.

Early detection of prostate cancer. PSA testing by itself is not effective in the screening or detection of early prostate cancer because PSA is specific for prostate tissue but not for prostate cancer. BPH is a common disease in men 50 years of age and older. Studies have shown that the PSA values in individuals with BPH are similar yet statistically different than those associated with early prostate cancer (that is, those of individuals with organ-confined cancer). The use of serum PSA together with digital rectal examination is recommended.

The clinical sensitivity of PSA is 78% at a cutoff value of 4.0 μg/L. As the cut-off value is lowered to 2.8 μg/L, sensitivity increases to 92%, whereas specificity decreases from 33% to 23%. Raising the cutoff value to 8 μg/L improves the specificity to 90%. Through ROC analysis (see Figure 23-1), PSA is a better predictor than PAP for the diagnosis of prostate cancer.

To improve the ability of PSA testing to detect early prostate cancer, several approaches have been suggested. One approach is to use age-adjusted reference intervals: 0 to 2.5 μg/L for men ages 40 to 49 years, 0 to 3.5 μg/L for those 50 to 59 years, 0 to 4.5 μg/L for those 60 to 69 years, and 0 to 6.5 μg/L for those 70 to 79 years. By lowering the upper limit of the reference interval, more cancer is detected in younger men for whom potential cure by radical prostatectomy is most beneficial. Another approach is to use PSA density (that is, divide PSA concentration by the prostate volume determined by transrectal ultrasonography). Men with PSA levels between 4 and 10 μg/L, a negative digital rectal examination result, and elevated PSA density have increased risk for prostate cancer. The third approach is use of PSA velocity (that is, the rate of PSA increase as a function of time). By establishing a baseline level of PSA in each individual, the rate of increase of PSA is calculated. The increase of PSA in healthy men, those with BPH, and those with prostate cancer appears to be different, with the highest rate (>0.75 μg/L/y) observed in individuals with prostate cancer.[16] The specificity improves to 90% for those with BPH, whereas sensitivity is 72% for men with prostate cancer. A 1996 study of free PSA velocity demonstrated that percent free PSA is the earliest serum marker for prediction of subsequent diagnosis of prostate cancer.[16] The fourth approach is the use of a neural network that uses multiple factors, including PSA, PAP, and CK isoenzymes, to derive an index. The sensitivity of the index is about 80%, and specificity is about 90%.[20] Finally, the percent free PSA can be used to improve the sensitivity and specificity in prostate cancer detection, particularly for individuals in the diagnostic "gray" zone of PSA between 4 and 10 μg/L or 2 and 20 μg/L.[2]

Staging of prostate cancer. PSA correlates with clinical stages A to D2 of prostate cancer. Higher PSA levels and higher percentages of individuals with elevated PSA concentrations are associated with advanced stages of the disease. However, PSA testing is not sufficiently reliable to determine stages on an individual basis. PSA also correlates with pathological stages of tumor extension and metastases. Advanced pathological stages are associated with higher PSA levels in the serum. Individuals with organ-confined disease seldom have PSA levels greater than 50 μg/L, suggesting that those with these elevated levels are most likely to have extracapsular tumor extension. Because significant overlap occurs in PSA values among stages, PSA cannot be used to determine the pathological stage in a given individual. Therefore PSA by itself should not be used to decide whether an individual has prostate cancer confined to the organ and therefore is a likely candidate for radical prostatectomy. The level of PSA can serve as a guide and is more useful in evaluating the presence of metastases. Individuals with PSA levels less than 20 μg/L rarely have bone metastases. Studies have shown that PSA could replace the radionuclide bone scan in individuals with newly diagnosed, untreated prostate cancer who have low serum PSA concentrations (<10 μg/L) and whose symptoms do not relate to the skeletal system.

Monitoring of treatment. The greatest clinical use of PSA is in the monitoring of definitive treatment of prostate cancer. This treatment includes radical prostatectomy, radiation therapy, and antiandrogen therapy. The surgery removes all prostate tissue. Because PSA is produced exclusively by the prostate tissue, after radical prostatectomy the PSA level should fall below the detection limit of the assay. This drop may require 2 to 3 weeks because of the 2- to 3-day half-life of PSA. If the half-life is longer than normal, a residual tumor is assumed to be present.

PSA levels should be measured every 3 months during the first year after surgery, every 4 months in the second year, and every 6 months thereafter. The clinical threshold of an elevated PSA varies with each institution and ranges from 0.1 to 0.3 μg/L. The test's analytical sensitivity and biological variation of serum PSA affect the clinical threshold. In any case an increasing PSA level after radical prostatectomy is a strong indication of disease recurrence. The time between PSA concentration elevation and clinical recurrence is between 1 and 5 years.

The role of PSA in the monitoring of patients after definitive radiation therapy is less well defined, compared with after radical prostatectomy. The majority of patients show an initial decrease of PSA level after radiation therapy. After 1 year half of the patients demonstrate increasing PSA levels. Most of these individuals have positive prostate biopsy results and develop metastatic disease.

Antiandrogen therapy includes bilateral orchiectomy and treatment with luteinizing hormone-releasing hormone analogue, diethylstilbestrol, and flutamide. PSA testing is useful for prognosis prediction and monitoring of treatment response to this type of therapy in individuals with stage D2 prostate cancer. The level of PSA is inversely proportional to the survival time and increases with cancer progression, decreases in remission, and remains unchanged in stable disease states. PSA could replace the radionuclide bone scan for monitoring of individuals with advanced disease. Androgen deprivation therapy may have a direct effect on the PSA level that is independent of the antitumor effect. The production of PSA may be under the influence of hormones such as dihydrotestosterone. Thus the PSA levels in patients who receive antiandrogen therapy may have a different meaning than they do in those receiving other types of therapies.

Hormones

The production of hormones in cancer involves two separate routes. First, the endocrine tissue that normally produces the hormone can produce excess amounts. Second, a hormone may be produced at a distant site by a nonendocrine tissue that normally does not produce the hormone. The latter condition is called **ectopic syndrome.** For example, the production of adrenocorticotropic hormone (ACTH) normally is produced by the pituitary and ectopically produced by the small cell of the lung. Consequently, elevation of a given hormone is not diagnostic of a specific tumor because a particular hormone may be produced by a variety of cancers.

APUDoma is a group of embryologically related tumors of endocrine organs. The acronym *APUD* refers to **a**mine **p**recursor **u**ptake and **d**ecarboxylase. APUD cells have properties of both neural and endocrine tissues. These tissues synthesize a number of polypeptide hormones, such as ACTH, calcitonin, gastrin, glucagon, insulin, melanocyte-stimulating hormone, secretin, and vasoactive intestinal polypeptide. Increasing frequency of hormone production correlates with the degree of embryological relationship of the cancer origin to other tissues in the APUD system. Several hormones that are used as tumor markers are listed in Table 21-5. Three of these hormones (ACTH, calcitonin, and CG) are discussed in more detail in the following sections.

TABLE 21-5	Hormones as Tumor Markers
Hormone	Type of Cancer
ACTH	Cushing's syndrome, lung (small cell)
Antidiuretic hormone	Lung (small cell), adrenal cortex, pancreatic, duodenal
Bombesin	Lung (small cell)
Calcitonin	Medullary thyroid
Gastrin	Glugagonoma
Growth hormone	Pituitary adenoma, renal, lung
CG	Embryonal, choriocarcinoma, testicular (nonseminomas)
Human placental lactogen	Trophoblastic, gonads, lung, breast
Neurophysins	Lung (small cell)
Parathyroid hormone	Liver, renal, breast, lung, various
Prolactin	Pituitary adenoma, renal, lung
Vasoactive intestinal peptide	Pancreas, bronchogenic, pheochromocytoma, neuroblastoma

ACTH, Adrenocorticotropic hormone; *CG,* chorionic gonadotropin.

Adrenocorticotropic hormone

ACTH is a polypeptide hormone with 39 amino acids and a molecular mass of 4.5 kD that is produced by the corticotropic cells of the anterior pituitary gland. In 1928, Brown described a patient with small-cell carcinoma of the lung who had the signs and symptoms of what is now known as cortisol excess. A small number of these carcinomas can produce pro-ACTH, the precursor to ACTH. This precursor has a molecular mass of 22 kD, a 5% bioactivity, and most of the immunoactivity of ACTH. Traditional RIA measures both the precursor and the hormone. One immunometric assay in use is specific for ACTH.

Elevated serum levels of ACTH could be the result of pituitary or ectopic production. A high level of ACTH (>200 ng/L) is suggestive of ectopic origin. Failure of the dexamethasone suppression test also indicates ectopic production. About half of the ectopic production of ACTH is a result of small-cell carcinoma of the lung. Other conditions that elevate ACTH levels have been reported, including pancreatic, breast, gastric, and colon cancer and benign conditions, such as chronic obstructive pulmonary disease, mental depression, obesity, hypertension, diabetes mellitus, and stress. The value of ACTH in the monitoring of therapy is still unclear.

Calcitonin

Calcitonin is a polypeptide with 32 amino acids and a molecular mass of about 3.4 kD. The C cells of the thyroid produce this hormone. Normally, calcitonin is secreted in response to increased serum calcium. It inhibits the release of calcium from bone and thus lowers the serum calcium level. The serum half-life is about 12 minutes. The level in healthy individuals is less than 0.1 μg/L. An elevated level usually is associated with medullary carcinoma of the thyroid.

Calcitonin is most useful in the detection of familial medullary carcinoma of the thyroid, an autosomal dominant disorder. Asymptomatic family members of the affected individuals benefit from screening with computed tomography because basal levels are increased in such populations. Provocative testing with intravenous administration of calcium and pentagastrin also produces increased calcitonin levels. Microscopic or occult malignancy has been detected in individuals with negative radioisotopic scans and normal thyroid glands on physical examination.

Increased levels of calcitonin appear to correlate with such indicators of extent of disease as tumor volume and tumor involvement in local and distant metastases. Calcitonin is useful for monitoring of treatment and detection of disease recurrence. Calcitonin levels also are elevated in some individuals with carcinoid, and cancer of the lung, breast, kidney, or liver. The usefulness of calcitonin as a tumor marker in these malignancies has not been proven. Calcitonin elevation has been reported in other nonmalignant conditions, such as pulmonary disease, pancreatitis, hyperparathyroidism, pernicious anemia, Paget's disease of bone, and pregnancy.

Chorionic gonadotropin

CG is a useful tumor marker for tumors of the placenta (trophoblastic tumors) and some tumors of the testes. It is also useful for diagnosing and monitoring of pregnancy (see Chapter 43). Although the terms *human chorionic gonadotropin* and *hCG* have been used extensively, the preferred terms are *chorionic gonadotropin* and *CG*.

CG is a glycoprotein secreted by the syncytiotrophoblastic cells of the normal placenta. CG consists of two dissimilar α- and β-subunits. The α-subunit is common to several other hormones, including luteinizing hormone (LH), follicle-stimulating hormone (FSH), and thyroid-stimulating hormone (TSH). The β-subunit is unique to CG, and the 28 to 30 amino acids that compose the carboxyl terminal are antigenically distinct. CG has a molecular mass of 45 kD. The upper reference limit in men and nonpregnant women is 5.0 IU/L.

Elevated CG levels are seen in pregnant women and individuals with trophoblastic diseases and germ-cell tumors. The highest level of CG (>1 million IU/L) is present in individuals with trophoblastic tumors. Moderate elevations occur in those with germ-cell tumors, mainly nonseminomatous testicular carcinoma.

The production of subunits of CG is under separate genetic control. In early pregnancy the free β-subunit is produced together with intact (a whole molecule of) CG; in late pregnancy the free α-subunit predominates. Differential production of the subunits has been observed in individuals with cancer. However, the number of individuals who produce only the free subunit is very small. Most individuals with cancer produce both free β-subunits and intact molecules.

In studies the measurement of serum CG improved significantly with the use of an antibody to the β-subunit of CG that had little cross-reactivity with other glycoprotein hormones, LH, FSH, and TSH. Currently, most CG assays use an immunometric assay ("sandwich") format. The CG assay measures the intact (whole) molecule when an antibody for the α-subunit and an antibody for the β-subunit are used in the immunometric format. This type of assay does not measure free α- or β-subunits because free subunits cannot form a sandwich with both antibodies. The total CGβ assay measures both the intact CG and free β-subunits. A total CGβ assay may be preferred as a tumor marker because cancer patients produce significant amounts of free β-subunit. None of the commercially available CG assays have been approved by the Food and Drug Administration (FDA) for use as a tumor marker assay.

CG is elevated in nearly all individuals with trophoblastic tumors, in 70% of those with nonseminomatous testicular tumors, and less frequently in those with seminoma. Lower percentages of elevation have been reported in cases of melanoma and carcinoma of the breast, gastrointestinal tract, lung, and ovary and in benign conditions, such as cirrhosis, duodenal ulcer, and inflammatory bowel disease. CG helps identify individuals with trophoblastic tumors and, together with AFP, detect nonseminomatous testicular tumors. Increasing levels of CG correlate with the tumor volume and disease prognosis. The presence of CG in seminoma may indicate the presence of choriocarcinoma. Because CG does not cross the blood-brain barrier, the normal cerebrospinal fluid-to-serum (CSF-to-serum) ratio is 1:60. Higher levels in CSF may indicate metastases to the brain. Furthermore, monitoring of the CSF CG level may indicate the response to therapy for patients with central nervous system metastases.

CG is most useful in monitoring of the treatment and progression of trophoblastic disease. Increasing levels of CG correlate with tumor volume. An individual with an initial CG level of more than 400,000 IU/L is considered at high risk for treatment failure. After surgical removal of the tumor, CG level is expected to decline. The normal half-life of serum CG is about 12 to 20 hours. Slowly decreasing or persistent levels of CG may indicate the presence of residual disease. During chemotherapy, weekly CG measurement is recommended. After remission is achieved, yearly CG measurement is recommended to detect relapse. The detection limit of the assay is important because any residual CG activity may indicate the presence of tumor. Specificity for β-subunit of CG is also a factor because low levels of cross-reactivity with LH or FSH can cause false-positive results.

Oncofetal Antigens

Oncofetal antigens are proteins produced during fetal life. These proteins are present in high concentrations in the sera of fetuses and decrease to low levels or disappear after birth. These proteins reappear in individuals with cancer. The production of oncofetal antigens demonstrates that certain genes are reactivated as the result of the malignant transformation of cells. Several oncofetal antigens, in addition to AFP and CEA, are listed in Table 21-6. Serum AFP and CEA usually are determined by immunometric assay with automated immunoassay systems.

Alpha-fetoprotein

AFP is a marker for hepatocellular and germ-cell (nonseminoma) carcinoma. AFP is a glycoprotein with a molecular mass of 70 kD. It consists of a single polypeptide chain and is 4% carbohydrate. AFP is synthesized in large quantities during embryonic development by the fetal yolk sac and liver. It is one of the major proteins in the fetal circulation, but its maximum concentration is about 10% that of albumin. AFP is related closely both genetically and structurally to albumin, having extensive homologies in amino acid sequence. The genes coding for both proteins have been localized to chromosome 4q. As albumin synthesis increases

TABLE 21-6 Oncofetal Antigens as Tumor Markers

Name	Nature	Type of Cancer
AFP	Glycoprotein, 70 kD, 4% carbohydrate	Hepatocellular, germ cell (nonseminoma)
β-Oncofetal antigen	80 kD	Colon
Carcinofetal ferritin	Glycoprotein, 600 kD	Liver
CEA	Glycoprotein, 22 kD, 50% carbohydrate	Colorectal, gastrointestinal, pancreatic, lung, breast
Pancreatic oncofetal	Glycoprotein, 40 kD	Pancreatic
Squamous cell antigen	Glycoprotein, 44 to 48 kD	Cervical, lung, skin, head and neck (squamous)
Tennessee antigen	Glycoprotein, 100 kD	Colon, gastrointestinal, bladder
Tissue polypeptide antigen	Cytokeratins 8, 18, 19	Various (breast, colorectal, ovarian, bladder)

AFP, α-Fetoprotein; *CEA*, carcinoembryonic antigen.

during the later stages of fetal development, AFP concentrations in fetal serum begin to decline. They finally reach the trace concentrations found in normal adults 18 months after birth.

For tumor-derived AFP the composition of carbohydrate on AFP depends on the activity of saccharide transferase in the tumor cells. Differences in carbohydrate side chains on AFP may be determined by the binding of AFP to lectins, such as concanavalin A (Con A) and lens culinaris (LCA). Molecular variants of AFP are separated into liver and the yolk-sac types; they differ from each other in their carbohydrate moiety. The yolk sac type of AFP contains an additional sugar, N-acetylglycosamine, linked to the β-mannose; this sugar blocks the Con A binding site on the AFP. Therefore the yolk-sac type of AFP shows a high percentage (50% to 70%) of Con A nonreactive (CNR) fraction, whereas the liver type, which lacks this additional sugar, shows a low CNR fraction (10% to 20%). LCA binds to the fucosylated form of the first core N-acetylglucose that is present in both liver and yolk-sac types of tumor-derived AFP but not in AFP generated by benign liver diseases.

In healthy adults the serum AFP level is less than 10 μg/L.[11] During pregnancy, maternal AFP levels increase from 12 weeks of gestation to a peak of about 300 μg/L during the third trimester. The fetal AFP reaches a peak of 2 g/L at 14 weeks and then declines to about 70 mg/L at term. (The use of AFP to detect fetuses with neural tube defects will be discussed in Chapter 43.) In addition to pregnancy, elevated levels of serum AFP also are associated with noncancerous liver diseases, such as hepatitis and cirrhosis. About 95% of individuals with these diseases have AFP levels lower than 200 μg/L.

Except in the pregnant woman, AFP levels greater than 1000 μg/L indicate cancer. At these levels of AFP, about half of hepatocellular carcinomas may be detected. However, because the serum level of AFP correlates with the size of the tumor, detection of hepatocellular carcinoma is more useful at the earlier stages, when the tumor is small enough to be resectable (<5 cm) than when the tumor is large. To detect small tumors, the cutoff level for AFP must be set at a much lower level than either 200 or 1000 μg/L. A cutoff

point of 10 to 20 μg/L has been recommended, but at this level, hepatitis and cirrhosis must be considered as possible causes of elevation.

Screening for hepatocellular carcinoma has been attempted in high-incidence areas, such as Africa, China, Taiwan, Japan, and Alaska. Initial large-scale screening in China using less sensitive techniques (for example, agglutination and immunodiffusion, which have cutoff values of 400 to 1000 μg/L) was able to detect significant numbers of new cases of this type of cancer. More sensitive immunoassay methods (10 to 20 μg/L) and ultrasonography have been used in Taiwan and Japan with better success in detection of hepatocellular carcinoma at earlier stages.

AFP also is useful to determine prognosis and monitor therapy for hepatocellular carcinoma.[11] The level of AFP is a prognostic indicator of survival. Elevated AFP levels (>10 μg/L), as well as serum bilirubin levels greater than 2 mg/dL, are associated with shorter survival times.

AFP level helps monitor therapy and changes in clinical status. Elevated AFP levels after surgery may indicate incomplete removal of the tumor or the presence of metastasis. Falling or rising AFP levels after therapy may determine the success or failure of the treatment regimen. Individuals considered free of metastatic tumor and who have significant increases in AFP levels may be developing metastasis.

Combined use of AFP and CG is useful in classification and staging of germ-cell tumors. Germ-cell tumors may be predominantly of one cell type or a mixture of seminoma, yolk-sac, choriocarcinomatous elements (embryonal carcinoma), or teratoma. AFP is elevated in individuals with yolk-sac tumors, whereas CG is elevated in those with choriocarcinoma. Both are elevated in cases of embryonal carcinoma. In those with seminomas, AFP is not elevated, whereas CG is elevated in 10% to 30% of individuals who have syncytiotrophoblastic cells in the tumor. Neither marker is elevated in cases of teratoma. One or both markers are elevated in about 90% of individuals with nonseminomatous testicular tumor. Elevations have been found in fewer than 20% of those with stage I disease, 50% to 80% with stage II disease, and 90% to 100% with stage III disease.

Increasing serum levels of these markers correlate with tumor volume and the prognosis of disease.

The combined use of both markers also is useful in monitoring of individuals with germ-cell tumors; elevation of either marker indicates recurrence of disease or development of metastasis. The success of chemotherapy is assessed by calculation of the decrease of the levels of both markers through the use of the half-lives of AFP (5 days) and CG (12 to 20 hours).

Carcinoembryonic antigen

CEA is a marker for colorectal, gastrointestinal, lung, and breast carcinoma. Gold and Freeman discovered CEA in 1965. Rabbits were immunized with extracts of human colonic cancer tissue, and the resultant antisera were absorbed with extracts of normal human colon. Some antisera reacted with the tumor extracts but not with the extracts of normal tissue. The antigen, which also was found in embryonic tissue, was named *carcinoembryonic antigen.*

CEA consists of a large family of related cell-surface glycoproteins. About 10 genes located on chromosome 19 encode the CEA proteins. Up to 36 different glycoproteins have been identified in the CEA family. The major proteins are the CEA and nonspecific cross-reacting antigen (NCA) 50. The domain structure of CEA, NCA 50, and the γ-heavy chain of the immunoglobulin IgG are very similar. Thus CEA is part of the immunoglobulin gene "superfamily."

CEA is a glycoprotein with a molecular mass of 150 to 300 kD; it contains 45% to 55% carbohydrate. It is a single polypeptide chain consisting of 641 amino acids, with lysine in the N-terminal position. The heterogeneity of CEA has been demonstrated through use of isoelectric focusing electrophoresis to separate the variants.

In the healthy population the upper limit of CEA is about 3 μg/L for nonsmokers and 5 μg/L for smokers. Because the level of CEA measured is method dependent, values should always be compared with values obtained with the same method. When methods are changed, all individuals being monitored should be tested in parallel with both the old and the new methods. CEA levels are elevated in some individuals with benign conditions, such as cirrhosis (45%), pulmonary emphysema (30%), rectal polyps (5%), benign breast disease (15%), and ulcerative colitis (15%).

CEA levels are elevated in individuals with a variety of cancers, such as colorectal (70%), lung (45%), gastric (50%), breast (40%), pancreatic (55%), ovarian (25%), and uterine (40%) carcinoma. Because of the elevations associated with benign disease (that is, false-positive results) and number of tumors that do not produce CEA (that is, false-negative results), CEA testing is not recommended for screening.

CEA testing may be useful as an adjunct to clinical staging. Persistently elevated levels that are 5 to 10 times the upper reference limit strongly suggest the presence of colon cancer but may be associated with other cancers. With colon cancer, CEA levels correlate with the stage of the disease. CEA level is elevated in 28% of individuals with Duke's stage A colorectal cancer and in 45% of those with stage B. The pretreatment CEA level is prognostic of the development of metastasis with a high level of CEA associated with a greater likelihood that metastasis will develop. Evidence suggests that CEA is a cellular adhesion molecule that may enhance invasion and metastasis.

After successful initial therapy, CEA levels decline. During remission, CEA levels are stable. Rising CEA values may indicate recurrence of disease. The lead time from CEA elevation to clinical recurrence is about 5 months. A repeat laparotomy can be performed to confirm the relapse, which is detected in 90% of cases. In the monitoring of metastatic colon cancer, CEA is useful to follow patients throughout therapy and the clinical course of the disease. For breast cancer, CEA is being replaced by other, more specific markers, such as CA 15-3. With lung cancer, CEA determination is helpful in diagnosis of non–small-cell lung carcinoma (>65% of individuals with elevated CEA) and monitoring of lung cancer.

Carbohydrate Markers

Carbohydrate-related tumor markers either are antigens on the tumor cell surface or secreted by the tumor cells.[8,10] Monoclonal antibodies have been developed against these antigens. These markers represent a new generation of clinically useful tumor markers. They tend to be more specific than naturally secreted markers, such as enzymes and hormones. Carbohydrate markers are high-molecular-weight mucins (Table 21-7) or blood group antigens (Table 21-8). They usually are abbreviated *CA* for carbohydrate antigen.

CA 15-3, CA 549, and CA 27.29 assays detect a high-MW glycoprotein mucin, known as *episialin,* which is produced by the mammary epithelium of the breast. The circulating episialin antigen is a heterogeneous molecule. CA 15-3, CA 549, and CA 27.29 assays detect similar, yet different epitopes on the surface of episialin molecules. Thus some differences are seen in the results of these tests, but all three are useful as markers for breast carcinoma.

CA 15-3

CA 15-3 is detected through use of two antibodies. The first is a murine monoclonal antibody (MAb) DF3 produced against a membrane-enriched extract of a human breast cancer metastatic to liver. The second monoclonal antibody, 115D8, was developed against human milk fat globule membrane. The circulating DF3-reactive antigen is a heterogeneous molecule with a molecular mass of 300 to 450 kD. The gene for this molecule is located on chromosome 1q. The DF3 antibody recognizes a repeating sequence of 20 amino acids within a peptide core. The recognition of the epitope is affected by glycation.[9]

TABLE 21-7　Carbohydrate Markers: Mucin Type

Name	Antigen and Source	Antibody	Type of Cancer
CA 125	Glycoprotein, 200 kD, OVCA 433	OC 125	Ovarian, endometrial
Episialin			
CA 15-3	Glycoprotein, 400 kD, membrane-enriched breast cancer extract	DF3 and 115D8	Breast, ovarian
CA 549	High-MW glycoprotein	BC4E549, BC4N154	Breast, ovarian
CA 27.29	High-MW glycoprotein	B27.29	Breast
MCA	350-kD glycoprotein	b-12	Breast, ovarian
DU-PAN-2	Mucin, 1000-kD peptide epitope	DU-PAN-2	Pancreatic, ovarian, gastrointestinal, lung

CA, Carbohydrate antigen; *MW,* molecular weight.

TABLE 21-8　Carbohydrate Markers: Blood Group Antigen Type

Name	Antigen and Source	Antibody	Type of Cancer
CA 19-9	Sialylated Le^{xa}, SW-1116 colon CA	19-9	Pancreatic, gastrointestinal, hepatic
CA 19-5	Le^a and sialylated Le^{ag}	19-5	Gastrointestinal, pancreatic, ovarian
CA 50	Sialylated Le^a and afucosyl form	C50	Pancreatic, gastrointestinal, colon
CA 72-4	Sialylated Tn	B27.3, cc49	Ovarian, breast, gastrointestinal, colon
CA 242	Sialylated carbohydrate	C242	Gastrointestinal, pancreatic

CA, Carbohydrate antigen.

In healthy subjects the upper limit of CA 15-3 concentration is 25 kU/L (1 kU/L = 1000 U/L). At this level, 5.5% of 1050 normal subjects, 23% of those with primary breast cancer, and 69% of those with metastatic breast cancer show elevated CA 15-3 levels.[9] Elevated CA 15-3 levels also are found in individuals with other malignancies, including pancreatic (80%), lung (71%), breast (69%), ovarian (64%), colorectal (63%), and liver (28%) cancer. In addition, CA 15-3 is elevated in individuals with benign diseases, although with less frequency (for example, benign liver [42%] and benign breast diseases [16%]).

CA 15-3 should not be used to diagnose primary breast cancer because the incidence of elevation (23%) is fairly low. CA 15-3 is most useful in monitoring of therapy and disease progression in metastatic breast cancer patients. A significant change must be at least 25% and correlates with disease progression in 90% of patients, with its regression in 78%. No change correlates with disease stability in 60%. CA 15-3 could replace CEA in metastatic breast cancer because of its sensitivity and specificity.

CA 549

CA 549 is an acidic glycoprotein with an isoelectric point of pH 5.2. By sodium dodecyl sulfate/polyacrylamide gel electrophoresis under reducing conditions, CA 549 is separated into two species with molecular masses of 400 and 512 kD. Immunizing mice with partially purified membrane preparations from T$_4$17 human breast tumor cell line produced a monoclonal IgG$_1$ antibody termed *BC4E549.* The other antibody, *BC4N154* (a murine IgM), was developed against human milk fat globule membranes.

The CA 549 assay is an immunometric assay. The BC4E 549 antibody is labeled with ^{125}I, and the BC4N154 is attached covalently to polystyrene beads. The first incubation allows binding of CA 549 to BC4N154 antibodies on the beads. After washings and aspirations the tracer antibody, BC4E549, is added.

In a population of healthy women, 95% have CA 549 values below 11 kU/L. Pregnancy and benign breast disease show minimal elevation. Some individuals with benign liver disease show a slight elevation (see Table 21-3). CA 549 is elevated in individuals with a variety of nonbreast metastatic carcinomas, including ovarian (50%), prostate (40%), and lung (33%) carcinomas.

Similar to CA 15-3, CA 549 is not useful in detecting early breast carcinoma because the proportion of individuals with elevated CA 549 levels is low. When ROC analysis is used, CA 549 is better than CEA at identifying active breast cancer (see Figure 21-2). CA 549 is useful in detecting recurrence of breast cancer in patients after initial therapy and followed by adjuvant therapy. An increasing CA 549 value after an initial decrease or stabilization indicates the development of metastases (see Figure 21-3). In the monitoring of advanced breast cancer patients, CA 549 correlates with disease progression and regression and helps detect metastases.[4]

CA 27.29

CA 27.29 is detected by a monoclonal antibody, B27.29, that is produced against an antigen in ascites of individuals with metastatic breast carcinoma. The minimum epitope to which B27.29 reacts is an 8-amino acid sequence within the 20-amino acid tandem repeating sequence of the mucin core. The reactive sequence of the B27.29 overlaps with the sequence of DF3 used in the CA 15-3 assay. In inhibition studies that use labeled MAb, B27.29 effectively competes with DF3 for binding to both CA 27.29 and CA 15-3 antigens.

CA 27.29 is measured through use of a solid-phase competitive RIA. A prediluted sample is added to a polystyrene tube coated with B27.29 antigen and incubated with the ^{125}I-labeled murine antibody for B27.29. A calibration curve is constructed with five calibrators that vary from 0 to 200 kU/L.

CA 27.29 has been approved by the FDA for clinical use in the detection of recurrent breast cancer in individuals with stage II or stage III disease. In a multicenter study over 2 years monitoring 166 breast cancer subjects, 26 of them developed recurrent disease. When two consecutive CA 27.29 antigen test results above 37.7 kU/L (99th percentile) were considered positive, the CA 27.29 assay had a sensitivity of 57.7%, specificity of 97.9%, positive predictive value of 83.3%, and negative predictive value of 92.6% for the detection of recurrent breast cancer. The performance appeared to be better than that of CA 15-3 in detection of recurrent breast cancer.[5] In a group of individuals with metastatic breast cancer, CA 27.29 and CA 15-3 performed similar clinically.

CA 125

CA 125 is a marker for ovarian and endometrial carcinomas.[11] CA 125 is a high–molecular-mass (>200 kD) glycoprotein recognized by the monoclonal antibody OC 125. It contains 24% carbohydrate and is expressed by epithelial ovarian tumors and other pathological and normal tissues of mullerian duct origin. Its physiological function is unknown.

MAb OC 125 was developed through use of a cell line (OVCA 433) from a patient with a serous papillary cystadenocarcinoma of the ovary. The OC 125 clone was selected for its reactivity with the OVCA 433 cell line and its lack of reactivity with a B-lymphocyte line from the same patient. An immunoradiometric assay for CA 125 has been approved by the FDA for the quantitative measurement of CA 125 in serum of women with primary epithelial invasive ovarian cancer.

In a healthy population the upper limit of CA 125 is 35 kU/L. CA 125 is elevated in individuals with nonovarian carcinoma, including endometrial, pancreatic, lung, breast, and colorectal and other gastrointestinal tumors. CA 125 is useful for determination of the prognosis of endometrial carcinoma. It also is elevated in women in the follicular phase of the menstrual cycle and in those with benign conditions, such as cirrhosis, hepatitis, endometriosis, pericarditis, and early pregnancy. CA 125 may help evaluate the disease status in women with advanced endometriosis but is not useful in screening for ovarian cancer in asymptomatic populations. CA 125 cannot be used to differentiate ovarian cancer from other malignancies.

In ovarian carcinoma, CA 125 is elevated in 50% of individuals with stage I disease, 90% with stage II, and more than 90% with stages III and IV. Increasing levels of CA 125 correlate with tumor size and staging. CA 125 also helps differentiate benign from malignant disease in women with palpable ovarian masses. This differentiation is important because surgical intervention for malignant ovarian masses is far more extensive than that for benign masses. In one study, 100 patients underwent diagnostic laparotomy for palpable lower abdominal masses; of these, 23 were found to have malignancies. With 35 kU/L as the cut-off value, the predictive values for malignant disease were 78% sensitivity, 95% specificity, 82% positive predictive value, and 91% negative predictive value. Tumor differentiation does not affect the CA 125 level.

A preoperative CA 125 level of less than 65 kU/L is associated with a significantly greater 5-year survival rate (42%) than is a level greater than 65 kU/L (5%). Postoperative CA 125 levels and the rate of decline also help predict survival. The half-life of CA 125 is normally 4.8 days. In one study a group of patients with a CA 125 half-life of 22 days responded poorly to chemotherapy, compared with another group with a CA 125 half life of 9 days.

CA 125 helps detect residual diseases in cancer patients after initial therapy. The sensitivity of CA 125 to detect tumors before repeat laparotomy is 50%, and the specificity is 96%. After chemotherapy, the CA 125 level provides an indication of disease prognosis. A factor of 10 decrease in the CA 125 level after the first cycle of chemotherapy can indicate improvement. Persistent elevation of CA 125 levels after three cycles of chemotherapy indicates a poor prognosis.

In the detection of recurrent metastasis, use of CA 125 level as an indicator is about 75% accurate. The lead time from CA 125 elevation to clinically detectable recurrence is about 3 to 4 months. Increasing levels of CA 125 correlate with disease progression or regression in 80% to 90% of cases.

Blood Group Antigens

Blood group carbohydrates identified by monoclonal antibodies that have been used as markers of cancers are listed in Table 21-8. These include CA 19-9 (sialylated Le^{xa}), CA 50 (sialylated Le^{x-1}, afucosyl forms), CA 72-4 (sialyl Tn), and CA 242 (sialylated carbohydrate coexpressed with CA 50).

TABLE 21-9	Proteins as Tumor Markers	
Name	Nature	Type of Cancer
β_2-Microglobulin	11 kD	Multiple myeloma, B-cell lymphoma, chronic lympho-cytic leukemia, Waldenström's macroglobulinemia
C-peptide	3.6 kD	Insulinoma
Ferritin	450 kD iron-binding protein	Liver, lung, breast, leukemia
Immunoglobulin	160 to 900 kD, 3% to 12% carbohydrate	Multiple myeloma, lymphomas
Melanoma-associated antigen	90 to 240 kD	Melanoma
Pancreas-associated antigen	100 kD, 20% carbohydrate	Pancreatic, stomach
Pregnancy-specific protein 1	10 kD, 30% carbohydrate	Trophoblastic, germ cell
Prothrombin precursor	Des-r-carboxy prothrombin	Hepatocellular
Tumor-associated trypsin inhibitor	6-kD polypeptide	Lung, gastrointestinal, ovarian

CA 19-9

CA 19-9 is a marker for both colorectal and pancreatic carcinoma. This carbohydrate antigen is a glycolipid, specifically, sialylated lacto-N-fucopenteose II ganglioside, which is a sialylated derivative of the Le^a blood group antigen and is denoted as Le^{xa}. The expression of the antigen requires the Lewis gene product, 1,4-fucosyl transferase. CA 19-9 is synthesized by normal human pancreatic and biliary ductular cells and by gastric, colonic, endometrial, and salivary epithelia. In serum, it exists as a mucin, a high–molecular-mass (200 to 1000 kD) glycoprotein complex. Individuals who are genotypically Le^{a-b-} (about 5%) do not express CA 19-9. A monoclonal antibody against CA 19-9 from a human colon carcinoma cell line, SW-1116 has been developed.

An immunoradiometric assay is available that uses the CA 19-9 antibody both as the capture and the signal antibody. A calibration curve extends from 0 to 120 kU/L. The upper reference limit is 37 kU/L. Of 1500 healthy blood bank donors tested, 99% had CA 19-9 values below this limit. Elevated levels (>37 kU/L) were seen in subjects with pancreatic (80%), hepatobiliary (67%), gastric (40% to 50%), hepatocellular (30% to 50%), colorectal (30%), and breast (15%) cancer. Some individuals (10% to 20%) with pancreatitis and other benign gastrointestinal diseases have elevated levels up to 120 kU/L. CA 19-9 levels correlate with pancreatic cancer staging. With the cutoff of 37 kU/L, 67% of individuals with resectable and 87% of those with unresectable pancreatic cancer have elevated values. By raising the cutoff to 1000 kU/L, 35% of individuals with unresectable tumors and only 5% of those with resectable tumors have elevated CA 19-9 values. CA 19-9 is useful in monitoring of pancreatic and colorectal cancer. Elevated levels can indicate recurrence 1 to 7 months before a recurrence is detected by radiographs or clinical findings. Unfortunately, early detection of relapse may not be useful because of the lack of effective therapy for pancreatic cancer.

CA 72-4

CA 72-4 is a marker for carcinomas of the gastrointestinal tract and ovary. B72.3 is a monoclonal antibody developed from the membrane-enriched fraction of breast carcinoma in an individual with liver metastasis. The B72.3 reactive antigen was purified and called *TAG-72* (tumor-associated glycoprotein). Further purification of TAG-72 from LS-174T human colon carcinoma xenograft produced a new generation of monoclonal antibodies with higher affinity. These antibodies, denoted *cc* for *colon carcinoma*, were used in subsequent studies.

CA 72-4 is measured with an immunoradiometric assay. It uses two monoclonal antibodies that were developed at the National Cancer Institute. B72.3 is the conjugate, whereas cc49 is the capture antibody.

A cutoff of 6 kU/L is used in the CA 72-4 assay. The following percentages of elevation were observed: in healthy subjects, 3.5%; in those with benign gastrointestinal diseases, 6.7%; in those with gastrointestinal carcinoma, 40%; in those with lung cancer, 36%; and in those with ovarian cancer, 24%. A poor clinical correlation between CEA and CA 72-4 levels was found in individuals with gastric cancer. CEA and CA 72-4 values may be complementary. The plasma clearance of TAG-72 was studied by measurement of serial TAG-72 values in subjects with primary carcinoma of the breast, as well as gastric, colorectal, and ovarian cancer. After removal of the tumor, the average time required for the level to decrease to 4 kU/L was 23.3 days. This time suggests that TAG-72 may be useful in detection of residual tumor in such cancer patients.

Proteins

Several proteins have been proposed as tumor markers (Table 21-9). Included in this group are proteins that are not enzymes or hormones and are not high in carbohydrate content. Additional research is required to assess the clinical usefulness of most such markers.

Immunoglobulin

Monoclonal immunoglobulin has been used as marker for multiple myeloma for more than 100 years. Monoclonal paraproteins (also known as myeloma components [MCs]) appear as sharp bands in the globulin area of the serum elec-

TABLE 21-10   Other Tumor Markers

Name	Nature	Type of Cancer
Estrogen and progesterone receptors	(Tissue)	Breast
Catecholamine metabolites	(Urine) VMA, HVA, metanephrines	Neuroblastoma, pheochromocytoma
Hydroxyproline	(Urine)	Bone metastasis (breast), multiple myeloma
Lipid-associated sialic acid	Sialic acid bound to lipid	Gastrointestinal, lung, rheumatoid
Polyamine	(CSF)	Brain
	(Urine)	Various

VMA, Vanillylmandelic acid; *HVA,* homovanillic acid; *CSF,* cerebrospinal fluid.

trophoretic patterns. More than 95% of individuals with multiple myeloma demonstrate this electrophoretic pattern. Appearance of nonmalignant monoclonal immunoglobulins increases with age, reaching 5% in individuals older than 75 years of age. These nonmalignant monoclonal bands usually are lower in concentration than malignant bands and not associated with Bence-Jones protein. Bence-Jones protein is a free monoclonal immunoglobulin light chain in the urine. The level of monoclonal immunoglobulin at the time of initial diagnosis is a prognostic indicator of disease progression. During treatment the serum concentration of urinary Bence-Jones protein may reflect the success of therapy. Lower levels are associated with more favorable outcomes (see Chapter 19).

NMP22

An enzyme immunoassay (EIA) for the measurement of a nuclear matrix protein, NMP22, called *nuclear mitotic apparatus protein* in urine sample, has been approved by the U.S. FDA for the management of patients with transitional cell carcinoma (TCC) of the urinary tract. Nuclear matrix proteins make up the internal structure of the nucleus. Their function has been associated with regulation of key reactions in the nucleus, such as DNA replication and RNA synthesis. The NMPs released by the cancer cell are different from the normal cell. Furthermore, different cell types may have different NMPs. Soluble NMPs are detected in the sera of individuals with cancer in higher concentrations than in the sera of those without cancer. In a multicenter follow-up study (125 cystoscopies) of 90 subjects with 33 pathologically confirmed TCCs, 70% of the 33 recurrences had NMP levels of more than 10 U/mL. Of those with NMP levels of less than 10 U/mL, 86% had no malignancy at subsequent cystoscopy.[19]

Bladder tumor-associated antigen

A qualitative test for bladder tumor-associated (BTA) antigen in urine has been developed. BTA antigens are high-MW polypeptides composed of complexes of basement membrane proteins. The presence of BTA in urine is thought to involve either invasion of the basement membrane by tumor, production by the tumor itself, or a combination of these, which may be linked with the body's im-

mune response. If BTA antigens are present in significant levels, they combine with latex particles to produce an agglutination reaction, which produces a visible color change on the BTA test strip. A multicenter trial compared the BTA test to voided urine cytology studies in 499 patients undergoing surveillance cystoscopy for recurrent bladder cancer. The BTA test identified 40% of patients with positive cystoscopy results, whereas cytology detected 17%. A positive test may encourage a higher degree of suspicion for recurrence.[17]

Receptors and Other Markers

Other tumor markers—including catecholamines, polyamines, lipid-associated sialic acid, and receptors—have been used clinically with various degrees of success (Table 21-10). Receptors are probably the most successful of this group of markers. (The catecholamines and their metabolites will be discussed in Chapter 27.)

Estrogen and progesterone receptors

Estrogen and progesterone receptors are used in breast cancer assessments as indicators for hormonal therapy. Patients with positive estrogen and progesterone receptors tend to respond to hormonal treatment. Those with negative receptors are treated with other therapies, such as chemotherapy. Hormone receptors also serve as prognostic factors in breast cancer. Patients with positive receptors in the tumor population are treated with hormones. These patients tend to survive longer than those with negative receptors. For additional information, the reader should consult a review on the clinical significance and assay of estrogen and progesterone receptors.[21]

Biochemistry

The first step in steroid hormone action is the binding of the hormone to specific cell receptors. An estrogen receptor is a specific cellular protein with high affinity and great specificity for estrogen. The estrogen-receptor protein is found in target tissue cells, such as in the uterus, pituitary gland, hypothalamus, and breast. Because estrogen stimulates biochemical processes in target cells that normally contain estrogen-receptor protein, a reduction in blood estrogen levels is expected to reduce the biochemical activity of these cells. This is the accepted rationale for use of endocrine therapy in women with breast carcinoma.

Methods

Although various methods have been used to estimate steroid hormone receptors, including centrifugation analysis, chromatographic methods, and titration Scatchard-plot assays, only two currently are used—EIAs and immunocytochemical assays. The College of American Pathologists offers a proficiency survey for external evaluation of hormone receptor methods (Survey Set HR).

Enzyme immunoassays. The classic methods employed techniques that measured the binding of steroids to the receptors. The availability of monoclonal antibodies against estrogen- and progesterone-receptor proteins led to the development of receptor assays based on direct antigenic recognition rather than on steroid-binding activity. Currently, solid-phase EIAs are available commercially to measure both estrogen and progesterone receptors in tissue cytosols. These assays are based on the use of two monoclonal antibodies directed to different portions of the purified receptor so that the receptor protein is "sandwiched" between the antibodies. In comparison with the classic assays, EIAs are preferred. Not only do they cost less, but from a technical point of view they also are simpler, require less time, and are performed in less tissue. Specimens with values greater than 15 fmol/mg of cytosol protein are considered positive for estrogen and progesterone receptors.

Immunocytochemical assays. Monoclonal antibodies also are used to detect steroid receptor proteins in frozen tissue sections, paraffin-imbedded tissues, fine-needle aspirates, and malignant effusions with immunocytochemical techniques. These methods make it possible to evaluate very small lesions when adequate tissue is not available to perform the EIA method or tissues have been fixed or imbedded. In these procedures the primary monoclonal antibody is incubated with a thin section of tissue mounted on a microscope slide. Localization and visualization of receptor material subsequently are accomplished by an indirect immunoperoxidase technique. Specimens with nuclear staining in at least 20% of malignant cells usually are considered receptor positive. Immunocytochemical assays are not influenced by the presence of estrogens, antiestrogens, or steroid-binding proteins. In addition, immunocytochemical methods make possible the study of receptor content specifically in malignant cells.

Clinical application

Cytoplasmic estrogen receptors now are measured routinely in samples of breast tissue after surgical removal of a tumor. Of individuals with carcinoma of the breast, 60% have tumors that are estrogen-receptor positive. Approximately two thirds of individuals with estrogen–receptor-positive tumors respond to endocrine therapy; 95% of those

with estrogen–receptor-negative tumors fail to respond. The greater the estrogen-receptor content of the tumor, the higher the response rate to endocrine therapy. Approximately one third of women with metastatic breast carcinoma obtain an objective remission after various types of endocrine therapy directed at lowering their estrogen levels. Such therapy includes oophorectomy, hypophysectomy, and adrenalectomy (ablative therapy), as well as administration of antiestrogens and androgens (additive therapy).

Occasionally a tumor is defined as estrogen-receptor negative, but the patient responds to endocrine therapy (thus, a false-negative result of the estrogen-receptor assay). The following are explanations for false-negative results:

1. Incorrect handling and storage of tissue sample leading to thermolabile receptor protein degradation
2. Inadvertent biopsy of neighboring nonmalignant tissue
3. Low protein concentration in the assayed sample

False-positive results of estrogen-receptor assays (estrogen–receptor-positive tumor but no response to endocrine therapy) are more common than are false-negative results. The most frequent explanation is heterogeneity of the tumor with biopsy of a site that is not representative of the other tumor deposits. In addition to this problem, evidence exists that some tumor cells have receptor defects distal to the initial binding step (for example, variant cells that are able to bind steroid in the cytoplasm but not transport the receptor to the nucleus).

Progesterone-receptor assay is a useful adjunct to the assay of estrogen receptors. Because progesterone-receptor synthesis apparently depends on estrogen action, measurement of progesterone-receptor activity provides confirmation that all the steps of estrogen action are intact. Indeed, metastatic breast cancer patients with both estrogen– and progesterone–receptor-positive tumors have a response rate of 75% to endocrine therapy, whereas those with estrogen-receptor-positive and progesterone–receptor-negative tumors have a 40% response rate. Only 25% of estrogen-receptor-negative/progesterone–receptor-positive patients respond to endocrine therapy, whereas fewer than 5% of estrogen–receptor-negative/progesterone–receptor-negative patients respond. The percentage of positive specimens is greater in postmenopausal women than in those who are premenopausal.

Genetic Markers

Cancer is an inheritable characteristic of cells and must be the outcome of genetic changes. Multiple genetic alterations may be necessary for the transformation of a cell from a normal state to a cancerous one and finally, for metastatic spread. Therefore the evaluation of chromosomal changes may fill the gap left by the traditional serum biochemical markers in establishment of cancer risk and screening (see Chapter 11).

TABLE 21-11 Some Oncogenes Found in Human Tumors

Oncogene	Function	Product	Type of Cancer
N-*ras* mutation	Signal transduction	GDP/GTP binding protein	Acute myeloid leukemia, neuroblastoma
K-*ras* mutation	Signal transduction	GDP/GTP binding protein	Leukemia, lymphoma
c-*myc* translocation	Transcription regulation	Binding with DNA	B- and T-cell lymphoma, small-cell lung carcinoma
c-*erb* B-2 amplification	Growth factor receptor	Tyrosine kinase	Breast, ovarian, gastrointestinal
c-*abl/bcr* translocation	Signal transduction	Tyrosine kinase	Chronic myelocytic leukemia
N-*myc* amplification	Transcription regulation	Binding with DNA	Neuroendocrine
bcl-2	Blocks apoptosis	Mitochondrial membrane protein	Leukemia, lymphoma

GDP, Guanosine diphosphate; *GTP,* guanosine triphosphate.

Two classes of genes are implicated in the development of cancer—oncogenes (cell activation genes; see Table 21-11) and suppressor genes (genes involved in the recognition and repair of damaged DNA; see Table 21-12).

Oncogenes

Proto-oncogenes are normal cellular genes related to tumor virus genes. Activation of proto-oncogenes is associated with cancer. These genes code for products that are involved in normal cellular processes, such as growth factor signaling pathways. Overexpression of the oncogene leads to abnormal cell growth, resulting in malignancy. Of the more than 40 proto-oncogenes recognized, only a few are useful as tumor markers[18] (Table 21-11).

ras Genes

The *ras* genes first were identified as those responsible for the tumorigenic properties of the Harvey (H-*ras*) and Kirsten (K-*ras*) sarcoma viruses, which produce tumors in animals, and provided the first evidence that cellular counterparts in human cells might be involved in development of human tumors. The *ras* gene products are proteins located at the inner face of the plasma membrane. They bind to guanine nucleotides and function as molecular switches that regulate mitogenic signals from growth factors to the nucleus via signal-transduction pathways.[6]

Ras proteins are activated in association with protein-tyrosine kinase receptors and are required for growth-factor proliferation or differentiation of a number of cell types. *Ras* activates the serine/threonine kinase *Raf,* sending positive signals down a kinase cascade (mitogen-activated kinases). The activated cells move through G_1 of the cell cycle. Normally excessive signaling by *ras/Raf* induces p21 and blocks entry into the S phase. However, *ras* also activates a GTPase, *Rho,* which suppresses the expression of p21 and overcomes the cell-cycle block. This step appears to be critical in carcinogenesis.

N-*ras* is found on the short arm of human chromosome 1. The mutated N-*ras* gene is found in individuals with neuroblastomas and acute myeloid leukemia. Mutated K-*ras* is present in 95% of those with pancreatic cancers, 40% of those with colon cancers, 30% of those with lung and bladder cancers, and in lower percentages in those with other tumors. A single point mutation at the 12th K-*ras* codon changes the coded amino acid from glycine to valine in the p21 protein. This mutation is by far the most frequently found in cancers. K-*ras* mutations appear to correlate with poor prognosis and shorter disease-free survival in individuals with adenocarcinoma of the lung and endometrial carcinoma.

However, overall, the presence of *ras* mutations has little practical application to determination of prognosis. Activated *ras* is detected by expression of the *ras* gene product, p21, in cancer tissues. By immunohistochemistry, the *ras* product is found not only in about 40% of individuals with colon cancers, but also in those with colonic polyps believed to be premalignant. A higher relative intensity of staining for p21-*ras* may discriminate malignant from normal tissues or benign lesions in breast, pancreas, stomach, lung, uterus, or thyroid tissues. An increasing level of expression in tissue appears to correlate with the stage or grade of the tumor, but p21-*ras* also may be present in some normal tissues and other studies show no significant difference between benign and malignant tumors. The use of p21 as a tumor marker in tissue or serum is not well established. Mutations of *ras* oncogenes have been detected in the DNA in the stools of 9 of 15 individuals with curable colorectal tumors.

c-*myc* Gene

The c-*myc* gene, located on chromosome 8, is the proto-oncogene of avian myelocytoma virus. It binds to DNA and is involved in transcription regulation. The gene product, p62, is located in the nucleus of transformed cells, and levels of c-*myc* correlate with the rate of cell division. The c-*myc* protein is essential for DNA replication and enhances mRNA transcription. Activation of the c-*myc* gene is associated with B- and T-cell lymphoma, sarcomas, and endotheliomas. In leukemias and lymphomas, increased c-*myc* expression may be due to amplification or chromosomal translocation of the gene. In acute T-cell leukemias, a translocation, (8:14)(q24:q11), results in activation of the gene, and activation of the gene is associated with a poor progno-

TABLE 21-12   Tumor-Suppressor Genes: Chromosome Location and Tumor Types

Chromosome Region	Tumor Type	Gene
3p	Kidney (von Hippel-Lindau syndrome)	*VHL* mutation
5q21	Colorectal	*APC* mutation
9p21	Bladder, glioblastoma, melanoma	*CDKN₂A* mutation (tumor protein p16)
11p13	Wilms tumor	*WT₁* mutation
11p15	Wilms, breast, hepatoblastoma, rhabdomyosarcoma, bladder	Loss of heterozygosity
13q	Breast	*BRCA2, RB1*
13q14	Retinoblastoma, osteosarcoma, small-cell lung	*RB1* mutation
16q	Breast	*CDH1* mutation
17q	Neurofibromatosis 1, melanoma, breast	*BRCA1* mutation
17p13	Breast, colorectal, lung, liver, renal cell, bladder, sarcomas (Li-Fraumeni syndrome)	*TP53* mutation (tumor protein p53)
18q21	Colorectal	*DCC* mutation
22q	Neurofibromatosis 2, meningioma	*NF2* mutation

Other genes indicated by loss of heterozygosity include 1p, 8p, 9q, 10q, and others. From http://www.gene.ucl.ac.uk/nomenclature/guidelines.html.

sis. A decrease in expression of c-*myc* after initiation of chemotherapy suggests a favorable response. Overexpression of p62 may be present in 70% to 100% of primary breast cancers with use of immunohistochemistry, and the intensity of staining is greater with the increasing stage of the tumor. Amplification in lung carcinomas and gliomas correlates with clinical aggressiveness. A fivefold to fortyfold higher expression of c-*myc* may be present in individuals with colon cancers, compared with those with normal mucosa, but the level of expression does not correlate with progression. A similar relationship has been found for cervical, gastric, liver, and other cancers. Serum levels of c-*myc* have been used to detect recurrence but not differentiate cancer and benign conditions. In addition, c-*myc* expression may be activated by the adenomatous polyposis coli gene.

c-*erb* B-2, HER-2/*neu* gene

The c-*erb* B-2 gene also is called *HER-2/neu* because of its association with neural tumors *(neu)*. In addition, its gene product, a 185-kD transmembrane protein expressed on epithelial cells, is similar to the epidermal growth factor receptor. Amplification of c-*erb* B-2 is found in individuals with breast, ovarian, and gastrointestinal tumors. In breast cancer, the gene is as useful a prognostic indicator of overall survival as tumor size or estrogen- and progesterone-receptor expression but not as good as the number of lymph nodes involved in metastases. Elevated serum c-*erb* B-2 antigen levels have demonstrated correlation with decreased response to hormone therapy for breast cancer. Of the three oncogenes—c-*erb* B-2, *ras*, and c-*myc*—c-*erb* B-2 has the strongest prognostic value in breast cancer. Elevated serum levels of a truncated form (p105) of the protein product are found in individuals with lung cancer. Reports have speculated that elevation may precede development of lung cancer by as much as 5 years, but further studies are needed to define clinical utility.

bcl-2

The product of the *bcl*-2 oncogene is a novel 239-amino acid, 25-kD integral membrane protein that localizes primarily to mitochondrial and other cellular membranes. This protein is known to inhibit apoptosis (programmed cell death) and contribute to survival of cancer cells, especially lymphoma and leukemic cells. The *bcl*-2 proto-oncogene was identified in follicular lymphomas, in which a 14:18 translocation results in formation of a *bcl*-2-immunoglobulin heavy-chain fusion gene. Activation of the *bcl*-2 gene through the immunoglobulin promoter results in production of high levels of *bcl*-2-protein.

The protein normally is expressed on cells that have a long life spans (for example, neurons) and the proliferative cells in rapidly renewing cell lineages, such as basal epithelial cells. The *bcl*-2 oncogene is expressed highly in individuals with a variety of hematological malignancies, including lymphomas, myelomas, and chronic leukemias (malignancies characterized by prolonged cell survival). In the normal colon, *bcl*-2- positive cells are restricted to basal epithelial cells, whereas with dysplastic polyps and carcinomas, many positive cells may be found in parabasal and superficial regions. Abnormal expression of the *bcl*-2 gene appears to be an early event in colorectal carcinogenesis. In addition, overexpression of the *bcl*-2 gene is associated with development of resistance to cytotoxic cancer chemotherapy with a variety of tumors, including epithelial tumors and lymphomas. Thus detection of the *bcl*-2-gene product in tumors indicates progression. Future studies may determine its usefulness in prediction of resistance to chemotherapy.

Suppressor genes

A summary of some suppressor genes in human cancer is shown in Table 21-12. Historically, evidence for tumor-suppressor genes was derived from study of hybrid cells of normal and malignant cells that behaved normally. The study concluded that normal cells contained a gene that suppressed the expression of malignancy. Reversion to malignancy occurred when the cultured cells lost normal chromosomes.

The study of suppressor genes may provide a clue as to the development of cancer from normal cell status to benign and cancerous statuses and metastasis. The development of colon cancer requires multiple steps that involve several mutations. The loss of a chromosome 5 gene leads to an increase in cell growth. Early adenoma is associated with the loss of methyl groups on the DNA strand. With the *ras* gene mutation and the loss of the "Deleted in Colon Cancer" (DCC) gene on chromosome 18, adenoma advances to the late stage. Carcinoma is found with the loss of the p53 gene on chromosome 17. Finally, metastasis occurs with other chromosome losses.[7] The clinical usefulness of detection of mutations in tumor-suppressor genes lies not only in the diagnosis and prognosis of cancer, but also in prediction of susceptibility when the mutation is carried in the germline, such as with the breast cancer genes *BRCA1* and *BRCA2*.

Retinoblastoma gene

The retinoblastoma (RB) gene was the first tumor-suppressor gene discovered. RB is a rare tumor in children that occurs both in families and sporadically. Knudson's brilliant analysis of the familial-specific incidence of RB led to development of the two-hit hypothesis. He reasoned that in the inherited form of the tumor, one mutation was present in the germline and all cells of the body, and the other mutational event occurred somatically in one of the cells of the developing retina. In the sporadic form, both mutations occur somatically in the same developing retinoblast, a relatively rare event.

The two-hit hypothesis has served as a model for other tumor-suppressor genes. The RB gene has been localized to chromosome 13q. Most tumors do not have gross deletions but point mutations or small insertions and deletions that result in premature truncation of the protein product. The protein product of the RB gene is a nuclear phosphoprotein with a molecular mass of about 105 kD (p105-RB). When p105-RB is hypophosphorylated, it is active; when hyperphosphorylated, it is inactive. In its active state the p105-RB blocks cells at the G_1 to S phase of the cell cycle. Inactivation or loss of p105-RB deregulates DNA syntheses and increases cellular proliferation. Thus RB is a tumor-suppressor gene when it suppresses DNA synthesis. Detection of mutations in RB are useful in determination of the susceptibility of an individual to development of RB in the familial form, but it is not used as a tumor marker.

p53 (TP53) gene

Of particular interest is the p53 gene, which lies on chromosome 17q. Native or wild-type p53 is believed to control cell division by regulating entry into the S phase. In addition, wild-type p53 enhances the expression of bax proteins, which inhibit the apoptosis-inhibiting effect of *bcl*-2. Because *bcl*-2 promotes cell survival, blocking of this function allows apoptosis to proceed in cells with DNA injury. Deletion of the gene or production of a competing mutant protein causes loss of these controlling effects. Nearly 75% to 80% of colon carcinomas show deletion in one p53 allele and a point mutation in the other allele; thus no wild-type p53 protein is expressed in these tumors. Allelic deletion of p53 occurs only rarely in adenomas (10%), suggesting that p53 inactivation may be a relatively late event in colon carcinogenesis. In addition, up to 70% of breast cancers also have deleted p53.

Mutations in p53 produces proteins that inactivate wild-type p53 protein and allow cells to move through the cell cycle and contribute to the autonomous growth of cancer. A number of different mutations of p53 have been found in human cancers. Most point mutations are localized in four regions of the protein—amino acid residues 117-142, 171-181, 134-158, and 270-286; three "hot spots" affect residues 175, 248, and 273. In addition, selective guanine-to-thymine mutations are found at codon 249 in hepatocellular carcinomas taken from subjects in high-incidence areas of Africa and Asia associated with aflatoxin exposure. Mutations at codons 245 and 258 are found in cases of Li-Fraumeni syndrome, a rare autosomal dominant syndrome characterized by diverse neoplasms at many different sites in the body.

Monoclonal antibodies to mutated p53 proteins are available, and assays for mutant p53 proteins may be applied to the analysis of tumor tissue in the future. Wild-type p53 normally is present in very small amounts that are not detected by immunohistochemistry, whereas the mutant protein accumulates to easily detectable levels. Overexpression of the mutant proteins has been detected in up to 70% of primary colorectal cancers. Overexpression of p53 in breast cancers is associated with poor prognosis, but this association is not as strong as the association with c-*erb* B-2. Up to 75% of small-cell lung carcinomas appear to overexpress a mutant (missense mutation) protein. Finally, circulating antibodies to mutant p53 proteins have been found in sera from individuals with breast and lung cancer and B-cell lymphomas. This antibody response may help monitor relapse in this subset of patients.

p21 *(WAF1/CIP1)*

The wild-type p53 protein activates transcription of a number of genes, including the *WAF1/CIP1* gene. The p21 protein product of this gene binds to and inhibits the cyclin-dependent protein kinases that are active in the G_1 phase of the cell cycle. Thus p21 inhibits apoptosis (programmed cell death). The cell-cycle arrest function of p53 in response to DNA damage is mediated by p21. Monoclonal antibodies to the p21 protein now are available and are being used to determine whether expression of p21 in tumors is clinically useful.

Adenomatous polyposis coli

One of the first events in the putative steps of progression of precursor lesions to colon cancer is loss of the adenomatous polyposis coli (APC) gene in premalignant polyps. The APC gene encodes a 300-kD protein that may be truncated in cancer cells. The normal function of the APC gene product is not known, but it interacts with proteins, such as α- and β-catenin, involved in cell-cell interactions in epithelial cells. This gene is mutated in hereditary colorectal cancer syndromes, polyposis and nonpolyposis types. In the polyposis types, hundreds and even thousands or more benign tumors (polyps) arise before cancer develops. In the nonpolyposis types, very few polyps are seen but the elevated risk of cancer is essentially similar. The APC gene was detected by an interstitial deletion on chromosome 5q in a patient with hundreds of polyps. More than 80% of individuals with hereditary colorectal cancer have germline mutations in one of the APC alleles, including gross deletions or localized mutations. The hereditary forms of colorectal cancer are relatively uncommon, but somatic mutations appear to be of great importance in the development of nonhereditary colorectal cancers. More than 70% of colorectal tumors, regardless of size or histology, have a specific mutation in one of the two APC alleles; mutation also may be found in individuals with other tumor types, including breast, esophageal, and brain tumors.

BRCA1 and *BRCA2*

A subset of breast cancer patients have been shown to possess a predisposition to developing breast and ovarian cancer that is inherited as an autosomal dominant trait.[12] Two genetic loci have been identified—*BRCA1* on chromosome 17q and *BRCA2*, which localizes to 13q12-13. *BRCA1* encodes for an 1863 amino acid protein, which may act as a transcription factor. Breast cancers with a *BRCA1* phenotype have an exceptionally high proliferation rate and frequent p53 overexpression. Those with a *BRCA2* phenotype also demonstrate a higher proliferation rate than *BRCA* negative tumors.

The ability to detect mutations in *BRCA1* and *BRCA2* in somatic cells permits the identification of individuals in breast cancer families who carry the mutated gene. An estimated 1 in 200 women in the United States may have a germline mutation in the *BRCA1* gene. This has created a new ethical dilemma for physicians, patients, and their families, as well as for insurance companies and health maintenance organizations. Prediction, with reasonable certainty, is now possible that an individual who carries a mutant in one of these genes will develop breast and/or ovarian cancer. What should be done if an otherwise healthy individual is shown to carry a *BRCA* gene mutation? Carriers of a *BRCA1* gene mutation have an 85% risk of developing breast cancer and a 45% risk of developing ovarian cancer by 85 years of age. Should such a carrier have a preventive mastectomy or ovariectomy? The goal of cancer research always has been to identify individuals at risk. Although detection of the mutation is not useful as a tumor marker per se, further understanding of how the mutated gene products act may help clinicians understand the molecular events for development of some breast and ovarian cancers.

References

1. Bonfrer JMG: Working group on tumor marker criteria (WGTMC). Tumour Biol 1990; 11:287-288.

2. Catalona WJ, Partin AW, Slawin KM et al: Use of the percentage of free prostate-specific antigen to enhance differentiation of prostate cancer from benign prostatic disease: a prospective multicenter clinical trial. JAMA 1998; 279:1542-1547.

3. Chan DW, Sokoll LJ: Prostate-specific antigen: advances and challenges. Clin Chem 1999; 45:755-756.

4. Chan DW, Beveridge RA, Bhargava A et al: Breast cancer marker CA 549: a multicenter study. Am J Clin Pathol 1994; 101:465-470.

5. Chan DW, Beveridge RA, Muss H et al: Use of TRU-QUANT BR RIA for early detection of breast cancer recurrence in patients with stage II and stage III disease. J Clin Oncol 1997; 15:2322-2328.

6. Clark GJ, Der CJ: *ras* proto-oncogene activation in human malignancy. In Garret G, Sell S (eds): Cellular Cancer Markers, pp 17-52, Totowa, NJ, Humana Press, 1995.

7. Fearon ER, Vogelstein B: A genetic model for colorectal tumorigenesis. Cell 1990; 61:759-767.

8. Hakomori SI: Tumor-associated carbohydrate markers. In Sell S (ed): Serological Cancer Markers, pp 207-232, Totowa, NJ, Humana Press, 1992.

9. Hayes DF, Tondini C, Kufe DW: Clinical applications of CA 15-3. In Sell S (ed): Serological Cancer Markers, pp 281-307, Totowa, NJ, Humana Press, 1992.

10. Jacobs I, Bast RC: The CA 125 tumor-associated antigen: a review of the literature. Hum Reprod 1989; 4:1-12.

11. Kelsten ML, Chan DW, Bruzek DJ et al: Monitoring hepatocellular carcinoma by using a monoclonal immunoenzymo metric assay for alpha-fetoprotein. Clin Chem, 1988; 34:76-81.

12. King MC, Rowell S, Love SM: Inherited breast and ovarian cancer. JAMA 1993; 269:1975-1980.

13. Kurian KM, Watson CJ, Wyllie AH: DNA chip technology. J Pathol 1999; 187:267-271.

14. Landis SH, Murray T, Bolden S et al: Cancer statistics 2000. CA Cancer J Clin 2000; 50:7-33.

15. Partin AW, Piantadosi S, Subong ENP et al: Clearance rate of serum free and total PSA following radical retropubic prostatectomy. Prostate Supp 1996; 7:35-39.

16. Pearson JD, Uderer AA, Metter EJ et al: Longitudinal analysis of serial measurements of free and total PSA among men with and without prostatic cancer. Urology 1996; 48:4-9.

17. Sarosdy MF, DeVere White RW, Soloway MS et al: Results of a multicenter trial using the BTA test to monitor for and diagnose recurrent bladder cancer. J Urol 1995; 154:379-384.

18. Sell S: Cancer markers of the 1990s. Clin Lab Med 1990; 10:27-31.

19. Soloway MS, Briggman JV, Carpinito GA et al: Use of a new tumor marker, Urinary NMP22, in the detection of occult or rapidly recurring transitional cell carcinoma of the urinary tract following surgical treatment. J Urol 1996; 156:363-367.

20. Stamey TA, Barnhill SD, Zhang Z et al: Effectiveness of ProstAsure in detecting prostate cancer and benign prostatic hyperplasia in men age 50 or older. J Urol 1996; 155:436A.

21. Wittliff KL, Pasic R, Bland KI: Steroid and peptide hormone receptors identified in breast tissue. In Kirby KI, Copeland EM (eds): The Breast, pp 900-936, Philadelphia, WB Saunders, 1990.

22. Zhang WM, Leinonen J, Kalkkinen N et al: Purification and characterization of different molecular forms of prostate-specific antigen in human seminal fluid. Clin Chem 1995; 41:1567-1573.

23. Sobin LH, Wittekind CH (eds): TNM Classification of Malignant Tumours, 5th edition, New York, Wiley-Liss, 1997.

Additional Reading

Boyd JC: Mathematical tools for demonstrating the clinical usefulness of biochemical markers. Scand J Clin Lab Invest Supp 1997; 227:46-63.

Nakamura RM, Wu JT: Human Circulating Tumor Markers: Current Concepts and Clinical Applications, Chicago, American Society of Clinical Pathology, 1998.

Saad E: Tumor Markers, Philadelphia, Lippincott Williams & Wilkins, 1998.

CHAPTER 22

Nonprotein Nitrogen Metabolites

DAVID J. NEWMAN, MSc, PhD, MCB, MRCPath, and
CHRISTOPHER P. PRICE, PhD, FRSC, FRCPath

Objectives

1. List the nonprotein nitrogen metabolites analyzed by a clinical chemistry laboratory.
2. Discuss the clinical utility nonprotein nitrogen metabolite assessment.
3. Outline the biosynthesis of urea, creatine, creatinine, uric acid, and ammonia.
4. State the importance of creatinine clearance measurement and, with appropriate information, calculate a creatinine clearance.
5. List the methods of analysis, principles, and possible interferences for each of the clinically important nonprotein nitrogen metabolites.

Key Words

Creatinine Clearance A test that measures the renal clearance of endogenous creatinine; used to estimate the GFR as an indicator of kidney function

Glomerular Filtration Rate (GFR) The rate in milliliters per minute that substances, such as creatinine and urea, are filtered through the kidney's glomeruli; a measure of the number of functioning nephrons

Gout A group of disorders of purine and pyrimidine metabolism

Hyperammonemia A condition of elevated levels of ammonia or its compounds in blood

Hyperuricemia An excess of uric acid or urates in the blood; a prerequisite for the development of gout; may lead to renal disease

Hyperuricuria An excess of uric acid or urates in the urine

Hypouricemia Deficiency of uric acid in the blood due to a deficiency of xanthine oxidase, the enzyme required for conversion of hypoxanthine to xanthine and xanthine to uric acid

Nonprotein Nitrogen Metabolites Catabolites of protein and nucleic acid metabolism that include urea, ammonia, creatinine, creatine, and uric acid

Renal Clearance The volume of plasma from which a substance is cleared completely by the kidneys per unit of time

---

Catabolism of proteins and nucleic acids results in the formation of the so-called **nonprotein nitrogenous metabolites.** Of interest to the clinical laboratory are urea, ammonia, creatinine, creatine, and uric acid.

◼ UREA

Urea is a metabolic product derived sequentially from the catabolism of either exogenous (dietary) or endogenous (tissue) proteins, as follows:

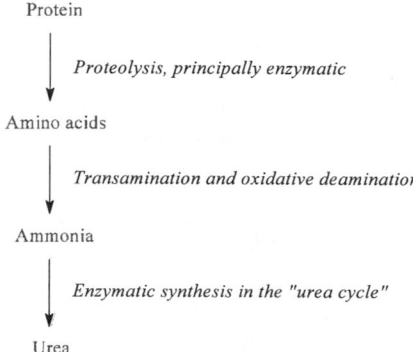

Biochemistry and Physiology

Urea is the major nitrogen-containing metabolic product of protein catabolism in humans, accounting for more than 75% of the nonprotein nitrogen eventually excreted. The biosynthesis of urea from amino nitrogen-derived ammonia is carried out exclusively by hepatic enzymes of the urea cycle. During protein catabolism, amino acid nitrogen is converted to urea in the liver by the action of the urea cycle enzymes (Figure 22-1).

The rate of hepatic urea synthesis depends on exogenous intake of nitrogen and endogenous protein catabolism. Newly synthesized urea equilibrates throughout the total body water compartment, and most is excreted in the urine. A small portion of it diffuses into the intestine, where bacterial enzymes hydrolyze urea and produce ammonia. Carbon dioxide is excreted, whereas ammonia is reabsorbed and must be recycled through the liver. Thus if total body water and the extent of gastrointestinal (GI) hydrolysis of urea are known, the rate of urea synthesis is calculated through analysis of urinary urea excretion and the blood urea nitrogen level. In individuals with cirrhosis the Krebs-Henseleit pathway is unable to incorporate excess ammonia nitrogen into urea.

More than 90% of urea is excreted through the kidneys, with the remainder excreted through the GI tract and skin. In a normal kidney, 40% to 70% of the highly diffusible urea moves passively out of the renal tubule ultimately to reenter plasma. The back-diffusion of urea is inversely related to urine flow rate. In cases of chronic renal failure the osmotic diuresis in the remaining functional nephrons limits the

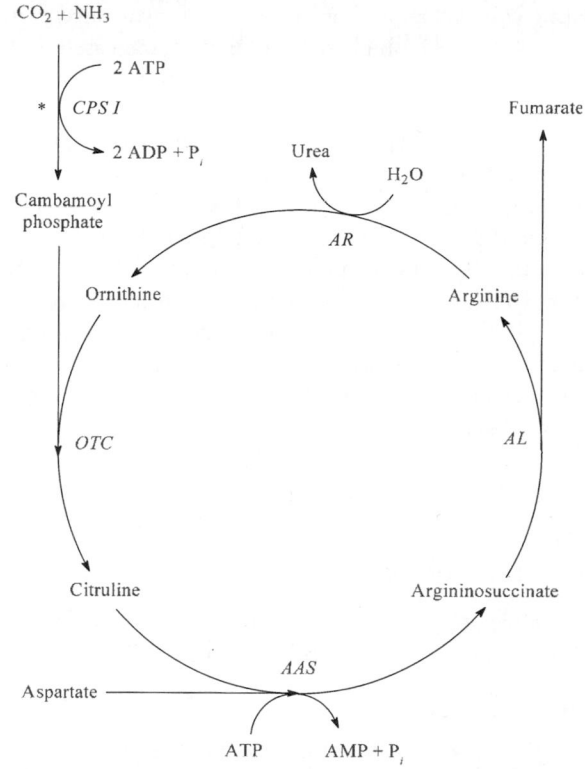

Figure 22-1 The urea cycle pathway. *CPS I,* Carbamoyl phosphate synthetase I; *,* *N*-acetylglutamate as positive allosteric effector; *OTC,* ornithine transcarbamoylase; *AAS,* argininosuccinate synthetase; *AL,* argininosuccinate lyase; *AR,* arginase; *ADP,* adenosine diphosphate; *ATP,* adenosine triphosphate; *P_i,* inorganic phosphate.

back-diffusion of urea so that urea clearance approaches inulin clearance (see Chapter 34).

Clinical Utility

The principal clinical utility of the determination of plasma/serum urea level lies in its measurement in conjunction with the measurement of the level of plasma/serum creatinine. Clinicians then calculate the ratio between the two ratios (urea nitrogen ratio/creatinine ratio) and use it to discriminate between prerenal and postrenal uremia. For a normal individual on a normal diet the reference interval for the ratio is between 12 and 20, with values for most individuals between 12 and 16. Lower ratios usually denote acute tubular necrosis, low protein intake, starvation, or severe liver disease. High ratios with normal creatinine levels may occur in individuals with hypercatabolic states, prerenal uremia, or high protein intake (especially in those with uremia) and after GI hemorrhage. High ratios associated with elevated creatinine concentrations may denote either postrenal obstruction or prerenal uremia superimposed on renal disease.

Measurements of the plasma or serum urea concentration or renal clearance no longer are considered measures of the **glomerular filtration rate (GFR)** (see Chapter 34) because of the number of nonrenal factors influencing the circulating concentration. For instance, the urea concentration is increased by (1) a high-protein diet; (2) increased protein catabolism; (3) muscle wasting (as in starvation); (4) digestion of blood proteins after a GI hemorrhage; and (5) some cases of chronic liver disease. Plasma urea also depends on the state of hydration of the individual, and dehydration should be considered when the urea is elevated to 24 mg/dL (9.0 mmol/L), but the plasma creatinine is normal. In postrenal conditions in which obstruction to the flow of urine is present (for example, malignancy, nephrolithiasis, and prostatism), both the plasma creatinine and urea levels are increased; in these situations a greater increase often is present in the plasma urea than in the plasma creatinine because of increased back-diffusion. Plasma urea levels in an individual with untreated chronic renal failure typically reach 108 to 135 mg/dL (38 to 48 mmol/L).

Analytical Methodology

Both enzymatic and chemical methods have been developed and used to quantify urea in body fluids.

Enzymatic methods

Enzymatic methods are considered indirect because they use an enzyme to convert urea to products that subsequently are quantified. For example, in one popular approach, urea is hydrolyzed to ammonia and water by urease (urea amidohydrolase, EC 3.5.1.5, main source Jack Bean meal), as follows:

$$\underset{\text{Urea}}{\overset{H_2N}{\underset{H_2N}{>}}C=O} + 2\,H_2O \xrightarrow{\text{Urease}} 2\,NH_4^{\oplus} + CO_3^{\ominus\ominus}$$

The resultant ammonium ion then is quantified through either the Berthelot reaction or a glutamate dehydrogenase enzymatic assay, as follows:

Berthelot method

With the Berthelot method, after urea is hydrolyzed with urease, the ammonium formed is reacted with phenol and hypochlorite in alkaline medium to form indophenol. Nitroprusside is used to catalyze the reaction. The absorbance of the dissociated indophenol, a blue chromogen, is measured at 560 nm and related to the concentration of ammonia formed.

Glutamate dehydrogenase methods

Glutamate dehydrogenase [EC 1.4.1.3] is used in these methods to catalyze the conversion of ammonium ion and 2-oxoglutarate to glutamate and water. Coupled with this conversion is the oxidation of NADH to NAD or another reaction that produces an optical change, as follows:

$$NH_4^{\oplus} + \text{2-Oxoglutarate} \xrightarrow[\substack{NADH \quad NAD^{\oplus} \\ + H^{\oplus}}]{\text{Glutamate dehydrogenase}} \text{Glutamate} + H_2O$$

For serum or plasma assays the reaction system usually is formulated so that the addition of sample starts the reaction. A decrease in absorbance resulting from the glutamate dehydrogenase reaction is monitored at 340 nm in either an equilibrium or kinetic mode. In another example of a coupled-enzyme assay system for urea, ammonia reacts with glutamate and adenosine triphosphate (ATP) in the presence of glutamine synthetase (EC 6.3.1.2). Adenosine diphosphate (ADP) produced in this second enzymatic reaction then is quantified in a third and fourth step through use of pyruvate kinase (EC 2.7.1.40) and pyruvate oxidase (EC 1.2.3.3), respectively, thus generating peroxide. In the final step, peroxide reacts with phenol and 4-aminophenazone, catalyzed by peroxidase (EC 1.11.1.7), to yield a quinone-monoamine dye that then is quantified spectrophotometrically.

Other indirect methods used to measure urea include dry chemistry assays that use a variety of detection methods and biosensors that use electrochemical measurements (see Chapter 6).

The specificity of all the enzymatic methods is acceptable, particularly for the urease/glutamate dehydrogenase procedure; however, endogenous ammonia interference must be expected when the protocol uses the sample to initiate the reaction. This fact may be relevant in aged samples, some urines, and particular metabolic disorders. In the methods with a photometric end point, the potential for interference must be considered (for example, ascorbic acid in the Berthelot and aminophenazone/phenol reactions, and bilirubin in the latter).

Chemical methods

In chemical methods, urea is measured directly. In the popular Fearon method, diacetyl condenses with urea to form the chromogen diazine. Because diacetyl is unstable, it usually is generated in the reaction system from diacetyl monoxime and acid. The reaction of diacetyl and urea gives diazine, as follows:

$$\underset{\text{Urea}}{\overset{H_2N}{\underset{H_2N}{>}}C=O} + \underset{\text{Diacetyl}}{\overset{H_3C}{\underset{H_3C}{>}}\overset{C=O}{\underset{C=O}{|}}} \xrightarrow[\text{heat}]{H^{\oplus}} \underset{\text{Diazine}}{\overset{H_3C}{\underset{H_3C}{>}}\overset{C=N}{\underset{C=N}{|}}C=O} + 2\,H_2O$$

Diazine absorbs strongly at 540 nm. Thiosemicarbazide and ferric ions are added to the system to enhance and stabilize the color. The method has been automated on various systems. Urea must be used as a calibrator for a direct method.

Reference intervals

The reference interval for urea nitrogen in the plasma or serum of healthy, ambulatory adults is 6 to 20 mg/dL (2.1 to 7.1 mmol/L expressed as urea).[8] The interval for a 1-week-old newborn is 3 to 25 mg/dL (1.1 to 8.9 mmol/L). In adults over 60 years of age the reference interval is 8 to

23 mg/dL (2.9 to 8.2 mmol/L). Plasma concentrations also tend to be slightly higher in men than in women. On an average protein diet, urinary excretion expressed as urea nitrogen is 12 to 20 g/day.

Comments

The long-established habit of reporting and expression of results of a urea assay in units of urea nitrogen appears to be entrenched strongly in the United States, although the Système International d'Unites (SI) recommends use of urea, expressed in millimoles per liter. Thus students of clinical chemistry should have in mind the conversion factors for urea to urea nitrogen. Because 60 g (1 g × molecular weight) of urea contains 28 g (2 g atomic weight) of nitrogen, the factor is 0.467 for conversion of urea mass units to those of urea nitrogen, and 2.14 for conversion of urea nitrogen mass units to those of urea. The factor for conversion of urea nitrogen in milligrams per deciliter to urea in millimoles per liter or millimoles per liter is 0.357.

■ AMMONIA

Biochemistry and Physiology

The major source of circulating ammonia is the GI tract. Plasma ammonia concentration in the hepatic portal vein is typically fivefold to tenfold higher than that in the systemic circulation. It is derived from the action of bacterial proteases, ureases, and amine oxidases on the contents of the colon, as well as from the hydrolysis of glutamine in both the small and the large intestines. Under normal circumstances, most of the portal vein ammonia load is metabolized to urea in hepatocytes through the Krebs-Henseleit urea cycle during the first pass through the liver; this process includes intramitochondrial and cytosolic enzyme-catalyzed steps (Figure 22-2).[6]

Ammonia enters tissue of the central nervous by passive diffusion. The rate of entry increases in proportion to the plasma concentration and depends on pH. As pH increases, the rate of entry of ammonia into the central nervous tissue increases. This increase is thought to be due to an increase in pH that produces a shift to the right in the equilibrium, as follows:

$$NH_4^{\oplus} + H_2O \rightleftharpoons NH_3 + H_3O^{\oplus}$$

This equilibrium shift results in an increased ammonia base concentration. Ammonia crosses the blood-brain barrier membranes more readily than ammonium ion. Given that the pK_a of ammonia is 8.9 at 37 °C, at the normal physiological pH of 7.4, approximately 3% of blood ammonia is NH_3. An increase in pH to 7.6 produces an increase in NH_3 to approximately 5% of total blood ammonia—a 67% increase in concentration.

Clinical Significance

Animal and human studies have shown that elevated levels of ammonia (**hyperammonemia**) exert toxic effects on the central nervous system. Several causes, both inherited and acquired, of hyperammonemia exist. The inherited deficiencies of urea cycle enzymes are the major cause of hyperammonemia in infants. The two major inherited disorders are those involving the metabolism of the dibasic amino acids lysine and ornithine and those involving the metabolism of organic acids, such as propionic acid, methylmalonic acid, isovaleric acid, and others (see Figure 22-2).

The acquired causes of hyperammonemia are advanced liver disease and renal failure. Severe or chronic liver failure (as occurs in individuals with fulminant hepatitis and cirrhosis, respectively) leads to a significant impairment of normal ammonia metabolism. Reye's syndrome, primarily a central nervous system disorder with minor hepatic dysfunction, also is associated with hyperammonemia (see Chapter 36). Hepatic encephalopathy, in individuals with cirrhosis, is precipitated by GI bleeding that enhances ammonia production by bacterial metabolism of the blood proteins in the colon and subsequent increases in blood ammonia levels. Other precipitating causes of encephalopathy include excess dietary protein, constipation, infections, drugs, or electrolyte and acid-base imbalance. When cirrhosis is accompanied by reduced hepatic portal blood flow, ammonia clearance is impaired, leading to increases in blood ammonia levels. Impaired renal function also causes hyperammonemia. As blood urea nitrogen increases, more of it diffuses into the GI tract, where it is converted to ammonia.

The fasting venous plasma ammonia concentration is useful in the differential diagnosis of encephalopathy when the clinician is uncertain whether encephalopathy is of a hepatic origin. It is especially helpful in the diagnosis of Reye's syndrome and inherited disorders of urea metabolism. However, the concentration is not a useful test for patients with known liver disease.

Analytical Methodology

As discussed previously, both enzymatic and chemical methods are used to measure ammonia in body fluids.[4] Enzymatic assay with glutamate dehydrogenase is the most frequently used method.

Sampling precautions

Reliable measurements of ammonia levels are achieved only when meticulous precautions are used to avoid false elevations. The following four concerns are of paramount importance:

1. *Smoking* is a source of ammonia contamination, both of the patient and of the specimen. The patient must not smoke after midnight before the morning when the fasting blood specimen is drawn. One cigarette smoked

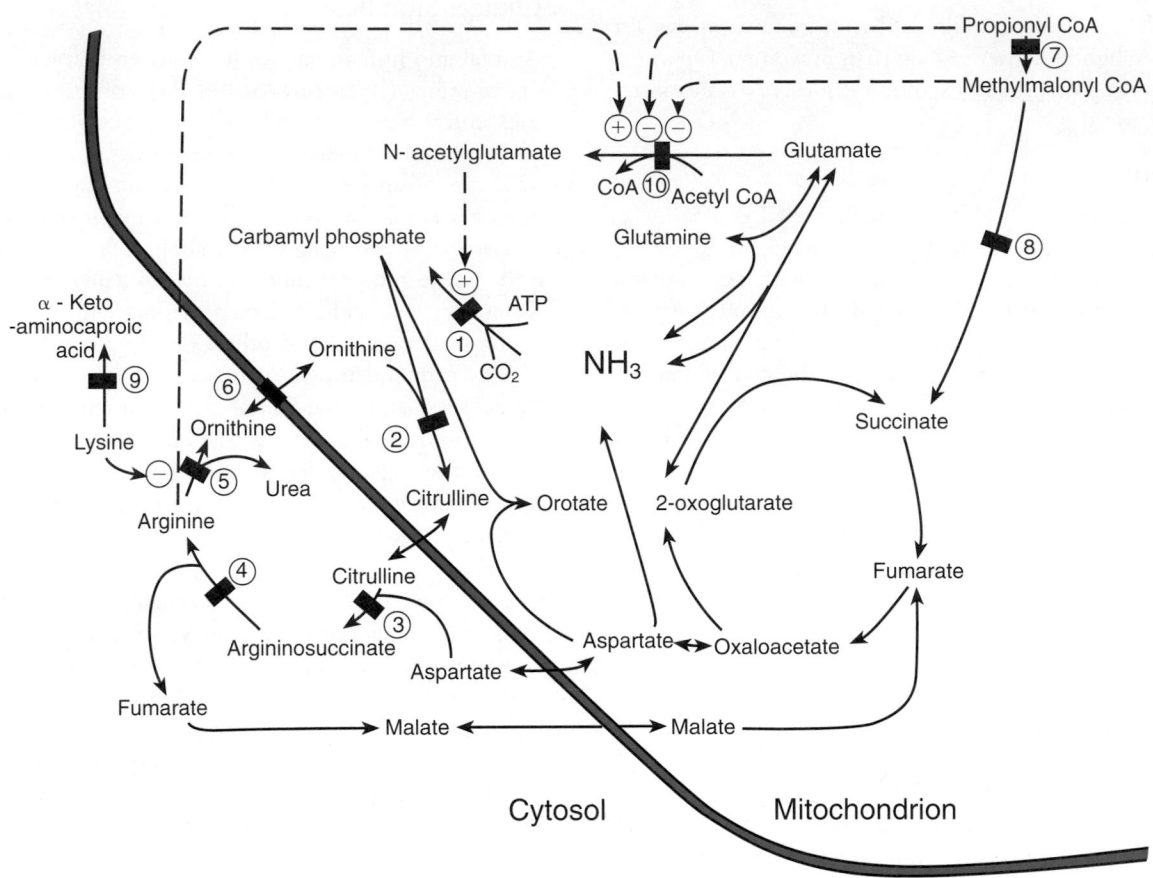

Figure 22-2 The major metabolic pathways for the utilization of ammonia by the hepatocyte. Note the sites of primary enzyme defects *(solid lines)* in various metabolic disorders associated with hyperammonemia— (1) carbamyl phosphate synthetase I, (2) ornithine transcarbamylase, (3) argininosuccinate synthetase, (4) argininosuccinate lyase, (5) arginase, (6) mitochondrial ornithine transport, (7) propionyl CoA carboxylase, (8) methylmalonyl CoA mutase, (9) L-lysine dehydrogenase, (10) *N*-acetylglutamine synthetase. Note also the site of pathway activation (+) or inhibition (−). *CoA,* Coenzyme A; *ATP,* adenosine triphosphate. (Modified from Flannery OB, Hsia YE, Wolf B: Current status of hyperammonemic syndromes. Hepatology 1982; 2:495-506.)

1 hour before venipuncture increases fasting venous blood ammonia concentration by 100 to 200 μg/L.[3] Patients who are heavy smokers should shower before the test. All patients should put on fresh pajamas before the blood specimen is taken. The technologist performing the test also should be a nonsmoker.

2. *Laboratory atmosphere* is a source of ammonia contamination for the specimen and for the assay method. To minimize contamination of specimens and glassware by ammonia in the laboratory atmosphere, blood collection for the ammonia analysis, as well as the performance of the analysis itself, ideally should be done in a special laboratory. Traffic in and from this laboratory should be restricted. Glassware must be chemically clean; it should be soaked in a solution of hypochlorite, 52.5 g/L, and rinsed thoroughly with deionized water the day before use.

3. *Poor venipuncture* technique may result in increased ammonia levels. Use of a heparin lock; probing for a vein; drawing of blood into a syringe and transfer of that blood to a tube containing an anticoagulant; or partial filling of the evacuated tube, which allows subsequent entry of air, may cause elevation of ammonia levels by 100 to 200 μg/L. Ethylenediaminetetraacetic acid (EDTA) and heparin are acceptable anticoagulants. Ammonia values in serum are significantly but variably higher than the corresponding plasma values.

4. *Metabolism of nitrogenous constituents* in the specimen is another source of ammonia contamination. Production of ammonia by deamination of amino acids in the blood specimen may occur once the specimen has been drawn. The specimen must be put on ice immediately and centrifuged without delay; the analysis also must be performed immediately. Even at 0 °C, delays exceeding 15 minutes between blood sampling and the start of centrifugation can increase ammonia concentrations.

Reference intervals

For the enzymatic method the reference interval is 15 to 45 μg of ammonia nitrogen (N) per day or 11 to 32 μmol N/L.[8] If values in normal subjects are significantly higher, consideration should be given to the existence and correction of sources of the preanalytical error identified previously.

CREATININE AND CREATINE

Biochemistry and Physiology

Creatine is synthesized in the kidneys, liver, and pancreas by two enzymatically-mediated reactions. In the first, transamidation of arginine and glycine forms guanidinoacetic acid; in the second, methylation of guanidinoacetic acid occurs with S-adenosylmethionine as the methyl donor. Creatine then is transported in blood to other organs, such as muscles and the brain, where it is phosphorylated to phosphocreatine, a high-energy compound, as follows:

Interconversion of phosphocreatine and creatine is a particular feature of the metabolic processes of muscle contraction. A proportion of the free creatine in muscle ($\sim$ 1% to 2%/day) spontaneously and irreversibly converts to creatinine, its anhydride. Thus the amount of creatinine produced each day is related to the muscle mass (and body weight) and does not vary greatly from day to day. The level of creatinine in the bloodstream is reasonably constant. However, depending on the individual's meat intake, diet may influence the value by about 10%. The free creatinine is a waste product of creatine metabolism, is present in all body fluids and secretions, and is freely filtered by the glomerulus. A small but significant amount of creatinine is secreted by the proximal tubule and increases with increasing levels of plasma creatinine. Creatinine production also decreases as the circulating level of creatinine increases.

Clinical Utility

Because creatinine is produced endogenously and released into body fluids at a constant rate and its plasma levels are maintained within narrow limits, its **renal clearance** (see

Chapter 34) is measured as an indicator of GFR.[10] Because of tubular secretion (see previous discussion), creatinine clearance usually exceeds inulin GFR by a factor of 1.1 to 1.2 at clearances above 80 to 90 mL/min. As GFR falls, the plasma creatinine rises disproportionately and the creatinine clearance reaches more than twice that of inulin. Treatment with cimetidine, which inhibits tubular secretion of creatinine, corrects this discrepancy and forms the basis of a modified creatinine clearance protocol.

To measure creatinine clearance, a timed urine specimen and a blood specimen are obtained. The volume (V) of the urine is measured (mL), urine flow rate is calculated (mL/min), and creatinine is measured in mg/dL or mmol/L in both the urine (U) and serum (S) specimens. The formula for the **creatinine clearance** is as follows:

$$\text{Clearance (mL/min)} = U(\text{mg/dL}) \times \frac{V(\text{mL/min})}{S(\text{mg/dL})}$$

Note that the units for the urinary and serum concentrations must be identical because they cancel each other. Note also that a customary practice is to standardize the calculated clearance by 1.73/A, which represents the external surface area (m^2) of the average-sized individual (standard surface area) divided by the individual's body surface area (A) as determined from a nomogram or formula that relates weight and height to surface area. A common practice is to use the standard surface area, and clearance therefore is reported in units of mL/min/1.73 m^2.

Because the accurate collection of urine is very difficult in clinical practice and even in research studies, the actual measurement of creatinine clearance is decreasing in clinical practice.[9] Serum or plasma creatinine is measured more accurately and reproducibly and, despite many confounding factors, is used to predict the creatinine clearance (GFR) with one of several algorithms. Because creatinine production is related closely to muscle mass, men have higher serum creatinine levels than do women. Muscle mass and GFR also change independently with age, both tending to fall with increasing age. Creatinine clearance (C_{Cr}) is estimated with the following Cockcroft and Gault algorithm:

$$\text{Creatinine clearance} = \frac{(140 - \text{age}) \times \text{weight(kg)} \times K}{72 \times \text{serum creatinine(mg/dL)}}$$

where $K = 0.85$ for women and 1.00 for men.

Analytical Methodology

Both chemical and enzymatic methods are used to measure creatinine in body fluids.[2]

Chemical methods

Most chemical methods used to measure creatinine are based primarily on the reaction with alkaline picrate. In this reaction, first described by Jaffe in 1886, creatinine reacts with picrate ion in an alkaline medium to yield an orange-red complex.[7] Despite the considerable literature that exists on the subject, the reaction mechanism and the structure of the product remain unclear.

The Jaffe reaction is not specific for creatine because many compounds have been reported to produce a Jaffe-like chromogen, including protein, glucose, ascorbic acid, acetone, acetoacetate, pyruvate, guanidine, and cephalosporins. The degree of interference from these compounds depends on the reaction conditions chosen, and consequently several approaches have been used in an attempt to improve the specificity of the Jaffe reaction.[7]

Kinetic assays were developed in a quest both for specificity and for faster and automated analyses. The importance of temperature control to ensure reproducibility of rate measurements was recognized early in the development of such assays. In early studies of interferences in the kinetic methods, two kinds of noncreatinine chromogens were identified—those with rates of adduct formation that were very rapid in the first 20 seconds after reagent and sample are mixed and those with rates that did not become rapid until 80 to 100 seconds after mixing. Thus improvement of specificity in the kinetic assays was achieved through selection of times for rate measurements 25 to 60 seconds after initiation of the reaction (mixing).

Despite all of these attempts to improve the specificity of the Jaffe method, the greatest success in terms of common usage and specificity has come from careful choice of reactant concentrations and use of a kinetic measurement approach. A massive amount of literature exists on the choice of reactant concentrations and reading intervals, as well as on the choice of wavelength and reaction temperature. Consider the following aspects:

Picrate concentration The Jaffe reaction is pseudo-first order with respect to picrate up to 30 mmol/L picrate.

Hydroxide concentration The initial rate of reaction is pseudo-first order with respect to hydroxide concentrations above 0.5 mmol/L.

Wavelength Although the absorbance maximum of the Jaffe reaction is between 490 and 500 nm, improved method linearity and reduced blank values have been reported at other wavelengths, the choice varying with hydroxide concentration.

Temperature The rate of the Jaffe complex formation and absorptivity of the complex are temperature dependent, measurable differences being observed even between 25 and 37 °C.

Reading interval The choice of the reading interval is the main determinant of the specificity of the Jaffe reaction. For example, some interferents act quickly (for example, acetoacetate), others slowly (for example, protein), and others change as a function of time (for example, bilirubin). In addition, interferents may exist that influence the creatinine picrate reaction itself without producing a change in absorbance (that is, inhibitors or activators). The majority of kinetic methods choose an interval between 20 and 80 seconds.

Addition of ferricyanide Ferricyanide oxidizes bilirubin, thereby reducing its interference.

Extent of interference The effect of ketones and ketoacids is probably of the greatest significance, although the effect is very method dependent. Thus reports on acetoacetate interference vary from a negligible increase to an increase of 3.5 mg/dL (310 μmol/L) in the apparent creatinine value at an acetoacetate concentration of 8 mmol/L.

Bilirubin is a negative interferent with the Jaffe reaction. However, the choice of reactant concentrations and the addition of buffering ions, such as borate and phosphate, together with surfactant, have been used to minimize the effects of this interference.

Enzymatic methods

Enzymes from a number of metabolic pathways have been investigated for the measurement of creatinine. All the methods involve a multistep approach, leading to a photometric end point. Enzymes that have been applied include creatininase, creatininase, creatinase, and creatinine deaminase.

Creatininase

Creatininase (EC 3.5.2.10; creatinine amidohydrolase) catalyzes the conversion of creatinine to creatine. The creatine then is detected through a series of enzyme-mediated reactions involving creatine kinase, pyruvate kinase, and lactate dehydrogenase, with monitoring of the decrease in absorbance at 340 nm:

$$ADP + Phosphoenolpyruvate \xrightarrow{\textit{Pyruvate kinase}} Pyruvate + ATP$$

$$Pyruvate \xrightarrow[\substack{NADH \\ +H^{\oplus}}]{\textit{Lactate dehydrogenase}} Lactate + NAD^{\oplus}$$

The approach has not been popular, partly due to poor sensitivity and precision and the relatively high cost of reagents.

Creatininase and creatinase

An alternative approach to the quantification of creatine is to use enzyme creatinase (EC 3.5.3.3; creatinine amidinohydrolase), which yields sarcosine and urea, the former being measured with further enzyme-mediated steps through use of sarcosine oxidase and peroxidase. Hydrogen peroxide is detected with a variety of methods:

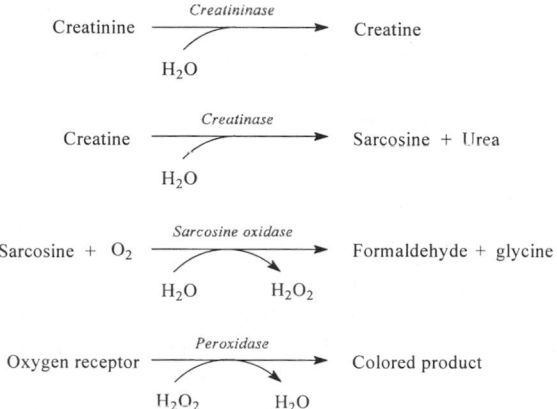

Care must be taken to prevent interference (for example, by bilirubin) in the final reaction sequence. This problem has been addressed with the addition of potassium ferricyanide (with limited success) or bilirubin oxidase. The potential interference due to ascorbic acid is overcome by the inclusion of ascorbate oxidase. The influence of endogenous intermediates, creatine and urea, is overcome by a preincubation step and initiation of the reaction with creatininase.

Creatinine deaminase

A promising approach to the enzymatic measurement of creatinine is to use creatinine deaminase (EC 3.5.4.21; creatinine iminohydrolase), which catalyzes the conversion of creatinine to N-methylhydantoin and ammonia. Early methods concentrated on the detection of ammonia through either glutamate dehydrogenase or the Berthelot reaction. However, a more innovative approach involves the enzyme N-methylhydantoin amidohydrolase, as follows:

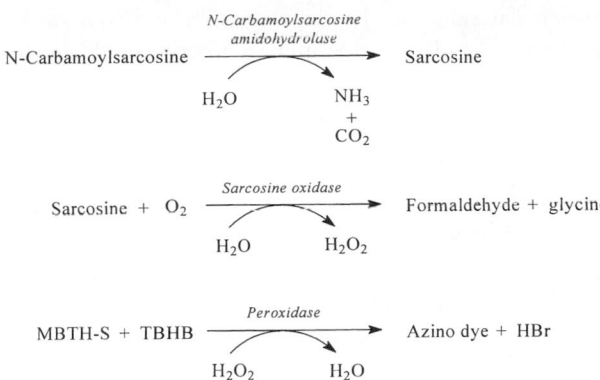

Electrochemical methods have been described for the latter two of the enzymatic approaches outlined previously, utilizing, respectively, a polarographic electrode to detect hydrogen peroxide and an ammonia gas-sensing electrode.

Dry chemistry systems

A number of dry reagent methods have been described for the measurement of creatinine that use an enzyme-mediated reaction. For example, a multilayer film system uses the creatinine deaminase approach, with the ammonia diffusing through a semipermeable and optically opaque layer to react with bromophenol blue to provide an increase in absorbance at 600 nm. A second multilayer film lacking the enzyme is used to quantify the endogenous ammonia. An alternative approach encompassing a means by which plasma is separated from red cells uses the creatininase-creatinase approach outlined previously. In both examples the color produced in the film is quantified by reflectance spectrophotometry. A third dry chemistry system uses a nonenzymatic approach based on the reaction with 3,5-dinitrobenzoic acid.

Comments

Although the enzymatic methods are more expensive, they are used commonly in the dry chemistry systems (with their lower reagent requirement). However, the Jaffe approaches still predominate in the wet chemistry analyzer systems. Any clinical laboratorian assessing a new creatinine method (for example, as part of an analyzer purchase) should review the data for that method concerning interference due to bilirubin, protein, glucose, and ketones/ketoacids; bilirubin also is particularly important in enzymatic procedures that generate hydrogen peroxide. Despite criticism of the Jaffe methods, invariably a good correlation exists between them and enzymatic procedures, with the differences likely due as much to calibration as to interference. The linearity of methods varies, but a range of up to even 1000 mg/dL (88.4 mmol/L) is possible. Within-run imprecision of less than 2% is obtainable with automated analyzers at levels above 200 mg/dL (17.6 mmol/L), with a slightly lower level of precision at the upper limit of the reference interval.

Between-day values in the range of ±3% to 5% are obtainable. Serum or plasma creatinine methods should be calibrated with a serum- or protein-based material if a Jaffe procedure is used. A definitive method that uses gas chromatography/mass spectrometry (GC/MS) also has been described.

Reference intervals

The reference intervals for creatinine clearance and plasma creatinine in healthy adults are method dependent. For a kinetic Jaffe or enzymatic assay the reference interval for men is 0.7 to 1.3 mg/dL (62 to 115 μmol/L) and for women, 0.6 to 1.1 mg/dL (53 to 97 μmol/L). Typical values for serum creatinine in individuals with acute renal failure reach 4 to 6 mg/dL (360 to 530 μmol/L), whereas values in excess of 10 mg/dL (886 μmol/L) are present in those with untreated chronic renal failure. Urinary creatinine excretion typically is 14 to 26 mg/kg/day (124 to 230 μmol/kg/day) in men and 11 to 20 mg/kg/day (97 to 177 μmol/kg/day) in women. The reference interval for creatinine clearance for men is 94 to 140 mL/min/1.73 m^2 and 72 to 110 mL/min/1.73 m^2 for women.

Creatine in Biological Fluids

Creatine constitutes only a small fraction of the total nonprotein nitrogen of plasma and urine. It is unstable at both alkaline and acidic pH and rapidly undergoes conversion to creatinine. Creatine in urine usually is measured as the difference between preformed creatinine in the sample and total "creatinine chromogens" found after the specimen has been subjected to acid condensation. The methods used are the same as those used for creatinine determination. Determination of creatine in plasma or urine has little clinical utility for evaluation of renal disease.

▮ URIC ACID

Biochemistry and Physiology

In humans, uric acid is the major product of the catabolism of the purine nucleosides, adenosine and guanosine (Figure 22-3). Purines from catabolism of dietary nucleic acid are converted to uric acid directly.[1] However, the bulk of purines ultimately excreted as uric acid in the urine originate from degradation of endogenous nucleic acids. The daily synthesis rate of uric acid is approximately 400 mg; dietary sources contribute another 300 mg. Men who consume purine-free diets have an estimated total body pool of exchangeable urate of 1200 mg; in women, this value is estimated as 600 mg. By contrast, individuals with gouty arthritis and tissue deposition of urate may have urate pools as large as 18,000 to 30,000 mg.

Overproduction of uric acid may result from increased synthesis of purine precursors. Synthesis and metabolism of

the major precursors are illustrated in Figure 22-3. Approximately 75% of the uric acid excreted by humans is excreted in the urine; most of the remainder is secreted into the GI tract, where it is degraded to allantoin and other compounds by bacterial enzymes.

Renal handling of uric acid is complex and involves four sequential steps: (1) glomerular filtration; (2) reabsorption of about 98% to 100% in the proximal convoluted tubule; (3) secretion into the lumen of the distal portion of the proximal tubule; and (4) further reabsorption in the distal tubule. The net urinary excretion of uric acid is 6% to 12% of the amount filtered.

The physicochemical properties of uric acid are important in consideration of uric acid concentrations in the circulation, tissues, and kidneys. The first pK_a of uric acid is 5.57; above a pH of 5.57, uric acid exists chiefly as urate ion, which is more soluble than uric acid.

Clinical Significance

Hyperuricemia most commonly is defined by serum or plasma uric acid concentrations greater than 7.0 mg/dL (0.42 mmol/L) in men or greater than 6.0 mg/dL (0.36 mmol/L) in women. The major causes of hyperuricemia are summarized in Table 22-1. Asymptomatic hyperuricemia frequently is detected through biochemical screening; long-

TABLE 22-1	Causes of Hyperuricemia

Increased Formation
PRIMARY
Increased purine synthesis
Inherited metabolic disorder

SECONDARY
EXCESS DIETARY PURINE INTAKE
Increased nucleic acid turnover
Malignancy
Psoriasis
Cytotoxic drugs

ALTERED ATP METABOLISM
Tissue hypoxia
Alcohol

Decreased Excretion
PRIMARY (IDIOPATHIC)
SECONDARY
CHRONIC RENAL FAILURE
Increased renal reabsorption
Reduced secretion
Lead poisoning
Organic acids (for example, lactate, acetoacetate)
Salicylate (low doses)
Thiazide diuretics

ATP, Adenosine triphosphate.

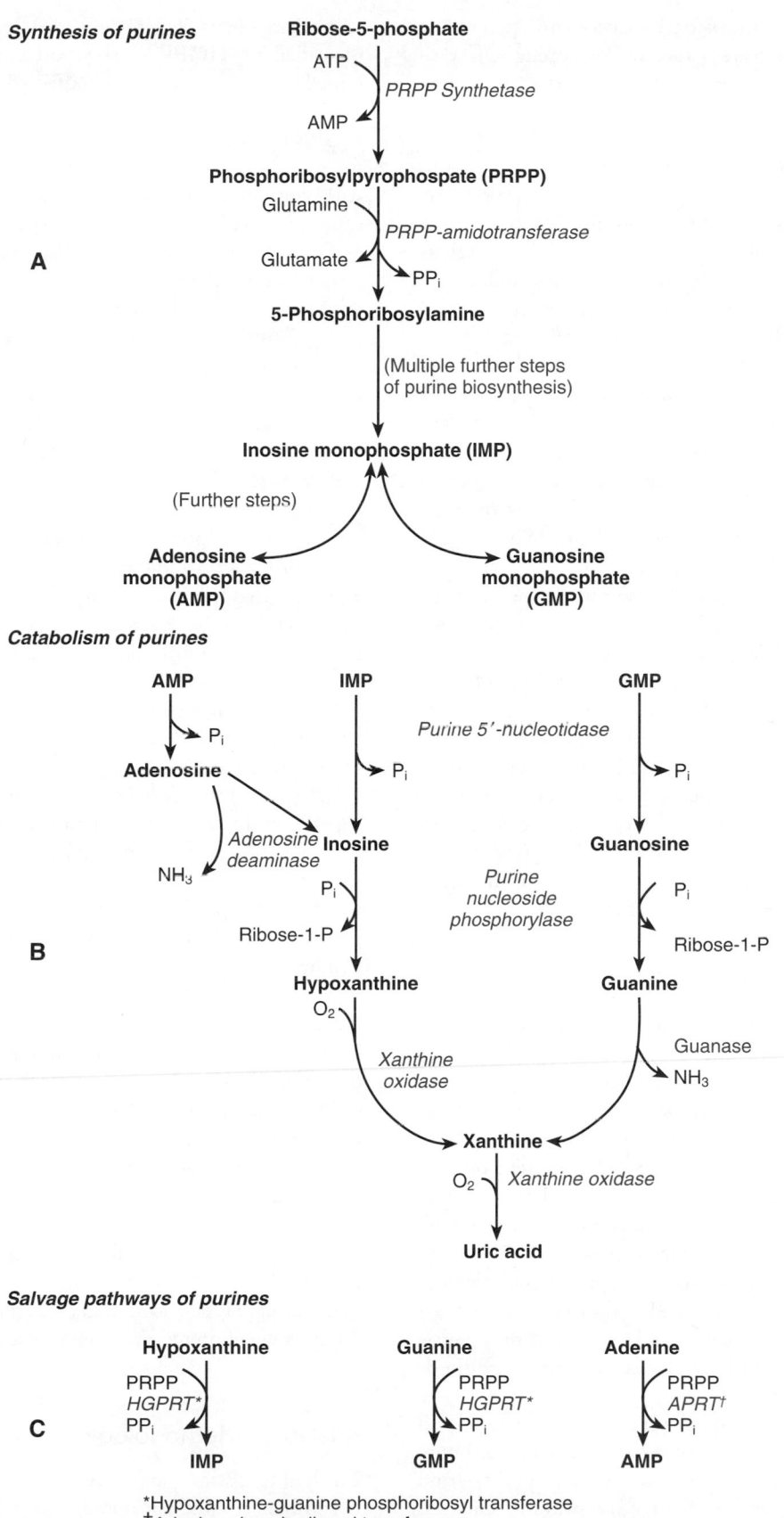

Figure 22-3   Metabolism of purines. **A,** Synthesis pathway. **B,** Catabolism pathway. **C,** Salvage pathway. *ATP,* Adenosine triphosphate, P_i, inorganic phosphate; PP_i, pyrophosphate.

term follow-up of asymptomatic hyperuricemic patients is performed because many are at risk for developing renal disease as a result of hyperuricemia and **hyperuricuria;** few such patients ever develop the clinical syndrome known as *gout*.

Gout occurs when monosodium urate precipitates from supersaturated body fluids; the deposits of urate are responsible for the clinical signs and symptoms. Gouty arthritis may be associated with urate crystals in joint fluid, as well as with deposits of crystals (tophi) in tissues surrounding the joint. The deposits may also occur in other soft tissues, and wherever they occur, they elicit an intense inflammatory response mediated by polymorphonuclear leukocytes and macrophages. Renal disease associated with hyperuricemia may take one or more of several forms—(1) gouty nephropathy with urate deposition in renal parenchyma, (2) acute intratubular deposition of urate crystals, and (3) urate nephrolithiasis. Medical treatment of sustained asymptomatic hyperuricemia is justified to prevent urate-induced renal damage.

Primary gout is associated with "essential" hyperuricemia due to metabolic overproduction of purines or underexcretion of uric acid. Secondary gout is a result of hyperuricemia attributable to several identifiable causes. Renal retention of uric acid may occur in cases of acute or chronic renal disease of any type or as a consequence of administration of drugs; diuretics, in particular, are implicated in the latter instance. Organic acidemia caused by increased acetoacetic acid in individuals with diabetic ketoacidosis or lactic acidosis may interfere with tubular secretion of urate. Increased nucleic acid turnover and a consequent increase in catabolism of purines may be encountered in cases of rapid proliferation of tumor cells, as well as those involving massive destruction of tumor cells during therapy with certain chemotherapeutic agents.

Hyperuricemia also is attributable to primary defects of enzymes in the pathways of purine metabolism. The Lesch-Nyhan syndrome is characterized by complete deficiency of hypoxanthine-guanine phosphoribosyl transferase (HGPRT), the major enzyme of the purine salvage pathways (see Figure 22-3). This sex-linked genetic disorder is manifested clinically by mental retardation, abnormal muscle movements, and behavioral problems (self-mutilation and pathological aggressiveness). Biochemically, it is characterized by hyperuricemia, hyperuricaciduria, and markedly decreased levels of HGPRT in erythrocytes, fibroblasts, and other cells. Intracellular levels of phosphoribosylpyrophosphate (PRPP) and rates of purine synthesis are increased (see Figure 22-3).

Neurological symptoms of this syndrome may be related to decreased availability of purines to the developing brain, which has limited capacity for de novo purine synthesis and therefore relies on the purine salvage pathways to supply it with most of the purine nucleotides it requires. Less severe deficiency of HGPRT displays a clinical spectrum of mild to moderate neurological defects. Affected fetuses have been identified by HGPRT assays on cultured fibroblasts obtained by amniocentesis; unaffected heterozygous female carriers of the defective gene are identified by observation of HGPRT mosaicism in cultured fibroblasts or individual hair follicles. Increased levels of intracellular PRPP production, with consequent increased uric acid levels, also occur because of mutations in PRPP synthetase, which are inherited as X-linked recessive traits. Glucose-6-phosphatase deficiency also leads to hyperuricemia as a result of both overproduction and underexcretion of uric acid.

Quantification of urinary uric acid excretion aids in selection of appropriate treatment for individuals with asymptomatic hyperuricemia. Hyperuricemic patients excreting less than 600 mg of uric acid daily are candidates for treatment with uricosuric drugs, such as probenecid or sulfinpyrazone; uricosuric drugs enhance renal excretion of uric acid by blocking the carriers in the tubular cells that mediate reabsorption. Individuals who excrete more than 600 mg/day are candidates for treatment with allopurinol, a drug that decreases intracellular concentrations of PRPP and inhibits xanthine oxidase activity, thereby suppressing purine synthesis and degradation of hypoxanthine to uric acid.

About one in five individuals with clinical gout also has urinary tract uric acid stones. Although formation of urinary tract stones is a complex process, about 50% of those with uric acid stones have either hyperuricuria, excretion of a persistently acid urine, or both. Undissociated uric acid (pK_a 5.57) is relatively insoluble, whereas urate at pH 7.0 is more than 10 times more soluble. Thus in individuals with urinary pH persistently less than 6.0, relatively small amounts of uric acid in urine may produce supersaturating conditions.

Hypouricemia, often defined as serum urate concentrations less than 2.0 mg/dL (0.12 mmol/L), is much less common than hyperuricemia. It may be secondary to any one of a number of underlying conditions. Severe hepatocellular disease with reduced purine synthesis is one possibility; another is defective renal tubular reabsorption of uric acid. Defective reabsorption may be congenital, as in generalized Fanconi's syndrome, or acquired. Overtreatment of hyperuricemia with allopurinol or uricosuric drugs and cancer chemotherapy with 6-mercaptopurine or azathioprine (inhibitors of de novo purine synthesis) also have caused hypouricemia. Hypouricemia in combination with xanthinuria rarely is encountered and suggests a deficiency of xanthine oxidase.

Analytical Methodology

Phosphotungstic acid (PTA), uricase, and high-performance liquid chromatography (HPLC) methods have been described to measure uric acid. Dry chemistry methods also have been developed that utilize uricase.[5]

Phosphotungstic acid methods

PTA methods are based on the development of a blue reaction (tungsten blue) as PTA is reduced by urate in alkaline medium; the color is read at wavelengths of 650 to 700 nm. In methods for plasma uric acid, protein removal is an obligatory step and a variety of precipitants have been used, including trichloroacetic acid, tungstic acid, and PTA. Methods that use PTA are subject to many interferences, including endogenous compounds, such as glucose, ascorbic acid, glutathione, and cysteine (spilled into plasma from hemolyzed erythrocytes) and exogenous compounds, such as acetaminophen, acetylsalicylic acid, and purines, such as caffeine, theobromine, and theophylline. All these compounds reduce PTA and thus introduce a positive error. The reader is referred to the review by Price and James for a more detailed analysis of interferences.[5]

Uricase methods

Uricase methods are more specific than the PTA versions because they use uricase ([urate:oxygen] oxidoreductase; EC 1.7.3.3), either as a single step or as the initial step to oxidize uric acid, as follows:

Urate   Allantoin

Uricase methods became feasible and popular as a result of the availability of high-quality, low-cost preparations of the bacterial enzyme. Preliminary precipitation of protein is not required except for the 282-nm method. In a majority of uricase methods, only guanine, xanthine, and a few other structural analogues of uric acid interfere, and then only at concentrations not expected in biological fluids. Uricase methods have replaced PTA methods in most current instrumentation.

The reaction is measured in either the kinetic or the equilibrium mode. The decrease of absorbance as urate is converted has been measured at wavelengths varying from 282 to 292 nm. A reference procedure has been suggested in which a protein-free filtrate is used with uricase, the reduction in absorbance at 293 nm monitored, and the result calculated from the molar extinction coefficient.

Most current enzymatic assays for uric acid in serum involve a peroxidase system coupled with one of a number of oxygen acceptors to produce a chromogen. For example, one popular method measures hydrogen peroxide with the aid of horseradish peroxidase and an oxygen acceptor (4-aminophenazone or a substituted phenol) to yield a chromogen in the visible spectrum. The benefit from use of substituted phenols is the enhanced molar absorptivity. Alternative oxygen acceptors include 3-methyl-1-benzothiazoline hydrazone (MBTH), 2,2'-azino-di-(3-ethyl-benzothiazoline)-6-sulphonate (ABTS), and o-dianisidine.

The use of a substituted phenol yielding a highly absorbing product helps to reduce the potential interference by reducing the sample volume requirement. The major interferents to minimize are ascorbic acid and bilirubin. In general, use of ascorbate oxidase to minimize ascorbic acid interference is necessary. Use of aminophenazone with a substituted phenol generally minimizes bilirubin interference. In addition, unknown metabolites in sera of individuals with renal failure, thought to be phenolic compounds, interfere by competing with the reagent phenol, providing a low recovery of urate. The interference is overcome with use of a substituted phenol.

High-performance liquid chromatography methods

HPLC methods using ion-exchange or reversed-phase columns are used to separate and quantify uric acid. The column effluent is monitored at 293 nm to detect the eluting uric acid. HPLC methods are specific and fast, mobile phases are simple, and the retention time for uric acid is less than 6 minutes. A proposed method for the assay of uric acid in serum uses isotope-dilution mass spectrometry.

Dry chemistry systems

Devices that utilize uricase in a dry reagent format to measure uric acid also have been described. For example, a multilayer film system uses uricase and peroxidase separated by a semipermeable membrane from a leuco dye that is oxidized to form a colored product. A cellulose matrix pad system uses uricase, peroxidase, and MBTH as the oxygen acceptor; the system uses a diluted serum sample, which helps to reduce interferences. A third system incorporates separation of plasma from red cells and uricase, peroxidase, and a substituted phenol to measure uric acid content. All three systems use a reflectance meter system to facilitate accurate and precise quantification of the color change. Electrochemical and biosensor systems also have been described for the measurement of uric acid.

Reference intervals

The reference interval for uric acid, measured by the phosphotungstate method, has been reported as 4.4 to 7.6 mg/dL (262 to 452 μmol/L) for men and 2.3 to 6.6 mg/dL (137 to 393 μmol/L) for women. However, reference intervals are method dependent; reference intervals using enzymatic methods are 3.5 to 7.2 mg/dL (208 to 428 μmol/L) for men and 2.6 to 6.0 mg/dL (155 to 357 mmol/L) for women. The level of plasma uric acid increases gradually with age, rising about 10% between 20 and 60 years of age. Women demonstrate a significant rise after the onset of menopause, reaching levels similar to those in men.

An alternative approach to the interpretation of serum uric acid levels is to consider the degree of hyperuricemia in relation to the risk of gout development. Men with plasma uric acid concentrations exceeding 9.0 mg/dL (540 μmol/L) are approximately 150 times more likely to have coexisting gouty arthritis than are men with uric acid concentrations less than 6.0 mg/dL (360 μmol/L). Urinary uric acid excretion in individuals on a diet containing purines is 250 to 750 mg/day (1.5 to 4.5 mmol/day). Excretion may decrease by 20% to 25% on a purine-free diet to less than 400 mg/day.[8]

References

1. Becker MA, Roessler BJ: Hyperuricemia and gout. In Scriver CR, Beaudet AL, Sly WS et al (eds): The Metabolic and Molecular Bases of Inherited Disease, 7th edition, pp 1655-1677, New York, McGraw-Hill, 1995.
2. Fossati P, Ponti M, Passoni G et al: A step forward in enzymatic measurement of creatinine. Clin Chem 1994; 40:130-137.
3. Gerron GG, Ansley JD, Isaacs JW et al: Technical pitfalls in measurement of venous plasma NH_3 concentration. Clin Chem 1976; 22:663-666.
4. Huizenga JR, Tangerman A, Gips CH: Determination of ammonia in biological fluids. Ann Clin Biochem 1994; 31:529-543.
5. Price CP, James DR: Analytical reviews in clinical biochemistry: the measurement of urate. Ann Clin Biochem 1988; 25:484-498.
6. Raushel FM, Thoden JB, Holden HM: The amidotransferase family of enzymes: molecular machines for the production and delivery of ammonia. Biochemistry 1999; 38:7891-7899.
7. Spencer K: Analytical reviews in clinical biochemistry: the estimation of creatinine. Ann Clin Biochem 1986; 23:1-25.
8. Tietz NW (ed): Clinical Guide to Laboratory Tests, 3rd edition, Philadelphia, WB Saunders, 1995.
9. Toto RD, Kirk KA, Coresh J et al: Evaluation of serum creatinine for estimating glomerular filtration rate in African Americans with hypertensive nephrosclerosis: results from the African-American study of kidney disease and hypertension (AASK) pilot study. J Am Soc Nephrol 1997; 8:279-287.
10. Walser M: Assessing renal function from creatinine measurements in adults with chronic renal failure. Am J Kidney Dis 1998; 32:23-31.

Additional Reading

Batshaw ML: Inborn errors of urea synthesis. Ann Neurol 1994; 35:133-141.

Brusilow SW, Horwich AL: Urea cycle enzymes. In Scriver CR, Beaudet AL, Sly WS et al (eds): The Metabolic and Molecular Bases of Inherited Disease, 7th edition, pp 1187-1232, New York, McGraw-Hill, 1995.

Newman DJ, Price CP: Renal function and nitrogen metabolites. In Burtis CA, Ashwood ER (eds): Tietz Textbook of Clinical Chemistry, 3rd edition, pp 1204-1270, Philadelphia, WB Saunders, 1998.

Rossiter BJF, Caskey CT: Hypoxanthine-guanine phosphoribosyltransferase deficiency: Lesch-Nyhan syndrome and gout. In Scriver CR, Beaudet AL, Sly WS et al (eds): The Metabolic and Molecular Bases of Inherited Disease, 7th edition, pp 1679-1706, New York, McGraw-Hill, 1995.

Schrier RW, Gottschalk CW: Diseases of the Kidney, 6th edition, Philadelphia, Lippincott Williams & Wilkins, 1996.

Thoene JG: Treatment of urea cycle disorders. J Pediatr 1999;134:255-256.

CHAPTER 23

Carbohydrates

DAVID B. SACKS, MB, ChB, FACP, FRCPath

Objectives

1. Define the following terms:

    Carbohydrate

    Monosaccharide, disaccharide, and polysaccharide

    Ketone

    Insulin

    Diabetes mellitus

    Glycogen

    Glycogenesis

    Glycogenolysis

    Glycolysis

    Gluconeogenesis

    Glucose tolerance

    Hyperglycemia and hypoglycemia

    Glycation

2. Provide examples of a monosaccharide, disaccharide, and polysaccharide.
3. Discuss the regulation of glucose concentration in the body and state the healthy reference interval of glucose.
4. Compare type 1 and type 2 diabetes mellitus with regard to prevalence, causes, age at onset, symptoms, and laboratory values.
5. State the basic criteria for the diagnosis of diabetes mellitus, including American Diabetes Association guidelines.
6. Discuss the abnormal metabolic relationships among glucose, ketones, fatty acids, and metabolic acids in an insulin-deficient individual.
7. Outline the procedure for administration of an oral glucose tolerance test and interpret the results.
8. List the laboratory procedures involved in assessment of diabetes mellitus in a nonpregnant individual.
9. List three causes of hypoglycemia.
10. List four methods of serum glucose analysis, state the specimen requirements and principles of each, and list the known interferences in each.
11. Define *glycohemoglobin,* state the clinical utility of its measurement, and list three methods of glycohemoglobin analysis.
12. Resolve case studies regarding carbohydrate analysis in the assessment of carbohydrate disorders.

Key Words

Advanced Glycation End Products (AGE) Proteins that have been irreversibly modified by nonenzymatic attachment of glucose; may contribute to the chronic complications of diabetes

Carbohydrates Neutral compounds composed of carbon, hydrogen, and oxygen (in a ratio of 1:2:1) that constitute a major food class

Diabetes Mellitus A group of metabolic disorders of carbohydrate metabolism in which glucose is underutilized, producing hyperglycemia

Diabetogenes Genes that contribute to the development of diabetes; fewer than 5% of individuals with type 2 diabetes have an identified genetic defect

Gestational Diabetes Mellitus (GDM) Carbohydrate intolerance that arises during pregnancy

Glucose A six-carbon simple sugar that is the premier fuel for most organisms and an important precursor of other body constituents

Glycated Hemoglobin Hemoglobin that has a sugar residue attached; Hb A_{1c} being the major fraction

(~80%) of glycated hemoglobin; also known as *glycohemoglobin* or *Hb A₁*

Glycogen A polysaccharide having a formula of $(C_6H_{10}O_5)n$ used by muscle and liver for carbohydrate storage

Hyperglycemia Increased glucose concentrations in the blood

Hypoglycemia Decreased glucose concentrations in the blood

Insulin A protein hormone produced by the β-cells of the pancreas that decreases blood glucose concentrations

Ketones Compounds that arise from free fatty acid breakdown; insulin deficiency leads to increased serum ketones, which are the major contributors to the metabolic acidosis that occurs in individuals with diabetic ketoacidosis

Lactate An intermediary product in carbohydrate metabolism that accumulates in the blood predominantly when tissue oxygenation is decreased; increased blood lactate concentrations result in lactic acidosis

Urinary Albumin Excretion (UAE) A rate of excretion of albumin in the urine (20 to 200 μg/min) that is between normal and overt proteinuria; increased UAE precedes and is highly predictive of diabetic nephropathy; also known as *microalbuminuria*

Carbohydrates, including sugar and starch, are widely distributed in plants and animals. They perform multiple functions, ranging from structural components of RNA and DNA (ribose and deoxyribose sugars) to a source of energy (glucose). **Glucose** is derived from the breakdown of carbohydrates in the diet (grains, starchy vegetables, and legumes) and body stores (glycogen), as well as by endogenous synthesis from protein or from the glycerol moiety of triglycerides. When energy intake exceeds expenditure, the excess is converted to fat and glycogen for storage in adipose tissue and liver or muscle, respectively. When energy expenditure exceeds calorie intake, endogenous glucose formation occurs from the breakdown of carbohydrate stores and from noncarbohydrate sources (for example, amino acids, lactate, and glycerol).

Regulatory hormones, such as insulin, glucagon, and epinephrine, maintain the glucose concentration in the blood within a fairly narrow range under diverse conditions (feeding, fasting, or severe exercise). Measurement of glucose is one of the most commonly performed procedures in hospital chemistry laboratories. The most frequently encountered disorder of carbohydrate metabolism is high blood glucose due to diabetes mellitus, which affects approximately 5% of the U.S. population. The incidence of hypoglycemia (low blood glucose) is unknown but is substantially lower.

◼ CHEMISTRY OF CARBOHYDRATES

Carbohydrates are aldehyde or ketone derivatives of polyhydroxy (more than one −OH group) alcohols, or compounds that yield these derivatives on hydrolysis.

Monosaccharides

A monosaccharide, or simple sugar, consists of a single polyhydroxy aldehyde or ketone unit and cannot be hydrolyzed to a simpler form. The backbone is made up of several carbon atoms. Sugars containing three, four, five, six, and seven carbon atoms are known as *trioses, tetroses, pentoses, hexoses,* and *heptoses,* respectively. One of the carbon atoms is double-bonded to an oxygen atom to form a carbonyl group. An aldehyde has the carbonyl group at the end of the carbon chain, whereas if the carbonyl group is at any other position, a **ketone** is formed (Figure 23-1). The simplest carbohydrate is glycol aldehyde, the aldehyde derivative of ethylene glycol. The aldehyde and ketone derivatives of glycerol are, respectively, glyceraldehyde and dihydroxyacetone (see Figure 23-1). Aldehyde derivatives are termed *aldoses,* and ketone derivatives are called *ketoses,* as shown in Figure 23-2.

Compounds that are identical in composition and differ only in spatial configuration are called *stereoisomers.* The carbon atoms in the unbranched chain are numbered 1 to 6, as shown by the numbers at the left of the formula for D-glucose in Figure 23-2. The designation D- or L- refers to the position of the hydroxyl group on the carbon atom adjacent to

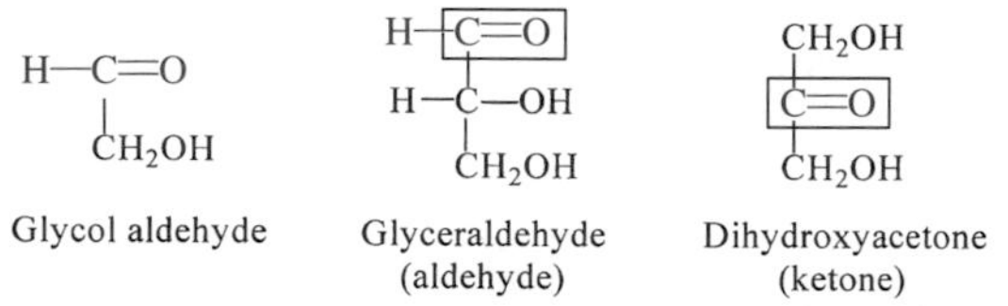

Figure 23-1　Two- and three-carbon carbohydrates.

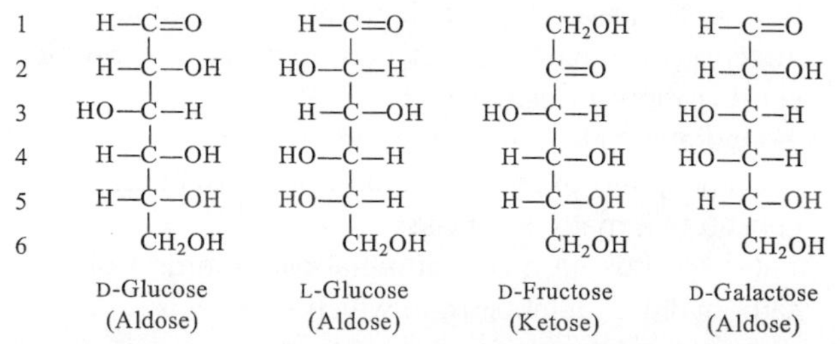

Figure 23-2　Typical six-carbon sugars.

the last (bottom) CH_2OH group. In general, the designation of D- and L- for a sugar molecule refers to the stereoisomeric forms of the highest-numbered asymmetrical carbon atom.* By convention the D-sugars are written with the hydroxyl group on the right, and the L-sugars are written with the hydroxyl group on the left (see Figure 23-2). Most sugars in the human body are of the D-configuration. A number of different structures exist, depending on the relative positions of the hydroxyl groups on the carbon atoms.

The formula for glucose can be written in the form of either aldehyde or enol, a short-lived reactive species. Shift to the enol anion is favored in alkaline solution, as follows:

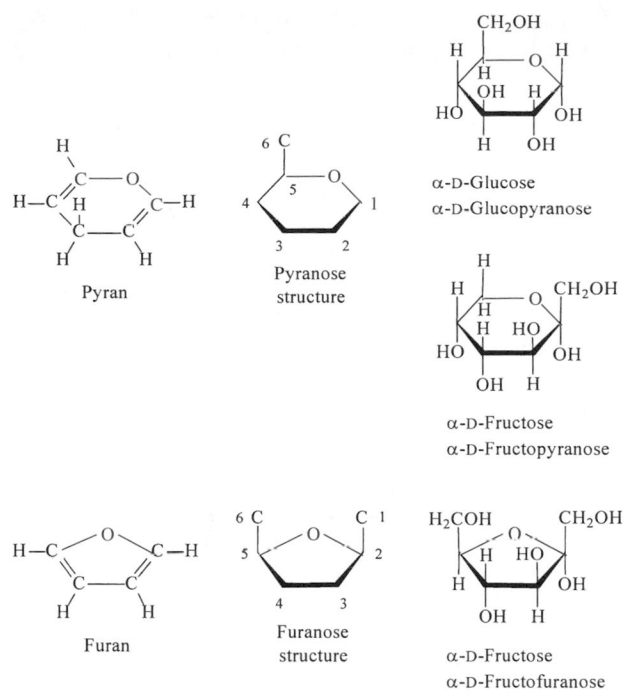

Figure 23-3   The Haworth formula for sugars.

The presence of a double bond and a negative charge in the enol anion makes glucose an active reducing substance that can be oxidized by relatively mild oxidizing agents, such as cupric (Cu^{2+}) and ferric (Fe^{3+}) ions. Glucose in hot alkaline solution readily reduces cupric ions to cuprous ions. The color change can be used as a presumptive indication for the presence of glucose, and for many years, blood and urine glucose were measured this way. Other sugars also can reduce cupric ions in alkaline solution, and these are collectively referred to as *reducing sugars*.

The aldehyde group reacts with the hydroxyl group on carbon 5, represented by a symmetrical ring structure and depicted by the Haworth formula, in which glucose is considered as having the same basic structure as pyran (Figure 23-3). In this formula the plane of the ring is considered to be perpendicular to the plane of the paper, with the heavy lines pointing toward the reader. Hydroxyl groups in position 1 are then below the plane (α-configuration) or above the plane (β-configuration). A six-member ring sugar, containing five carbons and one oxygen, is a derivative of pyran and is called a *pyranose*. When linkage occurs with formation of a five-member ring, containing four carbons and one oxygen, the sugar has the same basic structure as furan and is called a *furanose*. Fructose is shown in two cyclical forms. Fructopyranose is the configuration of the free sugar, and fructofuranose occurs whenever fructose exists in combination with disaccharides and polysaccharides, as in sucrose and inulin.

Disaccharides

Two monosaccharides join covalently by an *O*-glycosidic bond, with the loss of a molecule of water, to form a disaccharide. The chemical bond between the sugars always involves the aldehyde or ketone group of one monosaccharide joined to an alcohol group (for example, maltose) or an aldehyde or ketone group (for example, sucrose) of the other monosaccharide (Figure 23-4). The most common disaccharides are as follows:

Maltose = glucose + glucose
Lactose = glucose + galactose
Sucrose = glucose + fructose

If the linkage between two monosaccharides is between the aldehyde or ketone group of one molecule and a hydroxyl group of another molecule (as in maltose and lactose), one potentially free ketone or aldehyde group remains on the second monosaccharide. Consequently, the second glucose residue can be oxidized and is capable of existing in α- or β-pyranose forms. Thus the disaccharide is a reducing sugar, but its reducing power is only approximately 40% of the reducing power of the two single monosaccharides added together. On the other hand, if the linkage between two monosaccharides involves the aldehyde or ketone groups of both molecules (as in sucrose), a nonreducing sugar results because no free aldehyde or ketone group remains.

Polysaccharides

The linkage of multiple monosaccharide units results in the formation of polysaccharides. The major storage carbohydrates are starch in plants and glycogen in animals, both of which form granules inside cells. Polysaccharides can provide structural support. Cellulose is used by plants, whereas

---

*Although the D and L designations are retained in this chapter, readers should be aware that in the Cahn-Ingold-Prelog system a series of rules determines configurations. In this new system the symbols R and S are used to designate configurations, instead of D and L.

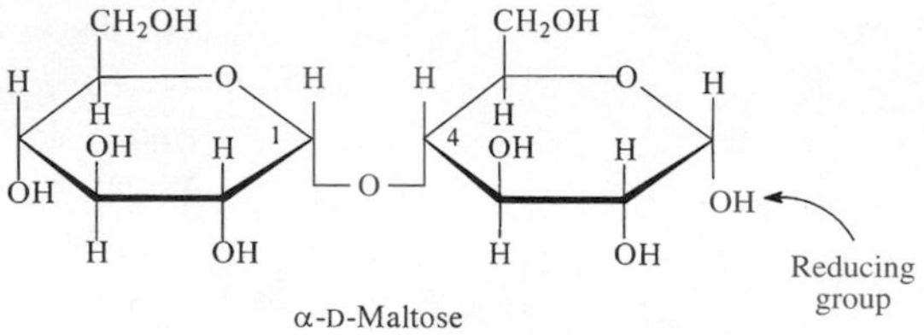

α-D-Maltose
O-α-D-Glucopyranosyl-(1→4)-α-D-glucopyranose

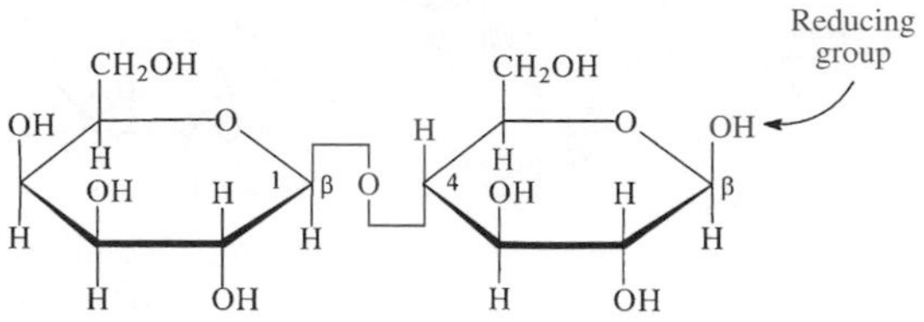

β-D-Lactose
O-β-D-Galactopyranosyl-(1→4)-β-D-glucopyranose

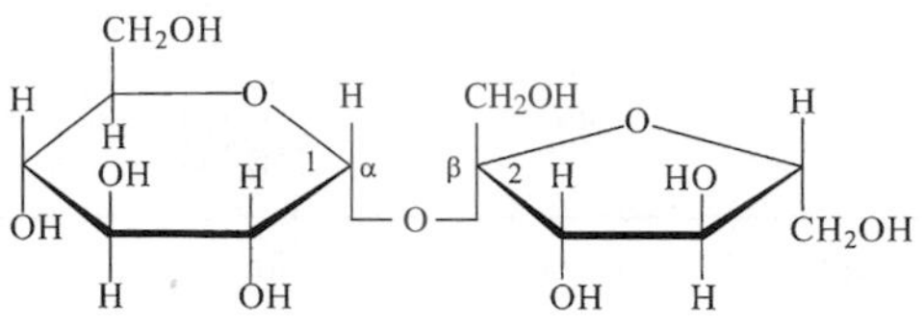

Sucrose
O-α-D-Glucopyranosyl-(1→2)-β-D-fructofuranose

Figure 23-4 Structural formulas of disaccharides.

chitin is the principal component of the exoskeleton of arthropods (insects and crustacea).

Starch and glycogen

Nearly all starches are composed of a mixture of amyloses and amylopectins. The relative proportions of these vary from approximately 20% amylose and 80% amylopectin in wheat and potato starch to nearly 100% amylopectin in the starch of waxy corn. On the other hand, a few corn starches are known to contain as much as 75% amylose. Both amylose and amylopectin consist of glucose residues, but their structures exhibit one significant difference. Amylose consists of one long unbranched chain of glucose units linked together by α-1,4-linkages, with only the terminal aldehyde group free. In amylopectin, most of the units are joined by α-1,4-links, but α-1,6-glycosidic bonds also exist every 24 to 30 residues, producing side chains. Amylopectin contains up to 1 million glucose residues. The structure of **glycogen** is similar to that of amylopectin, but branching is more extensive and occurs every 8 to 12 glucose residues. These branches enhance the solubility of glycogen and allow the glucose residues to be more readily mobilized. Glycogen is most abundant in the liver and also is found in skeletal muscle. The difference in structure between amylose and amylopectin is important in selection of the appropriate starch substrate for amylase determinations (see Chapter 20). The rate of hydrolysis is affected by structural differences in the starch.

Cellulose

Cellulose, an important structural polysaccharide in plants, is an unbranched polymer of glucose residues joined by β-1,4-linkages. The β-configuration facilitates the formation of long straight chains, producing fibers of high tensile strength. The β-1,4-linkages are not hydrolyzed by α-amylases. Because humans do not have cellulases, they are unable to digest vegetable fiber.

Glycoproteins

Many integral membrane proteins have oligosaccharides covalently attached to the extracellular region, forming glycoproteins. In addition, most proteins that are secreted, such as antibodies, hormones, and coagulation factors, are glycoproteins. The number of attached carbohydrate residues varies among proteins and constitutes 1% to 70% of the weight of the glycoprotein. The oligosaccharides are attached by *O*-glycosidic linkages to the side chain oxygen of serine or threonine residues. Alternatively, attachment is by *N*-glycosidic linkages to the side chain nitrogen of asparagine residues.

One biological function of the carbohydrate chains is to regulate the lifespan of proteins. For example, loss of sialic acid residues from the end of oligosaccharide chains on erythrocytes results in the removal of red blood cells from the circulation. Carbohydrates also have been implicated in cell-cell recognition and secretion and targeting of proteins to specific subcellular domains.

METABOLISM OF CARBOHYDRATES

Glucose is the primary energy source for the human body. After absorption (see Chapter 37), the metabolism of all hexoses proceeds according to the body's requirements. This metabolism results in (1) energy production by conversion to carbon dioxide and water, (2) storage as glycogen in the liver or triglyceride in adipose tissue, or (3) conversion to keto acids, amino acids, or protein.

The complete picture of intermediary metabolism of carbohydrates is complex and interwoven with the metabolism of lipids and amino acids. For details, readers should consult a biochemistry textbook.

Regulation of Blood Glucose Concentration

The concentration of glucose in the blood is regulated by a complex interplay of multiple pathways, modulated by several hormones. *Glycogenesis* is the name for the conversion of glucose to glycogen, the most important storage polysaccharide in liver and muscle. The reverse process, namely the breakdown of glycogen to glucose and other intermediate products, is termed *glycogenolysis*. The formation of glucose from noncarbohydrate sources, such as amino acids, glycerol, or lactate, is termed *gluconeogenesis*. The conversion of glucose or other hexoses into lactate or pyruvate is called *glycolysis*. Further oxidation to carbon dioxide and water occurs through the Krebs (citric acid) cycle and the mitochondrial electron transport chain coupled to oxidative phosphorylation, generating energy in the form of adenosine triphosphate (ATP). Oxidation of glucose to carbon dioxide and water also occurs through the hexose monophosphate shunt pathway, which produces the reduced form of nicotinamide-adenine dinucleotide phosphate (NADPH).

During a brief fast a precipitous decline in blood glucose concentration is prevented by breakdown of glycogen stored in the liver and synthesis of glucose in the liver. A small amount of glucose also may be derived from synthesis within the kidneys. These organs contain glucose-6-phosphatase, which is necessary to convert glucose-6-phosphate (derived from either gluconeogenesis or glycogenolysis) to glucose. Skeletal muscle lacks this enzyme, and muscle glycogen therefore cannot directly contribute to blood glucose. In cases of more prolonged fasting (>42 hours), gluconeogenesis accounts for essentially all the glucose production. In contrast, after a meal the absorbed glucose is converted to glycogen (for storage in the liver and skeletal muscle) or fat (for storage in adipose tissue).

Despite large fluctuations in the supply and demand of carbohydrates, the concentration of glucose in the blood is normally maintained within a narrow range by hormones that modulate the movement of glucose within the body. These include insulin, which decreases blood glucose, and the counterregulatory hormones (glucagon, epinephrine, cortisol, and growth hormone), which increase blood glucose concentrations (see Figure 23-5). Normal glucose disposal depends on (1) the ability of the pancreas to secrete insulin, (2) the ability of insulin to promote uptake of glucose into peripheral tissues, and (3) the ability of insulin to suppress hepatic glucose production. The major insulin target organs are the liver, skeletal muscle, and adipose tissue. These organs exhibit some differences in their responses to insulin. For example, insulin stimulates glucose uptake through a specific glucose transporter, GLUT4, in muscle and fat cells but not liver cells.

Regulation by Insulin of Blood Glucose Concentration

Insulin is a protein produced by the β-cells of the islets of Langerhans in the pancreas. Insulin was the first protein hormone to be sequenced, the first substance to be measured by radioimmunoassay (RIA), and the first compound produced by recombinant DNA technology for practical use. It is an anabolic hormone that stimulates the uptake of glucose into fat and muscle, promotes the conversion of glucose to

glycogen or fat for storage, inhibits glucose production by the liver, stimulates protein synthesis, and inhibits protein breakdown. The release and mechanism of action of insulin are more fully discussed in an expanded version of this chapter (pp 756-760).[26]

Human insulin (molecular mass 6000 D) consists of 51 amino acids in two chains (A and B) joined by two disulfide bridges, with a third disulfide bridge within the A chain.[21] Insulin from most animals is similar immunologically and biologically to human insulin, and in the past all insulin-dependent patients were treated with insulin purified from beef or pig pancreas. Virtually all patients are now treated with recombinant human insulin.

Preproinsulin, a protein of about 100 amino acids, is not detectable in the circulation under normal conditions because it is enzymatically cleaved and converted enzymes to proinsulin. Proinsulin is stored in secretory granules in the Golgi complex of the β-cells, where proteolytic cleavage to insulin and connecting peptide (C-peptide) occurs.[21] This posttranslational processing is catalyzed by two Ca^{2+}-regulated endopeptidases, namely prohormone convertase 1 and 2 (PC1 and PC2). The split proinsulin intermediates, split 32,33 proinsulin and split 65,66 proinsulin, are further hydrolyzed to insulin and C-peptide. At the cell membrane the insulin and C-peptide are released into the portal circulation in equimolar amounts. In addition, small amounts of proinsulin and intermediate cleavage forms enter the circulation.

Proinsulin, which has relatively low biological activity (approximately 10% of insulin potency), is the major storage form of insulin. Normally, only small amounts (about 3% of the amount of insulin, on a molar basis) of proinsulin enter the circulation. Because the hepatic clearance of proinsulin is only 25% of insulin clearance, the half-life of proinsulin is twofold to threefold longer and concentrations in the fasting state are approximately 10% to 15% of insulin concentrations.

C-peptide is devoid of biological activity but appears necessary to ensure the correct structure of insulin. Although insulin and C-peptide are secreted into the portal circulation in equimolar amounts, fasting concentrations of C-peptide are fivefold to tenfold higher than those of insulin due to the longer half-life of C-peptide (about 35 minutes). The liver does not extract C-peptide, which is removed from the circulation by the kidneys and degraded, with a fraction excreted unchanged in the urine.

Glucose transport

The molecular mechanism of insulin action is extremely complex. One of the fundamental effects of insulin is to increase glucose uptake into cells. The transport of glucose into cells is modulated by two families of proteins.[6] The intestinal sodium/glucose cotransporter promotes the uptake of glucose and galactose from the lumen of the small bowel and their reabsorption from the urine in the kidney. The

TABLE 23-1	Facilitative Human Glucose Transporters	
Name	Tissue	Function
GLUT1 (erythrocyte)	Wide distribution, especially brain, kidney, colon, and fetal tissues	Basal glucose transport
GLUT2 (liver)	Liver, β-cells of pancreas, small intestine, and kidney	Non–rate-limiting glucose transport
GLUT3 (brain)	Wide distribution, especially neurons, placenta, and testis	Glucose transport in neurons
GLUT4 (muscle)	Skeletal muscle, cardiac muscle, and adipose tissue	Insulin-stimulated glucose transport
GLUT5 (small intestine)	Small intestine, kidney, skeletal muscle, brain, and adipose tissue	Fructose transport (not glucose)
GLUT6	—	Pseudogene that is nonfunctional
GLUT7 (microsomal)	Liver	Release of glucose from endoplasmic reticulum

second family of glucose carriers, termed *facilitative glucose transporters (GLUT)*, is located on the surface of all cells (Table 23-1). These transporters are designated GLUT1 to GLUT7, based on the order in which they were identified. GLUT1 is widely expressed and provides many cells with their basal glucose requirement. GLUT1 in the blood-brain barrier and GLUT3 in neuronal cells provide the constant high concentrations of glucose required by the brain. GLUT2 is expressed in hepatocytes, β-cells of the pancreas, and basolateral membranes of intestinal and renal epithelial cells. It is a low-affinity, high-capacity transport system that allows non–rate-limiting movement of glucose into and from these cells. GLUT4 catalyzes the rate-limiting step for glucose uptake and metabolism in skeletal muscle, the major organ of glucose consumption. When circulating insulin concentrations are low, most of the GLUT4 is localized in intracellular compartments and is inactive. After a meal the pancreas releases insulin, which stimulates the translocation of GLUT4 to the plasma membrane, thereby promoting glucose uptake into skeletal muscle and fat. Insulin-stimulated glucose transport into skeletal muscle is impaired in individuals with type 2 diabetes mellitus, but the mechanism of the defect has not been established. GLUT6 is a pseudogene that is not expressed at the protein level. GLUT7 allows the diffusion of free glucose from the endoplasmic reticulum of gluconeogenic tissues.

Counterregulatory hormones

Several hormones have actions opposite those of insulin. These counterregulatory hormones are catabolic and increase hepatic glucose production initially by enhancing the breakdown of glycogen to glucose (glycogenolysis) and later by stimulating the synthesis of glucose (gluconeogenesis).[11] The body's initial response (within minutes) to low blood glucose is an increase in glucose production, stimulated by glucagon and epinephrine. With time (3 to 4 hours), growth hormone and cortisol increase glucose mobilization and decrease glucose use (see Figure 23-5). Evidence also suggests that glucose production by the liver is an inverse function of ambient glucose concentration, independent of hormonal factors (glucose autoregulation). The role of other hormones or neurotransmitters is not clear but appears

relatively unimportant. The multiple counterregulatory hormones exhibit both redundancy and hierarchy. Glucagon is the most important, and epinephrine becomes critical when glucagon is deficient. The other factors have lesser roles. (These hormones, briefly described in the text that follows, will be discussed further in Chapters 27, 37, and 41.)

Glucagon

Glucagon is a 29-amino-acid polypeptide secreted by the α-cells of the pancreas. The major target organ for glucagon is the liver, where it binds to specific receptors and increases intracellular adenosine 5′-monophosphate (AMP) and calcium. Glucagon stimulates the production of glucose in the liver by glycogenolysis and gluconeogenesis (Figure 23-5). In addition, glucagon enhances ketogenesis in the liver. A minor target organ for glucagon is adipose tissue, where the hormone increases lipolysis. Glucagon secretion is primarily regulated by plasma glucose concentrations, low and high plasma glucose concentrations being stimulatory and inhibitory, respectively. Long-standing diabetes mellitus results in an impaired glucagon response to hypoglycemia, increasing the incidence of hypoglycemic episodes. Stress, exercise, and amino acids also induce glucagon release. Insulin inhibits glucagon release from the pancreas and decreases glucagon gene expression, thereby decreasing its biosynthesis. Increased glucagon concentrations, secondary to insulin deficiency, are thought to contribute to the hyperglycemia and ketosis of diabetes.

Epinephrine

Epinephrine, a catecholamine secreted by the adrenal medulla, stimulates glycogen breakdown (glycogenolysis) and decreases glucose use, thereby increasing blood glucose concentrations. It also stimulates glucagon secretion and inhibits insulin secretion by the pancreas (see Figure 23-5). Epinephrine appears to play a key role in glucose counterregulation when glucagon secretion is impaired (for example, in cases of type 1 diabetes mellitus). Physical or emotional stress increases epinephrine production, releasing glucose for energy. Tumors of the adrenal medulla, known as *pheochromocytomas*, secrete excess epinephrine or norepi-

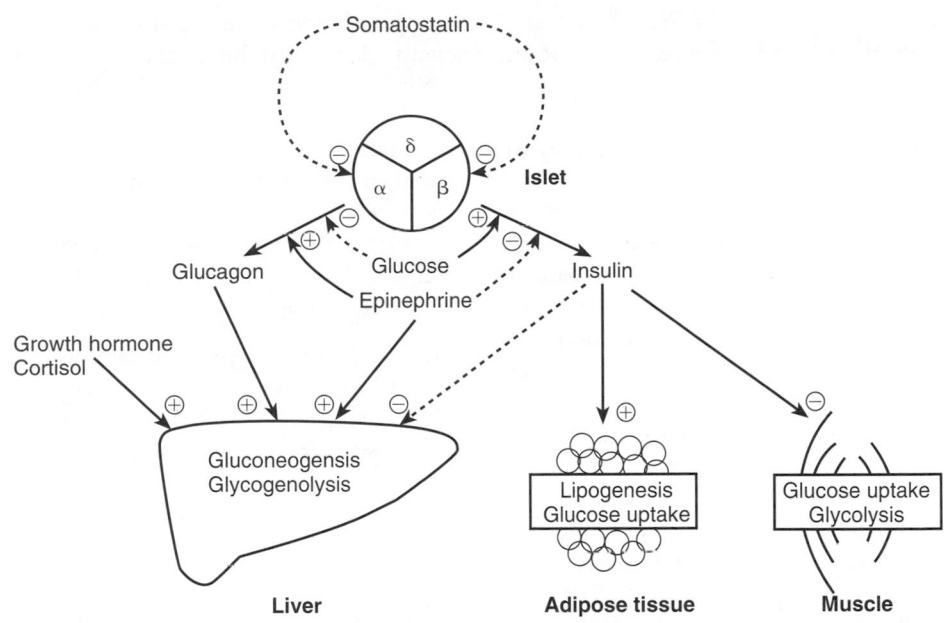

Figure 23-5   Hormonal regulation of blood glucose. Cortisol, growth hormone, and epinephrine also antagonize the effect of insulin. +, Stimulation; −, inhibition.

nephrine and produce moderate hyperglycemia as long as glycogen stores are available in the liver.

Growth hormone

Growth hormone is a polypeptide secreted by the anterior pituitary gland. It stimulates gluconeogenesis, enhances lipolysis, and antagonizes insulin-stimulated glucose uptake.

Cortisol

Cortisol, secreted by the adrenal cortex in response to adrenocorticotropic hormone (ACTH), stimulates gluconeogenesis and increases the breakdown of protein and fat. Individuals with Cushing's syndrome have increased cortisol concentrations because of a tumor or hyperplasia of the adrenal cortex and may become hyperglycemic. In contrast, those with Addison's disease demonstrate adrenocortical insufficiency because of destruction or atrophy of the adrenal cortex and may exhibit hypoglycemia.

Other hormones influencing glucose metabolism

Thyroxine

Thyroxine, secreted by the thyroid gland, is not directly involved in glucose homeostasis but stimulates glycogenolysis and increases the rate of gastric emptying and intestinal glucose absorption. These factors may produce glucose intolerance in thyrotoxic individuals, but such a person usually has a normal fasting plasma glucose concentration.

Somatostatin

Somatostatin, also called *growth hormone-inhibiting hormone*, is a 14-amino-acid peptide found in the gastrointestinal tract, hypothalamus, and the δ-cells of the pancreatic islets. Although somatostatin does not appear to have a direct effect on carbohydrate metabolism, it inhibits release of growth hormone from the pituitary. In addition, somatostatin inhibits secretion of glucagon and insulin by the pancreas, thus modulating the reciprocal relationship between these two hormones.

Measurement of Insulin, Proinsulin, C-Peptide, and Glucagon

A brief overview is provided in this chapter. Readers should consult an expanded version of this chapter (pp 761-766) for more details.[26] Insufficient data are available to recommend the general use of insulin, proinsulin, C-peptide, or glucagon measurements in individuals with diabetes mellitus. A point worth emphasis is that the diagnostic criteria for diabetes mellitus do not include measurements of hormones. However, although not clinically useful for diabetes cases, these hormone tests are useful for other disorders, such as hypoglycemia, suspected insulin overdose, and hormone-secreting tumors.

Insulin

The primary clinical application of insulin measurement is in the evaluation of individuals with fasting hypoglycemia (discussed in more detail later in this chapter). Insulin determination has been proposed as valuable in the identification of patients with diabetes mellitus who require insulin treatment and differentiation from those who can be controlled with diet alone. Large-scale epidemiological studies reveal that insulin concentrations predict the development of type 2 diabetes and may be useful in the prediction of diabetes susceptibility. In individuals with type 1 diabetes, plasma insulin concentrations have been used to provide an estimate of residual endogenous insulin secretion as a measure of β-cell activity. However, fasting or stimulated C-peptide measurements have replaced the insulin assay to make these distinctions.

Although insulin has been assayed for more than 35 years, no highly accurate, precise, and reliable procedure is available to measure the amount of insulin in a patient sample. RIA is the technique of choice for measurement of insulin in biological fluids. Enzyme-linked immunosorbent assay (ELISA) is used by a few laboratories and has lower imprecision than RIA.[24] Bioassays, although more physiologically relevant because they measure biological activity, are labor intensive and not widely used. Unless a patient's insulin requirements dramatically change, total endogenous insulin concentrations usually remain constant in those with type 1 diabetes, and repeated assays are not necessary.

The principle and general procedures of RIA are described in Chapter 10. Briefly, ^{125}I-labeled insulin competes with insulin in a patient sample for binding to an insulin-specific antibody immobilized on the walls of a polypropylene tube. The supernatant is decanted, and the bound ^{125}I is quantified in a gamma counter. The amount of insulin in the sample is established by comparison with a calibration curve obtained when the percent of radioactivity bound (B/T%) is plotted on logit-log graph paper against the concentration of the calibrators. Various commercial kits for insulin measurement are now available.

The term *immunoreactive insulin* is used in reference to assays that may recognize, in addition to insulin, substrates that share antigenic epitopes with insulin. Examples include proinsulin, proinsulin conversion intermediates (for example, split 32,33 proinsulin), and insulin derivatives produced by glycation or dimerization. Antisera raised against insulin show some cross-reactivity with proinsulin but not with C-peptide. Specificity is not a problem in healthy individuals because the low proinsulin concentrations do not appreciably affect the absolute values of insulin. In certain situations (for example, individuals with islet cell tumors or diabetes), proinsulin is present at high concentrations and direct assay of plasma may falsely overestimate the true insulin concentration. Monoclonal antibodies that are specific for insulin and do not measure proinsulin, although theoretically advantageous, are not superior to nonspecific assays. The presence of antibodies to insulin results in falsely increased or decreased (depending on the method used) insulin values.

The American Diabetes Association (ADA) appointed a task force to standardize the insulin assay.[24] Evaluation of unknown samples by 17 different laboratories revealed a wide range of insulin values, with interlaboratory variance of up to threefold.[24] Large differences were observed even among laboratories using the same assays. Use of a common calibrator did not decrease variance among laboratories. Assay coefficients of variation (CVs) ranged from 2% to 30%, with ELISAs exhibiting the best precision. Certain characteristics of some assays, including commercial kits, were unacceptable. The task force judged available proficiency and certification programs for insulin to be inadequate and recommended the establishment of a central laboratory to provide certification for insulin assays. Complete interlaboratory standardization was deemed neither practical nor universally acceptable. The ADA recommendations[24] for analysis of insulin are as follows:

1. Each laboratory should carefully evaluate its insulin assay to ensure acceptable assay performance.
2. Each laboratory should compare the performance of its assay with others, using common calibrators and unknown samples.
3. Because assay performance may change with time or new reagents or equipment, performance characteristics must be periodically remeasured.

Reference intervals vary with the specificity of the assay. After an overnight fast, insulin concentrations in healthy, normal, nonobese individuals range from 2 to 25 μIU/mL (12 to 150 pmol/L). More specific assays that have minimal cross-reactivity with proinsulin reveal a fasting plasma insulin concentration of less than 9 μIU/mL (60 pmol/L). Concentrations up to 200 μIU/mL can be reached during a glucose tolerance test. Fasting insulin concentrations are higher in obese, nondiabetic individuals and lower in trained athletes.

Proinsulin

High proinsulin concentrations are usually noted in individuals with benign or malignant β-cell tumors of the pancreas. Most of them have increased insulin, C-peptide, and proinsulin concentrations, but occasionally only proinsulin is increased. Despite its low biological activity, proinsulin may be sufficiently increased to produce hypoglycemia. In addition, a rare form of familial hyperproinsulinemia caused by impaired conversion to insulin has been described. Measurement of proinsulin can help determine the extent of proinsulin-like material that cross-reacts in an insulin assay. Some individuals with type 2 diabetes demonstrate increased proportions of proinsulin and proinsulin conversion intermediates; high concentrations are associated with cardiovascular risk factors. Even relatively mild **hyperglycemia** produces hyperproinsulinemia, with concentrations exceeding 40% of insulin concentration in those with type 2 diabetes. Increased proinsulin concentrations also may be detected in individuals with chronic renal failure, cirrhosis, or hyperthyroidism.

Accurate measurement of proinsulin has been difficult for the following reasons:

1. The blood concentrations are low.
2. Antibody production is difficult.

3. Most antisera cross-react with insulin and C-peptide, which are present in much higher concentrations.
4. The assays measure intermediate cleavage forms of proinsulin.
5. Reference preparations of pure proinsulin were previously not readily available.

Older assays initially removed either insulin or C-peptide, then measured proinsulin with antibodies. The availability of biosynthetic proinsulin has resulted in the production of monoclonal antibodies that do not cross-react with insulin and provide reliable proinsulin calibrators and reference preparations. Even this assay, however, does not discriminate between split proinsulins, and the assay sensitivity is barely adequate for fasting normal subjects.

With one immunoassay, measurement with a monoclonal antibody to proinsulin gave a fasting range of 2.0 to 2.6 pmol/L, with a maximum glucose-stimulated range of 8.5 to 11.3 pmol/L. The reference intervals are highly dependent on the method of analysis, degree of cross-reactivity of the antisera, and purity of proinsulin calibrators. Each laboratory should establish its own reference intervals.

C-Peptide

Measurement of C-peptide offers some advantages over insulin measurement. Because hepatic metabolism is negligible, C-peptide concentrations are better indicators of β-cell function than is peripheral insulin concentration. Furthermore, C-peptide assays do not measure exogenous insulin and do not cross-react with insulin antibodies, which interfere with the insulin immunoassays.

The primary indication for measurement of C-peptide is the evaluation of fasting hypoglycemia. Some individuals with insulin-producing β-cell tumors, particularly if hyperinsulinism is intermittent, may exhibit increased C-peptide concentrations with normal insulin concentrations. When hypoglycemia is due to surreptitious insulin injection, insulin concentrations are high but C-peptide concentrations are low; this difference occurs because C-peptide is not found in commercial insulin preparations, and exogenous insulin suppresses β-cell function.

Basal or stimulated (by glucagon or glucose) C-peptide concentrations can provide an estimate of an individual's insulin secretory capacity and rate. Although valuable in clinical research, C-peptide measurement plays a negligible role in routine management of patients with diabetes.

Measurement of C-peptide can be used to monitor individual responses to pancreatic surgery. C-peptide should be undetectable after a radical pancreatectomy and should increase after a successful pancreas or islet-cell transplant.

C-peptide assays do not react with antiinsulin antibodies. However, several methodological problems produce large between-method variations. These difficulties include variable specificity among different antisera, variable cross-reactivity with proinsulin, and the type of C-peptide prepa-

ration used as a calibrator. A comparison, in the clinically relevant range, using four commercial kits and four commercial C-peptide antisera, yielded values ranging from 0.54 to 1.06 nmol/L on the same sample. A number of RIA methods have been described for the measurement of C-peptide, and several kits are commercially available.

Fasting serum concentrations of C-peptide in healthy people range from 0.78 to 1.89 ng/mL (0.25 to 0.6 nmol/L). After stimulation with glucose or glucagon, values range from 2.73 to 5.64 ng/mL (0.9 to 1.87 nmol/L), three to five times the prestimulation value. Urinary C-peptide is usually in the range of 74 ± 26 μg/L.

Glucagon

Extremely high concentrations of glucagon are present in individuals with glucagonomas, which are tumors of the α-cells of the pancreas. Individuals with this type of tumor frequently experience weight loss, necrolytic migratory erythema, diabetes mellitus, stomatitis, and diarrhea. Most tumors have metastasized at the time of diagnosis. Low glucagon concentrations are associated with chronic pancreatitis and long-term sulfonylurea therapy.

A competitive RIA is available to measure glucagon.[26] With it an ^{125}I-labeled glucagon competes with glucagon in the patient specimen for binding to polyclonal glucagon antibody. Bound glucagon is separated from free glucagon with polyethylene glycol (PEG) and a second antibody. Bound radioactivity for the specimen is compared with that of glucagon calibrators. The calibrator values are assigned at the manufacturer by use of the World Health Organization (WHO) Glucagon International Standard (69/194).

Fasting plasma concentrations of glucagon vary from 70 to 180 ng/L (20 to 52 pmol/L). Values up to 500 times the upper reference limit may be found in individuals with autonomously secreting α-cell neoplasms.

■ DIABETES MELLITUS

Diabetes mellitus is a group of metabolic disorders of carbohydrate metabolism in which glucose is underutilized, producing hyperglycemia. Some individuals may experience acute life-threatening hyperglycemic episodes, such as ketoacidosis or hyperosmolar coma. As the disease progresses, individuals are at increased risk for the development of specific complications, including retinopathy leading to blindness, renal failure, neuropathy (nerve damage), and atherosclerosis.[19] The latter condition may result in stroke, gangrene, or coronary artery disease.

The prevalence of diabetes is unknown. The most recent published information is from the Third National Health and Nutrition Examination Survey, 1988 to 1994.[13] Nearly 10.2 million people in the United States were identified by a physician as having diabetes. With ADA criteria, the prevalence of undiagnosed diabetes was 5.4 million, yielding a total of more than 15 million.

The prevalence of diabetes mellitus increases with age, and approximately half of all cases occur in individuals older than 55 years. A racial predilection also exists, and by 65 years of age, 33%, 25%, and 17% of Hispanics, blacks, and whites, respectively, in the United States have diabetes mellitus. In 1997, diabetes mellitus was estimated to be responsible for $98 billion in health-care expenditures in the United States.[3] The direct costs were more than $44 billion, with 62% of that spent on patients admitted to hospitals. Indirect costs were $54 billion, 31% of which was due to the estimated 150,000 deaths annually from the disease. In fact, American women are twice as likely to die from diabetes mellitus as from breast cancer. Approximately one in seven health-care dollars is spent on individuals with diabetes mellitus.

Classification

Diabetes was initially diagnosed by the oral glucose tolerance test (OGTT). In 1979 a work group of the National Diabetes Data Group[20] proposed modified criteria for diagnosis. This classification scheme recognized two major forms of diabetes—type I (insulin-dependent) diabetes mellitus (IDDM) and type II (non–insulin-dependent) diabetes mellitus (NIDDM).[20] The terms *juvenile-onset diabetes* and *adult-onset diabetes* were abolished. To base the classification on etiology rather than treatment, in 1995 the ADA established a workgroup to reexamine the classification and diagnosis of diabetes mellitus. The revised classification, published in 1997,[1] eliminates the terms *insulin-dependent diabetes mellitus* and *non-insulin-dependent diabetes mellitus,* which now are termed *type 1 diabetes* and *type 2 diabetes,* respectively (Table 23-2). Another significant change is the elimination of the categories of previous abnormality of glucose tolerance and potential abnormality of glucose tolerance.

TABLE 23-2	Classification of Diabetes Mellitus and Other Categories of Glucose Intolerance

Type 1 diabetes
  Immune mediated
  Idiopathic
Type 2 diabetes
Other specific types of diabetes
Gestational diabetes mellitus (GDM)
Impaired glucose tolerance (IGT)
Impaired fasting glucose (IFG)

From the American Diabetes Association: Report of the expert committee on the diagnosis and classification of diabetes mellitus. Diabetes Care 1997; 20:1183-1201.

Type 1 diabetes mellitus

Type 1 diabetes mellitus was formerly known as insulin-dependent diabetes mellitus (IDDM), type I, or juvenile-onset diabetes. Approximately 5% to 10% of all individuals with diabetes mellitus have type 1 diabetes. Symptoms (for example, polyuria, polydipsia, and rapid weight loss) usually present acutely; diabetic individuals have insulinopenia (a deficiency of insulin) because of loss of pancreatic islet β-cells and depend on insulin to sustain life and prevent ketosis. Most individuals have antibodies that identify an autoimmune process (see later discussion); some have no evidence of autoimmunity and are classified as *type 1 idiopathic.* The peak incidence of this disease is in childhood and adolescence. Approximately 75% acquire the disease before 30 years of age, but the onset in the remaining percentage of individuals may occur at any age. Age at presentation is not a criterion for classification.

Type 2 diabetes mellitus

Type 2 diabetes mellitus, formerly non–insulin-dependent diabetes mellitus (NIDDM), type II, or adult-onset diabetes, comprises approximately 90% of all individuals with diabetes. Individuals have minimal symptoms, are not prone to ketosis, and do not depend on insulin to prevent ketonuria. Insulin concentrations may be normal, decreased, or increased, and most people with this form of diabetes have impaired insulin action. Obesity is commonly associated with the condition, and weight loss alone frequently ameliorates the hyperglycemia. However, many individuals with type 2 diabetes may require dietary manipulation, an oral hypoglycemic agent, or insulin to control hyperglycemia. The disease usually develops after 40 years of age, but type 2 diabetes may occur in young people, particularly those who are obese.

Other specific types of diabetes mellitus

This subclass includes uncommon individuals in whom hyperglycemia is due to a specific underlying disorder, such as genetic defects of β-cell function; genetic defects in insulin action; disease of the exocrine pancreas; endocrinopathies (for example, Cushing's disease, acromegaly, glucagonoma); the administration of hormones or drugs known to induce β-cell dysfunction (for example, dilantin, pentamidine) or impair insulin action (for example, glucocorticoids, thiazides, β-adrenergics); infections; uncommon forms of immune-mediated diabetes; or other genetic syndromes (for example, Down's, Klinefelter's, porphyria; see ADA[1] for a detailed list). This category was formerly termed *secondary diabetes.*

Impaired glucose tolerance

Impaired glucose tolerance is diagnosed in people who have fasting blood glucose concentrations less than those required for a diagnosis of diabetes mellitus but have plasma glucose response during the OGTT between normal and diabetic.

An OGTT is required to assign an individual to this class. Development of overt diabetes occurs at a rate of 1% to 5% per year, but a large proportion of cases spontaneously revert to normal glucose tolerance. Microvascular disease is quite rare in this group, and individuals usually do not experience the renal or retinal complications of diabetes. An increased prevalence of atherosclerotic disease is reported, but a consensus has not been reached and the predictive risk value for a given individual is limited.

Impaired fasting glucose

This new category is analogous to impaired glucose tolerance but is diagnosed by a *fasting* glucose concentration between normal and diabetic. It is a metabolic stage between normal glucose homeostasis and diabetes. As with impaired glucose tolerance, individuals with impaired fasting glucose are at increased risk for the development of diabetes and cardiovascular disease.

Gestational diabetes mellitus

The condition known as **gestational diabetes mellitus (GDM)** is defined as glucose intolerance with onset or first recognition during pregnancy; that is, diabetic women who become pregnant are not included in this category. Estimates of the frequency of abnormal glucose tolerance during pregnancy range from 1% to 20%, but the true incidence of GDM is probably 3% to 5%. In the United States, about 135,000 women with GDM give birth each year, and as many as 50% may remain unidentified. Women with GDM are at increased risk for the subsequent development of diabetes mellitus. The reported incidence rates range from 19% to 87% for diabetes plus impaired glucose tolerance, and 6% to 62% for diabetes alone.

Pathogenesis of Type 1 Diabetes Mellitus

Type 1 diabetes mellitus results from a cellular-mediated autoimmune destruction of the insulin-secreting cells of pancreatic β-cells (see Chapter 37).[5] The α, δ, and other islet cells are preserved. The islet cells have a chronic mononuclear cell infiltrate, called *insulitis*. The autoimmune process leading to type 1 diabetes begins years before the clinical presentation, and an 80% to 90% reduction in the volume of the β-cells is required to induce symptomatic type 1 diabetes. The rate of islet cell destruction is variable and usually more rapid in children than in adults.

Antibodies

The most practical markers of β-cell autoimmunity are circulating antibodies that can be detected in the serum years before the onset of hyperglycemia.[5] The most important antibodies are islet cell cytoplasmic antibodies (ICA), insulin autoantibodies (IAA), and antibodies to glutamic acid decarboxylase (anti-GAD).

ICAs react with a sialoglycoconjugate antigen present in the cytoplasm of all endocrine cells of the pancreatic islets and are believed to lead to cell destruction. These antibodies are detected in the serum of 0.5% of normal individuals and 70% to 80% of those with newly diagnosed type 1 diabetes. The antibodies are detected by immunofluorescence microscopy, and the recent development of a reference material has significantly decreased interlaboratory variation.

IAAs are present in 50% of newly diagnosed type 1 diabetic individuals and 0.5% of nondiabetic individuals. The presence of both IAA and ICA in an individual confers a significantly higher risk of the development of type 1 diabetes than either antibody alone.

GAD is a 64-kD enzyme required for the production of the neurotransmitter γ-aminobutyric acid (GABA). Anti-GAD antibodies have been identified in individuals up to 10 years before the clinical onset of type 1 diabetes and are present in a high percentage of those with newly diagnosed diabetes. Anti-GAD antibodies also may help identify individuals with apparent type 2 diabetes who will subsequently progress to type 1. Several different assay formats have been used for the measurement of anti-GAD antibodies, including enzymatic immunoprecipitation assay, radiobinding assay, ELISA, immunofluorescence, and Western blotting. The Second International GADAb Workshop significantly reduced the considerable variability in anti-GAD measurement among laboratories. Assay sensitivities ranged from 36.5% to 76%, with the radiobinding assay exhibiting the highest sensitivity. Specificity was 90% for all the assays. A monoclonal antibody MICA 3 was suggested as a reference material. These developments should facilitate interpretation of data from multicenter trials to establish the clinical utility of anti-GAD antibodies.

Genetics

Susceptibility to type 1 diabetes is inherited, but the mode of inheritance is complex and has not been defined. It is a multigenic trait. The major locus is the major histocompatibility complex on chromosome 6, but at least 11 other loci on 9 chromosomes also contribute. The concordance rate between identical twins is approximately 30%, and approximately 95% of whites with type 1 diabetes express either HLA-DR3 or -DR4 histocompatibility antigens. However, up to 40% of the nondiabetic population also express these alleles. The risk of a sibling becoming diabetic is 1%, 5%, and 10% to 20% if the number of haplotypes shared is none, one, and two, respectively. However, only 10% of individuals with type 1 diabetes have an affected first-degree relative. The multiplicity of independent chromosomal regions associated with a predisposition to type 1 diabetes suggests that other susceptibility genes will be identified.

Environment

Various studies have indicated that environmental factors are involved in the initiation of diabetes. Viruses, such as rubella, mumps, and coxsackievirus B, have been implicated. Other environmental factors that have been suggested include chemicals and cow's milk. Autoimmunity to β-cells initiated by a viral protein (that shares amino acid sequence with a β-cell protein) or some other environmental insult seems likely. Genetic susceptibility and other host factors (for example, HLA type) determine the progression of the β-cell destruction.

Pathogenesis of Type 2 Diabetes Mellitus

At least two major identifiable pathological defects exist in individuals with type 2 diabetes.[27] One is a decreased ability of insulin to act on the peripheral tissues. This defect is called *insulin resistance* and is thought by many investigators to be the primary underlying pathological process. The other is β-cell dysfunction, which is an inability of the pancreas to produce sufficient insulin to compensate for the insulin resistance. Thus a relative deficiency of insulin occurs early in the disease, and an absolute insulin deficiency is present later in the disease. The debate over whether type 2 diabetes is primarily due to a defect in β-cell secretion, peripheral resistance to insulin, or both has raged for decades. However, data support the concept that insulin resistance is the primary defect, preceding the derangement in insulin secretion and clinical diabetes by as much as 20 years.[27] Despite the lack of consensus, type 2 diabetes mellitus clearly is an extremely heterogeneous disease, and no single cause can adequately explain the progression from normal glucose tolerance to diabetes. The fundamental molecular defects in insulin resistance and insulin secretion result from a combination of environmental and genetic factors.

Diabetogenes

That genetic factors contribute to the development of type 2 diabetes is widely acknowledged.[27] For example, the concordance rate for type 2 diabetes in identical twins approaches 100%. Moreover, type 2 diabetes is 10 times more likely to occur in an obese individual with a diabetic parent than in an equally obese individual without a diabetic family history. However, the mode of inheritance is unknown, and type 2 diabetes has been described as a "geneticist's nightmare." Many less common diseases (for example, cystic fibrosis or Duchenne's muscular dystrophy) are caused by mutations at a single locus. More common diseases, such as diabetes mellitus, schizophrenia, atherosclerosis, hypertension, and osteoporosis, are not inherited according to Mendelian rules. These conditions are genetically more complex, and multiple genetic factors interact with exogenous influences (such as environmental factors) to produce the phenotype.

Multiple factors complicate the search for **diabetogenes** in type 2 diabetes.[27] A variety of different approaches have produced several genes that are associated with type 2 diabetes. However, despite considerable investigative efforts to identify the genetic basis of type 2 diabetes

mellitus, genetic defects identified to date account for fewer than 5% of individuals with type 2 diabetes. Therefore the gene or genes causing the common forms of type 2 diabetes remain unknown. The known genes affect insulin secretion, participate in insulin action, or regulate body weight.

Environment

Environmental factors, such as diet and exercise, are important determinants in the pathogenesis of type 2 diabetes. Convincing evidence links obesity to the development of type 2 diabetes, but the association is complex. Although 60% to 80% of those with type 2 diabetes are obese, diabetes develops in fewer than 15% of obese individuals. In contrast, virtually all obese people, even those with normal carbohydrate tolerance, have hyperinsulinemia and are insulin resistant. Other factors, such as family history of type 2 diabetes (genetic predisposition), the duration of obesity, and the distribution of fat, also are important.

An inverse relationship exists between the level of physical activity and the prevalence of type 2 diabetes. The risk of type 2 diabetes decreases by 6% for every 500-kcal increase in daily energy expenditure. The mechanism of the protective effect of exercise is thought to be an increased sensitivity to insulin in skeletal muscle and adipose tissue.

Loss of β-cell function

The increased β-cell demand induced by insulin resistance is ultimately associated with a progressive loss of β-cell function that is necessary for the development of fasting hyperglycemia. The major defect is a loss of glucose-induced insulin release that is termed *selective glucose unresponsiveness.* Hyperglycemia appears to render the β-cells increasingly unresponsive to glucose (a condition called *glucotoxicity*), and the extent of dysfunction correlates with both the glucose concentration and the duration of hyperglycemia. Restoration of euglycemia rapidly resolves the defect. Other insulin secretory abnormalities in individuals with type 2 diabetes include disruption of the normal pulsatile release of insulin and an increased ratio of plasma proinsulin to insulin.

Insulin resistance

Insulin resistance is defined as a decreased biological response to normal concentrations of circulating insulin and is found in both obese, nondiabetic individuals and those with type 2 diabetes. Measuring insulin resistance in a routine clinical setting is difficult, and surrogate measures, namely fasting insulin concentration or the insulin response to glucose, are used to provide an indirect assessment of insulin function. A broad clinical spectrum of insulin resistance exists, ranging from normal blood glucose concentrations (although marked elevations in endogenous insulin) to hyperglycemia, despite large doses of exogenous insulin. Several rare clinical syndromes are associated with insulin resistance. The prototype is the type A insulin resistance syndrome, which is characterized by hyperinsulinemia, acanthosis nigricans, and ovarian hyperandrogenism.

Diagnosis of Diabetes Mellitus

The diagnosis of diabetes mellitus depends solely on the demonstration of hyperglycemia (Table 23-3). For type 1 diabetes, the diagnosis is usually easy because hyperglycemia appears abruptly, is severe, and is accompanied by serious metabolic derangements. Diagnosis of type 2 diabetes may be difficult because the hyperglycemia is often not severe enough for the individual to notice symptoms of diabetes. Nevertheless, the development of complications makes identification of people with the disease important.

The previously recommended diagnostic criteria were (1) classic symptoms of diabetes with unequivocal increase of plasma glucose, (2) fasting plasma glucose of 140 mg/dL or greater on more than one occasion, or (3) a 2-hour and one other postload glucose concentration of 200 mg/dL or greater during an OGTT.[20] These criteria were widely adopted but are imperfect. The OGTT is more sensitive than fasting glucose early in the course of type 2 diabetes, resulting in a lack of equivalence between the fasting and 2-hour glucose values. Virtually all individuals with fasting plasma glucose concentrations of 140 mg/dL or greater have 2-hour glucose values of 200 mg/dL or greater in an OGTT. In contrast, in individuals without previously identified diabetes, a fasting glucose of 140 mg/dL or greater is present in only 25% of those who have a 2-hour glucose value of 200 mg/dL or greater. To address these and other

discrepancies the diagnostic criteria have been revised[1] (see Table 23-3). The major modification is that the diagnostic threshold for fasting glucose has been lowered from 140 to 126 mg/dL. The lower cut-off value should result in earlier diagnosis of diabetes, with consequent earlier therapeutic intervention. Although accepted in the USA, the revised classification has not been implemented in Europe, where the glucose concentration 2 hours after oral ingestion of a glucose load is used (WHO criteria). The two methods do not yield identical results.[13]

Fasting plasma glucose concentrations

Fasting plasma glucose concentrations more than 126 mg/dL on more than one occasion are diagnostic of diabetes mellitus (see Table 23-3). The diagnosis of most cases of diabetes mellitus can be established with this criterion. However, some investigators believe that hyperglycemia may be a relatively late development in the course of type 2 diabetes, delaying the diagnosis and underestimating the prevalence of diabetes mellitus in the population. Complications of diabetes, such as retinopathy, proteinuria, and neuropathy, are present in approximately 30% of individuals at clinical diagnosis of type 2 diabetes. Estimations are that the onset of type 2 diabetes probably occurs at least 10 years before clinical diagnosis. Population screening for diabetes, previously controversial, is now recommended.[1] Fasting glucose should be measured in all asymptomatic individuals at 45 years of age (or younger in those at increased risk), with subsequent follow-up testing every 3 years.

Oral glucose tolerance test

Serial measurement of plasma glucose before and after oral administration of a specific amount of glucose should provide a standard method to evaluate individuals and establish values for healthy and diseased subjects. Although more sensitive than fasting plasma glucose determinations, the OGTT is affected by multiple factors that result in poor reproducibility (see an expanded version of this chapter,[26] Table 24-6, p 770). Moreover, approximately 20% of OGTTs fall into the nondiagnostic category (for example, only one blood sample exhibiting increased glucose concentrations). The OGTT should be performed on two separate occasions before the results are considered abnormal.

The following conditions should be met in the performance of an OGTT:

- Discontinue, when possible, medications known to affect glucose tolerance.[29]
- Perform in the morning after 3 days of unrestricted diet (containing at least 150 g of carbohydrate/day) and activity.
- Perform the test after a 10- to 16-hour fast only in ambulatory subjects (bed rest impairing glucose tolerance), who should remain seated during the test without smoking cigarettes.

TABLE 23-3 **Criteria for the Diagnosis of Diabetes Mellitus**

Diabetes Mellitus
Any one of the following is diagnostic:*
1. Classic symptoms of diabetes and casual† plasma glucose concentration ≥200 mg/dL
2. Fasting‡ plasma glucose ≥126 mg/dL
3. A 2-hour postload plasma glucose concentration ≥200 mg/dL during the OGTT

Impaired Fasting Glucose
Fasting plasma glucose between 110 and 125 mg/dL
Impaired Glucose Tolerance
The following two criteria must be met:
1. Fasting plasma glucose <126 mg/dL
2. A 2-hour OGTT plasma glucose concentration between 140 and 199 mg/dL

From the American Diabetes Association: Report of the expert committee on the diagnosis and classification of diabetes mellitus. Diabetes Care 1997; 20:1183-1201.
OGTT, Oral glucose tolerance test.
*If positive, confirm by repeat testing on a subsequent day.
†Regardless of the time of the preceding meal.
‡No caloric intake for at least 8 hours.
    NOTE: Whole-blood glucose concentrations are approximately 10% to 15% lower than plasma concentrations.

Glucose tolerance testing should not be performed on hospitalized, acutely ill, or inactive individuals. The test should begin between 0700 and 0900 hours. Plasma glucose should be measured during fasting, then every 30 minutes for 2 hours after an oral glucose load. For nonpregnant adults the recommended load is 75 g, which may not be a maximal stimulus; for children, 1.75 g/kg, up to a 75-g maximum is administered. The glucose should be dissolved in 300 mL of water and ingested over 5 minutes.

An OGTT is rarely necessary for the diagnosis of diabetes mellitus and is not recommended for routine clinical use. Most diabetic individuals demonstrate increased fasting blood glucose concentrations. A fasting plasma glucose concentration less than 100 mg/dL or a random glucose concentration less than 140 mg/dL is sufficient to rule out the diagnosis of diabetes mellitus. An OGTT may be indicated in the following four situations:

1. Diagnosis of GDM (discussed later)
2. Diagnosis of impaired glucose tolerance
3. Evaluation of a patient with unexplained nephropathy, neuropathy, or retinopathy, with random glucose concentration less than 140 mg/dL
4. Population studies for epidemiological data

Gestational Diabetes Mellitus

Normal pregnancy is associated with increased insulin resistance, especially in the late second and third trimesters. Euglycemia is maintained by increased insulin secretion, with GDM developing in those women who fail to sufficiently augment insulin. Risk factors for GDM include a family history of diabetes in a first-degree relative, obesity, advanced maternal age, glycosuria, and selected adverse outcomes in a previous pregnancy (for example, stillbirth or macrosomia). The recommendations for screening and diagnosis were formulated in 1984 at the Second International Workshop-Conference on Gestational Diabetes Mellitus and refined at the Third and Fourth International Workshop-Conferences in 1990 and 1997, respectively.[23] Screening should be performed between 24 and 28 weeks of gestation on all pregnant women 25 years of age or older not identified as having glucose intolerance.[23] Women younger than 25 years of age should be screened if they are obese, have family histories of diabetes in a first-degree relative, or are members of an ethnic/racial group with a high prevalence of diabetes.

Although GDM is usually asymptomatic and not life threatening to the mother, the condition is associated with an increased incidence of neonatal morbidity, including hypocalcemia, hypoglycemia, polycythemia, jaundice, and macrosomia.[23] The maternal hyperglycemia causes the fetus to secrete more insulin, resulting in stimulation of fetal growth and macrosomia. Recognition is important because therapy can reduce the perinatal morbidity and mortality. Maternal complications include a high rate of cesarean delivery and chronic hypertension. Mothers are at increased

risk of diabetes, predominantly type 2, reaching an incidence of 60% by 15 years after parturition.

Distinct from GDM is pregnancy in a woman with preexisting diabetes (~19,000 per year in the United States). This condition is associated with an increased incidence of congenital malformations, but meticulous glycemic control during the first 8 weeks of pregnancy can significantly decrease the risk of congenital malformations. Tight control results in an increased incidence of maternal hypoglycemia, which is teratogenic in animals but does not cause malformations in humans.

Screening for GDM is performed by glucose measurement in the plasma 1 hour after a 50-g oral glucose load administered without regard to the time of day or last meal (Table 23-4). Approximately 15% of patients have a 1-hour venous plasma glucose concentration of 140 mg/dL or greater and require a full diagnostic glucose tolerance test.

Diagnosis of GDM in North America is based on criteria established by the National Diabetes Data Group. A 100-g oral glucose load is administered in the morning after an overnight fast, and venous plasma glucose is measured during fasting and at 1, 2, and 3 hours. The criteria for diagnosis are different from those for nonpregnant individuals (see Table 23-4).[23] International agreement is lacking, and criteria proposed by the WHO, based on the 75-g OGTT, are frequently used outside North America. The WHO criteria are more sensitive and result in a higher proportion of pregnancies classified as GDM. Evidence exists that even mild maternal hyperglycemia currently accepted to be within the reference interval is associated with an increased incidence of congenital malformations and complications of pregnancy. After giving birth, women with GDM should be evaluated 6 to 12 weeks postpartum. If glucose concentra-

---

TABLE 23-4   **Screening and Diagnosis of Gestational Diabetes Mellitus**

Screening
1. Perform between 24 and 28 weeks of gestation on all pregnant women ≥25 years of age (or <25 years of age with one risk factor).
2. Administer 50-g oral glucose load without regard to time of day or time of last meal.
3. Measure venous plasma glucose at 1 hour.
4. If glucose is ≥140 mg/dL, perform glucose tolerance test.

Diagnosis
1. Perform in the morning after an 8- to 14-hour fast.
2. Measure fasting venous plasma glucose.
3. Administer 100 g of glucose orally.
4. Measure plasma glucose hourly for 3 hours.
5. At least two values must exceed the following:

Fasting	105 mg/dL
1 hour	190 mg/dL
2 hours	165 mg/dL
3 hours	145 mg/dL

6. If results are normal in a clinically suspect situation, repeat during the third trimester.

tions have returned to normal, glycemia should be assessed at a minimum of 3-year intervals.

Role of the Clinical Laboratory in Diabetes Mellitus

The clinical laboratory plays a vital role in both the diagnosis and management of diabetes mellitus. Some of the important parameters assayed are outlined in Table 23-5.

Diagnosis

Preclinical

Immune intervention therapy before the appearance of clinical symptoms may be able to delay the onset of type 1 diabetes or prevent its development. Detecting cases at this stage therefore may be beneficial. The ADA now recommends that first-degree relatives of individuals with type 1 diabetes be screened by measurement of immune-related

TABLE 23-5	Role of the Laboratory in Diabetes Mellitus
Diagnosis	
Preclinical	Clinical
Immunological markers	Blood glucose
Islet cell antibodies (ICA)	Oral glucose tolerance test
Insulin autoantibodies (IAA)	Urine ketones
Glutamic acid decarboxylase	Other (for example, insulin,
antibodies (GAD)	C-peptide, stimulation tests)
Protein tyrosine phosphatase	
antibodies (IA-2)	
Genetic markers (for example,	
HLA)	
Insulin secretion	
Fasting	
Pulses	
Response to a glucose chal-	
lenge	
Management	
Acute	Chronic
Glucose	Glucose
Blood	Blood (fasting/random)
Urine	Urine
Ketones	Glycated proteins
Blood	Glycated hemoglobin
Urine	Fructosamine
Acid-base status (pH, bicarbon-	Urinary protein
ate)	Urinary albumin excretion
Lactate	(microalbuminuria)
Other abnormalities related to	Proteinuria
cellular dehydration or	Evaluation of complications (for
therapy (for example, potas-	example, renal function, cho-
sium, sodium, phosphate,	lesterol, triglycerides)
osmolality)	Evaluation of pancreas trans-
	plant (C-peptide, insulin)

ICA, Islet cell cytoplasmic antibodies; *IAA,* insulin autoantibodies; *GAD,* antibodies to glutamic acid decarboxylase.

markers.[2] Screening by determination of HLA type is not currently warranted, except in research studies. A decrease in glucose-stimulated insulin secretion is the first functional abnormality in both type 1 and type 2 diabetes cases. Preliminary evidence in the offspring of individuals with type 2 diabetes suggests that hyperinsulinemia and an increased second-phase response to an intravenous glucose load occur before the onset of clinical diabetes. In addition, individuals who have family histories of type 2 diabetes and mild glucose intolerance demonstrate loss of normal pulsatile insulin secretion. These findings require further validation, and tests of insulin secretion are not currently recommended for routine clinical use.

Clinical

The diagnosis of diabetes is solely determined by the demonstration of hyperglycemia. Other assays, such as the OGTT, may contribute to the classification. Although other tests (for example, C-peptide and insulin concentrations) have been proposed to assist in the diagnosis and classification of the disease, they do not currently have a role outside research studies.

Management

Acute

The clinical laboratory plays an essential role in both diagnosis of and monitoring of therapy in individuals with diabetic ketoacidosis, hyperosmolar nonketotic coma, and hypoglycemia. A number of analytes are frequently measured to guide clinicians in treatment regimens to restore euglycemia and correct other metabolic disturbances. The metabolic abnormalities of these conditions are beyond the scope of this textbook, and interested readers are referred to a standard textbook of medicine for detailed information.

Chronic

The Diabetes Control and Complications Trial (DCCT)[10] and the United Kingdom Prospective Diabetes Study (UKPDS)[31] demonstrated a correlation between blood glucose concentrations and the development of long-term complications of diabetes. Measurement of glucose and glycated proteins provides an index of short- and long-term glycemic control, respectively. The detection and monitoring of complications are achieved by assaying of urea, creatinine, urinary albumin excretion (microalbuminuria), and serum lipids. The success of newer therapies, such as islet cell or pancreas transplantation, can be monitored by measurement of serum C-peptide or insulin concentrations.

■ HYPOGLYCEMIA

Hypoglycemia is a blood glucose concentration below the fasting value, but definition of a specific limit is difficult.[28] A transient decline may occur 1.5 to 2 hours after a meal, and a plasma glucose concentration as low as 50 mg/dL may be observed 2 hours after ingestion of an oral glucose load. Similarly, extremely low fasting blood glucose values may be occasionally noted without symptoms or evidence of underlying disease.

Symptoms of hypoglycemia vary among individuals, and none is specific. Epinephrine produces the classic signs and symptoms of hypoglycemia, namely trembling, sweating, nausea, rapid pulse, lightheadedness, hunger, and epigastric discomfort. These autonomic symptoms may be noted in other conditions, such as hyperthyroidism, pheochromocytoma, or even anxiety. Although controversial, some investigators have proposed that a rapid decrease in blood glucose may trigger the symptoms even though the blood glucose itself may not reach hypoglycemic concentrations, whereas gradual onset to a similar glucose concentration may not produce symptoms.

The brain is completely dependent on blood glucose for energy production under physiological conditions, and approximately two thirds of glucose utilization in resting adults occurs in the central nervous system (CNS). Very low concentrations of plasma glucose (<20 or 30 mg/dL) cause severe CNS dysfunction. During prolonged fasting or hypoglycemia, ketones may be used as an energy source. The broad spectrum of symptoms and signs of CNS dysfunction range from headache, confusion, blurred vision, and dizziness, to seizures, loss of consciousness, and even death; these symptoms are known as *neuroglycopenia*. Restoration of plasma glucose usually produces a prompt recovery, but irreversible damage may occur.

The age of onset of hypoglycemia is a convenient way to classify the disorder, but some overlap occurs among the various groups. For example, some glycogen storage disorders may arise in the third decade of life and hormone deficiencies occur in childhood.

Hypoglycemia in Neonates and Infants

Neonatal blood glucose concentrations are much lower than those of adults (mean ~35 mg/dL) and decline shortly after birth when liver glycogen stores are depleted. Glucose concentrations as low as 30 mg/dL in a term infant and 20 mg/dL in a premature infant may occur without clinical evidence of hypoglycemia. The more common causes of hypoglycemia in the neonatal period include prematurity, maternal diabetes, GDM, and maternal toxemia (for a review, see Haymond[14]). These are usually transient. Hypoglycemia with onset in early infancy is usually less transitory and may be due to inborn errors of metabolism or ketotic hypoglycemia; this type of hypoglycemia usually develops after fasting or a febrile illness.

Fasting Hypoglycemia in Adults

Hypoglycemia may result from a decreased rate of hepatic glucose production or an increased rate of glucose utilization. Symptoms suggestive of hypoglycemia are fairly common, but hypoglycemic disorders are rare. However, true hypoglycemia usually indicates serious underlying disease and may be life threatening. An exact threshold for the establishment of hypoglycemia is not always possible, and values as low as 30 mg/dL may be encountered in healthy, premenopausal women after a 72-hour fast. Symptoms usually begin at plasma glucose concentrations below 55 mg/dL, and impairment of cerebral function begins when glucose is less than 50 mg/dL.

The classic diagnostic test is the 72-hour fast, which should be conducted in a hospital.[28] During the fast the patient should be allowed a liberal intake of calorie-free and caffeine-free fluids. Samples should be drawn for analysis of plasma glucose, insulin, C-peptide, and proinsulin every 6 hours. When plasma glucose concentration is 60 mg/dL or less, analysis should be performed every 1 to 2 hours. The fast should be concluded when plasma glucose concentration falls to 45 mg/dL or less, the patient exhibits signs or symptoms of hypoglycemia, or after 72 hours. Most patients with true hypoglycemia show an abnormally low value within 12 hours of beginning a fast. Women exhibit significantly lower glucose concentrations than men. Low plasma glucose alone is not sufficient to establish the diagnosis, and the absence of signs or symptoms of hypoglycemia during the fast excludes the diagnosis of a hypoglycemic disorder.

More than 100 causes of hypoglycemia have been reported. Drugs are the most prevalent cause, and a wide variety, including propranolol, salicylates, and disopyramide, can produce hypoglycemia. Oral hypoglycemic agents, which have long half-lives (35 hours for chlorpropamide), are the most frequent cause of drug-induced hypoglycemia and may be directly measured in blood or urine. Surreptitious administration of insulin can be detected by a discovery of low C-peptide concentrations with increased insulin concentrations.

Ethanol produces hypoglycemia by inhibiting gluconeogenesis, and this inhibition is aggravated by malnutrition (low glycogen stores) in individuals with chronic alcoholism. Individuals with hepatic failure (for example, viral hepatitis, toxins) have impaired gluconeogenesis or glycogen storage, which may result in hypoglycemia. Because decreased hepatic glucose production requires dysfunction of more than 80% of the liver, growth hormone (especially with coexistent ACTH deficiency), glucocorticoids, thyroid hormone, or glucagon may also produce hypoglycemia. Although a deficiency of glucocorticoids (for example, Addison's disease) is most consistently associated with hypoglycemia, most glucocorticoid-deficient adults are not hypoglycemic. Hormonal deficiency causes hypoglycemia in children more frequently than in adults.

Demonstration of a low plasma glucose concentration in the presence of a high plasma insulin value is highly suggestive of an insulin-producing pancreatic islet cell tumor. Because a wide range of insulin concentrations are found in healthy people, absolute hyperinsulinemia occurs in fewer than 50% of individuals with insulinomas. Serum insulin concentrations inappropriately high for concurrent plasma glucose values denote autonomous insulin secretion. Provocative tests (glucagon, tolbutamide, or calcium) or suppression tests (infusion of insulin and measurement of C-peptide), although strongly recommended in the past, are generally not necessary.

Nonpancreatic neoplasms that cause hypoglycemia are often extremely large mesenchymal neoplasms that appear to overutilize glucose but may also have an inhibitory effect on glucose mobilization.

Hypoglycemia due to septicemia should be relatively easy to diagnose. The mechanism is not well defined, but depleted glycogen stores, impaired gluconeogenesis, and increased peripheral use of glucose may all be contributing factors. Glucose tolerance is commonly depressed in individuals with renal disease, and hypoglycemia may occur in those with end-stage renal failure.

Some conditions that produce fasting hypoglycemia are readily apparent, but others require a lengthy diagnostic workup. Once fasting hypoglycemia is demonstrated, specific tests should be performed to establish the underlying etiology. The OGTT is not an appropriate study for evaluation of a patient suspected of having hypoglycemia.

Postprandial Hypoglycemia

Drugs, antibodies to insulin or the insulin receptor, and inborn errors (for example, fructose-1,6-diphosphatase deficiency) may produce hypoglycemia in the postprandial (fed) state.[15] Reactive hypoglycemia (also referred to as *functional hypoglycemia*), may also produce hypoglycemia in the postprandial state. Many commentaries and editorials have been published regarding the existence of reactive hypoglycemia.[15] The general consensus is that no scientific evidence supports the existence of "functional hypoglycemia." For individuals with vague symptoms after food ingestion the proposed terms include *idiopathic reactive hypoglycemia*[15] or *idiopathic postprandial syndrome.*[28]

At the Third International Symposium on Hypoglycemia, reactive hypoglycemia was defined as a clinical disorder in which the individual has postprandial symptoms that occur in everyday life and are accompanied by a blood glucose concentration less than 45 to 50 mg/dL, as determined by a specific glucose measurement on capillary or arterialized venous blood. Individuals complain of autonomic symptoms occurring approximately 1 to 3 hours after eating and seem to obtain relief, lasting 30 to 45 minutes, by eating. Rarely, these symptoms are due to low blood glucose concentrations (for example, diabetes mellitus, gastrointestinal dysfunction, or hormonal deficiency states). Most of these individuals have postprandial autonomic symptoms without neuroglycopenia in the postprandial state. Some experts in the field state that true hypoglycemic disorders are not solely charac-

terized by autonomic symptoms.[28] The OGTT should not be used in the diagnosis of reactive hypoglycemia.

Postprandial hypoglycemia is infrequent, and the demonstration of hypoglycemia during spontaneously occurring symptomatic episodes is necessary to establish the diagnosis. If this demonstration is not possible, a 5-hour meal tolerance test can be performed. This test is preferable to a 5-hour glucose tolerance test in that the meal simulates the composition of a normal diet.

A diagnosis of hypoglycemia has also been used to explain a wide variety of disorders that appear unrelated to blood glucose abnormalities. These nonspecific symptoms include fatigue, muscle spasms, palpitations, numbness, tingling, pain, sweating, mental dullness, sleepiness, weakness, and fainting. Behavior abnormalities, poor school performance, and delinquency have been incorrectly attributed to low blood glucose concentrations. The widespread use of the insensitive and nonspecific 5-hour glucose tolerance test caused overdiagnosis of hypoglycemia that led the ADA to publish a statement to discourage the inappropriate use of the OGTT for the diagnosis of hypoglycemia. Important considerations are to reassure such patients that low blood glucose is not the cause of their symptoms and deal with specific abnormalities that might underlie patients' complaints or problems. A diagnosis of hypoglycemia should not be made unless a patient meets the criteria of Whipple's triad—low blood glucose concentration with typical symptoms alleviated by glucose administration. Demonstration of a normal plasma glucose concentration when the individual exhibits symptoms excludes the possibility of a hypoglycemic disorder.

Hypoglycemia in Cases of Diabetes Mellitus

Hypoglycemia frequently occurs in both type 1 and type 2 diabetic individuals.[11] Those using insulin experience approximately one to two episodes of symptomatic hypoglycemia per week, and severe hypoglycemia (that is, requiring assistance from others or associated with loss of consciousness) affects about 10% of this population per year. In individuals who practice intensive insulin therapy (for example, multiple injections or continuous subcutaneous insulin infusion), these figures are increased twofold to sixfold. Similarly, hypoglycemia occurs in those with type 2 diabetes (due to oral hypoglycemic agents or insulin) but is less frequent than in those with type 1 diabetes. Two pathophysiological mechanisms, discussed in the following sections, contribute to hypoglycemia in patients with diabetes.

Defective glucose counterregulation

Counterregulatory responses become impaired in individuals with type 1 diabetes, increasing the risk of hypoglycemia. The response of glucagon to hypoglycemia is impaired by an unknown mechanism early in the course of type 1 diabetes. Epinephrine secretory response to hypoglycemia becomes deficient later in the course of the disease. These defects are selective because other stimuli continue to elicit glucagon and epinephrine secretion. Glucose counterregulation does not appear to be markedly defective in individuals with type 2 diabetes.

Hypoglycemia unawareness

Up to 50% of individuals with long-standing type 1 diabetes do not experience neurogenic warning symptoms and are prone to more severe hypoglycemia. The mechanism is thought to be associated with a decreased epinephrine response to hypoglycemia. Intensively treated patients with type 1 diabetes require lower plasma glucose concentrations to elicit symptoms of hypoglycemia.

■ MEASUREMENT OF GLUCOSE IN BODY FLUIDS

Many analytical procedures are used to measure blood glucose concentrations. In the past, analyses were often performed with relatively nonspecific methods that resulted in falsely increased values. Almost all techniques commonly used are now enzymatic (for example, hexokinase or glucose oxidase), and older methods, such as photometric or oxidation-reduction techniques, are rarely used. Results from a recent survey conducted by the College of American Pathologists (CAP) show that automated hexokinase methods are used in slightly more than half the participating laboratories. The extensive use of the hexokinase method is a reflection of the procedures adopted by the manufacturers of automated equipment. Glucose oxidase is the only other method that is widely used. It is also the most commonly used manual procedure. Reference to CAP surveys demonstrates that all the methods exhibit a CV less than 5% for glucose values on liquid control serum.

Specimen Collection and Storage

In individuals with normal hematocrits, fasting whole-blood glucose concentration is approximately 12% to 15% lower than plasma glucose. Although the glucose concentration in the water phase of red blood cells and plasma is similar (the erythrocyte plasma membrane being freely permeable to glucose), the water content of plasma (93%) is approximately 12% higher than that of whole blood. In most clinical laboratories, plasma or serum is used for most glucose determinations, whereas most methods for self-monitoring of glucose use whole blood. During fasting, the capillary blood glucose concentration is only about 2 to 5 mg/dL higher than that of venous blood. After a glucose load, however, capillary blood glucose concentrations are 20 to 70 mg/dL greater than concurrently drawn venous blood samples.

Glycolysis decreases serum glucose by approximately 5% to 7% per hour (5 to 10 mg/dL) in normal uncentrifuged coagulated blood at room temperature.[8] The rate of in vitro glycolysis is higher in the presence of leukocytosis or bacterial contamination. In separated, nonhemolyzed sterile serum, the glucose concentration is generally stable as long as 8 hours at 25 °C and up to 72 hours at 4 °C; variable stability is observed with longer storage periods. Plasma, removed from the cells after moderate centrifugation, contains leukocytes that also metabolize glucose, although cell-free sterile plasma has no glycolytic activity.

Glycolysis can be inhibited and glucose stabilized for as long as 3 days at room temperature by addition of sodium iodoacetate or sodium fluoride (NaF) to the specimen.[8] Fluoride ions prevent glycolysis by inhibiting enolase, an enzyme that requires Mg^{2+}. The inhibition is due to the formation of an ionic complex consisting of Mg^{2+}, inorganic phosphate, and fluoride ions; this complex interferes with the interaction of enzyme and substrate. Fluoride is also a weak anticoagulant because it binds calcium; however, clotting may occur after several hours, and a combined fluoride-oxalate mixture, such as 2 mg of potassium oxalate ($K_2C_2O_4$) and 2 mg of NaF per milliliter of blood, is advisable to prevent late clotting. Fluoride ions in high concentration inhibit the activity of urease and certain other enzymes; consequently, the specimens are unsuitable for determination of urea in procedures that require urease and for direct assay of some serum enzymes. $K_2C_2O_4$ causes a loss of cell water, thereby diluting the plasma. Samples collected in these tubes therefore should not be used for measurement of other analytes.

Although fluoride maintains long-term blood glucose stability, the rate of decline in the first hour after sample collection is not altered.[8] In routine analysis the use of a fluoride-containing tube is probably not necessary if plasma is separated from cells or glucose is measured within 60 minutes of blood collection. However, inhibitors of glycolysis are necessary in individuals with markedly increased leukocyte counts because differences of up to 65 mg/dL have been observed between glucose values with and without glycolytic inhibitors after 1 to 2 hours of contact with the blood cells.

Cerebrospinal fluid (CSF) may be contaminated with bacteria or other cells and should be analyzed for glucose immediately. If a delay in measurement is unavoidable, the sample should be centrifuged and stored at 4 °C or −20 °C.

In 24-hour collections of urine, glucose may be preserved by addition of 5 mL of glacial acetic acid to the container before the collection is begun. Other preservatives that have been proposed include 5 g of sodium benzoate per 24-hour specimen or chlorhexidine and 0.1% sodium nitrate (NaN_3) with 0.01% benzethonium chloride. However, these preservatives may be inadequate for urine specimens. Urine specimens should be stored at 4 °C during collection because they may lose as much as 40% of their glucose after 24 hours at room temperature.

Hexokinase Methods

Glucose is phosphorylated by ATP in the presence of hexokinase and Mg^{2+}. The glucose-6-phosphate formed is oxidized by glucose-6-phosphate dehydrogenase (G-6-PD) to 6-phosphogluconate in the presence of nicotinamide-adenine dinucleotide phosphate ($NADP^+$). The amount of reduced NADP (NADPH) produced is directly proportional to the amount of glucose in the sample and is measured by the change in absorbance at 340 nm. G-6-PD derived from yeast is used in the assay, with $NADP^+$ as the cofactor. NAD^+ is the cofactor if bacterial *(Leuconostoc mesenteroides)* G-6-PD is used, and the NADH produced is also measured at 340 nm. The reaction is as follows:

$$\text{Glucose} + \text{ATP} \underset{}{\overset{\textit{Hexokinase}}{\rightleftharpoons}} \text{Glucose-6-phosphate} + \text{ADP}$$

$$\text{Glucose-6-phosphate} \underset{}{\overset{\textit{G-6-PD}}{\rightleftharpoons}} \text{6-Phosphogluconate}$$

$$\begin{array}{cc} NADP^{\oplus} & NADPH + H^{\oplus} \\ (\text{or } NAD^{\oplus}) & (\text{or } NADH) \end{array}$$

A generally accepted reference method based on this principle has been developed and validated. Serum or plasma is deproteinated by the addition of solutions of barium hydroxide ($Ba[OH]_2$) and zinc sulfate ($ZnSO_4$). The clear supernatant is mixed with a reagent containing ATP, NAD^+, hexokinase, and G-6-PD, incubated at 25 °C until the reaction is complete, and NADH is measured. Calibrators and blanks are carried through the entire procedure, including the deproteination step.

Although highly accurate and precise, the reference method is too exacting and time consuming for routine use in a clinical laboratory. An alternative approach is to apply the reaction directly to serum or plasma and use a specimen blank to correct for interfering substances that absorb at 340 nm.

Either serum or plasma may be used. NaF, with an anticoagulant such as ethylenediaminetetraacetic acid (EDTA), heparin, oxalate, or citrate, may be used. Hemolyzed specimens containing more than 0.5 g of hemoglobin/dL are unsatisfactory because phosphate esters and enzymes released from red blood cells interfere with the assay. Other sources of interference include drugs, bilirubin, and lipemia (triglyceride ≥500 mg/dL causing a positive interference).

Absorbances of sample or calibrator reaction mixtures are measured after the reactions have continued to completion (equilibrium reaction). Although glucose concentrations may be directly calculated, based on the molar absorptivity of NADPH or NADH, inclusion of a set of calibrators is recommended to detect possible deterioration of enzymes, ATP, $NADP^+$, or NAD^+, all of which are unstable. Reagents may also contain substances that react with the coenzymes. Presence of these substances can be evaluated by measurement of the increase in absorbance observed in a reagent blank. The highest calibrator provides a check on the linearity of the response and adequacy of the enzyme reagent. The procedure is linear from 0 to 500 mg/dL. Glu-

cose concentrations that exceed 500 mg/dL should be diluted with isotonic saline and reassayed.

Also available are hexokinase procedures, in which indicator reactions produce colored products, enabling absorbance measurements in the visible range. An oxidation-reduction system containing phenazine methosulfate (PMS) and a substituted tetrazolium compound, 2-(*p*-iodophenyl)-3-*p*-nitrophenyl-5-phenyltetrazolium chloride (INT), is reacted with NADPH formed in the reaction. The reduced INT is colored, with maximal absorbance at 520 nm.

Glucose Oxidase Methods

The enzyme glucose oxidase catalyzes the oxidation of glucose to gluconic acid and hydrogen peroxide (H_2O_2), as follows:

$$\text{Glucose} + 2H_2O + O_2 \xrightarrow{\textit{Glucose oxidase}} \text{Gluconic acid} + 2H_2O_2$$

Addition of the enzyme peroxidase and a chromogenic oxygen acceptor, such as *o*-dianisidine, results in the formation of a colored compound that can be measured, as follows:

$$\underset{(\text{colorless})}{o\text{-Dianisidine} + H_2O_2} \xrightarrow{\textit{Peroxidase}} \underset{(\text{colored})}{\text{oxidized } o\text{-Dianisidine} + H_2O}$$

Glucose oxidase is highly specific for β-D-glucose. Because 36% and 64% of glucose in solution are in the α- and β-forms, respectively, complete reaction requires mutarotation of the α- to β-form. Some commercial preparations of glucose oxidase contain an enzyme, mutarotase, that accelerates this reaction. Otherwise, extended incubation time allows spontaneous conversion.

The second step, involving peroxidase, is much less specific than the glucose oxidase reaction. Various substances, such as uric acid, ascorbic acid, bilirubin, hemoglobin, tetracycline, and glutathione, inhibit the reaction (presumably by competing with the chromogen for H_2O_2), producing lower values. Some glucose oxidase preparations contain catalase as a contaminant; catalase activity decomposes peroxide and decreases the intensity of the final color obtained. Calibrators and unknowns should be simultaneously analyzed under conditions in which the rate of oxidation is proportional to the glucose concentration.

Glucose oxidase methods are suitable for measurement of glucose in CSF. Urine contains high concentrations of substances that interfere with the peroxidase reaction (such as uric acid), producing falsely low results. The glucose oxidase method therefore should not be used for urine. A method in which the urine is first pretreated with an ion-exchange resin to remove interfering substances has been described in the literature.

Some instruments use a polarographic oxygen electrode that measures the rate of oxygen consumption after the sample is added to a solution containing glucose oxidase. Because this measurement involves only the glucose oxidase reaction, interferences encountered in the peroxidase step are eliminated. To prevent formation of oxygen from H_2O_2 by catalase present in some preparations of glucose oxidase, H_2O_2 is removed by two additional reactions, as follows:

$$H_2O_2 + C_2H_5OH \xrightarrow{\text{Catalase}} CH_3CHO + 2\,H_2O$$

$$H_2O_2 + 2\,H^{\oplus} + 2\,I^{\ominus} \xrightarrow{\text{Molybdate}} I_2 + 2\,H_2O$$

The latter reaction is effective even when catalase activity has diminished on storage of reagents. The procedure can be applied directly to urine, serum, plasma, or CSF. However, this approach cannot be used for the determination of glucose in whole blood because blood cells consume oxygen.

In dry multilayer slide automated systems, glucose is measured by a glucose oxidase procedure. A 10-μL sample of serum, plasma, urine, or CSF is placed on a porous film on top of the layer containing the reagents. Glucose diffuses through the film and reacts with the reagents to produce a colored end product or dye. The intensity of this dye is measured through a lower transparent film by reflectance spectrophotometry. Advantages include small sample size, no liquid reagents, and improved stability on storage.

Glucose Dehydrogenase Method

The enzyme glucose dehydrogenase (β-D-glucose:NAD oxidoreductase, EC 1.1.1.47) catalyzes the oxidation of glucose to gluconolactone, as follows:

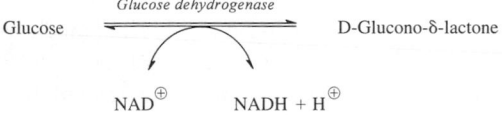

Mutarotase is added to shorten the time necessary to reach equilibrium. The amount of NADH generated is proportional to the glucose concentration. The reaction appears to be highly specific for glucose, shows no interference from common anticoagulants and substances normally found in serum, and provides results in close agreement with hexokinase procedures. The glucose dehydrogenase procedure is not widely used in the United States.

Self-Monitoring of Blood Glucose

Diabetic patients, especially those who require insulin, require careful monitoring to maintain control of blood glucose. This monitoring has become particularly important with the results of the DCCT[10] and the recommendation that such individuals use intensive insulin therapy regimens

to achieve nearly normal glycemia. These regimens include multiple daily insulin injections, insulin pumps, or continuous subcutaneous insulin infusion. Testing urine for glucose is not adequate for the monitoring of individuals on insulin therapy.[2]

Self-monitoring of blood glucose (SMBG), used by approximately 1 million diabetic patients, should be performed by all patients being treated with insulin. Optimum frequency of glucose monitoring varies among individuals, but SMBG is recommended three to four times a day for those with type 1 diabetes. SMBG is particularly important in the following cases:

1. Patients undergoing intensive insulin treatment programs (Their glucose levels should be measured at least four times a day.)
2. Hypoglycemia-prone patients, who may not experience the early warning signs
3. Avoidance of severe hyperglycemia, particularly in situations of increased risk (for example, medications that alter insulin secretion or action, intercurrent illness, or elderly people)
4. Patients with unstable diabetes
5. Pregnant women with diabetes

SMBG must not be used to diagnose diabetes mellitus, and its role in screening remains uncertain.

Individuals measure their own blood glucose concentrations and modify their insulin doses based on the glucose values obtained. Practically, individuals themselves cannot measure glucose by the laboratory methods described previously. However, a large number of simple test strips are now available that permit rapid and reasonably accurate measurements on a drop of whole blood.[2,17] Most strips use methods in which a dye is colored by the glucose oxidase-peroxidase chromogenic reaction. The reagents are combined in dry form on a small surface area of a test strip, and the colors that develop may be visually evaluated by comparison with a color chart or quantified in a specially designed meter. Visual reading with a color chart is not accurate enough for most clinical circumstances. At least 20 different blood glucose monitors are commercially available, and these vary in size, weight, calibration method, and other features.

Portable blood glucose monitors use reflectance photometry to measure the amount of light reflected from a test pad containing reagent. A sample of blood (from a fingerstick) is placed on the test pad, which is attached to a plastic support. Immediately after applying the sample, the operator presses a button on the meter to start the timer. An audible signal alerts the operator to remove excess blood from the strip by careful wiping or blotting. The test strip is then inserted into the meter. After a fixed time period the result appears on a digital display screen. A few devices use electrochemistry; the enzymatic reaction in an electrode incorporated on the test strip produces a flow of electrons. The current, which is directly proportional to the amount of glucose in the sample, is converted to a digital readout. Large variability exists among meters as to the test time (15 to 120 seconds) and reading range (40 to 400 mg/dL to 0 to 600 mg/dL). Calibration is automatic on some devices, whereas others use lot-specific code chips or strips. All manufacturers supply control solutions. Strict adherence to the instructions is necessary to obtain accurate results. The timing is critical, as is the wiping. Use of excessive force in wiping or blotting can decrease glucose concentrations by 50%.

The most common errors in SMBG are related to proper application, timing, and removal of the blood sample. The new generation of meters (for example, One Touch II, ExacTech, Accu-Check Easy, and Glucometer Encore) have eliminated the need for timing, blotting, and wiping. A drop of blood is applied to the reagent pad, the strip is inserted into the meter without wiping, and the results appear on a digital display screen 20 to 45 seconds later. A meter that automatically starts and times the test is a key component of such a device. Additional innovations include systems that abort testing if the sample volume is inadequate and built-in programs that simplify quality control. Some meters have memory that allows the instrument to store up to several hundred glucose readings that can be downloaded into a computer. The second-generation "no-wipe" devices exhibit improved accuracy and precision over the first-generation systems. Many such devices are also used in hospitals for point-of-care testing outside the central laboratory.

Several factors, including user variability and hematocrit, affect the accuracy and reproducibility of SMBG. These assays are unreliable at very high and very low glucose concentrations (<60 and >500 mg/dL). Because intramuscular volume depletion, a common feature of diabetic ketoacidosis, markedly increases blood viscosity, inaccurate low blood glucose results may be obtained. Test strips using whole blood result in glucose concentrations approximately 10% to 15% lower than plasma or serum. Adequate training is crucial for reliable performance of SMBG. The goal is to achieve variability of less than 10% at glucose concentrations of 30 to 400 mg/dL 100% of the time.[2]

Available SMBG devices, however, do not achieve the goal of the ADA for measurements within 15% of the reference measurement. Examination of a 1995 CAP survey revealed CVs ranging from 5% to 32%. An extensive 1994 study evaluated 11 different SMBG meters for reliability and accuracy.[17] With one exception the devices performed reasonably well. However, 19% to 48% of the analyses failed to achieve values of 15% or less of the value simultaneously determined by the laboratory. The failure rate for ±10% accuracy was 36% to 68%, and some variability existed among the different meters.

Minimally Invasive Monitoring of Blood Glucose

Fewer than 10% of individuals with diabetes routinely perform SMBG because it is painful and inconvenient. Since the 1960s, attempts have been made to develop a painless method for monitoring of blood glucose concentrations. Two general approaches have been used, namely implanted sensors and noninvasive monitoring.[16]

Implanted sensors

Several implanted biosensors have been developed and evaluated in both animals and humans. The most widely studied method is an electrochemical sensor that uses glucose oxidase. This sensor can be implanted intravenously or subcutaneously. Intravenous implantation in dogs for up to 3 months demonstrated the feasibility of this approach. Less success has been achieved with subcutaneous implants. Implantation of a needle-type sensor into the subcutaneous tissue induces inflammatory responses that alter the sensitivity of the device.

Noninvasive glucose monitoring

Noninvasive in vivo monitoring can be achieved with near-infrared spectroscopy. Devices of this type measure either the absorption or reflection of light from subcutaneous tissue. Although glucose has a specific absorption at 1035 nm, many substances interfere. An individually calibrated computer screens out interfering information to obtain the glucose result. The major problem with this technique is the lack of specificity for glucose. Another approach uses iontophoresis, in which an electrical current promotes movement of molecules across the skin. Analysis of glucose in transdermal fluid correlates well with serum glucose concentration in human subjects.

Continuous glucose sensing would be particularly important in the detection of hypoglycemia. Despite the obvious need for continuous or noninvasive monitoring, many technical challenges remain to be resolved.

Reference Intervals

Although glucose can be assayed by several different analytical procedures,[22] reference intervals do not vary significantly among methods. The following values are representative of virtually all glucose assays:

Sample Fasting Glucose (mg/dL)

Plasma/serum	
Adults	74 to 106 (4.5 to 5.9 mmol/L)
Children	60 to 100 (3.5 to 5.6 mmol/L)
Premature neonates	20 to 60 (1.1 to 3.3 mmol/L)
Term neonates	30 to 60 (1.7 to 3.3 mmol/L)
Whole blood	65 to 95 (3.5 to 5.3 mmol/L)
CSF	40 to 70 (60% of plasma value) (2.2 to 3.9 mmol/L)
Urine	
24 h	1 to 15 mg/dL (0.1 to 0.8 mmol/L)

No sex difference exists. Plasma glucose concentrations increase with age—fasting, approximately 2 mg/dL per decade; postprandial, 4 mg/dL per decade; and after a glucose challenge, 8 to 13 mg/dL per decade.

CSF glucose concentrations should be approximately 60% of the plasma concentrations and must always be compared with concurrently measured plasma glucose for adequate clinical interpretation.

Measurement of Glucose in Urine

Examination of urine for glucose is rapid, inexpensive, and noninvasive and can be used to screen large numbers of samples. However, urine glucose testing is not adequate for monitoring of glucose control in individuals with diabetes mellitus. The monitoring of urine glucose lacks sensitivity and specificity and provides no information about blood glucose concentrations below the renal threshold (usually 180 mg/dL). The older screening tests detect all sugars that reduce copper, producing a color and also react with reducing substances other than glucose. Specific tests for measurement of glucose that are quantitative or semiquantitative are widely available and have essentially replaced the nonspecific tests in adults. The copper reduction test is used to screen neonates and infants for inborn errors of metabolism that may result in the appearance of reducing sugars other than glucose (for example, galactose or fructose) in the urine.

Qualitative method for measurement of total reducing substances

Benedict's qualitative reagent contains cupric ion complexed to citrate in alkaline solution. Reducing substances convert cupric to cuprous ions, forming yellow cuprous hydroxide or red cuprous oxide. A convenient adaptation of the procedure is marketed in tablet form (Clinitest). The tablets contain anhydrous cupric sulfate, sodium hydroxide (NaOH), citric acid, and sodium bicarbonate ($NaHCO_3$). Five drops (0.25 mL) of urine are mixed with 10 drops of water in a test tube. One tablet is added, and the mixture is allowed to stand undisturbed for 15 seconds. It is then mixed and immediately observed for color. A chart provided by the manufacturer is used to interpret the result. Heat is generated by contact of NaOH and water. The initial reaction between citric acid and $NaHCO_3$ causes the release of carbon dioxide, which blankets the mixture and reduces contact with oxygen from the air to prevent reoxidation of cuprous ions. If large quantities (>2 g/dL) of sugar are present in the urine, the solution goes through the range of colors and returns to greenish-brown. This event may lead to an erroneous low reading unless the entire reaction is closely observed. Urine reacting this way should be retested with two drops of urine instead of five. False-positive interferences may be caused by other reducing substances that may appear in the urine.

Semiquantitative measurement of glucose in urine

Convenient paper test strips are commercially available from several manufacturers (Clinistix, Diastix, Chemstrip μG,

and Tes-Tape). All use the glucose-specific enzyme glucose oxidase in a chromogenic assay. For example, Clinistix has filter paper impregnated with glucose oxidase, peroxidase, and the dye o-tolidine. Other dyes, such as tetramethylbenzidine (TMB), can be used. The test end of the strip is moistened with freshly voided urine and examined after 10 seconds. A blue color develops if glucose is present at a concentration of 100 mg/dL or greater. The test is more sensitive for glucose than is the copper reduction test (Clinitest), which has a detection limit of 250 mg/dL.

False-positive results may be produced by contamination of urine with H_2O_2 or a strong oxidizing agent, such as hypochlorite (bleach). False-negative results may occur with large quantities of reducing substances, such as ketones, ascorbic acid, and salicylates. For routine examinations a negative result by the strip test is usually interpreted to mean that the urine specimen is negative for glucose.

Other strip tests (Keto-Diastix and Chemstrip μGK) are designed for the semiquantitative estimation of both glucose and ketone bodies. The glucose portion of the strip uses the glucose oxidase-peroxidase method. The hydrogen peroxide produced oxidizes iodide to iodine, yielding various intensities of brown that correspond to the concentration of glucose in the urine. The detection limit is 100 mg/dL.

Quantitative methods for determination of glucose in urine

Applications of various procedures for quantitative determination of glucose in urine were previously discussed in the section on the determination of glucose in body fluids. The hexokinase or glucose dehydrogenase procedures are recommended for greatest accuracy and specificity. Glucose oxidase procedures that depend only on the consumption of oxygen or production of H_2O_2 are also reliable. Glucose oxidase procedures that include the H_2O_2-peroxidase reaction are not acceptable.

■ KETONE BODIES

The development of ketosis requires changes in both adipose tissue and the liver. The primary substrates for ketone body formation are free fatty acids from adipose stores. Normally, long-chain fatty acids are taken up by the liver, reesterified to triglycerides, and stored in the liver or converted to very–low-density lipoproteins and returned to the plasma. In individuals with uncontrolled diabetes the low insulin concentrations result in increased lipolysis and decreased reesterification, thereby increasing plasma free fatty acids. The increased glucagon to insulin ratio enhances fatty acid oxidation in the liver. Thus increased hepatic ketone production and decreased peripheral tissue metabolism lead to acetoacetate accumulation in the blood. A small fraction undergoes spontaneous decarboxylation to form acetone, but the majority is converted to β-hydroxybutyrate, as follows:

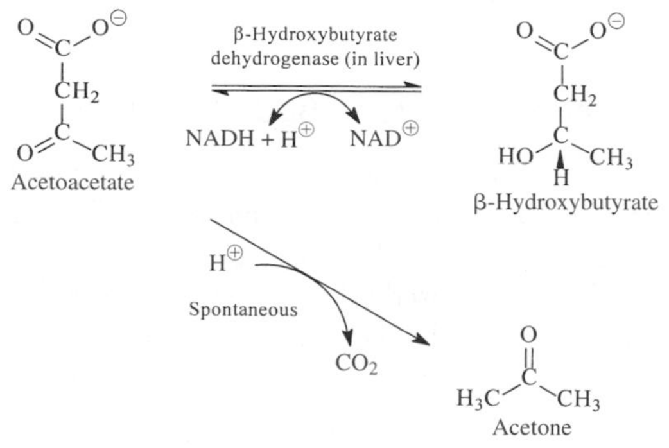

The relative proportions in which the three ketone bodies are present in blood vary, depending on the redox state of the cell. In healthy individuals, β-hydroxybutyrate and acetoacetate, which are present at approximately equimolar concentrations, constitute virtually all the serum ketones. Acetone is a minor component. In cases of severe diabetes the ratio of β-hydroxybutyrate to acetoacetate may increase up to 6:1 because of the presence of large amounts of NADH, which favors β-hydroxybutyrate production.

None of the commonly used methods for the detection and determination of ketone bodies in serum or urine reacts with all three ketone bodies. Gerhardt's ferric chloride test reacts with acetoacetate only. Tests using nitroprusside are at least 10 times more sensitive to acetoacetate than to acetone and give no reaction at all with β-hydroxybutyrate. Thus most of the tests to be described essentially detect or measure acetoacetate only. A paradoxical situation may result. When an individual is initially seen with ketoacidosis, the test for ketones may be only weakly positive. With therapy, β-hydroxybutyrate is converted to acetoacetate and the ketosis appears to worsen. Traditional tests for β-hydroxybutyrate are indirect; they require brief boiling of the urine to remove acetone and acetoacetate by evaporation (with acetoacetate initially undergoing spontaneous conversion to acetone), followed by gentle oxidation of β-hydroxybutyrate to acetoacetate and acetone with peroxide, ferric ions, or dichromate. The acetoacetate thus formed may be detected with Gerhardt's test or one of the procedures using nitroprusside (see discussion to follow). A quantitative enzymatic assay for β-hydroxybutyrate that can be directly performed on blood or serum is commercially available.

Clinical Significance

Excessive formation of ketone bodies results in increased blood concentrations (ketonemia) and increased excretion in the urine (ketonuria). This process is observed in conditions associated with decreased availability of carbohydrates (such as starvation or frequent vomiting) or decreased use of car-

bohydrates (such as diabetes mellitus, glycogen storage disease [von Gierke disease], and alkalosis). Diabetes mellitus and alcohol consumption are the common causes of ketoacidosis. Semiquantitative determination of ketone bodies in blood is more accurate than determination of these compounds in urine in the treatment of diabetic ketoacidosis. Although not always excreted in proportion to blood ketone concentrations, urine ketones are widely used for monitoring of control in patients with type 1 diabetes because of convenience. The ADA recommends urine testing for ketones in those with type 1 diabetes during acute illness or stress, with consistent increase of blood glucose exceeding 240 mg/dL; during pregnancy; or when symptoms of ketoacidosis are present.[2] Positive ketone readings may occur during fasting and pregnancy. False-positive tests may be produced by certain medications, whereas prolonged exposure of test strips to air can produce false-negative results.

Determination of Ketone Bodies in Serum

Although quantitative determination of individual ketone bodies is possible, these methods are not used as routine tests. The semiquantitative Acetest and Ketostix are frequently used but are insensitive to β-hydroxybutyrate. Therefore an important point to remember is that a negative nitroprusside test result does not rule out ketoacidosis.

Acetest

The Acetest tablets contain a mixture of glycine, sodium nitroprusside, disodium phosphate, and lactose. Acetoacetate or acetone (to a lesser extent) in the presence of glycine forms a lavender-purple complex with nitroprusside. β-Hydroxybutyrate does not react with nitroprusside. The disodium phosphate provides an optimal pH for the reaction, and lactose enhances the color.

A detailed procedure for the detection of ketone bodies by Acetest is supplied by the manufacturer with each package of tablets, and readers are referred to these instructions. After one drop of urine, serum, or blood is added, the color is read at 30 seconds, 2 minutes, or 10 minutes, respectively. Acetest was mainly designed for the detection of ketone bodies in urine. If serum is used, the tablets should be crushed and a drop of serum should be added to the powder. Failure to do so results in falsely decreased values. Positive and negative controls should be performed. This procedure has been reported to be more reliable than the Ketostix method.

A positive reaction (purple-lavender appearance) indicates the presence of ketone bodies at a concentration of 5 mg/dL (0.5 mmol/L) or greater and 10 mg/dL for urine and blood, respectively. A color chart provided with the package may be used to estimate actual concentrations of the ketone bodies. Semiquantitation is achieved by approximate values assigned to the color blocks, with 20 mg/dL (2 mmol/L) for "small," 30 to 40 mg/dL for "moderate," and 80 to 100 mg/dL for "large." If required, dilutions of serum with saline can be prepared to measure concentrations of ketone bodies exceeding 80 mg/dL. (Note that any dilution with saline introduces some error because the reaction is affected by proteins.) Ketones are not detected in blood or urine in individuals with normal carbohydrate metabolism.

Ketostix

Ketostix is a modification of the nitroprusside test in which a reagent strip is used instead of a tablet. The Ketostix test gives a positive reaction within 15 seconds in a specimen containing at least 50 mg of acetoacetate per liter. The accompanying color chart gives readings for ketone concentrations of 50, 150, 400, 800, and 1600 mg/L. Acetone also reacts, but the sensitivity is lower.

Determination of β-hydroxybutyrate

The KetoSite assay consists of a plastic card with a reagent pad in the center. β-Hydroxybutyrate in the presence of NAD^+ is converted to acetoacetate, producing NADH. Diaphorase catalyzes the reduction of nitroblue tetrazolium (NBT) by NADH to produce a purple compound. The color is read in a special meter that provides a digital readout. The reaction is as follows:

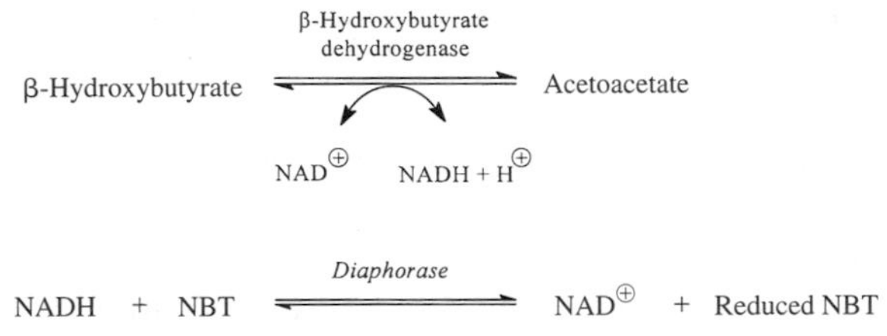

A cartridge is inserted into the meter to calibrate it to each specific lot of reagent. Low and high controls should be assayed daily. Acetoacetate has a negative interference, and increasing acetoacetate concentrations progressively decrease measured β-hydroxybutyrate values. For example, an 8 mmol/L solution of acetoacetate decreases measured β-hydroxybutyrate values by 60%. Samples with high acetoacetate concentrations should be diluted before analysis.

Considerable technical expertise is required to perform the assay, and it is not appropriate for self-monitoring. A card with a color chart that has readings of "normal," "small" (0.5 mmol/L), and "moderate" (1.5 mmol/L) is available for screening in physicians' offices or the emergency department of a hospital. A liquid assay that can be applied to several automated analyzers is also available. Clinical experience with the assay is limited. A short report in 1995 on individuals with diabetic ketoacidosis indicated that β-hydroxybutyrate levels correlated better than acetoacetate with changes in acid-base status. Despite the theoretical advantages the β-hydroxybutyrate assay has not achieved widespread clinical acceptance.

Reference interval

β-Hydroxybutyrate values range from 0.02 to 0.27 mmol/L (0.21 to 2.81 mg/dL) in healthy individuals after an overnight fast.

Determination of Ketone Bodies in Urine

Acetest and Ketostix also are suitable for detecting ketone bodies in urine. The sensitivity and specificity of the tests are the same as those outlined for serum.

Gerhardt's test is based on the reaction of ferric chloride with acetoacetate, producing a wine-red color. It is nonspecific, and other compounds, such as salicylates, phenol, and antipyrine give a similar color; thus a positive reaction merely signals the possible presence of acetoacetate. To confirm its presence, urine is heated to decompose acetoacetate to acetone and drive off the acetone. The test is then repeated. If the result is then negative, the original color can be assumed to indicate acetoacetate. This test has been replaced by the Acetest and Ketostix procedures.

■ LACTATE AND PYRUVATE

Lactic acid, an intermediary in carbohydrate metabolism, is predominantly derived from white skeletal muscle, brain, skin, renal medulla, and erythrocytes.[25] The blood lactate concentration depends on the rate of production in these tissues and the rate of metabolism in the liver and kidneys. The liver uses approximately 65% (75g) of the total basal lactate produced predominantly in gluconeogenesis. The Cori cycle is the conversion of glucose to **lactate** in the periphery and reconversion of lactate to glucose in the liver. Extrahepatic removal of lactate is by oxidation in red skeletal muscle and the renal cortex. A moderate increase in lactate production results in increased hepatic lactate clearance, but uptake by the liver is saturable when concentrations exceed 2 mmol/L. For example, during strenuous exercise, lactate concentrations may significantly increase, from an average concentration of about 0.9 to more than 20 mmol/L within 10 seconds. No concentration is uniformly accepted for the diagnosis of lactic acidosis, but lactate concentrations exceeding 5 mmol/L and with pH less than 7.25 indicate significant lactic acidosis.

Clinical Significance

Lactic acidosis occurs in two clinical settings—(1) type A (hypoxic), associated with decreased tissue oxygenation, such as shock, hypovolemia, and left ventricular failure; and (2) type B (metabolic), associated with disease (for example, diabetes mellitus, neoplasia, liver disease), drugs/toxins (for example, ethanol, methanol, salicylates), or inborn errors of metabolism.[25] Lactic acidosis is not uncommon and occurs in approximately 1% of those admitted to the hospital. It has a mortality rate greater than 60%, which approaches 100% if hypotension also is present. Type A is much more common.

An uncommon but often undiagnosed cause of lactic acidosis is D-lactic acidosis.[30] D-Lactate is not produced in human metabolism, but absorption and accumulation of D-lactate from abnormal intestinal bacteria may cause systemic acidosis. This condition occurs after jejunoileal bypass surgery and manifests as encephalopathy (confusion, ataxia, sleepiness) with increased blood concentrations of D-lactate. Virtually all the commonly used laboratory assays for lactate use L-lactate dehydrogenase, which does not detect D-lactate. D-Lactate can be measured by gas-liquid chromatography or, enzymatically, with a specific D-lactate dehydrogenase.

Lactate in CSF normally parallels blood concentrations. With biochemical alterations in the CNS, however, CSF lactate values change independently of blood values. Increased CSF concentrations are noted in individuals with cerebrovascular accidents, intracranial hemorrhage, bacterial meningitis, epilepsy, and other CNS disorders.

Measurement of pyruvate is useful in the evaluation of patients with inborn errors of metabolism who have increased serum lactate concentrations. A lactate to pyruvate ratio of less than 25 suggests a defect in gluconeogenesis, whereas an increased ratio ($\geq$35) indicates reduced intracellular conditions found in hypoxia. Inborn errors associated with an increased lactate to pyruvate ratio include pyruvate carboxylase deficiency and defects in oxidative phosphorylation. Pyruvate is also measured in clinical studies evaluating reperfusion after myocardial ischemia.

Determination of Lactate in Whole Blood

Lactate is oxidized to pyruvate by lactate dehydrogenase in the presence of NAD^+. The NADH formed in this reaction is measured spectrophotometrically at 340 nm and serves as a measure of the lactate concentration. The reaction is as follows:

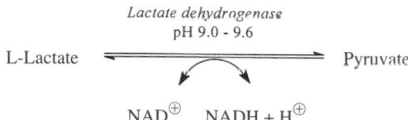

The equilibrium of the reaction normally lies far to the left. However, by buffering of the pH between 9.0 and 9.6, the addition of an excess of NAD^+, and trapping of the reaction product pyruvate with hydrazine, the equilibrium can be shifted to the right. Pyruvate can also be removed through reaction with L-glutamate in the presence of alanine aminotransferase.

Because of its high specificity and simplicity, the enzymatic method is the method of choice for the measurement of lactate, although other methods may also be used (for example, gas chromatography and photometry).

The Vitros analyzer, formerly the Ektachem, uses an assay in which lactic acid is oxidized to pyruvate by lactate oxidase. The H_2O_2 generated oxidizes a chromogen system, and the absorbance of the resulting dye complex, measured spectrophotometrically at 540 nm, is directly proportional to the lactate concentration in the specimen. Each mole of lactate oxidized produces 0.5 mol of dye complex.

Specimen collection and storage

Stringent sample preparation and handling techniques are necessary to prevent changes in lactate concentrations both during and after the blood is drawn. Patients should be fasting and at complete rest for at least 2 hours to allow lactate concentrations to reach steady state.

Venous specimens should be obtained without the use of a tourniquet or immediately after the tourniquet has been applied. Alternatively, the tourniquet should be removed after the puncture has been performed, and the blood should be allowed to circulate for several minutes before the sample is withdrawn. Arterial blood sampling, which prevents these potential pitfalls, may also be used. Patients should avoid exercise of the hand or arm immediately before and during the procedure.

Both venous and arterial blood may be collected in heparinized syringes and immediately delivered into a premeasured amount of chilled protein precipitant, such as trichloroacetic acid, metaphosphoric acid, or perchloric acid. The clear supernatant, after centrifugation, is stable at 4 °C for as long as 8 days. Meticulous attention to sample preparation is required. If blood is not preserved as directed, lactate rapidly increases in blood as a result of glycolysis. Increases may be as great as 20% within 3 minutes and 70% within 30 minutes at 25 °C. Specimens collected as described in this section are also suitable for determination of pyruvate.

If plasma is required as specimen, blood should be collected in a tube containing 10 mg of NaF and 2 mg of $K_2C_2O_4$ per milliliter of blood. The specimen should be immediately cooled and the cells separated within 15 minutes. Once the plasma is separated from the cells, lactate is stable.

Reference intervals

The reference intervals for lactate are as follows:

	Lactate	
Specimen	mmol/L	mg/dL
Venous Blood		
At rest	0.5 to 1.3	5 to 12
In hospital	0.9 to 1.7	8 to 15
Arterial Blood		
At rest	0.36 to 0.75	3 to 7
In hospital	0.36 to 1.25	3 to 11

Individuals in the hospital exhibit a wider range of values. Lactic acidosis occurs with blood lactate concentrations exceeding 5 mmol/L (45 mg/dL). Severe exercise dramatically increases lactate concentrations, and even movement of leg muscles by individuals at bed rest may result in significant increases. Plasma values are about 7% higher than those in whole blood, although differences depend on the procedure used. CSF values are usually similar to blood concentrations but may change independently in CNS disorders. Normal 24-hour urine output of lactate is 5.5 to 22 mmol/day.

Determination of Pyruvate in Whole Blood

The reaction involved in the determination of pyruvate is essentially the reverse of the reaction used in the lactate procedure, as follows:

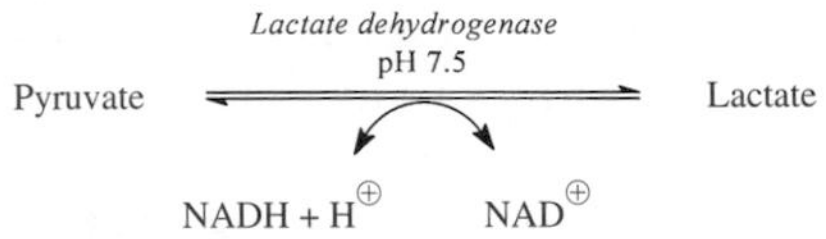

$$\text{Pyruvate} \underset{\substack{\text{Lactate dehydrogenase} \\ \text{pH 7.5}}}{\rightleftharpoons} \text{Lactate}$$

$$\text{NADH} + \text{H}^{\oplus} \qquad \text{NAD}^{\oplus}$$

At about pH 7.5 the equilibrium constant strongly favors the reaction to the right. The method is very specific, and 2-oxoglutarate, oxaloacetate, acetoacetate, and β-hydroxybutyrate do not interfere as they do with photometric methods. Pyruvate is extremely unstable in blood, and the same precautions detailed for lactate specimens should be observed.

Reference intervals

Fasting venous blood, drawn when the individuals is at rest, has a pyruvate concentration of 0.03 to 0.10 mmol/L (0.3 to 0.9 mg/dL). Arterial blood contains 0.02 to 0.08 mmol/L (0.2 to 0.7 mg/dL). Values for CSF are 0.06 to 0.19 mmol/L (0.5 to 1.7 mg/dL). Urine output of pyruvate is normally 1 mmol/day or less. Few clinical indications warrant the measurement of blood pyruvate concentrations.

■ GLYCATED PROTEINS

Measurement of glycated proteins is effective in the monitoring of long-term glucose control in individuals with diabetes mellitus. It provides a retrospective index of the integrated plasma glucose values over an extended period of time and is not subject to the wide fluctuations observed when assays of blood glucose concentrations are performed. Glycated protein concentrations therefore are a valuable and widely used adjunct to blood glucose determinations in the assessment of glycemic control. However, these analytes are not reliable for the diagnosis of diabetes mellitus.

Glycated Hemoglobin

Glycation is the nonenzymatic addition of a sugar residue to amino groups of proteins. Human adult hemoglobin (Hb)

usually consists of Hb A (97% of total), Hb A_2 (2.5%), and Hb F (0.5%). Hb A is made up of four polypeptide chains—two α- and two β-chains. Chromatographic analysis of Hb A identifies several minor hemoglobins, namely Hb A_{1a}, Hb A_{1b}, and Hb A_{1c}, which are collectively referred to as *Hb A_1, fast hemoglobins* (because they migrate more rapidly than Hb A in an electrical field), *glycohemoglobins,* or **glycated hemoglobins.** The Joint Commission on Biochemical Nomenclature of the International Union of Pure and Applied Chemistry recommends the term *neoglycoprotein* for such derivatives and the term *glycation* to describe the process. Therefore although the terms *glycosylated* and *glucosylated* have been widely used in the literature, the term *glycated* is preferred.

Hb A_{1c} is formed by the condensation of glucose with the *N*-terminal valine residue of each β-chain of Hb A to form an unstable Schiff base (aldimine, pre-Hb A_{1c}; Figure 23-6). The Schiff base may either dissociate or undergo an Amadori rearrangement to form a stable ketoamine, Hb A_{1c}. Hb A_{1a1} and Hb A_{1a2}, which make up Hb A_{1a}, have fructose-1,6-diphosphate and glucose-6-phosphate, respectively, attached to the amino terminal of the β-chain. The structure of Hb A_{1b} has been identified by mass spectrometry and contains pyruvic acid linked to the amino terminal valine of the β-chain, probably by a ketamine or enamine bond. Hb A_{1c} is the major fraction, constituting approximately 80% of Hb A_1.

Glycation may also occur at sites other than the end of the β-chain, such as lysine residues or the α-chain. These glycated hemoglobins, referred to as *glycated Hb A_0,* cannot be separated from nonglycated hemoglobin by methods based on charge but are measured by affinity chromatography (see later discussion).

Formation of glycated hemoglobin is essentially irreversible, and the amount in the blood depends on both the lifespan of the red blood cell (average 120 days) and the blood glucose concentration. Because the rate of formation of glycated hemoglobin is directly proportional to the concentration of glucose in the blood, the glycated hemoglobin concentration represents the integrated values for glucose over the preceding 6 to 8 weeks. This observation provides an additional criterion for assessment of glucose control because glycated hemoglobin values are free of day-to-day glucose fluctuations and are unaffected by exercise or recent food ingestion.

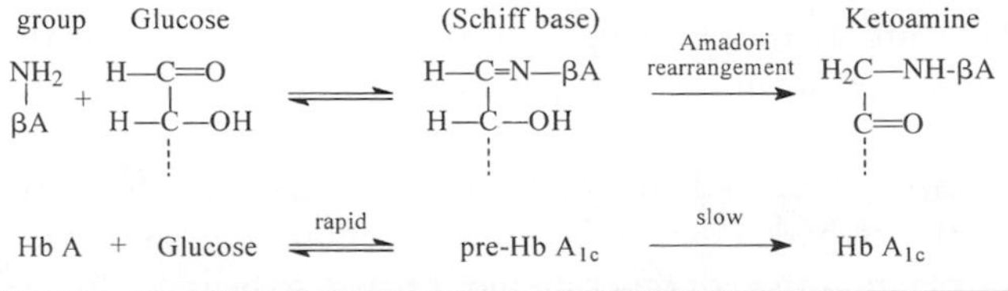

Figure 23-6 Formation of hemoglobin A_{1c}. *Hb,* Hemoglobin.

The interpretation of glycated hemoglobin depends on the red blood cells having a normal lifespan. Individuals with hemolytic disease or other conditions with shortened red blood cell survival exhibit a substantial reduction in glycated hemoglobin. Similarly, those individuals with recent significant blood loss have falsely low values because a higher fraction of young erythrocytes are present. Glycated hemoglobin concentrations can still be used to monitor these individuals, but values must be compared with previous values from the same person, not published reference intervals. High glycated hemoglobin concentrations have been reported in cases of iron deficiency anemia, probably because of the high proportion of old erythrocytes. The effect of hemoglobin variants (such as Hb F, Hb S, and Hb C) depends on the specific method of analysis (see later discussion). Another source of error in selected methods is carbamylated hemoglobin, which is formed by attachment of urea and is present in significant amounts in individuals with renal failure, which is common in individuals with diabetes.

Labile intermediates (pre-Hb A_{1c}, Schiff base) may produce artifact, especially in methods based on charge differences. The labile fraction rapidly changes with acute changes in blood glucose concentration and may spuriously alter glycated hemoglobin values. Pre-Hb A_{1c} amounts to 5% to 8% of total Hb A_1 in healthy individuals and ranges from 8% to 30% in those with diabetes, depending on the degree of control of blood glucose concentrations. In the absence of excess glucose, pre-Hb A_{1c} reverts to glucose and Hb A (see Figure 23-6). This observation provides the basis for some procedures to eliminate the labile fraction through incubation of washed red blood cells in saline. If the analytical method measures both fractions, the labile pre-Hb A_{1c} should first be removed to prevent falsely increased results.

Glycated hemoglobin should be routinely monitored at least every 3 months in all insulin-treated patients. In certain clinical situations, such as diabetic pregnancy or a major change in therapy, more frequent monitoring (every 4 weeks) is recommended. Although monitoring of glycated hemoglobin has been proposed as a diagnostic test, it does not have a role in the diagnosis of diabetes mellitus in children, nonpregnant adults, or individuals with GDM.

Clinical utility

Although the supposition that better glycemic control would decrease long-term complications of diabetes mellitus was held for years, not until the publication of the DCCT in 1993[10] was this hypothesis verified. The DCCT was a multicenter, randomized trial that compared intensive and conventional therapy with regard to their effects on complications in 1441 patients with type 1 diabetes. During the study period, which averaged 7 years, intensively managed patients maintained lower mean blood glucose concentrations. Compared with conventional therapy, intensive therapy reduced the risk of retinopathy, nephropathy, and neuropathy by 40% to 75%.[10] Intensive therapy delayed the onset and slowed the progression of these three complications, regardless of age, gender, or duration of diabetes. Although intensive therapy reduced the development of hypercholesterolemia, major cardiovascular and peripheral vascular disease were not significantly decreased. Glycated hemoglobin was a cornerstone of the study. For example, the risk of retinopathy continuously increased with increasing Hb A_{1c}, and a single measure of Hb A_{1c} predicted the progression of retinopathy 4 years later. In fact, subsequent analysis revealed that the mean Hb A_{1c} was the dominant predictor of retinopathy progression, and a 10% lower Hb A_{1c} concentration was associated with a 45% lower risk.

The effect of improved glucose control on the incidence of complications in patients with type 2 diabetes was reported at the end of 1998. The UKPDS recruited 5102 individuals with newly diagnosed type 2 diabetes in 23 centers and followed them for an average of 10 years.[31] The results establish that decreasing blood glucose concentrations by intensive therapy (diet and oral medications or insulin) reduced microvascular disease (retinopathy, nephropathy and perhaps neuropathy). No significant effect was observed on cardiovascular complications. For every percentage point decrease in Hb A_{1c}, a 35% reduction occurred in the risk of complications. These data, combined with the results of the DCCT, indicate that aggressive treatment of diabetes can diminish the morbidity and mortality of the disease by lowering its chronic complications.

Based on the DCCT the ADA recommended that a primary treatment goal in individuals with type 1 diabetes should be blood glucose control at least equal to that achieved in the intensively treated group.[2] The recommendations included Hb A_{1c} of approximately 7.2%. Glycated hemoglobin has been firmly established as an index of long-term blood glucose concentrations in individuals with diabetes mellitus. The more frequent use of this test by physicians is reflected in the increased number of laboratories participating in CAP glycated hemoglobin surveys. In 1985, approximately 300 laboratories participated; in 1990, 707; and in 2000, 2590 laboratories participated in the survey.

Methods for the determination of glycated hemoglobins

Methods for the determination of glycated hemoglobins use separation based on charge differences (ion-exchange chromatography, high-performance liquid chromatography [HPLC], electrophoresis, and isoelectric focusing), structural differences (affinity chromatography and immunoassay), or chemical analysis (photometry, spectrophotometry).[12] Regardless of the method, the result is expressed as a percentage of total hemoglobin. Most assays have acceptable precision when they are properly performed. The selection of a method by a laboratory is influenced by several factors, including sample volume, patient population, and cost. Consultation with clinicians in this selection is advisable.

Results from laboratories participating in quality control surveys conducted by CAP reveal that affinity chromatography is the technique most widely used in the United States. Most of the participating laboratories measure Hb A_{1c}. The CV exhibits wide variability among assays, ranging from 3.5% to 16.5%.

Ion-exchange chromatography

Ion-exchange chromatography separates hemoglobin variants on the basis of charge. The cation exchange resin (negatively charged), packed in a disposable minicolumn, has an affinity for hemoglobin, which is positively charged. The patient's sample is hemolyzed, and an aliquot of the hemolysate is applied to the column. A buffer is applied and the eluent collected. The ionic strength and pH of the eluent buffer are selected so that glycated hemoglobins are less positively charged than Hb A, do not bind as well to the negatively charged resin, and therefore are eluted first. The glycated hemoglobins (that is, $A_{1a} + A_{1b} + A_{1c}$, expressed collectively as Hb A_1) are measured in a spectrophotometer. A second buffer, of different ionic strength, can be added to the column to elute the more positively charged main hemoglobin fraction. This value is read in the spectrophotometer (total hemoglobin), and glycated hemoglobin is expressed as a percentage of total hemoglobin. Alternatively, only the Hb A_1 is eluted, and a separate dilution of the original hemolysate is made, against which the Hb A_1 is compared. Numerous commercial modifications have been developed, but they are all manual.

In all ion-exchange column methods, control of the temperature of the reagents and columns is important to obtain accurate and reproducible results. This control is best performed by thermostating of the columns. Alternatively, a temperature correction factor can be applied if the room temperature differs from the specified optimum. In addition, rigid control of pH and ionic strength must be maintained. Sample storage conditions are also important. These factors account for the large CVs obtained with this method. Results with three commonly used, commercially available column-chromatographic methods were found to satisfactorily correlate with an HPLC method, but the different minicolumns exhibited wide variability in performance.

The labile pre-Hb A_1 fractions elute with the stable ketoamine and produce increased results unless destroyed by pretreatment of the red blood cells (see later discussion). Hb F (fetal hemoglobin), present in normal neonates, typically also elutes with Hb A_1 and produces falsely increased results. Spuriously higher values are also obtained when the charge on hemoglobin is altered by the attachment of noncarbohydrate moieties, which may co-chromatograph with glycated hemoglobins, as in uremia, alcoholism, lead poisoning, or chronic treatment with large doses of aspirin. These substances interfere predominantly with Hb $A_{1a + b}$, and assays that measure Hb A_{1c} have only slight alterations

(<1% glycated hemoglobin). In contrast, Hb S, Hb C, and their glycated derivatives, if present, remain on the column; hence, misleading low values for Hb A_1 would be obtained in the presence of Hb S and Hb C because the relative concentration of Hb A is decreased.

High-performance liquid chromatography

Hb A_{1c} and other hemoglobin fractions can be separated by HPLC. The principle of the HPLC assay is cation-exchange chromatography. A hemolysate prepared from the patient's sample is injected onto a column packed with cation-exchange resin. Phosphate buffers of increasing ionic strength are used for stepped elution of the hemoglobins, which are detected by absorbance at 415 and 690 nm. The method can be fully automated, and several systems are commercially available. Both Hb A_{1c} and Hb A_1 are reported. Variant hemoglobins—Hb F, Hb S, and Hb C—are resolved. All HPLC methods have excellent precision. Hb A_{1c} by HPLC was used for analysis of all patient samples in the DCCT and has been recommended as the reference method.

Electrophoresis

Agar gel electrophoresis on whole-blood hemolysates at pH 6.3 provides good resolution of Hb A and Hb A_1. Quantification is performed by scanning densitometry at 415 nm. Results generally agree well with those obtained by HPLC or column chromatography but are less precise. Minor variations in pH, ionic strength, or temperature have little effect on results. Hb F migrates to the same region as Hb A_1 and causes a falsely increased Hb A_1 value, but Hb S and Hb C do not. The labile form should be removed before assaying.

Isoelectric focusing

The hemoglobin variants separate on isoelectric focusing on the basis of their migration in gel containing a pH gradient. Hb A_{1c} is adequately resolved from Hb A_{1a}, A_{1b}, S, and F. Results from isoelectric focusing have shown close agreement with other methods. The equipment is expensive and is not widely used in the United States; the technique is more popular in Europe.

Immunoassay

An early immunoassay for glycated hemoglobin used sheep antiserum that was raised against column-purified human Hb A_{1c}. This RIA exhibited some cross-reactivity with Hb A_{1a}. Subsequently, assays for Hb A_{1c} have been developed using antibodies raised against the Amadori product of glucose (ketoamine linkage) plus the first few (four to eight) amino acids at the N-terminal end of the β-chain of hemoglobin. Both polyclonal- and monoclonal-based techniques have been developed.

Enzyme immunoassays using monoclonal antibodies are commercially available and exhibit excellent precision. The antibodies do not recognize labile intermediates or other glycated hemoglobins, such as Hb A_{1a} or Hb A_{1b}, because both the ketoamine with glucose and the specific amino acid sequences are required for binding. Similarly, other hemoglobin variants, such as Hb F, Hb A_2, and Hb S and carbamylated hemoglobin are not detected. These assays have been shown to correlate well with HPLC, but they exhibit lower values. The lower values are thought to result from different calibration or, more likely, from the detection by HPLC of substances other than Hb A_{1c}. The procedure has been adapted for capillary blood samples by the use of a benchtop analyzer with reagent cartridges designed for use in physicians' office laboratories.

Affinity chromatography

Affinity gel columns are used to separate glycated hemoglobin, which binds to the column, from the nonglycated fraction (see Chapter 8). *m*-Aminophenylboronic acid is immobilized by its cross-linking to beaded agarose or another matrix (for example, glass fiber). The boronic acid reacts with the *cis*-diol groups of glucose bound to hemoglobin to form a reversible five-member ring complex, thus selectively holding the glycated hemoglobin on the column (Figure 23-7). The nonglycated hemoglobin does not bind. Sorbitol is then added to dissociate the complex and elute the glycated hemoglobin. Absorbance of the bound and unbound fractions, measured at 415 nm, is used to calculate the percentage of glycated hemoglobin.

With affinity chromatography, nonglycated hemoglobins do not interfere, and the labile intermediate form of Hb A_{1c} produces negligible interference. It is unaffected by variations in temperature and has reasonably good precision. Hemoglobin variants, such as Hb F, Hb S, or Hb C, produce little effect. A major disadvantage with affinity chromatography is that it produces higher values than HPLC. The higher results occur because affinity chromatography methods measure total glycated hemoglobin, which includes components other than Hb A_{1c}.

The assay detects ketoamine structures on lysine and valine residues on both α- and β-chains of hemoglobin. Re-

sults are reported as total glycated hemoglobin, but several commercially available systems are calibrated to also report an Hb A_{1c} standardized value. These values are derived from an equation obtained from correlation between total glycated hemoglobin and Hb A_{1c} analysis by HPLC. Columns and reagents are readily available from a number of manufacturers, several of which have automated the procedure.

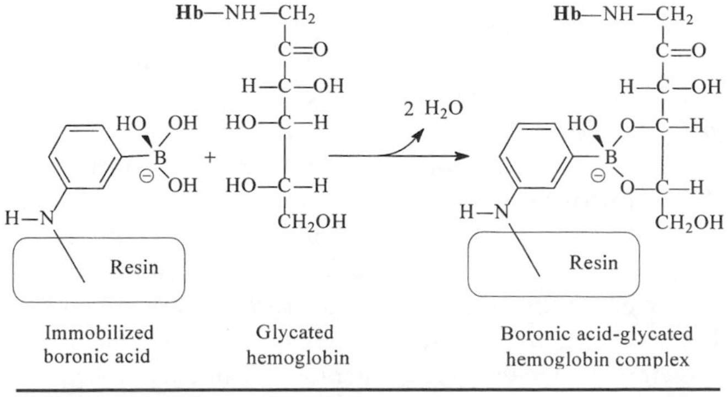

Removal of labile glycated hemoglobin from red blood cells

The concentration of the labile form of Hb A_{1c} (Schiff base) fluctuates rapidly in response to acute changes in plasma glucose concentrations and should be removed before analysis by charge-based assays. This removal may be accomplished by incubation of red blood cells in saline, in buffer solutions at pH 5 to 6, or by dialysis or ultrafiltration of hemolysates. Most kits for column assays contain reagents to remove this labile component.

Assay standardization

The DCCT results have provided a strong impetus for standardization of glycated hemoglobin assays. Clinical laboratories measure glycated hemoglobin with diverse assays that use multiple methods and quantify different components. The absence of a reference method and single glycated hemoglobin reference material have generated confusion. Interlaboratory comparisons are not possible, and even a single quality-control sample analyzed by a single method exhibited a CV as high as 16.5%. Similar large variability among laboratories has been observed in Europe.

Calibration, by use of a common set of calibrators, has been shown to significantly improve precision and facilitates direct comparison of results obtained by different methods. In these studies, calibrators were lyophilized hemolysates that were assayed by a precise HPLC method for Hb A_{1c}. Committees, established under the auspices of the American Association for Clinical Chemistry (the National Glycohemoglobin Standardization Program) and the International Federation of Clinical Chemistry, are working to standardize glycated hemoglobin determinations to allow individual laboratories to relate their assay results to those of the DCCT. The objectives are to establish a definitive reference method and develop a purified hemoglobin standard. The HPLC assay used in the DCCT is the interim reference method. However, even this method includes hemoglobin adducts other than Hb A_{1c}. CAP began proficiency testing in 1996 with whole blood and lyophilized samples. At the time of this writing, whole blood is the sample used for proficiency testing. Adoption of a universal standard ultimately should enhance the clinical utility of glycated hemoglobin.

Reference intervals

Values for glycated hemoglobins are expressed as a percentage of total blood hemoglobin. One of three major glycated hemoglobin species, namely Hb A_1, Hb A_{1c} or total gly-

Figure 23-7 Reaction of glycated hemoglobin with immobilized boronic acid. *Hb*, Hemoglobin.

cated hemoglobin, is usually measured. Reference intervals vary, depending on the method, as to the glycated hemoglobin component measured and whether the labile fraction is included in the assay. A consensus, based on several studies of apparently healthy subjects, suggests the following reference intervals:

Hemoglobin Species	Mean (%)	Interval (%)
Hb A_1 (A_{1a+b+c})	6.5	5.0 to 8.0
Hb A_{1c} only	4.5	3.0 to 6.0
Total glycated Hb ($A_1 + A_0$)	5.5	4.5 to 7.0

Reference intervals demonstrate some increase with age, in agreement with similar observations of fasting blood glucose concentrations. In individuals with poorly controlled diabetes mellitus, values may extend to twice or more the upper limit of the reference interval, but rarely exceed 20%. Values greater than 20% should prompt further studies to determine the possible presence of Hb F if it is known to interfere in the method.

No specific value of Hb A_{1c} exists below which the risk of diabetic complications is completely eliminated. The DCCT group recommended that the goal of treatment should be to lower Hb A_{1c} to as close to nondiabetic concentrations (<6.05%) as possible.[2] Each laboratory should establish its own nondiabetic reference interval. Assay precision is important because each 1% change in glycated hemoglobin represents an approximate 25 to 35 mg/dL change in average blood glucose.

Glycated Serum Protein

Selected individuals with diabetes mellitus (for example, GDM or major change in therapy), may require assays that are more sensitive than glycated hemoglobin to shorter-term alterations in average blood glucose concentrations. Nonenzymatic attachment of glucose to amino groups of proteins other than hemoglobin (for example, serum proteins, membrane proteins, lens crystallins) to form ketoamines also occurs. Because serum proteins turn over more rapidly than hemoglobin (the circulating half-life for albumin being about 20 days), the concentration of glycated albumin reflects glucose control over a period of 2 to 3 weeks. Therefore evidence of both deterioration of control and improvement with therapy is evident earlier than with glycated hemoglobin. Several methods are available to measure glycated proteins, but none is popular because of lack of suitability for routine clinical laboratories. The development of monoclonal antibodies to glycated albumin, although theoretically advantageous, has not resulted in the widespread availability of commercial glycated albumin assays.

Fructosamine is the generic name for plasma protein ketoamines.[4] The name refers to the structure of the ketoamine rearrangement product formed by the interaction of glucose with the (ε-amino group on lysine residues of albumin. Although the fructosamine assay can be automated,

provides better precision, and is cheaper than glycated hemoglobin, a lack of consensus exists as to its clinical value. Early work with the original assay, introduced in 1983, indicated that fructosamine concentrations were significantly higher in diabetic individuals than in healthy subjects. Several artifacts, including an apparent lack of specificity for glycated proteins (up to 60% of the value being due to nonfructosamine reducing substances), were identified that rendered the data from the first generation fructosamine assay difficult to interpret. Substantial modifications produced second-generation assays, and an industry standard was adopted. These improvements resulted in average values in nondiabetic individuals that are approximately 10% of those obtained with the first-generation assay. Preliminary clinical evaluation tends to support the validity of the new assay as a means to monitor glycemic control. However, the second-generation fructosamine assay has not been evaluated in the chronic complications of diabetes.

Because fructosamine determination monitors short-term glycemic changes different from glycated hemoglobin, it may have a role in conjunction with glycated hemoglobin. In addition, fructosamine may be useful in individuals with hemoglobin variants, such as Hb S or Hb C, that are associated with decreased erythrocyte lifespan, where glycated hemoglobin is of little value. Gross changes in protein concentration and half-life may produce large effects on the proportion of protein that is glycated. Results may be invalid in individuals with nephrotic syndrome, cirrhosis of the liver, or dysproteinemias, or after rapid changes in acute-phase reactants. The test should not be performed when serum albumin is less than 30 g/L. Whether fructosamine results should be corrected for protein concentrations in the absence of significant alterations in serum protein levels remains to be resolved. Although the fructosamine assay was initially postulated to replace the OGTT, no role exists for the fructosamine assay in the diagnosis of diabetes mellitus. A recent report indicated that the second-generation fructosamine assay achieved a sensitivity and specificity of close to 80% in screening of patients for GDM, but this study requires verification.

Determination of fructosamine

Under alkaline conditions, products with Amadori rearrangements (such as fructosamine) have reducing activity that can be differentiated from other reducing substances. In the presence of carbonate buffer, fructosamine rearranges to the eneaminol form, which reduces NBT to a formazan. The absorbance at 530 nm is measured at two time points, and the absorbance change is proportional to the fructosamine concentration. The assay is easily automated and has excellent between-batch analytical precision. Hemoglobin (>100 mg/dL) and bilirubin (>4 mg/dL) interfere; therefore moderate to grossly hemolyzed and icteric samples should not be used. Ascorbic acid concentrations greater than 5 mg/dL may cause negative interference. Kits are commercially available.

Reference intervals

Values in a nondiabetic population range from 205 to 285 μmol/L. The reference interval corrected for albumin is 191 to 265 μmol/L.

Advanced Glycation End Products

The molecular mechanism by which hyperglycemia produces toxic effects is unknown. Evidence suggests that glycation of tissue proteins may be important. Nonenzymatic attachment of glucose to long-lived proteins, such as collagen, produces stable Amadori early-glycated products. These products undergo a series of additional rearrangements and dehydration and fragmentation reactions, resulting in irreversible **advanced glycation end products (AGE)**. The amounts of these products do not return to normal when hyperglycemia is corrected, and they accumulate continuously over the lifespan of the protein. Hyperglycemia accelerates the formation of protein-bound AGE, and individuals with diabetes mellitus thus have higher concentrations than healthy people. Through effects on the functional properties of protein and extracellular matrix, AGE may contribute to the microvascular and macrovascular complications of diabetes mellitus. Moreover, the AGE inhibitor, aminoguanidine, has been shown to prevent several complications of diabetes in experimental animal models.

Several assays for AGE have been developed. An early method, AGE-dependent relative fluorescence, suffered from spurious contributions to total fluorescence by non-AGE protein adducts (such as glucose- or lipid-derived oxidation products) that have similar fluorescence spectra. A radioreceptor assay was developed, based on the presence of AGE receptors on the surface of a macrophage-like tumor cell line, and was capable of quantifying AGE on both circulating (albumin) and tissue proteins. A competitive ELISA using polyclonal anti-AGE antibody was developed to measure hemoglobin-AGE. With this assay a linear correlation was demonstrated between Hb A_{1c} and hemoglobin-AGE. In healthy people, hemoglobin-AGE accounts for 0.4% of circulating hemoglobin, with significantly higher values in those individuals with diabetes mellitus. After an acute change in glycemia, hemoglobin-AGE concentrations change, but the rate of alteration is 23% slower than that of Hb A_{1c}.[32] Thus hemoglobin-AGE provides a measure of diabetic control longer than that indicated by glycated hemoglobin, reflecting blood glucose concentrations over a greater proportion of the life of red blood cells. Whether knowledge of hemoglobin-AGE values offers clinical benefit remains to be established.

■ URINARY ALBUMIN EXCRETION

Individuals with diabetes mellitus are at high risk of suffering renal damage. End-stage renal disease requiring dialysis or transplantation develops in approximately one third of individuals with type 1 diabetes, and diabetes is the most common cause of renal failure in the United States. Although nephropathy is less common in individuals with type 2 diabetes, approximately 60% of all cases of diabetic nephropathy occur in these people because of the higher incidence of this form of diabetes. Persistent proteinuria detectable by routine screening tests (equivalent to a **urinary albumin excretion [UAE]** rate ≥200 μg/min) indicates overt diabetic nephropathy. This condition is usually associated with long-standing disease and is unusual less than 5 years after the onset of type 1 diabetes. Once diabetic nephropathy occurs, renal function rapidly deteriorates and renal insufficiency evolves. Treatment at this stage can retard the rate of progression but not stop or reverse the renal damage. Preceding this stage is a period of increased UAE not detected by routine methods. This range of 20 to 200 μg/minute (or 30 to 300 mg/24 hours) of increased UAE defines microalbuminuria.[7] The term *microalbuminuria*, although generally accepted, is misleading. It implies a small version of the albumin molecule rather than an excretion rate of albumin greater than normal but less than previously detected levels. A more accurate term would be *paucialbuminuria*.

The presence of increased UAE indicates an increase in the transcapillary escape rate of albumin and is therefore a marker of microvascular disease. Persistent UAE greater than 20 μg/minute represents a twentyfold greater risk for the development of clinically overt renal disease in individuals with type 1 and type 2 diabetes. Prospective studies have demonstrated that increased UAE precedes and is highly predictive of diabetic nephropathy, end-stage renal disease, and proliferative retinopathy in individuals with type 1 diabetes.[7] Tight glycemic control in both type 1 and type 2 diabetes retards progression to nephropathy. In individuals with type 2 diabetes, increased UAE is an independent predictor of progressive renal disease, atherosclerotic disease, and cardiovascular mortality. Increased UAE is often detected at the time of diagnosis of type 2 diabetes, probably because the diabetes has been present for some time. In addition, increased UAE, both independently and in conjunction with hyperinsulinemia, identifies a group of nondiabetic individuals at increased risk for the development of coronary artery disease. Interventions, such as control of blood glucose concentrations and blood pressure and restriction of protein intake, can decrease UAE in type 1 diabetic individuals and slow the rate of decline in renal function.

Specimen Collection and Storage

The method for the collection of a urine sample lacks consensus. Variations in urine flow rate in a person may be corrected by the expression of albumin as a ratio to creatinine (that is, albumin/creatinine). UAE is increased by physiological factors (for example, exercise, posture, diuresis), and the method of urine collection must be standardized. Samples should not be collected after exertion, in the presence of urinary tract infection, during acute illness, immediately after surgery, or after an acute fluid load. All the following urine samples are currently acceptable:

1. 24-hour collection
2. Overnight (8- to 12-hour) collection
3. 1- to 2-hour collection (in laboratory or clinic)
4. First-morning sample for simultaneous albumin and creatinine measurement

The timed specimens (24-hour or overnight) are the most sensitive, but the albumin-to-creatinine ratio is more practical and convenient for the patient. At least three separate samples should be assayed because of the high intraindividual variation (CV of 30% to 50%) and diurnal variation (50% to 100% higher during the day). Urine should be stored at 4 °C after collection. Alternatively, 2 mL of 50 g/L sodium azide can be added per 500 mL of urine, but preservatives are not recommended for some assays. Bacterial contamination and glucose have no effect.

Semiquantitative Assays

A number of semiquantitative assays for screening for increased UAE are available. These test strips, most of which are optimized to read "positive" at a predetermined albumin concentration, are suitable for screening programs. Because of the wide variability in UAE, a "normal" value does not rule out renal disease. Because these assays measure albumin concentration, dilute urine may yield a false-negative result. Refrigerated urine samples should be allowed to reach at least 10 °C before analysis. Albu Screen and Albu Sure detect urinary albumin concentrations exceeding 20 and 30 mg/L, respectively. The assay is a latex agglutination inhibition test. Briefly, one drop of urine is mixed with one drop of goat antihuman albumin, the titer of which is adjusted so that all antibody-binding sites are occupied at urinary albumin concentrations of 30 mg/L or greater. Excess albumin-binding sites are detected by the addition of one drop of albumin-coated latex microspheres and subsequent rocking for 2 minutes. Albumin concentrations less than 20 mg/L produce agglutination. Sensitivity and specificity are reported to be approximately 90% to 95%. Micro-Bumintest uses bromophenol blue in an alkaline matrix to detect albumin concentrations exceeding 40 mg/L. The assay sensitivity is approximately 95%, but because other proteins are also detected, the specificity is approximately 80%.

In the Micral test strip (Roche Diagnostics, Branchburg, N.J.) a monoclonal antialbumin IgG is complexed to β-galactosidase.[18] The albumin in the urine binds to the antibody-enzyme conjugate in the test strip. Excess conjugate is retained in a separation zone containing immobilized albumin, and only albumin bound to the antibody-enzyme immunocomplex diffuses to the reaction zone. There it reacts with a buffered substrate (chlorophenol red galactoside) to produce a red color when the β-galactosidase hydrolyzes galactose. The test strip is dipped into the urine for 5 sec-

onds, and the intensity of the color after 5 minutes is proportional to the urinary albumin concentration. Direct visual comparison is made with printed color blocks—yellow, light brown, medium brown, brick red, and burgundy, representing 0, 10, 20, 50, and 100 mg/L, respectively. No interference is observed with drugs, glucose, urea, or other proteins. Comparison with a reference method demonstrates a sensitivity and specificity of approximately 100% and 91%, respectively. Both the time the stick is in contact with the urine and the time of reading are critical. A modification (Micral II) uses gold-labeled instead of enzyme-labeled antibody. This method enhances the stability, allowing the strip to be read at any time from 1 to at least 60 minutes. Urine specimens with albumin concentrations greater than 100 to 300 mg/L may be diluted and reassayed. The assigned concentration of the color block is multiplied by the dilution factor to obtain the concentration in the sample. These semiquantitative assays are suitable for screening only and are not sufficiently accurate for regular monitoring of patients.

Quantitative Assays

All the sensitive, specific assays for urine albumin use immunochemistry with antibodies to human albumin. Four methodologies are available—RIA, ELISA, radioimmunodiffusion, and immunoturbidimetry. Each method has advantages and disadvantages, and the choice depends on local experience and technical support. All methods have similar precision, sensitivity, and range. Although dye-binding and protein precipitation assays have been described, these are insensitive and nonspecific and should not be used.

Radial immunodiffusion

Radial immunodiffusion is a reliable and inexpensive method but is unlikely to gain wide acceptance because it requires a long incubation period and high level of technical skill and cannot be automated. The antibody is incorporated into an agar gel. Aliquots of samples and calibrators are added to wells and allowed to diffuse into the agar. Antigen-antibody complexes precipitate at equilibrium, and the distance of migration is measured after staining.

Radioimmunoassay

Standard RIA is performed in the liquid phase in the presence of excess antigen. ^{125}I-labeled albumin and antialbumin antiserum are used, with separation of bound from free by the double-antibody technique. The sample values are determined by comparison with a calibration curve. Assays are sensitive, precise, and inexpensive, but reagents are radioactive and have short shelf lives. Commercial kits are available.

Enzyme-linked immunosorbent assay

Both competitive and "sandwich" ELISAs are available. Although the competitive ELISA is faster because it uses only one incubation with antibody, it is reportedly less sensitive and exhibits large variance. ELISA can be performed on a microplate reader, allowing semiautomation. In the sandwich assay the primary antibody (antialbumin antiserum) is fixed on the plastic plate, which is then washed. Samples, controls, and calibrators are added, and the complexes detected and quantified by a second antibody are conjugated to an enzyme label.

Immunoturbidimetry

Albumin in the urine sample forms an insoluble complex with antibodies to human albumin. PEG accelerates complex formation. The turbidity caused by the complexes is spectrophotometrically measured at 340 nm and provides a measure of albumin concentration. The background absorbance of the initial urine sample is automatically subtracted. This method is simple and less expensive than RIA, and rapid analysis of large numbers of samples is possible. The assays may be performed as either kinetic or equilibrium reactions. Kits are commercially available for use on automated analyzers.

High antigen concentrations may cause a "hook" effect, resulting in falsely low concentrations. This effect can be avoided by the screening of urine samples with a dipstick but may not be necessary if the analyzer automatically tests for antigen excess.

A urinary tract infection or contamination with seminal or menstrual fluid may produce false-positive results. High physiological Ca^{2+} concentrations in the urine falsely increase albumin values. The interference is abolished by the addition of EDTA, which has been incorporated into a commercial assay.

Reference intervals

Condition	Urinary Albumin Excretion		
	µg/min	mg/24 h	Corrected(mg/g urine creatinine)
Normal	<20	<30	<30
Increased UAE	20 to 200	30 to 300	30 to 300
Macroalbuminuria	>200	>300	>300

The ADA position statement[2] recommends initial UAE measurement in pubertal and postpubertal type 1 diabetic individuals who have had diabetes for at least 5 years, followed by routine estimates once a year. In those with type 2 diabetes, screening should be performed at the time of diagnosis and annually thereafter. Screening may be performed with a semiquantitative assay. If the screen is positive, UAE should be evaluated by a quantitative assay.

If the confirmatory test is positive, treatment with an angiotensin-converting enzyme (ACE) inhibitor (see Chapter 20) should be initiated. ACE inhibitors reduce UAE, and the National Kidney Foundation recommends their use in both normotensive and hypertensive type 1 and 2 diabetic patients.[7] Patients undergoing therapy should be monitored

every 3 to 6 months. If left untreated, the UAE increases 10% to 30% per year, whereas the albumin to creatinine ratio in individuals on ACE inhibitors should stabilize or decrease by up to 50%.

INBORN ERRORS OF CARBOHYDRATE METABOLISM

Deficiency or absence of an enzyme that participates in carbohydrate metabolism may result in accumulation of monosaccharides, which overflow into the urine. Most such conditions are inherited as autosomal recessive traits (see an expanded version of this chapter,[26] pp 801-802). Sugars frequently appear in the urine as a result of excessive consumption, without the presence of underlying disease.

Techniques used to separate and identify sugars have included fermentation, optical rotation, osazone formation with phenylhydrazine, specific chemical tests, and paper or thin-layer chromatography. The availability of glucose oxidase test strips, specific for glucose, has greatly simplified the differentiation of glucose from other reducing substances. For practical purposes the urinary sugars of clinical interest are glucose and galactose. Urine from infants and children should be routinely tested by both the glucose oxidase and copper reduction tests to identify individuals with inborn errors of metabolism. Reducing substances other than glucose should be further identified by chromatographic procedures (see an expanded version of this chapter[26]).

GLYCOGEN STORAGE DISEASE

Glycogen, although present in most tissues, is predominantly stored in the liver and skeletal muscle. During fasting, liver glycogen is converted to glucose to provide energy for the whole body. In contrast, skeletal muscle lacks glucose-6-phosphatase, and muscle glycogen can be used only locally for energy. Glycogen storage disease is a generic name encompassing at least 10 rare inherited disorders of glycogen storage in tissues. The different forms of glycogen storage disease are categorized by numerical type in the chronological sequence in which these defects were identified. Each form is due to a deficiency of a specific enzyme in glycogen metabolism, producing either a quantitative or qualitative defect of glycogen storage.

Because the liver and skeletal muscle have the highest rates of glycogen metabolism, these are the structures most affected. The liver forms (types I, III, IV, and VI) are marked by hepatomegaly (due to increased liver glycogen stores) and hypoglycemia (due to the inability to convert glycogen to glucose). The hypoglycemia is manifested by autonomic clinical symptoms (sweating, shakiness, lightheaded feeling), growth retardation, and laboratory findings of decreased insulin and increased glucagon concentrations in the blood. The muscle forms (types II, IIIa, V, and VII), in contrast, have mild symptoms that usually appear in young adulthood during strenuous exercise because of the body's inability to provide energy for muscle contraction. Other muscle disorders may exhibit similar symptoms but can be readily differentiated by examination of glycogen stores. The specific diagnosis of each type is directly made by demonstration of the enzyme defect in tissue. For a detailed description, readers should consult Chen and Burchell.[9]

References

1. American Diabetes Association: Report of the expert committee on the diagnosis and classification of diabetes mellitus. Diabetes Care 1997; 20:1183-1201.

2. American Diabetes Association: Clinical practice recommendations 1999. Diabetes Care 1999; 22(Suppl 1):S1-S114.

3. American Diabetes Association: Economic consequences of diabetes mellitus in the U.S. in 1997. Diabetes Care 1998; 21:296-309.

4. Armbruster DA: Fructosamine: structure analysis and clinical usefulness. Clin Chem 1987; 33:2153-2163.

5. Atkinson MA, MacLaren NK: The pathogenesis of insulin-dependent diabetes mellitus. N Engl J Med 1994; 331:1428-1436.

6. Bell GI, Burant CF, Takeda J et al: Structure and function of mammalian facilitative sugar transporters. J Biol Chem 1993; 268:19161-19164.

7. Bennett PH, Haffner S, Kasiske BL et al: Screening and management of microalbuminuria in patients with diabetes mellitus: recommendations to the Scientific Advisory Board of the National Kidney Foundation from an Ad Hoc Committee of the Council on Diabetes Mellitus of the National Kidney Foundation. Am J Kidney Dis 1995; 25:107-112.

8. Chan AYW, Swaminathan R, Cockram CS: Effectiveness of sodium fluoride as a preservative of glucose in blood. Clin Chem 1989; 35:315-317.

9. Chen Y-T, Burchell A: Glycogen storage diseases. In Scriver CR, Beaudet AL, Sly WS et al (eds): The Metabolic and Molecular Bases of Inherited Disease, 7th edition, vol 1, pp 935-965, New York, McGraw-Hill, 1995.

10. The DCCT Research Group: The effect of intensive treatment of diabetes on the development and progression of long-term complications in insulin-dependent diabetes mellitus. N Engl J Med 1993; 329:977-986.

11. Gerich JE: Glucose counterregulation and its impact on diabetes mellitus. Diabetes 1988; 37:1608-1617.

12. Goldstein DE, Little RR, Wiedmeyer H-M et al: Glycated haemoglobin estimation in the 1990s: a review of assay methods and clinical interpretation. In Marshall SM, Home PD (eds): The Diabetes Annual, pp 193-212, New York, Elsevier Science BV, 1994.

13. Harris MI, Flegal KM, Cowie CC et al: Prevalence of diabetes, impaired fasting glucose, and impaired glucose tolerance in U.S. adults. Diabetes Care 1998; 21:518-524.

14. Haymond MW: Hypoglycemia in infants and children. Endocrinol Metab Clin North Am 1989; 18:211-252.

15. Hofeldt FD: Reactive hypoglycemia. Endocrinol Metab Clin North Am 1989; 18:185-201.

16. Khalil OS: Spectroscopic and clinical aspects of noninvasive glucose measurements. Clin Chem 1999; 45:165-177.

17. Li K-L, Huang H-S, Lin J-D et al: Comparing self-monitoring blood glucose devices. Lab Med 1994; 25:585-591.

18. Marshall SM, Shearing PA, Alberti KG: Micral-test strips evaluated for screening for albuminuria. Clin Chem 1992; 38:588-591.

19. Nathan DM: Long-term complications of diabetes mellitus. N Engl J Med 1993; 328:1676-1685.

20. National Diabetes Data Group: Classification and diagnosis of diabetes mellitus and other categories of glucose intolerance. Diabetes 1979; 28:1039-1057.

21. Orci L, Vassalli JD, Perrelet A: The insulin factory. Sci Am 1988; 259:85-94.

22. Passey RB, Gillum RL, Fuller JB et al: Evaluation and comparison of 10 glucose methods and the reference method recommended in the proposed product class standard (1974). Clin Chem 1977; 23:131-139.

23. Proceedings of the Fourth International Workshop Conference on Gestational Diabetes Mellitus. Diabetes Care 1998; 21(Suppl 2):B1-B168.

24. Robbins DC, Andersen L, Bowsher R et al: Report of the American Diabetes Association's Task Force on Standardization of the Insulin Assay. Diabetes 1996; 45:242-256.

25. Robinson BH: Lactic acidemia (disorders of pyruvate carboxylase, pyruvate dehydrogenase). In Scriver CR, Beaudet AL, Sly WS et al (eds): The Metabolic and Molecular Bases of Inherited Disease, 7th edition, vol 1, pp 1479-1499, New York, McGraw-Hill, 1995.

26. Sacks DB: Carbohydrates. In Burtis CA, Ashwood ER (eds): Tietz Textbook of Clinical Chemistry, 3rd edition, Philadelphia, WB Saunders, 1999.

27. Sacks DB, McDonald JM: The pathogenesis of type II diabetes mellitus: a polygenic disease. Am J Clin Pathol 1996; 105:149-156.

28. Service FJ: Hypoglycemic disorders. N Engl J Med 1995; 332:1144-1152.

29. Tietz NW (ed): Clinical Guide to Laboratory Tests, 3rd edition, pp 274-276, Philadelphia, WB Saunders, 1995.

30. Thurn JR, Pierpont GL, Ludvigsen CW et al: D-Lactate encephalopathy. Am J Med 1985; 79:717-721.

31. UK Prospective Diabetes Study Group: Intensive blood-glucose control with sulphonylureas or insulin compared with conventional treatment and risk of complications in patients with type 2 diabetes (UKPDS 33). Lancet 1998; 352:857-863.

32. Wolffenbuttel BHR, Giordano D, Founds HW et al: Long-term assessment of glucose control by haemoglobin-AGE measurement. Lancet 1996; 347:513 515.

Additional Reading

Benjamin RJ, Sacks DB: Glycated protein update: implications of recent studies, including the Diabetes Control and Complications Trial. Clin Chem 1994; 40:683-687.

Johnson R, Jeppsson J-O, Kobold U et al: Standardization of hemoglobin A_{1c}. Clin Chem 1998; 44:1066-1067.

Kahn SE, Andrikopoulos S, Verchere CB: Islet amyloid: a long-recognized but underappreciated pathological feature of type 2 diabetes. Diabetes 1999; 48:241-253.

Little RR, Wiedmeyer H-M, England JD et al: Interlaboratory standardization of measurements of glycohemoglobins. Clin Chem 1992; 38:2472-2478.

O'Sullivan JB, Mahan CM: Criteria for the oral glucose tolerance test in pregnancy. Diabetes 1964; 13:278-285.

Sacks DB: Amylin: a glucoregulatory hormone involved in the pathogenesis of diabetes mellitus? Clin Chem 1996; 42:494-495.

Sacks DB: Implications of the revised criteria for the diagnosis and classification of diabetes mellitus. Clin Chem 1997; 43:2230-2232.

Vlassara H: Recent progress in advanced glycation end products and diabetic complications. Diabetes 1997; 46(Suppl 2):S19-S25.

Weykamp CW, Penders TJ, Miedema K et al: Standardization of glycohemoglobin results and reference values in whole blood studied in 103 laboratories using 20 methods. Clin Chem 1995; 41:82-86.

CHAPTER 24

Lipids, Lipoproteins, and Apolipoproteins*†

NADER RIFAI, PhD, PAUL S. BACHORIK, PhD, and JOHN J. ALBERS, PhD

Objectives

1. Define the following terms:
   Lipid | Lipoprotein
   Fatty acid | Chylomicron
   Prostaglandin | Atherosclerosis
   Apolipoprotein
2. Discuss the metabolism of cholesterol and triglyceride and state the healthy reference interval of each.
3. State the significance of the apolipoproteins in health and disease.
4. Compare and contrast the five lipoprotein classes based on chemical makeup and clinical significance.
5. List the hyperlipoproteinemias and state the laboratory findings associated with each.
6. List the hypolipoproteinemias and state the laboratory findings associated with each.
7. State the basic assay procedures for serum cholesterol and triglyceride and the specimen requirements, principles, and interferences in each.
8. State the procedures available to determine high-density and low-density lipoprotein concentration in blood.
9. State the Friedewald calculation for low-density lipoprotein.
10. Resolve case studies regarding lipid analysis in the assessment of lipid pathologies.

Key Words

Apolipoproteins   Any of the protein constituents of lipoproteins

Atherosclerosis   A condition in which deposits of yellowish plaques containing cholesterol, lipoid material, and lipophages are formed within the intima and inner media of large- and medium-sized arteries

Cholesterol   A steroid alcohol, $C_{27}H_{45}OH$, that is an essential component of lipid metabolism; often found esterified with a fatty acid

Chylomicron   A particle of the class lipoproteins responsible for the transport of exogenous cholesterol and triglycerides from the small intestine to tissues after meals; a spherical particle with a core of triglyceride surrounded by a monolayer of phospholipids, cholesterol, and apolipoproteins

Essential Fatty Acid   A fatty acid that cannot be synthesized by the human body; for example, linoleic, linolenic, and arachidonic acids

---

*The authors gratefully acknowledge the contributions of Drs. Evan A. Stein and Gary L. Myers, on which portions of this chapter are based. Additional portions have been adapted from Rifai N, Kwiterovich PO Jr: Disorders of lipid and lipoprotein metabolism in children and adolescents. In Soldin SJ, Rifai N, Hicks JMB (eds): Biochemical Basis of Pediatric Diseases, Washington, DC, AACC Press, 1998.

†This work was supported in part by the Lipid/Research/Atherosclerosis Unit, Department of Pediatrics, Johns Hopkins University, School of Medicine, Baltimore, MD, 21287-3654. The authors thank Dr. Moseley Waite of the Bowman Gray School of Medicine and Dr. Santica Marcovina of the University of Washington for their reviews and corrections, as well as Kathleen L. Lovejoy, Nicole Maxey, and Dorthy Westmorland for their assistance in preparing the manuscript.

Fatty Acid   Any straight-chain monocarboxylic acid generally classified as follows: saturated fatty acids—those with no double bonds; monounsaturated fatty acids—those with one double bond; and polyunsaturated fatty acids—those with multiple double bonds

Lipid   Any of a heterogeneous groups of fats and fatlike substances characterized by their insolubility in water and solubility in nonpolar solvents, such as alcohol, ether, chloroform, benzene, etc.

Lipoprotein   Any of the lipid-protein complexes in which lipids are transported in the blood; lipoprotein particles consisting of a spherical hydrophobic core of triglycerides or cholesterol esters surrounded by a monolayer of phospholipids, cholesterol, and apolipoproteins

Phospholipid   Any lipid that contains phosphorous, including those with glycerol backbone (phosphoglycerides) and sphingosine or related substances (sphingomyelins); the major form of lipid in cell membranes

Prostaglandin   Any of a group of compounds derived from unsaturated 20-carbon fatty acids (primarily arachidonic acid) via the cyclooxygenase pathway; potent mediators of a diverse group of physiological processes

Triglyceride   An organic compound consisting of up to three molecules of fatty acids esterified to glycerol

---

Lipids play an important role in virtually all aspects of biological life, serving as hormones or hormone precursors, aiding in digestion, providing energy storage and metabolic fuels, acting as functional and structural components in biomembranes, and forming insulation to allow nerve conduction or prevent heat loss. The causative relationship between plasma lipids and lipoproteins and atherosclerosis was established conclusively in the past decade. As a result, large national public health programs have been developed to detect, evaluate, and treat individuals with certain plasma lipid abnormalities.

In this chapter, lipids are categorized into basic lipids, lipoproteins, and apolipoproteins. The basic biochemistry, clinical significance, and analytical considerations of each are discussed. The role of lipid metabolism in various diseases, including coronary heart disease (CHD), also is discussed.

■ BASIC BIOCHEMISTRY

In this section the basic biochemistry of lipids, lipoproteins, apolipoproteins, and their metabolism are discussed.

Lipids

The term **lipid** applies to a class of compounds that are soluble in organic solvents and nearly insoluble in water. Chemically, lipids are either compounds that yield fatty acids on hydrolysis or complex alcohols that can combine with fatty acids to form esters. Some lipids contain nonlipid groups, such as sialic, phosphoryl, amino, or sulfate groups. The presence of these groups gives lipid molecules an affinity for both water and organic solvents. This affinity is important in the formation of biological membranes. Lipids

can be subdivided broadly into five groups based on their chemical structure (Table 24-1).

Cholesterol

Chemistry

Cholesterol is a steroid alcohol with 27 carbon atoms that are arranged in a tetracyclical perhydrocyclopentanophenanthrene (sterane) skeleton (Figure 24-1). It is found almost exclusively in animals, in which virtually all cells and

---

TABLE 24-1   Classification of Clinically Important Lipids

Sterol Derivatives
Cholesterol and cholesteryl esters
Steroid hormones
Bile acids
Vitamin D

Fatty Acids
Short chain (2 to 4 carbon atoms)
Medium chain (6 to 10 carbon atoms)
Long chain (12 to 26 carbon atoms)
Prostaglandins

Glycerol Esters
Triglycerides, diglycerides, and monoglycerides (acylglycerols)
Phosphoglycerides

Sphingosine Derivatives
Sphingomyelin
Glycosphingolipids

Terpenes (Isoprene Polymers)
Vitamin A
Vitamin E
Vitamin K

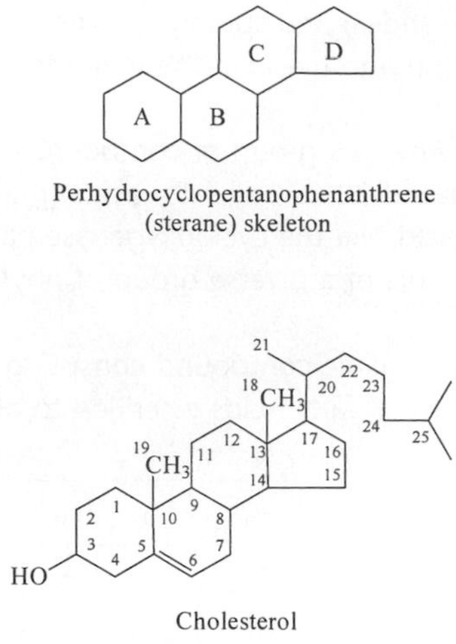

Figure 24-1   Structure of cholesterol.

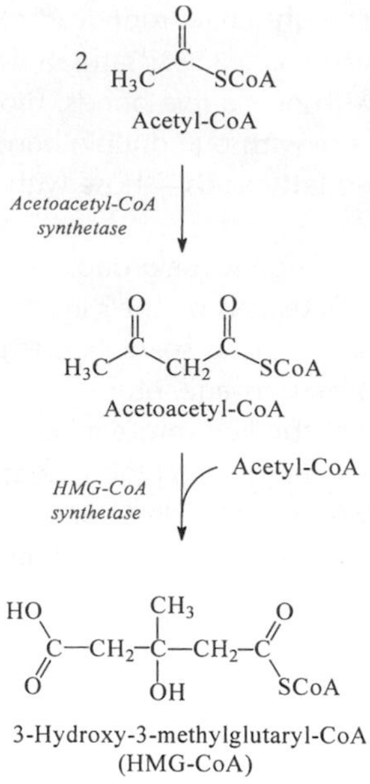

Figure 24-2   Cholesterol biosynthesis (stage 1). *CoA*, Coenzyme A.

body fluids contain some cholesterol. Knowledge of the numbering system of carbon atoms found in cholesterol is important because it is the initial starting point in other metabolic pathways, including vitamin D (see Chapter 38), steroid hormones (see Chapters 41 and 42), and bile acid synthesis (see Chapter 36). Because the enzymes modifying the sterane ring or its radicals in each metabolic pathway are known by both their site and their type of reaction (for example, 21-hydroxylase in cortisol synthesis), the diagnosis of many disease states consequently depends on isolation of the site of enzyme dysfunction (for example, 21-hydroxylase deficiency in adrenogenital syndrome).

Absorption

Cholesterol enters the intestine from three sources—the diet, bile and intestinal secretions, and cells. Animal products, especially meat, egg yolk, seafood, and whole-fat dairy products, provide the bulk of dietary cholesterol. Although cholesterol intake varies considerably according to an individual's dietary intake of animal products, the average American diet is estimated to contain approximately 300 to 450 mg of cholesterol per day. A similar amount of cholesterol is present in the gut from biliary secretion and the turnover of intestinal mucosal cells. Practically all cholesterol in the intestine is present in the nonesterified (free) form. Esterified cholesterol in the diet is hydrolyzed rapidly in the intestine to unesterified cholesterol and free fatty acids by cholesterol esterases secreted from the pancreas and small intestine.

Before being absorbed, unesterified cholesterol first is solubilized. This process occurs through the formation of mixed micelles that contain unesterified cholesterol, fatty acids, monoglycerides (derived from triglycerides), **phospholipids** (lysolecithin), and conjugated bile acids. Forma-

tion of mixed micelles aids cholesterol absorption by both solubilizing the cholesterol and facilitating its transport to the surface of the luminal cell, where it is absorbed. The bile acids act as detergents and are the most important factor affecting micelle formation. In their absence, digestion and absorption of both cholesterol and triglyceride are impaired severely. The quantity of dietary cholesterol that can be absorbed appears to depend on the amount that can be solubilized by micelles. On the average, 30% to 60% of dietary and intestinal cholesterol is absorbed daily. With increments in dietary cholesterol, additional cholesterol is absorbed to a maximum of approximately 1 g/day when oral intake reaches 3 g/day. The ability of cholesterol to form micelles also is influenced by the quantity of dietary fat. Increased amounts of fat in the diet result in expansion of mixed micelles, which in turn allows for more cholesterol to be solubilized and absorbed. Most cholesterol absorption occurs in the small intestine (jejunum and proximal ileum). As fat and cholesterol absorption occurs, the micelles break up, thus reducing further cholesterol absorption.

In addition to animal cholesterol, approximately 200 to 300 mg of plant sterols are ingested daily. The most common plant sterol is β-sitosterol. Plant sterols differ from cholesterol only by small variations on the sterol side chain. Despite their close similarity to cholesterol, plant sterols are absorbed poorly, but when plant sterols are administered in amounts of 5 to 15 g/day, they significantly inhibit the absorption of cholesterol. Although the mechanism for their reducing cholesterol absorption has not been determined, plant sterols have been used therapeutically to treat patients with elevated plasma cholesterol levels.

Once it enters the intestinal mucosal cell, cholesterol is packaged with triglycerides, phospholipids, and several specific apolipoproteins into a large lipoprotein called the

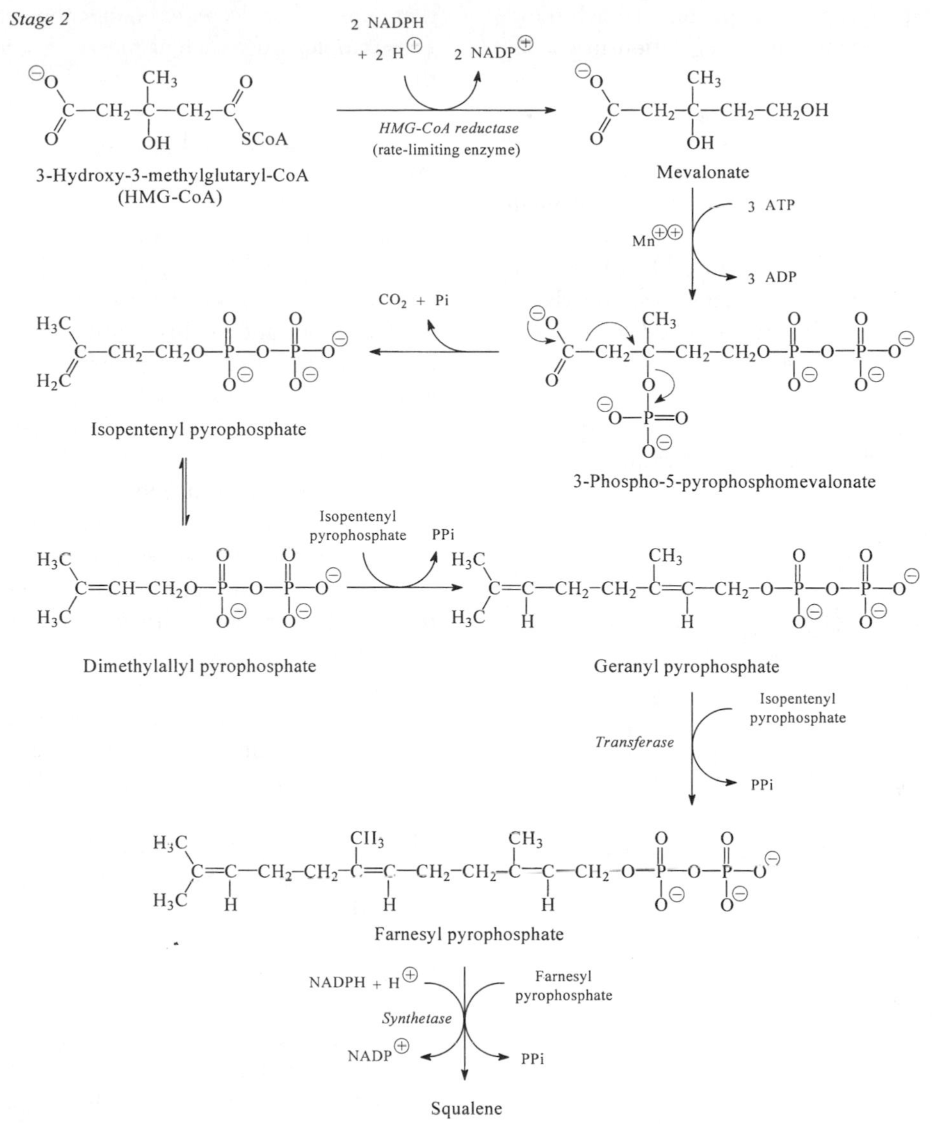

Stage 2

3-Hydroxy-3-methylglutaryl-CoA
(HMG-CoA)

2 NADPH
+ 2 H$^{\oplus}$ 2 NADP$^{\oplus}$

HMG-CoA reductase
(rate-limiting enzyme)

Mevalonate

Mn$^{\oplus\oplus}$ 3 ATP

3 ADP

Isopentenyl pyrophosphate

CO_2 + Pi

3-Phospho-5-pyrophosphomevalonate

Dimethylallyl pyrophosphate

Isopentenyl
pyrophosphate   PPi

Geranyl pyrophosphate

Transferase

Isopentenyl
pyrophosphate

PPi

Farnesyl pyrophosphate

NADPH + H$^{\oplus}$ Farnesyl
pyrophosphate

Synthetase

NADP$^{\oplus}$ PPi

Squalene

Figure 24-3   Cholesterol biosynthesis (stage 2). *CoA,* Coenzyme A; *NADP,* nicotinamide-adenine dinucleotide phosphate; *NADPH,* reduced NADP.

chylomicron (see discussion on lipoprotein metabolism, exogenous pathway). One apoprotein component known as *apolipoprotein (apo) B-48* is vital to the formation of chylomicrons, and in people with a rare deficiency of apo B-48 synthesis, chylomicron formation, and consequently cholesterol and fat absorption, are impaired severely. Chylomicrons enter the lymphatics, which empty into the thoracic duct and eventually enter the systemic venous circulation at the junction of the left subclavian and left internal jugular vein.

Synthesis

In addition to its absorption from the intestine, cholesterol can be synthesized endogenously by the liver and other tissues from smaller molecules, particularly acetate. Although essentially all cells have the capacity to synthesize cholesterol, almost 90% of its synthesis occurs in the liver and gut; peripheral cells and other organs depend on cholesterol delivery from the circulation.

Cholesterol biosynthesis occurs in three stages. In the first stage, acetyl-CoA (coenzyme A), a key metabolic intermediate derived from carbohydrates, amino acids, and fatty acids, forms the six-carbon thioester HMG-CoA (3-hydroxy-3-methylglutaryl-CoA; Figure 24-2). In the second stage, HMG-CoA is reduced to mevalonate, then decarboxylated to five-carbon isoprene units. These isoprene units are condensed to form first a 10-carbon (geranyl pyrophosphate) and then a 15-carbon intermediate (farnesyl pyrophosphate). Two of these C_{15} molecules combine to produce the final product of the second stage—squalene, a 30-carbon acyclic hydrocarbon (Figure 24-3). The second stage is important because it contains the step involving the microsomal enzyme HMG-CoA reductase, which is the rate-limiting enzyme in cholesterol biosynthesis. The enzyme that forms farnesyl pyrophosphate, geranyl transferase, is an important second site of regulation in cholesterol synthesis, and inhibition at this level permits the formation of physiologically important intermediate isoprenoids in the absence of cholesterol synthesis. The third and final stage of synthesis (Figure 24-4) occurs in the endoplasmic reticulum, with many of the intermediate products being bound to a specific carrier protein. Squalene, after an initial oxidation forms the 4-ring, 30-carbon intermediate, lanosterol. In a series of oxidation-decarboxylation reactions a number of side chains are removed from the pentanophenanthrene structure to form the 27-carbon molecule of cholesterol.

Knowledge of the endogenous cholesterol synthetic pathway has led to the development of therapeutic agents that suppress or decrease endogenous cholesterol synthesis For example, drugs such as mevastatin, lovastatin, simvastatin, pravastatin, and atorvastatin selectively suppress the rate-limiting enzyme HMG-CoA reductase and thereby lower serum cholesterol levels.

Figure 24-4 Cholesterol biosynthesis (stage 3). *NADP,* Nicotinamide-adenine dinucleotide phosphate; *NADPH,* reduced NADP.

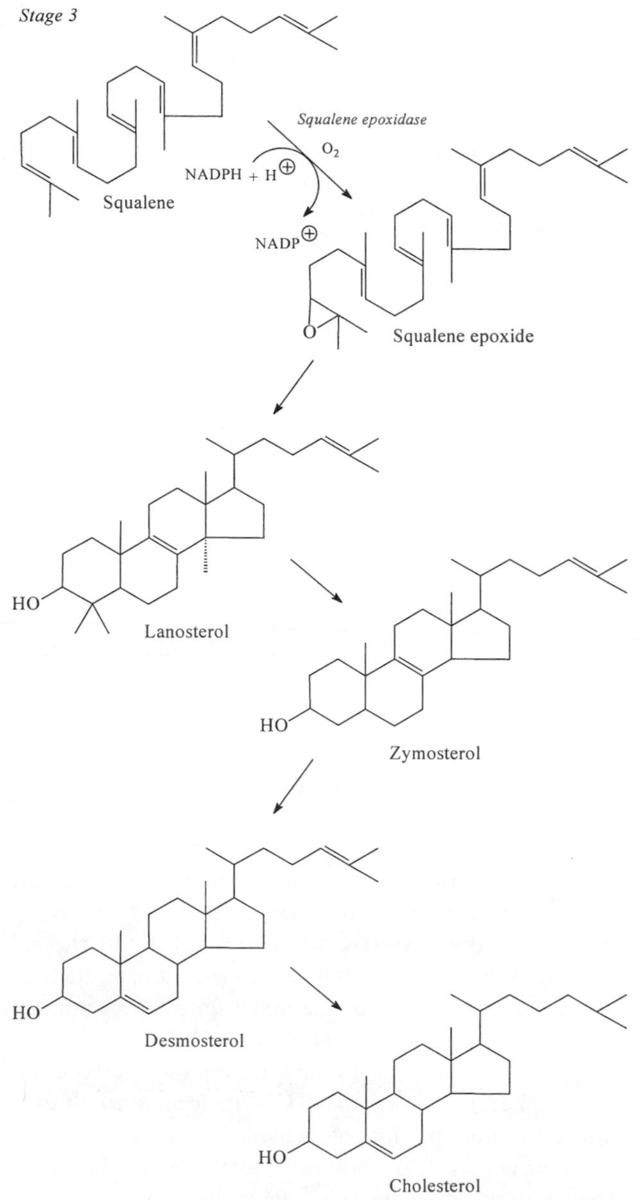

Esterification

Cholesterol is released into the circulation in the form of lipoprotein, primarily very–low-density lipoprotein (VLDL; see exogenous pathway discussion). Esterification of cholesterol is important in this process because it enhances the lipid-carrying capacity of the lipoprotein in plasma and prevents intracellular toxicity by unesterified cholesterol. The reaction is catalyzed by lecithin cholesterol acyltransferase (LCAT) in the plasma and acylcholesterol acyltransferase (ACAT) within the cell. The intracellular ACAT pathway is the major pathway in the liver, intestine, adrenal cortex, and probably in the arterial wall. This is an energy-requiring pathway, and the initial reaction (Figure 24-5) involves activation of a fatty acid with thio coenzyme A (CoASH) to form an acyl-CoA, which in turn reacts with cholesterol to form an ester. The LCAT reaction does not require CoASH and results from fatty-acid transfer from the second carbon position of lecithin to cholesterol (see Figure 24-5). Cholesteryl esters account for about 70% of the cholesterol in plasma, and LCAT is responsible for the formation of virtually all this cholesteryl ester. LCAT is synthesized in the liver, released into the circulation, and primarily activated by apo A-I.

Plasma LCAT activity may have some significance analytically because the enzyme continues to esterify plasma cholesterol even after the blood sample is drawn and stored at room temperature. If distinction between esterified and unesterified cholesterol is necessary, analysis should be carried out as soon as possible or the samples should be cooled to at least 4 °C or frozen, preferably at −70 °C or lower.

Catabolism

Once lipoprotein cholesterol enters the cell, the cholesteryl esters are hydrolyzed by lysosomal acid lipase. As

Intracellular:

Fatty acid + CoASH —(*Acyl-CoA synthetase*; ATP → PPi + AMP)→ Acyl-CoA

Acyl-CoA + cholesterol —(*ACAT*)→ Cholesterol ester + CoASH

Intravascular:

Lecithin + cholesterol —(*LCAT*)→ Cholesterol ester + lysolecithin

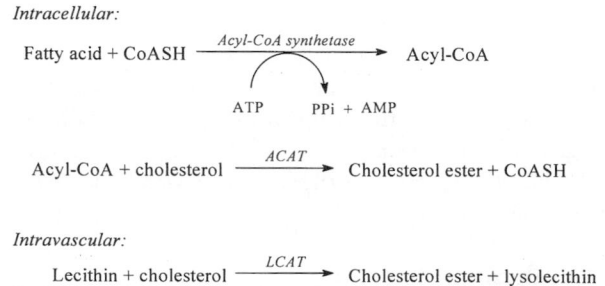

Figure 24-5 Intracellular and intravascular esterification of cholesterol mediated by acylcholesterol acyltransferase (ACAT) and lecithin cholesterol acyltransferase (LCAT), respectively. *ATP,* Adenosine triphosphate; *CoA,* coenzyme A; *AMP,* adenosine monophosphate; *CoASH,* thio coenzyme A.

will be discussed later, the lack or malfunction of this enzyme results in intracellular accumulation of cholesterol esters and produces a clinical disorder known as *cholesteryl ester storage disease.*

Cholesterol reaching the liver is either secreted unchanged into bile or metabolized to bile acids. Approximately one third of the daily production of cholesterol, or about 400 mg/day is converted into bile acids (Figure 24-6). The conversion of cholesterol to cholic and chenodeoxycholic acids, the major bile acids in humans, involves the shortening of the cholesterol side chain and hydroxylation of the sterol nucleus (see Chapter 36). The first step, which is the rate-limiting step, is the hydroxylation of the 7-position of the sterol nucleus, catalyzed by the enzyme 7-α-hydroxylase (see Figure 24-6). The bile acids then are conjugated with either glycine or taurine and enter the bile canaliculi. After reaching the small intestine, the conjugated bile acids play an active part in cholesterol and fat absorption, as discussed previously. Some of the bile acids are deconjugated and converted by bacteria in the intestine to secondary bile acids. Cholic acid is converted to deoxycholic acid, and chenodeoxycholic acid is metabolized to lithocholic acid. About 90% of the bile acids, except lithocholic, are reabsorbed in the lower third of the ileum and returned to the liver by the portal vein, thus completing the enterohepatic circulation.

A significant amount of cholesterol also is excreted directly into the biliary system, where it is solubilized to form mixed micelles with bile acids and phospholipids. If the amount of cholesterol in bile exceeds the capacity of these solubilizing agents, however, excess cholesterol can precipi-

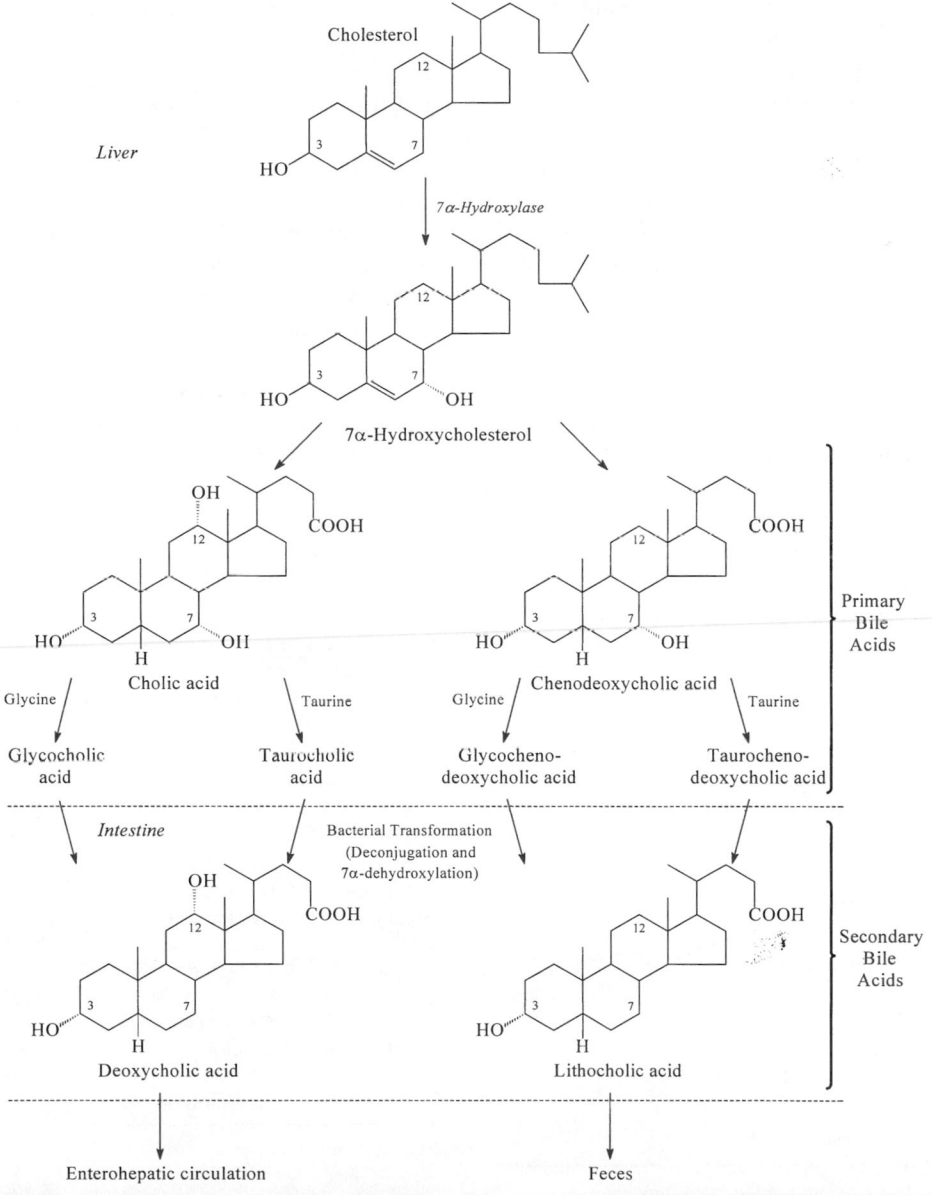

Figure 24-6 Bile acid synthesis.

tate, forming cholesterol gallstones. In Westernized societies, approximately 80% of all gallstones are cholesterol-containing stones.

Fatty acids

Chemistry

RCOOH is the general chemical formula for a **fatty acid,** where "R" is an alkyl chain. Fatty acid chain lengths vary and commonly are classified according to the number of carbon atoms present. Three somewhat arbitrarily defined groups of fatty acids are those containing 2 to 4 carbon atoms (short chain), 6 to 10 carbon atoms (medium chain), and 12 to 26 carbon atoms (long chain). Those of importance in human nutrition and metabolism are of the long-chain class containing an even number of carbon atoms (see Chapter 45).

Fatty acids are classified further according to their degree of saturation. Saturated fatty acids have no double bonds between carbon atoms; monounsaturated fatty acids contain one double bond; and polyunsaturated fatty acids contain more than one double bond (Figure 24-7). The double bonds in polyunsaturated fatty acids of both animal and plant origin are usually three carbon atoms apart. Some oils from marine fishes living in deep, cold waters (for example, salmon) possess numerous (up to six) unsaturated bonds and are usually more than 20 carbon atoms long. These oils can be oxidized easily because of their high degree of unsaturation.

The labeling of the carbon atoms in fatty acids can be either from the carboxyl terminal (Δ-numbering system) or methyl terminal (η- or ω-numbering system; Table 24-2). In addition, the carbon atoms may be labeled with Greek symbols, with α being adjacent to the carboxyl group and T being farthest away. In the (Δ-system, fatty acids are abbreviated according to the number of carbon atoms, number of double bonds, and position(s) of double bond(s). For example, linoleic acid, which contains 18 car-

bons and two unsaturated bonds between carbons 9 and 10 and between carbons 12 and 13, can be written as $C_{18}:2^{9,12}$. By use of the η- or ω-system, linoleic acid would be abbreviated to $C_{18}:2n\text{-}6$, in which only the first carbon forming the unsaturated pair is written. A third system of nomenclature is known as the *Geneva* or *systematic classification* (see Table 24-2).

In saturated fatty acids the chain is extended and flexible. (That is, the carbon atoms can rotate freely around the longitudinal axis.) Unsaturated fatty acids, however, have fixed 30-degree bends in their chains at each double bond. Depending on the plane in which this bend occurs, either the *cis* or *trans* isomer is produced. In mammals, all naturally occurring unsaturated fatty acids are of the *cis* variety. *Trans* fatty acids result from catalytic hydrogenation, a process used to "harden" fats in the manufacture of certain foods, such as margarine. Most fats in the human body are derived from the diet, which contains up to 40% fat, 90% of which is triglyceride. In addition, humans can synthesize most fatty acids, including saturated, monounsaturated, and some polyunsaturated fats. However, some fatty acids cannot be synthesized. One such fatty acid is linoleic acid ($C_{18}:2^{9,12}$), which is found only in plants. Because it is not synthesized but is vital for health, growth, and development, it is termed an **essential fatty acid.** Linoleic acid also can be converted to arachidonic acid, which plays an important role in prostaglandin synthesis and perhaps in myelinization of the central nervous system.

Circulating forms

Fatty acids circulate in esterified and free forms.* Much of the fatty acid in plasma is esterified with cholesterol or

---

*The term *free fatty acid* is a misnomer because fatty acids are transported complexed to albumin.

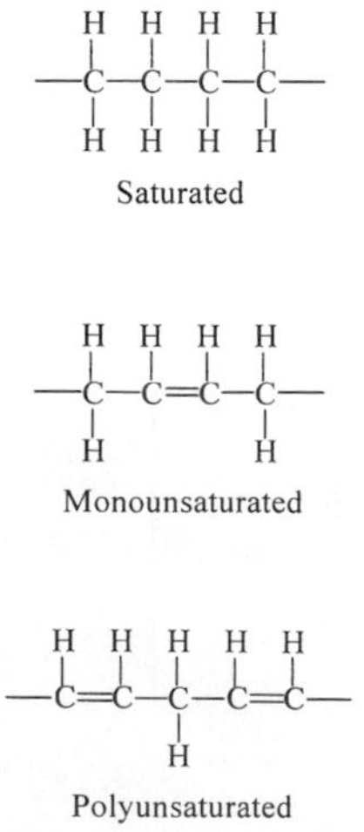

Figure 24-7 Saturated and unsaturated fatty acids.

TABLE 24-2	Fatty Acids Commonly Found in Human Tissue		
Common Name	Systematic Name	Δ-Numbering	η-(ω-) Numbering
Lauric	Dodecanoic	12:0	12:0
Myristic	Tetradecanoic	14:0	14:0
Palmitic	Hexadecanoic	16:0	16:0
Palmitoleic	9-Hexadecenoic	$16:1^9$	16:1n-7
Stearic	Octadecanoic	18:0	18:0
Oleic	9-Octadecenoic	$18:1^9$	18:1n-9
Linoleic*	9,12-Octadecadienoic	$18:2^{9,12}$	18:2n-6
Linolenic*	9,12,15-Octadecatrienoic	$18:3^{9,12,15}$	18:3n-3
Arachidic	Eicosanoic	20:0	20:0
Arachidonic	5,8,11,14-Eicosatetraenoic	$20:4^{5,8,11,14}$	20:4n-6

*Essential fatty acid.

glycerol or is transported as a fatty acid-albumin complex. One molecule of albumin can carry as many as 20 molecules of fatty acid. The free fatty acid carboxyl group has a pK_a of approximately 4.8; thus free fatty acid molecules in both plasma and intracellular fluid (pH of 7.4 and 7.0, respectively) exist in ionized form. The normal level of free fatty acids in human blood is 0.3 to 0.9 mmol/L, or about 8 to 25 mg/dL of plasma. The flux of free fatty acids through the plasma is very large and quite sensitive to physiological energy demands (exercise and physical work), the level of blood glucose, and psychological stresses that cause liberation of epinephrine.

Catabolism

Long-chain fatty acids are oxidized in the mitochondria and produce energy by a series of reactions that operate in a repetitive manner to shorten the fatty acid chain by two carbon atoms at a time from the —COOH terminal of the molecule, a process known as β-oxidation. For example, one mole of C_{16} fatty acid is converted to eight moles of acetyl-CoA. Acetyl-CoA does not normally accumulate in the cell

but is condensed enzymatically with oxaloacetate, derived largely from carbohydrate metabolism (Figure 24-8), to give citrate, which is a major component of the tricarboxylic acid cycle (Krebs cycle). The Krebs cycle is a common pathway for the final oxidation of nearly all food material, whether derived from carbohydrate, fat, or protein. An important consideration is that efficient operation of the Krebs cycle depends on the availability of sufficient oxaloacetate to serve as acceptor for acetyl-CoA.

A large quantity of energy can be produced from a single fatty-acid molecule; for instance, the complete oxidation of one mole of palmitic acid to carbon dioxide and water produces 16 moles of CO_2, 16 moles of H_2O, and 129 moles of adenosine triphosphate (ATP), or 2340 Cal.* Thus the standard free energy for oxidation of palmitic acid is 2340 Cal, whereas the free energy liberated by hydrolysis of 129 moles of ATP is 940 Cal, indicating that the efficiency of

---

*The unit used to discuss energy value of food is the Calorie (Cal), equal to 1000 calories or 1 kilocalorie (kcal). In the SI system the unit of energy is the joule (J), and 1 calorie is equal to 4.1868 J.

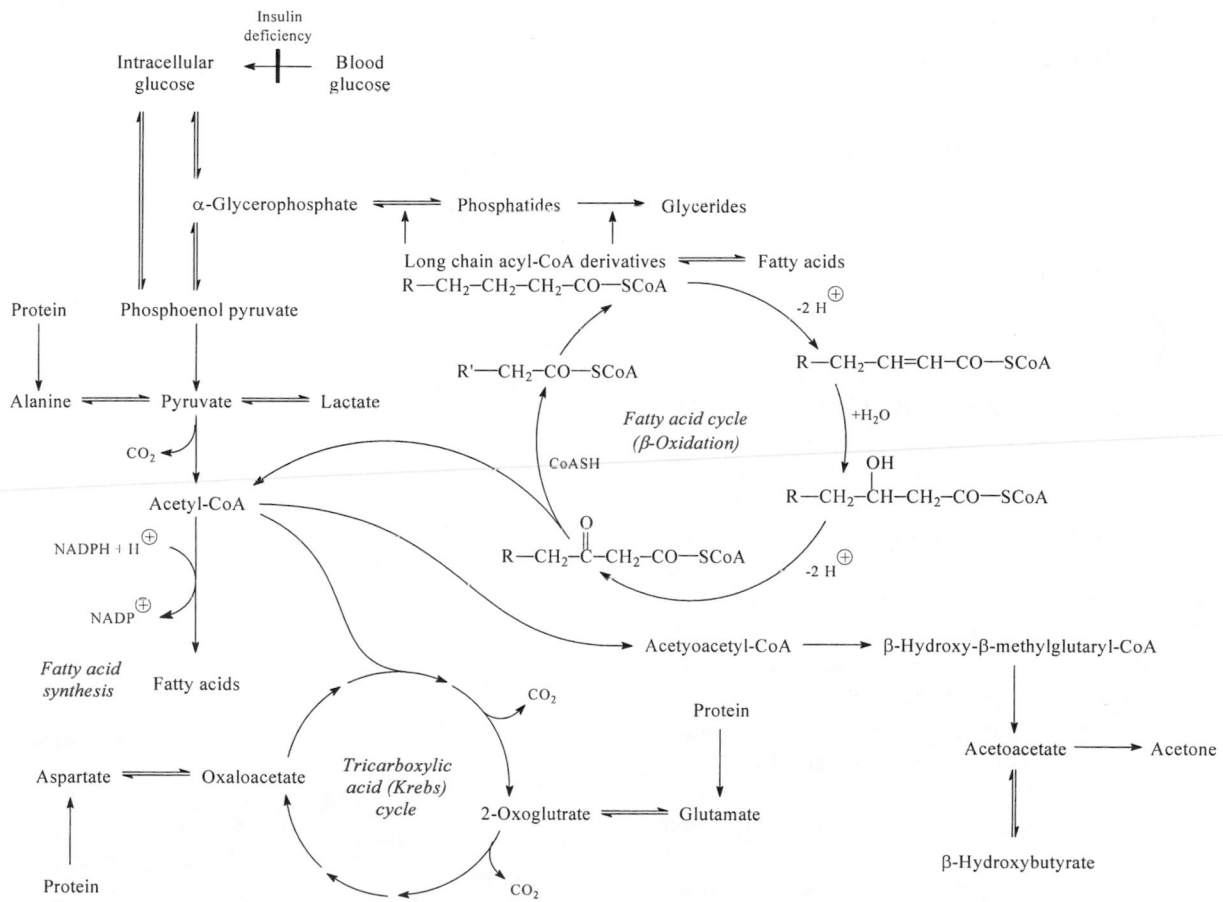

Figure 24-8 Metabolic relationships among intermediates of carbohydrate, fat, and protein metabolism. Note that acetyl-CoA is produced from both carbohydrate and fat. The glucogenic amino acids, derived from protein metabolism, enter glycolytic paths as 2-keto acids. Keto-genic amino acids enter as acetyl-CoA. *CoA,* Coenzyme A; *CoASH,* thio coenzyme A; *NADP,* nicotinamide-adenine dinucleotide phosphate; *NADPH,* reduced NADP.

energy conservation in fatty acid oxidation is approximately 40% under standard conditions.

By means of suitable enzyme reactions the chemical energy stored in fatty acids can be released for metabolic processes or stored in the form of high-energy compounds, such as ATP. Triglycerides that contain three fatty-acid molecules therefore are an efficient storage form for metabolic energy. The amount of energy produced by metabolism of 1 mol of palmitic acid (16 carbon atoms) is approximately twice that produced by metabolism of an equivalent amount (2.5 mol) of glucose (6 carbon atoms per molecule). Carbohydrate storage requires water for hydration; triglyceride storage does not. In addition to their high intrinsic energy content, triglycerides have a low density (<1 g/mL) and, because of their hydrophobic nature and peripheral distribution in the body, provide excellent insulation.

Ketone formation

During prolonged starvation or when carbohydrate metabolism is impaired severely, as it is in cases of uncontrolled diabetes mellitus, the formation of acetyl-CoA exceeds the supply of oxaloacetate. The abundance of acetyl-CoA results from excessive mobilization of fatty acids from adipose tissue and excessive degradation of the fatty acids by β-oxidation in the liver. The resulting acetyl-CoA excess is diverted to an alternative pathway in the mitochondria and forms acetoacetic acid, β-hydroxybutyric acid, and acetone—three compounds known collectively as *ketone bodies* (Figure 24-9). The presence of ketone bodies is a frequent finding in individuals with severe, uncontrolled diabetes mellitus.

The first step in the production of ketone bodies is the condensation of two molecules of acetyl-CoA to form acetoacetyl-CoA, which condenses in the mitochondria with a third molecule of acetyl-CoA to yield HMG-CoA (see Figure 24-9). This pool of HMG-CoA is distinct from that in the cytosol, which is an intermediate in cholesterol synthesis. The HMG-CoA produced in the mitochondria then is cleaved enzymatically to yield acetoacetate and acetyl-CoA. A portion of the acetoacetate formed in liver cells usually is reduced to β-hydroxybutyrate. Because acetoacetate is unstable, a further portion decomposes to form carbon dioxide and acetone, the third ketone body found in those with severe, untreated diabetes mellitus. Ketosis therefore develops from excessive production of acetyl-CoA as the body attempts to obtain necessary energy from stored fat in the absence of an adequate supply of carbohydrate metabolites (see Chapter 23).

Inadequate incorporation of acetyl-CoA into the Krebs cycle may be aggravated further by inhibition of the oxaloacetate-generating enzyme system by excess accumulation of palmityl-CoA and other long-chain fatty acyl-CoA derivatives in the liver. Skeletal muscle and the heart (and brain, in cases of prolonged fasting) can use ketone bodies by resynthesizing their CoA derivatives of the acids and

subsequently oxidizing them to produce energy. Although liver cells are largely responsible for converting fatty acids, they cannot metabolize acetoacetate because the liver lacks 3-ketoacid CoA transferase, the enzyme required for transfer of CoA from succinyl-CoA.

The entire process of ketosis can be reversed through restoration of an adequate level of carbohydrate metabolism. In cases of starvation, restoration consists of adequate carbohydrate ingestion; with diabetes mellitus, ketosis can be reversed by insulin administration, which permits circulating blood glucose to be taken up by the cells. With production of oxaloacetate, the acceptor of acetyl-CoA, normal metabolism is restored, and the release of fatty acids from adipose tissues slows and finally is reversed. A graphical view of these metabolic reactions is outlined in Figure 24-8, which illustrates the interrelationship between carbohydrate, fatty acid, and protein metabolism.

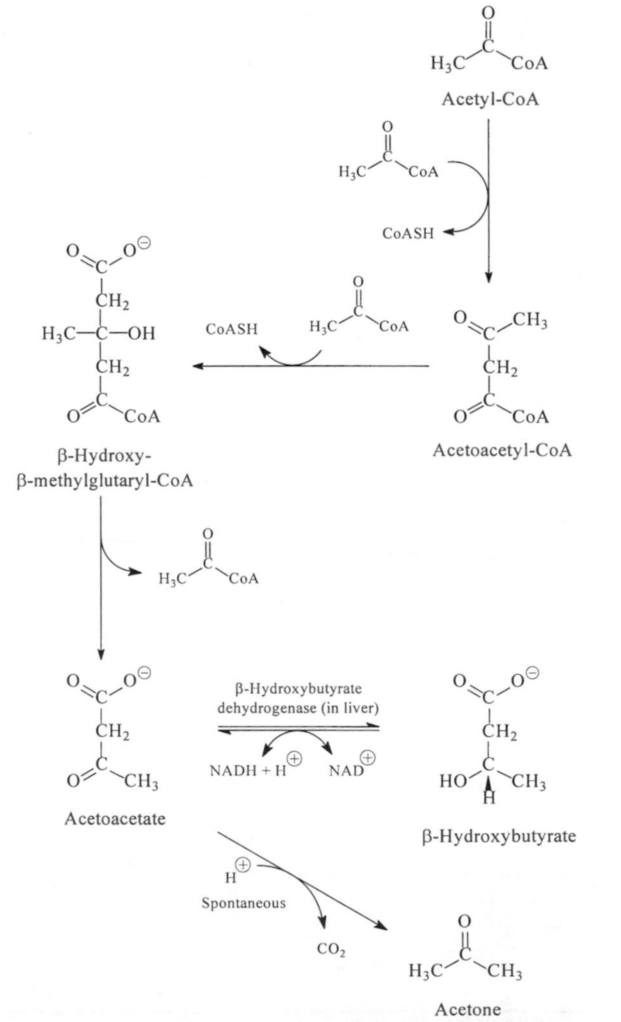

Figure 24-9 Formation of ketone bodies. *CoA,* Coenzyme A; *CoASH,* thio coenzyme A; *NADH,* nicotinamide-adenine dinucleotide (reduced); *NAD$^+$,* nicotinamide-adenine dinucleotide (oxidized).

Prostaglandins

Prostaglandins and related compounds are derivatives of fatty acids, primarily arachidonate. The group consists of prostaglandins, thromboxanes, some hydroperoxy- and hydroxy-fatty acid derivatives, and leukotrienes. Although their full physiological role is not completely known, they exert diverse biological actions. They are extremely potent, producing physiological actions at concentrations as low as 1 μg/L.

Chemistry

The prostaglandins are a series of C_{20} unsaturated fatty acids containing a cyclopentane ring; the parent fatty acid has been given the trivial name *prostanoic acid*. The seven-carbon chain linked to C-8 of prostanoic acid (R_1) projects below the plane of the ring, whereas the eight-carbon chain attached to C-12 (R_2) projects above the ring.

By convention, prostaglandins are abbreviated *PG*, with the class designated by a capital letter (A, B, E, F, G, H, and I) followed by a number and then in some cases a Greek letter (Figure 24-10). With the exception of PGG and PGH, which have the same ring structure (cyclopentane endoperoxide), the letters refer to different ring structures. PGA and PGB have keto groups at C-9, with the A series having a double bond between C-10 and C-11 and the B series having a double bond between C-8 and C-12. PGE also has a C-9 keto bond but a hydroxyl group at C-11. The F series has hydroxyl groups at both C-9 and C-11. The difference between PGG and PGH, which have identical ring struc-

tures, occurs in the side chain at C-15 in R_2; the G series has a peroxide group, whereas the H series has a hydroxyl group. The I series has a double-ring formation, C-9 of the cyclopentane ring being linked to C-6 of the side chain by an oxygen molecule to form a second five-sided ring (see Figure 24-10). The endoperoxide PGs (G and H series) are intermediates in the formation of other PGs, such as the A, B, E, F, and I series.

The number following the capital letter usually is written as a subscript and used to designate the number of unsaturated bonds in the PG side chains and not within the ring structure itself. In PGE_1, for example, a double bond exists between C-13 and C-14; in the 2 series (PGE_2), a double bond exists between C-13 and C-14 and between C-5 and C-6; and in the 3 series (PGE_3), an additional double bond occurs between C-17 and C-18. The 2 series is most common. The bond between C-13 and C-14 is always *trans*, whereas those between C-5 and C-6 and between C-17 and C-18 are always *cis*. At C-15, all naturally occurring prostaglandins have a hydroxyl group that projects below the plane of the ring. The use of the Greek letter (α or β) applies only to the F series and refers to the hydroxyl group found at C-9. In the α-series the hydroxyl group projects below the ring plane in the same direction as the C-11 hydroxyl group, whereas the β-series denotes that the hydroxyl at C-9 is above the plane of the ring. Sixteen naturally occurring prostaglandins have been described (Table 24-3), but only seven, along with two thromboxanes, are found commonly throughout the body. These are termed the *primary prostaglandins*.

Although prostaglandins appear hormonelike in action, they are different from hormones in at least two respects; they are synthesized at the site of action and are made in almost all tissues. Linoleic acid ($C_{18}:2^{9,12}$) is the precursor of two of the three 20-carbon fatty acids that form prostaglandins; linolenic acid ($C_{18}:3^{9,12,15}$) is the other precursor. Both these fatty acids are considered essential because they cannot be synthesized in the body and therefore must be present in the diet. The three C_{20} fatty acids subsequently

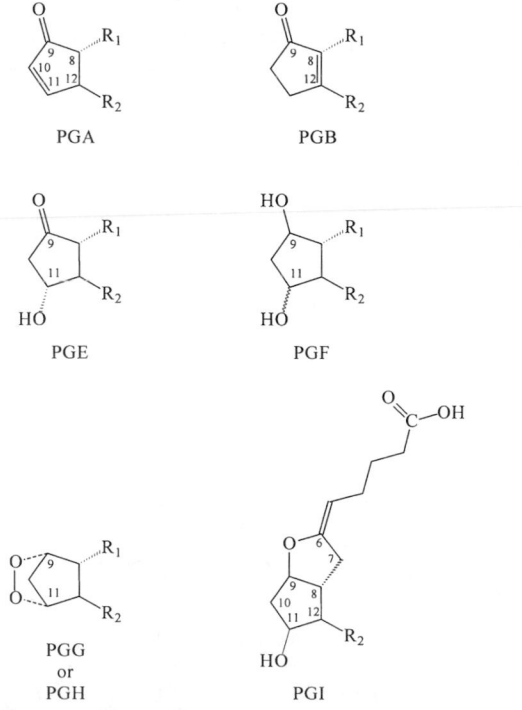

Figure 24-10 Major prostaglandin (PG) classes (series). R_1 and R_2 are prostaglandin side chains.

TABLE 24-3   Naturally Occurring Prostaglandins

Primary PG	Other PG
PGE_1	PGA_1
$PGF_{1\alpha}$	PGA_2
PGE_2	19α-OHPGA$_1$
$PGF_{2\alpha}$	19α-OHPGA$_2$
PGG_2	PGB_1
PGH_2	PGB_2
PGI_2	19α-OHPGB$_2$
Thromboxane A_2	PGE_3
Thromboxane B_2	$PGF_{3\alpha}$

PG, Prostaglandin; OHPGA, hydroxy-prostaglandin A; OHPGB, hydroxy-prostaglandin B.

formed are $C_{20}:3^{5,8,11}$ (eicosatrienoic acid), $C_{20}:4^{5,8,11,14}$ (eicosatetraenoic or arachidonic acid), and $C_{20}:5^{5,8,11,14,17}$ (e: cosapentaenoic acid). These three fatty acids form the PG_1, PG_2, and PG_3 series, respectively.

Once formed, prostaglandins exert very short-lived effects and are catabolized rapidly (their half-life being expressed in seconds). Inactivation of prostaglandin appears to be mediated by two enzymes, 15α-hydroxy-prostaglandin dehydrogenase and Δ^{13}-prostaglandin reductase. Prostaglandins are not stored; instead the precursor C_{20} fatty acids are present in tissues attached to the C-2 (see discussion on glycerol esters) of phosphoglycerides. When needed, the C_{20} precursor is hydrolyzed by phospholipase A_2, which is specific for the C-2 atom of the phosphoglyceride. The release of the C_{20} fatty acid appears to be the rate-limiting step in prostaglandin synthesis and is stimulated by the effect of bradykinin, thrombins, or angiotensin II.

Synthesis

Although the probability exists that all prostaglandins follow a similar synthetic pathway, $C_{20}:4$ (arachidonic acid) has been the most intensively studied and is used to illustrate the pathway (Figure 24-11). Once released, arachidonic acid can follow one of two pathways. The lipooxygenase route produces 12-L-hydroperoxy-5,8,10,14 eicosatetraenoic acid (HPETE); HPETE spontaneously

decomposes to 12-L-hydroxy-5,8,10,14 eicosatetraenoic acid (HETE), which is thought to be a chemotactic agent. The alternative pathway is that mediated by cyclooxygenase (COX) to produce the endoperoxides PGG_2 and PGH_2. The latter can be degraded to 12-L-hydroxy-5,8,10-heptadecatrienoic acid. Nonsteroidal antiinflammatory drugs (NSAIDs), such as aspirin, ibuprofen, and indomethacin, inhibit the COXs, thereby decreasing prostaglandin synthesis. Two isoforms of COX are known—COX-1 and COX-2. COX-1 levels are in general rather constant in cells, whereas COX-2 is synthesized in response to inflammation. Certain drugs that inhibit both COXs have nephrotoxic and ulcerogenic side effects. Therefore newer NSAIDs are being tested to inhibit preferentially COX-2 to reduce side effects while maintaining the desirable antiinflammatory therapy.

Prostaglandin I_2, or prostacyclin, is derived from arachidonic acid (see Figure 24-11) in the vascular endothelium. It has a powerful vasodilatory action, especially on the coronary arteries, and also is responsible for inhibiting platelet aggregation. Thromboxane A_2 is synthesized from arachidonic acid but also is produced by platelets. It has the opposite effect of prostacyclin; that is, it stimulates the contraction of arterial smooth muscle and enhances platelet aggregation. It has a very short half-life, about 30 seconds, and is converted rapidly to its inactive metabolite, thromboxane B_2. The thromboxanes are slightly different from the other prostaglandins in that they contain six-sided rings of five carbon atoms and one oxygen atom (Figure 24-12). Table 24-4 lists some of the reported functions of the various prostaglandins. With increasing knowledge of the physiological role of the prostaglandins, discrete disorders of prostaglandin metabolism likely will be discovered, and prostaglandins, prostaglandin analogues, or prostaglandin antagonists likely will be used in clinical practice.

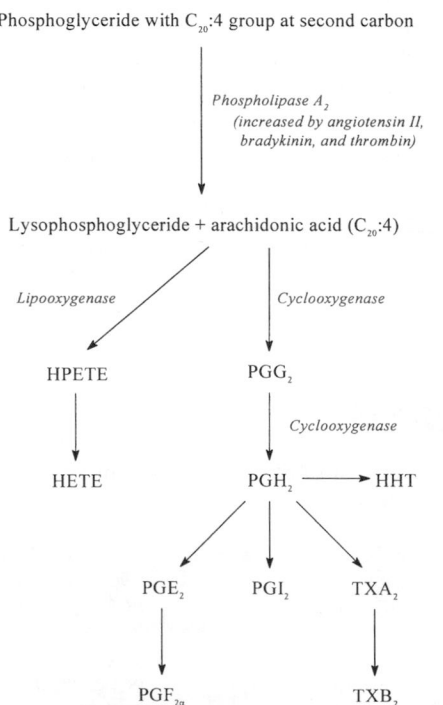

Figure 24-11 Synthesis of prostaglandins from arachidonic precursor. *PG,* Prostaglandin; *TX,* thromboxane; *HPETE,* 12-L-hydroperoxy-5,8,10,14 eicosatetraenoic acid; *HETE,* 12-L-hydroxy-5,8,10,14 eicosatetraenoic acid; *HHT,* 12-L-hydroxy-5,8,10-heptadecatrienoic acid.

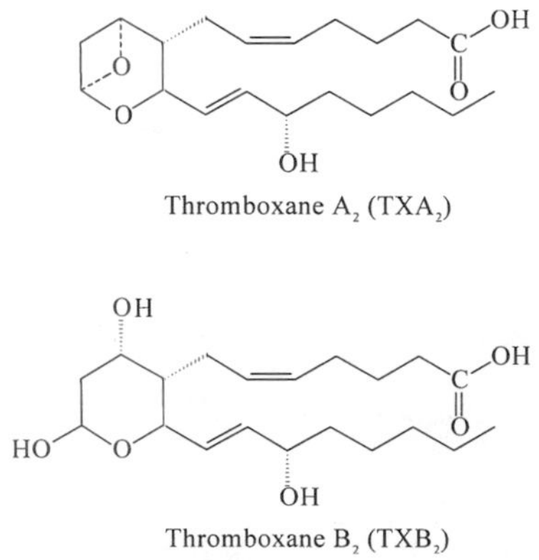

Figure 24-12 Structures of thromboxanes.

Glycerol esters (acylglycerols)

Chemistry

Glycerol is a three-carbon alcohol that contains a hydroxyl group on each of its carbon atoms. Each hydroxyl can be esterified with a fatty acid (Figure 24-13). The two terminal carbon atoms in the glycerol molecule are chemically equivalent and designated α and α'. The center carbon is labeled β. A common alternative labeling system uses the numeral 1 for the α-carbon, 2 for the β-carbon, and 3 for the α'-carbon.

The class of acylglycerol (glyceride) is determined by the number of fatty acyl groups present—one fatty acid, monoacylglycerols (monoglycerides); two fatty acids, diacylglycerols (diglycerides); three fatty acids, triacylglycerols (**triglycerides**). In a monoacylglycerol the fatty acid may be linked

TABLE 24-4	Prostaglandin-Mediated Effects
Site of Action	Physiological Response
Arterial smooth muscle	Alters blood pressure
Uterine muscle	Induces labor, therapeutic abortion
Lower gastrointestinal tract	Increases motility
Bronchial smooth muscle	Induces bronchospasm
Platelets	Increases coagulability
Capillaries	Increases permeability
Stomach	Enhances gastric-acid secretion
Adipose tissue	Inhibits triglyceride lipolysis

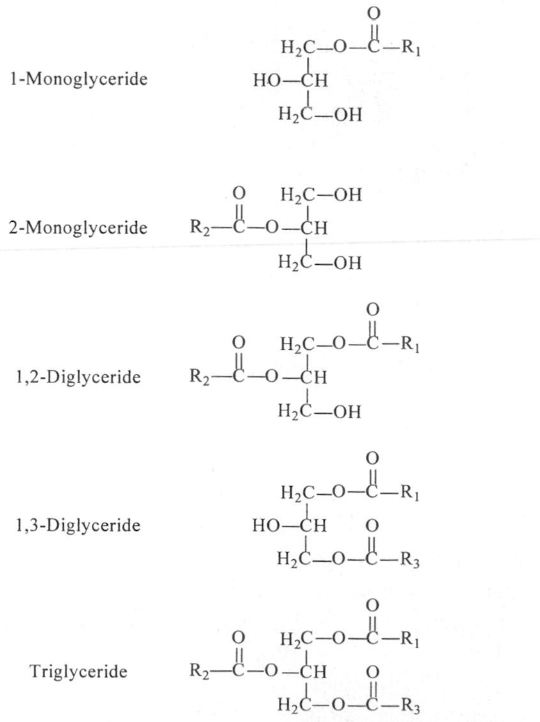

to any of the three carbon atoms. By convention the number system is used to indicate the carbon position (for example, 1-monoglyceride indicating a fatty acid attachment to the α-carbon). This numbering system applies to all acylglycerols, including the phosphoglycerides. Diglycerides can be either 1,2- or 1,3-diglycerides (see Figure 24-13).

In human nutrition, triglycerides constitute 95% of tissue storage fat and are the predominant form of glyceryl ester found in plasma. The fatty acid residues found in monoglycerides, diglycerides, or triglycerides vary considerably and usually include combinations of the long-chain fatty acids (see Table 24-2). Triglycerides from plants (for example, corn, sunflower seed, and safflower oils) tend to have large amounts of $C_{18}:2$ or linoleic residues and are liquid at room temperature. Triglycerides from animals, especially ruminants, tend to have $C_{12}:0$ through $C_{18}:0$ fatty-acid residues (saturated fats) and are solids at room temperature. Some plant triglycerides, such as coconut oil, are highly saturated and may be solid at room temperature.

Another major class of glycerol esters consists of those containing phosphoric acid at the third (α') carbon atom; these esters are called *phosphoglycerides* (Figure 24-14). In their simplest form the A group is a hydrogen atom and the molecule therefore is a diacylphosphoglyceride. Usually, however, the A is an alcohol-derived group, such as choline, serine, inositol, or ethanolamine (see Figure 24-14). If A is choline, the molecule is referred to as *phosphatidylcholine*; if A is ethanolamine, it is referred to as *phosphatidylethanolamine*. Phosphatidylcholines also have been collectively referred to as the *lecithins*, whereas phosphatidylethanolamine, phosphatidylethanolserine, and phosphatidylethanolinositol have been called the *cephalins*. As the fatty acid residues (R_1 and R_2 in Figure 24-14) vary, several different lecithins and cephalins are formed. These phosphoglycerides are named

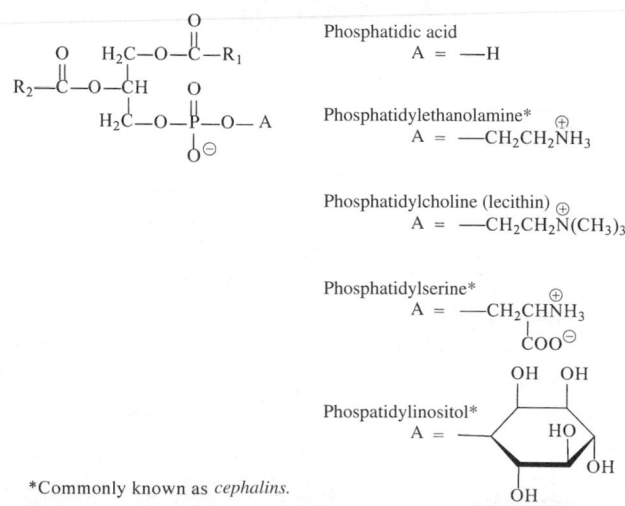

*Commonly known as *cephalins*.

Figure 24-13 Structure and classification of glycerol esters (acylglycerols). R_1, R_2, and R_3 are fatty acid(s) of varying chain lengths.

Figure 24-14 Structures of phosphoglycerides and common alcohol groups associated with them. R_1 and R_2 are fatty acid(s) of varying carbon atom lengths.

TABLE 24-5 Characteristics of Human Plasma Lipoproteins

Variable	Chylomicron	VLDL	IDL	LDL	HDL	Lp(a)
Density (g/mL)	<0.95	0.95 to 1.006	1.006 to 1.019	1.019 to 1.063	1.063 to 1.210	1.040 to 1.130
Electrophoretic mobility	Origin	Pre-β	Between β and pre-β	β	α	Pre-β
Molecular weight (daltons)	0.4 to 30 × 10^9	5 to 10 × 10^6	3.9 to 4.8 × 10^6	2.75 × 10^6	1.8 to 3.6 × 10^5	2.9 to 3.7 × 10^6
Diameter (nm)	>70	25 to 70	22 to 24	19 to 23	4 to 10	25 to 30
Lipid-protein ratio	99:1	90:10	85:15	80:20	50:50	75:25 to 64:36
Major lipids	Exogenous triglycerides	Endogenous triglycerides	Endogenous triglycerides, cholesteryl esters	Cholesteryl esters	Phospholipids	Cholesteryl esters, phospholipids
Major Proteins						
	A-I	B-100	B-100	B-100	AI	(a)
	B-48	C-I	E	—	AII	B-100
	C-I	C-II	—	—	—	—
	C-II	C-III	—	—	—	—
	C-III	E	—	—	—	—

VLDL, Very–low-density lipoproteins; *IDL,* intermediate-density lipoproteins; *LDL,* low-density lipoproteins; *HDL,* high-density lipoprotein; *Lp(a),* lipoprotein(a).

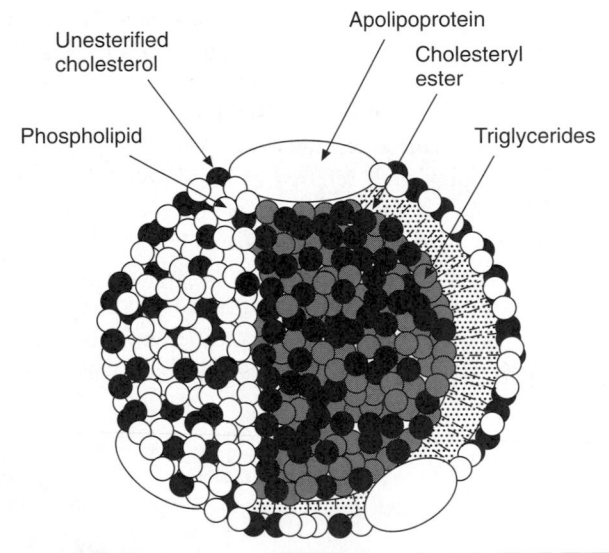

Figure 24-15 Structure of a typical lipoprotein particle.

according to the fatty acid acyl ester attached at C-1 and C-2 of the glycerol. The saturated fatty acid attaches to the C-1, whereas (poly)unsaturated fatty acid attaches primarily at C-2. Phosphatidylcholine is the precursor of the potent lipid mediator, platelet-activating factor.

In inner mitochondrial membranes, more complex phosphoglycerides, known as *cardiolipins,* can be found. They are derived from two phosphoglyceride molecules joined by a glycerol bridge.

Metabolism

Triglycerides are digested in the duodenum and proximal ileum. Through the action of pancreatic and intestinal lipases and in the presence of bile acids, they are hydrolyzed to glycerol, monoglycerides, and fatty acids. After absorption, triglycerides are resynthesized in the intestinal epithelial cells and combined with cholesterol and apo B-48 to form chylomicrons. Chylomicrons then are secreted to the lymphatic system, travel through the thoracic duct, and eventually reach the bloodstream through the jugular vein.

Lipoproteins

As discussed earlier, lipids synthesized in the liver and intestine must be transported to the various tissues to accomplish their metabolic functions. Because of their insolubility, they are transported in the plasma in macromolecular complexes called **lipoproteins.**

Chemistry

Lipoproteins are spherical particles with nonpolar lipids (triglycerides and cholesterol esters) in their core and more polar lipids (phospholipids and free cholesterol) oriented near the surface (Figure 24-15). They also contain one or more specific proteins, called *apolipoproteins,* that are located on their surfaces.[23] The association of the core lipids with the phospholipid and protein coat is noncovalent, occurring primarily through hydrogen bonding and van der Waals forces. This binding of lipid to protein is loose enough to allow the ready exchange of lipids among the plasma lipoproteins and between cell membranes and lipoprotein, yet strong enough to allow the various classes and subclasses of lipoprotein to be isolated by a variety of analytical techniques.

Classification

Historically, lipoproteins have been categorized into six major classes according to their physical and chemical properties (Table 24-5). Lipoprotein complexes contain different

TABLE 24-6   Chemical Composition (%) of Normal Human Plasma Lipoproteins

Lipoprotein	Surface Components*			Core Lipids*	
	Cholesterol	Phospholipids	Apolipoproteins	Triglycerides	Cholesteryl Esters
Chylomicrons	2	7	2	86	3
VLDL	7	18	8	55	12
IDL	9	19	19	23	29
LDL	8	22	22	6	42
HDL$_2$	5	33	40	5	17
HDL$_3$	4	25	55	3	13

From Havel RJ, Kane JP: Introduction: structure and metabolism of plasma lipoproteins. In Scriver CR, Beaudet AL, Sly WS et al (eds): The Metabolic and Molecular Bases of Inherited Diseases, 7th edition, pp 1841-1850, New York, McGraw-Hill, 1995.
VLDL, Very–low-density lipoprotein; *IDL,* intermediate-density lipoprotein; *LDL,* low-density lipoprotein; *HDL,* high-density lipoprotein.
*Surface components and core lipids given as percentage of dry mass.

proportions of lipids and proteins (Table 24-6). They can be separated by ultracentrifugation based on differences in their hydrated densities into chylomicrons, VLDL, intermediate-density lipoprotein (IDL), low-density lipoprotein (LDL), and high-density lipoprotein (HDL). HDL can be divided further by density into two subpopulations—HDL$_2$ and HDL$_3$. As discussed later in this chapter, the two subfractions of HDL seem to differ in their metabolic roles and clinical significance. Lipoprotein(a) [Lp(a)] is a distinct class of lipoprotein (see Table 24-5) that is structurally related to LDL because both lipoprotein classes possess one molecule of apo B-100 per particle and have similar lipid compositions.[18] However, unlike LDL, Lp(a) contains a carbohydrate-rich protein [apo(a)] that is covalently bound to the apo B-100 through a disulfide linkage. The available evidence suggest that Lp(a) contains one molecule of apo(a) and one molecule of apo B-100 per Lp(a) particle.[2] Apo(a) is the unique protein component of Lp(a) and exhibits a significant sequence homology with plasminogen and a high degree of variation in polypeptide chain length. Apo(a) is composed of a serine proteaselike domain* and a kringle-containing domain (Figure 24-16). Apo(a) contains 10 distinct classes of kringle 4-like domains that differ from one another in amino acid sequence. Kringle 4 type 1 and kringle 4 types 3 to 10 are present as a single copy on apo(a) particles. In contrast, kringle 4 type 2 is present in variable number of repeats (3 to >40) and therefore is primarily responsible for the size heterogeneity of apo(a) and consequently of Lp(a). Unlike plasminogen the serine protease domain cannot be converted to an active protease.

In the fasting state, most plasma triglyceride is present in VLDL. In the nonfasting state, chylomicrons appear transiently and contribute significantly to the total plasma tri-

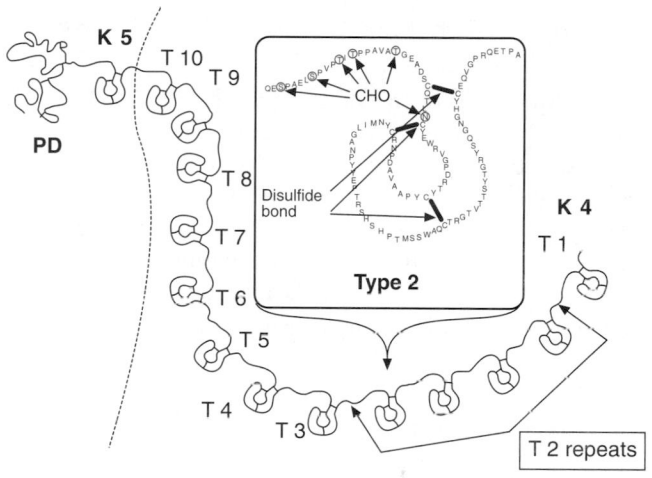

Figure 24-16   Structure of lipoprotein(a). *K,* Kringle; *PD,* protease domain; *T,* type.

glyceride level. LDL carries about 70% of total plasma cholesterol but very little triglyceride (see Table 24-6). HDL contains about 20% to 30% of plasma cholesterol.

Lipoproteins also can be separated from each other by electrophoresis on agarose, cellulose acetate, and paper, as well as polyacrylamide gels. At a pH of 8.6, HDL migrates with the α-globulins, LDL with the β-globulins, and VLDL and Lp(a) between the α- and β-globulins, in the pre-β-globulins region. IDL forms a broad band between β- and pre-β-globulins. Chylomicrons remain at the point of application. The lipoproteins have been referred to by their electrophoretic locations; pre-β-lipoprotein, VLDL; β-lipoprotein, LDL; and α-lipoprotein, HDL.

Apolipoproteins

Apolipoproteins are the protein components of lipoprotein. The characteristics and main known functions of the major apolipoproteins are summarized in Table 24-7.[15,23] Each class of lipoprotein has several apolipoproteins in differing proportions, except LDL, which contains only apo

---

*A domain is a compact globular structure composed of one section of a polypeptide chain that constitutes a recognizable unit of the tertiary structure of a protein. A kringle is a type of domain found in some proteins in which a cysteine-rich triply disulfide-bonded sequence of amino acids is folded into the characteristic "kringle" shape.

TABLE 24-7   Classification and Properties of Major Human Plasma Apolipoproteins

Apolipoprotein	Molecular Weight (daltons)	Chromosomal Location	Function	Lipoprotein Carrier(s)
Apo A-I	29,016	11	Cofactor LCAT	Chylomicron, HDL
Apo A-II	17,414	1	Not known	HDL
Apo A-IV	44,465	11	Activation of LCAT	Chylomicron, HDL
Apo B-100	512,723	2	Secretion of triglyceride from liver-binding protein to LDL receptor	VLDL, IDL, LDL
Apo B-48	240,800	2	Secretion of triglyceride from intestine	Chylomicron
Apo C-I	6630	19	Activation of LCAT(?)	Chylomicron, VLDL, HDL
Apo C-II	8900	19	Cofactor LPL	Chylomicron, VLDL, HDL
Apo C-III	8800	11	Inhibition of apo C-II; activation of LPL	Chylomicron, VLDL, HDL
Apo E	34,145	19	Facilitation of uptake of chylomicron remnant and IDL	Chylomicron, VLDL, HDL
Apo(a)	187,000 to 662,000	6	Unknown	Lp(a)

VLDL, Very–low-density lipoprotein; *IDL,* intermediate-density lipoprotein; *LDL,* low-density lipoprotein; *HDL,* high-density lipoprotein; *Lp(a),* lipoprotein(a); *LCAT,* lecithin cholesterol acyltransferase; *LPL,* lipoprotein lipase.

B-100. Apo A-I is the major protein in HDL. Apo C-I, -II, -III, and E are present in various proportions in all lipoproteins but LDL. Apolipoproteins collectively have three major physiological functions. They are involved in (1) activating important enzymes in the lipoprotein metabolic pathways, (2) maintaining the structural integrity of the lipoprotein complex, and (3) facilitating the uptake of lipoprotein into cells through their recognition by specific cell surface receptors.

Lipoprotein Metabolism

The pathways of lipoprotein metabolism are complex and include (1) exogenous, (2) endogenous, (3) intracellular LDL receptor, and (4) HDL reverse-cholesterol pathways.[5,12,23]

Exogenous pathway

Lipoproteins in this pathway are of dietary origin. Thus nascent chylomicrons are assembled from dietary triglyceride and cholesterol in secretory vesicles in the Golgi apparatus and introduced into circulation through the intestinal villi. The lipid content of nascent chylomicrons consists mainly of triglyceride (90% by mass), whereas the protein components include apo B-48 and the A apolipoproteins (2% by mass). Shortly after entering the circulation, these particles acquire the C apolipoproteins and apo E from circulating HDL (Figure 24-17). Apo C-II, now present on the surface of chylomicrons, activates the LPL attached to the luminal surface of endothelial cells, which rapidly hydrolyzes the triglycerides to free fatty acids. The fatty acids are associated with albumin and can either be taken up by muscle cells as an energy source or into adipose cells for storage. Simultaneously, some of the phospholipids and the A apolipoproteins are transferred from the chylomicron particle onto HDL. The newly formed particle, the chylomicron remnant, contains 80% to 90% of the triglyceride content of the original chylomicron. Because of the presence of apo B-48 and apo E on its surface, the chylomicron remnant can be recognized by specific hepatic remnant receptors and internalized by endocytosis. The components of the particle then are hydrolyzed in the lysosomes. The cholesterol released can form bile acids, be incorporated into newly synthesized lipoprotein, or be stored as cholesteryl ester. Furthermore, the cholesterol from these remnants can down-regulate HMG-CoA reductase, the rate-limiting enzyme of cholesterol biosynthesis.

Endogenous pathway

Lipoproteins in this pathway are of hepatic origin because hepatocytes have the ability to synthesize triglycerides from carbohydrates and fatty acids. In addition, when dietary cholesterol is insufficient, hepatocytes also synthesize their own cholesterol by increasing the activity of HMG-CoA reductase. The endogenously made triglycerides and cholesterol are packaged in secretory vesicles in the Golgi apparatus, transported by exocytosis into the extracellular space, and introduced into circulation in the form of nascent VLDL (Figure 24-18). This triglyceride-rich particle (55% by mass) contains apo B-100, apo E, and small amounts of C apolipoproteins on its surface. Additional C apolipoproteins are transferred after secretion from circulating HDL. As with chylomicron metabolism, apo C-II present on the surface of VLDL activates LPL on endothelial cells, which leads to the hydrolysis of VLDL triglycerides and the release of free fatty acids.

During the hydrolysis of VLDL triglycerides, the C apolipoproteins are transferred back to HDL. VLDL particles are converted to VLDL remnants, some of which are taken up by the liver. The rest are converted to smaller, denser particles called *IDL*. Large IDL particles, which also have several molecules of apo E, bind the hepatic remnant receptors

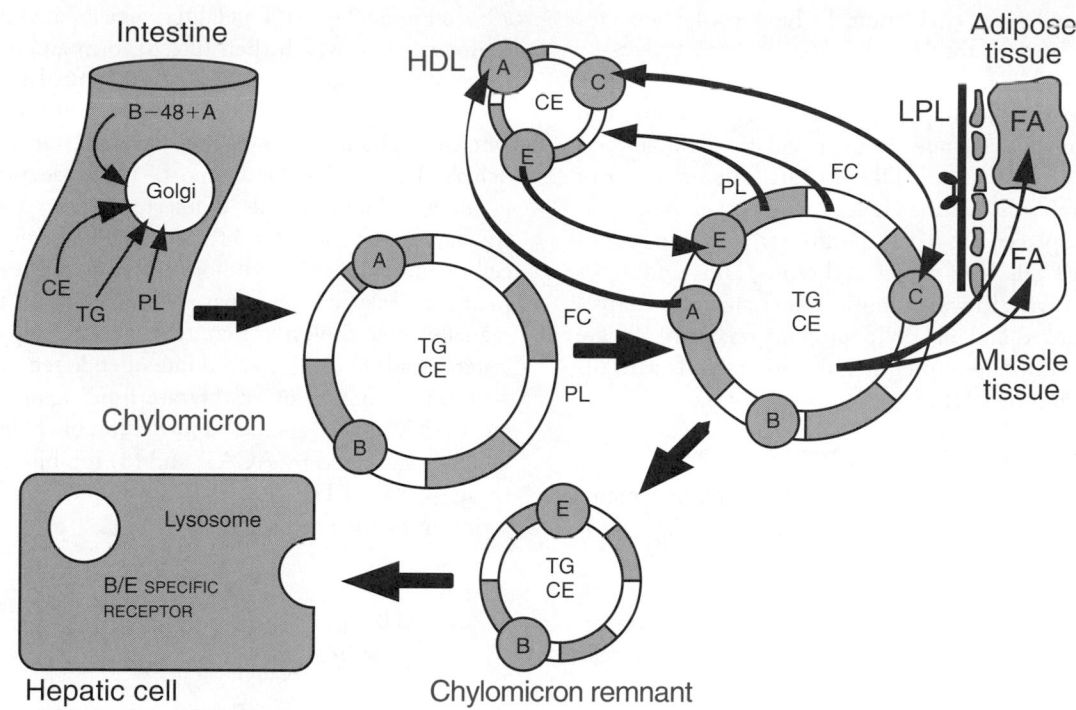

Figure 24-17   Exogenous lipoprotein metabolism pathway. *TG*, Triglyceride; *CE*, cholesterol ester; *FC*, free cholesterol; *PL*, phospholipids; *HDL*, high-density lipoproteins; *FA*, fatty acid; *LPL*, lipoprotein lipase; *B*, apolipoprotein B-48; *A*, apolipoprotein A-I; *C*, apolipoprotein C-II; *E*, apolipoprotein E.

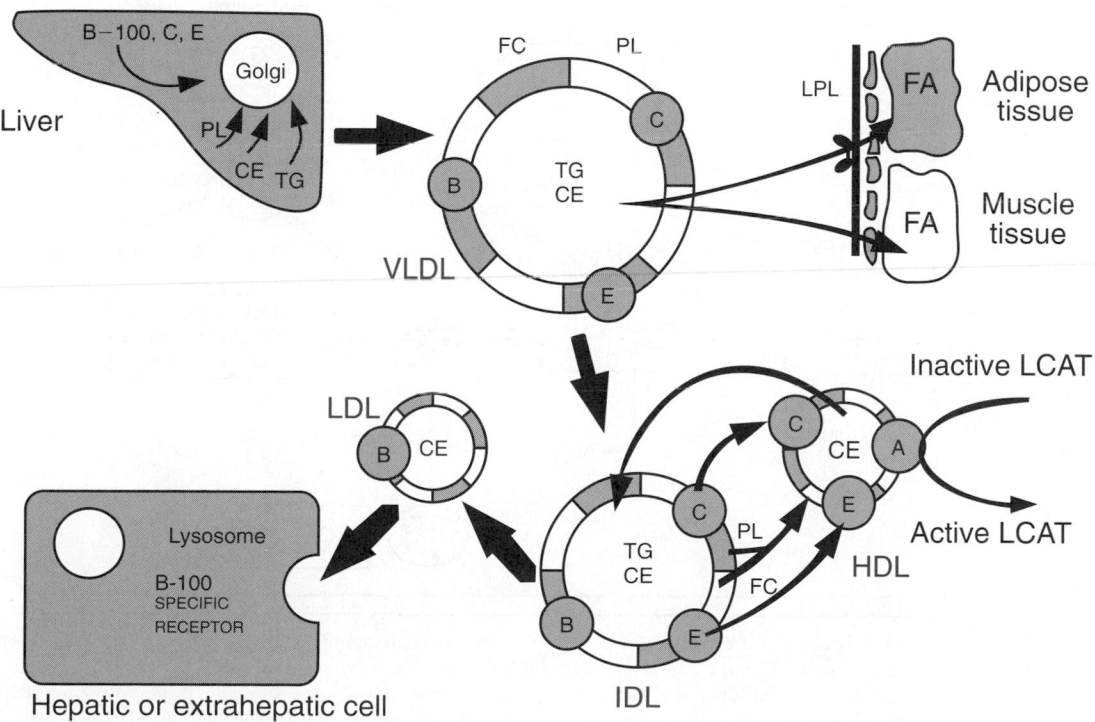

Figure 24-18   Endogenous lipoprotein metabolism pathway. *TG*, Triglyceride; *CE*, cholesterol ester; *FC*, free cholesterol; *PL*, phospholipids; *HDL*, high-density lipoproteins; *LDL*, low-density lipoproteins; *IDL*, intermediate-density lipoproteins; *VLDL*, very–low-density lipoproteins; *FA*, fatty acid; *LPL*, lipoprotein lipase; *LCAT*, lecithin cholesterol acyltransferase; *B*, apolipoprotein B-100; *A*, apolipoprotein A-I; *C*, apolipoprotein C-II; *E*, apolipoprotein E.

and are removed from circulation. In humans, hepatocytes remove about 50% of the IDL.

Surface materials from IDL, including some phospholipids, free cholesterol, and apolipoproteins, are transferred to HDL, or form HDL de novo in the circulation. Cholesteryl esters are transferred from HDL to LDL. The net result of the coupled lipolysis and the cholesteryl esters exchange reaction is the replacement of much of the triglyceride core of the original VLDL with cholesteryl esters. IDL undergoes a further hydrolysis, in which most of the remaining triglycerides are removed and all apolipoproteins except B-100 are transferred to other lipoproteins. This process ends with ultimate formation of LDL.

Low-density lipoprotein receptor pathway

Specific receptors present in coated pits on plasma membranes recognize and bind apo B-100 of LDL (Figure 24-

19; see Figure 24-18). The LDL particles are internalized in coated vesicles, which then fuse to form an endosome. Because of the acidic milieu of the endosome, LDL dissociates from the receptor, which returns to the cell surface for reuse, whereas LDL migrates to the lysosome. Once the LDL is delivered to the lysosome, apo B-100 is degraded to small peptides and amino acids. Cholesterol esters also are hydrolyzed, with the cholesterol then available for the synthesis of cell membranes, steroid hormones in tissues that make them, and bile acids in hepatocytes. Cells have the ability to regulate their cholesterol content. Oversupply of free cholesterol leads to (1) decreased rate of endogenous cholesterol synthesis by inhibition of the rate-limiting enzyme HMG-CoA reductase; (2) increased formation of cholesteryl esters, which is catalyzed by ACAT; and (3) inhibition of the synthesis of new LDL receptors by suppression of the transcription of the receptor gene.

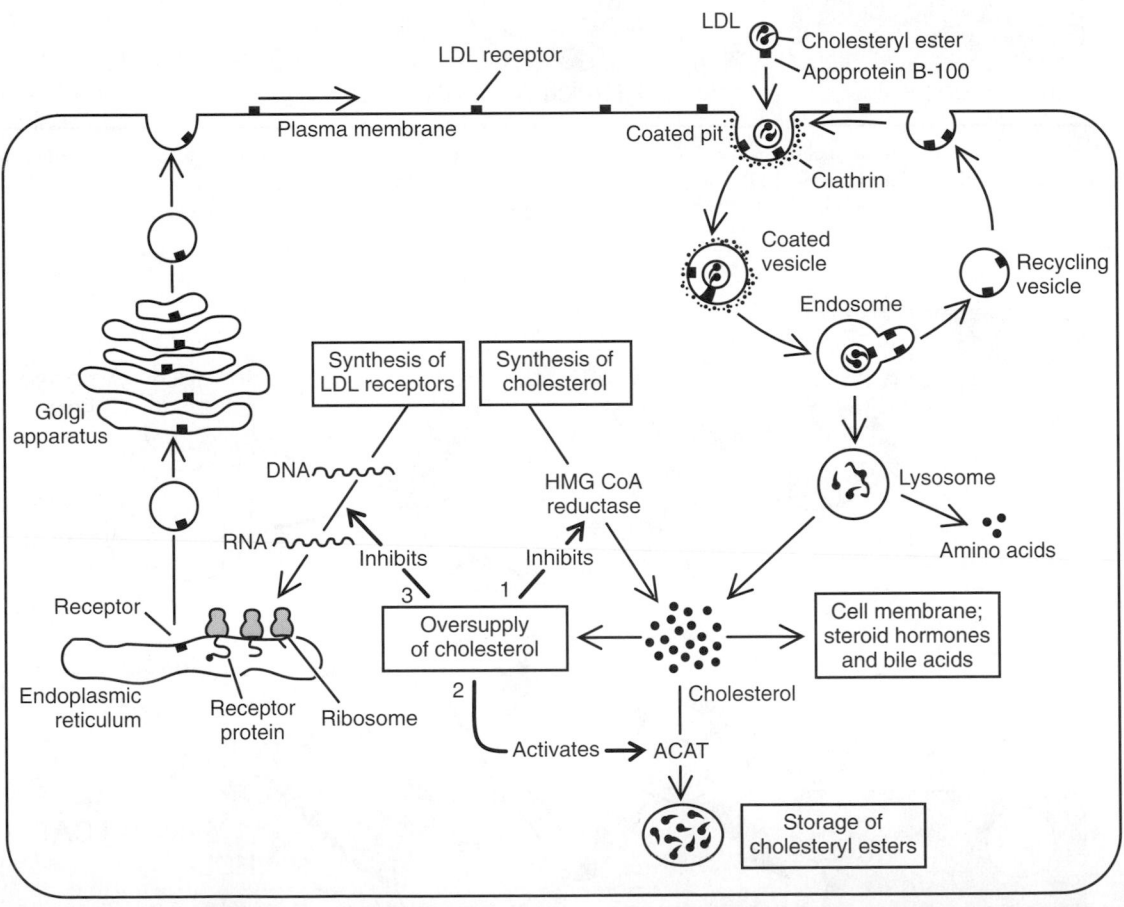

Figure 24-19 LDL receptor pathway. Because of the presence of apolipoprotein (apo) B-100 on its surface, the LDL particle is recognized by a specific receptor in a coated pit and taken into the cell in a coated vesicle *(top right)*. Coated vesicles fuse together to form an endosome. The acidic environment of the endosome causes the LDL particle to dissociate from the receptors, which return to the cell surface. The LDL particles are taken to a lysosome, where apo B-100 is broken down into amino acids and cholesterol ester is converted to free cholesterol for cellular needs. The cellular cholesterol level is self-regulated. Oversupply of cholesterol leads to (1) decreased rate of cholesterol synthesis by inhibition of HMG-CoA reductase, (2) increased storage of cholesteryl esters by activation of ACAT, and (3) inhibition of manufacture of new LDL receptors by suppression of the transcription of the receptor gene into messenger RNA. *LDL,* Low-density lipoproteins; *ACAT,* acyl-CoA cholesterol acyltransferase; *HMG-CoA reductase,* 3-hydroxy-3-methylglutaryl coenzyme A reductase. (Modified from Brown MS, Goldstein JL: How LDL receptors influence cholesterol and atherosclerosis. Sci Am 1984; 251:58-66. Copyright 1984 by Scientific American, Inc.)

LDL also can be taken up by extrahepatic tissues through scavenger receptors or nonreceptor-mediated pinocytosis. The nonreceptor-mediated uptake becomes significant as plasma LDL concentrations increase, as is the case with familial hypercholesterolemia (FH). Nonreceptor-mediated uptake cannot be saturated and is not regulated. Scavenger receptors are unregulated as well and recognize LDL that has been modified in various ways. They are found in macrophages and other cells. Macrophages that become engorged with cholesteryl esters are called "foam cells" and are considered the earliest components of the atherosclerotic lesion. Two thirds of LDL normally is removed by LDL receptors and the remainder by the scavenger cell system.

High-density lipoprotein reverse cholesterol transfer pathway

HDLs are secreted from the liver or intestine as disk-shaped nascent particles that consist primarily of phospholipids and apo A-I. Through the extracellular addition of surface components of triglyceride-rich particles, such as phospholipids, cholesterol, and certain apolipoproteins, nascent HDL is converted to spherical particles (Figure 24-20). Cholesterol is esterified by the action of lecithin cholesterol acyltransferase (LCAT) in the presence of its cofactor, apo A-I. The size of the HDL particle depends strongly on the amount of accumulated cholesteryl esters and the activity of LCAT. HDL cholesteryl esters are delivered to the liver by one of the following mechanisms:

1. Cholesteryl esters are selectively taken up from HDL, probably by hepatic HDL receptors, and HDL particles are returned to circulation for further transport.
2. Cholesteryl esters are transferred from HDL to apo B-100-containing lipoprotein, a process mediated by cholesterol ester transfer protein, then taken up by the liver through receptors for these lipoproteins.
3. HDL apo E can be recognized by the hepatic remnant receptors.[12]

These processes constitute the reverse cholesterol transport system, by which cellular and lipoprotein cholesterol is delivered back to the liver for reuse or disposal.

Although LDL is the major product resulting from the catabolism of VLDL, some conversion of HDL subfractions also occurs during this process. The surface materials from triglyceride-rich particles that have been transferred to the small circulating HDL_3 subsequently are esterified by LCAT, as described previously, to create the larger cholesteryl ester-rich HDL_2. In vitro HDL_2 has been shown to convert back to HDL_3 in the presence of hepatic LPL.[22] HDL_2 contains twice as many cholesterol molecules per unit of apolipoproteins as does HDL_3.

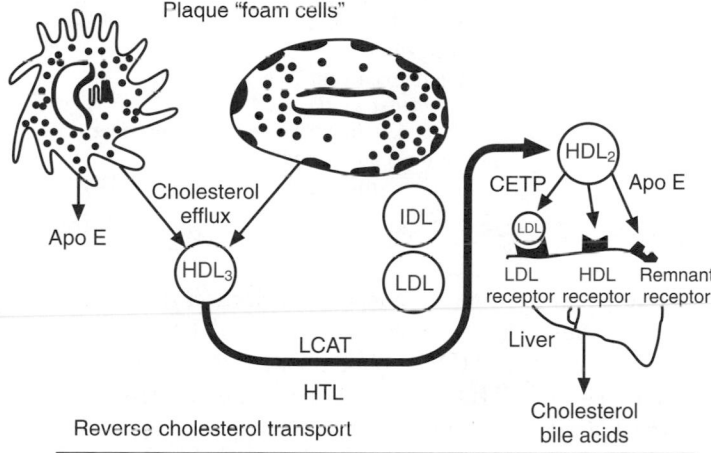

Figure 24-20   Reverse cholesterol transport pathway. Cholesterol is removed from macrophages and other arterial wall cells by an HDL-mediated process. The LCAT esterifies the cholesterol content of HDL to prevent it from reentering the cells. Cholesterol esters are delivered to the liver by one of three pathways—(1) cholesterol esters are transferred from HDL to LDL by CETP and enter the liver through the specific LDL receptor pathway; (2) cholesterol esters are selectively taken from HDL by HDL receptors, and HDL particles are returned to circulation for further transport; or (3) HDL have accumulated apo E, and therefore the particles can enter the liver through remnant receptors. *HDL*, High-density lipoproteins; *LDL*, low-density lipoproteins; *IDL*, intermediate-density lipoproteins; *HTL*, hepatic lipoprotein lipase; *LCAT*, lecithin cholesterol acyltransferase; *CETP*, cholesteryl ester transfer protein; *apo E*, apolipoprotein E. (Modified from Gwynne JT: High-density lipoprotein cholesterol levels as a marker of reverse cholesterol transport. Am J Cardiol 1989; 64:10G-17G. Copyright 1989, with permission from Excerpta Medica Inc.)

Reference Values

At birth, plasma cholesterol concentration is about 66 mg/dL (1.71 mmol/L), equally distributed among LDL and HDL, with a very small amount in VLDL. Triglyceride concentration is only about 36 mg/dL (0.41 mmol/L).[24] Umbilical cord blood apo A-I, apo B-100, and Lp(a) show mean concentrations of about 80, 33, and 4 mg/dL, respectively. Lipid, lipoprotein cholesterol, and apolipoprotein concentrations rise sharply during the first few months of life, with LDL becoming the major carrier of plasma cholesterol, and then remain relatively unchanged until puberty. A profile consisting of a total cholesterol of about 155 mg/dL (4.01 mmol/L), LDL cholesterol of 90 mg/dL (2.33 mmol/L), HDL cholesterol of 53 mg/dL (1.38 mmol/L), triglycerides of 55 mg/dL (0.62 mmol/L), apo B-100 of 86 mg/dL, and apo A-I of about 130 mg/dL is typical for a normal prepubertal individual.

After puberty an increase in triglycerides, LDL cholesterol, and apo B-100 occurs in both sexes, and a decrease in HDL cholesterol and apo A-I occurs in men. Lipid concentrations continue to increase throughout adult life, with total and LDL cholesterol and apo B-100 being higher in men than in women up to 55 years of age. Thereafter, women who are not receiving estrogen supplementation have higher total and LDL cholesterol and apo B-100 than their age-matched male counterparts. In contrast to the other lipids, lipoproteins, and apolipoproteins, Lp(a) concentration increases gradually to reach Lp(a) adult values after the third year of life.

CLINICAL SIGNIFICANCE

In clinical chemistry the use of the term *lipids* generally refers to lipoprotein metabolism and **atherosclerosis**, a cause of CHD. Much of this association has been recognized through the conduct of large national and international collaborative epidemiological and clinical studies. In the early 1980s, findings from the Coronary Primary Prevention Trial first demonstrated that lowering of plasma cholesterol concentration reduces the incidence of CHD. Since then this fact has been confirmed in various other clinical trials. Based on such trials and other evidence the National Heart, Lung and Blood Institute established the National Cholesterol Education Program (NCEP) to increase public awareness about cholesterol; devise strategies for diagnosis and treatment of hypercholesterolemia in adults, children, and adolescents; and improve the laboratory measurement of lipids. The European Atherosclerosis Society and other individual countries have established similar programs to address these issues.

In addition, lipids also are associated with a variety of specific disorders that result from hyperlipidemia and dyslipoproteinemia (Table 24-8).[1]

Coronary Heart Disease

Evidence clearly indicates that atherosclerosis is a major cause of CHD. It is a process that begins early in life and progresses silently for decades. The identification and treatment of individuals who may be at high risk for development of CHD at early ages offers the possibility to prevent or delay the progression of this disease.

The association between serum cholesterol and atherosclerosis in humans first was suggested in 1938, when Thanhauser and Muller each demonstrated familial aggregation of hypercholesterolemia and CHD. Further studies showed a positive association between increased levels of total cholesterol and the incidence and prevalence of CHD. The relationship between cholesterol and atherosclerotic coronary disease is not linear; if a risk ratio of 1.0 is assigned at a cholesterol value of 200 mg/dL (5.18 mmol/L), the risk ratio increases to 2.0 at 250 mg/dL (6.48 mmol/L) and 4.0 at 300 mg/dL (7.77 mmol/L).

When 60% of the surface of coronary arteries is covered with plaque, an individual enters a critical phase in which an increased serum cholesterol concentration markedly increases coronary disease risk.[11] Studies now have demonstrated the benefit of cholesterol lowering even in people with normal or moderately increased cholesterol concentrations (185 to 240 mg/dL; 4.79 to 6.21 mmol/L) and those with established disease. In contrast, fasting triglyceride has

TABLE 24-8	Causes of Secondary Hyperlipidemia and Dyslipoproteinemia
Disorder	**Cause**
Exogenous	Drugs: corticosteroids, isotretinoin (Accutane), thiazides, anticonvulsants, β-blockers, anabolic steroids, certain oral contraceptives
	Alcohol
	Obesity
Endocrine and metabolic	Acute intermittent porphyria
	Diabetes mellitus
	Hypopituitarism
	Hypothyroidism
	Lipodystrophy
	Pregnancy
Storage disease	Cystine storage disease
	Gaucher disease
	Glycogen storage disease
	Juvenile Tay-Sachs disease
	Niemann-Pick disease
	Tay-Sachs disease
Renal	Chronic renal failure
	Hemolytic-uremic syndrome
	Nephrotic syndrome
Hepatic	Benign recurrent intrahepatic cholestasis
	Congenital biliary atresia
Acute and transient	Burns
	Hepatitis
	Acute trauma (surgery)
	Myocardial infarction
	Bacterial and viral infections
Others	Anorexia nervosa
	Starvation
	Idiopathic hypercalcemia
	Klinefelter syndrome
	Progeria (Hutchinson-Gilford syndrome)
	Systemic lupus erythematosus
	Werner syndrome

not been shown to be an independent risk factor of CHD. Several studies demonstrated that increased LDL cholesterol and decreased HDL cholesterol are associated with increased risk of CHD. A reduction in LDL cholesterol is correlated with regression in the atherosclerotic lesion in individuals with CHD. Apo B-100 values were increased and apo A-I values were decreased in people with CHD, compared with those without disease. In most studies, apo A-I and apo B-100 were somewhat better discriminators of those with CHD than were HDL and LDL cholesterol, respectively. (The association of CHD risk with Lp(a) and apo E concentrations, as well as the various apo E phenotypes, will be discussed in subsequent sections of this chapter.)

Disorders of Lipoprotein Metabolism

Historically, lipoprotein disorders were classified according to Fredrickson and co-workers. However, these disorders are approached more functionally based on the four metabolic pathways discussed previously (see Figures 24-17 through 24-20). Defects in these pathways, leading to hyperlipidemia, may be related to (1) increased production of lipoproteins, (2) abnormal intravascular processing (for example, enzymatic hydrolysis of triglyceride), and (3) defective cellular uptake of lipoproteins. Finally, a significant decrease in production or an increase in the removal of lipoproteins can lead to a marked reduction in lipid and lipoprotein concentrations.

Deficiency in lipoprotein lipase activity

Deficiency in lipoprotein lipase activity is a disorder characterized by marked hyperchylomicronemia and a corresponding hypertriglyceridemia (triglyceride as high as 10,000 mg/dL; 113.0 mmol/L).[6] As indicated previously, LPL is essential for the hydrolysis of triglyceride and conversion of chylomicrons to chylomicron remnants. The massive accumulation of chylomicrons in the circulation indicates an inability to catabolize dietary fat. The concentration of VLDL cholesterol usually is normal and the concentrations of HDL cholesterol and LDL cholesterol are low (type I pattern). Furthermore, the concentration of apo C-II, the activator of LPL, is normal.

This disorder is expressed in childhood and usually detected after recurrent episodes of severe abdominal pain and repeated attacks of pancreatitis. Eruptive xanthomas usually are present when plasma triglyceride concentrations exceed 2000 mg/dL (22.6 mmol/L). The acuteness of the symptoms is directly proportional to the degree of hyperchylomicronemia. Individuals with this disorder *do not* appear to be predisposed to atherosclerotic disease. The diagnosis is made by the determination of LPL activity in postheparin plasma. This disorder is inherited in an autosomal recessive mode and is rare.

Deficiency in apolipoprotein C-II

Deficient or defective apo C-II impairs chylomicron catabolism and increases the concentrations of triglycerides in plasma (500 to 10,000 mg/dL; 5.65 to 113.0 mmol/L). Although the clinical symptoms are similar to those seen in individuals with LPL deficiency, they usually are milder and expressed at a later age. The predominant symptom usually is recurrent abdominal pain due to attacks of pancreatitis. As with LPL deficiency, individuals with apo C-II deficiency *are not* predisposed to atherosclerosis.

The diagnosis is made by the documentation of low LPL activity in postheparin plasma in the absence of added apo C-II. Normal enzymatic activity is restored by the addition of normal apo C-II to the assay mixture. The defective apo C-II disorder is inherited in an autosomal recessive mode, but at a lower frequency than LPL deficiency.

Familial combined hyperlipidemia

About 10% to 15% of individuals with premature CHD actually have familial combined hyperlipidemia (FCHL).[10]

Families with FCHL can have increased plasma concentrations of total and LDL cholesterol (type IIa), or triglyceride (type IV), or both (type IIb). In all cases, apo B-100 concentrations are increased. The presentation of lipoprotein patterns also can vary in an individual with time. Furthermore, those with hypertriglyceridemia with normal partners tend to produce offspring with hypercholesterolemia, and vice versa.

FCHL appears to result from the overproduction of VLDL and apo B-100. When increased, LDL cholesterol is about 190 mg/dL (4.92 mmol/L) but is lower than that present in individuals with heterozygous FH (350 mg/dL; 9.07 mmol/l). Triglycerides levels usually are between 200 and 400 mg/dL (2.26 and 4.52 mmol/L), but can be significantly higher. The concentration of HDL cholesterol usually is depressed mildly, particularly in the presence of hypertriglyceridemia. The association of FCHL with CHD incidence is high. The biochemical basis for FCHL remains unknown.

Hyperapobetalipoproteinemia

The disorder known as *hyperapobetalipoproteinemia* is characterized by increased LDL-apo B-100 concentrations with normal or moderately increased concentrations of LDL cholesterol.[30] The ratio of LDL cholesterol to apo B-100 therefore is reduced in these individuals (≤1.2). Total cholesterol and triglyceride levels may be normal but usually are increased, and HDL cholesterol and apo A-I levels are decreased. This disorder apparently is caused by an overproduction of VLDL and apo B-100 in the liver. The exact mode of inheritance and prevalence of the disorder remain unclear.

Familial hypertriglyceridemia

A moderate increase in the concentration of serum triglycerides is characteristic of familial hypertriglyceridemia (FHTG). The production of large VLDL with abnormally high triglyceride content appears to be responsible for this disorder.[13] The cholesterol content of VLDL also is increased, but plasma LDL cholesterol and apo B-100 concentrations are within their reference intervals. This finding suggests that the conversion of VLDL to LDL is not increased in these individuals. Furthermore, plasma HDL cholesterol in those with FHTG often is decreased dramatically, probably secondary to the hypertriglyceridemia.

The cause of the overproduction of VLDL triglyceride currently is unknown. The diagnosis of FHTG requires study of other family members to differentiate this disorder from FCHL. This disorder appears to be inherited in an autosomal dominant pattern.

Type V hyperlipoproteinemia

Type V hyperlipoproteinemia is characterized by an increase in both chylomicrons and VLDL. Although its exact etiology is unknown, the disorder may be caused by an increased production or decreased removal of VLDL, or to a combination of both. The activity of LPL in these individuals is either normal or low, and the plasma concentration of apo C-II is normal.

Clinical presentations include eruptive xanthomas, lipemia retinalis, pancreatitis, and abnormal glucose tolerance with hyperinsulinism. Premature atherosclerotic complications are not seen commonly. This heterogeneous syndrome appears to be inherited in an autosomal dominant mode.

Dysbetalipoproteinemia (type III)

Type III dysbetalipoproteinemia, also termed *type III hyperlipoproteinemia*, is caused by a primary genetic defect in the removal of remnants of both intestinal chylomicrons and hepatic VLDL.[16] As indicated previously, apo E present on the surface of lipoprotein remnants interacts with specific hepatic receptors and facilitates the removal of these particles from the circulation. As a result of amino acid substitutions, apo E exists in three common variants—designated E_2, E_3, and E_4. Individuals with dysbetalipoproteinemia are homozygous for a mutant form of apo E (apo E_2) that cannot bind the specific hepatic receptors efficiently, leading to the accumulation of lipoprotein remnants and a cholesterol-enriched lipoprotein of density less than 1.006 g/mL, commonly referred to as β-VLDL or floating β-lipoprotein, in plasma.

The disease is characterized in part by increased plasma cholesterol and triglycerides, and the concentrations of the two lipids are about the same when expressed in milligrams per deciliter. β-VLDL present in type III dysbetalipoproteinemia is related to triglyceride-rich lipoprotein remnants of both hepatic and intestinal origins. Both LDL and HDL cholesterol are lower than normal in these individuals.[16]

Type III dysbetalipoproteinemia has a late onset; it rarely manifests itself in childhood. The most distinctive clinical presentation of dysbetalipoproteinemia is the presence of palmar xanthomas, the yellow deposits that occur in the creases of the palms. Premature atherosclerosis develops in 30% to more than 50% of these individuals, particularly in the lower extremities.

The incidence of type III hyperlipoproteinemia is approximately 0.1% in the general population. Apo E_2 homozygosity, however, occurs in about 1% of the population in North America. Thus the occurrence of the defective alleles is necessary but not sufficient to produce clinical type III hyperlipoproteinemia. The development of overt hyperlipoproteinemia in these individuals is modulated by genetic, hormonal, or environmental factors, such as hypothyroidism, glucose intolerance, decreased estrogen levels after menopause, obesity, and diet.

Familial hypercholesterolemia

FH is caused by a primary genetic defect in the LDL receptor gene. As discussed previously, this cell surface receptor is responsible for the recognition and removal of LDL from circulation. The defects seen in individuals with FH include reduced LDL binding because of defective or absent LDL receptors or inefficient internalization of the LDL particles.[5] FH is characterized clinically by increased plasma LDL cholesterol concentration; cholesterol deposition in skin, tendons, and arteries; and autosomal dominant transmission that is expressed in heterozygous or homozygous mode.

Heterozygous FH is one of the most common genetic disorders, with an incidence of 1 in 500 people in the United States. The prevalence of homozygous FH is about one in a million people. The mean plasma LDL cholesterol in children and adult heterozygotes usually is two to three times that of normal individuals of similar age, whereas the mean plasma LDL cholesterol of homozygotes is four to six times that of normal individuals. Apo B-100, the main protein in LDL, is increased in proportion to LDL cholesterol. Triglyceride concentration is either normal or slightly increased, and HDL cholesterol concentration is slightly decreased in both heterozygotes and homozygotes.

Hypercholesterolemia is present at birth in most individuals with FH and persists throughout life. In heterozygotes, xanthomas appear toward the end of the second decade, and clinical manifestations of atherosclerotic disease appear during the fourth decade. In homozygotes, the unique yellow-orange cutaneous xanthomas develop by 4 years of age if they are not already present at birth. Tendon xanthomas and atherosclerotic complications begin during childhood. Death from myocardial infarction generally occurs in homozygotes before the end of the second or third decade of life.

Familial defective apolipoprotein B-100

Familial defective apo B-100 is the result of a mutation in the apo B-100 gene rather than in the LDL receptor. The defective apo B-100 has a decreased affinity for the LDL receptor, thus causing plasma LDL cholesterol to be increased. These individuals have an increased incidence of CHD. Triglyceride and HDL cholesterol concentrations are unaffected. Clinical differentiation between individuals with familial defective apo B-100 and those with heterozygous FH is difficult. However, because the management of patients with the two disorders is similar, the distinction is not clinically important.

Familial hypoalphalipoproteinemia

The disorder known as *familial hypoalphalipoproteinemia* is characterized by normal plasma lipids and LDL cholesterol and reduced HDL cholesterol, below the 5th percentile.[28] Although individuals with this disorder clinically are normal, they have a high incidence of CHD. The molecular basis of familial hypoalphalipoproteinemia is unknown. This disorder is the result of either the decreased biosynthesis or the increased catabolism of HDL or apo A-I.

Defects in the synthesis of apolipoprotein A-I

In individuals with homozygous familial hypoalphalipoproteinemia, only traces of HDL cholesterol are found in plasma, and apo A-I is undetectable. These individuals have corneal clouding and are at increased risk for development of premature CHD. Heterozygotes exhibit no clinical signs but have about half the normal concentrations of HDL cholesterol and apo A-I as those without the disorder.

Defects in catabolism of apolipoprotein A-I (Tangier disease)

Tangier disease results from defects in the catabolism of apo A-I. It is a disorder characterized by (1) severely reduced plasma HDL concentration, (2) abnormal HDL composition, and (3) accumulation of cholesteryl esters in many tissues throughout the body.[27] Increased catabolism of HDL, rather than a defect in biosynthesis, causes Tangier disease. Plasma cholesterol is decreased to about 70 mg/dL (1.82 mmol/L) in homozygotes and about 160 mg/dL (4.14 mmol/L) in heterozygotes. Triglyceride concentrations vary, depending on the diet. In homozygotes, plasma HDL cholesterol and apo A-I concentrations are almost zero, and apo A-II is present at less than 10% of its normal concentration in apo B–100-containing lipoproteins. Heterozygotes are characterized by half-normal concentrations of HDL cholesterol, apo A-I, and apo A-II.

The clinical symptoms of Tangier disease result from the deposition of cholesteryl esters in various tissues of the body. The three major clinical signs are hyperplastic orange tonsils, splenomegaly, and peripheral neuropathy. Other possible clinical signs include hepatomegaly and corneal opacities. The severely reduced HDL cholesterol and enlarged orange tonsils are pathognomonic. Current evidence suggests that these individuals have an increased incidence of CHD. Heterozygotes exhibit no clinical manifestations and can be identified only biochemically.

Diagnosis of Lipoprotein Disorders

The diagnosis of dyslipoproteinemia in most patients requires plasma lipid and lipoprotein cholesterol analysis. Hyperlipidemia must be evaluated to determine whether it results from a primary lipoprotein disorder or is secondary to one or more several other metabolic disorders. The diagnosis of primary hyperlipidemia is made after secondary causes have been ruled out.

Hypercholesterolemia in adults now is defined in terms of CHD risk. The NCEP Adult Treatment Panel (ATP)[8,19] defined cholesterol values below the 50th percentile as "desirable," whereas those more than the 75th percentile are considered "high risk" (Table 24-9). Values between the 50th and 75th percentiles are considered "borderline-high risk." According to this definition, 50% of the American adult population is at increased risk for development of premature CHD by virtue of having an increased plasma cholesterol. Cutoffs for LDL cholesterol concentrations in adults also have been established at the same percentiles (see Table 24-9). In addition, the NCEP defined low HDL cholesterol concentration as below 35 mg/dL (0.91 mmol/L). This level of HDL cholesterol corresponds to the 25th percentile in men and the 10th percentile in women and is considered a CHD risk factor.

Cholesterol screening to diagnose hypercholesterolemia now is recommended for all adults over 20 years of age.[19] The recent NCEP guidelines (ATP II) suggest the measurement of both total and HDL cholesterol at the initial screening. The guidelines for diagnosis and treatment of hypercholesterolemia in adults without evidence of CHD are illustrated in Figure 24-21. Note that the aggressiveness of treatment of hypercholesterolemia depends on the number of other risk factors the patient has. The major risk factors are listed in Table 24-10. Therapy is indicated for those with evidence of CHD when LDL cholesterol exceeds 100 mg/dL (2.59 mmol/L).[19]

The NCEP/Expert Panel on Blood Cholesterol Levels in Children and Adolescents[20] and the American Academy of Pediatrics[3] defined "high cholesterol" as concentrations more than the 95th percentile for total and LDL cholesterol in children and adolescents from families with hypercholesterolemia or premature vascular disease (see Table 24-9). "Borderline" total and LDL cholesterol concentrations are defined as values between the 75th and 95th percentiles. The NCEP panel referred to total and LDL cholesterol values below the 75th percentile as "desirable." Low HDL cholesterol also was defined as a concentration below 35 mg/dL (0.91 mmol/L). According to the NCEP and the American Academy of Pediatrics, only children over 2 years of age should be screened for hypercholesterolemia when they have a parent with hypercholesterolemia (>240 mg/dL; 6.22 mmol/L) or positive family history (mother, father, uncle,

| TABLE 24-9 | NCEP Classification of Total and LDL Cholesterol in Adults, Children, and Adolescents* |

| Category | Adults | | Children and Adolescents | |
	Total Cholesterol	LDL Cholesterol	Total Cholesterol	LDL Cholesterol
Desirable	<200	<130	<170	<110
Borderline	200 to 239	130 to 160	170 to 199	110 to 120
High	≥240	≥160	≥200	≥130

NCEP, National Cholesterol Education Program; *LDL*, low-density lipoproteins.
*All values are in mg/dL; to convert to mmol/L, multiply by 0.0259.

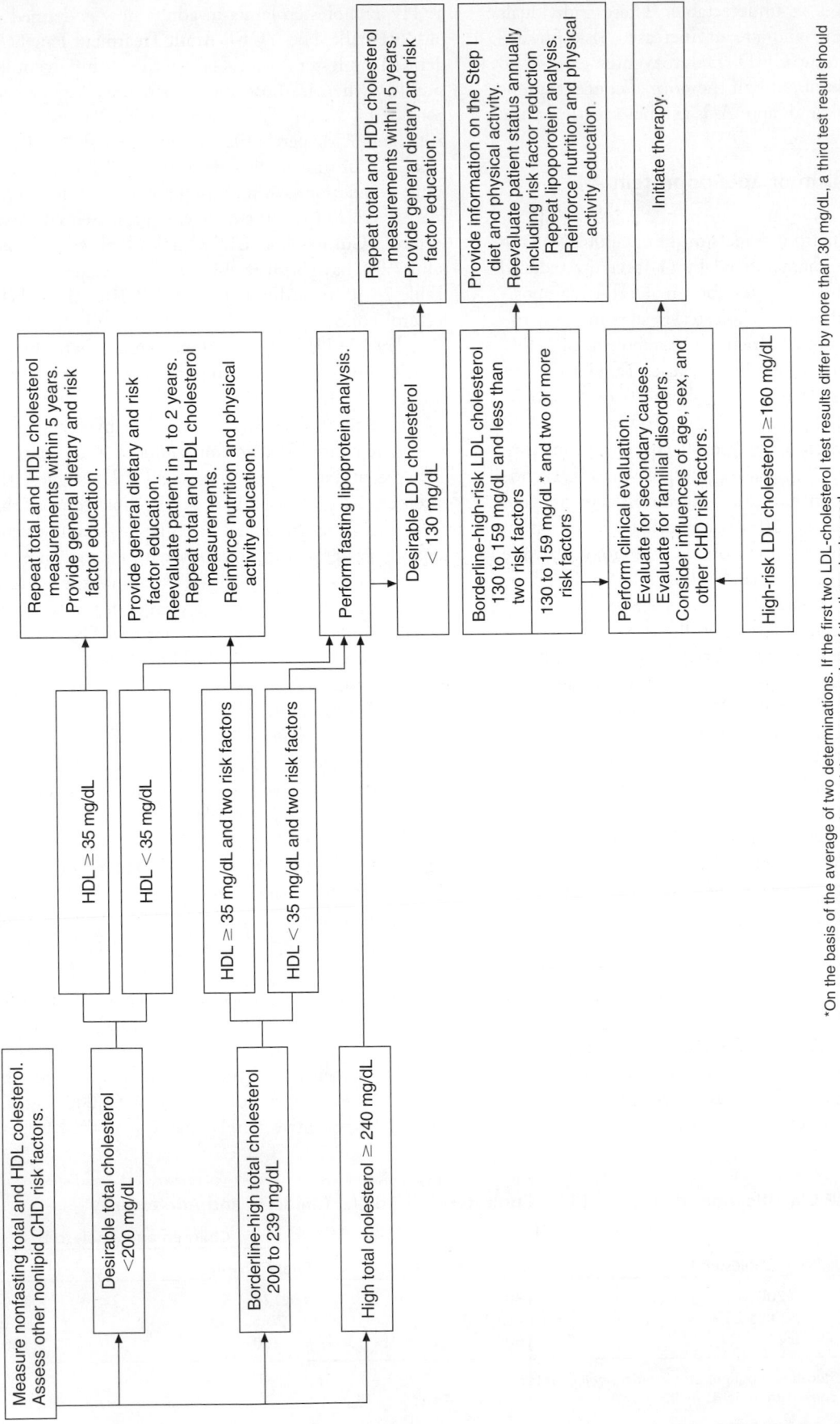

Figure 24-21 Risk assessment and clinical management of hypercholesterolemia as recommended by the National Cholesterol Education Program Expert Panel on Detection, Evaluation, and Treatment of High Blood Cholesterol in Adults II. *CHD*, Coronary heart disease; *HDL*, high-density lipoprotein; *LDL*, low-density lipoprotein. (Compiled from the Expert Panel on Detection, Evaluation, and Treatment of High Blood Cholesterol in Adults [ATP II]: National Cholesterol Education Program. Lipid Metabolism Branch, Division of Heart, Lung, and Blood Institute. U.S. Department of Health and Human Services, Public Health Service, National Institutes of Health. Bethesda, Md, National Institutes of Health, 1993.)

TABLE 24-10	CHD Risk Factors

Male sex
High LDL cholesterol
Hypertension
Cigarette smoking (>10 cigarettes/day)
Low HDL cholesterol (<35 mg/dL)
Diabetes mellitus
Severe obesity (>30% overweight)
Family history of premature CHD
Physical inactivity
Stress
Age

CHD, Coronary heart disease; *LDL,* low-density lipoprotein; *HDL,* high-density lipoprotein.

TABLE 24-11 Goals for LDL Cholesterol Concentration According to the NCEP-ATP II

Patient Category	Initiation Level	Goal of Therapy
Dietary Treatment		
Without CHD and <2 risk factors	≥160 mg/dL	<160 mg/dL
Without CHD and ≥2 risk factors	≥130 mg/dL	<130 mg/dL
With CHD	>100 mg/dL	≤100 mg/dL
Drug Treatment		
Without CHD and <2 risk factors	≥190 mg/dL	<160 mg/dL
Without CHD and ≥2 risk factors	≥160 mg/dL	<130 mg/dL
With CHD	>130 mg/L	≥100 mg/dL

LDL, Low-density lipoprotein; *NCEP-ATP II,* National Cholesterol Education Program Adult Treatment Panel II; *CHD,* coronary heart disease.
NOTE: To convert to mmol/L, multiply by 0.0259.

aunt, or grandparent) for early documented CHD (at 55 years of age or less), myocardial infarction, angina pectoris, peripheral vascular disease, cerebrovascular disease, or sudden cardiac death.

Management of Lipoprotein Disorders

Dietary and drug therapies are the cornerstones of the treatment of lipid disorders, such as hypercholesterolemia and hypertriglyceridemia. As presented in Table 24-11,[19] adult patients with no CHD who have LDL cholesterol levels of 130 mg/dL or higher (3.37 mmol/L) and two or more risk factors, or LDL cholesterol levels of 160 mg/dL or higher (4.15 mmol/L) and less than two risk factors, should receive dietary counseling and eliminate excess fat from their diets. If the patients comply with the dietary intervention yet do not respond, or have CHD and LDL cholesterol levels of 100 mg/dL or higher (2.59 mmol/L), they then should be placed on a low-fat diet. If dietary therapy fails again to produce the desired reduction in LDL cholesterol, the patient then is considered for drug therapy. Dietary therapy should be tried for at least 6 months before pharmacotherapy is initiated. Candidates for drug therapy include those with LDL cholesterol levels of 130 mg/dL or higher (3.37 mmol/L) with documented CHD, patients with LDL cholesterol levels of 160 mg/dL or higher (4.15 mmol/L) without CHD but with two or more risk factors, and patients with LDL cholesterol levels of 190 mg/dL or higher (4.92 mmol/L) without CHD and with less than two risk factors (see Table 24-11).

Only children older than 2 years of age and adolescents identified by the selective screening process are candidates for treatment. Those with average LDL cholesterol concentrations between 110 to 129 mg/dL (2.85 to 3.34 mmol/L) should be counseled about their diet and other heart disease risk factors and reevaluated after 1 year. Those with average LDL cholesterol concentrations of more than 130 mg/dL (3.37 mmol/L) also should receive dietary counseling, be evaluated for secondary causes, and have their family members screened. If 3 months after initiation of dietary therapy the LDL cholesterol concentration remains higher than 130 mg/dL (3.37 mmol/L), the patient should be placed on a low-fat diet, which entails further reduction of the saturated fatty acid and cholesterol intake. Drug therapy was recommended by the NCEP in children 10 years of age and older if after careful adherence to dietary therapy (6 months to 1 year) the LDL cholesterol concentration still exceeds 190 mg/dL (4.92 mmol/L). However, the action level is lower (160 mg/dL; 4.15 mmol/L) for patients who have positive family histories of premature CHD or those with two or more other risk factors.

Most FH homozygotes are resistant to drug therapy. Several alternative treatments that have been used include (1) plasmapheresis every 2 weeks, (2) partial ileal bypass or portacaval shunt to lower total and LDL cholesterol in these patients, and (3) transplantation of the liver from a donor with functional LDL receptors.

The classification of triglycerides according to the NCEP-ATP II is listed in Table 24-12.[19] Patients with mild primary hypertriglyceridemia but without hypercholesterolemia are advised to cut excess fat from their diet, control their blood glucose, exercise, lose weight, and abstain from alcohol intake. Those with severe primary hypertriglyceridemia, however, are placed on a very–low-fat diet or treated with medications.

MEASUREMENT OF LIPIDS, LIPOPROTEINS, AND APOLIPOPROTEINS

Many analytical techniques and methods have been developed to measure lipids, lipoproteins, and apolipoproteins in body fluids. They include chemical, enzymatic, and immunochemical methods, as well as physical methods, such as

TABLE 24-12	Classification of Triglycerides Concentration According to the NCEP-ATP II
Category	Serum Triglycerides (mg/dL)
Normal	<200
Borderline high	200 to 400
High	400 to 1000
Very high	>1000

NCEP-ATP II, National Cholesterol Education Program Adult Treatment Panel II.
NOTE: To convert to mmol/L, multiply by 0.0113.

ultracentrifugation, electrophoresis, column chromatography, precipitation methods, and others.

Lipids and Lipoproteins

Both reference and routine methods have been developed to measure lipids and lipoproteins in body fluids.

Reference methods

The Centers for Disease Control and Prevention (CDC) has developed reference methods for measurement of cholesterol, triglycerides, and HDL cholesterol. A reference method for LDL cholesterol currently is being developed. These reference methods establish the accuracy base for the measurement of these analytes. In practice, reference methods are involved, time consuming, and require a high level of expertise for proper operation. Consequently, simpler methods have been adopted for routine clinical use.

Cholesterol

The CDC reference method for cholesterol is based on a chemical method devised by Abell, Levy, and Brodie. In the CDC version of this method, serum is treated with alcoholic KOH to hydrolyze the cholesteryl esters. Total cholesterol then is extracted from the mixture with hexane. An aliquot of the extract is dried, and the dry residue is treated with a mixture of acetic acid, acetic anhydride, and sulfuric acid (Liebermann-Burchard reagent) for color development. Absorbance is read at 620 nm, and pure cholesterol is used as the calibrator. This method is performed according to a strict protocol requiring replicate measurements in multiple analytical runs. The method exhibits an approximate 1.6% positive bias, compared with isotope dilution mass spectrometry, which is considered the definitive method for cholesterol and used by the National Institute of Standards and Technology (NIST).

Triglycerides

In the CDC reference method for triglycerides, the triglycerides first are extracted quantitatively with chloroform to remove water-soluble interfering substances, such as glucose and glycerol, from the serum. The extract is treated with silicic acid to remove phospholipids, and the triglycerides in the extract are subjected to alkaline hydrolysis to produce unesterified fatty acids and glycerol. The glycerol is oxidized to produce formaldehyde, which then is reacted with chromotropic acid for color development. The absorbance of the chromogen in the reaction mixture is measured at 570 nm.

High-density lipoprotein cholesterol

Because HDL consists of several populations of particles that vary somewhat in their cholesterol content, HDL is defined in terms of the method used to prepare the HDL-containing fraction. The CDC reference method uses a combination of ultracentrifugation to remove chylomicrons and VLDL and precipitation with heparin-$MnCl_2$ to remove IDL, LDL, and Lp(a), leaving HDL in the supernatant. The cholesterol in this fraction then is quantitated by use of the CDC reference method for cholesterol.

Routine methods

A number of routine methods that have been developed to measure cholesterol, triglycerides, and HDL cholesterol are discussed in the following sections.

Cholesterol

Enzymatic methods for cholesterol measurement have been used for more than two decades. They are accurate, precise, and easy to use. Commercially available cholesterol reagents commonly combine all the enzymes and other required components into a single reagent. The reagent usually is mixed with a 3- to 10-μL aliquot of serum or plasma, incubated under controlled conditions for color development, and absorbance usually is measured in the visible portion of the spectrum, generally at about 500 nm. The reagents typically use a bacterial cholesteryl ester hydrolase to hydrolyze cholesteryl esters, as follows:

$$\text{Cholesterol ester} + H_2O \xrightarrow{\substack{\textit{Cholesteryl} \\ \textit{ester hydrolase}}} \text{cholesterol} + \text{fatty acid} \qquad (1)$$

The 3-OH group of cholesterol then is oxidized to a ketone in an oxygen-requiring reaction catalyzed by cholesterol oxidase, as follows:

$$\text{Cholesterol} + O_2 \xrightarrow{\substack{\textit{Cholesterol} \\ \textit{oxidase}}} \text{cholest-4-en-3-one} + H_2O_2 \qquad (2)$$

H_2O_2, one of the reaction products, is measured in a peroxidase catalyzed reaction that forms a dye. The reaction is as follows:

$$H_2O_2 + \text{phenol} + \text{4-aminoantipyrine} \xrightarrow{\textit{Peroxidase}} \qquad (3)$$
$$\text{quinoneimine dye} + 2\,H_2O$$

Triglycerides

A number of enzymatic methods have been developed to measure triglycerides directly in plasma or serum. A single reagent that combines all the required enzymes, cofactors, and buffers generally is used. In all the methods the first step is the lipase-catalyzed hydrolysis of triglycerides to glycerol and fatty acids, as follows:

$$\text{Triglyceride} + 3\,H_2O \xrightarrow{\textit{Lipase}} \text{glycerol} + 3\,\text{fatty acids} \qquad (4)$$

Glycerol then is phosphorylated in an ATP-requiring reaction catalyzed by glycerokinase, as follows:

$$\text{Glycerol} + ATP \xrightarrow{\textit{Glycerokinase}} \text{glycerolphosphate} + ADP \qquad (5)$$

In the most commonly used methods, glycerophosphate is oxidized to dihydroxyacetone and H_2O_2 in a glycerophosphate oxidase-catalyzed reaction, as follows:

$$\text{Glycerolphosphate} + O_2 \xrightarrow{\textit{Glycerophosphate oxidase}} \qquad (6)$$
$$\text{dihydroxyacetone} + H_2O_2$$

The H_2O_2 formed in the reaction subsequently is measured as described in equation (3).

Alternatively, glycerophosphate can be measured in an NADH-producing reaction and the NADH measured spectrophotometrically at 340 nm or in a diaphorase-catalyzed reaction to form a reaction product that can be measured at 500 nm.

Because glycerol is a product of normal metabolic processes, it is present endogenously as glycerol in serum. Thus the measured quantity of triglyceride in serum is overestimated slightly if not corrected for this endogenous glycerol. In normal individuals, endogenous glycerol represents the equivalent of less than 10 mg/dL (0.11 mmol/L) triglyceride. The errors usually are not clinically significant. However, in certain conditions, such as diabetes mellitus, emotional stress, intravenous administration of drugs or nutrients containing glycerol, contamination of blood collection devices by glycerol, and prolonged storage of whole blood under nonrefrigerated conditions, endogenous glycerol concentrations are significantly higher and can impart greater error.

High-density lipoprotein cholesterol

HDL cholesterol has been measured commonly in the supernatant after the precipitation of the apo B–100-containing lipoprotein directly from plasma or serum by use of a polyanion in the presence of a divalent cation.[4] The apo B–100-containing lipoproteins include VLDL, IDL, Lp(a), LDL, and, when present, chylomicrons (see Table 24-5). As indicated previously, LDL and HDL are the largest contributors to total cholesterol in normal individuals. On aver-

age, IDL and Lp(a) each account for only about 2 to 3 mg/dL (0.05 to 0.08 mmol/L) of the total cholesterol, although their concentrations can be considerably higher in some people.

Polyanions react with positively charged groups on lipoproteins; their action is facilitated in the presence of divalent cations, which interact with negatively charged groups. When polyanions are added to an aliquot of plasma or serum, an immediate heavy precipitate is formed. Precipitation is complete within 10 to 15 minutes at room temperature. The precipitate then is sedimented by centrifugation for at least 45,000 g-minutes (the equivalent of $1500 \times g$ for 30 minutes), and HDL cholesterol is measured in the clear supernatant. Several polyanion-divalent cation combinations have been used, including heparin sulfate-$MnCl_2$, dextran sulfate-$MgCl_2$, and phosphotungstate-$MgCl_2$.

In practice, precipitation methods can be inaccurate in samples containing high triglyceride concentrations (generally those above 400 mg/dL; 4.52 mmol/L). To minimize this problem, the following actions may be taken:

1. The sample can be ultracentrifuged and the triglyceride-rich lipoprotein removed.
2. A turbid supernatant sometimes can be cleared by centrifuging for a longer period of time.
3. The sample can be diluted to reduce the concentration of triglyceride-rich lipoproteins before the precipitant is added.
4. The turbid supernatant can be passed through a 0.45-μm filter to remove the unsedimented precipitate, and HDL cholesterol may be measured in the filtrate.

A new method used to measure HDL cholesterol is a variation of the dextran sulfate method for precipitation of apo B–100-containing lipoprotein.[32] In this method the precipitant is complexed with magnetic particles. Once the lipoprotein-precipitant-magnetic particle complex has been formed, it can be removed rapidly without centrifugation by placement in the reaction vessel on a magnetic disk that is supplied with the kit. The HDL-containing supernatant then is removed, and HDL cholesterol is measured enzymatically.

In yet another approach, HDL cholesterol is measured directly in serum without the preliminary separation of the HDL-containing fraction. This method depends on certain modifications of cholesteryl esterase and cholesterol oxidase, as well as on the presence of α-cyclodextrin in the reaction mixture. The overall effect is to render the cholesterol in HDL more reactive than that in the other lipoproteins, and under the conditions of the cholesterol assay, HDL cholesterol is measured selectively. This method is becoming more widely used and is expected to replace the older precipitation methods over the next few years.

Low-density lipoprotein cholesterol: indirect methods

Methods to measure LDL cholesterol assume that total cholesterol is composed primarily of cholesterol in VLDL, LDL, and HDL.* In practice, LDL can be measured indirectly by use of either the Friedewald equation or by β-quantification.

Friedewald equation. In the most widely used indirect method, cholesterol, triglyceride, and HDL cholesterol are measured and LDL cholesterol is calculated from the primary measurements by use of the empirical equation of Friedewald et al:[9]

$$[\text{LDL cholesterol}] = [\text{Total cholesterol}]$$
$$- [\text{HDL cholesterol}] - \frac{[\text{triglyceride}]}{5} \qquad (7)$$

where all concentrations are given in milligrams per deciliter. (Triglyceride/2.22 is used when LDL cholesterol is expressed in millimoles per liter.) The factor [triglyceride]/5 is an estimate of the VLDL cholesterol concentration and is based on the average ratio of triglyceride to cholesterol in VLDL.

NOTE: The Friedewald equation should not be used in samples that have triglyceride concentrations above 400 mg/dL (4.52 mmol/L), in those that contain significant amounts of chylomicrons (nonfasting specimen), or in patients with type III hyperlipoproteinemia. These individuals have abnormal VLDL compositions, and the factor [triglyceride]/5 does not apply.

β-Quantification. This method usually is used in samples for which the Friedewald equation is inappropriate. Ethylenediaminetetraacetic acid (EDTA) plasma is the specimen of choice. It uses a combination of preparative ultracentrifugation and polyanion precipitation.

In β-quantification an accurately measured aliquot of plasma (density [d] = 1.006 g/mL) is ultracentrifuged at 105,000 × g for 18 hours at 10 °C. Under these conditions, VLDL and, if present, chylomicrons and β-VLDL (characteristic of type III hyperlipoproteinemia), accumulate in a floating layer, with the d greater than 1.006 g/mL infranatant containing primarily LDL and HDL. This fraction also contains any IDL and Lp(a) that may be present. The floating layer is removed with the aid of a tube slicer. The infranate is remixed, reconstituted to known volume, and its cholesterol content measured. HDL cholesterol usually is measured in a separate aliquot of plasma (see previous discussion), but when necessary, an aliquot of the d greater than 1.006 g/mL infranate can be treated to remove the apo B−100-containing lipoproteins [IDL, LDL, and Lp(a)] and the HDL cholesterol then measured in the clear supernate. VLDL and LDL cholesterol are calculated as follows:

$$[\text{VLDL cholesterol}] = [\text{total cholesterol}]$$
$$- [\text{d} > 1.006 \text{ g/mL cholesterol}] \qquad (8)$$

---

*This actually may not be the case in all samples because some individuals may have high concentrations of IDL or Lp(a).

$$[\text{LDL cholesterol}] = [\text{d} > 1.006 \text{ g/mL cholesterol}]$$
$$- [\text{HDL cholesterol}] \qquad (9)$$

LDL cholesterol measured in this way is unaffected by the presence of either chylomicrons, other triglyceride-rich lipoproteins, or β-VLDL. VLDL cholesterol usually is calculated from equation (8) rather than measured directly in the ultracentrifugal supernate. This method is used because recovery of this fraction quantitatively, particularly when triglyceride concentrations are high, can be difficult.

The ratio of VLDL cholesterol to plasma triglyceride, expressed in terms of mass, is 0.2 or lower in normal samples and in those from individuals with lipoprotein disorders other than type III hyperlipidemia. In those with type III hyperlipoproteinemia this ratio is 0.3 or higher because of the presence of β-VLDL, and the elevated ratio persists even after treatment is initiated. In addition, β-VLDL can be observed directly after the separation of the VLDL fraction by agarose gel electrophoresis because it has the mobility of LDL rather than of VLDL. The combination of a VLDL cholesterol to plasma triglyceride ratio of 0.3 or higher, and the observation of β-VLDL in the ultracentrifugal supernatant, establishes the type III lipoprotein pattern.

Lipoproteins included in the indirect measurement of LDL cholesterol. From the preceding discussion, what is apparent is that whether the Friedewald equation or β-quantification is used, the term *LDL cholesterol* actually includes the contributions of cholesterol in IDL and Lp(a), as well as that in LDL. Although IDL and Lp(a) cholesterol usually contribute only a few milligrams per deciliter to the "LDL cholesterol" measurement, their contributions can be significant in individuals with high IDL or Lp(a) concentrations. One suggestion is that a more specific measure of LDL cholesterol could be obtained by correction of the measured LDL cholesterol value for the contribution of Lp(a) cholesterol;[26] a similar argument might be made for IDL. Elevated concentrations of both IDL and Lp(a) appear to be related to increased risk for CHD [see later section on Lp(a)], however, and although such corrections might increase the specificity of the methods for LDL cholesterol per se, they also may give LDL cholesterol values that underestimate cardiovascular risk because they exclude some atherogenic lipoproteins. This instance might be expected to occur more frequently in individuals with CHD or those at risk for CHD based on their "LDL cholesterol" levels. For this reason the NCEP Working Group on LDL cholesterol measurement decided that LDL cholesterol values should *not* be corrected for the contribution of other atherogenic lipoproteins and also recommended that further research be conducted to establish the individual contributions of IDL, Lp(a), and LDL cholesterol to CHD risk as reflected in current LDL cholesterol measurements that include all three lipoprotein classes.

Low-density lipoprotein cholesterol: direct methods

Several "direct" approaches have been developed to measure LDL. In several of these, LDL is precipitated selectively with polyvinyl sulfate or heparin at low pH. LDL cholesterol then is calculated as the difference between total cholesterol and that in the supernatant or in another variation, directly in the LDL precipitate. Whether atherogenic lipoproteins other than LDL itself also are detected is unclear, and these methods might be subject to sources of error similar to those encountered with precipitation methods for HDL separation.

An immunochemically based method that takes advantage of the fact that apo B-100 is essentially the only apolipoprotein in LDL has been developed. A mixture of polyclonal antibodies to apo A-I and apo E is used to precipitate VLDL, IDL, and HDL, and LDL cholesterol is measured in the supernatant enzymatically. The available information regarding its performance so far suggests that the method may be useful for measurement of LDL cholesterol directly but does require further validation. The nature of the lipoprotein species contributing to the LDL cholesterol measurement has not been specified, but because the antibodies used would be expected to remove at least some of the IDL, the major non-LDL contributor would be Lp(a), as expected. Thus the "LDL cholesterol" fraction detected by this method may differ somewhat from that measured with the Friedewald equation or ultracentrifugation-polyanion precipitation. One major drawback of the method is that it cannot be applied to frozen plasma or sera, which may limit its usefulness because quality control requires the ability to make repetitive measurements over extended time periods in one or more control pools.

Total lipoprotein

Several approaches have been used to quantitate total lipoprotein, and in some cases lipoprotein subclasses, in a single operation. The most rapid of these methods is nuclear magnetic resonance spectroscopy.[21] This method detects lipoprotein-associated fatty acyl methyl and methylene groups, and the signals from a number of subfractions of VLDL, LDL, and HDL are resolved mathematically. The values can be reported in terms of lipoprotein cholesterol concentrations by use of assumptions about the average cholesterol compositions of the different major classes of lipoprotein. A single sample can be analyzed in a few minutes with about 0.5 mL of serum. The method requires specialized equipment and expertise, although it is amenable to automation.

Another approach has been to use density gradient ultracentrifugation in a vertical rotor and measure cholesterol continuously in the fractions eluted from the gradient.[7] A mathematical curve resolution procedure is used to derive the component lipoprotein curves and calculate their cholesterol concentrations. The method is capable of deriving the concentrations of VLDL, IDL, LDL, Lp(a), and HDL cholesterol. LDL cholesterol can be expressed separately or combined with IDL and Lp(a) to give a measurement similar to that provided by the Friedewald equation or β-quantitation. This approach is demanding technically and requires instrumentation that is not usually available in clinical laboratories.

In another approach the lipoproteins are separated by gradient gel electrophoresis of unfractionated serum. The electropherogram is scanned densitometrically, and the areas under the various lipoprotein peaks are integrated and converted to equivalent lipoprotein cholesterol concentrations through use of assumed average cholesterol compositions for the lipoprotein. The calculations are performed with a computer program supplied by the manufacturer. Electrophoretic quantitation of lipoproteins in unfractionated samples has not gained wide acceptance because of the inherent limitations of these methods, such as the incomplete resolution of VLDL and LDL, the co-migration of β-VLDL with LDL and Lp(a) with VLDL, differences in staining intensity of different lipoprotein, and other methodological difficulties.

None of the lipoprotein methods described in this section has been used widely enough to have been validated in independent studies to the same extent as have been the Friedewald and β-quantitation methods. In most cases the identities of the lipoproteins contributing to the "LDL cholesterol" measurement have not been established adequately. Further evaluations should better define the relationships among these new methods and current reference and routine methods.

Sources of variation in lipid and lipoprotein measurements

Lipid and lipoprotein concentrations vary within individuals when measured on several occasions. The sources of variation are categorized broadly as *analytical and physiological*.[25] Analytical variations are inherent in the measurements themselves and arise from variations in sample collection procedures, volume measurements, instrument function, reagent formulations, uncertainties in the assignment of values to calibration materials, and other such factors. Normal physiological variation occurs independently of analytical error and reflects the actual changes in concentration that occur through the course of normal, day-to-day living. Such variations result from factors including a change in posture that causes the redistribution of water between the vascular and nonvascular space, thereby changing the concentrations of nondiffusible plasma components. Recent food intake produces transient increases in plasma triglycerides of 50% or more and decreases of up to 10% or 15% in LDL and HDL cholesterol, depending on the fat content of the meal. This change results from changes in the lipid composition of these lipoproteins that occur as chylomicrons are metabolized. Seasonal changes also have been observed, probably resulting from changes in dietary and exercise patterns throughout the year. Normal physiological variations tend to occur in both directions, causing the lipid or lipoprotein concentration to vary somewhat about a mean value for a particular individual. Other kinds of physiological changes occur when the individual's steady-state concentrations change, through acute illness or stress, pregnancy, dietary changes that result in weight loss or gain, or changes in saturated fat intake. In these cases the changes tend to either increase or decrease and are not considered normal physiological fluctuations. Lipoprotein concentrations eventually return to the original steady-state levels when the individual recovers or a new steady-state level is achieved.

The role of the laboratory is to provide accurate measurements in the particular sample being measured. For this reason the laboratory is concerned primarily with minimization of analytical error. From the physician's standpoint, however, the goal is to establish the patient's usual range of concentration for purposes of diagnosis and judgment of the effects of treatment. This aim is affected primarily by physiological variation because physiological variation contributes the larger proportion of the specimen-to-specimen variation observed in serial samples from the same patient.

The NCEP Laboratory Standardization Panel issued specific recommendations to minimize the effect of preanalytical factors on lipid and lipoprotein testing. The panel recommends the following:

1. An individual's lipid and lipoprotein profile should be measured only when the individual is in a metabolic steady state.
2. Subjects should maintain their usual diet and weight for at least two weeks before the determination of their lipids or lipoproteins.
3. Multiple measurements within two months, at least one week apart, should be performed before a medical decision about further action is made.
4. Subjects should not perform vigorous physical activity within the 24 hours before testing.
5. Fasting or nonfasting specimens can be used for total cholesterol testing. A 12-hour fasting specimen is required, however, for triglycerides and lipoproteins.
6. Individuals should be seated for at least 5 minutes before specimen collection.
7. The tourniquet should not be kept on more than 1 minute during venipuncture.
8. Total cholesterol, triglyceride, and HDL-C concentrations can be determined in either serum or plasma. When EDTA is used as the anticoagulant, plasma should be cooled immediately to 2 to 4 °C to prevent changes in composition, and values should be multiplied by 1.03.
9. For total cholesterol testing, serum can be transported either at 4 °C or frozen. Storage of specimens at −20 °C is adequate for total cholesterol measurement. However,

specimens must be stored frozen at −70 °C or lower for triglyceride, lipoprotein, and apolipoprotein testing.
10. Blood specimens always should be considered potentially infectious and therefore handled accordingly.

No specific recommendations were made by the panel concerning apolipoprotein testing. However, steps similar to those described should be taken to help minimize preanalytical sources of variation in apolipoprotein measurements.

A laboratory can estimate its conformance to the total error recommendations fairly closely with the following equation:

$$\text{Total error} = \%\text{ bias} + 1.96\,(CVa) \qquad (10)$$

where % *bias* is the mean laboratory difference between the measured value for a serum control pool and the reference value for the pool, and *CVa* is the overall analytical coefficient of variation for the pool, including within- and among-run variation. It is calculated as follows:

$$\frac{\text{Standard deviation}}{\text{laboratory mean}} \times 100 \qquad (11)$$

Bias should be calculated from reference values rather than from manufacturers' stated values when these two values differ. The NCEP recommendations for lipids and lipoproteins are listed in Table 24-13. A laboratory with less bias can tolerate slightly greater imprecision without exceeding the total error criteria. Conversely, imprecision must be lower if bias increases. For example, a laboratory operating with a bias of 3% and a CV of 3% for cholesterol would have a total error of 3% + (1.96 × 3%), or 8.9%. If, however, bias is only 1%, the coefficient of variation could be as high as 4% without exceeding the criteria for total error (1% + [1.96 × 4%] = 8.8%). (In practice, many laboratories can achieve total errors in the range of less than 6%, assuming a bias of 2% and CV of 2%.)

TABLE 24-13   **NCEP Recommendations for Analytical Performance of Lipid and Lipoprotein Measurements**

		Consistent With	
	Total Error (%)	Bias (%)	CV (%)
Cholesterol	8.9	≤ ±3	≤3
Triglycerides	≤15	≤ ±5	≤5
HDL cholesterol			
Before 1998*	≤22	≤ ±10	≤6
By 1998	≤13	≤ ±5	≤4
LDL cholesterol	≤12	≤ ±4	≤4

NCEP, National Cholesterol Education Program; *CV*, coefficient of variation; *HDL*, high-density lipoprotein; *LDL*, low-density lipoprotein.
*At HDL cholesterol concentrations >42 mg/dL. Because standard deviation (SD) tends to be constant at lower HDL cholesterol concentrations, an SD ≤1.7 mg/dL was recommended.

Apolipoproteins

Apolipoproteins are measured by a wide variety of immuno assays, including radioimmunoassay (RIA), enzyme-linked immunosorbent assay (ELISA), radial immunodiffusion (RID), immunoturbidimetric assay, and immunonephelometric assay.[14] The concentration of a particular apolipoprotein usually determines the immunotechnique used for its measurement. Immunoturbidimetry and immunonephelometry are used widely to measure apo A-I and apo B-100, which are present at relatively high concentrations. Alternatively, more sensitive techniques, such as ELISA and RIA, are perhaps more suitable for those apolipoproteins present at significantly lower concentrations, such as apo C-I and apo C-II.

Apolipoprotein measurements can aid further in the detection of CHD risk and the diagnosis of hyperlipoproteinemia. For example, the measurement of apo B-100 provides a reliable clinical tool to identify subjects with increased risk for CHD who may not be identified readily by the conventional cholesterol or lipoprotein cholesterol measurements (for example, individuals with borderline elevations of LDL cholesterol or those with hypertriglyceridemia without LDL cholesterol elevations). In addition, apo B-100 measurements can assess whether lipid-lowering drugs are effective in lowering the number of atherogenic apo B-containing lipoproteins.

However, for apolipoprotein measurements to be used in routine clinical practice, meaningful cutoff values for clinical decision making must be established and more information regarding their clinical utility is needed. The use of cutoff values for apo A-I and apo B-100, similar to those recommended by the NCEP for HDL and LDL cholesterol, respectively, has been suggested. An apo A-I concentration of less than 120 mg/dL may be associated with increased risk of CHD, whereas apo A-I concentrations of 160 mg/dL or greater may be protective. The apo B-100 cutoff points of 100 and 120 mg/dL approximately correspond to the LDL cholesterol cutoff points of 130 and 160 mg/dL (3.37 and 4.15 mmol/L), which fall at approximately the 50th and 75th percentiles, respectively. Therefore suggestions have been made that apo B-100 values greater than the 75th percentile should be regarded as high risk and those greater than the 50th percentile as moderate risk.[31]

Lipoprotein(a)

The structural heterogeneity of Lp(a) as a consequence of the apo(a) size heterogeneity has important implications for the accurate measurement of Lp(a) in human plasma.[17] Repeated antigenic determinants are present in variable numbers in different Lp(a) particles, and the immunoreactivity of the antibodies directed to these repeated epitopes can vary as a function of apo(a) size. As a consequence, immunoassays using polyclonal antibodies or monoclonal antibodies specifically directed to kringle 4 type 2 epitopes tend to underestimate apo(a) concentration in samples with apo(a) of smaller size than the apo(a) present in the assay calibrator and overestimate the apo(a) concentration in samples with larger apo(a).

A variety of methodological approaches, such as turbidimetric, nephelometric, radiometric, and enzymatic, currently are used for Lp(a) measurement. Most of these assays, except the enzyme immunoassays (ELISA), are based on the use of polyclonal antibodies from various animal species. Commercially available, direct-binding, sandwich-type ELISAs usually are based on the use of a combination of monoclonal and polyclonal antibodies. One approach takes advantage of the presence of both apo(a) and apo B in Lp(a) particles. In this approach, Lp(a) particles are "captured" by use of a polyclonal or monoclonal antibody to apo(a) and an enzyme-conjugated antibody to apo B-100 as the detection antibody. In another approach, both the capture and detection antibodies are specific for apo(a). At present, the best approach with respect to risk estimation for CHD or stroke is unclear because the pathogenic mechanisms involved have not yet been elucidated. Thus whether risk is associated simply with an elevated number of Lp(a) particles in the circulation (as measured by use of an anti-apo B antibody) or also related to the presence of particular size polyforms (as might be detected more readily with anti-apo(a) detection antibodies) is unknown. Both factors likely influence risk.

Historically, Lp(a) concentrations have been reported in terms of total Lp(a) particle mass, or, alternatively, in terms of Lp(a) protein. If the aim is to provide Lp(a) values that are independent of apo(a) size, the Lp(a) assay should use antibodies directed to an apo(a) domain other than kringle 4 type 2 or to the apo B-100 component of Lp(a). This use allows the values to be expressed in nanomoles per liter.

At present, Lp(a) measurements are not standardized, and Lp(a) values reported in clinical studies are difficult to compare. However, a value of about 30 mg/dL of total Lp(a) particle mass traditionally has been used as a cutoff above which elevated levels of Lp(a) are associated with increased risk of CHD. Lp(a) concentrations also can be expressed in terms of particle number, the mass of apo(a), apo B-100, or Lp(a) cholesterol. Which approach best predicts the risk for CHD is yet to be determined.

In view of the current lack of reference methods or standardization procedures for Lp(a), definition of precise cutoffs that can be used to make clinical decisions is difficult. Although less than ideal, one approach is to establish a reference interval for each assay and report individual results in terms of percentile values within these intervals. In Caucasians, individuals with Lp(a) values above the 80th percentile can be considered at increased risk for coronary atherosclerosis. However, because Lp(a) values can vary among ethnic groups, reference values need to be population based. Furthermore, such cutoffs also may have to be racially specific. For example, African Americans in general have significantly higher Lp(a) concentrations than Caucasians but do not manifest a higher incidence of CHD.

Virtually all retrospective case-control studies in Caucasians have reported a strong association between elevated Lp(a) and the risk of CHD. In contrast, prospective studies have provided contradictory results, although more recent studies tend to support the predictive value of Lp(a) measurement. Interestingly, the few clinical studies in which Lp(a) was evaluated as a CHD risk factor in African Americans suggest that elevated Lp(a) is not an important risk factor in this group.

Several recent studies have suggested that apo(a) size isoforms may be related to a high prevalence of CHD. The procedure with the highest resolution and sensitivity for determination of apo(a) phenotypes involves separation of apo(a) on agarose gel electrophoresis, immunoblotting with specific antibody, and detection with ^{125}I-labeled protein A. This approach identifies at least 34 apo(a) polymorphs and can be used to express apo(a) size in terms of kringle number.

Apolipoprotein E

Traditionally, the determination of apo E isoforms was assessed by isoelectric focusing (IEF) techniques that permit identification of charge variations of the different isoforms. In the early studies, IEF was performed on VLDL that had been extracted to remove the lipids. The separated proteins then were stained for protein. This approach is not used as frequently today because it requires a relatively large volume of plasma and the expensive and time-consuming step of ultracentrifugation to isolate VLDL. Apo E phenotypes now are assessed best by molecular biological methods that readily distinguish the three variants of the apo E gene.

As discussed previously, homozygosity for apo E_2 is characteristic of type III familial hyperlipoproteinemia. Homozygosity for apo E_2 is a necessary but not sufficient condition for expression of the type III hyperlipoproteinemia; a second gene defect appears to be required. The study of apo E variants has assumed greater importance in the last few years because of the association between the apo $\epsilon4$ allele and Alzheimer's disease and dementia.[29] How apo E_4 is related to these disorders is unknown.

References

1. A joint statement for physicians by the Committee on Atherosclerosis and Hypertension in Childhood of the Council on Cardiovascular Disease in the Young and the Nutrition Committee, American Heart Association: Diagnosis and treatment of primary hyperlipidemia in childhood. Circulation 1986; 74:1181-1188A.

2. Albers JJ, Kennedy H, Marcovina SM: Evidence that Lp(a) contains one molecule of apo(a) and one molecule of apo B: evaluation of amino acid analysis data. J Lipid Res 1996; 37:192-196.

3. American Academy of Pediatrics Committee on Nutrition: Indication for cholesterol testing in children. Pediatrics 1989; 83:141-142.

4. Bachorik PS, Albers JJ: Precipitation methods for quantification of lipoprotein. Methods Enzymol 1986; 129:78-100.

5. Brown MS, Goldstein JL: A receptor-mediated pathway for cholesterol homeostasis. Science 1986; 232:34-47.

6. Brunzell JD: Familial lipoprotein lipase deficiency and other causes of the chylomicronemia syndrome. In Scriver CR, Beaudet AL, Sly WS et al (eds): The Metabolic and Molecular Bases of Inherited Diseases, 7th edition, vol II, pp 1913-1932, New York, McGraw-Hill, 1995.

7. Chung BH, Wilkinson T, Geer JC et al: Preparative and quantitative isolation of plasma lipoproteins: rapid, single discontinuous density gradient ultracentrifugation in a vertical rotor. J Lipid Res 1980; 21:284-291.

8. Expert Panel: Report of the National Cholesterol Education Program Expert Panel on Detection, Evaluation and Treatment of High Blood Cholesterol in Adults. Arch Intern Med 1988; 148:36-69.

9. Friedewald WT, Levy RI, Fredrickson DS: Estimation of the concentration of low-density lipoprotein cholesterol in plasma, without use of the preparative ultracentrifuge. Clin Chem 1972; 18:499-502.

10. Goldstein JL, Scrott HG, Hazzard WR et al: Hyperlipidemia in coronary artery disease: II. Genetic analysis of lipid levels in 176 families and delineation of a new inherited disorder, combined hyperlipidemia. J Clin Invest 1973; 52:1544-1568.

11. Grundy SM: Cholesterol and coronary heart disease: a new era. JAMA 1986; 256:2849-2858.

12. Gwynne JT: High-density lipoprotein cholesterol levels as a marker of reverse cholesterol transport. Am J Cardiol 1989; 64:10-17G.

13. Kane JP, Havel RJ: Disorders of the biogenesis and secretion of lipoproteins containing the B apolipoproteins. In Scriver CR, Beaudet AL, Sly WS et al (eds): The Metabolic and Molecular Bases of Inherited Diseases, 7th edition, vol II, pp 1853-1886, New York, McGraw-Hill, 1995.

14. Labeur C, Shepherd J, Rosseneu M: Immunological assay of apolipoproteins in plasma: methods and instrumentation. Clin Chem 1990; 36:591-597.

15. Mahley RW, Innerarity TL, Rall SC et al: Plasma lipoproteins: apolipoprotein structure and function. J Lipid Res 1984; 25:1277-1294.

16. Mahley RW, Rall SC Jr: Type III hyperlipoproteinemia (dysbetalipoproteinemia): the role of apolipoprotein E in normal and abnormal lipoprotein metabolism. In Scriver CR, Beaudet AL, Sly WS et al (eds): The Metabolic and Molecular Bases of Inherited Diseases, 7th edition, vol II, pp 1953-1980, New York, McGraw-Hill, 1995.

17. Marcovina SM, Albers JJ: Lipoprotein Lp(a) quantification: comparison of methods and strategies for standardization. Curr Opin Lipidol 1994; 5:417-421.

18. Marcovina SM, Albers JJ, Gabel B et al: The effect of the number of apo(a) kringle 4 domains on the immunochemical measurements of Lp(a). Clin Chem 1995; 41:246-255.

19. National Cholesterol Education Program: Second Report of the Expert Panel on Detection, Evaluation, and Treatment of High Blood Cholesterol in Adults (Adult Treatment Panel II). Circulation 1994; 89:1329-1445.

20. National Cholesterol Education Program: Report of the Expert Panel on Blood Cholesterol Levels in Children and Adolescents. U.S. Department of Health and Human Services. NIH Publication No. 91-2732. Bethesda, Md, National Institutes of Health, 1991.

21. Otvos JD, Jeyarajah EJ, Bennett DW et al: Development of a proton NMR spectroscopic method for determining plasma lipoprotein concentrations and subspecies distributions from a single, rapid measurement. Clin Chem 1992; 38:1632-1638.

22. Patsch JR, Prasad S, Gotto AM Jr et al: Post prandial lipemia: a key for the conversion of HDL$_2$ into HDL$_3$ by hepatic lipase. J Clin Invest 1984; 74:2017-2023.

23. Rifai N: Lipoproteins and apolipoproteins: composition, metabolism, and association with coronary heart disease. Arch Pathol Lab Med 1986; 110:694-701.

24. Rifai N, Kwiterovich PO Jr: Disorders of lipid and lipoprotein metabolism in children and adolescents. In Soldin SJ, Rifai N, Hicks JMB (eds): Biochemical Bases of Inherited Disease, 3rd edition, p 457, Washington, DC, AACC Press, 1998.

25. Rifai N, Dufour R, Cooper GR: Preanalytical variation in lipid, lipoprotein and apolipoprotein testing. In: Rifai N, Dominiczak M, Warnick GR (eds): Handbook of Lipoprotein Testing, 2nd edition, Washington, DC, AACC Press, 2000.

26. Sandkamp M, Funke H, Schulte H et al: Lipoprotein (a) is an independent risk factor for myocardial infarction at a young age. Clin Chem 1990; 36:20-23.

27. Schaefer EJ, Blum CB, Levy RI et al: Metabolism of high-density lipoprotein, apolipoproteins in Tangier disease. N Engl J Med 1978; 299:905-910.

28. Schaefer EJ: Clinical, biochemical, and genetic features of familial disorders of high density lipoprotein deficiency. Arteriosclerosis 1984; 4:303-322.

29. Siest G, Pillot T, Regis-Bailly A et al: Apolipoprotein E: an important gene and protein to follow in laboratory medicine. Clin Chem 1995; 41:1068-1086.

30. Sniderman A, Shapiro S, Marpole D et al: The association of coronary atherosclerosis and hyperapobetalipoproteinemia (increased protein but normal cholesterol content in human plasma low-density lipoprotein). Proc Natl Acad Sci USA 1980; 97:604-608.

31. Sniderman AD, Cianlone K: Measurement of apoproteins: time to improve the diagnosis and treatment of atherogenic dyslipidemias. Clin Chem 1996; 42:489-491.

32. Sugiuchi H, Uji Y, Okabe H et al: Direct measurement of high-density lipoprotein cholesterol in serum with polyethylene glycol-modified enzymes and sulfated alpha-cyclodextrin. Clin Chem 1995; 41:717-723.

Additional Reading

Bradley WA, Gianturco SH, Segrest JP et al (eds): Methods in Enzymology: Plasma Lipoproteins: Quantitation, vol 263, part C, San Diego, Academic Press, 1995.

Rifai N, Dominiczak M, Warnick GR (eds): Handbook of Lipoprotein Testing, 2nd edition, Washington, DC, AACC Press, 2000.

Robins SJ: Management of Lipid Disorders: A Basis and Guide for Therapy, New York, Igaku-Shoin Medical Publishers, 1997.

Schettler G, Habenicht AJ: Principles and Treatment of Lipoprotein Disorders, New York, Springer-Verlag, 1994.

Sebedio J-L, Perkins EG: New Trends in Lipid and Lipoproteins Analysis, Champaign, Ill, AOCS Press, 1995.

CHAPTER 25

Electrolytes and Blood Gases*

MITCHELL G. SCOTT, PhD, JONATHAN W. HEUSEL, MD, PhD,
VICKY A. LEGRYS, DA, MT(ASCP), CLS(NCA), and OLE SIGGAARD-ANDERSEN, MD, PhD

Objectives

1. Define the following terms:
   Electrolyte   Blood gas
   Osmolality   Oxygen saturation
   Sweat testing P_{50}
2. List the major physiological electrolytes.
3. Discuss the physiological functions and regulation of sodium, potassium, and chloride in the body and list the healthy reference interval for each.
4. State the principle of the ion-selective electrode method specifically for sodium, potassium, and chloride analysis.
5. List the four colligative properties of a solution.
6. State the principle of the quantitative sweat test for cystic fibrosis.
7. State the Henderson-Hasselbalch equation.
8. State the methods used to assess blood pH, CO_2, O_2, and oxygen saturation.
9. List the sources of preanalytical error in blood gas analysis.

Key Words

Acid-Base Measurement   The measurement of whole blood pH and blood gases

Blood Gases PCO_2 and PO_2 (the partial pressures of carbon dioxide and oxygen), usually in whole blood

Cystic Fibrosis   An inherited disorder of a transmembrane conductance regulator protein (CFTR) that leads to chronic pancreatic and obstructive pulmonary disease

Electrolytes   Charged low–molecular-mass molecules present in plasma and cytosol, including ions of sodium, potassium, calcium, magnesium, chloride, bicarbonate, phosphate, sulfate, and lactate

Electrolyte Exclusion Effect   A situation in which electrolytes are excluded from the fraction of total plasma volume occupied by solids, which leads to underestimation of electrolyte concentration by some methods

Hemoglobin   An oxygen-carrying, heme-containing protein abundant in red blood cells

Henderson-Hasselbalch Equation   An equation that defines the relationship between pH, bicarbonate, and the partial pressure of dissolved carbon dioxide gas:

$$pH = pK' + \log \frac{CHCO_3^-}{\alpha \times PCO_2}$$

Osmometry   The technique used to measure the concentration of dissolved solute particles in a solution

Oxygen Dissociation Curve   The sigmoidal curve obtained when SO_2 of blood is plotted against PO_2

---

*The authors acknowledge the original contributions by Norbert W. Tietz, PhD, Elizabeth L. Pruden, PhD, and Esther F. Freier, MT(ASCP), MS, on which portions of this chapter are based.

Oxygen Saturation   The fraction (percentage) of the functional hemoglobin that is saturated with oxygen, abbreviated So_2

P_{50} The Po_2 for a given blood sample at which the hemoglobin of the blood is half saturated with O_2; reflects the affinity of hemoglobin for O_2

Partial Pressure   The substance (mole) fraction of gas times the total pressure; that is, the partial pressure of oxygen, Po_2, being the fraction of oxygen gas times the barometric pressure

pH   The negative logarithm of the hydrogen ion activity

Pilocarpine Iontophoresis   A technique in which electricity is used to force the drug pilocarpine into the skin to induce sweating at the site

Point-Of-Care Testing   Clinical testing that occurs next to the patient, usually with a handheld device and a unprocessed specimen collected immediately before testing

Sweat Chloride   The concentration of chloride in sweat; increased sweat chloride being characteristic of cystic fibrosis

---

Maintenance of water homeostasis is fundamental to life for all organisms. In mammals the maintenance of osmotic pressure and water distribution in the various body fluid compartments is primarily a function of the four major **electrolytes**—Na^+, K^+, Cl^-, and HCO_3^-. In addition to their function in water homeostasis, these electrolytes play an important role in the maintenance of pH, regulation of heart and muscle function, and electron transfer reactions, as well as serving as cofactors for enzymes. Thus abnormal levels of electrolytes may be either the cause or the consequence of a variety of disorders, and determination of electrolytes is an important function of the clinical laboratory. Interpretation of abnormal osmolality and results of **acid-base measurement** depends on specific knowledge of the electrolytes. Because of their physiological and clinical interrelationship, this chapter discusses the determination of electrolytes, osmometry, and acid-base/blood gas values.

ELECTROLYTES

Electrolytes are classified as either anions, negatively charged ions that move toward the anode, or cations, positively charged ions that move toward the cathode in an electrical field. Physiological electrolytes include Na^+, K^+, Ca^{2+}, Mg^{2+}, Cl^-, HCO_3^-, $H_2PO_3^-$, HPO_4^{2-}, and SO_4^{2-} as well as some organic anions, such as lactate, and trace elements. Although amino acids and proteins in solution also carry electrical charges, they usually are considered separately from electrolytes in clinical chemistry. The major electrolytes (Na^+, K^+, Cl^-, HCO_3^-) occur primarily as free ions, whereas significant amounts (>40%) of Ca^{2+}, Mg^{2+}, and trace elements occur associated with proteins such as albumin.

This section discusses Na^+, K^+, Cl^-, and HCO_3^-. Determinations of body fluid concentrations of these four electrolytes commonly are grouped in the familiar test order for an "electrolyte profile." Other substances that are also elec-trolytes but have special functions in particular contexts are discussed elsewhere in this text. (The interactions of electrolytes and acid-base status, including the use of the "anion gap," will be explained in Chapter 35.)

Sodium

Sodium is the major cation of extracellular fluid, representing almost one-half the osmotic strength of plasma. It therefore plays a central role in maintaining the normal distribution of water and osmotic pressure in the extracellular fluid compartment. The normal daily diet contains 8 to 15 g (130 to 260 mmol) of NaCl, which is absorbed nearly completely from the gastrointestinal tract. The body requires only 1 to 2 mmol/day. The kidneys, which are the ultimate regulators of the amount of Na^+ (and thus water) in the body, excrete the excess.

Sodium initially is filtered freely by the glomeruli. Then, 70% to 80% of the filtered Na^+ load is reabsorbed actively in the proximal tubules, with Cl^- and water passively following in an iso-osmotic and electrically neutral manner. Another 20% to 25% is reabsorbed in the loop of Henle along with Cl^- and more water. In the distal tubules, interaction of the adrenocortical hormone aldosterone with the coupled Na^+-K^+ and Na^+-H^+ exchange systems results directly in the reabsorption of Na^+, and indirectly, of Cl^-, from the remaining 5% to 10% of the filtered load. The regulation of this latter fraction of filtered Na^+ determines the amount of Na^+ excreted in the urine. (The mechanisms of these processes will be discussed in Chapters 34 and 35.)

Specimens

Serum or heparinized plasma, obtained from blood collected by venipuncture into an evacuated tube, are the usual specimens used for assays of electrolytes. Capillary blood, collected in either microsample tubes or capillary tubes or applied directly from a fingerstick to some point-of-care devices also is analyzed commonly. Heparinized (lithium or NH_4^+ salt) arterial specimens obtained for blood gas and pH determinations also may be presented for analysis. Urine collection for Na^+, K^+, or Cl^- assay should be made without addition of preservatives. Timed collections of urine or feces are preferable to allow comparison of values with reference intervals and determine rates of electrolyte loss. Serum, plasma, and urine may be stored at 2 to 4 °C or frozen for delayed analysis. Hemolysis of blood does not cause significant errors in serum or plasma Na^+ values. Lipemic samples should be ultracentrifuged unless Na^+ is measured with a direct ion-selective electrode (ISE).

Fecal and gastrointestinal fluid specimens require preparation before assay. Only liquid stools justify the trouble of analysis because it is only when liquid feces are passed that those losses of electrolytes are significant. Liquid stool specimens should be clarified of particulate matter by filtration or centrifugation. The fluid should be frozen if it is not analyzed immediately. Because even filtered or centrifuged liquid samples contain bacteria, the sampling systems of automated instruments should be cleaned and flushed after fecal analysis.

Determination of sodium in body fluids

Sodium may be determined by atomic absorption spectrophotometry (AAS), flame emission spectrophotometry (FES), electrochemically with a Na^+-specific ISE, or spectrophotometrically. (Because sodium and potassium are assayed routinely together, these methods will be described together after the potassium section of this chapter.)

Reference intervals

The reference interval for serum Na^+ is 135 to 145 mmol/L from infancy throughout life. Urinary sodium excretion varies with dietary intake, but for individuals on average diets containing 8 to 15 g/day, an interval of 40 to 220 mmol/day is typical. A large diurnal variation exists in Na^+ excretion, with the rate of Na^+ excretion during the night being only 20% of the peak rate during the day. The Na^+ concentration of cerebrospinal fluid is 136 to 150 mmol/L. Mean fecal Na^+ excretion generally is cited as less than 10 mmol/day.

Potassium

Potassium is the major intracellular cation. In tissue cells, its average concentration is 150 mmol/L, and in erythrocytes the concentration is 105 mmol/L (~23 times its concentration in plasma). High intracellular concentrations are maintained because K^+ diffuses very slowly outward through the cell membrane, while the Na, K-ATPase pump, which is fueled by oxidative energy, continually transports K^+ into the cell against the concentration gradient. This pump is a critical factor in the maintenance and adjustment of the ionic gradients on which nerve impulse transmission and contractility of cardiac and skeletal muscle depend. Diffusion of K^+ from the cell into the plasma exceeds pump-mediated K^+ uptake whenever pump activity is decreased.

The body's requirement for K^+ is satisfied by a dietary intake of 50 to 150 mmol/day. Potassium absorbed from the gastrointestinal tract is distributed rapidly, with a small amount taken up by cells and most excreted by the kidneys. Potassium filtered through the glomeruli is reabsorbed almost completely in the proximal tubules and then secreted in the distal tubules in exchange for Na^+ under the influence of aldosterone.

Factors that regulate distal tubular secretion of K^+ include intake of Na^+ and K^+, water flow rate in the distal tubules, plasma level of mineralocorticoids, and acid-base balance. Diminished glomerular filtration rate is typical of renal failure, and the consequent decrease in distal tubular flow rate is an important factor in the retention of K^+ present in individuals with chronic renal failure. Renal tubular acidosis, as well as metabolic and respiratory acidoses and alkaloses, also affect renal regulation of K^+ excretion. (see Chapters 34 and 35).

Specimens

Comments discussed previously concerning specimens for Na^+ analysis generally are applicable to those for K^+ analysis. However, some additional points must be considered. Potassium levels in plasma and whole blood are 0.1 to 0.7 mmol/L lower than those in serum. The extent of this difference depends on the platelet count because the additional K^+ in serum is primarily a result of platelet rupture in the coagulation process.[17] Nevertheless, stated reference intervals for serum K^+ are 0.2 to 0.5 mmol/L higher than those for plasma K^+. The variability in the amount of additional K^+ in serum makes plasma the specimen of choice; in addition, the report should note whether serum or plasma was assayed.

Specimens for determination of K^+ concentrations in serum or plasma must be collected in such a way as to minimize hemolysis because release of K^+ from as few as 0.5% of the erythrocytes can increase K^+ values by 0.5 mmol/L. An increase in K^+ of 0.6% has been estimated for every 10 mg/dL of plasma **hemoglobin (Hb)** due to hemolysis. Thus slight hemolysis (~50 mg Hb/dL) can be expected to raise K^+ values approximately 3%, marked hemolysis (~200 mg Hb/dL) 12%, and gross hemolysis (>500 mg Hb/dL) as much as 30%. Therefore any visible hemolysis must be noted on a reported K^+ value. If K^+ levels are determined on whole-blood specimens, increases in actual K^+ levels caused by hemolysis may be overlooked easily. When hemolysis is suspected, a portion of the specimen should be centrifuged and inspected visually.

Clinically significant preanalytical errors can occur in K^+ determinations if blood samples are not processed expediently. Maintenance of the intracellular-extracellular K^+ gradient depends on the activity of the energy-dependent Na, K-ATPase. If a whole-blood specimen is chilled before separation, glycolysis is inhibited and the energy-dependent Na, K-ATPase does not maintain this gradient. Thus false increases in plasma K^+ occur as a result of K^+ leakage from erythrocytes and other cells. The increase of K^+ in serum is of the order of 0.2 mmol/L in 1.5 hours at 25 °C, whereas at 4 °C, the increase is considerably greater and has been reported to be as much as an increase of 2 mmol/L after 5 hours at 4 °C.[18]

The opposite effect, namely a falsely decreased K^+ value, initially is observed if an unseparated sample is stored at 37 °C because glycolysis occurs and K^+ shifts intracellularly. Even at room temperature, leukocytosis can cause falsely decreased K^+ levels. The extent of this decrease depends on leukocyte count, temperature, and glucose concentrations. This effect is, however, biphasic. Initially, plasma K^+ decreases as a result of glycolysis, but subsequently K^+ increases after the glucose substrate is exhausted and K^+ leaks from cells. Taken together, the recommendation for the most reliable K^+ determinations is to collect blood with heparin, maintain it between 25 and 37 °C, and separate the plasma within minutes by high-speed centrifugation without cooling. However, in practical terms, separation within 1 hour at room temperature is unlikely to introduce great error.

Finally, skeletal muscle activity, because it draws its energy from anaerobic glycolysis (which has limited capacity for adenosine triphosphate [ATP] production), causes K^+ efflux from muscle cells into plasma and can cause a marked elevation in plasma K^+ values under one particular circumstance. In practice, an upper-arm tourniquet should be released before the phlebotomist begins to draw blood after a patient clenches the fist repeatedly to increase the prominence of veins for venipuncture. If it is not released, plasma K^+ values can increase artifactually as much as 2 mmol/L because of this muscle activity.[7]

Reference intervals

Reported reference intervals for serum K^+ in adults vary from 3.5 to 5.1 and 3.5 to 5.0 mmol/L; for plasma, frequently cited ranges are 3.5 to 4.5 and 3.3 to 4.9 mmol/L. Cerebrospinal fluid values are approximately 70% of plasma values.[30] Urinary excretion of K^+ varies with dietary intake, but a typical range observed for individuals on average diets is 25 to 125 mmol/day. In cases of severe diarrhea, fecal loss may be as much as 60 mmol/day.

Methods for the determination of sodium and potassium

Although AAS, FES, or spectrophotometric methods may be used for Na^+ and K^+ analysis, most laboratories now use ISE methods. For example, of approximately 6000 laboratories reporting College of American Pathologists (CAP) proficiency data for Na^+ and K^+, more than 5900 used ISE methods in 1996.

Ion-selective electrodes

Analyzers fitted with ISEs[15] usually contain Na^+ electrodes with glass membranes and K^+ electrodes with liquid ion-exchange membranes that incorporate valinomycin.

(Typical electrodes and the principles of potentiometry are described in detail in Chapter 6.) The principle of potentiometry can be stated simply as determination of change in electromotive force (E, potential) in the potential-measuring circuit between a measurement electrode (the ISE) and a reference electrode as the selected ion interacts with the membrane of the ISE. In instrument applications the measuring system is calibrated by introduction of calibrator solutions containing known quantities of Na^+ and K^+. The potentials of the calibrators are determined, and the $\Delta E/\Delta$ log concentration is stored in microprocessor memory as a factor for calculation of unknown concentration when E of the unknown is measured. Frequent calibration, initiated either by keyboard command or an automatic, microprocessor-controlled sample uptake from a reservoir of calibrator, is characteristic of most systems.

Two types of ISE methods can be distinguished. In the indirect methods, sample is introduced into the measurement chamber mixed with a rather large volume of diluent of high ionic strength. In the direct methods, sample is presented to the electrodes without dilution. Most whole-blood analyzers and those that incorporate single-use ISEs are direct ISE methods. During 1996 the number of laboratories reporting CAP proficiency sample results in the United States was divided equally between indirect and direct methods. Important differences exist between direct and indirect methods that can result in significant differences in results. (These will be discussed later in the section on the electrolyte exclusion effect.)

Errors observed in the use of ISEs fall into three categories. The first are errors due to lack of selectivity. For instance, many Cl^- electrodes lack selectivity against other halide ions. Second are errors introduced by repeated protein coating of the ion-sensitive membrane, and third is the contamination of the membrane or salt bridge by ions that compete or react with the selected ion. These errors necessitate periodic changes of the membrane as part of routine maintenance.

Flame emission spectrophotometry

Although at one time the most common method for Na^+ and K^+ analysis, FES no longer is a common laboratory method. Advances in ISE technology, combined with the high level of maintenance and safety procedures for FES, essentially have led to the demise of this method for electrolyte analysis. In 1996 less than 1% of CAP reporting laboratories in the United States used FES for Na^+ and K^+ analysis.

Principle.   Samples are diluted in a diluent containing known amounts of lithium or cesium and aspirated into a propane-air flame. Sodium, potassium, lithium, and cesium ions, when excited, emit spectra with sharp, bright lines at 589, 768, 671, and 852 nm, respectively. Light emitted from the thermally excited ions is directed through separate interference filters to photodetectors. The Li^+ or Cs^+ emission signal is used as an internal standard (usually 15 mmol/L) against which the Na$^+$ and K$^+$ signals are compared. The system is calibrated relative to low and high concentrations of each analyte, and the relation of signal to concentration is defined by an associated microprocessor.

Spectrophotometric methods

Spectrophotometric methods fall into two categories—those based on enzyme activation and those that detect the spectral shift produced when either Na$^+$ or K$^+$ binds to a macrocyclic chromophore. Both approaches have been applied to smaller automated instruments. However, the high cost of reagents for these methods and the fact that few problems exist with ISE methods has resulted in "niche" use of these methods, primarily in the smaller instruments used in physicians' offices or clinics. An example of a kinetic spectrophotometric assay for Na$^+$ is based on activation of the enzyme β-galactosidase by Na$^+$ to hydrolyze *o*-nitrophenyl-β-D-galactopyranoside (ONPG).[20] The rate of production of *o*-nitrophenol (the chromophore) is measured at 420 nm.

Macrocyclic ionophores are molecules with atoms that are organized to form a cavity into which metal ions fit and bind with high affinity. Such compounds also are called *polycyclic ethers, crown ethers, cryptands,* or *cryptahemispherands*. Different macrocyclics can be made with cavities tailored to fit the ionic radii of different elements. When chromogenic properties are imparted to these ionophores, spectral shifts occur when the cation is bound. The specificity of many of these ionophores clearly is sufficient for clinical purposes.[13]

Electrolyte Exclusion Effect

The **electrolyte exclusion effect**[2] is the exclusion of electrolytes from the fraction of total plasma volume that is occupied by solids. The volume of total solids (primarily protein and lipid) in an aliquot of plasma is approximately 7%; thus approximately 93% of the plasma volume is water. The main electrolytes (Na$^+$, K$^+$, Cl$^-$, HCO$_3^-$) essentially are confined to the water phase. When a fixed volume of total plasma, for example, 10 μL, is diluted before flame photometry or indirect ISE analysis, only 9.3 μL of plasma water containing the electrolytes actually is added to the diluent. Thus a concentration of Na$^+$ determined by flame photometry or indirect ISE to be 145 mmol/L is the concentration in the total plasma volume, not the plasma water volume. For example, if the plasma contains 93% water, the concentration of Na$^+$ in plasma water is 145 × (100/93), or 156 mmol/L.

This negative "error" in plasma electrolyte analysis has been recognized for many years, and even though the electrolyte concentration in plasma water is physiological, the tacit assumption is that the volume fraction of water in plasma is sufficiently constant that this difference could be ignored. In fact, all electrolyte reference intervals are based

on this assumption and reflect concentrations in total plasma volume. Indeed, virtually all concentrations measured in the clinical chemistry laboratory are related to the total sample volume rather than to the water volume. The electrolyte exclusion effect becomes problematic when pathophysiological conditions are present that alter the plasma water volume, such as hyperlipidemia or hyperproteinemia. In these settings, falsely low apparent electrolyte values occur whenever samples are diluted before analysis, as is done for flame photometry or indirect ISE[2] (Figure 25-1).

Because the indirect ISE method and flame photometry both involve sample dilution before measurement, they give essentially identical results for any particular sample, regardless of plasma water volume in that sample. However, the reason for the similarity is that both methods are subject equally to the electrolyte exclusion effect. In disorders such as ketoacidosis, with severe hyperlipidemia or multiple myeloma with severe hyperproteinemia, the effect can be quite large. The laboratory results may lead clinicians to believe that electrolyte concentrations are normal or low when their concentrations in the water phase may be high or normal, respectively. This result can lead to inappropriate electrolyte replacement therapy. For grossly lipemic samples, centrifugation at 100,000 × *g* and analysis on the chylomicron-poor infranate is the most common approach to overcome this effect.

The direct ISE methods still determine concentration relative to activity but do not require sample dilution. Because no dilution is required, activity is directly proportional to the concentration in the water phase, not the concentration in the total volume. To make results from direct ISEs equivalent to flame photometry and indirect ISEs, most di-

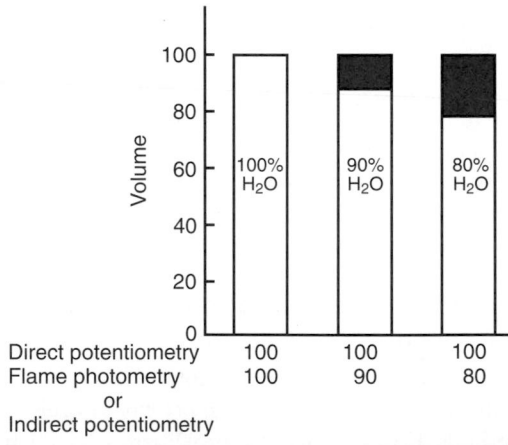

Figure 25-1 Predicted influence of water content on sodium measurements for a 100-mmol/L NaCl solution by direct ion-selective electrode (ISE) versus flame emission photometry or indirect ISE. Blue areas represent nonaqueous volumes, which could consist of lipids, proteins, or even a slurry of latex or sand particles. (Modified from Apple FS, Koch DD, Graves S et al: Relationship between direct-potentiometric and flame-photometric measurement of sodium in blood. Clin Chem 1982; 28:1931-1935.)

rect ISE methods operate in what commonly is referred to as the "flame mode." In this mode the directly measured concentration in plasma water is multiplied by the average volume fraction of water in total plasma (0.93). Although the latter may vary widely, as long as the activity of the specific ion is constant, the concentration of the ion in the water phase becomes independent of the relative proportions of water and total solids as long as proteins do not bind the ion. Therefore direct ISE methods are free of the electrolyte exclusion effect, and the values determined by direct ISE methods, even in the flame mode, are directly proportional to activity in the water phase and define electrolyte concentrations in a more physiological and physicochemical sense than methods that involve a sample dilution. Table 25-1 summarizes methods that are not subject to the electrolyte exclusion effects.

Chloride

Chloride is the major extracellular anion, with a plasma and interstitial fluid concentration of approximately 103 mmol/L. Together, sodium and chloride represent the majority of the osmotically active constituents of plasma. Therefore chloride is involved significantly in the maintenance of water distribution, osmotic pressure, and anion-cation balance in the extracellular fluid compartment. In contrast to its high extracellular concentrations, the concentration of Cl^- in the intracellular fluid of erythrocytes is 45 to 54 mmol/L, and in intracellular fluid of most other tissue cells, it is only about 1 mmol/L.

Chloride ions in food are absorbed almost completely from the intestinal tract. They are filtered from plasma at the glomeruli and passively reabsorbed, along with Na^+, in the proximal tubules. In the thick ascending limb of the loop of Henle, the chloride pump—the action of which promotes passive reabsorption of Na^+—actively reabsorbs Cl^-. Loop diuretics, such as furosemide and ethacrynic acid, inhibit the chloride pump. Surplus Cl^- is excreted in the urine and also can be lost in the sweat.

TABLE 25-1	Methods Measuring the Activity, Molality, or Concentration in the Water Phase and Thus Not Subject to Electrolyte Exclusion Effect
Method	Analytes
Ion-selective electrodes with undiluted sample	H^+ (pH), Na^+, K^+, Ca^{2+}, Cl^-, Li^+
Gas electrodes	CO_2, (P_{CO_2}), O_2 (P_{O_2}) HCO_3^- (calculated from pH and P_{CO_2})
Freezing point depression	H_2O (osmolality)

P_{CO_2}, Partial pressure of carbon dioxide; P_{O_2}, partial pressure of oxygen.

Specimens

Chloride most often is measured in serum, plasma, and urine. Specimen requirements were described in the section on sodium. Occasionally sweat Cl^- is determined. Because of the many factors that influence sweat collection and sweat-chloride measurements, this topic is presented separately later in the chapter. Cl^- is quite stable in serum and plasma. Even gross hemolysis does not alter significantly serum or plasma Cl^- concentration because the erythrocyte concentration of Cl^- is approximately half of that in plasma. Because little Cl^- is protein bound, changes in an individual's posture, in stasis, or in the use of tourniquets also have little effect on its plasma concentration. Fecal Cl^- determination can be clinically useful for the diagnosis of congenital hypochloremic alkalosis with hyperchloridorrhea (increased excretion of Cl^- in stool).

Methods for determination of chloride in body fluids

Chloride may be determined by mercurimetric titration, spectrophotometry, coulometric-amperometric titration, or, most commonly, ISE.

Mercurimetric titration

Mercurimetric titration is one of the earliest methods used to determine Cl^- in biological fluids and is mentioned in this chapter for historical purposes. With this method a tungstic acid, protein-free filtrate of specimen is titrated with mercuric nitrate solution in the presence of diphenyl-carbazone as an indicator. Free Hg^{2+} combines with Cl^- to form soluble but essentially nonionized mercuric chloride:

$$2\ Cl^- + Hg(NO_3)_2 \longrightarrow HgCl_2 + 2\ NO_3^-$$

Excess Hg^{2+} reacts with diphenylcarbazone to form a blue-violet color complex.

Spectrophotometric methods

Spectrophotometric methods based on the reaction of Cl^- with mercuric thiocyanate have been implemented on a number of automated analyzers. The principle is illustrated in the following equation:

$$Hg(SCN)_2 + 2\ Cl^- \longrightarrow HgCl_2 + 2\ SCN^-$$
$$3\ SCN^- + Fe^{3+} \longrightarrow Fe(SCN)_3$$

Chloride ions react with undissociated mercuric thiocyanate to form undissociated mercuric chloride and free thiocyanate ions. The thiocyanate ions react with ferric ion (Fe^{3+}) to form the highly colored, reddish complex of ferric thiocyanate with an absorption peak at 480 nm.

Automated spectrophotometric methods applied to high-volume testing for chloride present the problem of disposal of reagent waste containing a significant amount of toxic mercury. The ferric perchlorate method eliminates mercurial reagent entirely. Ferric perchlorate and Cl^- react in dilute perchloric acid to form a color complex with absorption maxima at 344 and 562 nm. The absorbance/concentration relationship is linear and the reaction more specific for Cl^- than many other spectrophotometric methods. The analytical range of these automated spectrophotometric methods generally is limited to concentrations of Cl^- in serum, plasma, or spinal fluid. Thus these methods often are not applicable to Cl^- analysis of other body fluids in which Cl^- concentrations may be much less than 80 or much more than 125 mmol/L. Strategies for measurement outside the usual interval include the dilution of the sample before analysis. Taken together, the mercuric thiocyanate, mercuric nitrate, and ferric perchlorate methods constituted about 4% of the laboratories reporting Cl^- results on a 1996 CAP survey report.

Coulometric-amperometric titration

Another method sometimes used to measure Cl^- is coulometric-amperometric titration (often called a *Cotlove chloridometer*). In this approach, determinations of Cl^- depend on the generation of Ag^+ from a silver electrode at a constant rate and the reaction of Ag^+ with Cl^- in the sample to form insoluble silver chloride,[5] as follows:

$$Ag^+ + Cl^- \longrightarrow AgCl$$

After the stoichiometric point is reached, excess Ag^+ in the mixture triggers shutdown of the Ag^+ generation system. A timing device records the elapsed time between start and stop of Ag^+ generation. Because the time interval is proportional to the amount of Cl^- present in the sample, the concentration of Cl^- can be calculated.

Unfortunately, this method is subject to interferences by other halide ions, CN^- and SCN^- ions, sulfhydryl groups, and heavy metal contamination. Because samples are prediluted before analysis, these methods also are subject to the electrolyte exclusion effect. Only 1% of laboratories in a 1996 CAP survey used coulometry. However, many laboratories still maintain these instruments as back-up analyzers and for sweat analysis.

Ion-selective electrode methods

Solvent polymeric membranes that incorporate quaternary ammonium salt-anion exchangers, such as tri-*n*-octylpropylammonium chloride decanol, are used to construct Cl^- selective electrodes in clinical analyzers. These electrodes, although exhibiting greatly improved linear responses since 1985, still suffer from membrane instability and lot-to-lot inconsistency in selectivity to other anions.[29] Anions that tend to be problematic are other halides and organic anions, such as SCN^-. Approximately 47% of 6017 U.S. laboratories in a 1996 CAP proficiency survey used indirect ISE methodology, whereas 48% used direct ISEs for Cl^-.

Reference intervals

Reported reference intervals for Cl^- in serum or plasma generally are 98 to 107 mmol/L, with some minor method-dependent variability. Spinal fluid Cl^- concentrations are approximately 15% higher than those in serum.[30] Urinary excretion of Cl^- varies with dietary intake, but an interval of 110 to 250 mmol/day is typical. Fecal excretion of Cl^- (for eight healthy subjects) has been reported as 2 to 3 mmol/day. (Sweat-chloride values will be discussed in a later section of the chapter.)

Bicarbonate (Total Carbon Dioxide)

Total carbon dioxide is used in this chapter to describe the quantity that is measured after acidification of a serum or plasma sample and measurement of the carbon dioxide released by acidification or by alkalinization and measurement of total bicarbonate. Under certain conditions of collection and specimen handling, total carbon dioxide values determined in this manner may be almost identical to values for the calculated concentration of total carbon dioxide obtained in blood gas analysis (see later section in this chapter on blood gas methods). (The pathophysiology of bicarbonate in acid-base disorders will be discussed in detail in Chapter 35.)

Specimens

Either serum or heparinized plasma may be assayed. The usual specimen is venous blood drawn into an evacuated tube, although capillary blood also may be presented for analysis. The concentration of total CO_2 is determined most accurately when the assay is done immediately after the tube is opened and as promptly as possible after collection and centrifugation of unopened tubes. Ambient air contains far less CO_2 than does plasma. Gaseous dissolved CO_2 escapes from the specimen into the air, with a consequent decrease in CO_2 value of up to 6 mmol/L in the course of 1 hour. In practical terms the logistics of high-volume processing and automated analysis of specimens almost ensures that most CO_2 measurements are done on specimens that have lost some dissolved, gaseous CO_2. Preservation of anaerobic conditions is not practical between the time plasma is placed on an instrument and the time it is sampled. On a comparative basis the result of a stat specimen, promptly introduced by an interrupt mode into an automated analyzer, probably has a much smaller error.

Methods for determination of serum or plasma total carbon dioxide

The first step in automated methods is acidification or alkalinization of the sample. Acidifying the sample converts the various forms of CO_2 in plasma to gaseous CO_2 by dilution with an acid buffer. Alkalinizing the sample converts all CO_2 and carbonic acid to bicarbonate HCO_3^-. Total CO_2 measurements use either electrode-based or enzymatic methods. In indirect electrode-based methods the released gaseous CO_2 after acidification is determined by a P_{CO_2} electrode (see Chapter 6). About 40% of laboratories reporting CAP data used one of these indirect ISE approaches in 1996. Direct ISE methods for total CO_2 have had problems with specificity and are not yet common, with only 7% of laboratories reporting CAP data in 1996 using them. Indeed, one direct total CO_2 electrode was found to react in an almost equivalent response to nitrate.[6] In enzymatic methods for CO_2 the specimen first is alkalinized to convert all CO_2 and carbonic acid to HCO_3^-. The enzymatic reactions are as follows:

Phosphoenolpyruvate   Oxaloacetate

Oxaloacetate   Malate

Decrease in absorbance of reduced nicotinamide-adenine dinucleotide (NADH) at 340 nm is proportional to the total CO_2 content. In 1996 these enzymatic methods were the most common methods used to report total CO_2 values on CAP surveys.

Reference intervals

Reference intervals for blood can be instrument dependent but generally vary from 24 to 31 mmol/L.

■ PLASMA AND URINE OSMOLALITY

Determination of plasma and urine osmolality can be useful in the assessment of electrolyte and acid-base disorders. Comparison of plasma and urine osmolalities can determine the status of renal water regulation in settings of severe electrolyte disturbances, as may occur in cases of diabetes insipidus or the syndrome of inappropriate secretion of antidiuretic hormone (SIADH) (see Chapters 23 and 39). The major osmotic substances in normal plasma are Na^+, Cl^-, glucose, and urea; thus expected plasma osmolality can be calculated from the following empirical equation:

$$mOsm/kg = 2.0\ Na^+\ (mmol/L)$$
$$+\ glucose\ (mmol/L) + urea\ (mmol/L)$$

or

$$mOsm/kg = 2.0\ Na^+\ (mmol/L) + 0.056$$
$$glucose\ (mg/dL) + 0.36\ urea\ N\ (mg/dL)$$

This empirical equation accounts for the contribution of other osmotically active substances in plasma, such as K^+, Ca^{2+}, and proteins. The reference interval for plasma osmolality is 275 to 300 mOsm/kg. Comparison of measured osmolality to the calculated value can help identify the presence of an "osmolal gap," which can be important in determination of the presence of exogenous osmotic substances in acid-base disturbances and toxic ingestions (see Chapter 32 and Chapter 35). Comparison of calculated and measured osmolalities also can confirm suspected pseudohyponatremia caused by the previously discussed electrolyte exclusion effect.

Principles of Osmotic Pressure and Osmosis

Osmometry is a technique used to measure the concentration of solute particles that contribute to the osmotic pressure of a solution. Osmotic pressure governs the movement of solvent (water in biological systems) across membranes that separate two solutions. Examples of biologically important selective membranes are those enclosing the glomerular and capillary vessels that are permeable to water and essentially all small molecules and ions but not to macromolecular colloids, such as proteins. Differences in the concentrations of osmotically active molecules that cannot cross a membrane cause those that can cross to move in order to establish an osmotic equilibrium. This movement of solute and permeable ions exerts what is known as *osmotic pressure*. Osmosis is the process that constitutes the movement of solvent across a membrane in response to differences in osmotic pressure across the membrane. Water migrates across the membrane toward the side containing more concentrated solute.

As an example, consider an aqueous solution of sucrose placed within a membranous sac that is permeable only to water, with an open vertical glass tube (a crude manometer) attached to the sac. If the sac is placed into a beaker of distilled water, water moves from the beaker across the membrane into the sucrose solution. The pressure of this solvent movement causes the sucrose solution to rise some distance up the tube.

At equilibrium the gravitational pressure of the column of solution in the tube equals the osmotic pressure and prevents further net movement of water from the beaker. The height of the rise of the sucrose solution in the manometer tube is a measure of the osmotic pressure of the sucrose solution. This measure is the pressure that would need to be exerted on the sucrose side of the membrane to prevent the flow of water across the membrane.

If the sucrose solution in the membrane sac were replaced with a sodium chloride solution of the same molarity, the solution in the manometer would reach equilibrium at a point almost twice as high as that observed with sucrose because sodium chloride dissociates into two ions per molecule.

In addition to increasing osmotic pressure when solute is added to solvent, the vapor pressure of the solution also is lowered. As a result of this change in vapor pressure, the boiling point of the solution is elevated and the freezing point of the solution depressed.

Colligative properties

The colligative properties of solutions are those that vary according to how much solute is in the solution. For example, the colligative properties of solutions include osmotic pressure, vapor pressure lowering, boiling point elevation, and freezing point depression. All these properties are related directly to the total number of solute particles per mass of solvent.

For example, a 1 molal solution in water boils at a temperature 0.52 °C higher and freezes at a temperature 1.858 °C lower than pure water. The term *osmolality* expresses concentrations relative to mass of solvent (1 osmolal solution containing 1 osmol/kg H_2O), whereas the term *osmolarity* expresses concentrations per volume of solution (1 osmolar solution containing 1 osmol/L solution). Although the term *osmolarity* often is used in medical literature, osmolality is what the clinical laboratory measures and is a more informative term.

An electrolyte in solution dissociates into two (in the case of NaCl) or three (in the case of $CaCl_2$) particles, and therefore the colligative effects of such solutions are multiplied by the number of dissociated ions formed per molecule. However, because of incomplete electrolyte dissociation, as well as associations between solute and solvent molecules, many solutions do not behave in the ideal case. For example, a 1 molal solution may give an osmotic pressure lower than theoretically expected. The osmotic activity coefficient is a factor used to correct for the deviation from the ideal behavior of the system

$$\text{Osmolality} = \text{osmol/kg } H_2O = \phi nC$$

where:

ϕ = Osmotic coefficient
n = Number of particles into which each molecule in the solution potentially dissociates
C = Molality in mol/kg H_2O

Glucose and ethanol have osmotic coefficients of 1.00, whereas the ϕ for sodium chloride is 0.93 at the concentrations found in serum. However, because NaCl contributes two osmotically active particles, its ϕ is 1.86 (2 × 0.93). The total osmolality or osmotic pressure of a solution is equal to the sum of the osmotic pressures or osmolalities of all solute species present. The electrolytes Na^+, Cl^-, and HCO_3^-, which are present in relatively high concentrations, make the greatest contribution to serum osmolality. Nonelectrolytes, such as glucose and urea, which are present normally at lower molal concentrations, contribute less, and serum proteins contribute less than 0.5% of the total serum osmolality because even the most abundant protein is present at millimolar concentrations.

Theoretically, any of the four colligative properties (vapor pressure, boiling point, freezing point, or osmotic pressure) could be used as a basis for the measurement of osmolality. However, the freezing-point depression property is used most commonly in clinical laboratories because of its simplicity.

Freezing-point depression osmometer

The instrument used most commonly to measure osmolality is a freezing-point depression osmometer,[1] but it often is referred to simply as an *osmometer*. To operate a freezing-point depression osmometer, the sample, in which a thermistor probe and stirring wire are centered, is placed into a cooling bath. The sample is supercooled to a temperature several degrees below its freezing point (−7 °C) through gentle stirring. When this supercooling has occurred, the sample is raised to a point above the liquid in the cooling bath and the wire stirrer is changed from a gentle stir rate to a momentary vigorous amplitude that initiates freezing of the super-cooled solution. This freezing is only to the slush stage, with about 2% to 3% of the solvent solidifying. The released heat of fusion initially warms the solution, and then the temperature plateaus and remains stationary, indicating the equilibrium temperature at which both freezing and thawing of the solution is occurring. At the end of the equilibrium temperature plateau, the thermistor again detects decreasing temperature as the sample freezes further toward a complete solid. More than 94% of the laboratories in the 1996 CAP surveys used freezing-point depression osmometers.

An example of the calculation to obtain osmolality follows. Suppose the observed freezing point of a serum specimen is −0.53 °C, then

$$\text{mosmol/kg } H_2O = \frac{-0.53}{-1.86} \times 1000 = 285$$

where −1.86 °C is the molal freezing-point depression of pure water.

Vapor-pressure osmometer

Another type of osmometer used to measure total osmolality in the clinical laboratory is the vapor-pressure osmometer. In reality, osmolality measurement in these instruments is not related directly to a change in vapor pressure (in millimeters of mercury), but to the decrease in the dew-point temperature of the pure solvent (water) caused by the decrease in vapor pressure of the solvent by the solutes. An important clinical difference between the vapor-pressure technique and the freezing-point depression osmometer is the failure of the former to include in the measurement of total osmolality any volatile solutes present in the serum. Substances such as ethanol, methanol, and isopropanol are volatile, and thus escape from the solution and increase the vapor pressure instead of lowering the vapor pressure of the solvent (water). Thus vapor pressure osmometers are impractical for identification of osmolal gaps in acid-base disturbances (see Chapter 35) and are not recommended for most clinical laboratories.

SWEAT TESTING

The analysis of sweat for increased electrolyte concentration is used to confirm the diagnosis of **cystic fibrosis (CF)**. CF is the most common, lethal genetic disorder of the Caucasian population with a wide spectrum of clinical presentations, including chronic obstructive pulmonary disease and pancreatic insufficiency. CF is associated with a defect in the cystic fibrosis transmembrane conductance regulator protein (CFTR), a protein that normally regulates electrolyte transport across epithelial membranes. Several hundred mutations of CFTR have been identified (see Chapter 37). Although direct mutational analysis is available, it is not informative in all cases, and the sweat test remains the standard for diagnostic testing.[21] In an effort to standardize testing, the National Committee for Clinical Laboratory Standards (NCCLS) developed the guidelines document C34-A2: Sweat Testing: Sample Collection and Quantitative Analysis. In addition, the Cystic Fibrosis Foundation has produced a videotape detailing the performance and interpretation of the sweat test.

The sweat test is performed in three phases—sweat stimulation by pilocarpine iontophoresis; collection of the sweat; and qualitative or quantitative analysis of **sweat chloride,** sodium, conductivity, or osmolality.

Sweat Stimulation and Collection

Because of transient increases in sweat electrolytes shortly after birth, individuals should be at least 48 hours of age before a sweat test is performed. The subject should be physiologically and nutritionally stable, well hydrated, and free of acute illness. The skin should be free of cuts, rashes, and inflammation to avoid contamination of the sweat sample with serous fluid. For example, sweat testing never should be performed over an area of eczema.

Stimulation

Localized sweating is produced by **pilocarpine iontophoresis** of a cholinergic drug, pilocarpine nitrate, into an area of the skin. Iontophoresis uses a small electric current to deliver pilocarpine into the sweat glands from the positive electrode, while an electrolyte solution at the negative electrode completes the circuit. After iontophoresis, sweat is collected onto preweighed gauze pads or filter paper or into Macroduct coils, with techniques used to minimize evaporation and contamination. Although the Occupational Safety and Health Administration (OSHA) does not list sweat as a potentially infectious, laboratory personnel should practice the same universal precautions they would use with any other body fluid.

Collection

If sweat is collected onto gauze or filter paper, the electrodes usually are made of copper and are slightly smaller than the stimulation and collection area. The composition of the electrolyte solution should be selected to avoid contamination with the sweat sample. Before collection is performed the gauze or filter paper used for sweat collection should be placed into a weighing vial with a secure sealing lid, and the vial should be labeled and weighed with an analytical balance. For a detailed procedure for stimulation and collection, the reader should refer to NCCLS document C34-A2.

Alternatively for sweat stimulation, the electrodes and current source can be integrated, as they are in the Wescor Macroduct system, which uses gel reagents containing pilocarpine. The battery-powered iontophoresis system delivers a current of 1.5 mA for 5 minutes. With this stimulation system, sweat is collected into a disposable microbore-tubing coil collector. After sufficient sweat has been collected, the sweat is transferred from the coil into a sealable microsample cup.

Critical issues associated with sweat collection

The proper collection of sweat is difficult. The analyst must avoid evaporation and contamination of the sample, collect a sufficient amount of sample, and minimize skin reactions. When gauze or filter paper collection pads are used, the collector should observe the following guidelines:

1. Use gauze or filter paper that is low in electrolyte content.
2. Wash and dry the patient's skin thoroughly after stimulation and before collection with type I distilled, deionized water,
3. Do not touch the weighing vial, wax film, collection site, or collection pad. (Always use forceps or powder-free gloves.)
4. Use two pieces of waterproof adhesive tape on all sides of the paraffin-wax film or wrap with a disposable stretch bandage to produce an airtight seal.
5. Blot back into the collection pad any condensate that may have formed on the wax film during collection. (Failure to collect the condensate can result in false-positive test results.)
6. After collection is complete, quickly transfer the specimen pad to the weighing vial and reweigh promptly.

When collecting sweat into Macroduct coils, the analyst should apply the following guidelines:

1. Wash and dry the patient's skin thoroughly after stimulation and before collection with type I distilled, deionized water.
2. Avoid touching the collecting surface of the coil.
3. Fasten the collector to the extremity with firm strap pressure; test for proper attachment after sweat appears in the coils.
4. Do not attempt to remove the entire collector assembly from the patient's extremity before separating the coil from the main body. (Loss of specimen may occur.)
5. Do not contaminate the nippers or sweat-dispensing needle with sweat sample.

Determination of and adherence to a minimum sweat weight or volume are critical to obtain valid sweat-testing results. The requirement for a minimum amount is to ensure an appropriate sweat rate and sweat-electrolyte concentration. It is independent of the instrument used to measure sweat electrolytes. Unfortunately, many analysts misunderstand the necessity of collecting the correct volume, leading to false-positive and false-negative sweat tests, which have a significant implication for patient care. Sweat-electrolyte concentration is related to sweat rate. At low sweat rates, sweat-electrolyte concentration decreases and the opportunity for sample evaporation increases. To ensure a valid result the average sweat rate should exceed 1 g/m^2/minute. To standardize and simplify the collection process, the size of the electrodes, reagent pads, and collection material must be approximately the same. Insufficient samples must not be pooled for analysis.

When the acceptable rate is applied to the parameters described in the NCCLS document, the minimum acceptable sample for analysis from a single site with use of 2- by- 2-inch gauze or filter paper for stimulation and collection is 75 mg of sweat collected within 30 minutes. With the Macroduct system the electrodes and stimulation area are smaller, and the minimum acceptable sample is 15 μL collected within 30 minutes.

When the collection process deviates from standard parameters, the minimum acceptable sweat volume or weight changes. Sweat should be collected for only 30 minutes. If the collection time exceeds 30 minutes, the requirement for the amount of sweat needed to ensure adequate stimulation must increase. Extending the collection time can allow additional opportunity for sweat evaporation, and, practically, does not increase the sweat yield significantly.[14] Acquiring the minimum sample should not be a problem if both the procedure in the NCCLS document and the manufacturer's recommendations are followed. On average in the collection process the percentage of insufficient samples should not exceed 5%. Insufficient sweat samples can be due to several factors, such as age, race, skin condition, and collection system. Burns to the patient's skin after iontophoresis are ex-

tremely rare but can occur at either electrode. If the burn occurs at the site of pilocarpine stimulation, sweat should not be collected. The reader should refer to NCCLS document C34-A2 for techniques to minimize the potential for burns.

Qualitative tests

A qualitative sweat test represents a screening test for CF. Individuals having positive or borderline results should have quantitative sweat testing. Screening tests may or may not measure the amount of sweat collected and may report a result as positive, negative, or borderline or give an actual concentration of sweat analytes. Although a variety of systems are used for sweat testing, several of the methods have documented problems, making them inappropriate for clinical use. For example, older conductivity analyzers using unheated collection cups are not recommended as diagnostic procedures because problems have been reported with sample evaporation and condensation and the ability to quantify sweat samples adequately.

The Cystic Fibrosis Foundation has approved the Wescor Macroduct Sweat-Chek for screening at clinical sites, such as community hospitals, using the criteria that an individual having a sweat conductivity 50 mmol/L or greater should be referred to an accredited CF care center for a quantitative sweat-chloride test. Note that sweat-conductivity methods produce results that are approximately 15 mmol/L higher than sweat-chloride concentration. The difference most likely is caused by the presence of unmeasured anions, such as lactate and bicarbonate.[10] Because of this difference, laboratories should not report conductivity results as if they were chloride results. In addition to the conductivity results (in mmol/L), the report should include sweat-conductivity reference intervals.

Quantitative Tests

According to the NCCLS C34-A2 document, a quantitative sweat test consists of three steps—collection of sweat into gauze, filter paper, or Macroduct coils; evaluation of the amount collected either in weight (milligrams) or volume (microliters); and subsequent measurement of the sweat chloride or sodium concentration. Chloride provides more diagnostic discrimination, as compared with sodium, making it the preferred analyte.[9] Chloride concentration can be determined either by coulometric titration with a chloridometer or manual titration with mercuric nitrate (see previous section in this chapter). If a laboratory chooses to quantitate sweat chloride with an automated analyzer that employs an ISE, these methods must be validated systematically for accuracy, precision, and lower limit of detection. In the context of clinically significant findings, a sweat-chloride level greater than 60 mmol/L is consistent with CF; concentrations between 40 and 60 mmol/L are considered borderline, and values less than 40 mmol/L in general are considered normal.[21] Some mutations of the CF gene are associated with borderline or normal sweat-chloride concentrations.[27]

Quality Assurance

Laboratories that wish to provide high-quality sweat testing should select appropriate methods, have sufficient testing volumes to ensure familiarity with the test, and limit the testing personnel to a small number of well-trained individuals. To monitor the accuracy and precision of the analytical process, two levels of controls should be performed every day when patient samples are analyzed. The reportable range for sweat chloride is 1 to 165 mmol/L. The laboratory, following acceptable validation protocol for the analytical method, periodically should confirm the reportable range. Sweat chloride concentrations greater than 165 mmol/L are not physiologically possible and can represent specimen contamination or analytical error. An important part of a quality-assurance plan includes the external validation of sweat-analysis accuracy through participation in proficiency testing, such as that offered by the CAP.

Sources of Error in Sweat Testing

Unreliable methodology, technical errors, and errors in interpretation all can lead to erroneous sweat-test results. Methods that do not measure the amount of sweat collected or do not have an established minimum amount are subject to false-negative results because an adequate sweat rate cannot be ensured. Other problems with sweat testing include errors of evaporation and contamination and those in dilution, instrument calibration, sample identification, and re-

TABLE 25-2 **Diseases Other Than CF Associated with Elevated Sweat-Electrolyte Concentrations**

Anorexia nervosa	Klinefelter's syndrome
Atopic dermatitis	Long-term prostaglandin
Autonomic dysfunction	E1 infusion
Ectodermal dysplasia	Mauriac's syndrome
Environmental deprivation	Mucopolysaccharidosis type 1
Familial cholestasis	Nephrogenic diabetes insipidus
Fucosidosis	Nephrosis
Glucose-6-phosphate	Protein calorie malnutrition
dehydrogenase deficiency	Pseudohypoaldosteronism
Glycogen storage disease:	Psychosocial failure to thrive
type 1	Untreated adrenal insufficiency
Hypogammaglobulinemia	Untreated hypothyroidism

From National Committee for Clinical Laboratory Standards: Sweat Testing: Sample Collection and Quantitative Analysis: Approved Guideline. NCCLS Document C34-A2. Wayne, Pa, National Committee for Clinical Laboratory Standards, 2000.
CF, Cystic fibrosis.

sult reporting. These errors occur more frequently in institutions performing relatively few tests. Laboratories with low testing volumes for sweat analysis should consider discontinuing the test and referring patients to accredited CF care centers for testing and evaluation. Interpretation errors are caused by inadequate technical knowledge, failure to repeat borderline and positive results, failure to repeat negative test results when they are inconsistent with the clinical setting, and failure to repeat testing in patients diagnosed with CF who do not follow the expected clinical course. Malnutrition, dehydration, eczema, and rash can increase sweat electrolytes, whereas edema and the administration of mineralocorticoids can decrease sweat electrolytes. Several conditions other than CF are associated with elevations in sweat electrolytes; however, these conditions usually are distinguishable from CF based on the patient's clinical presentation (Table 25-2).

■ BLOOD GASES AND pH

Clinical management of respiratory and metabolic disorders often depends on rapid, accurate measurement of the partial pressures of oxygen and carbon dioxide in blood **(blood gases)**. Vigorous measures to preserve and support life in individuals with cardiopulmonary impairment depend largely on assisted ventilation through use of mixtures of gases that are tailored in response to laboratory blood gas and acid-base results. Determination of blood gases also plays an important part in the detection of acid-base imbalance and in monitoring of the effect of therapy (see Chapter 35). Modern instruments for blood-gas determinations are simple to operate and, with meticulous maintenance and quality control, are capable of rapid turnaround of very reliable laboratory data.

The recommended nomenclature in this area of analysis was finalized in 1994 by the NCCLS (C12-A), but because alternative nomenclatures exist and are in common use, some of them also are summarized in Table 25-3.

Behavior of Gases

Determination of gas pressures in expired air or blood depends on the application of certain physical principles (Table 25-4). The **partial pressure** of a gas in a gas mixture is defined as the substance (mole) fraction of gas times the total pressure. The partial pressure of a gas dissolved in blood is defined as the partial pressure of the gas in an imaginary ideal gas phase in equilibrium with the blood. The tension of a gas in a liquid is in fact a measure of the chemical activity of the gas in the liquid.

Various spaces where gases are present with respect to blood gas analysis include the ambient space, the bronchial tree and alveoli of the individual, and the measuring chamber of a laboratory instrument. In all these spaces, atmo-

TABLE 25-3	Conversion Factors, Prefixes, Symbols, and Descriptors Used in Discussions of Gases Measured in Blood and Expired Air*

Conversion Factors

1 mm Hg = 0.133 kPa

1 kPa = 7.5 mm Hg

kPa: 1 kilopascal = 1000 pascal (The pascal is the SI-derived unit of pressure; it equals 1 Newton/m².)

General Prefixes

P: partial pressure or tension

    Usage: P_{O_2}, P_{CO_2}, P_{H_2O}

    Alternative: p_{O_2}

S: saturation fraction

    Usage: S_{O_2}

    Alternative: s_{O_2}

c: Substance concentration

    Usage: ct_{O_2} for concentration of total O_2

        ct_{CO_2} for concentration of total CO_2

        $cHCO_3^-$ for concentration of bicarbonate

d: Dissolved gas, used with substance concentration (c)

t: Total, used with substance concentration (c), thus $ct_{CO_2} = cHCO_3^- + cd_{CO_2}$

Specimen origin is indicated by lowercase letters. Whole blood and plasma are distinguished by capitals.

    a: arterial

    v: venous

    c: capillary

    B: blood

    P: plasma

    Usage: $P_{O_2}(aB)$, for partial pressure of O_2 in arterial blood

Prefixes Associated with External Respiration

V: volume of air or blood (unit: L)

$\dot{V}$: volume rate (unit, L/minute)

F: substance fraction; also known as *mole fraction*

E: expired air

I: inspired air

A: alveolar air

Other Descriptors

BTPS: **B**ody **T**emperature (37 °C or 310.16 K) and ambient **P**ressure, fully **S**aturated (P_{H_2O} = 47 mm Hg or 6.25 kPa)

STPD: **S**tandard **T**emperature (0 °C or 273.16 K) and standard **P**ressure (760 mm Hg or 101.08 kPa) of **D**ry gas

Amb: ambient atmosphere (unit: Atm [atmosphere])

B: barometric (atmospheric)

    Usage: P(amb), P(Amb)

SVP: **S**aturated **V**apor **P**ressure, the vapor pressure of water

    SVP_T means SVP at a specified temperature (for example, $SVP_{37 °C}$ = 47 mm Hg; P_{H_2O} [saturated]).

SI, International System of Units.

*This list is not complete but is presented to facilitate interpretation of terms used in the text and illustrate various forms that the reader may encounter in the literature.

spheric (barometric) pressure, P(Amb), is the prevailing pressure, and partial pressures of each of the gases present in these spaces must add up to the value of P(Amb), which varies with altitude and weather. Scientific convention reduces measurements of gas volumes made at P(Amb) to

standard *t*emperature (0 °C or 273.16 K) and *p*ressure (760 mm Hg or 101.325 kPa) for *d*ry gas (STPD) in order to make experimental data transferable. However, in blood-gas work, this conversion usually is not done.

For blood-gas analysis, measurements of partial pressure in biological specimens always are made at body temperature (usually 37 °C), at P(Amb), and in the presence of saturated water vapor (P_{H_2O} = 47 mm Hg). This convention is known as BTPS (*b*ody *t*emperature and ambient *p*ressure, fully *s*aturated; see Table 25-3). Use of BTPS has the following practical effects:

1. It relates laboratory data for blood gases strictly to the geographical location of the patient so that reference intervals become altitude dependent.

2. It assumes that the standard body temperature of a normal individual is exactly 37 °C and that the measuring device also holds the sample of blood at exactly 37 °C. This assumption requires special concern for thermal stability of the instrument and in instances when a patient's temperature is not 37 °C.

3. It recognizes that the partial pressures of measured gases in the blood coexist with a constant standard water vapor pressure (SVP), which is identical for both the calibration conditions of the instrument and measurement conditions of the blood sample.

Boyle's and Charles's laws and Avogadro's hypothesis are combined into what is called the *general gas equation*:

$$P = \frac{(nRT)}{V}$$

where:

    P = Pressure in units of millimeters of mercury (mm Hg) or kilopascals (kPa)

    V = Volume in liters in which an ideal gas is contained

    T = Temperature in degrees kelvin (0 °C = 273.16 K)

    n = Number of moles of gas

    R = Gas constant

Use of the Système International d'Unites (SI) units has an advantage in that 1 atm almost equals 100 kPa (1 atm = 101.325 kPa); however, the unit of millimeters of mercury (also called *torr*) has continued to be more popular (see Table 25-3 for conversion factors). Partial pressures expressed in kilopascals therefore are very close estimates of percentages of the gases in the mixture at 1 atm. Pressure, P (or p), may mean either total pressure, as in the expression P(Amb) for the mixture of gases in ambient air, or partial pressure in blood, as in $P_{O_2}(aB)$.

Dalton's law (see Table 25-4) may be written for room air as

$$P(Amb) = P_{O_2} + P_{CO_2} + P_{N_2} + P_{H_2O} + P_X$$

where P_{H_2O} is the partial pressure of water vapor, and P_X is that of any other gas in the air sample. Dalton's law of partial pressures, although not always applicable to gases in so-

TABLE 25-4	Physical Principles Applied to Blood Gas Measurements	
Principle	Description	Expression
Boyle's law	The volume (V) of an ideal gas at a constant temperature varies inversely with the pressure (P) exerted to contain it.	$V \propto 1/P$
Charles's (Gay-Lussac's) law	The volume (V) of an ideal gas at a constant pressure varies directly with its absolute temperature (T).	$V \propto T$
Avogadro's hypothesis	Equal volumes (V) of different ideal gases at the same temperature and pressure contain the same number of molecules (n).	$n_i/V_i = n_j/V_j$
Dalton's law	The total pressure (P) exerted by a mixture of ideal gases is the sum (Σ) of the partial pressures (P_i) of each of the gases in the mixture.	$P = \Sigma P_i$
Henry's law	The amount of a sparingly soluble gas dissolved in a liquid is proportional to the partial pressure of a the gas over the liquid.	$c = \alpha \times P$

lution, remains important for calibration and control of the measuring devices.

Consider a calibrator gas certified to contain 15% O_2 (L/L or mol/mol) and 5% CO_2, the remainder being N_2. This mixture, after saturation with water vapor at 37 °C (to mimic an individual's blood or alveolar air), is introduced into the instrument's measuring chamber (held at 37 °C to mimic an individual's body temperature) for the purpose of calibration of the instrument for subsequent measurements of gases in subjects' samples. If the local barometric pressure, $P(\text{Amb})$, on this occasion is 747 mm Hg, then the humidified calibrator gas is present in the chamber at ambient, barometric pressure, such that

$$P(\text{Amb}) = 747 \text{ mm Hg} = P_{O_2} + P_{CO_2} + P_{N_2} + P_{H_2O}$$

To set the instrument to the P_{O_2} and P_{CO_2} of the calibrator gas, P_{H_2O} at 37 °C, which is 47 mm Hg, first must be taken into account. Therefore

$$P(\text{Amb}) - P_{H_2O} = P_{O_2} + P_{CO_2} + P_{N_2}$$
$$747 - 47 = 700 \text{ mm Hg}$$

The $P(\text{Amb})$ corrected for P_{H_2O} represents the sum of partial pressures for the dry gases. The exact P_{O_2} and P_{CO_2} values for the calibration of the instrument are

$$P_{O_2} = 700 \times 0.15 = 105 \text{ mm Hg}$$
$$P_{CO_2} = 700 \times 0.05 = 35 \text{ mm Hg}$$

The law of partial pressure also is applied in definition of gas mixtures used to determine $P_{O_2}(0.5)$ or P_{50} and other derived quantities and to control instrumentation with tonometered samples.

Henry's law predicts the amount of dissolved gas in a liquid in contact with a gaseous phase (see Table 25-4). For gas in blood at 37 °C the solubility coefficient for O_2, αO_2, is 0.00140 (mol/L)/mm Hg so that when arterial P_{O_2} is normal (100 mm Hg) the concentration of dissolved O_2 in arterial blood, cdO_2, is 0.140 mmol/L (100 × 0.00140). This value represents a very small proportion of the total oxygen content (ctO_2) in blood (~9 mmol/L), of which the bulk of O_2 is bound by hemoglobin. Increasing the O_2 fraction of inspired air to 100% or increasing the pressure of inspired air, as in a hyperbaric chamber, forces more O_2 into solution.

Prediction of levels of cdO_2 in these therapies is useful because tissue oxygenation by dissolved O_2 becomes increasingly important when hemoglobin-mediated O_2 delivery is impaired. The $cdCO_2$ can be calculated in the same way: a CO_2 at 37 °C in plasma = 0.0306 mmol/L/mm Hg. Thus at a P_{CO_2} of 40 mm Hg, the $cdCO_2$ = 40 × 0.0306 = 1.224 mmol/L.

Application of the Henderson-Hasselbalch Equation in Blood Gas Measurements

Carbon dioxide and water react to form carbonic acid, which in turn dissociates to hydrogen ions and HCO_3^-, as follows:

$$CO_2 + H_2O \underset{}{\overset{K_{hydration}}{\rightleftarrows}} H_2CO_3 \underset{}{\overset{K_{dissociation}}{\rightleftarrows}} H^{\oplus} + HCO_3^{\ominus}$$

In the classic 1908 formulation, Henderson used concentrations (c) for bicarbonate, CO_2, and H^+ and assumed the concentration of water to be constant, to arrive at the K'

$$K' = \frac{cH^+ \times cHCO_3^-}{cdCO_2}$$

The concentration of dissolved CO_2 ($cdCO_2$) includes the small amount of undissociated (dissolved) carbonic acid. It can be expressed as $cdCO_2 = \alpha \times P_{CO_2}$, where α is the solubility coefficient for CO_2. The symbol $cHCO_3^-$ represents the concentration of total CO_2 ($ctCO_2$) minus the concentration of dissolved CO_2 ($cdCO_2$), which includes carbonic acid. The "bicarbonate" concentration by this definition includes undissociated sodium bicarbonate, carbonate (CO_3^{2-}, and carbamate (carbamino-CO_2; $RCNHCOO^-$), which are present in exceedingly small amounts in plasma.

If the Henderson equation is rearranged and $cdCO_2$ is replaced by $\alpha \times P_{CO_2}$, the following equation results:

$$cH^+ = \frac{K' \times \alpha \times P_{CO_2}}{cHCO_3^-}$$

In 1916, Hasselbalch demonstrated that a logarithmic transformation of the equation was a more useful form, and used the symbols pH (= $-\log cH^+$) and pK' (= $-\log K'$). **pH** is defined as the negative log of the activity of H^+ (aH^+), which is the entity actually measured with pH meters. The resulting **Henderson-Hasselbalch equation** becomes

$$pH = pK' + \log \frac{cHCO_3^-}{\alpha \times P_{CO_2}}$$

or

$$pH = pK' + \log \frac{ctCO_2 - \alpha \times P_{CO_2}}{\alpha \times P_{CO_2}}$$

K' is the apparent, overall (combined) dissociation constant for carbonic acid. K' depends not only on the temperature but also on the ionic strength of the solution. For an aqueous sodium bicarbonate solution at 37 °C, the following approximate relationship exists between K' and ionic strength (I) measured in moles per kilogram of water:

$$pK' = 6.33 - 0.5 \sqrt{(I)}$$

For blood at 37 °C the normal mean value is $pK'(P) = 6.103$, with a normal biological standard deviation (SD) of about ±0.0015, mainly due to normal variations in ionic strength. The solubility coefficient for CO_2 gas, in normal plasma at 37 °C, is 0.0306 mmol $\times$ L^{-1} $\times$ mm Hg^{-1}. When pK' and α are inserted for normal plasma at 37 °C, the Henderson-Hasselbalch equation takes the following form:

$$pH = 6.103 + \log \frac{cHCO_3^-}{0.0306 \times P_{CO_2}}$$

or

$$pH = 6.103 + \log \frac{ctCO_2 - 0.0306 \times P_{CO_2}}{0.0306 \times P_{CO_2}}$$

where P_{CO_2} is measured in millimeters of mercury, and $cHCO_3^-$ and $ctCO_2$ are measured in millimoles per liter. Taking the antilogarithm, combining the constants, and expressing cH^+ in nmol/L provides the following equation:

$$cH^+ = 24.1 \times \frac{P_{CO_2}}{cHCO_3^-}$$

If normal values are substituted in the equation,

$$cH^+ = 24.1 \times \frac{40}{25.4} \text{ nmol/L} = 38.0 \text{ nmol/L}$$

Clearly, by measurement of any two of the four parameters, P_{CO_2} or $cdCO_2$, pH, $ctCO_2$, or $cHCO_3^-$, and use of the Henderson-Hasselbalch equation with appropriate values for pK' and α, the other two parameters may be calculated. The values used for pK' and α are 6.103 and 0.0306, respectively, in the microprocessors of modern blood-gas instruments.

One advantage of such a calculated value is that it essentially reflects the activity of $cHCO_3^-$ (that is, bicarbonate concentration being reported as if measured with an ISE) in the water phase of plasma. Thus it is not affected by the electrolyte exclusion effects, as other nondirect measurements of $cHCO_3^-$ may be.

Oxygen in Blood

The total O_2 content (ctO_2) of a blood sample is the sum of concentrations of hemoglobin-bound O_2 and of cdO_2, and thus $ctO_2 = O_2Hb + cdO_2$. With a normal blood ctO_2 of 9 mmol/L, the cdO_2 is only approximately 0.14 mmol/L, and the rest of the O_2 is associated with hemoglobin as oxyhemoglobin (O_2Hb). The O_2Hb is defined as hemoglobin with O_2 reversibly bound to Fe^{2+} of the heme group of hemoglobin. Each mole of hemoglobin-Fe^{2+} binds 1 mol of O_2. In addition, 1 g of hemoglobin is capable of binding 1.39 mL (0.062 mmol) of O_2. This value is referred to as the *specific O_2 binding capacity of hemoglobin* when defined in terms of hemoglobin A (HbA, the normal adult gene product), which reversibly binds O_2 at its heme moiety. When this hemoglobin is not bound to O_2, it is termed *reduced hemoglobin (HHb)*. Methemoglobin (MetHb), carboxyhemoglobin (COHb), sulfhemoglobin (SulfHb), and cyanmethemoglobin are forms of hemoglobin that are not capable of reversible associations with O_2 because their heme moieties are altered chemically. These nonfunctional hemoglobins collectively are termed *dyshemoglobins*. Hemoglobins with genetically altered protein sequences that alter the O_2-binding properties of the molecule collectively are referred to as *hemoglobin variants* or *hemoglobinopathies*. More than 400 hemoglobin variants have been described,[4] with sickle cell hemoglobin (HbS) as just one example.

Uptake of O_2 by the blood in the lungs is governed primarily by the P_{O_2} of alveolar air and the ability of O_2 to diffuse freely across the alveolar membrane into the blood. At the P_{O_2} normally present in alveolar air (~102 mm Hg) and with a normal membrane and normal hemoglobin, more than 95% of the hemoglobin binds O_2. At a P_{O_2} greater than 110 mm Hg, more than 98% of normal hemoglobin binds O_2. When all hemoglobin capable of binding O_2 is saturated, further increase in the P_{O_2} of alveolar air simply increases the cdO_2 in arterial blood. Delivery of O_2 by the blood to the tissues is governed by the large diffusion gradient between P_{O_2} of the blood and that of the tissue cells, resulting in dissociation of O_2Hb from Hb at the lower P_{O_2} of the blood-tissue cell interface.

The following three properties of arterial blood are essential to ensure adequate O_2 delivery to the tissues:

1. Arterial P_{O_2} must be sufficiently high (~90 mm Hg) to create a diffusion gradient from the arterial blood to the tissue cells. Low arterial P_{O_2} (hypoxemia) results in tissue hypoxia (O_2 starvation).
2. The O_2-binding capacity of the blood must be normal. (That is, the concentration of hemoglobin capable of binding and releasing O_2 must be normal.) Decreased Hb concentration may cause so-called anemic hypoxia.

3. The hemoglobin must be able to bind O_2 in the lungs yet release it at the tissues. In other words the affinity of hemoglobin for O_2 must be normal. Too great an affinity of hemoglobin for O_2, as is the case with some hemoglobinopathies, may cause "affinity-based" tissue hypoxia, in which O_2 is not released at the capillary-tissue interface.

The PO_2 at the venous end of the capillaries should stay around 38 mm Hg, and thus the normal arteriovenous difference in PO_2 is 50 to 60 mm Hg.

Hemoglobin oxygen saturation

Before the factors that affect Hb affinity for O_2 are discussed, definition of the concept of hemoglobin **oxygen saturation** is important, as follows:

$$SO_2 = \frac{Hb\ oxygen\ content}{Hb\ oxygen\ capacity}$$

This value is the fraction (percentage) of the functional hemoglobin that is saturated with oxygen and is essentially an indirect means used to estimate the PO_2. Currently, however, at least three different approaches exist to determine oxygen "saturation," and each is a distinct entity. Unfortunately, the three approaches often are used interchangeably for the generic term, *oxygen saturation*. The three terms, *hemoglobin oxygen saturation* (SO_2), *fractional oxyhemoglobin* (FO_2Hb), and *estimated oxygen saturation* (O_2Sat), have distinct definitions set by the NCCLS (C12-A and C25-A). The ambiguous use of these three terms is due to the fact that in healthy subjects the values for all three are very similar. However, assumptions made for healthy subjects through use of these values interchangeably can lead to erroneous conclusions in seriously ill individuals and those with dyshemoglobins or hemoglobinopathies. Spectrophotometric methods are used to determine O_2Hb and HHb specifically so that SO_2 is calculated according to the following equation:

$$SO_2 = \frac{cO_2Hb}{cO_2Hb + cHHb}$$

where cO_2Hb is the concentration of oxyhemoglobin, $cHHb$ is the concentration of deoxyhemoglobin (reduced Hb), and the sum of oxyhemoglobin and deoxyhemoglobin represents the amount of hemoglobin capable of reversibly binding O_2. SO_2 usually is expressed as a percent in the United States. SO_2 most often is determined either by simple oximetry, a spectrophotometric approach that can determine oxyhemoglobin and reduced hemoglobin (HHb) but not COHb, MetHb, or by SulfHb. These devices are often bedside monitors used to monitor HbO_2 saturation and serve this purpose extremely well. However, use of SO_2 in the initial evaluation of an individual with dyshemoglobins or other abnormal hemoglobins can be misleading. For instance, in a comatose individual with 15% COHb, the SO_2 by simple oximetry might read

0.95, whereas the fraction of oxyhemoglobin in reality would be only 0.80. For this reason, the NCCLS (C25-A) recommends an assessment of the presence of dyshemoglobins before the use of SO_2 for clinical purposes.

Another expression of oxygen saturation is the fractional oxyhemoglobin, FO_2Hb, which is calculated as follows:

$$FO_2Hb = \frac{cO_2Hb}{ctHB}$$

where the concentration of total hemoglobin ($ctHb$) equals the sum of O_2Hb, HHb, and the dyshemoglobins COHb, MetHb, and SulfHb. This value requires determination of all hemoglobin species and usually is performed on a co-oximeter. The instrument prepares a hemolysate from whole blood by sonication and spectrophotometrically determine the percent of each Hb species. This determination is accomplished by use of monochromatic light at six fixed wavelengths between 535 and 670 nm and measurement of absorbance at each of the six wavelengths. Newer co-oximeters use diode arrays. Because each species of hemoglobin has its own absorbance pattern, a microcomputer can calculate the percent of each one.

The microprocessors of blood-gas instruments sometimes estimate the oxygen saturation (SO_2) from measured pH, PO_2, and hemoglobin with the use of empirical equations. If used at all, this value clearly should be referred to as an *estimated* SO_2, but it frequently is reported and referred to as "O_2Sat." Calculated values, such as O_2Sat, should be interpreted with reservations because the algorithm assumes normal O_2 affinity of the hemoglobin, normal 2,3-diphosphoglycerol (2,3-DPG) concentrations, and the absence of dyshemoglobins (see following discussion). Such calculated estimates have been found to vary by as much as 6% from measured values.[22]

Decreases in arterial FO_2Hb indicate either a low arterial PO_2 or an impaired ability of hemoglobin to bind as an O_2 carrier. Decreased PO_2 indicates a reduced ability of O_2 to diffuse from alveolar air into the blood because of hypoventilation, increased venoarterial shunting, or both. Low total hemoglobin can result from a decreased number of erythrocytes that contain normal concentrations of hemoglobin (normochromic anemia) or a decreased mean cell concentration of hemoglobin in the erythrocytes (hypochromic anemia). Decreased FO_2Hb hemoglobin also can occur as a result of poisonings that convert part of the hemoglobin into the species COHb, MetHb, SulfHb, or cyanmethemoglobin, which are unable to bind or exchange O_2. Clinically, distinguishing between arterial hypoxemia (decreased arterial PO_2 and decreased SO_2 or FO_2Hb is important because of decreased availability of O_2) and cyanosis (decreased FO_2Hb) because of abnormally high concentrations of reduced hemoglobin or chemically altered hemoglobin incapable of carrying O_2. Note that in the cyanosis setting, measurement of SO_2 or an estimated SO_2 (O_2Sat) may be normal if the cyanosis is due to the presence of MetHb or COHb.

The oxygen concentration of blood (ctO_2) is the sum of O_2 bound to hemoglobin and cdO_2. Most blood gas analyzers determine ctO_2 by the following calculation:

$$ctO_2(mL/dL) = FO_2Hb \times bO_2 \times ctHb(g/dL) + (\alpha O_2) \times (PO_2)$$

where bO_2 equals 1.39 mL/g and αO_2, the solubility coefficient of O_2, equals 0.0031. This calculation is based on FO_2Hb and $ctHb$. If SO_2 is used, use of the effective hemoglobin concentration is necessary (that is, to subtract the concentration of any dyshemoglobins present from the concentration of $ctHb$). Thus on initial patient presentation, determination of any dyshemoglobins may be necessary to obtain an accurate value for ctO_2 for its use in subsequent calculations.

Hemoglobin oxygen dissociation

The degree of association or dissociation of O_2 with hemoglobin is determined by PO_2 and the affinity of hemoglobin for O_2. When the SO_2 of blood is determined over a range of PO_2 and plotted against PO_2, a sigmoidal curve called the **oxygen dissociation curve** is obtained. The shape of the curve arises from the increasing efficiency with which HHb molecules bind more O_2 once some O_2 has been bound. The location of the curve relative to the PO_2 required to achieve a particular level of SO_2 in the blood is a function of the affinity of the hemoglobin for O_2.

The affinity of hemoglobin for O_2 depends on five factors—(1) temperature, (2) pH, (3) PCO_2, (4) concentration of 2,3-DPG, and (5) the presence of minor hemoglobins, such as COHb and metHB. 2,3-DPG is an intermediate in the process of glycolysis, the primary energy source for the erythrocyte. The graph in Figure 25-2 illustrates the effect of plasma pH on the O_2 dissociation curve (the Bohr effect). If a similar graph were made for variations of PCO_2 from 40

mm Hg (with pH at 7.4, 2,3-DPG at 5.0 mmol/L, and temperature at 37 °C) and another for variations of temperature from 37 °C (with pH at 7.4, PCO_2 at 40 mm Hg, and 2,3-DPG at 5.0 mmol/L), the locations of the curves would shift to the right (less O_2 affinity), with decreasing pH, higher temperature, higher PCO_2, and higher 2,3-DPG.

Determination of P_{50}

P_{50} is defined as the PO_2 for a given blood sample at which the hemoglobin of the blood is half saturated with O_2 and reflects the affinity of Hb for O_2. The measured value of P_{50} differs from the standard value of P_{50} by some amount determined by the effect that factors different from pH = 7.40, PCO_2 = 40 mm Hg, T = 37 °C, and 2,3-DPG = 5.0 mmol/L have to shift the dissociation line from the reference line. The value of P_{50} therefore becomes a measure of change imposed on hemoglobin affinity by the individual or multiple factors that affect it.

Procedure. The simplest method used to determine P_{50} consists of measurement of PO_2 potentiometrically and SO_2 spectrophotometrically on an anaerobically collected venous whole-blood sample.[26] pH and PCO_2 should be measured along with the other parameters. The following equation is used to calculate P_{50}:

$$\log P_{50} = \log PO_2 - \frac{\text{logit } SO_2}{2.7}$$

where logit $SO_2 = \log[SO_2/(1 - SO_2)]$, and 2.7 is the Hill slope constant. This equation is a useful approximation, provided that the measured SO_2 is in the interval 0.4 to 0.8 (40% to 80%, SO_2%), thus requiring the use of venous blood in most instances. Here, SO_2 and not FO_2Hb must be used in the calculations because P_{50} refers to 50% SO_2 (that is, the only hemoglobin capable of binding and releasing O_2).

The standard P_{50} thus defined may be interpreted as an indirect measure of the 2,3-DPG concentration in erythrocytes because an increase or decrease in 2,3-DPG concentration is the most common cause of an increase or decrease in P_{50}. However, other causes should be kept in mind, such as increases in COHb, MetHb, or HbF (decreased standard P_{50}) or congenital hemoglobin variants (causing both increased and decreased standard P_{50}).[26]

Clinical significance. Increased values for P_{50} indicate displacement of the O_2 dissociation curve to the right, which indicates a decreased affinity of the hemoglobin for O_2. The chief causes are hyperthermia, acidemia, hypercapnia, high concentrations of 2,3-DPG, or the presence of an abnormal hemoglobin with decreased O_2 affinity. 2,3-DPG concentrations tend to be increased in individuals with chronic alkalemia, anemia, and chronic hypoxemia. An example of hemoglobin with decreased O_2 affinity is hemoglobin Seattle.

Low values for P_{50} signify displacement of the O_2 dissociation curve to the left and an increased affinity of hemoglobin. The main causes are hypothermia, acute alkalemia, hypocapnia, low concentration of 2,3-DPG, increased

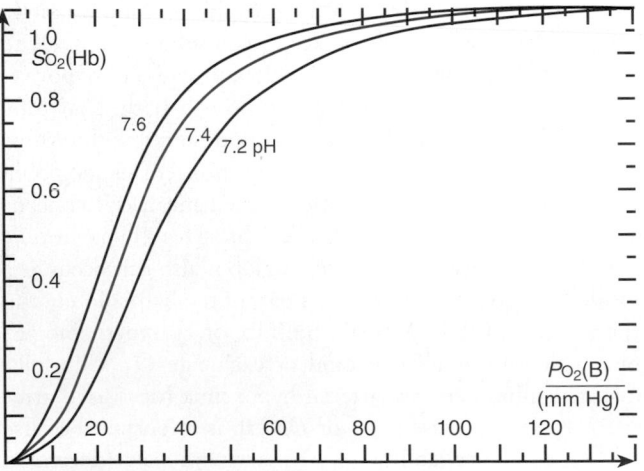

Figure 25-2　Oxygen dissociation curves for human blood with different plasma pH values, but constant PCO_2 values of 40 mm Hg, a 2,3-diphosphoglycerol concentration in erythrocytes of 5.0 mmol/L, and temperature at 37 °C. SO_2(Hb), Hemoglobin oxygen saturation; PO_2(B), partial pressure of oxygen in blood.

COHb and MetHb, or an abnormal hemoglobin. Decreases of 2,3-DPG are observed commonly in acidemic states that have persisted for more than a few hours; the initial increase in P_{50} caused by the acidemia is compensated gradually for by a decrease in 2,3-DPG so that P_{50} then falls to lower-than-normal values.

Tonometry

Tonometry is the process by which a liquid is exposed to a gas phase in such a way that each gas in the gaseous phase partitions to an equilibrium between the liquid and gas. This equilibration, in effect, imparts the P_{CO_2} and P_{O_2} of the equilibrating gas to the blood that is exposed to it in a tonometer. Equilibration by tonometry uses gases of known fractional composition, humidified at 37 °C to give a saturated water vapor pressure of 47 mm Hg. The P_{CO_2} or P_{O_2} of such gases is calculated according to Dalton's law (see discussion on behavior of gases).

Tonometry is used to treat blood samples for various special studies that are requested only rarely in most hospital settings and to prepare quality control material in whole blood. Direct determination of P_{50} and standard bicarbonate are two applications of tonometry. Quality assurance applications include preparation of a blood sample for quality control of blood-gas measurements, determination of the liquid-gas difference for a P_{O_2} electrode, and verification of accuracy and linearity of P_{O_2} and P_{CO_2} electrodes.

Determination of P_{CO_2}, P_{O_2}, and pH

The measurements of P_{CO_2}, P_{O_2}, and pH are among the most frequently requested critical tests in hospitals. In the United States the testing is performed in larger central, "core" laboratories, smaller specialty laboratories, and sometimes at the point of care.

Specimens

Arterial or venous whole-blood specimens may be obtained from any site accessible to vascular catheterization or entry. These sites commonly are the vessels of the extremities, but when special studies are performed the chambers of the heart and great vessels of the chest may be accessed. Analysts should recognize that these specimens are difficult to obtain and should be handled with utmost care. Differences in measured blood-gas values between arterial and venous blood are most pronounced for P_{O_2}. In practice, P_{O_2} is the only clinical reason that the more difficult arterial collections are performed. P_{O_2} generally is 60 to 70 mm Hg lower in venous blood after O_2 is released in the capillary tissues.

Quality assurance of blood analysis for gases and pH depends largely on control of preanalytical error (that is, on proper collection and handling of the specimen). Guidelines used to control preanalytical error have been published in the NCCLS document C27-A. Laboratory personnel do not always control collection of arterial or venous specimens, and thus clinical laboratorians must work closely and cooperatively with physicians, nurses, respiratory therapists, and other personnel who obtain these samples and take active roles in developing interdepartmental mechanisms to guarantee their quality.

Arterial puncture carries a slight medical risk and under no circumstances should it be undertaken by anyone who has not been trained properly to perform it. Arterial puncture always is done with syringe and needle. No tourniquet is used, and no pull is applied to the plunger of the syringe because the arterial blood pressure pushes blood into the syringe. An NCCLS-approved standard, H-11A3, describes appropriate procedures and best practice.

Venous blood is collected best with a needle and syringe, although some laboratories also accept specimens drawn to a complete fill of an evacuated tube containing a dry heparin salt. When an arm vein is used, the specimen should be obtained after release of a tourniquet or in the first few seconds after application of the tourniquet and the patient should not be allowed to flex the fingers or clench the fist. Prolonged application of a tourniquet and/or muscular activity decreases venous P_{O_2} and pH. Placement of indwelling catheters with heparin locks for short- and long-term intravenous therapies now is fairly common, with the catheter serving as a port for specimen collection. The lock must be flushed thoroughly with blood (usually 5 times the catheter volume) before a specimen is drawn to measure blood gases and pH (or any other assay, for that matter). Failure to flush the lock properly has unpredictable effects on measured quantities and is indicated frequently by bizarre results.

Arterial or venous specimens are collected best anaerobically with lyophilized heparin anticoagulant in sterile syringes with capacities of 1 to 5 mL. If liquid heparin is used, the size of the syringe, the concentration and volume of liquid heparin (which can dilute the sample), and the volume of blood drawn into the syringe are important. Adequate anticoagulation (~0.05 mg heparin/mL blood) is achieved by drawing of enough liquid heparin solution into the syringe in such a way as to wet the interior of the barrel over the maximal inner surface area of the syringe and ejection of air and excess heparin in such a way as to leave the dead space of the syringe filled with heparin. Failure to expel liquid heparin from all but the syringe dead space, or filling of the syringe to less than full capacity can increase further the dilution of the specimen with liquid heparin. An increasing ratio of heparin to blood can have an increasingly marked effect on measured P_{CO_2} and the parameters calculated from it.

An anaerobic technique for collection has as its guiding principle either no exposure or minimal exposure of blood to atmospheric air. The P_{CO_2} of dry air is much less than that of blood so that the CO_2 content and P_{CO_2} of blood exposed to air decrease. The P_{O_2} of atmospheric air (~155 mm Hg) is approximately 60 mm Hg higher than that of arterial blood. Therefore blood from individuals breathing room air that is exposed to atmospheric air gains O_2. In contrast, blood with PO_2 exceeding 150 mm Hg, as might be obtained from patients undergoing O_2 therapy, loses O_2 on exposure to air. Even with care in sample handling, blood can be exposed to air simply from the air in the needle and syringe hub dead space. Error remains minimal if the resulting bubble is ejected immediately on removal of the needle from the puncture site and before the syringe tip is capped. The potential effect of small bubbles on blood-gas results was demonstrated clearly in one study in which a 100-μL bubble of room air was added to 10 2-mL blood samples with PO_2 values between 25 and 40 mm Hg. In these samples, PO_2 increased an average of 4 mm Hg in only 2 minutes, whereas PCO_2 decreased 4 mm Hg.[16]

Arterialized capillary blood sometimes is an acceptable alternative to arterial blood when blood losses must be minimized. Freely flowing cutaneous blood originates in the arterioles and corresponds closely to arterial blood in composition. However, arterialized capillary blood is not acceptable when systolic blood pressure is less than 95 mm Hg, in cases of vasoconstriction, in patients undergoing O_2 therapy, in newborns during the first few hours after birth, or in newborns with respiratory distress syndrome. These situations pose a particular risk of admixture with blood from the venules. Warming of the selected skin-puncture site to 45 °C for 10 minutes to achieve vasodilation and adequate blood flow must precede capillary puncture. The first blood drop to appear should be wiped away and subsequent free-forming drops taken up in a capillary collection tube containing lyophilized heparin.

Transport and analysis of specimens should be prompt. Physicians who use blood-gas and pH measurements in acute-care management often require turnaround times of less than 15 minutes between specimen acquisition and reporting of results. Ideally, specimens never should be stored, although analysis of properly preserved specimens may be delayed up to 1 hour. The pH of freshly drawn blood decreases on standing at a rate of 0.04 to 0.08 pH unit per hour at 37 °C, 0.02 to 0.03 per hour at 22 °C, and less than 0.01 per hour at 4 °C. Partial CO_2 pressure increases by approximately 5 mm Hg/hour at 37 °C, 1 mm Hg/hour at 22 °C, and only about 0.5 mm Hg/hour at 2 to 4 °C. A corresponding decrease in glucose and an equivalent increase in lactate accompany the decrease in pH. The primary cause of these changes is glycolysis by leukocytes, platelets, and reticulocytes.

In freshly drawn blood with a normal PO_2 that is maintained anaerobically, cell respiration causes PO_2 to decrease at a rate of approximately 2 mm Hg/hour at room temperature but 5 to 10 mm Hg/hour at 37 °C. Adverse effects of glycolysis and respiration can be avoided best by analysis within 30 minutes after collection. If analysis must be delayed or circumstances create a risk of delay, the syringe or tube containing the blood should be immersed in a mixture

of ice and water until analysis is possible. Under these conditions, changes are negligible because glycolysis is inhibited. These changes in values that can be expected with delays in analysis at different temperatures are true only when the white blood cell count (WBC) is normal or elevated only slightly. Glycolysis and the resulting effects on pH, PO_2, and PCO_2 increase dramatically with markedly elevated WBC, such as occurs in individuals with leukemia.

Instrumentation

A schematic diagram characteristic of a contemporary blood-gas analyzer is shown in Figure 25-3. Electrochemical principles and structural features of pH, PO_2, and PCO_2 electrodes are discussed in Chapter 6. HCO_3^- and SO_2 are calculated results. Recent developments in instrumentation have included "stat profile" equipment for point-of-care testing (POCT), or bedside testing.[8] Although design and construction may differ significantly from those used in traditional instruments, the principles of analysis—especially for blood pH and gases—are not novel. Additional information is available in manufacturers' literature and later in this chapter (see section on POCT).

The operation of a blood-gas instrument begins with the analyst presenting a blood specimen at the sample probe. A keyboard-entered command to sample a specimen initiates uptake of sample through the probe by a peristaltic pump that loads the chamber with 60 to 150 μL of fluid sample and empties it by pushing its contents to waste. The pump is under the microprocessor's control because it must pause after the admission of sample to let the sample reside in the chamber long enough to permit thermal equilibration to establish and to complete the measurements. On completion of measurement the pump pushes the sample to waste, while digital output is made available on a display, on a printed tape, and often to a laboratory information system through an interface.

Calibrations

Most instruments are designed to be self-calibrating. Under the command of the microprocessor, calibrator gases and buffers are cycled at short intervals through the chamber and electronic responses are monitored continually and reset to the constants initially entered for high and low PCO_2 and PO_2 and high and low pH of the calibrator materials. In the United States the regulations written for the Clinical Laboratory Improvements Amendments of 1988 (CLIA '88) mandate one point calibration every 30 minutes or within 30 minutes of every patient sample and two point calibrations every 8 hours.

pH

The pH measurement system is calibrated against primary standard buffers admitted either manually or automatically into the sample chamber. The buffers are phosphate solutions that should meet National Institute of

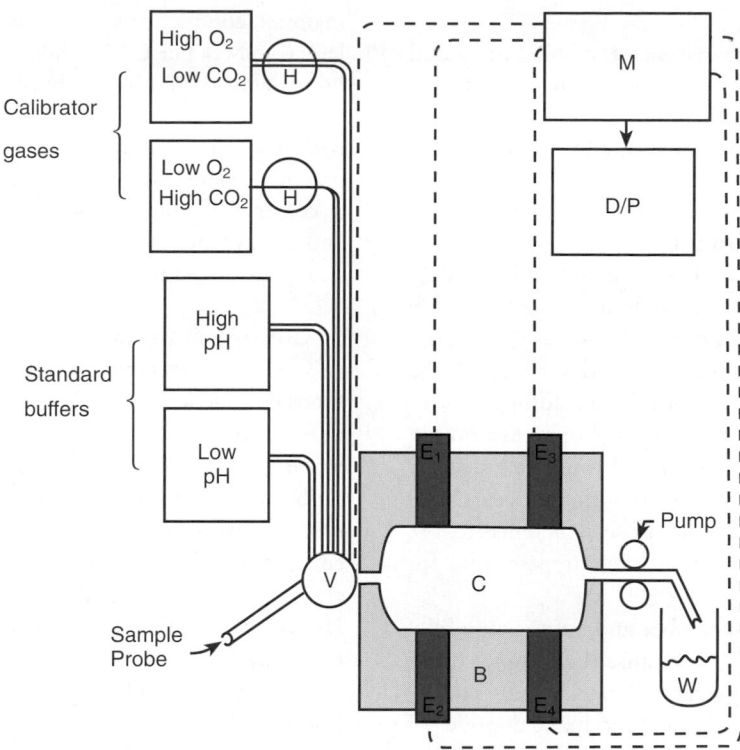

Figure 25-3   Diagram of blood-gas instrumentation. *H*, Humidification device; *V*, valve; *C*, chamber; *B*, constant temperature bath at 37 °C; *W*, waste; *M*, microprocessor; *D/P*, display/printer; *E*, electrodes, where E_1 is PO_2, E_2 PCO_2, E_3 is pH, and E_4 is the reference for pH.

Standards and Technology (NIST) specifications and are available readily from manufacturers. The pH values of the low and high calibrator buffers are set by the manufacturer but always lie close to 6.8 and 7.4 at 37 °C.

PCO_2 and PO_2

Calibration of the gas measurement systems is made against gases of known O_2 and CO_2 compositions. Compressed gases, with a certificate of analysis provided by the manufacturer, are used as primary standards. Pure O_2, CO_2, and N_2 may be obtained in individual tanks and mixed as desired with a precision gas mixer in the blood-gas laboratory, or gas mixtures of various fractional compositions also may be purchased. The "low gas" mixture for calibration usually has a fractional composition of 5% CO_2, 0% O_2, and 95% N_2. The "high gas" mixture has a fractional composition of 10% CO_2, 20% O_2, and 70% N_2. These compositions correspond roughly to a calibration range of 38 to 76 mm Hg for PCO_2 and 0 to 152 mm Hg for PO_2.

The mode of calibration is determined by the design of the instrument. Some instruments contain a barometer or transducer responsive to P(Amb) so that barometric pressure always is known to the microprocessor. With such instruments, only a keyboard entry of the fractional composition of O_2 and CO_2 in low and high calibrator gas mixtures must be made. The microprocessor calculated the values for PO_2 and PCO_2 (according to Dalton's law) for gases saturated with water vapor at 37 °C.

Liquid-gas difference of a PO_2 electrode

When calibration gases are used to calibrate an instrumental system for measurement of gases in blood samples, a particular property of the PO_2 electrode must be considered. This property is called the *liquid-gas* or *blood-gas difference*.

PO_2 and PCO_2 electrodes are alike in that gas diffusing from a liquid or gaseous sample passes through a gas-permeable membrane. In both electrodes the rate of diffusion of a gas through the membranes is slower from a liquid phase than from a gaseous phase. However, PCO_2 and PO_2 electrodes use different principles of measurement (see Chapter 6). Because O_2 passing through the membrane of a PO_2 electrode enters an irreversible reaction at a polarized cathode, the current generated by the reaction is proportional to the amount of O_2 reduced. A steady state is achieved when the rate of diffusion equals the rate of reduction. Thus the electrode responds to a greater degree to O_2 diffusing from a gaseous phase than that diffusing from a liquid phase.

The liquid-gas difference for a PO_2 electrode becomes significant when an electrode is calibrated with gas and used to measure PO_2 of blood. The difference usually is expressed as a ratio of PO_2 (gas sample) to PO_2 (liquid sample). For contemporary electrodes the ratio is commonly 1.02:1.00 to 1.06:1.00. For routine clinical work, a ratio of 1.04:1.00 frequently is assumed rather than determined.

Quality assurance

The elements of good quality assurance of blood-gas and pH measurements include proper maintenance of the instrument, use of control materials, verification of electrode linearity, checks of barometer accuracy, and accurate measurement of temperature.

Maintenance of instrumentation

Sophistication of contemporary equipment and availability of high-quality calibrator materials have made reliable and accurate determination of blood pH and gases primarily a matter of meticulous maintenance and control of the equipment and proper control of specimens admitted to it. Software programs of the instrument's microprocessor often provide display warnings and diagnostic routines that alert the operator and assist in the trouble-shooting process. Nevertheless, regular maintenance and close adherence to the manufacturer's recommended procedures are essential for satisfactory operation.

Cleanliness of the sample chamber and path is especially important. Automatic flushing to cleanse the sample chamber and path after each blood sample measurement is a feature of many instruments. When it is not, manual modes of flushing recommended by the manufacturer should be practiced faithfully. Despite proper flushing, however, complete or partial clogging of chamber, path, or both may occur. Frequency of clogging often is related to the number of heparinized capillary blood samples that are analyzed. Fibrin threads and small clots may be present in the specimen or form while the sample resides in the warm chamber.

Prompt and reliable service by the manufacturer or an in-house biomedical engineer is essential for a laboratory performing many analyses per day, even when back-up instruments are available. Also important is ready availability of goods from the manufacturer or laboratory supply houses, including calibrator materials (pH buffers and gases of certified quality), replacement membranes, and small parts for maintenance of electrodes. The NCCLS describes manufacturing standards and basic operational requirements for blood-gas instrumentation in publication C21-A.

Proficiency testing mandated by federal law in the United States (CLIA '88) has assumed new importance for quality control of blood-gas analysis. The rules that became effective in January 1991 set evaluation criteria for satisfactory interlaboratory performance as follows:

pH target value ±0.04

PO_2, target value ±3 SD

PCO_2, target value $\pm8\%$ or ±5 mm Hg, whichever is greater

The significance of proficiency testing and the penalties for failure place a new incentive on faithful performance of internal control measures and effective response to failures of quality control. However, pressures to control costs raise the question of how often and how many levels of control materials are necessary to monitor performance effectively. The facile answer is as often and as many levels as it takes to maintain confidence in the measurement systems. The regulatory answer per CLIA '88 is one level of control every 8 hours, with the entire range of control levels covered in every 24-hour period. The CAP requires at least two levels of controls every 8 hours. In many laboratories, however, the practical answer is to run on every instrument in use, at least once per shift, three levels of control for pH, PO_2, and PCO_2 and always on completion of maintenance and trouble-shooting procedures.

Control materials

Quality control materials can be commercial blood-based fluids or aqueous fluids. Alternatively, independent standard buffers can be used for pH control and tonometered whole blood for PCO_2 and PO_2 control.

Blood-based and fluorocarbon-based control materials. Commercial blood-base control material usually consists of tanned human erythrocytes suspended in buffered medium and sealed in vials with a gas mixture of known O_2 and CO_2 content. Blood-free fluorocarbon materials with O_2-carrying properties similar to those of blood also are available. These products usually are made at three levels of pH, PCO_2, and PO_2. Unopened, these types of control material have the advantages of long shelf life in the refrigerator—for the tanned erythrocytes, from 20 to 28 days and for the others, even longer.

Aqueous fluid control materials. An aqueous fluid control material consists of a buffered medium in a sealed vial containing a known gas mixture. The fluid is equilibrated with the gas through vigorous shaking by hand for a prescribed length of time immediately before the vial is opened. The disadvantages of aqueous controls stem from their dissimilarity to blood. Lower viscosity and surface tension confer different washout characteristics, greater electrical conductivity reduces their effectiveness to detect inadequate grounding, and lower thermal coefficients make them slower to detect failures of temperature control. These disadvantages are most apparent in respect to PO_2, where a fluorocarbon-based matrix is superior. Nevertheless, aqueous commercial controls are used commonly.

Tonometered whole blood. To prepare tonometered (gas-equilibrated) samples for use as controls, NCCLS document C27-A recommends a fresh, single-source blood specimen, free of recently transfused erythrocytes, with hemoglobin normal in both amount and type and with normal hematocrit and leukocyte count. When equilibrated against gas mixtures, a tonometered sample on a properly calibrated and properly operating instrument should give measured values for PCO_2 and PO_2 that are within 1% to 4% of those calculated for the equilibrating gas.

Quality control of PO_2 and PCO_2 by tonometered blood is considered the method of choice because the control material approximates most nearly patient samples in its interaction with gas electrodes. The disadvantages include the time required for tonometry, particularly if two or three levels of control are desired; difficulties in frequent obtaining of fresh, normal blood samples; the necessity for repeated calculation (and risk of miscalculation) of the equilibrating gases; the need to keep special gas mixtures; and the inapplicability to control pH measurement.

Linearity of electrodes

Linearity of new electrodes should be verified. Today, most manufacturers provide the linearity data obtained for a particular electrode before installation. To perform linearity verification, certified gases or tonometered blood must be used. For the PCO_2 electrode, linearity can be tested after calibration with 5% and 10% CO_2 by determination of PCO_2 on a gas containing 7% CO_2. A similar test of an intermediate point of the calibration range for a PO_2 electrode calibrated with 0% and 20% O_2 might use 10% O_2 or for a PO_2 electrode calibrated in the extended range, 50% O_2. The gases used in the initial verification can be used subsequently for periodic checks in the quality assurance program. In some laboratories, checks of linearity with tonometered whole-blood samples is preferred to use of gases.

Barometer

A barometer, whether built into the instrument or free standing, should be checked periodically for accuracy. The most reliable reference is local $P(Amb)$ as recorded by the nearest official meteorological station, obtained by a phone call or via the Internet, and corrected for any altitude difference.

Temperature control

Because an exact temperature of 37 °C is essential for the accurate measurement of blood gases and pH, state-of-the-art instrumentation is furnished with thermal sensors, embedded in the heat sink around the measuring chamber, that communicate to the microprocessor. Audible or visible alarms signal deviation of temperature outside preset tolerances (usually 37 ± 0.1 °C). Inclusion of temperature-sensitive piperazine buffers, such as HEPES or TES, in pH quality assurance procedures also helps in monitoring of temperature control.

Sources of error

With good control of analytical error the most probable source of error is in the collection and handling of a specimen. General causes of analytical error include calibration of the instrument with incorrect set points, failure of temperature control, a dirty sample chamber or path, and protein-clogged membranes. Incorrect calibration may arise from wrong entries made for buffer or gas values into the microprocessor, incorrect manual calculations of PCO_2 and PO_2 values for calibrator gases, or use of gases that are dry because the humidification device is not working properly.

A source of error for the PO_2 electrode is use of the electrode in a range above 500 mm Hg when it has not been calibrated for use in this range. Measurements of PO_2 are particularly sensitive to temperature error. To keep systematic error to 1% to 2%, the temperature control at 37 °C must be within ±0.1 °C. The PO_2 electrode liquid-gas difference can introduce a 2% to 6% error. This error is less if a liquid-gas correction factor is incorporated into the algorithm that generates results.

Reference intervals

Reference intervals for arterial blood PO_2, SO_2, PCO_2, and pH are listed in Chapter 46. Arterial blood PO_2, low at birth, rises to an adult level of 83 to 108 mm Hg. Saturation fraction, $SO_2(aB)$, may be as low as 0.40 at birth but thereafter is 0.95 to 0.98. The FO_2 is 0.90 to 0.95 in healthy adults. The P_{50} corrected to pH 7.40 is 18 to 24 mm Hg for newborns and 24 to 29 mm Hg for adults. Arterial blood PCO_2 ranges at sea level are somewhat lower for infants than for adults; the interval for men is 35 to 48 mm Hg and for women, 32 to 45 mm Hg. Values decrease with altitudes above sea level at a rate of 3 mm Hg/km (5 mm Hg/mile). During pregnancy, a woman's PCO_2 falls gradually to a mean of about 28 mm Hg just before term. Arterial blood pH in the first few hours of life may vary normally over a range of 7.09 to 7.50, but thereafter is 7.35 to 7.45.

Temperature correction of measured pH, PCO_2, and PO_2

In the Henderson-Hasselbalch equation, pK' and α are used as constants for a temperature of 37 °C. The temperature-controlled sample chamber of an instrument is specified to be 37 ± 0.1 °C, and at that temperature, all measurements of pH and partial pressure of gases are made. The body temperature of a febrile individual may be elevated to 40 to 41 °C, or an individual may be made hypothermic for cardiopulmonary bypass surgery and have a temperature as low as 23 °C. Most blood-gas instruments, on keyboard entry of an individual's actual temperature, can calculate and present temperature-corrected pH and PCO_2 using fairly complex equations.[3,11]

Correction of pH and PCO_2 to the actual temperature of the individual usually is omitted in states of hyperthermia. Disagreement exists with respect to hypothermic states. Pros and cons of management of acid-base balance of hypothermic individuals have been noted by several investigators.[3,11] The prudent policy for the laboratory may be to generate and report temperature-corrected results for pH and PCO_2 only on specific request of the physician. Furthermore, temperature-corrected results never should be reported without the original results measured at 37 °C.

Continuous and noninvasive monitoring of blood gases

Obtaining arterial, venous, or capillary blood is an invasive procedure, and test results reflect conditions pertaining only to a single point in time. Repetitive sampling in intensive acute-care management carries risks, including infection and vascular complications. Decisive action during intensive cardiopulmonary care or cardiac surgery often demands either continuous monitoring or discrete real-time data for blood gases. Systems to serve these demands use surface-applied or inline probes to return discrete or continuous data for evaluation of oxygenation and CO_2 retention.

Extensive discussion of noninvasive and continuous modes of monitoring is beyond the scope of this text. However, laboratorians must be aware of them because blood samples and standard analytical equipment remain the reference for monitoring of the effectiveness of such devices and responsibility for quality assessment and review for them often is assigned to the clinical laboratory. Readers are referred to several reviews[25,28] for descriptions of pulse and pulmonary artery oximetry and continuous in vivo monitoring with high-technology sensor probes. In most studies the correlations to arterial blood gases are reasonable (r values ranging from 0.7 to 0.8), and they are recommended for trending and monitoring. However, in most instances recommendations state that baseline arterial values should be obtained before noninvasive monitoring begins. A committee of the International Federation of Clinical Chemistry (IFCC) has published guidelines[12] for transcutaneous measurement of PO_2 and PCO_2.

■ POINT-OF-CARE TESTING

Besides glucometers, most **point-of-care testing,** or POCT, focuses on electrolytes and blood gases by use of miniaturized direct ISEs.[24] The goal of POCT is to provide rapid (<5-minute) test results that meet laboratory standards for validity, reliability, and precision in a manner that promotes effective and efficient patient care. This goal implies that valid results are available within a time frame that enhances diagnostic and treatment decisions, that testing is cost effective, and that POCT technology is integrated effectively into the total system of laboratory services. Common sites for POCT are the physician's office, operating suite, intensive care unit, emergency department, and at the bedside of suitable groups of patients. Devices based on disposable microelectrodes that measure electrolytes, PCO_2, PO_2, pH, urea, glucose, and hematocrit in small volumes of undiluted whole blood have been reported to provide sufficient reliability, precision, and accuracy for clinical use.[8,23]

Considerations for point-of-care testing

Several questions persist regarding POCT.[24] Management of patient data (for example, billing and entry into medical records and medical information systems) is not automatic or always straightforward for these devices. Thus their use may lead to problems, including lack of a permanent medical or billing record. In addition, nonlaboratory personnel, whose primary responsibilities may be in a very hectic environment such as the emergency department, operating room, or intensive care unit, usually operate POCT; these health-care providers may not be familiar, or always comply, with preanalytical procedures, quality control, quality assur-

ance, or regulatory policies. For instance, in one study that examined use of a POCT in an emergency-room setting, numerous clinically significant errors in hematocrit values were observed.[19] These errors were thought not to be due to the device itself but rather to failure of the operators to resuspend cells before analysis. Finally, the relationship between increased cost and a beneficial impact on patient care is unclear. Because these devices generally have reagent/disposable costs that are considerably higher per patient than the central laboratory's costs, determination of whether faster laboratory values will result in a positive clinical or economic outcome is necessary.

Quality assurance

Quality assurance of POCT raises several issues that do not apply to centralized laboratory testing. One obvious issue is that the operators of these devices, particularly if nonlaboratory personnel perform the actual quality control analysis. Thus the assessment of operator competency must be included in the institution's quality assessment manual. Another quality assurance issue that is as yet unresolved is how best to perform quality control analysis for the handheld devices that utilize single-use, disposable electrode cartridges. Some manufacturers have eschewed liquid control material in favor of an electronic "quality control cartridge" that provides a pass/fail analysis of the electronics and calibration of the device. However, this approach does not provide quantitative values to detect drifts or shifts in the traditional approach to quality control analysis, nor does it provide an assessment of operator competency. On the other hand, use of a traditional liquid quality control material on a device with disposable, single-use electrodes cannot assess the cartridge that actually is used to produce patient data.

Impact on patient care

Although the impact of laboratory value turnaround time on patient outcome or length of stay (LOS) is uncertain, the general perception seems to be that faster is better. One area of the health-care system in which faster laboratory results might result in beneficial patient outcome by facilitating faster clinical decisions and decreased LOS is the emergency department. Indeed, several studies suggested that POCT could improve emergency department LOS in 17% to 19% of patients, based on results of retrospective emergency department physician interviews.[23] However, two other studies, including one that prospectively compared LOS with and without a POCT device in the emergency department for more than 5000 patients, concluded that POCT had no impact on patient LOS.[19] Other settings in which POCT might benefit patient outcome and LOS are the operating room and the anesthesia recovery room. However, one note of caution is not always to extrapolate conclusions regarding POCT from one institution to another. Rather, studies such as those mentioned previously should be used as examples for design of studies that address the impact of POCT within a particular setting or institution.

References

1. Abel JE: The physical background to freezing-point osmometry and its medical-biological applications. Am J Med Elect 1963; 2:32-41.

2. Apple FS, Koch DD, Graves S et al: Relationship between direct-potentiometric and flame-photometric measurement of sodium in blood. Clin Chem 1982; 28:1931-1935.

3. Ashwood ER, Kost G, Kenny M: Temperature correction of blood gas and pH measurements. Clin Chem 1983; 29:1877-1885.

4. Bunn HF, Forget BG (eds): Hemoglobin: Molecular, Genetic and Clinical Aspects, Philadelphia, WB Saunders, 1986.

5. Cotlove E: Determination of chloride in biological materials. In Glick D (ed): Methods of Biochemical Analysis, vol 12, pp 277-391, New York, Interscience Publishers, 1964.

6. Daoud EWR, McClellan AC, Scott MG: Positive interferences with the Ektachem total CO_2 assay from therapy with topical cerous nitrate. Clin Chem 1990; 36:1521-1522.

7. Don BR, Sebastian A, Cheitlin M et al: Pseudohyperkalemia caused by fist clenching during phlebotomy. N Engl J Med 1990; 322:1290-1292.

8. Erickson KA, Wilding P: Evaluation of a novel point-of-care system, the I-STAT portable clinical analyzer. Clin Chem 1993; 39:283-287.

9. Gleeson M, Henry RL: Sweat sodium or chloride? Clin Chem 1991, 37:112.

10. Hammond KB, Turcios NL, Gibson LE: Clinical evaluation of the macroduct sweat collection system and conductivity analyzer in the diagnosis of cystic fibrosis. J Pediatr 1994; 124:255-260.

11. Hansen JE, Sue DY: Should blood gas measurements be corrected for patient's temperature? N Engl J Med 1980; 303:341.

12. International Federation of Clinical Chemistry, Committee on pH, Blood Gases and Electrolytes: Guidelines for transcutaneous PO_2 and PCO_2 measurement. Ann Biol Clin 1990; 48:39-43.

13. Kumar A, Chapoteau E, Czech BP et al: Chromogenic ionophore-based methods for spectrophotometric assay of sodium and potassium in serum and plasma. Clin Chem 1988; 34:1709-1712.

14. LeGrys VA: Sweat testing for the diagnosis of cystic fibrosis: practical considerations. J Pediatr 1996; 129:892-897.

15. Maas AH, Siggaard-Andersen O, Weisberg HF et al: Ion-selective electrodes for sodium and potassium: a new problem of what is measured and what should be reported. Clin Chem 1985; 31:482-485.

16. Mueller RG, Lang GE: Blood gas analysis: effects of air bubbles in syringe and delay in estimation. Br Med J (Clin Res Ed) 1982; 285:1659-1660.

17. Nijsten MWN, de Smet BJ, Dofferhoff ASM: Pseudohyperkalemia and platelet counts. N Engl J Med 1991; 325:1107.

18. Oliver TK, Young GA, Bates GD et al: Factitial hyperkalemia due to icing before analysis. Pediatrics 1966; 38:900-902.

19. Parvin CA, Lo SF, Deuser SM et al: Impact of point-of-care testing on patients' length of stay in a large emergency department. Clin Chem 1996; 42:711-717.

20. Quiles R, Fernandez-Romero JM, Fernandez E et al: Automated enzymatic determination of sodium in serum. Clin Chem 1993; 39:500-503.

21. Rosenstein BJ, Cutting GR: The diagnosis of cystic fibrosis: a consensus statement. J Pediatr 1998; 132:589-595.

22. Salyer JW, Chatburn RL, Dolcini DM: Measured vs calculated oxygen saturation in a population of pediatric intensive care patients. Respir Care 1989; 34:342-348.

23. Sands VM, Auerbach PS, Birnbaum J et al: Evaluation of a portable clinical blood analyzer in the emergency department. Acad Emerg Med 1995; 2:172-178.

24. Santrach PJ, Burritt MF: Point-of-care testing. Mayo Clin Proc 1995; 70:493-494.

25. Shapiro BA, Cane RD: Blood gas monitoring: yesterday, today, and tomorrow. Crit Care Med 1989; 17:573-580.

26. Siggaard-Andersen M, Siggaard-Anderson O: Oxygen status algorithm, version 3, with some applications. Acta Anaesthesiol Scand Suppl 1995; 107:13-20.

27. Stern RC: The diagnosis of cystic fibrosis. N Engl J Med 1997; 336:487-491.

28. Wahr JA, Tremper KK: Continuous intravascular blood gas monitoring. J Cardiothorac Vasc Anesth 1994 8:342-353.

29. Wang T, Diamandis EP, Lane A et al: Variability in selectivity of Hitachi ion-selective electrodes. Clin Biochem 1994; 27:37-44.

30. Watson MA, Scott MG: Clinical utility of biochemical analysis of cerebrospinal fluid. Clin Chem 1995; 41:343-360.

Additional Reading

Driscoll P, Brown T, Gwinnutt C et al: A Simple Guide to Blood Gas Analysis, London, BMJ Books, 1999.

Halperin ML, Goldstein MB: Fluid, Electrolyte, and Acid-Base Physiology: A Problem-Based Approach, Philadelphia, WB Saunders, 1998.

Rose BD, Post T, Rose B: Clinical Physiology of Acid-Base and Electrolyte Disorders, 5th edition, New York, McGraw-Hill, 2000.

CHAPTER 26

Hormones

RONALD J. WHITLEY, PhD

Objectives

1. Define the following terms:
Endocrinology	Adenohypophysis
Steroid hormone	Neurohypophysis
Peptide hormone	Hypothalamic-pituitary axis
Amino acid-derived hormone	Hormone receptor

2. List three physiological functions of hormones and discuss the mechanisms involved in the regulation of hormone secretion.
3. Discuss the significance of free and bound hormone.
4. State the two types of receptor-hormone interaction and the specific effect each type produces in a cell.
5. List the hormones synthesized in the hypothalamus and anterior pituitary gland and describe their principal physiological actions.
6. List the hormones stored in the posterior pituitary gland and describe their principal physiological actions.
7. List six major causes of endocrine disorders.
8. Discuss three analytical techniques used to measure hormones in body fluids.

Key Words

Adenohypophysis   The anterior lobe of the pituitary gland

Autocrine   A mode of hormone action in which a hormone binds to receptors on and affects the function of the cell type that produced it

Biorhythm   The cyclical occurrence of physiological events (for example, a circadian rhythm)

Endocrine System   The system of glands and tissues that synthesize and secrete hormones

Endocrinology   The scientific study of hormones and their roles in health and disease states

Half-Life   In endocrinology, the time required for a hormone to fall to half its original concentration in a specified fluid or blood

Homeostasis   The maintenance of equilibrium of the internal body functions in response to external changes

Hormone   A chemical substance produced in the body by specialized glands and tissues that elicits a regulatory response or action in target cells or organs

Hypothalamic Hormones   Hormones of the hypothalamus that exert control over other organs, primarily the pituitary gland

Hypothalamus-Hypophyseal System   A system of neurons, fiber tracts, endocrine tissue, and blood vessels that is responsible for the production and release of pituitary hormones into the systemic circulation

Neurohypophysis   The posterior lobe of the pituitary gland that produces various hormones

Paracrine   A mode of hormone action in which a hormone synthesized in and released from endocrine cells binds to its receptor in nearby cells of a different type and affects their function

Receptor   A molecular structure within a cell or on the cell surface characterized by (1) selective binding of a specific substance and (2) a specific physiological effect that accompanies the binding (for example, cell surface receptors for peptide hormones, neurotransmitters, antigens, complement fragments, and immunoglobulins and cytoplasmic receptors for steroid hormones)

Endocrinology is the study of intracellular and extracellular communication by messenger molecules known as *hormones*. Historically a **hormone** has been defined as a chemical substance that is produced by a specialized gland in one part of the body and carried to a distant target organ, where a regulatory response is elicited. What now is apparent is that hormones also are secreted by nonglandular tissues, produced in more than one site in the body, and transported by mechanisms other than the blood circulation. Moreover, a hormone may act on neighboring cells (**paracrine** action) and on the very cell in which it was produced (**autocrine** action) without entering the circulation. Figure 26-1 shows the location of several endocrine glands in the body, and Table 26-1 summarizes the types of hormone actions.

Most hormones can be grouped into one of the following several chemical categories:

1. Steroids
2. Polypeptides or proteins
3. Hormones derived from amino acids
4. Fatty acid derivatives

Steroid hormones generally are hydrophobic. Because they are insoluble in water, many steroid hormones circulate in plasma bound reversibly to transport proteins, leaving a small percentage of the hormone free for biological activity. The **half-lives** of these steroids generally vary from 30 to 100 minutes. In contrast, polypeptide hormones are water soluble, circulate unbound in plasma, and often undergo rapid fluctuations in their concentrations. Their plasma half-lives vary from 10 to 30 minutes. Half-lives of amino acid-derived hormones differ, depending on whether they are protein bound. Thyroxine, for example, circulates bound to three binding proteins and has a half-life of almost 1 week, whereas epinephrine circulates free and has a half-life of less than 1 minute.

Hormones possess a high degree of structural specificity. A slight alteration in the molecular composition of a hormone may result in significant changes in its physiological activity. For example, estradiol and estriol differ by only an α-hydroxyl group, but estradiol is a much more potent estrogen. Classifications of hormones, their sources, and a brief description of their principal actions are provided in Table 26-2.

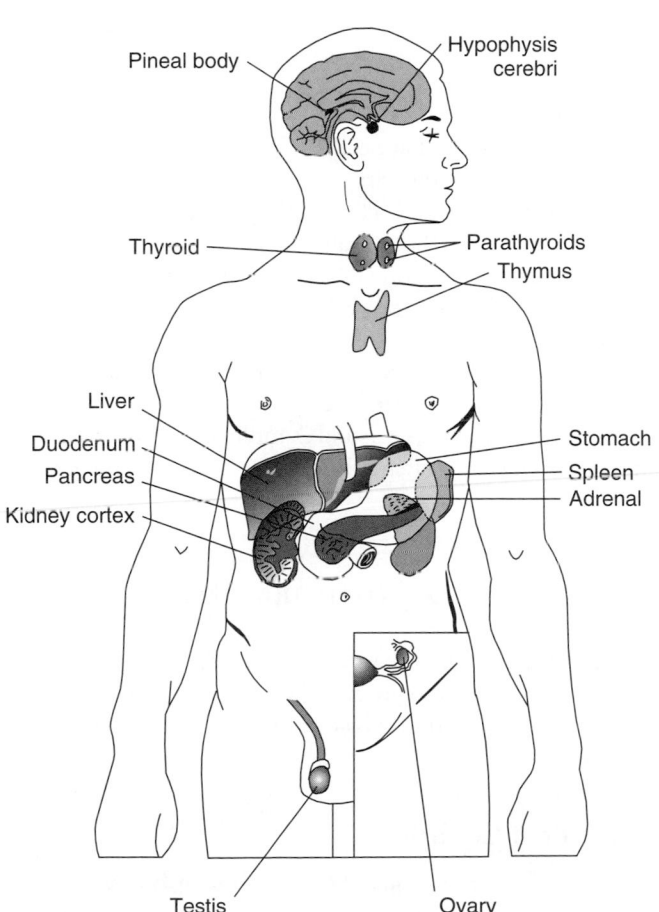

Figure 26-1   Location of the endocrine glands in humans. (Modified from Turner CD: General Endocrinology, 4th edition, Philadelphia, WB Saunders, 1966.)

ACTIONS OF HORMONES

The various actions of hormones can be divided broadly into regulatory functions, morphogenic functions, and integrative functions.

Regulatory Function

A major function of the **endocrine system** is to maintain the constancy of chemical composition (**homeostasis**) of extracellular and intracellular fluids. Homeostasis is maintained through the action of hormones that tightly regulate

---

TABLE 26-1 **Types of Hormone Action**

Hormone Type	Action	Example
Endocrine	Synthesized in one location and released into blood circulation; binds to specific receptor in cells at a distant site to elicit characteristic physiological response	Action of thyroid-stimulating hormone from the anterior pituitary gland on the thyroid
Paracrine	Synthesized in endocrine cells and released into interstitial space; binds to specific receptor in adjacent or neighboring cell and affects its function	Release of somatostatin from islet delta cells and its subsequent action on nearby α- and β-cells in the same pancreatic islet
Autocrine	Synthesized in endocrine cells and sometimes released into interstitial space; binds to specific receptor on cell of origin, thereby autoregulating its function	Action of somatostatin on its own secretion
Juxtacrine	Synthesized in endocrine cells and remains associated with plasma membrane; acts on immediately adjacent receptor cell by direct cell-to-cell contact	Actions of membrane-anchored epidermal growth factors on contiguous receptor cells
Exocrine	Synthesized in endocrine cells and released into lumen of gut; binds to cells lining gut at varying distances from endocrine cells, thereby affecting their function	Release of gastrin by mucosal cells and its action on gastric-acid secretion by the stomach
Neurocrine	Synthesized in neurons and released into extracellular space; binds to receptor in nearby cell and affects its function	Action on cardiac muscle cells of norepinephrine synthesized in nerve endings in the heart
Neuroendocrine	Synthesized in nerve endings and released into blood circulation; interacts with receptors of cells at distant site	Action of norepinephrine synthesized in splanchnic nerve ending on the heart
Neurotransmission	Synthesized in neurons and released from nerve endings; crosses synapse and binds to specific receptor in another neuron, affecting its action	Release of acetylcholine from preganglionic nerve fibers in sympathetic ganglia and binding to receptor in postganglionic neuron with liberation of norepinephrine

---

metabolism of salt, water, carbohydrate, fat, and protein. Other important regulatory functions of hormones are their responses to demands of starvation, infection, trauma, psychological stress, and sexual reproduction.

Morphogenesis

Hormones play an important role in the growth and development of an organism. For example, the development of the male and female sex characteristics is under the influence of testosterone and estradiol.

Integrative Action

A single hormone may act independently or in concert with other hormones to regulate a specific function. For example, normal carbohydrate metabolism requires the concerted action of the hormones produced by the pancreas (insulin and glucagon), pituitary gland (growth hormone), adrenal glands (glucocorticoids, epinephrine), thyroid gland (T_4), and gonads (estrogen). This interrelation is not limited to the endocrine glands but extends to the nervous system as well. For example, the influence of mineralocorticoids (deoxycorticosterone, aldosterone) on salt and water balance would fail without simultaneous adjustment of the rate of blood flow, blood pressure, and vasoconstriction by the nervous system.

The brain itself is an endocrine gland, and several **hypothalamic hormones** are synthesized within hypothalamic

neurons and released at nerve endings, where they act as local mediators or true circulating hormones. The immune system also has been linked to the endocrine and nervous systems as part of the overall control of body function.

Maintenance of homeostasis may require a single hormone to regulate several different biological functions. For example, cortisol enhances gluconeogenesis in the liver, inhibits glucose uptake and use in peripheral tissues, activates lipolysis, enhances protein breakdown, and decreases protein synthesis in fat, muscle, and lymphoid tissues. Together, these actions are integrative and increase blood glucose concentration.

▇ REGULATION OF HORMONE SECRETION

Several mechanisms exist to maintain the balance between production of hormones and the organism's need for hormones. For detailed discussions of these mechanisms, readers are referred to other texts.[1,3,5]

Hormonal Control

The anterior pituitary gland (**adenohypophysis**) occupies a central position in the control of hormone secretion through the production of so-called tropic hormones that regulate other target endocrine glands. Without these tropic hormones the target glands are unable to maintain normal rates of secretion. The main target organs of pituitary tropic

TABLE 26-2   Hormones—Sources and Actions

Endocrine Gland and Hormone	Nature of Hormone	Site of Action	Principal Actions
Hypothalamus			
Thyrotropin-releasing hormone (TRH)	Peptide (3 aa)	Anterior pituitary lobe	Release of TSH and PRL
Gonadotropin-releasing hormone (GnRH) or luteinizing hormone-releasing hormone (LHRH)	Peptide (10 aa)	Anterior pituitary lobe	Release of LH and FSH
Corticotropin-releasing hormone (CRH)	Polypeptide (41 aa)	Anterior pituitary lobe	Release of ACTH and β-LPH
Growth hormone-releasing hormone (GHRH)	Polypeptide (40 aa)	Anterior pituitary lobe	Release of GH
Somatostatin* (SS) or growth hormone-inhibiting hormone (GHIH)	Peptide (14 aa)	Anterior pituitary lobe	Suppression of GH and TSH; inhibition of gastrin, VIP, GIP, secretin, motilin, and insulin
Prolactin-releasing factors (PRF)	Peptide?	Anterior pituitary lobe	Release of PRL
Prolactin-inhibiting factor (PIF)	Dopamine	Anterior pituitary lobe	Suppression of PRL
Anterior Pituitary Lobe			
Thyrotropin or thyroid-stimulating hormone (TSH)	Glycoprotein† (α, 89 aa; β, 112 aa)	Thyroid gland	Stimulation of thyroid hormone formation and secretion
Follicle-stimulating hormone (FSH)	Glycoprotein† (α, 89 aa; β, 115 aa)	Ovary	Growth of follicles and, with LH, secretion of estrogens and ovulation
		Testis	Development of seminiferous tubules; spermatogenesis
Luteinizing hormone (LH)	Glycoprotein† (α, 89 aa; β, 115 aa)	Ovary	Ovulation; formation of corpora lutea; secretion of progesterone
		Testis	Stimulation of interstitial tissue; secretion of androgens
Prolactin (PRL)	Protein (198 aa)	Mammary gland	Proliferation of mammary gland; initiation of milk secretion; antagonist of insulin action
Growth hormone (GH) or somatotropin	Protein (191 aa)	Body as a whole	Growth of bone and muscle
β-Lipotropin (β-LPH)	Polypeptide (91 aa)	Unknown	Precursor of β-MSH and the endorphins
Corticotropin or adrenocorticotropin (ACTH)	Polypeptide (39 aa)	Adrenal cortex	Stimulation of adrenocortical steroid formation and secretion
β-Endorphin (β-END)*‡	Polypeptide (31 aa)	Brain	Endogenous opiate; raising of pain threshold and influence on extrapyramidal motor activity
α-Melanocyte-stimulating hormone (α-MSH)	Peptide (13 aa)	Skin	Dispersion of pigment granules; darkening of skin
Leu-enkephalin (LEK)†§ and met-enkephalin (MEK)†§	Peptide (5 aa)	Brain	Same as β-endorphin
Posterior Pituitary Lobe			
Vasopressin or antidiuretic hormone (ADH)	Peptide (9 aa)	Arterioles	Elevation of blood pressure
		Renal tubules	Water reabsorption
Oxytocin	Peptide (9 aa)	Smooth muscles (uterus, mammary gland)	Contraction; action in parturition and sperm transport; ejection of milk

aa, Amino acid.

*Also produced by the gastrointestinal tract and pancreas.

†Glycoprotein hormone composed of two dissimilar peptides. The α-chain is similar in structure or identical to other glycoprotein hormones; the β-chain differs for each hormone and confers specificity.

‡Also produced in the brain.

§Two chains linked by disulfide bonds: A, 21 aa; B, 30 aa.

Continued

TABLE 26-2	Hormones—Sources and Actions—cont'd		
Endocrine Gland and Hormone	Nature of Hormone	Site of Action	Principal Actions
Pineal Gland			
Serotonin or 5-hydroxytryptamine (5-HT)	Indoleamine	Cardiovascular, respiratory, and gastrointestinal systems; brain	Neurotransmitter; stimulation or inhibition of various smooth muscles and nerves; possible role in mental illness
Melatonin	Indoleamine	Hypothalamus	Suppression of gonadotropin and GH secretion; induction of sleep
Thyroid Gland			
Thyroxine (T_4) and triiodothyronine (T_3)	Iodoamino acids	General body tissue	Stimulation of oxygen consumption and metabolic rate of tissue
Calcitonin or thyrocalcitonin	Polypeptide (32 aa)	Skeleton	Inhibition of calcium resorption; lowering of plasma calcium and phosphate
Parathyroid Gland			
Parathyroid hormone (PTH) or parathormone	Polypeptide (84 aa)	Skeleton, kidney, gastrointestinal tract	Regulation of calcium and phosphorus metabolism
Adrenal Cortex			
Cortisol	Steroid	General body tissue	Metabolism of carbohydrates, proteins, and fats; inflammation; resistance to infection; hypersensitivity
Aldosterone	Steroid	Kidney	Salt and water balance
Adrenal Medulla			
Norepinephrine and epinephrine	Aromatic amines	Sympathetic receptors; liver and muscle; adipose tissue	Stimulation of sympathetic nervous system; glycogenolysis; lipolysis
Ovary			
Estrogens	Phenolic steroids	Female accessory sex organs	Development of secondary sex characteristics
Progesterone	Steroid	Female accessory reproductive structure	Preparation of the uterus for ovum implantation; maintenance of pregnancy
Relaxin	Polypeptide	Uterus	Inhibition of myometrial contraction
Inhibin	Polypeptide	Hypothalamus	Suspected role in control of FSH secretion
Testis			
Testosterone	Steroid	Male accessory sex organs	Development of secondary sex characteristics, maturation, and normal function
Inhibin	(See ovary)	(See ovary)	(See ovary)
Placenta			
Estrogens	(See ovary)	(See ovary)	(See ovary)
Progesterone	(See ovary)	(See ovary)	(See ovary)
Relaxin	(See ovary)	(See ovary)	(See ovary)
Chorionic gonadotropin (CG) or choriogonadotropin	Glycoprotein† (α, 92 aa; β, 144 aa)	Same as LH	Same as LH; prolongation of corpus luteal function; suspected role in steroidogenesis during fetal life
Chorionic somatomammotropin (CS) or placental lactogen (PL)	Protein (191 aa)	Same as PRL	Same as PRL
Pancreas			
Insulin	Polypeptide§	Most cells	Regulation of carbohydrate metabolism; lipogenesis
Glucagon	Polypeptide (29 aa)	Liver	Glycogenolysis
Pancreatic polypeptide (PP)	Polypeptide (36 aa)	Gastrointestinal tract	Increased gut motility and gastric emptying; inhibition of gallbladder contraction
Somatostatin (SS)	Peptide (14 aa)	Pancreas	Inhibition of insulin, glucagon

TABLE 26-2   Hormones—Sources and Actions—cont'd

Endocrine Gland and Hormone	Nature of Hormone	Site of Action	Principal Actions
Gastrointestinal Tract			
Gastrin§	Peptide (17 aa)	Stomach	Secretion of gastric acid; gastric mucosal growth
Secretin	Polypeptide (27 aa)	Pancreas	Secretion of pancreatic bicarbonate and digestive enzymes
Cholecystokinin-pancreozymin (CCK-PZ)‡	Polypeptide (33 aa)	Gallbladder and pancreas	Stimulation of gallbladder contraction; secretion of pancreatic enzymes
Motilin	Polypeptide (22 aa)	Gastrointestinal tract	Stimulation of gastrointestinal motility
Vasoactive intestinal peptide (VIP)‡	Polypeptide (28 aa)	Gastrointestinal tract	Neurotransmitter; relaxation of smooth muscles of gut and of circulation; increased release of hormones and secretion of water and electrolytes from pancreas and gut
Gastric inhibitory polypeptide (GIP)	Polypeptide (42 aa)	Gastrointestinal tract	Inhibition of gastric secretion and motility; increase of insulin secretion
Bombesin‡	Peptide (14 aa)	Gastrointestinal tract	Stimulation of release of various hormones and pancreatic enzymes, smooth muscle contractions and hypothermia; changes in cardiovascular and renal function
Neurotensin‡	Peptide (13 aa)	Gastrointestinal tract and hypothalamus (gut and brain)	Uncertain
Substance P (SP)‡	Peptide (11 aa)	Gastrointestinal tract and brain	Sensory neurotransmitter, analgesic; increase in contraction of gastrointestinal smooth muscle; potent vasoactive hormone; promotion of salivation; increased release of histamine
Kidney			
1,25-(OH)$_2$ vitamin D	Sterol	Intestine; bone; kidney	Facilitation of calcium and phosphorus absorption; increase in bone resorption in conjunction with PTH; increase in reabsorption of filtered calcium
Erythropoietin	Glycoprotein	Bone marrow	Stimulation of red-cell formation
Liver			
Insulin-like growth factor I	Peptide (70 aa)	Most cells	Stimulation of cellular and linear growth
Insulin-like growth factor II	Peptide (67 aa)	Most cells	Insulin-like activity
Thymus			
Thymosin and thymopoietin	Peptides (49 and 28 aa)	Lymphocytes	Maturation of T lymphocytes
Heart			
Atrial natriuretic factor (ANF, Atriopeptin)	Peptide (28 aa)	Vascular, renal, and adrenal tissue	Regulation of blood volume and blood pressure
Adipose Tissue			
Leptin	Protein (165 aa)	Hypothalamus and other tissues	Control of body weight; regulation of energy expenditure; possible role in onset of puberty

Continued

TABLE 26-2 Hormones—Sources and Actions—cont'd

Endocrine Gland and Hormone	Nature of Hormone	Site of Action	Principal Actions
Multiple Cell Types			
Parathyroid hormone-related peptide (PTH-RP)	Peptide (141 aa)	Kidney, bone	Conjectural; PTH-like actions; tumor marker
Growth factors (for example, epidermal growth factor, fibroblast growth factor, transforming growth factor family, platelet-derived growth factor, nerve growth factors)	Polypeptides		Stimulation of cellular growth
Monocytes/Lymphocytes/Macrophages			
Cytokines (for example, interleukins I-18, tumor necrosis factor, interferons)	Polypeptides		Stimulation or inhibition of cellular growth

hormones are the thyroid gland, adrenal cortex, and gonads.

The production of most hormones is regulated by the metabolic activity of the hormone itself through either a positive- or a negative-feedback system. In a positive-feedback system an increase in the product increases the activity of the system, which in turn increases the rate of production of the product itself. In a negative-feedback system an increase in the product decreases the activity of the system, resulting in a decrease in the level of the product. Negative feedback is the principal mechanism for the control of adrenocortical, gonadal, and thyroidal hormone secretions. When levels of these target organ hormones fall, the pituitary senses the decline and increases production of the appropriate tropic hormone, which then enters the circulation and stimulates additional production of the target organ hormone.

In contrast to negative feedback, positive feedback does not operate in isolation but constitutes an integral part of a control system. Stimulation of luteinizing hormone (LH; lutropin) release by a progressive increase in estradiol before ovulation is an example of positive-feedback regulation.

Central Nervous System Control

Hormones secreted by the **neurohypophysis** (for example, vasopressin and oxytocin) and adrenal medulla (for example, epinephrine) are controlled primarily by the nervous system.

The importance of the relationship between the nervous system and the endocrine system is apparent through various feedback-control mechanisms that involve the **hypothalamus-hypophyseal system.** Because the hypothalamus receives signals from higher centers in the brain, one feature of the regulation of pituitary hormone release is the ability of the brain to override or fine-tune other control mechanisms. This type of control by higher centers of the brain is called an *open-loop control system;* the hormonal response to stress is an example of this type of control system.

■ BIORHYTHMS

A **biorhythm** is the cyclical occurrence of a physiological event, and many examples exist in endocrinology. Rhythmic secretion of hormones is an important regulatory feature of endocrine systems.[2] Rhythms with 24-hour time intervals are termed *circadian,* or *diurnal,* and usually are synchronized by the dark/light cycle and sleep. Biorhythms that occur more frequently than once a day are referred to as *ultradian rhythms,* whereas infradian rhythms have time periods that are longer than 24 hours.

Some of the most remarkable endocrine rhythms involve pulsatile and circadian release of pituitary hormones. For example, pulses of LH can be detected about every 90 minutes; these pulses are triggered by pulsatile secretory bursts of gonadotropin-releasing hormone released by the hypothalamus. Superimposed on this ultradian rhythm of pituitary LH secretion is an endogenous circadian rhythm that increases during sleep in most pubertal children. In adult women this 24-hour variation in LH is modulated markedly by the menstrual cycle.

All pituitary hormones have characteristic circadian rhythms. For example, adrenocorticotropic hormone (ACTH) levels rise early in the morning, peak at about 0800 hours, and gradually fall over the course of the day, with a nadir around midnight. Thyroid-stimulating hormone secretion (TSH) is highest just before midnight, whereas large surges of growth hormone occur during periods of rapid-eye-movement sleep.

The remarkable reproducibility of endocrine rhythms and their relative ease of measurement have resulted in their frequent use in laboratory medicine. Samples taken at appropriate times of the day or night provide useful dynamic indicators of endocrine function. For example, loss of the diurnal rhythm of cortisol secretion serves as a diagnostic screening test for Cushing's syndrome (see Chapter 41).

HORMONE RECEPTORS

The biological response to a hormone is initiated by binding of the hormone to target cell **receptors.** The receptor provides the target cell with a mechanism for recognizing and concentrating the hormone, and the hormone-receptor complex activates the target cell to begin the chain of events that constitutes the biological effects of that hormone. The hormone-receptor complex has several characteristics, as follows:

1. It is highly *specific;* the target tissue is affected only by the active hormone and not by the innumerable other substances to which the cells are exposed.
2. It is an *equilibrium system* in which the hormone and receptor react reversibly to form the hormone-receptor complex; the reaction is assumed to reach equilibrium.
3. It is *saturable* due to the presence of a finite number of receptors in cells. The degree of a biological response of a target tissue is proportional to the number of hormone-receptor complexes; a maximum response is obtained when all sites are filled.
4. It is of high *affinity,* which allows hormone-receptor complexes to form in the presence of very low levels of circulating hormones. For most hormones the equilibrium dissociation constant (K_d) falls approximately in the concentration range of the circulating hormone.

Regulation of Receptors

The quantity and quality of receptors may increase or decrease in response to various stimuli, and receptor properties may change with varying physiological conditions. The exposure of responsive cells to high concentrations of hormones decreases the number and binding affinity of surface membrane receptors. In addition, the binding of a hormone to its receptor also influences the affinity of neighboring binding sites. Such a mechanism modulates hormone action by enhancing cell sensitivity at low hormone concentrations and reducing cell sensitivity at high hormone concentrations.

Receptors also are modulated by other hormones. Furthermore, one hormone may have a strong affinity for its own receptor and some affinity for the receptor of another hormone. Such a spillover, or cross-reaction, generally occurs between hormones with structural similarities. If one hormone is produced in excess, that hormone not only shows an excessive biological effect of its own but also elicits the response of a structurally similar hormone through receptor interactions. Thus high concentrations of glucocorti-

coids produce both excess glucocorticoid and mineralocorticoid effects.

Dysfunction of receptors also causes a variety of endocrine diseases. For example, androgen resistance observed in some male pseudohermaphrodites results from the presence of abnormal receptors or the absence of normal receptors.

MECHANISM OF ACTION OF HORMONES

Two general models of hormone action prevail at present—one for peptide hormones and catecholamines that act at the cell surface via membrane receptors and the other for steroids and iodothyronines that bind to receptors within the cell.

Peptide Hormones and Catecholamines

Peptide hormones and catecholamines elicit their responses by binding to receptors located on or in the cell membrane. Two major classes of membrane-bound receptors exist for peptide hormones and neurotransmitters—the G-protein family and protein kinases.

Receptors of the G-protein class use guanine nucleotide-binding proteins (G proteins) to interface with target proteins, such as adenylate cyclase and phospholipase C. As shown in Figure 26-2, when a stimulatory hormone binds to the appropriate receptor, the hormone-receptor complex associates with a nearby G protein, thereby activating adenylate cyclase. This enzyme catalyzes the formation of cyclic adenosine monophosphate (cAMP) from adenosine triphosphate (ATP) at the inner membrane surface. cAMP diffuses through the cell and activates a group of closely related enzymes known as *cAMP-dependent protein kinases.* These kinases phosphorylate intracellular proteins, especially other enzymes, and thus regulate (activate or inactivate) the activity of these intracellular enzymes or proteins. The hormone-receptor activation of phospholipase C is analogous to the adenylate cyclase system and operates through a regulatory G protein (Figure 26-3).

Some membrane-bound receptors, such as protein kinase receptors, do not activate adenylate cyclase or generate second-messenger molecules. For example, insulin receptors contain an intrinsic, hormone-activated tyrosine kinase activity; these receptors serve as direct catalysts of phosphorylation reactions. Receptors for growth hormone, prolactin, and peptide growth factors are similar in structure to the receptor kinases.

Steroids and Thyroid Hormones

Steroid and thyroid hormones enter the target organ cells and bind with intracellular receptors. Most of these hormones are lipid soluble and transported in plasma bound to

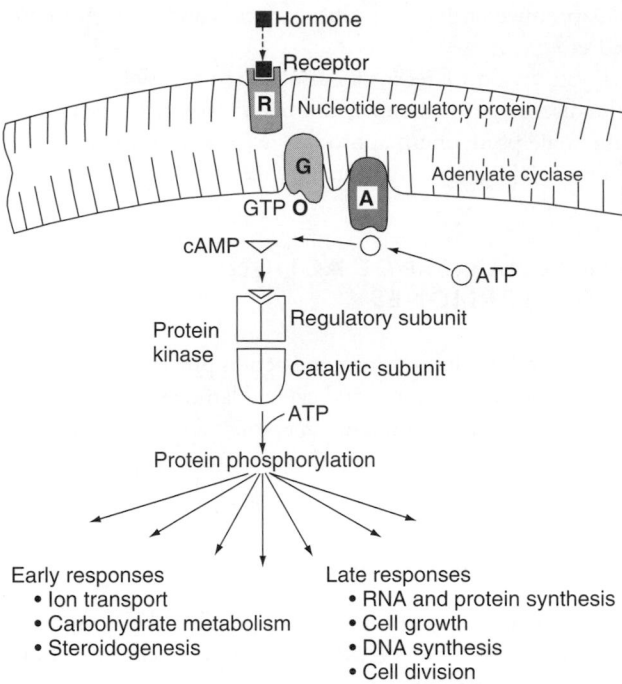

Figure 26-2 Cyclic adenosine monophosphate (cAMP) as a second messenger mediating the effects of extracellular chemical messengers, such as hormones and neurotransmitters. The ligand hormone binds to the receptor protein (*R*), and this reaction activates adenylate cyclase (*A*) through the guanine nucleotide regulatory protein (*G*), which binds GTP. Activation of adenylate cyclase converts ATP to cAMP. The cAMP binds to the regulatory subunit of protein kinase, resulting in dissociation of the catalytic subunit. The free catalytic subunit, in turn, phosphorylates enzymes and other proteins to produce a variety of effects. *GTP,* Guanosine triphosphate; *ATP,* adenosine triphosphate. (Modified from Catt KJ, Harwood JP, Clayton RN et al: Regulation of peptide hormone receptors and gonadal steroidogenesis. Recent Prog Horm Res 1980; 36:557-662.)

carrier proteins. The free hormone enters the cell by passive diffusion and binds to specific receptor proteins located in the cytoplasm or nucleus (Figure 26-4). The activated receptor binds to DNA and either enhances or represses the rate of gene transcription. The messenger RNA (mRNA) that is formed directs the synthesis of specific cytoplasmic proteins or enzymes that in turn mediate the hormone's effects.

Thyroid hormones act in a manner similar to that of steroids. They enter cells and bind to receptors in the target cell's nucleus. Nuclear triiodothyronine (T_3) is derived both from serum T_3 and from intracellular deiodination of thyroxine (T_4). The interaction of T_3 with its receptor stimulates the transcription of specific genes by mechanisms that are similar to those described for steroid hormones.

■ ENDOCRINE DISORDERS

Endocrine disorders are caused by (1) an excess or deficiency of hormones normally produced by the endocrine glands, (2) the production of abnormal hormones, (3) a resistance to

hormone action, (4) abnormalities of hormone action, (5) abnormalities of hormone transport or metabolism, and (6) multiple endocrine abnormalities. Assays now are available to measure most hormones found in body fluids. Recombinant DNA methods (for example, Southern blot, oligonucleotide specific hybridization, polymerase chain reaction, restriction fragment length polymorphisms) also are being applied to the study of endocrine disorders.[4]

■ MEASUREMENTS OF HORMONES AND RELATED ANALYTES

Hormones are measured by a variety of analytical techniques, including bioassay, receptor assay, and immunoassay.

Bioassay Techniques

Bioassays are based on observations of physiological responses specific for the hormone being measured. In vivo bioassays usually involve the injection of test materials into suitably prepared animals; target gland responses, such as growth or steroidogenesis, then are measured. In vitro bioassays involve the incubation of tissues, membranes, dispersed cells, or permanent cell lines in a defined culture medium, with subsequent measurement of an appropriate hormone response. Most in vitro bioassays measure responses proximal or distal to a second messenger, such as stimulation of cAMP formation.

Receptor Assays

Receptor assays depend on the in vitro interaction of a hormone with its biological receptor. In this type of assay, unlabeled hormone displaces trace amounts of radioactively labeled hormone from receptor sites. In general, receptor assays are simpler to perform and have greater sensitivity than bioassays. Receptor assays also have an advantage over immunoassays in that they reflect the biological function of a hormone, namely the capacity to combine with specific receptor sites. By contrast, immunoassays may measure active hormone and inactive prohormone, hormone polymer, and metabolites, all of which have the same antigenic determinant. In general, receptor assays are not as sensitive as immunoassays, and enzymes in the biological specimen may degrade the receptor or destroy the labeled tracer. The added complexity and lability of receptor preparations also contribute to the limited application of these assays in the routine clinical laboratory.

Immunoassay Techniques

Immunoassays are used widely to quantitate hormones (see Chapter 10). Currently, labeled-antibody (immunometric) assays with nonisotopic labels are the method of choice used to measure most hormones, especially peptides and proteins.

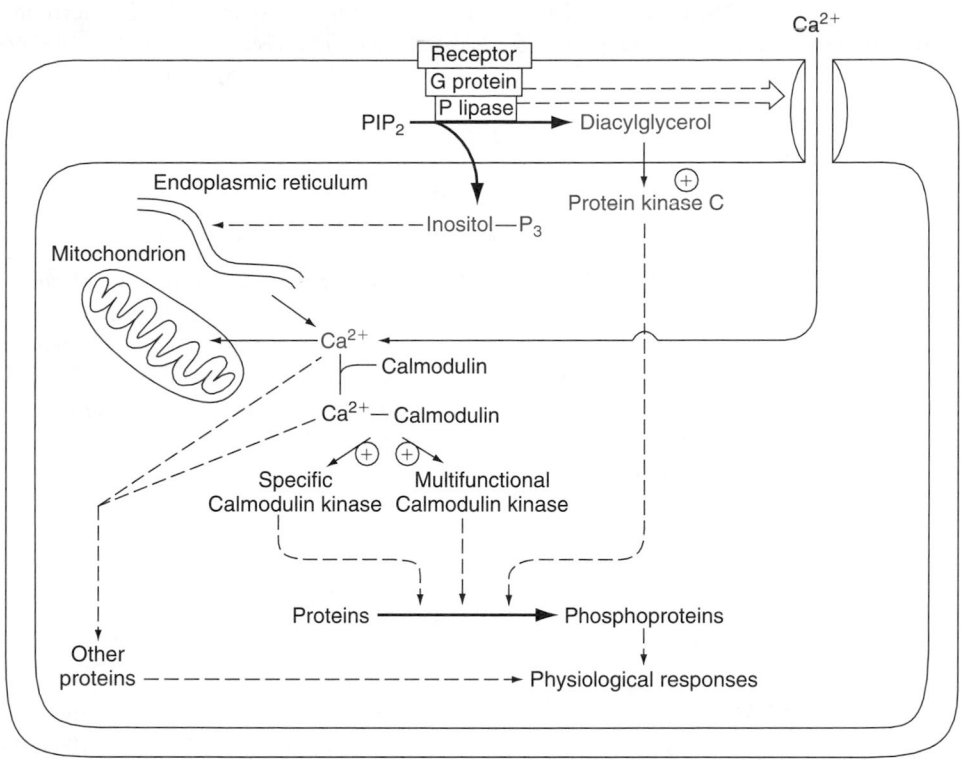

Figure 26-3   Phospholipase C activation. Hormone-receptor interactions result in the activation of phospholipase C. This process involves a specific G protein, which also may activate a calcium channel. Activation of phospholipase C results in the generation of inositol-P_3 (which liberates stored intracellular Ca^{2+}) and diacylglycerol (which activates protein kinase C). The Ca^{2+}-calmodulin complex also activates specific kinases. These actions result in the modification of substrates, which then alter physiological responses. (Courtesy Dr. J. Exton. Modified from Granner D: Hormone action. In Murray RK (ed): Harper's Biochemistry, 24th edition, p 519, Norwalk, Conn, Appleton and Lange, 1996.)

Molecular pathway of steroid hormone action

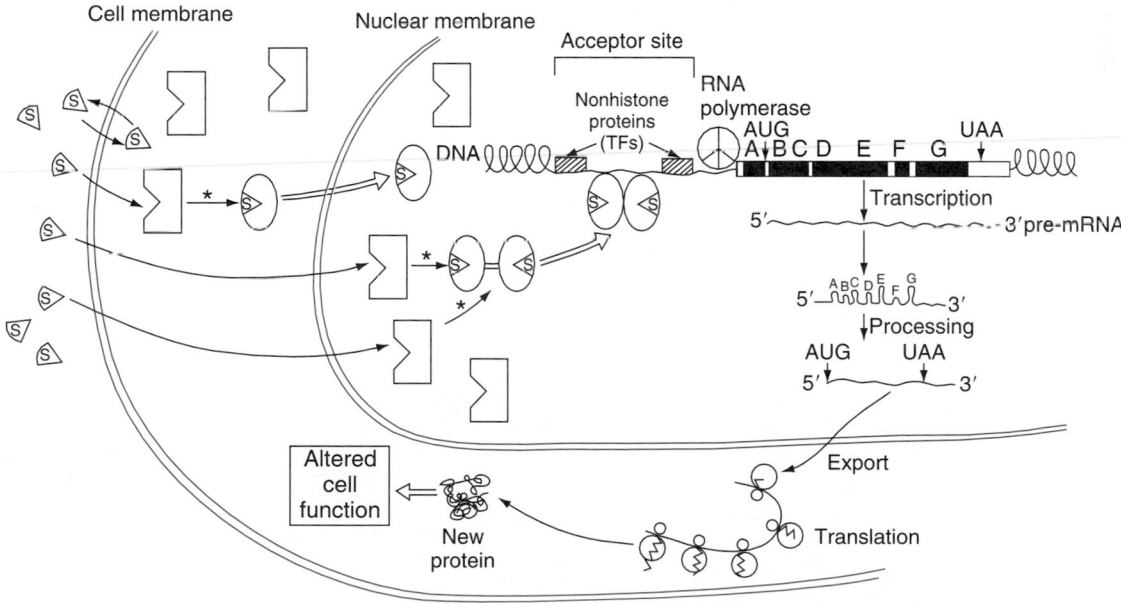

Figure 26-4   General model of steroid (S) or thyroid hormone action. Binding of hormone to an inactive receptor in the cytoplasm or nucleus causes a conformational change in the receptor. The receptor is activated and binds to nuclear DNA as a dimer. This activated dimer binds upstream of genes to acceptor sites (hormone response elements) composed of DNA and nonhistone chromosomal protein. This interaction leads to activation or repression of gene transcription. (Modified from Clark J, Schrader W, O'Malley B: Mechanisms of action of steroid hormones. In Wilson JD, Foster DW, Kronenberg HM et al (eds): Williams Textbook of Endocrinology, 9th edition, p 56, Philadelphia, WB Saunders, 1998.)

Immunometric assays use saturating concentrations of two or more antibodies (often monoclonal) that are prepared against different epitopes of the protein molecule. One of the two antibodies usually is attached to a solid-phase separation system and extracts the hormone from the serum specimen. The second antibody is linked to a signal molecule, which then is measured. The resultant signal is used to quantify the bound hormone.

References

1. Becker KL (ed): Principles and Practice of Endocrinology and Metabolism, 2nd edition, Philadelphia, JB Lippincott, 1995.
2. Cauter E, Turek F: Endocrine and other biological rhythms. In DeGroot LJ (ed): Endocrinology, 3rd edition, pp 2487-2548, Philadelphia, WB Saunders, 1995.
3. DeGroot LJ, Jameson JL (eds): Endocrinology, 4th edition, Philadelphia, WB Saunders, 2000.
4. Jameson JL: Applications of molecular biology in endocrinology. In DeGroot, LJ (ed): Endocrinology, 3rd edition, pp 119-147, Philadelphia, WB Saunders, 1995.
5. Wilson JD, Foster DW, Kronenberg HM et al (eds): Williams Textbook of Endocrinology, 9th edition, Philadelphia, WB Saunders, 1998.

Additional Reading

Jialal I, Winter WE, Chan DW: Handbook of Diagnostic Endocrinology, Washington, DC, AACC Press, 1999.

Raging hormones: closing the loop from bench to bedside: Conference Proceedings from the 22nd Arnold O. Beckman Conference. Clin Chem 1999; 45:1321-1390.

CHAPTER 27

Catecholamines and Serotonin

THOMAS G. ROSANO, PhD, DABCC, DABFT, and RONALD J. WHITLEY, PhD

Objectives

1. List the hormones synthesized by the adrenal medulla, as well as the physiological actions, regulation of secretion, and clinical significance of each; state a method of analysis.
2. Define *pheochromocytoma* and the laboratory results obtained in the assessment of this disease.
3. Summarize the metabolic pathway of the catecholamines and state the clinical significance of the metabolites.
4. Discuss the clinical significance of serotonin and its metabolite; state a method of analysis.

Key Words

Carcinoid Syndrome A symptom complex associated with carcinoid tumors and characterized by attacks of severe cyanotic flushing of the skin lasting from minutes to days and diarrheal watery stools, bronchoconstrictive attacks, sudden drops in blood pressure, edema, and acites; symptoms being caused by secretion by the tumor of serotonin, prostaglandins, and other biologically active substances

Carcinoid Tumor A yellow circumscribed tumor arising from enterochromaffin cells, usually in the small intestine, appendix, stomach, or colon, and less commonly in the bronchus; sometimes used alone to refer to the gastrointestinal tumor (called also *argentaffinoma*)

Catecholamine One of a group of biogenic amines having a sympathomimetic action; the aromatic portion of the molecule being catechol, and the aliphatic portion an amine; examples including dopamine, norepinephrine, and epinephrine

Catecholamine Metabolites Products of catecholamine metabolism, such as homovanillic acid, 5-hydroxyindoleacetic acid, methoxyhydroxyphenylglycol, normetanephrine, and vanillylmandelic acid

Chromaffin Cell Cells that take up and stain strongly with chromium salts; said of certain cells occurring in the adrenal, coccygeal, and carotid glands, along the sympathetic nerves, and in various organs in which cytoplasmic granules give a brownish reaction with chromium salts; stores epinephrine

DOPA An amino acid, 3,4-dihydroxyphenylalanine, produced by oxidation of tyrosine by monophenol monooxgenase; the precursor of dopamine and an intermediate product in the biosynthesis of norepinephrine, epinephrine, and melanin

Dopamine A catecholamine formed in the body by the decarboxylation of DOPA; an intermediate product in the synthesis of norepinephrine; acts as a neurotransmitter in the central nervous system; also produced peripherally and acts on peripheral receptors (for example, in blood vessels)

Epinephrine (Adrenaline) A catecholamine hormone secreted by the adrenal medulla and a neurotransmitter released by some neurons

Homovanillic Acid (HVA) A product of catecholamine metabolism; elevated urinary levels occurring in individuals with pheochromocytoma or other catecholamine-secreting tumors

5-Hydroxyindoleacetic Acid (5-HIAA) A metabolite of serotonin (5-hydroxytryptamine) that is excreted in large amounts by individuals with carcinoid tumors

Metanephrine A pharmacologically and physiologically inactive metabolite of epinephrine resulting from O-methylation of epinephrine

3-Methoxy-4-Hydroxyphenylglycol (MHPG) A metabolite of epinephrine and norepinephrine found in brain, blood, cerebrospinal fluid, and urine, where its concentrations are used to measure catecholamine turnover

Neuroblastoma A sarcoma consisting of malignant neuroblasts, usually arising in the autonomic nervous system (sympathicoblastoma) or the adrenal medulla; considered a type of neuroepithelial tumor and affects mostly infants and children up to 10 years of age

Norepinephrine (Noradrenaline) A homologue of epinephrine that has one less methylene group; a neurohormone released by the postganglionic adrenergic nerves and some brain neurons; a major neurotransmitter that acts on α- and β$_1$-adrenergic receptors

Normetanephrine A methylated metabolite of norepinephrine that is excreted in the urine and found in certain tissues

Pheochromocytoma A usually benign tumor of chromaffin tissue of the adrenal medulla or sympathetic paraganglia.

Serotonin (5-Hydroxytryptamine) A monoamine vasoconstrictor synthesized in the intestinal chromaffin cells or central or peripheral neurons and found in high concentrations in many body tissues, including the intestinal mucosa, pineal body, and central nervous system

Vanillylmandelic Acid (VMA) The primary end product of catecholamine metabolism excreted in the urine; urinary levels being used in screening of patients for pheochromocytoma

---

The catecholamines and serotonin are organic amines that are produced in the body and serve as chemical signals for a wide range of essential biological functions. Epinephrine, norepinephrine and dopamine are the naturally occurring catecholamines. **Epinephrine** is produced primarily by the adrenal medulla (see Chapter 41), whereas **norepinephrine** is a neurotransmitter produced in the central nervous system (CNS) and postganglionic sympathetic nerves.[12] **Dopamine** is present in highest concentration in localized regions of the brain and also functions in the peripheral organs. **Serotonin** also is a physiologically important amine and functions as a signal transmitter in the CNS and peripheral organs, such as the gastrointestinal tract.[11] Abnormal production of the catecholamines or serotonin may result from a number of disorders, including tumors of neural origin. Amine overproduction results in clinical signs and symptoms that exaggerate the normal physiological effects of the overproduced amine, and measurement of specific amines and their metabolites therefore is important in the detection and treatment of these disorders

■ CATECHOLAMINES AND METABOLITES

Catecholamines are a group of similar compounds having a sympathomimetic action. Such compounds include dopamine, epinephrine, and norepinephrine.

Biochemistry and Physiology
Structure and function

Catecholamines are compounds that consist of monoamines attached to a benzene ring bearing two hydroxyl groups (catechol). The structure and nomenclature of the naturally produced catecholamines are shown in Figure 27-1. Both dopamine and norepinephrine are primary amines, whereas epinephrine is a secondary amine. Due to their catechol structure, the catecholamines are sensitive to oxidation in neutral and alkaline environments, and special collection procedures are used to ensure stability of specimens submitted to the clinical laboratory for testing.

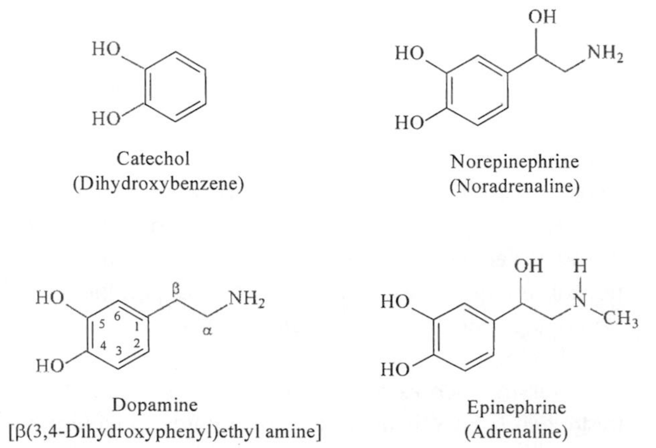

Catechol
(Dihydroxybenzene)

Norepinephrine
(Noradrenaline)

Dopamine
[β(3,4-Dihydroxyphenyl)ethyl amine]

Epinephrine
(Adrenaline)

Figure 27-1 Structure and numbering system of catecholamines.

In the CNS, dopamine and norepinephrine function as important transmitters of nerve signals. Dopamine, for example, is the neurotransmitter in a major system of the brain, including the extrapyramidal and mesolimbic system, as well as the hypothalamic-pituitary axis. Norepinephrine-containing neurons are present in the cerebellum, midbrain, cerebral cortex, and hypothalamus. In addition to their function in the CNS, dopamine and norepinephrine have a marked influence on the vascular system. In contrast to the neurotransmitter functions of norepinephrine and dopamine, epinephrine is considered to be a true adrenal medullary hormone and influences metabolic processes, especially carbohydrate metabolism.

Each of the catecholamines has characteristic physiological functions and pharmacological actions as a result of its interaction with adrenergic or dopaminergic receptors that are located on the surface of target cells throughout the body. The physiological actions are important in maintenance of normal body function, whereas the pharmacological actions produce clinical signs and symptoms in a number of disorders of catecholamine overproduction. The adrenergic receptors, which include α- and β-subtypes, bind epinephrine and norepinephrine. The α-receptors interact with both epinephrine and norepinephrine, while β-receptors respond to epinephrine but are relatively insensitive to norepinephrine. The physiological responses that are induced by both of these receptors are listed in Table 27-1. Different subtypes of the dopamine receptor also are known and involved in the signaling of nerve cells by binding dopamine. The unique distribution of catecholamine receptors throughout the body accounts for the wide range of effects on nervous, metabolic, endocrine, and cardiovascular function.

Biosynthesis, storage, and release

L-Tyrosine is the precursor of the catecholamines (Figure 27-2). The first and rate-limiting step in the biosynthetic pathway of catecholamines is hydroxylation of tyrosine by tyrosine hydroxylase in sympathetic nerve endings and the adrenal medulla. The product, dihydroxyphenylalanine **(DOPA)**, is converted in a variety of tissues to dopamine through the action of aromatic L-amino acid decarboxylase. Dopamine then is transported by an energy-dependent mechanism into storage particles present in both the sympathetic nerve endings and the adrenal medulla. These particles contain dopamine-β-hydroxylase, an enzyme responsible for final conversion of dopamine to norepinephrine, which then is stored in the particle. In the adrenal medulla, norepinephrine released from storage granules becomes the substrate for another cytosolic enzyme, phenylethanolamine-N-methyl transferase (PNMT). This enzyme transfers a methyl group from S-adenosylmethionine to norepinephrine, thus forming epinephrine, which reenters the granule for storage.

Biosynthesis and release of catecholamines are regulated both by intracellular compartmentalization and by feedback inhibition by the products on the rate-limiting steps in the biosynthetic pathway. The particles sequester the catecholamines, thus preventing premature degradation by cytoplasmic monoamine oxidase (MAO) until neurogenic stimulation commands their release. When norepinephrine is released, it inhibits tyrosine hydroxylase activity and transport of dopamine into the particles. Epinephrine is a potent noncompetitive inhibitor of PNMT.

Nerve stimulation is necessary for the release of catecholamines. The chemical mediation of catecholamine release is linked to the presence of acetylcholine and the influx of calcium ions. The process is energy dependent; it requires glycolysis or oxidative metabolism to produce adeno-

TABLE 27-1 Physiological Responses Induced by α– and β-Receptors

Site of Effect	α-Response	β-Response
Vascular beds	Vasoconstriction	Vasodilatation
Intestinal smooth muscle	Relaxation	Relaxation
Bronchial smooth muscle	None	Relaxation
Cardiac contraction	None	Increase
Heart rate	None	Increase
Pupils	Dilation	None
Piloerection	Stimulation	None
Insulin release	Inhibition	Stimulation
Blood glucose	Increase	Decrease

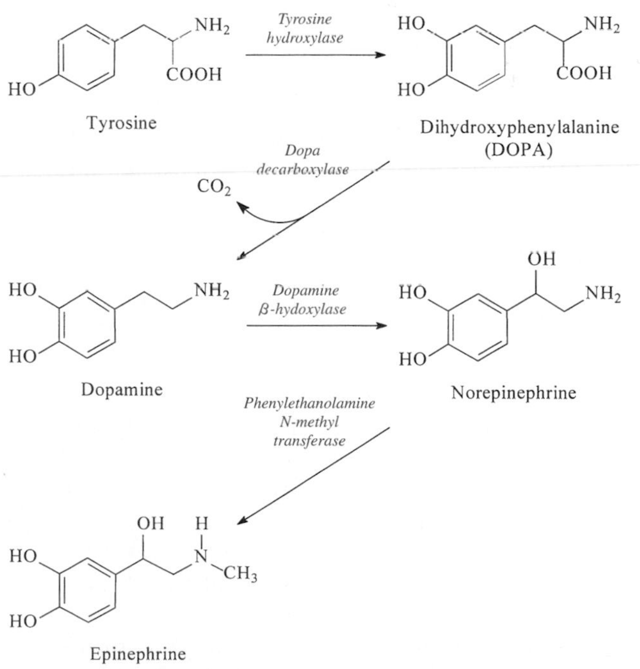

Figure 27-2   Biosynthesis of catecholamines.

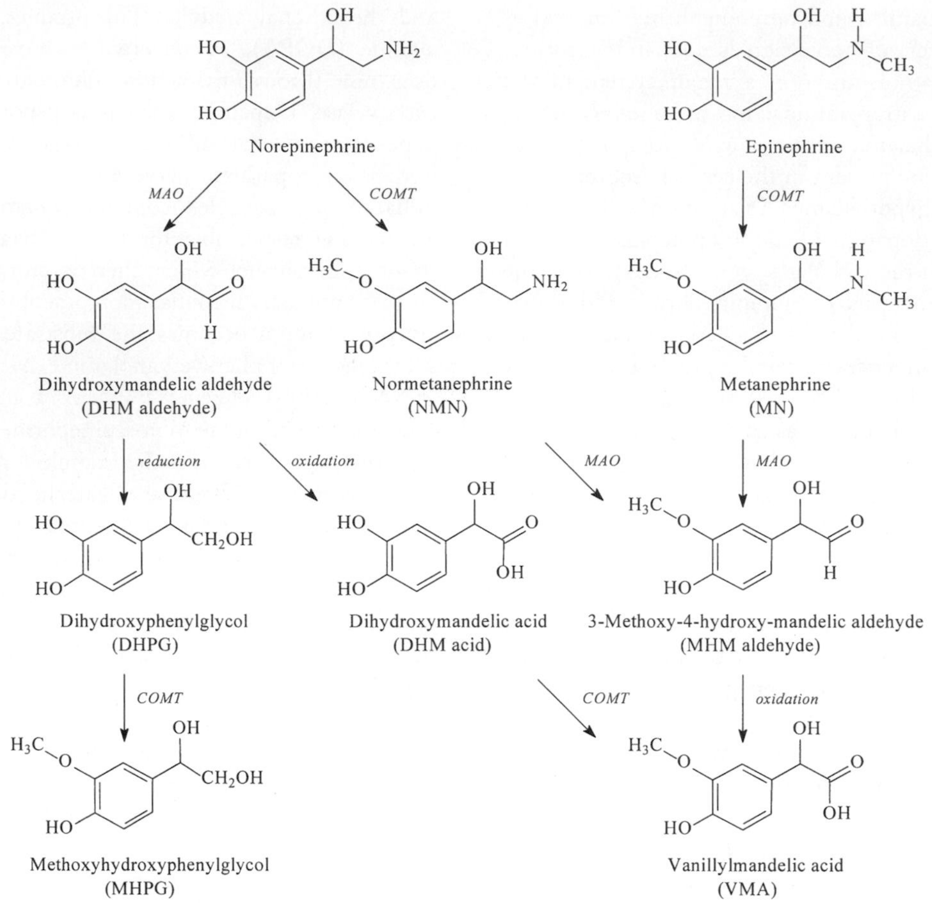

Figure 27-3 Metabolism of epinephrine and norepinephrine. Aldehyde intermediates exist only transiently. *COMT,* Catechol–*O*–methyl transferase; *MAO,* monoamine oxidase.

sine triphosphate (ATP). The catecholamines are released from their particles by the process of exocytosis. Other soluble contents are released along with the catecholamines, including chromogranin A, ATP, and opioid peptides (enkephalins).

Metabolism and excretion

After their release from storage particles, catecholamines act on effector cells through receptors on the cell surface. They then are inactivated rapidly through reuptake by storage particles, conversion to **catecholamine metabolites,** or excretion as free amines or conjugates. Catecholamines that escape the reuptake process are transported in blood, with a very short plasma half-life of approximately 2 minutes. Two important enzymatic pathways for the inactivation of catecholamines in the body involve catechol-*O*-methylation and oxidative deamination. Catechol-*O*-methyl transferase (COMT) is present in most tissues, and this cytoplasmic enzyme methylates the C-3 hydroxyl group of norepinephrine and epinephrine, resulting in the formation of **normetanephrine** and **metanephrine,** respectively (Figure 27-3).

However, most catecholamines under normal conditions undergo deamination by the ubiquitous mitochondrial MAO to 3-methoxy-4-hydroxymandelic aldehyde. This latter intermediate exists only transiently and is oxidized rapidly to vanillylmandelic acid (VMA) or reduced to **3-methoxy-4-hydroxyphenylglycol (MHPG),** both of which subsequently are excreted. When oxidative deamination of catecholamines occurs first, as in adrenergic nerve endings, dihydroxymandelic aldehyde results. Oxidation and reduction of this transient intermediate and subsequent *O*-methylation by COMT yield the excretory products VMA and MHPG, respectively (see Figure 27-3). Regardless of the nature of the initial enzymatic attack, the principal end product of both norepinephrine and epinephrine metabolism is VMA. MHPG is produced to a lesser degree, except in the brain, where it is the major metabolic end product of norepinephrine. Therefore urinary measurements of these acid metabolites, primarily VMA, reflect the total rather than the differential production of norepinephrine and epinephrine in the body. The final metabolite of dopamine after oxidative deamination and *O*-methylation is homovanillic acid (HVA; Figure 27-4).

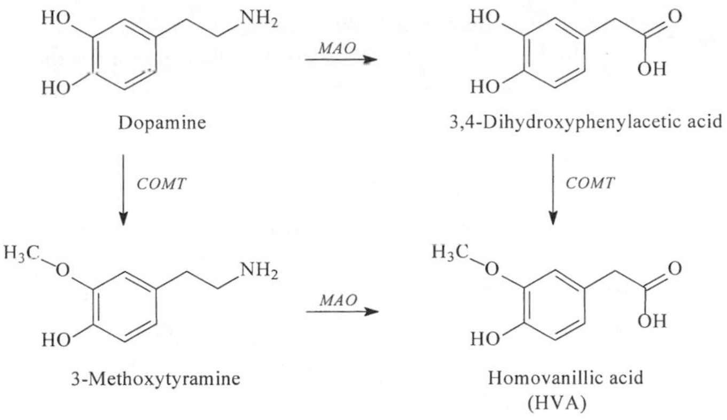

Figure 27-4 Metabolism of dopamine. *COMT,* Catechol–*O*–methyl transferase; *MAO,* monoamine oxidase.

Clinical Significance

Normal production and release of catecholamines play important roles in maintenance of health, whereas catecholamine excess or deficiency is associated with a number of disease states. For example, excess catecholamines are found with a fall in blood pressure or blood volume, thyroid hormone deficiency, congestive heart failure, arrhythmias, and stress; low levels of catecholamines are seen in individuals with idiopathic postural hypotension. Clinical laboratory measurements of epinephrine, norepinephrine, or their metabolites, however, are used primarily in the diagnosis of catecholamine-secreting neurochromaffin tumors (pheochromocytomas, paragangliomas, or neuroblastomas) as described in the following sections.[1]

Pheochromocytomas

Benign or malignant **pheochromocytomas** arise from neurochromaffin cells in the autonomic nervous system or the adrenal medulla. These tumors usually produce excessive amounts of catecholamines or catecholamine metabolites. Such tumors are rare, occurring in only 0.1% to 0.3% of the population; up to 75% of these tumors are found initially at autopsy, having gone undetected before death. However, when the classic findings of catecholamine excess occur (that is, sustained or paroxysmal hypertension, weight loss, "spells" of sweating, headache, palpitations, and anxiety), the clinical picture is obvious. Diagnosis requires a high degree of clinical suspicion, with confirmation by determination of elevated catecholamine levels, metabolite levels, or both in plasma or urine.[9] Although life threatening, this condition usually is curable with surgery.

In adults, 90% of pheochromocytomas occur in the adrenal medulla, and 10% of these adrenal tumors may be bilateral. The 10% that occur in extraadrenal sites are known as *paragangliomas.* Pheochromocytoma occurs at any age but is most common in the fourth and fifth decades of life. It is slightly more common in women than in men. In addition, 9 of 10 pheochromocytomas in adults are benign; hormonally "silent" tumors are more likely to be malignant. Malignant and bilateral tumors occur more frequently in children. Although hypertension is a common symptom in individuals with pheochromocytoma, this tumor is not a common cause of hypertension and accounts for less than 0.5% of all cases of hypertension. Pheochromocytomas are familial in about 10% of cases, usually occurring in families with histories of multiple endocrine neoplasia syndromes.

Because of a number of factors, the performance of one test of a single catecholamine or metabolite is unsatisfactory for biochemical detection or confirmation of a diagnosis of pheochromocytoma.[5] For example, circulating catecholamines, such as norepinephrine, have short half-lives, and their levels in plasma usually reflect only a small fraction of the concentration of norepinephrine at the synaptic nerve ending. Rapid and noticeable increases in plasma catecholamine concentration may be induced by stress, upright posture, exercise, hypoglycemia, hypovolemia, cold, hypoxia, hypercapnia, or the mental states of anxiety and anger. In addition, a diurnal variation of catecholamine level exists, with the zenith occurring in the morning and the nadir at night. Medications also may change catecholamine concentrations through their usual pharmacological mechanisms of action. For example, α- and β-adrenergic blockers, vasodilators, and theophylline increase norepinephrine levels, whereas adrenergic neuron blockers, clonidine, α-methyldopa, bromocriptine, and phenothiazines decrease the levels of norepinephrine. Other factors that further complicate the selection of these tests include drug interference with specific assay procedures and the conditions of sample collection. In individuals with pheochromocytoma the release of catecholamines by the tumor may be intermittent, or the uptake and degradation of catecholamines by the tumor may be so great that normal or near-normal concentrations of catecholamines are measured in blood and urine when striking increases in catecholamine metabolites are observable in urine.

The measurement of urinary metanephrines is considered the single most sensitive screening test for pheochromocytoma. Several large studies have found this test produces almost no false-negative results (nearly 100% clinical sensitivity). This high degree of clinical sensitivity may be due to preferential metabolism of tumor-secreted catecholamines through the extraneuronal pathway catalyzed by COMT. Therefore tumor-secreted catecholamines may be metabolized preferentially to metanephrines through the extraneuronal pathway, whereas normal metabolism leads primarily to VMA. Although this action leads to a sensitive diagnostic test, the measurement of urinary metanephrines is not specific for pheochromocytoma. False-positive test results often are seen in times of severe stress, such as in individuals with critical illnesses. To maximize diagnostic sensitivity and specificity, measurements of VMA and free catecholamines in urine also usually are included in the initial assessment. These tests are slightly less sensitive and yield more false-negative results but are more specific and yield fewer false-positive results than do metanephrine measurements. For urinary assays, a 24-hour collection is desirable and provides an "integrated" picture of catecholamine production over time. Overnight or untimed (random) collections also are useable, provided that results are expressed per gram of creatinine.

Measurement of plasma catecholamines and metanephrines also has been used in the detection of pheochromocytoma. Some clinicians have advocated the measurement of plasma catecholamines as an alternative initial test before urinary measurements.[3] Conditions of sampling, however, are very important and should be standardized. Impaired renal function may affect the specificity of plasma metanephrine test results and should be considered in the interpretation of plasma test results. If measurements of basal catecholamines and metabolites fail to establish or exclude the diagnosis of pheochromocytoma, pharmacological tests to suppress catecholamines may be considered.

Neuroblastomas

Neuroblastoma is one of the most common malignant tumors in children. Approximately 80% of these neoplasms are found in children younger than 5 years of age. Rapid growth and widespread metastasis are characteristic manifestations of neuroblastomas. More than 90% of these tumors are associated with excessive production of catecholamines and catecholamine metabolites. Consequently, assays of urinary catecholamine excretion are helpful in (1) screening, (2) establishment of a diagnosis, and (3) following of the results of treatment. Norepinephrine (but not epinephrine), VMA, HVA, and dopamine may be excreted in increased amounts, and increased dopamine excretion is particularly characteristic of neuroblastoma.

Orthostatic (postural) hypotension

Orthostatic hypotension is a drop in blood pressure that is precipitated by changes in body position. Under normal circumstances, postural stress is not associated with a significant decrease in blood pressure. However, when blood pressure drops excessively after the individual assumes an upright posture, a dysfunction of the sympathetic nervous system should be considered. Measurements of plasma norepinephrine levels provide a means for diagnosis and classification of patients with orthostatic hypotension. Normally, the supine norepinephrine concentration increases twofold to threefold when the individual assumes a standing position. A decrease in blood pressure, coupled with a failure to increase plasma norepinephrine on standing, suggests a sympathetic nervous system disorder.

Psychopathology

The clinical significance of determination of norepinephrine and its metabolites in depressed individuals results from the hypothesis that a norepinephrine deficiency at critical CNS synapses underlies the cyclical emergence of depression in many individuals with affective disorders. Abnormal levels of catecholamines and their metabolites have been reported in a number of mood affective disorders. For example, MHPG, a major metabolite of norepinephrine in the brain, has been evaluated in plasma, urine, and cerebrospinal fluid for the diagnosis of anxiety disorders, as a possible marker for depression, and for prediction of the outcome of treatment with tricyclic antidepressants. Several investigators have demonstrated that individuals with low urinary excretion of MHPG exhibit favorable therapeutic responses to antidepressant drug therapy.

Analytical Methodology

Numerous methods have been developed for the determination of catecholamines and their metabolites in biological fluids.[9] They include fluorometric and spectrophotometric assays and chromatographic methods, such as gas chromatography/mass spectrometry and high-performance liquid chromatography (HPLC) with electrochemical detection. Of these, HPLC is the most widely used in clinical laboratories. Consequently, this chapter discusses HPLC methods used to measure various catecholamines and their metabolites in plasma and urine.

Plasma catecholamines

Highly sensitive, specific, and reliable assay methods are required for measurement of the normally low concentrations of epinephrine, norepinephrine, and dopamine in plasma. Both unconjugated (free) and sulfoconjugated catecholamines circulate in human plasma and are increased in plasma of individuals with pheochromocytoma. Clinical measurement of the active free form is the preferred method because of the potential influence of diet on the conjugated fraction. Earlier assays included fluorometric and radioenzymatic, details of which are provided in an expanded version of this chapter.[10] However, few laboratories now use these methods. HPLC with electrochemical detection currently is the method of choice.

Principle

Preliminary extraction and concentration of plasma is required to measure the very low levels of catecholamines found in normal subjects. The most common pretreatment involves alumina extraction, with or without an anion-exchange step. Many HPLC procedures analyze the extract with reversed-phase chromatography with ion-pairing reagents; others use cation-exchange HPLC columns to separate the extracted amines. Electrochemical detection using amperometric or coulometric measurement is used most commonly to quantify the catecholamines. With amperometric detection the catecholamines present in a portion of the column effluent in contact with the electrode surface are oxidized, resulting in a current flow and detector response. In coulometric detection the effluent passes through a reaction matrix that allows a high-efficiency oxidation of catecholamines eluted from the column.

Specimen collection and storage

Different methods of blood collection have been reported, and variations in collection techniques include the choice of anticoagulant, addition of antioxidants, and various sample-processing techniques. Standardization of posture is essential because plasma catecholamine levels increase twofold to threefold when a supine subject assumes an upright position. Most procedures recommend that morning specimens be drawn from subjects who have been resting quietly for 30 minutes in the recumbent position after insertion of a venous catheter. In addition, subjects should refrain from eating, using tobacco, or drinking coffee or tea for at least 4 hours before venipuncture. If possible, specimens should be obtained from individuals who are drug free. Most antihypertensive drugs (other than clonidine) and many other drugs have produced false-positive results (see expanded chapter for list of interfering drugs).[10] Use of these drugs should be discontinued 3 to 7 days before the sample is obtained. If hypertension must be treated before measurement of catecholamines, then clonidine is the preferred drug because it does not produce a false-positive result.

Catecholamines in general are unstable compounds that are oxidized readily. To prevent oxidation, many procedures recommend that blood samples be transported to the laboratory on ice and centrifuged at 4 °C within 30 minutes of collection. The plasma is removed and frozen at −70 °C until analysis. Two anticoagulants are used commonly, heparin and ethylenediaminetetraacetic acid (EDTA), with or without the addition of antioxidants, such as glutathione or metabisulfite. At −70 °C, catecholamines in heparin or EDTA plasma are stable for at least 8 months without the addition of preservatives.

Reference intervals

As the following table demonstrates, normal physiological levels of plasma catecholamines are affected by body position.

Position	Norepinephrine pg/mL (pmol/L)	Epinephrine pg/mL (pmol/L)	Dopamine pg/mL (pmol/L)
Supine (30 min)	110 to 410 (650-2423)	<50 (<273)	<87 (<475)
Sitting (15 min)	120 to 680 (709-4019)	<60 (<328)	<87 (<475)
Standing (30 min)	125 to 700 (739-4137)	<90 (<491)	<87 (<475)

Urinary catecholamines

Catecholamines are excreted in the urine as free amines and glucuronide and sulfate conjugates. As with plasma measurements, total urinary catecholamines (conjugated and unconjugated forms) may be measured by hydrolysis of the sample before assay. However, free amines relate more closely to the tumor load of pheochromocytoma than do conjugated catecholamines and are least affected by dietary catechols. Therefore measurement of the free hormone is recommended. Consequently, most methods omit the hydrolysis step and measure only the free hormone.

HPLC procedures are used in routine practice because of their sensitivity and ability to quantitate specific catecholamines. HPLC methods use either reversed-phase chromatography with ion-pair reagent or ion-exchange chromatography, and electrochemical detection using either amperometric or coulometric measurement are used most commonly. All methods require removal of interfering substances before the catecholamines are quantitated. Ion-exchange chromatography, absorption chromatography, or a combination of both are the most common extraction techniques.

Principle

After protein precipitation with perchloric acid, an aliquot of a 24-hour urine collection (preserved in acid) first is applied to a weak-acid cation-exchange resin. Unconjugated catecholamines are adsorbed selectively at pH 6.5 and then eluted with dilute boric acid (pH 4.0). An intermediate water wash removes interfering urine impurities. Subsequent resolution of the individual catecholamines is achieved by reversed-phase, paired-ion HPLC under optimized isocratic conditions. Alkyl-bonded silica is used as the nonpolar stationary phase, and an organic/aqueous buffer mixture (pH 2.8) is used as the polar mobile phase. To enhance the affinity of the polar catecholamines for the hydrophobic stationary phase, an ion of opposite charge (octyl sodium sulfonate) also is included in the mobile phase. This "counter-ion" is capable of forming uncharged ion pair conjugates with catecholamine cations before partitioning into the lipophilic stationary phase. The reversed-phase column then has the physical characteristics of a conventional ion-exchange resin.

A thin-layer glassy carbon or carbon-paste working electrode, in conjunction with a silver-silver chloride reference electrode and a stainless steel auxiliary electrode, are used as the amperometric detection system. Each catecholamine passing through the detector cell undergoes a rapid two-electron oxidation at a fixed potential to form an o-quinone, as follows:

The resulting current is converted to a voltage signal and monitored as a function of time. At a constant temperature and flow rate, this oxidation current is directly proportional to the concentration of the analyte.

Catecholamine reference materials that have been checked previously for purity are used to calibrate the system on the basis of peak heights and retention times. To calculate sample concentrations, peak height ratios relative to an internal standard (for example, dihydroxybenzylamine) for unknowns are compared with those of the calibrations.

Specimen collection and storage

All antihypertensive medications should be withheld from the individual for at least 2 days before and during specimen collection. If the subject cannot be removed completely from a drug regimen, the test still may be performed as long as the results are evaluated with an understanding of the expected physiological response to the drug or drugs.

A complete 24-hour urine sample is collected in a container with 10 mL of hydrochloric acid (HCl), 6 mol/L, added as a preservative. The specimen should be refrigerated during collection. The total urine volume is measured and recorded; a 100-mL aliquot is stored in the refrigerator until the test is performed or frozen and stored indefinitely.

Reference intervals

Reference intervals depend on age and are expressed as daily output or normalized for creatinine excretion.[8] Normalized excretion data are used frequently during testing of newborns and children but also may be used when random specimens are collected after an adult's hypertensive episode.

Age (y)	Urinary Daily Excretion µg/day (nmol/day)		
	Norepinephrine	Epinephrine	Dopamine
Children			
0 to 1	0 to 10 (0-59)	0 to 2.5 (0-14)	0 to 85 (0-555)
1 to 2	1 to 17 (6-100)	0 to 3.5 (0-19)	10 to 140 (65-914)
2 to 4	4 to 29 (24-171)	0 to 6.0 (0-33)	40 to 260 (261-1697)
4 to 7	8 to 45 (47-266)	0.2 to 10 (1-55)	65 to 400 (424-2612)
7 to 10	13 to 65 (77-384)	0.2 to 10 (1-55)	65 to 400 (424-2612)
10 to 15	15 to 80 (89-473)	0.5 to 20 (3-109)	65 to 400 (424-2612)
Adults >15	15 to 80 (89-473)	0.5 to 20 (3-109)	65 to 400 (424-2612)

Age (y)	Daily Excretion Relative to Creatinine µg/g Creatinine		
	Norepinephrine	Epinephrine	Dopamine
0 to 1	up to 0.31	up to 0.38	up to 1.29
1 to 4	up to 0.29	up to 0.08	up to 1.22
4 to 10	up to 0.11	up to 0.09	up to 0.72
10 to 18	up to 0.11	up to 0.06	up to 0.45
>18	up to 0.11	up to 0.04	up to 0.35

Urinary metanephrine and normetanephrine

Metanephrines are excreted in urine as free amines and glucuronide and sulfate conjugates. Unlike the catecholamines, metanephrine excretion is not influenced significantly by diet, and most procedures measure total metanephrine level (including conjugated and unconjugated forms) by hydrolysis of the urine before assay. An initial purification step is required to isolate the hydrolyzed metanephrines from the sample matrix. Weak cation-exchange resins are used predominantly in sample cleanup, although some procedures use a combination of strong and weak cation exchange to enhance recovery. Differential solvent extraction methods (for example, use of ethyl acetate, cyclohexane) also have been applied to remove potential interferences. Although photometric, fluorometric, radioenzymatic, and gas chromatography methods have been used to measure metanephrine and normetanephrine, HPLC has become the most commonly used technique.

Procedures based on HPLC techniques offer practical alternatives to other methods. Although native fluorescence and ultraviolet absorption have been used to quantify metanephrine concentrations, most HPLC procedures are based on electrochemical detection. Column conditions and stationary phases vary; typical applications include reversed-phase chromatography with ion-pairing reagents and silica-based cation-exchange chromatography. The combination of a preliminary extraction procedure, HPLC separation, and electrochemical detection makes these analyses highly selective.

Principle

An aliquot of urine is combined with an internal standard (4-O-methyldopamine), and the mixture is hydrolyzed with acid to convert all the metanephrines to their free, unconjugated forms. Isolation of metanephrines from the sample matrix is accomplished with two disposable minicolumns. The hydrolyzed urines, diluted with an ammonium pentaborate buffer, first are applied to a weak acid cation-exchange resin. The adsorbed metanephrines then are eluted with ammonium hydroxide directly onto a strong quaternary amine anion-exchange column, which separates the metanephrines from nonphenolic amines and more hydrophobic phenolic compounds. The final elution uses a weak ammonium acetate buffer; the eluate then is injected onto a reversed-phase HPLC system. Electrochemical detection is used to quantify metanephrine and normetanephrine separately.

Specimen collection and storage

A complete 24-hour urine specimen is collected in a clean container that has acid as a stabilizing preservative (for example, 10 mL of HCl, 6 mol/L). The specimen should be refrigerated during collection. Overnight or untimed (random) urine collections should be acidified to a pH between 1 and 3 immediately after collection. The total urine volume is measured and recorded after collection, and a 50-mL aliquot is reserved for analysis. Samples are refrigerated until the test is performed or frozen for long-term storage.

Reference intervals

Reference intervals depend on age and are expressed as daily output and also normalized for creatinine excretion in the newborn and pediatric population.

Age	Normetanephrine*		Metanephrine*	
	μg/Day	μg/g Creatinine	μg/Day	μg/g Creatinine
0 to 3 mo	47 to 156	1535 to 3355	5.9 to 37	202 to 708
4 to 6 mo	31 to 111	737 to 2194	6.1 to 42	156 to 572
7 to 9 mo	42 to 109	592 to 1046	12 to 41	150 to 526
10 to 12 mo	23 to 103	271 to 1117	8.5 to 101	148 to 651
1 to 2 y	32 to 118	350 to 1275	6.7 to 52	40 to 526
2 to 6 y	50 to 111	104 to 609	11 to 99	74 to 504
6 to 10 y	47 to 176	103 to 452	54 to 138	121 to 319
10 to 16 y	53 to 290	96 to 411	39 to 242	46 to 307
Adult	105 to 354		74 to 297	

* Free plus conjugated.

Vanillylmandelic acid in urine

Vanillylmandelic acid (VMA) is a major catecholamine metabolite that represents about 60% of the total excretion products derived from norepinephrine and epinephrine. Unlike metanephrines, VMA is not conjugated significantly and is measured without a hydrolysis step. Immunoassay methods have been developed, and photometric, chromatographic, and electrophoretic methods also have been used to measure VMA in urine. Historically, the direct vanillin method has been used extensively to measure VMA in urine, but HPLC is the most frequently used method in current practice.

Most HPLC procedures for measurement of VMA in urine use reversed-phase separation with a variety of monitoring systems, including ultraviolet, fluorometric, electrochemical, or postcolumn reaction. HPLC procedures are relatively free of interferences and do not require the stringent dietary restrictions necessary for the less specific photometric methods. The HPLC method may be adapted for simultaneous measurement of other catecholamine metabolites, such as HVA, metanephrines, or MHPG. For overall sensitivity, accuracy, reproducibility, and speed of analysis, HPLC with electrochemical detection is the method of choice.[2]

Principle

An aliquot of urine is mixed with an internal standard (isovanillylmandelic acid [iso-VMA]) and then applied to a strongly basic anion-exchange resin that has been preconditioned with an acetate buffer. Uric acid and hydrophobic acids, such as HVA, are removed from the cleanup column during an acetic acid-ethanol wash step. VMA and iso-VMA are eluted with a phosphoric acid solution and subsequently resolved by reversed-phase HPLC under isocratic conditions. The VMA concentration is determined electro-

chemically with an amperometric or coulometric detection system.

Specimen collection and storage

A complete 24-hour urine collection is recommended because variations in VMA excretion occur throughout the day. Shorter collection times may be useful, provided that VMA results are expressed per milligram of creatinine. The urine should be collected in a clean container with acid as a stabilizing preservative (for example, 10 mL of HCl, 6 mol/L, for a 24 hour collection). The specimen should be refrigerated during and after collection. The total urine volume is measured and recorded; a 50-mL aliquot is stored at 4 °C until the test is performed or may be frozen for long-term storage. No dietary restrictions during urine collection are necessary.

Reference intervals

Age (y)	mg VMA/Day	mg VMA/g Creatinine
3 to 6	1.0 to 2.6	4.0 to 10.8
6 to 10	2.0 to 3.2	4.0 to 7.5
10 to 16	2.3 to 5.2	3.0 to 8.8
16 to 83	1.4 to 6.5	

Homovanillic acid in urine

Homovanillic acid (HVA) is the principal urinary metabolite of DOPA and dopamine. Tests for urinary HVA excretion have been used for the diagnosis and management of neuroblastomas. Several spectrophotometric and chromatographic methods are used to assay HVA. Most of the earlier photometric procedures were based on the nonspecific reaction of nitrosonaphthol with biogenic amines. Chromatographic methods, such as gas chromatography, gas chromatography/mass spectrometry, and HPLC have been used to measure HVA in biological fluids. HPLC methods are the most popular, and most use a reversed-phase HPLC column and detection of the HVA peak by ultraviolet or fluorescence spectrometry or amperometry.

HPLC methods with electrochemical detection are sensitive, show little interference from endogenous or exogenous organic acids, and may provide simultaneous measurement of VMA and other metabolites. However, the speed of analysis usually is increased if HVA is analyzed separately. (An HPLC/electrochemical method, using the hydrophobic extract from the VMA procedure described in the previous section, will be described in the following section.)

Principle

An aliquot of urine is mixed with an internal standard (iso-VMA) and then applied to a strongly basic anion-exchange resin preconditioned with an acetate buffer. HVA is eluted with acetic acid in ethanol and subsequently resolved by reversed-phase HPLC under optimized isocratic conditions. The HVA concentration is determined electrochemically through an amperometric detection system.

Specimen collection and storage

A complete 24-hour urine collection is recommended because variations in HVA excretion occur throughout the day. Shorter collection times may be useful, provided that HVA results are expressed per milligram of creatinine. The urine should be collected in a clean container that has acid as a stabilizing preservative (for example, 10 mL of HCl, 6 mol/L, for a 24-hour collection). The specimen should be refrigerated during and after collection. The total urine volume is measured and recorded; a 50-mL aliquot is stored at 4 °C until the test is performed or may be frozen and stored indefinitely. No dietary restrictions are necessary.

Reference intervals

Age (y)	mg HVA/Day	mg HVA/g Creatinine
3 to 6	1.4 to 4.3	5.4 to 15.5
6 to 10	2.1 to 4.7	4.4 to 11.5
10 to 16	2.4 to 8.7	3.3 to 10.3
16 to 83	1.4 to 8.8	

3-Methoxy-4-hydroxyphenylglycol in urine

As discussed previously, MHPG is an important metabolite of norepinephrine that may have particular relevance to the disposition of norepinephrine in the brain. In humans, MHPG is found in cerebrospinal fluid, urine, and plasma. In urine, MHPG is present mainly in the form of sulfate and glucuronide conjugates, and only a small proportion of it is in the unconjugated form. Various techniques have been used to measure MHPG in urine and other body fluids, including gas chromatography with electron capture or mass spectrometric detection; HPLC with spectrophotometric, fluorescence, or electrochemical detection; and fluorescence polarization immunoassay. In most early clinical studies, MHPG was measured in urine by use of gas chromatography, but liquid chromatography is more suited for routine analysis of urine and plasma samples.

Principle

Reliable HPLC procedures have been described for measurement of total MHPG levels. Most require enzyme hydrolysis of urinary conjugates, followed by a multistep organic solvent extraction, isocratic separation on a reversed-phase column, and quantification using electrochemical detection (amperometry or coulometry). In general, HPLC assays provide a high degree of recovery, reproducibility, and specificity.

Specimen collection and storage

Plasma is obtained more easily than is urine or cerebrospinal fluid and is becoming the preferred specimen for the determination of MHPG. Plasma contains both free (20% to 30%) and conjugated MHPG, and several methods have been described for measurement of the free hormone.

Reference intervals

The adult reference interval for total MHPG (free and conjugated) in a 24-hour urine sample collected without preservatives is 0.9 to 3.5 mg/day. The reference values for free (unconjugated) MHPG in heparin or EDTA plasma are, for the adult man, 3.57 ± 0.97 µg/L ($\pm$SD) and, for the adult woman, 3.68 ± 0.90 µg/L ($\pm$SD).

■ SEROTONIN AND 5-HYDROXYINDOLEACETIC ACID

Serotonin (5-hydroxytryptamine [5-HT]) is found in various animals, from coelenterates to vertebrates, in bacteria, and in many plants. In humans, it is synthesized in the intestinal **chromaffin cells** in central or peripheral neurons and is found in high concentrations in many body tissues, including the intestinal mucosa, pineal gland, and CNS.

Biochemistry and Physiology

Serotonin is a derivative of tryptophan and functions as a powerful smooth-muscle stimulant and vasoconstrictor. It is transported in the blood by platelets. The formation and breakdown of serotonin is depicted in Figure 27-5. As indicated, tryptophan first is hydroxylated to form 5-hydroxytryptophan (5-HTP). Approximately 1% to 3% of dietary tryptophan normally is metabolized by this pathway. The 5-HTP then is decarboxylated to 5-HT. The enzymatic decarboxylation is very active in carcinoid tumors. Pharmacologically, 5-HT is the most active indole amine; however, its biological activity apparently is lost when it is bound to tissues or platelets.[11] It rapidly undergoes oxidative deamination in a tumor or in the blood after release from a tumor.

The oxidative deamination of serotonin by the enzyme MAO leads to the formation of **5-hydroxyindoleacetic acid (5-HIAA),** which is quantitatively the most significant metabolite of the 5-hydroxyindole pathway. Most of the 5-HIAA is excreted in the free form, although a small amount may be conjugated as the *o*-sulfate ester before excretion.

Clinical Significance

Clinically, serotonin plays a role in depression and carcinoid tumors.

Depression

The most important physiological role of serotonin is that of a transmitter in serotoninergic neurons within the brain. In humans, serotonin has been implicated in a variety of behavioral patterns, including sleep, perception of pain, social behavior, schizophrenia, and mental depression. Many studies have indicated that alterations in serotonin-

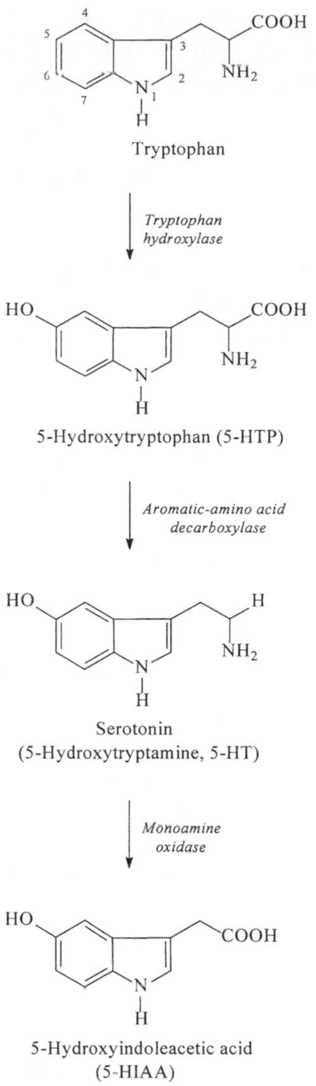

Figure 27-5 Biosynthesis and metabolism of serotonin.

ergic neuronal function in the CNS occur in individuals with major depression.[6] Evidence for this relationship comes from (1) numerous reports of diminished levels of 5-HIAA in the cerebrospinal fluid of depressed individuals, (2) reduced concentrations of 5-HT and 5-HIAA in postmortem brain tissue of depressed individuals, and (3) the observation that 5-HTP, a precursor of 5-HT, is an effective antidepressant only in depressed subjects with decreased cerebrospinal fluid 5-HIAA concentrations. Furthermore, in such serotonin-deficient individuals, treatment with antidepressant drugs, such as amitriptyline and trazodone, elicits a favorable clinical response. These pharmacological agents inhibit the reuptake of 5-HT by the presynaptic neurons, thereby increasing the concentration of 5-HT at serotoninergic synapses. Drugs that selectively inhibit serotonin reuptake are used with increasing frequency in the treatment of depression and

are a safer alternative to earlier tricyclic antidepressant drugs.

Carcinoid tumors

A **carcinoid tumor** is a serotonin-secreting neoplasm. In a large study, carcinoid tumors were found in 1% of individuals at autopsy, but 90% of the tumors found had not been suspected premortem. Carcinoid tumors usually arise in the small intestine, appendix, or rectum; individuals often have bleeding, obstruction, or metastases, but humoral manifestations vary with the site of origin of the tumor.

Carcinoid tumors develop from enterochromaffin cells, which are distributed widely throughout the gastrointestinal tract, biliary tract and gallbladder, pancreatic ducts, and bronchial tree. These cells also are found in the thymus, thyroid gland, ovary, uterus, and salivary glands. Carcinoid tumors occur in any of these sites.

The production and metabolism of serotonin varies in relation to the tissue of origin of the tumor. Tumors from midgut cells, such as ileal carcinoid tumors, usually contain and release large quantities of 5-HT, and individuals with these tumors have elevated urinary 5-HIAA levels. Tumors derived from foregut cells (bronchial, pancreatic, duodenal, or biliary carcinoid cells) secrete primarily 5-HTP, which may be converted to serotonin and its metabolites by other tissues in the body. Tumors derived from hindgut cells (rectal carcinoid) only rarely produce excess 5-HTP, 5-HT, or 5-HIAA.

The classic clinical presentation of **carcinoid syndrome** includes pronounced flushing, bronchial constriction, diarrhea, and cardiac valvular lesions and often is associated with right-sided heart failure.[7] Not all such manifestations are explained by serotonin excess, but carcinoid tumors often produce excesses of other substances as well, including histamine, bradykinin, prostaglandins, and vasoactive peptides called *tachykinins*. In some instances, carcinoid tumors may coexist with other endocrine tumors that produce gastrin, insulin, adrenocorticotropic hormone, and catecholamines. Carcinoid tumors also may be associated with multiple endocrine neoplasia type 1 (MEN-1), an inherited predisposition to hyperparathyroidism and pituitary and pancreatic adenomas.

Individuals with functioning carcinoid tumors usually have large increases in urinary excretion of 5-HIAA (>25 mg/day, compared with normal levels of <6 mg/day). If a borderline elevation of 5-HIAA is found (6 to 15 mg/day), repeat collections should be made and care taken that the individual avoid foods and medications that might elevate 5-HIAA (for example, pineapples, avocados, bananas, walnuts, chocolate, guaifenesin, and reserpine). Nontropical sprue may cause a slight increase in urinary 5-HIAA concentration. 5-HIAA levels are lowered by phenothiazines, in cases of renal insufficiency, and after small-bowel resection.

When an individual strongly suspect for carcinoid syndrome shows normal or only borderline increases of 5-HIAA, one of the following two possibilities should be considered

1. The large amounts of serotonin produced are not being metabolized, in which case measurement of 5-HTP or 5-HT is necessary to document the diagnosis.[4]
2. Secretion of 5-HIAA by the tumor is intermittent, in which case repeat specimen collections and serial measurements are needed to demonstrate the abnormality.

Analytical Methodology

A variety of methods have been developed to measure serotonin and 5-HIAA in blood and urine.

Serotonin measurement

Spectrophotometry, fluorometry, immunoassay, gas chromatography, and HPLC have been used to measure 5-HT in body fluids and platelets, with the latter being the method of choice.

Principle

For sensitive and specific determination of 5-HT, HPLC is the preferred method; systems using fluorometric, spectrophotometric, and electrochemical detection have been described for platelet-rich plasma, serum, and whole blood. Both reversed-phase and cation-exchange stationary phases have been used.

Specimen collection and storage

Whole-blood serotonin is unstable and should be preserved by mixing of blood (10 mL) with 10 mg EDTA and 75 mg ascorbic acid and immediate freezing of the mixture. Platelets contain almost all the serotonin found in blood. To obtain platelet-rich plasma, venous blood is collected with EDTA and promptly centrifuged at $150 \times g$ for 20 minutes at 4 °C. Preparation of platelet pellets from the platelet-rich plasma, which then is stored frozen until assayed, also is possible.

Reference intervals

The reference interval for serotonin in whole blood is 50 to 200 ng/mL (0.28 to 1.14 μmol/L); in platelets, it is 125 to 500 ng/10^9 platelets (0.7 to 2.8 micromol/platelet).

5-Hydroxyindoleacetic acid

Estimation of the parent hormone (5-HT) in blood and urine has been limited severely in the clinical laboratory because of its very low concentration and methodological complications. As a result, the urinary determination of 5-HIAA is available more readily and continues to be the most frequently used test for the diagnosis of carcinoid tumors. In such cases this serotonin metabolite is excreted in

very large amounts, often exceeding 350 mg/day, and a positive result is obtained on simple qualitative (screening) tests. However, for early diagnosis when tumors are small and have not metastasized, and in some carcinoid tumors for which the excretion values barely exceed 8 mg, the more sensitive and specific quantitative test is required.

Screening method for 5-hydroxyindoleacetic acid

Historically, photometric methods have been used for qualitative screening methods with nitrosonaphthol/nitrous acid or dimethylaminobenzaldehyde (Ehrlich's aldehyde) reagent.

Principle

This test is based on the development of a purple color when 5-hydroxyindoles react with 1-nitroso-2-naphthol and nitrous acid. Other interfering chromogens are extracted into ethylene dichloride.

Specimen collection and storage

A random urine specimen usually is suitable for this screening method. For quantitative analysis a 24-hour urine specimen is collected without preservatives. The specimen should be refrigerated during and after collection. When it is received in the laboratory, the urine specimen is mixed thoroughly and the total volume measured and recorded. If desired, aliquots may be removed at this time for determination of acid-labile substances (for example, MHPG). The pH of the urine then is adjusted to between 2 and 3 by addition of HCl, 6 mol/L. The acidified urine can be kept at 4 °C for 2 weeks and for longer periods of time at −20 °C. False-negative results may occur in individuals taking phenothiazine drugs. The ingestion of foods high in hydroxyindole content (for example, bananas, avocados, red plums, eggplants, pineapples, kiwi fruit, walnuts, hickory nuts, tomatoes) or cough medications containing glycerol guaiacolate may lead to false-positive results. Therefore individuals should be restricted from using these drugs and foods 3 to 4 days before and during the collection.

Reference interval

A test result is considered negative when the 5-HIAA urine level is less than 25 mg/day (<131 μmol/day).

Quantitative 5-hydroxyindoleacetic acid methods

For quantitative measurement of 5-HIAA a number of techniques are available, including photometry, fluorometry, gas chromatography, radioimmunoassay, fluorescence polarization immunoassay, and HPLC. Many variations of the latter are available; some use fluorometric detection, with or without derivatization, but most use electrochemical detection. Liquid chromatography with electrochemical detection is preferred for specific measurement of very small quantities of 5-HIAA.

Principle of photometric method

With this method, 5-HIAA, other phenolic acids, and drug metabolites are extracted into diethyl ether from acidified urine; a saturating amount of sodium chloride is added to promote quantitative transfer into the ether phase. The 5-HIAA then is back-extracted into a phosphate buffer (0.1 mol/L, pH 7) and reacted with nitrosonaphthol and nitrous acid at 37 °C to form a violet color. Phosphate buffer at pH 7 is chosen for efficient extraction because 5-HIAA becomes progressively more unstable at higher pH values. Urinary phenols lacking an acid group are not ionized at pH 7 and remain behind in the ether layer, thereby providing a relatively clean extract. An intense blue chromophore is formed rapidly on subsequent addition of 2-mercaptoethanol, as follows:

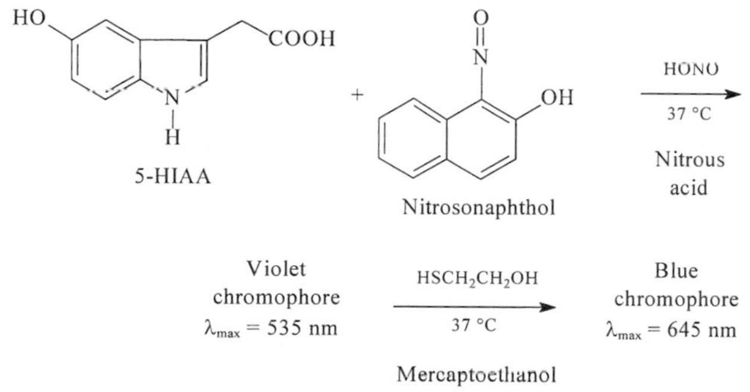

Extraneous absorbance, caused by reactive phenols and indoleacetic acid, is removed by treatment with the mercaptoethanol and extraction into ethyl acetate. The absorbance maximum of the remaining blue solution occurs at 645 nm, but measurements usually are made at 590 nm, at which Beer's law is obeyed through a suitable range of 5-HIAA concentration.

Principle of high-performance liquid chromatography method

Diluted urine samples are analyzed without sample preparation by use of reversed-phase HPLC with electrochemical detection.

Specimen collection and storage

The collection and storage procedure described previously for the screening method for 5-HIAA is applicable for the quantitative analysis of 5-HIAA.

Reference interval

The 5-HIAA reference interval for adults is 2.0 to 7.0 mg/day (10.4 to 35.6 μmol/day).

References

1. Benowitz NL: Pheochromocytoma. Adv Intern Med 1990; 35:195-219.
2. Bonfigli AR, Coppa G, Testa R et al: Determination of vanillylmandelic, 5-hydroxyindoleacetic and homovanillic acid in urine by isocratic liquid chromatography. Eur J Clin Chem Clin Biochem 1997; 35:57-61.
3. Bravo EL: Evolving concepts in the pathophysiology, diagnosis, and treatment of pheochromocytoma. Endocr Rev 1994; 15:356-368.
4. Kema IP, deVries EGE, Schellings AMJ et al: Improved diagnosis of carcinoid tumors by measurement of platelet serotonin. Clin Chem 1992; 38:534-540.
5. Klee GG: Maximizing efficacy of endocrine tests: importance of decision-focused testing strategies and appropriate patient preparation. Clin Chem 1999; 45(8 Part 2):1323-1330.
6. Owens MJ, Nemeroff CB: Role of serotonin in the pathophysiology of depression: focus on the serotonin transporter. Clin Chem 1994; 40:288-295.
7. Roberts LJ, Anthony LB, Oates JA: Disorders of vasodilator hormones: the carcinoid syndrome and mastocytosis. In Wilson JD, Foster DW, Kronenberg HM et al (eds): Williams Textbook of Endocrinology, 9th edition, pp 1711-1732, Philadelphia, WB Saunders, 1998.
8. Rosano TG: Liquid-chromatographic evaluation of age-related changes in the urinary excretion of free catecholamines in pediatric patients. Clin Chem 1984; 30:301-303.
9. Rosano TG, Swift TA, Hayes LW: Advances in catecholamine and metabolite measurements for diagnosis of pheochromocytomas. Clin Chem 1991; 37:1854-1867.
10. Rosano TG, Whitley RJ: Catecholamine and Serotonin. In Burtis CA, Ashwood ER (eds): Tietz Textbook of Clinical Chemistry, 3rd edition, pp 1570-1600, Philadelphia, WB Saunders, 1999.
11. Saxena PR: Serotonin receptors: subtypes, functional responses and therapeutic relevance. Pharmacol Ther 1995; 66:339-368.
12. Young JB, Landsberg L: Catecholamines and the adrenal medulla. In Wilson JD, Foster DW, Kronenberg HM et al (eds): Williams Textbook of Endocrinology, 9th edition, pp 665-728, Philadelphia, WB Saunders, 1998.

Additional Reading

Goldstein DS: Stress, Catecholamines and Cardiovascular Disease. New York, Oxford University Press, 1995.

Kotulak R: Inside the Brain: Revolutionary Discoveries of How the Mind Works, Kansas City, Mo, Andrews & McMeel, 1996.

Robin NL: Clinical Handbook of Endocrinology and Metabolic Disease, Pearl River, NY, Parthenon, 1996.

Wilson JD, Foster DW, Kronenberg HM et al (eds): Williams Textbook of Endocrinology, 9th edition, Philadelphia, WB Saunders, 1998.

CHAPTER 28

Vitamins

DONALD B. McCORMICK, PhD, and GEORGE G. KLEE, MD, PhD

Objectives

1. Define *vitamin* and *vitamer*.
2. Classify the vitamins according to solubility.
3. List the natural forms of each vitamin, as well as the physiological functions, metabolism, causes, and symptoms of vitamin excess and deficiency.
4. State the methods of analysis for each vitamin, the principle of the reactions, and the possible interferences in each.

Key Words

Apoenzyme A protein moiety of an enzyme that requires a coenzyme

Avitaminosis A disease condition, described as a deficiency syndrome, resulting from lack of a vitamin

Coenzyme An organic molecule, generally derived from a vitamin, that functions catalytically in an enzyme system

Cofactor A natural reactant, usually either a metal ion or a coenzyme, required in an enzyme-catalyzed reaction

Holoenzyme A catalytically active enzyme constituted by coenzyme bound to apoenzyme

Hypervitaminosis An unhealthy condition resulting from excess of a vitamin

Hypovitaminosis An unhealthy condition resulting from too little of a vitamin; interchangeable with avitaminosis

Vitamin An essential organic micronutrient that must be supplied exogenously and in many cases is the precursor to a metabolically derived coenzyme

Vitamer A term used to describe any of a number of compounds that possess a given vitamin activity

---

Vitamins are essential nutrients that affect the health and development of humans. The word *vitamine* was coined in 1911 by Polish chemist Casimir Funk, who discovered a nutrient that was capable of curing beriberi in pigeons. He found the nutrient to be an amine and suggested that it was representative of a group of chemicals in foods that prevented various diseases when eaten in small amounts. He named them *vitamines* (*vita* meaning *life,* so *vitamines* being amines necessary for life). More vitamines were identified later and, because most of them were not amines, the *e* was dropped and these compounds have subsequently been called *vitamins.*

Although deficiency of a single vitamin is relatively uncommon in humans, it can occur because of an inborn error of metabolism or unusual restriction in dietary intake. More frequently encountered are complex deficiencies that arise because of (1) food fads; (2) complications of certain diseases, especially those affecting food absorption; (3) massive losses of blood or hemodialysis; and (4) the use of certain drugs.

Instances exist in which excessive use of vitamins is encountered. These and other influences that cause vitamin imbalances have led to an increased demand for laboratory tests for the evaluation of the vitamin status of individuals. This demand in turn has advanced the improvement and interpretation of results obtained by use of newer methods.

This chapter begins with an introduction of the definition and classification of vitamins and continues with a discussion of each vitamin individually.

■ DEFINITION OF VITAMINS

Vitamin is a general term for a number of unrelated organic substances that occur in many foods and are required in trace amounts (in microgram to milligram quantities per day) for the normal metabolic functioning of the body. They may be water or fat soluble. **Vitamer** is a term used to describe any of a number of compounds that possess a given vitamin activity. They are categorized into subclasses under the parent common or chemical name for the respective vitamin group.

TABLE 28-1   Vitamins Required by Humans*

Common Name	Trivial Chemical Name	General Roles	Symptoms of Deficiency or Disease	Direct and Indirect Assays
Fat Soluble				
Vitamin A₁ A₂	Retinol 3-Dehydroretinol	Vision, growth, reproduction	Nyctalopia, xerophthalmia, keratomalacia	Photometric, fluorometric, dark adaptation, RIA, HPLC
Vitamin D₂ D₃	Ergocalciferol Cholecalciferol	Modulation of Ca^{+2} metabolism, calcification of bone and teeth	Rickets (older infants and children), osteomalacia (adult)	CPB, HPLC, RIA
Vitamin E	Tocopherols, α, β, γ, δ Tocotrienols	Antioxidant for unsaturated lipids	Lipid peroxidation, including red-blood cell fragility, hemolytic anemia (premature, newborn)	Photometric, HPLC, erythrocyte hemolysis
Vitamin K₁ K₂	Phylloquinones Menaquinones	Blood clotting, osteocalcins	Increased clotting time, hemorrhagic disease (infant)	Photometric, HPLC, prothrombin time, RIA (abnormal prothrombin)
Water Soluble				
Vitamin B₁	Thiamine	Carbohydrate metabolism, nervous function	Beriberi, Wernicke-Korsakoff syndrome	Fluorometric, microbiological, transketolase, HPLC
Vitamin B₂	Riboflavin	Oxidation-reduced reactions	Angular stomatitis, dermatitis, photophobia	Fluorometric, HPLC, microbiological, glutathione reductase
Vitamin B₆	Pyridoxine, pyridoxal, pyridoxamine	Amino acid, phospholipid, and glycogen metabolism	Epileptiform convulsions, dermatitis, hypochromic anemia	Microbiological, HPLC, tyrosine decarboxylase
Niacin Niacinamide	Nicotinic acid Nicotinamide	Oxidation-reduction reactions	Pellagra	Microbiological, fluorometric
Folic acid	Pteroylglutamic acid	Nucleic acid and amino acid biosynthesis	Megaloblastic anemia	CPB, microbiological, immunoassay
Vitamin B₁₂	Cyanocobalamin	Amino acid and branched-chain keto acid metabolism	Pernicious and megaloblastic anemia, neuropathy	CPB, microbiological, immunoassay
Biotin	—	Carboxylation reactions	Dermatitis	Microbiological, photometric, carboxylases, avidin binding
Pantothenic acid	—	General metabolism	Burning feet syndrome	Microbiological, photometric, enzymatic, HPLC-avidin binding, CPB/HPLC
Vitamin C	Ascorbic acid	Connective tissue formation	Scurvy	Photometric, HPLC

RIA, Radioimmunoassay; *HPLC,* high-performance liquid chromatography; *CPB,* competitive protein binding.
*Only one vitamer from a vitamin group (for example, A₁ for vitamin A or pyridoxine for vitamin B₆) is sufficient for that vitamin.

Table 28-1 provides a current list of vitamins and vitameric groups essential to humans. For most of these, well-discerned levels of requirements have led to daily recommended dietary allowances (RDA) in the United States.[3,13] However, RDAs are being renamed as *Dietary Reference Intakes (DRIs)* to recognize the broad application of the information contained. The DRIs take into consideration the relationship between nutrient intake and the development of chronic diseases, creating recommendations approaching the definition of optimal intakes. This new approach differs markedly from the previously approach, which set the RDAs at levels to prevent nutrient deficiency. Guidelines that have been established for vitamins are listed in the Additional Reading section of this chapter.

CLASSIFICATION OF VITAMINS

Historically, vitamin groups, such as A, B, and D, bear an Arabic subscript number following the letter either to (1) designate structural and functional similarity (for example, A_1, [retinol] and A_2 [3-dehydroretinol]) or (2) indicate the approximate order in which they were identified as the members of the so-called B-complex (for example, B_1 [thiamine] and B_2 [riboflavin]). Common chemical names provide a better indication of the types of compounds involved. These names often reflect the presence of some specific atom (*thia*mine), the prime functional group (pyridox-*amine*), or even a larger portion of the molecular structure (phyllo*quinone*). Parts of some names reflect functional properties (for example, chole*calciferol*).

Another classification pertains to relative solubility of vitamins. Those of the "fat-soluble" group (A, D, E, and K) are more soluble in organic solvents, whereas others, such as the B-complex group vitamins and vitamin C, are "water soluble." This general separation based on solubility is useful not only for gross physical properties but also as a reminder that the fat-soluble vitamins are absorbed, transported, and stored for longer periods of time and in a manner generally similar to that for fats. Most water-soluble vitamins share the fate of other solutes more compatible with an aqueous, physiological medium; this classification includes a tendency to be retained for shorter periods of time in the body and a more rapid loss by way of urinary excretion. In addition, a general functional difference also exists because the water-soluble vitamins function as **coenzymes** for numerous important enzymatic reactions in both mammals and microorganisms. By contrast, the fat-soluble vitamins generally do not function as coenzymes and are used rarely by microorganisms.

Some vitamins have been designated in earlier or more restricted literature under other names (for example, vitamin H for biotin); in other cases, the term *vitamin* has been ap-plied incorrectly to material not proven essential and even potentially toxic (for example, Laetrile and B_{17}).

FAT-SOLUBLE VITAMINS

Vitamins A, D, E, and K are the principle fat-soluble vitamins required by humans.

Vitamin A

Vitamin A serves many important functions in the body, with its role in vision being particularly significant.

Chemistry and sources

A number of vitaminic forms of vitamin A exist, including alcohols (retinols), aldehydes (retinals), and retinoic acids (Figure 28-1). Retinol (A_1) and 3-dehydroretinol (A_2) are the two natural forms of vitamin A. They are C_{15}-isoprenoid alcohols that have a substituted β-ionone and 3-dehydro-β-ionone ring, respectively (see Figure 28-1). These compounds are yellowish oils or low-melting-point solids (depending on isomeric purity) that are practically insoluble in water but soluble in organic solvents and mineral oil. Vitamin A is sensitive to oxygen and ultraviolet light, which induces a greenish fluorescence. When they are scanned spectrophotometrically, absorbance peaks are observed at 325 and 351 nm for A_1 and A_2, respectively. Vitamin A_1 predominates, especially as a long-chain fatty acid ester, in the livers of mammals and saltwater fish (cod liver), whereas vitamin A_2 is found in freshwater fish oils. Although higher primates are unable to synthesize the β-ionone-type ring structure, they derive the retinal from intestinal dioxygenase-catalyzed cleavage of plant-derived carotenes and cryptoxanthin, which are provitamins. Retinal then is reduced reversibly by pyridine nucleotide-dependent enzymes to retinol or irreversibly oxidized to retinoic acid.

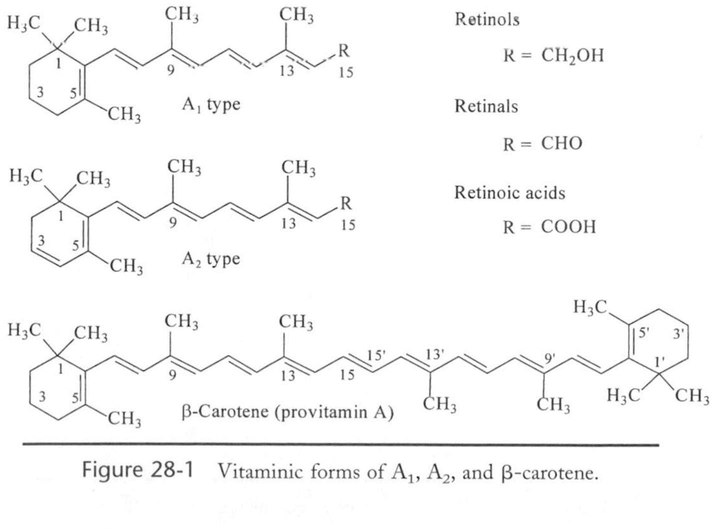

Figure 28-1   Vitaminic forms of A_1, A_2, and β-carotene.

The structure for the most common and effective provitamin A, β-carotene, also is provided in Figure 28-1. This compound is an orange-to-purple, water-insoluble solid that is oxidized in air to inactive products. The other carotenes yield less vitamin A_1 activity. These carotenoid compounds constitute the yellow-to-orange pigments of most vegetables and fruits and often are the main dietary source of what ultimately becomes vitamin A.

Functions

Vitamin A has a significant function in vision. On transport to the retina, all-*trans*-retinol is isomerized to the 11-*cis* alcohol, which then is dehydrogenated reversibly to 11-*cis* retinal. This sterically hindered geometrical isomer of the aldehyde combines as a lysyl-linked Schiff base with suitable proteins, such as opsin, to generate photosensitive pigments, such as rhodopsin. Illumination of such pigments causes photoisomerization and release of all-*trans*-retinal and the protein, a process that couples the large conformational change to ion flux and optic nerve transmission. The all-*trans*-retinal can be isomerized to the 11-*cis* isomer, which again combines with the liberated protein to reconstitute the photo pigment in a visual cycle shown in Figure 28-2. The pyridine nucleotide-dependent dehydrogenase (reductase) also reduces the all-*trans*-retinal to all-*trans*-retinol.

Broader functions of vitamin A include a role in reproduction and growth. Systemic effects that reflect a requirement for vitamin A are the stabilization of cellular and intracellular membranes, maintenance of the integrity of epithelial tissue, and synthesis of glycoproteins. All-*trans*-retinyl-1-β-phospho-D-mannose is formed from retinyl phosphate and uridine diphospho-mannose and is an in vitro donor of mannose to certain glycoproteins. Retinoic acid has been reported to be able to maintain normal growth in humans but unable to replace vitamin A in reproduction or vision. Nuclear receptors exist for the acid and other retinoids. These receptors function as ligand-dependent transcription factors and account for many of the pleiotrophic effects of retinoids.

Absorption, transport, and metabolism

The emulsification of vitamin A and provitamin A forms to the micellar level by bile salts enhances their uptake by mucosal cells of the small intestine and, for retinyl esters, facilitates hydrolysis by pancreatic retinyl ester hydrolase. The remaining ester is hydrolyzed by a brush border enzyme. Intestinal cell absorption of the free retinol is followed by reesterification with long-chain fatty acids, predominantly palmitic and stearic, within the mucosal cell. Those carotenoids capable of being cleaved by the cellular dioxygenase system are converted in part to retinal, which is reduced primarily to retinol and then esterified. Retinyl esters in association with chylomicrons then pass via the lymphatic system to the liver, where uptake by parenchymal cells again involves hydrolysis. Cellular retinol-binding proteins bind retinol, which, when adequately supplied, may be reesterified by acyl donors—mainly palmitoyl-CoA (coenzyme A), stearyl-CoA, and oleyl-CoA—and stored in a lipoglycoprotein complex. Retinol released from the complex by esterases allows association with plasma retinol-binding protein, which is synthesized by the rough endoplasmic reticulum of hepatocytes. Release from hepatocytes via secretory vesicles presents holo-retinol-binding protein (molecular weight [MW] ~21,000) for further association with circulating prealbumin (MW ~55,000) to form a molecular aggregate of sufficient size to avoid loss by glomerular filtration.

In addition to retinal, other products from cleavage of β-carotene include the 8′-, 10′-, and 12′-apo-β-carotenals, which are degraded further in intestinal mucosal cells to retinal. Although most of the aldehyde is reduced reversibly to retinol, lesser amounts are oxidized to retinoic acid in the intestine, liver, and kidney. Retinoic acid from the intestinal mucosa is transported bound to serum albumin via the portal vein. Retinoic acid is not reduced significantly to retinal but is metabolized rapidly in tissue, such as in the liver, to yield more polar catabolites (for example, 5,6-epoxyretinoic acid and conjugates such as retinoyl β-glucuronide, which is excreted). A small amount of retinoic acid undergoes enterohepatic circulation after intestinal hydrolysis of the glucuronide excreted in bile.

Deficiency

Clinically, degenerative changes in eyes and skin are observed commonly in individuals with vitamin A deficiency.[18] Poor dark adaptation, or night blindness (nyctalopia), is an early symptom that is followed by degenerative changes in the retina. More serious effects of deficiency are known as *keratomalacia* and cause ulceration and necrosis of the cornea, which lead to perforation, prolapse, endophthalmitis, and blindness. Usually, associated skin changes

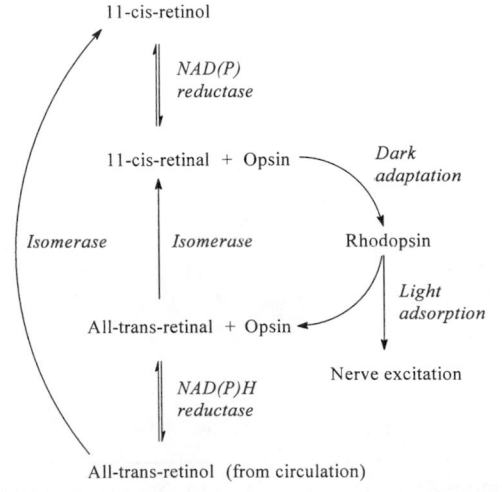

Figure 28-2   Participation of A vitamers in the visual cycle.

also occur, including dryness, roughness, papular eruptions, and follicular hyperkeratosis.

Because maternal hepatic accumulation of vitamin A occurs during the last trimester of pregnancy, preterm infants are relatively deficient in vitamin A at birth. Therefore provision of a daily oral intake of vitamin A that meets the RDA of 375 RE* is important. Infants with birth weights of less than 1500 g (those less than 30 weeks gestation) have virtually no hepatic vitamin A stores and are at risk for vitamin A deficiency.

Toxicity

Toxic effects occur with **hypervitaminosis** A as a result of ingestion of excess vitamin or as a side effect of inappropriate therapy.[18] One of the most important factors relating to toxicity is the form of vitamin A administered. For example, symptoms appear more rapidly after administration of aqueous emulsions rather than oily solutions. Hypervitaminosis A occurs after the liver storage of retinol and its esters exceeds 10,000 IU/g of tissue, a level 10 times the estimated RDA for adult men, or if plasma vitamin A levels exceed 140 µg/dL.

Acute toxicity from a single massive dose manifests as abdominal pain, nausea, vomiting, severe headaches, dizziness, sluggishness, and irritability, followed within a few days by desquamation of the skin and finally, recovery. Chronic toxicity from moderately high doses taken for protracted periods is characterized by bone and joint pain, hair loss, dryness and fissures of the lips, anorexia, benign intracranial hypertension, weight loss, and hepatomegaly. Carotenemia results from a chronic excessive intake of carotene-rich foods, principally carrots. This condition, in which yellowing of skin is observed, is benign because the excess carotene is deposited rather than converted to vitamin A.

Methods for the determination of vitamin A and β-carotene

Many methods are used to measure serum vitamin A and carotenoid concentrations. Of historical interest is the photometric Carr-Price method, which uses antimony trichloride in chloroform as an analytical reagent. It was replaced subsequently by the Neeld-Pearson procedure, in which trifluoroacetic acid is reacted with the conjugated double-bond system of the organic solvent-extracted compounds to produce a blue color (A_{620}). Both methods are imprecise, tedious, and nonspecific. Consequently, several other photometric/spectrophotometric, fluorometric, and chromatographic methods have been developed and used to quantify carotenoids and retinoids in biological specimens.

Currently, high-performance liquid chromatography (HPLC) is the technique of choice used to measure vitamins (see Chapter 8). In practice, HPLC methods have improved

markedly the laboratory's ability to measure vitamin A because they are rapid, sensitive, and allow for the simultaneous determination of vitamin A and E. Both normal-phase and reversed-phase techniques are used. In the former, compounds to be separated are adsorbed to microparticulate silica gel and eluted in the order of least polar to most polar. Reversed-phase HPLC is preferable for acid-sensitive compounds, such as 5,6-epoxyretinoic acid. Photometric, electrochemical, and mass spectrophotometric[17] detectors have been used.

Reference intervals

Reference intervals[7] for vitamin A in serum or plasma are 20 to 43 µg/dL (0.70 to 1.50 µmol/dL) for 1- to 6-year-old children; 26 to 49 µg/dL (0.91 to 1.71 µmol/dL) for 7- to 12-year-old children; 26 to 72 µg/dL (0.91 to 2.51 µmol/dL) for 13- to 19-year-old teenagers; and 30 to 80 µg/dL (1.05 to 2.80 µmol/dL) for adults. Values above 30 µg/dL are associated with appreciable reserves in the liver and correlate well with vitamin-A intake. Within the reference interval, values for men are generally about 20% higher, when compared with those for women. Values above 100 µg/dL indicate toxicity.

With HPLC methods the reference interval for serum β-carotene is 10 to 85 µg/dL (0.19 to 1.58 µmol/L). Elevated levels are found in hypothyroid individuals in whom conversion to vitamin A is decreased and in individuals with hyperlipemia associated with diabetes mellitus.

Plasma retinol-binding protein (see Chapter 19) has been used to assess the nutritional status of individuals. Its reference interval is 3 to 6 mg/dL (30 to 60 mg/L). Liver, thyroid, and kidney diseases (with protein loss), cystic fibrosis, and protein-calorie malnutrition cause decreases in serum the concentration of this protein.

Vitamin D

Vitamin D plays an essential role as a hormone in the control of calcium and phosphorous metabolism. It is produced by UV irradiation of the skin.

Chemistry and sources

The two major forms of vitamin D are ergocalciferol (D_2) and cholecalciferol (D_3), and both are steroid-derived compounds (Figure 28-3).[6] D_2 does not occur naturally but is produced by ultraviolet irradiation of ergosterol, which occurs in molds, yeast, and plants. The action of light causes ring cleavage to yield an intermediate preergocalciferol (plus lumisterol and other related congeners), which rearranges under thermal conditions to ergocalciferol. Vitamin D_3 occurs in humans but similarly derives from irradiation of provitamin 7-dehydrocholesterol in skin to produce, via thermal arrangement of precholecalciferol, the natural cholecalciferol. Structurally, the only chemical difference between the two vitamin and provitamin forms is in the side chain (see

---

*One retinol equivalent (RE) equals 1 µg of all-*trans*-retinol, 6 µg of all-*trans*-carotene, or 12 µg of other provitamin A carotenoids.

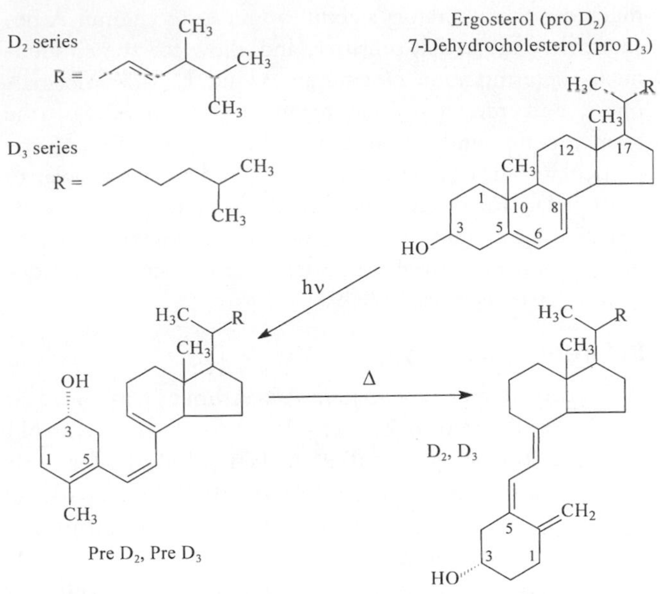

D₂ series

R =

D₃ series

R =

Ergosterol (pro D₂)
7-Dehydrocholesterol (pro D₃)

hv

Pre D₂, Pre D₃

Δ

D₂, D₃

Figure 28-3   Provitamin, previtamin, and vitamins D₂ and D₃.

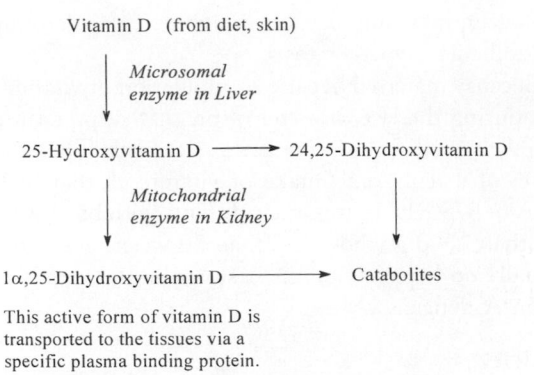

Vitamin D   (from diet, skin)

*Microsomal
enzyme in Liver*

25-Hydroxyvitamin D ⟶ 24,25-Dihydroxyvitamin D

*Mitochondrial
enzyme in Kidney*

1α,25-Dihydroxyvitamin D ⟶ Catabolites

This active form of vitamin D is
transported to the tissues via a
specific plasma binding protein.

Figure 28-4   Transport and metabolism of vitamin D.

Figure 28-3). At least 10 compounds exist that are known to yield vitamin D-active compounds on irradiation. Most differ only in the side chain at C-17 of the sterol nucleus.

The extent to which ultraviolet irradiation converts 7-dehydrocholesterol to vitamin D₃ in skin depends on (1) seasonal variations in sunlight, (2) amount of clothing worn, (3) degree of skin pigmentation, and (4) other factors. Availability and consumption of such vitamin D₃-containing animal foods as fatty fish, eggs, liver, and butter also are variable.

Therefore widespread fortification of food has been adopted to ensure a more secure supply. Because dairy foods in the United States supply about 75% of dietary calcium in a calcium/phosphorus ratio near optimal for bone growth, milk and infant formulas were judged to be desirable vehicles for vitamin D fortification. Although a poor source of vitamin D itself, milk now is routinely marketed to contain 10 μg (400 IU) of added vitamin D per quart. Both ergocalciferol and cholecalciferol are converted about equally in humans to hormonally active dihydroxy forms.

Functions

A detailed discussion of the functions of vitamin D may be found in Chapter 38.

Absorption, transport, and metabolism

Vitamin D is absorbed efficiently from the gastrointestinal tract. When absorbed, the vitamin is bound directly to chylomicrons and transported initially via the lymphatics. To exert its biological activity, vitamin D must be altered metabolically. Much of the prohormone-like vitamin initially supplied to the liver is hydroxylated at the terminal side-chain position to yield 25-hydroxy-D.

The 25-hydroxycholecalciferol, which represents the major metabolite of D₃ in plasma, circulates bound to a vitamin D-binding α-globulin (MW ~52,000). In the kidneys a second hydroxylation at the α-position results from the action of a cytochrome P₄₅₀-mediated, mixed-function oxidase located on the inner mitochondrial membrane. The kidney 1α-hydroxylase is regulated by vitamin D status and calcium/phosphate levels, which are controlled by parathyroid hormone and calcitonin.

An outline of the transport and metabolism of vitamin D is provided in Figure 28-4. More detailed treatment of the influence of 1α,25-dihydroxycholecalciferol on calcium and phosphorus metabolism; the regulatory interplay of parathormone, calcitonin, and prolactin; and the clinical significance of insufficient and excess vitamin D may be found in Chapter 38.

Methods for the measurement of vitamin D and its metabolites

Many methods are used to measure vitamin D and its metabolites. A general discussion of these methods may be found in Chapter 38.

Reference intervals

The reference interval[7] for 1,25-dihydroxy vitamin D is 16 to 65 pg/mL (42 to 169 pmol/L) and 14 to 60 ng/mL (35 to 150 nmol/L) for 25-hydroxy vitamin D.

Vitamin E

Vitamin E is an antioxidant that acts as a scavenger for molecular oxygen and free radicals. It also plays a role in cellular respiration.

Chemistry and sources

The form of vitamin E that is biologically most active and on which units are based is d-α-tocopherol.[6] This vitaminic group contains eight related natural compounds that are biosynthesized in plants and are abundant especially in vegetable oils (Figure 28-5). Members of the vitamin E group are viscous oils at room temperature. They are soluble in fat

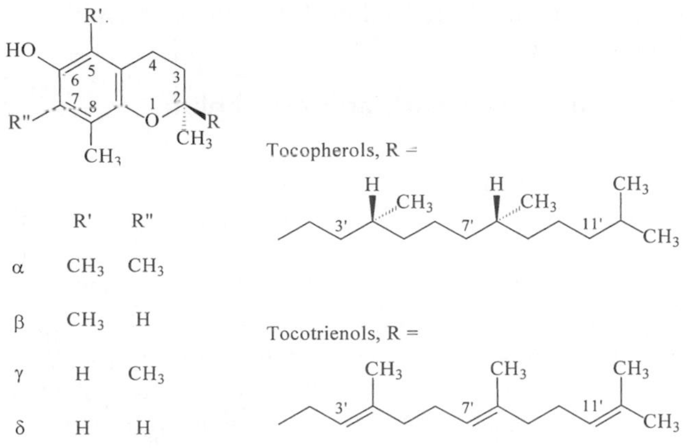

Figure 28-5   Vitaminic forms of E.

solvents, insoluble in water, and stable to acid and heat in the absence of oxygen but labile to oxygen in alkaline solutions and to ultraviolet light. The absorption maximum for α-tocopherol is 294 nm.

Functions

The major function of vitamin E is as an antioxidant for unsaturated fatty acyl moieties of lipids within membranes. Without it, oxidative damage to polyunsaturated fatty acyl parts of membrane phospholipids occurs as a result of hydrogen peroxide production by flavoprotein oxidases. Interactions among vitamin E, selenium (Se), and sulfur amino acids have been rationalized on the basis that although vitamin E is oxidized in lieu of unsaturated fatty acyl functions, the Se-containing glutathione peroxidase helps reduce such lipid peroxidases as they are formed, thereby decreasing peroxidative auto-catalysis. In addition, in the mammal, decreases in liver microsomal drug hydroxylation and increases in net synthesis of xanthine oxidase have been found in vitamin E-deficient animals.

Absorption, transport, and metabolism

In the presence of bile, vitamin E is absorbed from the small intestine. Most tocopherol enters the bloodstream via lymph, where the tocopherol is associated with chylomicrons and very–low-density lipoproteins. The vitamin is stored in most tissues, with the largest amount stored in adipose tissue. Some of the deposition is in association with lipoproteins in cellular membranes. Rapid exchange of tocopherol occurs between the erythrocyte membranes and plasma lipoproteins. When physiological amounts are administered, only a small fraction of the dose appears in urine.

Deficiency

Premature and low-birth-weight infants are particularly susceptible to development of vitamin E deficiency, because placental transfer is poor and these infants have limited adipose tissue, where much of the vitamin nor-

mally is stored. Signs of deficiency include irritability, edema, and a hemolytic anemia. The anemia reflects the shortened life span of erythrocytes with fragile membranes; it does not respond to iron therapy, which may aggravate the condition. Deficiency symptoms rarely occur in children or adults except in cases of severe malabsorption, as, for example, in cystic fibrosis.

Health claims for large dietary supplements of vitamin E are largely unconfirmed. However, support from animal experiments does indicate that supplements of tocopherol protect against chemical oxidants that constitute a portion of atmospheric pollutants, such as ozone and nitrous oxide. In addition, vitamin E therapy may provide some benefit for individuals with intermittent lameness resulting from arteriosclerotic peripheral vascular disease. A reduction in low-density lipoprotein oxidation also may occur in at-risk, diabetic individuals who consume 400 mg/day of vitamin E.

Toxicity

Toxicity from chronic high intake of vitamin E has been noted in animals, in which competition for absorption may increase requirements for other fat-soluble vitamins, notably D and K. This problem appears to be the case in individuals who already have limited vitamin K levels because of anticoagulant therapy after coronary infarcts and who also have ingested large amounts of vitamin E, which additionally may suppress vitamin K absorption. Malaise, intestinal distress, depressed prothrombin, and ecchymoses have been reported. In general, however, relatively high doses of vitamin E (for example, 300 mg/day) appear to be tolerated in most adults.

Methods for the determination of vitamin E and E status

Physical methods used to determine vitamin E involve solvent extraction of vitamin E forms after saponification of plasma samples. Molecular distillation and paper, thin-layer, and column chromatographic techniques have been used to measure vitamin E. Gas chromatography and HPLC methods permit rapid separation of the different tocopherols and tocotrienols. HPLC methods are used widely and are specific for α- and γ-tocopherol. They also measure vitamin A and related compounds.

Chemical methods are based on an oxidation-reduction reaction. Following specific elution techniques, fractions are subjected commonly to the Emmerie-Engel procedure, in which tocopherol is oxidized to tocopheryl quinone by $FeCl_3$, and the Fe^{+2} in the resultant $FeCl_2$ forms a complex with α,α′-dipyridyl to produce a red color.

Evaluation of vitamin E status should be based on measurements of tocopherol and the degree of erythrocyte hemolysis after treatment of cells with hydrogen peroxide (preferred), dialuric acid, or isotonic saline phosphate buffer.

Reference intervals

Reference intervals[7] for serum or plasma (heparin) vitamin E are 0.1 to 0.5 mg/dL (2.3 to 11.6 μmol/L) for premature neonates; 0.3 to 0.9 mg/dL (7 to 21 μmol/L) for children (1 to 12 years of age); 0.6 to 1.0 mg/dL (14 to 23 μmol/L) for teenagers (13 to 19 years of age); and 0.5 to 1.8 mg/dL (12 to 42 μmol/L) for adults.

Vitamin K

Vitamin K promotes blood clotting and is required for the conversion of several clotting factors and prothrombin.

Chemistry and sources

The two principal natural classes of vitamin K are the phylloquinones (K_1 type) synthesized in plants and the menaquinones (K_2 type) of bacterial origin (Figure 28-6).[6] Several synthetic analogues and derivatives exist; most relate to or derive from menadione (K_3), which lacks a side-chain substituent at position 3. The K vitamins are insoluble in water but dissolve in organic fat solvents. They are destroyed by alkaline solutions and reducing agents and also are sensitive to ultraviolet light.

Functions

Vitamin K is recognized as a dietary antihemorrhagic factor necessary for liver syntheses of plasma clotting factors II (prothrombin), VII (proconvertin), IX (plasma thromboplastin component), and X (Stuart factor). Vitamin K also is needed for the synthesis of protein S and protein C. These and other factors, including Ca^{+2}, are known to initiate a process whereby an aggregate composed of several proteins with prothrombin, calcium ion, and phosphatide react to form thrombin, which then catalyzes the proteolytic conversion of fibrinogen ultimately to a polymerized fibrin clot.

Bis-4-hydroxycoumarin (dicumarol), the anticlotting compound derived from spoiled sweet clover, and synthetic 4-hydroxycoumarins, such as warfarin, have been used as anticoagulants. They have been found to interfere with the reductase-catalyzed conversion of epoxide to quinone forms

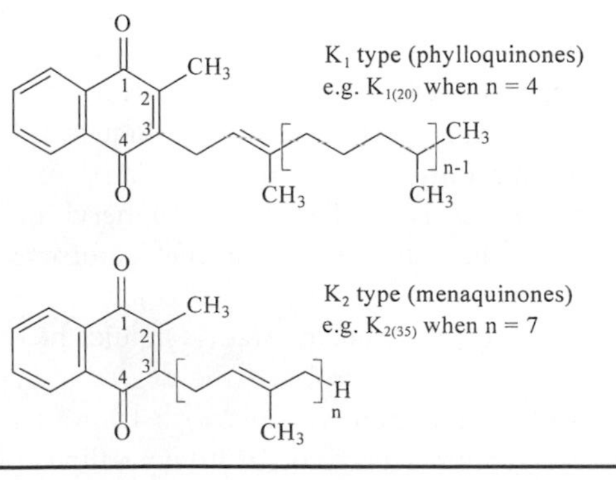

Figure 28-6 Vitaminic forms of K.

of vitamin K and the reduction of the latter to the functional hydroquinone.

Absorption, transport, and metabolism

The absorption of natural vitamin K from the small intestine is facilitated by bile. Efficiency of absorption varies from 15% to 65%, as reflected by recovery in lymph within 24 hours. Vitamins K_1 and K_2 are bound to chylomicrons for transport from mucosal cells to the liver. Menadione (K_3) is absorbed more rapidly and completely from the gut before entering the portal blood. In liver, intracellular distribution is mostly in the microsomal fraction, where phenylation of menadione to form K_2 occurs. Release of vitamin K to the bloodstream allows association with circulating β-lipoproteins for transport to other tissues. Significant levels of vitamin K have been noted in spleen and skeletal muscle. Because only traces of urinary metabolites of vitamins K_1 and K_2 appear in urine, a considerable portion of menadione is conjugated at the hydroquinone level to form β-glucuronide and sulfate esters, which are excreted.

Deficiency

Hemorrhagic disease of the newborn develops readily because the menaquinone-synthesizing intestinal flora have not become established within the first week after birth and early breast milk is low in vitamin K. Prothrombin levels during this period are only about 25% of adult levels. Severe diarrhea and antibiotics used to suppress diarrhea readily exacerbate the situation; prothrombin levels consequently drop below 5% of the adult level and bleeding can occur. Development of vitamin K deficiency in the adult may require both reduction of dietary intake and antibiotic inhibition of intestinal microflora or 4-hydroxycoumarin-type anticoagulant therapy. Thus deficiency is relatively uncommon in the adult and is found only in cases of chronic malabsorption of fats, including fat-soluble vitamins, or during long-term antibiotic or anticoagulant treatments.[18] Defective blood coagulation and demonstration of abnormal noncarboxylated prothrombin are signs of vitamin K deficiency.

Toxicity

The use of high doses of naturally occurring vitamin K (K_1 and K_2) does not appear to be toxic; however, menadione treatment can lead to the formation of erythrocyte cytoplasmic inclusions, known as *Heinz bodies*, and hemolytic anemia. In cases of severe hemolysis, increased bilirubin formation and undeveloped capacity for its conjugation may produce kernicterus in the newborn.

Methods for the determination of vitamin K and K status

After extraction and chromatographic separations,[10] spectrophotometric[11] direct methods have been used to measure the different forms of vitamin K. Photometric determinations based on reactivity of the quinoid nucleus of K vitamins include reactions with acidic phenylhydrazine, 2,6-dichloroindophenol, active methylene compounds, alkalis, and piperidine. In addition, spectrophotometric determination of chemically reduced vitamin K has been used. HPLC methods also are available.

Conventional assessment of vitamin K status relies on the clotting ability of plasma as reflected by the prothrombin time. In this procedure, tissue thromboplastin is added to recalcified plasma and the time required for clot formation is compared with that for a normal control. When the prothrombin concentration declines below 30% of normal, prothrombin time rises above 30 seconds. Deficiency of vitamin K can be distinguished from hypoprothrombinemia of liver disease by measurement with radioimmunoassay (RIA) of the non-γ-carboxylated prothrombin precursor (that is, "abnormal prothrombin") that accumulates in plasma when the vitamin is deficient. Alternatively, if a vitamin K deficiency exists, parenteral administration of the vitamin results in prompt correction of an abnormal prothrombin or clotting time. Wilson has suggested that routine determination of prothrombin time should be performed before all surgical procedures and deliveries.[18]

Reference intervals

The reference interval[7] for vitamin K is 0.13 to 1.19 ng/mL (0.28 to 2.64 nmol/L).

■ WATER-SOLUBLE VITAMINS

Water-soluble vitamins that are important in human metabolism include vitamin B_1 (thiamine), vitamin B_2 (riboflavin), vitamin B_6, niacin, vitamin B_{12}, folic acid, biotin, pantothenic acid, and vitamin C.

Thiamine

Thiamine forms the coenzyme thiamine pyrophosphate (TPP). It is required for the essential reactions catalyzed by decarboxylase subunits of dehydrogenase complexes for pyruvate, 2-oxoglutarate, and branched-chain keto acids and for transketolase.

Chemistry and sources

Thiamine (vitamin B_1) is a pyrimidyl-substituted thiazole (3-[4-amino-2-methyl-pyrimidyl-5-methyl]-4-methyl-5-[β-hydroxyethyl]thiazole) (Figure 28-7). The basic vitamin is isolated or synthesized and handled as a solid thiazolium salt (for example, thiamine chloride hydrochloride). The principal if not sole coenzyme form is the pyrophosphate ester, TPP, formed at the β-hydroxyethyl substituent (see Figure 28-7). Monophosphate and triphosphate esters occur naturally. Small amounts of thiamine and its phosphates are present in most plant and animal tissue, but more abundant food sources include unrefined cereal grains, liver, heart, kid-

ney, and lean cuts of pork.[6] The enrichment of flour and derived food products has increased considerably the availability of this vitamin. Thiamine is somewhat thermolabile, particularly in alkaline solutions, where base attack occurs at carbon 2 of the thiazolium ring.

Functions

TPP functions as the Mg^{+2}-coordinated coenzyme for so-called active aldehyde transfers in the oxidative decarboxylation of α-keto acids catalyzed by dehydrogenase complexes and the formation of α-ketols (ketoses) as catalyzed by transketolase.

Absorption, transport, and metabolism

Thiamine is absorbed readily in the small intestine by an active transport process that is probably carrier-mediated as long as intake is less than 5 mg/day; at higher intake levels, passive diffusion increasingly contributes to absorption.[18] Phosphorylation takes place in the jejunal mucosa to yield TPP. Thiamine is carried by the portal blood to the liver. The free vitamin occurs in the plasma, but the coenzyme, TPP, predominates in the cellular components. About half the body's stores is found in skeletal muscles, with much of the remainder in the heart, liver, kidneys, and nervous tissue (including the brain, which contains most of the triphosphate). Thiamine, and several of its catabolites (Figure 28-8), is excreted into the urine by the renal tubules.

Deficiency

As thiamine deficiency develops, all tissues except the brain experience a rather rapid loss of the vitamin. The decrease of TPP in the erythrocyte roughly parallels the decrease of this coenzyme in other tissues. During this time the thiamine in urine falls to near zero; the urinary metabolites remain high for some time before decreasing.

Beriberi is the disease resulting from thiamine deficiency. The causes for deficiency[1,13] include inadequate intake because of a diet largely dependent on milled, nonenriched grains, such as rice and wheat, or the ingestion of raw fish containing microbial thiaminases. Chronic alcoholism is a common contributor to deficiency because of a low intake of thiamine (and other B vitamins) and impaired absorption and storage. Several thiamine-responsive inborn errors of

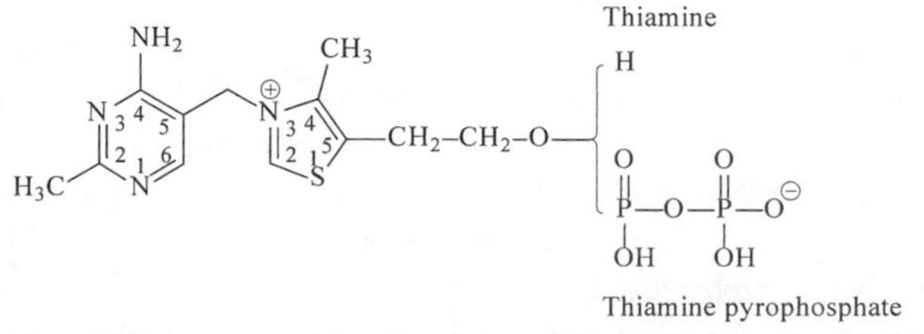

Figure 28-7   Thiamine and the pyrophosphate coenzyme.

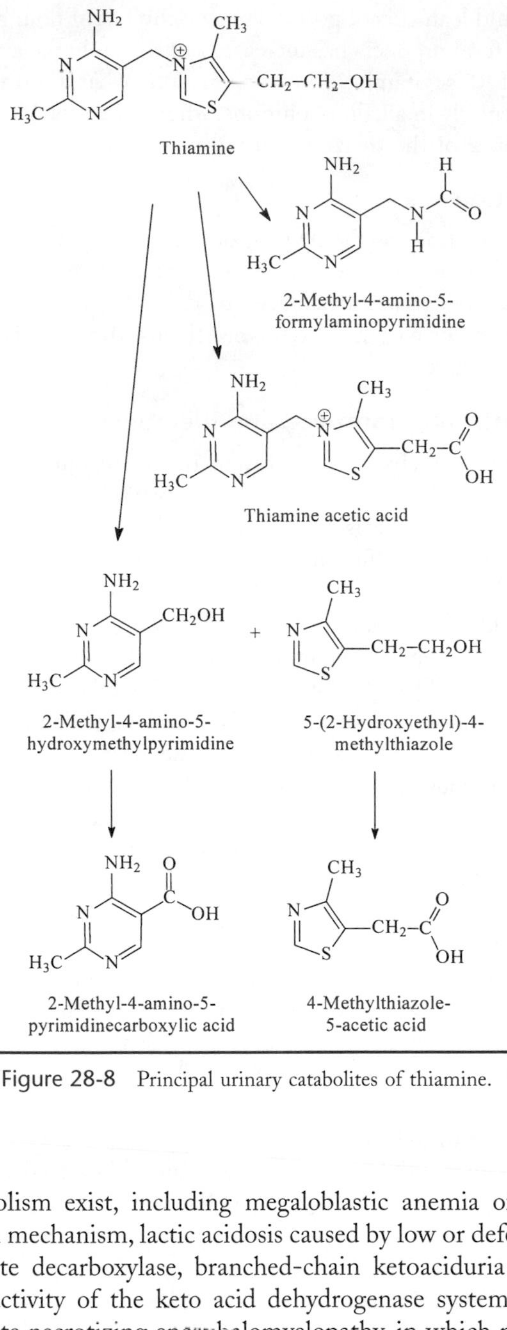

Figure 28-8　Principal urinary catabolites of thiamine.

metabolism exist, including megaloblastic anemia of unknown mechanism, lactic acidosis caused by low or defective pyruvate decarboxylase, branched-chain ketoaciduria with poor activity of the keto acid dehydrogenase system, and subacute necrotizing encephalomyelopathy, in which neural tissues demonstrate a lack of thiamine triphosphate. Therapeutic doses of 5 to 20 mg of thiamine daily have proved beneficial. Other at-risk individuals are those undergoing long-term renal dialysis or intravenous feeding and those with chronic febrile infections.[13]

Clinical signs of thiamine deficiency primarily involve the nervous and cardiovascular systems.[13,18] In the adult, symptoms most frequently observed are mental confusion, anorexia, muscular weakness, ataxia, peripheral paralysis, ophthalmoplegia, edema (wet beriberi), muscle wasting (dry beriberi), tachycardia, and an enlarged heart. In infants, symptoms appear suddenly and severely, often involving cardiac failure and cyanosis.

Methods for the determination of thiamine and thiamine status

Earlier microbiological methods and the chemical conversion of thiamine to fluorometrically determined thiochrome were the principal means used to determine the vitamin in various biological fluids. Now, electrophoretic, ion-exchange, and HPLC techniques are used to determine the free vitamin and its phosphate esters. Determination of the urinary excretion of thiamine in a 4-hour specimen, especially with comparison of excretion before and after a test load, is helpful in differentiation among extremes of thiamine status. However, as is the case in most assessments based on the amount of water-soluble vitamins in urine, excretion is influenced considerably by dietary intake, absorption, and other factors. Measurements of certain urinary metabolites, notably thiamine acetic acid, also have been suggested as being reflective of thiamine status.

The measurement of whole blood or erythrocyte transketolase—requiring TPP as a coenzyme—is a useful and reliable method used to assess thiamine status (Figure 28-9). The TPP effect is measured by assaying of enzyme activity before and after TPP supplementation. The percent increase in activity is defined as the TPP effect.

Transketolase activity in blood usually is measured by determination of the rate of disappearance of D-ribose-5-phosphate with the orcinol reagent (orcinol and ferric chloride in concentrated hydrochloric acid). Transketolase activity in blood also can be measured by determination of the amount of fructose-6-phosphate formed.

Reference intervals

The reference interval[7] for transketolase levels in whole blood is 9 to 12 μmol/hour/mL (150 to 200 U/L). The reference interval for erythrocyte transketolase activity is 0.75 to 1.30 U/g of hemoglobin (48.4 to 83.9 kU/mol Hb). The reference intervals for percent TPP effect are normal, 0% to 15%; marginally deficient, 15% to 25%; severely deficient with clinical signs, greater than 25%.

Riboflavin

Riboflavin, also known as vitamin B_2, is an essential component of flavin adenine dinucleotide (FAD) and flavin mononucleotide (FMN), both of which are coenzymes involved in many redox reactions.

Chemistry and sources

Riboflavin (7,8-dimethyl-10-[1'-D-ribityl]isoalloxazine) is a yellow fluorescent compound that is distributed widely throughout the plant and animal kingdoms.[6] Numerous naturally occurring flavins now are known to have the vitamin or closely related derivatives as an integral part of their structures. Principal among these are the coenzymes FMN and FAD (Figure 28-10). The liver, kidney, and heart are rich sources of these coenzymes. Many vegetables also are

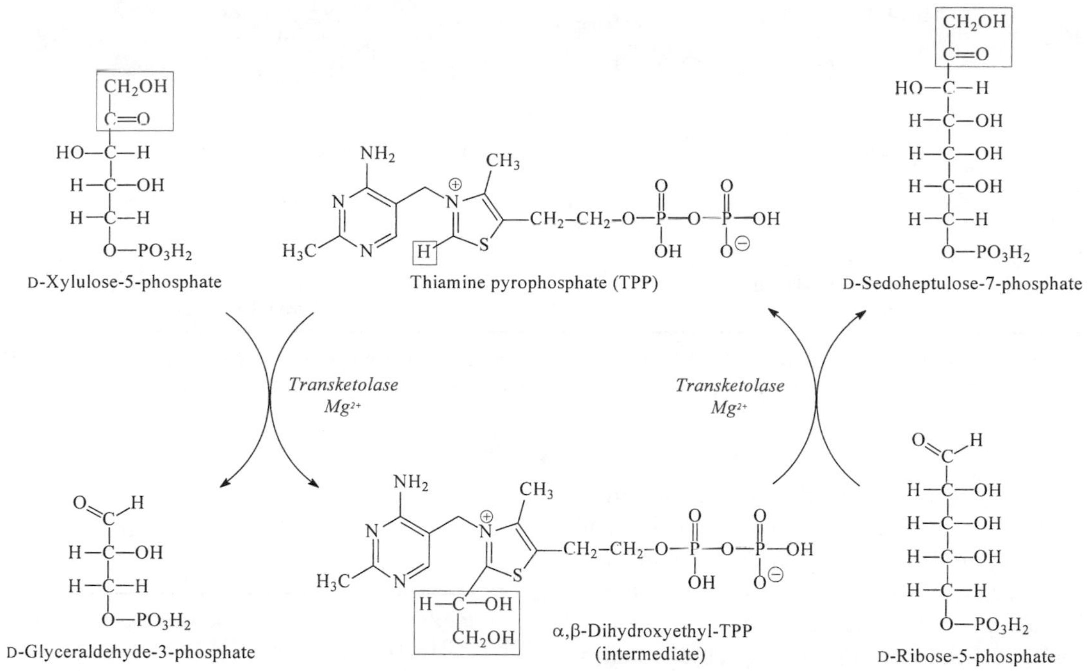

D-Xylulose-5-phosphate   Thiamine pyrophosphate (TPP)   D-Sedoheptulose-7-phosphate

Transketolase
Mg²⁺

Transketolase
Mg²⁺

D-Glyceraldehyde-3-phosphate   α,β-Dihydroxyethyl-TPP
(intermediate)   D-Ribose-5-phosphate

Figure 28-9   The transketolase reaction. In this reaction a two-carbon fragment *(boxed area)* is transferred from a donor ketose (D-xylulose-5-phosphate) to thiamine pyrophosphate (TPP) and then finally to an ac- ceptor aldose (D-ribose-5-phosphate). The products of this reaction are D-glyceraldehyde-3-phosphate and D-sedoheptulose-7-phosphate.

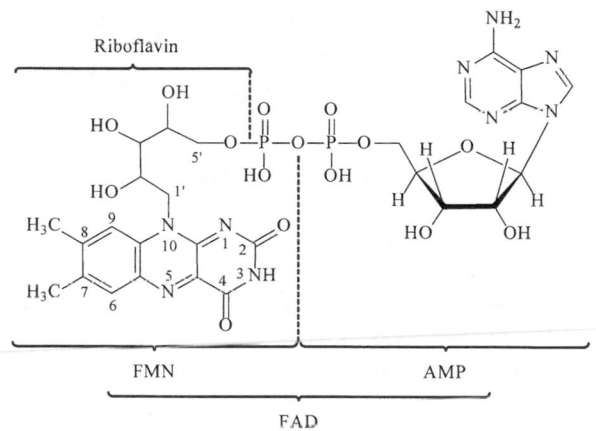

Figure 28-10   Riboflavin and FMN as components of FAD. *FMN,* Flavin mononucleotide; *FAD,* flavin adenine dinucleotide; *AMP,* adenosine monophosphate.

good sources, but cereals are rather low in flavin content. Milk is a good source of the vitamin, but considerable loss occurs from exposure to light during pasteurization and bottling or as a result of irradiation to increase the vitamin D content. Flavins are stable during exposure to heat but are decomposed by light.

Functions

In bound coenzymic form, riboflavin participates in oxidation-reduction reactions in numerous metabolic path- ways and in energy production via the respiratory chain.[3] Flavins serve as redox carriers on differential binding to proteins, participate in both one- and two-electron transfers, and react rapidly with oxygen—in the reduced (1,5-dihydro) form.

Absorption, transport, and metabolism

During digestion, coenzyme forms of the vitamin (mainly FAD and some FMN) are released from noncovalent attachment to proteins as a consequence of gastric acidification. Nonspecific action of pyrophosphatase and phosphatase on the coenzyme forms occurs in the upper gut. The vitamin is absorbed primarily in the proximal small intestine by a saturable transport system that is rapid and proportional to intake before leveling off at doses near 25 mg of riboflavin per day. Bile salts appear to facilitate the uptake. After transport through blood plasma in protein-bound complexes,[12] conversion of riboflavin to coenzymes (Figure 28-11) occurs within the cellular cytoplasm of most tissue, but particularly in the small intestine, liver, heart, and kidney.

Thyroxine and triiodothyronine stimulate FMN and FAD synthesis in mammalian systems. FAD is the predominant flavocoenzyme present in tissues, where it forms complexes mainly with numerous flavoprotein dehydrogenases and oxidases. Because only small amounts of riboflavin are stored in this manner, the urinary excretion reflects dietary intake.

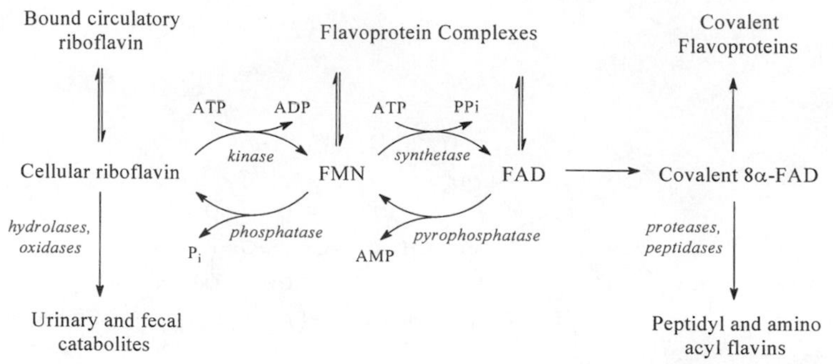

Figure 28-11　Cellular interconversions of flavins. *ATP,* Adenosine triphosphate; *ADP,* adenosine diphosphate; *P*$_i$, inorganic phosphate; *PP*$_i$, inorganic pyrophosphate; *FMN,* flavin mononucleotide; *FAD,* flavin adenosine dinucleotide; *AMP,* adenosine monophosphate.

Deficiency

Although riboflavin has a wide distribution in foodstuffs, many people live for long periods of time on low intakes, and consequently minor signs of deficiency are common in many parts of the world. Several diseases affect riboflavin status. Moreover, deficiency is encountered almost invariably in combination with deficit of other water-soluble vitamins. The deficiency syndrome **(avitaminosis)** is characterized by sore throat, hyperemia and edema of the pharyngeal and oral mucous membranes, cheilosis, angular stomatitis, glossitis (magenta tongue), seborrheic dermatitis, and normochromic, normocytic anemia associated with pure red blood cell (RBC) aplasia of the bone marrow. Severe riboflavin deficiency also can affect the conversion of vitamin B_6 to its coenzyme and even curtail conversion of tryptophan to niacin.

Methods for the determination of riboflavin and flavin status

Numerous biochemical methods are used to separate and quantify the diverse natural flavins.[9] Among the more sensitive are those that invoke specific binding, for example, riboflavin with egg white riboflavin-binding protein, FMN with apoflavodoxin, and FAD with apoproteins D-amino acid oxidase or glucose oxidase. However, nutritional status is assessed commonly by measurement of urinary excretion of the vitamin in fasting, random, or 24-hour specimens or by load return tests, measurement of erythrocyte riboflavin concentration, or determination of the erythrocyte glutathione reductase activity coefficient.

Urinary riboflavin can be measured by use of fluorometric and microbiological procedures, but for specificity, HPLC combined with fluorometric detection is the method of choice. Under conditions of adequate intake, the amount excreted per day is more than 120 µg or 80 µg/g of creatinine. The rate of excretion expressed as µg/g of creatinine is greater for children than for adults. Conditions causing negative nitrogen balance and the administration of antibiotics and certain psychotropic drugs (phenothiazine) increase urinary riboflavin as a consequence of tissue depletion and displacement. A load-return test augments the reliability in a given case.

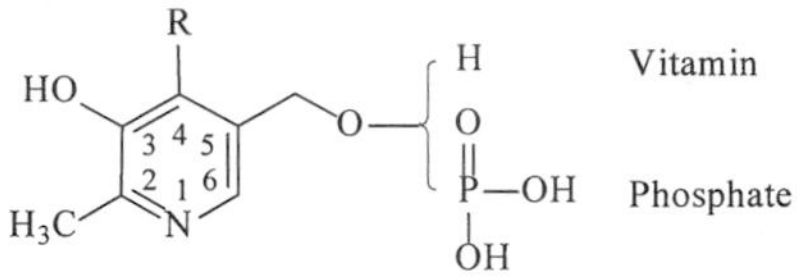

Figure 28-12　Free and phosphorylated forms of vitamin B_6. R = CH_2OH for pyridoxine, CH_2NH_2 for pyridoxamine, and CHO for pyridoxal.

Erythrocyte riboflavin also can be determined by either fluorometric or microbiological means. Values below 15 µg/dL of cells are considered to reflect low or deficient status.

A commonly used method for assessment of riboflavin status uses the determination of FAD-dependent glutathione reductase activity in freshly lysed erythrocytes. However, individuals who have received relatively large quantities of replacement blood, such as very–low-birth-weight infants (<1500 g), should have their blood level of the vitamin quantitatively measured through use of HPLC.

Reference intervals

The reference interval[7] for erythrocyte riboflavin by use of the fluorometric method is 10 to 50 µg/dL (266 to 1330 nmol/L). The reference interval for serum or plasma levels of riboflavin is 4 to 24 µg/dL (106 to 638 nmol/L).

Vitamin B_6

Pyridoxine (pyridoxol), pyridoxamine, and pyridoxal are the three natural forms of vitamin B_6. They are converted to pyridoxal phosphate, which is required for the synthesis, catabolism, and interconversion of amino acids.

Chemistry and sources

The three natural forms of vitamin B_6 are 4-substituted 2-methyl-3-hydroxyl-5-hydroxymethyl pyridines (Figure 28-12). Both pyridoxamine-5′-phosphate (PLP) and pyridoxal-5′-phosphate (P-5′-P) interconvert as coenzyme forms during aminotransferase (transaminase)-catalyzed reactions. Vitamin B_6 is distributed widely in animal and plant tissues, where the phosphorylated forms, and particularly

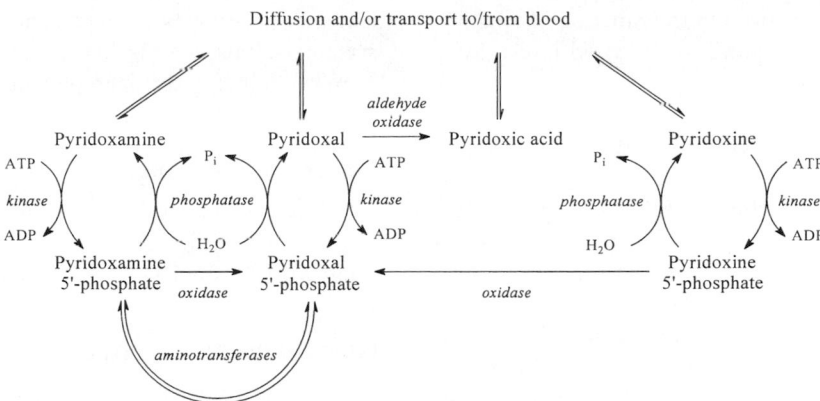

Figure 28-13   Metabolism of vitamin B_6. *ATP,* Adenosine triphosphate; *ADP,* adenosine diphosphate; P_i, inorganic phosphate.

PLP, predominate. Meats, poultry, and fish are good sources, as are yeast, certain seeds, and bran; somewhat more limited sources are milk, eggs, and green, leafy vegetables.[6,13] The common commercial form of the vitamin is pyridoxine hydrochloride, which is a water-soluble, white, crystalline solid. Solutions of the B_6 vitamers are decomposed by light, especially in the ultraviolet region at neutral to alkaline pH. The reactive aldehyde function of PLP leads to significant loss during thermal processing of foods.

Functions

As a coenzyme PLP, vitamin B_6 functions in numerous reactions that embrace the metabolism of proteins, carbohydrates, and lipids. Especially diverse are PLP-dependent enzymes that are involved in amino acid metabolism. Biochemically, PLP has the ability to condense its 4-formyl substituent with the α-amino group of an amino acid to form an azomethine (Schiff base) linkage. Aminotransferases affect rupture of the α-hydrogen bond with the ultimate formation of an α-keto acid and PLP; this reversible reaction provides an interface between amino acid and ketogenic and glucogenic reactions. Amino acid decarboxylases lead to formation of amines, including several that are functional in nervous tissue (for example, epinephrine, norepinephrine, serotonin, and γ-aminobutyrate). The biosynthesis of heme depends on the early formation of 5-aminolevulinate from PLP-dependent condensation of glycine and succinyl-CoA, followed by decarboxylation. Many examples of enzymes, such as cysteine desulfhydrase and serine hydroxymethyltransferase, use PLP to effect the loss or transfer of amino acid side chains. PLP is the essential coenzyme for phosphorylase, which catalyzes phosphorolysis of the α-1,4-linkages of glycogen. An important role in lipid metabolism is the PLP-dependent condensation of L-serine with palmitoyl-CoA to form 3-dehydrosphinganine, a precursor of sphingomyelins.

Absorption, transport, and metabolism

The three B_6 vitamers are released effectively from their 5'-phosphate esters by intraluminal action of intestinal alkaline phosphatase, but pyridoxine-5'-β-D-glucoside from plant foods is hydrolyzed less effectively by nonspecific glycosidase within cells.[20] The vitamers are absorbed readily by the mucosal cells, which contain cytoplasmic pyridoxal kinase responsible for catalyzing the adenosine triphosphate (ATP)-dependent phosphorylation of all three vitamin forms (Figure 28-13). Most cells contain a cytosolic FMN-dependent, pyridoxine (pyridoxamine)-5'-phosphate oxidase responsible for catalyzing the oxygen-dependent conversion of pyridoxine phosphate and pyridoxamine phosphate to PLP (and hydrogen peroxide). The coenzyme can enter directly into subcellular organelles, such as hepatocyte mitochondria. PLP binds for catalytic function with numerous specific **apoenzymes** throughout the cell. The erythrocyte, in addition, traps PLP as a conjugate Schiff base with hemoglobin. Glycogen phosphorylase contains most of the PLP in skeletal muscle.

Release of free vitamin (mainly pyridoxal), when physiological nonsaturating levels of vitamin are absorbed, occurs when the phosphates are hydrolyzed by nonspecific alkaline phosphatase located on the plasma membranes of cells. However, some PLP also is released into the circulation by the liver. Although PLP is the principal tissue form of vitamin B_6 and pyridoxal constitutes much of the circulating vitamin, the main catabolite excreted in urine is 4'-pyridoxic acid, which is formed by the action of the FAD-dependent general liver aldehyde oxidase and especially by NAD-specific aldehyde dehydrogenase found in most tissues.

Deficiency

A vitamin B_6 deficiency usually occurs in association with deficits in other vitamins of the B-complex. Chemotherapeutic or fortuitous ingestion of antagonists has led to **hypovitaminosis** B_6.[1,18] Antagonists include the tuberculostatic drug isoniazid (isonicotinic acid hydrazide), and several naturally occurring substituted hydrazines and hydroxylamines, among them D-cycloserine. Penicillamine (β-dimethyl cysteine), used in treatment of patients with Wilson's disease to decrease the damaging levels of copper found in the liver, inactivates PLP. Several genetic conditions exist in which abnormalities in the function of vitamin B_6 occur, but they usually respond to increased levels (5 to 50 mg/day) of administered vitamin B_6.

Biochemical changes occur early in deficiency states and become more marked as deficiency of B_6 progresses.[1,18] Plasma levels of PLP and urinary output of B_6 and 4′-pyridoxic acid decrease within 1 week of the removal of vitamin B_6 from the diet. Increased amounts of xanthurenic acid appear in urine. Transaminase activity in serum and RBCs also decreases. Electroencephalographic abnormalities appear within 3 weeks. Epileptiform convulsions are a common finding in young vitamin B_6-deficient subjects. In addition, skin changes include a dermatitis. Hematological manifestations may include a decrease in the number of circulating lymphocytes and possible normocytic, microcytic, or sideroblastic anemia.

Methods for the determination of vitamin B_6 and B_6 status

Several functional and chemical methods have proved useful for assays of vitamin B_6 and PLP. These assays involve PLP-dependent enzymes and metabolites of vitamin B_6 and those amino acids that reflect vitamin B_6 status in humans.

Direct assessment of all or separate vitaminic forms of B_6 in urine and blood involves microbiological assays with specific strains of bacteria. Fluorometric assays of urinary 4′-pyridoxic acid and blood PLP after conversion of the latter to the cyanide complex or condensation with a fluorophore, such as methyl anthranilate followed by reduction, also have found application. HPLC is an excellent technique for measurement of 4′-pyridoxic acid and PLP levels in plasma, tissues, and urine. During deficiency the level of 4′-pyridoxic acid decreases well below the normal level of at least 0.8 mg/day in urine. The PLP concentration in plasma has been judged the most reliable indicator of B_6 status.

Activities of blood transaminases have been used frequently as indirect measurements of vitamin B_6 status. Although the enzyme activity in serum is depressed in B_6-deficient individuals, a considerable variability results because release of these enzymes reflects cell death and breakdown in various tissues. Erythrocyte levels of aspartate and alanine aminotransferases provide a better reflection of vitamin B_6 status. Enzymatic assays are run best before and after the addition in vitro of PLP to yield an activity coefficient. Activity coefficients of less than approximately 1.5 for aspartate aminotransferase and 1.2 for alanine aminotransferase are considered normal but may depend somewhat on the assay method used.

Measurement of urinary tryptophan metabolites, particularly xanthurenic acid, after an oral load (2 to 5 g) of tryptophan, is a common test used in studies of vitamin B_6 nutriture. Amounts of xanthurenate well above the normal (near 25 mg/day) are present in B_6-deficient individuals. Levels of other metabolites, such as kynurenic acid and 3-hydroxykynurenine, also are increased. The methionine

load test also has been used. The ratio of cystathionine to cysteine sulfinic acid is elevated in a 24-hour urine sample from vitamin B_6-deficient patients who have received 3-g methionine loads.

Reference intervals

The reference interval[7] for plasma levels of vitamin B_6 is 5 to 30 ng/mL (20 to 121 nmol/L). Plasma levels less than 5 ng/mL (20 nmol/L) are considered deficient.

Niacin and Niacinamide

Niacin (nicotinic acid) and niacinamide (nicotinamide, nicotinic acid amide) are converted to the ubiquitous redox coenzymes nicotinamide adenine dinucleotide (NAD) and nicotinamide adenine dinucleotide phosphate (NADP).

Chemistry and sources

Structures of nicotinic acid and nicotinamide and the two coenzyme forms containing the nicotinamide moiety are presented in Figure 28-14. NAD and NADP represent most of the niacin activity found in good sources, such as yeast, lean meats, liver, and poultry. Milk, canned salmon, and several leafy green vegetables contribute lesser amounts but still are sufficient to prevent deficiency. Additionally, some plant foodstuffs, especially cereals such as corn and wheat, contain niacin bound in forms that are not available readily for nutritional purposes. At least part of such material appears to be constituted by nicotinic acid that is amide-linked to the ε-amino lysyl groups of peptides.

Because of its tryptophan content, protein provides a considerable portion of niacin equivalent. As much as two-thirds the niacin required by adults can be derived from tryptophan. Studies have found that 60 mg of tryptophan is equivalent to 1 mg of niacin in the adult. Free forms of the vitamin are white, stable solids that are quite soluble in water. The oxidized coenzymes are labile to alkali, whereas the

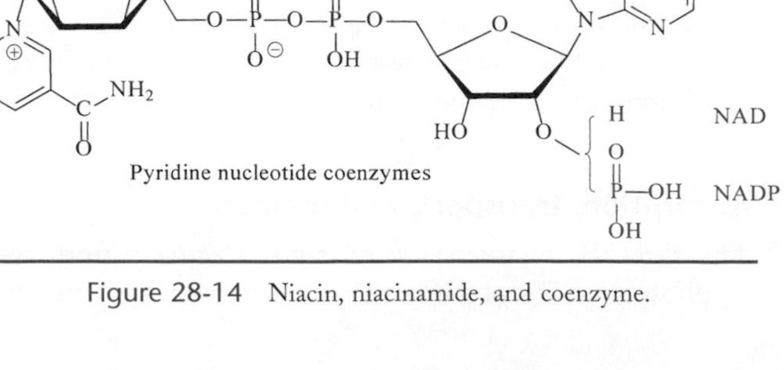

Figure 28-14   Niacin, niacinamide, and coenzyme.

reduced (dihydro) coenzymes are labile to acid. Reduction of the oxidized coenzymes commonly occurs by addition of a hydride ion to the *para* (4) position of the nicotinamide ring, with simultaneous formation of a solvated proton. Reduced NAD (NADH) and reduced NADP (NADPH) absorb light in the near-ultraviolet region (339 nm).

Functions

Hundreds of enzymes require either NAD or NADP. Most of these oxidoreductases function as dehydrogenases and catalyze such diverse reactions as the (1) conversion of alcohols (often sugars and polyols) to aldehydes or ketones, (2) hemiacetals to lactones, (3) aldehydes to acids, and (4) certain amino acids to keto acids. The common mechanism for such conversions involves the stereospecific abstraction of a hydride ion from substrate, with *para* addition to one or the other side of carbon 4 in the pyridine ring of the nucleotide coenzyme. The second hydrogen of the substrate group oxidized is removed concomitantly as a proton and ultimately exchanges in water as a hydronium ion. Most dehydrogenases using NAD or NADP function reversibly. Glutamate dehydrogenase, for example, favors the oxidative direction, whereas others, such as glutathione reductase, preferentially catalyze reduction. Most NAD-dependent enzymes are involved in catabolic reactions, whereas NADP systems are more common to biosynthetic reactions.

Absorption, transport, and metabolism

The coenzymes of niacin are hydrolyzed in the intestinal tract, and both the acid and amide forms of the vitamin are absorbed readily. Nicotinic acid and nicotinamide both are present in blood and move between it and cerebrospinal fluid. Both compounds are converted to the coenzyme forms in the blood cells, kidney, brain, and liver. In the tissues, most of the vitamin is present as nicotinamide in NAD and NADP, although the liver may contain a significant fraction of the free vitamin.

Although nicotinamide can be converted to nicotinic acid by a rather widespread microsomal deamidase, no direct reamidation of nicotinic acid exists. Humans excrete 1-methyl-nicotinamide and 1-methyl-3-carboxamido-6-pyridone as the primary urinary metabolites of niacin.[1]

Deficiency

Lack of niacin may lead to pellagra, a classic deficiency disease in humans that has been most often found among those who subsist chiefly on corn. The typical presentation of pellagra is that of a chronic wasting disease associated with dermatitis, dementia, and diarrhea. The characteristic erythematous dermatitis is bilateral and symmetrical and occurs on skin areas exposed to sunlight. Mental changes include fatigue, insomnia, and apathy, which precede an encephalopathy characterized by confusion, disorientation, hallucination, loss of memory, and eventually frank organic psychoses. The diarrhea, when it occurs, reflects a widespread inflammation of the intestinal mucosal surfaces; other gastrointestinal manifestations include achlorhydria, glossitis, stomatitis, and vaginitis. Although its pathogenesis has been attributed to a deficiency of niacin (and tryptophan), other associated complicating factors may include an imbalance of amino acid intake, particularly the ingestion of high levels of leucine,[1,18] and the presence of mycotoxins elaborated by mold infestations.[18]

Pellagra also is an occasional secondary manifestation of carcinoid syndrome, in which up to 60% of tryptophan is catabolized by what is ordinarily a minor pathway of metabolism, and Hartnup disease, an autosomal recessive disorder in which several amino acids, including tryptophan, are absorbed poorly.

Toxicity

Although relatively large daily intakes of niacin (40 to 200 mg/day) may be required in treatment of Hartnup disease and carcinoid syndrome,[1,18] the use of pharmacological doses is of doubtful value for other dysfunctions and may even prove harmful. Nicotinic acid (but not the amide) in large doses, ranging from 1.3 to 3 g/day, produces vascular dilation or "flushing," with an accompanying sensation of burning or stinging of the face and hands. Pruritus, nausea, vomiting, and diarrhea have been reported commonly but often abate with continued therapy. Varying degrees of hyperpigmentation and acanthosis nigricans occur in rare cases. Additional effects include abnormal glucose tolerance, hyperuricemia, peptic ulcer, hepatomegaly, jaundice, and increased serum transaminases. Therefore high chronic doses of nicotinic acid may be potentially hepatotoxic and should be administered only by physicians.

Methods for the determination of niacin

The measurement of the excretion of N^1-methyl-nicotinamide and N^1-methyl-3-carboxamide-6-pyridone (also named N^1-*methyl-2-pyridone-5-carboxamide*) has been used continually in the biochemical assessment of niacin nutriture. Normally, adults excrete 20% to 30% of their niacin in the form of methylnicotinamide and 40% to 60% as the pyridone. An excretion ratio of pyridone to methylnicotinamide of 1.3 to 4.0 is acceptable, but latent niacin deficiency is indicated by a value below 1.0. As depletion occurs, the pyridone is absent for weeks before clinical signs are noted, while the methylnicotinamide excretion falls to a minimum at about the time that clinical signs are evident. The pyridone-to-methylnicotinamide ratio is determined best with HPLC methods.

Several efficient means exist to separate and quantify both vitaminic and coenzymic forms. Some methods rely on the absorbance of reduced pyridine nucleotides at 340 nm in coupled-enzyme systems, whereas others use fluorescent properties, especially of addition products (for example, with methyl ethyl ketone).

Reference intervals

The reference interval[7] for the excretion rate of N^1-methylnicotinamide is 2.4 to 6.4 mg/day (17.5 to 46.7 μmol/day) or 1.6 to 4.3 mg/g of creatinine (11.7 to 31.4 μmol/g of creatinine).

Vitamin B_{12}

Vitamin B_{12}, also known as *cyanocobalamin*, is a water-soluble hematopoietic vitamin that is required for the maturation of erythrocytes and is involved in general somatic cell metabolism.

Chemistry and sources

The generic term *vitamin B_{12}* refers to a group of physiologically active substances chemically classified as cobalamins or corrinoids. They are composed of tetrapyrrole rings surrounding central cobalt atoms and nucleotide side chains attached to the cobalt atom (Figure 28-15). Cyanocobalamin is a stable compound that forms dark-red, needlelike crystals; it is the reference compound used to measure serum cobalamin concentration. The predominant physiological form of cobalamin in serum is methylcobalamin, whereas that in cytosols is 5'-deoxyadenosylcobalamin.

Vitamin B_{12} is associated closely with animal proteins, and the only significant dietary sources of vitamin B_{12} are

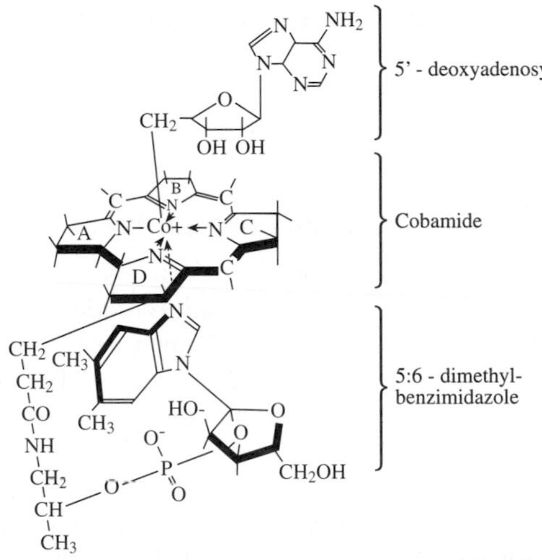

Figure 28-15 The structure of 5'-deoxyadenosyl cobalamin, a physiologically important form of vitamin B_{12}. All the active cobalamins contain a corrin ring (a ring similar to that in heme, but with no bridging carbon atom between rings A and D and with cobalt rather than iron at its center), labeled *cobamide* in this illustration, a purine nucleotide (5:6-dimethylbenzimidazole), and an organic ligand, in this case 5'-deoxyadenosine. The various cobalamins differ principally in the moiety linked to the cobalt above the plane of the corrin nucleus in this illustration. Methylcobalamin is the simplest of these, with a methyl group bound to the cobalt atom. Cyanocobalamin, commercial vitamin B_{12}, has CN^- at this same position. In hydroxocobalamin and aquocobalamin, OH^- and H_2O groups, respectively, are linked to cobalt at this position. (Modified from Chanarin I: The Megaloblastic anaemias, 2nd edition, Oxford, Blackwell Scientific, 1979.)

meats, milk or milk products, and eggs. It is not found in vegetables.

Functions

Vitamin B_{12} is a coenzyme for the synthesis of methionine and conversion of methylmalonic acid to succinic acid (Figure 28-16). The synthesis of methionine requires methylcobalamin, whereas the conversion of methylmalonyl CoA requires deoxyadenosylcobalamin. In reaction *(1)*, methylcobalamin serves as an intermediate in the transfer of a methyl group from N^5-methyltetrahydrofolate to homocysteine for the formation of methionine. Methionine is required for the synthesis of formate and S-adenosylmethionine. Formate is essential for purine synthesis, the conversion of deoxyuridylate to thymidylate, and the production of the active folate coenzyme. S-adenosylmethionine is thought to be important in neuronal metabolism. Reaction *(2)* plays an important role in the metabolism of fatty acids and aliphatic amino acids; deficiency of vitamin B_{12} causes accumulation of abnormal lipids.

Absorption, transport, and metabolism

In the upper gastrointestinal tract, vitamin B_{12} is bound to haptocorrin, a salivary protein, and travels with it into the intestine, where the haptocorrin is digested by pancreatic enzymes. The liberated vitamin B_{12} then binds to intrinsic factor (IF), a glycoprotein secreted by the parietal cells of the stomach with an MW of approximately 50,000. When the vitamin B_{12}-IF complex reaches the distal ileum, it is bound by receptors on the surface of mucosal epithelial cells and then enters the cells. Within the mucosal epithelial cells the vitamin B_{12}-IF complex is dissociated, and the vitamin then passes into the plasma of the mucosal capillaries and then to the portal vein. Almost all the vitamin B_{12} is taken up by hepatocytes as the portal vein blood passes through the liver.

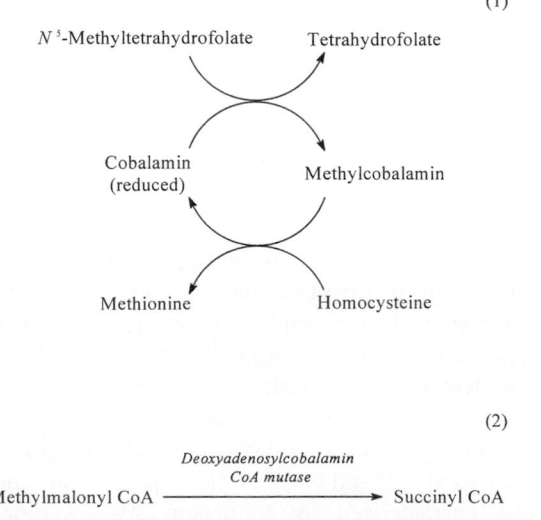

(1)

(2)

Figure 28-16 Role of vitamin B_{12} in the synthesis of methionine and succinyl CoA. *CoA*, Coenzyme A.

It is stored in the liver and released to plasma to meet physiological demands. If the quantity of vitamin B_{12} exceeds the capacity of hepatocyte receptors, most of the excess is excreted by the kidneys. Normally, approximately 1 mg of vitamin B_{12} is stored in the liver, a quantity equivalent to the daily metabolic requirement for 2000 days. Thus when the dietary supply of vitamin B_{12} is interrupted or mechanisms of absorption are impaired, vitamin B_{12} deficiency does not become evident for 5 years or more.

Deficiency

Among the causes of vitamin B_{12} deficiency are lack of IF secretion by the stomach and intestinal malabsorption. In the absence of IF (pernicious anemia), vitamin B_{12} is not absorbed from food. Pernicious anemia most commonly occurs in young black women or in middle-aged to elderly whites. Pernicious anemia also may occur in children because of either failure of IF secretion or secretion of biologically inactive IF. In addition, vitamin B_{12} deficiency may occur many years after partial gastrectomy.

Intestinal malabsorption of vitamin B_{12} may be caused by gastrectomy or ileal resection. Other causes of malabsorption include tropical sprue, inflammatory disease of the small intestine, and intestinal stasis with overgrowth of colonic bacteria.

Deficiency of vitamin B_{12} in humans is associated with megaloblastic anemia, neuropathy, and often irreversible neurological disorders, such as burning pain or loss of sensation in the extremities, weakness, spasticity and paralysis, confusion, disorientation, and dementia.[2] This condition has been given the name *subacute combined degeneration of the spinal cord*. Neurological symptoms may occur without any discernible hematological changes in the blood.

Methods for the determinations of vitamin B_{12} and B_{12} status

Both indirect and direct methods are available to measure vitamin B_{12} acid in body fluids.

Indirect methods

Indirect tests used to assess vitamin B_{12} deficiency include assays for measurement of the urinary and serum levels of methylmalonic acid and plasma homocysteine and the vitamin B_{12} absorption test. Cytochemical staining of RBC precursors and the test for IF-blocking antibodies also are ancillary methods used to assess vitamin B_{12} status.

Methylmalonic acid assay.   Because vitamin B_{12} is necessary for the conversion of methylmalonic acid to succinic acid, individuals deficient in vitamin B_{12} excrete excess amounts of methylmalonic acid in the urine. Methylmalonic acid can be measured reliably by a gas chromatograph-mass spectrometer operated in the selective ion-monitoring mode. For serum specimens this technique can detect as little as 0.026 μmol/L, with a normal reference interval of 0.08 to 0.56 μmol/L and a coefficient of variation (CV) of less than $\pm 8\%$. This test is useful to confirm tissue cobal-

amin deficiency in individuals with low serum cobalamin concentrations.

Measurement of homocysteine.   Homocysteine is increased in the plasma of individuals who are deficient in vitamin B_{12} because their cells do not metabolize homocysteine to methionine at a normal rate. The increase in plasma homocysteine may precede the typical signs of macrocytic anemia and decreased serum cobalamin concentrations. The homocysteine concentration returns to normal on administration of therapy with cobalamin. The measurement of homocysteine is discussed in Chapter 18.

Vitamin B_{12} absorption (Schilling) test.   The B_{12} absorption (Schilling) test permits differentiation of causes of vitamin B_{12} deficiency (pernicious anemia or intestinal malabsorption). The proportion absorbed from orally administered [57]Co- or [58]Co-labeled vitamin B_{12} can be measured by determination of the radioactivity in feces, urine, or serum or by externally scanning of the liver. The usual procedure is to measure radioactivity in a 24-hour urine sample, which is collected after oral administration of 0.5 μg of radioactive cobalt-labeled vitamin B_{12} after an overnight fast. The patient also is injected intramuscularly with a "flushing dose" of 1000 μg of unlabeled vitamin B_{12} to cause urinary excretion of the absorbed vitamin B_{12}. In normal individuals, 8% or more of the administered dose is excreted in the urine, whereas in those with pernicious anemia, less than 7% (often 3% or less and sometimes none) is excreted.

A confirmatory test for lack of IF requires ingestion of B_{12} and IF and a repeat of the flushing dose 1 or 2 days after the initial vitamin B_{12} absorption tests. When gastric secretion of IF is lacking, oral administration of IF simultaneously with vitamin B_{12} increases the absorption of vitamin B_{12} by the intestinal tract; thus the urinary excretion increases to 8% or more of the administered dose. In patients with malabsorption, oral administration of IF does not increase the percentage of the excreted dose. However, approximately 25% of individuals with pernicious anemia also have intestinal malabsorption secondary to vitamin B_{12} deficiency, which is reversible after weeks or months of vitamin B_{12} therapy. Thus a low value for vitamin B_{12} absorption when it is administered with IF does not rule out pernicious anemia.

Tests for intrinsic factor-blocking antibodies.   IF-blocking antibodies have been observed in the serum of nearly 50% of individuals with pernicious anemia but rarely in those with any other condition. Demonstration of these antibodies in the serum is valuable for confirmation of pernicious anemia. However, negative results do not rule out pernicious anemia. A kit for detection of IF-blocking antibody in serum is available commercially.

Direct tests

Microbiological, competitive protein binding (CPB), and immunometric assays are direct methods used to quantify vitamin B_{12}. The microbiological assays have been replaced largely by the other, more convenient and precise methods.

Competitive protein binding assay.   Commercial kits are available for the CPB assays of vitamin B_{12} and folic acid. Most provide for simultaneous measurement of both substances in the same reaction tube. A different binder is needed for each vitamin. Nonhuman IF and β-lactoglobulin are used as binders for vitamin B_{12} and folate, respectively. To measure only metabolically active vitamin B_{12} ("true B_{12}") in CPB assays, either the IF must be highly purified or cobinamide (a vitamin B_{12} analogue) must be added to the IF. The addition of cobinamide eliminates interferences in the assay caused by B_{12} analogues that may be present in the sample or by other binders that may be present in the IF preparation.

Immunometric assay.   Most immunometric methods use solid-phase separation by immobilization of the IF and folate binder on beads or magnetic particles. For simultaneous folate/vitamin B_{12} measurement, a (γ-scintillation counter that discriminates between the energy levels of ^{57}Co (for vitamin B_{12}) and ^{125}I (for folate) must be used. Two dose-response curves are constructed by use of calibrators with known concentrations of vitamin B_{12} and folate, and the concentrations of assayed samples are determined by interpolation from the calibration curves.

Reference intervals

The reference interval[7] for serum vitamin B_{12} for adults in the fasting state is 200 to 835 pg/mL (148 to 616 pmol/L). Individuals with untreated pernicious anemia usually have serum vitamin B_{12} concentrations of less than 100 ng/L. Because deficiency disorders develop gradually, individuals with results in the indeterminate range should have the serum reassayed in a few months, except when a diagnosis is established clearly by other means.

Folic Acid

Folic acid serves as a carrier of one-carbon groups in many metabolic reactions. It is required for the biosynthesis of such compounds as choline, serine, glycine, purines, and deoxythymidine monophosphate (dTMP, also known as *deoxythymidylic acid*).

Chemistry and sources

Folic acid and *folate* are general terms used to describe a family of compounds related to pteroic acid (abbreviated *Pte* in combination forms). Pteroic acid is composed of a pteridine ring joined to a *p*-aminobenzoic acid residue (Figure 28-17). In basic solution this substance is fluores-

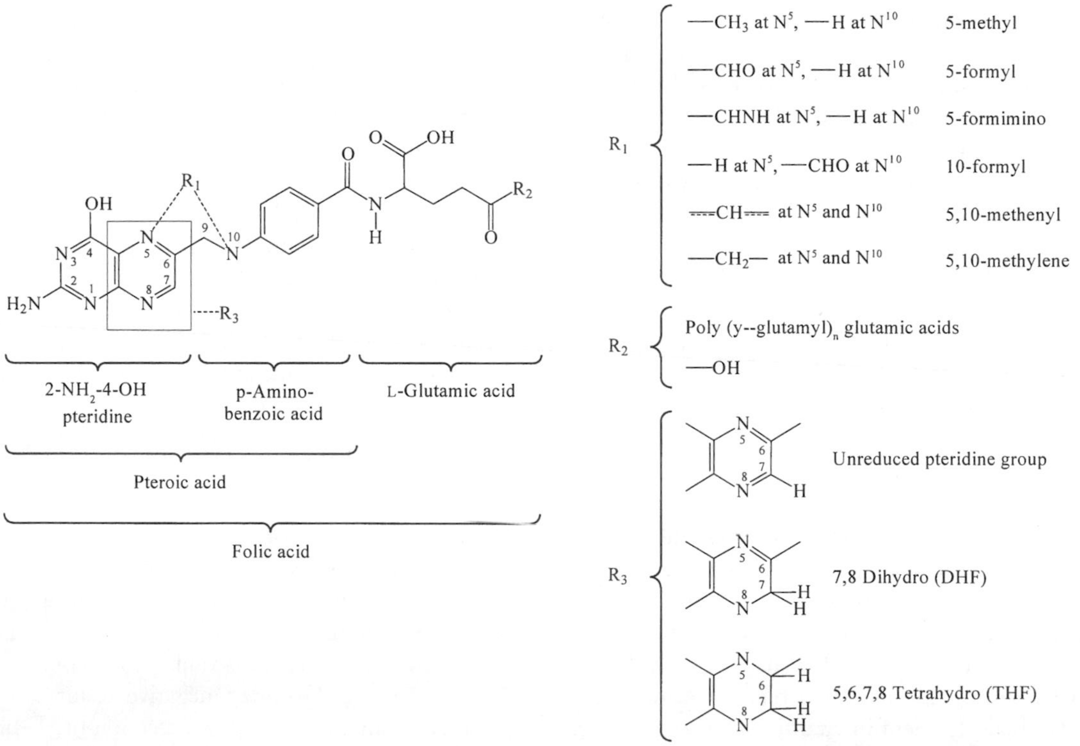

Figure 28-17   Structure and relationships of folic acid and its derivatives. The three basic subunits of folic acid are indicated. Biologically active derivatives have substituent groups at positions R_1, R_2, or R_3. For example, the physiologically active compound N^5,N^{10}-methylene tetrahydrofolate heptaglutamate has a methylene bridge between N^5 and N^{10}; four additional protons at positions 5, 6, 7, and 8 in the pteridine ring (R_3 and six additional glutamate residues attached at position R_2 in the glutamic acid side chain). (Modified from Row PB: Inherited disorders of folate metabolism. In Stanbury JB, Wyngaarden DS (eds): The Metabolic Bases of Inherited Disease, 5th edition, New York, McGraw-Hill, 1983.)

cent and has absorption maxima at 256, 282, and 365 nm. Pterolyglutamic acid (PteGlu) is formed when pteroic acid is conjugated with one molecule of L-glutamic acid. It can be reduced to dihydrofolic acid ($H_2PteGlu$ or FH_2) or to tetrahydrofolate ($H_4PteGlu$ or FH_4). Only the reduced forms are biologically active. Although various forms of folic acid normally are present in human serum and other body fluids, the principal form is N^5-methyltetrahydrofolate.

Folate is found in green vegetables, potatoes, cereals and cereal products, fruits, and organ meats.

Functions

Folate coenzymes are essential for the transfer of single carbon units. Five of the major reactions involve the conversion of serine to glycine; catabolism of histidine; and synthesis of thymidylate, methionine, and purine (Figure 28-18). As indicated in Table 28-2, different folates are involved in these

TABLE 28-2   Reactions in which Folic Acid Derivatives Are Involved

Reaction	Group Transferred	Folic Acid Derivative
Serum/glycine metabolism	Methylene (–CH$_2$–)	N^5, N^{10}-methylene FH$_4$
Histidine catabolism	Formimino (–CHNH)	N^5-Formimino FH$_4$
Thymidylate synthesis	Methylene (–CH$_2$–)	N^5,N^{10}-methylene FH$_4$
Methionine synthesis	Methyl (–CH$_3$)	N^5,N^{10}-methylene FH$_4$
Purine synthesis	Methenyl (=CH–) Formyl (–CHO)	N^5,N^{10}-methenyl FH$_4$ N^5,N^{10}-formyl FH$_4$

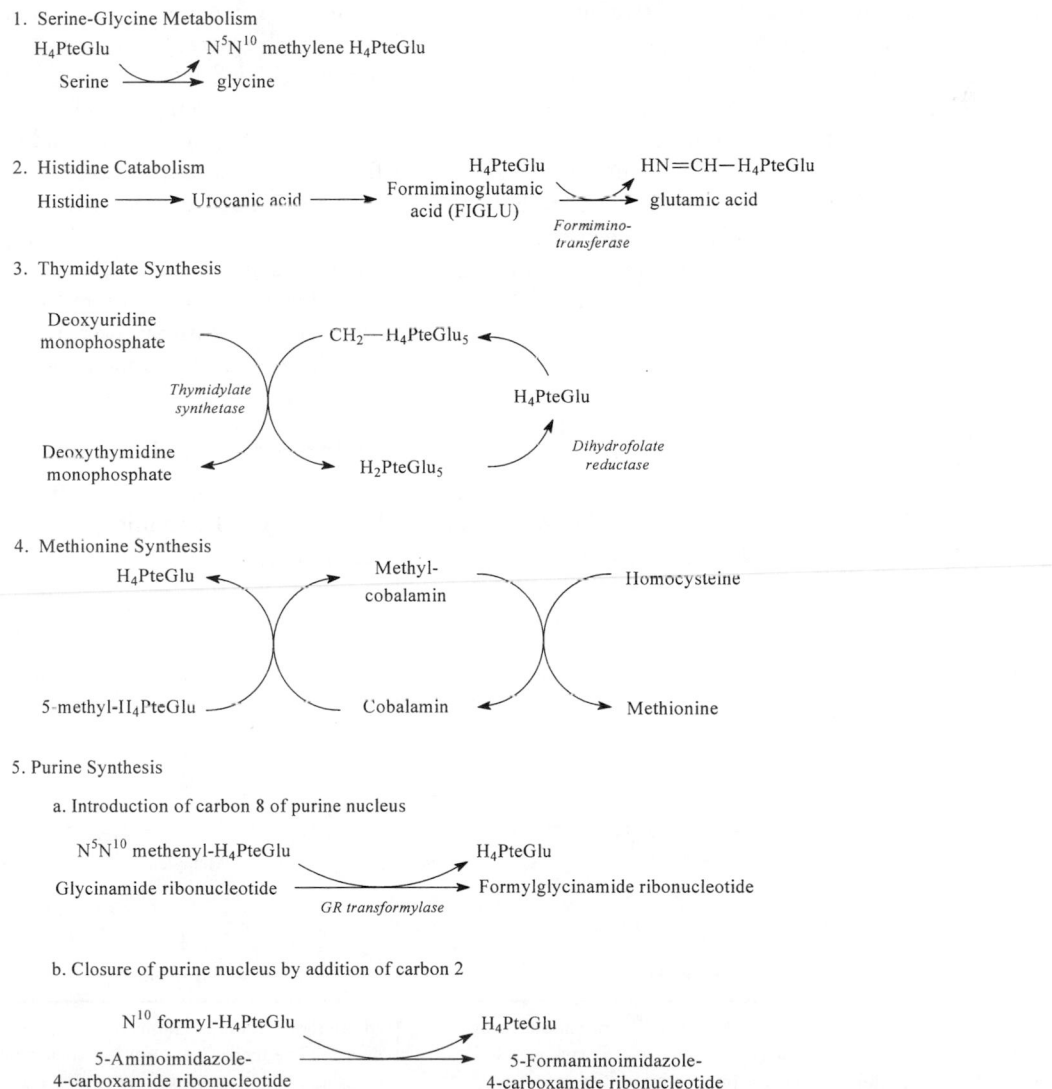

Figure 28-18   The five major metabolic functions of folate in human cells (see text for details). *PteGlu*, Pterolyglutamic acid.

reactions, depending on the chemical state of the single carbon fragments transferred.

The interconversion of these forms of folic acid takes place through various electron-transfer reactions facilitated by specific enzyme systems and coenzymes, such as the reduced forms of flavin adenine dinucleotide ($FADH_2$) and NADPH (Figure 28-19). The conversion between the N^5,N^{10}-methylene form and N^{10}-formyl forms is reversible readily, but the reduction of methylene to methyl and reduction of free tetrahydrofolate to formyltetrahydrofolate essentially is irreversible. Conversion of N^5-methyltetrahydrofolate back to free tetrahydrofolate may require cobalamin.

Absorption, transport, and metabolism

Folate is absorbed from dietary sources such as green, leafy vegetables. Polyglutamate forms of folate present in food first are converted to monoglutamates, by pteroylpolyglutamate hydrolase in the intestinal mucosa. After cellular uptake, most folate is reduced and methylated and enters the circulation as N^5-methyltetrahydrofolate

In blood, folate is transported bound to high- and low-affinity folate protein binders found in plasma. The functional role of these binders is unknown, but they may serve to reduce folate loss from renal filtration and they possibly could play a role in bacterial defense. Serum folate-binding capacity increases in individuals with chronic granulocytic leukemia, acute hepatitis, cirrhosis, and uremia and in pregnant women. Unlike vitamin B_{12}, no clinical disorders have been reported that relate to the absence of absorption or transport-binding proteins for folic acid.

Folate and vitamin B_{12} metabolism are linked by the reaction that transfers a methyl group from N^5-methyltetrahydrofolate to cobalamin. In cases of cobalamin deficiency, folate is "trapped" as N^5-methyltetrahydrofolate. It is "metabolically dead" in the absence of vitamin B_{12} and is not recycled as tetrahydrofolate back into the folate pool

to serve as the main one-carbon unit acceptor for many biochemical reactions. Cellular depletion of methylenetetrahydrofolate eventually ensues, causing a reduction in thymidylic acid synthesis, which in turn results in megaloblastic anemia and neuropathies.

Deficiency

Deficiency of folate may result from (1) absence of intestinal microorganisms (gut sterilization), (2) poor intestinal absorption (for example, after surgical resection or in celiac disease or sprue), (3) insufficient dietary intake, and (4) excessive demands (as in pregnancy, liver disease, and malignancies). Administration of antifolate drugs (for example, methotrexate), and anticonvulsant therapy (which increases folate requirements, especially during pregnancy) also can result in folate deficiency.

Megaloblastic anemia is the major clinical manifestation of folate deficiency, although sensory loss and neuropsychiatric changes also may occur. Combined deficiency of both folate and iron commonly occurs in malnourished individuals. In such cases, macrocytosis of RBCs, otherwise typical of folic acid deficiency, is not observed. Lower-than-normal serum folate concentrations have been reported in individuals with psychiatric disorders and in pregnant women whose fetuses have neural-tube defects.

Several rare inborn errors of folate metabolism include congenital folate malabsorption, dihydrofolate reductase deficiency, forminotransferase deficiency, 5,10-methylenetetrahydrofolate reductase deficiency, tetrahydrofolate methyltransferase deficiency, and hereditary aplastic anemia caused by abnormal cellular folate uptake or retention.[15]

Methods for the determination of folic acid

Similar to those methods described for vitamin B_{12}, microbiological, CPB, and immunometric assays are used to measure folic acid.

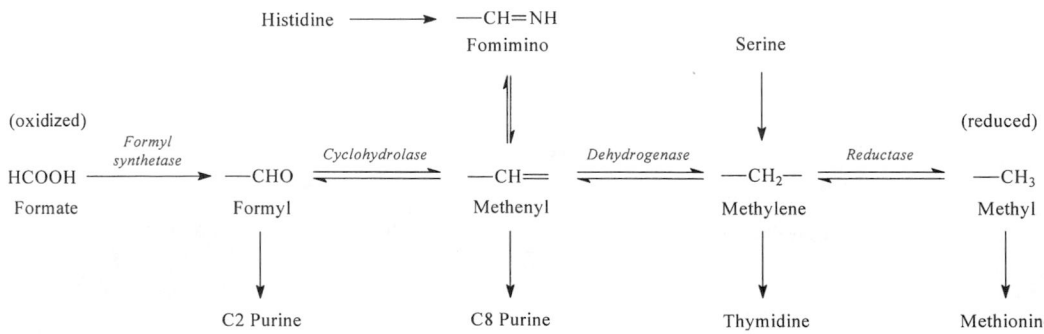

Figure 28-19   The metabolism and interconversion of various forms of folate. Formate is the most oxidized form, and the formyl, methenyl, methylene, and methyl forms represent progressive reduction states. These various forms are related directly to the metabolic functions illustrated in Figure 28-18. The formyl form closes the purine nucleus by addition of carbon 2. The methenyl form adds carbon 8 to the purine nucleus. The methylene form is a coenzyme in thymidylate synthesis, and the methyl forms are coenzymes in methionine synthesis. (Modified from Chanarin I, Deacon R, Lumb M et al: Vitamin B_{12} regulates folate metabolism by the supply of formate. Lancet, 2:505, 1980.)

Reference intervals

The representative reference interval[7] for adults in the fasting state for serum folate is 3 to 20 ng/mL (7 to 45 nmol/L).

Biotin

Biotin is the prosthetic group for a number of carboxylation reactions (for example, pyruvate, acetyl-CoA, and propionyl Co-A decarboxylases).

Chemistry and sources

Biotin was known formerly as *vitamin H*. Its chemical structure is *cis*-tetrahydro-2-oxothieno[3,4-*d*]-imidazoline-4-valeric acid (Figure 28-20). In most organisms, biotin is found mainly bound to protein. In addition, some biotin is linked noncovalently as a complex with avidin, a protein in egg white. Good sources of biotin include liver, kidney, pancreas, eggs, yeast, and milk.[6] Cereal grains, fruit, and meat are regarded as poor sources of the vitamin.[13]

Functions

Biotin-dependent enzymes include carboxylases, decarboxylases, and transcarboxylase. Four carboxylases found in human tissue are for acetyl-CoA, propionyl-CoA, β-methylcrotonyl-CoA, and pyruvate. The biotin-dependent carboxylases operate via a common mechanism, which involves phosphorylation of bicarbonate by ATP to form carbonyl phosphate, followed by transfer of the carboxyl group to the sterically less hindered nitrogen of the biotin moiety. The resulting N(1)-carboxybiotinyl enzyme then exchanges the carboxylate function with a reactive center in a substrate. With cytosolic acetyl-CoA carboxylase, the product is malonyl-CoA, which is used for fatty acid biosynthesis. In mitochondria, pyruvate carboxylase catalyzes formation of oxaloacetate, which together with acetyl-CoA forms citrate. The other carboxylases are involved in the metabolism of odd-numbered fatty acids and branched-chain fatty acids.

Absorption, transport, and metabolism

Digestion of dietary proteins containing bound biotin yields biocytin (ε-N-biotinyl-L-lysine). Biocytin and biotin both are absorbed readily. Biotin is cleared from the circulating blood and taken up by such tissues as liver and muscle. Because of microfloral biosynthesis, urinary excretion of biotin-like substances often exceeds dietary intake, with fe-

cal excretion as much as three to six times greater than dietary intake.[13]

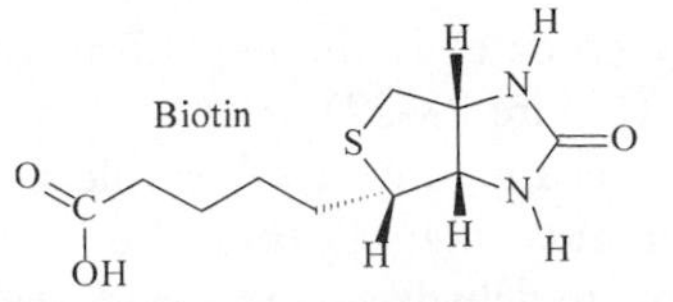

Deficiency

Dietary deficiency of biotin is seen infrequently and is produced in the adult usually only after ingestion of diets that include large amounts of raw egg white (containing avidin).[13] Symptoms include anorexia, nausea, vomiting, glossitis, pallor, depression, and a dry, scaly dermatitis. A seborrheic dermatitis in infants under 6 months of age is caused by inadequate biotin, but the condition responds promptly to biotin therapy. Significantly lowered urinary excretion or circulating blood levels also have been found in pregnant women, alcoholics, individuals with achlorhydria, the elderly, and some athletes. In addition, rather rare genetic enzyme defects, such as in **holoenzyme** synthetase (reflected in inadequate conversion of apocarboxylases to holocarboxylases) and proprionyl-CoA carboxylase (reflected in a distinguishing acidemia), also occur.

Methods for the determination of biotin

Biotin can be quantified with microbiological assays. Bound biotin first is liberated by proteolytic digestion of the sample through use of a protease, such as papain. Aliquots then are added to a biotin-deficient medium inoculated with a test organism, such as *Lactobacillus plantarum*. Calibration curves are derived from growth in calibrators containing known amounts of biotin. Isotopic dilution, avidin-binding, HPLC-avidin binding,[8,19] chemiluminescent, and photometric methods also are available. In the photometric assay, biotin forms a red Schiff base with acidic p-dimethylaminocinnamaldehyde.

Reference intervals

The reference interval[7] for biotin in whole blood or serum is 200 to 500 pg/mL (0.82 to 2.05 nmol/L).

Pantothenic Acid

Pantothenic acid is a component of CoA and the 4′-phosphopantotheinyl moiety of the acyl carrier protein of the fatty acid synthase complex. This vitamin is necessary for the metabolism of fat, protein, and carbohydrate via the citric acid cycle.

Chemistry and sources

Pantothenic acid (pantothenate) occurs ubiquitously in nature, where it is synthesized by most microorganisms and plants from pantoic acid. It is an integral part of 4′-phosphopantetheine, which serves as a covalently attached prosthetic group of acyl carrier proteins (ACPs), and within the structure of CoA (Figure 28-21). The vitamin is distributed widely in foods, mostly within CoA-containing compounds, and is particularly abundant in animal sources, legumes, and whole-grain cereals.[6,13] Egg yolk, kidney, liver,

Figure 28-20   Biotin.

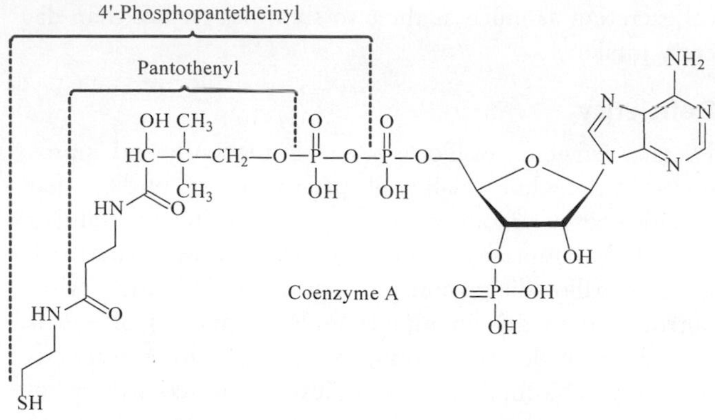

Figure 28-21 Pantothenate and 4′-phosphopantetheine as components of coenzyme A.

and yeast are excellent food sources, containing 100 to 200 μg/g of dry weight. Broccoli, lean beef, skim milk, sweet potatoes, and molasses are fair sources (35 to 100 μg/g) of the vitamin. Over one-half the pantothenate in wheat may be lost during the manufacture of flour, and up to one-third is lost during cooking of meat. Pantothenic acid is a hygroscopic, viscous oil that is destroyed easily by heat, especially at extremes of pH. The most common commercial synthetic form is the calcium salt.

Functions

Pantothenic acid is a constituent of acyl thiol esters of CoA. These esters are central to the metabolism of numerous compounds, especially lipids and the ultimate catabolic disposition of carbohydrates and ketogenic amino acids. The chemical properties of the thiol ester, which has a high group-transfer potential, permits acylations and facilitates condensation reactions. For example, acetyl-CoA, which results from the metabolism of carbohydrates, fats, and amino acids, acetylates compounds such as choline and hexosamines to produce essential biochemicals; it also condenses with other metabolites, such as oxaloacetate, to supply citrate and cholesterol.

Another essential role of pantothenic acid is its participation in the 4′-phosphopantetheine moiety of ACP, where the phosphodiester-linked prosthetic group uses the sulfhydryl terminus to exchange with malonyl-CoA to form a malonyl thioester derivative, which can chain-elongate during fatty acid biosynthesis.

Absorption, transport, and metabolism

CoA, the form in which much of the pantothenic acid is ingested, is hydrolyzed by intestinal pyrophosphatase and phosphatase to pantetheine (pantothenyl cysteamine), which together with pantothenate is absorbed into the portal circulation. About 80% of the vitamin in animal tissues is in CoA form, with the rest existing mainly as phosphopantetheine and phosphopantethenate. Enzymes hydrolyze the phosphate moieties from pantothenate releasing

β-mercaptoethylamine, which is excreted in the urine. Only a small fraction of pantothenate is secreted into milk and even less into colostrum.

Deficiency

With its widespread occurrence in foods, a dietary deficiency of pantothenate is rare in humans.[1,13] Symptoms have been produced in a few volunteers who have received ω-methylpantothenic acid as an antagonist and in individuals fed semisynthetic diets virtually free of pantothenate. Such individuals become irritable and develop a postural hypotension and rapid heart rate on exertion, epigastric distress with anorexia and constipation, numbness and tingling of the hands and feet, hyperactive deep tendon reflexes, and weakness of finger extensor muscles.

Methods for the determination of pantothenic acid

Pantothenic acid usually is measured by microbiological procedures, often by use of *Lactobacillus plantarum. Pediococcus acidilactici* NCIB 6990 has been found to be especially sensitive as an assay organism. Radioimmunoassay, gas chromatographic, HPLC, capillary electrophoretic methods also have been used to quantify pantothenic acid in infant milk formulas[14] and pharmaceutical preparations,[5] respectively. Enzymatic assays are available for measurement of CoA and ACP.

Because urinary output is directly proportional to dietary intake, it can be used to assess pantothenate status. Urinary excretion of less than 1 mg/day is considered abnormally low. Suspicion of inadequate intake is supported further if whole blood levels are less than 100 μg/dL. Functional tests based on acetylation of sulfanilamide by RBCs and urinary excretion of acetylated *p*-aminobenzoic acid after a load test of the acid also are available.

Reference intervals

The reference interval[7] for pantothenic acid in whole blood or serum is 0.2 to 1.8 μg/mL (0.9 to 8.2 μmol/L). The reference interval for its urinary excretion rate is 1 to 15 mg/day (5 to 68 μmol/day).

Ascorbic Acid

Vitamin C (L-ascorbic acid) serves as a reducing agent in several important hydroxylation reactions in the body.

Chemistry and sources

L-Ascorbic acid (ascorbate) is the enol form of 2-oxo-L-gulofuranolactone (Figure 28-22). It is a white, crystalline solid that is soluble readily in water. Ascorbic acid is a relatively strong reductant with an E_0' (pH 7) of +0.58 volt. It is oxidized reversibly to dehydroascorbic acid, also known as *ascorbone* (see Figure 28-12). The dehydro form is more la-

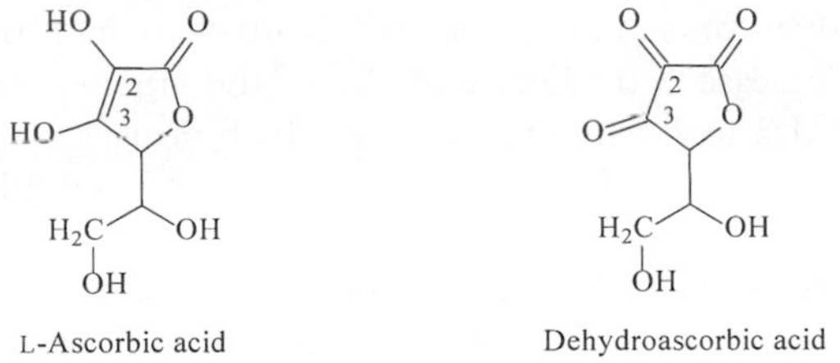

Figure 28-22 L-Ascorbic and dehydroascorbic acids.

bile than the reduced form.[13] Plants and most animals possess the ability to synthesize the vitamin from D-glucose via the lactones of D-glucuronic and L-gulonic acids; however, some mammals, including the human, lack L-gulonolactone oxidase, the enzyme that catalyzes the formation of 2-keto-L-gulonolactone, which spontaneously tautomerizes to L-ascorbic acid. The best sources of the vitamin are citrus fruits, berries, melons, tomatoes, green peppers, raw cabbage, and leafy, green vegetables. Losses during processing, especially with heat and aerobic conditions, can be considerable.

Functions

The most clearly established and critical functional role for ascorbic acid is as a **cofactor** for protocollagen hydroxylase, the enzyme responsible for hydroxylation of prolyl and lysyl residues within nascent peptides in connective tissue proteins. Among these are collagen and related proteins, which comprise intercellular material of cartilage, dentin, and bone. Vitamin C functions similarly in the hydroxylation of γ-butyrobetaine to carnitine. Vitamin C also may be involved in tyrosine metabolism, microsomal drug metabolism, synthesis of epinephrine and antiinflammatory steroids by the adrenals, folic acid metabolism, and leukocyte functions. These roles seem to relate to the favorable reductive properties of L-ascorbic acid, especially on Fe^{+2}-enzyme systems. Iron absorption, as Fe^{+2}, also is enhanced by simultaneous ingestion of the vitamin.

Absorption, transport, and metabolism

Absorption of vitamin C occurs readily from the stomach, where some of the ascorbic acid is converted to the dehydro form. At physiological pH, the uncharged dehydroascorbic acid passes across cell membranes faster than the monoanionic L-ascorbate. Passive diffusion of vitamin C may account largely for entry into some cells, such as leukocytes and erythrocytes, but an active transport mechanism also may operate, especially for platelets, adrenals, and retina. The free diffusion of dehydroascorbic acid into cells, followed by intracellular reduction into the less diffusible ascorbate ion, may explain the occurrence of the higher concentration of ascorbate in leukocytes than in plasma. Vitamin C is found in most tissues, but glandular tissues, such as the pituitary, adrenal cortex, corpus luteum, and thymus, have the highest amounts, and the retina has 20 to 30 times

the plasma concentration. The half-life for vitamin C in the human is approximately 16 days. In addition to the presence of ascorbate and dehydroascorbic acid, lesser amounts of a number of catabolites also are present in urine.

Deficiency

Prolonged deficiency of vitamin C leads to scurvy. Inability to form adequate intercellular substance in connective tissue is reflected in swollen, tender, and often bleeding or bruised loci at joints and in other areas where structurally weakened tissue cannot withstand stress.[6] Infantile scurvy, also known as *Barlow's disease*, exhibits a bayonet-rib syndrome. The gums are livid and swollen, particularly in the regions of the papillae between the teeth; sometimes "scurvy buds" develop, which may project beyond the biting surface. Cutaneous bleeding often begins on the lower thighs as perifollicular hemorrhages; these then may spread to the buttocks, abdomen, legs, and arms. Petechial hemorrhages caused by the rupture of capillaries often appear. Thereafter, large spontaneous bruises (ecchymoses) may arise almost anywhere on the body. Ocular hemorrhages, drying of salivary and lacrimal glands, parotid swelling, femoral neuropathy, edema of the lower extremities, and psychological disturbances also have been described. Some scorbutic individuals may develop anemia, display radiological changes characteristic of osteoporosis, or die suddenly from heart failure. A daily dose of 10 mg of vitamin C is sufficient to alleviate and cure the clinical signs of scurvy.

Toxicity

The use of "megadoses" of vitamin C for the prevention or amelioration of the common cold is controversial. As reviewed elsewhere,[13,16] large doses of ascorbic acid generally have been considered nontoxic, except for gastrointestinal symptoms, which some individuals do experience. However, more serious adverse effects have been observed and suspected as potential hazards; these include reductive destruction of concomitantly ingested vitamin B_{12}, facilitation of too much iron absorption, reduced catabolism leading to higher requirements (dependency), increased production of oxalate favoring deposition of calcium oxalate stones in the kidney and bladder (particularly by those who are congenital familial hyperoxalurics), and uricosuria. Both the benefits, indicated epidemiologically for some cancers and heart disease, and hazards from high levels of vitamin C seem minimal for most people, who simply excrete the excess.

Methods for the determination of ascorbic acid

Ascorbic acid can be determined photometrically with 2,4-dinitrophenylhydrazine to form the red *bis*-hydrazone or with 2,4-dichlorophenol-indophenol, which is reduced to a colorless form. Fluorometric and HPLC methods also have been developed.[4,8] Vitamin C status generally is assessed by measurement of serum (plasma) and leukocyte levels of the vitamin. Urinary excretion and RBC concentrations have not been found to be specific and useful indicators of vitamin C status; however, urinary levels of ascorbic acid, especially after a load test, are helpful in the clinical diagnosis of scurvy.

Reference intervals

In individuals who ingest adequate amounts of vitamin C, plasma concentrations of total vitamin (ascorbic acid plus dehydroascorbic acid) are between 0.4 and 1.5 mg/dL (23 to 85 µmol/L).[7] The lower limit value may be seen in some cases with subclinical vitamin C deficiency and in older individuals. A value lower than 0.2 mg/dL (11 µmol/L) is considered deficient. The reference interval for vitamin C levels in leukocytes is 20 to 53 µg/10^8 leukocytes (1.14 to 3.01 fmol/leukocyte). A value in leukocytes of less than 10 µg/10^8 leukocytes (0.57 fmol/leukocyte) is considered deficient.

Plasma (or serum) levels of ascorbate demonstrate a linear increase with dietary intake of the vitamin up to a level of 1.2 to 1.4 mg/dL, beyond which urinary excretion rapidly increases. Plasma values above 0.3 mg/dL are considered acceptable, those from 0.2 to 0.29 are "at risk," and those below 0.2 indicate deficiency. Leukocyte ascorbate levels are somewhat more difficult to measure but are more representative of tissue stores. Values ranging from 0 to 7 mg/dL of leukocytes suggest deficiency, whereas values greater than 15 indicate satisfactory vitamin C status. Values also may be expressed as 20 to 50 µg/10^8 WBCs (white blood cells). The urinary excretion of ascorbic acid by healthy adults ranges from 8 to 27 mg/day; this level declines to undetectable levels after depletion.

References

1. Brown ML (ed): Present Knowledge in Nutrition, 6th edition, Washington, DC, International Life Sciences Institute-Nutrition Foundation, 1990.
2. Chanarin I, Metz J: Diagnosis of cobalamin deficiency: the old and the new. Br J Haematol, 1997; 97:695-700.
3. Curti B, Ronchi S, Zanetti G (eds): Flavins and Flavoproteins, New York, de Gruyter, 1990.
4. Esteve MJ, Farre R, Frigola A et al: Determination of ascorbic and dehydroascorbic acids in blood plasma and serum by liquid chromatography. J Chromatogr B Biomed Sci Appl 1997; 688:345-349.
5. Fotsing L, Fillet M, Bechet I et al: Determination of six water-soluble vitamins in a pharmaceutical formulation by capillary electrophoresis. J Pharm Biomed Anal 1997; 15:1113-1123.
6. McCormick DB: Vitamins, structure, and function. In Meyers RA (ed): Encyclopedia of Molecular Biology and Molecular Medicine, vol 6, pp 244-252, New York, VCH, 1997.
7. McCormick DB, Greene HL: Vitamins. In Burtis CA, Ashwood, ER (eds): Tietz Textbook of Clinical Chemistry, 3rd edition, pp 999-1029, Philadelphia, WB Saunders, 1999.
8. McCormick DB, Suttie JW, Wagner C (eds): Vitamins and coenzymes. In Methods in Enzymology, vol 280, part I, San Diego, Academic Press, 1997.
9. McCormick DB, Suttie JW, Wagner C (eds): Vitamins and coenzymes. In Methods in Enzymology, vol 280, part J, San Diego, Academic Press, 1997.
10. McCormick DB, Suttie JW, Wagner C (eds): Vitamins and coenzymes. In Methods in Enzymology, vol 280, part L, San Diego, Academic Press, 1997.
11. McCormick DB, Wright LD (eds): Vitamins and coenzyme. In Methods in Enzymology, vol 67, part F, San Diego, Academic Press, 1980.
12. Merrill AH Jr, Froehlich JA, McCormick DB: Isolation and identification of alternative riboflavin-binding proteins from human plasma. Biochem Med 1981; 25:198-206.
13. National Research Council, Committee on Dietary Allowances: Recommended Dietary Allowances, 10th revised edition, Washington, DC, National Academy of Sciences, 1989.
14. Romera JM, Ramirez M, Gil A: Determination of pantothenic acid in infant milk formulas by high performance liquid chromatography. J Dairy Sci 1996; 79:523-526.
15. Rosenblatt DS: Inherited disorders of folate transport and metabolism. In Scriver CR, Beaudet AL, Sly WS et al (eds): The Metabolic and Molecular Bases of Inherited Disease, 7th edition, vol 2, pp 3111-3128, New York, McGraw-Hill, 1995.
16. Sauberlich HE: Pharmacology of vitamin C. In Olson RE (ed): Annual Review of Nutrition, vol 14. Palo Alto, Calif, Annual Reviews, 1994.
17. Van Breeman RB: Innovations in carotenoid analysis using LC/MS. Anal Chem 1996; 68:299A-304A.
18. Wilson JD: Vitamin deficiency and excess. In Fauci AS, Braunwald E, Isselbacher KJ et al (eds): Harrison's Principles of Internal Medicine, 14th edition, pp 480-492, New York, McGraw-Hill, 1998.
19. Zempleni J, Mock DM: Advanced analysis of biotin metabolites in body fluids allows a more accurate measurement of biotin bioavailability and metabolism in humans. J Nutr 1999; 129:494S-497S.
20. Zhang Z, McCormick DB: Pyridoxine-5'-β-D-glucoside competitively inhibits uptake of vitamin B_6 into isolated rat liver cells. J Nutr 1993; 123:85-89.

Additional Reading

Basu TK, Dikerson JW: Vitamins in Human Health and Disease, Oxford, Oxford University Press, 1996.

Dietary Reference Intakes for Calcium, Phosphorus, Magnesium, Vitamin D, and Fluoride, Washington, DC, National Academy Press, 1997.

Dietary Reference Intakes for Thiamine, Riboflavin, Niacin, Vitamin B6, Folate, Vitamin B12, Pantothenic Acid, Biotin, and Choline, Washington, DC, National Academy Press, 1999.

Dietary Reference Intakes for Vitamin C, Vitamin E, Selenium, Beta-Carotene, and Other Carotenoids, Washington, DC, National Academy Press, 2000.

Gunter EW, Lewis BL, Koncikowski SM: Laboratory methods used for the Third National Health and Nutrition Examination Survey (NHANES III), 1988-1994. Hyattsville, Md, Centers for Disease Control and Prevention, 1996.

Klee GG: Cobalamin and folate evaluation: measurement of methylmalonic acid and homocysteine vs vitamin B12 and folate. Clin Chem 2000; 46:1277-1283.

McCormick DB, Chen H: Update on interconversions of vitamin B-6 with its coenzyme. J Nutr 1999; 129:325-327.

Newman P, Shearer MJ: Vitamin K metabolism. Subcell Biochem 1998; 30:455-488.

Traber MG, Sies H: Vitamin E in humans: demand and delivery. Ann Rev Nutr 1996; 16:321-347.

CHAPTER 29

Trace Elements

DAVID B. MILNE, PhD

Objectives

1. Define *trace element* and *ultratrace element*.
2. List the characteristics of trace elements.
3. List seven physiologically essential trace elements and state the clinical significance of each.
4. State the basic functions of the seven essential trace elements.
5. List the analytical methods available for the assessment of trace elements.
6. State the specimen collection requirements for trace elements.

Key Words

Essential Nutrients   Those nutrients (proteins, minerals, carbohydrates, lipids, vitamins) necessary for growth, normal functioning, and maintenance of life; must be supplied by food because they cannot be synthesized by the body

Nutriture   The status of the body in relation to nutrition, generally or in regard to a specific nutrient, such as a trace element

Trace Elements   Inorganic molecules found in human and animal tissues in milligram-per-kilogram amounts or less

Ultratrace Elements   Inorganic molecules found in human and animal tissues in microgram-per-kilogram amounts or less

Trace elements are inorganic molecules that are essential for life. They occur in human and animal tissues in milligram-per-kilogram amounts or less. Intake requirements of trace elements for humans are reported in milligrams per day. Since the 1970s the term **ultratrace elements** has been used to refer to elements present in tissues in microgram-per-kilogram amounts or less and with estimated dietary requirements indicated as micrograms per day.

■ BASIC CONCEPTS AND DEFINITIONS

An element is considered essential when a deficient intake produces an impairment of function, and physiological amounts of only that element prevent or alleviate the impairment. Ultimately, a biochemical basis for the element's essential function must be demonstrated. For trace metals this basis is often the identification of a unique metalloenzyme that contains the metal as an integral part or as an enzyme activator.

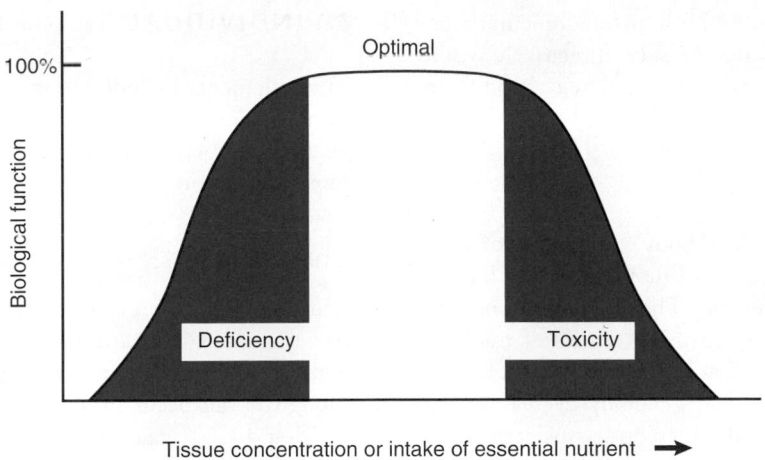

Figure 29-1   Model of the relationship between tissue concentration or intake of an essential nutrient and dependent biological function.

A simple model of the relationship between the intake of an **essential nutrient** and a dependent biological function is shown in Figure 29-1. In states of absolute deficiency, death results. With limited intake the organism may survive, but biological functions are impaired (thus defining a *deficiency state*). The plateau of the curve reflects homeostatic regulation that ensures optimal health over a wide range of intake. As the nutrient is consumed in excess, marginal toxicity is attained, followed by mortal toxic response (see Chapter 32). The basic curve holds true for most essential elements, although the curve may vary quantitatively for each. For many elements, only a 10-fold to 100-fold range exists between survival and the appearance of toxic effects.

Both defined biochemical functions and signs of deficiency in humans are known for only seven trace or ultratrace elements. These include iron, zinc, copper, cobalt (as vitamin B_{12}), iodine, molybdenum, and selenium. Signs of deficiency for chromium and boron have been described in humans, but their biochemical functions have not been defined conclusively. Essential functions for manganese have been described. However, unequivocal signs of deficiency of this element in humans have not been identified. Four other trace or ultratrace elements likely are essential for humans based on findings in animals—nickel, silicon, vanadium, and arsenic. Several elements, such as bromine, cadmium, lead, strontium, and tin, have been suggested as essential, but controversial or limited data have limited the acceptance of an essential classification. Two elements with beneficial pharmacological properties are lithium (antimanic) and fluorine (anticariogenic).

■ TRACE ELEMENT CHARACTERISTICS

Known characteristics of trace element function include (1) amplification of trace element action, (2) specificity, (3) homeostasis, and (4) interactions.

Amplification of Action

Because the action is amplified, only milligram amounts of a trace element are necessary for optimal performance of the whole organism. For example, lack of a small amount of a trace element, such as iron, can result in a clinical abnormality (anemia) seemingly disproportionate to the amount of element missing. This amplification is thought to result from trace elements being constituents of, or interacting with, enzymes and hormones that regulate the metabolism of much larger amounts of biochemical substrates.

Specificity

Essential trace elements are specific for their in vivo functions; they cannot be replaced effectively by chemically similar elements. The essential trace metal or element interacts with electron donor atoms, such as nitrogen, sulfur, and oxygen; the types of interaction depend on configurational preferences and bond types. Certain trace elements are stable in more than one valence state (for example, iron, copper, molybdenum), which allows for a biological oxidation-reduction function, whereas others are stable in only a single state (for example, Zn^{2+}, Ni^{2+}), which allows for more of a conformation or substrate-binding role.

Transition metals with partially filled d electron orbitals (for example, Fe, Cu, Co) tend to coordinate with a larger number of electron donor atoms than metals with filled d-orbitals (Zn^{2+}) and exhibit qualitatively different preferences for the donor atoms. Each transition metal tends to coordinate with the donor atoms in a specific geometrical configuration that depends on the number of d-orbital electrons and the valence state. Nonmetals, such as selenium and iodine, and metalloids, such as silicon and boron, have strong tendencies to form covalent bonds with carbon and oxygen and may be incorporated as part of the organic matrix of a structural protein or enzyme (for example, selenium in selenocysteine and silicon in connective tissue). Elements such as fluorine, magnesium, and lithium are ionic in nature. They are present mainly as free ions, bind relatively weakly to proteins and substrates, and often regulate or modify enzyme activity.

Homeostasis

Mechanisms that ensure optimal body distribution of an element over a range of intakes constitute a system of homeostatic regulation for that element. They include absorption, storage, and excretion. Although many details of trace element absorption processes still are being elucidated, the rate of absorption of a trace element generally decreases as its concentration in the intestinal lumen and associated tissues increases. Active transport mechanisms involving absorption by specific metal binders and feedback inhibition have been postulated for iron, zinc, and copper. Storage proteins, such as metallothionein and ferritin, are important in the regulation of zinc, copper, and iron through their ability to buffer against excess free metal.

The principal excretory route for elimination of most trace metals is via the feces. Fecal excretion reflects dietary intake and homeostatic regulatory mechanisms, such as gastrointestinal absorption and endogenous metal secretion into the intestine. Relatively small amounts of trace metals are excreted via the urine, but halides (iodide and fluoride), selenium, chromium, and boron are eliminated effectively through the urine. The loss of trace elements through other routes, such as hair, nails, skin-cell desquamation, and sweat, generally is relatively minor. Body-surface losses of some trace metals, particularly zinc, selenium, and iron, can be appreciable in hot climates or in certain stressful conditions. Menstrual iron loss and seminal zinc loss also are minor but can be significant in some cases.

Interactions

An overabundance of one trace element can interfere with the metabolic use of another element present in normal or marginal concentrations. Alternatively, the effect of a toxic trace element may be ameliorated by another "protective" trace element. The addition of large amounts of zinc to a diet interferes with intestinal copper absorption, resulting in copper deficiency despite an otherwise adequate copper intake. Hence, zinc is said to antagonize copper absorption. Copper deficiency, in turn, is known to provoke iron deficiency and anemia. Molybdenum deficiency is much easier to produce in animals when the chemically similar element tungsten is administered simultaneously in large amounts. Interactions that involve toxic elements include the increased retention of cadmium and lead associated with iron deficiency and the protective effect of selenium against cadmium and mercury toxicity.

◾ INDIVIDUAL TRACE ELEMENTS

Trace elements include chromium, cobalt, copper, fluoride, iron, magnesium, manganese, molybdenum, selenium, and zinc. Of these, iron, zinc, and copper are considered the most important.

Chromium

Chromium (Cr) is a transitional element with many industrial uses. It occurs naturally in various crustal materials and is discharged into the environment as industrial waste. Although it can occur in a number of oxidation states, only Cr^{+3} and Cr^{+6} valence states are found in biological systems. The biological behavior of chromium is largely a function of its oxidation state. The biochemical and clinical aspects of chromium nutrition have been reviewed.[27]

Biochemistry

Chromium functions in the control of glucose and lipid metabolism. Studies have shown that a low molecular weight (MW) chromium compound potentiates insulin action. Insulin resistance may be a consequence of chromium deficiency, and insulin apparently is ineffective as a glucose regulator without chromium.

Low-molecular weight chromium binding substance (LMWCr) is a naturally occurring chromium-related substance that potentiates the action of insulin.[30] LMWCr is a mammalian oligopeptide of about 1500 Da that binds four chromic ions and potentiates the ability of insulin to stimulate the conversion of glucose into lipids and carbon dioxide by isolated rat adipocytes. A proposed biological role for LMWCr is the stimulation of insulin receptor tyrosine kinase activity after the receptor is activated by insulin.[30]

Metabolism

The site and mechanism of intestinal chromium absorption in humans have not been determined. However, animal studies indicate that chromium is absorbed in the upper small intestine. Trivalent chromium is absorbed poorly; estimates of absorption of dietary chromium range from 0.3% to about 2%, depending on dietary intake.

After absorption, trivalent chromium binds to the β-globulin fractions of serum proteins, specifically to transferrin. Transferrin apparently is the protein involved in chromium transport to the tissues; chromium has about the same affinity as iron toward transferrin.

The regulation of chromium homeostasis is still obscure, although urinary excretion seems to be important. The majority of orally absorbed inorganic chromium is excreted via the kidneys in an unknown form.

Trivalent chromium has a low order of toxicity. A wide margin of safety, about 1:10,000, exists between supplementation used to cure deficiency and toxicity. Cr^{+6} is considerably more toxic than Cr^{+3}. Occupational exposure to chromate occurs in electroplating, steel making, leather tanning, photography, dyeing, and chemical manufacture operations. Acute exposure may produce an allergic reaction, conjunctivitis, nasal septum ulceration, dermatitis, edema, and ulcer. Chronic exposure may produce gastrointestinal symptoms, hepatitis, and lung cancer. Gastric lavage followed by administration of demulcents and close monitoring of fluid and electrolyte balance are useful in the treatment of acute chromium poisoning. For dermatitis, topical aluminum acetate or 10% ethylenediaminetetraacetic acid (EDTA) ointment may be useful. British antilewisite (BAL; 2,3-dimercaptopropanol) may be used to treat systemic poisoning.

Clinical significance

The clinical significance of chromium rests primarily with its relation to glucose metabolism. Few definitive studies of human chromium deficiency have been performed, mainly because of analytical difficulties in the determination of ultratrace amounts of chromium in tissue. Evidence of human chromium deficiency is mostly indirect, based on the improvement of insulin-resistant glucose intolerance after supplementation with chromium-containing compounds.

In the United States, the simple addition of 150 μg of Cr^{+3} to the daily diet improved glucose tolerance of type 2 diabetics and middle-aged and elderly subjects. Malnourished children in Jordan and Turkey showed normalization of intravenous glucose tolerance tests after supplementation of their diet formulas with 250 μg of chromium per day. However, malnourished children in Egypt demonstrated no beneficial response to dietary chromium supplementation. In a different study a group of hypoglycemic women responded to chromium supplements with increased serum glucose values 2 to 4 hours after administration of a glucose load and increased insulin receptor numbers.[27]

Deficiencies of chromium have been documented in cases of total parenteral feeding.[27] In one such case, severe chromium deficiency was described in a female patient fed intravenously with a chromium-deficient (8 μg/day) solution for more than 5 years. Low blood and hair chromium concentrations, negative chromium balance, weight loss, glucose intolerance, decreased respiratory quotient, and peripheral neuropathy all were corrected by intravenous administration of 250 μg/day of chromium for 2 weeks. In a second case, glucose intolerance, insulin resistance, and central nervous system disorder of a totally parenterally fed patient was corrected after chromium—but not after insulin—administration.

The potentiation of insulin action with dietary supplementation of chromium-rich brewer's yeast has been demonstrated in a number of human studies.[27] In insulin-dependent diabetics a daily insulin requirement was lowered, from 60 to 133 U/day to 20 to 45 U/day after 1 to 2 months of supplements. On supplementation with brewer's yeast, elderly diabetics required less insulin within 24 hours, and their need for insulin progressively declined 1 to 2 U every 2 to 3 days. The complete elimination of insulin requirements by chromium-rich yeast supplements has not been achieved, probably because of a deficit in endogenous insulin production. A risk of hypoglycemia during the initial brewer's yeast-supplementation period has been emphasized.

Several conditions that affect glucose metabolism have been shown to increase urinary excretion of chromium. Insulin-dependent diabetics and individuals with Turner's syndrome excrete about threefold more chromium than do control subjects. Urinary excretion of chromium also is increased by high amounts of simple sugars in the diet, glucose loads, or various stressors, such as heavy exercise or physical trauma. Whether the increased excretion in these conditions is the result of increased intestinal absorption of chromium or the loss of chromium stores remains unclear.

Methods

Flameless atomic absorption spectrophotometry (AAS) is recommended as a practical analytical technique to measure chromium in biological samples. Flame AAS methods using enhanced background correction capability to determine serum and urinary chromium have been described.[31] Nitric acid/peroxide digestion of samples in quartz tubes with threaded Teflon caps provides an organically clean digest that can be used for chromium quantification in a graphite analyzer. Losses of volatile organo-chromium components of biological specimens during analytical procedures have been reported. Use of techniques to avoid contamination and loss, such as closed-tube digestions, are recommended.

Cobalt

Cobalt is essential for humans only as an integral part of vitamin B_{12} (cobalamin). No other function for cobalt in the human body is known. Details of vitamin B_{12} biochemistry and function are discussed in Chapter 28. Microflora of the human intestine cannot utilize cobalt to synthesize physiologically active cobalamin. The human vitamin B_{12} requirement must be supplied by the diet. Free (nonvitamin B_{12}) cobalt does not interact with the body vitamin B_{12} pool.

Copper

Copper (Cu) is an important trace element associated with a number of metalloproteins. It is present in biological systems in both the Cu^{+1} and Cu^{+2} valence states. The biochemical and clinical aspects of human copper nutrition have been reviewed.[12,19]

Biochemistry

The major functions of copper metalloproteins involve oxidation-reduction reactions; most known copper-containing enzymes bind and react directly with molecular oxygen. Copper is an integral component of many metalloenzymes, including ceruloplasmin, cytochrome c oxidase, superoxide dismutase, dopamine-β-hydroxylase, ascorbate oxidase, lysyl oxidase, and tyrosinase.

A number of pathological conditions have been attributed to the loss of cuproenzyme activity. Failure of skin pigmentation has been attributed to depressed tyrosinase activity required in the first step in the biosynthesis of melanin. A variety of connective tissue cross-linking defects (cardiac, vascular, and skeletal) are believed to be caused by a loss of amine oxidase activity, particularly that of lysyl oxidase. Ataxia may result from depressed cytochrome c oxidase activity in motor neurons. Depressed dopamine-β-hydroxylase activity can result in abnormal catecholamine conversions.

Copper plays an important role in iron metabolism. Copper deficiency impairs iron absorption, and anemia accompanies severe copper deficiency. Ceruloplasmin, the major copper-containing protein in plasma, has a ferroxidase activity that oxidizes ferrous iron to the ferric state before its binding by plasma transferrin.

Metabolism

Copper absorption is maximal in the duodenum and may be absorbed from the stomach, with both active and passive components to the system. Within the intestinal mucosal cells, copper can react with metallothionein, a sulfhydryl group-rich protein that binds copper through the formation of mercaptide bonds. Whether metallothionein has a role in the normal absorptive process and whether it can prevent excessive absorption when copper intake is high are unclear. Other metal ions, particularly zinc and cadmium, compete with copper for sulfhydryl-binding sites, thus explaining the antagonism of these metals toward copper absorption.

The amount of orally ingested copper absorbed from the intestine is between 50% and 80% of ingested copper. Factors affecting copper absorption include sex (women absorbing a greater percentage than men), amount ingested, chemical form, and certain dietary constituents. The latter include other trace elements, sulfate, various amino acids, fiber, and phytates. Copper absorption may be impaired in individuals with diffuse diseases affecting the small bowel, such as sprue, lymphosarcoma, and scleroderma.

Absorbed copper is transported rapidly as copper-albumin or copper-histidine complexes to the liver, where it is stored, mostly as metallothionein-like cuproproteins. Copper is released from the liver, mainly as ceruloplasmin, a multifunctional cuproprotein that accounts for more than 95% of the total copper in plasma. Copper may be transported to cells for incorporation into copper-containing enzymes by several identified transport mechanisms, including ceruloplasmin, transcuprein, copper-albumin, and copper-amino acid complexes. Evidence suggests that the movement of copper within the cell and its incorporation into cu-

proproteins is regulated by both glutathione and metallothionein.[2]

The adult human body contains between 80 and 150 mg of copper. Tissue concentrations range from 1.5 to 2.5 μg/g. The liver is the main storage site for copper and has copper concentrations in the interval of 30 to 50 μg/g of dry tissue. Relatively high amounts also are found in the heart, brain, and kidneys. Muscle and bone copper concentrations are low but constitute about 50% of the total-body copper because of their large mass.

Copper is excreted primarily in the feces; this copper includes that unabsorbed from the diet and that arising from biliary and gastrointestinal secretions. Biliary copper excretion ranges from 0.5 to 1.3 mg/day. Gastrointestinal sources include copper from gastric juice and from desquamated mucosal cells. Copper losses in urine and sweat amount to less than 3% of dietary intake. Menstrual losses of copper apparently are minor—0.1 to 0.8 mg per period.

The liver is the key organ for copper regulation. There copper is stored, incorporated, and released as ceruloplasmin to maintain blood levels. Intestinal absorption mechanisms and regulation of biliary excretion also seem to play major roles in regulating copper homeostasis.

Clinical significance

Copper deficiency in infants has been observed in cases of prematurity, malnutrition, malabsorption, chronic diarrhea, hyperalimentation, and prolonged feeding with low-copper, total-milk diets. The susceptibility of premature infants to copper deficiency is related to their lower stores of liver and spleen copper (which accumulates rapidly during the last trimester of gestation) and the probability of longer maintenance on exclusively milk formulas. A deficit in protein **nutriture** sufficient to impair copper transport and storage also may be a causal factor.

Signs of copper deficiency include (1) neutropenia and hypochromic anemia in the early stages, both of which are responsive to oral copper but not to iron; (2) osteoporosis and various bone and joint abnormalities that reflect deficient copper-dependent cross-linking of bone collagen and connective tissue; (3) decreased pigmentation of the skin and general pallor, which are attributed to tyrosine-required melanin synthesis; and (4) in the later stages, possible neurological abnormalities (hypotonia, apnea, psychomotor retardation), probably caused by a cytochrome c oxidase deficit. Signs of copper deficiency in infants generally are reversed by copper supplementation. The concentrations of plasma copper and ceruloplasmin reflect the degree of copper-deficient and replete states.

Long-term hyperalimentation with infusates deficient in trace minerals has been shown to produce copper deficiency in both infants and adults. Observed signs are those usually associated with copper deficiency, including lowered plasma copper and ceruloplasmin, anemia, neutropenia, leukopenia, and hypocellular bone marrow. Parenteral infusates often have been found to contain little or no copper. Delivery of 0.5 to 1.5 mg of copper daily is recommended.[1] Human copper deficiency also has been associated with zinc therapy for sickle cell disease and treatment with copper-chelating agents, such as penicillamine.

Copper depletion is thought to contribute an increased risk of coronary heart disease through instability of heart rhythm and hyperlipidemia. Experimental animals fed copper-deficient diets and humans fed diets believed to be marginal in copper have exhibited many signs closely related to those of coronary heart disease. These include abnormal electrocardiograms, hypercholesterolemia, glucose intolerance, and hypertension. Diseases known to be related to copper nutriture include Menkes' syndrome, Wilson's disease, and others.

Menkes' syndrome

An extreme form of copper deficiency is seen in Menkes' steely-hair syndrome, an X-linked genetic defect in copper transport and storage. Clinical manifestations occur early in life and include kinky or twisted brittle hair (steely), depigmentation of the skin and hair, hypothermia, seizures, cerebral degeneration, and vascular defects. The formation of steely hair is attributed to loss of copper-catalyzed disulfide bond formation and also is found in sheep grazing in copper-deficient pastures. The affected infants have been shown to be copper deficient, with low serum, hepatic, and cerebral copper concentrations; low ceruloplasmin; and little or no cytochrome *c* oxidase activity in nerve tissue. Symptoms usually appear by 3 months of age, with death occurring by 5 years. Affected infants exhibit an accumulation of copper in the duodenal mucosal tissue as the result of defective copper absorption. Intravenous administration of copper may help raise plasma copper concentrations; however, urinary copper excretion increases accordingly, and the course of vascular and cerebral degeneration is irreversible. The copper content of erythrocytes is not decreased, and neutropenia and anemia, two usual signs of copper deficiency, do not appear.

Wilson's disease

Wilson's disease (hepatolenticular degeneration) is a genetically determined copper accumulation disease that usually occurs between 6 and 40 years of age. Disease signs include neurological disorders, cirrhosis of the liver, and Kayser-Fleischer rings (green-brown discoloration) in the cornea caused by copper deposits. Copper accumulates in the liver, brain, kidney, and cornea. The hemolysis, necrosis, and other cellular damage that occur may be caused by lipid peroxidation, a known effect of copper toxicity. Urinary copper excretion is increased. The hepatic synthesis of copper-containing ceruloplasmin is decreased, which results in a low serum concentration of this enzyme (<20 mg/dL). Although free and albumin-bound copper are increased, total serum copper generally is decreased because of low cerulo-

plasmin concentrations. Thus the simultaneous measurements of serum copper, ceruloplasmin, and urinary copper are useful in the diagnosis of this disease. Wilson's disease can be controlled—and in some cases halted—by early and persistent treatment with zinc acetate or with copper chelators, such as penicillamine and BAL.

Other conditions

Estrogens increase serum copper concentrations, probably by increasing hepatic ceruloplasmin synthesis. Serum copper normally is higher in women than in men. This difference increases further in women taking estrogenic oral contraceptives. Serum copper during pregnancy is increased twofold to threefold over normal concentrations during the last trimester. Testosterone and progesterone administration also has been reported to increase plasma copper.

During infections or inflammatory stress, serum copper concentrations rise because of the acute-phase action of interleukin-1. The action of interleukin-1 may cause the elevated serum copper and decreased serum zinc concentrations present during the acute phase of myocardial infarction. Increases in ceruloplasmin have also been observed in the serum and synovial fluid of individuals with rheumatoid arthritis.

Because the liver is an important organ for copper storage and homeostatic regulation, abnormal copper metabolism is seen in individuals with liver disease. Elevated serum copper concentrations are present in those with portal cirrhosis, biliary tract disease, and hepatitis, probably because excess copper that normally would be excreted in the bile is retained in the circulation. Hypocupremia has been observed in cases of hemolytic jaundice, hemochromatosis, and some types of hepatic cirrhosis because of the inability of the damaged liver to synthesize ceruloplasmin.

Laboratory assessment

A number of indices are useful in the diagnosis of human copper deficiency, including concentrations of serum or plasma copper and ceruloplasmin and enzymatic activity of superoxide dismutase and cytochrome *c* oxidase.

Serum or plasma copper concentrations

Serum or plasma copper provides a relatively easy routine test for the clinical assessment of copper nutriture; low concentrations may indicate severely depleted copper stores. However, plasma concentrations are relatively poor indicators of short-term marginal copper status in humans. Plasma copper concentrations are regulated by strong homeostatic mechanisms and maintained within a relatively narrow range within an individual; plasma copper falls only after stores are depleted severely.[16] As with zinc, circulating copper concentrations are sensitive to factors not directly related to copper nutriture. Plasma copper concentration has a diurnal variation, with peak values found in the morning. Pregnancy, birth control pills, estrogen therapy, and infections or inflammatory conditions increase plasma or serum copper, whereas corticosteroids and adrenocorticotropic hormone tend to lower serum copper. Thus conditions that elevate serum copper may obscure changes in copper status.

Ceruloplasmin

Ceruloplasmin is a copper-containing protein that accounts for more than 95% of the copper found in plasma (see Chapter 19). It is sensitive to the same factors that affect plasma copper and can be measured immunochemically or by its oxidase activity. A copper-depleted apoceruloplasmin likely is present in normal and copper-deficient serum. Thus assays of the oxidase activity may be preferred to immunological methods. Studies of experimental copper depletion in humans suggest that the specific enzymatic activity of ceruloplasmin, estimated by the ratio of enzymatically measured to immunoreactive ceruloplasmin, may be a more sensitive indicator of copper status than either plasma copper or erythrocyte superoxide dismutase.[13]

Superoxide dismutase and cytochrome *c* oxidase activities

Measurement of the activities of the cuproenzymes erythrocyte superoxide dismutase and cytochrome *c* oxidase in platelets or leukocytes also can provide useful information in the assessment of copper status.[13] The activities of both enzymes are reduced significantly in severely copper-deficient animals and were lower in some humans fed diets low in copper.[15]

Methods

AAS, after direct dilution, is the method of choice used to measure serum copper. Photometric methods are available, such as those using diethyldithiocarbamate, biscyclohexanone, oxaldihydrazone (cuprizone), and bathocuproine as chromogens. Hemolysis is not a great concern for copper determinations because concentrations of copper in plasma and erythrocytes are nearly equal.

Serum ceruloplasmin can be determined by a photometric oxidase reaction or immunonephelometry. Its reference interval of 180 to 450 mg/L varies slightly, depending on the method used.

Fluoride

In the form of fluoride, fluorine (F) is incorporated into the structure of teeth and bone and provides protection against dental caries. The biochemistry, metabolism, and anticariogenic properties of fluoride have been reviewed.[20]

Metabolism

Inorganic fluoride is absorbed readily in the stomach and small intestine and distributed almost entirely to bone and teeth. Fluoride enters into calcified tissues either by substituting for the hydroxyl ion or bicarbonate ion in hydroxyapatite in bone or enamel to form fluoroapatite, or by ionic exchange within the hydration shell of the crystalline surface. Renal excretion is most important for regulation of body fluoride content, with about 50% of the daily intake being cleared by the kidneys.

Clinical significance

The exact form of fluoride treatment that provides maximal anticariogenic effect is not known definitively. Supplemental fluoride generally is most effective during the period of tooth eruption and immediately thereafter. Some evidence suggests that high fluoride intake is associated with decreased risk of osteoporosis and that sodium fluoride combined with calcium supplementation may stimulate bone formation. The mechanism responsible for the cariostatic effects of fluoride is not known exactly. Elements of the action may include alteration of the tooth crown morphology, greater integrity of apatite crystal formation, stimulation of enamel surface processes, decreased enamel solubility, and decreased bacterial enzyme activity.

Excessive fluoride intake produces mottled or pitted enamel in growing teeth. Chronic fluorosis may produce osteosclerosis, calcification of ligaments and tendons, and crippling deformities, such as kyphosis, stiffness of the spine, and bony exostoses.

Methods

Ion-specific potentiometry has been used to measure fluoride in plasma and urine.

Iron

Iron (Fe) is the most important of the essential trace elements. An appreciable number of human diseases are related to iron deficiency or disorders of iron metabolism. Iron is present in biological systems in either the Fe^{+2} or Fe^{+3} valence state. (Biochemical, clinical, and analytical aspects of iron will be discussed in Chapter 30.)

Magnesium

Magnesium (Mg) is not technically a trace element; it is the fourth most abundant cation in the body and is second only to potassium within the cell. However, magnesium often is considered a trace element. The adult human body (70 kg) contains 21 to 28 g of magnesium (approximately 1 mol). Of this, about 60% is in bone, 20% in skeletal muscle, 19% in other cells, and 1% in extracellular fluid.

Biochemistry

The best-defined manifestation of magnesium deficiency is impairment of neuromuscular function; examples include hyperirritability, tetany, convulsions, and electrocardiographic changes.

Human magnesium deficiency, as indicated by reduced serum magnesium amounts (hypomagnesemia), occurs with either normal or reduced serum calcium concentrations. Hypomagnesemia may be a secondary effect in individuals with hypocalcemic or calcium-deficient tetany. Yet, a hypomagnesemic-normocalcemic tetany has been described that can be treated effectively with magnesium supplementation alone. During tetany, serum magnesium concentrations of 0.15 to 0.5 mmol/L, accompanied by normal serum calcium and pH, have been reported. Evidence exists that tetany, accompanied by hypocalcemia and hypomagnesemia, may not be treated optimally with calcium administration alone. Decreased serum potassium concentrations (hypokalemia) also have been found to accompany magnesium depletion. The occurrence of otherwise unexplained hypokalemia or hypocalcemia suggests magnesium deficiency.

Clinical significance

Magnesium deprivation has been associated with cardiovascular disease through epidemiological evidence that relates low magnesium intake to (1) a high incidence of cardiac deaths, particularly in soft-water areas, where water-borne magnesium is low, and (2) a low incidence of cardiac deaths in hard-water areas, where magnesium intakes are higher. Hypertension, myocardial infarction, cardiac dysrhythmias, coronary vasospasm, and premature atherosclerosis also have been linked to magnesium depletion.

Other conditions that have been associated with hypomagnesemia include chronic alcoholism, childhood malnutrition, lactation, malabsorption, acute pancreatitis, hypothyroidism, chronic glomerulonephritis, aldosteronism, digitalis intoxication, and prolonged intravenous feeding. Magnesium depletion occurs in conditions that disrupt the normal renal conservation of magnesium (for example, in individuals with renal tubular reabsorption defects and those taking chlorothiazides, ammonium chloride, or mercurial diuretics for congestive heart failure).

Increased serum magnesium concentrations have been observed in individuals with dehydration, severe diabetic acidosis, and Addison's disease and immediately after a myocardial infarction. Conditions that interfere with glomerular filtration (for example, uremia) result in retention of magnesium and, hence, elevation of serum concentrations. Hypermagnesemia leads to an increase in the atrioventricular conduction time of the electrocardiogram.

Methods

The analytical aspects of magnesium are discussed in Chapter 38 and have been reviewed elsewhere.[7,24]

Manganese

Manganese (Mn) is present in biological systems bound to protein in either the Mn^{+2} or Mn^{+3} valence state. It is associated mainly with the formation of connective and bony tissue, growth and reproductive functions, and carbohydrate and lipid metabolism. The biochemical and clinical aspects of manganese nutrition have been reviewed.[8]

Biochemistry

The biochemical basis for manganese essentiality is its function as a constituent of metalloenzymes and an enzyme activator. Important manganese-containing enzymes include arginase, pyruvate carboxylase, and mitochondrial manganese superoxide dismutase. As an enzyme activator, manganese binds to the substrate (such as adenosine triphosphate [ATP]) or directly to the protein, causing conformational changes. Manganese-activated enzymes include hydrolases, kinases, decarboxylases, and transferases. Many of these activations are nonspecific in that other metal ions, such as magnesium, iron, or copper, can replace manganese as the activator. Such activation can mask the effects of manganese deficiency and make observation of the biochemical or clinical effects of manganese deficiency difficult. Exceptions to the nonspecific manganese activation of enzymes are the manganese-specific activations of glycosyltransferases, phosphoenolpyruvate carboxykinase, and glutamine synthetase.

Metabolism

Dietary manganese is absorbed poorly, mainly from the small intestine by mechanisms that largely are unknown. Reported absorption from ^{54}Mn-labeled meals ranged from 2% to 15%. The efficiency of manganese absorption declines with increased manganese intake and increases with low manganese intake.[6] On the other hand, endogenous excretion of manganese does not seem to be influenced by manganese intake or status. Dietary factors that affect manganese absorption include iron, calcium, phosphates, fiber, and phytate. Absorbed manganese entering the portal blood may be bound rapidly to α_2-macroglobulin or albumin or remain in hydrated complexes before rapid transport to the liver, where it is removed almost completely. Most of the manganese then is excreted rapidly in the bile and pancreatic secretions.

Clinical significance

Iron, zinc, and copper are considered essential because clinical evidence of their importance exists; however, manganese is accepted as essential for humans mainly on the basis of its proven role in manganese-dependent enzymes and the production of manganese deficiency in experimental animals, rather than on direct evidence of human deficiency. Blood-clotting defects, hypocholesterolemia, dermatitis (miliaria crystallina), elevated serum calcium and phosphorus concentrations, and alkaline phosphatase activity have been reported in some subjects experimentally depleted of manganese.

However, manganese supplementation was not shown to correct these signs completely. Although manganese deficiency has not been documented in humans consuming natural diets, some disease states have been linked to possible disturbances in manganese metabolism. Children with seizure disorders without head trauma have low blood manganese concentrations, thus raising the possibility that manganese deficiency may contribute to childhood epilepsy. Low tissue manganese concentrations were reported in children with maple syrup urine disease and phenylketonuria. A pyrolidase deficiency, evident in some cases of chronic ulcers, is accompanied by a decreased concentration of manganese in serum and urine. Additionally, manganese deficiency was suggested as an underlying factor in the development of hip abnormalities, joint disease, and congenital malformations.[8] Serum manganese concentrations are increased after industrial exposure, acute hepatitis, and myocardial infarction. Increased erythrocyte concentrations have been found in individuals with rheumatoid arthritis.

Methods

Flameless AAS with Zeeman background correction is the method of choice for manganese detection because of the low amounts in blood, hair, and urine. Instrumental parameters, pitfalls, and references to published methods for the flameless AAS determination of manganese in biological specimens have been reviewed.[16]

The most common method used to estimate changes in manganese metabolism and status is to measure its concentration in whole blood or serum. Whole-blood manganese, or manganese in blood cells, may reflect best manganese stores in tissue. Evidence suggests that the manganese concentration and manganese superoxide dismutase activity in lymphocytes are sensitive to changes in manganese status.[6]

Molybdenum

The essential need for molybdenum (Mo) by animals and humans is based on its incorporation into metalloenzymes. The biochemical and clinical aspects of molybdenum nutrition have been reviewed.[18,21]

Biochemistry

Molybdenum is incorporated into xanthine oxidase, aldehyde oxidase, and sulfite oxidase. Xanthine oxidase participates in the degradation of purines to uric acid; aldehyde oxidase catalyzes the oxidation of aldehydes; and sulfite oxidase catalyzes the final stage of sulfur-containing amino acid oxidation.

Metabolism

In humans, between 25% and 80% of ingested molybdenum is absorbed, mainly in the stomach and small intestine by mechanisms that are unclear. Dietary copper and sulfate decrease molybdenum retention. The highest amounts of molybdenum are retained in the liver. The skeleton and kidney also retain significant amounts. After it is absorbed, most of the molybdenum is turned over rapidly and eliminated via the urine, which indicates that this form of clearance may be the major homeostatic mechanism for this element; however, significant amounts also are excreted in the bile.

Molybdenum is relatively nontoxic to humans. Biochemical manifestations of acute molybdenum poisoning in mammals are similar or identical to copper deficiency or indicate abnormal sulfur metabolism. The copper-dependent enzymes ceruloplasmin and cytochrome oxidase, in addition to glutaminase, cholinesterase, and sulfite oxidase activities are inhibited. High dietary and occupational exposures to molybdenum have been linked to elevated uric acid in blood and an increased incidence of gout.

Clinical significance

Defined cases of dietary human molybdenum deficiency have not been reported. A possible congenital defect in molybdenum metabolism was suggested for an infant who exhibited feeding difficulties, mental retardation, skull asymmetry, dislocation of the left lens, and biochemical defects in xanthine- and sulfite-oxidase activities. A patient receiving prolonged parenteral nutrition therapy acquired a syndrome characterized by hypermethioninemia, hypouricemia, hyperoxypurinemia, hypouricosuria, and low urinary sulfate excretion. Additionally, the patient had mental disturbances that progressed to coma. The symptoms were indicative of sulfite- and xanthine-oxidase deficiencies. Supplementation of the patient's therapy with ammonium molybdate improved the clinical condition, reversed the sulfur-handling defect, and normalized uric acid production.

Methods

Current methods for the determination of molybdenum in biological specimens are inadequate. The methods have used mostly emission spectroscopy (ES), neutron activation analysis (NAA), and AAS techniques. Use of a high-temperature nitrous oxide-acetylene flame has been suggested for molybdenum determinations by AAS. However, molybdenum concentrations in biological specimens are so low that preconcentration or prior extraction of the sample is necessary for flame AAS determinations.

Selenium

Selenium (Se) is an essential element for humans. The relation of selenium to human health and disease has been reviewed.[11]

Biochemistry

Selenium is a constituent of glutathione peroxidase and iodothyronine deiodinases. Most of the selenium in tissues is present in two forms—selenocysteine (Secys) and selenomethionine. Selenomethionine cannot be synthesized in the body and must be supplied by the diet. It can replace methionine in a variety of proteins. Selenomethionine is regarded as an unregulated storage compartment for selenium; when the dietary selenium supply is interrupted, this pool turns over and supplies selenium to the organism.

Secys is a selenium-containing analog of cysteine that is recognized as the 21st amino acid encoded by DNA.[26] It is the biologically active form of selenium and is regulated tightly. It is found in the prokaryotic and eukaryotic kingdoms in active sites of enzymes involved in oxidation-reduction reactions. Secys is present in selenoproteins, such as glutathione peroxidase, iodothyronine deiodinases, selenoprotein P, selenoprotein W, and thioredoxin reductase.

Selenium helps defend the organism against oxidant stress, is involved in the synthesis and metabolism of thyroid hormones, and has a reproductive function in rats. A number of selenoproteins have been identified and found to have defined functions.[11] They include four different glutathione peroxidases, three different iodothyronine deiodinases, and thioredoxin reductase. Glutathione peroxidase catalyzes the breakdown of hydrogen peroxide, phospholipid hydroperoxides, and other free hydroperoxides. Erythrocyte glutathione peroxidase contains four selenium atoms in the form of selenocysteine that are essential for its biological activity. In individuals with long-term selenium deficiency, all body tissues show decreased glutathione peroxidase activity. Thioredoxin reductase is thought to have an immunological function.

Types I, II, and III iodothyronine deiodinases are selenoproteins.[11] These enzymes remove iodine from thyroid hormone molecules, thereby activating thyroxine (T_4) and inactivating triiodothyronine (T_3). Type I iodothyronine deiodinase, present in liver, kidney, and thyroid tissue, provides T_3 to peripheral tissue made from T_4 secreted by the thyroid gland. The activity of the type I enzyme declines during selenium deficiency. Type II iodothyronine deiodinase is found in the brain, brown fat, pituitary gland, and placenta. It regulates intracellular T_3 in these tissues and controls thyroid-stimulating hormone secretion. Type III iodothyronine deiodinase inactivates T_3 and degrades other thyroid hormones; little is known about its function in selenium deficiency. Animal studies have demonstrated that combined selenium and iodine deficiencies lead to more severe hypothyroidism than does iodine deficiency alone. In addition, cretinism in newborns has been suggested as the consequence of combined deficiencies of these two elements in the mothers.

Selenoprotein P, a selenocysteine-containing protein, has been isolated from plasma. Concentrations fall to less than 10% of reference values in selenium deficiency. The function of selenoprotein P is unknown. However, one suggestion is that selenoprotein P transports selenium from the liver to the testes and is an extracellular oxidant defense enzyme. Selenoprotein W, found in muscle, also contains Secys. The concentration of selenoprotein W decreases during selenium deficiency; it may be involved in the pathogenesis of muscular degeneration present in combined selenium and vitamin E deficiencies.[11]

Metabolism

The principal dietary forms of selenium are selenoamino acids; selenomethionine is derived from plants and Secys from animal sources. Inorganic forms of selenium often are supplied as supplements and in experimental diets. More than 50% of selenium is absorbed from the gastrointestinal tract, but the absorption apparently is not regulated. Little is known about the mechanisms of absorption, but selenomethionine is absorbed by the same mechanism as methionine. Selenium homeostasis is achieved by regulation of its excretion via the urine. In addition, very high intakes of selenium lead to exhalation of volatile forms of selenium.

Clinical significance

Selenium deficiency has been associated in China with Keshan and Kashin-Beck diseases. Keshan disease is an endemic cardiomyopathy that primarily affects children and women of childbearing age in certain areas of China. Its most common symptoms include dizziness, malaise, loss of appetite, nausea, chills, abnormal electrocardiograms, cardiogenic shock, cardiac enlargement, and ultimate congestive heart failure. Diets in these regions are very low in selenium, and individuals demonstrate glutathione peroxidase activities and hair and serum selenium concentrations that are 30% to 40% lower than controls. Selenium supplementation has been shown, in large population trials, to control Keshan disease effectively.

Kashin-Beck disease is an endemic osteoarthritis that occurs during adolescent and preadolescent years. The exact cause of this disease is unknown, and other factors, such as mineral imbalance, mycotoxins in grain, or organic contaminants in drinking water, may be involved.

Cardiomyopathy and skeletal muscle weakness have been observed in a few intravenously fed patients who were not supplemented with selenium.[29] Several cases of low plasma or blood selenium concentrations and low glutathione peroxidase activities without the previously mentioned symptoms were reported in patients receiving liquid total parenteral nutrition without added selenium.[10]

Epidemiological studies have related low selenium status and intake with increased incidences of cancer and cardiomyopathies. Experiments with rodent models and human trials have demonstrated a protective effect of nonnutritive amounts of selenium against tumorigenesis. However, more research is necessary to clarify any role that selenium may play in either cancer or heart disease.

Chronic selenosis, or selenium toxicity, is characterized by loss of hair and nails, skin lesions, tooth decay, and nervous system abnormalities (see Chapter 32). The most common signs of acute selenium poisoning are nausea, vomiting, hair loss, nail changes, irritability, fatigue, and peripheral neuropathy.

Laboratory assessment

The determinations of urinary and blood selenium are useful measures of human selenium status. Plasma or serum selenium concentration may be a more sensitive indicator of selenium status than whole-blood concentration. In China, hair selenium concentrations were found to correlate with blood concentrations, and hair selenium was used to assess an individual's risk for selenium deficiency. Levels of erythrocyte glutathione peroxidase activity have been shown to correlate with blood selenium and has some usefulness as a functional test of selenium status. The determination of selenoprotein P, the major selenium-containing protein in plasma, also is a useful and sensitive test for determination of selenium nutritional status.

Methods

Methods used to determine selenium in biological specimens include flameless AAS, either with deuterium-arc or Zeeman-effect background correction, and spectrofluorometry.[23] Selenium has the capability to form covalent organocompounds that can lead to two analytical problems. First, the organo-selenium forms are likely to be quite volatile and therefore can be lost in certain sample preparation steps, such as high temperature ashing. Second, the easy reduction of sample selenium to the volatile hydride form allows for the determination of selenium by the AAS hydride-generation technique. Factors influencing blood selenium values have been reviewed.[22]

Zinc

The discovery of a variety of zinc-related clinical disorders has demonstrated the importance of zinc in human nutrition. It is second to iron as the most abundant trace element in the body. The metabolic interactions of zinc in humans and animals have been reviewed.[5]

Biochemistry

Zinc is an integral component of nearly 300 enzymes in different species of all phyla. Important zinc-containing metalloenzymes in humans include carbonic anhydrase, alkaline phosphatase, RNA and DNA polymerases, thymidine kinase, carboxypeptidases, and alcohol dehydrogenase. The zinc atoms are an integral, firmly bound part of the metalloprotein molecule and often are involved in the active site; they also contribute to the conformation and structural stability of many metalloenzymes.

Loss of zinc metalloenzyme activity with zinc depletion varies with different zinc enzymes. Activity loss depends on the tissue, enzyme turnover rate, and affinity of the enzyme for zinc. Pancreatic carboxypeptidase A, thymidine kinase, and alkaline phosphatase activities are reduced appreciably by zinc depletion, whereas the activities of some dehydrogenases are not compromised immediately. Carbonic anhydrase activity also is lowered in the blood, stomach, and intestines of zinc-deficient animals, and in the blood of individuals with sickle cell anemia, whose erythrocytes have decreased zinc content.

Zinc plays a major role in protein synthesis and has an important function in gene expression; the involvement in gene expression is both a structural and an enzymatic role. Metal binding by DNA and RNA affects the chemical and physical properties of the macromolecules in ways that may be related to replication and protein synthesis. Thymidine kinase and various RNA and DNA polymerases require zinc for their activity. Zinc finger proteins bind to specific domains of DNA molecules. These proteins require zinc for their conformation and DNA-binding abilities. Details of these proteins have been reviewed.[9]

In addition to its roles in catalysis and gene expression, zinc stabilizes the structures of proteins and nucleic acids, preserves the integrity of subcellular organelles, participates in transport processes, and has important roles in viral and immune phenomena.

Zinc is an important element in wound healing. Several studies have implicated zinc as a necessary factor in the biosynthesis and integrity of connective tissue. For this reason, adequate zinc nutriture is especially important for the postsurgical patient.

Metabolism

Approximately 20% to 30% of ingested dietary zinc is absorbed. Zinc absorption occurs mostly in the duodenum and proximal jejunum. The absorption process is active, energy dependent, and apparently mediated by specific transport (binding) ligands. Evidence indicates that the zinc absorption mechanism plays a significant role in homeostatic regulation. Zinc absorption is variable and depends on a variety of factors.

Zinc is transported in blood plasma mostly by albumin (60% to 70%) and α_2-macroglobulin (30% to 40%), with a small amount associated with transferrin and free amino acids. The major route of zinc excretion is via the feces. Pancreatic secretion accounts for about 25% of total excretion. Biliary losses are small. Urinary losses of zinc, about 0.6 mg/day in an adult who consumes about 12 mg/day, seem to be related directly to zinc intake and status. Sweat losses are similar to those in urine but can be appreciable in individuals living in tropical climates or who are under physical stress. In men, semen losses of 0.4 to 0.6 mg of zinc per ejaculum may be significant only at very low intakes of zinc.

Clinical significance

Nutritional zinc deficiency in humans is fairly prevalent throughout the world. Clinical features include retardation of growth and skeletal maturation, testicular atrophy, and hepatosplenomegaly. Growth failure, reduced taste acuity, and hypogonadism in young adults have been ascribed to zinc deficiency. Old age, pregnancy, lactation, and alcoholism also are associated with a higher incidence of poor zinc nutrition.

As zinc deficiency progresses, the clinical manifestations exist as a spectrum. In individuals with experimentally induced mild zinc deficiency, oligospermia, weight loss, hyperammonemia, and lowered ethanol tolerance have been observed. Moderate zinc deficiency is characterized by growth retardation in children and adolescents, hypogonadism in males, mild dermatitis, poor appetite, delayed wound healing, abnormal dark adaptation, mental lethargy, and impaired immune responses. Manifestations of severe cases of zinc deficiency include bullous-pustular dermatitis, alopecia, weight loss, diarrhea, neuropsychiatric disorders, recurrent infection, and ultimate death if the deficiency is not treated.

Causes of human zinc deficiency other than deficient dietary intake also exist. Besides nutritional factors, many diseases and medical treatments may produce conditioned zinc deficiency. Zinc deficiency in individuals with hepatic cirrhosis (for example, alcoholism, viral hepatitis) is characterized by low serum and hepatic zinc concentrations, along with increased urinary excretion of zinc. Increased urinary zinc excretion and low serum zinc concentrations also have been reported in alcoholics without cirrhosis. Lowered zinc status has been documented in individuals with gastrointestinal disorders, such as ulcers, ulcerative colitis, Crohn's disease, sprue, intestinal bypass, gluten-sensitive enteropathy, and regional enteritis. The occurrence of zinc deficiency in individuals with renal disease has been attributed to a loss of protein-zinc complexes in proteinuria or to decreased tubular reabsorption of zinc. In burned patients, loss of zinc in exudates and zinc requirements for healing are likely causes of observed zinc deficiencies. Supplemental zinc sulfate has been effective in healing of pilonidal sinus lesions, bedsores, and leg ulcers, although the findings have been inconsistent.

Therapeutic causes of conditioned zinc deficiency include administration of anabolic and metal-chelating drugs, such as corticosteroids and penicillamine, and synthetic diet treatments. Synthetic oral diets and total parenteral alimentation fluids are often trace-element deficient and have been shown to produce zinc and other trace-element deficiencies in patients receiving long-term treatment.

Zinc deficiencies in individuals with neoplastic and inflammatory diseases (arthritis, lupus erythematosus) have been attributed to anorexia, starvation, loss of zinc from catabolized tissue, and increased urinary excretion of zinc subsequent to its mobilization by interleukin-1. This polypeptide cytokine, released by granulocytes, mediates a redistribution of body zinc during the acute-phase reaction, which results in increased hepatic zinc sequestration and urinary excretion of zinc. The long-term effect of interleukin-1 in cases of chronic infection or injury is to-

ward increased body zinc loss through hyperzincuria. Some parasitic infections also contribute to zinc deficiency as the result of intestinal blood loss of zinc.

Pregnant women are at higher risk of acquired zinc deficiency because of the high uptake of zinc by the fetus and associated tissues. Zinc is required for normal fetal development and influences pregnancy outcome. Excessive iron and folic acid supplements, often prescribed during pregnancy, may interfere with zinc absorption and utilization and exacerbate the effects of marginal zinc intakes.[25] In addition, the use of oral contraceptives produces a decrease in plasma zinc, with an increase in erythrocyte zinc.

The most clearly defined genetic disorder of zinc metabolism is acrodermatitis enteropathica. Manifestations of the disease are similar with those of zinc deficiency, including retarded growth, hypogonadism, dermatological and ophthalmic lesions, and gastrointestinal disturbances. Affected individuals exhibit lowered plasma zinc concentrations. Symptoms are completely alleviated with zinc sulfate supplementation. Zinc deficiency also often is associated with sickle cell anemia; zinc supplementation may be beneficial in helping to decrease symptoms and crises of some individuals with sickle cell anemia.

Laboratory assessment

Laboratory tests used to assess zinc nutriture can be classified into those involving the analysis of zinc in a body tissue or fluid and those testing a zinc-dependent function. Useful tests in the first group include determinations of the zinc content of plasma or serum, blood cells, urine, and saliva. Functional tests include measurement of activities of zinc-containing enzymes and assessment of taste acuity. All such indices have been shown to decrease with zinc deficiency. Other tests that are either too complex for routine diagnostics or not well investigated include skin and fingernail zinc determinations, [65]Zn uptake by erythrocytes, measurement of changes of plasma zinc content during exercise, blood ethanol clearance, [65]Zn retention and turnover, and zinc balance.

Plasma or serum zinc

Although circulating zinc in plasma and serum often has been shown to indicate human zinc deficiency, it does not always accurately reflect whole-body zinc status. Circulating zinc concentrations closely correlate with the major carrier protein, albumin. Thus lowered plasma zinc concentrations observed in hypoalbuminemic conditions, such as hepatic cirrhosis and malnutrition, may reflect depressed plasma binding of zinc. Many forms of steroids depress circulating concentrations of zinc (for example, exogenous cortical steroids, exogenous gonadal steroids in the form of oral contraceptives, and endogenous gonadal hormones during pregnancy). Depressed plasma zinc has been associated with infection and inflammation. In addition, plasma zinc exhibits a diurnal variation; it declines significantly after meals, and short-term fasting elevates plasma zinc concentrations. Because the zinc concentrations of erythrocytes are 10 times higher than those of serum, hemolysis of the sample during sampling or processing may invalidate the determination of circulating zinc.

Zinc in hair

Lowered hair zinc concentrations have been documented in zinc-deficient Egyptian dwarfs, in marginally deficient U.S. infants and children, and in conditions associated with zinc deficiency, including acrodermatitis enteropathica, sickle cell anemia, and celiac disease. However, in some cases of severe zinc deficiency, above-normal concentrations of hair zinc were attributed to accumulation of zinc in hair in which growth was stunted as a result of the deficiency. Environmental contamination of hair also apparently can lead to high zinc concentrations. Correlations between hair zinc and blood or tissue zinc usually are poor.

Zinc in urine

Decreased urinary zinc excretion usually accompanies human zinc deficiency. However, certain conditions associated with zinc depletion, such as hepatic cirrhosis, high alcohol intake, viral hepatitis, sickle cell anemia, postsurgical periods, and total parenteral nutrition, often result in increased urinary zinc excretion. The utility of urinary zinc determinations as a measure of zinc status is also limited by the difficulties encountered in the collection of a 24-hour urine specimen without exogenous zinc contamination.

Zinc in leukocytes

Studies have indicated reductions in the apparent zinc content of peripheral blood leukocytes in individuals with experimental zinc depletion and other conditions related to zinc deficiency. Additionally, correlations between the zinc concentration, on a dry-weight basis, of blood leukocytes and the zinc concentrations in muscle have been reported in pregnant women and in individuals with liver disease. However, other investigators using different cell-separation techniques were unable to confirm these findings, apparently because of the degree of contamination by blood platelets.[14]

Zinc-containing enzyme activities and metallothionein

Zinc-dependent enzymes, such as alkaline phosphatase, carbonic anhydrase, nucleoside phosphorylase, and ribonuclease are useful indicators of zinc deficiency. Depression of alkaline phosphatase activity in either serum or neutrophils has been observed in a number of animal species and human zinc-deficient conditions. A study of zinc-deficient patients receiving zinc supplementation showed increases in alkaline phosphatase activity that paralleled the degree of zinc repletion. However, as with serum zinc, alkaline phosphatase activities are nonspecific and are affected by conditions unrelated to zinc status. In individuals with sickle cell anemia whose zinc nutriture was impaired, carbonic anhydrase and nucleoside phosphorylase activities were related to zinc status and responded to zinc supplementation. Zinc metalloenzyme test methods that contain zinc in the reagents are not suitable tests for zinc status. Metallothionein I concentrations in plasma or erythrocytes, plasma or white cell 5′-nucleotidase, and extracellular superoxide dismutase also may be useful in the assessment of zinc status in humans.

Methods

The determination of plasma or serum zinc concentrations by AAS is the simplest and analytically most reliable test for the routine assessment of zinc nutriture. Photometric methods are available for laboratories without an AAS instrument and provide results that are comparable to those obtained by AAS. Other methods used to determine plasma zinc include ES and NAA.

■ INDIVIDUAL ULTRATRACE ELEMENTS

Nickel (Ni), vanadium (V), silicon (Si), arsenic (As), and boron (B) also are considered the "new" trace or ultratrace elements, with their tissue concentrations in the nanogram-per-gram amounts and dietary requirements of about 50 ng/g or less (excepting silicon and boron). These elements have been shown to be most likely essential to animals and thus may be essential for humans. However, no conclusive cases of deficiency of these elements have been described in humans. Thus no human requirements or allowances have been set. The evidence for the essentiality and proposed functions of these elements has been reviewed.[17,18]

■ LABORATORY ASSESSMENT OF TRACE METAL STATUS

Few completely satisfactory clinical laboratory methods to assess metal status in humans have been established. Currently, the only definitive test of human deficiency of trace metals is the clinical response to therapeutic supplementation, with the trace metal in question.

Measurements of metalloenzyme activities have been proposed as useful assessment tests because plasma trace metal concentrations often are affected by factors not related to the whole-body metal status. Although hair is relatively easy to sample and analyze for trace metal content, its chief problem as a tissue for the assessment of metal nutriture is its susceptibility to environmental contamination. Thus its use as an indicator of nutritional status is limited; low metal concentration in hair may indicate metal depletion, but "normal" or high amounts do not necessarily preclude depletion or indicate the presence of toxic amounts.

A simultaneous battery of tests involving body tissue or body fluid metal determinations, metalloenzyme assays, and functional-morphological indices would provide the most reliable assessment of metal status.

Sample Collection and Testing

Special precautions are required for the accurate determination of trace elements in biological specimens. In practice, sampling procedures must be considered carefully because heterogeneity of trace element distributions in tissues is the rule rather than the exception. Analysis of seemingly homogeneous specimens, such as blood, saliva, and sweat, can be affected significantly by sampling and sample processing procedures. For example, zinc concentrations can be 5% to 15% higher in serum than in plasma because of the release of zinc from erythrocytes and platelets during clotting. Conversely, the choice of anticoagulant affects plasma values by osmotic influences on fluid shifts from blood cells. Hemolysis or microhemolysis of a sample can lead to erroneously high plasma or serum values for iron, zinc, and manganese because red blood cell concentrations are tenfold or greater than those in plasma for these elements. Special blood collection tubes are available for trace element determination (see Chapter 2).

The primary analytical problem encountered in trace element analysis is external contamination. Many trace elements are present in the laboratory environment in nanogram and even microgram amounts; hence a significant portion of an analytical value for a trace element may be the result of contamination unless extraordinary measures are taken. This is a major reason for the wide variation in reported reference values. A laboratorian contemplating trace element analysis must be prepared to take precautions, to the point of fanaticism, through all sampling, preparation, and analytical procedures to ensure that contamination is minimized. Details on sources of contamination have been outlined.[14]

Analytical Methods

A variety of analytical techniques are used to determine trace elements in biological specimens, including photometry, AAS and ES, which includes inductively coupled atomic plasma emission spectrometry (ICP-AES). Other techniques used include NAA, mass spectrometry (MS), inductively coupled plasma mass spectrometry (ICP-MS), x-ray fluorescence spectrometry (XRF), and electrochemical techniques, such as anodic stripping voltametry (ASV). High-performance liquid chromatography (HPLC) of metal complexes and polarographic techniques also have been described.

ES, ICP-MS, and NAA offer simultaneous multielement determination. The NAA technique is one of the most sensitive, and the analysis can be performed uniquely without sample preparation, destruction, or contamination. Many ES techniques also require minimal sample preparation but lack sensitivity for some ultratrace element determinations and are susceptible to spectral interferences. The ICP-AES, MS, and XRF techniques also provide multielement detection. Considerable sample preparation, such as digestion, is required to remove interfering organic matrices and convert the samples to soluble forms for most ICP-ES and MS procedures. Because method requirements are not the same for all minerals and all specimens, the analytical method of choice depends on the sample type and element to be determined.

Reference intervals for most of the trace minerals are listed in Chapter 46 and elsewhere.[4,28]

Atomic absorption spectrophotometry

AAS has replaced photometric techniques as the method of choice for trace metal analysis. The principles of AAS are detailed in Chapter 3. The detection limits of the AAS methods used to determine the various elements depend on the element of interest and the technique used. The flame AAS mode is simpler and less tedious to perform than the flameless mode. Generally, if analyte concentrations of a specimen are below 50 ng/g, flameless AAS techniques are necessary.

Inductively coupled atomic plasma emission spectrometry

The ICP-AES technique is a multielement method that is replacing AAS as the method of choice for many trace metal applications because it provides simultaneous multielement determinations over a wide analytical range. The principles of ICP-AES and its applications to biological and clinical samples have been reviewed.[3]

Quality Control of Trace Element Determinations

Because methods for trace element analysis are affected by matrix effects and contamination problems, effective measures of quality assurance must be incorporated into trace element analysis schemes. An effective quality assurance scheme for trace or ultratrace element analysis requires incorporation of the following into each batch of analyses:

1. Reagent blanks
2. Replicate analyses to assess precision
3. Calibrators of the trace elements of interest in the expected concentration range of the specimens analyzed
4. A control or reference solution with known or certified concentrations of the trace elements to be determined to assess accuracy and batch-to-batch precision

The reference material should be of the same matrix type and contain approximately the same amounts of analyte as the specimens.

References

1. American Medical Association: Guidelines for essential trace element preparations for parenteral use. JAMA 1979; 241:2051-2054.
2. Anonymous: Copper-glutathione: a key intermediate in cellular copper metabolism? Nutr Rev 1991; 49:95-96.
3. Chaudhri MA, Hannaker P: Reliability of the ICP-AES for trace elements studies of biological materials. Biol Trace Elem Res 1987; 13:417.
4. Chiba M: Concentrations of essential trace elements in blood and introduction of analytical techniques. Nippon Rinsho 1996; 54:179-185.
5. Cousins RJ: Zinc. In Ziegler EE, Filer FF Jr (eds): Present Knowledge in Nutrition, 7th edition, pp 293-306, Washington, DC, ILSI Press, 1996.
6. Davis CD, Greger JL: Longitudinal changes of manganese-dependent superoxide dismutase and other indexes of manganese and iron status in women. Am J Clin Nutr 1992; 55:747-752.
7. Elin RJ: Magnesium: the fifth but forgotten electrolyte. Am J Clin Pathol 1994; 102:616-622.
8. Keen CL, Zidenberg-Cherr S: Manganese. In Ziegler EE, Filer FF Jr (eds): Present Knowledge in Nutrition, 7th edition, pp 334-343, Washington, DC, ILSI Press, 1996.
9. Klug A, Schwabe JW: Protein motifs 5. Zinc fingers. FASEB J 1995; 9:597-604.
10. Lane HW, Barroso AO, Englert D et al: Selenium status of seven chronic intravenous hyperalimentation patients. JPEN 1982; 6:426-431.
11. Levander OA, Burk RF: Selenium. In Ziegler EE, Filer FF Jr (eds): Present Knowledge in Nutrition, 7th edition, pp 320-328, Washington, DC, ILSI Press, 1996.
12. Linder MC: Copper. In Ziegler EE, Filer FF Jr (eds): Present Knowledge in Nutrition, 7th edition, pp 307-319, Washington, DC, ILSI Press, 1996.
13. Milne DB: Assessment of copper nutritional status. Clin Chem 1994; 40:1479-1484.
14. Milne DB: Trace elements. In Burtis CA, Ashwood ER (eds): Tietz Textbook of Clinical Chemistry, 3rd edition, pp 1029-1055, Philadelphia, WB Saunders, 1999.
15. Milne DB, Johnson PE, Klevay LM et al: Effect of copper intake on balance, absorption, and status indices of copper in men. Nutr Res 1990; 10:975.
16. Neve J, Leclercq N: Factors affecting determinations of manganese in serum by atomic absorption spectrometry. Clin Chem 1991; 37:723-728.
17. Nielsen FH: Nutritional requirements for boron, silicon, vanadium, nickel, and arsenic: current knowledge and speculation. FASEB J 1991; 5:2661-2667.
18. Nielsen FH: Other trace elements. In Ziegler EE, Filer FF Jr (eds): Present Knowledge in Nutrition, 7th edition, pp 353-377, Washington, DC, ILSI Press, 1996.
19. O'Dell BL: Copper. In Ziegler EE, Filer FF Jr (eds): Present Knowledge in Nutrition, 7th edition, pp 261-267, Washington, DC, ILSI Press, 1996.
20. Phipps KR: Fluoride. In Ziegler EE, Filer FF Jr (eds): Present Knowledge in Nutrition, 7th edition, pp 329-333, Washington, DC, ILSI Press, 1996.
21. Rajopalan KV: Molybdenum: an essential trace element in human nutrition. Ann Rev Nutr 1988; 8:401-427.
22. Robberecht H, Deelstra H: Factors influencing blood selenium concentration values: a literature review. J Trace Elem Electrolytes Health Dis 1994; 8:129-143.
23. Sheehan TMT, Halls DJ: Measurement of selenium in clinical specimens. Ann Clin Biochem 1999; 36:301-315.
24. Shils ME: Magnesium. In Ziegler EE, Filer FF Jr (eds): Present Knowledge in Nutrition, 7th edition, pp 256-264, Washington, DC, ILSI Press, 1996.
25. Simmer K, Iles CA, James C et al: Are iron-folate supplements harmful? Am J Clin Nutr 1987; 45:122-125.
26. Stadtman TC: Selenium biochemistry. Ann Rev Biochem 1996; 65:83-100.
27. Stoeker BJ: Chromium. In Ziegler EE, Filer FF Jr (eds): Present Knowledge in Nutrition, 7th edition, pp 344-352, Washington, DC, ILSI Press, 1996.
28. Tietz NW (ed): Clinical Guide to Laboratory Tests, 3rd edition, Philadelphia, WB Saunders, 1995.
29. van Rij AM, Thompson CD, McKenzie JM et al: Selenium deficiency in total parenteral nutrition. Am J Clin Nutr 1979; 32:2076-2085.
30. Vincent JB: Mechanisms of chromium action: low-molecular-weight chromium-binding substance. J Am Coll Nutr 1999; 18:6-12.
31. Veillon C, Patterson KY, Bryden NA: Determination of chromium in human serum by electrothermal atomic absorption spectrometry. Anal Chim Acta 1984; 164:67.

Additional Reading

Evans S: Metals & the Immune System, New York, Chapman & Hall, 1998.
Miller GD (ed): Nutrition and Toxicology. In Massaro EJ (ed): Handbook of Human Toxicology, Boca Raton, Fla, CRC Press, 1997.

National Committee for Clinical Laboratory Standards: Control of Preanalytical Variation in Trace Element Determinations: Approved Guideline C38-A. Wayne, Pa, National Committee for Clinical Laboratory Standards, 1997.

O'Dell RA, Sunde RA: Handbook of Nutritionally Essential Minerals, New York, Marcel Dekker, 1997.

Roe DA, Dwyer JT: Nutrition and Chronic Disease, New York, Chapman & Hall, 1997.

Somer E: The Essential Guide to Vitamins & Minerals, New York, Harper Collins, 1996.

The USP Guide to Vitamins & Minerals, New York, Avon Books, 1996.

Vandecasteele C, Block CB: Modern Methods for Trace Element Determination, New York, John Wiley & Sons, 1997.

CHAPTER 30

Analytes of Hemoglobin Metabolism— Porphyrins, Iron, and Bilirubin*

KERN L. NUTTALL, MD, PhD, and GEORGE G. KLEE, MD, PhD

Objectives

1. Define the following terms:

Porphyrin	Ferritin	Hemosiderosis
Heme	Hemosiderin	Bilirubin (conjugated and unconjugated)
Porphobilinogen (PBG)	Transferrin	Urobilinogen
Porphyria	Hemochromatosis	Jaundice
Hemoglobin		

2. Summarize the biosynthetic pathway of porphyrin and heme and state the physiological functions of porphyrins and heme.
3. List and describe the symptoms of the seven porphyrias and state the major elevated intermediates involved in each.
4. Discuss the clinical laboratory analysis of the porphyrin disorders, including screening tests, methods of analysis, and possible interferences in each.
5. State the clinical utility of analysis of erythrocyte protoporphyrin and zinc protoporphyrin in the assessment of lead toxicity.
6. State the physiological functions of iron, transferrin, and ferritin.
7. Describe iron absorption, transport, and metabolism.
8. List and describe the symptoms of three disorders of iron metabolism.
9. List five conditions that affect serum iron concentration and how it is affected in each.
10. Describe the methods of analysis of serum iron, ferritin, and total iron binding capacity; state the formula used to calculate percent iron saturation.
11. Describe the biosynthetic pathway of bilirubin, including conjugation in the liver.
12. State the clinical utility of the analysis of unconjugated and conjugated serum bilirubin levels and urobilinogen.
13. Describe the methods of analysis for bilirubin; state the principles of and possible interferences in each.

Key Words

Conjugated Bilirubin (Direct Bilirubin)   Bilirubin that has been taken up by the liver cells and conjugated to form the water-soluble bilirubin diglucuronide

Coproporphyrin   A porphyrin with four methyl and four propionic acid side chains attached to the tetrapyrrole backbone

Direct Bilirubin (Conjugated Bilirubin)   Bilirubin that has been taken up by the liver cells and conjugated to form the water-soluble bilirubin diglucuronide

---

*The authors gratefully acknowledge the original contributions of Virgil F. Fairbanks, Robert Rej, and Keith J. Tolman, on which portions of this chapter are based.

584

Ferritin The iron-apoferritin complex, which is one of the chief forms in which iron is stored in the body; occurs in the gastrointestinal mucosa, liver, spleen, bone marrow, and reticuloendothelial cells

Heme Any quadridentate chelate of iron with the four pyrrole groups of a porphyrin, further distinguished as *ferroheme* or *ferriheme*, referring to the chelates of Fe (II) and Fe (III), respectively

Hemochromatosis A disorder caused by deposition of hemosiderin in the parenchymal cells, causing tissue damage and dysfunction of the liver, pancreas, heart, and pituitary; also called *iron overload disease*

Hemoglobin The oxygen-carrying pigment of the erythrocytes, formed by the developing erythrocyte in bone marrow; a conjugated protein containing four heme groups and globin

Hemosiderin An intracellular storage form of iron, the granules consisting of an ill-defined complex of ferric hydroxides, polysaccharides, and proteins having an iron content of about 33% by weight

Hemosiderosis A focus or general increase in tissue iron stores without associated tissue damage; hepatic and pulmonary hemosiderosis being characterized by abnormal quantities of hemosiderin in the liver and lungs, respectively

Hyperbilirubinemia Excessive concentrations of bilirubin in the blood, which may lead to jaundice; the hyperbilirubinemias being classified as conjugated or unconjugated, according to the predominant form of bilirubin in the blood

Indirect Bilirubin Free bilirubin that has not been conjugated with glucuronic acid

Jaundice A syndrome characterized by hyperbilirubinemia and deposition of bile pigment in the skin, mucous membranes, and sclera, with resulting yellow appearance of the patient; called also *icterus*

Kernicterus A clinical syndrome of the neonate, resulting from high levels of unconjugated bilirubin, which pass the immature blood-brain barrier of the newborn and causes degeneration of cells of the basal ganglia and hippocampus

Myoglobin A heme containing protein found in red skeletal muscle

Neurological Porphyrias Inherited porphyrin disorders characterized by acute attacks of neurological and/or psychiatric symptoms; potentially life threatening and diagnosed by elevated urine porphobilinogen

Porphobilinogen (PBG) The immediate precursor of the porphyrins, a pyrrole ring with acetyl, propionyl, and aminomethyl side chains; four molecules of porphobilinogen being condensed to form one molecule of uroporphyrinogen III, which then is converted successively to coproporphyrinogen III, protoporphyrin IX, and heme

Porphyrins Any of a group of compounds containing the porphyrin structure—four pyrrole rings connected by methylidyne bridges in a cyclic configuration—to which a variety of side chains are attached

Porphyrias A group of metabolic disorders that result from a disturbance in porphyrin metabolism, causing increased formation and excretion of porphyrins and its precursors; acute intermittent porphyria being a rare inherited (autosomal dominant) form that results in abdominal pain and neurological disturbances; the various forms being differentiated by measurement of porphyrins and porphyrin intermediates

Porphyrin Precursors Aminolevulinic acid and porphobilinogen, the biosynthetic intermediates that produce porphyrinogens and porphyrins

Protoporphyrin A porphyrin with four methyl, two vinyl, and two propionic acid side chains attached to the tetrapyrrole backbone; found in hemoglobin, myoglobin, most of the cytochromes, and a variety of other enzymes

Transferrin A β-globulin that carries iron in the blood

Unconjugated Bilirubin Free bilirubin that has not been conjugated with glucuronic acid

Uroporphyrin A porphyrin with four acetic acid and four propionic acid side chains attached to the tetrapyrrole backbone

Zinc Protoporphyrin (ZPP) A normal but minor product of the heme pathway in the red blood cell that increases its formation when insufficient Fe (II) is available to the developing erythrocyte

---

Hemoglobin is the iron-containing pigment of the red blood cells (RBCs) that carries oxygen. Each molecule of hemoglobin contains a central heme (iron-porphyrin) group that is the site of O_2 uptake and release.

Heme is an essential component of hemoglobin and a variety of other molecules and plays a central role in the metabolism of porphyrins, iron, and bilirubin. Porphyrins are synthesized from small precursors, with atoms of iron inserted to produce molecules of heme. As RBCs age, they are removed from the circulation by phagocytic cells of the reticuloendothelial system. On phagocytosis, hemoglobin is released and catabolized to globin, iron, and bilirubin. The globin and iron are recycled and the bilirubin excreted.

To summarize, heme (1) is synthesized via the porphyrin pathway, (2) provides a controlled environment for iron in a variety of biomolecules and enzymes, and after fulfilling its function, (3) is degraded into bilirubin. The basic chemistry of porphyrins, the synthesis of heme via the porphyrin pathway, the iron cycle, and the degradation of heme into bilirubin are discussed in this chapter.

■ PORPHYRINS

Porphyrins are derivatives of porphyrin, a compound composed of four pyrrole rings connected by methine bridges (Figure 30-1). This structure often is described as a *tetrapyrrole* to emphasize its four-rings-within-a-ring pattern. Many porphyrin compounds are known, but only a limited number typically are of clinical interest. The porphyrin compounds relevant to the present discussion primarily are

uroporphyrin, coproporphyrin, and protoporphyrin, and they differ in the substituents occupying the peripheral positions 1 through 8 (Table 30-1).

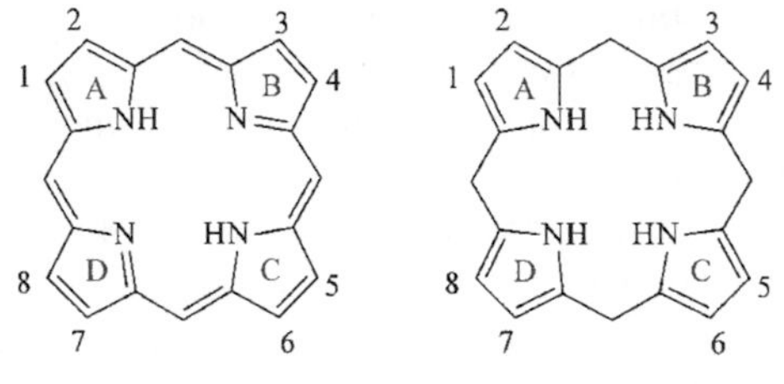

Porphyrin Chemistry

Metal chelation

The arrangement of four nitrogen atoms in the center of the porphyrin ring enables porphyrins to chelate various metal ions. Protoporphyrin that contains iron is known as **heme;** ferroheme refers specifically to the Fe^{2+} complex and ferriheme to Fe^{3+}. Heme functions as a prosthetic group in various proteins in which, depending on the function of the protein, the iron shifts freely between the 2+ and 3+ valence states.

In mammals, heme-containing proteins participate in a variety of biochemical processes, most of which are associated with some aspect of oxidative metabolism. Included are the following:

1. Oxygen transport (by hemoglobin) and storage (by **myoglobin**)
2. Mitochondrial respiration (by cytochromes b, c_1, c, a, and a_3)
3. The enzymatic destruction of peroxides (by catalase and peroxidases)
4. Drug metabolism (by cytochrome P_{450} monooxygenases)
5. The desaturation of fatty acids (by microsomal cytochrome b_5)
6. Tryptophan catabolism (by tryptophan oxygenase)

Figure 30-1   Representations of porphyrin and porphyrinogen. Numbering system and ring designations are based on the Fischer system.

TABLE 30-1   **Trivial Names for Substituted Porphyrins**

Porphyrin	Substituent Ring Position							
IUPAC-IUB Numbering	2	3	7	8	12	13	17	18
Fischer Numbering	1	2	3	4	5	6	7	8
Protoporphyrin	Me	Vn	Me	Vn	Me	Cet	Cet	Me
Deuteroporphyrin	Me	H	Me	H	Me	Cet	Cet	Me
Mesoporphyrin	Me	Et	Me	Et	Me	Cet	Cet	Me
III Isomers								
Uroporphyrin	Cm	Cet	Cm	Cet	Cm	Cet	Cet	Cm
Heptacarboxylate porphyrin*	Cm	Cet	Cm	Cet	Cm	Cet	Cet	Me
Hexacarboxylate porphyrin*	Me	Cet	Cm	Cet	Cm	Cet	Cet	Me
Pentacarboxylate porphyrin*	Me	Cet	Me	Cet	Cm	Cet	Cet	Me
Coproporphyrin	Me	Cet	Me	Cet	Me	Cet	Cet	Me
Isocoproporphyrin*	Me	Vn	Me	Cet	Me	Cet	Cet	Me
I Isomers								
Uroporphyrin	Cm	Cet	Cm	Cet	Cm	Cet	Cm	Cet
Coproporphyrin	Me	Cet	Me	Cet	Me	Cet	Me	Cet

IUPAC-IUB, International Union of Pure and Applied Chemistry-International Union of Biochemistry; *Cm,* $-CH_2CO_2H$; *Cet,* $-CH_2CH_2CO_2H$; *Et,* $-CH_2CH_3$; *Me,* $-CH_3$; *Vn,* $-CH=CH_2$.
*Unapproved trivial name.

The actions of nitric oxide (NO) often are mediated by NO binding with heme in control enzymes, such as guanylate cyclase. Other naturally occurring tetrapyrroles include vitamin B_{12} and chlorophyll, each of which contain an atom of chelated cobalt and magnesium, respectively.

Optical properties

Porphyrins were named from the Greek root for "purple" *(porphyra)*. Crystalline and concentrated solutions of porphyrins typically are dark red to purple in color because of the highly conjugated double-bond structure of the tetrapyrrole ring. Porphyrins show a particularly strong absorbance near 400 nm, often called the *Soret band.* When exposed to light in the 400-nm region, porphyrins display a characteristic orange-red fluorescence in the range of 550 to 650 nm. Absorbance and fluorescence are altered by substituents around the porphyrin ring and metal binding. Zinc chelation shifts the fluorescence peak of protoporphyrin to longer wavelengths and reduces the fluorescence intensity. The strong binding of iron alters the character of protoporphyrin to the extent that heme lacks significant fluorescence.

Solubility

Solubility determines much of the behavior of porphyrins, which are only marginally soluble in water. At pH 7, the only charges on the porphyrin derivatives are on the carboxyl groups, which behave as typical weak organic acids. At physiological pH, the number of its substituent carboxyl groups determines the solubility of a given porphyrin. **Uroporphyrin** has eight carboxylate groups and is the most soluble porphyrin in aqueous media. Protoporphyrin has only two carboxylate groups and is essentially insoluble in water, but it dissolves readily in lipid environments and binds readily to the hydrophobic regions of proteins such as albumin.

Coproporphyrin, with four carboxylate groups, has intermediate solubility. Because of its water solubility, uroporphyrin concentrates in the urine, although it also is found at lower concentrations in the blood and feces. Protoporphyrin is not found in the urine but is located in the blood and excreted entirely in the bile and feces. Coproporphyrin is excreted either in the urine or feces, depending on its rate of formation or the pH of the urine, with more alkaline urine favoring the urinary route.

Extraction

Extraction is a time-tested technique used for porphyrin analysis and is based on porphyrin solubility characteristics. The traditional extraction methods have two steps—(1) an extraction into an acidified organic solvent, followed by (2) a second or back-extraction into aqueous acid. The initial extraction takes advantage of the fact that at pH 3 to 5 porphyrins are less soluble in aqueous media and move into the organic phase. The back-extraction induces porphyrin compounds to move back into an aqueous solution by decreasing the pH to less than 2. This pH shift causes the protonation of the pyrrolenine nitrogen atoms, thereby reversing the solubility characteristics of porphyrins. Compounds such as heme, in which the pyrrolenine nitrogen atoms are bound to iron, remain uncharged at low pH and trapped in the organic layer. Many newer chromatographic procedures for porphyrin analysis also are based on the characteristic solubility of the porphyrin.

Porphyrin precursors

Aminolevulinic acid (ALA) and **porphobilinogen (PBG)** are the **porphyrin precursors** (see Figure 30-2). ALA also is known as *5-aminolevulinic acid* and *δ-aminolevulinic acid* (the latter being an older term). The compound is ionized at physiological pH and often called *aminolevulinate* to emphasize its ionic nature. PBG is a pyrrole derivative that sometimes is referred to as a *monopyrrole* to emphasize that four PBG molecules are used in the pathway to synthesize porphyrins (tetrapyrroles). PBG polymerizes readily, particularly at high concentrations in acid solution, and spontaneously forms primarily the type I isomer of uroporphyrin. ALA and PBG are highly water soluble, and the renal threshold for both compounds is low. Consequently, porphyrin precursors concentrate in the urine and remain at low levels in the circulation.

Biosynthesis of Porphyrins and Heme

The biosynthetic pathway of porphyrins and heme is shown in Figure 30-2. Each step in the pathway produces progressively less water-soluble molecules until, with protoporphyrin and heme, the compounds are insoluble in aqueous solutions. For this reason, excess intermediates early in the pathway tend to accumulate in the urine, whereas intermediates late in the pathway, particularly protoporphyrin, are found in the blood, bile, and feces but not the urine.

Eight enzymes are required to synthesize heme—four in the mitochondria and four in the cytosol (see Figure 30-2). The recommended names for these enzymes, associated porphyrin disorders, and elevated intermediates are listed in Table 30-2. In addition, other clinical conditions associated with these intermediates are listed in Table 30-3.

Aminolevulinic acid synthase

ALA synthase catalyzes the formation of ALA from glycine and succinyl CoA. The enzyme functions in the mitochondrial matrix, with pyridoxal phosphate being a required cofactor. ALA synthase catalyzes the rate-determining step in nonerythroid cells and is controlled tightly by a number of mechanisms acting in concert. At the enzyme level, as well as at the level of translation and transcription, heme is a negative feedback control agent. Given the unique require-

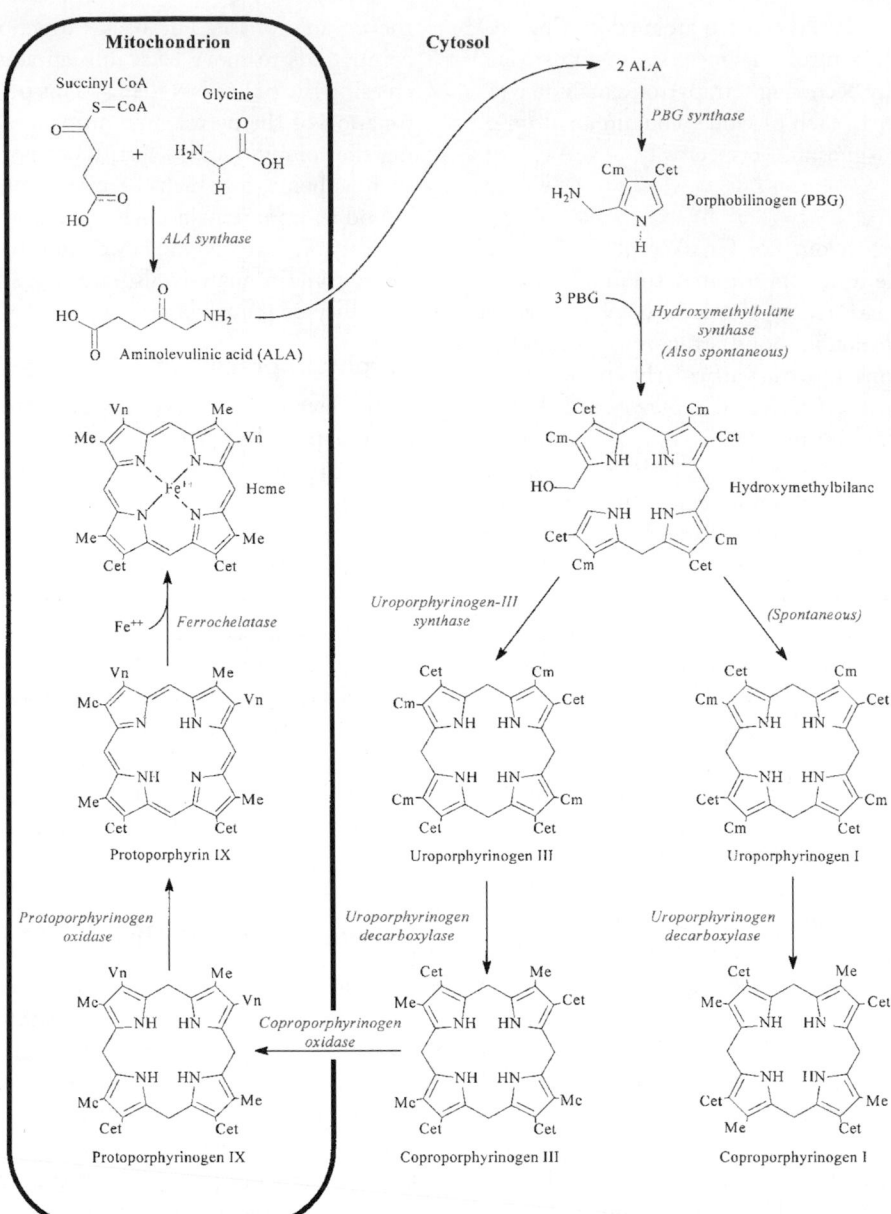

Figure 30-2   Biosynthetic pathway of porphyrins and heme. (Excess concentrations of coproporphyrinogen and protoporphyrinogen inhibit hydroxymethylbilane synthase.) *CoA*, Coenzyme A; *Cet*, $-CH_2CH_2CO_2H$; *Cm*, $-CH_2CO_2H$; *Me*, $-CH_3$; *Vn*, $-CH=CH_2$.

ments of RBCs, the control mechanism is different, and ALA synthase does not catalyze the rate-limiting step in this cell type (see later section on control of heme biosynthesis).

Porphobilinogen synthase

PBG synthase catalyzes the second step of heme synthesis in which PBG is formed from two molecules of ALA. Because the enzyme removes water during the reaction, it previously was called *ALA dehydratase* (see Table 30-2). ALA is produced in the mitochondrial matrix and moves to the cytosol, its site of action; whether the process is active or passive is unknown. The enzyme requires Zn^{2+} and reduced sulfhydryl groups for activity; enzyme activity is lost when zinc is displaced from the active site or when the critical sulfhydryl groups are oxidized.

Hydroxymethylbilane synthase

Hydroxymethylbilane synthase catalyzes the sequential combination of four molecules of PBG to form hydroxymethylbilane, a linear tetrapyrrole. The addition of each successive PBG releases an amino group, accounting for the older name, *PBG deaminase*. This enzyme also previously was named *uroporphyrinogen-I synthase* before the enzyme product was recognized as hydroxymethylbilane.

TABLE 30-2 Enzymes of Porphyrin and Heme Biosynthesis		
Enzyme* EC Number (Other Names)	Associated Inherited Porphyria	Major Elevated Intermediates†
1. ALA synthase 2.3.1.36 (ALA synthetase)	None	
2. PBG synthase 4.2.1.24 (ALA dehydrase) (ALA dehydratase) (ALA hydrolase)	PBG synthase deficiency porphyria	ALA (more common in acquired disorders)
3. Hydroxymethylbilane synthase 4.3.1.8 (PBG deaminase) (Uroporphyrinogen-I synthase)	Acute intermittent porphyria	PBG (and ALA)
4. Uroporphyrinogen-III synthase 4.2.1.75 (Uroporphyrinogen cosynthase) (Uroporphyrinogen isomerase)	Congenital erythropoietic porphyria	Uroporphyrin-I (diagnosis by history)
5. Uroporphyrinogen decarboxylase 4.1.1.37	Porphyria cutanea tarda Hepatoerythropoietic porphyria	Uroporphyrin and heptacarboxylate porphyrins
6. Coproporphyrinogen oxidase 1.3.3.3 (Coproporphyrinogenase)	Hereditary coproporphyria	PBG; coproporphyrin
7. Protoporphyrinogen oxidase 1.3.3.4	Variegate porphyria	PBG; protoporphyrin
8. Ferrochelatase 4.99.1.2 (Heme synthase) (Heme synthetase) (Protoheme ferrolyase)	Erythropoietic protoporphyria	Protoporphyrin (PBG normal)

ALA, Aminolevulinic acid; *PBG*, porphobilinogen.
*Enzyme names recommended by the Nomenclature Committee of the International Union of Biochemistry, 1992.
†Concentrations of intermediates are elevated during symptomatic episodes and may be normal in remission.

Uroporphyrinogen-III synthase

In the fourth step of heme synthesis, uroporphyrinogen-III synthase catalyzes the conversion of hydroxymethylbilane to uroporphyrinogen. In addition to closing the structure, the enzyme rotates the D ring, producing the type III isomer. In the absence of synthase the hydroxymethylbilane substrate spontaneously condenses to produce primarily the type I isomer. Only the type III isomer contributes to heme synthesis.

Uroporphyrinogen decarboxylase

Uroporphyrinogen decarboxylase catalyzes the decarboxylation of uroporphyrinogen to coproporphyrinogen. Each uroporphyrinogen molecule contains eight carboxyl groups—four as methylcarboxylate and four as ethylcarboxylate groups. Uroporphyrinogen decarboxylase catalyzes the sequential decarboxylation of the four methylcarboxylate groups to produce the more lipophilic coproporphyrinogen; the four ethylcarboxylate groups are left unaltered.

Coproporphyrinogen oxidase

Coproporphyrinogen oxidase is the sixth enzyme in the heme pathway and is found in the intermembrane space of the mitochondria. This enzyme catalyzes the oxidation of two of the four ethylcarboxylate groups to vinyl groups, producing the more lipophilic protoporphyrinogen. Oxygen is required as the oxidant. The mechanisms for the transport of the reactant and product across the outer and inner mitochondrial membranes are not understood well. The enzyme requires sulfhydryl groups for activity, making it a target for metal-induced inhibition.

Protoporphyrinogen oxidase

The seventh step in heme biosynthesis is catalyzed by the enzyme protoporphyrinogen oxidase, which is found in the inner mitochondrial membrane. It involves the oxidation of protoporphyrinogen to protoporphyrin. The protoporphyrin produced by the enzymatic oxidation is the only porphyrin that functions in the heme pathway. The other porphyrins are produced by nonenzymatic oxidation and represent porphyrinogens that have escaped irreversibly from the heme biosynthetic pathway.

Ferrochelatase

The last step in the pathway to heme is the insertion of Fe^{2+} into protoporphyrin. This insertion is catalyzed by the enzyme ferrochelatase, which is located on the inner membranes of the mitochondria. Ferrochelatase is specific for Fe^{2+} and does not insert Fe^{3+} into the porphyrin molecule. However, the enzyme is capable of inserting other metal ions in the 2+ valence state. For example, Zn^{2+} is present at relatively high concentrations in the developing RBCs and competes directly with Fe^{2+} for enzymatic insertion into protoporphyrin. The resulting **zinc protoporphyrin (ZPP)** is an indirect measure of iron availability in the developing erythroblast.

Porphyrin Disorders

The **porphyrias** are a group of diseases associated with hereditary and acquired deficiencies in the biosynthetic pathway of heme.[15,18,20] Porphyrin disorders are classified as either primary or secondary. Primary conditions are inherited,

TABLE 30-3 Conditions Associated with Elevated Porphyrin Intermediates

Elevated Intermediate (Associated Enzyme)	Conditions*
ALA (PBG synthase)	Ethanol
	Lead
	Some malignancies
	Hereditary tyrosinemia
	PBG synthase deficiency porphyria
PBG and ALA (hydroxymethylbilane synthase)	Acute intermittent porphyria
	Variegate porphyria
	Hereditary coproporphyria
	PBG synthase deficiency porphyria
	Some malignancies
Uroporphyrin (uroporphyrinogen decarboxylase)	Chronic renal failure
	Porphyria cutanea tarda
	Elevated PBG
	Some malignancies
	Congenital erythropoietic porphyria
Coproporphyrin (coproporphyrinogen oxidase)	Diet
	Liver disease
	Chronic renal failure
	Hexachlorobenzene
	Lead, mercury, arsenic
	Some malignancies
	Hereditary coproporphyria
	Alagille's syndrome
Protoporphyrin (protoporphyrinogen oxidase and ferrochelatase)	Variegate porphyria
	Erythropoietic protoporphyria
Zinc protoporphyrin (ferrochelatase)	Early iron deficiency
	Anemia of chronic disease
	Lead
	Aluminum in hemodialysis

ALA, Aminolevulinic acid; PBG, porphobilinogen.
*In approximate order of decreasing incidence; list not exhaustive.

and secondary conditions are acquired, with the acquired disorders much more common than the inherited ones (see Table 30-3). Laboratory support for the diagnosis of the porphyrin disorders is based primarily on the measurement of excess porphyrins and porphyrin precursors (Table 30-4).[2,7,13] Supplemental information may be available from the activity of individual biosynthetic enzymes and from gene-based testing. However, with reference to the porphyrias, the diagnostic tools of molecular biology still are confined primarily to research laboratories.

Primary porphyrin disorders

The metabolic abnormalities observed in the primary porphyrin disorders result from inherited deficiencies of specific enzymes in the heme biosynthetic pathway (see Table 30-2). The primary porphyrin disorders are divided into two broad categories based on clinical manifestation—(1) the neurological and/or psychiatric forms of porphyria, which often present as acute episodes, and (2) the forms associated with cutaneous photosensitivity. This classification has the advantage of relating the clinical presentation to important diagnostic information. For example, symptoms of the **neurological porphyrias** invariably are associated with elevations of the porphyrin precursors, primarily PBG but also ALA, whereas symptoms of the photosensitive porphyrias invariably are associated with an accumulation of porphyrins. Neurological symptoms and photosensitivity may be present simultaneously when PBG and porphyrin concentrations are elevated at the same time. These basic principles apply even to those cases in which more than one enzymatic defect is present.

Acute neuropsychiatric porphyrias

PBG and ALA are excreted in excess during symptomatic episodes of the neurological/psychiatric forms of porphyria. These include acute intermittent porphyria, hereditary coproporphyria, and variegate porphyria, the neurological manifestations of which are essentially identical.[7] During the acute phase, PBG is excreted in the urine in marked excess, but during asymptomatic intervals this abnormality may resolve. Although PBG levels typically are elevated, normal results during quiescent periods do not exclude a diagnosis.

Episodes of the neurological/psychiatric forms of porphyria are characterized by attacks of autonomic dysfunction. An acute episode may include symptoms of abdominal pain, limb or chest pain, nausea, paresthesias, weakness, confused thoughts, depression, hallucinations, and psychosis. Signs often include hypertension and tachycardia; constipation or diarrhea may occur, with the former more common; nausea is accompanied by vomiting. Fever, leukocytosis, the syndrome of inappropriate antidiuretic hormone secretion, convulsions, and respiratory paralysis are less common.

About 5% of attacks requiring hospitalization result in fatal outcomes. Acute attacks usually have a relatively brisk onset of hours to days, but characterization of a typical prodrome is impossible. The spectrum of symptoms and signs, as well as the duration and intensity of symptoms, is variable among individuals. Those individuals with recurrent attacks often experience similar symptoms with each recurrence. An attack may last several days, to weeks and months, and may have chronic sequelae. Recurrent abdominal pain has been noted in some cases for years after an acute attack.

Fewer than 10% of individuals carrying a predisposing gene defect ever experience an active episode of an acute porphyria.[7,13] An acute attack often is precipitated by a drug exposure, dietary restriction, or some other event. Drugs associated with attacks include ethanol, barbiturates, and anticonvulsants. However, such drugs do not inevitably induce attacks in susceptible individuals, and the regular use of many precipitating drugs often is not associated with attacks. Active disease is influenced by hormonal status, with the disease more often remaining latent before puberty

TABLE 30-4   Selection of Laboratory Tests

Clinical Presentation	Primary Test	Supplemental Tests
1. Acute neuropsychiatric porphyria	Random urine PBG	Second urine PBG Urine ALA
2. Chronic neuropsychiatric porphyria	Urine PBG	Fecal porphyrins
3. Differentiation among the neurological porphyrias	Fecal porphyrins	Serum and urine porphyrins Enzyme- and gene-based tests
4. Latent neurological porphyria	None	Urine PBG and porphyrins Fecal and serum porphyrins Enzyme- and gene-based tests
5. Acute photosensitivity	Serum or fecal porphyrins	Liver function tests Urine porphyrins
6. Bullous skin lesions	Urine porphyrins	Serum and fecal porphyrins Urine PBG
7. Monitoring of porphyria cutanea tarda	Urine porphyrins	Serum porphyrins
8. Elevated coproporphyrin	None	Evaluation of diet Liver function tests
9. Identification of iron disorders	ZPP	Serum ferritin Other iron studies
10. Lead exposure	Whole-blood lead	ZPP

ALA, Aminolevulinic acid; *PBG,* porphobilinogen; *ZPP,* zinc protoporphyrin.

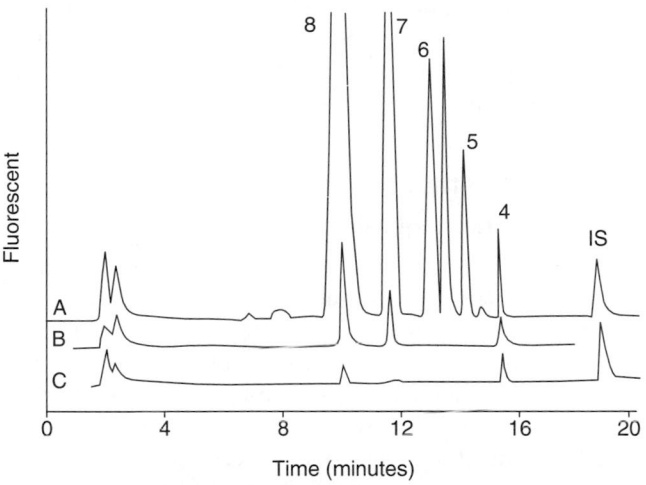

Figure 30-3   Representative urine porphyrin chromatograms from (*a*) patient with overt porphyria cutanea tarda; (*b*) patient with successfully treated (subclinical) porphyria cutanea tarda; and (*c*) normal individual. Numbers next to peaks refer to the number of carboxyl groups in the porphyrin molecule (*8* corresponds to uroporphyrin; *7, 6,* and *5,* to heptacarboxylate, hexacarboxylate, and pentacarboxylate porphyrins, respectively; and *4* to coproporphyrin). The unlabeled peak between *5* and *6* corresponds to isocoproporphyrin. Early peaks are due to normally occurring fluorescent compounds in urine. *IS,* Mesoporphyrin, the internal standard. (Modified from Nuttall KL, Pingree SS, Ashwood ER: Reference intervals for 24-hour and random urine porphyrins. Ann Clin Lab Sci 1996; 26:313-322.)

and becoming manifest after the onset of puberty. Episodes occur in children, not uncommonly in association with anticonvulsant medications. Acute attacks are more common in women, may occur in association with menses, and may cease with menopause. Individuals with neurological por-

phyria appear to experience an increased incidence of hypertension, chronic renal failure, and hepatocellular carcinoma.

Porphyrias with photosensitivity

Porphyrins deposited in skin and exposed to sunlight cause considerable skin damage. The most common porphyrin disorder associated with photosensitivity is porphyria cutanea tarda, which typically presents in middle age, with characteristic blistering on sun-exposed areas. As shown in Figure 30-3, individuals with porphyria cutanea tarda demonstrate a highly characteristic pattern of porphyrin intermediates. Erythropoietic protoporphyria usually presents in childhood, with relatively mild photosensitivity in which blistering is less common and less severe than with porphyria cutanea tarda. Congenital erythropoietic porphyria is a very rare disorder typically presenting as severe bullous photosensitivity at birth. Variegate porphyria and coproporphyria may manifest with photosensitivity, as neurological porphyria, or with both, as may dual porphyrias. Acquired disorders, such as sideroblastic anemia, also may demonstrate photosensitivity as a consequence of abnormal porphyrin deposition.

Dual porphyrias

In addition to porphyrias characterized by both neurological presentations and photosensitivity, porphyrias have been reported in which two inherited enzyme defects are present. The pattern of porphyrin excretion in such cases is complex and requires repeated studies for unambiguous characterization. Examples include coexistent acute intermittent porphyria with (1) porphyria cutanea tarda, (2) coproporphyria, and (3) variegate porphyria (also called *Chester porphyria*), and variegate porphyria with porphyria cutanea tarda. Other similar diagnostic problems include homozygous acute intermittent porphyria, porphyria cutanea tarda (also called *hepatoerythropoietic porphyria*), variegate porphyria, and erythropoietic protoporphyria. The homozygous conditions often present earlier and have more severe manifestations.

Secondary (acquired) porphyrin disorders

In the secondary, or "acquired," porphyrias the disturbances of porphyrin metabolism are not the result of an inherited enzyme deficiency, but rather an enzyme inhibition secondary to a superimposed toxin or drug. Lead poisoning and hereditary tyrosinemia are examples of diseases in this category. Lead inhibits the enzyme PBG synthase, among others,[14] resulting in increased excretion of ALA. ZPP concentration also is increased, and urine coproporphyrin often becomes elevated as a delayed response. In practice, chronic lead poisoning is one of the many causes of significant coproporphyrinuria. Hereditary tyrosinemia also produces an acute porphyria-like illness, and although it is an inherited disease, the effect on porphyrin metabolism is secondary to the production of succinylacetone. This abnormal metabolite is a potent inhibitor of PBG synthase and produces markedly increased concentrations of ALA.

Identification of iron disorders

ZPP concentrations in whole blood are elevated in individuals with three relatively common conditions—iron deficiency, the anemia of chronic disease, and lead poisoning. ZPP is an early indicator of reduced iron stores.[3,10]

ZPP levels also increase in individuals with the anemia of chronic disease. This classification includes malignant diseases, such as acute lymphoblastic leukemia, Hodgkin's disease, and non-Hodgkin's lymphoma, as well as other conditions, such as sideroblastic anemia (in which iron is not utilized properly), hemolytic anemia (in which erythropoiesis is accentuated greatly), and secondary polycythemia (in which a stimulus exists to erythropoiesis extrinsic to the marrow).

Lead exposure

The primary test for lead exposure in children is whole-blood lead, but ZPP measurements are potentially useful in any situation in which lead exposure reaches whole-blood concentrations above 25 μg/dL (1.2 μmol/L). Blood porphyrin concentrations become elevated within days of exposure to significant levels of lead. Without additional lead exposure, the blood lead level decreases, with a half-life of approximately 30 days, whereas the blood porphyrin concentrations remain elevated for the lifetime of the involved erythrocytes. Specimens collected for lead testing, particularly blood collected by fingersticks, are notoriously prone to contamination by exogenous lead; contamination should be suspected in specimens with elevated whole-blood lead levels that do not show concordance with ZPP measurements.

In 1985 the Centers for Disease Control and Prevention (CDC) defined an elevated blood lead level in children as 25 μg/dL (1.2 μmol/L) or greater and recommended the erythrocyte protoporphyrin assay as a screening test for lead exposure. Such testing has the added advantage of screening children for iron deficiency, a condition that is more common than lead poisoning and produces similar developmental problems. In 1991 the CDC lowered the acceptable blood lead levels in children to less than 10 μg/dL (0.48 μmol/L). ZPP and erythrocyte protoporphyrin methods are not considered adequate biological indicators of less than 25 μg/dL (1.2 μmol/L) of whole-blood lead and therefore currently are not recommended by the CDC for lead screening in children 6 years of age and younger.

Other toxic exposures

The heme pathway is sensitive to a wide variety of environmental influences. For example, exposure to chemicals, such as hexachlorobenzene, polyhalogenated aromatic hydrocarbons, vinyl chloride, and dioxin, alters the heme pathway functionally. This functional alteration may serve as a sensitive index for chemical exposure and occupational diseases. The measurement of urine porphyrins has been suggested as a biomarker for mercury exposure. The results of a study of smelter employees suggest that long-term exposure to arsenic is associated with increased urine coproporphyrin.

Analytical Methods

Analysis of hemoglobin

Hemoglobin and related compounds are measured by several different types of methods, including spectrophotometry, electrophoresis, immunoassay, molecular techniques, and sensitive separation techniques, such as high-performance liquid chromatography (HPLC), capillary electrophoresis (CE), and mass spectrometry (MS).

Measurement of hemoglobin concentration in venous or capillary blood is one of the most frequently performed clinical laboratory tests. The cyanmethemoglobin method is used widely for this purpose and has been adopted internationally as the approved reference method for hemoglobin measurement. With this method the Fe^{2+} of hemoglobin is oxidized to the Fe^{3+} of methemoglobin by ferricyanide, and the methemoglobin is converted into stable cyanmethemoglobin by addition of potassium cyanide (KCN), as follows:

$$HbFe^{2+} + Fe^{3+}(CN)_6^{3-} \longrightarrow HbFe^{3+} + Fe^{2+}(CN)_6^{4-}$$
$$HbFe^{3+} + CN^- \longrightarrow HbFe^{3+}CN$$

where $HbFe^{2+}$ represents a hemoglobin monomer, $HbFe^{3+}$ a methemoglobin monomer, and $HbFe^{3+}CN$ a monomer of cyanmethemoglobin; nonreactive ions are omitted. The absorbance of cyanmethemoglobin is measured at 540 nm, at which it exhibits a broad absorbance peak.

The procedure requires a minimum of 0.02 mL of whole blood. Blood may be anticoagulated with disodium-ethylenediaminetetraacetic acid (EDTA) or taken directly from a finger (or heel) puncture without use of an anticoagulant.

Analysis of porphyrin precursors

PBG and ALA are water soluble and concentrate in the urine and therefore are measured almost exclusively in urine in the clinical laboratory. PBG is in general the more important of the precursors, and ALA is used more as a supplemental test (see later section on ALA). Assays for both PBG and ALA include the traditional color reaction with Ehrlich's aldehyde reagent, an acidic solution of p-dimethylaminobenzaldehyde (DMAB). PBG reacts with Ehrlich's reagent to form a colored product variously described as "rose red" or "magenta." Several modifications of Ehrlich's reagent are used, each varying in the concentration of DMAB and kind and concentration of the acid solvent.

Porphobilinogen

Both screening and quantitative tests are available to measure PBG. Screening tests include the generic Watson-Schwartz and Hoesch tests and a commercial test. The screening tests are qualitative, relatively insensitive, and prone to both false-positive and false-negative results. Whenever screening procedures are used, most specimens warrant additional testing at a later time with a quantitative method.

Watson-Schwartz screening test. Historically the Watson-Schwartz test was the best known screening method for the detection of PBG. Although it is essentially obsolete and insufficiently sensitive for routine screening, it still is used in a variety of settings.

This test uses pH adjustment and solvent extractions to separate the PBG chromogen from other interfering substances. Equal volumes of urine and "modified" Ehrlich's reagent (0.7 g DMAB, 150 mL of concentrated HCl, and 100 mL of water) are mixed, and two volumes of saturated sodium acetate are added. To maximize extraction efficiency the pH of the solution should be adjusted to a range of 4 to 5. An equal volume of chloroform is added, and the solution is shaken vigorously for at least 1 minute to achieve adequate equilibrium. If color is absent in the aqueous (upper) layer, the result is negative and no further testing is needed. A red color in the organic (lower) phase suggests urobilinogen. The color from urobilinogen is not always limited to the organic layer, so when color is present in the aqueous layer, the aqueous layer is separated and extracted with an equal volume of butanol. With butanol a "rose-red" color in the aqueous (lower) layer indicates a positive result and suggests a concentration of PBG that is several times the upper limit of the reference interval. A clear aqueous layer suggests PBG levels within the reference interval, thereby excluding an episode of an acute neuropsychiatric

porphyria. Both false-positive and false-negative results are relatively common.

Interpretation of some results may be ambiguous, particularly for the inexperienced analyst. In the Watson-Schwartz test, PBG and the chromogen that it forms always remain in the aqueous phase. The extractions with chloroform and butanol remove frequently occurring substances that interfere with the test. The most common interfering substance is urobilinogen, which is chloroform soluble and produces a red color with Ehrlich's reagent, similar to PBG. Other red colors in urine from agents such as beet juice also have been reported as false-positive results. Substances that sometimes are present in urine produce a variety of colors when they are combined with Ehrlich's reagent, including green, yellow, and orange, all of which tend to make the positive identification of PBG difficult.

Hoesch screening test. The Hoesch screening test is easier to perform but not as specific as the Watson-Schwartz version. Consequently, false-positive and false-negative results are common with its use. The Hoesch test uses Ehrlich's reagent in the original formulation (2 g DMAB in 100 mL of 6 mol/L HCl) but in a manner described as a "reverse" reagent that does not react as quickly with urobilinogen. Several milliliters of this Ehrlich's reagent are placed in a test tube, and one to two drops of fresh urine are added. If PBG levels are increased, a red color should develop immediately at the interface of the mixing solutions. Colors that develop after more than a few seconds likely are due to interfering compounds. Many of the same problems that exist with color interpretation in the Watson-Schwartz also apply to the Hoesch test.

PBG Test Kit. The PBG Test Kit is available from Trace (Miami, Fla.) and uses a syringe filled with an anion-exchange resin to trap PBG and remove interfering compounds, the principle being much like that for the quantitative PBG procedure described later in the chapter. This test may represent a better screening method than the older Watson-Schwartz and Hoesch tests, although it still must rely on a color change that is not entirely specific.

Quantitative test for porphobilinogen in urine. This procedure uses a commercially available ion-exchange column and is the most commonly used method for PBG quantitation.

In practice, urine is adjusted to a pH between 8 and 10, and an aliquot is introduced into an anion-exchange column. PBG adsorbs to the resin, whereas many interfering substances are flushed from the column with repeated water washes. PBG then is eluted with acetic acid. A modified Ehrlich's aldehyde reagent is added to the eluate, which produces the classic rose-red color with pyrroles, similar to PBG. The reaction is quantified with a spectrophotometer, and elevated results are scanned for evaluation of possible interferences.

A random urine specimen associated with a symptomatic episode is preferred as long as the urine is not too dilute (for example, creatinine <25 mg/dL). A first-morning specimen represents a relatively concentrated sample, although concern has been expressed that PBG is not stable in the environment of the bladder. A 24-hour urine collection is appropriate when the overall excretion rate is to be measured. For most purposes, a 24-hour urine specimen is preserved adequately if it is refrigerated during collection, transport, and storage.

PBG is more stable around pH 8 to 9 (whereas ALA is more stable at pH 3 to 4), but pH adjustment runs the risk of a decrease in stability because it can overshoot the optimum pH range, dilute the specimen, and otherwise interfere with the analytical procedure. When properly refrigerated at 4 °C in the dark, PBG tolerates acid solutions for several days. The recovery of PBG from a solution at pH 5.5 was 90% after 3 days and 80% after 6 days. Older recommendations for PBG preservation specify the use of 0.5 g of sodium carbonate per 100 mL of urine, although this addition causes foaming problems. An appropriate goal is a pH of 8 to 9 by use of indicator paper, with the addition of base when necessary.

The reference interval for PBG for a random urine specimen is 0 to 2.0 mg/L (0 to 8.8 μmol/L). For a 24-hour urine specimen the reference interval is 0 to 3.4 mg/day (0 to 15 μmol/day). Episodes of the neuropsychiatric porphyrias often are associated with massive elevations more than 10 times the upper limit of the reference interval, and normal results exclude an episode with a high degree of confidence. Scanning the optical spectrum of the reaction mixture is necessary if interferences are to be identified. Imipenem, for example, often gives a peak at 580 nm with Ehrlich's reagent. Interferences occur commonly, particularly those that give modest elevations less than two or three times the reference cutoff, and particularly when the urine specimen is concentrated (for example, creatinine >150 mg/dL). The coefficient of variation (CV) at the cutoff of 8.8 μmol/L is approximately ±10%, but the methods become imprecise at lower concentrations.

Aminolevulinic acid

For diagnosis of the acute neurological porphyrias, testing for ALA sometimes is performed along with PBG. Both PBG and ALA are elevated in individuals with the acute porphyrias, although ALA typically is less so. ALA is an appropriate test for the evaluation for hereditary tyrosinemia and the very rare PBG synthase deficiency porphyria. Acute and chronic ethanol exposure and lead exposure also produce elevations of ALA (see Table 30-3).

Assays for ALA are similar to those for PBG. However, they require an additional reaction with a reagent such as acetylacetone to convert ALA into a pyrrole derivative, which then produces the characteristic color reaction with Ehrlich's reagent. Compared with PBG procedures, interferences are more common with ALA. For example, the acetylacetone derivatization step forms a compound with penicillin that reacts with Ehrlich's reagent, thereby providing a false-positive result.

As for PBG, prompt refrigeration is required for specimen preservation. Urine specimens have been stored at 4 °C in the dark for at least 2 weeks without significant loss of ALA, and frozen specimens are stable for weeks. Whereas PBG is more stable around pH 8 to 9, ALA is more stable around pH 3 to 4, although more acidic environments markedly reduce ALA stability. The reference interval for ALA in a random urine specimen is 0 to 4.5 mg/L (0 to 34 μmol/L), and for a 24-hour urine collection is 0 to 7.5 mg/day (0 to 57 μmol/day).

Analysis of porphyrins

Most porphyrin compounds have a strong absorption band in the vicinity of 400 nm that is referred to as the *Soret band*. The exact location of the Soret peak with a given porphyrin depends on a variety of factors, including concentration of the porphyrins, solvent type, pH, and ionic strength. Illumination of the Soret band typically produces a characteristic fluorescence in the orange-red region between 550 to 650 nm. The fluorescence intensity is pH dependent and is most intense in acid solutions. This fluorescence allows porphyrins to be detected at nanomolar concentrations. Most definitive methods for porphyrin identification are based on HPLC methodology through use of fluorescence detection.[11] In addition, CE[5] and MS[22] have been used for the analysis of porphyrins. Porphyrins and related products are available from Porphyrin Products (Logan, Utah) and Sigma Chemical Co. (St. Louis, Mo.).

Measurement of porphyrins in urine

To measure porphyrins in urine a urine specimen is centrifuged briefly and an aliquot of the supernatant then injected into a reverse-phase C_{18} column of an HPLC system. The initial mobile phase is a mixture of equal parts of phosphate buffer and methanol. Porphyrins are trapped in the hydrophobic C_{18} stationary phase and sequentially eluted with a solvent of increasing methanol concentration. The order of elution depends on the increasing lipophilicity of the individual porphyrins and the number of carboxyl functional groups on their porphyrin ring. Uroporphyrin is the most hydrophilic and elutes first, followed by the increasingly lipophilic heptacarboxylate, hexacarboxylate, and pentacarboxylate porphyrins, and coproporphyrin (see Figure 30-3). The column eluent passes through a flow cell of a fluorometer, where the eluting porphyrins are identified through comparison of their characteristic elution times with those obtained from reference porphyrins. The magnitude of the resulting fluorescence signal is proportional to the concentration (μmol/L) of the eluting porphyrin. In practice, a creatinine ratio is calculated to compensate for diuresis. Older methods involve calculation of the daily porphyrin output (for example, μmol/day) based on the volume of a 24-hour urine collection, although the 24-hour volume is often a value that has been determined less accurately than the associated porphyrin concentrations.

Either a random urine or 24-hour collection is used. The specimen must be refrigerated as soon as possible. Porphyrins are stabilized further by adjustment of the pH to an alkaline range, freezing, and by protection from intense light. An additional factor with porphyrins is that they are only marginally soluble in aqueous solutions. Minimum solubility in aqueous solutions occurs in the pH range 3 to 5, and decreased solubility induces porphyrins to precipitate or adsorb to precipitates in the specimen. Because phosphate salts form precipitates easily, some laboratorians have suggested that phosphate salts not be used for porphyrin preservation.

The reference limits for both 24-hour and random urine collections are as follows:

- Uroporphyrin: 3.9 mmol/mol of creatine
- Heptacarboxylate porphyrin: 2 mmol/mol of creatine
- Coproporphyrin: 22 mmol/mol of creatine

For 24-hour urine collections, the reference limits are as follows:

- Uroporphyrin: 37 nmol/day
- Heptacarboxylate porphyrin: 20 nmol/day
- Coproporphyrin: 221 nmol/day

Porphyrin output typically peaks in the afternoon and evening, although a strictly circadian rhythm is not seen. Although men normally excrete slightly higher concentrations of urine porphyrins, the differences between male and female values are small. Hexacarboxylate and pentacarboxylate porphyrins also are seen on abnormal chromatograms, although their quantitation is of little clinical significance.

Measurement of porphyrins in serum and plasma

Serum and plasma porphyrins often provide excellent diagnostic information on several porphyrin disorders.[11] The porphyrin present at highest concentrations in whole blood and erythrocytes is ZPP, which is not found in serum and plasma unless hemolysis also is present. ZPP is produced in the developing erythrocyte and is trapped along with heme in the binding sites in hemoglobin, where it remains for the lifetime of the erythrocyte. The ZPP in whole blood and erythrocytes is measured by two techniques in the clinical laboratory—front-surface fluorometry and more cumbersome extraction methods.

Serum and plasma porphyrins are measured easily with scanning fluorometry.[8] This method is not as conclusive as HPLC analysis, but the ease of the procedure and quality of the information obtained recommend it to the clinical laboratory setting. The need for a more sophisticated analytical method to diagnose or exclude erythropoietic protoporphyria seldom is needed, assuming the serum specimen is protected properly from light. Scanning fluorometry is also useful in the search for the marker often associated with variegate porphyria. Although the marker has not been characterized fully, it has a fluorescence emission peak at 626 nm and appears to be a protein-bound porphyrin.

In practice, serum is diluted with phosphate-buffered saline, transferred to a fluorometric cuvet, and examined in a scanning fluorometer with the excitation wavelength set at 400 nm. The emission spectrum is scanned between 550 to 650 nm. Abnormal porphyrins demonstrate fluorescence proportional to the concentration present, and the wavelength of peak fluorescence provides some information on the specific porphyrin species present.

Protoporphyrin produces a fluorescence emission peak at 633 nm, the marker for variegate porphyria at 626 nm, and uroporphyrin at 620 nm. Heptacarboxylporphyrin and uroporphyrin cannot be distinguished by this peak at 620 nm, but this peak has been used to follow the progress of treatment for porphyria cutanea tarda. ZPP, which is not seen normally in plasma, has a peak emission at 595 nm. Intermediate peak wavelengths suggest mixtures of porphyrins that require a separation method (for example, HPLC) to resolve.

Serum usually is the specimen of choice but plasma, whole blood, and amniotic fluid also have been analyzed through use of this method. Because protoporphyrin is very sensitive to light degradation, specimens should be protected carefully from light. Other porphyrins are much less light sensitive and are unlikely to be affected by moderate light exposure. Porphyrins are stable in refrigerated serum specimens for more than 1 week.

Measurement of whole blood zinc protoporphyrin

Guidelines for measurement of ZPP in erythrocytes are available from the National Committee for Clinical Laboratory Standards (NCCLS).[17] Routinely a hematofluorometer is used to measure ZPP fluorescence. The hematofluorometer is a simple filter-type fluorometer that measures the surface fluorescence of whole blood and washed erythrocytes. Instrumental parameters are set so that the fluorescence signal is presumed to be caused by the presence of ZPP.

Hematofluorometers use filter-type optics with excitation centered about 415 nm and emission about 595 nm. These parameters are optimized to measure ZPP. However, other compounds also may fluoresce, including bilirubin, riboflavin, and drugs such as doxorubicin, spironolactone, amoxicillin, methotrexate, and doxycycline. For example, for each 1 mg/L rise in plasma bilirubin, the hematofluorometer signal increases by approximately 8 μmol of ZPP/mol heme. Many of these interferences are removed when the cells are washed and the measurement repeated. Elevated ZPP values are evaluated further with tests such as serum ferritin and other iron studies, whole-blood lead, other acute-phase reactants, and so on, depending on clinical circumstances.

Only several drops of anticoagulated whole blood is required. Heparin is adequate when the specimen is analyzed promptly. When specimens are stored for more than a day, EDTA is preferred to heparin to avoid the formation of microclots as the heparin activity declines. ZPP is stable in a refrigerated specimen at 4 °C for up to 5 weeks. Moderate hemolysis of 5% lowers the ZPP reading slightly. Because of the massive hemolysis that occurs on thawing, frozen specimens are not suitable.

The reference interval for ZPP is 30 to 70 μmol of ZPP/mol heme. Low levels have no known clinical significance, and some laboratories may prefer simply to list a cutoff value. ZPP levels also are reported in micrograms per deciliter when a simple assumption is made about the hemoglobin concentration.[17] The rationale for conversion to micrograms per deciliter is that it allows hematofluorometer results to resemble the older and more familiar erythrocyte protoporphyrin testing results (see following section).

Measurement of erythrocyte protoporphyrin

Extraction of protoporphyrin from whole blood and erythrocytes is an example of the traditional method for porphyrin analysis. The recommended name is *erythrocyte protoporphyrin*, although a variety of similar names and acronyms have been used, including *whole-blood porphyrins*, *total erythrocyte protoporphyrin*, *free erythrocyte porphyrins*, and *free erythrocyte protoporphyrin*. The NCCLS has published a recommended method.[17] With this procedure, porphyrins are extracted with a mixture of 4:1 ethyl acetate and acetic acid, back-extracted into a 1.5-mol/L hydrochloric acid solution, and the acid extract is quantified fluorometrically against a protoporphyrin calibrator. The acid extraction removes the zinc ion from ZPP, leaving uncomplexed, "free" protoporphyrin.

In 1989 a corrected value for the absorptivity of protoporphyrin of 297 L/mmol-cm was published. Historically, proficiency programs have used the older, "traditional" millimolar absorption coefficient of 241 L/mmol-cm for the protoporphyrin calibrator.[17] Careful note should be made of which value is used, particularly because it also affects the reference interval. The reference interval based on the more accurate protoporphyrin absorptivity of 297 L/mmol-cm is 30 to 70 μmol/mol of heme (which also corresponds to ≤30 μg/dL of whole blood when those units are used). Also of note is that the hematofluorometer determination of ZPP and the extraction method for erythrocyte protoporphyrin are not equivalent.

Analysis of fecal porphyrins

Fecal analysis traditionally is used to differentiate among the acute neurological porphyrias, although fecal testing often provides ambiguous results. The porphyrins in stool most relevant to the diagnosis of porphyrin disorders are coproporphyrin and protoporphyrin. Uroporphyrin and the intermediate series of heptacarboxylate through pentacarboxylate porphyrins have been identified in fecal specimens. How-ever, the quantification of these compounds is easier and more appropriate in urine specimens, where bacterial decomposition is less of a factor. Bile specimens collected by duodenal aspiration are superior to fecal specimens for diagnostic purposes, although they are not a popular specimen type. Serum or plasma also should be considered in searches for protoporphyrin and the disorders variegate porphyria and erythropoietic protoporphyria. Some analysts may find initial screening procedures useful as a cost-saving measure, but screening should be used only to exclude those specimens that do not need more extensive analysis. HPLC-type methods are necessary to identify common interferences.

Bacterial modification of the fecal specimen is extensive. A variety of porphyrins, such as mesoporphyrin and deuteroporphyrin, are produced by gastrointestinal (GI) bacteria and contribute significantly to total fecal porphyrin levels, confusing the diagnosis of porphyrin disorders. Diet also introduces a variety of confounding compounds into the fecal specimens. Chlorophyll, for example, has a strong fluorescence similar to that of the closely related porphyrins. A red-meat diet increases fecal porphyrin concentrations into the range suggestive of porphyrin disorders. Dietary supplements, such as brewer's yeast, are rich in porphyrins and their use has led to the misdiagnosis of porphyria.

■ IRON

The metabolism of iron in many respects resembles that of a trace element (see Chapter 29). Normally, very small quantities are present in most cells of the body, in plasma, or in other extracellular fluids, and the body rigorously conserves its hoard of iron so that less than 1000th part of the body iron content is lost daily. Reviews on iron metabolism have been published.[1,9]

Biochemistry and Physiology

Iron is distributed in the body in a number of different compartments, including hemoglobin, tissue iron, myoglobin, and a labile pool (Figure 30-4). Approximately 2.5 g of iron is in hemoglobin, an iron protein that contains 0.34% iron by weight. Normally, virtually all hemoglobin iron is contained within RBCs or their precursors in the bone marrow. A total of approximately 2.5 mg of iron typically is in plasma. Transferrin also is found within the cytosol of many cells and is thought to serve as an intracellular iron transport protein within the cells.

Transport

A plasma iron transport protein called *apotransferrin* transports iron from one organ to another. This β_1-globulin with an MW of 75,000 has two iron binding sites per molecule. Each of these sites may bind one Fe^{3+} ion together with one

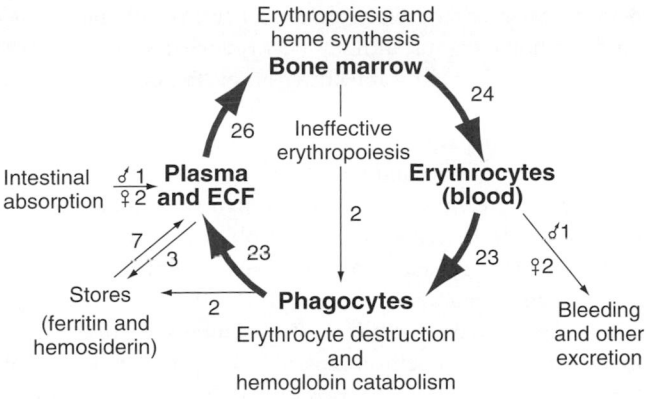

Figure 30-4   Principal pathways of iron metabolism in humans. Numbers indicate approximate number of milligrams that enter or leave the various compartments daily. Omitted from this diagram for simplicity are the very small "tissue iron" compartment, which is also in equilibrium with the plasma iron pool, and the hypothetical "labile iron pool." *ECF,* Extracellular fluid.

ion of HCO_3^-. The apotransferrin-Fe^{3+} complex is called **transferrin.**

Storage

Ferritin is the major iron storage compound and is a very efficient iron trap, as well as a readily available source of iron for metabolic requirements. It is a spherical molecule consisting of an apoferritin shell and an interior ferric oxyhydroxide $(FeOOH)_x$ crystalline core. The apoferritin shell is composed of 24 subunits or monomers. As Fe^{2+} ions enter the molecule, they are oxidized to FeOOH and released to be added to the surface of the core crystal. Release of iron from ferritin is probably nonenzymatic and may involve reduction by reduced flavin mononucleotide or other reducing substances. The resultant Fe^{2+} leaves the crystal and diffuses through a pore of the ferritin shell. The oxidation or reduction of iron takes place rapidly.

Ferritin is found in nearly all cells of the body. In hepatocytes of the liver and in the macrophage system of the bone marrow and other organs, ferritin provides a reserve of iron readily available for formation of hemoglobin and other heme proteins. In men the total body content of stored iron, mostly as ferritin, is approximately 800 mg; in healthy women, it varies from 0 to 200 mg. Minute quantities of ferritin also are present in serum in concentrations proportional to total body stored iron. Liver injury results in the release of relatively large amounts of ferritin into plasma.

Hemosiderin, the other form of stored iron, is aggregated, partially deproteinized ferritin. In contrast to ferritin, hemosiderin is insoluble in aqueous solutions, a difference that traditionally has been used to distinguish these two iron storage compounds. Iron is released only slowly from hemosiderin, probably because it occurs in relatively large aggregates and therefore has a much smaller surface/volume ratio.

Similar to ferritin, hemosiderin normally is found predominantly in cells of the liver, spleen, and bone marrow.

Absorption and excretion

The average American diet provides 10 to 15 mg of iron daily, mostly in the form of hemoglobin and myoglobin from meat. Normally, approximately 1 mg of iron is absorbed each day. Absorption occurs principally in the duodenum. Heme is absorbed directly; inorganic iron is absorbed in the ferrous state (Fe^{2+}).

Both ferritin and transferrin are present in the absorptive cells of the intestinal mucosa and are believed to function together to regulate iron absorption. When body iron stores are high, the ferritin content of mucosal epithelium also is high and the transferrin content is low. Iron that enters mucosal cells is trapped in ferritin and lost when the mucosal cell is sloughed into the intestinal lumen. This mechanism reduces iron absorption when body stores of iron already are increased. Conversely, with iron deficiency the mucosal cell content of apoferritin is diminished, the transferrin (and apotransferrin) content is increased, and iron absorption is accelerated.

The major pathway of iron metabolism (see Figure 30-4) is a virtually closed cycle in which iron passes from plasma transferrin to the RBC precursors in the bone marrow, where it is incorporated into hemoglobin; these cells then enter the circulation as mature RBCs, where they remain nearly 4 months before they become metabolically "worn out" and are engulfed by phagocytes; the iron is released from hemoglobin and returns to plasma transferrin, thus completing one cycle and beginning another. From this iron cycle, small quantities of iron are diverted for use in other iron compartments; a slow, continuous exchange also takes place between the storage and transport compartments.

Each day, approximately 1 to 2 mg of iron absorbed from the intestinal tract enters this cycle to compensate for the 1 to 2 mg of iron lost each day from the body. Most of the iron loss is due to minute quantities of iron present in epithelial cells and RBCs in urine and feces. With each menstrual cycle, women lose approximately 40 to 80 mL of blood, which is equivalent to 20 to 40 mg of iron. This loss must be made up by increased absorption of iron by the intestinal mucosa. Similarly, approximately 600 to 900 mg of iron is lost as a consequence of each pregnancy. Compensation for iron loss from pregnancy and menstruation often is difficult, particularly because many women consume iron-poor diets. Thus iron deficiency is very common in women, even women whose diets may seem adequate.

Disorders of Iron Metabolism

Iron deficiency and iron overload are the major disorders of iron metabolism. However, altered iron metabolism has been observed or shown to be related to a number of other diseases, including anemia, cardiovascular disease, chronic hepatitis, end-stage renal disease, HIV infection, and infection.

Iron deficiency

Iron deficiency is one of the most prevalent disorders of humans. It is particularly a disease of children, young women, and older people, but it occurs in individuals of all ages and social strata. Infants, children, and pregnant women have increased requirements for iron, and dietary deficiency of iron leads to iron deficiency. In women, iron deficiency occurs as a result of blood loss during their menstrual cycles. Chronic blood loss into the GI tract is the usual reason for iron deficiency in men.

Measurements of serum iron concentration and total iron binding capacity (TIBC) have been used widely as aids in the diagnosis of iron deficiency. However, assay of serum ferritin concentration is considered a much more sensitive and reliable means of demonstration of this disorder. Free erythrocyte protoporphyrin concentration is increased in individuals with iron deficiency or lead poisoning but within normal levels in those with thalassemia minor, a condition often confused with iron deficiency. Measurement of erythrocyte protoporphyrin is used as a diagnostic aid and performed rapidly on small samples of blood. The most reliable method for diagnosis of iron deficiency is cytochemical staining of bone marrow aspirate by the Prussian blue reaction, which demonstrates the presence or absence of hemosiderin. The cytochemical stain for hemosiderin is evaluated microscopically. An individual's diet history also is useful in screening for iron deficiency.

Iron overload

Hemosiderosis, hemochromatosis, and sideroblastic anemia are conditions associated with iron overload.

Hemosiderosis
Hemosiderosis is a term that has been used to imply iron overload without associated tissue injury.

Hemochromatosis
Hemochromatosis[4] implies iron overload with injury to involved organs, as manifested by cellular degeneration and fibrosis. In practice, however, hemochromatosis is a generic synonym for iron overload, regardless of the presence or absence of evidence of tissue injury. Iron overload most commonly results from chronic excessive absorption of iron from a normal diet. It is rarely the result of protracted ingestion of iron medication or inappropriate injections of iron. Chronic alcohol abuse once was thought to be a cause of iron overload; however, this concept now is considered inaccurate.

Hereditary hemochromatosis is the classic disorder of iron overload. It is due to an inborn error of iron absorption. Approximately 10% of whites of Northern European origin are carriers of a gene conferring susceptibility to hereditary hemochromatosis; between three and five people per thousand are homozygous, although only a portion of these individuals have the clinical features of severe hemochromatosis, such as diabetes mellitus, arthritis, cardiac arrhythmia or heart failure, hepatic cirrhosis, impotence, hypothyroidism, liver cancer, or hyperpigmentation.

Routine screening for hemochromatosis is indicated for all individuals 20 years of age and older except those with limited life expectancies from other serious lethal diseases or those of advanced age (for example, >80 years). Screening also is appropriate for all family members of individuals known to have hemochromatosis. Although several cases of hemochromatosis have been reported in children younger than 15 years of age, systematic screening of children for hemochromatosis does not seem warranted. For those individuals whose screening tests are negative, repeat screening at more often than at 5-year intervals does not seem warranted.

Sideroblastic anemia
Sideroblastic anemia is a group of iron-loading disorders of unknown cause. In a hereditary type of this disorder, deficiency of ALA synthase exists in RBCs. Iron accumulates in mitochondria because of this metabolic bottleneck.

Analytical Methodology

A number of methods are used to measure iron and related analytes. These include methods for serum iron, TIBC, transferrin saturation, and serum ferritin. In addition to these direct methods, hemoglobin, hematocrit, and RBC measurements are used as indirect screening tests for determination of iron deficiency.

Determination of serum iron, total iron binding capacity, and serum transferrin

Serum iron is measured with a variety of techniques, including photometry and atomic absorption spectrophotometry. Through modification of the serum iron method, TIBC and serum transferrin are determined.

Principle

Iron is released from transferrin through a decrease in the pH of the serum; it is reduced from Fe^{3+} to Fe^{2+} and then forms a complex with a chromogen. The resultant iron-chromogen complex has an extremely high absorptivity. Absorbance is proportional to iron concentration. Two chromogens that have been used widely for this purpose are bathophenanthroline and ferrozine (Figure 30-5).[16] Characteristics of these and of alternative chromogens are shown in Table 30-5.

Reference intervals for serum iron, by use of an International Council for Standardization in Haematology reference method, are 65 to 175 µg/dL (11.6 to 31.3 µmol/L) for men and 50 to 170 µg/dL (9.0 to 30.4 µmol/L) for women. Reference intervals for neonates and children are listed in Chapter 46. Because reference intervals for serum iron are very method dependent, a laboratory should define independently its own reference intervals.

The serum unsaturated iron binding capacity and TIBC are determined by addition of sufficient Fe^{3+} to saturate iron binding sites on transferrin. The excess Fe^{3+} is removed, for example, by adsorption with light magnesium carbonate ($MgCO_3$) powder, and the assay for iron content then is repeated. From this second measurement the TIBC is obtained.

Serum transferrin concentration is estimated from the TIBC through use of the following relationship:

$$\text{Serum transferrin} = 0.007 \times \text{TIBC } (\mu g/dL)$$

The relationship, however, is not entirely linear because a small portion of iron in serum is bound to other proteins. Therefore the calculated TIBC values are a few micromoles per liter higher than the amount of transferrin-bound iron. These small differences are of no practical consequence. Immunoassays are available for assay of serum transferrin concentration. Results of the immunological measurement of

Figure 30-5 Bathophenanthroline and ferrozine are two chromogens that have been used widely for iron assays. Each exhibits a marked color change when Fe^{2+} is chelated between the two nitrogens.

transferrin concentration correlate with those of the TIBC assay.

Transferrin saturation is calculated as follows:

$$\text{Transferrin saturation (\%)} = \frac{100 \times \text{serum iron}}{\text{TIBC}}$$

Comments and precautions

Except when atomic absorption spectroscopy is used, hemolysis has very little effect on the serum iron assay results. However, when serum specimens show marked hemolysis, a small amount of iron may be liberated from hemoglobin. Such sera should be rejected.

Many factors influence serum iron concentration and TIBC. Changes that may be observed in various physiological or pathological conditions are listed in Table 30-6. Day-to-day variation is quite marked in healthy individuals. A distinct diurnal variation results in serum iron concentrations being lower in the afternoon than in the morning and quite low in the evening (as low as 2 to 4 μmol/L [10 to 20 μg/dL] in healthy individuals). Because of the numerous causes of low serum iron concentration, results must be interpreted with caution. Furthermore, many individuals with iron deficiency have normal values for serum iron concentration and TIBC. Results exceeding 35 μmol/L (200 μg/dL) have been observed in women who are taking progesterone-related contraceptive medication or in instances when iron has contaminated the syringe or specimen container.

Because of the large quantities of iron in the environment, scrupulous care is necessary to ensure that glassware, water, and reagents do not become contaminated with iron.

Clinical significance

Serum iron concentration is decreased in many but not all individuals with iron deficiency anemia and those with chronic inflammatory disorders, such as acute infection, immunization, and myocardial infarction (see Table 30-6). Serum iron concentration diminishes markedly in individuals who are beginning to respond to specific hematinic therapy for anemias of other causes, such as treatment of pernicious

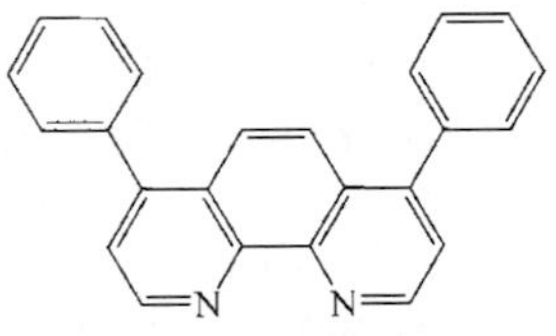

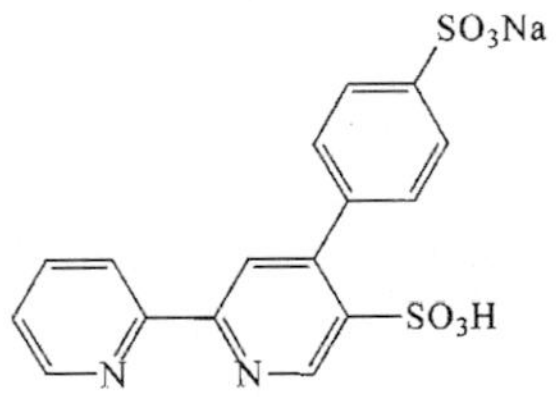

TABLE 30-5   Characteristics of Some Chromogens Used in Iron Assays

	Chromogen		
Common Name	Chemical Name	Absorptivity Maximum of Fe^{2+} Complex (nm)	Molar Absorptivity of Fe^{2+} Complex
Bathophenanthroline disulfonate, sodium	4,7-bis(4-phenyl sulfonic acid)-1,10-phenanthroline, disodium salt	534	22.14×10^3
Tripyridyl triazine	2,4,6-tripyridyl-s-triazine	593	22.6×10^3
Ferrozine	3-(2-pyridyl)-5,6-bis(4-phenyl sulfonic acid) 1,2,4 triazine, sodium salt	562	28.0×10^3
Terosite	2,6-bis(4-phenyl-2,2-pyridyl)-4-phenyl pyridine	583	30.2×10^3

Modified from Carter P: Spectrophotometric determination of serum iron at the submicrogram level with a new reagent [ferrozine]. Anal Biochem 1971; 40:450-458.

TABLE 30-6 Conditions Known to Affect Serum Iron Concentration, TIBC, and Transferrin Saturation

Condition	Effect
Diurnal variation	Normal values in morning; low values in midafternoon; very low values near midnight
Menstrual cycle	Premenstrually, elevated values (SI increased by 10% to 30%); at menstruation, low values (SI decreased by 10% to 30%)
Pregnancy	Possible elevation of SI because of increased progesterone; possible lowering of SI because of iron deficiency
Ingestion of iron (including iron-fortified vitamins)	High values; possible increase of SI by +54 μmol/L (+300 μg/dL) and Tsat to 100%
Oral contraceptives (progesterone-like)	High values; possible increase of SI to >36 μmol/L (>200 μg/dL) and Tsat to 75%; also elevation of TIBC
Iron contamination of syringe, Vacutainer tube, or other glassware (may be rare, sporadic, very difficult to prove phenomenon)	High values (SI >30 μmol/L [>170 μg/dL]); Tsat of 75% to 100%
Iron dextran injection	Very high values; possible SI of >180 μmol/L (>1000 μg/dL), Tsat 100%, probably from circulating iron dextran; effects possibly lasting for several weeks
Hepatitis	Very high values; possible SI of >180 μmol/L (>1000 μg/dL) because of hyperferritinemia from hepatocyte injury
Acute inflammation (respiratory infection), abscess, immunization, myocardial infarction	Low or normal SI; normal or low Tsat
Chronic inflammation or malignancy	Low or normal SI; normal or low Tsat
Iron deficiency	Low or normal SI; low or normal Tsat; increased TIBC
Iron overload (hemochromatosis)	High SI; high Tsat; normal or low TIBC

Modified from Fairbanks VF: Laboratory testing for iron status. Hosp Pract 1991; 26:19.
TIBC, Total iron binding capacity; *SI*, serum iron concentration; *Tsat*, transferrin saturation.

anemia with vitamin B_{12}. Acute or recent hemorrhage, including that due to blood donation, results in a low serum iron concentration. Serum iron concentration decreases during menstruation. Use of hormonal contraceptives raises serum iron concentration, but on cessation of contraceptive hormone intake, serum iron concentration decreases as much as 30% concurrent with uterine bleeding.

Greater-than-normal concentrations of serum iron occur in iron loading disorders such as hemochromatosis, in acute

iron poisoning in children, and after oral ingestion of iron medication or parenteral iron administration or acute hepatitis. For example, one 0.3-g tablet of ferrous sulfate ingested by an adult may raise the serum iron concentration by 50 to 90 μmol/L (300 to 500 μg/dL).

Because normally only about one third of the iron binding sites of transferrin are occupied by Fe^{3+}, serum transferrin has considerable reserve iron binding capacity. This capacity is called the *serum unsaturated iron binding capacity*. The TIBC is a measurement of the maximum concentration of iron that is bound by serum proteins, principally transferrin. The serum TIBC varies in disorders of iron metabolism. It often is increased in cases of iron deficiency and decreased in those of chronic inflammatory disorders or malignancies; in addition, it often is decreased in cases of hemochromatosis.

Measurement of serum iron, iron binding capacity, and transferrin saturation should not be used as a test for iron deficiency. The assays of serum iron, iron binding capacity, and percent transferrin saturation are useful only in screening for chronic iron overload diseases and for confirmation and monitoring of acute iron poisoning in children.

Determination of serum ferritin

Numerous methods exist to measure serum ferritin, including immunoradiometric assay, enzyme-linked immunosorbent assay (ELISA), and immunochemiluminescent and immuofluorometic methods. Reagents for this assay are available in kit form and in automated immunoassay instruments from several manufacturers. The reference intervals for serum ferritin are 20 to 250 ng/mL for men and 10 to 120 ng/mL for women. In cases of iron overload, serum ferritin levels are more than 400 ng/mL for men and 200 ng/mL for women. Because considerable variation in reference values has been observed with different methods for serum ferritin assay, each laboratory should determine its own reference intervals.

Comments and precautions

Replicate same-day assays on the same specimen each should have a CV of $\pm$4% for ferritin concentrations of 100 to 300 μg/L and $\pm$10% for ferritin concentrations of 10 to 20 μg/L.

Because precision decreases at very high serum ferritin concentration, all specimens with results exceeding 80 μg/L must be diluted with diluting sera to the 200- to 400-μg/L range and repeated in the next assay. Any specimen with greater than 7% difference between duplicate assay results should be reassayed.

Clinical significance

Plasma ferritin concentrations decline very early in the development of iron deficiency, long before changes are observed in blood hemoglobin concentration, RBC size, or serum iron concentration. Thus measurement of serum ferritin concentration serves as a very sensitive indicator of iron deficiency that is uncomplicated by other concurrent disease. Alternatively, a large number of chronic diseases result in increased serum ferritin concentration. These diseases include chronic infections; chronic inflammatory disorders, such as rheumatoid arthritis or renal disease; heart disease; and numerous malignancies, especially lymphomas, leukemias, breast cancer, and neuroblastoma. In individuals who demonstrate any of these chronic disorders together with iron deficiency, serum ferritin concentration often is within the reference interval. An increase in plasma ferritin concentration occurs in cases of viral hepatitis or after toxic liver injury as a result of release of ferritin from damaged liver cells. Plasma ferritin concentration also is increased in individuals with hemosiderosis or hemochromatosis. However, as a screening test for detection of early iron overload, measurement of serum ferritin concentration appears to be less sensitive than measurement of serum iron concentration, TIBC, and percent transferrin saturation.

■ BILIRUBIN

Bilirubin is the orange-yellow pigment derived from the catabolism of heme. The majority of bilirubin comes from senescent RBCs. It is extracted and biotransformed in the liver and excreted in bile and urine.

Chemistry

Protoporphyrin is a linear tetrapyrrolic molecule (Figure 30-6) that is insoluble in water and readily soluble in a variety of nonpolar solvents. X-ray crystallographic studies of crystalline bilirubin have confirmed both trans and cis isomers. When exposed to light, bilirubin in the trans configuration is converted to the cis conformation, which is more water soluble. In practice, this is the clinical justification for exposure of neonates who have clinically significant jaundice to light in order to reduce plasma **unconjugated bilirubin** concentrations.

The following four bilirubin fractions have been isolated from serum:

1. Unconjugated bilirubin (α-bilirubin)
2. Monoconjugated bilirubin (β-bilirubin)
3. Diconjugated bilirubin (γ-bilirubin)
4. A fraction irreversibly bound to protein (δ-bilirubin)

The δ-bilirubin fraction has been shown to react directly with diazotized sulfanilic acid. HPLC analyses of sera from individuals with various liver disorders revealed the following proportions of bilirubin in the four fractions

*   27% unconjugated bilirubin
*   24% monoconjugated bilirubin
*   13% diconjugated bilirubin
*   37% protein-bonded bilirubin

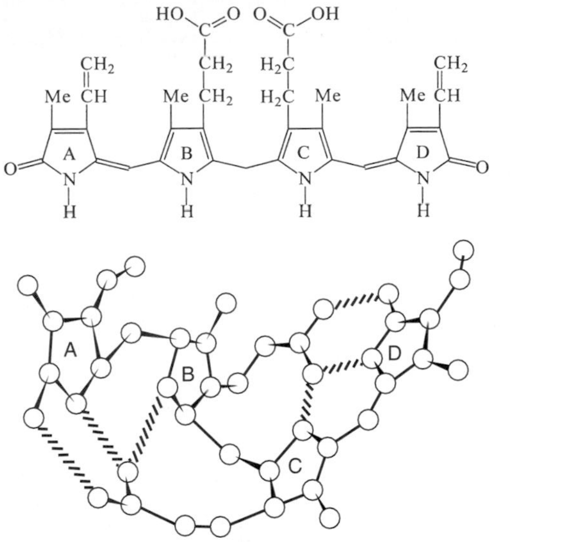

Figure 30-6   Bilirubin IXα structure. The unfolded or linear tetrapyrrole structure shows the Z bonds (*top*). The folded conformation shows extensive internal hydrogen bonding (*bottom*). (From Schmid R: Bilirubin metabolism: state of the art. Gastroenterology 1978; 74:1307-1312; and copyright 1978 by the American Gastroenterological Association.)

Biochemistry and Physiology

Bilirubin IXα is produced from protoporphyrin by microsomal heme oxygenase. The tetrapyrrolic product of the ring opening at the α-methene bridge is the green pigment biliverdin, which subsequently is hydrogenated to bilirubin by the NADPH-dependent, cytosolic enzyme biliverdin reductase (Figure 30-7). For each mole of heme catabolized by this pathway, 1 mole each of carbon monoxide, bilirubin, and Fe^{2+} is produced. Daily bilirubin production from all sources in the human averages 250 to 300 mg. Approximately 85% of the total bilirubin produced is derived from the heme moiety of hemoglobin released from aging erythrocytes that are destroyed in the reticuloendothelial cells of the liver, spleen, and bone marrow. The remaining 15% is produced from RBC precursors destroyed in the bone marrow (so-called ineffective erythropoiesis) and from the catabolism of other heme-containing proteins, such as myoglobin, cytochromes, and peroxidases.

Bilirubin is bound to albumin and transported to the liver. Bilirubin then dissociates from albumin at the sinusoidal membrane of the hepatocyte and is transported across the membrane (Figure 30-8). Once inside the liver cells, bilirubin is bound reversibly to soluble proteins known as *ligandins* or *protein Y*. Ligandins are cytosolic proteins of the glutathione-S-transferase gene family and constitute approximately 5% of the total protein of human liver cytosol. Ligandin also binds a variety of other compounds, such as steroids, bromsulfophthalein, indocyanine green, and some carcinogens.

Inside the hepatocytes, bilirubin is conjugated rapidly with glucuronic acid to produce bilirubin monoglucuronide and diglucuronide, which then are excreted into bile (see

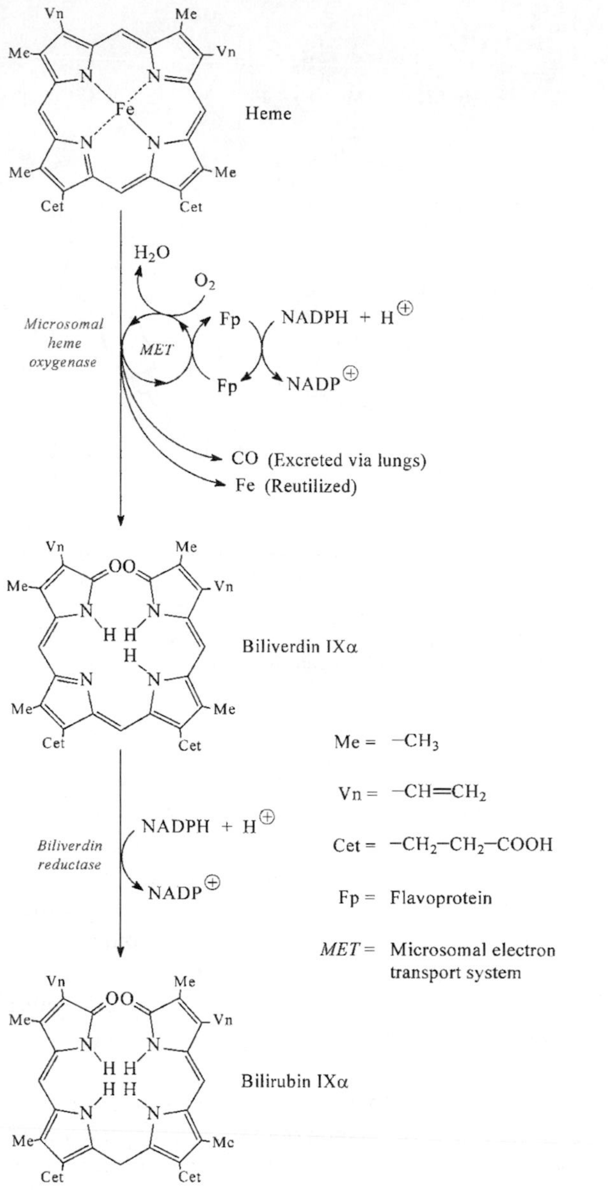

Figure 30-7   Catabolism of heme to bilirubin IXα. (From Berlin NI, Berk PD: Quantitative aspects of bilirubin metabolism for hematologists. Blood 1981; 57:983-999.)

Me = —CH₃ rendered as $Me = -CH_3$

$Me = -CH_3$

$Vn = -CH=CH_2$

$Cet = -CH_2-CH_2-COOH$

$Fp = $ Flavoprotein

$MET = $ Microsomal electron transport system

TABLE 30-7   Physiological Classification of Jaundice

Unconjugated Hyperbilirubinemia
INCREASED PRODUCTION OF UNCONJUGATED BILIRUBIN FROM HEME
Hemolysis
  Hereditary
  Acquired
Ineffective erythropoiesis
Rapid turnover of increased red blood cell mass (in the neonate)

DECREASED DELIVERY OF UNCONJUGATED BILIRUBIN (IN PLASMA) TO HEPATOCYTE
Right-sided congestive heart failure
Portacaval shunt

DECREASED UPTAKE OF UNCONJUGATED BILIRUBIN ACROSS HEPATOCYTE MEMBRANE
Competitive inhibition
  Drugs
  Others?
Gilbert's syndrome
Sepsis, fasting

DECREASED STORAGE OF UNCONJUGATED BILIRUBIN IN CYTOSOL (DECREASED Y AND Z PROTEINS)
Competitive inhibition
Fever

DECREASED BIOTRANSFORMATION (CONJUGATION)
Neonatal jaundice (physiological)
Inhibition (drugs)
Hereditary (Crigler-Najjar)
  Type I (complete enzyme deficiency)
  Type II (partial deficiency)
Hepatocellular dysfunction
Gilbert's syndrome?

Conjugated Hyperbilirubinemia (Cholestasis)
DECREASED SECRETION OF CONJUGATED BILIRUBIN INTO CANALICULI
Hepatocellular disease
  Hepatitis
  Cholestasis (intrahepatic)
Dubin-Johnson and Rotor syndromes
Drugs (estradiol)

DECREASED DRAINAGE
Extrahepatic obstruction
  Stones
  Carcinoma
  Stricture
  Atresia
Sclerosing cholangitis
Intrahepatic obstruction
  Drugs
  Granulomas
  Primary biliary cirrhosis
  Bile-duct paucity
  Tumors

Figure 30-8). The microsomal enzyme bilirubin UDP-glucuronyltransferase (EC 2.4.1.17) catalyzes the formation of bilirubin monoglucuronide. The excretion of **conjugated bilirubin** into bile against a marked concentration gradient is thought to be an energy-dependent, active-transport process.

In adults, approximately 95% of all bilirubin is excreted in bile in the form of glycuronide conjugates; glucosides and xylosides constitute the remainder. Of the glucuronides, di-glucuronide is the major fraction (~90%) and monoglucu-ronide the minor fraction (~10%).

Bilirubin glucuronides are not reabsorbed substantially in the intestine. Rather, they are hydrolyzed by the catalytic action of β-glucuronidase from the liver, intestinal epithelial

cells, and bacteria. This unconjugated bilirubin then is re-duced by anaerobic intestinal microbial flora to form a group of three colorless tetrapyrroles collectively called *urobilino-gens*. In each of these three bilirubin reduction products, all bridge carbons are in the saturated (methylene) form. The

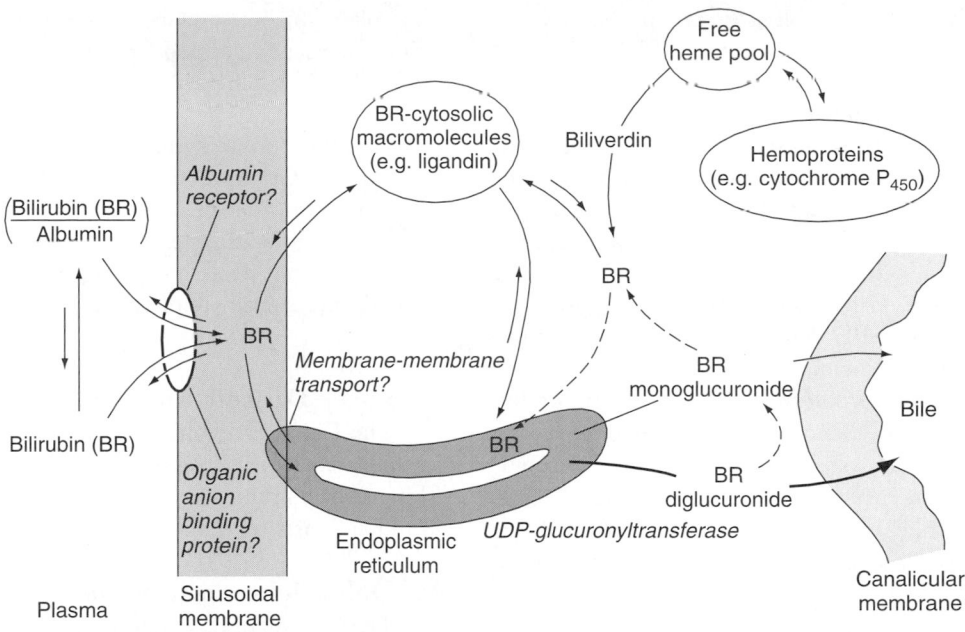

Figure 30-8 Bilirubin uptake, metabolism, and transport in the hepatocyte. (Modified from Gollan JL, Schmid R: Progress in Liver Diseases, vol 7, chapter 15, Philadelphia, WB Saunders, 1982.)

urobilinogens differ from one another in the degree of hydrogenation of the vinyl side chains, as well as in the two end pyrrole rings. Urobilinogens containing 6, 8, or 12 more hydrogen atoms than bilirubin are named *stercobilinogen, mesobilinogen,* and *urobilinogen,* respectively. Up to 20% of the urobilinogen produced daily is reabsorbed from the intestine and enters the enterohepatic circulation. Most of the reabsorbed urobilinogen is taken up by the liver and reexcreted in the bile; a small fraction (2% to 5%) enters the general circulation and appears in urine. In the lower intestinal tract the three urobilinogens spontaneously oxidize at the middle methylene bridge to produce the corresponding bile pigments stercobilin, mesobilin, and urobilin, which are orange-brown and the major pigments of stool. Approximately 50% of the conjugated bilirubin excreted in bile is metabolized to products other than the urobilinogens.

Disorders of Bilirubin Metabolism

Defects in bilirubin metabolism resulting in **jaundice** can occur at each step in the metabolic pathway (see Figure 30-7). The disorders are classified as (1) jaundice in the newborn and (2) inherited disorders of bilirubin metabolism. All these disorders are characterized by predominant elevations in either conjugated or unconjugated bilirubin in the absence of other abnormal liver tests. Only in these disorders is bilirubin fractionation clinically useful.

Jaundice in the neonate

Disorders that cause jaundice in the neonate are classified as either unconjugated or conjugated hyperbilirubinemia

(Table 30-7).[21] Thus fractionation of bilirubin in neonates is a useful diagnostic tool.

The significance of unconjugated **hyperbilirubinemia** is the potential for development of kernicterus, especially in low-birth-weight infants. **Kernicterus** is a necrotic syndrome that occurs from bilirubin neurotoxicity. Affected infants become lethargic, with gradual progression to opisthotonos with seizures. Nearly 70% of infected infants die within the first week, and the remaining have severe brain damage. This syndrome is prevented by phototherapy and exchange transfusion.

Unconjugated hyperbilirubinemia

Causes of unconjugated hyperbilirubinemia in the neonate are physiological jaundice of the newborn, hemolytic disease, and breast milk hyperbilirubinemia.

Physiological jaundice of the newborn. Infants frequently become jaundiced within a few days of birth. This condition is known as *physiological jaundice of the newborn,* and bilirubin levels reach a peak within 1 to 7 days of birth and last for approximately 2 weeks. Bilirubin is less than 5 mg/dL, with 90% unconjugated. Hyperbilirubinemia exceeding 5 mg/dL in the first day or 10 to 12 mg/dL later is pathological. Physiological jaundice generally is not harmful, but bilirubin levels above 10 mg/dL may be complicated by kernicterus. This situation is of special concern in the premature infant.

Physiological jaundice of the newborn is treated by phototherapy, in which the infant is exposed to light of approximately 450 nm. This light converts bilirubin to a stable, nontoxic isomer by uncoupling internal hydrogen bonding in the bilirubin molecule. Exchange transfusions rarely are necessary.

Hemolytic disease.   Hemolytic disease in the newborn results from maternal-fetal incompatibility of Rhesus blood factors, in which the maternal Rh-negative blood becomes sensitized by either a previous pregnancy with an Rh-positive baby or an Rh-positive blood transfusion. The infant becomes jaundiced with unconjugated bilirubin in the first 2 days of life and is susceptible to kernicterus. Diagnosis is confirmed by Coomb's test in the infant and confirmation of Rh-positive blood in the infant and Rh-negative blood in the mother. Other rare inherited hemolytic anemias, such as glucose-6-PD deficiency also may lead to unconjugated hyperbilirubinemia.

Breast-milk hyperbilirubinemia.   This type of hyperbilirubinemia affects about 30% of breast-fed newborns. It is due to β-glucuronidase in breast milk, which deconjugates bilirubin in the intestine. The deconjugated bilirubin, being more lipophilic, is absorbed passively. The condition lasts for a few weeks and is treated by discontinuation of breast feeding.

Conjugated hyperbilirubinemias

The conjugated hyperbilirubinemias are characterized by hyperbilirubinemia in which the conjugated bilirubin is more than 30% of the total. The most important are idiopathic neonatal hepatitis and biliary atresia. The diagnosis of the cholestatic syndromes is difficult.

Idiopathic neonatal hepatitis.   About 75% of cases of hepatitis in the neonate are idiopathic giant cell hepatitis, a disorder of unknown etiology characterized by cholestatic jaundice.

Biliary atresia.   This is a heterogeneous group of acquired disorders that involve either the extrahepatic or intrahepatic bile ducts. Possible etiologies include cytomegalovirus, Reovirus III, Epstein-Barr virus, rubella virus, α_1-antitrypsin deficiency, Down's syndrome, and trisomy 17 or 18.

Inherited disorders of bilirubin metabolism

Gilbert's syndrome

Gilbert's syndrome is a heterogeneous group of disorders characterized by increases of less than 3 mg/dL (51 μmol/L) in unconjugated bilirubin.[12] This benign condition occurs in approximately 2% of the population and probably is inherited in an autosomal recessive fashion.

Crigler-Najjar syndrome (type 1)

The type 1 Crigler-Najjar syndrome is a rare disorder caused by complete absence of uridine diphosphate (UDP) glucuronyl transferase and manifested by very high levels of unconjugated bilirubin (25 to 50 mg/dL). It is inherited as an autosomal recessive disorder. Most affected individuals die of severe brain damage caused by kernicterus (encephalopathy related to increased bilirubin that leads to permanent brain damage) within the first year of life. Phlebotomy

and plasmapheresis reduce the serum bilirubin, but encephalopathy usually develops. Early liver transplantation is the only effective therapy.

Crigler-Najjar syndrome (type 2)

Type 2 Crigler-Najjar syndrome is a rare autosomal dominant disorder characterized by a partial deficiency of UDP glucuronyl transferase. Unconjugated bilirubin is usually 5 to 20 mg/dL. Unlike Crigler-Najjar type 1, type 2 responds dramatically to phenobarbital, and a normal life then is expected.

Lucey-Driscoll syndrome

The Lucey-Driscoll syndrome is a familial form of unconjugated hyperbilirubinemia caused by a circulating inhibitor of bilirubin conjugation. The hyperbilirubinemia is mild and lasts for 2 to 3 weeks.

Dubin-Johnson syndrome

The Dubin-Johnson syndrome is a benign, autosomal recessive condition characterized by jaundice with predominantly elevated conjugated bilirubin and a minor elevation of unconjugated bilirubin.

Rotor syndrome

Rotor syndrome is another form of conjugated hyperbilirubinemia similar to the Dubin-Johnson syndrome. Total urinary coproporphyrins are elevated, with about two-thirds being coproporphyrin I. The prognosis is excellent.

Analytical Methodology

Several analytical techniques are used to measure bilirubin and metabolites in serum, urine, and feces.

Serum Bilirubin

Bilirubin and related compounds are measured in body fluids through use of a variety of chromatographic, capillary electrophoretic, and photometric methods. Reference intervals for bilirubin and related compounds are listed in Chapter 46.

The most widely used chemical methods for bilirubin measurement are those based on the diazo reaction, first described by Ehrlich in 1883. In this reaction, diazotized sulfanilic acid (the diazo reagent) reacts with bilirubin to produce two azodipyrroles (Figure 30-9), which are reddish purple at neutral pH and blue at low or high pH values. Subsequent laboratorians established that alcohol accelerates the diazotization reaction of unconjugated bilirubin. The fraction of bilirubin that reacted with the diazo reagent in the absence of alcohol was termed **direct bilirubin. Indirect bilirubin** is considered as the difference between total bilirubin (found after the addition of alcohol to the reaction mixture) and the direct bilirubin fraction. Later variations all have utilized one of a variety of "accelerators"

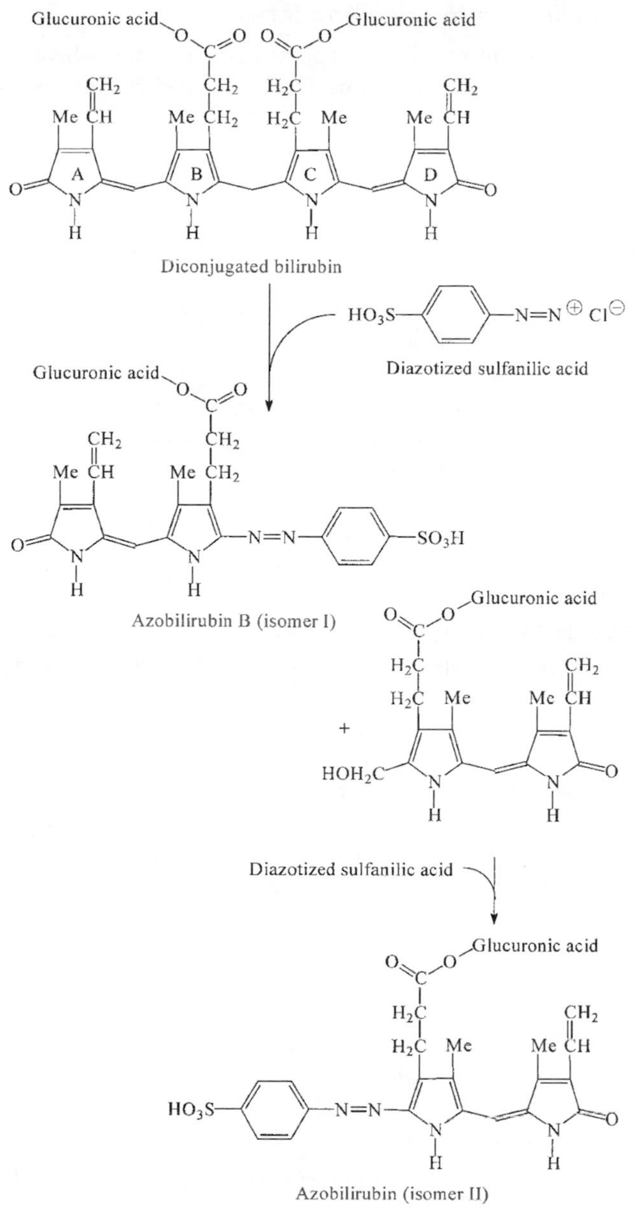

Figure 30-9 The reaction of bilirubin glucuronide with diazotized sulfanilic acid to produce isomers I and II of azobilirubin B. Unconjugated bilirubin reacts in the same way to produce isomers I and II of azobilirubin A. *Me,* –CH$_3$.

that facilitate the reaction of unconjugated (indirect) bilirubin with the diazo reagent.

In practice, direct-reacting bilirubin is considered primarily conjugated bilirubin and indirect bilirubin the unconjugated species, whereas total bilirubin consists of a mixture of the two. As discussed previously, at least four distinct bilirubin species exist in serum. Direct-reacting bilirubin consists of monoconjugated and diconjugated bilirubin (β- and γ-bilirubin) and the δ-fraction, which is bilirubin tightly bound to albumin. Unconjugated α-bilirubin, which is water insoluble and bound to albumin, reacts with the

diazo reagent only after the addition of an accelerator, such as alcohol or caffeine.

The diazo method of Malloy and Evelyn, which uses methanol as an accelerator, has substantial matrix effects, interference by hemoglobin, turbidity due to protein precipitation by methanol, and a relatively long reaction time. The diazo method described by Jendrassik and Gróf in 1938 and later modified by Doumas and colleagues[6,19] gives results for serum bilirubin that are as reliable as those produced by a reference HPLC method. In this procedure, total bilirubin in serum or plasma is measured through the addition of caffeine reagent (accelerator) to the specimen, followed by the addition of diazotized sulfanilic acid. During the incubation period, both conjugated and unconjugated bilirubin react with the diazo reagent to produce azobilirubin. Then, 10 minutes after the addition of diazotized sulfanilic acid, solutions of ascorbic acid, alkaline tartrate, and dilute hydrochloric acid are added to the reaction mixture. The absorbance of the resulting blue-green azobilirubin solution is measured at 600 nm.

To measure conjugated bilirubin the serum or plasma is acidified with dilute hydrochloric acid and then mixed with diazotized sulfanilic acid to produce azobilirubin. Only the conjugated forms of bilirubin react with the diazo reagent in the absence of the accelerator, caffeine-benzoate. The reaction is halted by the addition of an ascorbic-acid solution. Then, an alkaline tartrate solution is added to the reaction mixture, followed by the addition of an aliquot of the caffeine reagent. The latter shifts the absorbance peak of azobilirubin from 585 to 600 nm; at 600 nm the absorbance is measured. The tartrate reagent provides an alkaline pH to produce the blue and more intense color of azobilirubin.

In the conjugated bilirubin method, either serum or plasma is used as the specimen. A morning specimen from a fasting subject is preferred to avoid lipemia. Hemolysis should be avoided because it produces falsely low values with diazo methods. Because both conjugated and unconjugated bilirubin are photo-oxidized when exposed to white or ultraviolet light, specimens should be protected from direct exposure to either artificial light or sunlight as soon as they are drawn. The sensitivity to light is temperature dependent; for optimal stability, storage of specimens in the dark and at low temperatures is essential. When specimens are stored in the refrigerator, stability is maintained for 3 days. Specimens are stable for 3 months when stored frozen at −70 °C in the dark.

Bilirubin is determined in infants by direct spectrophotometry. When bilirubin is present in the sample, the absorbance at 454 nm is increased and is proportional to the concentration of bilirubin. Subtraction of the absorbance at 540 nm, if present in the sample, corrects for oxyhemoglobin. The serum of newborns does not contain carotene and other pigments that increase the absorbance at 454 nm. However, these pigments may be present in serum from older children and adults, and thus use of the direct spectrophotometric method should be restricted to newborns.

Urine bilirubin

Bilirubin also is present in urine. Because only conjugated bilirubin is excreted in urine, use of urine is an indirect test for increased concentrations of conjugated bilirubin in serum. The most popular method used to detect bilirubin in urine involves the use of a dipstick impregnated with a diazo reagent. Dipstick methods detect concentrations of 0.5 mg/dL or greater.

A fresh urine specimen is required because bilirubin is very unstable when exposed to light and room temperature. If the test must be delayed, the sample should be protected from light and stored in a refrigerator at 2 to 8 °C for no longer than 24 hours. The reagent strip (Chemstrip [Roche Diagnostic Systems, Inc., Branchburg, N.J.]) is inserted into the urine specimen for no longer than 1 second. After 60 seconds the bilirubin reacts with 2,6-dichlorobenzene-diazonium-tetrafluoroborate at an acidic pH. A pink to red-violet color is produced, the intensity of which is proportional to the bilirubin concentration. The reaction mechanism for urinary conjugated bilirubin is the same as that described in Figure 30-9 with diazotized sulfanilic acid, except that the diazo reagent is 2,6-dichlorobenzene-diazonium-tetrafluoroborate.

Urobilinogen in urine and feces

An increase in urobilinogen in the urine occurs whenever hepatocellular function is decreased or an excess of urobilinogen in the GI tract exceeds the liver's capacity to reexcrete it. Examples of such conditions are viral hepatitis, cirrhosis, and hemolysis (see Chapter 36). In contrast, when biliary excretion of bilirubin (for example, cholestasis) is impaired, urinary excretion of urobilinogen decreases due to the limited delivery of bilirubin to the gut and the low rate of urobilinogen production. The clay-colored or chalky-white stool of individuals with cholestatic jaundice results from decreased bilirubin reaching the GI tract and the subsequent low quantities of metabolites produced. These disturbances of urobilinogen excretion are the basis for the historical use of urobilinogen analysis in urine and feces as an index of liver disease.

Urobilinogen is measured in freshly collected urine by reaction with DMAB in concentrated hydrogen chloride (Ehrlich's reagent) to produce a red-colored product. To maintain urobilinogen in a reduced state and prevent reformation of urobilin, ascorbic acid is added as a reducing agent. Sodium acetate is added to reduce the acidity after reaction of the urobilinogen with Ehrlich's reagent The principle of the method for the determination of fecal urobilinogen is the same as that described for urinary urobilinogen, except that an aqueous extract of fresh feces first is treated with alkaline ferrous hydroxide (to reduce urobilin to urobilinogen) before Ehrlich's reagent is added.

References

1. Aisen P, Wessling-Resnick M, Leibold EA: Iron metabolism. Curr Opin Chem Biol 1999; 3:200-206.
2. Bonkovsky HL, Barnard GF: Diagnosis of porphyric syndromes: a practical approach in the era of molecular biology. Semin Liver Dis 1998; 18:57-65.
3. Braun J: Erythrocyte zinc protoporphyrin. Kidney Int Suppl 1999; 69:S57-60.
4. Camaschella C, Piperno A: Hereditary hemochromatosis: recent advances in molecular genetics and clinical management. Haematologica 1997; 82:77-84.
5. Chiang SC, Li SF: Separation of porphyrins by capillary electrophoresis in fused-silica and ethylene vinyl acetate copolymer capillaries with visible absorbance detection. Biomed Chromatogr 1997; 11:366-370.
6. Doumas BT, Perry BW, Sasse EA et al: Standardization in bilirubin assays: evaluation of selected methods and stability of bilirubin solutions. Clin Chem 1973; 19:984-993.
7. Elder GH, Smith SG, Smyth SJ: Laboratory investigation of the porphyrias. Ann Clin Biochem 1990; 27:395-412.
8. Enriquez de Salamanca R, Sepulveda P, Morgan MJ et al: Clinical utility of fluorometric scanning of plasma porphyrins for the diagnosis and typing of porphyrias. Clin Exp Dermatol 1993; 18:128-130.
9. Fodinger M, Sunder-Plassmann G: Inherited disorders of iron metabolism. Kidney Int Suppl 1999; 69:S22-34.
10. Hastka J, Lasserre JJ, Schwarzbeck A et al: Laboratory tests of iron status: correlation or common sense? Clin Chem 1996; 42:718-724.
11. Hindmarsh JT, Oliveras L, Greenway DC: Plasma porphyrins in the porphyrias. Clin Chem 1999; 45:1070-1076.
12. Iyanagi T, Emi Y, Ikushiro S: Biochemical and molecular aspects of genetic disorders of bilirubin metabolism. Biochem Biophys Acta 1998; 1407:173-184.
13. Kushner JP: Laboratory diagnosis of the porphyrias. N Engl J Med 1991; 324:1432-1434.
14. Labbe RF: Lead poisoning mechanisms. Clin Chem 1990; 36:1870-1871.
15. Murphy GM: The cutaneous porphyrias: a review. Br J Dermatol 1999; 140:573-581.
16. National Committee for Clinical Laboratory Standards: Determination of Serum Iron, Total Iron Binding Capacity and Percent Transferrin Saturation: Approved Standard (1998). NCCLS Document H17-A. Wayne, Pa, National Committee for Clinical Laboratory Standards, 1998.

17. National Committee for Clinical Laboratory Standards: Erythrocyte protoporphyrin testing: Approved Guideline. NCCLS document C42-A. Wayne, Pa, NCCLS, 1996.

18. Nordmann Y, Puy H, Deybach JC: The porphyrias. J Hepatol 1999; 30(Suppl 1):12-16.

19. Perry BW, Doumas BT, Bayse DD et al: A candidate reference method for determination of bilirubin in serum: test for transferability. Clin Chem 1983; 29:297-301.

20. Scarlett YV, Brenner DA: Porphyrias. J Clin Gastroenterol 1998; 27:192-198.

21. Schwoebel A, Sakraida S: Hyperbilirubinemia: new approaches to an old problem. J Perinat Neonatal Nurs 1997; 11:78-97.

22. Vandell VE, Limbach PA: Electrospray ionization mass spectrometry of metalloporphyrins. J Mass Spectrom 1998; 33:212-220.

Additional Reading

Bothwell TH, Charlton RW, Motulsky AG: Hemochromatosis. In Scriver CR, Beaudet AL, Sly WS et al (eds): The Metabolic and Molecular Bases of Inherited Disease, 7th edition, pp 2103-2159, New York, McGraw-Hill, 1995.

Chowdhury JR, Wolkoff AW, Chowdhury NR, Arias IM: Hereditary jaundice and disorders of bilirubin metabolism. In Scriver CR, Beaudet AL, Sly WS et al (eds): The Metabolic and Molecular Bases of Inherited Disease, 7th edition, pp 2161-2210, New York, McGraw-Hill, 1995.

Elder GH: Update on enzyme and molecular defects in porphyria. Photodermatol Photoimmunol Photomed 1998; 14:66-69.

Harthoorn-Lasthuizen EJ, Lindemans J, Langenhuijsen MM: Zinc protoporphyrin as screening test in female blood donors. Clin Chem 1998; 44:800-804.

Kappas A, Sassa S, Galbraith RA et al: The porphyrias. In Scriver CR, Beaudet AL, Sly WS et al (eds): The Metabolic and Molecular Bases of Inherited Disease, 7th edition, pp 2103-2159, New York, McGraw-Hill, 1995.

Zaider E, Bickers DR: Clinical laboratory methods for diagnosis of the porphyrias. Clin Dermatol 1998; 16:277-293.

CHAPTER 31

Therapeutic Drug Monitoring

THOMAS P. MOYER, PhD

Objectives

1. Define the following terms:

Therapeutic index	Pharmacokinetics
Mechanism of action	Dose-response
Peak and trough drug concentration	Drug half-life
Steady state	Bioavailability
Pharmacodynamics	First-pass metabolism

2. List and describe the five factors that affect the pharmacokinetics of drugs.
3. State the rationale for monitoring of therapeutic drug concentrations.
4. List the methods of analysis available for the assessment of therapeutic drug concentration.
5. List five antiepileptic drugs, their specific uses, their active metabolites (if applicable), and a proprietary name for each.
6. List five cardioactive drugs, their specific uses, their active metabolites (if applicable), and a proprietary name for each.
7. List five antidepressant drugs and state their modes of action.
8. State the clinical use of lithium.
9. State the clinical use of antineoplastic drugs, immunosuppressant drugs, and antibiotics and describe their modes of action.
10. Identify possible drug interactions when given appropriate information.

Key Words

Antiarrhythmic Agents   Agents used for the treatment or prevention of cardiac arrhythmias; often classed into four main groups according to their mechanism of action—sodium channel blocker, β-adrenergic blocker, repolarization prolongation, or calcium channel blocker

Antiepileptic   A substance used to prevent or alleviate convulsive seizures

Beta (β-) Adrenergic Agonists   Drugs that bind to and activate β-adrenergic receptors

Beta (β-) Blocker   A drug that induces adrenergic blockade at either β1- or β2-adrenergic receptors, or at both

Calcium Channel Blocker   One of a group of drugs that inhibit the entry of calcium into cells or the mobilization of calcium from intracellular stores, resulting in slowing of atrioventricular and sinoatrial conduction and relaxation of arterial smooth and cardiac muscle; used in the treatment of angina, cardiac arrhythmias, and hypertension

Dose-Response Relationship   The relationship between the dose of an administered drug and the response of the organism to the drug

Drug Half-Life   Time required for one-half an administered drug to be lost through metabolism and elimination

Drug Interactions   The action of one drug on another

Drug Monitoring   The process used to study the effects of a chemical substance administered to an individual

Enzyme Induction   Increased synthesis of an enzyme in response to an inducer or other stimulus

First-Pass Metabolism   Extensive metabolism of a drug with a high hepatic extraction rate by the liver before it reaches the systemic circulation

Gamma (γ-) Aminobutyric Acid (GABA)   An amino acid that inhibits neurotransmitter activity in the central nervous system

Generic Drug   A drug not protected by a trademark; also, the scientific name, as opposed to the proprietary, or brand, name

Immunosuppressant   An agent capable of suppressing immune responses

Pharmacodynamics   The study of the biochemical and physiological effects of drugs and the mechanisms of their actions, including the correlation of actions and effects of drugs with their chemical structures; also, such effects on the actions of a particular drug or drugs

Pharmacokinetics   The activity or fate of drugs in the body over a period of time, including the processes of absorption, distribution, localization in tissues, biotransformation, and excretion

Xenobiotics   A chemical substance foreign to the biological system

---

Therapeutic drug monitoring (TDM) is an important function of a modern clinical laboratory.[2,3,7,11] The rapid development of TDM has evolved from a conjunction of several events that occurred in the 1960s to 1970s, including the following:

1. Development of drugs with significant therapeutic efficacy but narrow therapeutic index
2. Development of analytical technologies that were accurate, precise, sensitive, and specific for measurement of drugs in biological fluids
3. Use of computers with pharmacokinetic data analysis to predict dose regimen design

When used correctly, TDM improves drug therapy. If used incorrectly, it increases the cost of laboratory operations and ultimately the cost of care without improving that care. To be effective, TDM requires the acquisition of a valid specimen, timely and reliable determination of the drug concentration in the specimen, and interpretation of results in the context of dose, time of last dose, and other drugs present. Results should be reported or collated with the dosing schedule so that they may be interpreted in a pharmacokinetic context.

Clinical pharmacokinetics is the study of the action of drugs in the body over a period of time, including the processes of absorption, distribution, localization in tissues, biotransformation, and excretion. It applies mathematical relationships to drug measurement. These mathematical relationships are used to predict dosage adjustments in either amount or dosing interval to attain an optimal response to the drug as quickly as possible. Therefore laboratorians must understand not only how to measure drugs in biological specimens but also how to use the results to achieve effective therapy.

TDM calls for a multidisciplinary approach because it relies on cooperative efforts of the physician, nurse, pharmacologist, pharmacist, and laboratorian. This chapter focuses on the laboratory's role in this discipline. Excellent descriptions of the roles of the physician and consulting pharmacologist are presented in the textbooks listed in the Additional Reading section at the end of this chapter.

■ BASIC CONCEPTS AND DEFINITIONS

The pharmacologic effect of a drug is elicited by direct interaction of the drug with a receptor controlling a specific function or by a drug-mediated alteration of the physiological process regulating the function. For most drugs the intensity and duration of the observed pharmacologic effect are proportional to the concentration of the drug at the receptor. In a given tissue the site at which a drug acts to initiate events leading to a specific biological effect is called the *site of action* of the drug.

Mechanism of Action

The mechanism of action of a drug is the biochemical or physical process occurring at the site of action to produce the pharmacologic effect. Drug action usually is mediated through a receptor. Cellular enzymes, as well as structural or transport proteins, are important examples of drug receptors. Nonprotein macromolecules also may bind drugs, resulting in altered cellular functions controlled by membrane permeability or DNA transcription. Some drugs are chemically similar to important natural endogenous substances and may compete for binding sites. In addition, some drugs may block formation, release, uptake, or transport of essential substances. Others may produce effects by interacting with relatively small molecules to form complexes that actively bind to receptors.

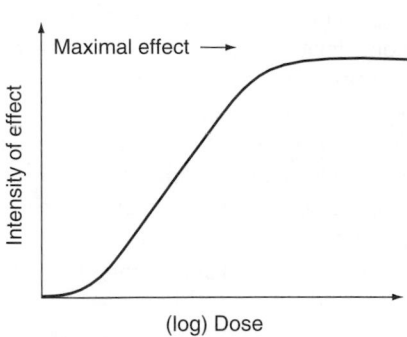

Figure 31-1   The log dose-effect relationship. The plateau (maximum effect) likely is due to saturation at the receptor.

Although the exact molecular interactions that describe the mechanism of action remain obscure for many drugs, theoretical models have been developed to explain them. One concept postulates that a drug binds to intracellular macromolecular receptors through ionic and hydrogen bonds and van der Waals forces. This theoretical model further postulates that if the drug-receptor complex is sufficiently stable and able to modify the target system, an observable pharmacologic response will occur. As Figure 31-1 illustrates, the response is dose dependent until a maximal effect is reached. The plateau in response may be due to saturation at the receptor or overload of a transport process.

The utility of drug concentration monitoring is based on the premise that a pharmacologic response correlates with the concentration of the drug at the site of action (receptor). Measurement of the concentration at the receptor site in a patient is technically impractical, if not impossible. However, studies have shown that for many drugs, a strong **dose-response relationship** exists among the serum drug concentration, concentration at the receptor, and observed pharmacologic effect.

In practice, changes in blood or serum drug concentration versus time are assumed to mirror changes in local concentrations at the receptor site or in body tissues. This assumption is sometimes called the *property of kinetic homogeneity* and is applicable to all pharmacokinetic models in postabsorptive and postdistributive phases of the time course.

The property of kinetic homogeneity is an important assumption in TDM because it is the basis on which all therapeutic and toxic concentration ranges are established. Measurable concentration ranges collectively define a therapeutic range, which, as illustrated in Figure 31-2, represents the relationship between minimum effective concentration (MEC) and minimum toxic concentration (MTC). In the optimal dosing cycle the trough blood concentration (the lowest concentration achieved immediately before the next dose) should not fall below the MEC, and the peak

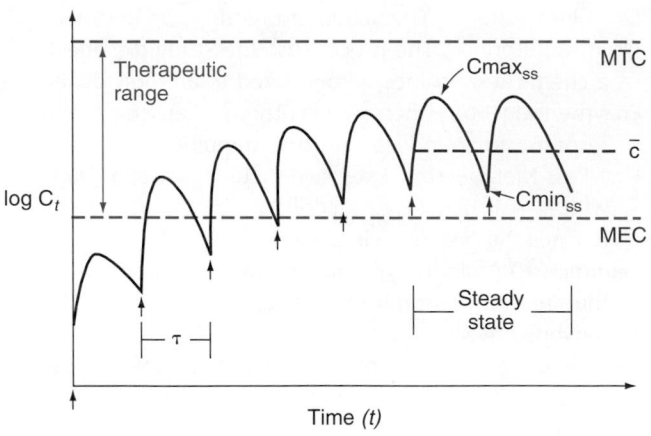

Figure 31-2   The drug concentration changes with multiple identical doses. Note that steady-state, peak and trough concentrations lie below the MTC and above the MEC; these limits often are referred to as the *therapeutic range*. Also note that five to seven half-lives passed to reach steady state. $Cmax_{ss}$ and $Cmin_{ss}$, Maximum and minimum steady-state concentrations; $\bar{C}$, average steady-state concentration; t, dosing interval; τ, dose; *MTC*, minimum toxic concentration; *MEC*, minimum effective concentration. (Modified from Gilman AG, Goodman L, Gilman A (eds): The Pharmacologic Basis of Therapeutics, 6th edition, New York, Macmillan, 1980.)

blood concentration (the highest concentration achieved within the dosing cycle) should not rise higher than the MTC. Such a cycle usually is achieved by administration of the drug once every half-life (see Figure 31-2).

Multiple dosing regimens should achieve steady-state serum drug concentrations consistently within the therapeutic range (greater than the MEC and less than the MTC). Steady state is the point at which the body concentration of the drug is in equilibrium with the rate of the dose administered and the rate of elimination. Blood concentrations greater than the MTC put patients at risk for toxicity; concentrations less than the MEC put them at risk for treatment failure. MTC and MEC are useful guidelines in therapy; these concepts are incorporated into tables presented later in this chapter that summarize specific drug data. Doses must be planned to achieve therapeutic concentrations, and these drug concentrations must be monitored to guide adjustment of the dose, if necessary. The smaller the difference between the MEC and MTC, the smaller is the therapeutic index and the more likely TDM will be necessary. The key concept to remember is that the MEC and MTC define the therapeutic range for most drugs.

Definitions

Drug monitoring is the process by which the concentration of a chemical substance administered to an individual therapeutically or diagnostically is observed, recorded, or detected. **Drug half-life** ($t_{1/2}$) is the time required for the amount of drug in the blood to decline to one-half a measured value. *Pharmacology* comprises that body of knowledge

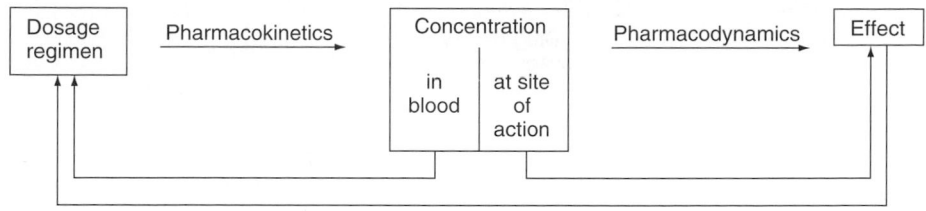

Figure 31-3 Conceptual relationship between pharmacodynamics and pharmacokinetics.

describing the effects of drugs useful in the prevention, diagnosis, and treatment of disease. *Pharmacotherapeutics* is that part of pharmacology concerned primarily with the application or administration of drugs to patients for the purpose of prevention and treatment of disease. For this aspect of medical practice to be effective, the pharmacodynamic and pharmacokinetic properties of drugs should be understood.

Pharmacodynamics encompasses the processes of interaction of pharmacologically active substances with target sites, and the biochemical and physiological consequences leading to therapeutic or adverse effects. For many drugs the ultimate effect or mechanism of action at the molecular level is understood poorly, if at all. However, effects at the cellular or organ system level or in the whole body are relatively well understood and usually related to dose of the drug.

Pharmacokinetics describes the processes of the uptake of drugs by the body, the biotransformations they undergo, the distribution of the drugs and their metabolites in tissues, and the elimination of drugs and their metabolites from the body. Clinical pharmacokinetics is the discipline that applies the principles of pharmacokinetics to safe and effective therapeutic management of individual patients. It strongly influences the interpretation of TDM results.

Figure 31-3 illustrates the conceptual relationship between pharmacodynamics and pharmacokinetics. Pharmacodynamics relates drug concentration at the site of action to the observed magnitude of the effect. Pharmacokinetics relates dose, dosing interval, and route of administration (regimen) to drug concentration in the blood. Figure 31-4 depicts the many factors affecting drug concentration and pharmacologic response.

In pharmacokinetics, mathematical approaches are used to predict or describe certain events, usually for calculation of a dosing regimen or prediction of the serum drug concentration after a given drug dose. The mathematical tools most often used in clinical pharmacokinetics are compartmental models and model-independent relationships.

Compartmental models are defined by the blood drug concentration and time data. The vascular fluid compartment (blood) usually is the anatomical reference compartment. The advantage of vascular fluid as the reference compartment is the ease with which it may be sampled to provide a definitive profile of blood concentration of drug versus time. The actual number of compartments are extensive but have no true anatomical reality. However, for the sake of simplicity, one- or two-compartment models are used most often.[9]

Drug Disposition

A large number of factors influence the pharmacokinetics of drugs and a patient's pharmacologic response and disposition of drugs (Table 31-1). Some important factors include the manner in which a drug is absorbed, distributed, metabolized, cleared by the liver, biotransformed, and excreted.

Absorption

Most drugs administered chronically to patients are administered extravascularly. Although intravenous, intramuscular, and subcutaneous routes are used, the oral route accounts for most of the extravascular doses administered. The absorption process depends on the drug's dissociating from its dosing form, dissolving in gastrointestinal (GI) fluids, and then diffusing across biological membrane barriers into the bloodstream. The rate and extent of drug absorption may vary considerably, depending on the nature of the drug itself on the matrix in which it is present and the physiological environment.

The fraction of a drug that is absorbed into the systemic circulation is referred to as its *bioavailability*. The bioavailability *(f)* of a given drug usually is calculated by comparison, in the same subjects, of the area under the plasma concentration-time curve (AUC) of an equivalent dose of the intravenous form (IV) and oral form (ORAL).

$$f = \frac{AUC_{ORAL}}{AUC_{IV}}$$

The bioavailability of a particular useful drug must be great enough so that the active component passes in sufficient amount and in a desirable time from the gut into the systemic circulation. Bioavailability typically must be greater than 70% for drugs to be orally useful. An exception would be a case in which the lumen of the GI tract is the site of drug action (for example, antibiotics used to sterilize the gut). Low bioavailability then would be considered advantageous.

Some drugs that are absorbed rapidly and completely nevertheless have low bioavailability to the systemic circulation. This low bioavailability is true of drugs with high hepatic extraction rates. After oral administration, drugs that are absorbed in the lumen of the small intestine are carried by the portal vein directly to the liver. A drug with a high

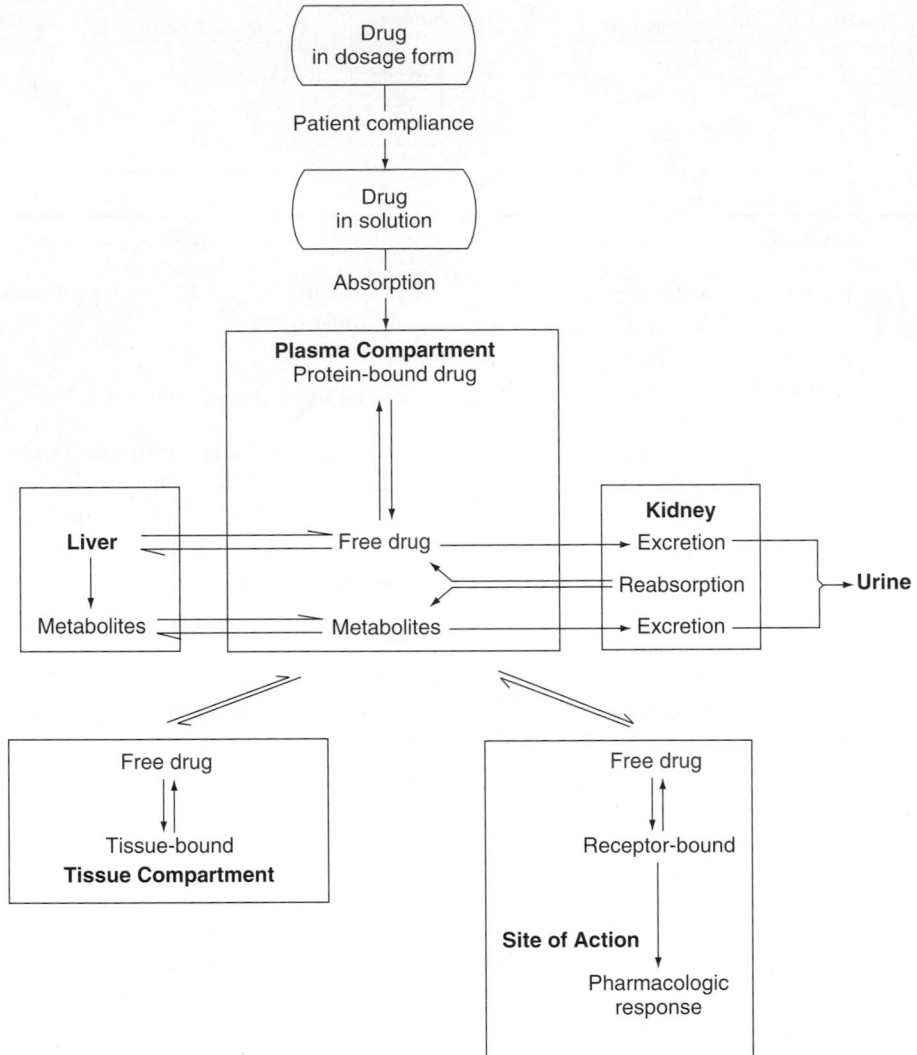

Figure 31-4 Factors affecting plasma drug concentration. *Absorption:* Drug must be formulated to ensure bioavailability for absorption from the GI tract or other administration site. *Metabolism:* Drug is converted to a more soluble compound (metabolite) that may be pharmacologically active or inactive. Metabolism may occur in tissues other than the liver. *Excretion:* The more water-soluble drugs and their metabolites usually are excreted in urine. Excretion also may occur via bile, feces, saliva, and expired air. *Tissue storage:* The drug may be stored in tissues that exhibit no pharmacologic response to it; side effects may occur from drug interaction with a specific physiological system. *Site of action:* Free drug binds to the receptor and produces pharmacologic response. The number and type of receptors to which the drug is bound determine the intensity and duration of the observed response. (Modified from Pippenger CE: TDM: Principles of drug utilization. Syva Monitor, November, 1978; 1,3-5. [pamphlet by Syva Corp., San Jose, Calif.])

hepatic extraction rate may be metabolized extensively by the liver before it reaches the systemic circulation. This phenomenon is called **first-pass metabolism** or *effect.*

In addition to the extent of absorption, the rate of absorption is important. To minimize this effect the pharmaceutical industry has decreased the apparent rate of absorption of many drugs by manipulating their formulations to produce "slow-" or sustained-release products. Formulations that provide sustained release permit drugs taken orally to be taken at less frequent intervals. Conditions that may influence the extent or rate of drug absorption include abnormal GI motility, diseases of the stomach and of the small and large intestine, GI infections, radiation, food, and interac-

tion with other substances in the GI tract. In addition, drug absorption also is affected by coadministered drugs that directly affect gut absorption, such as antacids, kaolin, sucralfate, cholestyramine, opiates, and antiulcer medications.

Distribution

After entering the vascular compartment, a drug interacts with various blood constituents and is carried by various transport processes to different body organs and tissues. The overall process is referred to as *distribution.* The factors determining the distribution pattern of a drug are (1) binding of the drug to circulating blood components, (2) binding to fixed receptors, (3) passage of the drug through membrane

TABLE 31-1   Factors that Influence Drug Disposition in Humans

Demographic Factors

Age category (premature infant, neonate, infant, prepubescent and postpubescent child, adult, elderly adult)
Weight
Sex
Race
Genetic constitution

Disease-Related Factors

Liver disease (cirrhosis, hepatitis, cholestasis)
Kidney disease
Thyroid disorders (hypothyroidism or hyperthyroidism)
Cardiovascular disease (arrhythmias, congestive heart failure)
Gastrointestinal disease or disorder (sprue or other malabsorption syndromes, peptic ulcer, colitis)
Cancer
Surgery
Burns
Nutritional status (cachectic or anorexic states)

Extracorporeal Factors

Hemodialysis
Peritoneal dialysis
Cardiopulmonary bypass
Hypothermia or hyperthermia

Chemical and Environmental Factors Influencing Drug Properties

ABSORPTION OF DRUG

Food or coadministered drug affecting extent and rate of absorption

DISTRIBUTION OF DRUG

Coadministered drug affecting binding to plasma proteins or tissue receptors

METABOLISM OF DRUG

Food intake (carbohydrates, proteins, lipids) competing for metabolizing systems
Coadministration of drug that induces metabolizing enzymes (for example, phenobarbital)
Coadministration of drug that inhibits metabolizing enzymes (for example, cimetidine)

EXCRETION OF DRUG

Coadministration of drug that competes for renal tubular secretory paths (for example, probenecid or penicillin)
Changes in urinary flow rate
Coadministration of compounds that enhance tubular reabsorption (for example, sodium bicarbonate or phenobarbital)

barriers, and (4) the ability to dissolve in structural or storage lipids. Molecular weight, pK_a, lipid solubility, and other physical and chemical properties of the drug are important determinants of distribution.

Once a drug enters the systemic circulation, it distributes and equilibrates with many blood components, such as plasma proteins. An equilibrium then exists between free and protein-bound drug, with the free fraction being available for distribution and elimination. In addition, only the free drug is available to cross cellular membranes or interact with the drug receptor to elicit a biological response. Therefore changes in the protein-binding characteristics of a drug have a profound influence on the distribution and elimination of the drug and interpretation of its steady-state concentrations. Each drug has its own characteristic protein-binding pattern that depends on its physical and chemical properties. As a general rule, however, acidic drugs are bound primarily to albumin, and basic drugs primarily to globulins, particularly α_1-acid glycoprotein (AAG). Some drugs bind to both albumin and globulins.

Depending on its affinity, a drug is bound either tightly or loosely to plasma proteins. A weakly bound drug is displaced from its protein sites by a drug with a greater affinity for the same plasma protein-binding sites. For example, phenytoin and valproic acid compete with each other as they bind to albumin. Because valproate is present at a higher concentration, its mass causes a significant shift of phenytoin from bound to free form. Protein binding of a drug also depends on the physical characteristics of the plasma proteins and the presence or absence of fatty acids or other drugs in the blood. Free fatty acids also displace a drug from its protein-binding sites. Thus even though the total drug concentration may remain unchanged, displacement of a drug from its plasma protein-binding sites elevates free drug concentrations and results in clinical toxicity. In addition, because the free fraction is the form that crosses biological membranes and is available to bind to the receptor, increasing the free fraction produces significant toxicity.

Anything that alters the concentration of free drug in the plasma ultimately alters the amount of drug available to enter the tissues and interact with specific receptor systems. For example, some disease states, such as uremia, alter free-drug concentrations. In individuals with uremia the composition of plasma is altered by an increase in nonprotein nitrogen compounds, by acid-base and electrolyte imbalances, and often by a decrease in albumin. Under these conditions, free-drug concentrations frequently are elevated. Patients may experience adverse effects that are a direct consequence of the increased free-drug concentrations. If the total plasma drug concentration is monitored in these patients, no change is noted because the total concentration remains unchanged and may not be dramatically different from that observed in healthy individuals. For example, phenytoin is 90% bound and 10% free in healthy subjects. In uremic individuals, 20% to 30% of the total plasma concentration of phenytoin may be free. If a healthy individual has a total plasma phenytoin concentration of 15 μg/mL, the free phenytoin concentration is likely to be 1.5 μg/mL. If a uremic individual has a total concentration of 15 μg/mL, the free drug concentration may be 4.5 μg/mL. A free phenytoin concentration of 4.5 μg/mL is sufficient to precipitate severe phenytoin side effects. Consequently, in uremic individuals, quantification of free phenytoin concentrations and adjustment of the drug dose are advisable to maintain free phenytoin concentration at approximately 2.0 μg/mL.

Alteration of protein concentration in response to acute stress also alters free-drug concentration. For example, after myocardial infarction, an individual's AAG concentration rises rapidly. Lidocaine is the drug of choice for control of arrhythmias caused by the infarction, but lidocaine is a basic drug that is bound to AAG. Doses of lidocaine adequate to control arrhythmia immediately after infarction are likely to become ineffective 48 to 72 hours later because the higher concentration of AAG that occurs after infarction diminishes the amount of free drug available to tissue. The arrhythmia reappears and because the total lidocaine plasma concentration necessary to control the arrhythmia appears to be in the toxic range, the lidocaine dose is decreased when it should be increased to maintain the optimal free concentration.

Some drugs exhibit saturation of the available plasma protein-binding sites at optimal total drug concentrations. For example, disopyramide binding is concentration dependent and varies widely from patient to patient. Consequently, its total concentration and the observed clinical responses vary markedly from patient to patient. Valproic acid is also a drug that shows saturation at concentrations greater than 100 μg/mL. Thus an increase of total plasma valproate concentration from 100 to 125 μg/mL represents a significant increase in the free valproate concentration.

Changes in normal physiological status also can alter free-drug concentrations and thus change the distribution of drugs between plasma and tissue. For example, geriatric patients often exhibit hypoalbuminemia with a marked decrease in protein-binding sites for drugs and thus an increase in the concentration of free drugs. This occurrence may lead to drug intoxication in elderly individuals that manifests as impaired cognitive function—particularly confusion. Thus an elderly patient may be considered senile when in reality an increased free drug concentration is affecting the individual's cognitive ability. Reduction of drug dose to decrease the free-drug concentrations often results in dramatic improvements in these patients' personalities.

Estimation of the free-drug concentration continues to be of interest to TDM through use of techniques such as ultrafiltration. However, a point to remember is that laboratory measurements now only *estimate* the free drug concentration in circulating blood. Artifacts introduced in drawing, processing, and storing of blood can modify dissociation equilibria for some drugs. Despite these drawbacks, free-drug estimations by ultrafiltration are superior to estimations of free-drug concentration based on measurements in saliva. Few drugs show a strong correlation between salivary concentration and free-drug concentration in plasma. In addition, collection of saliva from acutely ill patients is difficult.

Biotransformation

The liver is the principal organ responsible for drug metabolism (see Chapter 36). It does so by converting the lipophilic nonpolar drugs to more polar, water-soluble forms using either phase I or phase II reactions. Phase I reactions modify chemical structure by oxidation, reduction, or hydrolysis. Phase II reactions conjugate the drug (glucuronidation or sulfation) to water-soluble forms. These reactions take place in the microsomal fraction of the hepatocytes, where many environmental chemicals and endogenous biochemicals **(xenobiotics)** also are processed, and by the same mechanisms.

Synthesis and secretion of the enzymes of the hepatic microsomal system are increased by a process known as **enzyme induction.** In this process the production of hepatic enzymes is increased in response to an environmental signal, such as a drug. Specifically, the enzymes of the cytochrome P_{450} system are responsible for metabolism of drugs and induced by the presence of drugs in the liver. However, the isoenzymes of this system are affected variably by different enzyme-inducing drugs. For example, phenobarbital and polycyclic hydrocarbons induce different enzymes of the cytochrome P_{450} system.

Phenobarbital represents a type of enzyme inducer with broad induction effects. After a latency period, production of cytochrome P_{450}, cytochrome P_{450} reductase, and related enzymes is increased. In addition, liver weight, hepatic blood flow, bile flow, and production of hepatic proteins also increase. This enzyme subsystem is referred to as *cytochrome P_{450}-2D6.* Phenobarbital induction has little effect on theophylline clearance, suggesting a different isoenzyme for theophylline metabolism.

Polycyclic hydrocarbons found in tobacco smoke (3-methylcholanthrene) are a second type of enzyme inducer with broad induction effects. They induce cytochrome P_{450}-1A, in which no change in P_{450} reductase occurs, and a different terminal oxidase appears. After this type of induction the clearance of theophylline, but not of antipyrine, is increased. These substances have served as prototypes for the classification of enzyme inducers. Obviously, when a patient is receiving a drug with a narrow therapeutic index, the dosing regimen should be adjusted if a known enzyme-inducing drug is added to or deleted from therapy.

The drug-metabolizing enzymes of the liver are nonspecific and interact with a wide variety of endogenous and exogenous substances, so the presence of one drug inhibits the metabolism of a second drug that is coadministered. Mechanisms proposed to describe this inhibition include substrate competition, competitive or noncompetitive inhibition, product inhibition, and repression (in which the amount of enzyme is reduced by either decreased synthesis or increased degradation). Examples of such inhibition include the inhibition of (1) warfarin by chloramphenicol, resulting in excess bleeding, (2) theophylline metabolism by cimetidine and erythromycin, causing theophylline toxicity, and (3) cyclosporine metabolism by erythromycin and itraconazole, resulting in renal toxicity. As with enzyme inducers, the addition or deletion of an inhibitory drug in a patient's drug therapy requires appropriate TDM and dose adjustment of the affected drug. TDM allows these processes to be monitored and dosing adjusted accordingly.

The role of TDM becomes particularly apparent for drugs that undergo hepatic metabolism. Wide variability in the rate of metabolism of any given drug exists not only in different individuals in the general population but also in the same individual at different times and in different circumstances. This variability is due to factors such as age, weight, sex, genetics, exposure to environmental substances, diet, coadministered drugs, and disease. Furthermore, no biochemical marker is available to assess routinely an individual's hepatic function and drug clearance before drug therapy is initiated.

The biotransformation of drugs may produce metabolites that are pharmacologically active. In such instances the metabolite also should be measured because it contributes to the effect of the drug on the patient. Primidone and procainamide are examples of such drugs. If the metabolite is inactive, it need not be measured, but steps should be taken to ensure that it does not interfere with the analytical process.

Excretion

Excretion of drugs or chemicals from the body occurs through biliary, intestinal, pulmonary, or renal routes. Although each route represents a possible mechanism of drug elimination, renal excretion is a major pathway for the elimination of most water-soluble drugs or metabolites and is important in TDM. In addition, alterations in renal function may have a profound effect on the clearance and apparent half-life of the parent compound or its active metabolite(s). Thus decreased renal function causes elevated serum drug concentrations and increases the pharmacologic response.

Kidney function, in contrast to liver function, is evaluated readily and reliably by estimation of creatinine clearance (see also Chapter 34). Renal clearance of creatinine at 120 mL/minute approximates the glomerular filtration rate of 90 to 130 mL/minute. Therefore routine measurement of creatinine clearance provides an effective tool to evaluate kidney function. A strong correlation has been demonstrated between creatinine clearance and the total body clearance or elimination rate constant of those drugs primarily dependent on the kidneys for their elimination. Examples of drugs with which therapeutic use is adjusted to account for changes in creatinine clearance include gentamicin, tobramycin, amikacin, digoxin, vancomycin, and cyclosporine.

Clinical Utility

TDM has been proven clinically useful to both the clinician and patient and is most valuable when the drug in question is used chronically and has a narrow therapeutic index. Features of its clinical utility include the following:

1. *Recognition of noncompliance* Many patients, especially those with chronic disease, require prolonged drug therapy. The problem of noncompliance is particularly evident with patients who are characteristically free of pain or unusual discomfort, as with epilepsy, asthma, hypertension, mild heart disease, and transplantation. Patients may develop a sense that their disease has been cured and they no longer need the drug. The end result of noncompliance is treatment failure and an exacerbation of the existing disorder. Drug concentration values provide positive feedback to physicians regarding the compliant and noncompliant patients.

2. *Recognition when patients undergo changes in drug disposition characteristics* Occasionally, the disposition pattern of drugs in particular individuals may change from the average patient population parameters. Aberrant disposition may be attributed to an effect of a drug or disease state not recognized previously. The clinical condition and individual metabolism of patients may not only differ from one individual to another but may change in the same patient during treatment. Both the pharmacokinetic disposition and pharmacodynamic response to a given drug dose in individual patients may vary widely as a direct consequence of genetic influences. Studies of these genetic factors (pharmacogenetics) have demonstrated clearly that all aspects of pharmacokinetics and pharmacodynamics are under genetic control. One frequent example of such a change can be seen when adolescents progress through puberty; most drug disposition parameters change, requiring frequent dose and dosing interval adjustment, guided by TDM.

3. *Provision of rationale to adjust therapeutic drug regimens during periods of continuous physiological change* Normal alterations in physiological state, as in cases of pregnancy or aging, or continuous pathophysiologic or hemodynamic changes as consequences of disease, surgical treatment of disease, and the healing process, complicate assessment of drug dose needs.

4. *Identification of baseline concentrations associated with an optimal therapeutic regimen* After a patient has undergone an extensive workup to define an appropriate therapeutic regimen, a physician establishes a baseline drug concentration at which the patient responds well. If the patient's response changes significantly in the future, the physician then is able to document rapidly whether the patient has been compliant or whether a new disease state may be altering the pharmacodynamics or pharmacokinetics of a drug.

5. *Initiation and maintenance of the most appropriate drug-dosing regimens for a particular patient*

Analytical and Practical Requirements

The value and quality of a TDM service are only as good as the data produced. Routine analyses for drug concentrations are subject to many problems that can cause misinterpretation. Issues of continuing concern include the following:

1. Assay methods used for TDM should be accurate and reproducible. All clinical laboratories with a TDM service should be involved actively in an internal quality control and external proficiency testing program. In addition, sample volume and assay turnaround time should be considered in the selection of the most appropriate analytical method.

2. Each laboratory should inform the medical staff members about therapeutic and toxic concentration ranges, analytical methods (when appropriate), action values, required sample volume, and collection tube specifications.

3. Guidelines should be available outlining ideal sample schedules for each drug monitored. Steady-state trough concentrations usually are most desirable; however, other sample schedules often are invoked, depending on the properties of the drug or the individual needs of the patient.

4. The time and date of collection of the drug sample and last dose should be noted. To assess steady-state conditions, the length of time a patient has been on a particular regimen should be documented. In vitro conditions affecting stability of the drug in a sample (for example, penicillin or heparin and aminoglycoside antibiotics) or the assay specificity (for example, presence of hemolysis) should be considered for sample handling procedures.

5. Because laboratory reports become part of a patient's chart, creation of a reporting format that incorporates all the data necessary for interpretation (drug formulation, frequency and amount, plasma concentration, time of dose, time of draw, and other drugs coadministered) is useful.

■ ANALYTICAL TECHNIQUES

The evolution of TDM has depended on the development of rapid, sensitive, and specific analytical techniques. They include both instrumental and immunoassay methods.

Instrumental Methods

The application of gas-liquid chromatography (GLC) for TDM has been a major breakthrough over early spectro-photometric methods of drug analysis because it permits separation of parent drug from metabolite(s) and differentiation from coadministered drugs and endogenous compounds. Early disadvantages of GLC included the complexity of the instrumentation and need for a relatively large volume of sample. However, newer instruments are automated and easy to operate and require only microliter volumes of plasma.

Other chromatographic techniques, such as high-performance liquid chromatography (HPLC) and capillary electrophoresis (CE), offer versatility with minimal sample preparation. Specificity and sensitivity have made these techniques extremely effective tools. In addition, the relatively small sample requirements and ease of operation make HPLC and CE appealing alternatives to GLC. (See Chapters 7 and 8 for more details on these techniques.)

Immunoassay

Radioimmunoassay (RIA) techniques have permitted quantification of drug concentrations in microliter volumes of serum, at nanograms-per-milliliter concentrations. However, the complexity of this technique, long turnaround time, and lack of RIA for a wide variety of drugs have prevented its widespread adoption for routine drug assays. Few RIAs are used routinely for TDM.

Proliferation of TDM to all laboratories and physicians was achieved with the development of the nonisotopic immunoassay (see Chapter 10). Numerous systems have evolved to provide this technology in both the clinical laboratory and physician's office. The major advantages of these systems are their microcapability, specificity, rapidity, ease of performance, and adaptation to automated analyzers (see Chapter 12). Today, most TDM is carried through use of such techniques.

Common laboratory procedures for TDM are described in detail in an expanded version of this chapter.[9]

■ SPECIFIC DRUG GROUPS

Drugs that are monitored routinely are classified conveniently by the kind of therapy they support (for example, control of epilepsy, management of respiratory or cardiac function, suppression of immune response). Such a classification is used in the following discussion of specific drugs. (Note that some drugs, such as salicylate and nitroprusside [as thiocyanate], will be discussed in Chapter 32.)

Cardioactive Drugs

Cardioactive drugs that are monitored routinely by TDM include amiodarone, digoxin, disopyramide, flecainide, lidocaine, mexiletine, procainamide, propafenone, propranolol, quinidine, tocainide, and verapamil. Pharmacokinetic parameters of digoxin and other cardioactive drugs are summarized in Table 31-2.

Amiodarone

Amiodarone (Cordarone) is used to control supraventricular and ventricular tachyarrhythmias. The drug is of interest as a substitute for other class I antiarrhythmics (such as procainamide or quinidine) because it has a very long elimination half-life (35 days). The effective serum concentration of the drug, measured 24 hours after a single daily dose, varies from 1.0 to 2.0 µg/mL. The drug is indicated for control of ventricular tachycardia and fibrillation resistant to other forms of therapy.

Amiodarone is a structural analog of thyroxine, and much of its toxicity is related to interactions that occur at thyroid hormone receptors. Pulmonary fibrosis is a frequent adverse effect that is related to dose and drug level; doses less than 200 mg/day and maintenance of peak levels less than 2 µg/mL can help avoid this life-threatening side effect.

Digoxin

Digoxin (Lanoxin) is one of a group of cardiac glycosides obtained from digitalis plants (for example, *Digitalis lanata*). It restores the force of cardiac contraction in individuals with congestive heart failure and also is used to help manage supraventricular tachycardias. The drug binds to the extracytoplasmic side of the α-subunit of membrane-bound Na, K-ATPase, inhibiting both cellular Na^+ efflux and K^+ influx in myocardial cells. This inhibition reduces the sodium/potassium gradient in the Purkinje's fibers of the atrial, junctional, and ventricular myocardium, resulting in a decreased transmembrane potential. Inhibition of Na, K-ATPase is postulated to enhance movement of calcium ions in the cell, increasing calcium ion availability and improving cardiac contractility.

At low concentrations, digoxin causes the atrium to be less electrically excitable. Moderate concentrations of digoxin are required to reduce the rate of depolarization in the spontaneously depolarizing conductive fibers (Purkinje's fibers), and toxic concentrations of digoxin are necessary to diminish depolarization of the ventricular myocardium. Disagreement over the clinical value of digoxin measurements and the failure of the digoxin concentration to correlate with clinical toxicity usually are related to aberrations in serum and tissue concentrations of sodium, potassium, magnesium, and calcium. Increased sensitivity to digoxin has been noted in states of hypokalemia, hypomagnesemia, and hypercalcemia, which make establishment of the true therapeutic concentration of digoxin difficult because all parameters are interactive.

Absorption of digoxin is variable and dependent on the drug formulation. The U.S. Pharmacopeia requires more than 65% of digoxin in tablet form to dissolve in 60 minutes. In plasma, digoxin is 25% protein bound. Digoxin is concentrated in tissues, and at a steady-state the concentration of digoxin in cardiac tissue is 15 to 30 times that of plasma. Accumulation of digoxin in tissue lags behind the plasma concentration; the peak plasma concentration occurs 2 to 3 hours after the oral dose, whereas the peak tissue concentration occurs 6 to 10 hours after administration of an oral dose. Although pharmacologic effects and toxicity correlate with tissue concentration rather than with plasma concentration, the effective and safe therapeutic plasma concentration of digoxin varies from 0.8 to 2.0 ng/mL. This effective range is not determined at the peak plasma concentration but rather at the time of peak tissue concentration. Thus to ensure a correlation between plasma concentration and tissue concentration, the appropriate time to collect the specimen is 8 hours or more after administration of the dose. Results from specimens collected earlier than 8

TABLE 31-2   Pharmacokinetic Parameters of Cardioactive Drugs

Drug	MEC (unit/mL)	MTC (unit/mL)	Average Half-Life (h)	Average Volume of Distribution (L/kg)	Average Oral Bioavailability (%)	Average Protein Binding (%)
Amiodarone	1.0 µg	2.0 µg	35 days*	60	45	99
Digoxin	0.8 ng	2.0 ng	40	5	70	25
Disopyramide	2.0 µg	5.0 µg	8	0.6	83	45 to 70*
Flecainide	0.2 µg	1.0 µg	14	5	70	45
Lidocaine	1.5 µg	6.0 µg	1.8	1.1	35	70
Mexiletine	0.7 µg	2.0 µg	19	5	90	60
Procainamide	4.0 µg	12.0 µg	6	1.9	83	20
N-Acetylprocainamide	12.0 µg	18.0 µg	8	NA	NA	NA
Propafenone	0.2 µg	1.0 µg	6	2.0	40	90
Propranolol	20 ng	100 ng	4	4.0	25	90
Quinidine	2.0 µg	5.0 µg	6	2.7	80	85
Tocainide	6.0 µg	15.0 µg	14	3	90	10
Verapamil	50 ng	250 ng	4	5	20	90

MEC, Minimum effective concentration; *MTC*, minimum toxic concentration; *NA*, not available.
*See text.

hours after the dose administration are misleading because they do not correlate with tissue concentrations.

The toxic effect of digoxin is characterized by nonspecific symptoms of nausea, vomiting, anorexia, and predominance of green/yellow visual distortion. Cardiac symptoms of intoxication include multiform premature ventricular contractions (PVCs), ventricular bigeminy, ventricular tachycardia, and ventricular fibrillation. Combinations of decreased conduction and increased automaticity may result in paroxysmal atrial tachycardia with atrioventricular node block and nonparoxysmal junction tachycardia. These symptoms are observed frequently when the blood concentration exceeds 2 ng/mL in adults. Children tolerate higher concentrations and do not usually exhibit toxicity until the digoxin concentration exceeds 4 ng/mL. The relationship between blood level of digoxin and clinical and toxic response was described by Lewis[5] and is presented in Figure 31-5.

Elimination of digoxin follows first-order kinetics; 50% to 70% is excreted unchanged or in the form of digoxigenin monosaccharides or disaccharides in the urine. A small amount is metabolized to dihydrodigoxin and also excreted by the kidneys. The remainder is found in the stool as digoxigenin and its saccharides. As a result, digoxin toxicity develops more frequently and lasts longer in individuals with renal impairment. Dose requirements are decreased in those with renal disease. Bresnahan and Vlietstra[1] have developed a simple method to calculate dose that is based on creatinine clearance. Coadministration of cyclosporine, quinidine, or verapamil prolongs the rate of clearance of digoxin, requiring dose adjustment.

Decreased GI absorption occurs in individuals with sprue and small intestinal resections, high-fiber diets, hyperthyroidism, and situations of increased GI motility. A more dangerous situation develops secondary to the interaction of quinidine and digoxin, resulting in an increase in the digoxin concentration. The actual mechanism of this interaction has

not been defined clearly, although quinidine has been shown to decrease the rate of clearance and volume of distribution of digoxin.

In practice, digitoxin is prescribed infrequently today; however, serum levels should be evaluated in patients suspected of having digitalis intoxication with nondetectable digoxin levels. Digoxin immunoassay procedures cross-react only minimally with digitoxin, requiring that a digitoxin-selective antibody be substituted in the assay.

Disopyramide

Disopyramide (Norpace) is used to maintain sinus rhythm in individuals with atrial flutter and atrial fibrillation and to prevent ventricular tachycardia and fibrillation. The mechanism of action of disopyramide is similar to that of quinidine, and the drug is used as replacement therapy for quinidine when quinidine side effects are intolerable.

Disopyramide is absorbed almost completely, and a small fraction undergoes first-pass hepatic metabolism. In the blood, disopyramide binds to plasma proteins. Binding is highly variable among individuals and also depends on the concentration of disopyramide—the higher the concentration, the greater the free fraction. Thus toxicity develops rapidly as the drug concentration increases. The elimination half-life averages 8 hours. Elimination is by renal clearance and hepatic metabolism. Metabolism has a minor role in elimination, but with renal insufficiency, clearance is prolonged, causing accumulation of disopyramide.

An optimal antiarrhythmic effect is accomplished at plasma concentrations of 2.0 to 5.0 μg/mL. The relationship between clinical response and optimal therapeutic concentration is confused by a decrease in protein binding that occurs as plasma concentration of disopyramide rises. Disopyramide binds variably to serum proteins; binding varies from 45% to 70% at 2 μg/mL total serum concentration and 30% to 45% at 5 μg/mL.

Metabolism of disopyramide is by dealkylation. The principal metabolite is nordisopyramide (monodealkylated), a compound reported to have antiarrhythmic activity approximately 25% that of disopyramide. Under normal circumstances, nordisopyramide accumulates to concentrations ranging from 0.2 to 1.0 μg/mL, and the compound accumulates in proportion to disopyramide in situations of reduced hepatic or renal function. Therefore little additional therapeutic information is gained by monitoring of nordisopyramide.

The predominant side effects of disopyramide are anticholinergic, including dry mouth, urinary hesitancy, and constipation. These symptoms occur at plasma concentrations exceeding 4.5 μg/mL. Cardiac toxicity usually is associated with blood concentrations greater than 10 μg/mL and characterized by atrioventricular node blockage, bradycardia, and asystole. Because of the wide degree of variability of protein binding, interindividual differences are high in the blood concentration at which these symptoms develop.

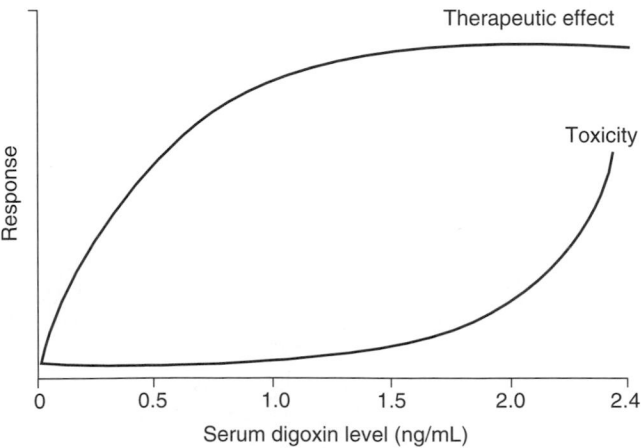

Figure 31-5 Relationship between digoxin dose and response, showing that the therapeutic effect occurs at low concentration, whereas the onset of toxicity occurs exponentially as the concentration increases.

Flecainide

Flecainide (Tambocor) is a sodium channel blocker with cardiac activity similar to disopyramide. The drug has significant toxicity in individuals with myocardial infarction and therefore has fallen from favor. For those patients who do not respond to other sodium channel blockers, it may be a drug of last resort.

Flecainide is absorbed completely. It has an elimination half-life of 10 to 17 hours. Elimination occurs by hepatic metabolism and renal clearance. Drugs affecting the cytochrome P_{450}-2D6 enzyme system interfere with flecainide metabolism. Optimal response occurs when serum levels are in the range of 200 to 1000 ng/mL.

Lidocaine

Lidocaine (Xylocaine) is the drug of choice for the initial therapy of PVCs and the prevention of ventricular arrhythmias. Lidocaine is contraindicated when bradycardias and severe atrioventricular node block appear after myocardial infarction. Lidocaine shortens the action potential refractory period in these fibers and does so at concentrations less than those required to exert pharmacologic effects at other sites, such as the ventricular myocardium.

Because lidocaine undergoes almost complete first-pass hepatic metabolism when administered orally, it typically is administered only as an intravenous or intramuscular injection. Once in the blood, lidocaine is bound 50% to protein, mainly to AAG and albumin. Clearance of lidocaine is very rapid. The distribution half-life is approximately 0.5 hours, and the elimination half-life is 1.5 to 2.0 hours. Reduced hepatic function impairs clearance and causes prolonged elimination and accumulation of the drug. These effects are due both to reduced blood flow to the liver (seen in heart failure) and to decreased metabolism of lidocaine. Consequently, lidocaine intoxication occurs if the dose is not adjusted to account for this decreased metabolic rate.

The greatest likelihood of therapeutic success, therapeutic failure, or toxicity for lidocaine depends on increments of its concentration.[10] For example, blood concentrations less than 1.5 µg/mL rarely are effective. Concentrations ranging from 1.5 to 6.0 µg/mL usually are effective and are associated only rarely with any form of central nervous system (CNS) or cardiovascular toxicity. Concentrations ranging from 4 to 6 µg/mL may be necessary for suppression of arrhythmias but may be associated with mild CNS depression and slight QRS widening on the electrocardiogram. Concentrations ranging from 6 to 8 µg/mL have been associated with significant CNS depression and atrioventricular node blockage and are acceptable only if alternative therapy is not possible. Concentrations exceeding 8 µg/mL commonly are associated with seizure activity, significant hypotension, and life-threatening decreased cardiac output.

Monoethylglycinexylidide (MEGX) and glycinexylidide (GX) are the two metabolites of lidocaine commonly found in plasma. MEGX and lidocaine have nearly identical toxic equivalency, and the sum total of lidocaine and MEGX concentration averaged 18.7 µg/mL (ranging from 17.9 to 28.0 µg/mL) in patients experiencing lidocaine-induced convulsions. Substitution of MEGX for lidocaine resulted in the same mean concentration for the equivalent convulsive activity. The metabolite GX was shown to be unimportant because it does not accumulate to significant concentrations. Measurement of MEGX has been proposed as a marker of hepatic function.

Because lidocaine is administered most commonly as a constant infusion after a loading dose, the time to collect the specimen is determined by the reason for monitoring. If the blood concentration is intended to document an adequate concentration early in therapy, the specimen should be collected 30 minutes before the loading dose, or 5 to 7 hours after therapy is initiated if no loading dose is given (five half-lives after start of therapy) to monitor the trough concentration. If a patient demonstrates diminished mental status, QRS widening, or other toxic symptoms, the specimen should be collected as close to the episode as possible and analysis performed immediately because these symptoms present a potentially life-threatening situation (onset of severe lidocaine intoxication). This situation is more likely to occur at the peak concentration.

The total plasma concentration of lidocaine is a result of clearance of the drug and is modulated by hepatic function. Little impact on clearance is noticed in renal disease. In situations of decreased organ perfusion, clearance is reduced and increased blood concentrations of lidocaine should be expected; reduced dosing is appropriate in these circumstances. AAG is the principal binding protein of lidocaine and has been demonstrated to accumulate after myocardial infarction. The result of accumulation of this protein is reduction of free lidocaine, which reduces the pharmacologic effect of the drug. Another interaction of interest is the decreased clearance of lidocaine associated with a concomitant dose of cimetidine or propranolol. Accumulation of lidocaine in this situation could result in toxicity.

Mexiletine

Mexiletine (Mexitil) is used for control of ventricular dysrhythmias. Mexiletine has the advantage of a long half-life (7 to 14 hours) compared with other antiarrhythmic agents. Mexiletine undergoes hepatic metabolism by the cytochrome P_{450}-2D6 enzyme system. The therapeutic concentration has been identified as ranging from 0.7 to 2.0 µg/mL. The drug exhibits a high degree of oral bioavailability, is approximately 60% protein bound, and is predominantly cleared by the kidneys. Mexiletine has a large volume of distribution (5 L/kg), indicating that it is highly tissue bound. Myocardial infarction and uremia reduce renal clearance, resulting in an increase in half-life. Mexiletine toxicity occurs at concentrations greater than 2 µg/mL and is characterized by tremor, dizziness, ataxia, dysarthria, diplopia, nystagmus, confusion, and hypotension.

Procainamide

Procainamide (Pronestyl) is used for therapy of PVCs, ventricular tachycardia, atrial fibrillation, and paroxysmal atrial tachycardia. Its mechanism of action is similar to that of quinidine in that it increases the threshold membrane potential by blocking potassium outflow, reducing excitability and contraction velocity in Purkinje's fibers and ventricular muscle.

Absorption of procainamide is rapid and complete. Peak plasma concentrations after oral administration are reached within 0.75 to 1.5 hours if the drug is given in capsule form, or within 1 to 3 hours if it is given in tablet form. Once absorbed, procainamide is about 20% bound to plasma proteins. Excretion of procainamide depends on hepatic metabolism and renal clearance; therefore alteration in either organ function leads to accumulation of procainamide and its metabolites. Its half-life is 3 to 9 hours in healthy adults.

The concentration at which procainamide blocks PVCs and inhibits ventricular tachycardia varies from 4 to 12 μg/mL, although individuals tolerate concentrations higher than this for short periods of time. Studies suggest that individuals experiencing chronic PVCs are able to tolerate blood concentrations as high as 16 μg/mL to reduce PVCs to a reasonable number.[8] Minimum plasma concentrations of 8 μg/mL were required for protection against sustained ventricular tachycardia.

The ideal therapeutic concentration for procainamide is complicated by the fact that N-acetylprocainamide (NAPA), an acetylated metabolite, has antiarrhythmic activity similar to procainamide. Consequently, coanalysis of NAPA is necessary to provide a complete assessment of therapy or define metabolic status. However, the optimal therapeutic concentration of NAPA is not well defined.

Patients receiving procainamide are classified as "slow" or "fast" acetylators to indicate the degree to which they acetylate procainamide. NAPA has been shown to accumulate in fast acetylators or those with impaired renal function. NAPA is used in Europe, where the maximum tolerable concentration of NAPA in the absence of procainamide is 30 μg/mL. Fast acetylators have concentrations of NAPA equal to or exceeding those of procainamide in a specimen collected 3 hours after administration, whereas slow acetylators have procainamide present at greater than twice the NAPA concentration in a specimen collected during the same time interval. Because the effects of procainamide and NAPA are cumulative, peak plasma concentrations of procainamide should be limited to 8 to 12 μg/mL, and peak concentrations of procainamide plus NAPA should not exceed 30 μg/mL. Interpretation of results requires knowledge of a patient's cardiac status; given concentrations may be intolerable in some patients, whereas others may require higher levels for control of PVCs.

Symptoms of intoxication include bradycardia, prolongation of the QRS interval, atrioventricular block, and induced arrhythmias. These symptoms occur at blood concentrations of procainamide and NAPA exceeding 30 μg/mL. Hypotension sometimes encountered in procainamide therapy is not related to excessive plasma concentration. The development of systemic lupus erythematosus associated with procainamide therapy is not related to plasma concentration but is associated with the acetylator status of the patient; slow acetylators predominate in the group in whom the syndrome develops. Because some degree of erythematosus develops in most patients, and because the short half-life requires frequent dosing, use of procainamide is limited to those patients who experience poor response from other therapies.

Propafenone

Propafenone (Rythmol) is an antiarrhythmic drug that has β-adrenergic receptor blocking properties and minor calcium antagonistic activity. It undergoes extensive first-pass metabolism, with a half-life of approximately 6 hours. Its clinical efficacy is maintained through formation of metabolites (primarily 5-hydroxypropafenone) that are more pharmacologically active than the parent drug and have longer plasma half-lives (11 to 24 hours). Occasionally, measurement of the serum concentration of propafenone is useful to document patient compliance. Normal response to the drug occurs when the serum concentration is in the range of 0.2 to 1.0 μg/mL. Toxicity related to propafenone occurs when the blood concentration exceeds 2 μg/mL and is expressed as GI upset, CNS irritability, and skin reactions.

Propranolol

Propranolol is used in the treatment of arrhythmias of atrial and ventricular origin, angina pectoris, myocardial infarction, and hypertension. It is a nonselective **beta (β-) blocker** with action on cardiac receptors (β_1) and vascular and bronchial smooth muscle receptors (β_2). Its principal effect is to reduce the heart rate, thus relieving angina, and to slow conduction at the atrioventricular node, reducing the ventricular rate in individuals with atrial fibrillation. It is included in this chapter's discussion as representative of other β-blockers, such as acebutolol, aprindolol, esmolol, flestolol, metoprolol, nadolol, and sotalol, which are similar to propranolol.

Although propranolol is absorbed rapidly, it undergoes such a high degree of first-pass hepatic metabolism that its final bioavailability is low (20% to 40%), widely variable between individuals, and dose dependent (the higher the dose, the greater the bioavailability). In the plasma, propranolol is highly protein bound (95%) to albumin and AAG. Elimination half-life is 3 to 4 hours. Elimination is predominantly by metabolism; therefore reduced hepatic function or reduced blood flow to the liver causes accumulation of propranolol.

A correlation exists between slowing of the heart rate and increasing of blood concentrations of propranolol. However, virtually no relationship exists between plasma concentration of propranolol and the hypotensive effect of the drug.

Quinidine

Quinidine, available as either quinidine sulfate or quinidine gluconate, is used in the treatment of atrial premature contraction, paroxysmal supraventricular tachycardia, supraventricular tachyrhythmia, PVCs, and ventricular tachycardia and in prophylactic treatment after myocardial infarction. It also is used with care in the treatment of atrial fibrillation and atrial flutter, although this treatment commonly is accompanied by the administration of either digoxin or a (β-blocker (propranolol) to provide atrioventricular node blockade.

Absorption of quinidine is complete and rapid. Peak serum concentrations are reached in 1.5 to 2 hours after oral intake, unless the "slow-release" preparation (quinidine gluconate) is used. Peak plasma concentrations are attained 4 to 5 hours after quinidine gluconate administration, and the trough concentration occurs 1 to 2 hours after the next administration. Once absorbed, quinidine is 80% protein bound. Clearance of quinidine depends on both adequate hepatic function and adequate renal function. Reduction of either of these two functions results in accumulation of the drug. Renal clearance is a function of urine pH. If the urine is alkaline or if a patient has renal tubular acidosis, clearance is reduced.

The optimum therapeutic concentration for quinidine is 2 to 5 μg/mL. Quinidine toxicity usually is observed at concentrations exceeding 8 μg/mL and characterized by symptoms of cinchonism, tinnitus, lightheadedness, giddiness, and cardiovascular toxicity, including PVCs and atrioventricular node block. The predominant toxic effect is GI distress, including nausea, vomiting, anorexia, and abdominal discomfort. Hypersensitivity reactions associated with quinidine are not related to blood concentration.

Clearance of quinidine depends on an active cytochrome P_{450}-2D6 enzyme system in the liver. Induction of this system by barbiturates leads to enhanced clearance of quinidine. Diminished organ perfusion results in decreased clearance. Quinidine itself has been reported to dilate peripheral blood vessels, resulting in mild to moderate hypotension and reduced clearance over the short term. Quinidine affects the rate of clearance of digoxin.

Tocainide

Tocainide (Tonocard) has electrophysiological properties similar to lidocaine. It is useful in the management of ventricular arrhythmias typified by a prolonged QT interval of the electrocardiogram. Tocainide has the advantage over lidocaine in that it can be taken orally and has a relatively long half-life (13 to 16 hours). Optimal response to tocainide occurs when the blood concentration is in the range of 6 to 15 μg/mL. At therapeutic concentrations, tocainide is 10% protein bound, does not undergo significant first-pass metabolism, and has a volume of distribution of 3 L/kg, but it undergoes significant hepatic metabolism and renal clearance. Toxicity associated with tocainide occurs at concentra-tions in excess of 15 μg/mL and is characterized by GI disturbance, CNS irritability culminating in convulsions, and cardiopulmonary depression.

Congestive heart failure and uremia reduce renal clearance and the volume of distribution and increase the clearance half-life. Because tocainide is not highly protein bound, it does not exhibit the protein-binding phenomenon described for lidocaine after myocardial infarction.

Verapamil

Verapamil (Calan) is a **calcium channel blocker** that is effective in the treatment of various cardiovascular disorders, including angina (classic and variant), arrhythmias (paroxysmal supraventricular tachycardia), atrial flutter, atrial fibrillation, hypertrophic cardiomyopathy (idiopathic hypertrophic subaortic stenosis), hypertension, congestive heart failure, and Raynaud's phenomenon, as well as in the preservation of ischemic myocardium and the treatment of migraine headaches.

The effective blood concentration of verapamil varies from 50 to 250 ng/mL. In studies, toxic symptoms were characterized by sinus bradycardia and heart block occurring at blood concentrations exceeding 250 ng/mL. All subjects studied showed atrioventricular block at concentrations exceeding 450 ng/mL.

Antiepileptic Drugs

Seizures are attacks of cerebral origin consisting of sudden and transitory abnormal phenomena of a motor, sensory, autonomic, or psychic nature resulting from transient dysfunction of the brain. Epilepsy is a seizure disorder in which paroxysmal transient disturbances of brain function are manifested as episodic impairment or loss of consciousness, abnormal motor phenomena, psychic or sensory disturbances, or perturbation of the autonomic nervous system. Types of seizures include generalized tonic-clonic, absence, and partial or focal seizures. A number of **antiepileptic** drugs are used to treat seizures (Table 31-3).

Phenobarbital

Phenobarbital is used in the treatment of all seizures except absence seizures and is known by a wide variety of proprietary names and found in combination with many other drugs. It is particularly useful for treatment of generalized tonic-clonic, partial, focal motor, temporal lobe, and febrile seizures. It also is known to reduce synaptic transmission, resulting in decreased excitability of the entire nerve cell and a consequent sedating effect. Phenobarbital potentiates synaptic inhibition through action on the γ-aminobutyric acid-A ($GABA_A$) receptor by increasing the duration of chloride flow into the synapse. This increase in results is an increase in seizure threshold and inhibition of the spread of discharges from the epileptic foci.

TABLE 31-3   Pharmacokinetic Parameters of Antiepileptic Drugs

Drug	MEC (μg/mL)	MTC (μg/mL)	Average Half-Life (h)	Average Volume of Distribution (L/kg)	Average Oral Bioavailability (%)	Average Protein Binding (%)
Bromide	750	1500	290	NA	NA	0
Carbamazepine	4	12	18	1.4	70	75
Clonazepam	0.015	0.06	25	3.2	98	85
Ethosuximide	40	100	45	0.7	NA	0
Felbamate	40	120	18	0.8	90	25
Gabapentin	2	12	8	0.8	60	0
Lamotrigine	1	8	25	1.2	98	60
Mephobarbital	1	5	30	NA	NA	50
Methsuximide	0.01	0.04	3	NA	NA	NA
Normethsuximide	10	40	30	NA	NA	NA
Phenobarbital	15	40	85	1.0	90	50
Phenytoin	10	20	~20	0.6	90	90
Primidone	5	12	10	0.7	92	20
Valproic acid	40	100	16	0.2	100	93

MEC, Minimum effective concentration; *MTC*, minimum toxic concentration; *NA*, data not available.

Absorption of oral phenobarbital is slow but complete. The time at which peak plasma concentrations are reached is widely variable and ranges from 4 to 10 hours after administration of the dose. Phenobarbital is 40% to 60% bound to plasma proteins. Its elimination half-life varies from 70 to 100 hours and is age dependent. (Children average about 70 hours, whereas geriatric patients average 100 hours.) Because hepatic metabolism is one of the prime routes of elimination, reduced liver function increases the drug's half-life.

The effective concentration of phenobarbital is between 15 and 40 μg/mL. The predominant side effect observed in adults at blood concentrations greater than 40 μg/mL is sedation, although tolerance to this effect develops with long-term therapy.

Phenobarbital is metabolized in the liver to *p*-hydroxyphenobarbital, which is excreted largely as the glucuronide or sulfate ester. When renal and hepatic functions are decreased, patients experience decreased clearance of the drug. Elimination of phenobarbital may be decreased in the presence of valproic acid and salicylate if reduction in urinary pH occurs. During long-term administration of either valproate or salicylate, the concentration of phenobarbital may increase 10% to 20%, and a dose adjustment may be necessary to prevent intoxication. Phenobarbital induces mixed-function oxidative enzymes, resulting in increased metabolism of other xenobiotics after approximately 1 to 2 weeks of therapy.

Because of the long elimination half-life of phenobarbital, the blood concentration does not change rapidly. Therefore a serum specimen collected late in the dose interval (trough) is representative of the overall effect. Results from specimens collected 2 to 4 hours after the dose is administered can be misleading; such a result may be construed to be the peak concentration when in actuality it precedes the peak.

Phenytoin

Phenytoin (diphenylhydantoin), most commonly available as *Dilantin* but also available in its **generic drug** form, is used to treat primary or secondary generalized tonic-clonic seizures, partial or complex-partial seizures, and status epilepticus. The drug is not effective in the treatment of absence seizures. Phenytoin modulates the synaptic sodium channel by prolonging inactivation, which reduces the ability of the neuron to respond at high frequency. The physiological effect of this action is reduction in central synaptic transmission, which aids in the control of abnormal neuronal excitability.

Phenytoin is not readily soluble in aqueous solutions. When the drug is administered by intramuscular injection, most of the dose precipitates at the site of injection and then is absorbed slowly. A prodrug called *fosphenytoin (Cerebyx)* is available as a therapeutic form of phenytoin. Fosphenytoin has increased aqueous solubility for intramuscular injection. After injection, it is converted rapidly to phenytoin.

Absorption of oral phenytoin is slow and sometimes incomplete. Variations in the drug preparation have been blamed for low bioavailability. Once absorbed, phenytoin is bound tightly to protein (90% to 95%). As with all drugs the pharmacologic effect of phenytoin is related directly to the amount present in the free (unbound) state. Only free phenytoin is available to cross biological membranes and interact at biologically important binding sites. The degree of protein binding is reduced by the presence of other drugs, anemia, and hypoalbuminemia, which often are present in elderly individuals. In these conditions an increased effect is observed at the same total drug concentration as in plasma from normal individuals.

The optimum therapeutic concentration for seizure control without side effects is 10 to 20 μg/mL. A 50% response rate was observed in patients with plasma concentrations greater than 10 μg/mL, and an 86% suppression of seizure activity was observed in those with concentrations exceeding 15 μg/mL. These concentrations also serve as reasonable guidelines when the drug is used as a cardiac **antiarrythmic agent.** Free phenytoin concentrations of 1 to 2 μg/mL are optimum. Total phenytoin concentrations in excess of 20 μg/mL usually do not enhance seizure control and often are associated with nystagmus and ataxia. Total phenytoin plasma concentrations in excess of 35 μg/mL have been shown to precipitate seizure activity. A side effect of phenytoin not related to plasma concentration is development of gingival hyperplasia.

Phenytoin is metabolized by hepatic microsomal hydroxylating enzymes. The principal metabolite is 5-(*p*-hydroxyphenyl)-5-phenylhydantoin, which is excreted principally as a glucuronide ester. Other minor metabolites are of minimal clinical importance. Hepatic metabolism of phenytoin may become saturated within the therapeutic range. Once metabolism is saturated, small-dose increments result in large changes in blood concentration; this phenomenon partially explains the wide variation in dose among patients that is required to achieve a therapeutic effect. Because of this saturation phenomenon, first-order kinetics do not apply to phenytoin at blood concentrations in excess of 5 μg/mL.

The time to collect the specimen for phenytoin analysis is dictated by the reason for monitoring. If a patient displays any symptoms of intoxication, then the peak blood concentration is of interest. This specimen is collected 4 to 5 hours after administration of the dose, although the peak level may be delayed up to 8 hours if the drug is given in conjunction with substances that increase stomach acidity. If the principal question at hand is adequate therapy, then the trough concentration is most useful and the specimen is collected directly before the next dose is administered.

A number of **drug interactions** result in alteration of the disposition of phenytoin. Alcohol, barbiturates, and carbamazepine induce oxidative enzymes; this induction results in increased metabolism of phenytoin, reduced serum concentration of both total and free phenytoin, and reduced pharmacologic effect. Drugs such as chloramphenicol, cimetidine, disulfiram, isoniazid, and dicumarol compete with phenytoin metabolism, resulting in an increase of both total and free phenytoin concentrations and enhancement of the pharmacologic effect. Salicylate, valproic acid, phenylbutazone, sulfisoxazole, and sulfonylureas compete with phenytoin for serum protein-binding sites. This competition results in diminished total serum concentration of phenytoin, whereas the free phenytoin concentration and pharmacologic effect remain approximately the same. The interest in monitoring of the free phenytoin concentration is in response to these altered disposition states.

Primidone

Primidone (Mysoline) is effective in the treatment of tonic-clonic and partial seizures. The mechanism of action of this drug is similar to that described for phenobarbital, and the therapeutic effect is partially due to the accumulation of its major metabolite, phenobarbital. A second metabolite of primidone, phenylethylmalonamide, also has some antiepileptic activity.

Primidone is absorbed rapidly and completely after oral administration. Once absorbed, the drug is not highly protein bound and has a half-life of approximately 10 hours. Disposition of the drug is not known to be significantly altered by other disease states or drugs.

The optimum therapeutic concentration of primidone has been established as 5 to 12 μg/mL. Because phenobarbital is an active metabolite of primidone, concurrent analysis of phenobarbital is required for complete result interpretation. The previously defined therapeutic range for phenobarbital applies to adequate primidone therapy. The phenobarbital concentrations rise gradually over a period of 1 to 2 weeks after therapy is initiated. Toxicity because of accumulation of primidone occurs at serum concentrations in excess of 15 μg/mL and usually is associated with symptoms of sedation, nausea, vomiting, diplopia, dizziness, ataxia, and a phenobarbital concentration greater than 40 μg/mL. Specimen collection is dictated by the same rules that apply for phenobarbital; the trough concentration is most useful.

Coadministration of acetazolamide with primidone results in decreased GI absorption of primidone and subsequent diminished plasma concentrations. Primidone administered in association with phenytoin produces a modest elevation of the phenobarbital/primidone ratio because phenytoin competes with the hepatic hydroxylating enzymes associated with phenobarbital's metabolism. Coadministration of valproic acid, for the same reasons outlined for phenobarbital, causes a modest increase in both primidone and phenobarbital serum concentrations.

Carbamazepine

Carbamazepine (Tegretol) is used in the treatment of generalized tonic-clonic, partial, and partial-complex seizures. It also is used to treat pain associated with trigeminal neuralgia. Like phenytoin, carbamazepine modulates the synaptic sodium channel, which prolongs inactivation, reducing the ability of the neuron to respond at high frequency. The physiological effect of this action is reduction in central synaptic transmission, which helps control abnormal neuronal excitability. Carbamazepine also has an antidiuretic effect, reducing concentrations of antidiuretic hormone.

After oral administration, carbamazepine is absorbed slowly and erratically with wide individual variability. The drug is highly protein bound (80%). The elimination half-life with continued therapy is approximately 18 hours. With long-term therapy the enzymes responsible for metabolism are induced, and the elimination half-life is reduced to 15 to 20 hours. Because hepatic metabolism is the principal means by which plasma levels are reduced, any reduction in liver function results in drug accumulation.

The therapeutic concentration range for optimal pharmacologic effect of carbamazepine is 4 to 12 μg/mL. Toxicity associated with excessive carbamazepine ingestion occurs at plasma concentrations in excess of 15 μg/mL and is characterized by symptoms of blurred vision, paresthesia, nystagmus, ataxia, drowsiness, and diplopia. Side effects unrelated to plasma concentration include development of an urticarial rash, which usually disappears on discontinuation of the drug, and hematological depression (leukopenia, thrombocytopenia, and aplastic anemia).

The active metabolite of carbamazepine is carbamazepine-10,11-epoxide. This metabolite has been found to accumulate in children to concentrations equivalent to carbamazepine. It may contribute to symptoms of intoxication in children who have therapeutic plasma concentrations of the parent drug. Because carbamazepine is metabolized through the hepatic oxidative enzyme system, drugs that induce this system (phenytoin, phenobarbital) increase the rate of clearance of carbamazepine.

Coadministration of phenobarbital, phenytoin, or valproic acid increases the rate of metabolism of carbamazepine, reducing the blood concentration. Erythromycin and propoxyphene interfere with metabolism, increasing carbamazepine levels.

Because of carbamazepine's relatively long half-life, the specimen yielding the most useful information is the one representing the trough concentration. However, in the case of suspected mild intoxication the peak value of the plasma concentration correlates more closely with toxicity. The peak specimen should be collected 4 to 8 hours after the oral dose is administered.

Ethosuximide

Ethosuximide (Zarontin) is used to treat absence seizures characterized by brief loss of consciousness. It is absorbed readily from the GI tract. The half-life of ethosuximide is approximately 45 hours, although this time may be prolonged in adults. The drug is cleared mainly by metabolism as either the hydroxyethyl compound or the glucuronide ester of the hydroxyethyl metabolite. The trough specimen yields the most useful information regarding therapeutic efficacy. The optimum therapeutic concentration of ethosuximide is 40 to 100 μg/mL. Toxicity related to an excessive blood concentration of ethosuximide is rare. Symptoms of GI distress, lethargy, dizziness, and euphoria may be encountered early in therapy, but patients usually become tolerant to these symptoms.

Valproic acid

Valproic acid (Depakene or Depakote) is used to treat absence seizures. It also has demonstrated usefulness in the treatment of tonic-clonic and partial seizures when used in conjunction with other antiepileptic agents, such as phenobarbital or phenytoin. The drug inhibits the enzyme GABA transaminase, resulting in an increase in the concentration of GABA in the brain. GABA is a potent inhibitor of presynaptic and postsynaptic discharges in the CNS. Valproic acid also modulates the synaptic sodium channel by prolonging inactivation, which reduces the ability of the neuron to respond at high frequency.

Valproic acid is absorbed rapidly and almost completely after oral administration. Peak concentrations occur 1 to 4 hours after an oral dose. The principal metabolite, 2-*n*-propyl-3-ketopentanoic acid, has anticonvulsant activity comparable to that of valproic acid, although this metabolite does not accumulate in plasma. The single-dose half-life is 16 hours in healthy adults, but this time reduces to 12 hours on long-term therapy and may be as short as 8 hours in children. In neonates and individuals with hepatic disease, when metabolism is reduced, the half-life becomes prolonged. Valproic acid is highly protein bound (93%). In circumstances in which competition for protein binding increases, such as in uremia, cirrhosis, or concurrent drug therapy, the percent of free valproic acid increases.

The MEC of valproic acid is 40 μg/mL. Concentrations that exceed 100 μg/mL have been associated with hepatic toxicity and acute toxic encephalopathy. Glycine has been observed to accumulate in patients undergoing valproic acid therapy.

Clearance of valproic acid is rapid, presenting a dosing dilemma. The dose must be adequate to provide a plasma concentration greater than 40 μg/mL without exceeding concentrations more than 100 μg/mL. The ideal specimen used to monitor the blood concentration is that drawn directly before the next dose, usually early in the morning, to confirm that an adequate dose has been prescribed before bedtime. Dosing is particularly problematic in young children, who may sleep for more than one complete half-life of the drug.

Valproic acid modulates concentrations of other common antiepileptic drugs. For example, it inhibits the nonrenal clearance of phenobarbital, resulting in elevated phenobarbital levels. It also competes with phenytoin for protein-binding sites. The free phenytoin concentration remains approximately the same, but the total phenytoin in the plasma decreases. Because the free phenytoin concentration remains unchanged, the pharmacologic effect is retained. Other common antiepileptic drugs that induce hepatic oxidative enzymes result in increased valproic acid clearance; this increased clearance rate requires a higher dose to maintain effective therapeutic levels.

Bromide

Since the discovery in 1857 that potassium bromide proved useful in the management of epilepsy, bromide has been used widely for seizure control. The advent of new, more directed therapies has reduced significantly the common use of bromide, although it still is used occasionally in combination therapy.

Bromide intoxication, which occurs easily, happens because of its slow excretion. The half-life in the blood is approximately 290 days. Consequently, bromide accumulates if it is taken daily, and over a period of weeks a toxic level may be attained. In toxicity, delirium, delusions, hallucinations, mania, lethargy, or coma may occur; electroencephalographical changes accompany the intoxication. Neurological disturbances are manifested as tremors, fixed speech, motor incoordination, decreased superficial reflexes, and positive Babinski's great toe sign. CNS pressure may rise, and in cases of severe intoxication, papilledema may be present. In normal therapy, serum concentrations of 750 to 1500 μg/mL are attained.

Gamma aminobutyric acid analogs/agonists

Studies of benzodiazepines have led to knowledge of the **gamma (γ-) aminobutyric acid (GABA)** receptor, a membrane-bound protein complex on the surface of dedicated neural and glial cells. Inhibition of these cells restrains neuronal excitation. Absence of or decreased GABA control of neurotransmission is one cause of seizure activity. These studies led to the development of drugs that increase the activity of GABA receptors, either by increasing GABA concentration or by directly interacting with the GABA receptor. Felbamate, gabapentin, and lamotrigine (Figure 31-6) are examples of such drugs.

Felbamate

Felbamate (Felbatol) is used for primary or adjunctive therapy for partial seizures. Its use is limited to those patients who fail other drug treatments because felbamate carries with it a substantial risk of aplastic anemia and liver failure that is not related to blood level. Biweekly monitoring of complete blood count, serum aminotransferases, and bilirubin is recommended to detect early onset of these side effects. Felbamate is particularly effective in control of Lennox-Gastaut syndrome.

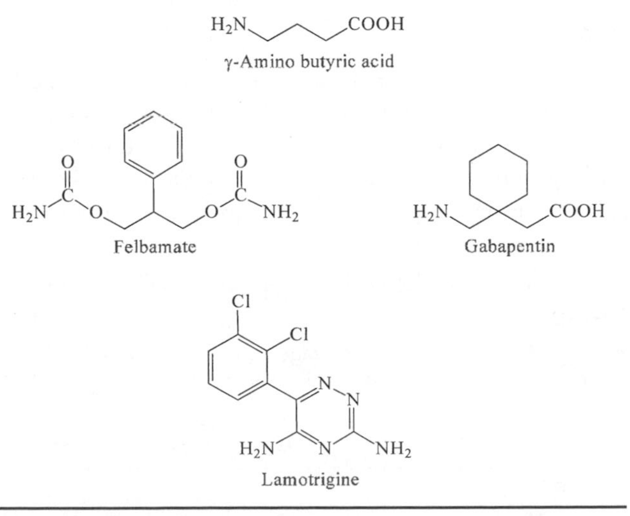

Felbamate is absorbed completely from the GI tract. The drug is 30% bound to plasma proteins, and optimum blood concentrations for felbamate range from 40 to 120 μg/mL. It is eliminated by hepatic metabolism, with a half-life ranging from 14 to 21 hours. Felbamate saturates metabolism when the concentration exceeds 120 μg/mL; at that concentration, metabolism converts from first order to zero-order kinetics.

Gabapentin

Gabapentin (Neurontin) is a chemical analog of GABA that promotes the release of GABA by an as yet unknown mechanism. It does not interact directly with the GABA receptor, nor does it inhibit glutamic acid decarboxylase, the enzyme that usually controls cellular concentration of GABA. Gabapentin has been proven effective for treatment of drug-resistant partial seizures.

Gabapentin is absorbed completely from the GI tract after oral administration. It is 10% bound to plasma proteins, and its elimination half-life is 5 to 9 hours. The optimum effective therapeutic concentration of gabapentin is between 2 and 12 μg/mL. The predominant side effects observed in adults at blood concentrations greater than 12 μg/mL are somnolence, ataxia, dizziness, and fatigue. The drug does not undergo hepatic metabolism, and it does not activate any metabolic enzymes, so coadministration of gabapentin with other drugs does not affect their concentrations. Coadministration with antacids is known to reduce absorption of gabapentin by approximately 20%.

Lamotrigine

Lamotrigine (Lamictal) binds to the GABA receptor and is considered a GABA agonist. Lamotrigine acts similar to phenytoin and carbamazepine, blocking repetitive nerve firings induced by depolarization of spinal cord neurons. It is used for adjunctive therapy for partial and absence seizures.

Lamotrigine is well tolerated and absorbed completely from the GI tract after oral administration. It is 60% bound to plasma proteins. Optimal response occurs when the trough blood level is between 1 and 2 μg/mL, and the peak level ranges from 5 to 8 μg/mL. Half-life varies from 20 to 30 hours. Elimination occurs through hepatic metabolism; the primary metabolite is the glucuronide ester. Coadministration with P_{450}-inducing drugs, such as phenobarbital, phenytoin, or carbamazepine, results in reduced lamotrigine levels; dosage increases of approximately 30% are required to maintain optimal blood levels. Dizziness, ataxia, diplopia, blurred vision, nausea, and vomiting are signs of toxicity that occur when the blood level exceeds 10 μg/mL.

Lamotrigine is a potent inhibitor of dihydrofolate reductase. Folate levels are decreased when this drug is administered. If replacement is not implemented, rash and anemia may develop when lamotrigine is at its therapeutic concentration.

Figure 31-6   Chemical structures of selected antiepileptic drugs showing chemical analogy to γ-aminobutyric acid (GABA).

Miscellaneous, infrequently used antiepileptic drugs

Benzodiazepines, mephobarbital, and succinimides all demonstrate antiepileptic activity. However, they are prescribed infrequently for this purpose.

Benzodiazepines

Benzodiazepines interact at the $GABA_A$ receptor to increase the duration of chloride flow into the synapse. The end result is an increase in seizure threshold and inhibition of the spread of discharges from the epileptic foci.

Diazepam (Valium) is used frequently in emergency situations to gain control in cases of status epilepticus. Unfortunately, tolerance to diazepam at the GABA receptor develops rapidly, and diazepam becomes ineffective within 2 to 3 days. Diazepam therefore is not used for long-term control of seizure disorders, but as an anxiolytic drug.

Clonazepam (Clonopin) is a benzodiazepine with chemical structure closely related to diazepam. The mechanism of action is the same as that described for diazepam, but tolerance does not develop as rapidly as with diazepam. Clonazepam currently is used to treat individuals with absence seizures, infantile spasms, akinetic seizures, and Lennox-Gastaut syndrome. Plasma concentrations associated with maximal effectiveness of the drug range from 15 to 60 ng/mL. At concentrations higher than 80 ng/mL, no additional seizure protection is observed, and toxicity (drowsiness, ataxia) ensues.

Mephobarbital

Mephobarbital (Mebaral) owes most of its antiepileptic activity to its principal metabolite, phenobarbital. Metabolism is through hepatic demethylating mixed-function oxidases that are induced by phenobarbital. Thus long-term therapy results in multiphasic elimination profiles of the drug. Early in therapy, high concentrations (>5 μg/mL) of mephobarbital and low concentrations (<10 μg/mL) of phenobarbital may be observed. After enzymatic induction the pattern shifts to one in which phenobarbital predominates (20 to 40 μg/mL) and mephobarbital is a minor constituent (1 to 3 μg/mL) at equilibrium. Effective therapeutic monitoring is accomplished only after a steady-state concentration has been achieved by administration of a constant dose for at least 21 days. Mephobarbital concentration usu-

ally is determined by chromatography, as described for phenobarbital methods. In addition, mephobarbital in most immunoassays cross-reacts to some degree with phenobarbital.

Succinimides

Three succinimides have proved useful in the control of absence seizures—ethosuximide *(Zarontin)*, methsuximide *(Celontin)*, and phensuximide *(Milontin)*. Ethosuximide is used widely and is reviewed elsewhere in this chapter. Methsuximide and phensuximide are used and monitored less commonly.

Both methsuximide and phensuximide are active in control of absence seizures and seizures of temporal lobe origin, but phensuximide has been found less effective because of its short half-life. Methsuximide is effective because it is metabolized to an active metabolite that is stable and has a long half-life. Steady-state serum concentrations of methsuximide and normethsuximide on a standard adult dose of 900 mg/day range from 0.01 to 0.040 μg/mL and 10 to 40 μg/mL, respectively.

Bronchodilators

Drugs used as bronchodilators include the β-adrenergic agonists, caffeine, and theophylline (Table 31-4).

β-Adrenergic agonists

Beta (β-) adrenergic agonists, such as albuterol, bitolterol, isoproterenol, metaproterenol, pirbuterol, and terbutaline, in the inhaled form have become the treatment of choice for a short-acting approach to relief of asthma. These drugs are very effective at providing rapid bronchodilation without significant cardiac or systemic effects. Because they are administered in the vapor form, have short time of action, and produce little toxicity, measurement of blood concentration offers little clinical benefit; patient response provides a convenient form by which to monitor therapy.

Caffeine

A minor metabolite of theophylline in adults, caffeine has been shown to accumulate to significant concentrations in neonates. Caffeine itself is an effective inhibitor of apnea.[5] Therapy with caffeine alone has been effective in the treatment of neonatal apnea; such therapy is gaining popularity

TABLE 31-4	**Pharmacokinetic Parameters of Bronchodilator Drugs**					
Drug	MEC (μg/mL)	MTC (μg/mL)	Average Half-Life (h)	Average Volume of Distribution (L/kg)	Average Oral Bioavailability (%)	Average Protein Binding (%)
Caffeine	3	15	5*	0.6	100	35
Theophylline	8	20	7	0.5	95	55

MEC, Minimum effective concentration; *MTC,* minimum toxic concentration.
*20 to 100 hours in neonates.

because of caffeine's long half-life in neonates (>30 hours). The optimum therapeutic concentration of caffeine in this situation varies from 8 to 14 μg/mL.

Theophylline

Theophylline, available under many proprietary names, relaxes bronchial smooth muscles to relieve or prevent asthma. The therapeutic effect of theophylline likely is due to antagonism of adenosine receptors in smooth muscle, whereas the toxic effects are due to inhibition of cyclic nucleotide phosphodiesterase. With increased use of β-adrenergic agonists and because of the considerable toxicity associated with such use, theophylline now is considered a second-level approach used only to treat individuals with persistent asthma.

Theophylline is absorbed readily after oral, rectal, or parenteral administration. If the drug is taken orally without food, the blood concentration peaks within 2 hours. If it is administered with food or as the slow-release formula, peak concentrations occur 3 to 5 hours after the dose administration. Once absorbed, theophylline is 50% protein bound. The drug is cleared rapidly in children and in adults who smoke. In these individuals the half-life varies from 4 to 6 hours. Nonsmoking adults in good health have an elimination half-life of about 5 to 9 hours. The half-life in neonates and in adults with congestive heart failure can be prolonged to 20 to 40 hours, depending on the degree of liver immaturity or loss of liver function. Coadministration of erythromycin, troleandomycin, and fluvoxamine also has been shown to reduce significantly the clearance of theophylline. Cimetidine reduces hepatic metabolism of theophylline, resulting in increased serum concentrations.

The relationship between serum concentration and prevention of symptoms of chronic asthma is well documented. A proportional relationship exists between forced expiratory volume and theophylline concentration, with the optimal therapeutic effect occurring at concentrations ranging from 8 to 20 μg/mL. Suppression of exercise-induced bronchospasm in asthmatic patients occurs at concentrations exceeding 10 μg/mL and is optimal at 15 μg/mL. Neonatal apnea treated with theophylline responds to slightly lower concentrations, ranging from 5 to 10 μg/mL. Relaxation of bronchial smooth muscle is directly proportional to blood concentration and continues at concentrations greater than 20 μg/mL. When the blood level exceeds 20 μg/mL, the secondary side effects become significant.

Theophylline clearance is a function of a metabolic process that is dose dependent. At serum concentrations greater than 20 μg/mL, small dose increases lead to disproportionately large increases in serum concentration and intoxication. Symptoms of theophylline toxicity include nausea, vomiting, headache, diarrhea, irritability, and insomnia. Transient CNS stimulation occurring at initial administration is not related directly to blood concentration. This effect diminishes with chronic use. Serious toxicity characterized by cardiac arrhythmias and seizures usually is associated with serum concentrations in excess of 30 μg/mL. Once seizure activity begins, the final prognosis is very poor. Morbidity is reported in nearly all patients, and mortality can be as high as 50%.

Antibiotics

Antibiotics that require TDM include aminoglycosides, chloramphenicol, sulfonamides, vancomycin, trimethoprim, β-lactams, and tetracyclines. Pharmacokinetic details of these antibiotics are summarized in Table 31-5.

Aminoglycosides

Aminoglycosides are polycationic agents that kill aerobic gram-negative bacteria. They bind to the 30S ribosomal subunit of bacterial messenger RNA (mRNA), thereby inhibiting protein synthesis. They are inactive under anaerobic conditions because an oxygen-dependent active transport mechanism is involved in the transfer of aminoglycosides across the bacterial cell wall. The aminoglycoside class of drugs includes amikacin, gentamicin, kanamycin, neomycin, netilmicin, sisomycin, streptomycin, and tobramycin. Structures of the common aminoglycosides are shown in Figure 31-7.

TABLE 31-5	Pharmacokinetic Parameters of Antibiotic Drugs					
Drug	MEC* (μg/mL)	MTC (μg/mL)	Average Half-Life (h)	Average Volume of Distribution (L/kg)	Average Oral Bioavailability (%)	Average Protein Binding (%)
Amikacin	25	35	2.5	0.3	NA	5
Chloramphenicol	10	25	3	0.9	75 to 90	53
Gentamicin	<5	8	2.5	0.3	NA	5
Kanamycin	25	35	2.1	0.25	NA	0
Sulfonamides, all	75	125	6 to 10	0.2	100	70 to 90
Tobramycin	<5	8	2	0.3	NA	<10
Vancomycin	20	40	6	0.5	NA	<10

MEC, Minimum effective concentration; MTC, minimum toxic concentration; NA, not applicable.
*Organism sensitivity studies (minimum inhibitory concentration; see text) define the minimum effective level.

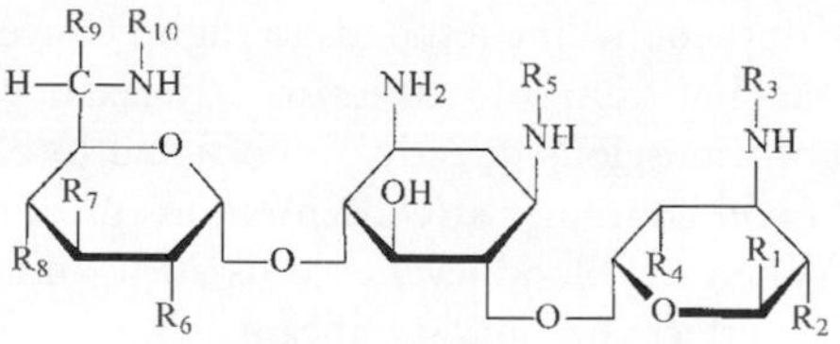

R₉ R₁₀ structure diagram (aminoglycoside backbone with substituents R₁–R₁₀)

	Amikacin	Gentamicin* (C₁, C₂, C₁ₐ)	Kanamycin* (A, B)	Tobramycin
R_1	—CH₂OH	—H	—CH₂OH	—CH₂OH
R_2	—OH	—CH₃	—OH	—OH
R_3	—H	—CH₃	—H	—H
R_4	—OH	—OH	—OH	—OH
R_5	$\overset{O}{\overset{\|}{—C}}—\overset{OH}{\underset{\|}{CH}}CH_2\overset{NH_2}{\underset{\|}{CH_2}}$	—H	—H	—H
R_6	—OH	—NH₂	(—OH, —NH₂)	—NH₂
R_7	—OH	—H	—OH	—H
R_8	—OH	—H	—OH	—OH
R_9	—H	(—CH₃, —CH₃, —H)	—H	—H
R_{10}	—H	(—CH₃, —H, —H)	—H	—H

Figure 31-7　Aminoglycoside structures. *, Gentamicin is a mixture of isomers, the major constituents being C_1, C_2, and C_{1a}, which differ at R_9 and R_{10}. Kanamycin is a mixture of two isomers, A and B, which differ at R_6.

The aminoglycosides are a very polar group of compounds but are absorbed poorly from the intestinal tract. They are administered routinely via intravenous or intramuscular injection to achieve a high degree of bioavailability. When administered directly into the blood, aminoglycosides rapidly distribute to the extracellular fluid but do not cross cell membranes or bind to plasma proteins; this behavior is consistent with their unusually low volume of distribution. Most tissues and nonrenal or hepatic secretions contain very small concentrations of aminoglycosides, the exceptions being the renal cortex, where the drug is concentrated, and bile, because of active hepatic secretion. The drugs are excreted mainly by glomerular filtration. Elimination half-lives are short, ranging from 2 to 3 hours. Because clearance is highly dependent on renal function, any impairment of glomerular filtration causes accumulation of these drugs.

Therapy with antimicrobial agents differs from the approach used for most other drugs discussed in this chapter. The goal is to achieve a concentration in plasma such that the bacteria are killed but the host remains undamaged. Because the organisms treated are variable and can become resistant to certain drugs, treatment with specific aminoglycoside agents always should be directed by susceptibility testing.

Numerous studies recommend a limit to the blood concentration of aminoglycosides. Renal tubular necrosis and degeneration of the auditory nerve are the side effects most frequently experienced after exposure to high concentrations of aminoglycosides. Both peak and trough specimens are required to monitor toxicity. In a large surgical patient survey in which dosing was performed under controlled conditions, limited nephrotoxicity was experienced when the peak serum concentration of gentamicin was maintained below 8 μg/mL.

Dose corrections must be made in patients with compromised renal function because these patients have prolonged half-lives and slower elimination rates. Guidelines have been prepared for estimation of adequate initial dose.[12] This dose then should be followed up by quantification of the blood concentration and dose adjustment.

Toxicity associated with aminoglycosides manifests as delayed-onset vestibular and cochlear sensory cell destruction and acute renal tubular necrosis. The degree and severity of cell damage are variable among the various drugs, but they all cause cell damage if the concentrations exceed the specified limit. Unfortunately, the available guidelines[12] do not guarantee the prevention of toxicity; a small number of patients experience toxic effects regardless of the concentration. Fortunately, most patients reverse the toxic effects without direct intervention if the toxicity is associated with reasonable blood concentrations. Irreparable loss of vestibular, cochlear, or renal function usually correlates with administration of an aminoglycoside at elevated blood concentrations for a period longer than 2 weeks.

Heparin has been implicated as a deactivator of gentamicin by formation of an inactive complex. This complex, although biologically inactive, retains some structural resemblance to the initial aminoglycoside and cross-reacts with antibodies to the specific aminoglycoside. Heparin concentrations encountered in therapeutic antithrombotic therapy are less than 3 units/mL, making an in vivo complication unlikely. However, specimen collection tubes containing heparin (1000 units/mL) may lead to complex formation, a phenomenon that could interfere with some immunoassay procedures.

Chloramphenicol

Chloramphenicol (Chloromycetin) is used as a bactericidal agent. It binds to the 50S ribosomal subunit of bacteria mRNA, and inhibits protein synthesis in prokaryotic organisms. Use of this drug depends on its relative toxicity against the microorganism versus the host. The drug is used against gram-negative bacteria, such as *Hemophilus influenzae*, *Neisseria meningitidis*, *Neisseria gonorrhoeae*, *Salmonella typhi*, all *Brucella* species, *Bordatella pertussis*, *Vibrio cholerae*, and *Shigella*. These organisms all are susceptible to a serum concentration of 6 μg/mL. Organisms that are susceptible to a concentration of 12 μg/mL are *Escherichia coli*, *Klebsiella pneumoniae*, *Pseudomonas pseudomallei*, *Chlamydia*, and *Mycoplasma*.

Chloramphenicol is absorbed rapidly in the GI tract. Peak serum concentrations occur 1 to 2 hours after the oral dose. In plasma, chloramphenicol is approximately 50% protein bound and is cleared with a half-life of 2 to 4 hours. Peak serum concentrations after administration of chloramphenicol palmitate or succinate occur 4 to 6 hours after administration of the dose. Chloramphenicol distributes to all tissues and concentrates in the cerebrospinal fluid. The drug is metabolized actively by the liver by *N*-acetylation and glucuronidation. Thus chloramphenicol accumulates in cases of hepatic disease. Renal disease does not reduce clearance dramatically.

Indicators of chloramphenicol toxicity include blood dyscrasias and cardiovascular collapse that correlate with increasing concentrations of the drug. Other blood concentration-related toxicities include anemia, characterized by maturation arrest in the marrow; cytoplasmic vacuolation of early erythroid and myeloid cells; reticulocytopenia; and increases in both serum iron and serum iron-binding capacity. These symptoms all are associated with serum concentrations in excess of 25 µg/mL. Development of aplastic anemia is not related to dose or blood concentration. Cardiovascular collapse, which occurs primarily in newborns, has been related to a total serum chloramphenicol concentration in excess of 50 µg/mL. An oral dose of 50 mg/kg/day results in an optimum peak serum concentration of 10 to 25 µg/mL in a healthy adult.

Sulfonamides

Sulfonamides competitively antagonize bacterial use of *p*-aminobenzoic acid, which is important in the synthesis of folic acid. Therefore organisms dependent on self-synthesized folic acid for growth are susceptible to sulfonamides. Sulfonamides are used to treat common urinary tract pathogens, such as *E. coli, Klebsiella, Enterobacter, Proteus mirabilis,* and indole-positive *Proteus* species. They are not used for infections due to *Pseudomonas aeruginosa.* The sulfonamides are active against *H. influenzae, Streptococcus pneumoniae, Shigella flexneri,* and *Shigella sonnei* isolated from the middle ear or bronchial secretions. Chemical structures of various sulfonamides are shown in Figure 31-8.

The sulfonamides are absorbed nearly completely from the GI tract. Once absorbed, they are bound to protein (60% to 90%), mainly to albumin, and are distributed to all tissues. Metabolism is by *N*-acetylation, the products having no antimicrobial activity.

Blood dyscrasias associated with sulfonamide use are not related to dose or blood concentration of the drug. The predominant toxicity associated with sulfonamide use is the formation and deposition of crystalline aggregates in the kidneys, ureters, and bladder. The safe and effective peak concentration of these drugs in serum (75 to 125 µg/mL) is separated well from the serum concentration at which crystallization in the urinary tract occurs. Serum concentrations in excess of 300 µg/mL maintained for prolonged periods of time have been associated with such crystal formation.

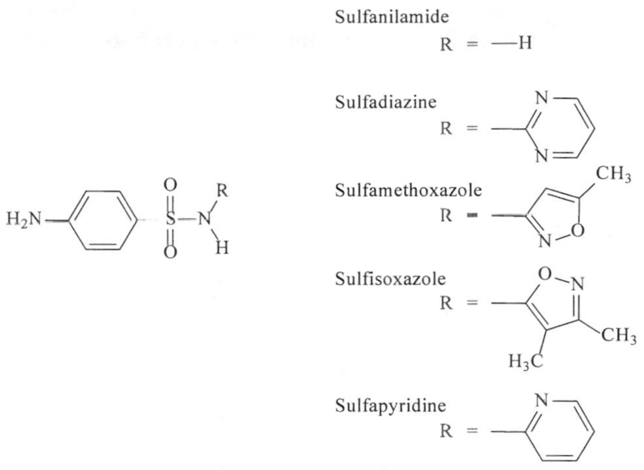

Figure 31-8   Structures of sulfonamides.

Vancomycin

Vancomycin is a glycopeptide that is bactericidal against gram-positive bacteria and some gram-negative cocci. Vancomycin is used because of its activity against methicillin-resistant staphylococci and corynebacteria. It is used widely for treatment of endocarditis and sepsis caused by these organisms.

Although vancomycin is absorbed poorly when it is administered orally, a 1-g intravenous dose every 12 hours accomplishes a peak blood concentration of 20 to 40 µg/mL and a trough concentration of 5 to 10 µg/mL. It has an average elimination half-life of 5 to 6 hours. Blood concentration-related toxicity involves the auditory nerve. Concentrations less than 30 µg/mL are associated rarely with this development. Toxicities not related to dose or blood concentration are rare and include fever, phlebitis, and pain at the infusion site. In patients with impaired renal function, the serum concentration may increase to toxic levels because of reduced clearance. Immunoassay is the standard approach to monitoring of drug levels.

Antipsychotic Drugs

Drugs used in psychiatric care that are monitored commonly include antidepressants, some neuroleptics, and lithium. Pharmacokinetic parameters of these antipsychotic drugs are shown in Table 31-6.

Antidepressants

The antidepressants, such as amino ketones (bupropion [Wellbutrin]), cyclohexanols (venlafaxine [Effexor]), dibenzoxazepines (amoxapine [Asendin]), diphenylamines (fluoxetine [Prozac]), naphthalenamines (sertraline [Zoloft]), tetracyclics (maprotiline [Ludiomil]), triazoles (nefazodone [Serzone], paroxetine [Paxil], and trazodone [Desyrel]), and tricyclics (amitriptyline [Elavil], chlorimipramine [Anafranil], desipramine [Norpramin], doxepin [Sinequan], imip-

TABLE 31-6 Pharmacokinetic Parameters of Antipsychotic Drugs

Drug	MEC (ng/mL)	MTC (ng/mL)	Average Half-Life (h)	Average Volume of Distribution (L/kg)	Average Oral Bioavailability (%)	Average Protein Binding (%)
Amitriptyline	80	250	21	15	50	95
Amoxapine	200	600	8	NA	NA	90
Bupropion	25	100	15	7	NA	84
Clozapine	100	600	8	NA	NA	97
Doxepin	150	250	17	20	27	90
Fluoxetine	90	300	55	35	60	95
Haloperidol	1	10	18	18	60	65
Imipramine	150	250	12	18	40	90
Lithium	0.6 mmol/L	1.2 mmol/L	22	0.8	100	0
Maprotiline	200	600	40	NA	NA	NA
Nefazodone	25	2500	3	NA	95	99
Nortriptyline	50	150	30	18	50	92
Olanzapine	10	1000	30	15	90	93
Paroxetine	30	70	21	13	90	95
Protriptyline	70	260	80	22	75	92
Sertraline	NA	300	26	76	NA	98
Trazadone	800	1600	7	1	75	93
Trimipramine	100	300	NA	NA	NA	90
Venlafaxin	?	?	5	6.5	92	27

MEC, Minimum effective concentration; *MTC,* minimum toxic concentration; *NA,* data not available.

ramine [Tofranil], nortriptyline [Pamelor], protriptyline [Vivactil], and trimipramine [Surmontil]), are used to treat endogenous depression characterized by depressed mood, feelings of guilt, appetite suppression, insomnia, weight change, diminished ability to concentrate, loss of interest or pleasure in usual activities, and decreased sexual drive. Endogenous depression implies that no apparent organic or societal cause exists to precipitate these behavior changes. Treatment of depression with the tricyclic or tetracyclic depressants results in pharmacologic activity through inhibition of the reuptake of catecholamines in the CNS. The end result is a positive effect on mood. The optimum therapeutic concentrations and important pharmacokinetic parameters of antidepressants are listed in Table 31-6.

Bupropion

Bupropion is a weak blocker of serotonin, norepinephrine, and dopamine. Bupropion is absorbed rapidly, reaching its peak level within 2 hours of oral administration. It is thought to undergo considerable first-pass metabolism, although studies have not been done to confirm this because the drug is not available in intravenous form. Bioavailability is estimated to vary from 5% to 20%. Major metabolites include the hydroxylated morphinol metabolite and the *threo*-amino alcohol metabolite. The half-life of bupropion varies from 10 to 20 hours. On a typical daily dose (100 to 250 mg), increasing bupropion serum concentrations correlate with dose and are in the range of 25 to 100 ng/mL.

Fluoxetine

Fluoxetine (and other serotonin-selective reuptake inhibitors [SSRI]) inhibits serotonin uptake in the CNS. The drug has fewer antagonistic effects on muscarinic, histaminic, and β-adrenergic receptors than the tricyclic antidepressants, allowing it to be used with fewer side effects. Fluoxetine has a very long half-life (55 hours), and its active metabolite, norfluoxetine, is eliminated with a half-life of 180 hours. Optimal response to fluoxetine occurs when the plasma concentration is in the range of 90 to 300 ng/mL. Norfluoxetine usually is present at approximately the same concentration as fluoxetine. The drug undergoes significant hepatic metabolism, and blood levels are affected by liver disease. Compromised renal function has little effect on the excretion rate of fluoxetine.

Nefazodone

Nefazodone is an SSRI that inhibits neuronal uptake of serotonin and norepinephrine. Nefazodone is a 5-HT$_2$ antagonist that is absorbed rapidly and has low bioavailability (20%) because it undergoes first-pass metabolism. Nefazodone and its metabolite, hydroxynefazodone, exhibit zero-order kinetics, with blood levels increasing exponentially, compared with the dose. On a typical daily dose (150 mg twice daily), nefazodone is highly protein bound (99%), has a half-life of 3 hours, and is present in blood serum in the concentration range of 25 to 2500 ng/mL at steady state.

Paroxetin

Paroxetin is an SSRI with demonstrated clinical utility as an antidepressant. Paroxetine is absorbed completely after oral ingestion and reaches peak steady-state levels of 30 to 70 ng/mL in approximately 5 hours. It undergoes hepatic metabolism and has a half-life of 21 hours; its metabolites are inactive. Steady-state levels of paroxetine on a typical dose of 20 mg/day are achieved in 10 days. Clinical response appears to be related to serum level.

Tricyclic antidepressants

Tricyclic antidepressants are absorbed nearly completely from the GI tract but undergo first-pass hepatic metabolism, so their ultimate bioavailability is variable. Because these drugs have slow GI activity and gastric emptying, their absorption may be delayed. Once absorbed, they are highly protein and tissue bound, resulting in large apparent volumes of distribution. Peak plasma concentrations are reached from 2 to 12 hours after administration of the oral dose. Metabolism is by N-demethylation and aromatic ring hydroxylation, followed by conjugation with glucuronic acid. If the drug administered is the tertiary tricyclic amine (amitriptyline, doxepin, imipramine), metabolism causes accumulation of the respective secondary amine (nortriptyline, nordoxepin, desipramine). These substances generally have equal pharmacologic activity and accumulate to concentrations approximately (but variably) equal to the parent drug. The hydroxylated metabolites have little pharmacologic activity.

Drugs such as cimetidine, chloramphenicol, haloperidol, methylphenidate, and phenothiazines inhibit hepatic oxidative enzymes. Inhibition of end-product metabolism of the tertiary tricyclic antidepressants results in a greater accumulation of the metabolite (amitriptyline being metabolized to nortriptyline, doxepin to nordoxepin, imipramine to desipramine) because conversion to the aromatic ring-hydroxylated metabolites is blocked. Coadministration of perphenazine with a tricyclic antidepressant causes accumulation of the metabolite to concentrations two to four times normal, with onset of toxicity occurring at the expected blood concentrations.

Tricyclic antidepressants show a good correlation between therapeutic response and serum concentration. A linear relationship between clinical improvement and serum concentration is noted for most of these drugs, the exception being nortriptyline, which has a specific therapeutic window. A serum concentration of nortriptyline below or above the concentration range of 50 to 150 ng/mL correlates with worsening of moods. The other antidepressants do not display this effect; the upper limit of the optimum blood concentration for these other antidepressants is limited by the onset of toxicity.

Toxicity is expressed as dry mouth and perspiration, signs that also may occur with depression. Thus differentiation between mild toxicity due to the drug and the disease that is being treated is difficult. More serious toxicity is expressed as atrioventricular node block, characterized by a widening of the electrocardiographic QRS interval. Onset occurs at serum concentrations ranging from 800 to 1200 ng/mL, and the severity of intoxication is related to the serum concentration. The relationship between serum concentration and cardiac toxicity diminishes with time after intoxication as the drug is absorbed into tissues. Despite this toxicity, the tricyclic antidepressants remain very important drugs in the treatment of depression.

Serotonin-release inhibitors

The antidepressants amoxapine, fluoxetine, sertraline, trazodone, and venlafaxin do not have the same degree of cardiac toxicity as the tricyclic and tetracyclic antidepressants. Treatment with doses slightly greater than normal does not predispose the patient to major toxicity. Therefore monitoring levels of these drugs are not required to prevent toxic side effects. However, if the patient does not respond to the drug as expected, monitoring may be useful to demonstrate noncompliance.

Other antipsychotic drugs

Psychotic patients most often are treated with clozapine, haloperidol, lithium, olanzapine, or one of the phenothiazines, or a combination of these drugs. Because response to these drugs is unpredictable and patients are difficult to control, monitoring of serum concentration may aid in therapy adjustments.

Clozapine

Clozapine (Clozaril) is an effective antipsychotic drug that inhibits dopamine binding at the D-1 and D-2 receptors and binds more actively at limbic binding sites than at striatal sites. Clozapine undergoes hepatic phase I metabolism to yield numerous, inactive metabolites; the serum half-life of clozapine is 4 to 12 hours. On a typical daily dose (100 mg twice daily), clozapine is 97% bound to plasma proteins. Patients respond to the drug when trough serum levels of clozapine are in the range of 100 to 600 ng/mL.

Clozapine is likely to produce agranulocytosis in approximately 1% of patients who receive the drug. This toxicity is an exposure-related event that occurs regardless of blood level. For this reason, use of clozapine is limited to schizophrenic patients who do not respond to conventional treatment. Biweekly monitoring of white cell count is required in all patients prescribed this drug.

Lithium

Lithium (Eskalith, Lithane, Lithonate) is administered as lithium carbonate and used to treat the manic phase of affective disorders, mania, and manic-depressive illness. It is postulated to enhance reuptake of catecholamines, thereby reducing their concentration in the neuronal junction. This reduction produces a sedating effect on the CNS. Lithium also modulates the distribution of sodium, calcium, and magnesium in nerve cells, which reduces the rate of glucose metabolism that affects nerve function.

Absorption of lithium from the GI tract is complete, and the peak plasma concentration is reached 2 to 4 hours after the administration of an oral dose. This cation does not bind to protein. Lithium elimination is biphasic; during the first phase, 30% to 40% of the dose of lithium is cleared, with an apparent half-life of 22 hours. During the second phase the remainder of lithium incorporated into the cellular ion pool is cleared, exhibiting a half-life of 48 to 72 hours. Clearance is predominantly a function of the kidneys, where active reabsorption occurs. Reduced renal function causes prolonged clearance times.

The optimal therapeutic response to lithium has not been related to a specific serum concentration; however, toxicity is related to serum concentration. Serum lithium concentrations are monitored to ensure patient compliance and prevent intoxication. One recommendation is that a standardized 12-hour postdose serum lithium concentration should be used to assess adequate therapy. The interval of 1.0 to 1.2 mmol/L is the optimum trough therapeutic concentration. Concentrations of 1.2 to 1.5 mmol/L signify a warning range, and a concentration in excess of 1.5 mmol/L in a specimen drawn 12 hours after the dose indicates a significant risk of intoxication. Early symptoms of intoxication include apathy, sluggishness, drowsiness, lethargy, speech difficulties, irregular tremors, myoclonic twitchings, muscle weakness, and ataxia. These symptoms, although not life threatening, are uncomfortable for patients and indicate that the onset of life-threatening seizures is imminent.

Lithium excretion parallels that of sodium. It readily passes the glomerular membrane and is reabsorbed in the proximal convoluted tubules. In situations in which patients are vulnerable to dehydration (fever, watery stools, vomiting, loss of appetite, hot weather), the potential for lithium intoxication is increased. In cases of dehydration the proximal tubular response to reabsorption of sodium (and lithium) is reduction of clearance. Increased reabsorption of lithium leads to increased blood concentration of lithium. Severe intoxication, characterized by muscle rigidity, hyperactive deep tendon reflexes, and epileptic seizures, usually is associated with lithium concentrations in excess of 2.5 mmol/L.

Olanzapine

Olanzapine, a thienobenzodiazepine with the proprietary name *Zyprexa*, is a serotonin and dopamine antagonist with antimuscarinic activity. It also blocks histamine receptors. Olanzapine is absorbed completely to reach peak concentrations in the range of 1000 ng/mL in 6 hours; it has a half-life averaging 30 hours. It is 93% protein bound. Olanzapine is cleared by hepatic cytochrome P_{450}-1A2 and -2D6 metabolism to inactive desalkyl amine and N-glucuronide metabolites.

Antineoplastic Drugs

Several drugs used to treat neoplastic diseases require TDM. They include methotrexate and purines and pyrimidines.

Methotrexate

Methotrexate has proved useful in (1) the management of acute lymphoblastic leukemia in children; (2) choriocarcinoma and related trophoblastic tumors in women; (3) carci-

nomas of the breast, tongue, pharynx, and testes; (4) maintenance of remission in leukemia; and (5) treatment of severe, debilitating psoriasis. High-dose methotrexate administration followed by leucovorin rescue is effective in treatment of carcinoma of the lung and osteogenic sarcoma. Intrathecal administration is effective in treatment of meningeal leukemia or lymphoma. Table 31-7 lists the pharmacokinetic parameters for methotrexate.

Methotrexate inhibits DNA synthesis by decreasing availability of pyrimidine nucleotides. Methotrexate competitively inhibits the enzyme dihydrofolate reductase, thus decreasing the concentrations of the tetrahydrofolate essential to the methylation of the pyrimidine nucleotides and consequently the rate of pyrimidine nucleotide synthesis. Leucovorin, a folate analog, is used to rescue host cells from methotrexate inhibition; as a synthetic substrate for dihydrofolate reductase, leucovorin, when administered, allows resumption of tetrahydrofolate-dependent synthesis of pyrimidines and reinitiation of DNA synthesis. Methotrexate is a nonspecific cytotoxin, and prolongation of blood levels appropriate for killing of tumor cells may lead to severe, unwanted cytotoxic effects, such as myelosuppression, GI mucositis, and hepatic cirrhosis.

Serum concentrations of methotrexate are monitored commonly during high-dose therapy (>50 mg/m^2) to identify the time at which active intervention by leucovorin rescue should be initiated. Criteria for blood concentrations indicative of a potential for toxicity after single-bolus high-dose therapy are as follows:

1. Methotrexate concentration greater than 10 μmol/L 24 hours after dose
2. Methotrexate concentration greater than 1 μmol/L 48 hours after dose
3. Methotrexate concentration greater than 0.1 μmol/L 72 hours after dose

Blood concentrations typically are monitored at 24, 48, and 72 hours after administration of the single dose. Leucovorin is administered when methotrexate levels are inappro-

TABLE 31-7 **Pharmacokinetic Parameters of Methotrexate**

Parameter	Value
Volume of distribution	0.4 L/kg
Bioavailability, oral	65%
Protein bound	45 ± 14%
Half-life, at concentrations:	
>100 μmol/L	1.8 h
<100 μmol/L	8.4 h
<0.1 μmol/L	>10 h
Potentially toxic concentrations	
24 h after dose (single bolus)	>10 μmol/L
48 h after dose	>1 μmol/L
72 h after dose	>0.1 μmol/L

priately high for a postdose phase. The route of elimination for methotrexate is primarily renal excretion. During the period of high blood levels, particular attention must be paid to maintenance of output of a large volume of alkaline urine. The pK_a of methotrexate is 5.5; thus small decreases in urine pH result in significant reduction in its solubility. Keeping urinary pH alkaline diminishes the risks of intratubular precipitation of the drug and obstructive nephropathy during the treatment period. Monitoring blood levels therefore provides the basis for decisions that involve timing of initiation and continuance of leucovorin treatment and for management of urinary pH.

Purines and pyrimidines

For various reasons, other antineoplastic drugs are not monitored routinely outside clinical trials. Cytosine arabinoside, 5-fluorouracil, 5-fluorodeoxyuridine and its monophosphate, 5-azacytidine, and 2,2 difluorodeoxycytidine, which are all antimetabolites like methotrexate, have been studied extensively. Analytical methods also have been developed, but no relationship between circulating blood level and therapeutic efficacy has been proven sufficiently firm to justify routine monitoring. Alkylating agents, such as cyclophosphamide, are converted metabolically to active compounds, with lifespans of only seconds before they interact with tissue and are destroyed. Measurement of active metabolites would be extremely useful but is impractical. Actinomycin and doxorubicin have toxic effects (bone marrow suppression and dermatitis) that are both immediate and long acting and that appear to relate not to a circulating blood concentration but to dose mass and length of exposure. Definition of specific dosing regimens for these drugs currently is of more concern than is control of circulating concentration. Cisplatin, easily measurable by platinum analysis, causes renal toxicity that may be related to both blood levels and length of exposure, although monitoring is not common.

Immunosuppressants

Survival rates of transplant patients have increased significantly with the introduction of **immunosuppressant** drugs, such as cyclosporine, mycophenolic acid, tacrolimus, and sirolimus; pharmacokinetic data for these drugs are listed in Table 31-8.

Cyclosporine

Cyclosporine (Sandimmune [Cyclosporin A] and Neoral) is a cyclic peptide composed of 11 amino acids, some of novel structure, isolated from the fungus *Trichoderma polysporum* (Figure 31-9). The compound has demonstrated effectiveness in suppressing host-versus-graft rejection in individuals who have undergone heterotopic organ transplants. Cyclosporine is approved for use in cases of renal, cardiac, hepatic, pancreatic, and bone marrow transplants.

Cyclosporine inhibits synthesis of certain cytokines (particularly interleukin-2) that control lymphocyte proliferation. This action is initiated when cyclosporine enters the lymphocyte to form a complex with cytoplasmic receptors that bind to calcineurin; this process interferes with normal calcium-initiated cytokine transcription. Reduced levels of cytokines, which are the normal promoters of lymphocyte proliferation, lead to reduced cellular response to antigens—immunosuppression.

Absorption of cyclosporine in the form of Sandimmune is highly variable, ranging from 5% to 40%. A poor relationship exists between dose and blood concentration, but the whole-blood concentration correlates with the degree of immunosuppression and toxicity. A microemulsion form of cyclosporine, Neoral, has more reproducible absorption, averaging 40%, and correlates with dose, blood concentration, and clinical response.

Immunosuppression requires trough whole-blood concentrations of at least 100 ng/mL. Trough whole-blood concentrations exceeding 600 ng/mL were associated with hepatic, renal, neurological, and infective complications.[4] Therapeutic trough blood concentrations of cyclosporine for renal transplants are 100 to 300 ng/mL, whereas 200 to 350 ng/mL is used as the target concentration for individuals who have undergone cardiac, hepatic, and pancreatic transplants. Simultaneous immunosuppression with low-dose prednisone and either azathioprine or mycophenolate mofetil (MMF) allows the patient to enjoy a good response to cyclosporine at lower levels; some renal transplant pa-

---

TABLE 31-8   **Pharmacokinetic Parameters of Immunosuppressant Drugs**

Drug	MEC (ng/mL)	MTC (ng/mL)	Average Half-Life (h)	Average Volume of Distribution (L/kg)	Average Oral Bioavailability (%)	Average Protein Binding (%)
Cyclosporin A*	100	350†	8.4	3 to 5	30	90
Mycophenolic acid	2 μg/mL	12 μg/mL	18	4	94	97
Sirolimus	10	60†	13	2.6	NA	NA
Tacrolimus	2	40	21	0.85	15	85

MEC, Minimum effective concentration; *MTC*, minimum toxic concentration; *NA*, data not available.
*Refers to data for Neoral.
†Trough level.

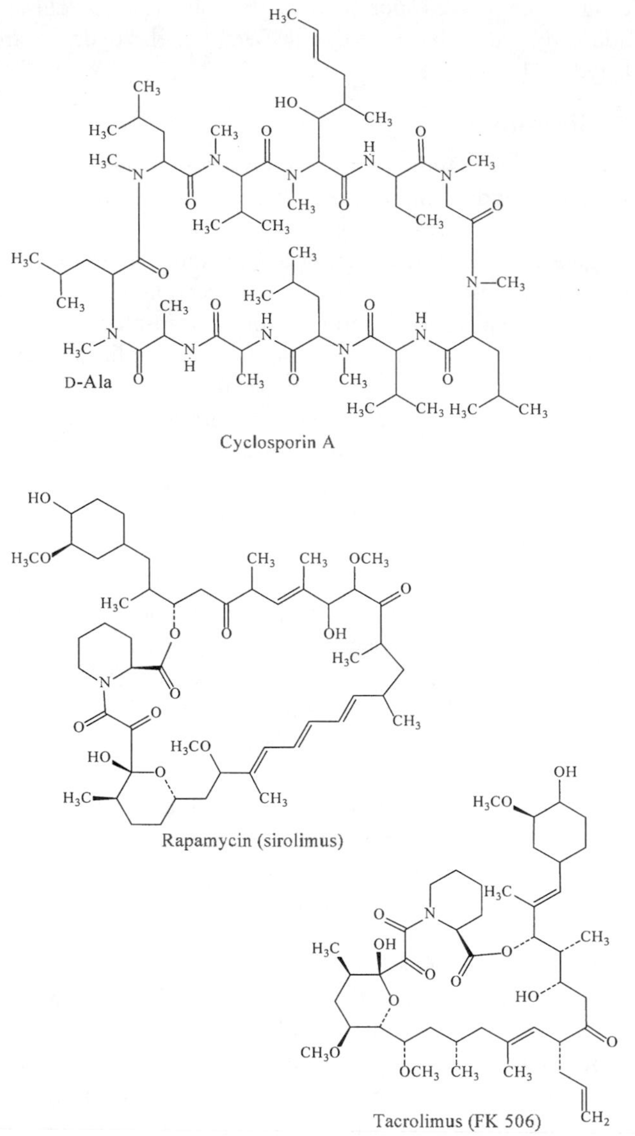

Figure 31-9   Chemical structures of cyclosporine, rapamycin, and tacrolimus.

tients obtain a satisfactory response with trough cyclosporine levels of 70 ng/mL.

Cyclosporine is absorbed slowly, and peak concentrations are reached in 4 to 6 hours. Cyclosporine is 90% protein bound and concentrated in erythrocytes. The degree of concentration in erythrocytes is temperature dependent in vitro; thus measurement of plasma concentration requires strict attention to specimen temperature if reproducible results are to be obtained. Because of this effect the best specimen for analysis is whole blood. The elimination profile of cyclosporine is biphasic. An early elimination phase with an apparent half-life that typically varies from 3 to 7 hours is followed by a slower elimination phase with an apparent half-life ranging from 18 to 25 hours. The volume of distribution is 17 L/kg. Many of the 31 known metabolites of cyclosporine are inactive.

One of the major metabolites, hydroxylated at the number 1 amino acid, retains approximately 10% of the immunosuppressive activity of the parent compound.

Several drugs alter the disposition of cyclosporine. Ketoconazole, erythromycin, melphalan, amphotericin B, and aminoglycoside antibiotics all prolong metabolism of cyclosporine sufficiently to increase the risk of nephrotoxicity. Coadministration of phenytoin, phenobarbital, carbamazepine, and rifampin results in induction of cytochrome P_{450} enzymes, which increase the rate at which cyclosporine is metabolized. Intravenous administration of sulfadimidine and trimethoprim decreases cyclosporine concentrations.

Mycophenolic acid

Mycophenolic acid (MPA) is a product of *Penicillium* species that exhibits antitumor, antiviral, antifungal, antibacterial, and immunosuppressive activity. MPA is administered as MMF, its morpholinoethyl ester. MMF is considered a prodrug because its immunosuppressive activity is expressed only after its hydrolysis to MPA in the liver. MPA inhibits inosine monophosphate dehydrogenase, an important enzyme in the purine metabolic pathway. T lymphocytes rely on this pathway for purine synthesis, whereas other cells use the hypoxanthine-guanosine ribosyl transferase salvage pathway for purine biosynthesis. Thus MPA selectively inhibits purine synthesis, and consequently transcription in T lymphocytes. Because MPA has immunosuppressive activity similar to azathioprine but without the side effects, it is anticipated that to replace azathioprine in most clinical applications.

MMF is absorbed completely and rapidly and metabolized completely to MPA. It is metabolized in the liver by phase II enzymes to form the major metabolite, mycophenolic acid glucuronide (MPAG). The elimination half-life of MPA averages 18 hours, the volume of distribution averages 4 L/kg, and typical serum levels range from a peak of 12 μg/mL to a trough level of 2 μg/mL. Monitoring serum levels of MPA and MPAG have been proposed as useful because some patients have impaired phase II enzymes, causing decreased conversion to MPAG and accumulation of MPA; this accumulation predisposes the patient to overimmunosuppression, which may increase the opportunity for infection. Optimal response is indicated by trough serum levels of MPA in the range of 2 to 4 μg/mL and MPAG levels of 60 to 100 μg/mL.

Sirolimus (rapamycin)

Sirolimus, also known as *rapamycin*, is a macrolide antibiotic with immunosuppressive activity. It is structurally similar to tacrolimus (see Figure 31-9), and its mechanism of action is believed to be the same. It is administered intravenously at a dose of 0.8 mg/kg/day to yield trough blood levels in the range of 10 to 60 ng/mL. The drug has a half-life of 10 to 15 hours and a volume of distribution averaging 2.6 L/kg.

Complications associated with levels above 60 ng/mL include muscle wasting and an increased infection rate. Blood is the specimen of choice for monitoring because rapamycin is highly sequestered in erythrocytes.

Tacrolimus

Tacrolimus (Prograf; formerly called *FK-506*) is a macrolide antibiotic isolated from a strain of *Streptomyces tsukubaensis* that has significant immunosuppressant properties (see Figure 31-9). The mechanism of action of this compound is thought to be through blockade of the induction of lymphocyte proliferation by inhibition of interleukin production. The mechanism of action is similar to that described for cyclosporine; when tacrolimus enters the lymphocyte, it binds to a receptor (FK-binding protein) that interacts with calcineurin to interfere with calcium-mediated transcription of cytokines.

Tacrolimus is an effective immunosuppressant in organ transplantation, particularly in liver transplantation; however, coadministration of it and cyclosporine is contraindicated. Adverse reactions of nausea, vomiting, and headaches similar to those with cyclosporine were experienced by some recipients. Approximately 5% of patients receiving tacrolimus experience neurotoxicity, typified by light sensitivity, tingling in the palms, and tinnitus.

The dosage of tacrolimus is significantly less than that of cyclosporine (0.3 mg/kg/day, bid), and nephrotoxicity is significantly less than with cyclosporine. No hypertension has been noted. Blood concentrations in patients showing good response to the drug range from 3 to 15 ng/mL.[6]

References

1. Bresnahan JF, Vliestra RE: Digitalis glycosides. Mayo Clin Proc 1979; 54:675-684.
2. Gilman AG, Goodman LS, Gilman A: The Pharmacologic Basis of Therapeutics, 8th edition, New York, Macmillan, 1990.
3. Goodman LS, Limbird LE, Milinoff PB et al (eds): Goodman & Gilman's The Pharmacologic Basis of Therapeutics, 9th edition, New York, McGraw-Hill, 1996.
4. Kahan BD, Van Buren CT, Lin SN et al: Immunopharmacologic monitoring of cyclosporin A-treated recipients of cadaveric kidney allografts. Transplantation 1982; 34:36-45.
5. Lewis RP: Digitalis. In Leier CV (ed): Cardiotonic Drugs: A Clinical Survey, pp 85-150, New York, Marcel Dekker, 1987.
6. Mandell GL, Bennett JE, Dolin R (eds): Principles and Practice of Infectious Diseases, 4th edition, New York, Churchill Livingstone, 1995.
7. Melmon MF, Morelli HF, Hoffman BB et al (eds): Melmon & Morelli's Clinical Pharmacology: Basic Principles in Therapeutics, 3rd edition, New York, McGraw-Hill, 1992.
8. Meyerburg RJ, Kessler KM, Kiem I et al: Relationship between plasma levels of procainamide suppression of premature ventricular complexes and prevention of recurrent ventricular tachycardia. Circulation 1981; 64:280-290.
9. Moyer TP: Therapeutic Drug Monitoring. In Burtis CA, Ashwood, ER (eds): Tietz Textbook of Clinical Chemistry, 3rd edition, pp 862-905, Philadelphia, WB Saunders, 1999.
10. Rodman JH: Lidocaine. In Evans WE, Schentag JJ, Jusko WJ (eds): Applied Pharmacokinetics: Principles of Therapeutic Drug Monitoring, pp 358-359, San Francisco, Applied Therapeutics, 1980.
11. Rowland M, Tozer TN: Clinical Pharmacokinetics: Concepts and Application, Philadelphia, Lea & Febiger, 1995.
12. Sarubbi FA, Hull JH: Amikacin serum concentrations: prediction of levels and dosage guidelines. Ann Intern Med 1978; 89:612-618; *and* Gentamicin serum concentrations: pharmacokinetic predictions. Ann Intern Med 1976; 85:183-189.

Additional Reading

Drug Monitoring Data Pocket Guide II, Washington, DC, AACC Press, 1994.

Hallworth M, Capps N: Therapeutic Drug Monitoring and Clinical Biochemistry, Washington, DC, AACC Press, 1994.

Koren G: Therapeutic drug monitoring principles in the neonate. Clin Chem 1997; 43:222-227.

Schumacher GE: Therapeutic Drug Monitoring, Stamford, Conn, Appleton & Lange, 1995.

Warner A, Annesley T: Guidelines for the Therapeutic Drug Monitoring Services: National Academy of Clinical Biochemistry, Washington, DC, AACC Press, 1999.

Wong SHY, Sunshine I (eds): Handbook of Analytical Therapeutic Drug Monitoring and Toxicology, Washington, DC, AACC Press, 1997.

CHAPTER 32

Clinical Toxicology

WILLIAM H. PORTER, PhD, and THOMAS P. MOYER, PhD

Objectives

1. Define the following terms:
   Toxicology
   Toxicokinetics
   Toxin
2. State the physiological factors that affect the toxicity of a substance.
3. List two analgesics that are toxic in overdose form, as well as their active metabolites (if applicable), toxic effects, and antidotes.
4. List three alcohols that are toxic in overdose form, as well as their active metabolites (if applicable), toxic effects, and antidotes.
5. Describe the manifestations of barbiturate, carbon monoxide, cyanide, and ethylene glycol intoxication and list appropriate antidotes.
6. List the toxic effects of amphetamine, cannabinoid, cocaine, opiates, phencyclidine, as well as their active metabolites (if applicable) and antidotes.
7. List the toxic effects of overexposure to five metals, including lead, and their antidotes.
8. State the methods of analysis for the toxic drugs, including ancillary drug tests.

Key Words

Amphetamine   A sympathomimetic amine that has a stimulating effect on both the central and peripheral nervous systems

Analgesics   Agents that relieve pain without causing a loss of consciousness

Antihistamines   Antagonists of the H_1 or H_2 histamine receptors that are used to treat allergic reactions

Barbiturate   Any of a class of sedative-hypnotic agents derived from barbituric acid or thiobarbituric acid and classified into long-, intermediate-, short-, and ultrashort-acting classes

Benzodiazepines   Any of a group of minor tranquilizers, having a common molecular structure and similar pharmacologic activity, including antianxiety, sedative, hypnotic, anticonvulsant, and muscle-relaxing effects

Clinical Toxicology   A subdivision of toxicology involving the analysis of drugs, heavy metals, and other chemical agents in body fluids and tissues for the purpose of patient care

Cocaine   A crystalline alkaloid, obtained from leaves of *Erythroxylon coca* (coca leaves) and other species of *Erythroxylon,* or by synthesis from ecgonine or its derivatives; used as a local anesthetic applied topically to mucous membranes; abuse of cocaine or its salts leads to dependence

Confirmatory Test   A second analytical procedure used to identify the presence of a specific drug or metabolite; independent of the initial screening test and uses a different technique and chemical principle from that of the initial test to ensure reliability and accuracy; gas chromatography/mass spectrometry (GC/MS) typically being the confirmation technique of choice

Diuresis   Increased excretion of urine

Ethylene Glycol   An ethylene compound that is a common ingredient in antifreeze and is very toxic if ingested

Forensic Drug Testing   The application of drug testing to questions of law

Half-Life ($t_{1/2}$)   The amount of time taken for one-half an administered drug or toxin to be lost through biological processes

Heavy Metals   Metallic elements with high atomic weights, generally toxic in low concentrations to plant and animal life; often residual in the environment and exhibit biological accumulation; for example, mercury, chromium, cadmium, arsenic, and lead

Illegal Drug   A controlled substance, as specified in Schedules I through V of the Controlled Substances Act, 21 U.S.C. 811, 812, except when used in accordance with terms of a valid prescription or when authorized by law

Intoxication   A state of impaired mental or physical functioning resulting from ingestion of drugs or alcohol

Lysergic Acid Diethylamide (LSD)   A hallucinogenic derivative of an alkaloid found in certain fungi

Marijuana   A crude preparation of the leaves and flowering tops of *Cannabis sativa* (male or female plants), usually used in cigarettes and inhaled as smoke for its euphoric properties

Methadone   A synthetic narcotic, possessing pharmacologic actions similar to those of morphine and heroin and almost equal addiction liability; used as an analgesic and a narcotic abstinence syndrome suppressant in the treatment of heroin addiction

Phencyclidine (PCP)   A potent analgesic and anesthetic used in veterinary medicine, the abuse of which may lead to serious psychological disturbances

Random Testing   An unscheduled, unannounced urine drug testing of randomly selected individuals; uses a process designed to ensure that selections are made in a nondiscriminatory manner

Screening Test   An initial test, such as immunoassay or thin-layer chromatography, that is used to "screen" urine specimens to eliminate "negative" ones from further consideration and identify the presumptively positive specimens that then require confirmation testing

Toxin   A poison, frequently used to refer specifically to a protein produced by some higher plants, certain animals and pathogenic bacteria, which is highly toxic for other living organisms

---

Toxicology is a broad, multidisciplinary science, the goal of which is to determine the effects of chemical agents on living systems. **Clinical toxicology**, a subdivision of toxicology, is the analysis of drugs, heavy metals, and other chemical agents in body fluids and tissues for the purpose of patient care.

■ SPECIFIC DRUGS AND TOXIC AGENTS

The toxic, pharmacologic, biochemical, and analytical characteristics of several individual drugs and **toxins** are discussed in this section.

Agents that Cause Cellular Hypoxia

Carbon monoxide and methemoglobin-forming agents reduce the oxygen supply to tissues to less than physiological levels (cellular hypoxia). Cyanide interferes with oxygen utilization and also causes an apparent cellular hypoxia.

Carbon monoxide

Carbon monoxide is a colorless, odorless, tasteless gas that is a product of incomplete combustion of carbonaceous material. Common exogenous sources of carbon monoxide include cigarette smoke, gasoline engines, and improperly ventilated home-heating units. Small amounts of carbon monoxide are produced endogenously in the metabolic conversion of heme to biliverdin. This endogenous production of carbon monoxide is accelerated in cases of hemolytic anemias.

Toxic effects

Carbon monoxide combines reversibly with hemoglobin to form carboxyhemoglobin. However, the binding affinity of hemoglobin for carbon monoxide is about 250 times greater than that for oxygen. Therefore high concentrations of carboxyhemoglobin limit the oxygen content of blood. Moreover, the binding of carbon monoxide to a hemoglobin subunit increases the oxygen affinity for the remaining subunits in the hemoglobin tetramer. Thus carbon monoxide not only decreases the oxygen content of blood, but also decreases oxygen availability to tissues, thereby producing a greater degree of tissue hypoxia than would an equivalent reduction in oxyhemoglobin caused by hypoxia alone. Carbon monoxide also binds to other heme proteins, such as myoglobin and mitochondrial cytochrome oxidase a_3, which limits oxygen use when tissue PO_2 is very low.

The toxic effects of carbon monoxide are a result of hypoxia. Organs with high oxygen demand, such as the heart and brain, are most sensitive to hypoxia and account for the major clinical sequelae of carbon monoxide poisoning. A general correlation between blood carboxyhemoglobin concentration and clinical symptoms is provided in Table 32-1. However, carboxyhemoglobin concentration does not always correlate with the clinical findings or prognosis. Factors other than carboxyhemoglobin concentration that contribute to toxicity include length of exposure, metabolic activity, and underlying disease, especially cardiac or cerebrovascular disease. Moreover, low carboxyhemoglobin concentrations relative to the severity of poisoning may be observed if the individual was removed from the carbon monoxide-contaminated environment several hours before blood sampling was performed.

An insidious effect of carbon monoxide poisoning is the delayed development of neuropsychiatric sequelae, which may include personality changes, motor disturbances, and memory impairment. These manifestations do not correlate either with the length of exposure or the maximum blood carboxyhemoglobin concentration but are more likely to occur if individuals experienced deep coma.

Treatment for carbon monoxide poisoning involves removal of the individual from the contaminated area and administration of oxygen. The **half-life ($t_{1/2}$)** of carboxyhemoglobin is 5 to 6 hours when the individual breathes room air; it is reduced to about 1.5 hours when the individual breathes 100% oxygen. In severe cases, hyperbaric oxygen treatment at 2 to 3 atmospheres is recommended. In the latter instance the carboxyhemoglobin half-life is reduced to about 25 minutes. Hyperbaric oxygen therapy has been shown to reduce the incidence of neurological manifestations after exposure. Hyperbaric oxygen therapy has been recommended when the carboxyhemoglobin concentration exceeds 25%.

TABLE 32-1	Carboxyhemoglobin Effects	
Carboxy-hemoglobin (%)	Response
10	Shortness of breath on vigorous muscular exertion
20	Shortness of breath on moderate exertion; slight headache
30	Decided headache, irritation, ready fatigue, and disturbance of judgment
40 to 50	Headache, confusion, collapse, and fainting on exertion
60 to 70	Unconsciousness, respiratory failure, and death if exposure is continued
80	Rapid fatality
More than 80	Immediate fatality

From Deichmann WB, Gerarde HW: Symptomatology and Therapy of Toxicological Emergencies, New York, Academic Press, 1964.

Analytical methodology

After it is released from hemoglobin, carbon monoxide is measured directly by gas chromatography (GC) or indirectly as carboxyhemoglobin by spectrophotometry. GC methods are accurate and precise even for very low concentrations of carbon monoxide; in practice, however, they are considered reference methods. The spectrophotometric methods are rapid and convenient, as well as accurate and precise, except at very low concentrations of carboxyhemoglobin (<2% to 3%).

The spectrophotometric methods are based on the characteristic absorption bands of hemoglobin and its derivatives in the visible light region. These bands are utilized to measure carboxyhemoglobin. Oxyhemoglobin and carboxyhemoglobin have similar double bands in alkaline solution. If a weakly alkaline dilution of blood is treated with sodium hydrosulfite, oxyhemoglobin (and any methemoglobin present) is converted to deoxygenated hemoglobin. Carboxyhemoglobin is unaffected by such treatment.

Many spectrophotometric methods are based on automated, multiwavelength measurements of several hemoglobin species. Commercially available co-oximeters perform absorption measurements on blood specimens at several wavelengths and then compute the concentrations of deoxyhemoglobin, oxyhemoglobin, carboxyhemoglobin, and methemoglobin based on a series of matrix coefficients.

Reference values

Reference values for carboxyhemoglobin in nonsmokers who live in rural areas are about 0.5%; for urban nonsmokers, 1% to 2%; and for smokers, 5% to 6%. Values may be increased by about 3% in individuals with hemolytic anemias.

Fetal hemoglobin has slightly different spectral properties than does adult hemoglobin. Consequently, falsely high (by 4% to 7%) carboxyhemoglobin values have occurred when blood from neonates is measured by some spectrophotometric methods. Moreover, erroneous results may occur with lipemic specimens and in the presence of methylene blue (see later section on methemoglobin-forming agents).

Cyanide

Hydrocyanic acid, often referred to as *prussic acid* or as *cyanide* when in the ionized state (CN^-), is a colorless, odorless gas released when any substance containing ionically bound or complexed CN^- is exposed to acid. Burning of urea foam produces formaldehyde and hydrocyanic acid; fires in homes with urea foam insulation represent a significant source of exposure.

Toxic effects

When inhaled, hydrocyanic acid is absorbed rapidly across alveolar capillaries into blood and binds to hemoglobin. Cyanide in serum readily crosses all biological membranes and avidly binds to heme iron in the ferric state

(Fe^{+3}) in the cytochrome $a\text{-}a_3$ complex within mitochondria. When bound to cytochrome $a\text{-}a_3$, CN^- is a competitive inhibitor and causes uncoupling of oxidative phosphorylation. Individuals exposed to toxic levels of CN^- exhibit rapid onset of symptoms typical of cellular hypoxia—flushing, headache, tachypnea, dizziness, and respiratory depression—which progress rapidly to coma, seizure, complete heart block, and death if the dose is sufficiently large. Symptoms are usually dose related and correlate strongly with CN^- concentration. Treatment requires rapid identification of CN^- as the intoxicant, followed by administration of sodium nitrite to cause formation of methemoglobin, which avidly binds and clears CN^-, and thiosulfate (a sulfur donor) to enhance clearance via metabolism.

Cyanide is metabolized by the ubiquitous enzyme rhodanase to thiocyanate (SCN^-), drawing on the body's sulfur-donor pool for substrate to convert CN^- to SCN^-. Thiocyanate is relatively inert and cleared by the kidney. The conversion of CN^- to SCN^- occurs slowly, relative to the pharmacologic action of CN^-, and SCN^- is measured to monitor clearance. However, its measurement is not very useful in assessment of acute CN^- exposure. In a case of acute exposure the individual experiences symptoms of toxicity with high blood CN^- levels, but the serum SCN^- level remains low until 12 to 24 hours later.

Analytical methodology

After microdiffusion, whole-blood CN^- is measured either by photometric analysis or ion-selective electrode analysis.

In one photometric method a sealed, two-well microdiffusion cell is used to separate hydrocyanic acid released from a blood and strong acid mixture in the first well. The hydrocyanic acid gas generated is absorbed into strong base located in the second well of the sealed chamber.[15] The first well of the cell contains the blood specimen and strong acid (unmixed until the cell is sealed), and the other well contains strong base to absorb the hydrocyanic acid gas. After the hydrocyanic acid is collected in the aqueous base medium, pyridine, barbituric acid, and chloramine-T are added to generate a red complex, the intensity of the color of which is proportional to the concentration of CN^-.

Reference values

The normal CN^- concentration is less than 0.2 µg/mL of whole blood because of the presence of CN^- in such foods as dark-green vegetables and nuts that contain cyanogenic glycosides (for example, amygdalin) and the use of tobacco products that contain CN^-. Normal SCN^- concentration in serum is less than 4 µg/mL of serum, but smokers may have serum SCN^- levels as high as 10 µg/mL. Individuals with acute CN^- exposure are likely to have high blood CN^- levels and low serum SCN^- concentrations. The individual is likely to become comatose when the blood CN^- level exceeds 2 µg/mL, and levels greater than 5 µg/mL are lethal. Administration of nitroprusside to control acute hypertension contributes to the total body pool of CN^- and complicates the interpretation of the blood CN^- levels. For example, hypertensive individuals may have blood CN^- concentrations as high as 50 to 100 µg/mL without symptoms of toxicity. Therefore the measurement of SCN^-, rather than CN^-, should be used to monitor nitroprusside therapy.

Methemoglobin-forming agents

The heme iron in hemoglobin is normally in the ferrous state (Fe^{+2}). When oxidized to the ferric state (Fe^{+3}), methemoglobin is formed and this form of hemoglobin does not bind oxygen. The principle physiological system to maintain hemoglobin iron in the reduced state is reduced nicotinamide-adenine dinucleotide (NADH)-methemoglobin reductase (diaphorase I) (Figure 32-1) or reduced nicotinamide-adenine dinucleotide phosphate (NADPH)-methemoglobin reductase (diaphorase II).

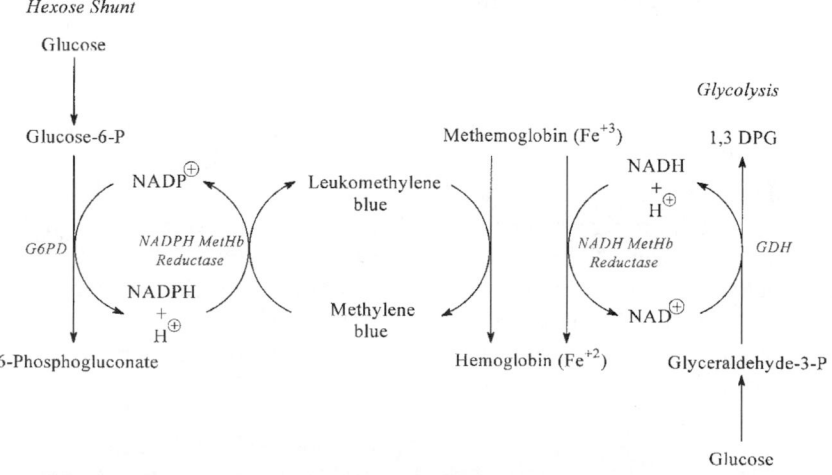

Figure 32-1   Enzymatic pathways for methemoglobin reduction.

TABLE 32-2 Acquired Causes of Methemoglobinemia

Drugs	Chemical Agents
Amyl nitrite	Aniline
Benzocaine	Aniline dyes
Chloroquine	Butyl nitrite
Dapsone	Chlorobenzene
Lidocaine	Nitrates
Nitroglycerin	Nitric oxide
Phenacetin	Nitrites
Phenazopyridine	Nitrophenol
Primaquine	Nitrous oxide
Sulfonamides	

Congenital methemoglobinemia results from a deficiency of NADH methemoglobin reductase or more rarely from hemoglobin variants (hemoglobin M) in which heme iron is both more susceptible to oxidation and more resistant to reduction by the methemoglobin reductase system. More commonly an acquired (toxic) methemoglobinemia may be caused by a number of drugs and chemicals (Table 32-2).

Toxic effects

The toxic effects of methemoglobin are a consequence of hypoxia associated with the diminished O_2 content of the blood and with a decreased O_2 dissociation from hemoglobin species in which some, but not all, subunits contain heme iron in the ferric state (that is, shift of dissociation curve to the left). The PO_2 is normal in these individuals and therefore so is the calculated hemoglobin oxygen saturation. Thus a normal PO_2 in a cyanotic individual is a significant indication for the possible presence of methemoglobinemia. Specific therapy for toxic methemoglobinemia involves the administration of methylene blue.

Analytical methodology

Methemoglobin is measured with a manual spectrophotometric method[7] or by automated multiwavelength measurements with a co-oximeter (see previous section on carbon monoxide). However, methylene blue and sulfhemoglobin cause spectral interference in the measurement of methemoglobin with some co-oximeters but not with the manual spectrophotometric method.

Methemoglobin is not stable at room temperature; therefore specimens should be kept on ice or refrigerated but not frozen. The stability of methemoglobin at 4 °C has not been studied well. Some sources indicate significant decreases in methemoglobin concentrations after 4 to 8 hours, whereas others report little or no change after 24 hours. Freezing results in an increase in methemoglobin concentration.

Reference values

The normal concentration of methemoglobin is less than 1.5% of total hemoglobin. In otherwise healthy individuals,

methemoglobin levels up to 20% cause only cyanosis. Concentrations between 20% and 50% may cause dyspnea, exercise intolerance, fatigue, weakness, and syncope. More severe symptoms of dysrhythmias, seizures, metabolic acidosis, and coma are associated with methemoglobin concentrations of 50% to 70%, and levels greater than 70% may be lethal.

Alcohols

Ethanol is considered the most often used and abused chemical substance. Consequently, the measurement of ethanol is one of the more frequently performed tests in the toxicology laboratory. Although they are encountered less frequently, methanol, isopropanol, and acetone (a metabolite of isopropanol) should be included in a test battery for alcohols for proper evaluation of the acutely intoxicated individual.

Ethanol

The principal pharmacologic action of ethanol is depression of the central nervous system (CNS). The CNS effects vary, depending on the blood ethanol concentration, from euphoria and decreased inhibitions ($\leq$50 mg/dL) to increased disorientation and incoordination (100 to 300 mg/dL) and finally to coma and death (>400mg/dL) (Table 32-3).

A blood alcohol concentration of 100 mg/dL has been established as the statutory limit for operation of a motor vehicle in most states in the United States. This limit is established at 80 mg/dL in 17 states. Not all individuals experience the same degree of CNS dysfunction at similar blood alcohol levels. Moreover, the CNS actions of ethanol are more pronounced when the blood ethanol concentration is increasing (absorptive phase) than when it is declining (elimination phase), partly because of the phenomenon of acute tolerance. In addition, heavy alcohol use leads to a more chronic form of tolerance. When consumed with other CNS-depressant drugs, ethanol exerts a potentiation or synergistic depressant effect. This effect occurs at relatively low alcohol concentrations, and a number of deaths have resulted from combined ethanol and drug ingestion.

Ethanol is metabolized principally by liver alcohol dehydrogenase (ADH) to acetaldehyde, which is oxidized subsequently to acetic acid by aldehyde dehydrogenase. The rate of elimination of ethanol from blood generally approximates a zero-order process. Although this rate varies among individuals, it averages about 15 mg/dL/hour (ranging from 11 to 22 mg/dL/hour) for men and 18 mg/dL/hour (ranging from 11 to 22 mg/dL/hour) for women. At both low (<20 mg/dL) and high (>300 mg/dL) ethanol concentrations the elimination becomes more nearly first-order and is accelerated at high concentrations (for example, ~22 mg/dL/hour at ~300 mg/dL). The elimination rate also is influenced by drinking practice. (For example, alcoholics have average elimination rates of about 30 mg/dL/hour.)

TABLE 32-3	Stages of Acute Alcoholic Influence/Intoxication	
Blood-Alcohol Concentration (g/100 mL)	Stage of Alcoholic Influence	Clinical Signs/Symptoms
0.01 to 0.05	Subclinical	Influence/effects not apparent or obvious; behavior nearly normal by ordinary observation; impairment detectable by special tests
0.03 to 0.12	Euphoria	Mild euphoria, sociability, talkativeness; increased self-confidence; decreased inhibitions; diminution of attention, judgment, and control; some sensory-motor impairment; slowed information processing; loss of efficiency in finer performance tests
0.09 to 0.25	Excitement	Emotional instability; loss of critical judgment; impairment of perception, memory, and comprehension; decreased sensory response; increased reaction time; reduced visual acuity, peripheral vision, and glare recovery; sensory-motor incoordination; impaired balance; drowsiness
0.18 to 0.30	Confusion	Disorientation, mental confusion; dizziness; exaggerated emotional states (fear, rage, grief, etc.); disturbances of vision (diplopia, etc.), perception of color, form, motion, dimensions; increased pain threshold; increased muscular incoordination; staggering gait; slurred speech; apathy, lethargy
0.25 to 0.40	Stupor	General inertia; approaching loss of motor functions; markedly decreased response to stimuli; marked muscular incoordination; inability to stand or walk; vomiting; incontinence of urine and feces; impaired consciousness; sleep or stupor
0.35 to 0.50	Coma	Complete unconsciousness; coma; anesthesia; depressed or abolished reflexes; subnormal temperature; impairment of circulation and respiration; possible death
0.45+	Death	Death from respiratory arrest

Courtesy KM Dubowski, Oklahoma City, 1997.

Methanol

Methanol is used as a solvent in a number of commercial products, as a constituent of antifreeze and window cleaning fluids, and as a component of canned fuel. It has been consumed by alcoholics intentionally as an ethanol substitute or accidentally when present as a contaminant in illegal whisky. Accidental ingestions also have occurred in children.

The CNS effects of methanol are substantially less severe than those of ethanol. Methanol is oxidized by liver ADH (at about one-tenth the rate of ethanol) to formaldehyde. Formaldehyde in turn is oxidized rapidly by aldehyde dehydrogenase to formic acid, which may cause serious acidosis and optic neuropathy, resulting in blindness or death. Serum formate concentrations correlate better with the degree of acidosis and the severity of CNS and ocular toxicity than do serum methanol concentrations. Therefore some toxicologists recommend the measurement of serum formate to assess the severity of toxicity and guide appropriate therapy in cases of methanol ingestion.

Treatment for methanol intoxication may include the administration of ethanol or 4-methylpyrazole to inhibit the metabolism of methanol, sodium bicarbonate therapy to help alleviate the metabolic acidosis, folate administration to enhance folate-mediated metabolism of formate, and the use of hemodialysis to enhance clearance of methanol and formate.

Isopropanol

Isopropanol is available readily to the general population as a 70% aqueous solution for use as rubbing alcohol. It has about twice the CNS-depressant action as ethanol, but it is not as toxic as methanol.

Isopropanol has a short half-life of 3 to 6 hours because it is metabolized rapidly by ADH to acetone, which is eliminated much more slowly (half-life = 22 hours), primarily in alveolar air and urine. Therefore concentrations of acetone in serum often exceed those of isopropanol during the elimination phase after isopropanol ingestion (Figure 32-2). Acetone has CNS-depressant activity similar to that of ethanol, and because of its longer half-life, it prolongs the apparent CNS effects of isopropanol.

Severe isopropanol intoxication, similar to that of ethanol, has resulted in coma or death. Appropriate therapy in such cases includes hemodialysis. The therapeutic administration of ethanol is not indicated for treatment of isopropanol intoxication.

Analysis of alcohols

Similar techniques are used to measure alcohol in blood, serum, saliva, or urine. Determination of ethanol in expired air requires specialized breath alcohol analyzers (see later section on breath alcohol).

Blood alcohol

Suitable specimens for the determination of alcohols are serum, plasma, or whole blood. The venipuncture site should be cleansed with an alcohol-free disinfectant, such as aqueous benzalkonium chloride (Zephiran).

Alcohol distributes into the aqueous compartments of blood, and because the water content of serum (~93%) is

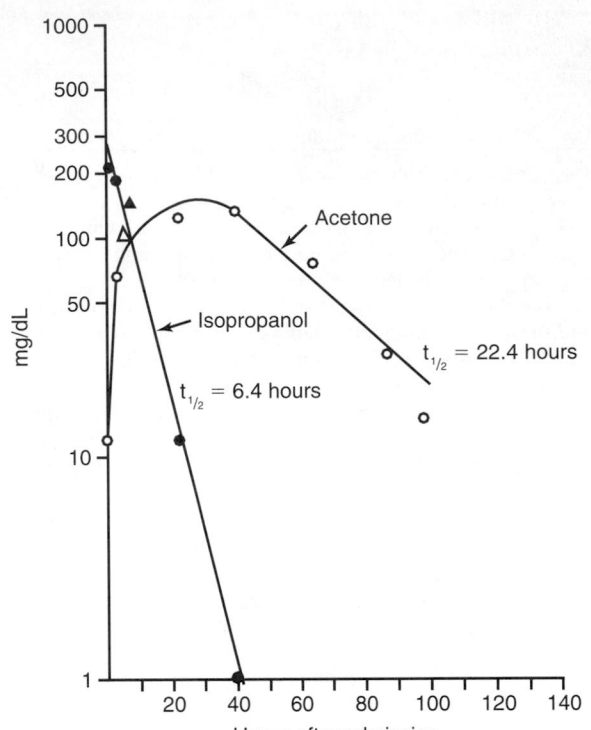

Figure 32-2 Isopropanol and acetone concentrations in serum after an acute overdose of isopropanol. Closed and open circles indicate serum isopropanol and acetone concentrations, respectively. Isopropanol and acetone concentrations in spinal fluid are indicated by closed and open triangles, respectively. $t_{1/2}$, Half-life. (Modified from Natowicz M, Donahue J, Gorman L et al: Pharmacokinetic analysis of a case report of isopropanol intoxication. Clin Chem 1985; 31:326-328.)

greater than that of whole blood (~85%), results indicating higher alcohol levels are obtained with serum. Experimentally, the serum to whole blood ethanol ratio is 1.14 (1.09 to 1.18) and varies slightly with hematocrit. Several states have enacted laws that define **intoxication** during operation of a motor vehicle under the influence of alcohol based on whole-blood ethanol concentrations. Some states do not specify the specimen type. Therefore laboratories that perform alcohol determinations should make clear the choice of specimen.

Because of the volatile nature of alcohols, specimens must be kept capped to avoid evaporative loss to the atmosphere. Blood may be stored, when properly sealed, for 14 days at room temperature or at 4 °C, with or without preservative. For longer storage or for nonsterile postmortem specimens, sodium fluoride should be used as a preservative to prevent a decrease or an occasional increase (via fermentation) in ethanol concentration.

Head-space analysis is used to measure the alcohol content of blood. Enzymatic analysis is used widely to measure ethanol in a variety of body fluids.

Head-space analysis of alcohols. In a closed system, short-chain aliphatic alcohols (ethanol, methanol, isopropanol) and acetone are sufficiently volatile to be present in eas-

ily measurable concentrations in the air space (head space) above a liquid specimen. A portion of this head space is injected into a gas chromatograph for analysis. Head space sampling provides an extremely clean specimen, resulting in prolonged column performance and no clogging of syringe needles.

For the analysis of alcohols in blood or serum, dilutions are made with saturated sodium-chloride containing *n*-propanol as the internal standard. Sodium chloride increases the vapor pressure of the alcohols and eliminates matrix differences between aqueous calibrators and blood or serum specimens. For quantitation the peak height ratio of the analyte alcohol to the internal standard is compared with the ratio for calibrators.

Enzymatic determination of ethanol. To measure ethanol in blood, urine, or saliva, enzymatic analysis is the method of choice for many clinical laboratories. In this method, ethanol is measured by oxidation to acetaldehyde with NAD, a reaction catalyzed by ADH, as follows:

$$\underset{\underset{CH_3}{|}}{CH_2OH} \quad \xrightarrow[\text{NAD}^+ \quad \text{NADH} + H^+]{\textit{Alcohol dehydrogenase}} \quad \underset{\underset{CH_3}{|}}{\overset{O}{\underset{}{H-C}}}$$

Formation of NADH, measured at 340 nm, is proportional to the amount of ethanol in the specimen. The reaction is driven almost completely to the right by use of excess oxidized NAD (NAD^+) and ADH and agents such as semicarbazide or Tris (hydroxymethyl) aminomethane to trap acetaldehyde as it is formed.

Under most assay conditions, ADH is more than 90% specific for ethanol. However, isopropanol, methanol, and ethylene glycol have interferences of 7%, 3%, and 4%, respectively. Reagent kits for use with manual spectrophotometers or automated analyzers are available from several manufacturers.

Serum (or plasma) is the most common specimen for ethanol analysis by ADH methods; the method also performs well with urine or saliva. In some methods, whole blood may be used directly, but in others, a precipitation step may be required before analysis is performed to avoid interference from hemoglobin. These methods generally compare closely with GC methods.

Ethanol measurements have been used in conjunction with the osmolal gap to screen for the possible presence of significant quantities of methanol, isopropanol, or ethylene glycol (see later section on determination of volatiles by serum osmolal gap).

Breath ethanol

Statutory laws for driving under the influence of alcohol originally were based on the measurement of the concentration of ethanol in venous whole blood. Because the collection of blood is invasive and requires intervention by medical personnel, the determination of alcohol in expired air now is the preferred method for evidential alcohol measurements. This method is based on the rapid equilibration of alcohol in capillary alveolar blood with alveolar air in a ratio of approximately 2100:1 (blood to breath). Therefore breath alcohol expressed as g/210 L is approximately equivalent to g/dL of alcohol in whole blood. To alleviate the confusion and uncertainty surrounding the conversion from breath to blood alcohol concentration, the traffic laws in the United States have been amended to read "Alcohol concentration shall mean either grams of alcohol per 100 milliliters of blood or grams per 210 liters of breath." Before breath analysis is performed a waiting period of 15 minutes is required to allow for clearance of any residual alcohol that may have been present in the mouth (for example, very recent drinking, the use of alcohol-containing mouthwash, or vomiting alcohol-rich gastric fluid).

During the period of active alcohol absorption (30 to 120 minutes before peak venous blood alcohol concentration), the alcohol concentration in arterial blood may be higher than that in peripheral venous blood. Consequently, breath alcohol concentration also may be higher than that in venous blood during this absorption phase because end-expiratory air equilibrates with pulmonary arterial blood. The potential consequences of breath alcohol analysis performed during the absorption phase is controversial.

In the interest of public safety the U.S. Department of Transportation (DOT) has mandated breath alcohol testing, in addition to screening for drugs of abuse in urine (see later section on drugs of abuse), for commercial transportation employees.[3,4] If the breath alcohol concentration is between 0.02 and 0.04 g/210 L for duplicate measurements (within 30 minutes), an employee is not allowed to resume safety-sensitive duties for 8 hours (24 hours for motor vehicle drivers); if the concentration is 0.04 g/210 L or greater, the employee is suspended from duty until evaluation by substance abuse professionals has been obtained and appropriate follow-up testing initiated.

Several commercial evidential breath alcohol measurement devices are available. The principle of measurement is either infrared absorption spectrometry (most common), dichromate-sulfuric acid oxidation-reduction (photometric), GC (flame ionization or thermal conductivity detection), electrochemical oxidation (fuel-cell), or metal-oxide semiconductor sensors.

Saliva ethanol

Because saliva may be collected easily and noninvasively, interest is growing in its use for ethanol measurements and for the detection of drugs of abuse (see later section on drugs of abuse). Ethanol distributes between blood and saliva by passive diffusion largely according to the water content of these fluids (85% w/v for whole blood; 99% w/v for saliva). Experimentally the ethanol concentration in saliva is about 9% higher than that in whole blood. The concentration time

profiles for ethanol in blood, breath, and saliva are all similar.

A small test device has been developed to measure ethanol in saliva. Saliva is absorbed onto a swab, which then is inserted into the test cartridge. Ethanol measurement is based on an ADH reaction with visual end-point detection on a thermometer-like scale after a 2-minute incubation.

A test-card device has been developed for the qualitative measurement of ethanol in saliva or urine that is also based on an ADH-mediated detection scheme. This test card is designed to produce a positive response for ethanol concentrations greater than 20 mg/dL.

Urine alcohol

Urine has been used as an alternate, less invasive specimen for the determination of alcohol. During the post absorptive phase after alcohol ingestion, the concentration of alcohol in urine is roughly 1.3 times that in blood. Calculations of blood alcohol concentration from that determined in urine based on this average urine-blood alcohol ratio are admissible in some jurisdictions. However, the use of urine alcohol measurements for this purpose has been questioned because the ratio of 1.3 is highly variable and the urine alcohol concentration represents an average of the blood alcohol concentration during the time period in which urine is collected in the bladder. A better correlation of urine to blood alcohol concentration is obtained by initial emptying of the bladder and subsequent collection of urine 20 to 30 minutes later.

Renewed interest exists in urine alcohol testing in conjunction with testing of urine for drugs of abuse (see later section on drugs of abuse). For this purpose the detection of alcohol in urine represents ingestion of alcohol within the previous 8 hours.

Analgesics

Analgesics are substances that relieve pain without causing a loss of consciousness. When used in excess, analgesics, such as acetaminophen and salicylate, often produce a toxic response.

Acetaminophen

Acetaminophen is the generic name for a common nonprescription medication useful in the treatment of mild pain or fever. It also is known as *paracetamol*.

Toxic effects

When consumed in overdose quantities, acetaminophen may cause severe hepatic toxicity or death. Less frequently, nephrotoxicity also may occur. The initial clinical findings in acetaminophen toxicity are relatively mild and nonspecific (nausea, vomiting, abdominal discomfort) and thus do not predict impending hepatic necrosis, which typically is not evident until 3 to 5 days after ingestion. Although uncom-

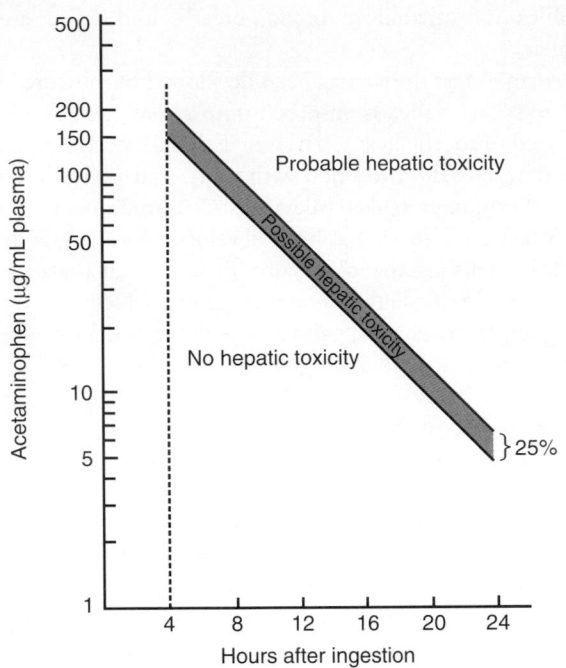

Figure 32-3 Rumack-Matthew nomogram. (Modified from Rumack BH, Matthew H: Acetaminophen poisoning and toxicity. Pediatrics 1975; 55:871-876.)

mon, coma and metabolic acidosis may occur before hepatic necrosis develops. For the more typical presentation the measurement of serum acetaminophen concentration is necessary for proper assessment of the severity of overdose and for determination of appropriate decisions for antidotal therapy (see following text).

A useful nomogram is available that relates serum acetaminophen concentration and time after acute ingestion to the probability of hepatic necrosis (Figure 32-3). However, the following factors must be considered when this nomogram is used:

1. Blood samples should not be obtained earlier than 4 hours after ingestion to ensure that absorption is complete.
2. The nomogram applies only to acute and not to chronic ingestions. Toxicity from chronic ingestion of acetaminophen or other drugs is cumulative and typically occurs at blood concentrations lower than those of acute overdose.
3. The nomogram is not useful if the time of ingestion is unknown (within ±2 hours) or is considered unreliable. In this case, two or more samples taken at 2- to 3-hour intervals may be used to estimate the elimination half-life of acetaminophen. Hepatotoxicity is more probable when the acetaminophen half-life is greater than 4 hours, and hepatic coma is likely when the half-life is more than 12 hours.
4. Serial determination of serum levels (for example, every 2 hours) is warranted if extended-release medication

has been ingested because the time required to reach peak serum concentration may be delayed beyond 4 hours. Serial serum levels also are required when co-ingestion of drugs that may delay gastric emptying (for example, propoxyphene, present in combination with acetaminophen) has occurred. In this case, if the individual's history is known reliably, clinical presentation and/or drug screen results should alert the physician to the need for serial monitoring.

5. Alcoholic individuals, fasting or malnourished individuals, and those individuals undergoing chronic therapy with microsomal enzyme-inducing drugs (anticonvulsants) may exhibit increased susceptibility to acetaminophen hepatotoxicity. In these cases, some physicians recommend that the decision line in the nomogram be lowered by 50% to 70%.

Acetaminophen normally is metabolized in the liver to glucuronide (50% to 60%) and sulfate conjugates (~30%). A smaller amount (~10%) is metabolized by a cytochrome P_{450} mixed-function oxidase pathway that is thought to involve formation of *N*-acetylbenzoquinoneimine, a highly reactive intermediate (Figure 32-4). This intermediate normally undergoes electrophilic conjugation with glutathione and subsequent transformation to cysteine and mercapturic acid conjugates of acetaminophen.

In the case of acetaminophen overdose the sulfation pathway becomes saturated, and consequently a greater portion is metabolized by the P_{450} mixed-function oxidase pathway. When the tissue stores of glutathione become depleted, acylation of cellular molecules by the benzoquinoneimine intermediate leads to hepatic necrosis. Specific therapy for acetaminophen overdose is to administer *N*-acetylcysteine (NAC; Mucomyst), which probably acts as a glutathione substitute. NAC also may provide substrate to replenish hepatic glutathione, enhance sulfate conjugation, or both. The time of administration of NAC is critical. Maximal efficacy is observed when NAC is administered within 8 hours of ingestion, but efficacy then declines sharply between 18 and 24 hours after ingestion. An initial loading dose (140 mg/kg) of NAC should be followed by 17 maintenance doses (70 mg/kg) at 4-hour intervals. If the serum acetaminophen results are not available locally within 8 hours of suspected ingestion, treatment with NAC should begin. This treatment may be discontinued if belated assay results indicate that it is not warranted.

Analytical methodology

Many photometric methods are available for the determination of acetaminophen. Although these methods are relatively easy to perform, they are prone to a number of interferences. Some methods measure the nontoxic metabolites and potentially toxic parent acetaminophen and thus may produce especially misleading results. Therefore only methods specific for parent acetaminophen should be used.

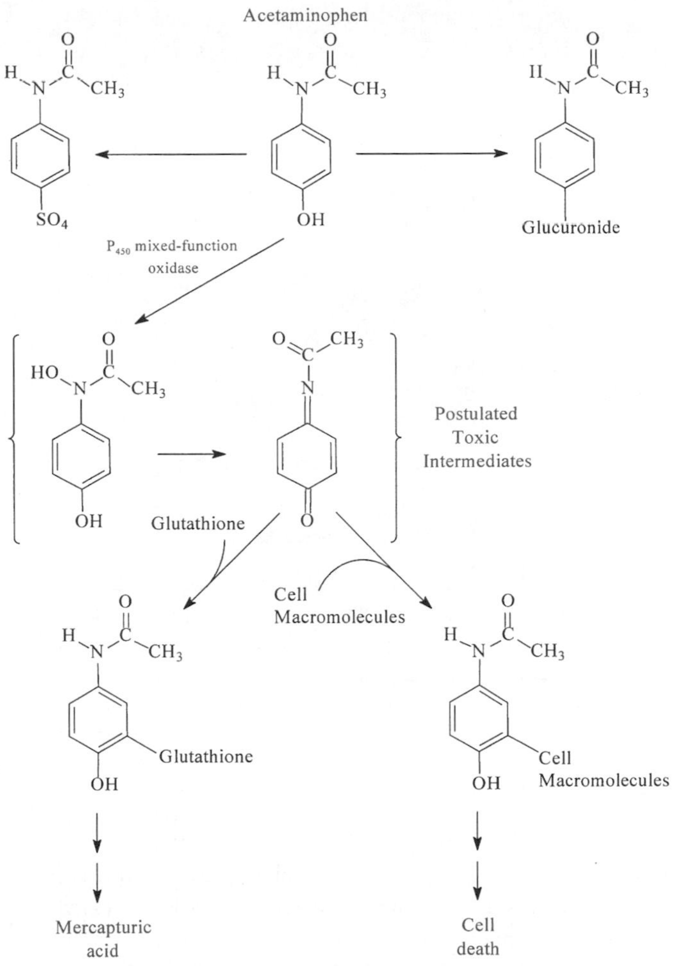

Figure 32-4   Pathways of acetaminophen metabolism. (Modified from Mitchell JR, Thorgeirsson SS, Potter WZ et al: Acetaminophen-induced hepatic injury: protective role of glutathione in man and rationale for therapy. Clin Pharmacol Ther 1974; 16:676.)

Immunoassays for acetaminophen, such as enzyme-multiplied immunoassay technique (EMIT) and fluorescence polarization immunoassay, are used widely because they are rapid, easily performed, and accurate (see Chapter 10). An alternative enzyme assay uses aryl acylamide amidohydrolase for hydrolysis of acetaminophen (but not conjugates) to *p*-aminophenol and acetate. Subsequent color formation depends on reaction of the generated *p*-aminophenol with 8-hydroxyquinoline. Most chromatographic methods are highly accurate and therefore may be considered reference procedures; however, they are more difficult to execute, especially on an emergency basis.

Aspirin (acetylsalicylic acid)

Aspirin (acetylsalicylic acid) has analgesic, antipyretic, and antiinflammatory properties. Because of these therapeutic benefits and the general lack of serious side effects at normal doses, aspirin is available widely and consumed frequently. Therapeutic serum salicylate concentrations are generally

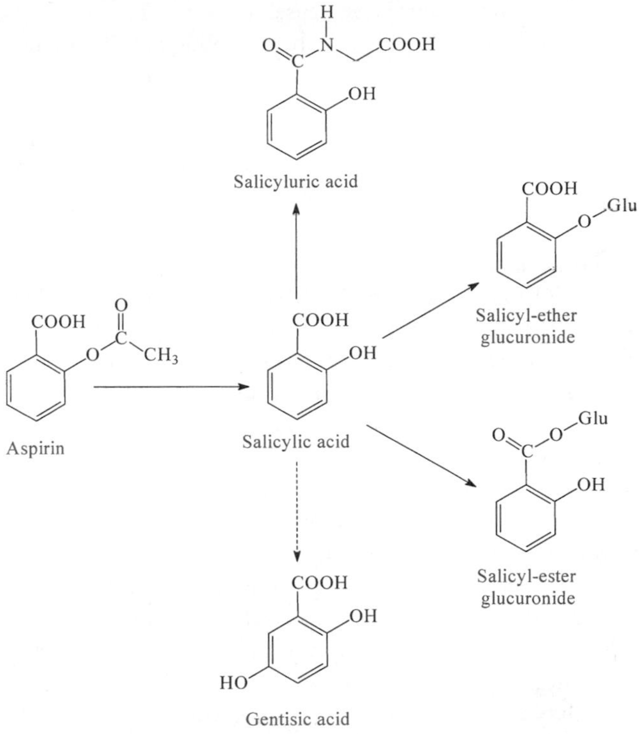

Figure 32-5   Metabolism of aspirin. *Glu*, glucuronide.

lower than 60 mg/L for analgesic-antipyretic effects, and 150 to 300 mg/L for antiinflammatory actions.

The absorption of normal doses of regular aspirin from the gastrointestinal (GI) tract generally is rapid, with peak serum concentration achieved within 2 hours of ingestion. This peak value may be delayed for 12 hours or longer for enteric-coated or slow-release formulations. Moreover, toxic doses of aspirin may produce pylorospasm and thereby delay absorption. Serum salicylate in such instances may not reach maximum concentration for 6 hours or longer, an important consideration when the assessment of the severity of toxicity is based on such measurements.

Once absorbed, aspirin has a very short, 15-minute half-life because it is hydrolyzed rapidly to salicylate. With the exception of irreversible platelet inhibition, the pharmacologic actions of aspirin are due primarily to salicylate. Salicylate is eliminated mainly by conjugation with glycine to form salicyluric acid and to a lesser extent with glucuronic acid to form phenol and acyl glucuronides. A very small amount is hydroxylated to gentisic acid (Figure 32-5). These metabolic pathways may become saturated even at high therapeutic doses. Consequently, the serum salicylate concentration may increase disproportionately with dosage. At high therapeutic or toxic doses, the salicylate elimination half-life is prolonged (15 to 30 hours, versus 2 to 3 hours at low doses), and a much larger portion of the dose is excreted in urine as salicylate.

Salicylates directly stimulate the central respiratory center and thereby cause hyperventilation and respiratory alkalosis. Moreover, salicylates cause uncoupling of oxidative phosphorylation. As a result, heat production (hyperthermia), oxygen consumption, and metabolic rate may be increased. In addition, salicylates enhance anaerobic glycolysis but inhibit Krebs tricarboxylic acid cycle and transaminase enzymes, all of which lead to accumulation of organic acids and thus to metabolic acidosis.

Toxic effects

The primary acid-base disturbance observed with salicylate overdosage depends on age and severity of intoxication. Respiratory alkalosis predominates in children older than 4 years of age and in adults, except in very severe cases that may progress through a mixed respiratory alkalosis-metabolic acidosis to metabolic acidosis. In children under 4 years of age the initial period of respiratory alkalosis is very brief and therefore may not be observed; in such cases, metabolic acidosis predominates. CNS depression is more pronounced when acidemia is severe, a consequence of increased brain uptake of unionized salicylic acid. Respiratory acidosis, a result of severe CNS depression or pulmonary edema, sometimes may occur and indicates a poor prognosis.

The symptoms of salicylate intoxication include tinnitus, diaphoresis, hyperthermia, hyperventilation, nausea, vomiting, and acid-base disturbances. CNS effects include lethargy, disorientation, and in severe cases, coma and seizures. Tinnitus may occur at salicylate concentrations greater than 200 mg/L, but more serious toxic manifestations generally are not evident unless the salicylate concentration exceeds 300 mg/L.

Measurement of serum salicylate concentration is important for assessment of the severity of intoxication. A nomogram that relates serum salicylate concentration and time after ingestion with the severity of intoxication has been developed (Figure 32-6) primarily for use with pediatric patients. The nomogram applies only to acute ingestion of salicylate and should not be used to estimate severity of chronic toxicity. Salicylate absorption may be delayed when overdose quantities are consumed, especially of enteric-coated or slow-release preparations. This instance must be considered in the interpretation of serum salicylate values, especially for specimens obtained earlier than 6 hours after ingestion. Repeat testing within 2 to 3 hours is recommended to ensure that absorption is complete; subsequent testing indicates the effectiveness of therapeutic intervention. The nomogram may be less useful for adults, who tend to have less severe acidemia (mixed respiratory alkalosis-metabolic acidosis) than young children (acidosis). Moreover, interpretation of the nomogram is complicated in instances of mixed drug ingestion. For these reasons, use of the nomogram is discouraged by some toxicologists.

Treatment for salicylate intoxication is directed toward the decrease of further absorption, increase in elimination, and correction of acid-base and electrolyte disturbances. Syrup of ipecac induces vomiting, and activated charcoal

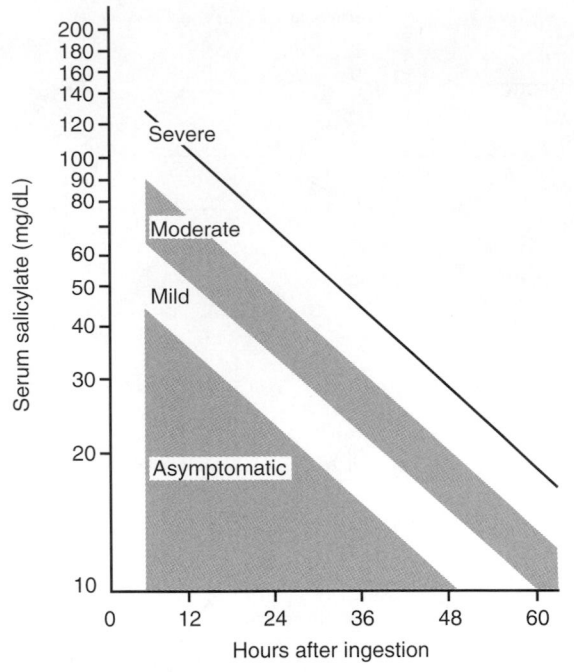

Figure 32-6   Nomogram used to estimate the severity of acute salicylate intoxication. (Modified from Done AK: Salicylate intoxication: significance of measurements of salicylate in blood in cases of acute ingestion. Pediatrics 1960; 26:800.)

binds salicylate and prevents its absorption. Elimination may be enhanced by alkaline **diuresis** and in severe cases by hemodialysis. Sodium bicarbonate may be administered to alleviate metabolic acidosis. Indications for hemodialysis include serum salicylate levels greater than 1000 mg/L, severe CNS depression, intractable metabolic acidosis, hepatic failure with coagulopathy, and renal failure.

Analytical methodology

A urine drug screen may be helpful to recognize the presence of drugs from combination medications with salicylate (for example, antihistamines, sympathomimetic amines, propoxyphene) or that otherwise are coingested with salicylate.

The most popular methods for the measurement of salicylate in serum are based on the photometric method of Trinder. These procedures rely on the reaction between salicylate and Fe^{+3} to form a colored complex that is measured at 540 nm. To lessen endogenous background interference, either a protein precipitation step or serum blank is necessary. Nevertheless, blank readings equivalent to about 20 to 25 mg/L generally are observed. Moreover, interference by endogenous compounds and some drugs—especially structurally related drugs, such as diflunisal (difluorophenyl salicylate)—may occur. Azide, present as a preservative in some commercial control sera, also causes interference. Despite these limitations, photometric methods continue to be used successfully to assess salicylate overdose.

Other methods used for salicylate quantification include fluorescent polarization immunoassay and a salicylate monooxygenase-mediated photometric procedure. These procedures are subject to some of the same interferences as the Trinder method, but the salicylate monooxygenase method is probably more specific. GC and liquid chromatographic methods are the most specific methods for salicylate, but their general availability, especially for emergency use, is limited and probably unnecessary.

Anticholinergic Drugs

Tricyclic antidepressants, the phenothiazines, and the antihistamines have similar toxic effects. These overlapping toxicities likely are related in part to their common methyl or dimethyl-aminoethyl ($-CH_2CH_2N[CH_3]_2$; $-CH_2CH_2NHCH_3$) moieties, which are related structurally to similar groups in acetylcholine ($-CH_2CH_2N[CH_3]_3$) and histamine ($-CH_2CH_2NH_2$).

Tricyclic antidepressants

Tricyclic antidepressants represent a class of drugs widely prescribed for the treatment of endogenous depression (see Chapter 31). Tricyclic antidepressants include imipramine, amitriptyline, and their *N*-demethylated derivatives, desipramine and nortriptyline (Figure 32-7). Other cyclic antidepressant drugs include doxepin, amoxapine, maprotiline, trazodone, and fluoxetine.

Toxic effects

Because of their widespread use, narrow therapeutic range, and the nature of the illness for which they are prescribed most often, tricyclic antidepressants are a frequent culprit in accidental or intentional overdoses, which may be fatal. The clinical features of tricyclic antidepressant overdose are largely extensions of their normal pharmacologic effects and involve principally the CNS, cholinergic nervous system (peripheral and central), and cardiovascular system.

The anticholinergic actions of tricyclic antidepressants are responsible for side effects frequently experienced even at therapeutic doses and therefore are present commonly in cases of overdose. These effects include tachycardia, hyperpyrexia, dilated pupils, dry skin and mouth, flushing, decreased GI motility, and urinary retention.

The CNS manifestations of tricyclic antidepressant overdose may vary from mild agitation or drowsiness to delirium, coma, respiratory depression, or seizures. These manifestations are thought to result in part from central anticholinergic and antihistaminic actions of these drugs.

Cardiovascular toxicity is the most serious manifestation of tricyclic antidepressant overdose and accounts for the majority of fatalities. Tricyclic antidepressants inhibit Na^+ entry via sodium channels in the myocardium, which results in decreased conductivity, decreased contractility, and arrhythmia (quinidine-like effect). In addition, their anticholinergic

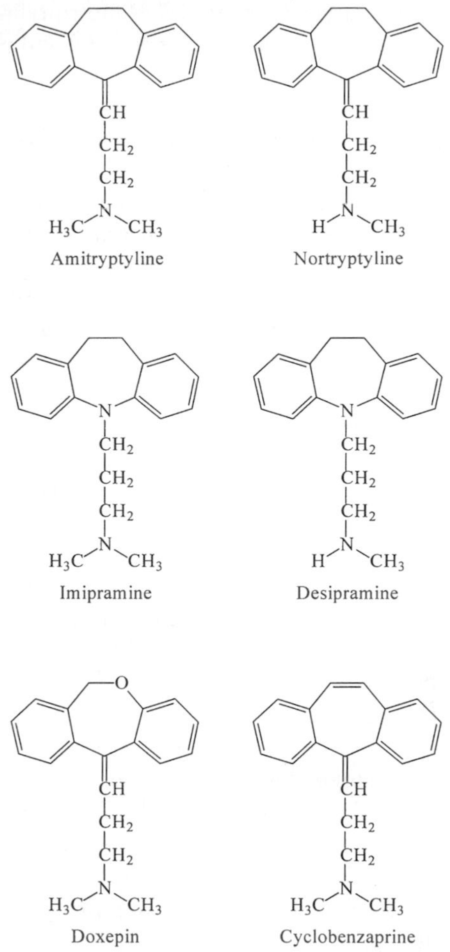

Figure 32-7   Structures of some tricyclic antidepressants and the muscle relaxant, cyclobenzaprine.

and sympathomimetic (inhibition of norepinephrine uptake) effects contribute to dysrhythmias. In situations of mild overdose these effects result in tachycardia and slight increases in blood pressure. With more severe overdose, serious arrhythmias and conduction delays may develop, of which the most distinct feature is prolongation of the QRS interval in the electrocardiogram (see Chapter 33). In addition, cardiac output decreases, which, coupled with peripheral vasodilatation (α_1-adrenergic blockade), leads to life-threatening hypotension. Death often results from arrhythmias or hypotension. The cardiotoxic manifestations may occur within a few hours of overdose, or they may be delayed for 24 hours or longer. An important point to recognize is that a patient's symptomology (perhaps initially only mild anticholinergic effects) is caused by tricyclic antidepressants so that a proper period of monitoring for delayed and possibly catastrophic cardiotoxicity may be followed. Thus laboratory identification of these drugs, especially in the absence of a reliable history, provides crucial information.

Cyclobenzaprine, a tricyclic amine structurally very similar to amitriptyline (see Figure 32-7), is used as a centrally acting skeletal muscle relaxant. Like amitriptyline, cyclobenzaprine causes sedation, produces central and peripheral muscarinic blockade, and potentiates adrenergic actions. In overdose situations, cyclobenzaprine may cause a typical anticholinergic toxidrome and cardiac arrhythmias, hypotension, and coma. However, cyclobenzaprine overdose is not as frequent nor as lethal as amitriptyline overdose.

In addition to general supportive measures (gastric lavage, activated charcoal, intravenous [IV] fluids), therapy for tricyclic antidepressant overdose includes administration of NaHCO₃ for dysrhythmias. (Alkalinization causes tricyclic antidepressants to dissociate from the membrane sodium channels.) Physostigmine, a reversible cholinesterase inhibitor, effectively reverses the central and peripheral anticholinergic manifestations of tricyclic antidepressant toxicity. However, its use generally is contraindicated in cases of tricyclic antidepressant overdose because of the risk that cardiac conduction delays may be enhanced, which can result in asystole. Hemodialysis and hemoperfusion are not beneficial because the tricyclic antidepressant drugs have a large volume of distribution and are bound extensively to plasma proteins.

Analytical methodology

Tricyclic antidepressants are quantified in serum by use of either chromatographic methods (most commonly high-performance liquid chromatography [HPLC]) or immunoassay (EMIT, fluorescence polarization immunoassay; see Chapters 10 and 31). These immunoassays also are used for qualitative or semiquantitative screening for the presence of tricyclic antidepressants. Immunoassays are rapid and relatively easy to perform but may be subject to interference by

other drugs, such as chlorpromazine, thioridazine, cyproheptadine, cyclobenzaprine, and diphenhydramine. Tricyclic antidepressants are detected adequately in urine by use of thin-layer chromatography (TLC) and colloidal gold immunoassay. In cases of overdose, qualitative identification (serum or urine) is sufficient because the severity of intoxication is indicated more reliability by an increase in the QRS interval of an electrocardiogram (>100 ms) than by the serum concentration.

The analytical distinction between amitriptyline and cyclobenzaprine often is difficult. Cyclobenzaprine cross-reacts with immunoassays for tricyclic antidepressants and generally co-elutes with amitriptyline in HPLC and TLC. However, cyclobenzaprine and amitriptyline have different ultraviolet spectra; therefore they may be distinguished by HPLC with a diode array detector. Although these two drugs co-elute using commercial TLC kit methodology, they may be distinguished by differences in fluorescence. (Amitriptyline produces pink fluorescence, whereas cyclobenzaprine fluoresces orange.) Finally, amitriptyline and cyclobenzaprine are resolved by use of capillary column GC and may be distinguished by careful examination of their respective mass spectra.

Phenothiazines

Phenothiazines are tricyclic compounds (see Chapter 31) that have chemical and pharmacologic properties in common with tricyclic antidepressant drugs (Figure 32-8). They are used primarily for their neuroleptic (behavior-modifying) properties in the treatment of severe psychiatric illness (psychoses and mania). In addition, phenothiazines

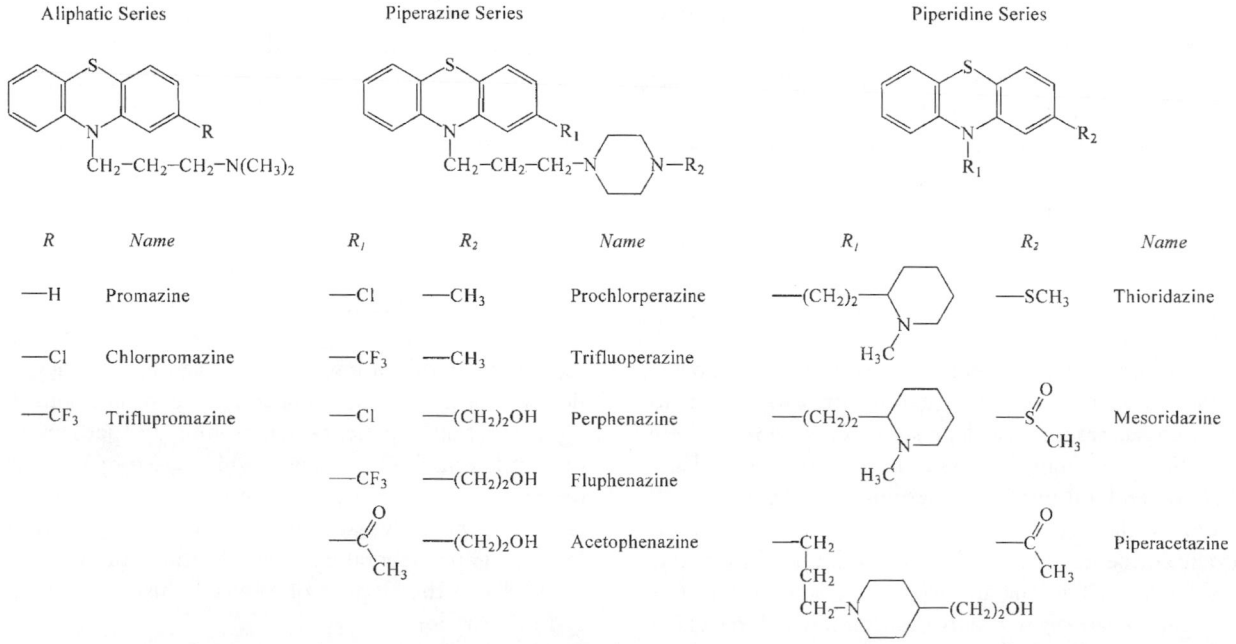

Figure 32-8 Chemical structures of representative phenothiazines.

are administered to control nausea and vomiting, to sedate, and to potentiate analgesia and general anesthesia.

The phenothiazines inhibit dopaminergic receptors in the CNS, a property thought to account for their neuroleptic effect. In addition, phenothiazines inhibit cholinergic, α-adrenergic, histaminic, and serotonergic receptors, which accounts for many of their toxic or undesirable side effects.

Toxic effects

The principle manifestations of phenothiazine toxicity involves the CNS and cardiovascular system. Signs of CNS toxicity include sedation, coma, respiratory depression (uncommon), seizures, hypothermia or hyperthermia, and extrapyramidal movement disorders (acute dystonia, parkinsonism, akathisia, tardive dyskinesia, neuroleptic malignant syndrome); the extrapyramidal symptoms result from an imbalance between inhibitory dopamine and excitatory acetylcholine responses within the extrapyramidal motor system. The cardiovascular effects include orthostatic or frank hypotension and arrhythmias, a consequence of the quinidine-like depressant action on the myocardium and α-adrenergic blockade. Additional peripheral anticholinergic manifestations include decreased bowel sounds, urinary retention, skin flushing, blurred vision, and dry mouth.

The cardiovascular, CNS, and anticholinergic symptoms of phenothiazine toxicity are similar to but generally much less severe than those for the tricyclic antidepressants. Phenothiazines are relatively safe, and few deaths have occurred when individuals have ingested toxic doses alone. A more severe toxicity occurs when phenothiazines are co-ingested with tricyclic antidepressant drugs or other CNS depressant drugs, such as ethanol, opioids, barbiturates, or benzodiazepines.

Therapy for phenothiazines generally is supportive and similar to that for tricyclic antidepressant overdose. Physostigmine reverses the central and peripheral anticholinergic manifestations of phenothiazines; however, physostigmine may cause severe bradycardia or asystole and therefore is not used if cardiac conduction delay is evident. Because of the large volume of distribution and extensive protein binding, hemodialysis and hemoperfusion are not beneficial for phenothiazine overdose.

Analytical methodology

The phenothiazines are metabolized extensively by the liver to a number of metabolites, some of which are pharmacologically active. Less than 1% of a dose is excreted unchanged in the urine. Qualitative detection of phenothiazines or their metabolites in urine is sufficient to document ingestion for symptomatic individuals. Suitable methods of detection include TLC and the spot test, through use of the Forrest reagent (see later section on spot tests). The ability also to detect other co-ingested drugs, such as opioids, tricyclic antidepressants, barbiturates, and benzodiazepines, is important to alert the

physician to the enhanced potential for severe toxicity from the combined ingestion.

Antihistamines

The **antihistamines** (Figure 32-9) are classified as H_1 or H_2 antagonists, based on their principle receptor site binding. The therapeutic actions of H_1 antagonists include smooth muscle relaxation, decreased bronchial secretions, decreased allergic response, and sedation. They therefore are used (1) to treat immediate hypersensitivity reactions, (2) as cold remedies, (3) to suppress motion sickness, and (4) for sedation. (The second-generation H_1 antagonists, [for example, fexofenadine] do not penetrate the blood-brain bar-

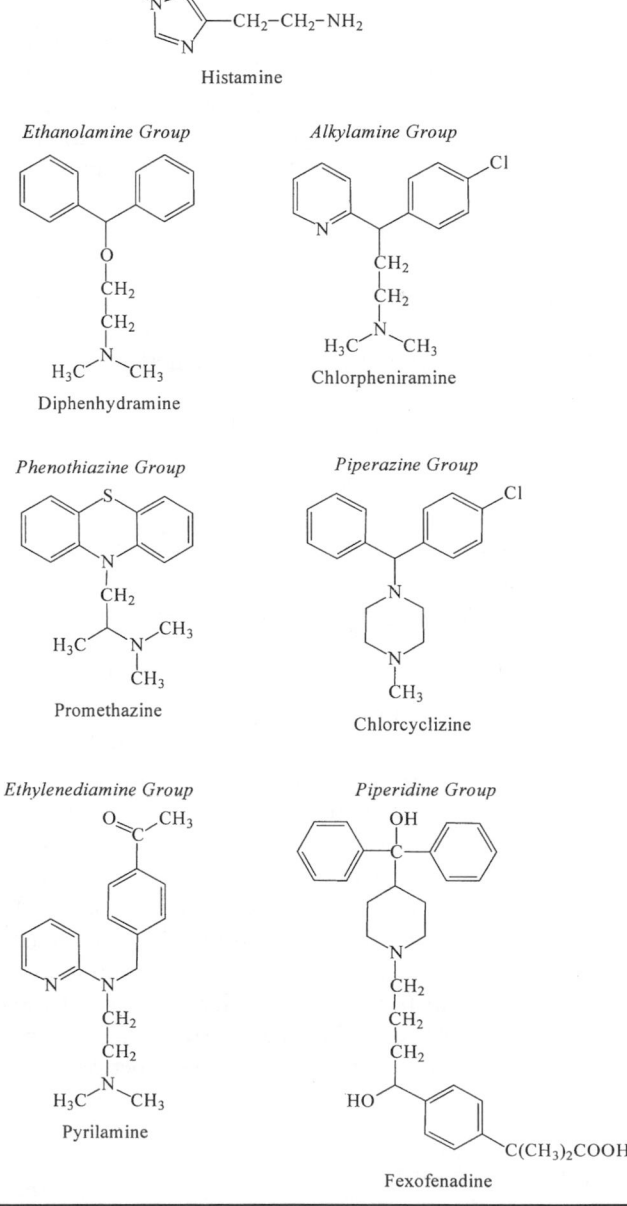

Figurer 32-9 Chemical structures of histamine and representative H_1-antagonists.

rier well and therefore do not cause sedation). The H_2 antagonists are used widely to treat peptic ulcer disease. The most prominent H_2 antagonists are cimetidine (Tagamet), ranitidine (Zantac), and famotidine (Pepcid).

Toxic effects

The principle manifestations of overdose of H_1 antagonists are CNS depression or stimulation and anticholinergic symptoms. Symptoms of CNS depression include sedation, drowsiness, ataxia, and coma. CNS stimulation, more common in children, results in excitement, hallucinations, toxic psychosis, delirium, and convulsions. The anticholinergic toxidrome includes dry mouth, flushed dry skin, urinary retention, sinus tachycardia, dilated pupils, blurred vision, and fever. Death may occur, caused by respiratory depression or cardiovascular collapse.

Treatment for H_1-antagonist overdose is general and supportive (for example, gastric lavage and activated charcoal). Hemodialysis and hemoperfusion are not beneficial because these drugs have a large volume of distribution and are highly protein bound. Physostigmine may be used cautiously if central and peripheral anticholinergic symptoms are prominent and no evidence of cardiac conduction delays exists. (Evidence includes an electrocardiogram or a history or drug screen that provides proof of exposure to drugs that cause conduction delays, such as cocaine, tricyclic antidepressants, phenothiazines, and procainamide.)

Overall the antihistamines are relatively safe. However, their CNS-depressant actions are enhanced by co-ingestion of ethanol, sedative-hypnotic drugs, and opioids; their anticholinergic actions are potentiated by co-ingestion of tricyclic antidepressants and phenothiazines. Therefore the detection of any such drugs in combination on a urine drug screen should alert the physician to a potentially more serious intoxication.

Analytical methodology

Antihistamines are present in prescription and nonprescription forms, alone or in combination with analgesics, such as aspirin and acetaminophen. In instances of overdose a urine drug screen that detects acetaminophen and the antihistamines, plus a spot test for salicylate, is helpful, especially when the source of intoxication is unknown. The detection of either analgesic in the urine of a symptomatic individual should lead to its quantitation in serum to assess its potential toxicity (see previous sections on salicylates and acetaminophen). Quantitation of antihistamines in serum is not useful because a poor correlation exists between dose, drug level, and degree of toxicity.

Other Toxic Agents

Ethylene glycol and organophosphate insecticides are discussed in the following sections.

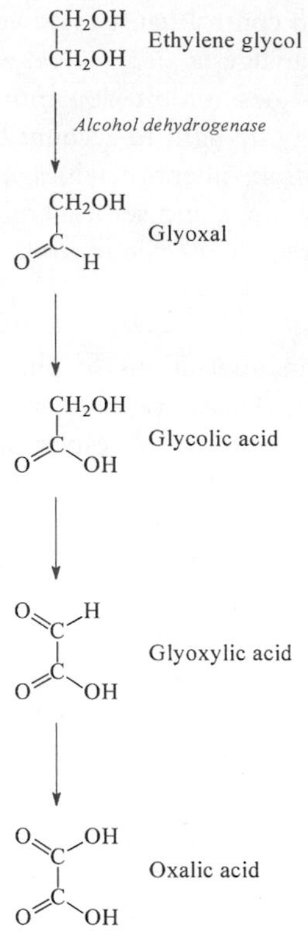

Figure 32-10   Metabolism of ethylene glycol.

Ethylene glycol

Ethylene glycol is present in antifreeze products and is ingested either accidentally or for the purpose of inebriation or suicide.

Toxic effects

Ethylene glycol itself is relatively nontoxic, and its initial CNS effects resemble those of ethanol. However, metabolism of ethylene glycol by ADH results in the formation of a number of acid metabolites, including oxalic acid and glycolic acid (Figure 32-10).

These acid metabolites are responsible for much of the toxicity of ethylene glycol, the clinical manifestations of which include neurological abnormalities (CNS depression; in severe cases, coma and convulsions), severe metabolic acidosis, acute renal failure, and cardiopulmonary failure. The serum concentration of glycolic acid correlates more closely with clinical symptoms and mortality than does the concentration of ethylene glycol. Because of the rapid elimination of ethylene glycol (half-life ~3 hours), its serum concentration may be low or undetectable at a time when that for glycolic acid remains elevated. Thus the determination of both ethylene glycol and glycolic acid provides useful clinical and confirmatory analytical information in cases of ethylene glycol ingestion. Other laboratory findings commonly observed with ethylene glycol poisoning include increased serum osmolal and anion gaps, decreased serum calcium, and the presence of calcium oxalate crystals in the urine. The decreased serum calcium results from calcium oxalate deposition in tissues, from a possible interference in normal parathyroid hormone response, or both.

Appropriate therapy for ethylene glycol intoxication includes administration of ethanol to saturate ADH and thereby inhibit metabolism of ethylene glycol or the administration of the ADH inhibitor, 4-methylpyrazole (Antizol [fomepizole]), aggressive therapy with sodium bicarbonate to help alleviate the acidosis, and hemodialysis or forced diuresis to enhance the removal of ethylene glycol and acid metabolites. A serum ethanol concentration of approximately 100 mg/dL is sufficient to saturate ADH and thus prolong the elimination half-life of ethylene glycol from approximately 3 hours (metabolism and renal excretion) to about 17 hours (renal excretion). Administration of ethanol or 4-methylpyrazole generally is recommended when the serum ethylene glycol concentration is greater than 20 mg/dL. Hemodialysis effectively removes ethylene glycol and glycolic acid and is recommended when the serum ethylene glycol concentration is greater than 50 mg/dL, in cases of severe metabolic acidosis, or in situations of vascular collapse, regardless of the serum ethylene glycol concentration.

Analytical methodology

Ethylene glycol intoxication is relatively rare, but when it does occur, the laboratory must provide rapid analytical support. The measurement of ethylene glycol and glycolic acid is performed best by GC. Ethylene glycol also may be measured rapidly in an enzymatic method with the use of glycerol dehydrogenase, but these methods are subject to interference by glycerol, propylene glycol, 2,3-butanediol, β-hydroxybutyrate, and high concentrations of lactate and lactate dehydrogenase.

Organophosphate and carbamate insecticides

Acetylcholine is an essential neurotransmitter that affects parasympathetic synapses (autonomic and CNS), sympathetic preganglionic synapses, and the neuromuscular junction. Hydrolysis of acetylcholine by acetylcholinesterase, present in nervous tissue, normally limits the duration of action of this neurotransmitter and allows for normal synaptic function. Organophosphate (for example, Malathion, Parathion, Diazinon, Dursban) and carbamate (for example, Sevin, Furadan) insecticides (Figure 32-11) exert their toxicity by inhibiting the action of acetylcholinesterase and thereby causing a pronounced cholinergic response. Enzyme inhibition is the consequence of phosphorylation (organophosphates) or carbamylation (carbamates) of the cholinesterase-active site serine residue. The resulting phosphoryl-serine bond is stable; therefore enzyme inhibition is physiologically irreversible, whereas the carbamyl-serine bond undergoes spontaneous hydrolysis with regeneration of enzyme activity (24 to 48 hours).

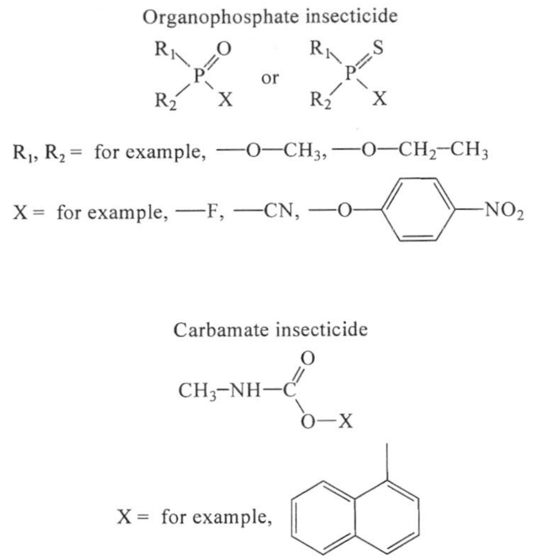

Figure 32-11 General chemical structures for organophosphate and carbamate insecticides.

Toxic effects

By inhibiting the action of acetylcholinesterase, organophosphate and carbamate insecticide poisoning results in the formation of excess acetylcholine. This excess of acetylcholine at the synapses results in the stimulation of muscarinic receptors (peripheral and CNS) and stimulates but then depresses or paralyzes nicotinic receptors. The CNS neurotoxic effects include restlessness, agitation, lethargy, confusion, slurred speech, seizures, coma, cardiorespiratory depression, or death. Stimulation or paralysis of nicotinic receptors at the neuromuscular junction causes muscle fasciculations, cramping, weakness, and respiratory muscle paralysis; stimulation of nicotinic receptors at sympathetic ganglia results in hypertension, tachycardia, pallor, and mydriasis.

Specific therapy for organophosphate and carbamate insecticide poisoning includes the administration of atropine to block the muscarinic (but not nicotinic) actions of acetylcholine. In addition, pralidoxime is administered to reactivate cholinesterase. Pralidoxime binds to the cholinesterase catalytic site and dephosphorylates or decarbamylates the serine group. The administration of pralidoxime may not be necessary in cases of carbamate insecticide poisoning because carbamylated cholinesterase spontaneously reactivates within a few hours. Acetylcholinesterase similar to that in nervous tissue also is present in erythrocytes, and its measurement is useful for the diagnosis of organophosphate or carbamate insecticide poisoning (see Chapter 20). A different cholinesterase, pseudocholinesterase, is present in serum and also is inhibited by these insecticides. The activity of pseudocholinesterase declines and returns to normal more rapidly than that for the red-cell enzyme.

Pseudocholinesterase is synthesized in the liver, and its serum activity is influenced by liver disease and other acute or chronic illness. Thus red-cell cholinesterase activity theoretically should correlate more closely with the degree of neurotoxicity. In cases of acute poisoning, symptoms generally begin when cholinesterase activity is inhibited by about 50% of normal. Moderate toxicity is associated with activities that are 10% to 20% of normal; severe toxicity is likely when activity is suppressed to less than 10% of normal. Interpretation of test results may be difficult because of considerable individual variability of normal levels.

Analytical methodology

Measurement of serum pseudocholinesterase activity is easier to perform than that for red-cell cholinesterase and thus is more likely to be performed in hospital clinical laboratories (see Chapter 20). These measurements are useful for the diagnosis of acute ingestions or for monitoring of chronic exposure. They may be less useful in instances of carbamate insecticide poisoning because of spontaneous enzyme activity regeneration.

Toxic Metals

Several metals are known to be toxic when humans are exposed to elevated levels of them (Table 32-4).[5] They include aluminum, arsenic, cadmium, chromium, cobalt, copper, iron, lead, manganese, mercury, nickel, platinum, selenium, silicon, silver, and thallium. Several of these metals also are considered trace elements, and their biochemistry is discussed in more detail in Chapter 29.

Diagnosis of metal toxicity requires demonstration of all three of the following features:

1. A source of exposure
2. Patient demonstration of the signs and symptoms typical of the metal
3. Abnormal concentration of the metal in the appropriate tissue

TABLE 32-4 Conditions in which Metal Toxicity Is a Causative Factor

Metal	Condition
Aluminum	Dialysis encephalopathy or dementia
Arsenic	Patient report of bilateral pain radiating from foot to leg
Cadmium	Renal disease in aerosol painters
Copper-zinc deficiency	Induced loss of wound healing
Lead	Children under 2 years of age living in older homes
Mercury	Acute changes in behavior
Manganese	Onset of parkinsonism under 50 years of age
Selenium (deficiency)	Patients undergoing total parenteral nutrition
Thallium	Acute hair loss
Zinc (deficiency)	Burn patients exhibiting erythema

Aluminum

Aluminum (Al) is an extremely light and versatile metal with many applications. Pharmacologically, aluminum compounds are used chiefly for their antacid and astringent properties. Under normal physiological conditions, the usual daily dietary intake of aluminum is 5 to 10 mg. This amount is filtered efficiently from the blood by the glomerulus of the kidney and eliminated completely. Individuals in renal failure lose this ability and become candidates for aluminum toxicity, especially when they undergo dialysis treatment. The use of dialysis fluid that contains aluminum further increases the aluminum burden of the patient receiving dialysis. In addition, a common practice is to administer aluminum-based gels orally to patients in renal failure to reduce the amount of phosphate absorbed from their diet and thus avoid excessive phosphate accumulation. Consequently, individuals in renal failure accumulate this aluminum. After dialysis treatment, albumin may be administered to replace that which is removed during dialysis. Some albumin products have high aluminum content. Efforts to reduce aluminum intake include the switch from aluminum-containing phosphate binders to calcium-containing phosphate binders, ensuring that dialysis water contains less than 10 μg/L of aluminum and that the albumin used during postdialysis therapy is aluminum free.

At higher levels of intake or in cases of renal malfunction, aluminum accumulates in the blood, where it binds avidly to proteins, such as albumin. It then is distributed rapidly throughout the body. Aluminum overload leads to the accumulation of aluminum at two significant sites—in bone and in the brain. In bone, aluminum replaces calcium at the mineralization front, disrupting normal osteoid formation. This occurrence is visualized readily histologically by use of Goldner's stain. Deposition of aluminum in bone also interrupts normal calcium exchange; the calcium in bone becomes unavailable for resorption back into blood under the physiological control of parathyroid hormone (PTH). This unavailability causes an abnormal physiological response by the parathyroid gland that results in an unusual biochemical profile that is virtually diagnostic of aluminum overload disease. However, the definitive test for aluminum-related bone disease is bone histomorphometry with special staining for aluminum.

In individuals with aluminum overload or renal failure, serum aluminum levels exceed 6 μg/L. In studies, those individuals with no signs or symptoms of osteomalacia or encephalopathy usually had serum aluminum levels lower than 60 μg/L and immunoreactive C-terminal PTH (icPTH) levels greater than 5 pmol/mL, which is typical of secondary hyperparathyroidism; individuals with signs and symptoms of osteomalacia or encephalopathy had serum aluminum levels greater than 100 μg/L and icPTH levels lower than 5 pmol/mL. Patients with serum aluminum levels greater than 60 μg/L but less than 100 μg/L were identified as candidates for possible onset of aluminum overload. This condition requires aggressive efforts to reduce daily aluminum exposure. A graphical presentation of these situations is presented in Figure 32-12.

Specimens for serum aluminum analysis must be collected carefully to avoid aluminum contamination. For example, many of the common evacuated blood-collection devices used in phlebotomy have rubber stoppers made of aluminum silicate. Simple puncture of the rubber stopper for blood collection is sufficient to contaminate the sample with aluminum sufficient to produce an abnormal concentration of aluminum. Typically, blood collected in standard evacuated blood tubes is contaminated by 20 to 60 µg/L of aluminum. Special evacuated blood-collection tubes are available and should be used for aluminum testing.[11]

Arsenic

Arsenic (As) is considered a **heavy metal** toxin and also is one of the more common toxicants found in insecticides.

Arsenic exists in a number of different forms (Figure 32-13). Some forms are toxic, whereas others are not. The toxic forms are the inorganic species As^{+3} (also denoted as As[III]), As^{+5} (As[V]), and their partially detoxified metabolites, monomethylarsine (MMA) and dimethylarsine (DMA). As^{+3} is more toxic than As^{+5}. Detoxification occurs as As^{+3} is oxidized to As^{+5} and then methylated by the liver to MMA and DMA. As a result of these detoxification steps, As^{+3} and As^{+5} are found in the urine shortly after ingestion, whereas MMA and DMA are the species that predominate more than 24 hours after ingestion. Urinary As^{+3} and As^{+5} levels peak at approximately 10 hours and return to normal 20 to 30 hours after ingestion. Urinary MMA and DMA levels normally peak at about 40 to 60 hours and return to baseline 6 to 20 days after ingestion. The blood half-life of inorganic arsenic is 4 to 6 hours, and the blood half-life of the methylated metabolites is 20 to 30 hours. Serum levels of arsenic are elevated for only a short time after administration, after which arsenic rapidly disappears into the large body phosphate pool. Abnormal serum arsenic levels are detected for only a few hours (<4 hours) after ingestion.

Nontoxic organic forms of arsenic are present in many foods, with arsenobetaine and arsenocholine being two most common forms. The foods that most commonly contain significant concentrations of organic arsenic are shellfish and other predators in the seafood chain, such as cod and haddock. The rate of arsenic excretion in normal individuals is 0 to 120 µg per 24-hour urine specimen. After ingestion, arsenobetaine and arsenocholine undergo rapid renal clearance to become concentrated in the urine. Organic arsenic is excreted completely within 1 to 2 days after ingestion, and no residual toxic metabolites remain. The apparent half-life of organic arsenic is 4 to 6 hours. Consumption of seafood before collection of a urine sample for arsenic testing is likely to result in an elevation of the concentration of arsenic reported in the urine. This elevation interferes with clinical interpretation. The toxic inorganic and nontoxic organic species of arsenic of seafood origin are separated with HPLC.[13]

The toxicity of arsenic is due to three different mechanisms, two of which are related to energy transfer. Arsenic avidly binds to dihydrolipoic acid, a necessary cofactor for pyruvate dehydrogenase. Absence of the cofactor inhibits the conversion of pyruvate to acetyl coenzyme A (CoA), the first step in gluconeogenesis. Arsenic also competes with phosphate for reaction with adenosine diphosphate (ADP), resulting in formation of the lower energy ADP-arsenate rather than adenosine triphosphate (ATP). Arsenic also binds with any hydrated sulfhydryl group on protein, distorting the three-dimensional configuration of the protein and thus causing it to lose activity. Arsenic also is a known carcinogen, but the mechanism of this effect is not definitively known. British antilewisite (BAL) is an effective antidote for treatment of arsenic intoxication; the active agent in BAL is dimercaprol, a sulfhydryl-reducing agent. This fact suggests that the primary mechanism of action of arsenic's toxicity is related to sulfhydryl binding. Arsenic also

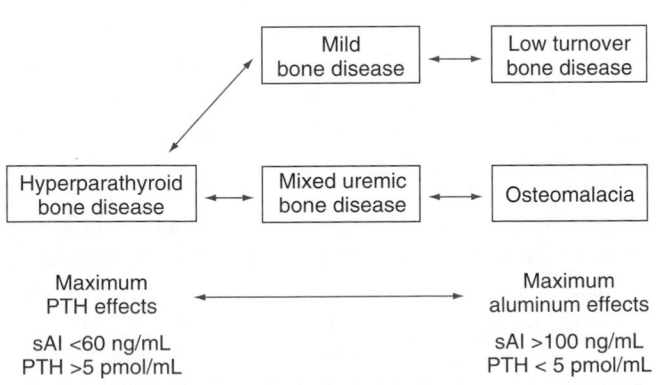

Figure 32-12 Aluminum's effect on bone physiology. *sAl,* Concentration of serum aluminum.

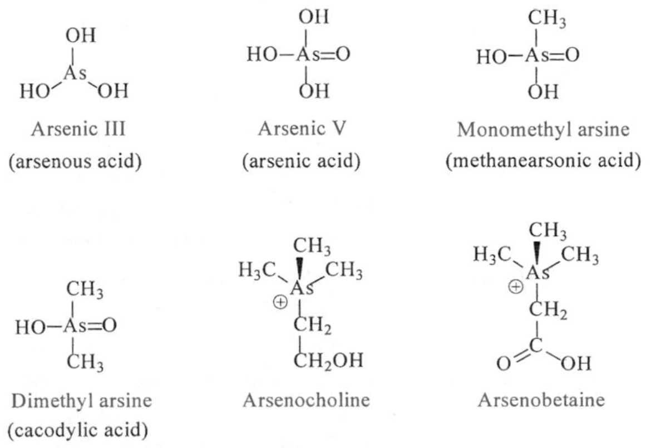

Figure 32-13 Structures of arsenic species.

interferes with the activity of several enzymes of the heme biosynthetic pathway.

Hair analysis is used frequently to document time of arsenic exposure. Arsenic circulating in the blood binds to protein by formation of a covalent complex with sulfhydryl groups of the amino acid cysteine. Because arsenic has a high affinity for hair keratin, which has high cysteine content, the concentration of arsenic in hair or nails is higher than in other tissues. Several weeks after exposure, transverse white striae, called "Mees' lines," may appear in the fingernails; this condition is caused by denaturation of keratin by heavy metals, such as arsenic, cadmium, lead, and mercury. Because hair grows at a rate of approximately 0.5 cm/month, hair collected from the nape of the neck can be used to document recent exposure. Axillary or pubic hair is used to document long-term exposure (6 months to 1 year). Hair arsenic greater than 1 µg/g of dry weight indicates excessive exposure. The highest hair arsenic observed by this chapter's author was 210 µg/g of dry weight in a case of chronic exposure that caused death.

Serum is not a useful specimen for identification of arsenic exposure because serum levels are elevated for only a short time after administration, after which arsenic is bound to protein and disappears rapidly into the large body phosphate pool. The body treats arsenic as it does phosphate, incorporating it wherever phosphate is incorporated. Absorbed arsenic is circulated rapidly and distributed into tissue storage sites. Abnormal serum arsenic levels are detected for only a few hours (<4 hours) after ingestion. This test is useful only during an acute event, when the arsenic is likely to exceed 100 ng/mL for a short period of time. Normally, serum arsenic is less than 35 ng/mL.

Cadmium

Cadmium (Cd) is obtained as a byproduct of zinc and lead smelting. It is used for industrial purposes in electroplating, in the production of nickel-based rechargeable batteries, and as a common pigment in organic-based paints; tobacco products also contain cadmium. A common source of chronic exposure is spray painting of organic-based paints without the use of a protective breathing apparatus. Auto-repair mechanics represent one group that has significant opportunity for exposure to cadmium.

Renal dysfunction with proteinuria of slow onset (over a period of years) is the typical presentation of cadmium toxicity. Chronic exposure to cadmium causes accumulated renal damage. Breathing the fumes of cadmium vapors leads to nasal epithelial deterioration and pulmonary congestion resembling chronic emphysema. Cadmium toxicity is expressed via formation of protein-Cd adducts that change the conformational structure of the protein, causing it to denature. This protein denaturation occurs in the alveoli if exposure is due to dust inhalation or in the proximal tubule of the kidney, which is a major route of excretion.

In 1992 the National Institute of Occupational Safety and Health (NIOSH) mandated that employees exposed to cadmium in the workplace be monitored by measurement of urine cadmium and creatinine and expression of the results of µg of cadmium per gram of creatinine.[14] Cadmium excretion greater than 3 µg Cd/g of creatinine indicates significant exposure to cadmium. Concentration exceeding 15 µg Cd/g of creatinine is considered indicative of severe exposure. Urine cadmium is a more specific measure of cadmium exposure than are other markers of renal function, such as β_2-microglobulin, retinol-binding protein, or N-acetyl glucosaminidase.

Normal blood cadmium level is less than 5 ng/mL, with most levels being in the interval of 0.5 to 2 ng/mL. Acute toxicity is observed when the blood level exceeds 50 ng/mL. Usual excretion of cadmium is less than 3 µg/day. Collection of urine samples with a rubber catheter has resulted in elevated results because rubber contains trace amounts of cadmium that are extracted as urine passes through it. Brightly colored plastic urine-collection containers should be avoided because the pigment in the plastic may be cadmium-based. Cadmium levels also increase with age, which may play a role in senescence.

Chromium

Occupational exposure to chromium (Cr) represents a significant health hazard. Chromium is used extensively in the manufacture of stainless steel, in chrome plating, in the tanning of leather, as a dye for printing and textile manufacture, as a cleaning solution, and as an anticorrosive in cooling systems. The toxic form is Cr^{+6} (Cr[VI]), which is quite rare; a strong oxidizing environment is required to convert the common form, Cr^{+3} (Cr[III]), to Cr^{+6}. These environments include high temperatures in the presence of oxygen or high-voltage electroplating. Inhalation of the vapors of Cr^{+6} causes erosion of the epithelium of the nasal passages and squamous-cell carcinomas of the lung. Cr^{+6} is very lipid soluble and crosses cell membranes readily, whereas Cr^{+3} is rather insoluble and does not cross membranes readily. The instant Cr^{+6} enters a cell, it is reduced to Cr^{+3}, which has no known toxicity. Thus monitoring biological specimens for Cr^{+6} is neither practical nor clinically useful to detect chromium toxicity. Rather, monitoring the air at the manufacturing site for Cr^{+6} is the usual way to test for Cr^{+6} exposure. However, measurement of total chromium in urine has been used to assess chromium exposure.

Cobalt

Cobalt (Co) is found in pigments and in metal alloys that are very hard, have high melting points, and are resistant to oxidation. Occupational exposure occurs during production and machining of these metal alloys and has lead to interstitial lung disease. Cardiomyopathy and renal failure are symptomatic of acute cobalt exposure. Measurement of urinary cobalt is an effective means by which to identify individuals with excessive exposure.

Copper

Excessive ingestion of copper (Cu) has been known to result in significant toxicity. It is used in pesticides, marine antifouling paints, and wood preservatives. Green "treated" wood contains high concentrations of copper and arsenic. Ingestion of either source produces severe GI upset with severe irritation of the epithelial layer of the GI tract, hemolytic anemia, centrilobular hepatitis with jaundice, and renal damage. Excess copper ingestion interferes with absorption of zinc and can lead to zinc deficiency typified by slow healing. The classic presentation of copper toxicosis is represented by the genetic disease of copper accumulation known as *Wilson's disease*. This disease is typified by hepatocellular damage (increased transferases) and/or changes in mood and behavior due to accumulation of copper in central neurons.

Iron

Acute iron (Fe) intoxication occurs most often accidentally in children, and severe intoxication has caused significant morbidity or death. The limited physiological regulation of iron absorption from the GI tract may become overwhelmed with acute ingestion of large doses of iron. Acute ingestion of more than 0.5 g of iron produces severe irritation of the epithelial lining of the GI tract and results in hemosiderosis, which may develop into hepatic cirrhosis. The presence of excessive amounts of iron in serum *and* urine supports this diagnosis.

In such instances the likelihood of iron toxicity is enhanced because no specific mechanisms exist for iron elimination. When the concentration of iron exceeds the iron-binding capacity of serum, unbound iron accumulates and may cause toxicity. The initial toxic effects on the GI tract are a result of a direct corrosive action of iron on the mucosa, which may cause mucosal edema, infarction, ulceration, or hemorrhage. As a result, clinical symptoms of nausea, vomiting, abdominal pain, diarrhea, hematemesis, and melena may be evident. The systemic actions of excess unbound iron affect the cardiovascular system, general metabolic functions, the liver, and the CNS. The cardiovascular effects of iron toxicity include decreased cardiac output, venous pooling of blood, and capillary leakage, all of which may lead to hypotension, shock, cyanosis, lethargy, tachycardia, and lactic acidosis. Within the liver, excess iron may cause swelling or necrosis of hepatocytes, resulting in abnormal liver function tests and a coagulopathy. Moreover, iron may accumulate within hepatic mitochondria and promote oxygen free radical formation, lipid peroxidation of mitochondrial membranes, and interference with the electron transport system. Consequently, dysfunction of the Krebs cycle and oxidative phosphorylation lead to metabolic acidosis and secondarily cause hyperglycemia. The effects on the CNS range from lethargy and obtundation to frank coma. These effects may be secondary to cardiovascular, hepatic, and metabolic toxicity and to a direct CNS action of iron.

Specific treatment for iron toxicity involves administration of deferoxamine to chelate unbound iron. The deferoxamine-Fe complex then is excreted in the urine, often resulting in a characteristic rose color. The decision to administer deferoxamine is based on the history, clinical symptoms, and measurement of serum iron. In general, only mild toxicity is evident when the serum iron is below 300 μg/dL, and deferoxamine administration normally is not necessary. When the serum iron reaches 500 μg/dL, serious toxicity is likely and may be fatal at concentrations of 1000 μg/dL or greater. Serum iron should be measured on admission and again 4 to 6 hours after ingestion, when absorption should be complete and the maximum serum level obtained.

Iron toxicity is more likely to occur when the total serum iron concentration exceeds the total iron-binding capacity (TIBC; see Chapter 30). However, measurement of TIBC is not practical because of methodological limitations. Because these limitations do not apply to the measurement of the unbound iron-binding capacity (UIBC), this test should be performed in cases of suspected iron intoxication. An elevated total serum iron and a very low or unmeasurable UIBC indicate potential iron toxicity.

Deferoxamine interferes with photometric measurements of iron and UIBC, an important consideration if serum iron and UIBC measurements are used to monitor therapy with deferoxamine. Deferoxamine has a short half-life (half-life ~1 hour); therefore a delay of at least 2 to 3 hours after deferoxamine administration is appropriate before measurements of serum iron and UIBC are repeated.

Lead

Lead (Pb) is a heavy metal commonly found in the environment. It is both an acute and chronic toxin. Exposure to lead by ingestion, inhalation, or dermal contact causes significant toxicity. Lead is present at high concentration (up to 35% w/w) in many paints manufactured before 1970. The lead content of paints intended for household use was limited to less than 0.5% in 1972, but lead still is found in paint products intended for nondomestic use and in artists' pigments. Occasionally ceramic products for use in homes, such as dishes or bowls, available from noncommercial suppliers (such as local artists) have been found to contain significant amounts of lead. Such lead has been found to leach from the ceramic by weak acids, such as vinegar and fruit juices. Leaded crystal contains up to 10% lead, which has been found to leach during long-term storage of acidic fluids, such as fruit juice. Lead also is found in dirt from areas adjacent to homes painted with lead-based paints and on highways where it has accumulated from the use of leaded gasoline in automobiles. Use of leaded gasoline has diminished significantly since the introduction of unleaded gasoline, which has been required in personal automobiles in the United States since 1978. In addition, lead is found in soil near abandoned industrial sites where lead may have been used. Water transported through lead or lead-soldered pipe contains some lead, with higher concentrations found in water that is weakly acidic. Some foods (for example, moonshine distilled in lead pipes) and some traditional home medicines also contain lead.

A typical diet in the United States contributes approximately 300 μg of lead per day, of which 1% to 10% is absorbed; children may absorb as much as 50% of the dietary intake, and the fraction of lead absorbed is enhanced by nutritional deficiency. The majority of the daily intake is excreted in the stool after direct passage through the GI tract. Although a significant fraction of the absorbed lead is incorporated rapidly into bone and erythrocytes, lead is distributed ultimately among all tissues. Lipid-dense tissues, such as those in the CNS, are particularly sensitive to organic forms of lead. All lead absorbed is excreted ultimately in bile or urine. Soft-tissue turnover of lead occurs within approximately 120 days.

Lead expresses its toxicity by several mechanisms (Figure 32-14). It avidly inhibits porphobilinogen (PBG) synthase, an enzyme necessary for heme synthesis, and a reductase, a heme-synthesis enzyme necessary to produce Fe^{2+}. Inhibition of the reductase causes accumulation of protoporphyrin in erythrocytes (see Chapter 30), which is a significant marker for lead exposure. Anemia due to lack of heme is observed frequently in cases of lead toxicity. Lead also is an electrophile that avidly forms covalent bonds with the sulfhydryl group of cysteine in proteins. Thus proteins in all tissues exposed to lead have lead bound to them. Keratin in hair contains a high fraction of cysteine relative to other amino acids and avidly binds lead; hair analysis for lead is a good marker for exposure. Some proteins become labile as lead binds with them because lead causes the tertiary structure of the protein to change; cells of the nervous system are particularly susceptible to this effect. Some lead-bound proteins change their tertiary configurations sufficiently so that

they become antigenic; renal tubular cells are particularly susceptible to this effect because they are exposed to relatively high lead concentrations during clearance.

The development of lead toxicity follows a progressive pattern. Figure 32-15 illustrates this progression through a series of symptoms. In children, lead poisoning has been found to contribute significantly to decreased intellectual capability. Young children are particularly prone to the toxic effects of lead because they have greater opportunity for exposure. In older homes that have been treated previously with lead-based paints, lead-laden paint chips and dust accumulate on the floor where children are likely to pick them up and put them in their mouths.

Whole-blood lead measurement has been declared the best test for detection of lead exposure by the Centers for Disease Control and Prevention (CDC).[16] Whole-blood lead levels lower than 10 μg/dL are considered normal in

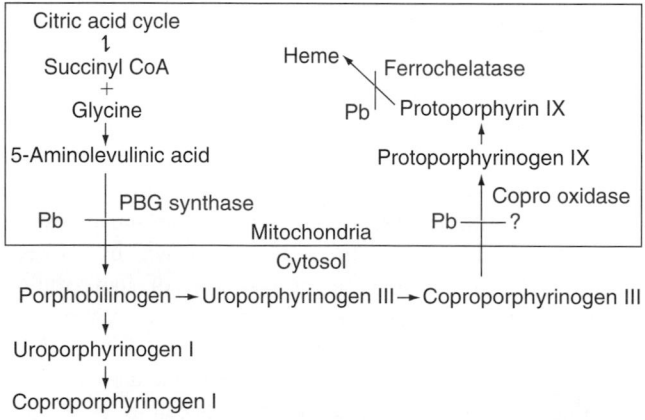

Figure 32-14 Erythropoietic effects of lead. *Pb*, Lead; *CoA*, coenzyme A; *PBG*, porphobilinogen.

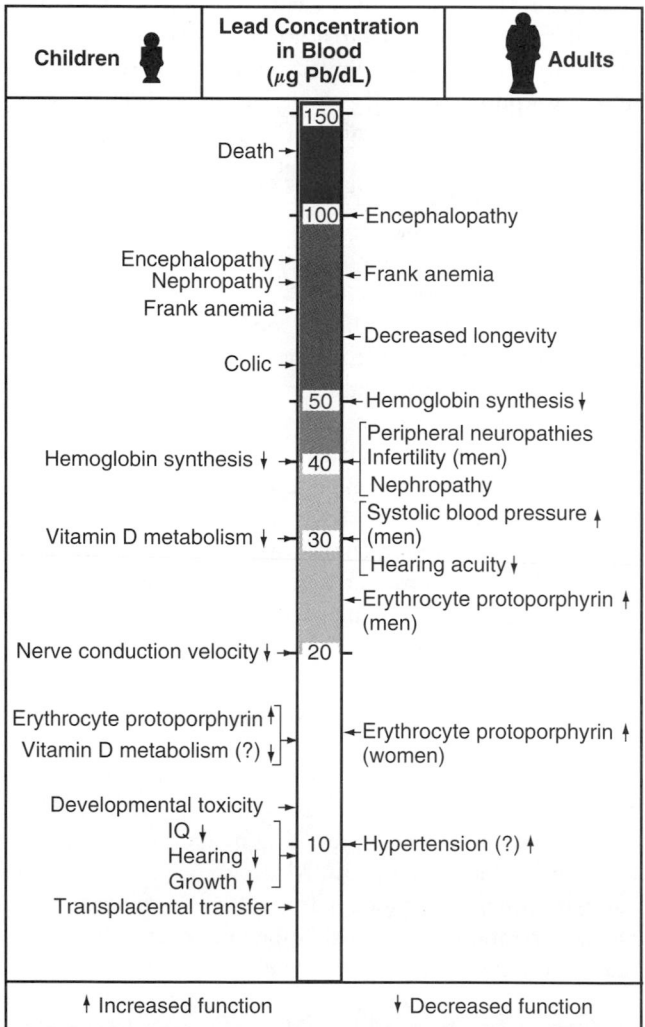

Figure 32-15 Effects of inorganic lead on children and adults (lowest observable adverse effect levels). (Modified from Royce SE, Needleman HL (eds): Case Studies in Environmental Medicine: Lead Toxicity. U.S. Public Health Service, ATSDR, 1990.)

children. The World Health Organization (WHO) has defined whole-blood lead levels greater than 30 μg/dL in adults as indicative of significant exposure. Lead levels greater than 60 μg/dL require chelation therapy.

Erythrocyte protoporphyrin levels are not a sensitive indicator of low-level lead exposure but are definitive markers for lead overdose; an erythrocyte protoporphyrin level greater than 60 μg/dL is a significant indicator of lead exposure. Serum PBG synthase levels also are useful indicators of medium to high levels of lead exposure; however, they do not correlate with low levels of lead exposure. Serum lead analysis is of very limited utility because serum lead levels are abnormal only for a short period of time after exposure. Normally, the hair lead content is lower than 5 μg/g; hair lead concentration greater than 25 μg/g indicates severe lead exposure. Measurement of urine excretion rates either before or after chelation therapy has been used as to indicate lead exposure.

Avoidance of continued exposure to lead is very important when blood lead levels exceed 100 μg/dL (4.83 μmol/L). Severe lead toxicity may require chelation therapy with BAL, administered intravenously. Oral dimercaprol also is used in the outpatient setting for all affected individuals except those with the most severe forms of lead poisoning.

Manganese

Manganese (Mn) is ubiquitous in the environment. Manganese is a binding agent in red brick, is present in most steel alloys as an anticorrosive, is used extensively in laboratories as a cleaning agent for glassware, and is a common pigment in paints and glazes. Humans exhibit toxicity to manganese when exposed to large quantities of dust containing the metal, which occurs in mining, ore crushing, the machining of manganese alloys, and the construction and destruction of brick. After chronic exposure occurs, manganese accumulates in the *substania nigra* of the brain, causing a Parkinson-like syndrome. Manganese toxicity also has been observed in children receiving long-term parenteral nutrition.

Blood or urine manganese concentrations are good indicators of exposure. Adult reference intervals for blood manganese are 0.4 to 1.1 ng/mL (7.0 to 20.0 nmol/L) for serum or plasma and 7.7 to 12.1 ng/mL (140 to 220 nmol/L) for whole blood. Typical excretion of manganese in urine is from 0.2 to 0.5 μg/day. However, approximately 5% of normal individuals excrete up to 2 μg of the metal per day, probably because of greater-than-average exposure.

Most of the manganese in daily diets is not absorbed. Because manganese-containing dust is common, contamination of urine with the metal has been known to occur. Trace contamination of acid preservatives used to stabilize the urine also has been observed.

Mercury

Considerable opportunity exists for mercury (Hg) exposure in our environment. For example, mercury is used as a conductor in many electrical switches, and older home thermostats contain elemental mercury. Mercury is used extensively in the pulp and paper industry as a whitener; the effluents from paper plants are a known source of mercury. Mercury is used commonly in the manufacturing industry as a catalyst in the synthesis of plastics and is found frequently in antifouling and latex paints because it is a potent fungicide. Mercury is present in small quantities (>1 μg/g) in some seafood; commercial fish considered safe for consumption contain less than 0.3 μg/g of mercury, but some game fish contain more than 2.0 μg Hg/g and if consumed on a regular basis, contribute to significant mercury accumulation in the body. Mercury is approximately 50% of the mass of dental amalgams. The single largest source of mercury in the environment is natural outgassing from granite rock; this source accounts for approximately 80% of all mercury accumulation in the environment.

Mercury is essentially nontoxic in its elemental form (Hg^0). In the absence of any chemical or biological system that chemically alters Hg^0, oral consumption does not result in significant side effects. However, Hg^0 becomes toxic when it is modified chemically to the ionized, inorganic species Hg^{+2}. Further bioconversion to an alkyl mercury, such as methyl mercury (CH_3Hg^+), yields a very toxic species of mercury that is highly selective for lipid-rich tissue, such as the neuron.

In industrial uses, mercury is converted chemically from the elemental state to the ionized state through exposure of Hg^0 to a strong oxidant, such as chlorine. Elemental mercury also is bioconverted to both Hg^{+2} and alkyl mercury by microorganisms that exist both in the normal human gut and in the bottom sediment of lakes and rivers. When Hg^0 enters bottom sediment, it is absorbed by bacteria, fungi, and related microorganisms; these organisms metabolically convert it to Hg^{+2}, CH_3Hg^+, $(CH_3)_2Hg$, and similar species. If these organisms are consumed by larger marine animals and fish, these toxic forms of mercury are passed up the food chain.

Mercury expresses its toxicity in the following three ways:

1. Hg^{+2} avidly reacts with sulfhydryl groups of protein, causing a change in the tertiary structure of the protein, with a subsequent loss of the biological activity associated with that protein. Because Hg^{+2} becomes concentrated in the kidney during the regular clearance processes, this is the target organ that experiences the greatest toxicity.
2. With a change in their tertiary structures, some proteins become immunogenic, eliciting a proliferation of B-lymphocytes that generate immunoglobulins to bind the new antigen. (Collagen tissues are particularly sensitive to this occurrence.)
3. Alkyl mercury species, such as CH_3Hg^+, are particularly lipophilic and avidly bind to proteins in lipid-rich

tissues, such as neurons. (Myelin is particularly susceptible to disruption by this mechanism.) Mercury also has been found to alter porphyrin excretion patterns.

Concern has been raised about the possibility of exposure to mercury from dental amalgams. Restorative dentistry has used a mercury-silver amalgam for approximately 90 years as a filling material. One study has shown a small (2 to 20 μg/day) release of Hg^0 from amalgam when it is manipulated mechanically, such as by chewing. The normal bacterial flora present in the mouth convert a fraction of this Hg^0 to Hg^{+2} and to CH_3Hg^+; the latter has been shown to be incorporated into body tissues. The WHO safety standard for daily exposure is 45 μg of mercury per day. Thus if an individual has no other source of exposure, the amount of mercury released from dental amalgams is not significant. However, many foods contain mercury, especially some game fish. If these mercury-containing foods are consumed on a regular basis, significant amounts of mercury accumulate in the body. The habit of gum chewing is thought to release mercury from dental amalgams at levels significantly above normal. For example, after chewing gum for 8 hours, up to 100 μg/day of mercury was found in several subjects who had the typical placement of dental amalgams.

The quantity of mercury found in blood and urine correlates with degree of toxicity (that is, higher quantities mean higher toxicity), and hair analysis also is used to document the time of peak exposure. Normal whole-blood mercury concentration is usually lower than 10 μg/L. Individuals who have mild occupational exposure (for example, dentists) routinely may have whole-blood mercury levels of up to 15 μg/L. Significant exposure is indicated when the whole blood mercury level is greater than 50 μg/L (if exposure is to alkyl mercury) or greater than 200 μg/L (if exposure is to Hg^{+2}). According to the WHO, urine excretion exceeding 50 μg/day indicates significant exposure. Normally, hair contains less than 1 μg/g of mercury; greater amounts indicate increased exposure. Treatment with BAL or penicillamine mobilizes mercury, allowing for its excretion in the urine. Therapy usually is monitored by following of urinary excretion of mercury; therapy may be terminated after the daily excretion rate falls below 50 μg/dL.

Nickel

Nickel (Ni) is used frequently in the production of metal alloys (popular for their anticorrosive and hardness properties), in nickel-based rechargeable batteries, and as a catalyst in the hydrogenation of oils. Elemental nickel is nontoxic except that it may induce inflammation at point of contact. Nickel likely is essential for life at very low concentrations. Nickel carbonyl ($Ni[CO]_4$), used in petroleum refining, is one of the most toxic chemicals known to humans. Nickel carbonyl is absorbed after inhalation, readily crosses all biological membranes, and noncompetitively inhibits ATPase and RNA polymerase. Individuals exposed to nickel car-

bonyl exhibit rapid onset of pulmonary congestion and inability to oxygenate hemoglobin, followed by development of lesions of the lung, liver, kidney, adrenal glands, and spleen. Patients undergoing dialysis are exposed to nickel and accumulate nickel in blood and other organs. No adverse health effects appear to result from this exposure.

Platinum

A variety of platinum-containing antineoplastic agents are used in chemotherapy, typified by cisplatin (*cis*–dichlorodiamineplatinum dihydrate). All these compounds have some nephrotoxicity that is related to the concentration of platinum (Pt) circulating in the blood. Measurement of platinum levels in individuals with reduced renal function is useful to identify whether the platinum is the cause of the compromised renal function. Peak serum levels greater than 1 μg/mL but less than 1.5 μg/mL correlate with little nephrotoxicity and good therapeutic response.

Selenium

Selenium (Se) is an essential element (see Chapter 29). The normal daily dietary intake of selenium is 0.01 to 0.04 ppm, which is similar to the typical content of the metal in soil (0.05 ppm) and sea water (0.09 ppm). Excessive exposure occurs when daily intake exceeds 0.4 ppm. Selenium accumulates in biological tissue so that the normal concentration in human blood serum is 95 to 160 ng/mL (0.15 ppm).

Selenium toxicity has been observed in animals when daily intake exceeds 0.44 ppm. Teratogenic effects are noted frequently in the offspring of animals living in regions where selenium soil content is high, such as in south-central South Dakota and the northern coastal regions of California. Selenium toxicity in humans is not known to create a significant problem except in acute overdose cases, and selenium is not classified as a human teratogen. Selenium is found in many over-the-counter vitamin preparations because its antioxidant activity is thought to be anticarcinogenic. However, no substantiating evidence exist to support the idea that selenium inhibits cancer development.

Silicon

Several forms of silicon (Si) are of toxicological interest, including amorphous oxides of silicon (for example, asbestos) and methylated polymers of silicon (for example, silicone).

Inhalation of asbestos-containing dust leads to deposition of asbestos fibers in the pulmonary alveoli. These fibers are needle-shaped spicules approximately 150 μm in length and up to 15 μm in diameter. When these fibers are inhaled, they deposit in the alveoli, where they are surrounded by macrophages and become coated with protein and mucopolysaccharide to form "asbestos bodies." The diagnosis of asbestosis is made by interpretation of a chest x-ray by a qualified radiologist, demonstration of asbestos in sputum, and documentation of asbestos bodies in a lung biopsy by electron microscopy. Direct analysis of lung tissue for silicon is not useful because all lung tissue is infiltrated with silicon, most of which is not asbestos. Thus direct analysis for silicon does not distinguish asbestosis from normal background silicon.

Silver

The clinical interest in silver (Ag) analysis is limited to two applications—(1) monitoring of burn patients treated with silver sulfadiazine and (2) monitoring of patients treated with silver-containing nasal decongestants. In both cases, silver deposits in many organs, including the subepithelium of skin and mucous membranes, producing a syndrome called *argyria* (graying of the skin). Argyria is associated with growth retardation, hemopoiesis, cardiac enlargement, degeneration of the liver, and destruction of renal tubules. The normal concentration of serum silver is less than 2 ng/mL. Typical silver levels observed in serum of unaffected patients during treatment range up to 300 ng/mL, and their urine output may be as high as 550 µg/day.

Thallium

Thallium (Tl) is a byproduct of lead smelting. Toxicological interest in thallium results from its use as a rodenticide; accidental exposure represents the most likely source of contact. Thallium is absorbed rapidly via ingestion, inhalation, and skin contact. It is considered as toxic as lead and mercury and has similar sites of action. The mechanism of thallium toxicity is (1) competition with potassium at cell receptors to affect ion pumps, (2) inhibition of DNA synthesis, (3) binding to sulfhydryl groups on proteins in neural axons, and (4) concentration in renal tubular cells to cause necrosis. Individuals exposed to high doses of thallium (>1 g) demonstrate alopecia (hair loss), peripheral neuropathy and seizures, and renal failure. Normal serum concentrations are less than 10 ng/mL, and normal urine excretion is less than 10 µg/day. Exposed individuals can exhibit serum levels as high as 50 µg/mL, with urine output in excess of 500 mg/day. The long-term prognosis from such exposure is poor.

Analytical methodology

Atomic absorption spectrophotometry (AAS) with flame or electrothermal atomization furnace, inductively coupled plasma-emission spectroscopy (ICP-ES), inductively coupled plasma-atomic emission spectrometry (ICP-AES), inductively coupled plasma-mass spectrometry (ICP-MS), and HPLC-MS are state-of-the-art analytical techniques used to measure metals in biological fluids.[12] They are specific and sensitive and provide the clinical laboratory with the capability to measure a broad array of metals at clinically significant levels. Photometric assays also are available but require large volumes of sample and have limited analytical performance. In addition, spot tests are available but are considered obsolete because they are error prone and often yield false-positive results.

■ DRUGS OF ABUSE

Governmental, industrial, and sports agencies increasingly are requiring drug testing of prospective and existing employees and participants in professional and amateur athletics. Drug abuse during pregnancy also is of concern. Consequently, **forensic drug testing** for these purposes represents a rapidly growing activity for toxicology laboratories.

General Information

Testing for drugs of abuse usually involves testing a single urine specimen for a number of drugs. It should be noted, however, that a single urine drug test detects only fairly recent drug use; it does not differentiate casual use from chronic drug abuse. The latter requires sequential drug testing and clinical evaluation. Also, urine drug testing does not determine the degree of impairment, the dose of drug taken, or the exact time of use. In addition to urine testing, alternate biological specimens have also been used for drug testing (see later section on alternative specimens).

Because of the serious consequences of a positive drug test, testing often is considered a forensic toxicology activity, requiring the highest standards of analytical methodology, specimen security, and documentation. In addition, many laboratories engaged in this testing are certified appropriately by the Substance Abuse and Mental Health Service Administration (SAMHSA)* of the U.S. Department of Health and Human Services (HHS) or the Forensic Urine Drug Testing program sponsored jointly by the American Association for Clinical Chemistry (AACC) and the College of American Pathologists (CAP).

Several tactics have been used by donors to alter the specimen to prevent drug detection, including the exchange of urine from a drug-free individual and adulteration of the specimen. For example, specimens have been diluted to below cutoff limits with tap or toilet water, and detergent, vinegar, bleach, salt, glutaraldehyde (previously commercially available as UrinAid), potassium nitrite (commercially available as Klear), pyridinium chlorochromate (commercially available as Urine Luck), alkali, or acid have been added to the specimen to interfere with immunoassay screening procedures. Nitrites also have been added to specimens to prevent confirmation by gas chromatography/mass spectrometry (GC/MS) for the principle metabolite of the psychoactive agent in marijuana. Pyridinium chlorochromate also may prevent confirmation by GC/MS for opiates.

Direct observation of urine collection is the most stringent means to guard against specimen exchange or adulteration. However, the need for the highest degree of certainty of specimen integrity must be weighed against individual privacy and dignity. Alternative measures to prevent specimen adulteration include a limitation on clothing or other

---

*Formerly named the National Institute on Drug Abuse (NIDA).

personal belongings allowed in the specimen collection area, addition of coloring agent to toilet water, and inactivation of the hot-water tap. In addition, the temperature of the urine specimen should be checked at the time of collection, and the pH, specific gravity, or creatinine level measured. If values are beyond physiological limits for these parameters, adulteration of the specimen should be suspected.

Urine specimens are collected in tamper-proof specimen cups that are often split (apportioned) into separate specimens identified with the same specimen number. One of these "split" specimens is designated as the primary, or "A," specimen and the other the secondary, or "B," specimen. In practice the primary specimen is analyzed first. The secondary specimen is analyzed only subsequently when a challenge is raised to the results obtained from the primary specimen.

A chain of custody is maintained to identify all individuals involved in specimen collection, transfer, and testing. Specimens that test positive should be stored frozen for a minimum of 1 year. Detailed information on the collection and processing of specimens for drug testing has been described in the federal rules for employee drug testing[17] and the federal regulations promulgated by the DOT[1] and the Nuclear Regulatory Commission (NRC).[8]

Workplace drug testing generally is restricted to detection of alcohol (see section on alcohols) and a few drugs that have a high abuse potential or are **illegal drugs.** Depending on the nature of the testing program, this procedure may involve testing for only one, two, or a select number of drugs or drug classes, including amphetamine/methamphetamine, cannabinoids, cocaine, opiates, and phencyclidine (PCP). (Collectively these five drugs are known as the "NIDA five.") Other drugs tested include barbiturates, benzodiazepines, lysergic acid diethylamide (LSD), methadone, methaqualone, and propoxyphene.

In many programs in which workplace drug testing is conducted, **random testing** is practiced. In this type of testing an unscheduled, unannounced urine drug testing of randomly selected individuals is conducted by a process designed to ensure that selections are made in a nondiscriminatory manner.

Testing programs for participants engaged in athletic competitions may be much more extensive and include assays for a larger group of drugs, including stimulants, β-blockers, diuretics, and anabolic steroids. A listing of the banned drugs included in the Olympic testing programs is found on the Internet at the homepage of the United State Olympic Committee (http://www.usoc.org/inside/drugadmin.html).

Initial **screening tests** for the previously listed drugs most often are immunoassays (see Chapter 10). These assays are calibrated at established cutoff concentrations. Specimens yielding responses greater than the cutoff (threshold) value are considered positive, whereas values below the cutoff are considered negative. Cutoff values are not synony-

TABLE 32-5 U.S. Government Drug Detection Cutoff Concentrations

Drug or Drug Class	Immunoassay (ng/mL) HHS/DOT	Immunoassay (ng/mL) DOD	GC/MS (ng/mL) HHS/DOT	GC/MS (ng/mL) DOD
Amphetamines	1000			
Amphetamine		500	500	500
Methamphetamine		500	500*	500*
Barbiturates		200		
Amobarbital				200
Butalbital				200
Pentobarbital				200
Secobarbital				200
Cannabinoids	50	50		
THC-COOH			15	15
Cocaine metabolites	300	150		
Benzoylecgonine			150	100
LSD		0.5		0.2
Opiates	2000‡	300†		
Morphine			2000‡	4000
Codeine			2000‡	2000
6-Acetylmorphine			10	10
PCP	25	25	25	25

Data from Fed Reg 1988; 53:11,963; 1994; 59:29,908-29,981; 1997; 62:51,118-51,120; Irving J: Drug testing in the military: technical and legal problems. Clin Chem 1988; 34:637-640; Liu RH: Evaluation of common immunoassay kits for effective workplace drug testing. In Liu RH, Goldberger BA (eds): Handbook of Workplace Drug Testing, p 70, Washington, DC, AACC Press, 1995.
HHS, Department of Health and Human Services; *DOT,* Department of Transportation; *DOD,* Department of Defense; *PCP,* phencyclidine; *LSD,* lysergic acid diethylamide; *THC-COOH,* 11-nor-Δ^9-tetrahydrocannabinol-9-carboxylic acid.
*Also requires presence of amphetamine (200 ng/mL).
†25 ng/mL if assay specific for free morphine.
‡Screening and confirmatory values recently changed (effective May 1998) from 300 to 2000 ng/mL.

mous with assay detection limits. Instead, the cutoff is established higher than the detection limit (to ensure reliable measurement) but low enough to detect drug use within a reasonable time frame.

Immunoassays may not be specific for the tested drug. Similar drugs may result in a positive test; for example, pseudoephedrine, present in cold medications, may produce a positive response in immunoassays designed to detect amphetamine and methamphetamine. Therefore positive screening tests must be confirmed by an alternate, more definitive **confirmatory test.** The most widely accepted method for drug confirmation is GC/MS (see Chapter 8).

For confirmation, quantitative drug measurements are performed by use of selective ion monitoring with GC/MS. (NOTE: Detailed GC/MS procedures for the drugs discussed in the following sections have been published elsewhere.)[15] Cutoff values for confirmation are established at or generally below cutoff values for the initial screening tests (Table 32-5). The result then is reported as positive or negative relative to the cutoff value. However, the actual concentration may be helpful in the interpretation of morphine and codeine results (see following sections) and in monitoring of individuals enrolled in drug-treatment programs. In the latter case, subjects who test positive but who demonstrate decreasing values on sequential testing may be judged abstinent, whereas those whose values suddenly increase are likely noncompliant. For this purpose, normalization of the drug concentration to urine creatinine level (nanograms of drug per milligram of creatinine) is necessary. This step compensates for fluctuations in absolute drug concentrations related to physiological variation in urine dilution or concentration.

Specific Drugs

The pharmacologic, biochemical, and analytical characteristics of several drugs that are abused commonly are discussed in this section.

Amphetamine and methamphetamine

Amphetamine and methamphetamine (Figure 32-16) are CNS-stimulant drugs that have been used to treat obesity, narcolepsy, and attention-deficit hyperactivity disorders. However, they produce an initial euphoria and thus have a high abuse potential. For this reason their use for appetite suppression has been discouraged. In addition to these conventional **amphetamines**, "designer" amphetamines, such as methylenedioxyamphetamine (MDA) and methylenedioxymethamphetamine (MDMA) also exist and are abused.

Pharmacologic response and metabolism

In addition to the initial euphoria, amphetamine and methamphetamine produce a feeling of increased well-being and self-esteem, with heightened mental and physical capacity. Appetite is suppressed. This initial state may be followed by restlessness, irritability, and especially in chronic users, paranoid psychosis. These unpleasant responses reinforce the continued use of the drugs to maintain the "high." In extreme cases, addicts may have "speed runs," in which large IV doses are used for several days during which they do not sleep or eat. This speed run is followed by prolonged sleep (1 to 2 days), after which the cycle is repeated. Tolerance and psychological dependence develop with repeated use of amphetamines.

The CNS-stimulatory effects of amphetamine and methamphetamine result from their ability to enhance the release of neurotransmitter catecholamines, such as norepinephrine and dopamine, from presynaptic terminals and inhibit their neuronal reuptake. Consequently, the neurotransmitter content in the synaptic cleft is increased, resulting in enhanced postsynaptic activation. As with cocaine the euphorigenic actions of amphetamine probably involve an increase in synaptic dopamine concentration. The duration of action of amphetamine is longer than that for cocaine, a

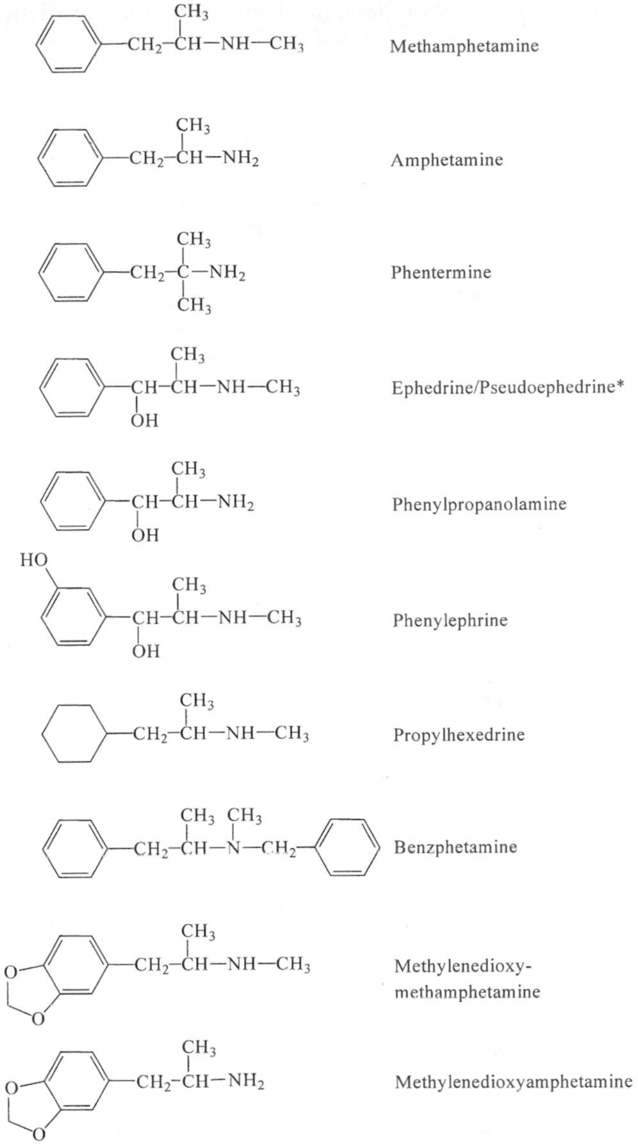

Figure 32-16   Chemical structures of sympathomimetic amines.
*Ephedrine and pseudoephedrine are diastereoisomers.

consequence of the more rapid metabolic elimination of cocaine. Peripheral adrenergic activation may result in increased blood pressure and cardiac arrhythmias.

The optical isomers (enantiomers) of amphetamine and methamphetamine exhibit stereoselective pharmacologic properties. The CNS activity of S(+)-amphetamine is three to four times greater than of R(−)-amphetamine, but the latter drug has more potent cardiovascular effects than the former.* Because of the minimal CNS activity and thus low abuse potential, R(−)-methamphetamine is included in

---

*Although the D and L designations still are used widely to designate enantiomers ("mirror images"), they are being replaced with the Cahn-Ingold-Prelog system, in which the symbols R and S are used to designate configurations instead of D and L.

some nonprescription nasal inhalants for its vasoconstrictive properties.

Amphetamine is metabolized primarily by oxidative deamination, a process that is stereoselective for S(+)-amphetamine. Consequently, the elimination half-life for R(−)-amphetamine may be as much as 40% longer than that for S(+)-amphetamine. In addition to hepatic metabolism, amphetamine is eliminated as unchanged drug in urine; the extent of such elimination depends on urine pH. Normally about 30% of a dose is excreted unchanged, but this amount may vary from as much as 70% in acid urine to as low as 1% in alkaline urine. The elimination half-life (renal excretion and hepatic metabolism) also varies with urine pH, from 7 to 14 hours at acid pH to 18 to 34 hours at alkaline pH. These effects of urine pH on the elimination of unchanged amphetamines are a consequence of tubular reabsorption of unionized but not ionized amphetamine.

A significant portion of a methamphetamine dose is eliminated unchanged in urine in a pH-dependent manner similar to that for amphetamine. In addition, methamphetamine is metabolized in liver primarily by hydroxylation and to a lesser extent by N-demethylation to amphetamine. After methamphetamine ingestion, amphetamine is present in urine at a concentration that is roughly 10% of that for methamphetamine. The overall rate of metabolism, including formation of amphetamine, is selective for the S(+)-methamphetamine enantiomer. Thus when racemic methamphetamine is ingested, urine specimens contain relatively more R(−)-methamphetamine than S(+)-methamphetamine, but a greater amount of S(+)-amphetamine than R(−)-amphetamine.

In cases of overdose, amphetamine and methamphetamine cause dizziness, tremor, irritability, hypertension, diaphoresis, mydriasis, cardiac arrhythmias, and if severe, hyperpyrexia, convulsions, coma, and cerebral hemorrhage. Treatment involves general supportive measures. Acid diuresis enhances the elimination of the amphetamines, but its use is controversial.

Analytical methodology

Immunoassays for amphetamine and methamphetamine have variable cross-reactivities with other sympathomimetic amines, such as ephedrine, pseudoephedrine, phenylpropanolamine, phentermine, MDA, and MDMA. Confirmation of positive test results determined by immunoassay therefore is mandatory. Moreover, chiral discrimination of methamphetamine isomers may be necessary to distinguish use of nonprescription nasal inhalants (R[−]-methamphetamine) from illicit use of S(+)-methamphetamine. Some immunoassays have high specificity for S(+)-methamphetamine. However, definitive discrimination of enantiomers requires the use of a chiral derivatization reagent to form diastereomers of R- and S-methamphetamine, which may be resolved by use of conventional GC/MS.

Several prescription drugs are metabolized to methamphetamine (and subsequently to amphetamine) or to amphetamine. For instance, selegiline (Eldepryl), used to treat Parkinson's disease, is metabolized to R(−)-methamphetamine and R(−)-amphetamine. The (+)-isomer of benzphetamine (Didrex), administered as an anorectic agent, also is metabolized to methamphetamine and amphetamine, and the metabolites are presumed to be the S(+)-isomers. Chiral discrimination can rule out illicit use of methamphetamine in the case of selegiline but not benzphetamine. However, benzphetamine is a schedule III drug, so its use without a prescription is illicit. Other prescription drugs, not legally available in the United States, that are metabolized to methamphetamine (and amphetamine) include dimethylamphetamine, famprofazone, fencamine, and furfenorex; those metabolized to amphetamine include amphetaminil, clobenzorex, ethylamphetamine, fenethylline, fenproporex, mefenorex, mesocarb, and prenylamine.

For GC/MS confirmation, a urine specimen that tests positive for amphetamine or methamphetamine by immunoassay is treated with periodate to remove possible interferences due to α-hydroxyamines, such as ephedrine, pseudoephedrine, norpseudoephedrine, and phenylpropanolamine. The periodate-treated urine is extracted at alkaline pH with organic solvent, and the isolated organic layer is reacted with 4-carbethoxyhexafluorobutyryl chloride to derivatize the amines. After addition of ethanol to destroy excess derivatizing reagent, the solvent is removed by evaporation, and the residue is dissolved in ethyl acetate and analyzed by GC/MS with selected ion monitoring detection.

Barbiturates

The **barbiturates** have a low therapeutic index and a relatively high abuse potential. Because of their rapid onset and short duration of action, the short- to intermediate-acting barbiturates* are used as sedative-hypnotics (amobarbital, butabarbital, butalbital, pentobarbital, secobarbital) and are abused most commonly. The longer-acting barbiturates (mephobarbital, phenobarbital), used primarily for their anticonvulsant properties, are abused rarely. Street names of barbiturates include barbs, sleepers, downers, yellow jackets, and rainbow.

Pharmacologic response and metabolism

Barbiturates suppress CNS neuronal activity and thus have sedative and hypnotic properties. The major manifestations of barbiturate intoxication are CNS, cardiovascular, and respiratory depression. Severe intoxication results in coma, hypothermia, hypotension, and cardiorespiratory arrest.

---

*The classification of barbiturates as "ultrashort-acting," "short-acting," "intermediate-acting," and "long-acting" refers to the duration of effect and not to the elimination half-life.

Because of their low therapeutic index and high potential for abuse, the barbiturates have been replaced largely by the safer benzodiazepines for sedative and hypnotic purposes. Nevertheless, they continue to be available for these purposes or in combination with other analgesic, antihypertensive, antiasthmatic, antispasmodic, or antidiuretic drugs. The combination of barbiturates such as butalbital with analgesic preparations is especially ironic. Not only do barbiturates lack analgesic properties, but at low doses they also antagonize the effects of analgesics. Phenobarbital is effective as an anticonvulsant drug (see Chapter 31), and short- and ultrashort-acting barbiturates (Table 32-6) are used for IV anesthesia. Anesthetic doses of barbiturates such as pentobarbital also are used to reduce intracranial pressure from cerebral edema associated with head trauma, surgery, or cerebral ischemia. However, barbiturates continue to be subject to abuse and are a source of intentional or less commonly, accidental drug intoxication. Measurement of the common barbiturates in serum aids in the diagnosis and management of barbiturate intoxication.

The general formula for barbiturates is provided in Table 32-6. Any change in the constituents at position five that confers an increase in lipid solubility typically results in increased onset of action, decreased duration of action, and increased potency. An increase in hydrophobic properties also leads to more rapid and extensive hepatic metabolic clearance and thus to decreased urinary elimination of unchanged drug.

The barbiturates undergo extensive hepatic metabolism, in which the C5 substituents are transformed to alcohols, phenols, ketones, or carboxylic acids; these metabolites may be excreted in urine in part as glucuronide conjugates. For some barbiturates (amobarbital, phenobarbital), *N*-glucosylation is an additional important metabolic transformation (Figure 32-17). As a result, only a relatively small amount of an administered barbiturate dose is excreted in urine as parent drug; notable exceptions are phenobarbital and aprobarbital (Table 32-7). Nevertheless, the parent drugs, rather than hydroxy or carboxylic acid metabolites, are targeted for detection in urine screening and confirmation procedures. This analytical approach generally is successful for barbiturates because these drugs are ingested in sufficiently high doses to allow detection of unmetabolized drug in urine.

Appropriate treatment for barbiturate intoxication includes general cardiopulmonary support and measures to prevent further drug absorption. Forced alkaline diuresis may enhance the elimination of long-acting barbiturates (for example, phenobarbital, barbital) but has little effect on intermediate-, short-, or ultrashort-acting barbiturates.

Analytical methodology

To detect barbiturate overdose, semiquantitative immunoassays are available and used to detect barbiturates in serum. All assays use secobarbital as a calibrator at a cutoff

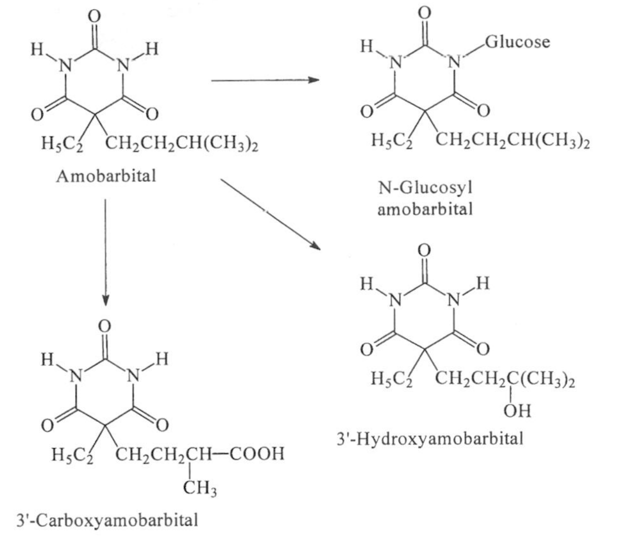

Figure 32-17   Metabolism of amobarbital.

concentration of either 200 or 300 ng/mL. The degree of cross-reactivity of other barbiturates varies with each assay. Little information is known concerning cross-reactivity with barbiturate metabolites, except for *p*-hydroxyphenobarbital, which is detected by several of the immunoassays. The detection period in urine after ingestion of barbiturates varies somewhat with different assays and depends on the pharmacologic properties of the drugs. The short- to intermediate-acting barbiturates generally may be detected for 1 to 4 days after use; long-acting barbiturates, such as phenobarbital, may be detected for several weeks after chronic use. Capillary GC also has been used to detect barbiturate overdose in serum. Barbiturate overdose is detected in urine by use of either TLC or immunoassay. When urine specimens are tested for detection of barbiturate abuse, immunoassay and GC/MS are the methods of choice for screening and confirmation, respectively.

For GC/MS confirmation a urine specimen that tests positive for barbiturates by immunoassay is extracted (liquid-liquid); the extract is dried and then treated with *N,N*-dimethylformamide dimethyl acetal to form methyl derivatives of the barbiturates. After buffer is added, the methylated barbiturates are extracted with hexane, which then is reduced in volume by evaporation (but not to dryness) before analysis by GC/MS.

Benzodiazepines

Benzodiazepines are a class of drugs widely used in medical practice as CNS depressants. They enhance the inhibitory action of γ-aminobutyric acid (GABA) by modulating $GABA_A$ receptors.

Pharmacologic response and metabolism

Benzodiazepines have anxiolytic, sedative-hypnotic, muscle relaxant, and anticonvulsant properties. They are

TABLE 32-6　Characteristics of Barbiturates

Barbiturate	Duration of Action (h)	Half-life (h)	Therapeutic Concentration (μg/mL)	Toxic Concentration (μg/mL)	% Protein Bound	% Excreted Unchanged in Urine	pK_a	R_1	R_2
Ultrashort Acting									
Thiopental*	0.5	6 to 7	1 to 5 (hypnotic); 7 to 130 (anesthesia)	>10	75 to 90	0.3	7.6	$-CH_2CH_3$	$-CHCH_2CH_2CH_3$ / $-CH_3$
Short Acting									
Butalbital	3 to 4	34 to 42	—	—	26	3	7.9	$-CH_2CH=CH_2$	$-CH_2CHCH_3$ / $-CH_3$
Secobarbital	3 to 4	19 to 34	1 to 2	>5	46 to 70	5	7.9	$-CH_2CH=CH_2$	$-CHCH_2CH_2CH_3$ / $-CH_3$
Pentobarbital	3 to 4	15 to 30	1 to 5	>10	65	1	7.9	$-CH_2CH_3$	$-CHCH_2CH_2CH_3$ / $-CH_3$
Intermediate Acting									
Amobarbital	6 to 8	8 to 42	1 to 5	>10	59	1 to 3	7.9	$-CH_2CH_3$	$-CH_2CH_2CHCH_3$ / $-CH_3$
Aprobarbital	6 to 8	14 to 34	—	—	55 to 70	13 to 24	8.1	$-CH_2CH=CH_2$	$-CHCH_3$ / $-CH_3$
Butabarbital	6 to 8	34 to 42	—	—	26	5 to 9	7.9	$-CH_2CH_3$	$-CHCH_2CH_3$ / $-CH_3$
Long Acting									
Phenobarbital	10 to 12	40 to 140	15 to 40	>65	45 to 50	25 to 33	7.2	$-CH_2CH_3$	$-C_6H_5$

From Baselt RC, Cravey RH (eds): Disposition of Toxic Drugs and Chemicals in Man, Chicago, Year-Book, 1989; Tietz NW (ed): Clinical Guide to Laboratory Tests, Philadelphia, WB Saunders, 1990; and Physician's Desk Reference, 46th edition, p. 534, Oradell, NJ, Medical Economics Data, 1991.
pK_a, Dissociation constant.
*Oxygen at position 2 is replaced by sulfur.

among the most commonly prescribed drugs in the Western hemisphere. However, despite their widespread use, abuse of benzodiazepines is relatively low and is more likely to occur in individuals who abuse other drugs or alcohol. Benzodiazepine CNS toxicity is generally mild to moderate and may manifest as drowsiness, slurred speech, ataxia, and occasionally coma. More serious toxic effects causing respiratory depression or cardiovascular compromise are infrequent. Indeed, few well-documented deaths have been attributed to benzodiazepine intoxication alone.

Currently, 13 benzodiazepines are approved for use in the United States (Table 32-8). Specific clinical applications are determined largely by differences in onset and duration of action and by quantitative differences in their clinical effects. One member of this class, alprazolam, has been used for the treatment of depression. Another benzodiazepine, flunitrazepam, is approved for use in many countries but not the United States. However, it recently has entered the United States illegally (especially Texas and Florida) and has been sold illicitly. Moreover, because of its sedative-hypnotic action and ability to induce short-term amnesia, it has gained notoriety as a "date-rape" pill.

Benzodiazepines are administered most often orally, and the rate of absorption is the principal determinant of rate of onset and intensity of action. Highly lipophilic benzodiazepines (diazepam, flurazepam) are absorbed rapidly (time to peak serum concentration of <1.2 hours), and less lipophilic compounds (oxazepam, temazepam) are absorbed more slowly (time to peak serum concentration of 2 to 3 hours).

After GI absorption or IV administration, benzodiazepines are distributed rapidly to the CNS. Subsequently, benzodiazepines are redistributed more slowly from the CNS to more poorly perfused tissues, such as adipose tissues and muscle. The rate of this redistribution is an important determinant of the duration of action of benzodiazepines and, similar to that for GI absorption, is determined largely by drug lipophilicity. For example, the more lipophilic drugs (midazolam, triazolam) have the shortest duration of action.

TABLE 32-7   Urinary Excretion of Barbiturates and Metabolites

Barbiturate	Single Dose Excreted in Urine (%)			
	Parent	Hydroxy Derivatives	N-Glucosyl Derivatives	Carboxylic Acids
Amobarbital	1 to 3	30 to 50	29	5
Aprobarbital	8 to 18			
Butabarbital	5 to 9	2 to 3		24 to 34
Butalbital*	3	60		
Pentobarbital	1	88		
Phenobarbital	25 to 33	18 to 19	24 to 30	
Secobarbital	5	50		

From Baselt RC, Cravey RH: Disposition of Toxic Drugs and Chemicals in Man, 4th edition, Foster City, Calif, Chemical Toxicology Institute, 1995.
*In dogs; excretion in humans is unknown.

TABLE 32-8   Benzodiazepine Characteristics

Compound (Trade Name)	Therapeutic Uses	Half-Life (h)	Main Urinary Metabolite
Alprazolam (Xanax)	Anxiety; depression	8 to 14	α-Hydroxy glucuronide
Chlordiazepoxide (Librium, others)	Anxiety; alcohol withdrawal; preanesthetic medication	6 to 27; active metabolites	Oxazepam glucuronide
Clorazepate (Tranxene, others)	Anxiety; seizure disorders	2 (prodrug)* active metabolite	Oxazepam glucuronide
Diazepam (Valium, others)	Anxiety; status epilepticus, muscle relaxation; preanesthetic medication	30 to 56	Oxazepam glucuronide
Lorazepam (Ativan)	Anxiety; preanesthetic medication	8 to 25	Lorazepam glucuronide
Oxazepam (Serax)	Anxiety	5 to 15	Oxazepam glucuronide
Estazolam (ProSom)	Insomnia	10 to 24	4-Hydroxy glucuronide
Flurazepam† (Dalmane)	Insomnia	2 to 3; active metabolite, 50 to 100	N^1-hydroxy ethyl glucuronide
Quazepam (Doral)	Insomnia	6 to 10	2-Oxo-3-hydroxy glucuronide
Temazepam (Restoril)	Insomnia	5 to 17	Temazepam glucuronide
Triazolam (Halcion)	Insomnia	2 to 3	α-Hydroxy glucuronide
Clonazepam (Klonopin)	Seizure disorders	20 to 60	7-Amino-3-hydroxy conjugates
Midazolam (Versed)	Preanesthetic and intraoperative medication	1 to 4	α-Hydroxy glucuronide

From Baselt RC, Cravey RH: Disposition of Toxic Drugs and Chemicals in Man, 4th edition, pp 251, 380, 384, 572, Foster City, Calif, Chemical Toxicology Institute, 1995; Hobbs WR, Rall TW, Verdoorn TA: Hypnotics and sedatives. In Hardman JG, Limbird LE, Molinoff PB (eds): Goodman and Gilman's The Pharmacological Basis of Therapeutics, 9th edition, pp 361-396, New York, McGraw-Hill, 1996.
*Converted to nordiazepam by gastric hydrochloric acid.
†Active metabolite, N-desalkylflurazepam.

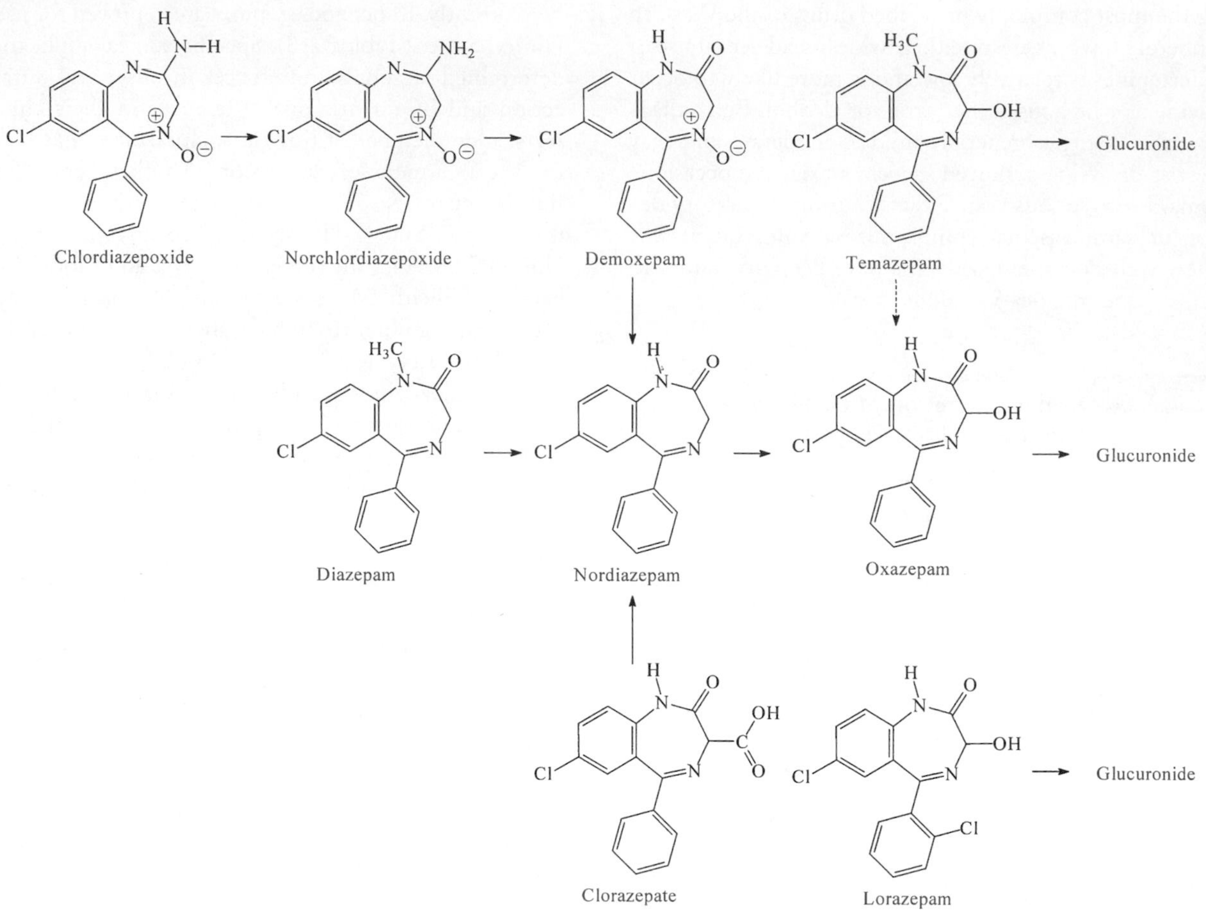

Figure 32-18   Metabolic transformations of chlordiazepoxide, diazepam, and related 1,4-benzodiazepines.

Additional factors that influence the duration of benzodiazepine action are hepatic metabolism and acute tolerance.

Benzodiazepines act on the CNS by potentiating the action of the major endogenous CNS inhibitory neurotransmitter, GABA. Benzodiazepines bind to $GABA_A$ receptor sites and thereby enhance $GABA_A$-mediated chloride transmembrane conductance, which results in diminished neural electrical discharge. The remarkable safety of benzodiazepines, compared with barbiturates, probably is related to their activation of the endogenous GABA effect. Conversely, barbiturates increase neural chloride conductance independent of GABA.

Benzodiazepines undergo hepatic oxidation and conjugation, often forming metabolites with pharmacologic activity (Figure 32-18). Several benzodiazepines are metabolized to oxazepam, which is excreted as the inactive glucuronide. Others are inactivated by glucuronidation as the only metabolic transformation (lorazepam) or the most important metabolic transformation (temazepam). Metabolic transformations can occur before the drug reaches significant concentrations in the systemic circulation. For example, clorazepate is decarboxylated to nordiazepam by stomach acid, and flurazepam and prazepam are converted to active metabolites by hepatic first-pass metabolism.

Benzodiazepines with the shortest elimination half-lives generally also have the shortest durations of action. In some cases an active metabolite may have a half-life longer than the parent drug and thus may contribute to a longer duration of action. For instance, flurazepam has a half-life of 2 to 3 hours, but its active metabolite, desalkylflurazepam, has a half-life of 50 to 100 hours. Benzodiazepines used to treat anxiety generally have intermediate to long elimination half-lives (alprazolam, diazepam), and those benzodiazepines used primarily as anticonvulsants (clonazepam) have long half-lives.

Individuals may develop some degree of tolerance and physical dependence after prolonged use of benzodiazepines. A withdrawal syndrome similar to that for barbiturates and alcohol may be observed, but it is generally less severe, less frequent, and not as prolonged. These symptoms may include anxiety, apprehension, tremors, muscle weakness, anorexia, nausea, vomiting, dizziness, hyperthermia, and convulsions. The frequency and severity of withdrawal symptoms are greater for the most rapidly eliminated benzodiazepines, as well as in cases of longer duration of therapy (>4 months), higher doses, and abrupt discontinuation of the drug. Withdrawal symptoms may be especially severe for individuals who have taken alprazolam. Tolerance to some effects of benzodiazepines may occur. Tolerance is believed to result from an adaptation of the GABA receptors to continued benzodiazepine exposure, in which case their response is diminished. This diminished response leads to a need for higher doses to achieve the desired effect.

Analytical methodology

Benzodiazepines have been quantified in serum, generally by HPLC, but such quantitative information is not warranted in cases of benzodiazepine overdose because serum levels are not predictive of severity of intoxication. However, a urine or serum immunoassay screening test for benzodiazepines is valuable to aid in the evaluation of patients with unknown causes of CNS depression. To detect abuse the initial screening test for benzodiazepines most often is immunoassay. Several commercial immunoassay systems are available for the detection of a wide variety of benzodiazepines and metabolites.

For confirmation of a presumptive positive a quantitative drug measurement is performed by use of GC/MS. In practice a urine specimen that tests positive for benzodiazepines by immunoassay is treated with β-glucuronidase, subjected to liquid-liquid extraction, and the extracts evaporated. The residue is treated with *N*-methyl-*N*-trimethylsilyl-trifluoroacetamide (MSTFA) to form trimethylsilyl (TMS) derivatives of the benzodiazepines, which are analyzed with selected ion monitoring.

Cannabinoids (marijuana)

Marijuana is a street drug that is derived from the hemp plant *(Cannabis sativa)*. It is a green or gray mixture of dried, shredded flowers and leaves. Hashish describes the dried, resinous secretions of the plant. Marijuana is the most often used illegal drug in the United States. Most users roll loose marijuana into a cigarette called a *joint*. Some users mix marijuana into foods or use it to brew tea. Hash users either smoke the drug in a pipe or mix it with tobacco and smoke it as a cigarette.

Pharmacologic response and metabolism

Marijuana contains a number of cannabinoids that are C_{21} compounds. The principal psychoactive cannabinoid is Δ^9-tetrahydrocannabinol (THC; Figure 32-19). Marijuana is metabolized extensively to a large number of compounds, most of which are inactive. The principal urinary metabolite is 11-nor-Δ^9-tetrahydrocannabinol-9-carboxylic acid (THC-COOH) and its glucuronide conjugate.

The major psychoactive effects of THC are euphoria and a sense of relaxation and well-being. These effects occur within minutes of marijuana smoking, reach a peak in about 15 to 30 minutes, and may persist for 2 to 4 hours. Associated with this "high" are a loss of short-term memory and impairment of intellectual performance (recall, reading comprehension, ability to concentrate, and mathematical problem solving). Moreover, psychomotor skills may be im-

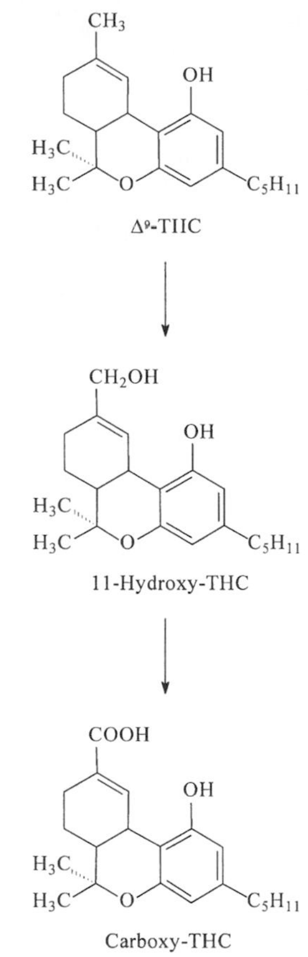

Figure 32-19   Principal metabolic route for THC in humans. *THC, Δ^9-tetrahydrocannabinol.*

paired sufficiently to affect adversely an individual's operation of an automobile or airplane. Some controversy exists concerning the degree of impairment of performance beyond 4 hours after marijuana use. Even greater uncertainty surrounds the long-term negative health effects of chronic marijuana use. Tolerance and a mild degree of physical dependence may develop after chronic marijuana and hashish use.

After an individual inhales marijuana smoke, THC is absorbed rapidly through the lungs and reaches peak blood concentration within minutes; thereafter, blood concentration rapidly declines to about 10% of peak levels within 1 to 2 hours. This rapid decline in THC concentration is a result of its facile distribution to tissues, such as brain, fat, and muscle. The rapid tissue distribution phase, a consequence of the lipophilic nature of THC, is followed by a slow redistribution of THC back into the bloodstream and subsequent hepatic elimination. The terminal elimination half-life of THC is about 1 day in casual marijuana users and 3 to 5 days in chronic users. The peak psychoactive effects of THC generally lag behind the peak blood concentration by about 20 to 30 minutes.

Although marijuana is the most frequently used illicit drug, it does have some limited legitimate medicinal uses.

For example, it is used to treat anorexia and nausea in AIDS patients, nausea and vomiting associated with chemotherapy, and asthma and glaucoma.

Analytical methodology

The initial screening test for marijuana is most often immunoassay. Immunoassays designed to screen urine samples for marijuana use measure THC-COOH and other THC metabolites. These assays are calibrated with THC-COOH, but because of cross-reactivity with many other THC metabolites, quantitative results based on them are 1.5 to 8 times greater than the actual concentration of THC-COOH as determined by GC/MS. Therefore immunoassay results are interpreted as THC-COOH equivalents. For confirmation of a presumptive positive a quantitative drug measurement is performed by use of GC/MS.

Because of the slow release of THC from tissue storage sites, urine may test positive for THC metabolites (>20 ng/mL THC-COOH equivalents) for 2 to 5 days after the last marijuana use by infrequent smokers; some individuals may test positive for as long as 10 days. Chronic smokers may test positive for 3 to 4 weeks after abstinence. Some heavy smokers may remain positive for up to 46 days and require as long as 77 days to test negative for 10 consecutive days. Therefore a positive urine test for THC-COOH is interpreted as past marijuana use (immediate to several weeks) and is unrelated to impairment.

Due to fluctuations in fluid excretion the concentration of THC metabolites in urine may vary between positive and negative values when it is measured sequentially after several days of abstinence. In this case an increase in metabolite concentration could imply falsely the reuse of marijuana. Therefore to monitor abstinence properly the concentration of THC-COOH should be expressed per milligrams of creatinine. An increase of 50% or more from the previous value implies reuse.

Concern has been raised about the possibility of passive inhalation of sufficient sidestream marijuana smoke from nearby users to result in a positive urine cannabinoid test. This does occur—but only under rather unrealistic conditions. Under more normal circumstances, passive inhalation has not resulted in a urine THC-COOH concentration in excess of 12 ng/mL. Nevertheless, as a precaution against passive inhalations resulting in a positive test, some laboratories screen for urine cannabinoids at a cutoff concentration of 100 ng/mL THC-COOH equivalents. However, at this cutoff value, test sensitivity in one study was only 47%, when compared with that for GC/MS (cutoff value of 15 ng/mL THC-COOH). Test sensitivity increased to 93% at a cutoff value of 20 ng/mL THC-COOH equivalents. The U.S. federally mandated screening cutoff has been reduced from 100 ng/mL to 50 ng/mL THC-COOH equivalents. One study that demonstrated such a reduction in screening cutoff resulted in a 23% to 54% increase in test sensitivity, depending on immunoassay, with only a slight decrease (1.0% to 2.6%) in test specificity.

Cocaine

Cocaine is an alkaloid present in the leaves of the coca plant that grows in South America. The drug has a long history of human consumption, beginning with its use by ancient South American civilizations, followed by its initial incorporation in a popular cola drink (discontinued in the early 1900s), and continuing to its current popularity as a recreational drug. "Crack" is the street name given to cocaine that has been processed from cocaine hydrochloride to a free base for smoking.

Pharmacologic response and metabolism

Cocaine is a potent CNS stimulant that elicits a state of increased alertness and euphoria. In this regard, its actions are similar to those of amphetamines but are of shorter duration. This euphoric response leads to recreational abuse of cocaine. Cocaine also blocks the reuptake of norepinephrine at presynaptic nerve terminals; this blocking produces a sympathomimetic response, including an increase in blood pressure, heart rate, and body temperature. Cocaine is effective as a local anesthetic and vasoconstrictor of mucous membranes and therefore is used clinically in nasal surgery, rhinoplasty, and emergency nasotracheal intubation. The psychomotor-stimulant effects of cocaine depend both on dose and on route of administration, with IV administration and smoking resulting in the most rapid rates of increase in concentration.

For recreational use, cocaine (hydrochloride salt) often is ingested by nasal insufflation ("snorting") or the free base inhaled by smoking. This latter route of administration results in a rapid onset of action.

Acute cocaine toxicity produces a sympathomimetic response that has resulted in mydriasis, diaphoresis, hyperactive bowel sounds, tachycardia, hypertension, hyperthermia, agitation, seizures, or coma. Sudden death due to cardiotoxicity may occur as a result of cocaine use.

Cocaine is hydrolyzed rapidly by separate liver esterases to the inactive metabolites ecgonine methyl ester and benzoylecgonine (Figure 32-20). Ecgonine methyl esters also are formed by the action of serum pseudocholinesterase, and cocaine is converted to benzoylecgonine by spontaneous hydrolysis. The formation of benzoylecgonine often has been attributed entirely to spontaneous hydrolysis, but it also is mediated by a liver carboxylesterase. This latter enzyme, in the presence of ethanol, catalyzes transesterification of cocaine (benzoylecgonine methyl ester) to cocaethylene (benzoylecgonine ethyl ester). Cocaethylene possesses the same CNS stimulatory activity as cocaine in experimental animals. Cocaethylene also has resulted in enhanced cardiotoxicity; it is more lethal than cocaine in experimental animals. Cocaethylene may be found in the urine or serum of hospital patients who test positive for benzoylecgonine. When "crack" cocaine is smoked, a pyrolysis product—anhydroecgonine methyl ester—is formed and has been detected in urine.

The elimination half-life varies from 0.5 to 1.5 hours for cocaine, 3 to 4 hours for ecgonine methyl ester, and 4 to 7

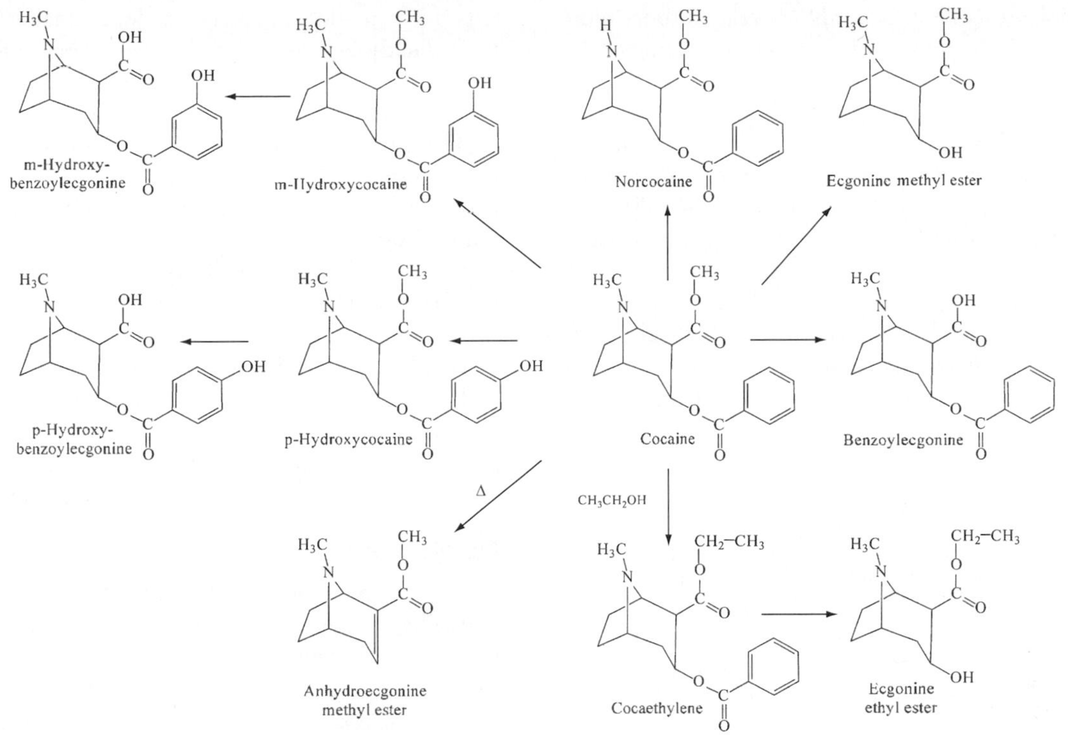

Figure 32-20   Metabolism and pyrolysis of cocaine.

hours for benzoylecgonine. The principal urinary metabolites are benzoylecgonine and ecgonine methyl ester. Only small amounts of cocaine are excreted in urine. The elimination half-life for cocaethylene is 2.5 to 6 hours, considerably longer than that for cocaine. This longer elimination half-life may contribute to cocaethylene's toxicity.

Analytical methodology

Commercial immunoassays detect benzoylecgonine. With these assays, benzoylecgonine excretion normally is detected at a cutoff of 300 ng/mL for 1 to 3 days after cocaine use. However, for chronic, heavy cocaine users, the detection time may extend to 10 to 22 days after the last use, apparently because of tissue storage of cocaine. Cocaine is detected in urine by chromatographic methods for only about 8 to 12 hours after use, but in heavy, chronic users, this detection period may be 4 to 5 days. Thus a positive urine drug test for benzoylecgonine beyond 3 days after the last dose does not necessarily indicate continued use. For such purposes, quantitative monitoring of the urinary excretion of benzoylecgonine, normalized to creatinine, over time is recommended. Drug abstinence is indicated by decrease in urinary excretion of cocaine metabolites. Minor metabolites of cocaine (*m*- and *p*-hydroxybenzoylecgonine) in adult urine may contribute significantly to the benzoylecgonine-immunoreactivity in meconium (see later section on meconium).

For GC/MS confirmation an internal standard (benzoylecgonine-D$_3$) first is added to the urine specimen. After liquid-liquid extraction and solvent evaporation, the residue is treated with MSTFA to form benzoylecgonine (and ecgonine methyl ester) TMS derivatives. The reaction mixture is analyzed by GC/MS through use of selected ion monitoring.

Lysergic acid diethylamide

Lysergic acid diethylamide (LSD) is a hallucinogenic chemical that may precipitate psychosis. A resurgence in the use of LSD, previously popular as a drug of abuse during the 1960s, has been seen. The U.S. Department of Defense (DOD) includes LSD among the drugs for which urine testing is required (see Table 32-5). Popular dose forms include powder, gelatin capsule, tablet, or LSD-impregnated sugar cubes, filter paper, or postage stamps.

Pharmacologic response and metabolism

LSD is an extremely potent psychedelic amine. It shares structural features with serotonin (5-hydroxytryptamine; Figure 32-21), a major CNS neurotransmitter and neuromodulator. LSD binds to serotonin receptors in the CNS and acts as a serotonin agonist. The principle psychological effects of LSD are perceptual distortions of colors, sound, distance, and shape; depersonalization and loss of body image; and rapidly changing emotions that swing from ecstasy to depression or paranoia. These hallucinogenic actions of LSD are stereoselective, elicited only by the D-isomer. LSD is absorbed rapidly from the GI tract; the effects begin within 40 to 60 minutes, peak at about 2 to 4 hours, and subside by 6 to 8 hours after ingestion. The elimination half-life is about 3 hours.

The physiological effects of LSD are related to its sympathomimetic actions and include excessive dilatation of the pupil of the eye (mydriasis), tachycardia, increased body temperature, profuse perspiration (diaphoresis), and hypertension; at higher doses, parasympathomimetic actions, such as salivation, lacrimation, nausea, and vomiting (muscarinic actions), have been observed. Neuromuscular effects include paresthesia, muscle twitches, and lack of coordination (nicotinic actions).

The most common adverse effects of LSD are panic attacks. In addition, unpredictable recurrence of hallucinations (flashbacks) may occur weeks or months after the last drug use, and LSD may elicit psychotic reactions (thought disorders, hallucinations, depression, depersonalization). LSD is used illicitly because of its hallucinogenic effects. No evidence exists that repeated LSD use results in dependence or withdrawal symptoms.

The clinical effects of LSD ingestion are usually benign and require no medical intervention. However, panic attacks may be severe and require treatment with diazepam; LSD-induced psychosis may be treated with haloperidol. Few, if any, well-documented deaths directly related to LSD ingestion have been reported.

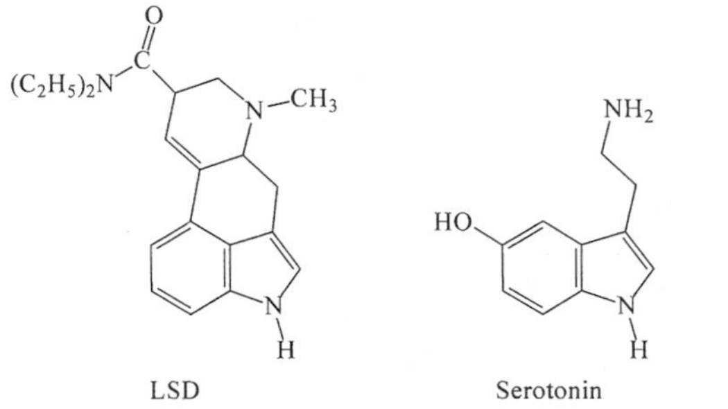

Analytical methodology

LSD is detected in urine by immunoassay. At a cutoff concentration of 0.5 ng/mL, LSD typically is detected for 24 to 120 hours after ingestion. For confirmation by GC/MS, LSD is converted to the TMS derivative.

Opioids/Opiates

Opioid is a general term applied to all substances with morphinelike properties. The term *opiate* is used to describe naturally occurring or semisynthetic analgesic alkaloids derived from opium, the dried, milky juice from the unripe seeds of the poppy plant. Morphine is the principal and prototypical analgesic alkaloid of opium. Opium also contains smaller amounts of codeine. Some important semisynthetic derivatives of morphine include heroin, oxycodone, and hydromorphone. Codeine also has been synthesized by

Figure 32-21 Chemical structures of LSD and serotonin. *LSD,* Lysergic acid diethylamide.

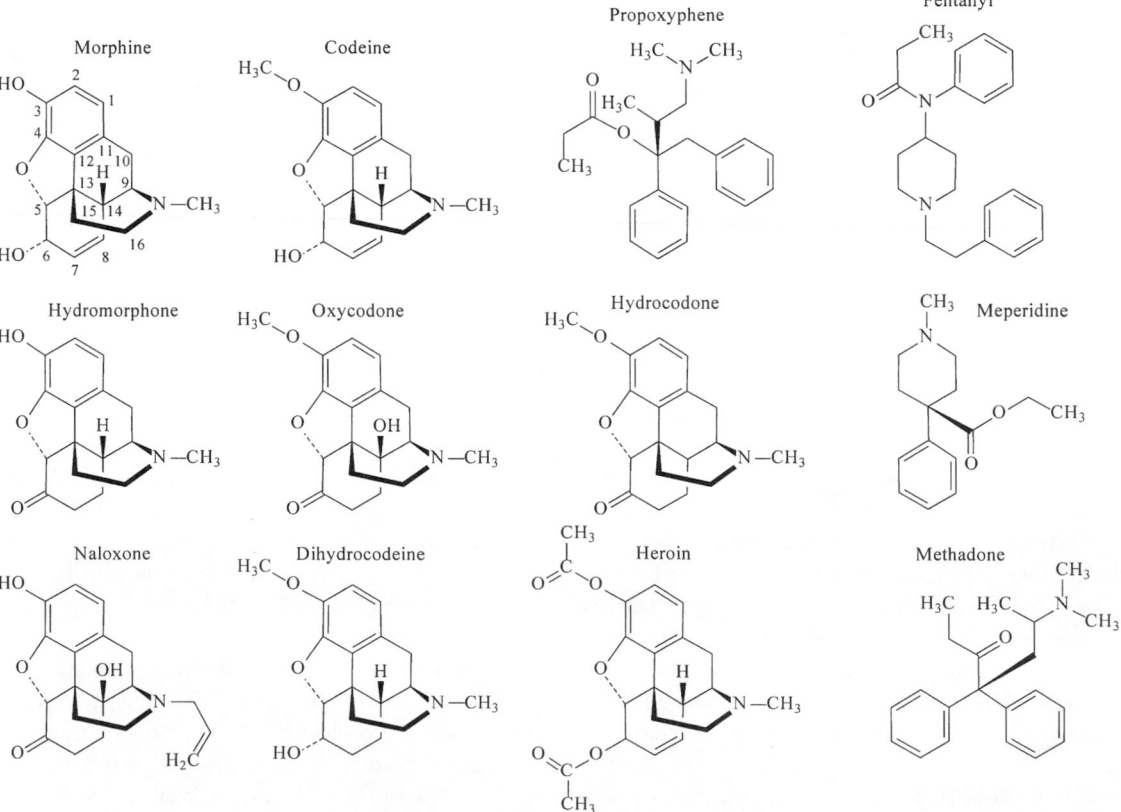

Figure 32-22 Chemical structures of representative opioids.

3-methylation of morphine. Synthetic agents with morphinelike properties include propoxyphene, methadone, meperidine, and fentanyl (Figure 32-22).

Pharmacologic response and metabolism

Opiates (morphine, codeine, dihydrocodeine, hydrocodone, hydromorphone, oxycodone) are used clinically for their analgesic properties. Opiates also cause sedation, euphoria, respiratory depression, orthostatic hypotension, diminished intestinal motility, nausea, and vomiting. The major manifestations of morphine overdose are coma, miosis (pinpoint pupils), and respiratory depression. Pulmonary edema often is a complication of morphine overdose, and death may result from cardiopulmonary arrest. Treatment for morphine overdose includes administration of the opiate antagonist naloxone (Narcan), which dramatically reverses the effects of morphine.

Because of their analgesic and euphorigenic properties, opiates have a high abuse potential. Chronic use of morphine leads to tolerance and both physical and psychological dependence. Withdrawal from morphine addiction may be treated by the administration of methadone, a long-lasting, orally active opiate. Other therapeutic agents used to treat morphine addiction include naltrexone, a long-acting opiate antagonist, and clonidine, a central α-adrenergic agonist antihypertensive agent.

Heroin (diacetylmorphine) is the form of morphine most favored by opiate abusers because of its rapid onset of action. It generally is administered by IV or subcutaneous injection or less frequently by smoking or nasal insufflation. Heroin itself is not active, but it is converted rapidly (half-life of <6 minutes) to 6-acetylmorphine, which in turn is hydrolyzed (half-life of <40 minutes) to morphine (Figure 32-23). Both 6-acetylmorphine and morphine are pharmacologically active. Morphine (average elimination half-life of 2 hours; range of 1 to 8 hours) is inactivated mainly by glucuronide conjugation at the 3- or phenolic hydroxyl group. The average elimination half-life for morphine-3-glucuronide is 3 to 4 hours after IV, 8 hours after intramuscular, and 9 to 10 hours after oral morphine ingestion. Of the total morphine in urine, about 90% is morphine-3-glucuronide (50% to 75% of a morphine dose) and about 10% is free morphine.

Codeine has only about one-tenth the analgesic potency of morphine. A small amount of codeine (10%) is converted to morphine (see Figure 32-23), which accounts for its analgesic properties. A similar amount of norcodeine is formed by *N*-demethylation. Thus both codeine and morphine have been detected in urine after codeine ingestion. Codeine is combined frequently with nonopiate analgesic agents (for example, aspirin and acetaminophen); it is also an effective antitussive agent in some cough medicines.

As a common contaminant of heroin, codeine may be detected frequently in urine after heroin use. In this case the concentration of morphine exceeds that of codeine, whereas the reverse is true within the first 24 hours after codeine use.

However, a reversal in the codeine-to-morphine ratio may occur in the late elimination period (>24 hours) subsequent to codeine administration. Thus distinguishing between legitimate codeine use (for example, from a cough preparation) and heroin abuse based on the codeine-to-morphine ratio in urine is not always possible.

The consumption of foods that contain poppy seeds (for example, cakes, muffins, rolls, and bagels) may result in significant urinary excretion of morphine and codeine. This excretion may result in false incrimination of illicit opiate use, as determined by drug-testing programs. Guidelines have been proposed to eliminate poppy seed ingestion as the source of a positive urine opiate test.[6] Adherence to these guidelines eliminates poppy seed ingestion as the principal opiate source in the following situations:

1. A morphine level greater than 5000 ng/mL
2. A codeine level greater than 300 ng/mL
3. A morphine-to-codeine ratio less than 2
4. A morphine level greater than 1000 ng/mL with no codeine

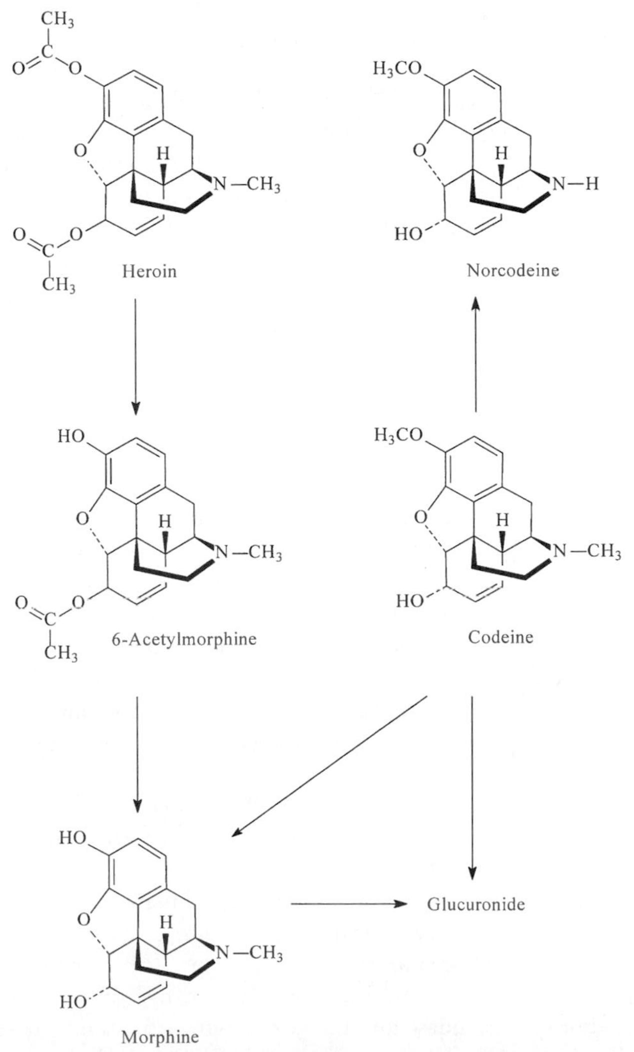

Figure 32-23   Metabolism of heroin and codeine.

In addition, detection of the heroin metabolite 6-acetylmorphine (see Figure 32-23) also eliminates poppy seed ingestion as a cause. However, 6-acetylmorphine is eliminated rapidly, so its detection in urine is limited to earlier than 24 hours (perhaps <8 hours) after heroin use. Therefore the absence of 6-acetylmorphine does not rule out heroin or morphine use. To avoid some of the issues concerning poppy seed ingestion and the legitimate use of opiate medications, the DOD established confirmatory cutoff concentrations of 4000 ng/mL morphine and 2000 ng/mL codeine and also requires testing for 6-acetylmorphine (see Table 32-5). The HHS likewise recently has increased the screening and confirmatory cutoff concentrations from 300 ng/mL to 2000 ng/mL for morphine and codeine, respectively, and also requires testing for 6-acetylmorphine (cutoff of 10 ng/mL).

Hydromorphone and oxymorphone are semisynthetic opiates that have about 8 to 10 times the potency of morphine. Hydromorphone has greater oral bioavailability than morphine; oxymorphone has limited IV use for postsurgical analgesia. Hydrocodone, oxycodone, and dihydrocodeine are 3 to 10 times more potent than codeine, and, like codeine, they have relatively good oral bioavailability. Hydrocodone is metabolized to hydromorphone and dihydrocodeine. The elimination half-life for all these opiates is slightly longer than that for morphine, ranging from about 2.5 to 5 hours. As for codeine, oxycodone is formulated frequently in combination with aspirin (Percodan) or acetaminophen (Percoset, Tylox). Therefore the detection of either salicylate or acetaminophen, along with codeine or oxycodone, in the urine of an individual who displays opiate toxicity should lead to the measurement of salicylate or acetaminophen in serum to assess potential toxicity.

Analytical methodology

Immunoassays are rapid, convenient procedures used to screen urine specimens for opiates. A cutoff point of either 300 ng/mL or 2000 ng/mL of morphine (or morphine equivalents) is used commonly to distinguish negative from positive urine specimens. The commercial immunoassays for opiates are designed primarily for the detection of morphine and codeine. The degree of cross-reactivity with morphine-3-glucuronide and other opiates varies among the immunoassays. In general, cross-reactivity with oxycodone and oxymorphone is low.

The detection period after morphine or codeine use varies somewhat with the cutoff concentration for the immunoassay and the degree of cross-reactivity with the glucuronide conjugates. In general, urine specimens test positive for 1 to 3 days after morphine (or heroin) or codeine use.

For GC/MS confirmation, urine specimens that test positive for opiates by immunoassay are hydrolyzed with acid or glucuronidase and then extracted with a solid-phase absorbent. After the extraction column is washed, the opiates are eluted with solvent, which subsequently is evaporated. The residue is treated with MSTFA to form TMS derivatives of the opiates, which are analyzed by selected ion monitoring GC/MS in which deuterated morphine-D_3 and codeine-D_3 are used as internal standards.

Methadone

Methadone is a synthetic opioid that has a chemical structure similar to propoxyphene (see Figure 32-22). It is used clinically for relief of pain, to treat opioid abstinence syndrome, and to treat heroin addicts to wean them from illicit IV drug use. However, prolonged use of methadone itself may result in dependence.

Pharmacologic response and metabolism

The major pharmacologic actions of methadone are similar to those of other opioids and include analgesia, sedation, respiratory depression, miosis, antitussive effects, and constipation. Methadone is administered as a racemic mixture ([±]-methadone), but the analgesic activity is due almost entirely to the (−)-isomer. When administered intramuscularly, methadone and morphine have equivalent analgesic potency.

Methadone is absorbed rapidly from the GI tract with an onset of action within 30 to 60 minutes. The elimination half-life is long (15 to 55 hours), compared with morphine (half-life of 1 to 8 hours). Because of its longer elimination half-life, methadone accumulates in blood and tissues after repeated doses, and this accumulation presumably contributes to its relatively long duration of action (6 to 8 hours).

Tolerance to the effects of methadone develops with repeated doses, but more slowly than with morphine. Likewise, withdrawal develops more slowly and is generally less intense but more prolonged than morphine withdrawal. Withdrawal symptoms include weakness, anxiety, insomnia, abdominal discomfort, sweating, and hot and cold flashes.

In cases of overdose, methadone causes CNS and respiratory depression, miosis, bradycardia, hypotension, circulatory collapse, hypothermia, coma, seizures, and pulmonary edema (although less frequently than does morphine). Treatment for methadone overdose includes supportive measures to maintain adequate respiration and blood pressure and the administration of the opioid antagonist, naloxone, to reverse the effects of methadone. Due to the prolonged elimination half-life, repeated administration of naloxone may be required, and patients should be monitored for 48 to 72 hours after overdose.

Methadone is metabolized in the liver primarily to 2-ethylidene-1,5-dimethyl-3,3-diphenylpyrrolidine (EDDP) and 2-ethyl-5-methyl-3,3-diphenylpyrroline (EMDP). The principle urinary excretion products are methadone (5% to 50% of dose) and EDDP (3% to 25% of dose); relatively more methadone than EDDP is excreted when urine is acidic.

Analytical methodology

Numerous immunoassays are available for screening for methadone. A typical assay cutoff concentration is 300 ng/mL. No cross-reactivity with EDDP or EDMP has been reported. Methadone generally may be detected in urine for up to 72 hours after ingestion.

For GC/MS confirmation a urine specimen that tests positive for methadone by immunoassay is extracted (liquid-liquid); the extract is evaporated, reconstituted with ethyl acetate, and analyzed by selected ion monitoring GC/MS.

Propoxyphene

Propoxyphene is an opioid structurally similar to methadone.

Pharmacologic response and metabolism

Propoxyphene is a widely prescribed narcotic analgesic with a potency approximately one-half that of codeine when each is administered orally. Typical oral doses of propoxyphene have about the same analgesic effect as 600 mg aspirin. Only the (+)-isomer (Darvon, others) has analgesic activity; the (−)-isomer (Novrad) is devoid of analgesic activity but is effective as an antitussive agent. Propoxyphene is prescribed most often as a combination with acetaminophen or salicylate.

Propoxyphene is absorbed rapidly and undergoes extensive hepatic first-pass metabolism to norpropoxyphene. The elimination half-life for propoxyphene is about 15 hours (8 to 24 hours), and that for norpropoxyphene is 27 hours (24 to 34 hours). Norpropoxyphene may contribute to the analgesic and cardiotoxic effects of propoxyphene.

Propoxyphene overdose has resulted in nausea, vomiting, and drowsiness or in more severe cases, CNS depression, convulsion, respiratory depression, and cardiovascular collapse. Cardiac arrhythmia atypical for opioid overdose is thought to be caused primarily by norpropoxyphene. Death, usually as a result of respiratory depression and cardiac arrhythmia, is more common when propoxyphene is ingested with another CNS depressant, such as alcohol.

Because propoxyphene and norpropoxyphene serum concentrations correlate poorly with the degree of impairment or prognosis, such quantitative information generally is not helpful in cases of propoxyphene overdose. However, their qualitative identification in urine may help confirm or establish the cause of a patient's symptomology. Because propoxyphene is taken frequently in combination with acetaminophen or aspirin, quantitation of the latter two drugs in serum is advisable to assess their possible toxicity.

Naloxone is effective in reversing the CNS- and respiratory-depressant actions of propoxyphene but has little effect on the cardiotoxicity. Because propoxyphene has a large volume of distribution (V_d: 10 to 18 L/kg) and is highly protein bound (70% to 80%), hemodialysis is of little value in instances of serious overdose. Forced diuresis likewise is of little value because only about 1% of the dose is eliminated in urine as unchanged propoxyphene.

Analytical methodology

Immunoassays for propoxyphene are designed to detect the parent drug; cross-reactivity with norpropoxyphene, present in much greater concentrations than the parent drug, is weak. In general, propoxyphene may be detected for about 2 days after use.

A positive screening result for propoxyphene obtained by immunoassay is confirmed by GC/MS analysis of the urine specimen for norpropoxyphene. Because norpropoxyphene is present in urine at considerably greater concentrations than propoxyphene and because the latter has poor GC characteristics, confirmation analysis by GC/MS is directed at the determination of norpropoxyphene after its conversion to norpropoxyphene amide.

For this GC/MS confirmation an aliquot of a urine specimen that tests positive for propoxyphene by immunoassay is treated with alkali to convert norpropoxyphene to norpropoxyphene amide. After liquid-liquid extraction is performed, the organic extract is evaporated to dryness; the residue is dissolved in ethyl acetate and then analyzed by selected ion monitoring. Norpropoxyphene-D_5 is used as the internal standard.

Phencyclidine

Phencyclidine (PCP) originally was introduced for use as a surgical anesthetic but subsequently was withdrawn from application because of adverse side effects. Because of its euphoric and hallucinogenic properties and ease of synthesis, illicit use of the drug continues. PCP is not found in smaller cities, nor is it found in many large ones, in contrast to cocaine or THC.

Pharmacologic response and metabolism

The pharmacologic actions of PCP are complex. For example, PCP has stimulant, depressant, hallucinogenic, and analgesic properties. Adverse effects are unpredictable and include euphoria, ataxia, diaphoresis, hypertension, tachycardia, nystagmus, muscle rigidity, hallucinations, delusions of grandeur, anxiety, agitation, hostility, paranoia, disorientation, stupor, coma, seizures, and respiratory depression. PCP-related deaths most often result from intentional or accidental trauma secondary to the adverse behavioral effects of the drug. With repeated use of PCP, psychological dependence may develop, but tolerance and withdrawal syndrome are not profound.

The drug is absorbed rapidly from the GI tract. This form of ingestion is difficult to regulate and therefore results in the highest probability of overdose, or "bad trips." Thus smoking (PCP sprinkled on tobacco, parsley leaves, or marijuana) is now the most popular mode of ingestion because users may self-titrate the most dangerous effects of PCP. Once absorbed, PCP is metabolized extensively by the liver (~90% of a dose); only 10% to 15% is excreted unchanged in the urine. The principle metabolites excreted in urine are the glucuronide conjugates of hydroxylated metabolites

(~25% to 30%), 5-(1-phenylcyclohexyl-amino) valeric acid (~15%), and unidentified polar metabolites (~40%).

PCP is a lipophilic weak base (pK_a ~8.5). It is secreted into and "trapped" in ionized form in the acidic gastric fluid, where concentrations may be 20 to 50 times greater than in serum; subsequently, PCP is reabsorbed in the alkaline duodenum. This gastroenterohepatic recirculation probably contributes to the typical waxing and waning of clinical effects of PCP and, along with its large V_d of 5 to 7 L/kg, partly explains PCP's long elimination half-life (20 to 50 hours), long duration of action (24 to 48 hours), and prolonged urinary excretion after last dose (1 to 2 weeks; longer with chronic use).

Analytical methodology

Quantitation of PCP in serum is not useful in the diagnosis or management of PCP toxicity because a low correlation exists between drug concentration and drug effects. However, qualitative identification of PCP in urine can help diagnose PCP toxicity. For this purpose, PCP-specific immunoassays are rapid and generally are more sensitive than TLC. Whether PCP is included in a general urine drug screen depends on the applicable regulations and the prevalence of PCP use in the local community. In some locations the prevalence of PCP use may be too low to warrant routine screening for PCP. Immunoassays for PCP are generally reliable; however, false-positive results have been reported due to high concentrations of dextromethorphan, diphenhydramine, and thioridazine.

Therefore confirmation of immunoassay-positive specimens by use of an alternate technique (for example, GC/MS) is necessary. For GC/MS confirmation a urine specimen that tests positive for PCP by immunoassay is subjected to liquid-liquid extraction. The organic extract is evaporated, reconstituted with ethyl acetate, and then analyzed by selected ion-monitoring GC/MS, with PCP-D_5 used as an internal standard.

Alternative Specimens

Urine currently is the preferred specimen for detection of drugs of abuse. However, the window in which drugs can be detected in urine generally is limited to a few days after drug use. Moreover, the collection of urine requires some invasion of privacy and dignity, and urine specimens are subject to adulteration or manipulation to evade detection. For these reasons, alternative biological specimens, such as meconium, hair, sweat, and saliva, are being investigated.

Meconium

Urine testing of the mother or newborn can detect only recent drug use (within a few days before the birth), and urine collection from newborns has been problematic. For these reasons, drug testing of meconium, the first stools of the newborn, offers an alternative means to determine drug use.

Meconium begins to form during the second trimester and continues to accumulate until birth. Drugs are believed to be deposited in meconium via fetal bile excretion and from swallowed amniotic fluid, which contains drug and drug metabolites eliminated in the fetal urine. Testing of meconium therefore provides evidence of maternal drug use any time during the last two trimesters.

Meconium is a heterogeneous, gelatinous material from which drugs must be extracted before analysis by immunoassay and confirmation by GC/MS are performed. Drug extraction from meconium by use of inorganic acids, methanol, or any other alcohol is protected by U.S. patents.

Hair

Increasing interest is developing in the analysis of hair to detect drug use.[9] Hair is advantageous as a biological specimen because it is obtained easily without loss of privacy or dignity (unless pubic hair is obtained), and it is not altered or manipulated easily to prevent drug detection. Moreover, once deposited in hair, drugs are very stable; therefore prior drug use may be detected for several months. Because hair grows at a relatively constant rate (0.3 to 0.4 mm/day), the potential exists for segmental hair analysis to provide a "chronicle" of prior drug use.

The mechanisms by which drugs are deposited in hair are not well understood but may include transfer from blood to the growing hair shaft, transfer from sweat (because some sweat glands empty into hair follicles), and environmental contamination. Factors that may affect the deposition of drugs in hair also are not well established but may include the rate of hair growth, anatomical location of hair, type of hair, effects of various hair treatments, and environmental contamination, especially for drugs that are smoked (marijuana, cocaine, heroin, PCP).

Drugs, when deposited in hair, generally are present in relatively low concentrations (pg/mg to ng/mg); thus sensitive analytical techniques are required for detection. Moreover, the parent drug generally is present in a greater concentration than are the metabolites. Parent drug-specific radioimmunoassay (RIA) procedures have been used most commonly for drug detection in hair. Some immunoassays designed primarily for urine drug testing—and therefore those that may have greatest reactivity with metabolites—are of limited use for hair analysis. Confirmation of immunoassay results, generally by GC/MS, remains a requisite for any forensic application of hair drug testing.

Sweat

Drugs may be excreted in sweat, and, as with hair, the parent drug generally is present in a greater amount than are the metabolites. Sweat-patch collection devices that resemble adhesive bandages have been developed. Such devices are worn for several days to several weeks, during which drug, if present, accumulates in the absorbent pad in the patch, while water vapor escapes through semipermeable covering. Thus sweat drug testing offers the possibility to monitor drug use over extended periods of time without the need for frequent urine collection. Sweat drug testing is particularly advantageous for monitoring of drug use in correctional institutions or in drug-rehabilitation programs.

Saliva

The measurement of drugs in saliva is of interest both for purposes of therapeutic drug monitoring and for the detection of illicit drug use. Saliva is easy to obtain, with less invasion of privacy and ease of adulteration, compared with urine. Saliva is an ultrafiltrate of plasma; therefore drug concentration in saliva reflects the free or active fraction and may reflect more closely the drug's effect than is possible with urine measurements. The transfer of drugs from blood to saliva is influenced by drug protein binding, pK_a, lipid solubility, and blood pH (saliva being more acidic than blood). In general, drugs are present in saliva in lower concentrations and may be detected for shorter time periods, compared with urine. Detection of drugs in saliva therefore indicates recent drug use. Moreover, saliva drug concentration may correlate with degree of impairment, except when buccal contamination may have occurred due to smoking or snorting of the drug.

■ ANALYTICAL TECHNIQUES

A number of analytical techniques are used to measure drugs and metals in biological specimens.

Drug Analysis

Because of the wide range of drugs of interest, no single analytical technique is adequate for broad-spectrum drug detection. Therefore several analytical approaches in combination generally are required. They include simple, inexpensive, and rapid spot tests; immunoassays (see Chapter 10); and chromatographic techniques (see Chapter 8).

Speed of analysis, or turnaround time, is a critical issue in clinical toxicology. A drug analysis that requires several hours to complete or is not available at all hours of the day is of little value in a clinical emergency. On the other hand, a rapid test that provides false information could result in erroneous diagnostic and therapeutic decisions. Quantitative determinations in serum are important for acetaminophen, salicylate, alcohols, ethylene glycol, anticonvulsant drugs, iron, lithium, theophylline, digoxin, and barbiturates (possibly) and in whole blood for carboxyhemoglobin and methemoglobin. For many other drugs, their serum concentrations do not correlate sufficiently with the severity of toxicity to warrant the obtaining of quantitative information. In these cases, qualitative identification in urine generally is sufficient.

The proper selection of analytical methods and interpretation of results require a knowledge of the pharmacology and pharmacokinetics of the toxins of interest. For example, the potential hepatotoxicity of acetaminophen is related to the concentration of unmetabolized drug. Therefore appropriate analytical methods for acetaminophen measure only parent drug and not inactive metabolites. Moreover, quantitation of serum acetaminophen or salicylate before completion of the absorptive phase may be misleading in instances of overdose. Morphine is excreted in urine largely as morphine-3-glucuronide. The most sensitive detection of morphine requires prior hydrolysis (acid or enzymatic) or methods that directly measure the conjugate (for example, immunoassay). Detection of the unique heroin metabolite, 6-acetylmorphine, distinguishes heroin use from ingestion of poppy seeds as the cause of a positive urine test for morphine.

Screening procedures are designed for the relatively rapid and generally qualitative detection of drugs or other toxic substances. In general, screening tests have adequate sensitivity but may not be highly specific. Thus a negative result yielded by a screening procedure rules out the presence of clinically significant concentrations of a particular analyte with reasonable certainty. Because of possible interferences a positive result should be considered "presumptive" positive and should be confirmed by an alternate procedure of greater specificity. Screening procedures may be designed to detect a particular drug or drug class. Tests for such purposes include simple visual color tests (spot tests) and determination of serum osmolal gap. Immunoassay and chromatographic techniques also are used for screening purposes.

Spot tests

Spot tests are rapid, easily performed, noninstrumental qualitative procedures that provide presumptive evidence for the presence of tested drugs. Any positive response must be followed by testing with a more specific method. They are valuable to rule out the presence of drugs or to suggest (but not prove) the presence of a drug of a particular group. Five of the most useful spot (color) tests for the visual detection of selected drugs in physiological fluids are presented in the following sections. Detailed procedures for each spot test have been published in an expanded version of this chapter.[15] A more extensive list of spot tests also has been published.[2]

Acetaminophen

Acetaminophen is not detected in some TLC procedures, and it generally demonstrates poor gas chromatographic properties unless it is derivatized. Therefore a relatively rapid screening procedure for acetaminophen may be advantageous. For this spot test, acetaminophen first is hydrolyzed to p-aminophenol, which then reacts with o-cresol and ammonium hydroxide to form an indophenol blue chromogen.

Salicylate

Salicylate normally is not detected by TLC, and its GC response is variable without derivatization. Therefore a spot test is useful to screen for the possible presence of salicylates. This test depends on the formation of a violet color between iron (Trinder's reagent) and salicylate. Diflunisal and labetalol produce a positive test response.

Phenothiazines

Phenothiazines are metabolized extensively to a large number of metabolites. The presence of these metabolites may lead to some confusion in the interpretation of thin-layer chromatograms. The ferric, perchloric, nitric (FPN) spot test is helpful when it is used in conjunction with TLC screening. Not all phenothiazines produce a positive test.

Imipramine, desipramine, and trimipramine

The presence of the tricyclic antidepressant drugs imipramine, its metabolite desipramine, and trimipramine may be detected in urine after oxidation to colored reaction products with acidic dichromate (Forrest's reagent). These tricyclic antidepressant drugs are metabolized to several metabolites that may increase the complexity of the interpretation of thin-layer chromatograms. The spot test with Forrest's reagent therefore may be helpful in conjunction with TLC. Other common antidepressants, including amitriptyline, clomipramine, doxepin, maprotiline, protriptyline, and trazodone, are not detected by this spot test.

Ethchlorvynol

Ethchlorvynol is not detected with some TLC procedures. When detected, ethchlorvynol may not be resolved completely from glutethimide. Thus a color test based on the reaction of diphenylamine and ethchlorvynol is useful in conjunction with TLC. The presence of a pink color indicates a positive test result for ethchlorvynol. Phenothiazines may produce a light-pink color that fades and cannot be extracted into chloroform.

Determination of volatiles by serum osmolal gap

The principal osmotically active constituents of serum are Na^+, Cl^-, HCO_3^-, glucose, and urea. Several empirical formulas based on the measurement of these substances have been used to calculate the serum osmolality. One commonly used formula is

$$mOsm/kg = 2\,Na^+\,(mmol/L) + 0.056\,glucose\,(mg/dL) + 0.36\,urea\,N\,(mg/dL)$$

The difference between the actual osmolality, measured by freezing-point depression, and the calculated osmolality is referred to as *delta-osmolality*, or the *osmolal gap*. Normally, the osmolal gap is zero (± 10 mOsm/kg). Alcohols, acetone, and ethylene glycol, when present in significant concentrations, increase actual serum osmolality and thus would result in an increased osmolal gap (>10 mOsm/kg). Volatile substances are not detected when osmolality is measured with a

	TABLE 32-9	Laboratory Findings Characteristic of Ingestion of Alcohols			
Alcohol	Osmolal Gap	Metabolic Acidosis with Anion Gap	Serum Acetone	Urine Oxalate
Ethanol	+	−	−	−
Methanol	+	+	−	−
Isopropanol	+	−	+	−
Ethylene glycol	+	+	−	+

+, Positive; −, negative.

vapor-pressure osmometer. Therefore to determine the osmolal gap, only osmolality measurements based on freezing-point depression are acceptable. The determination of the osmolal gap is a rapid means to detect exogenous osmolutes present in milligram-per-deciliter concentrations.

Each 100 mg/dL of ethanol in serum results in a delta-osmolality of 21.7 mOsm/kg. By considering this predictable effect of ethanol on the serum osmolality, determination of the portion of an increased osmolal gap that is due to ethanol is possible. A significant residual osmolal gap (>10 mOsm/kg) suggests the possible presence of isopropanol, methanol, acetone, or ethylene glycol. In addition, the contribution of ethanol to the measured osmolality can be calculated (0.217 ethanol, mg/dL) and included in the preceding formula for delta-osmolality. This information, in conjunction with the presence or absence of metabolic acidosis or serum acetone, is helpful to the clinician if specific measurements of alcohols other than ethanol and of ethylene glycol are not available on an emergency basis (Table 32-9). Substances, such as mannitol (osmotic diuretic) and propylene glycol (solvent for diazepam and phenytoin), administered to patients may increase serum osmolality. Moreover, this screening method is insensitive to low, yet clinically significant, concentrations of ethylene glycol (<50 mg/dL) and methanol (<30 mg/dL). After ingestion of methanol, some individuals may have increased osmolal gaps not entirely accounted for by the presence of methanol.

Immunoassay

Different types of immunoassay, such as EMIT, fluorescence polarization immunoassay, cloned enzyme donor immunoassay (CEDIA), kinetic microparticle immunoassay (Abuscreen Online), and RIA (see Chapters 10 and 31), are useful methods for both screening and quantitative purposes. In some cases these assays are relatively specific for a single drug (for example, for PCP or propoxyphene), but in others, several drugs of a similar class are detected (for example, opiates, barbiturates, β-phenylethylamines ["amphetamines"]). The detection limit for various members of a class of drugs or the degree of cross-reactivity for similar drugs varies, and each manufacturer of immunoassay reagents should be consulted for specific information. These assays are (1) easy to perform, (2) provide "semiquantitative" results (higher or lower than a predetermined calibrator cutoff concentration), and (3) generally have low detection limits (0.02 to 1.0 µg/mL). Several nonisotopic immunoassays (for example, EMIT, CEDIA, Online, and fluorescence polarization immunoassay) have been automated (see Chapter 12). A number of portable, noninstrumental immunoassay-based drug-detection devices are available for nonlaboratory, point-of-care testing (POCT). Test principles for these devices include solid-phase enzyme immunoassay, microparticle-capture immunochromatography, latex agglutination-inhibition, or gold microparticle-capture immunoassay.

For comprehensive clinical (emergency) drug screening, immunoassays complement chromatographic procedures (TLC and GC) because they detect the drugs that otherwise would require hydrolysis before chromatography (for example, morphine-3-glucuronide and oxazepam glucuronide), that may require a separate extraction (for example, benzoylecgonine), or that have high TLC detection limits (for example, PCP). For drug abuse detection, immunoassay is the method of choice for initial screening.

Chromatographic techniques

Several chromatographic techniques are used to screen or quantify drugs in biological specimens. They include TLC, GC, HPLC, and GC/MS.

Thin-layer chromatography

TLC, more correctly known as *planar chromatography,* is a versatile procedure that requires no instrumentation and thus is operationally relatively simple and inexpensive (see Chapter 8). However, its application to drug screening requires considerable skill to recognize drug and metabolite patterns. TLC detects a large number of drugs in a variety of body fluids, such as serum, gastric contents, or urine. Urine, however, is the specimen of choice because most drugs and drug metabolites are present in urine in relatively high concentrations. The detection limit varies for each drug but generally is in the range of 0.5 to 4.0 µg/mL. Most TLC plates used for drug detection are coated with silica gel. Although these plates may be prepared in the clinical laboratory, most clinical laboratorians find it advantageous to purchase commercial precoated plates. After extraction and specimen spotting, the TLC plates are developed with appropriate solvents to achieve chromatographic resolution. The drugs and metabolites then are visualized as spots by their fluorescence or ultraviolet absorbance and by their color development with a combination of reagent sprays or dip solutions. Identification is made by the inclusion of reference compounds with the unknowns, followed by comparison of their relative migration distances (known as R_f values) and detection characteristics with those of the unknowns.

Although some laboratories use a single TLC plate for drug screening, use of as many as three separate plates per urine specimen is advantageous. Different developing solvents then may be used to separate drugs more effectively in the acidic-neutral and basic drug classes. Moreover, the sequential application of multiple spray reagents to a single TLC plate results in diffusion of spots and increases the complexity of interpretation. Some commonly used drug-detection reagents and their preparations are as follows:

- **Ninhydrin**—reacts with drugs that contain primary or secondary amines, such as amphetamine and other sympathomimetic amines.
- **Mercuric sulfate**—forms white precipitate with barbiturates, glutethimide, and phenytoin.
- **Diphenylcarbazone**—reacts with barbiturates, glutethimide, and phenytoin to form blue or purple spots.
- **Iodoplatinate**—forms various colors with tertiary amine compounds.
- **Dragendorf's reagent**—methaqualone forms an orange color; most drugs form a brown color.
- **Absorption of ultraviolet light (254 nm)**—is used to determine benzodiazepines, barbiturates, and methaqualone.
- **Fluorescence of long ultraviolet light (366 nm)**—is used to determine benzodiazepines, quinine, and quinidine.

The TLC plates in commercial kits are made of glass microfibers impregnated with silicic acid. Specimen application is facilitated by the rapid evaporation of the solvent in the extract in the presence of a glass fiber disc. During evaporation, the specimen is absorbed onto the disc, which is then placed in a prepunched hole on the TLC strip. Discs containing reference drugs are already in place on the TLC strips. By combining two different plates and development solvents and a variety of color development and monitoring techniques, each sample can be screened for a large number of acidic, neutral, and basic drugs. The entire procedure may be completed in approximately 30 to 40 min.

Gas chromatography

GC is relatively rapid and is capable of resolving a broad spectrum of drugs; it is used widely for qualitative and quantitative drug analysis. Capillary columns, because of their high efficiency, have become the most commonly used analytical columns for drug detection by GC (see Chapter 8). In many instances, nonderivatized drugs have good GC properties when capillary columns are used; in some instances, derivatization to a less polar or more volatile compound is required. Common detectors for drug detection by GC are flame ionization and alkali flame ionization (nitrogen phosphorus) detectors and mass spectrometers.

High-performance liquid chromatography

Advantages of HPLC over GC for drug screening include the capability to analyze polar compounds without derivatization (for example, morphine and benzoylecgonine) and thermally labile drugs (for example, chlordiazepoxide). The introduction of "array" detectors that provide a spectral scan of compounds as they elute from the column has increased greatly the discriminatory power of this technique, and screening procedures for more than 200 drugs are available.[10]

Gas chromatography/mass spectrometry

Because of the innumerable drugs, metabolites, and endogenous substances that may be encountered, positive identification based on the results of a single analytical technique is generally not sufficiently definitive. Sound laboratory practice dictates the use of a second or confirmatory test that preferably is based on different analytical principles than the first. Currently, GC/MS is the most definitive confirmatory procedure and is legally mandatory for forensic drug testing (for example, workplace drug testing). Liquid chromatography/mass spectrometry (LC/MS) also is used for drug analysis.

Metal Analysis

AAS with flame or electrothermal atomization furnace, ICP-ES, ICP-AES, ICP-MS, and HPLC-MS are state-of-the-art analytical techniques used to measure metals in biological fluids.[12] They are specific and sensitive and provide the clinical laboratory with the capability to measure a broad array of metals at clinically significant levels. Photometric assays also are available but require large volumes of sample and have limited analytical performance. Spot tests are available but are considered obsolete because they are error prone and often yield false-positive results.

References

1. Allen MJ: Procedures for transportation workplace drug testing programs. Fed Reg 1989; 54:49,854-49,884.
2. Blanke RV, Decker WJ: Analysis of toxic substances. In Tietz NW (ed): Textbook of Clinical Chemistry, pp 1670-1744, Philadelphia, WB Saunders, 1986.
3. Department of Transportation, National Highway Traffic Safety: Procedures for transportation workplace drug and alcohol testing programs. Fed Reg 1994; 59:7340-7378.
4. Department of Transportation, National Highway Traffic Safety Administration: Highway safety programs: model specifications for devices to measure breath alcohol. Fed Reg 1996; 61:3078-3081.
5. Documentation of the Threshold Limit Values and Biological Exposure Indices, 6th edition, Cincinnati, Ohio, American Conference of Governmental Industrial Hygienists, 1991.
6. ElSohly HN, ElSohly MA, Stanford DF: Poppy seed ingestion and opiate urinalysis: a closer look. J Anal Toxicol 1990; 14:308-310.
7. Fairbanks VF, Klee GG: Biochemical aspects of hematology. In Burtis CA, Ashwood, ER (eds): Tietz Textbook of Clinical Chemistry, 3rd edition, pp 1676-1678, Philadelphia, WB Saunders, 1999.
8. Hoyle JC: Fitness-for-duty programs. Fed Reg 1988; 54:24,468-24,508.
9. Kintz P (ed): Drug Testing in Hair, Boca Raton, Fla, CRC Press, Inc, 1996.
10. Maier RD, Bogusz M: Identification power of a standardized HPLC-DAD system for systematic toxicological analysis. J Anal Toxicol 1995; 19:79-83.
11. Moyer TP, Mussman GV, Nixon DE: Blood-collection device for trace and ultra-trace metal specimens evaluated. Clin Chem 1991; 37:709-714.
12. Moyer TP: Toxic metals. In Burtis CA, Ashwood, ER (eds): Tietz Textbook of Clinical Chemistry, 3rd edition, pp 982-998, Philadelphia, WB Saunders, 1999.
13. Nixon DE, Moyer TP: Arsenic analysis II: rapid separation and analysis of inorganic arsenic plus metabolites and arsenobetaine from urine. Clin Chem 1992; 38:2479-2483.
14. Occupational exposure to cadmium. Fed Reg 1992; 57:42, 102-142, 462.
15. Porter WH: Clinical toxicology. In Burtis CA, Ashwood ER (eds): Tietz Textbook of Clinical Chemistry, 3rd edition, pp 906-981, Philadelphia, WB Saunders, 1999.
16. Roper WL, Houk VN, Falk H et al: Preventing lead poisoning in young children: a statement by the Centers for Disease Control. Atlanta, Ga, Centers for Disease Control, US Department of Health and Human Services publication PB92-155076/HDM, 1991.
17. Sullivan M: Mandatory guidelines for federal workplace drug testing programs. Fed Reg 1988; 53:11,970-11,989.

Additional Reading

Chang LW (ed): Toxicology of Metals, Boca Raton, Fla, Lewis Publishers, 1996.

Ellenhorn MJ, Schonwald S, Ordog G et al (eds): Ellenhorn's Medical Toxicology: Diagnosis and Treatment of Human Poisoning, 2nd edition, Baltimore, Williams & Wilkins, 1997.

Goldfrank LR, Flomenbaum NE, Lewin NA et al (eds): Goldfrank's Toxicologic Emergencies, 6th edition, Norwalk, Conn, Appleton & Lange, 1998.

Gosselin RE, Smith RP, Hodge HC et al (eds): Clinical Toxicology of Commercial Products, 5th edition, Baltimore, Williams & Wilkins, 1984.

Haddad LM, Winchester JF (eds): Clinical Management of Poisoning and Drug Overdose, 3rd edition, Philadelphia, WB Saunders, 1998.

Hardman JG, Limbird LE, Molinoff PB et al (eds): Goodman and Gilman's The Pharmacological Basis of Therapeutics, 9th edition, New York, McGraw-Hill, 1996.

Klaassen CD, Amdur MO, Doull J (eds): Casarett and Doull's Toxicology: The Basic Science of Poisons, 5th edition, McGraw-Hill, New York, 1996.

PART V

Pathophysiology

CHAPTER 33

Cardiac Function

FRED S. APPLE, PhD

Objectives

1. Define the following terms:

Acute coronary syndrome	Myocardium
Angina	Myocardial infarction
Coronary artery disease	Myoglobin
Creatine kinase	Plaque
Ischemia	Troponin
Lactate dehydrogenase	

2. Diagram blood flow through the heart and lungs.
3. State the events that lead to an acute myocardial infarction.
4. List the cardiac markers and their order of appearance after a myocardial infarction.
5. State the methods used to measure cardiac markers.

Key Words

Acute Coronary Syndrome (ACS) A sudden cardiac disorder that varies from angina (chest pain on exertion with reversible tissue injury), to unstable angina (with minor myocardial injury), and to myocardial infarction (with extensive tissue necrosis)

Acute Myocardial Infarction (AMI) Gross necrosis of the myocardium as a result of interruption of the blood supply to the area; almost always caused by atherosclerosis of the coronary arteries, on which coronary thrombosis usually is superimposed; commonly called a *heart attack*

Angina Chest pain often associated with a decrease in oxygen (ischemia) to the heart

Angiography Visualization of the coronary arteries by use of radiographic equipment after injection of a radiographically opaque dye

Angioplasty An angiographic procedure for elimination of areas of narrowing in blood vessels; usually performed through inflation of a balloon catheter at the site of the narrowing

Arrhythmia Any variation from the normal rhythm of the heart beat

Atherosclerosis The disease process that causes plaque formation within large and medium-sized arteries

Cardiac Marker A clinical laboratory test useful for the detection of acute myocardial infarction or minor myocardial injury

Coronary Arteries Small blood vessels that originate from the aorta above the aortic valve and provide the blood supply to the heart

Electrocardiogram (ECG) A graphical recording of the electrical activity produced by the heart muscle

Ischemia Deficiency of blood flow to part of the heart caused by functional constriction or actual obstruction of a coronary artery

Plaque A pearly white area within an artery that causes the intimal surface to bulge into the lumen;

composed of lipid, cell debris, smooth muscle cells, collagen, and sometimes calcium; also known as *atheromas*

Reperfusion   The restoration of blood flow to an area of the heart after an acute myocardial infarction

Thrombolysis   Dissolution of a thrombus (clot), often after injection of a drug such as streptokinase or tissue plasminogen activator (TPA)

Unstable Angina   Angina that is increasing in severity, duration, or frequency

The heart is a muscular organ responsible for moving blood through the vessels to all parts of the body. Through rhythmic contractions, the right side of the heart pumps deoxygenated blood into the lungs. The left side receives oxygenated blood from the lungs and in turn pumps it to all other parts of the body. It is an efficient and durable pump. For example, during 75 years of human life the heart contracts approximately 3 billion times. However, heart failure can and does occur. Although heart failure is precipitated by a number of factors, including anemia, arrhythmias, infection, and pulmonary embolism, most do not rely on laboratory tests for diagnosis. An exception is myocardial infarction, the major focus of this chapter.

As defined in the 28th edition of *Dorland's Illustrated Medical Dictionary*, **acute myocardial infarction (AMI)** is "gross necrosis of the myocardium as a result of interruption of the blood supply to the area: it is almost always caused by atherosclerosis of the coronary arteries upon which coronary thrombosis is usually superimposed." AMI occurs during the period when circulation to a region is obstructed and necrosis is occurring.

In the United States, approximately 1.5 million individuals suffer annually from AMI, which causes one fourth of all deaths. About 500,000 individuals with confirmed AMI are hospitalized yearly in the United States, and at least as many additional patients are admitted because of suspected AMI. Some 40% to 60% of deaths associated with AMI occur within 1 hour of the event and are attributable to **arrhythmias,** most often ventricular fibrillation. Mortality rates are approximately 10% for individuals during hospitalization and the year after the AMI. In the United States the yearly economic burden of coronary artery disease (CAD) exceeds $100 billion. Perhaps as much as half of this cost is related to AMI and its prevention and treatment.

ANATOMY AND PHYSIOLOGY

The average adult human heart weighs approximately 325 g in men and 275 g in women and is 12 cm in length (Figure 33-1). The heart is enclosed in a sac called the *pericardium*. The cardiac wall is composed of three layers—the outer epicardium, the middle myocardium, and the inner endocardium.

The heart has four internal chambers. The two upper chambers are termed the *right* and *left atria*, and the two lower chambers are known as the *right* and *left ventricles*. Each atrium is connected to its ventricle through a muscular atrioventricular (AV) valve, termed the *mitral valve* on the left side and the *tricuspid valve* on the right side. The right ventricle pumps blood into the pulmonary artery through a passive three-section pulmonary valve. The left ventricle pumps blood into the aorta through a passive three-section aortic valve. The right and left **coronary arteries** begin in two cusps of the aortic valve. They encircle the heart in the epicardium, and smaller arteries branch and enter the myocardium, thereby supplying oxygenated blood to its muscle fibers.

The myocardium contains bundles of striated muscle fibers. The alternating contraction and relaxation of these fibers generate the pumping action of the heart. The fibers are composed of the cardiac-specific contractile proteins—actin and myosin—and regulatory proteins—troponin and tropomyosin. They also contain proteins and enzymes that are vital for energy use, such as myoglobin, creatine kinase (CK), and lactate dehydrogenase (LD). Each of these proteins can be a marker for AMI.

Cardiac Cycle

A typical cardiac cycle (that is, one heartbeat) consists of two major time intervals known as *systole* and *diastole*. During diastole, oxygenated blood returns from the lungs to the left atrium, while deoxygenated blood from other parts of the body fills the right atrium. At the end of diastole the atria contract, forcing blood through the AV valves into the respective ventricles. During systole the ventricles contract, the AV valves close, and blood is pumped across the pulmonary and aortic valves into the pulmonary artery and aorta, respectively. The resting heart rate varies from 60 to 100 beats per minute, and the cardiac output typically ranges from 2.5 to 3.6 L/minute/m^2 of body surface area.

Cardiac Conducting System

The **electrocardiogram (ECG)** is an extremely useful test that identifies anatomical, metabolic, ionic, and hemodynamic changes of the heart. Occasionally, it is the only indi-

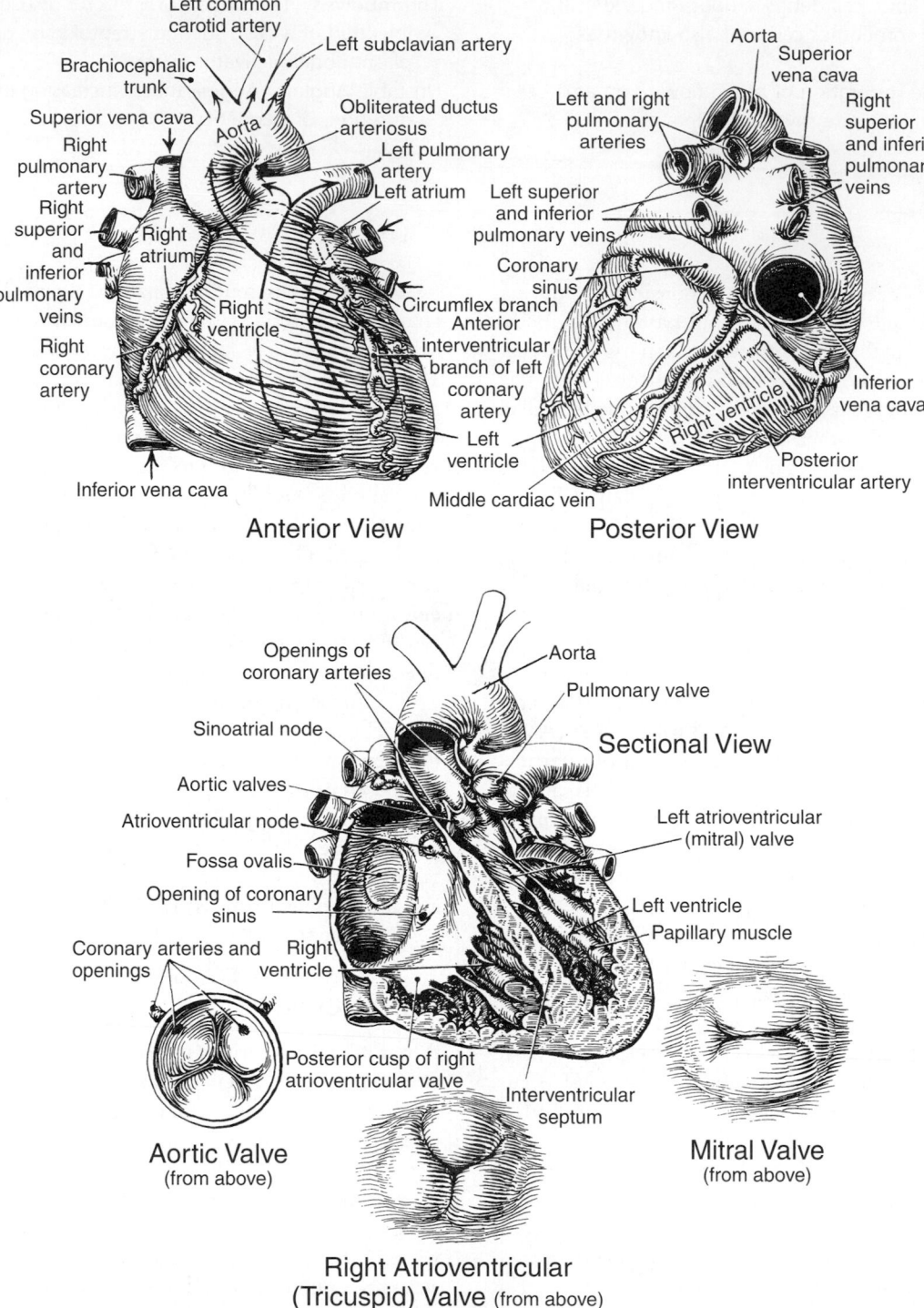

Figure 33-1   Anatomy of the heart. (From Dorland's Illustrated Medical Dictionary, p 737, 28th edition, Philadelphia, WB Saunders, 1994.)

cator of a pathological process. The ECG presents a visible record of the heart's electrical activity (Figure 33-2). In a normal ECG, all heartbeats appear as a similar pattern equally spaced, with three major parts—the P wave, QRS complex, and T wave. Each beat manifests as five major waves—P, Q, R, S, and T. The P wave reflects the impulse that produces atrial contraction. The QRS complex is the impulse that produces contraction of the ventricles. Finally, the T wave is produced by the electrical recovery of the ventricles. The QRS complex consists of three deflections—the Q wave, the downstroke before the R wave; the R wave, the first upward deflection; and the S wave, the downstroke after the R wave. However, not every QRS complex shows discrete Q, R, and S waves.

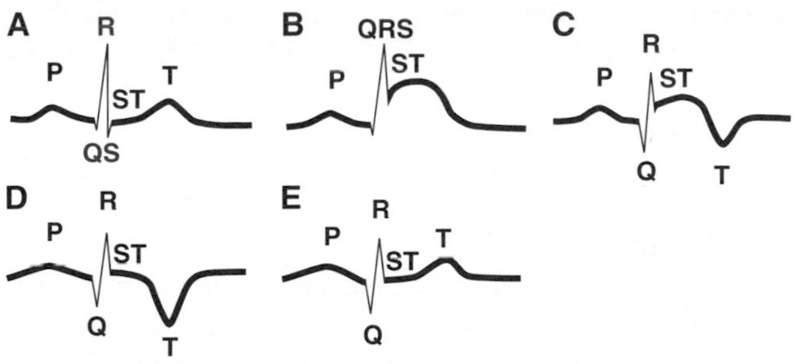

Figure 33-2   Electrocardiogram serial tracing of a patient with an acute myocardial infarction. **A,** Normal. **B,** Hours after infarction the ST segment becomes elevated. **C,** Hours to days later the T wave inverts and the Q wave becomes larger. **D,** Days to weeks later the ST segment returns to near normal. **E,** Weeks to months later the T wave becomes upright again, but the large Q wave may remain.

■ CARDIAC DISEASE

This chapter's discussion focuses on atherosclerosis, AMI, and heart failure. The vast number of other cardiac diseases are not discussed here because of the minor role of clinical laboratory tests in the diagnosis of such disorders.

Atherosclerosis

The major cause of CAD is **atherosclerosis.** This disease process causes plaque formation within large- and medium-sized arteries. A **plaque** is a pearly white area within an artery. In early plaque formation the lumen is spared, but as plaques age and expand, they sometimes bulge into the lumen. The internal portion of a plaque is composed of lipid, cell debris, smooth muscle cells, collagen, and sometimes calcium; externally the plaque is covered by a fibrous cap.

Arterial blood flow is reduced across plaques that narrow the arterial lumen. Some individuals with advanced atherosclerosis of the coronary arteries experience chest pain and shortness of breath with mild exertion. This is known as stable **angina.** The cause is myocardial **ischemia** resulting from the inability to increase coronary artery blood flow across the restrictions in the vessels. It is termed *stable*, because the myocardial injury is reversible. The ischemia and pain end shortly after the exertion is discontinued.

Sporadically the fibrous cap of a plaque can rupture, exposing the internal contents of a plaque to the bloodstream. These contents are highly thrombotic. The subsequent thrombus formation rapidly restricts downstream blood flow. When this phenomenon occurs within a coronary artery, an acute coronary syndrome (ACS) ensues. If blood flow is blocked completely and the affected downstream myocardium has insufficient collateral blood flow, acute myocardial ischemia and infarction occurs. If the thrombus causes partial occlusion, the reduced blood flow leads to milder ischemia and myocardial damage known as **unstable angina.** Why the fibrous cap ruptures is unknown,

but current theories stress inflammation as opposed to degeneration. Plaques that are predisposed to rupture are termed *vulnerable.*

Conditions associated with atherosclerosis

Atherosclerosis begins early in life and progresses silently for decades. Although the exact cause of atherosclerosis is unknown, it is thought to be an inflammatory response to injury of the arterial endothelium. Many conditions increase the risk of the disease, including increasing age, male sex, genetics, diabetes mellitus, hypertension, smoking, hyperlipidemia, and increased plasma homocysteine. Genetics plays an important but incompletely understood role in atherosclerosis. Plaque rupture may be caused by inflammation. The associations of mildly increased C-reactive protein (CRP) and chlamydia infection with ACS support this theory.

Prevention of atherosclerosis

The identification and treatment of individuals who may be at high risk for atherosclerosis can prevent or delay the progression of this disease. Those individuals with diabetes mellitus should attempt tight glycemic control (see Chapter 23). Children should be urged not to begin smoking cigarettes, and smokers should attempt to quit. Daily consumption of beverages containing 1 to 2 ounces of alcohol is protective of CAD, but higher consumption can lead to hyperlipidemia. Individuals with high blood pressure can lower their risk of CAD with drug therapy. Lipid screening is recommended for adults (see Chapter 24). Aerobic exercise has been shown to raise high-density lipoprotein (HDL) cholesterol. Those with high hyperlipidemia should reduce their body weight if they are obese. Diets low in fat and high in omega (ω)-3 fatty acids can be beneficial. Individuals who continue to have hyperlipidemia are candidates for drug therapy. In addition, lipoprotein (a), plasma homocysteine, and CRP are gaining physician support as CAD risk factors.

Acute Myocardial Infarction

As explained previously, AMI occurs during the period when circulation to a region of the heart is obstructed and necrosis (massive cell death) ensues. AMI is characterized by severe pain (angina pectoris), frequently associated with perspiration, nausea, shortness of breath, and dizziness. A precursor state of AMI is myocardial ischemia, in which obstruction of a coronary artery leads to severe oxygen deprivation of the myocardium before necrosis.

The major causes of AMI are atherosclerotic plaque rupture and thrombus formation. Myocardial ischemia and subsequent infarction usually begin in the endocardium and spread toward the epicardium. When the necrosis occurs through the full thickness of the myocardium, the infarct is termed *transmural.* Irreversible cardiac injury occurs if occlusion is complete for at least 15 to 20 minutes. Irreversible injury occurs maximally when occlusion is sustained for 4 to 6 hours, but most of the damage occurs within the first 2 to 3 hours. Restoration of flow within the first 4 to 6 hours is associated with salvage of myocardium, but the salvage is greater if restoration occurs in 1 to 2 hours. Coronary thrombosis undergoes spontaneous lysis in about 50% of cases within 10 days. Individuals who exhibit minimal myocardial damage may have experienced early spontaneous lysis, which may account for many cases of nontransmural infarction.

Precipitating factors

Although no precipitating factor can be identified in most individuals with AMI, the event is not random. Studies have shown that AMI occurs more frequently during physical exertion, after surgical procedures, early in the morning, in the winter months, during sexual activity, and during emotional stress. Trauma may precipitate an AMI in one of the following two ways:

1. Myocardial contusion and hemorrhage into the myocardium actually may cause cell necrosis.
2. The injury may involve a coronary artery, causing occlusion of that vessel with resultant AMI.

Neurological disturbances (transient ischemic attacks or strokes) also may precipitate AMI.

Studies have demonstrated that the early-morning peak in AMI parallels the peak incidence of death from ischemic heart disease, occurring at about 0800 to 0900 hours. In addition, a second peak occurs, at approximately 1700 hours. The reason this event occurs more often in the morning hours may be due to normal circadian rhythms. During the early morning, adrenergic activity, plasma fibrinogen levels, and platelet adhesiveness all increase naturally. Nontransmural infarction does not exhibit this circadian rhythm.

Silent myocardial infarction and atypical presentation

Studies suggest that between 40% and 50% of nonfatal AMIs are unrecognized by the affected individual and are discovered only on subsequent routine ECG or postmortem examinations. Of these unrecognized infarctions in individuals with diabetes and hypertension, approximately half are truly silent, with the individual unable to recall any symptoms. The other half of individuals with so-called silent infarction can recall an event characterized by symptoms compatible with AMI.

Diagnosis of acute myocardial infarction

The diagnosis of AMI, as formally established by the World Health Organization (WHO), requires at least two of the following criteria:

- A history of chest pain
- Evolutionary changes on the ECG
- Elevation of serial cardiac enzymes (proteins)

Often the examining physician is fairly certain that AMI has occurred after obtaining a patient's history, completing a physical examination, and performing ECG. When the ECG fails to demonstrate an AMI, cardiac markers are used.

Clinical history

The recent medical history of the patient greatly assists with the establishment of a diagnosis. The first symptom (prodrome) is usually angina occurring at rest or with less activity than usual. A prodromal history can be elicited in 40% to 50% of patients with AMI. The prodrome also may include undue fatigue or shortness of breath. Among patients who are hospitalized for angina, fewer than 15% develop AMI. Of the patients with AMI presenting with prodromal symptoms, approximately one-third have had symptoms from 1 to 4 weeks before hospitalization; in the remaining two-thirds, symptoms predate admission by a week or less, with one third of these patients having had symptoms for 24 hours or less.

The pain of AMI is variable in intensity; in most patients, it is severe and in some instances intolerable. The pain is prolonged, usually lasting for more than 30 minutes and frequently for many hours. The discomfort is described as constricting, crushing, or compressing; often the patient complains of feeling as though something is sitting on or squeezing the chest. Although usually described as a squeezing, choking, or heavy pain, it also may be characterized as a stabbing or burning discomfort. The pain is usually retrosternal in location, spreading frequently to both sides of the chest but favoring the left side. Often the pain radiates down the left arm, producing a tingling sensation in the left wrist, hand, and even fingers. Some patients note only a dull ache or numbness of the wrists in association with severe substernal discomfort. In some instances the pain of AMI may begin in the epigastrium, which often causes AMI to be misdiagnosed as indigestion. In patients with preexisting angina the pain of infarction usually resembles that of angina with respect to features and location. However, the pain of AMI is generally much more severe, lasts longer, and is not relieved by rest and nitroglycerin.

The pain of AMI may have disappeared by the time the physician first encounters the patient (or the patient reaches the hospital), or it may persist for many hours. With severe angina, nausea and vomiting occur in more than 50% of patients with transmural AMI.

Electrocardiogram

One of the most valuable contributions of the ECG is in the diagnosis of AMI. It is usually the first test performed and is often the cornerstone of the diagnosis. The initial ECG is diagnostic of AMI in slightly more than 50% of AMI patients. In about 15% of AMIs, no changes appear on the initial ECG tracing. Serial tracings over a 24-hour period increase its sensitivity to more than 75%. The ECG changes of an AMI are those of ischemia, injury, and cell death and are reflected by T-wave changes, ST-segment changes, and the appearance of enlarged Q waves, respectively (see Figure 33-2).

However, clear-cut differentiation may not be possible in every case. For example, T-wave changes may be due to ischemia, injury, or death of myocardial cells. The ST segment is elevated in AMI after myocardial injury. It is depressed when the heart is not receiving a sufficient supply of oxygen (for example, during an episode of angina). The cell necrosis in AMI produces a local area of electrically inert myocardium. When the necrosis is transmural, the electrically inert area produces an enlarged Q wave. These specific patterns sometimes can be obscured by prior heart disease, or they may not appear at all. This fact accounts for the diagnostic sensitivity of the ECG, ranging from only 50% to 75%, although the diagnostic specificity is about 100%. If the ECG pattern is equivocal, then the physician must depend on serum markers of myocardial damage.

Cardiac markers

A **cardiac marker** is a clinical laboratory test useful in the detection of AMI or minor myocardial injury.[8] Cardiac markers are most useful when individuals have nondiagnostic ECG tracings.[21] Individuals with AMI can be categorized into the following four groups:

1. The first is the group of patients who present early to the emergency room, within 0 to 4 hours after the onset of chest pain, without diagnostic ECG evidence of AMI. For laboratory tests to be clinically useful in this group of patients, markers of AMI must be released rapidly from the heart into the circulation. Further, the analytical assays must be sensitive enough to distinguish small changes within the serum reference interval.
2. The second group of patients are those presenting 4 to 48 hours after the onset of chest pain without clear evidence of AMI on the ECG. In this group of patients the diagnosis of AMI requires serial monitoring of both cardiac markers and ECG changes.
3. In the next group are patients who present more than 48 hours after the onset of chest pain with nonspecific ECG changes. The ideal marker of myocardial injury in this group would persist in the circulation for several days, providing diagnostic information of more remote infarction. A shortcoming of such a marker might be its inability to distinguish recurrent injury from old injury.
4. The last group of patients are those who present to the emergency department at any time after the onset of chest pain with clear ECG evidence of AMI. In this group, detection with serum markers of myocardial injury is not necessary but is confirmatory.

Treatment and prognosis

When untreated, transmural infarction is associated with a high in-hospital mortality rate and a highly vulnerable period lasting 6 to 12 weeks. In contrast, nontransmural infarction is associated with a lower acute mortality and complication rate but a longer period of vulnerability to reinfarction and death. As a result, 1- to 2-year survival rates are similar for transmural and nontransmural infarctions.

Patients who present quickly to the hospital with diagnostic ECG changes may be treated with intravenous thrombolytic drugs, a process termed **thrombolysis**. This treatment sometimes restores blood flow and often limits the extent of myocardial necrosis. The prognosis of transmural infarction after thrombolysis appears to be improved because the vulnerable period appears to be shorter.[10]

Emergent percutaneous transluminal coronary **angioplasty** (PCTA) can be life saving. A catheter is inserted in the femoral artery and threaded up into the aorta. The catheter tip is inserted into a coronary vessel. Radiographic dye is injected, a process known as **angiography,** so that the vessel blood flow can be observed. The catheter tip is advanced to the area of restricted flow, and a balloon is inflated. A stent can be inserted inside the vessel to help maintain blood flow.

Several weeks after recovery from AMI, patients are evaluated through use of exercise and ECG. If significant CAD remains, repeat PCTA or coronary artery bypass graft surgery is recommended. In addition, a daily dose of aspirin has been shown to reduce reinfarction.

Heart Failure

The ultimate complication of most forms of heart disease is heart failure. Heart failure is defined as the pathophysiological condition in which an abnormality of cardiac function is responsible for failure of the heart to pump blood at a rate necessary for the requirements of the metabolizing tissues. Encompassed in this definition is a wide spectrum of clinical conditions, ranging from impairment of pumping function, as during a massive AMI, to the gradual impairment of function observed when an individual's heart sustains a pressure or volume overload for a prolonged period.

Brain natriuretic peptide (BNP) is a cardiac hormone primarily synthesized in and secreted from the myocardial ventricles. This hormone has been shown as a sensitive and specific marker for changes in ventricular function. Circulating concentrations of BNP are increased in individuals with chronic heart failure and appear to correlate with its severity. Early studies have demonstrated that BNP secretion reflects regional wall stress in the ventricles and thus is associated with adverse ventricular remodeling and poor prognosis after AMI. Increased BNP in the early phase of infarction also has been proposed as an indicator of poor prognosis. The clinical usefulness of a laboratory test for BNP requires additional clinical studies, as well as the development of versatile and applicable immunoassays for its analysis.

TESTS USED TO ESTIMATE INCREASED RISK OF CARDIOVASCULAR DISEASE

Low-density lipoprotein (LDL) and HDL cholesterol, triglycerides, lipoprotein (a), CRP, homocysteine, and fibrinogen are laboratory tests that help indicate an individual's risk for CAD. The biochemistry and measurement of lipids, as well as the National Cholesterol Education Program (NCEP) guidelines, are discussed in Chapter 24. The use of CRP and homocysteine are reviewed is this chapter.

C-Reactive Protein

The biochemistry of CRP is discussed in Chapter 19. In addition to being a sensitive marker of systemic inflammation, plasma concentrations of CRP are increased among women and men at risk for future cardiovascular events. For example, prospective studies have indicated that when a sensitive CRP assay (analytical detection limit of 0.05 mg/L and upper reference limit of 0.20 mg/L) is used to measure CRP concentrations, individuals with increased baseline concentrations of CRP are at increased risk for AMI and stroke. This increased risk is associated also with individuals who are older, smoke, have symptomatic angina, or have had previous AMIs. In addition, the predictive value of CRP testing appears to add to those of total and HDL cholesterol measurements. This information suggests that screening with a method sensitive for CRP concentrations may play a role in cardiovascular risk prediction.

Homocysteine

The biochemistry of homocysteine is described in Chapter 18. This amino acid is a part of the synthetic pathway from methionine to cysteine. Most free homocysteine rapidly forms disulfide bridges with itself and free sulfhydryl groups on proteins. Total homocysteine is usually less than 15 μmol/L in plasma collected from fasting individuals. In rare cases an inborn error of homocysteine metabolism causes plasma levels to exceed 100 μmol/L. Affected individuals develop CAD in their teens. Mildly elevated levels increase the risk of CAD. Homocysteine may cause direct injury to the vascular endothelium or may be merely a marker of atherosclerosis. Ingestion of vitamins B_{12}, B_6, and folate at doses greater than the daily recommendations sometimes can lower homocysteine levels. Unlike in cases of hyperlipidemia, population screening for hyperhomocysteinemia is not recommended, but testing of individuals from families with unexplained premature CAD is useful.

Assays for homocysteine include a reduction step, which cleaves the disulfide bonds. The total homocysteine is measured (this fraction not including any homocysteine incorporated into proteins via peptide bonds). Techniques for measurement include gas chromatography-mass spectrometry, high-performance liquid chromatography (HPLC; with either electrochemical or fluorescence detection), and immunoassay (with fluorescence polarization or enzyme detection). The immunoassay techniques use S-adenosylhomocysteine (SAH) hydrolase to catalyze the production of SAH from homocysteine. The fluorescence polarization immunoassay then uses a monoclonal antibody to SAH and a fluorescent analog of SAH.

CARDIAC MARKERS

Many tests have been used to assess cardiac injury. The most commonly available tests, including CK isoenzymes, LD, myoglobin, and cardiac troponins, are discussed in this chapter.

Biochemistry and Tissue Distribution of Cardiac Markers

Although the cardiac markers are all myocardial proteins, they differ in their location within the myocyte, release after damage, and clearance from the serum, as noted in Table 33-1. Because they are markers of myocardial damage, the biochemistry of each is considered separately.

TABLE 33-1   Characteristics of Cardiac Markers and Time Course after Onset of AMI

Marker	Molecular Mass	Time (h) until Marker Increases above Upper Reference Limit	Time (h) until Peak Concentration	Time (Days) until Return to within Reference Interval
CK	86,000	3 to 8	10 to 24	3 to 4
CK-2	86,000	3 to 8	10 to 24	2 to 3
LD, LD-1	135,000	8 to 12	72 to 144	8 to 14
Myoglobin	18,000	1 to 3	6 to 9	1
Troponins I and T	23,000 (I)	3 to 8	24 to 48 (first peak)	3 to 5 (I)
	42,000 (T)		72 to 100 (second peak; T only)	5 to 10 (T)

AMI, Acute myocardial infarction; *CK*, creatine kinase; *LD*, lactate dehydrogenase.

Creatine kinase isoenzymes and isoforms

CK catalyzes the formation of phosphocreatine from creatine and adenosine triphosphate (ATP). Both cytosolic and mitochondrial isoenzymes have been identified. The cytosolic form of the enzyme is a dimer composed of two subunits (M and B) and thus has three isoenzymes—CK-3 (MM), CK-2 (MB), CK-1 (BB). The mitochondrial CK (CK-Mt) has two isoenzymes. Thus three different genes encode and are specific for CK-M, CK-B, and CK-Mt_1. CK-3 (CK-MM) is predominant in both heart and skeletal muscle, but CK-2 (CK-MB) is more specific for the myocardium. The total CK activity of the heart is from 10% to 20% CK-2, whereas skeletal muscle is less than 2% CK-2.

Electrophoresis of CK isoenzymes, with use of extended electrophoresis times or higher voltages, further separates the bands of CK-3 and CK-2. Three CK-3 and two CK-2 isoforms (subtypes of the individual isoenzymes) exist. The tissue isoform (gene product) of CK-3 is designated CK-3_3. When this enzyme is released into the circulation, a time-mediated carboxypeptidase hydrolysis of C-terminal lysine residue on the M subunits occurs, giving rise to two posttranslational products—CK-3_2 and CK-3_1. Similarly, after release of CK-2_2 (the tissue isoform of CK-2) into the circulation, carboxypeptidase cleavage of the CK-M C-terminal lysine residue gives rise to CK-2_1, the posttranslational product. The clearance rate of total CK activity from blood is a composite of the clearance rates of the individual isoforms. The more prolonged half-lives are associated with the posttranslational degradation isoforms. Thus the order of half-lives is CK-3_1 > CK-3_2 > CK-3_3, and CK-2_1 > CK-2_2. Posttranslational modifications of isoforms occur in blood, are unidirectional, and do not occur in the lymphatic system or necrotic tissue.

Studies involving animal hearts or specimens obtained at autopsy from human hearts suggested a uniform distribution of CK-3 and CK-2. The proportion of CK-2 varies from 5% to 50% of the total CK activity. In response to acute and chronic coronary artery occlusion in a dog model, myocardium showed twofold to threefold increases in CK-2 activity in both the ischemic and the nonischemic myocardium. In more complete studies in humans, CK-2 concentrations ranged from 15% to 24% of total CK in myocardial tissue obtained from individuals with CAD, enlarged hearts, or both. In contrast, individuals with normal cardiac tissue had a low percentage of CK-2.[14] These data suggest that the proportion of CK-2 increases in the hypertrophied and diseased human myocardium.

Normal skeletal muscle contains approximately 1% CK-2. Severe skeletal muscle injury after trauma or surgery can lead to absolute elevations of CK-2 above the upper reference limit in serum, with the percent CK-2 in serum less than 1% of the total CK activity. Increases in total CK and CK-2 in several patient groups often present a diagnostic challenge to the clinician. For example, persistent elevations of serum CK-2 resulting from chronic muscle disease occur in individuals with muscular dystrophy and polymyositis, as well as in healthy subjects who undergo extreme exercise or physical activities. The mechanism responsible for increased CK-2 in skeletal muscle after chronic muscle disease, injury, or exercise is thought to be due to the regeneration process of muscle, with reexpression of CK-B genes similar to those found in the heart. This reexpression gives rise to increased CK-2 levels in skeletal muscle.[1] Thus distressed skeletal muscle can become like diseased heart muscle in its CK isoenzyme composition, with up to 15% CK-2.

Lactate dehydrogenase isoenzymes

LD is localized in the cytoplasm of tissues. The highest activities of LD are found in skeletal muscle, liver, heart, kidney, and red blood cells. At least five isoenzymes exist, composed of four subunit peptides of two distinct types, designated M (for muscle) and H (for heart). LD-1 (H_4) moves the fastest toward the anode, whereas LD-5 (M_4) is closest to the cathode on an electrophoretic gel. LD-1 is found in the highest concentrations in the heart, kidney (cortex), and red blood cells. LD-5 is found in the highest concentrations in the liver and skeletal muscle. The hybrid LD isoenzymes LD-2 (H_3M), LD-3 (H_2M_2), and LD-4 (HM_3) also are found in the heart, kidneys, RBCs, and several other tissues.

Because LD is not a tissue-specific enzyme, serum total LD is increased in a wide variety of diseases, including heart disease. For example, the activities of total LD and LD-1 increase from the right to left ventricles, with the H subunit activity varying twofold between different locations of the heart. As with CK-2 in skeletal muscle, the heart-specific LD-1 isoenzyme in skeletal muscle can increase twofold (from 10% to 20% of total LD activity) during a 9-week period of exercise training, with parallel decreases in LD-5. Thus individuals must be aware that after exercise, increases in serum total LD, especially in LD-1 and a "flipped" ratio of LD-1 to LD-2 (≥ 1.0), can arise from skeletal muscle, as opposed to the myocardium.

Myoglobin

Myoglobin is an oxygen-binding protein of cardiac and skeletal muscle. The protein's low molecular weight and cytoplasmic location probably account for its early appearance in the circulation after muscle injury. Increases in serum myoglobin occur after trauma to either skeletal or cardiac muscle, as in crush injuries or AMI. Serum myoglobin methods are unable to distinguish the tissue of origin. Even minor injury to skeletal muscle may result in an elevated concentration of serum myoglobin, which may lead to the misdiagnosis of AMI.

Cardiac troponin I and T

The contractile proteins of all myofibrils include the regulatory protein troponin. Troponin is a complex of three protein subunits—troponin C (the calcium-binding component), troponin I (the inhibitory component), and troponin T (the tropomyosin-binding component). Troponin is localized primarily in the myofibrils (94% to 97%), with a smaller cytoplasmic fraction (3% to 6%). On injury, troponin is released into the circulation.

The troponin subunits exist in a number of isoforms. The distribution of these isoforms varies between cardiac muscle and slow- and fast-twitch skeletal muscle. Two major isoforms of troponin C are found in human heart and skeletal muscle. These are characteristic of slow- and fast-twitch skeletal muscle. The heart isoform is identical to the slow-twitch skeletal muscle isoform and thus is not a useful cardiac marker. However, cardiac-specific troponin T (cTnT) and troponin I (cTnI) isoforms have been identified.

Different genes encode the cardiac and skeletal troponin I. Human cTnI is 30 amino acid residues longer than skeletal muscle TnI isoforms, giving it unique cardiac specificity. Only one cardiac isoform has been identified. cTnI has never been shown to be expressed in normal, regenerating, or diseased human or animal skeletal muscle.[5]

cTnT also has separate genes encoding for the cardiac and skeletal isoforms. cTnT has an unique 11-amino acid sequence that gives this marker cardiac specificity. However, small amounts of cTnT are made by skeletal muscle during human fetal development, in regenerating muscle, and in diseased muscle.[18] Thus cTnT has been found in skeletal muscle specimens obtained from individuals with muscular dystrophy, polymyositis, and chronic renal disease.[18]

Analytical Measurement of Cardiac Proteins

The analytical techniques used to measure most cardiac markers are described elsewhere in this textbook. All the initial cardiac markers were enzymes, so the earliest techniques measured the catalytic activity of the marker. Many of the recently discovered markers have no enzymatic activity and are measured by immunoassay.

Creatine kinase-2

Although CK-2 was measured first by electrophoresis and enzymatic detection, it is commonly measured now by immunoassays that use monoclonal anti-CK-2 antibodies. Commercially available immunoassays that use monoclonal anti-CK-2 antibodies are available widely. Excellent concordance has been shown between mass concentration and activity assays. All have detection limits of approximately 1 µg/L, are 100% specific for CK-2, and are remarkably similar in clinical performance in the diagnosis of AMI. Analytical performance, linearity, and cost may vary among assays. One of the many impacts these new immunoassays provide is that serum CK-2 values can be determined conveniently at almost any time of day, without additional laboratory personnel and without known analytical or biochemical interferences. This availability improves the clinician's ability to triage patients in the emergency department and intensive care units.

Creatine kinase isoforms

At present, CK isoforms are analyzed rarely on a 24-hour basis in the clinical laboratory. Recent studies have shown dramatic improvements for a commercial high-voltage electrophoresis procedure, which provides rapid and sensitive enough results to permit CK-2 isoform measurement at all levels of total CK.[23] Collection of the specimen into ethylenediaminetetraacetic acid (EDTA) tubes stabilizes the isoforms and permits accurate measurement of CK-2_2 and CK-2_1.

Myoglobin

Myoglobin is measured most often in serum or plasma by rapid immunoassays (<30 minutes) that use monoclonal antibodies. Use of myoglobin permits the early identification of AMI and reperfusion, as well as the negative prediction of myocardial injury in an emergency department setting.

Cardiac troponin I

Several manufacturers have commercialized quantitative monoclonal antibody-based immunoassays for the measurement of cTnI in serum, plasma, and whole blood. Assay times range from 7 to 30 minutes. In addition, a qualitative, whole-blood cTnI assay is available commercially. This system shows a visible colored band for a positive test.

cTnI results from different assays vary because of calibration and antibody differences. Currently, no primary reference cTnI material is available for manufacturers to use to standardize their assays.[4,22] In addition, the assays fail to agree with each other because of the different epitopes recognized by the reagent antibodies used. cTnI is present in the circulation in the following three forms:

1. Free
2. Bound as a two-unit complex (cTnI-cTnC)
3. Bound as a three-unit complex (cTnT-cTnI-cTnC)

These three forms circulate in differing degrees of degradation. Thus the different assays do not produce equivalent results, and comparisons of absolute cTnI concentrations in clinical studies cannot be made. Until appropriate standardization is attained, comparisons must use changes relative to each assay's respective upper reference limit.

Cardiac troponin T

One manufacturer has commercialized a quantitative cTnT immunoassay. This system provides results from serum, plasma, or whole blood within 15 minutes, using third-generation reagents and antibodies that show no cross-reactivity with skeletal muscle troponin isoforms or cardiac troponin isoforms expressed in diseased skeletal tissue; thus the assay is 100% specific for the cTnT isoforms expressed in the heart. In addition, a qualitative screening assay has been developed with the same monoclonal antibodies specific against cTnT used in the quantitative assay. Thus in contrast to cTnI, no standardization bias exists for cTnT.

Clinical Utility of Cardiac Markers

Acute coronary syndrome (ACS) describes the clinical spectrum from angina (reversible tissue injury), to unstable angina (with minor myocardial injury), to AMI (with extensive tissue necrosis). The ideal marker of myocardial injury would provide early AMI diagnosis, assist in risk stratification, optimize management of the success of reperfusion after thrombolytic therapy, detect reocclusions and reinfarctions, determine infarct size, and detect perioperative AMI during cardiac or noncardiac surgery. For all presenting ACS patients, results of cardiac markers should be provided to clinicians within 60 minutes.

Detection of acute myocardial infarction

In practice, ruling out of AMI requires a test with high diagnostic sensitivity, whereas ruling in AMI requires a test with high diagnostic specificity. These diagnostic strategies often require different decision thresholds (cutoff points) for different biochemical markers. One of the laboratory's functions is to provide advice to physicians about these tests' characteristics. Recommendations have been made by the National Academy of Clinical Biochemistry to define two decision cutoffs.[21] The first, determined by use of the 97.5 percentile from a normal, healthy population, would define myocardial injury. The second, determined by receiver operating characteristic (ROC) curve analysis, would define optimally AMI. Manufacturers should provide this information on the package insert for each immunoassay.

Studies that assess the ability of a cardiac marker use two differing time intervals—the time from onset of chest pain and the time from presentation in the emergency department. Usually, 1 to 6 hours difference exists between these time intervals. This difference makes comparison of studies problematic and explains some of the disparate reported sensitivities and specificities. Both intervals are important for the clinician. Thrombolytic therapy is useful if administered within 12 hours of the onset of chest pain. Likewise, knowing which marker is more likely to be positive on presentation to the emergency department can assist in patient management.

Creatine kinase-2

The measurement of CK-2 in serum is still a frequently requested laboratory test for the diagnosis of AMI; however, its continued use is being challenged and questioned. The classic time versus CK-2 pattern observed after the onset of chest pain in AMI is illustrated in Figure 33-3. Although CK-2 (CK-MB) rises quickly in cases of AMI, it usually takes 4 to 6 hours to exceed the upper reference limit. Peak levels occur at approximately 24 hours. Return to normal (baseline) takes 48 to 72 hours. (The half-life of CK-2 is 10 to 12 hours.) Factors that can affect the classic pattern include the size of the infarction, CK-2 composition in the myocardium, concomitant skeletal muscle injury, and reperfusion. Differentiation of increased CK-2 due to the heart or skeletal muscle is sometimes difficult. A normal percent-

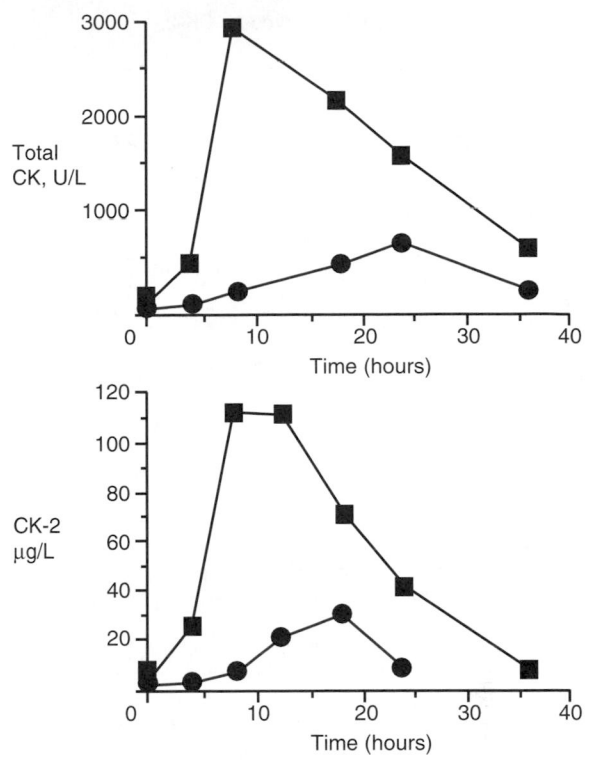

Figure 33-3 Serial total creatine kinase (CK) and creatine kinase 2 (CK-2) values for two patients after AMI occurred; one patient was reperfused successfully after tissue plasminogen activator therapy *(boxes)* and another without reperfusion *(circles)*. (Modified from Apple FS: Creatine kinase MB. Lab Med 1992; 23:299.)

age of CK-2 of total CK activity may be misleading if concomitant injury occurs in skeletal muscle and heart and the absolute amount of CK-2 is hidden due to the large release of total CK from skeletal muscle injury.

Nearly 50% of individuals with AMI present to the emergency department with a nondiagnostic ECG. Rapid and sensitive assays for the measurement of CK-2 help clarify the diagnosis in those patients. The clinical sensitivity of a single test (CK-2) result varies considerably for patients admitted to the emergency department. For the improved CK-2 mass immunoassays, the sensitivity is from 17% to 62% at the time of presentation. This sensitivity improves to 92% to 100% at 3 hours after presentation. ROC curves for CK-2 are shown in Figure 33-4. A sampling schedule of 0, 3 to 6, 6 to 9, and 12 to 24 hours after presentation would allow earlier detection of a rise in CK-2. Older electrophoretic assays for CK-2 cannot detect AMI as early as the mass immunoassays.

The percent relative index (%RI) is the CK-2 mass result (in μg/L) divided by total CK activity (in U/L) multiplied by 100%. Use of %RI aids in the interpretation of CK-2 concentrations for the detection of AMI. The diagnostic cutoff is assay dependent because of lack of CK-2 standardization among different manufacturers. Although it is not absolute, an increased %RI points toward the heart as the source of CK-2 in serum. However, the %RI should not be

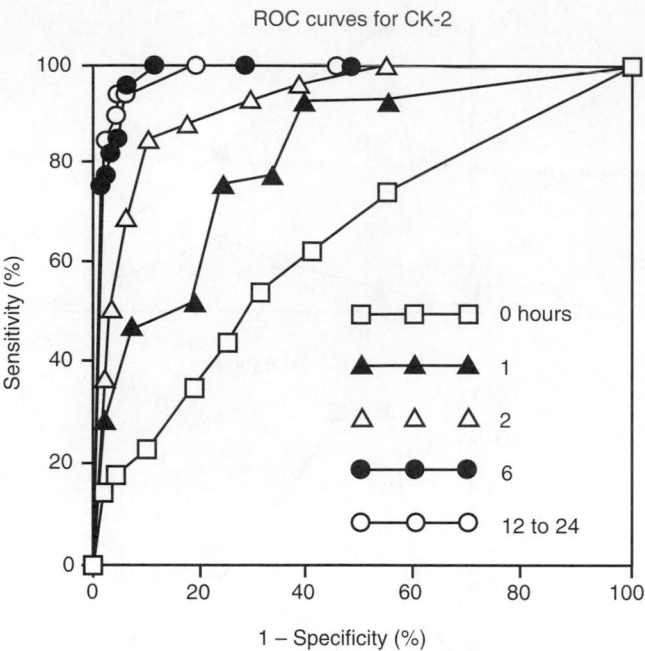

Figure 33-4 Receiver operating characteristic (ROC) curves to establish the best discriminator limits for acute myocardial infarction by use of creatine kinase 2 (CK-2). Each curve represents a different time interval after the onset of chest pain in 35 patients. (Data from Tucker JF, Collins RA, Anderson AJ et al: Early diagnostic efficiency of cardiac troponin I and cardiac troponin T for acute myocardial infarction. Acad Emerg Med 1997; 4:13-21.)

used for interpretation when the total CK activity remains within the reference interval because of the potential of falsely elevated values.

Creatine kinase-2 isoforms

Prospective studies (involving approximately 2000 patients, 240 of whom had AMI) have found that CK-2 isoforms are a reliable marker for triaging of patients in the first 6 hours after the onset of symptoms.[23] Clinical sensitivities of the CK-2 isoforms for detection of AMI at 6 hours after the onset of chest pain ranged from 90% to 95%, compared with 75% to 85% for myoglobin. However, no statistically significant difference appears to exist between myoglobin and CK-2 isoforms over the early 6-hour period. In comparison, diagnostic sensitivities are lower at 6 hours for cTnT, cTnI, and CK-2 (<60%) than for myoglobin or CK-2 isoforms. Little, if any differences were found for diagnostic specificities, ranging from 89% to 100%.

In practice, concentrations of CK-2 isoforms have been found to reliably detect AMI early, potentially reducing admissions to intensive care units by 50%. However, a shortcoming that often limits the routine use of CK-2 isoforms has been demonstrated in studies in which CK-2 isoforms were increased (similar to AMI findings) in most individuals with acute skeletal muscle injury and in subjects after ex-

treme physical exercise. In addition, the rapid electrophoretic assays used to measure CK-2 isoforms are not performed routinely in many clinical laboratories.

Lactate dehydrogenase isoenzymes

The use of LD and LD isoenzymes for detection of AMI is declining rapidly. Likely few, if any, laboratories will continue to offer these tests to detect AMI. The troponin tests are much more useful, as will be explained later in the chapter. For historical purposes the pattern of total LD and LD isoenzymes during AMI is reviewed briefly.

For patients having an AMI, serum total LD values become elevated at 12 to 18 hours after the onset of symptoms, peak at 48 to 72 hours, and return to below the upper reference limit after 6 to 10 days. LD-1 (the isoenzyme enriched in the heart) rises within 10 to 12 hours, peaks at 72 to 144 hours, and returns to normal approximately 10 days after AMI, paralleling total LD. Because of its prolonged half-life, LD-1 is a clinically sensitive (90%) marker for infarction when it is used more than 24 hours after the occurrence of an AMI.

The LD-1 increase over LD-2 in serum after AMI (the so-called flipped pattern, in which the LD-1/LD-2 ratio becomes ≥ 1.0) has a clinical sensitivity of about 75% in individuals suspected of having sustained an AMI. The clinical specificity of the flipped LD-1/LD-2 ratio is approximately 85% to 90% in these individuals. However, the measurement of LD isoenzymes often depends on the separation of isoenzymes by electrophoresis, which is time-consuming, and involves estimation of isoenzyme activity by scanning densitometry, which is marginally precise. Regardless of the assay used to determine LD-1 concentrations or the LD-1/LD-2 ratio, the optimum interval for analysis of LD isoenzymes is the 48- to 72-hour period after the onset of chest pain.

Myoglobin

The major advantage offered by myoglobin as a serum marker for myocardial injury is that it is released early from damaged cells. As shown in Figure 33-5, serum concentrations of myoglobin rise above the reference interval as early as 1 hour after the occurrence of an AMI, with peak activity in the range of 4 to 12 hours (demonstrating 90% to 100% sensitivity). This peak suggests that serum myoglobin reflects the early course of myocardial necrosis. Myoglobin is cleared rapidly and thus has a substantially reduced clinical sensitivity after 12 hours. The role for myoglobin in the detection of AMI is within the first 0 to 4 hours, the time period in which CK-2 and cardiac troponin are still within their reference intervals. However, the measurement of serum myoglobin has not been used extensively in clinical laboratories for the routine analysis of AMI. The main reason has been the poor clinical specificity (usually <80%) of the protein caused by the large quantities of myoglobin found in skeletal muscle.

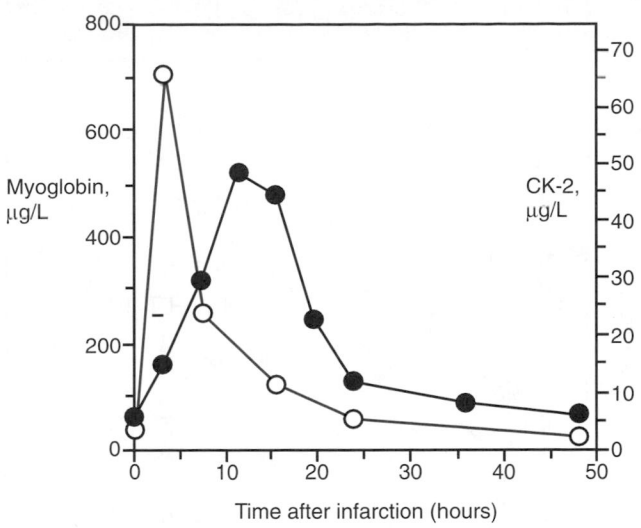

Figure 33-5   Temporal pattern of serum myoglobin *(open circles)* and creatine kinase-2 (CK-2; *closed circles*) in patients with acute myocardial infarction. (Modified from Vaidya HC: Myoglobin. Lab Med 1992; 23:307.)

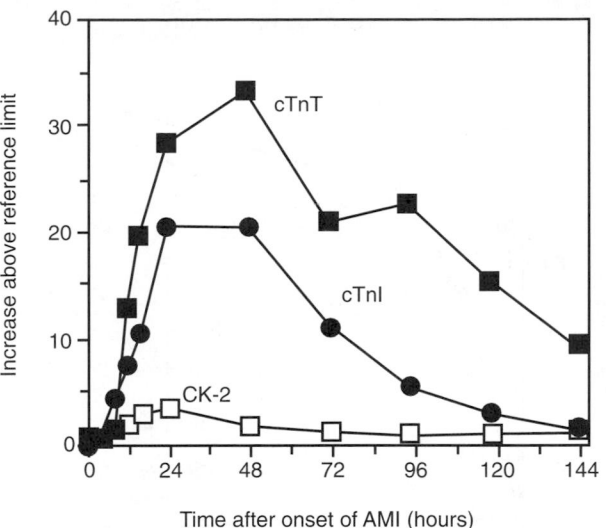

Figure 33-6   Serial serum creatine kinase-2 (CK-2), cardiac troponin I (cTnI), and cardiac troponin T (cTnT) profiles after acute myocardial infarction (AMI). Cardiac markers are plotted as multiples of the upper reference limit.

The best use of early serum myoglobin measurements after admission to emergency departments is as a negative predictor of AMI. If myoglobin concentrations remain unchanged and within the reference interval on multiple, early samplings within 2 to 4 hours after the onset of chest pain, certainty is 100% that muscle (either cardiac or skeletal) injury has not occurred recently.

Troponins

Several general clinical impressions can be made regarding cTnI and cTnT. First, the early release kinetics of both cTnI and cTnT are similar to those of CK-2 after AMI; increases above the upper reference limit are seen at 4 to 8 hours (Figure 33-6). This initial rise is due to the approximately 5% cytoplasmic fraction of troponin (CK-2 being 100% cytoplasmic). Second, cTnI and cTnT also can remain elevated up to 5 to 10 days, respectively, after an AMI occurs. The mechanism is likely the ongoing release of troponin from the approximately 95% myofibril-bound fraction. The long time interval of cardiac troponin increase means it can replace the LD isoenzyme assay in the detection of late-presenting AMI individuals. Third, the very low to undetectable cardiac troponin values in serum from individuals without cardiac disease permits the use of lower discriminator values, compared with CK-2, for the determination of myocardial injury and risk stratification. Finally, cardiac specificity of troponin I and T should eliminate a false diagnosis of AMI in patients with increased CK-2 concentrations after skeletal muscle injuries.

Direct comparisons of cTnI and cTnI measurements in serum from individuals with chronic renal failure have indicated that both troponin values were increased in 10% to 30% of individuals without documented myocardial inju-

ries.[16] One 12-month follow-up study of individuals undergoing chronic hemodialysis demonstrated that increases in both cTnT and cTnI predicted poor outcomes (fatal infarctions). The second-generation cTnT assay was associated with a considerably lower false positive rate (12% to 17%) than the first-generation assay (25% to 70%). Larger studies must be performed in this population because the mortality rate in individuals with end-stage renal disease within 2 years after an AMI is greater than 60%.

Clinical evidence is mounting that either cTnI or cTnT should replace CK-2 as the test of choice to rule in or rule out AMI. For more information, the reader should refer to two documents published in 1999, sponsored by the National Academy of Clinical Biochemistry[21] and the International Federation of Clinical Chemistry.[17] The following ordering patterns are recommended—myoglobin (early marker) and either cTnI or cTnT (definitive mid to late marker) at presentation and at 3 to 6 hours, 6 to 9 hours, and 12 to 24 hours after presentation. If the clinical decision algorithm does not include triage within 9 hours of presentation, myoglobin measurement is not recommended as a cost-effective test.

Troponin T

Numerous clinical studies involving cTnT have been published pertaining to AMI. The clinical sensitivity of cTnT (by use of a 0.1 μg/L decision cutoff) is similar to that of CK-2 during the first 48 hours after the onset of chest pain.[20,21] As an early marker for AMI, cTnT shows a clinical sensitivity of 50% to 65% from up to 6 hours after the onset of chest pain. Therefore like CK-2, cTnT is insufficient for effective early diagnosis. This insufficiency is exemplified in Figure 33-7 by ROC-curve analysis. However,

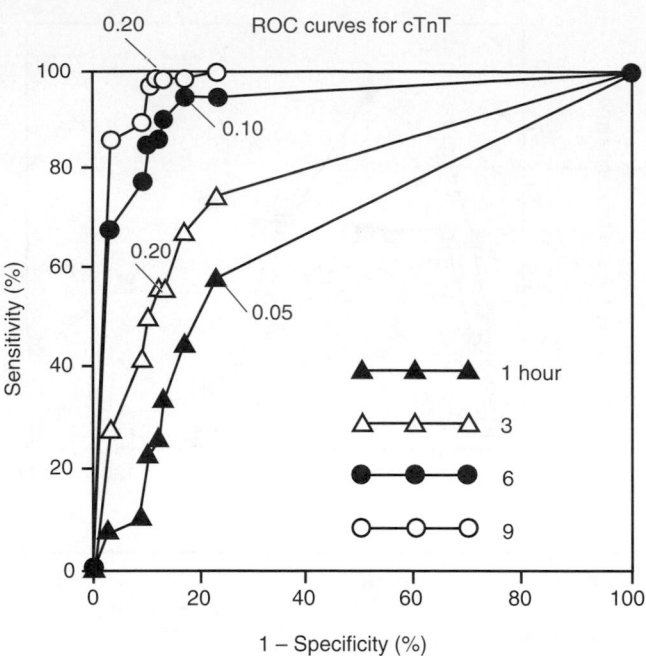

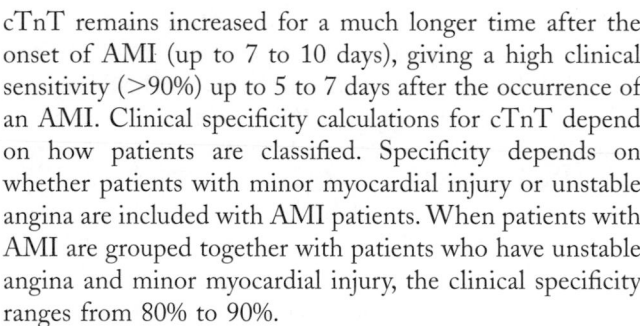

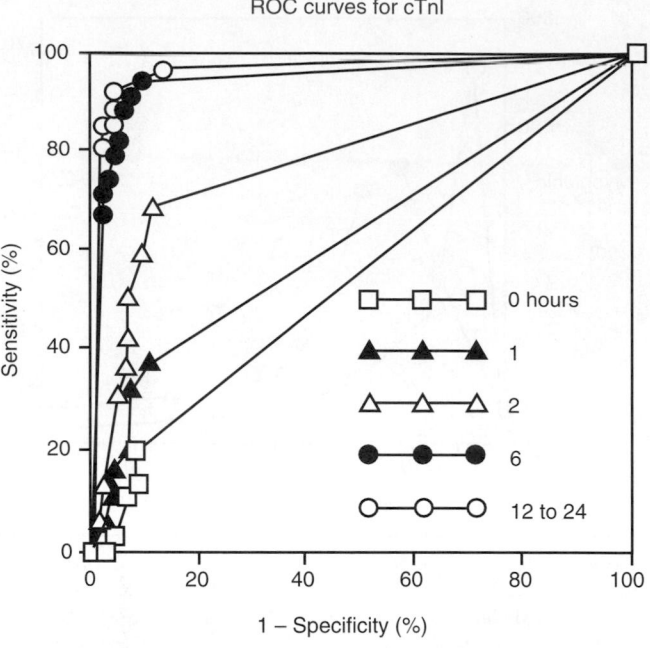

Figure 33-7 Receiver operating characteristic (ROC) curves at different times after the onset of symptoms. These curves help establish the best discriminator (time interval and cutoff) for cardiac troponin T (cTnT) for the prediction of acute myocardial infarction. The best discriminating point for cTnT is 0.20 μg/L at 9 hours after the onset of chest pain. (Reprinted by permission of Elsevier Science from Burlina A, Aaniotto M, Secchiero S et al: Troponin T as a marker of ischemic myocardial injury. Clinical Biochemistry 27:115; and copyright 1993 by Canadian Society of Clinical Chemists.)

Figure 33-8 Receiver operating characteristic (ROC) curves to establish the best discriminator limits for acute myocardial infarction by use of cardiac troponin I (cTnI). Each curve represents a different time interval after the onset of chest pain in 35 patients. (Data from Tucker JF, Collins RA, Anderson AJ et al: Early diagnostic efficiency of cardiac troponin I and cardiac troponin T for acute myocardial infarction. Acad Emerg Med 1997; 4:13-21.)

cTnT remains increased for a much longer time after the onset of AMI (up to 7 to 10 days), giving a high clinical sensitivity (>90%) up to 5 to 7 days after the occurrence of an AMI. Clinical specificity calculations for cTnT depend on how patients are classified. Specificity depends on whether patients with minor myocardial injury or unstable angina are included with AMI patients. When patients with AMI are grouped together with patients who have unstable angina and minor myocardial injury, the clinical specificity ranges from 80% to 90%.

Review of 1578 subjects during 1995 to 1998 from the Swedish Classification study showed that use of a 0.4 μg/L decision cutoff demonstrated 99% sensitivity and 94% specificity (755 AMI subjects). Within the 0.1- to 0.4-μg/L range, 43% had AMI and 57% were classified as minor myocardial damage subjects. The minor myocardial damage subjects were at increased risk of having a cardiac event at 30 days after an AMI.

cTnT has been shown to differentiate individuals with increased CK-2 due to skeletal muscle injury from those individuals with concomitant AMIs. Furthermore, cTnT has been an excellent marker of myocardial injury in the presence of sepsis, drug-induced toxicities, chronic dis-

eases, malignancies, hematological disorders, and noncardiac surgery.

Troponin I

Numerous studies have shown that cTnI is comparable to CK-2 for the sensitive detection of AMI.[11,20,21] cTnI has serial rise-and-fall kinetics similar to those of CK-2 after AMI during the initial 48 to 72 hours after onset (see Figure 33-6). Therefore like CK-2, cTnI is insufficient for effective, very early diagnosis of AMI. cTnI remains elevated 3 to 5 days after the occurrence of an AMI, also because of ongoing release from the large cTnI myofibril fraction. cTnI has been shown to have diagnostic sensitivity for AMI approximately equal to that of CK-2 during the initial 48 to 72 hours after an AMI occurs. Following 72 to 96 hours after AMI, cTnI exhibits an increased sensitivity.[3,6] As noted previously, cTnI is specific for myocardium, with studies showing clinical specificity of more than 85% for cTnI. However, the overall clinical sensitivity and specificity of AMI detection depend on cutoff values for cTnI, as shown in the ROC curve in Figure 33-8.

When cTnI, CK-2, and total CK in serum were compared in individuals with extreme skeletal muscle injury but without cardiac muscle injury, cTnI remained undetectable even when peak concentrations of CK-2 were greater than 200 µg/L and total CK reached more than 50,000 U/L. In individuals who had elevated CK-2 concentrations because of (1) acute skeletal muscle injury after marathon racing, (2) chronic myopathy of Duchenne's muscular dystrophy, or (3) chronic renal failure requiring dialysis, cTnI was not elevated unless myocardial injury was detected concomitantly.

The measurement of cTnI has been shown as a sensitive and specific method for the diagnosis of perioperative MI in noncardiac surgery, preventing the increased incidence of false diagnosis associated with elevated CK-2 concentrations. For example, 8 of 108 patients undergoing noncardiac-related vascular surgery showed new abnormalities on echocardiograms and were diagnosed subsequently as having sustained perioperative infarction. All 8 had increased cTnI. Of the other 100 individuals without perioperative infarction, 19 demonstrated elevations in CK-2 and 1 individual exhibited a slight elevation in cTnI.

Risk stratification

Of those patients who present with chest pain but who are not having an AMI, a large proportion have unstable angina with minor myocardial injury. Up to 30% of these patients progress to AMI or cardiac death within the first year of the initial presentation. Numerous prospective and retrospective clinical studies have evaluated and compared the utility of measurements of cTnI, cTnT, and CK-2 for the identification of those at risk.[9,12,13,15,19] This process is known as *risk stratification*. The goal of cardiac marker monitoring in ACS patients without AMI is to identify possible unstable coronary disease. This identification allows the clinician to offer the patient diagnostic alternatives, such as a coronary angiogram, an echocardiography, a radionuclide scan, or exercise stress testing. These tests help identify the pathological etiology responsible for the tissue release of markers of myocardial injury.

One quarter to one third of individuals with unstable angina have shown increased serum concentrations of cTnI, cTnT, or both.[7] From 18% to 34% of these individuals who have increased serum cTnI or cTnT within 24 hours of presentation progress to have an AMI or cardiac-related death within approximately 1 month. This statistic is compared with only 3% to 7% of individuals with serum negative marker results. From the largest meta-analysis published, measurement of either cTnT or cTnI within 24 hours of admission demonstrated a twofold to tenfold greater risk of AMI or cardiac-related death within approximately 1 month after presentation in ACS patients diagnosed without an AMI.[15] Use of either cTnT or cTnI appears to offer better risk assessment than use of CK-2.

Risk stratification should be examined critically in current practice guidelines regarding diagnosis and management of unstable angina. In today's environment of preventive and evidence-based medicine, cTnI or cTnT measurements in patients once at presentation and again at 12 hours thereafter allows clinicians to use markers both as exclusionary and prognostic indicators. For example, recent findings[12] indicate that an increased concentration of whole-blood troponin T identifies a high-risk subgroup of individuals with refractory unstable angina who particularly can benefit from early drug therapy with low-molecular-weight heparin or glycoprotein IIB and III A inhibitors. However, general population screening of hospitalized patients with use of cTnI or cTnT is not recommended.

Monitoring of reperfusion after thrombolytic therapy

Biochemical markers of myocardial injury are not needed routinely to assess patients with diagnostic ECG evidence of AMI but are useful for confirmation.[17,21] Furthermore, markers do not indicate which patients do or do not receive thrombolytic therapy. However, a growing body of evidence indicates that early monitoring of markers may be useful to determine **reperfusion** success in patients receiving thrombolytic therapy. Complete opening of diseased coronary arteries is an important therapeutic goal during the early hours after AMI. Markers may assist clinicians in patient management strategies.

The kinetics of myocardial protein appearance in the circulation after AMI depends on the infarct area perfusion status.[15] In the early hours, successful reperfusion is characterized by a rapid increase of markers and an early peak (see Figure 33-3).[2] Assessment of the amount of irreversible injury by biochemical infarct sizing is difficult because of the variability in the amount of protein washout that appears in the circulation after reperfusion. The laboratory can be used best to assess reperfusion status after thrombolytic therapy when early, frequent blood sampling is combined with rapid analysis of a marker of myocardial injury.

Several retrospective studies have demonstrated that the use of cardiac markers can predict the success or failure of reperfusion.[17,21] The pretherapy marker concentration is compared with its level 60 to 120 minutes after the initiation of therapy to determine the rate of increase, the absolute increase, or the ratio of the 90-minute value to the pretherapy value. A rapid increase of serum CK-2, myoglobin, cTnT, and cTnI have high sensitivities (>75%) to predict successful reperfusion. In addition, numerous studies now are appearing in the literature that demonstrate and validate the use of cardiac troponin monitoring to detect myocardial injury and determine risk in non-AMI and non-ACS individuals. These pathological processes include myocarditis, congestive heart failure, cardiac contusion, stunned myocardium chronic renal disease, and stroke.

References

1. Apple FS, Rogers MA, Casal DC et al: Skeletal muscle creatine kinase MB alterations in women marathon runners. Eur J Appl Physiol 1987; 56:49-52.

2. Apple FS, Sharkey SW, Henry TD: Early serum cardiac troponin I and T concentrations following successful thrombolysis for acute myocardial infarction. Clin Chem 1995; 41:1197-1198.

3. Apple FS, Falahati A, Paulson PR et al: Improved detection of minor ischemic myocardial injury with measurement of serum cardiac troponin I. Clin Chem 1997; 43:2047-2051.

4. Apple FS: Clinical and analytical standardization issues confronting cardiac troponin I. Clin Chem 1999; 45:18-20.

5. Bodor GS, Porterfield D, Voss E et al: Cardiac troponin I is not expressed in fetal and adult human skeletal muscle tissue. Clin Chem 1995; 41:1710-1715.

6. Falahati A, Sharkey SW, Christensen D et al: Implementation of cardiac troponin I for detection of acute myocardial infarction. Am Heart J 1999; 137:332-337; correction Am Heart J 1999; 138:798-800.

7. Galvanni M, Ottani F, Ferrini E et al: Prognostic influence of elevated values of cardiac troponin I in patients with unstable angina. Circulation 1997; 95:2053-2059.

8. Gibler WB, Runyon JP, Levy RC et al: A rapid diagnostic and treatment center for patients with chest pain in the emergency department. Ann Emerg Med 1995; 25:1-8.

9. Guest TM, Ramanthan AV, Tuteur PG et al: Myocardial injury in critically ill patients: a frequently unrecognized complication. JAMA 1995; 273:1945-1949.

10. GUSTO Angiographic Investigators: The effects of tissue plasminogen activator, streptokinase, or both on coronary artery patency, ventricular function, and survival after acute myocardial infarction. N Engl J Med 1993; 329:1615-1622.

11. Hamm CW, Goldmann BU, Heeschen C et al: Emergency room triage of patients with acute chest pain by means of rapid testing for cardiac troponin T or troponin I. N Engl J Med 1997; 337:1648-1653.

12. Hamm CW, Heeschen C, Goldmann B et al: Benefit of abciximab in patients with refractory unstable angina in relation to serum troponin T levels. N Engl J Med 1999; 240:1623-1629.

13. Hamm CW, Ravkilde J, Gerhardt W et al: The prognostic value of serum troponin T in unstable angina. N Engl J Med 1992; 327:146-150.

14. Ingwall JS, Kramer MF, Fifer MA et al: The creatine kinase system in normal and diseased human myocardium. N Engl J Med 1985; 313:1050-1054.

15. Kaski JC, Holt DW (eds): Myocardial Damage: Early Detection by Novel Biochemical Markers, Dordrecht, The Netherlands, Kluwer Academic, 1998.

16. McLaurin MD, Apple FS, Voss EM et al: Cardiac troponin I, cardiac troponin T, and creatine kinase MB in dialysis patients without ischemic heart disease: evidence of cardiac troponin T expression in skeletal muscle. Clin Chem 1997; 43:976-982.

17. Panteghini M, Apple FS, Christenson RH et al: Proposals from IFCC Committee on Standardization of Markers of Cardiac Damage (C-SMCD): recommendations on use of biochemical markers of cardiac damage in acute coronary syndromes. Scand J Clin Lab Invest Suppl 1999; 230:103-112.

18. Ricchiuti V, Voss EM, Ney A et al: Cardiac troponin T isoforms expressed in renal diseased skeletal muscle will not cause false positive results by the second generation cardiac troponin T assay by Boehringer Mannheim. Clin Chem 1998; 44:1919-1924.

19. Stubbs P, Collinson P, Moseley D et al: Prognostic significance of admission troponin T concentrations in patients with myocardial infarction. Circulation 1996; 94:1291-1297.

20. Tucker JF, Collins RA, Anderson AJ et al: Early diagnostic efficiency of cardiac troponin I and cardiac troponin T for acute myocardial infarction. Acad Emerg Med 1997; 4:13-21.

21. Wu AHB, Apple FS, Gibler WB et al: National Academy of Clinical Biochemistry Standards of laboratory practice: recommendations for use of cardiac markers in coronary artery disease. Clin Chem 1999; 45:1414-1423.

22. Wu AHB, Feng YJ, Moore R et al: Characterization of cardiac troponin subunit release into serum after acute myocardial infarction and comparison of assays for troponin T and I. Clin Chem 1998; 44:1198-1208.

23. Zimmerman J, Fromm R, Meyer D et al: Diagnostic marker cooperative study for the diagnosis of myocardial infarction. Circulation 1999; 99:1671-1677.

Additional Reading

Acute coronary syndromes: from bench to bedside—the Twenty-First Annual Arnold O. Beckman Conference in Clinical Chemistry. Clin Chem 1998; 44:1795-1881.

Braunwald E (ed): Heart Disease: A Textbook of Cardiovascular Medicine, 5th edition, Philadelphia, WB Saunders, 1997.

Canto JG, Shlipak MG, Rogers WJ et al: Prevalence, clinical characteristics, and mortality among patients with myocardial infarction presenting without chest pain. JAMA 2000; 283:3223-3229.

Chesebro MJ: Using serum markers in the early diagnosis of myocardial infarction. Am Fam Physician 1997; 55:2667-2674.

Gerhardt W, Nordin G, Ljungdahl L: Can troponin T replace CK MB mass as "gold standard" for acute myocardial infarction ("AMI)? Scand J Clin Lab Invest 1999; 230:83-89.

Ridker PM, Glynn RJ, Hennekens CH: C-reactive protein adds to the predictive value of total and HDL cholesterol in determining the risk of first myocardial infarction. Circulation 1998; 97:2007-2011.

Willerson JT, Cohn JN (eds): Atlas of Ischemic Heart Disease: Clinical and Pathologic Aspects, New York, Churchill Livingstone, 1996.

Wu AHB (ed): Cardiac Markers, Totowa, NJ, Humana Press, 1998.

Yellon DM, Rahimtoola SH, Opie LH (eds): New Ischemic Syndromes: Beyond Angina and Infarction, Philadelphia, Lippincott-Raven, 1997.

CHAPTER 34

Renal Function

DAVID J. NEWMAN, MSc, PhD, MCB, MRCPath,
and CHRISTOPHER P. PRICE, PhD, FRSC, FRCPath

Objectives

1. Describe the macroscopic and microscopic anatomy of the renal system.
2. Define the following terms:

   Nephron   Renin

   Glomerular filtration rate   Erythropoietin

   Plasma renal flow   Hemodialysis

   Clearance   Homeostasis
3. List the functions of the renal system and state the system's role in the maintenance of acid-base balance.
4. State the clinical laboratory tests used to assess renal function and the laboratory values associated with renal pathology.
5. Discuss the causes, symptoms, and pertinent laboratory results obtained with each of the following conditions:

   End-stage renal disease (uremic syndrome)   Nephrotic syndrome

   Acute renal failure   Pyelonephritis

   Acute nephritic syndrome   Urinary tract obstruction

Key Words

Antidiuretic Hormone (ADH; Vasopressin) A nonapeptide hormone formed by the neuronal cells of the hypothalamic nuclei and stored in the posterior lobe of the pituitary gland (neurohypophysis); has both antidiuretic and vasopressor actions

Azotemia An excess of urea or other nitrogenous compounds in the blood

Bence-Jones Protein An abnormal plasma or urinary protein, consisting of monoclonal immunoglobulin light chains, excreted in some neoplastic diseases and characterized by its unusual solubility properties; precipitates on heating at 50 to 60 °C and redissolves at 90 to 100 °C; on cooling, again precipitates and redissolves; characteristic protein found in the urine of most individuals with multiple myeloma

Diabetes Insipidus A metabolic disorder due to injury of the neurohypophyseal system, which results in a deficient quantity of antidiuretic hormone being released or produced, and thus in failure of tubular reabsorption of water in the kidney

End-Stage Renal Disease (ESRD) A condition in which renal function is inadequate to support life

Glomerular Filtration Rate (GFR) The rate in milliliters per minute that substances such as creatinine and urea are filtered freely through the kidney's glomeruli; a measure of the number of functioning nephrons

Glomerulonephritis Nephritis accompanied by inflammation of the capillary loops in the glomeruli of the kidney; occurs in acute, subacute, and chronic forms and may be secondary to hemolytic streptococcal infection; evidence suggesting possible immune or autoimmune mechanisms

Glomerulus A tuft of blood vessels found in the nephron of the kidney that are involved in the filtration of the blood

Hematuria   Blood in the urine

Hemodialysis   The removal of certain elements from the blood by virtue of the difference in the rates of their diffusion through a semipermeable membrane (for example, by means of a hemodialysis filter)

Lithotripsy   The destruction of a calculus within the urinary system or gallbladder, followed at once by the washing out of the fragments; may be done either surgically or by several different noninvasive methods

Nephritis   Inflammation of the kidney with focal or diffuse proliferation or destructive processes that may involve the glomerulus, tubule, or interstitial renal tissue

Nephrolithiasis   A condition marked by the presence of renal calculi (stones)

Nephron   The anatomical and functional unit of the kidney, consisting of the renal corpuscle, proximal convoluted tubule, descending and ascending limbs of Henle's loop, distal convoluted tubule, and collecting tubule

Nephrotic Syndrome   General name for a group of diseases involving increased glomerular permeability, characterized by massive proteinuria and lipiduria with varying degrees of edema, hypoalbuminemia, and hyperlipidemia

Peritoneal Dialysis   Hemodialysis through the peritoneum, the dialyzing solution being introduced into and removed from the peritoneal cavity as either a continuous or an intermittent procedure

Pyelonephritis   An inflammation of the kidney and its pelvis

Renal Clearance   The volume of plasma from which a given substance is cleared completely by the kidneys per unit time

Renal Failure   An acute or chronic decline in renal function

Tamm-Horsfall Protein   A mucoprotein produced by the ascending limb of the loop of Henle that is a normal constituent of urine and is the major protein constituent of urinary casts

Uremia   An excess in the blood of urea, creatinine, and other nitrogenous end products of protein and amino acid metabolism; more correctly referred to as *azotemia*

The kidneys play a central role in the homeostatic mechanisms of the human body, and reduced renal function strongly correlates with increasing morbidity and mortality. Biochemical measurements, both routine and specialized, are important diagnostic tools. Investigations from nephrology wards and clinics constitute a significant element of the workload of most clinical laboratories.

■ ANATOMY

The kidneys form a paired organ system located in the lumbar region. They (1) filter the blood; (2) regulate the concentrations of hydrogen, sodium, potassium, phosphate, and other ions in the extracellular fluid; and (3) excrete the end products of body metabolism in the form of urine. In an adult, each kidney is about 12 cm long and weighs about 150 g in men and 135 g in women. A kidney has a characteristic shape through which passes the vessels, nerves, and ureter (Figure 34-1).

A kidney consists of a cortex and a medulla. The medullary substance forms pyramids, the bases of which are in the cortex and the apices of which, called *papillae*, project into the calyces of the kidney. The renal pyramids number from 10 to 15. The parenchyma of each kidney is composed of nephrons held together by connective tissue. From the nephrons, urine collects in the pelvis and flows through the ureteropelvic junction into the ureter. The ureters carry urine from each kidney into the bladders, where it is stored until voided through the urethra. The kidneys have both sympathetic and parasympathetic nervous supplies and lymphatic drainage.

Nephron

The **nephron** is the functional unit of the kidney. Each kidney contains between 400,000 and 800,000 nephrons. Each nephron consists of a **glomerulus,** proximal tubule, loop of Henle, distal tubule, and collecting duct (see Figure 34-1).

The glomeruli are formed from a specialized capillary network. Each capillary develops into about 40 glomerular loops about 200 μm in size and consists of a variety of different cell types supported on a specialized basement membrane forming what is known as *Bowman's capsule* (Figure 34-2). Bowman's capsule forms the beginning of the proximal convoluted tubule (PCT).

The proximal tubule is the most metabolically active part of the nephron, facilitating the reabsorption of 60% to 80% of the glomerular filtrate volume, 70% of the filtered load of Na^+ and Cl^-, and most of the potassium, glucose, bicarbonate, phosphate, and sulfate, as well as secreting 90% of the H^+ excreted by the kidney. The proximal tubule drains into the descending thin loop of Henle, becoming first the ascending thin limb and then the thick ascending loop. The cells of the ascending thin limb are very similar to those in the descending loop, but important differences exist in their permeability to water and their capability for active transport. The main role of the loop of Henle is to provide the

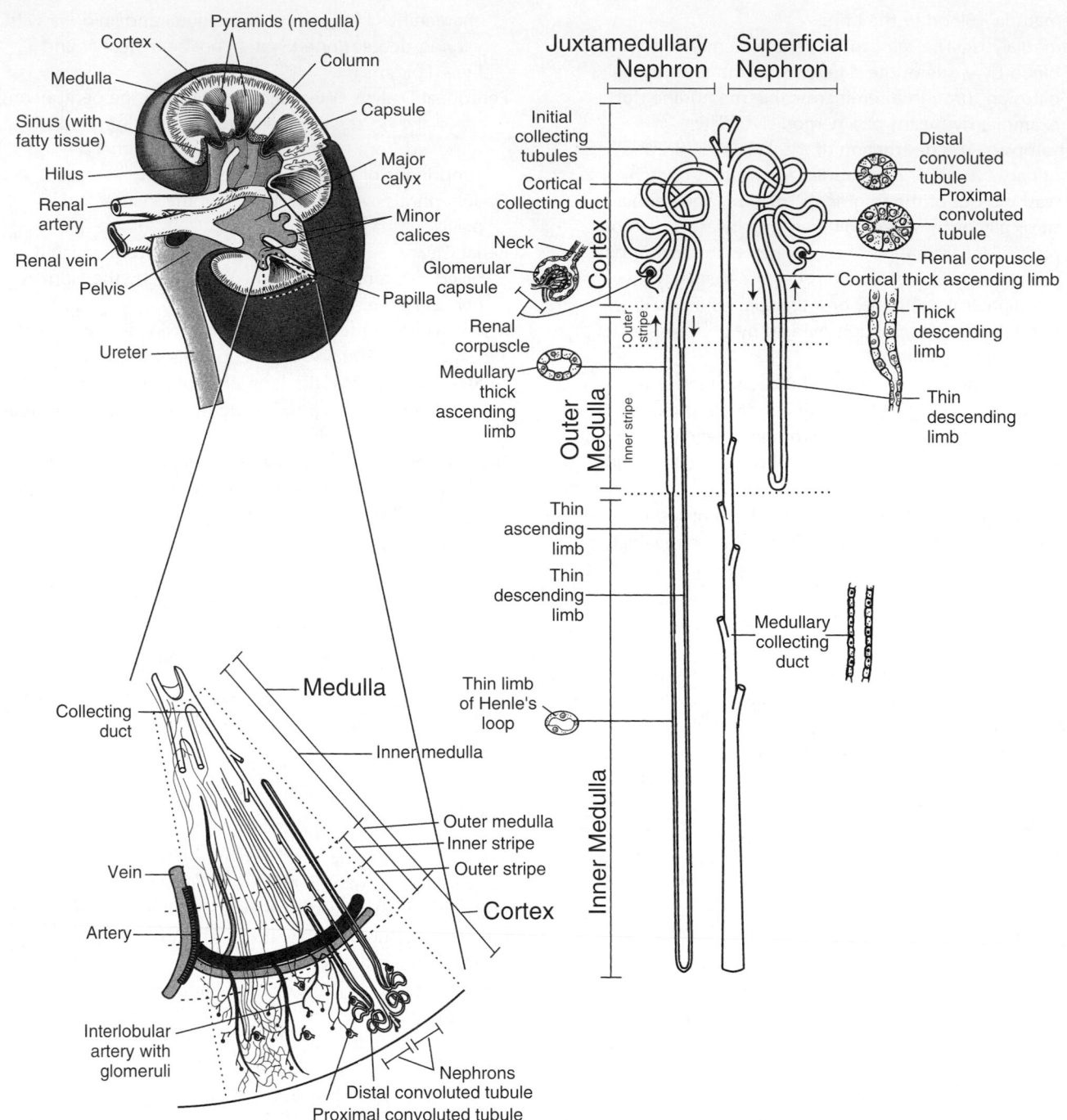

Figure 34-1   Anatomy of the kidney. (Modified from Dorland's Illustrated Medical Dictionary, 28th edition, p 883, Philadelphia, WB Saunders, 1994.)

ability to generate a concentrated urine, hypertonic with respect to serum. The distal tubule connects the ascending loop of Henle with the collecting tubule. It is involved with sodium, potassium, chloride and hydrogen ion excretion and reabsorption.

Where the ascending loop of Henle passes very close to the Bowman's capsule of its own nephron, the cells of the tubule and afferent arteriole show regional specialization. The tubule forms the macula densa, and the arteriolar cells are filled with granules (containing renin) and are innervated with sympathetic nerve fibers. This area is called the

juxtaglomerular apparatus (JGA). The JGA plays an important part in maintaining systemic blood pressure through regulation of the circulating intravascular blood volume and sodium concentration.

Blood Supply

The renal artery divides into the afferent arterioles, which expand into the highly specialized capillary bed that forms the glomerulus. These capillaries then rejoin to form the efferent arteriole, which supplies the rest of the nephron with

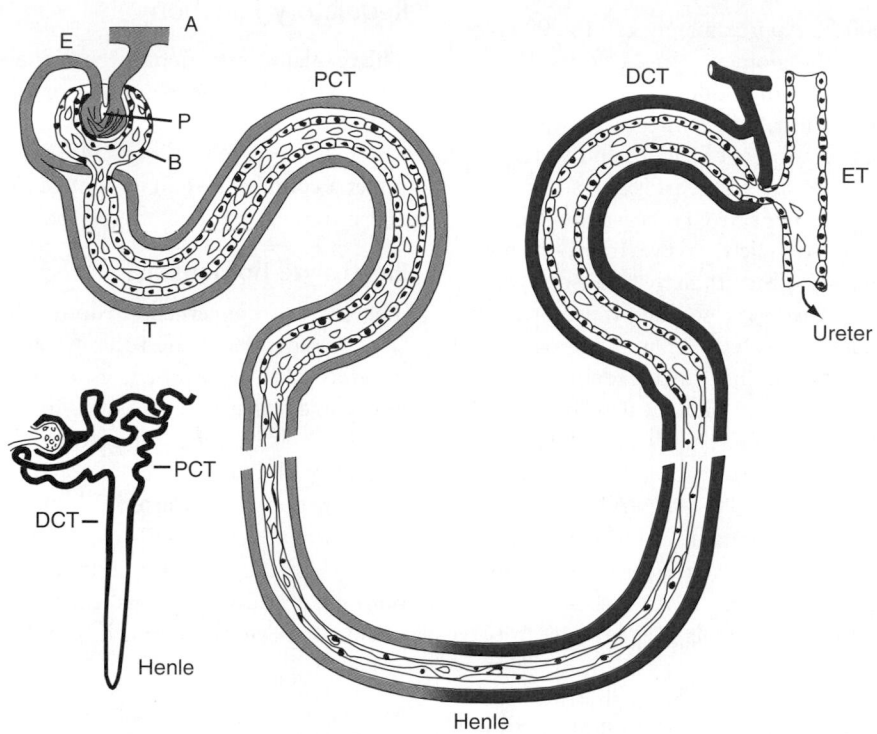

Figure 34-2   Schematic drawing of the glomerulus and tubular system of the nephron. The blood capillaries shown along the tubular system *(T)* gradually change to venous capillaries as they pass down the tubular system. *A,* Afferent arteriole; *E,* efferent arteriole; *P,* plexus of capillaries (glomerular tuft); *B,* Bowman's capsule; *T,* tubular blood supply; *PCT,* proximal convoluted tubule; *Henle,* loop of Henle; *DCT,* distal convoluted tubule; *ET,* excretory tubule or duct.

oxygen and nutrients and removing ions, molecules, and water, which are reabsorbed by the nephron. The efferent arteriole then merges with renal venules to form the renal veins, which emerge into the inferior vena cava.

In the adult the kidneys receive approximately 25% of the cardiac output; however, in the newborn infant this value is 5%, only reaching adult proportions by the end of the first year of life. About 90% of this blood flow supplies the renal cortex, maintaining the highly active tubular cells. The maintenance of renal blood flow is essential for renal function, and a complex array of intrarenal regulatory mechanisms help ensure that this flow is maintained across a wide range of systemic blood pressures. The renal glomerular perfusion pressure is relatively independent of the systemic pressure and is maintained at a constant 45 mm Hg.

■ BIOLOGICAL FUNCTIONS

Excretion, homeostatic regulation, and endocrine function are the main biological functions of the kidneys.

Excretion

The kidneys produce and excrete urine, which rids the body of the end products of metabolism and the excess of inorganic substances ingested in the diet.

Definitions

Urine is a fluid excreted by the kidneys, passed through the ureters, stored in the bladder, and discharged through the urethra. In healthy individuals, it is sterile and clear and has an amber color, a slightly acid pH, and a charactcristic odor. In addition to dissolved compounds, urine contains a number of cellular fragments, complete cells, proteinaceous casts, and crystals (formed elements). Changes in these formed elements are studied with urine microscopy. Urine from a healthy individual should be clear, with a pH of about 5.0 to 6.0 and a specific gravity of about 1.024 g/mL.

Urination, also termed *micturition,* is the discharge of urine. In healthy adults, adequate homeostasis is maintained with a daily urine output of about 500 mL. Alterations in urinary output are described as *anuria* (<100 mL/day), *oliguria* (<400 mL/day), or *polyuria* (<2 L/day). The most common disorder of micturition is altered frequency, which has been associated with increased urinary volume or partial urinary tract obstruction (for example, in cases of prostatic hypertrophy).

Formation of urine

The first step in urine formation is filtration of plasma water at the glomeruli. The filtrate is called an *ultrafiltrate* because its composition is essentially the same as that of plasma, with a notable reduction in molecules of molecular weight

(MW) exceeding 50,000 D. Approximately 170 to 200 L of ultrafiltrate pass through the glomeruli in 24 hours. Reabsorption of solutes and water in various regions of the tubules reduces the total volume, which ranges between 0.4 and 2 L of urine per day. Transport of solutes and water occurs both across and between the epithelial cells that line the renal tubules. Transport is either active (energy requiring) or passive, but many of the so-called passive transport processes depend on or are secondary to active transport processes, particularly those involving sodium transport. All known transport processes involve receptor or mediator molecules, many of which now have been identified and characterized by use of molecular biological techniques.[11] Direct coupling of adenosine triphosphate (ATP) hydrolysis is an example of an active transport process; the most important of these in the nephron is Na^+-K^+-ATPase. Renal epithelial cell membranes also contain proteins that act as ion channels. Ion channels enable much faster rates of transport than ATPases but are relatively fewer in number, approximately 100 Na^+ and Cl^- channels as against 10^7 Na^+-ATPase molecules per cell.

Different regions of the tubule have been shown to specialize in certain functions. In the proximal tubule, 60% to 80% of the ultrafiltrate is reabsorbed in an obligatory fashion, along with sodium, chloride, bicarbonate, calcium, phosphate, and other ions. Glucose, a high-threshold substance,* is reabsorbed virtually completely, predominantly in the proximal tubule by a passive but Na^+-dependent process that is saturated at a plasma glucose concentration of about 11 mmol/L. Uric acid also is reabsorbed in the proximal tubule by a passive Na^+-dependent mechanism, but an active secretory mechanism also exists.

In the loops of Henle, chloride and more sodium without water are reabsorbed, generating dilute urine. Water reabsorption in the more distal tubules and collecting ducts then is regulated by **antidiuretic hormone (ADH)**, also known as *vasopressin*. In the distal tubule, secretion is the prominent activity; organic ions, potassium ions, and hydrogen ions are transported from the blood in the efferent arteriole into the tubular fluid. This region also secretes H^+ and reabsorbs Na^+ and HCO_3^- to aid in acid-base regulation (see Chapter 35). Paracellular (between-cell) movement is driven predominantly by concentration, osmotic, or electrical gradients.

---

*Certain substances appear in the urine when their plasma levels are above certain set-point, or "threshold," levels. Creatinine is a low-threshold substance. High-threshold substances, such as glucose and amino acids, are reabsorbed almost completely by means of specific transport systems in the tubular cells. The appearance of a high-threshold substance in the urine is evidence that the filtered load of the substance is exceeding the maximal reabsorption rate of its transport system. The renal threshold of a filterable compound is its plasma concentration that exceeds the maximal reabsorption rate for it and it then "spills" into the urine.

Regulatory Function

The regulatory function of the kidneys plays a major role in homeostasis. The mechanisms of differential reabsorption and secretion, located in the tubule of a nephron, are the effectors of regulation (Figure 34-3). The mechanisms operate under a complex system of control in which both extrarenal and intrarenal humoral factors participate.

Electrolyte homeostasis

The PCT is concerned predominantly with reabsorption. In it, about 75% of the sodium, chloride, and water of the ultrafiltrate is reabsorbed, as is most of the bicarbonate, phosphate, calcium, and potassium. Water reabsorption in the PCT is termed "obligatory" because its volume is related to the heavy load of solutes being returned to the blood in the efferent arteriole. The amount of bicarbonate reabsorption is related to the glomerular filtration rate (GFR) and the hydrogen ion secretory rate; the amount of phosphate reabsorption is controlled in part by plasma calcium concentration and in part by the effect of parathy-

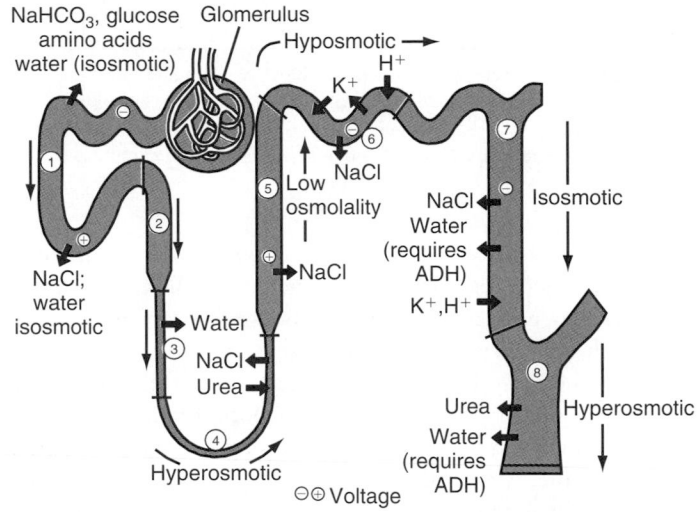

Figure 34-3 Schematic representation of the principal processes of transport in the nephron. In the convoluted portion of the proximal tubule *(1)*, salts and water are reabsorbed at high rates in isotonic proportions. Bulk reabsorption of most of the filtrate (65% to 70%) and virtually complete reabsorption of glucose, amino acids, and bicarbonate take place in this segment. In the pars recta *(2)*, organic acids are secreted and continuous reabsorption of sodium chloride takes place. The loop of Henle comprises three segments—the thin descending *(3)* and ascending *(4)* limbs and the thick ascending limb *(5)*. The fluid becomes hyperosmotic, because of water abstraction, as it flows toward the bend of the loop and hyposmotic, because of sodium chloride reabsorption, as it flows toward the distal convoluted tubule *(6)*. Active sodium reabsorption occurs in the distal convoluted tubule and cortical collecting tubule *(7)*. This latter segment is water impermeable in the absence of ADH, and the reabsorption of sodium in this segment is increased by aldosterone. The collecting duct *(8)* allows equilibration of water with the hyperosmotic interstitium when ADH is present. *ADH,* Antidiuretic hormone. (Modified from Burg MB: The nephron in transport of sodium, amino acids, and glucose. Hosp Pract 1978; 13:100; and modified from a drawing by A. Iselin.)

roid hormone (PTH) on the tubular cells. Normally, the high-threshold substances—glucose and to a great extent, amino acids—are reabsorbed in the PCT by means of specific intracellular active transport systems. Uric acid may be either reabsorbed or secreted in the PCT by a two-way, carrier-mediated process.

In the ascending loop of Henle, 20% to 25% of filtered sodium is reabsorbed without concomitant reabsorption of water. This process generates dilute urine with an osmolality of 100 to 150 mOsm/kg of water and helps establish the corticomedullary osmotic gradient. The resulting hypertonicity of the interstitium is important in the pathogenesis of renal infections because the hypertonic environment interferes with leukocyte function. Subsequent water reabsorption is regulated by ADH. Although the reabsorption of Na^+ in the loop of Henle is complex and incompletely understood, at least one mechanism consists of an active Cl^- pump with subsequent reabsorption of Na^+ along an electrochemical gradient. This mechanism is apparently the one inhibited by the powerful loop diuretics.

The distal tubule is functionally the most active region of the nephron for the homeostatic regulation of plasma electrolytes and plasma acid-base levels. In this location a combination of secretion and reabsorption takes place among Na^+, K^+, and H^+. Although excess plasma hydrogen ions are secreted all along the tubule, in the distal tubule is where the exchange of H^+ for Na^+ (which is reabsorbed) fine-tunes the balance between H^+ loss and retention (see Chapter 35). Potassium ions also are secreted in the distal tubule. Aldosterone is a potent modulator of Na^+ reabsorption in the distal tubule, particularly when the need arises to conserve Na^+. Production of aldosterone in the adrenal cortex is stimulated by the renin-angiotensin system and by high plasma potassium concentration. Renal secretion of renin is complex but is regulated at least partly by renal perfusion and plasma sodium concentration. Both inadequate perfusion and a low concentration of plasma sodium stimulate renin secretion. Organic anions, such as acetoacetate and β-hydroxybutyrate, also consume H^+ as they are eliminated, in part, in their nondissociated acid form. When H^+ must be conserved to maintain plasma pH, distal tubule cells reduce the secretion of H^+, reduce NH_4^+ generation, reduce Na^+-H^+ exchange, and increase bicarbonate excretion. The net effect is a reduction in plasma bicarbonate and restoration of normal plasma pH.

Water homeostasis

Approximately 70% of the water content of the tubular fluid is reabsorbed in the proximal tubule, 5% in the loop of Henle, 10% in the distal tubule, and the remainder in the collecting ducts. Plasma membranes of all mammalian cells are water permeable, but to variable degrees. Water homeostasis is linked intrinsically to renal urea handling; the urea transporter provides a very low-affinity but high-

capacity passive transport process linked to Na^+ reabsorption in the proximal tubule. The importance of urea to water reabsorption is that the cortical collecting ducts are impermeable to urea, as are the medullary collecting ducts, unless they are acted upon by ADH. ADH is a nonapeptide that binds to specific receptors on the basal membranes of renal collecting-duct cells. It increases water permeability in the cortical cells but increases both water and urea permeability in the medullary tubules.[20]

Endocrine Function

The kidneys synthesize hormones and also are a target site for hormones produced or activated elsewhere. In addition, the kidneys are a site of degradation for hormones such as insulin and aldosterone. Hormones produced by the kidneys include erythropoietin, renin, prostaglandins, thromboxanes, and 1,25(OH) vitamin D.

Erythropoietin

Erythropoietin is a glycoprotein (46 kD) hormone produced by specialized cells in the kidneys that regulates the production of red blood cells (RBCs) in the marrow. Both anemia and hypoxia are major stimuli for erythropoietin production. Recombinant human erythropoietin has proved very effective in the treatment of anemia of chronic renal failure, particularly among individuals who depend on dialysis.

Renin

Renin is produced within juxtaglomerular cells after processing and cleavage of prorenin, which is produced in the liver. The primary stimuli for renin release from juxtaglomerular cells is the reduction of renal perfusion pressure and hyponatremia. The JGA consists of specialized smooth muscle cells within the afferent glomerular arteriolar wall, which is in close proximity to the macula densa region of the ascending limb of the loop of Henle, emphasizing the relationship between tubular salt content and renin release. The juxtaglomerular cells also respond to stretch, thus serving as their own baroreceptor. Renin release also is influenced by the sympathetic nervous system and endocrine influences, including angiotensin II, ADH (vasopressin), endothelin, and prostaglandins. Atrial natriuretic peptide and endothelial cell-derived relaxation factor also are thought to influence renin secretion. Increased production of renin results in the formation of angiotensin II in the liver, which is a powerful intrarenal vasoconstrictor and a key stimulus of aldosterone release from zona glomerulosa cells in the adrenal glands. The net effect is systemic vasoconstriction, intrarenal vasoconstriction, and increased aldosterone release. Aldosterone controls salt and water balance in the kidney. Its effect is predominantly on the distal tubular network, facilitating an increase in sodium reabsorption in exchange for potassium.

Prostaglandins and thromboxanes

Prostaglandins and thromboxanes are synthesized from arachidonic acid by the cyclooxygenase enzyme system (see Chapter 24). This system is present in many parts of the kidneys. The predominant metabolite of its vascular endothelial activity is prostacyclin (PGI_2); prostaglandin E_2 (PGE_2) appears to be the major metabolite of mesangial and tubular cells. The production and activity of these biologically active compounds play an important role in regulation of the physiological action of other hormones on renal vascular tone, mesangial contractility, and tubular processing of salt and water.

Vitamin D

The active form of vitamin D, $1,25(OH)_2D$, is produced by 25(OH)D-1-hydroxylase, an enzyme found in the kidneys (see Chapters 28 and 38).

■ RENAL PHYSIOLOGY

The GFR and renal blood flow are important physiological components of renal function.

Glomerular Filtration Rate

The **glomerular filtration rate (GFR)** is the rate in milliliters per minute that substances such as creatinine and urea are filtered through the kidney's glomeruli. It is considered the most reliable measure of the functional capacity of the kidneys and often is thought of as indicative of the number of functioning nephrons. As a physiological measurement, it has proved the most sensitive and specific marker of changes in overall renal function. The rate of formation of the glomerular filtrate depends on the balance between hydrostatic and oncotic forces along the afferent arteriole and across the glomerular filter. The net pressure difference must be sufficient not only to drive filtration across the glomerular filtration barrier but also to drive the ultrafiltrate along the tubules against their inherent resistance to flow. In the absence of sufficient pressure the lumina of the tubules collapses. This balance of forces is expressed as follows:

$$\text{Rate of filtration} = K_f((P_{GCap} + II_{BC}) - (P_{BC} + II_{GCap}))$$

where

$$
\begin{aligned}
K_f &= \text{Hydraulic permeability} \times \text{surface area} \\
P_{GCap} &= \text{Glomerular-capillary hydrostatic pressure} \\
II_{BC} &= \text{Oncotic pressure* in Bowman's capsule} \\
P_{BC} &= \text{Hydrostatic pressure in Bowman's capsule} \\
II_{GCap} &= \text{Oncotic pressure in the glomerular capillary}
\end{aligned}
$$

---

*Oncotic pressure is defined in Dorland's Illustrated Medical Dictionary as "the osmotic pressure due to the presence of colloids in a solution."

TABLE 34-1	Summary of Factors that Influence the GFR	
	Major Influencing Factors	Effect on GFR
K_f	Increased glomerular surface area due to relaxation of mesangial cells	Increase
	Decreased glomerular surface area due to contraction of mesangial cells	Decrease
P_{GCap}	Altered renal arterial pressure	
	Afferent dilation	Increase
	Afferent constriction	Decrease
	Efferent constriction	Increase
	Efferent dilation	Decrease
P_{BC}	Increased intratubular pressure (for example, tubular obstruction)	Decrease
II_{GCap}	Altered plasma oncotic pressure: increased	Decrease
	Altered renal blood flow: decreased	Decrease

GFR, Glomerular filtration rate; K_f, hydraulic permeability $\times$ surface area; P_{GCap}, glomerular-capillary hydrostatic pressure; P_{BC}, hydrostatic pressure in Bowman's capsule; II_{GCap}, oncotic pressure in the glomerular capillary.

Because the oncotic pressure in Bowman's capsule (II_{BC}) is considered negligible (protein concentration usually 10 to 100 mg/L), the equation becomes the following:

$$\text{Rate of filtration} = K_f(P_{GCap} - P_{BC} - II_{GCap})$$

Changes in K_f are caused by drugs and by glomerular disease. However, K_f also is regulated by mesangial cell contraction, which causes a reduction in K_f that tends to reduce GFR. Net P_{GCap} represents a balance between renal arterial pressure and afferent and efferent arteriolar resistance. Although an increase in arterial pressure tends to increase P_{GCap}, the magnitude of the change is modulated by differential manipulation of afferent and efferent tone, which results in minimal change to the P_{GCap}. When the renal blood flow is low, oncotic pressure changes as the plasma passes along the renal capillaries. As filtrate is removed, the oncotic pressure rises, and by the end of the capillary the net filtration rate may become zero; thus GFR falls, which limits the amount of filtrate that is obtained from a given volume of plasma. The average filtration pressure is about 17 mm Hg.

Regulation of GFR

The factors involved in regulation of GFR are listed in Table 34-1. Autoregulation of renal blood flow and GFR is based on the myogenic principle that an increase in the wall tension of the afferent arterioles, brought about by an increase in perfusion pressure, causes automatic contraction of the arteriolar smooth muscle, thus increasing resistance and keeping the flow constant despite the increase in perfusion pressure.

The tubuloglomerular feedback mechanism, involving the macula densa and release of the vasodilator adenosine, appears also to regulate GFR, with changes in renal blood flow as a secondary consequence. The macula densa is

TABLE 34-2   Relative Glomerular Permeability of Molecules

Molecule	MW (daltons)	Molecular Radius (nm)	pI	GSC
Water	18	0.38	—	1.0
Urea	60	0.54	—	1.0
Creatinine	113	0.60	—	1.0
Potassium	39	0.66	—	1.0
Sodium	23	0.72	—	1.0
Glucose	180	0.90	—	1.0
Dextran	15,000	2.0	—	1.0
Inulin	5000	2.4	—	1.0
β_2-Microglobulin	11,800	1.6	5.6	0.7
Cystatin C	12,800	3.5	9.2	Not known
Retinol-binding protein	22,000	5.2	4.5	Not known
α_1-Microglobulin	30,000	?	4.5	Not known
Albumin	66,000	6.3	4.7	0.0002
Immunoglobulin G	150,000	8.5	7.3	0.0001

GSC, Glomerular sieving coefficient; *MW*, molecular weight; *pI*, isoelectric point.

thought to sense either the distal tubular sodium chloride content, its osmolality, or the rate at which sodium chloride is transported. The macula densa then signals the JGA to cause the release of adenosine and possibly angiotensin II and prostaglandins. Adenosine usually acts as a vasodilator in other vascular beds, but in the kidney it acts as an afferent arteriolar vasoconstrictor.

Nitric oxide (NO) has been identified as an important vasodilator produced by vascular endothelial cells.[17] NO is synthesized from L-arginine and oxygen by nitric oxide synthetase (NOS). NO synthesis plays an important role in the regulation of human vascular tone and a crucial role in control of blood pressure and kidney function.

Renal Blood Flow

Renal blood flow is regulated independently of GFR and provides an additional measure of renal function. However, the distribution of blood flow within the kidney is not homogeneous, and it is altered quickly in response to various factors.

Glomerular permeability

The glomerulus acts as a selective filter for the blood passing through its capillaries. The combination of a specialized endothelium, basement membrane, and epithelial cell barrier produces a filter that restricts the passage of macromolecules in a size-, charge-, and shape-dependent manner. The basement membrane is a compressible filter, becoming more permeable as the applied pressure decreases and the fibers separate.

Markers of permeability

The glomerular permeability of a number of different molecules is shown in Table 34-2. Linear dextran chains of varying MWs and charges were used in early experiments to delineate glomerular filtration characteristics. However, a linear carbohydrate chain does not behave in the same manner as a globular protein of equal MW or charge. Linear molecules have higher glomerular sieving coefficients (GSCs) than globular proteins.*

In general, proteins of MWs greater than albumin (66.3 kD) are retained by the healthy glomerulus and termed *high-molecular-weight proteins*. Proteins of lower MWs still are retained significantly. For example, β_2-microglobulin (BMG) at 11.8 kD is retained (GSC of 0.7).[1] Molecules become freely filtered at about the MW of insulin (5.0 kD).

The filtered load of protein depends on the product of the GSC and the free plasma concentration, and therefore the albumin load per nephron is much greater than that of the other filtered proteins. The urinary concentration of proteins depends on the filtered load and the efficiency of the proximal tubular reabsorptive process. As indicated in Table 34-3, the reabsorptive mechanism removes the vast bulk of the filtered protein, retaining most of the essential amino acid constituents for reuse.

Proteinuria

Proteinuria is defined as an increase in the amount of protein in urine. The pattern of urinary protein excretion is used to identify the cause and classify the proteinuria. Types include glomerular, tubular, overload, and postrenal proteinuria (Table 34-4). Details on these types of proteinuria are found in Chapter 19.

Investigation of proteinuria

Mixed proteinuria with the elevation of both high- and low-MW proteins is the most frequent pattern observed. The relative ratio between these two groups of proteins

*The glomerular sieving coefficient is defined as the ratio of the tubular fluid concentration/plasma concentration.

TABLE 34-3 Filtered Load and Reabsorption of Proteins

Protein	Free Plasma Concentration	GSC	Filtered Load	Urinary Concentration	% Reabsorbed
Immunoglobulin G	10 g/L	0.0001	1 mg/L	0.1 mg/L	99
Albumin	40 g/L	0.0002	8 mg/L	5 mg/L	99
Retinol-binding protein	25 mg/L	~0.7	17.5 mg/L	0.1 mg/L	99
α_1-Microglobulin	25 mg/L	~0.3	7.5 mg/L	5 mg/L	99
Cystatin C	1 mg/L	~0.7	0.7 mg/L	0.1 mg/L	99
β_2-Microglobulin	1.5 mg/L	0.7	1.1 mg/L	0.1 mg/L	99
Total protein	70 g/L	NA*	700 mg/L	150 mg/L	NA*

GSC, Glomerular sieving coefficient.

*Not applicable due to tubular secretion of proteins (for example, Tamm-Horsfall glycoprotein, which form approximately 50% of urinary total proteins).

TABLE 34-4 Characterization of Proteinuria

Increased Filtered Load

Glomerular—increased glomerular permeability; progressively increasing excretion of higher-molecular-weight proteins as permeability increases

Increased plasma concentration of relatively freely filtered protein "overflow proteinuria" (for example, of Bence-Jones protein)

Decreased glomerular number—increased filtered load per nephron

Decreased Tubular Reabsorptive Capacity

Proximal tubular damage (for example, from nephrotoxic drugs)

Decreased glomerular number—increased filtered load per nephron

Enzymuria (for example, NAG)

Postglomerular Secretion or Leakage

Tamm-Horsfall glycoprotein

Hematuria

NAG, N-acetylglucosaminidase.

gives an indication of the pathological process involved. Proteinuria also occurs because of functional or benign proteinuria (orthostatic) and exercise. These sporadic changes are not known to be pathological but have caused interpretative difficulties when a pathology is suspected.

Consequences of proteinuria

Studies have shown a strong correlation between the degree of proteinuria and the rate of progression of renal failure in a number of renal diseases. This correlation has led to the hypothesis that proteinuria itself may contribute to the progression of renal disease and not be simply a consequence of it. Cortical interstitial expansion results in impairment of tubular function caused by a tubular anoxia, which may lead to glomerular injury caused by an increase in glomerular hydrostatic pressure. Furthermore, slowing of the rate of progression of renal failure has been observed in animals and humans in whom proteinuria was reduced with the use of angiotensin-converting enzyme (ACE) inhibitors and/or ingestion of a low-protein diet, emphasizing the significance of proteinuria in the pathogenesis of renal failure.

RENAL PATHOPHYSIOLOGY

The symptoms and signs of **renal failure** are summarized in Table 34-5 and are a consequence of the loss of the important homeostatic regulation that the kidneys provide. Nephrons are lost via toxic, anoxic, or immunological injury that may initially injure either the glomerulus, the tubule, or both together.

The kidneys have considerable ability to increase their functional capacity in response to injury. Thus a significant reduction in functioning renal mass (50% to 60%) may occur before the onset of any significant symptoms or even before any major biochemical alterations appear. The most sensitive and specific measure of functional change is the GFR, which is reduced to less than 50 mL/minute/1.73 m^2 (Table 34-6) before even minor signs and symptoms of acute renal failure are observed.[16] This increase in workload per nephron is thought to be an important cause of progressive renal injury itself. A well-recognized hypothesis suggests that, independent of the primary renal injury, a point is reached in the decline in nephron number when further loss becomes inevitable and progressive as a consequence of a common pathway leading to interstitial fibrosis.[18]

Types of Renal Failure

Types of renal failure include acute renal failure (ARF) or chronic renal failure (CRF).

Acute renal failure

ARF most commonly occurs in a hospital setting, frequently as a result of ischemic or nephrotoxic insults. ARF is differentiated best from CRF by careful scrutiny of a patient's history, performance of a renal biopsy, and imaging of the kidneys; small, shrunken kidneys are a clear indication of chronicity.[7]

ARF develops rapidly, and therefore its sequelae are mainly a consequence of rapid electrolyte, acid-base, and fluid imbalances that are difficult to control, hence the high mortality. ARF also has been divided into three main categories—prerenal, intrarenal, and postrenal, depending

TABLE 34-5 Signs and Symptoms of Renal Failure

Symptoms of uremia (nausea, vomiting, lethargy)
Disorders of micturition (frequency, nocturia, retention, dysuria)
Disorders of urine volume (polyuria, oliguria, anuria)
Alteration in urinary composition (hematuria, proteinuria, bacteriuria, leukocyturia, calculi)
Pain (an inconsistent symptom)
Edema (hypoalbuminemia, salt and water retention)

TABLE 34-6 Symptoms Associated with Falling Glomerular Filtration Rate

GFR (mL/minute/ 1.73 m^2)	Symptoms
125 to 152	Symptomless except for those symptoms resulting from any underlying pathology
<45	Fatigue; diminished well-being; PTH elevated and 1,25-vitamin D reduced
<30	Anemia; metabolic abnormalities, such as acidosis; calcium homeostasis deterioration
<15	Nausea; vomiting; gastritis
<10	Cardiovascular and neurological symptoms
<5	End-stage renal failure; K$^+$ homeostasis failure

PTH, Parathyroid hormone.

TABLE 34-7 Causes of Acute Renal Failure

Cause	Agents
Prerenal	
Hypovolemia	Trauma, burns, surgery
Decreased effective plasma volume	Nephrotic syndrome, sepsis; shock
Decreased cardiac output	Congestive cardiac failure, pulmonary embolism
Renovascular obstruction	Atherosclerosis, stenoses
Interference with renal autoregulation	ACE inhibitors, cyclosporin
Renal	
Glomerular and small vessel disease	Aggressive glomerulonephritis (for example, poststreptococcal, preeclampsia)
Interstitial nephritis	Infection, infiltration, drugs/toxins
Tubular lesions	Postischemic, nephrotoxins, hypercalcemia
Postrenal	
Bladder outflow obstruction	Prostatism, neurogenic bladder
Ureteric obstruction	Stones, blood clots, tumors, radiotherapy, retroperitoneal fibrosis

ACE, Angiotensin-converting enzyme.

on where the damage has occurred (Table 34-7). Although the pathogenesis is uncertain, a well-recognized clinical pattern exists with anuria or oliguria and abnormalities indicate tubular dysfunction. If the patient recovers, recovery usually occurs within days or weeks of the removal of the initiating event. Although temporary replacement of renal function through hemodialysis has cut the mortality from ARF in half, it still remains high, at about 50%.[7]

The role of the clinical laboratory in the assessment and monitoring of ARF is limited to the measurement of electrolyte disturbance and fluid status. During the recovery period an initial polyuric phase occurs because glomerular function recovers before tubular function recovers. This polyuric phase recedes after a few days to weeks but requires careful monitoring to enable suitable fluid and electrolyte replacement.

Chronic renal failure

CRF is the progressive loss of functioning nephrons. However, the rate at which CRF progresses is exacerbated by episodes of ARF. The main causes of CRF from 1977 to 1991 were diabetes, renal vascular disease, and glomerulonephritis. In clinical practice the differential diagnosis of CRF is achieved by use of percutaneous renal biopsy linked with optical or electron microscopy in association with immunohistochemistry or, more recently, with in situ hybridization and polymerase chain reaction (PCR) techniques. The clinical laboratory plays a minimal role in establishing the diagnosis.

Uremic Syndrome

Uremia, or **azotemia,** is defined as an excess in blood of urea, creatinine, and other nitrogenous end products of amino acid and protein metabolism. The uremic syndrome is the terminal clinical expression of kidney failure and results from the failure of the kidneys to maintain adequate excretory, regulatory, and endocrine function.

The classic signs of the uremic syndrome include progressive weakness and easy fatigue, loss of appetite followed by nausea and vomiting, muscle wasting, tremors, abnormal mental function, frequent but shallow respirations, and metabolic acidosis. The syndrome then evolves to produce stupor, coma, and ultimately death unless support is provided by hemodialysis or successful renal transplantation. Renal disease also has been characterized as occurring in four stages, as defined by the percentage of renal function remaining and the plasma concentrations of creatinine and urea nitrogen (Table 34-8).

The most characteristic laboratory findings are increased concentrations of nitrogenous compounds in plasma (for example, urea nitrogen and creatinine) as a result of reduced GFR and decreased tubular function. Retention of these compounds and of metabolic acids is followed by progressive hyperphosphatemia, hypocalcemia, and potentially dangerous hyperkalemia. Biochemical characteristics of the uremic syndrome are summarized in Table 34-9.

End-stage renal disease (ESRD) and the resulting uremic syndrome results from any of a wide variety of renal diseases, including chronic glomerulonephritis, chronic py-

TABLE 34-8 Stages of Chronic Progressive Renal Disease

Stage	Renal Function Remaining (%)	Serum Creatinine (mg/dL)	Serum Urea Nitrogen (mg/dL)
1. Decreased renal reserve	50 to 75	1.0 to 2.5	15 to 30
2. Renal insufficiency	25 to 50	2.5 to 6.0	25 to 60
3. Renal failure	10 to 25	5.5 to 11.0	55 to 110
4. Uremic syndrome (end-stage)	0 to 10	>8.0	>80

TABLE 34-9 Biochemical Characteristics of the Uremic Syndrome

Retained Nitrogenous Metabolites
Urea
Cyanate
Creatinine
Guanidine compounds
"Middle molecules"
Uric acid

Fluid, Acid-Base, and Electrolyte Disturbances
Fixed urine osmolality
Metabolic acidosis (decreased blood pH, bicarbonate)
Hyponatremia or hypernatremia
Hypokalemia or hyperkalemia
Hyperchloremia
Hypocalcemia
Hyperphosphatemia
Hypermagnesemia

Carbohydrate Intolerance
Insulin resistance
  Plasma insulin normal or increased
  Delayed response to carbohydrate loading
  Hyperglucagonemia

Abnormal Lipid Metabolism
Hypertriglyceridemia
Decreased high-density lipoprotein cholesterol
Hyperlipoproteinemia

Altered Endocrine Function
Secondary hyperparathyroidism
Osteomalacia (secondary to abnormal vitamin D metabolism)
Hyperreninemia and hyperaldosteronism
Hyporeninemia
Hypoaldosteronism
Decreased erythropoietin production
Altered thyroxine metabolism
Gonadal dysfunction (increased prolactin and luteinizing hormone; decreased testosterone)

elonephritis, immunological diseases with renal involvement (for example, systemic lupus erythematosus [SLE]), hypertension, acute obstruction of the lower urinary tract, and toxic or ischemic damage to the kidney.

Glomerular Diseases

Many renal diseases are the result of glomerular injury. Among the more important are the acute nephritic syndrome,* rapidly progressive **glomerulonephritis,** autoim-

---

*Nephritis is defined in Dorland's Illustrated Medical Dictionary as "inflammation of the kidney with focal or diffuse proliferation or destructive processes that may involve the glomerulus, tubule, or interstitial renal tissue."

mune **nephritis,** chronic glomerulonephritis, and the nephrotic syndrome.

Acute nephritic syndrome

The acute nephritic syndrome (acute glomerulonephritis) is characterized by the rapid onset of **hematuria** (blood in urine), proteinuria (protein in urine), reduced GFR, and sodium and water retention with resulting hypertension and sometimes localized peripheral edema. Congestive heart failure and oliguria also may develop. Renal biopsy shows enlarged, inflamed glomeruli with narrowed capillary lumina.

In a number of individuals affected with the acute nephritic syndrome, the pathological process is related to recent group A β-hemolytic streptococcal infection of the pharynx or less commonly, the skin. Only certain strains of streptococci are capable of inducing acute nephritis. Involvement of the kidneys is diffuse. Electron microscopy reveals deposits, presumably immune complexes, on the epithelial side of the basement membrane. Glomerular injury with damage of the glomerular basement membrane leading to reduction of GFR is thought to be due to activation of the inflammatory response by immune complexes. Abnormal laboratory results usually are present early in the course of acute nephritis. Hematuria, gross or microscopic, and proteinuria, usually less than 3 g/day, are present almost always. RBC casts are highly suggestive of glomerulonephritis. The proteinuria is progressively more nonselective, with higher-MW species exhibiting greatly increased clearances (see Chapter 19). Clinically the degree to which selectivity is lost can indicate the severity of damage to the glomerular basement membrane. The urine protein also may have greatly increased amounts of fibrinopeptides (cleavage products of fibrinogen), although these may be elevated moderately in individuals with renal insufficiency of many causes.

In individuals suspected of having acute poststreptococcal glomerulonephritis, evidence of recent infection may be found in increased titers of antibodies to streptococcal extracellular products—antistreptolysin O (ASO), antihyaluronidase (AHase), and antideoxyribonuclease-B (ADNase-B).

Most individuals have moderate reductions in total hemolytic complement activity (CH_{50}) and in the C3 component of the complement cascade. Persistent and severe depression of C3 levels should suggest membranoproliferative glomerulonephritis, SLE, endocarditis, or other forms of sepsis. Although depressed levels of complement imply disease activity, they are not useful for grading of the severity or determination of the prognosis of the illness.

Other causes of acute nephritis include reactions to drugs, acute infection of the kidneys, systemic diseases with immune complexes such as SLE, bacterial endocarditis, and disease in which the antigen is unknown but possibly related to antecedent viral infections.

Rapidly progressive glomerulonephritis

Rapidly progressive glomerulonephritis (RPGN) is a heterogeneous group of disorders characterized by a fulminant clinical course that leads to renal failure in weeks to a few months. This group of diseases is characterized by a consistent histological picture of glomerular crescent formation. The glomerular epithelial crescent is a proliferation of blood-derived macrophages and parietal epithelial cells lining the Bowman's capsule. The proliferating epithelial cells and macrophages eventually compress the glomeruli and obstruct the PCTs, thus severely compromising nephron function. These crescents may develop rapidly, and thus the parameters of declining renal function show changes in a matter of days.

RPGN is classified as either idiopathic renal disease or a disease secondary to other conditions, such as infectious diseases, multisystem diseases, and on occasion, an adverse reaction to medication. RPGN also has been associated with infectious disease processes, such as streptococcal infection, endocarditis, or occult visceral bacterial sepsis. Multisystem diseases associated with RPGN include Goodpasture's syndrome, SLE, Henoch-Schönlein purpura, and systemic vasculitis.

Autoimmune nephritis

Autoimmune nephritis (also known as *antiglomerular basement membrane disease*) is an autoimmune disorder characterized by the presence of autoantibodies directed against basement membrane components. Its classic manifestation is a rapidly progressing nephritis with lung hemorrhage. Its antigen has been characterized and found to be the $\alpha 1,3$ chain of type IV collagen that forms part of the glomerular and alveolar basement membranes. Goodpasture's syndrome is an example of this type of nephritis.

Chronic glomerulonephritis

Chronic glomerulonephritis is a clinical syndrome that results from a number of glomerular diseases that have a prolonged downhill course with progressive loss of nephron mass. Many of these diseases remain entirely asymptomatic except for mild hematuria, proteinuria, and slightly reduced renal function. In some cases the first indication of disease is the gradual onset of the uremic syndrome. In the late stages of chronic glomerulonephritis, hypertension is frequently a complication and ESRD becomes apparent, regardless of the initial cause.

Many glomerular diseases lead to chronic glomerulonephritis. It also occurs as an idiopathic process. The kidneys are small, due to the loss of mass, but not as scarred and distorted as they appear in cases of chronic pyelonephritis. The remaining functional nephrons may undergo hypertrophy, giving the surface of the kidneys a granular appearance. Differentiation from nonglomerular diseases is not always possible, but heavy proteinuria or RBC casts suggest a glomerular process. Chronic glomerulonephritis ultimately becomes indistinguishable from chronic tubulointerstitial nephritis and chronic vascular diseases, such as hypertension.

Nephrotic syndrome

The **nephrotic syndrome** is characterized by heavy proteinuria (total protein >3 g/24 hours or albumin >1.5 g/24 hours), hypoalbuminemia, hypercholesterolemia and finally massive edema. The edema is a consequence of the decreased intravascular oncotic pressure due to the loss of protein. However, the concomitant transudation of salt and water into interstitial spaces causes a decrease in plasma volume that also triggers the kidneys to retain sodium. The proteinuria is a consequence of a reduction in the charge-selective properties of the filtration barrier, particularly the basement membrane and the podocytes (epithelial cells). Nephrotic syndrome results from a variety of causes, including minimal change glomerulonephritis; membranous glomerulonephritis, drugs, or infection; SLE; and diabetic nephropathy. The protein selectivity index may be used to complement plasma and urine total protein measurement to assess the type of damage. An index of less than 0.16 for the IgG albumin clearance ratio indicates high selectivity, whereas a value greater than 0.3 indicates poor selectivity. The use of the selectivity index may help to identify the cause of the renal disease.

The consequences of nephrotic syndrome include susceptibility to infection, venous and arterial thrombosis, and abnormalities in lipid metabolism, such as hepatic overproduction of very–low-density lipoprotein (VLDL). Synthesis of high-density lipoprotein (HDL) also is increased, but a selective loss of HDL_3 into the urine and reduced lecithin-cholesterol acyltransferase (LCAT) activity also occur, resulting in decreased transport of cholesterol from the tissues to the liver.

Interstitial Nephritis

A variety of chemical, bacterial, and immunological injuries to the kidney cause either generalized or localized changes that primarily affect the tubulointerstitium. This group of disorders is characterized by alterations in tubular function that lead to vascular and glomerular damage. **Pyelonephritis** is the term associated with a bacterial infection that causes this kind of damage and is the most common of the

TABLE 34-10 Development of Diabetic Nephropathy

Stage Designation	Functional Changes	Structural Changes	GFR (mL/minute/ 1.73 m^2)	Blood Pressure (mm Hg)
I Hyperfunction	Hyperfiltration	Glomerular hypertrophy	>150	Normal
II Normo-albuminuria	Normal AER	Basement membrane thickening	150	Normal
III Incipient diabetic nephropathy	Elevated AER	AER correlation with structural damage	125	Increased
IV Overt diabetic nephropathy	Clinical proteinuria	Advanced structural damage	<100	Hypertension

AER, Albumin excretion rate; *GFR,* glomerular filtration rate.

interstitial nephritides. It is a frequent cause of ESRD. Both acute and chronic types of pyelonephritis exist, with the acute type most commonly associated with urinary tract infection. Tubulointerstitial nephritis also is caused by a variety of drugs. Proteinuria is associated with interstitial nephritis; however, it is usually less severe than in cases of glomerular disease.

Cystic Renal Disease

Autosomal dominant polycystic kidney disease (APKD) is the second most common inherited monogenic disease after familial hypercholesterolemia and is by far the most frequently occurring inherited kidney disease. The prevalence of the disease ranges from 1 in 200 individuals to 1 in 1000, but many cases, possibly up to 50%, remain undiagnosed. The disease causes the development of multiple renal cysts, often associated with liver and cardiovascular abnormalities. Hypertension is an early and frequent manifestation, and gross hematuria is a common presenting symptom.

Progression to ESRD is not universal, with as many as 80% of individuals with APKD being free of dialysis even if they demonstrate evidence of renal impairment, such as increased levels of serum creatinine. This incidence now is known to be due to APKD being a genetically heterogeneous disorder. APKD1 mutation on chromosome 16 is the most frequent mutation and is found in 86% of cases. It codes for an abnormal form of the protein polycystin (460 kD), which has been shown to play a role in epithelial cell differentiation.

Nephropathies Secondary to Systemic Diseases
Diabetic nephropathy

Renal disease is a common microvascular complication of both type 1 and type 2 diabetes mellitus.[2] The clinical definition of diabetic nephropathy is the presence of persistent proteinuria (>0.5 g/24 hours) in a diabetic individual with concomitant retinopathy and elevated blood pressure. However, before the diagnosis is made, urinary tract infection, any other renal disease, and cardiac insufficiency first must be ruled out. Nephropathy in individuals with type 1 diabetes develops in four phases

(Table 34-10). (For more detailed information, the reader is referred to Chapter 23.)

Hypertensive nephropathy

Hypertension often develops as a consequence of renal failure due to alterations in salt and water metabolism.[4] It then acts as an accelerating force in the development of ESRD. However, hypertension per se may initiate the development of nephropathy (for example, in cases of preeclampsia and idiopathic essential hypertension). The most effective test used to identify the development of significant nephropathy in hypertensive individuals is to monitor urinary albumin excretion.

Vasculitides

Vasculitis or angiitis is an inflammatory reaction in the wall of any blood vessel. A range of systemic vasculitides exists, including Wegner's granulomatosis and microscopic polyarteritis; they cause microvascular damage leading to necrotizing glomerulonephritis. If unrecognized, these diseases progress very rapidly to ESRD.

Antineutrophil cytoplasmic antibodies (ANCA) and antiendothelial cell antibodies (AECA) are examples of autoantibodies that have been identified to have diagnostic and prognostic usefulness for vasculitides. The classic laboratory measurement used in diagnosis and prognostic risk assessment is the measurement of ANCA, which appear in the plasma of almost all individuals with active and generalized disease. In addition, measurement of C-reactive protein (CRP) has been used to monitor the acute phase reaction in active disease processes, together with tests for the general assessment of progressive renal disease, including proteinuria.

Miscellaneous Renal Disease
Renal tubular acidosis

Renal tubular acidosis (RTA) is characterized by hyperchloremia, a normal anion gap, and urinary HCO_3^- or H^+ excretion inappropriate for the plasma pH. Hyperchloremia is caused by enhanced Cl^- reabsorption stimulated by contraction of the extracellular volume. Other causes of hyperchloremic acidosis with normal anion gap must be ruled out, but this action generally is done on clinical grounds. RTA is the result of loss of bicarbonate or decreased reabsorption by the proximal renal tubules; it also can result from insufficient acidification of the distal tubular fluid due to various causes (see Chapter 35).

Renal calculi

Nephrolithiasis is a condition marked by the presence of renal calculi (typically known as "kidney stones").[9] The majority of these stones are composed of one or more of the following substances—calcium oxalate, calcium phosphate, uric acid, cystine, or a mixture of these with magnesium ammonium phosphate (struvite). These substances crystallize within an organic matrix. All the substances are poorly soluble in aqueous solution, with solubility influenced by the urinary pH. The mechanisms responsible for the multiple recurrences of renal stones in only certain individuals involve a multitude of factors, including (1) urine flow (fluid intake), (2) excretion of excess quantities of the relatively insoluble substances listed previously, and perhaps (3) the absence, in individuals who form stones, of a substance or substances in the urine that, under normal circumstances, inhibit(s) precipitation of some of these nearly insoluble agents.

Calcium oxalate stones are perhaps the most common stones encountered, and they occur in a worldwide "stone belt" that is confined mainly to the tropical and subtropical regions of the globe. They may be associated with either persistently concentrated urine or consistently increased excretion of urinary calcium or oxalate. Most commonly this type of stone is composed of predominantly calcium oxalate, with small quantities of calcium phosphate and uric acid also present. In many instances, finding of any abnormality in stone-forming individuals beyond a persistently small urine volume is impossible; however, obtaining of data on calcium and oxalate output in the urine to ascertain that the mechanism of urinary acidification is normal is useful.

Chemically, urine contains many mineral salts that are present in concentrations that approach their solubility products, and the solutions are metastable. Anyone who has seen a urine sample before and after refrigeration has witnessed the consequences of this occurrence in the massive crystal deposits that form on cooling. Crystals often form spontaneously if the salt concentrations are high enough or if preformed nuclei provoke their formation. Human urine contains a number of promoters of stone formation and a variety of inhibitors (Table 34-11), the concentrations of which are influenced by dietary factors. However, the predominant risk factor is poor hydration, a concentrated urine increasing the concentrations of the mineral salts further, predisposing them to crystallization.

Both qualitative and quantitative analyses of the chemical constituents of kidney stones may be useful in the establishment of the etiology and the planning of rational therapy. In some patients, however, two or more possible causes exist, and analysis of the calculus may help distin-

TABLE 34-11	Promoters, Inhibitors, and Predisposing Risk Factors of Stone Formation
Promoters	**URINARY**
Albumin	Increased Ca^+
Globulins	Increased urate
Matrix substance A	Increased oxalate
	Increased pH
Inhibitors	Decreased Mg^+
Magnesium	Decreased volume
Citrate	Decreased citrate
Pyrophosphate	
Tamm-Horsfall glycoprotein	**Metabolic Disorders**
RNA	Primary hyperparathyroidism
	Renal tubular acidosis type I
Predisposing Factors	Hereditary hyperoxaluria
PREURINARY	Medullary sponge kidney
Female sex	Cushing's disease
Hot climate	Milk-alkali syndrome
Stress	
Decreased fluid intake	
Protein-rich diet	
Immobilization	

guish among different diagnoses. For example, patients with hypercalciuria and calcium oxalate stones may develop renal infections with deposition of magnesium ammonium phosphate on the calcium oxalate stones, forming "mixed stones." Chemical analysis of these stones is needed to confirm this sequence of events. However, specialized physical techniques, such as infrared spectroscopy and x-ray diffraction, are replacing gradually less specific, qualitative chemical methods for stone analysis.

Ultrasonic **lithotripsy**, also known as *extracorporeal shock wave lithotripsy*, is used frequently to treat kidney stones. This procedure uses sound waves delivered inside a water bath to pulverize kidney stones painlessly inside the body. After treatment and successful removal of the stones, follow-up monitoring is required because many patients experience recurrent stone formation.

Diabetes insipidus

Diabetes insipidus is a rare form of diabetes in which the kidney tubules do not reabsorb sufficient amounts of water. This decreased reabsorption results from (1) the renal tubules having defective receptors for ADH, (2) defective aquaporin water channels in the collecting duct, or (3) an inadequate ADH production by the pituitary, leading to the excessive production of dilute urine. A number of similar disorders are listed in Table 34-12.

Obstructive uropathy

Benign prostatic hypertrophy (BPH) is one of the most common types of obstructive uropathy and an almost universal finding in aging men. Among the frequent symptoms are disorders of micturition, in particular an increased frequency, and in many cases this condition progresses to blad-

TABLE 34-12 Diseases Associated with Disturbances in the Renal Concentrating Mechanism

Marked Polyuria and Hypotonic Urine after Water Deprivation
Diabetes insipidus
Hereditary nephrogenic diabetes insipidus
Chronic lithium toxicity
Sickle cell nephropathy
Hypokalemia (rarely)

Moderate Polyuria and Inability to Produce Hypertonic Urine
Hypercalcemia
Hypokalemia
Chronic pyelonephritis
End-stage renal disease
Amyloidosis
Interstitial nephritis

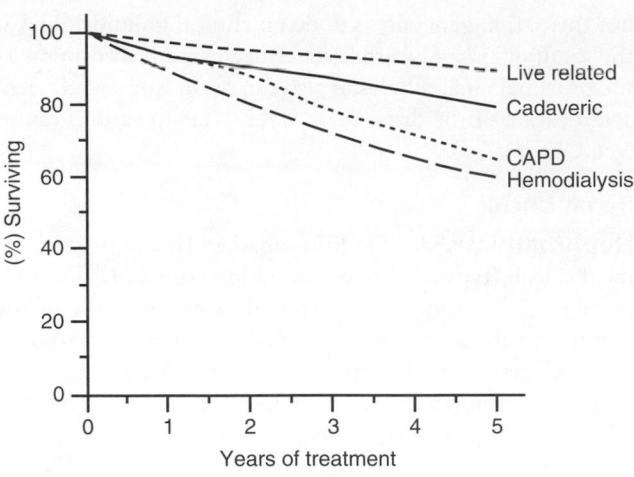

Figure 34-4 Comparison of survival rates of patients receiving different forms of renal replacement therapy—transplantation, hemodialysis, or continuous ambulatory peritoneal dialysis (CAPD). (Data from United Network for Organ Sharing, Richmond, Va, [http://www.unos.org].)

der outflow obstruction. Between 10% and 40% of men with bladder outflow obstruction due to BPH present in acute retention of urine. Approximately 5% of this same group have high-pressure chronic retention of urine, which may result in upper urinary tract obstruction and consequent renal impairment as a result of glomerular and tubular damage.

Pseudohypoparathyroidism

An unusual form of hypocalcemia of renal origin is pseudohypoparathyroidism, in which the serum PTH levels are elevated. The resistance to PTH is thought to be present in the kidney and is classified into types Ia-c and II, depending on the purported defect. The defects are thought to be caused by a reduced level of the protein Gsα in the cell plasma membrane (responsible for the complex that links the PTH receptor to the adenylate cyclase catalytic unit), a possible defect in the PTH receptor complex, or a defect in the protein kinase or second-messenger system.

Toxic nephropathy

A wide variety of nephrotoxins exist in the environment, many of which are associated with particular occupations.[3] A variety of heavy metals, such as cadmium and lead, long have been known to be associated with kidney disease, often causing proximal tubular dysfunction and glomerular damage (see Chapter 32). A summary of the drugs and environmental toxins known to cause renal damage is given in Table 34-13. Both glomerular nephritis and tubulointerstitial damage result from exposure to these toxins; detection of both requires biochemical monitoring of GFR and both tubular and glomerular proteinuria. Markers of damage have been used to set legislative limits of exposure to these toxins, and along with drug-induced damage, this exposure is the only clinically established use of markers of tubular protein-

uria. Analgesic nephropathy is a common cause of ESRD in a number of European countries, reaching 10% in Switzerland. However, it is essentially a preventable condition for which biochemical monitoring has proved useful.

RENAL REPLACEMENT THERAPY

Hemodialysis and peritoneal dialysis are used to treat renal failure and have extended the lives of hundreds of thousands of people, sometimes for 20 or 30 years. In addition, renal transplantation (Figure 34-4) also has become an effective form of renal replacement therapy. A wide variety of laboratory tests are required to support renal replacement therapy (Table 34-14).

Hemodialysis

Hemodialysis is the removal of certain elements from the blood by use of the difference in the rates of their diffusion through a semipermeable membrane. It is used to remove toxic substances from the blood when the kidneys are not able to remove them satisfactorily from the circulation. In this process, blood solutes diffuse down a concentration gradient, across a semipermeable membrane, and into a recipient fluid, the dialysate. Water molecules and small-MW molecules cross the membrane, but larger proteins and cellular elements are retained in the vascular space.

A typical modern hemodialyzer and its major components are shown in Figure 34-5. The most important functional part is the dialyzer membrane; a wide variety of membranes are available that vary in size (surface area), pore size, and constituents. All of these factors influence treatment efficiency and the nature of the secondary dialytic complications that might develop. Biocompatibility of the dialyzer

TABLE 34-13	Drugs and Environmental Toxins Associated with the Development of Nephropathy	
Drug	**Toxic Action**
ACE inhibitors	Drastic drop in GFR in patients with bilateral renal artery stenosis; high-dose captopril possible cause of proteinuria
NSAIDs	Drastic drop in GFR in patients with circulatory insufficiency (for example, cardiac failure); hypovolemia; can cause acute and chronic interstitial nephritis
Antirheumatoid drugs	
Gold salts	Membranous-type picture with nephrotic syndrome (mechanism unknown)
Mercury compounds	Membranous-type picture with nephrotic syndrome (mechanism unknown)
D-Penicillamine	Membranous-type picture with nephrotic syndrome (mechanism unknown)
Antitumor drugs	
Mitomycin	Hemolytic-uremic syndrome
Cisplatin	Acute tubular necrosis
Methotrexate	Intraluminal precipitation and acute tubular necrosis
Antibiotics/antifungals	
Aminoglycosides	Acute tubular necrosis and interstitial nephritis
Cephalosporins	Interstitial nephritis
Penicillin G	Interstitial nephritis
Ampicillin	Interstitial nephritis
Amoxicillin	Interstitial nephritis
Amphotericin	
Lithium	Distal tubular damage with nephrogenic diabetes insipidus
Allopurinol	Interstitial nephritis
Environmental toxins	
Heavy metals	
Mercury	Glomerulonephritis
Cadmium	Chronic interstitial nephritis
Lead	Hypertension and tubulointerstitial nephritis
Chromium	Increased tubular proteins and enzymuria
Vanadium	Increased tubular proteins and enzymuria
Nickel	Increased tubular proteins and enzymuria
Solvents—dry cleaning/paints	Glomerulonephritis

ACE, Angiotensin-converting enzyme; *GFR,* glomerular filtration rate; *NSAIDs,* nonsteroidal antiinflammatory drugs.

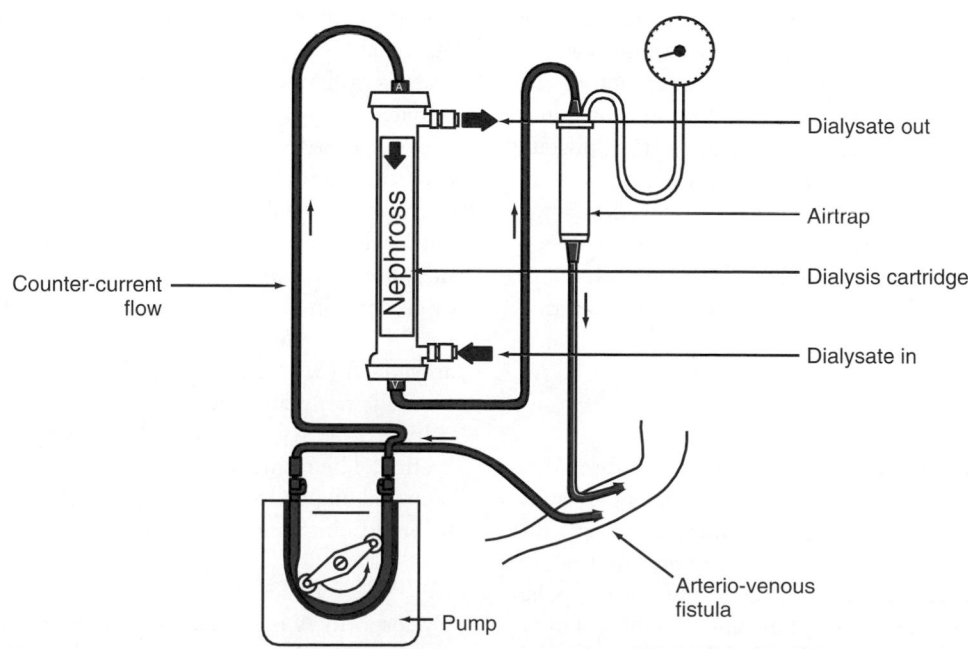

Figure 34-5   A modern hemodialyzer setup with an inset flow diagram.

TABLE 34-14 Laboratory Support for Renal Replacement Therapy

Factor	Laboratory Tests
Complications	
ACUTE	
Dialysis disequilibrium	Plasma electrolytes
Pyrexia	C-reactive protein
Bleeding	Clotting factors
CHRONIC	
Anemia	Hemoglobin, ferritin
Septicemia/peritonitis	C-reactive protein
Malnutrition	Albumin, prealbumin
Cardiovascular disease	Lipid profiles
Amyloidosis	Serum β_2-microglobulin
Osteodystrophy	Ca^{2+}, PO_4^-, bone alkaline phosphatase, intact PTH, aluminum
Adequacy of Dialysis	
Urea kinetic modeling	Predialysis and postdialysis urea
Weekly creatinine clearances (carbamylated hemoglobin)	Predialysis and postdialysis creatinine
Transplant Monitoring	
Immunosuppression	Trough whole blood cyclosporin A
Graft function	Serum creatinine, plasma and urine electrolytes

PTH, Parathyroid hormone.

membrane is an essential requirement because of high surface areas and long contact times with blood. The most important physiological interactions that occur, apart from protein fouling of tubing and membranes, are complement activation and induction of cytokine release. Particle release from silicone rubber pump tubing (spallation) and air microbubbles also have caused problems. By alteration of the applied pressure across the membrane, ultrafiltration (fluid removal) is regulated, and through alteration of the flow rate of dialysate and blood flow, solute removal is regulated. With the advent of techniques to assess dialysis adequacy, a patient is prescribed a certain dialysis "dose." Patients are dialyzed in home-based or hospital-based units, with dialysis usually performed three times a week for sessions lasting 3 to 5 hours.

Peritoneal Dialysis

In **peritoneal dialysis** a special solution is run through a tube into the peritoneum, a thin tissue that lines the cavity of the abdomen. Waste products are removed through the tube. Three types of peritoneal dialysis exist. Continuous ambulatory peritoneal dialysis (CAPD) is the most popular because it does not require a machine and is done at home. Continuous cyclical peritoneal dialysis (CCPD) uses a machine and usually is performed at night when the individual is sleeping. Intermittent peritoneal dialysis (IPD) uses the same type of machine as CCPD, but it usually is done in the hospital because treatment takes longer.

Renal Transplantation

Renal transplantation is an effective form of renal replacement therapy, with several thousand procedures performed per year in the United States alone. For example, kidney grafts have been transplanted successfully for over 30 years, with average survival of around 80% at 1 year and 60% at 4 years.

Preoperative assessment

Laboratory assessment of candidates for renal transplantation includes the measurement of indicators of general operative health (for example, electrolytes, acid-base status, clotting profile, full blood cell count, and cross-matching). In addition, full human leukocyte antigen (HLA) tissue typing is performed, along with a full screen for infectious diseases, particularly cytomegalovirus (CMV), hepatitis, herpes, and human immunodeficiency virus (HIV) status.

Postoperative assessment

Careful monitoring of plasma creatinine and urine output is required during the initial postoperative phase of 1 to 2 weeks to monitor graft function.[13] Most grafts produce measurable amounts of urine within a matter of hours, and this occurrence is a clear sign of a functioning graft. A small proportion of transplant patients, however, experience primary nonfunction. In this subgroup, continuing dialytic support is necessary. In some patients the condition resolves without treatment, but in others a percutaneous renal biopsy may be necessary to establish whether the graft is still viable and which form of therapy should be initiated.

In otherwise uncomplicated cases the serum creatinine concentration falls rapidly in the postoperative period (Figure 34-6), and subsequent changes in the rate of fall of creatinine are monitored to detect early episodes of acute rejection. However, creatinine is a relatively insensitive measure of changes in function, and a range of alternative markers have been evaluated, including BMG, neopterin, serum amyloid A (SAA), and CRP, alone or in combination; however, all transplant patients suffer from the common difficulty that both infection and rejection cause significant elevation. The ultimate arbiter of rejection versus infection is the renal biopsy, from which the decision regarding whether to modify immunosuppressive therapy is taken.

Immunosuppression

Cyclosporin A is used widely as an immunosuppressant to prevent rejection of renal transplants (see Chapter 31).

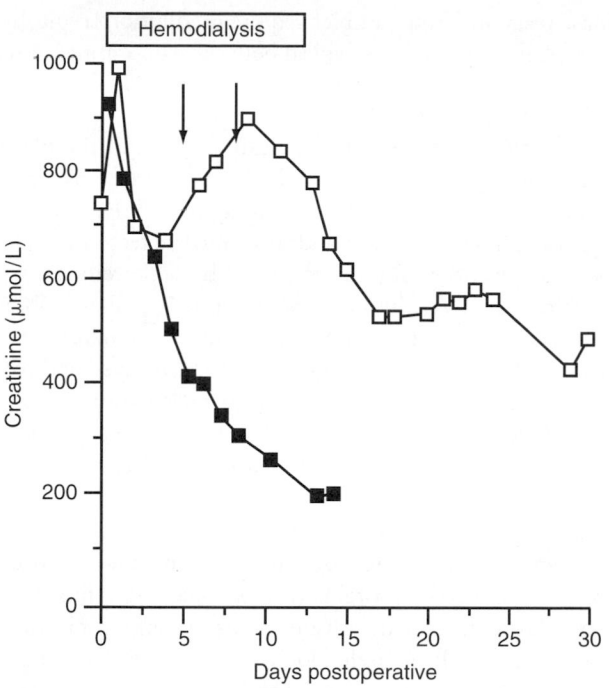

Figure 34-6   Posttransplantation biochemical profile, illustrating the course of a patient who experienced an early rejection episode (confirmed by biopsy, ↓) and requiring initial hemodialysis support *(open squares)* and the typical profile of an uncomplicated transplant recipient *(solid squares).*

Typically, it is used in combination with corticosteroids and azathioprine. Different regimens of dosage are used around the world. Because the main side effect of cyclosporin is nephrotoxicity, careful monitoring is essential to maintain sufficient immunosuppressive effect without significant nephrotoxicity (see Chapter 31). Both rejection/infection and nephrotoxicity cause a significant alteration in renal function, and this alteration has led the research activities designed to discover new, less nephrotoxic immunosuppressive agents. During acute graft rejection, additional immunosuppressive therapies are used, including intravenous corticosteroids, antilymphocyte globulin (ALG), and monoclonal antibodies, such as OKT3.

Later monitoring phases of a successfully transplanted graft require assessment of graft function (plasma creatinine), signs of nephrotoxicity, reactivation of viral infections (particularly CMV), reemergence of the primary renal disease, and monitoring for malignancy, particularly skin tumors and lymphomas.

New and less nephrotoxic immunosuppressive agents are being sought continually. Among the most hopeful recent candidates are tacrolimus (FK506), rapamycin, and mycophenolate mofetil. Even with these pharmacological advances, renal transplantation is limited currently by the availability of donor organs. This limitation has led recently to the consideration of xenotransplantation, an investigational therapeutic approach that uses cells, tissues, and organs of animal origin (xenografts).

■ ASSESSMENT OF KIDNEY FUNCTION

The composition of blood and urine reflects not only functional disorders of the nephron but also various systemic disorders. Practical evaluation of kidney status in individuals with renal disease includes examination of (1) circulating levels of nonprotein nitrogenous compounds, (2) nephron functions of glomerular filtration, (3) the secretory capacity for particular endogenous and exogenous compounds, and (4) the kidneys' reabsorptive capacity for water and electrolytes as manifested by their urine-concentrating ability. In addition, the nonprotein nitrogenous metabolites are measured in blood and urine and the results used to assess kidney function (see Chapter 22).

Glomerular Filtration Rate

The GFR is the rate in milliliters per minute that substances are cleared from the circulation through the kidneys' glomeruli. It is a measure of the number of functioning nephrons. A number of methods are used to measure the GFR (Table 34-15). Most involve the kidneys' ability to clear either an exogenous or endogenous marker (Table 34-16).

The **renal clearance** of a substance is defined as the volume of plasma from which the substance is completely cleared by the kidneys per unit time. The clearance of a substance S is given by the following equation:

$$C_S = \frac{(U_S \times V)}{P_S}$$

where

C_S = Clearance in units of milliliters of plasma cleared of a substance per minute

U_S = Urinary concentration of the substance

V = Volumetric flow rate of urine in milliliters per minute

P_S = Plasma concentration of the substance

In practice, all clearance estimates usually are adjusted to a standard body surface area (BSA) of 1.73 m^2.

Clinical measurement of glomerular filtration rate

Measurement of clearance requires an accurate measurement of the plasma and urine concentrations of the marker used plus a reliable urine collection. A molecule has to meet certain essential criteria to be considered a suitable marker of glomerular filtration. For example, it should be (1) freely filterable at the glomerular barrier, (2) not reabsorbed by the tubules, (3) not secreted by the tubules, and (4) present at a

TABLE 34-15 Methods Used to Assess Glomerular Filtration Rate

Exogenous Substances

RENAL CLEARANCE
- Bolus injection
  — Measure arteriovenous differences by direct cannulation of the renal artery and vein (for example, inulin, ^{51}Cr-EDTA, iohexol).
  — Choose a molecule that is cleared only by renal filtration and not via the GI tract or any other route, and measure the plasma disappearance curve.
- Constant infusion
  — After administration of a priming bolus injection, administer a constant intravenous infusion to maintain a steady-state concentration. Collect a blood sample and accurately timed urine samples during the constant infusion period (for example, inulin, ^{51}Cr-EDTA, iohexol).
- Plasma clearance
  — Bolus injection: Measure the plasma disappearance curve of a substance that is cleared predominantly by renal filtration (for example, inulin, ^{51}Cr-EDTA, iohexol).

Endogenous Substances
- Measure the plasma concentration of a substance that has a constant production rate and is cleared only by renal filtration; at the same time, collect an accurately timed urine sample. Calculate the clearance of substance x according to the following formula:

$$C_x = \frac{U_x V}{P_x}$$

- Measure the plasma concentration of a substance that meets the following requirements:
  — Is filtered freely at the glomerulus
  — Is neither secreted nor reabsorbed intact by renal tubules
  — Has a stable production rate
  — Has a clearance from the systemic circulation that depends only on glomerular filtration

^{51}Cr-EDTA, ^{51}Chromium-ethylenediaminetetraacetic acid.

stable plasma concentration. Both exogenous and endogenous markers are used to measure GFR (see Table 34-16).

Exogenous markers

Several compounds are used as exogenous markers to measure GFR (see Table 34-16). Inulin, considered the "gold standard," and iohexol are two examples.

Inulin clearance. Early methods used to measure inulin were based on the hydrolysis of inulin with concentrated sulfuric acid and condensation with anthrone to produce a green product measurable at 620 nm. More recent methods use the enzyme inulinase (EC 3.2.17), which converts inulin to fructose; the fructose then is determined with the aid of sorbitol dehydrogenase (EC 1.1.1.14). The amount of inulin present is determined from the reduction of nicotinamide-adenine dinucleotide (NADH) measured as a decrease in absorbance at 340 nm. The method is calibrated with either inulin or fructose; endogenous fructose in each sample is measured by incubation with an inactivated inu-

linase reagent. Urine samples require predilution (typically 1 in 40) before analysis. A typical between-run imprecision of less than $\pm2\%$ for plasma and less than $\pm4\%$ for urine is obtainable with an automated assay.

Iohexol clearance. The iohexol content of the plasma and urine samples collected is measured by high-performance liquid chromatography (HPLC) with reversed-phase separation and ultraviolet detection.[5] Before measurement, the samples first must be deproteinized with perchloric acid. Analytical imprecision is less than $\pm3\%$ intraassay and $\pm5\%$ interassay. The nonisotopic nature of iohexol enables the analysis of samples to be delayed and common reference centers to be used for multinational studies. A stable molecule such as iohexol also can enable quality assessment schemes to be developed for GFR analysis.

Endogenous markers

Examples of endogenous markers include creatinine, urea, and low-MW proteins (for example, cystatin C). Endogenous molecules are advantageous in that no injection is required and only a single blood sample is needed. The use of creatinine and urea as markers for the measurement of GFR is described in Chapter 22.

A number of proteins with MWs of less than 30 kD also are used to measure GFR. These include BMG, retinol-binding protein (RBP), α_1-microglobulin (A1M), and cystatin C. These proteins are filtered at the glomerulus, then reabsorbed in the proximal tubule or excreted into the urine; thus they are eliminated entirely from the circulation. However, apart from cystatin C, all the other proteins have been shown to have serum concentrations influenced by nonrenal factors, such as inflammation (BMG) and liver disease (RBP, A1M). The relationship among the circulating concentrations of these proteins shows the same curvilinear form as serum creatinine; however, recently several groups have demonstrated that cystatin C measurement may offer a more sensitive and specific monitoring of changes in GFR than serum creatinine.[6,14]

Cystatin C is a low-MW protein (13,000 D) with a physiological role of a cysteine protease inhibitor. With regard to renal function, its most important attributes are its small size and high pI of 9.2, which enable it to be filtered more freely than the aforementioned proteins. Cystatin C is measured by immunoassay; the most practical approach is to use a latex particle-enhanced turbidimetric or nephelometric immunoassay. Intraassay precision of less than $\pm3\%$ is obtainable at the upper limit of the reference interval (~1.00 mg/L), with less than $\pm4\%$ for the between-day value.[14]

Reference intervals

Clinically, kidney size and GFR are roughly proportional to body weight. As discussed previously, a measured GFR often is normalized to a standardized BSA of 1.73 m^2, which enables comparison of GFRs among individuals. Reference

TABLE 34-16	Markers of Glomerular Filtration Rate	
Marker	Advantages	Disadvantages
Exogenous		
Inulin (sinsitrin)	Gold standard	Time consumption
		Poor specificity of analysis
		Extrarenal clearance = 0.83 mL/min/10 kg
^{51}Cr-EDTA	Isotopic (simple measurement)	Time consumption
		Extrarenal clearance = 0.79 mL/min/10 kg
		^{51}Cr less readily available than ^{99m}Technetium (Tc)
^{131}I-iodoacetate	Isotopic	More time required
^{131}I-hippuran	Isotopic	30% protein binding
^{99m}Tc-DTPA	Isotopic	More time required
		Protein binding
Iohexol	Nonisotopic	Extrarenal clearance = 0.87 mL/min/10 kg
Endogenous		
Creatinine	Inexpensive	Poor sensitivity and specificity
Urea	Inexpensive	Poor sensitivity and specificity
β_2-Microglobulin	Not secreted/reabsorbed	Nonrenal influences on production rate
Retinol-binding protein (RBP)	Not secreted/reabsorbed	Nonrenal influences on production rate
		Filtration less free than β_2-microglobulin
α_1-Microglobulin	Not secreted/reabsorbed	Nonrenal influences on production rate
		Filtration less free than RBP
Cystatin C	Not secreted/reabsorbed	Immunoassay required
	Constitutively expressed	
	More sensitive and specific than creatinine	

^{51}Cr-EDTA, ^{51}Chromium-ethylenediaminetetraacetic acid; ^{99m}Tc-DTPA, ^{99m}technicium-diethylenetriaminepentaacetic acid.

values for the different techniques are similar and demonstrate a decline with increasing age (Table 34-17). However, demonstration of an influence of sex on GFR has proved difficult.

Measurement of Renal Blood and Plasma Flow

Renal blood flow and renal plasma flow (RPF) are measured by use of (1) dye- and gas-dilution methods with renal artery and vein catheterization, (2) electromagnetic flow meters on the renal artery, (3) the uptake of radioactive microspheres, or (4) the renal excretion rates of substances undergoing both glomerular filtration and tubular secretion. For example, by use of a marker such as p-aminohippurate (PAH), RPF is determined experimentally with the following equation:

$$RPF = \frac{U_S \times V_S}{A_S}$$

where U_S is the urinary concentration of the marker, and V_S and A_S are its venous and arterial concentrations, respectively.

The test is performed in a similar manner to a plasma clearance/GFR measurement, with a bolus injection and blood samples collected at 10- to 15-minute intervals over 1 to 2 hours. PAH is monitored by isotopic monitoring, HPLC, or the reaction, with a chromogenic aldehyde dimethylaminocinnamaldehyde.

In practice, PAH is the reference substance of choice for measurement of RPF. However, because plasma and urine assays for PAH often are not practical for use in routine clinical laboratories, plasma creatinine or creatinine clearance also is used for clinical assessment of RPF. As discussed in Chapter 22, plasma and urine creatinine values are measured easily and conveniently by either manual or automated methods.

The reference interval for effective RPF is 328 to 980 and 284 to 898 mL/minute/1.73 m^2 for men and women, respectively. A diurnal variation is thought to exist, analogous to that of GFR, and exercise and emotional stress decrease renal flow. Flow levels in infants are approximately 30% below those of adults. In adults, little change occurs with age until about 50 to 60 years, after which a gradual decline of about 70 mL/minute per decade is apparent.

Assessment of Glomerular Permeability

Glomerular integrity is assessed by measurement of the concentration of urine protein (either total and/or individual proteins) that is retained predominantly by the healthy glomerulus. For example, with one such technique the relative clearance of proteins of different molecular masses is measured to assess the degree of deterioration of the glomerular membrane. The determination of total and individual urinary proteins is covered in more detail in Chapter 19.

TABLE 34-17   Glomerular Filtration Rate Reference Values

Marker	Age (y)	GFR*(mean (range)mL/min/1.73 m²)
Inulin (constant infusion)	20 to 29	
	20	118 (90 to 146)
	25	115 (88 to 142)
	30 to 39	
	30	112 (86 to 138)
	35	109 (84 to 134)
	40 to 49	
	40	106 (82 to 130)
	45	104 (80 to 128)
	50 to 59	
	50	101 (78 to 124)
	55	99 (75 to 123)
	60	96 (73 to 119)
⁵¹Cr-EDTA (single injection)	20 to 63	103 ± 15
	20 to 63	112 ± 13
Iohexol (single injection)	20 to 50	100 (78 to 122)
	51 to 65	83 (58 to 108)
	66 to 80	72 (52 to 92)
Iohexol (constant infusion) triplicate determinations	19 to 30	116 ± 10
	19 to 30	117 ± 9
	19 to 30	110 ± 12
Inulin (single injection)	27 ± 6	104 ± 14
	27 ± 3	102 ± 20
	26 ± 8	95 ± 12
Inulin (constant infusion)	30 ± 5	100 ± 19
	26 ± 8	88 ± 12

⁵¹Cr-EDTA, ⁵¹Chromium-ethylenediaminetetraacebic acid.
*All values have been rounded to the nearest whole number.

Measurement of total urinary proteins

Sample collection

The appropriate urine sample to use for the investigation of protein excretion still is being debated. For example, a 24-hour sample, an overnight sample, a first-morning void, a second morning void, or just a random sample all have been recommended. In the case of the last three types of collection, the protein-to-creatinine ratio is used to correct for dilution effects, or the protein-to-osmolality ratio also has been used. In general the reference point is the accurately timed 24-hour specimen, but for most practical purposes the random albumin-to-creatinine ratio is an excellent screening test because the variability in protein excretion within an individual is high (50% to 100%).[19]

Methods

Numerous methods are used to measure protein in urine (see Chapter 19), including (1) the biuret method, (2) turbidimetry after mixture with trichloroacetic or sulfosalicylic assay, (3) turbidimetry with benzethonium chloride, (4) dye binding with Coomassie Brilliant Blue (CBB), and (5) dye binding with pyrogallol red molybdate. Many laboratories find the biuret methods too time consuming for routine use and prefer turbidimetric and dye-binding methods. Of the dye-binding methods, pyrogallol red, Ponceau S, and CBB are the most popular. The turbidimetric and dye-binding methods have nonlinear calibration curves and unequal sensitivities for individual proteins. Most such methods underestimate low-MW proteins in individuals with tubular proteinuria and immunoglobulin light chains in those with overload proteinuria. The reactivity of chemical methods to some of the globulins is enhanced by the inclusion of sodium dodecyl sulfate (SDS) in the reagent. The analytical range of the turbidimetric assays also has been a problem because high protein concentrations give lower signals. This problem is negated by monitoring of the early period of the turbidity formation.

Reference intervals

Normal urinary total protein excretion is less than 150 mg per 24 hours. The proteins excreted are predominantly albumin (50% to 60%) and some smaller proteins, together with proteins secreted by the tubules, of which Tamm-Horsfall protein is the major component. **Tamm-Horsfall protein** is a mucoprotein produced by the ascending limb of the loop of Henle. It is a normal constituent of urine and is the major protein constituent of urinary casts.

Measurement of specific urinary proteins

Bence-Jones protein

The presence of immunoglobulin light chains **(Bence-Jones protein)** in the urine is an important indication of the presence of myeloma and may occur in the absence of a paraprotein band in the serum. Although a variety of tests for Bence-Jones protein are available (see Chapter 19), electrophoresis is the most reliable test if the sample is concentrated and the test supplemented by immunofixation typing. Immunoturbidimetric and immunonephelometric methods also are available. However, the more sensitive tests can detect low levels of protein associated with benign proliferation of B cells.

Urinary myoglobin in crush injury

Muscle damage often causes a significant increase in plasma myoglobin, which, with a MW of approximately 14,000 D, is filtered freely at the glomerulus. As a heme-containing protein, myoglobin is toxic to the renal tubules and causes acute tubular necrosis with ARF. Urinary myoglobin is measured by immunochemical means, although preconcentration of urine often is necessary.

Lysozyme

Lysozyme is an enzyme that occurs in neutrophilic granulocytes, monocytes, and macrophages, as well as several organs of the body, including the spleen, kidney, and gastrointestinal tract. It is filtered freely by the kidney and absorbed by the proximal tubules.[10] Thus increases in the level of lysozyme in urine are seen in conditions associated with tubular damage and are associated particularly with increased endogenous synthesis (for example, monocytic leukemia and inflammatory bowel disease).

The urinary levels of lysozyme are measured by several methods, including catalytic activity and immunoassay. The reference interval for the excretion of lysozyme in healthy adults is 1.3 to 3.6 mg/day.

N-acetylglucosaminidase

N-acetylglucosaminidase (NAG) is an enzyme derived from the kidney and found in the urine of healthy individuals. Isoforms of this enzyme have been observed in individuals with different renal diseases. However, although it is a sensitive marker of renal damage, NAG has not been shown to provide any unique benefit over urine protein assays, such as albumin and A1M.

Although many enzymes are unstable or inhibited by other urine constituents, NAG is stable in urine. A number of photometric and fluorometric methods are used to measure NAG in urine.[15]

Markers of basement membrane damage

Several new markers now are available to monitor the breakdown of the glomerular basement membrane, including collagen breakdown products, laminin, and antiglomerular basement membrane antibodies. All markers are measured by immunological techniques.

Tubular proteinuria

The functional integrity of the renal tubule is assessed through the investigation of tubular proteinuria by the measurement of one of the low-MW proteins (see Chapter 19).

A suggested strategy for the assessment of glomerular proteinuria is provided in Table 34-18. For the identification of tubular damage, urinary RBP is probably more sensitive than A1M, but because of its lower concentration, it is more difficult to measure. Laboratory methods to measure both albumin and A1M are available now that facilitate screening and monitoring of both glomerular and tubular proteinuria. Panels of protein measurements, including albumin, A1M, immunoglobulin G (IgG), and α_2-macroglobulin, have been used in the differential diagnosis of prerenal and postrenal disease. This general strategy has been extended with the inclusion of dipstick tests for hematuria, leukocyturia, and proteinuria in the development of an expert system to achieve a concordance of 98% with clinical diagnosis.[8]

Assessment of Renal Concentrating Ability

The capacity of the kidneys to conserve water is assessed by demonstration that the solute concentration of the urine approaches the maximal range achievable in a healthy individual. The osmolality and specific gravity are used to assess this function.

TABLE 34-18   Protocol for Urinary Protein Measurement

1. Test random urine samples for protein with a Dipstix or Multistix. These show many false positive results but very few false negatives.
2. If a result is positive (trace or above), repeat on two further occasions over a period of 1 to 2 weeks.
3. If two or three tests are positive (trace or above), send a random sample for laboratory analysis of albumin and creatinine.
4. If two samples give albumin/creatinine ratios between 2 and 30 mg/mmol, send a plain 24-hour sample for determination of the albumin excretion rate.
5. In the absence of a systemic disease, such as diabetes or hypertension, a borderline elevation in albumin excretion (2 to 30 mg/mmol), without hematuria or a rise in serum creatinine, a serious primary renal pathology is unlikely.
6. If the urinary albumin/creatinine ratio is greater than 30 mg/mmol, refer the patient to a renal specialist.
7. In a diabetic patient, if the albumin/creatinine ratio is greater than 5 mg/mmol, detailed assessment of blood pressure, macrovascular risk factors, and optic fundi should be performed, with referral for specialist diabetic opinion if concern remains about the appropriate way to proceed.

Osmolality

Measurements of the osmotic concentration of urine are considered more valid than specific gravity measurements in the assessment of the concentrating ability of the kidneys because regulation of water excretion is determined in part by the osmolality of the fluid compartments of the body. Consequently, measurement of the urine osmolality, especially as part of a concentration test, is preferred. (Measurement of osmolality is described in more detail in Chapter 25.)

The urine osmolality of normal individuals varies widely, depending on the state of hydration. After excessive intake of fluids, for example, the osmotic concentration may fall as low as 50 mOsm/kg, whereas in individuals with severely restricted fluid intake, concentrations of up to 1200 mOsm/kg have been observed. In individuals on average fluid intakes, values of 300 to 900 mOsm/kg are found most frequently.

If a random urine specimen of an individual has an osmolality of 600 mOsm/kg water or higher (or >850 mOsm/kg water after 12 hours of fluid restriction), renal concentrating ability is assumed to be normal. The usual test used to assess renal concentrating ability of the kidneys entails withholding of fluids overnight, obtaining of the first voided specimen in the morning, and measurement of osmolality. Maximal urine concentration requires fluid deprivation for 36 to 48 hours; however, after fluid deprivation of 18 hours or more, urine osmolality that exceeds 850 mOsm/kg is considered to reflect a normal renal concentrating mechanism.

In individuals with either hypothalamic or pituitary disorders causing complete ADH deficiency or those who lack the normal renal response to ADH (nephrogenic diabetes insipidus), urine osmolality rarely exceeds 300 mOsm/kg.

Specific gravity

The simple specific gravity test measures the density of urine relative to the density of water, and in most circumstances, density bears a constant relationship to osmolality. However, in some conditions (for example, after intravenous administration of iodine-containing radiopaque compounds for radiological studies) a difference exists between osmolality and specific gravity. Glucose and protein also may contribute substantial increments to the density of urine, and semiquantitative determination of these substances is necessary for valid interpretation or correction of urine specific gravity measurements. Diabetic individuals with uncontrolled hyperglycemia and glucosuria may have high urine specific gravity even when the normal renal concentrating function is impaired seriously. A dipstick test used to determine specific gravity is described in a later section of this chapter.

Assessment for Renal Tubular Acidosis

Fractional bicarbonate excretion and ammonium chloride loading are tests used to assess for RTA.

Fractional bicarbonate excretion

The fractional bicarbonate excretion test may be helpful in the assessment of a patient with proximal RTA.[7] Plasma and urine samples are collected, and creatinine and bicarbonate are measured in each. The fractional excretion of bicarbonate then is calculated from the ratio of urine and plasma creatinine, expressed as a percentage. In individuals with proximal RTA the excretion is more than 10% to 15%, whereas in most cases of distal RTA the excretion is less than 10%.

Ammonium chloride loading test

The ammonium chloride loading test is used in the diagnosis of distal RTA; it is not necessary if the pH of the urine collected after an overnight fast is below 5.5. The patient is given a load of ammonium chloride (100 mg/kg of body weight), and the urine pH is measured in samples collected hourly for up to 8 hours. In normal subjects the urine pH falls below 5.5 in at least one sample; in an individual with RTA this decrease does not occur, and the urinary pH is unlikely to fall below 6.5. Ammonium chloride should not be given to patients with liver disease; in this situation, calcium chloride may be administered as an alternative.

Urinalysis

Examination of the urine is often the first step in the assessment of a patient suspected of having or confirmed to have a deterioration in renal function. The appearance (color and

odor) of urine itself is helpful, a darkening from the normal pale straw color indicating a more concentrated urine or the presence of another pigment. Hemoglobin and myoglobin in urine produce a pink-red-brown coloration, depending on the concentration. Turbidity in a fresh sample may indicate infection but also may be due to fat particles in an individual with nephrotic syndrome. Foaming of a urine when shaken suggests proteinuria.

The specific gravity provides an indication of the concentration of a urine. The measurement of urine pH is helpful in individuals with RTA and in stone formers.

Because proteinuria is one of the most common findings in individuals with renal disease, urine often is screened by use of simple, qualitative or semiquantitative dipstick tests.

The presence of leukocyte esterase is indicative of the production of urine containing white blood cells (WBCs; pyuria). The detection of nitrite is indicative of the presence of bacteria that degrade nitrate excreted in the urine. The combination of the two tests is valuable in individuals with urinary tract infections. The absence of both constituents is a valuable test used to rule out urinary tract infection, thereby reducing the number of samples sent to the laboratory for further tests. The nitrite test may be less helpful in young children, in whom the urine remains in the bladder for less time, which limits the time for nitrite production.

The presence of free hemoglobin or RBCs in the urine indicates the presence of renal or bladder disease. Hematuria is present in individuals with a range of renal diseases, including glomerular nephritis, polycystic disease, sickle cell disease, vasculitis, and a range of infections. A spectrum of urological diseases also may produce hematuria, including bladder, prostate, and pelvic/ureteric malignancy; renal stones; trauma; bladder damage; and ureteric stricture. To measure urinary analytes, urine often is evaluated chemically with the help of dipstick tests or examined under a microscope.

Dipstick testing

In the dipstick type of qualitative or semiquantitative testing, strips ("sticks") of cellulose or pads of cellulose on strips of plastic are coated or impregnated with reagents for the analyte in question. The strip is "dipped" into a test solution, such as urine. A color change occurs, which then is compared to a color chart for the test in question. A dipstick may contain reagents for just one test per stick or reagents for multiple tests on a single stick. With this type of test the different methods detect substances such as glucose, ketones, bilirubin diglucuronide, and urobilinogen that overflow into the urine. These dipstick tests also detect changes in constituents that are linked more directly to alterations brought about by some pathological process affecting the kidney or urinary tract.[12]

Urine samples for dipstick testing should be collected in sterile containers and dipstick testing performed on the fresh urine. Dipstick tests are available for a variety of analytes, including total protein, hemoglobin, glucose, nitrite, leukocytes, specific gravity, and pH. The method principles and comments on the performance of these tests are discussed in more detail in an expanded version of this chapter.[15]

Microscopic examination of urine

Microscopical examination of the sediment obtained from the centrifugation of a fresh urine sample shows the presence of a few cells (erythrocytes, leukocytes, and cells derived from the kidney and urinary tract), casts (composed predominantly of Tamm-Horsfall protein), and possibly fat or pigmented particles. An increase in RBCs or casts implies hematuria possibly due to glomerular disease; WBCs or casts imply the presence of white cells in the tubules. Inflammation of the upper urinary tract may result in polymorphonuclear leukocytes and various types of casts, whereas in lower urinary tract, inflammation of the casts is not present. In individuals with acute glomerulonephritis, hematuria may lead to coloration of the urine and the presence of large numbers of RBCs and WBCs; as the duration of the disease increases, the amount of sediment diminishes.

Renal Stone Analysis

Investigation of the individual with renal stones or suspected of being a stone former involves analysis of the urine and stone, if one can be obtained. The major types of stone found in the West include calcium oxalate, with or without phosphate (frequency 67%); magnesium ammonium phosphate and calcium phosphate, also known as *triple phosphate* (12%); calcium phosphate (8%); urate (8%); cystine (1% to 2%); and complex mixtures of the previous types (2% to 3%).

Both qualitative and quantitative analysis of the chemical constituents of kidney stones are used to establish the etiology and plan rational therapy. Analysis is not necessary for every urinary calculus, especially when other laboratory and clinical findings are diagnostic. In some patients, however, two or more possible causes exist, and analysis of the calculus may help distinguish among different diagnoses. For example, individuals with hypercalciuria and calcium oxalate stones may develop renal infections with deposition of magnesium ammonium phosphate on the calcium oxalate stones, forming "mixed stones." Chemical analysis of these stones is necessary to confirm this sequence of events.

Specialized physical techniques, such as infrared spectroscopy and x-ray diffraction, gradually are replacing less specific qualitative chemical methods for stone analysis.

References

1. Beetham R, Cattell WR: Proteinuria: pathophysiology, significance and recommendations in clinical practice. Ann Clin Biochem 1993; 30:425-434.

2. Bennett PH, Haffner S, Kasiske BL et al: Screening and management of microalbuminuria in patients with diabetes mellitus: recommendations to the scientific advisory board of the National Kidney Foundation from an Ad Hoc Committee of the Council on Diabetes Mellitus of the National Kidney Foundation. Am J Kidney Dis 1995; 25:107-112.

3. de Broe ME, D'Haese PC, Nuyts GD et al: Occupational renal disease. Curr Opin Nephrol Hyperten 1996; 5:114-121.

4. Freedman BI, Iskander SS, Appel RG: The link between hypertension and nephrosclerosis. Am J Kidney Dis 1995; 25:207-221.

5. Gaspari F, Perico N, Ruggenenti P et al: Plasma clearance of nonradioactive iohexol as a measure of glomerular filtration rate. J Am Soc Nephrol 1995; 6:257-263.

6. Grubb A: Diagnostic value of analysis of cystatin C and protein HC in biological fluids. Clin Nephrol 1992; 38(Suppl 1):S20-S27.

7. Humes HD: Acute renal failure: prevailing challenges and prospects for the future. Kidney Int 1995; 48(Suppl 50):S26-S32.

8. Ivandic M, Hofmann W, Guder WG: Development and evaluation of a urine protein expert system. Clin Chem 1996; 42:1214-1222.

9. Jaeger P: Genetic versus environmental factors in renal stone disease. Curr Opin Nephrol Hyperten 1996; 5:342-346.

10. Jung K, Mattenheimer H, Burchardt U (eds): Urinary Enzymes in Clinical and Experimental Medicine, p 9, Berlin, Springer-Verlag, 1992.

11. Molecular cell biology and physiology of solute transport. Curr Opin Nephrol Hyperten 1996; 5:B153-B166.

12. Murakami M: Screening for proteinuria and hematuria in school children: methods and results. Acta Paediatr Jpn 1990; 32:682-689.

13. Nankivell BJ, Allen RDM, O'Connell PJ et al: Renal dysfunction in acute rejection. Transplantation 1995; 60:28-36.

14. Newman DJ, Thakkar H, Edwards RG et al: Serum cystatin C measured by automated immunoassay: a more sensitive marker of changes in GFR than serum creatinine. Kidney Int 1995; 47:312-318.

15. Newman DJ, Price CP: Renal function and nitrogen metabolites. In Burtis CA, Ashwood ER (eds): Tietz Textbook of Clinical Chemistry, 3rd edition, pp 1204-1270, Philadelphia, WB Saunders, 1999.

16. Nyengaard J, Bendsten T: Glomerular number and size in relation to age, kidney weight, and body surface in normal men. Anat Rec 1992; 232:194-200.

17. Raij L, Bayki C: Glomerular actions of nitric oxide. Kidney Int 1995; 48:20-32.

18. Remuzzi G, Ruggenenti P, Benigni A: Understanding the nature of renal disease progression. Kidney Int 1997; 51:2-15.

19. Ricos C, Jimenez CV, Hernandez A et al: Biological variation in urine samples used for analyte measurements. Clin Chem 1994; 40:472-477.

20. Sands JM, Kokko JP: Current concepts of the countercurrent multiplication system. Kidney Int 1996; 57(Suppl): S93-S99.

Additional Reading

Brenner BM: Brenner's and Rector's The Kidney, 6th edition, Philadelphia, WB Saunders, 1999.

Davison AM, Cameron JS, Grunfeld J (eds): Oxford Textbook of Clinical Nephrology, 2nd edition, Oxford, Oxford University Press, 1997.

Lote CJ: Principles of Renal Physiology, 4th edition, London, Chapman & Hall, 2000.

Schrier RW, Gottschalk CW: Diseases of the Kidney, 6th edition, New York, Little, Brown, 1996.

Seldin DW: The Kidney: Physiology and Pathophysiology, 3rd edition, Philadelphia, Lippincott Raven, 1999.

CHAPTER 35

Physiology and Disorders of Water, Electrolyte, and Acid-Base Metabolism

JONATHAN W. HEUSEL, MD, PhD, OLE SIGGAARD-ANDERSEN, MD, PhD, and MITCHELL G. SCOTT, PhD

Objectives

1. Discuss total body water and electrolyte distributions.
2. Discuss the maintenance of homeostasis with regard to electrolyte concentrations.
3. State the Henderson-Hasselbalch equation.
4. List the physiological buffer systems and their role in the regulation of blood pH.
5. Describe the contribution of respiration to acid-base status.
6. List the conditions associated with abnormal acid-base status and abnormal anion-cation composition of blood; state the primary deficit, compensatory mechanism, laboratory values obtained for each.

Key Words

Acid-Base Balance   The homeostatic maintenance of acids and bases within the body to achieve a physiological pH (approximately 7.40)

Acidemia   An arterial blood pH less than 7.35

Alkalemia   An arterial blood pH greater than 7.45.

Anion Gap   The difference between the serum sodium concentration and the sum of the serum chloride and bicarbonate concentrations; high in some forms of metabolic acidosis

Compensation   The body's physiological response to an acid-base disorder (for example, hyperventilation compensation for metabolic acidosis)

Extracellular Fluid (ECF)   A general term for all the body fluids outside the cells, including the interstitial fluid and plasma, lymph, and cerebrospinal fluids; provides a constant external environment for the cells

Henderson-Hasselbalch Equation   An equation that defines the relationship between pH, bicarbonate, and the partial pressure of dissolved carbon dioxide gas

Hyperkalemia   A concentration of serum potassium above the reference limit of 5.0 mmol/L

Hypernatremia   A concentration of serum sodium above the reference limit of 150 mmol/L

Hypervolemia   An abnormal increase in the volume of circulating fluid (plasma) in the body

Hypokalemia   A concentration of serum potassium below the reference limit of 3.5 mmol/L

Hyponatremia   A concentration of serum sodium below the reference limit of 136 mmol/L

Hypovolemia   An abnormally decreased volume of circulating fluid (plasma) in the body

Intracellular Fluid (ICF)   The portion of the total body water and dissolved solutes that are within the cell membranes

Metabolic Acidosis   A pathological process that leads to the accumulation of acid, which lowers the bicarbonate concentration and decreases the pH or to the direct loss of alkali (primarily bicarbonate); also known as *primary bicarbonate deficit*

Metabolic Alkalosis   A pathological process that leads to the accumulation of base, which raises the bicarbonate concentration and increases the pH; also known as *primary bicarbonate excess*

Mixed Acid-Base Disturbance   The occurrence of more than one acid-base disorder simultaneously, in which the blood pH may be low, high, or within the reference interval

Respiration, Internal   Exchange of CO_2 for O_2 between the body cells and the blood

Respiration, External   Exchange of O_2 for CO_2 in the lungs between alveolar air and blood in the pulmonary capillaries

Respiratory Acidosis   A pathological process that leads to the accumulation of carbon dioxide, which raises the P_{CO_2} and decreases the pH; usually caused by emphysema or hypoventilation

Respiratory Alkalosis   A pathological process that leads to the excessive elimination of carbon dioxide, which lowers the P_{CO_2} and increases the pH; caused by hyperventilation

Total Body Water (TBW)   The amount of water in the body, usually expressed in liters

Mammalian adaptation to terrestrial life has involved the development of complex physiological systems that maintain the composition of their internal milieu. These systems include a variety of chemical buffers, as well as highly specialized mechanisms of the pulmonary and renal organs, that work together to regulate water, electrolytes, and pH. Perturbations in the dynamic equilibria that exist for water, electrolytes, and pH may arise from external (for example, trauma, changes in altitude, ingestion of toxic substances) or internal (for example, normal metabolism and disease states) sources. Correction of theses imbalances by buffers and the pulmonary and renal compensatory mechanisms may not always be adequate. The clinical laboratory can provide valuable diagnostic information for the implementation of appropriate therapy.

TOTAL BODY WATER—VOLUME AND DISTRIBUTION

At birth, approximately 75% of total body mass is water, and from roughly 1 year of age through middle age this value is approximately 60% for the average man (falling to ~50% thereafter; women averaging ~5% lower due to a relatively higher percentage of body fat). Approximately two thirds of

total body water (TBW) is distributed into the **intracellular fluid (ICF)** compartment, and one-third exists in the **extracellular fluid (ECF)** compartment. The ICF and ECF compartments are separated physically by the cellular plasma membrane. The ECF may be subdivided further into the interstitial (~75% of ECF) and intravascular (~25% of ECF) fluid compartments. These compartments are separated by the capillary endothelium. (The larger blood vessels contain additional layers of smooth muscle and connective tissue but constitute a relatively small surface area for exchange, compared with that of the capillary beds.) Within the intravascular (whole blood) compartment, plasma, the acellular (liquid) fraction, represents approximately 60%, or 3.5 L, for the average adult with a hematocrit of approximately 40%.

The minimum daily requirement for water can be estimated from renal (~1200 mL in urine) and "insensible" water losses (~200 mL due to evaporation from the skin and respiratory tract) minus a small amount of water that is produced from endogenous metabolism. Activity, environmental conditions, and disease all have dramatic effects on daily water (and electrolyte) requirements. However, on average, an adult must take in 1.0 to 1.5 L of water daily to maintain fluid balance. Because primary regulatory mechanisms are designed to maintain normal intracellular hydration status,

TABLE 35-1	Causes and Clinical Manifestations of Changes in ECF Volume	
Change	Clinical Manifestations	Causes
ECF loss	Thirst; anorexia; nausea; lightheadedness; orthostatic hypotension; syncope; tachycardia; oliguria; decreased skin turgor and "sunken eyes;" shock; coma; death	Trauma (and other causes of acute blood loss); "third-spacing" of fluid (for example, burns, pancreatitis, peritonitis); vomiting; diarrhea; diuretics; renal or adrenal (that is, sodium wasting) disease
ECF gain	Weight gain; edema; dyspnea (due to pulmonary edema); tachycardia; jugular venous distension; portal hypertension; esophageal varices	Heart failure; hepatic cirrhosis; nephrotic syndrome; iatrogenic treatment (intravenous fluid overload)

ECF, Extracellular fluid.

uncorrected imbalances in TBW are reflected initially in the ECF compartment. Table 35-1 lists common causes and clinical manifestations of expansion and contraction of the ECF compartment.

WATER AND ELECTROLYTES— COMPOSITION OF BODY FLUIDS

The electrolyte concentrations of the body fluid compartments are shown in Table 35-2. Sodium (Na^+), potassium (K^+), chloride (Cl^-), and bicarbonate (HCO_3^-) in the plasma or serum are analyzed commonly together in a metabolic panel because their concentrations provide the most relevant information about osmotic, hydration, and pH status of the body. Although the hydrogen ion (H^+) chemically is a cation, its concentration is approximately 1 million-fold lower in plasma than the major electrolytes in Table 35-2 and thus is negligible in terms of osmotic activity. However, the total number of positive ions (including H^+) *must* equal that of the negative ions to maintain electrical neutrality.

Extracellular Fluid Compartment

The ECF compartment is composed of plasma, interstitial fluid, lymph, and cerebrospinal fluid (CSF). The ECF provides a constant external environment for the cells and represents about 30% of the total body volume.

TABLE 35-2	Electrolyte and Water Composition of Body Fluid Compartments*		
Component	Plasma (L)	Interstitial Fluid (L)	ICF (L)†
Volume, H_2O	3.5L	10.5L	28 L (TBW = 42 L)
Na^+	142	145	12
K^+	4	4	156
Ca^{2+}	6	2 to 3	3
Mg^{2+}	2	1 to 2	26
Trace elements	1		
Total Cations	158.5		
Cl^-	103	114	4
HCO_3^-	27	31	12
Protein$^-$	16	—	55
Organic acids$^-$	5	—	—
HPO_4^{2-}	2		
SO_4^{2-}	1		
Total Anions	154		

ICF, Intracellular fluid; *TBW*, total body water.
*All electrolyte values are expressed in mmol/L of fluid; because the H_2O content of plasma is approximately 90% by volume, the corresponding electrolyte concentrations in plasma water are approximately 10% higher. Note that the molar concentration of divalent ions is one-half the depicted value.
†These values are derived from skeletal muscle.

Plasma

Plasma, which is of main interest in discussions of water and electrolytes, generally has a volume of 1300 to 1800 mL/m² of body surface and constitutes approximately 5% of the body volume (~3.5 L for a 66-kg individuals). Generally, body volume is derived from body mass by use of an estimated body density of 1.0 kg/L. (Because the density of bone is greater than that of tissue, a more accurate value is 1.06 kg/L.) The electrolyte composition of venous plasma is summarized in Table 35-2. The mass concentration of water in normal plasma is about 0.933 kg/L, depending on the protein and lipid content (see discussion on the electrolyte exclusion effect in Chapter 25). Thus a concentration of sodium in the plasma of 140 mmol/L would correspond to a molality of sodium in plasma water of 150 mmol/kg H_2O (that is, 140 mmol/L divided by 0.933 kg/L). The concentration of net protein ions in plasma is approximately 12 mmol/L, with the charge mainly due to albumin because the charge of globulins is negligible.

Interstitial fluid

Interstitial fluid is essentially an ultrafiltrate of blood plasma. When all extracellular spaces except plasma and CSF are included, the volume accounts for about 26% (~17 L) of the total body volume. Plasma is separated from the interstitial fluid by the endothelial lining of the capillaries, which acts as a semipermeable membrane and allows passage of water and diffusible solutes but not of compounds of large molecular mass, such as proteins. However, this "impermeability" is not absolute, as demonstrated by the low concentration of protein in interstitial fluids. In pathological conditions causing "shock," such as bacterial sepsis, the permeability of the vascular endothelium increases dramatically, resulting in leakage of albumin and a reduction in the effective circulating volume. The resulting hypotension may be fatal if not treated properly.

Intracellular Fluid Compartment

The exact composition of ICF is extremely hard to measure because most cells are inaccessible in their physiological milieu. Although erythrocytes are accessible easily, any generalizations based on the composition of these highly specialized cells would be inaccurate. Data on cell composition (see Table 35-2) therefore are considered only approximations. The volume of the ICF constitutes approximately 66% of the total body volume.

Reasons for Composition Differences of Body Fluids

The composition of ICF differs markedly from that of ECF. The separation of these compartments by a cell membrane allows the composition of these fluids to differ. The composition differences are a consequence of the Gibbs-Donnan equilibrium and the active and passive transport of ions.

Gibbs-Donnan equilibrium

Two solutions separated by a semipermeable membrane establish an equilibrium so that all ions are distributed equally in both compartments, provided that the solutes can move freely through the membrane. At the state of equilibrium the total ion concentration and therefore the total concentration of osmotically active particles (osmolals) are equal on both sides of the membrane. If the solution on one side of a membrane contains ions that cannot move freely through the membrane (for example, proteins), distribution of the diffusible ions at the steady state is unequal, but the product of the concentrations of diffusible ions in one compartment is equal to the product of the concentrations of diffusible ions in the other compartment (Gibbs-Donnan law). In addition, electrical neutrality is obeyed for both compartments. An example of the uneven distribution of an ion in two compartments with different protein contents (nondiffusible ions) is the concentration of chloride ions in plasma and CSF. As a result of the increased selectivity of the blood-brain barrier against proteins, Cl^- ions are approximately 15% higher in CSF than in plasma to establish electrical and osmotic equilibrium.

Cells that contain nondiffusible protein anions can withstand only a limited and temporary difference in osmotic pressure across the cell membrane. The osmotic pressure is normally identical inside and outside the cells because the cell membrane can correct concentration differences by excluding some small ions by active transport processes. If these processes cease, the cells gradually swell and eventually burst (osmotic lysis).

Distribution of ions by active and passive transport

Examination of Table 35-2 reveals that the electrolyte compositions of blood plasma and interstitial fluid (both ECFs) are similar, but their compositions differ markedly from that of ICF. The major extracellular ions are Na^+, Cl^-, and HCO_3^-, whereas the main ions in ICF are K^+, Mg^{2+}, organic phosphates, and protein. This unequal distribution of ions is due to an active transport of Na^+ from inside to outside the cell against an electrochemical gradient. This process requires energy supplied by the metabolic processes in the cell (for example, glycolysis). An active sodium pump deriving its energy from adenosine triphosphate (ATP) is present in most cell membranes, frequently coupled with the transport of K^+ in the opposite direction.[12] In addition to this so-called Na^+/K^+-ATPase, a ubiquitous Na^+-H^+ exchanger (often referred to as an *antiporter*) also actively pumps H^+ from the ICF in exchange for Na^+. This exchanger is critical for the maintenance of intracellular pH homeostasis (particularly in muscle cells), volume homeostasis, and cell growth.

■ ELECTROLYTES

Homeostasis and disorders of Na^+, K^+, Cl^-, and HCO_3^- are considered separately.

Sodium

Disorders of Na^+ homeostasis can by caused by excessive loss, gain, or retention of the Na^+ or excessive loss, gain, or retention of H_2O. Separating disorders of Na^+ and H_2O balance is difficult because of their close relationship in the establishment of normal osmolality in all three body water compartments.

As described in detail in Chapter 34, the primary organ used to regulate body water and extracellular Na^+ is the kidney. In the proximal tubules, 80% to 90% of the filtered Na^+ is reabsorbed actively with H_2O and Cl^- then filtered passively by diffusion. In the ascending loop of Henle, Cl^- is reabsorbed actively, with Na^+ then absorbed.

At the level of the distal tubule the first of the two primary Na^+/H_2O regulating processes occurs. Receptors located in the juxtaglomerular cells sense decreased arteriolar pressure or decreased Na^+ and stimulate the production of renin.[13] Renin stimulates the adrenal glands to produce the mineralocorticoid aldosterone (see Chapter 41). This steroid hormone stimulates the distal tubules to reabsorb Na^+ (with water then absorbed passively) and to secrete K^+ (and to a lesser extent, H^+). Thus when plasma Na^+ is low or when the kidneys are hypoperfused (as occurs when blood volume decreases or when a renal artery is obstructed), the distal tubules, under the influence of aldosterone, reclaim Na^+.

Water regulation in the kidney occurs from the distal tubule through the collecting duct, where tubular permeability to H_2O is under the influence of antidiuretic hormone (ADH) (see Chapters 34 and 39). ADH (also called *vasopressin*) is released by the posterior pituitary under the influence of baroreceptors in the aortic arch[13] and hypothalamic chemoreceptors that are responsive to circulating osmolality, the osmolality being primarily a reflection of Na^+ concentration. When blood volume is decreased or when plasma osmolality is increased, (1) ADH is secreted, (2) tubular permeability to H_2O increases, and (3) H_2O is reabsorbed in an attempt to restore blood volume or decrease osmolality. In contrast, when blood volume is increased or osmolality decreased, ADH secretion is inhibited, and more H_2O is excreted in the urine (diuresis).

The body's only other mechanism for restoring Na^+/H_2O homeostasis is ingestion of H_2O. Thirst is stimulated by either decreased blood volume or a hyperosmotic condition. The receptors that influence renal handling of Na^+ and H_2O (as well as the thirst reflex) sense changes only in the blood volume and not the total ECF. The clinician must assess the status of TBW and blood volume before interpreting laboratory values in the diagnosis of water electrolyte disorders. The physical findings and clinical manifestations of these disorders are as important as laboratory values (see Table 35-1).

Hyponatremia

Hyponatremia is defined as a decreased plasma Na^+ concentration (<136 mmol/L). Hyponatremia manifests itself clinically as generalized weakness and mental confusion at values less than 110 to 120 mmol/L and severe mental impairment between 90 and 105 mmol/L.[9] The central nervous system (CNS) symptoms primarily are due to intracellular shifting of H_2O to maintain osmotic balance, resulting in swelling of the CNS cells. The rapidity of the development of hyponatremia influences the levels of Na^+ at which these symptoms develop.

Hyponatremia can occur in the settings of hyperosmotic, isosmotic, and hypo-osmotic plasma; thus the measurement of plasma osmolality can be an important initial step in the assessment of hyponatremia. Of the previously mentioned settings the most common is hypo-osmotic hyponatremia because Na^+ is the primary determinant of plasma osmolality. Figure 35-1 describes an algorithm for laboratory measurements and physical examination findings in the differential diagnosis of a plasma Na^+ level less than 135 mmol/L.

Hyperosmotic hyponatremia

When hyponatremia occurs in the presence of an increased plasma osmolality, an increased amount of other solutes in the ECF results in a shift of extracellular water or

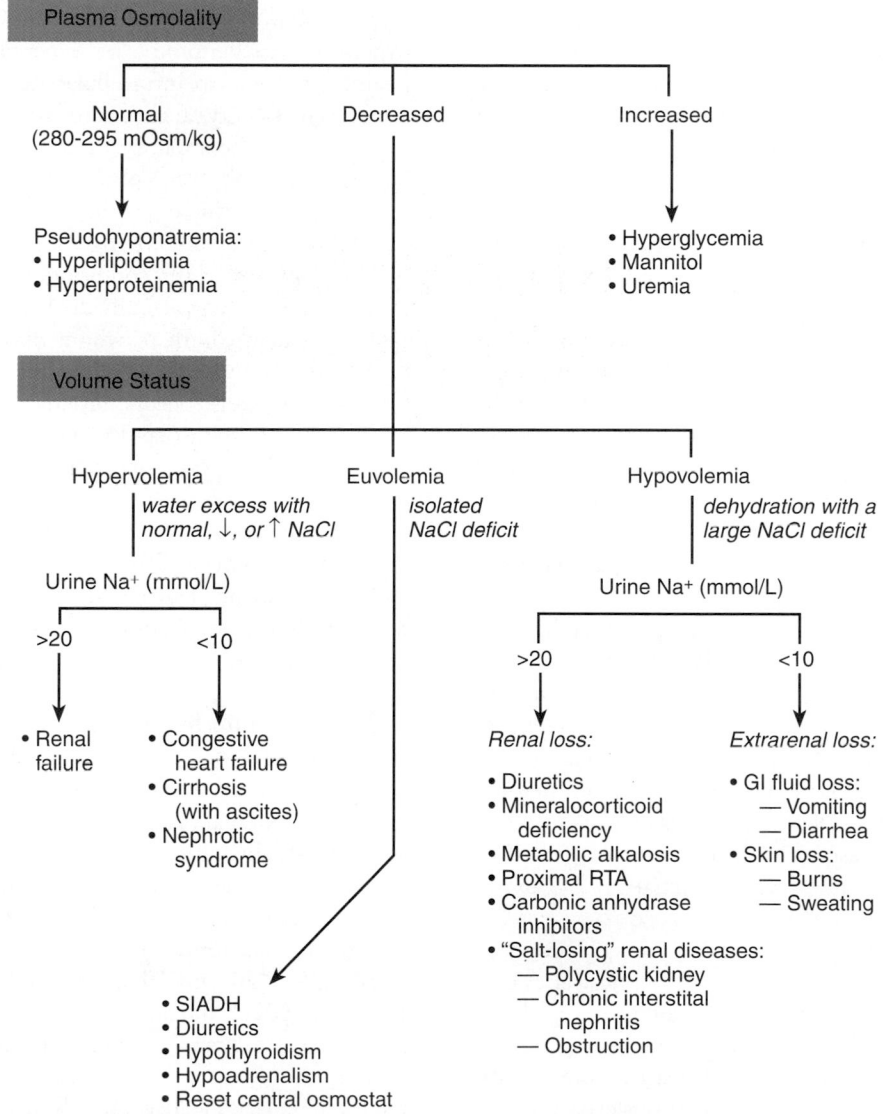

Figure 35-1   Algorithm for the differential diagnosis of hyponatremia. *NaCl*, Sodium chloride; *RTA*, renal tubular acidosis; *GI*, gastrointestinal; *SIADH*, syndrome of inappropriate antidiuretic hormone. (Modified from Kirkpatrick W, Kreisberg R: Acid-base and electrolyte disorders. In Lui P (ed): Blue Book of Diagnostic Tests, pp 239-254, Philadelphia, WB Saunders, 1986.)

intracellular Na^+ to maintain osmotic balance between the ECF and ICF compartments. The most common cause of this type of hyponatremia is severe hyperglycemia. As a general rule the Na^+ can be expected to decrease approximately 1.6 mmol/L for every 100 mg/dL increase of glucose above 100 mg/dL.

Isosmotic hyponatremia

If the measured Na^+ concentration in plasma is decreased but measured plasma osmolality, glucose, and urea are normal, the resultant pseudohyponatremia is caused by the electrolyte exclusion effect (see Chapter 25). This effect can occur in individuals with severe hyperlipidemia or in states of hyperproteinemia (for example, paraproteinemia of multiple myeloma) when Na^+ is measured by either flame emission spectrophotometry or an indirect ion-selective electrode (see Chapters 3 and 6).

Hypo-osmotic hyponatremia

Typically when the plasma Na^+ concentration is low, the calculated or measured osmolality also is low. This type of hyponatremia can be caused by either excess loss of Na^+ (depletional hyponatremia) or increased ECF volume (dilutional hyponatremia). Differentiating the causes of this type of hyponatremia initially requires a clinical assessment of TBW and ECF volume. A history and physical examination are useful in this assessment.

Depletional hyponatremia (excess loss of Na^+) is accompanied almost always by a loss of ECF water, but to a lesser extent than the Na^+ loss. Hypovolemia is apparent in the physical examination (orthostatic hypotension, tachycardia, decreased skin turgor). Loss of isosmotic or hypertonic fluid is the cause of hyponatremia, and this loss can occur through either renal or extrarenal routes. If urine Na^+ is low (generally <10 mmol/L), the loss is extrarenal, from the gastrointestinal tract or skin (see Figure 35-1).

If, alternatively, urine Na^+ is elevated (generally >20 mmol/L), renal loss of Na^+ is likely. Renal loss of Na^+ can occur with osmotic diuresis, thiazide diuretics, adrenal insufficiency (the absence of aldosterone and cortisone preventing reabsorption of Na^+), or "potassium-sparing" diuretics, such as spironolactone, that block aldosterone-mediated reabsorption of Na^+. Renal loss of Na^+ in excess of H_2O also occurs in cases of metabolic alkalosis caused by prolonged vomiting because increased renal HCO_3^- excretion is accompanied by Na^+ ions.

Dilutional hyponatremia is a result of excess H_2O retention and sometimes is detected during the physical examination when the clinician notices weight gain or edema. When ECF is increased but the blood volume is decreased, such as in individuals with congestive heart failure, hepatic cirrhosis, or the nephrotic syndrome, a vicious cycle is established. The decreased blood volume is sensed by peripheral baroreceptors and results in increased aldosterone and ADH, even though ECF volume is excessive. The kidneys properly reabsorb Na^+ and H_2O in response to the increased aldosterone and ADH to restore the blood volume, but this reabsorption simply results in further increases in the ECF and further dilution of Na^+ in the ECF.

In individuals with hypo-osmotic hyponatremia with normal volume status, the most common etiologies are the syndrome of inappropriate ADH (SIADH), primary polydipsia, hypothyroidism, and adrenal insufficiency (see Figure 35-1). SIADH is usually a result of ectopic or otherwise 'inappropriate" ADH production arising from a variety of conditions[7] (see Chapters 34 and 39) and results in excessive H_2O retention. SIADH often is diagnosed by a urine osmolality that is greater than plasma osmolality in the setting of hyponatremia, but only when renal, adrenal, and thyroid functions are normal.

Hypernatremia

Hypernatremia (plasma Na^+ >150 mmol/L) is always hyperosmolar. Symptoms of hypernatremia are primarily neurological, due to intracellular dehydration, and include tremors, irritability, ataxia, confusion, and coma.[9] As with hyponatremia the rapidity of the development of hypernatremia determines the plasma Na^+ value at which symptoms occur. In many cases the symptoms of hypernatremia may be masked by underlying conditions that contribute to the development of the condition. Clinically, most cases of hypernatremia occur in individuals with altered mental status or in infants, both of whom may have difficulty rehydrating themselves despite a normal thirst reflex. Thus hypernatremia rarely occurs in an alert individual with a normal thirst response and who has access to water.

In general, hypernatremia can arise from (1) excessive water loss or failure to replace normal water losses, (2) a net Na^+ gain in excess of water, or (3) decreased Na^+ excretion. Again, assessment of TBW status by physical examination and measurement of urine Na^+ and osmolality are important steps in the establishment of a diagnosis for hypernatremia (Figure 35-2).

Hypovolemic hypernatremia

Hypovolemia is an abnormal decrease in the plasma volume. Hypernatremia in the setting of hypovolemia is caused by the renal or extrarenal loss of hypo-osmotic fluid, leading to dehydration. Thus once hypovolemia is established, measurement of urine Na^+ and osmolality can determine the source of fluid loss. Extrarenal losses are characterized by a concentrated urine (>800 mosmol/L) with low urine Na^+ (<20 mmol/L), reflecting the proper renal conservation of Na^+ and water as a means to restore ECF volume. Extrarenal causes include diarrhea, skin losses (burns or excessive sweating), or respiratory losses coupled with failure to replace the lost water. Renal causes of water loss in excess of Na^+ include osmotic diuresis or thiazide diuretics with decreased water intake. In these settings, urine volume is high, urine osmolality low, and urine Na^+ high.

Normovolemic hypernatremia

Hypernatremia in the presence of normal ECF volume is normovolemic hypernatremia. It is often a prelude to hypovolemic hypernatremia. Insensible losses through the lung or skin again must be suspected and are characterized by concentrated urine as the kidneys function to conserve water. Another cause of normovolemic hypernatremia is water diuresis, which is manifested by polyuria (see Figure 35-2). The differential for polyuria (generally defined as >3 L urine output/day) is either a water or a solute diuresis. Solute diuresis is exemplified by the osmotic diuresis of diabetes mellitus and generally is characterized by urine osmolality greater than 300 mOsmol/L and hyponatremia (see previous section). A water diuresis is a manifestation of diabetes insipidus[11] and is characterized by dilute urine (osmolality <250 mosmol/L) and slight hypernatremia. Diabetes insipidus can be either central or nephrogenic.[11] Central diabetes insipidus is caused by decreased or total lack of ADH secretion as a result of head trauma, hypophysectomy, pituitary tumor, or granulomatous disease. Nephrogenic diabetes insipidus is due to renal resistance to ADH as a result of drugs (for example, lithium, demeclocycline, amphotericin) or diseases such as sickle cell anemia and Sjögren's syndrome, which affect collecting duct responsiveness to ADH. Central diabetes insipidus usually is treated with vasopres-

sin, whereas discontinuation of the offending drug or provision of easy and frequent access to drinking water treats nephrogenic diabetes insipidus.

Hypervolemic hypernatremia

The presence of excess TBW (**hypervolemia**) and hypernatremia indicates a net gain of water and Na^+, with Na^+ gain in excess of water (see Figure 35-2). This condition is observed commonly in hospitalized patients receiving hypertonic saline or sodium bicarbonate. Other causes of hypervolemic hypernatremia include hyperaldosteronism and Cushing's syndrome (see Chapters 34 and 41).

Potassium

The total body potassium of a 70-kg individual is approximately 3.5 mol (40 to 59 mmol/kg), of which only 1.5% to 2% is present in the ECF. Nevertheless, plasma K^+ is a relatively good indicator of total K^+. Disturbance of K^+ homeostasis has serious consequences. For example, muscle weakness, irritability, and paralysis characterize a decrease of extracellular K^+ (hypokalemia). At levels less than 2.5 mmol/L, tachycardia and specific cardiac conduction effects are apparent by electrocardiographic examination (flattened T waves) and can lead to cardiac arrest.[9] Plasma K^+ levels

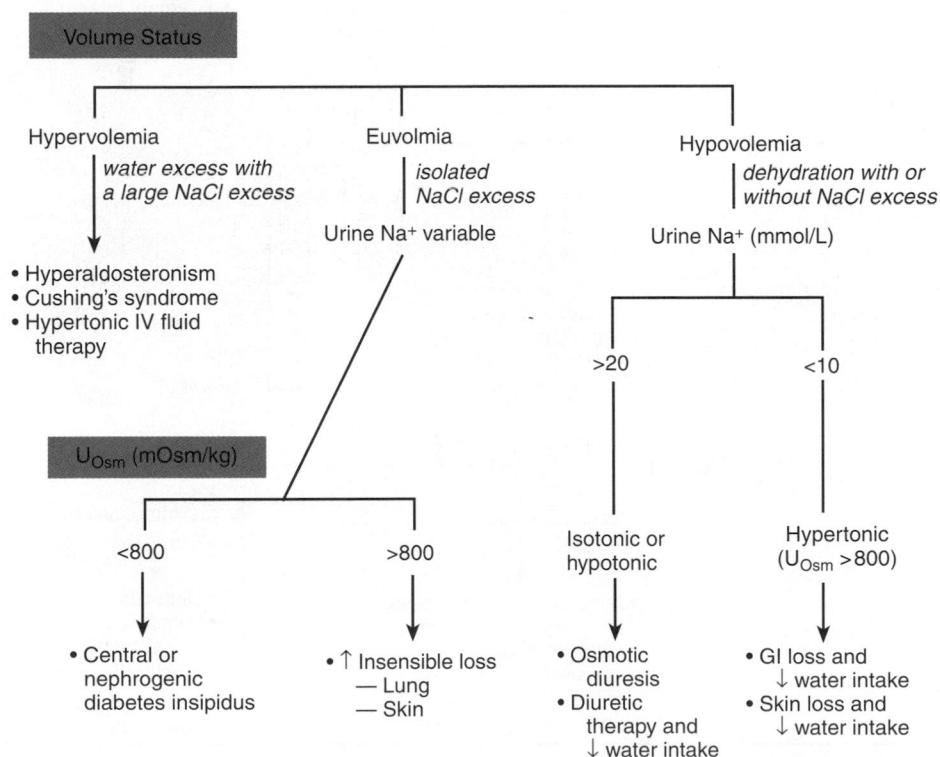

Figure 35-2   Algorithm for the differential diagnosis of hypernatremia. *NaCl,* Sodium chloride; *GI,* gastrointestinal. (Modified from Kirkpatrick W, Kreisberg R: Acid-base and electrolyte disorders. In Liu P (ed): Blue Book of Diagnostic Tests, pp 239-254, Philadelphia, WB Saunders, 1986.)

less than 3.0 mmol/L are associated with marked neuro-muscular symptoms and indicate a critical degree of intracellular depletion.

Abnormally high extracellular K^+ (hyperkalemia) levels produce symptoms of mental confusion, weakness, tingling, flaccid paralysis of the extremities, and weakness of the respiratory muscles.[9] Cardiac effects of hyperkalemia include bradycardia and conduction defects evident on the electrocardiogram by prolonged PR and QRS intervals and "peaked" T waves. Prolonged severe hyperkalemia greater than 7.0 mmol/L can lead to peripheral vascular collapse and cardiac arrest. Symptoms are present almost always at K^+ levels greater than 6.5 mmol/L, and levels of 10.0 mmol/L or more are fatal in most cases.

Hypokalemia

Causes of **hypokalemia** (plasma K^+ <3.5 mmol/L) can be classified as redistribution of extracellular K^+ into ICF, or true K^+ deficits, as a result of either decreased intake or a loss of potassium-rich body fluids (Figure 35-3).

Redistribution

Intracellular redistribution of K^+ is illustrated by the fall in plasma K^+ that can occur after the initiation of insulin therapy for diabetic hyperglycemia. The cells must take up K^+ as a consequence of glucose transport. Redistribution hypokalemia is also a feature of alkalosis, in which K^+ moves from ECF into the cells as H^+ moves in the opposite direction. Pseudohypokalemia is a feature of acute leuke-

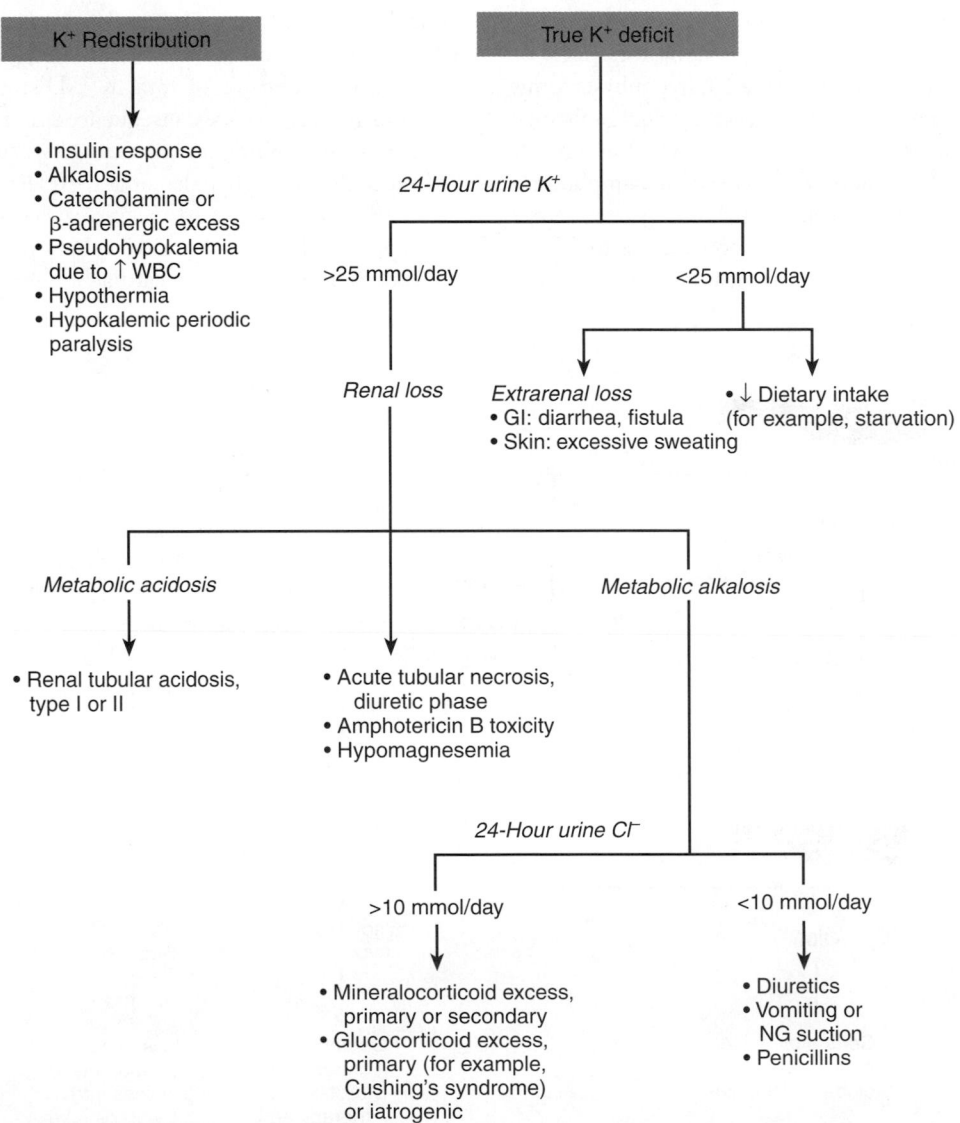

Figure 35-3   Algorithm for the differential diagnosis of hypokalemia. *WBC,* White blood cell; *GI,* gastrointestinal; *NG,* nasogastric. (Modified from Kirkpatrick W, Kreisberg R: Acid-base and electrolyte disorders. In Liu P (ed): Blue Book of Diagnostic Tests, pp 239-254, Philadelphia, WB Saunders, 1986.)

mias. The elevated white blood cell count can cause a time-dependent transport of K^+ into the leukemic cells after the blood sample is drawn. Other less common causes of intracellular redistribution are listed in Figure 35-3.

True potassium deficit

Hypokalemia reflecting true total body deficits of K^+ can be classified into renal and nonrenal losses based on daily excretion of K^+ in the urine (see Figure 35-3). If urine excretion of K^+ is less than 30 mmol/day, the conclusion can be reached that the kidneys are functioning properly and attempting to reabsorb as much K^+ as possible. Causes are either decreased K^+ intake or extrarenal loss of potassium-rich fluid. Situations of decreased intake include chronic starvation and postoperative intravenous fluid therapy with potassium-poor solutions. Gastrointestinal loss of K^+ occurs most commonly with diarrhea.

Urine excretion exceeding 25 to 30 mmol/day in a hypokalemic setting is inappropriate and indicates that the kidneys are the primary source of lost K^+. Renal losses of K^+ may occur during the diuretic (recovery) phase of acute tubular necrosis and during states of excess mineralocorticoid (primary or secondary aldosteronism) or glucocorticoid (Cushing's syndrome). Renal loss of K^+ also can be caused by thiazides and loop diuretics. In cases of contraction alkalosis, which can occur with prolonged vomiting or diuretic abuse, K^+ can be lost from the kidneys in exchange for reclaimed H^+ ions. This cause of hypokalemia is evident in low urine Cl^- and alkaline urine.

Hyperkalemia

Hyperkalemia (plasma $K^+ > 5.0$ mmol/L) can be a result of redistribution, increased intake, or increased retention. In addition, preanalytical conditions, such as hemolysis, thrombocytosis ($> 10^6/\mu L$), and leukocytosis ($> 10^5/\mu L$), can cause a marked pseudohyperkalemia, which is described in detail in Chapter 25 (Figure 35-4).

Redistribution

The transfer of intracellular K^+ into ECF invariably occurs in cases of acidosis as H^+ shifts intracellularly and K^+ shifts outward to maintain electrical neutrality. As a general rule, K^+ concentrations can be expected to rise 0.2 to 0.7 mmol/L for every 0.1 unit drop in pH. When the underlying cause of the acidosis is treated, normokalemia is restored. Extracellular redistribution of K^+ also may occur

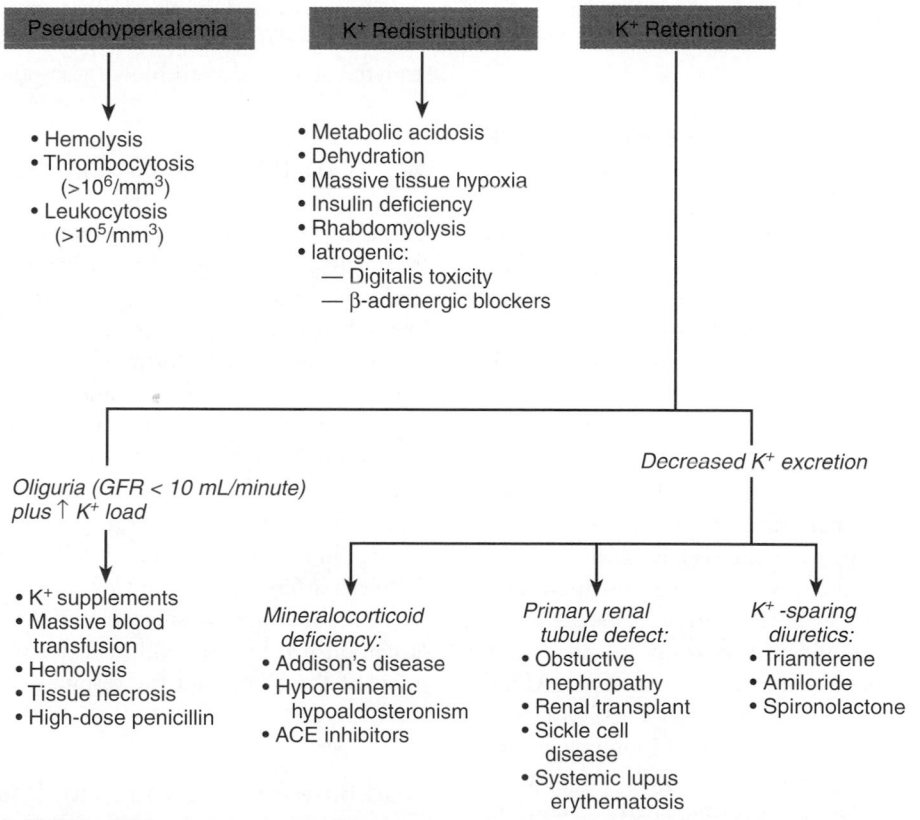

Figure 35-4　Algorithm for the differential diagnosis of hyperkalemia. *GFR,* Glomerular filtration rate; *ACE,* angiotensin-converting enzyme. (Modified from Kirkpatrick W, Kreisberg R: Acid-base and electrolyte disorders. In Liu P (ed): Blue Book of Diagnostic Tests, pp 239-254, Philadelphia, WB Saunders, 1986.)

in cases of dehydration, shock with tissue hypoxia, diabetic ketoacidosis, severe burns, and violent muscular activity, which accompanies epileptic seizures. Finally, important iatrogenic causes of redistribution hyperkalemia include digoxin toxicity and β-adrenergic blockade.[9]

Potassium retention

Acute renal disease (with decreased excretion of K^+) and end-stage renal failure (with oliguria or anuria and acidosis) are the most common causes of prolonged hyperkalemia (see Figure 35-4). In individuals with shock-induced renal failure and renal tubular acidosis (RTA), interference with Na^+-H^+ exchange in the tubules leads to K^+ retention. Indeed, in the absence of severe renal failure, hyperkalemia seldom is prolonged. Hyperkalemia occurs with Na^+ depletion in cases of adrenocortical insufficiency (for example, Addison's disease) because diminished Na^+ reabsorption and a concomitant decrease in Na^+-K^+ exchange results in decreased K^+ secretion. Drugs that block the production of aldosterone, such as the inhibitors of the angiotensin-converting enzyme (ACE inhibitors; for example, captopril) also may cause hyperkalemia. Other causes of hyperkalemia include the tumor lysis syndrome, salt-losing congenital adrenal hyperplasia, and excess administration of potassium-sparing diuretics that block distal tubular K^+ secretion (for example, triamterene, amiloride, and spironolactone).

Chloride

Chloride (Cl^-) ion is the most abundant anion in the ECF (see Table 35-2). In the absence of acid-base disturbances, Cl^- concentrations in plasma generally follow those of Na^+. However, determination of plasma Cl^- concentration can be useful in the differential diagnoses of acid-base disturbances and is essential for calculation of the anion gap. Clinically, fluctuations in serum or plasma Cl^- have little consequence but are signs of an underlying disturbance in fluid and acid-base homeostasis.

Hypochloremia

Decreased plasma Cl^- concentration is observed in individuals with salt-losing nephritis (for example, chronic pyelonephritis) when hyponatremia also is observed. The loss most likely is due to defective tubular reabsorption despite a body deficit of Cl^-. Other conditions associated with hypochloremia include bromide intoxication, so-called cerebral salt wasting that may occur after head injury, SIADH, and conditions associated with expansion of ECF, such as those described for hyponatremia. Hypochloremia is observed frequently in cases of metabolic acidoses that are caused by increased production or diminished excretion of organic acids (for example, diabetic ketoacidosis and renal failure). In such cases the fraction of total anion concentration represented by Cl^- is diminished because the complementary fraction of β-hydroxybutyrate, acetoacetate, lactate,

and phosphate is increased. Persistent gastric secretion and prolonged vomiting, whatever the cause, result in significant loss of Cl^- and ultimately in hypochloremia and depletion of total body Cl^-.

Hyperchloremia

Increased plasma Cl^- concentration accompanies dehydration, RTA, acute renal failure, metabolic acidosis associated with prolonged diarrhea and loss of sodium bicarbonate, diabetes insipidus, and states of adrenocortical hyperfunction. Hyperchloremic acidosis may be a sign of severe renal tubular disease. Extremely high dietary intake of salt and overtreatment with saline solutions are also causes of hyperchloremia.

Bicarbonate

Total carbon dioxide (CO_2) content of plasma consists of carbon dioxide dissolved in an aqueous solution ($cdCO_2$), CO_2 loosely bound to amine groups in proteins (carbamino compounds), HCO_3^-, and small amounts of CO_3^{2-} ions and carbonic acid (H_2CO_3). Bicarbonate ions compose all but approximately 2 mmol/L of the total carbon dioxide of plasma (22 to 31 mmol/L). Alterations of HCO_3^- and CO_2 dissolved in plasma are characteristic of acid-base imbalance, as discussed in the following section. Bicarbonate's value has the most significance in the context of other electrolyte values and with blood gases and pH values.

◼ ACID-BASE PHYSIOLOGY

Metabolic processes in the body result in the production of relatively large amounts of carbonic, sulfuric, phosphoric, and other acids. For example, during a 24-hour period an individual weighing 70 kg exhales about 20 mol of carbon dioxide (the volatile form of carbonic acid) through the lungs and about 70 to 100 mmol (or ~1 mEq/kg) of titratable, nonvolatile acids (mainly sulfuric and phosphoric acids) through the kidneys. These products of metabolism are transported to the excretory organs (lungs and kidneys) via the ECF and the blood without producing any appreciable change in the plasma pH and only a minimal pH difference between arterial (pH 7.36 to 7.44) and venous (pH 7.32 to 7.38) blood. This transportation and subsequent excretion is accomplished by the combined functions of the buffer systems of the blood and the respiratory and renal regulatory mechanisms.

Acid-Base Balance and Acid-Base Status

A description of **acid-base balance** involves an accounting of the carbonic (H_2CO_3, HCO_3^-, CO_3^{2-}, and CO_2) and noncarbonic acids and conjugate bases in terms of input (intake plus metabolic production) and output (excretion plus metabolic conversion) over a given time interval. The acid-base status of the body fluids typically is assessed by the measurements of plasma pH and P_{CO_2} because the bicarbonate/carbonic acid system is the most important buffering system of the plasma.

Clinical laboratorians should understand the clinical terms used to describe the acid-base status. **Acidemia** is defined as an arterial blood pH of less than 7.35; **alkalemia** indicates that an arterial blood pH is greater than 7.45. *Acidosis* and *alkalosis* refer to pathological states that can lead to acidemia or alkalemia. More than one type of pathological process can occur simultaneously, giving rise to a **mixed acid-base disturbance,** in which the blood pH may be low, high, or within the reference interval. If unrecognized and untreated, disturbances in acid-base balance can be fatal. These measurements reflect a static sampling of a dynamic process involving complex interactions between multiple buffering systems and the compensatory mechanisms of the kidneys and lungs. To understand how these and other perturbations of acid-base metabolism affect human physiology, a review of the concepts of acids, bases, pH, and buffers in relation to the relevant systems that function to maintain normal acid-base balance in the human body is necessary.

Acid-base parameters—definitions and abbreviations

Acids are chemical substances that can donate protons (H^+ ions) in solution, and bases are substances that accept protons. Strong acids readily give up H^+, whereas strong bases readily accept H^+. Thus the conjugate base of a strong acid is a weak base, and vice versa (see Chapter 1). Examples of acid and conjugate base are as follows:

$$acid \rightleftharpoons H^{\oplus} + conjugate\ base$$

$$HCl \rightleftharpoons H^{\oplus} + Cl^{\ominus}$$

$$NH_4^{\oplus} \rightleftharpoons H^{\oplus} + NH_3$$

$$glycine \rightleftharpoons H^{\oplus} + glycinate^{\ominus}$$

$$glycinium^{\oplus} \rightleftharpoons H^{\oplus} + glycine$$

Thus hydrochloric acid (HCl), ammonium ion (NH_4^+), and amine ions (glycinium$^+$) are acids, and free ammonia (NH_3), glycinate$^-$, and free (electrically neutral) amines are bases. Some hydrogen-containing anions, such as HCO_3^- and HPO_4^{2-} and all amino acids and proteins, can act as an acid or a base, as follows:

$$H_2PO_4^{\ominus} \rightleftharpoons H^{\oplus} + HPO_4^{\ominus\ominus}$$
$$(conjugate\ base)$$

$$HPO_4^{\ominus\ominus} \rightleftharpoons H^{\oplus} + PO_4^{\ominus\ominus\ominus}$$
$$(acid)$$

pH and pK

The pH of a solution is defined as the negative logarithm of the hydrogen ion activity (pH = -log aH^+). Thus pH is a dimensionless quantity so that a decrease of one pH unit represents a tenfold increase in the H^+ activity. The average pH of blood (7.40) corresponds to a hydrogen ion concentration of 40 nmol/L (Figure 35-5). Potentiometric determinations of blood pH measure H^+ activity and not H^+ concentration, although the activity is assumed to equal the concentration. The inverse and nonlinear relationship between hydrogen ion activity and pH is illustrated in Figure 35-5.

The pK (also, pK' and pK_a) represents the negative logarithm of the ionization constant of an acid (K_a). That is, the pK is the pH at which a buffer exists in equal proportions with its acid and conjugate base. Thus acids have pK values less than 7.0, whereas bases have pK values greater than 7.0. The lower the pK, the stronger the acid, and the higher the pK, the stronger the conjugate base.

The pH of the plasma may be considered a function of the following two independent variables:

1. The P_{CO_2}, which is regulated by the lungs and represents the acid component of the carbonic acid/bicarbonate buffer system
2. The concentration of titratable base, which is regulated by the kidneys

For a pure bicarbonate solution, changes in the concentration of titratable base equal the changes in the bicarbonate concentration. Thus the plasma bicarbonate concentration

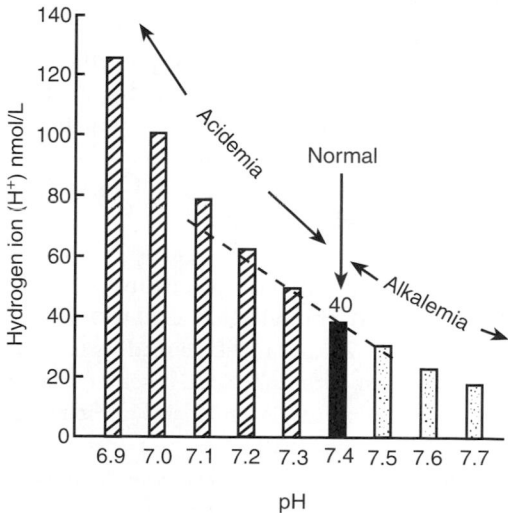

Figure 35-5 Relationship of pH to hydrogen ion concentration. Note the (approximate) linear relationship between hydrogen ion concentration and pH over the pH range of 7.2 to 7.5 (*broken line*). (Modified from Narins RG, Emmett M: Simple and mixed acid-base disorders: a practical approach. Medicine 1980; 59:161-187.)

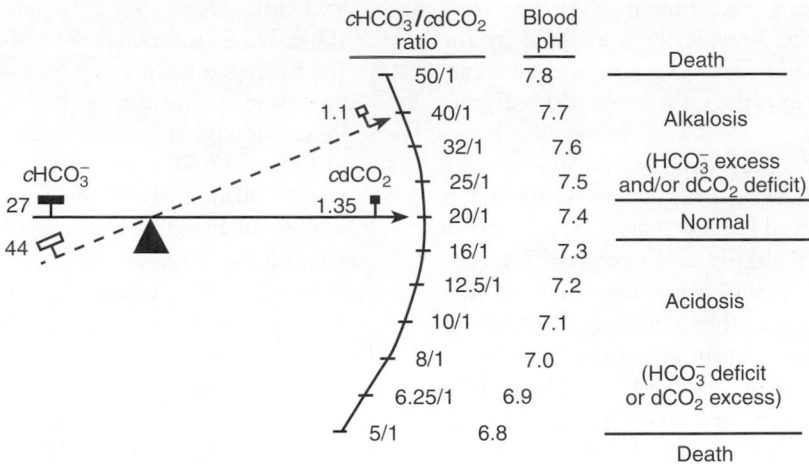

Figure 35-6 Schematic demonstration of the relationship between pH and ratio of bicarbonate concentration to the concentration of dissolved CO_2. If the ratio in blood is 20/1 ($cHCO_3^- = 27$ mmol/$cdCO_2 = 1.35$ mmol/L), the resultant pH is 7.4, as demonstrated by the *solid beam*. Note also a case of uncompensated alkalosis (bicarbonate excess) with a bicarbonate concentration of 44 mmol/L and a $cdCO_2$ of 1.1 mmol/L (*dotted line*). Therefore the ratio is 40/1, and the resultant pH is 7.7. In a case of uncompensated acidosis the pointer of the balance would point to a pH between 6.8 and 7.35, depending on the $cHCO_3^-/cdCO_2$ ratio. HCO_3^-, Bicarbonate; dCO_2, dissolved carbon dioxide. (Modified from Weisberg HF: A better understanding of anion-cation ("acid-base") balance. Surg Clin North Am 1959; 39:93-120; and Snively WD, Wessner M: ABC's of fluid balance. J Ind State Med Assoc 1954; 47:957-972.)

generally is taken as a measure of the base excess or deficit in plasma and ECF.

Bicarbonate and dissolved CO_2

Bicarbonate is the second largest fraction (behind Cl^-) of plasma anions (~25 mmol/L). As described in Chapter 25 the analyte usually measured in plasma is called *total CO_2*, which includes bicarbonate and dissolved CO_2 ($cdCO_2$). The dissolved CO_2 fraction includes both the undissociated carbonic acid and physically dissolved, free CO_2. At the pH of the blood the amount of dissolved CO_2 is 700 to 1000 times greater than the amount of carbonic acid, and therefore $cdCO_2$ is the term used to express their combined concentration. $cdCO_2$ is calculated from the solubility coefficient of CO_2 in blood at 37 °C ($\alpha = 0.0306$ mmol/L) multiplied by the PCO_2 measured in mm Hg. Thus at a PCO_2 of 40 mm Hg, $cdCO_2$ is 1.224 mmol/L (0.0306 mmol/L × 40 mm Hg).

Henderson-Hasselbalch equation

The **Henderson-Hasselbalch equation** is described in detail in Chapter 25. In practice, a reader's understanding of this equation is important because it helps explain the role of the body's compensatory mechanisms in the regulation of body pH in individuals with acid-base disturbances. The equation derived in Chapter 25 also can be written as follows:

$$pH = 6.1 + \log \frac{cHCO_3^-}{cdCO_2}$$

where $cdCO_2$ is equal to α (0.0306) × PCO_2 (mmHg), and 6.1 is the pK' for the carbonic acid/bicarbonate system (see Chapter 25).

The average normal ratio of the concentrations of bicarbonate and dissolved carbon dioxide in plasma is 25 (mmolL)/1.25 (mmol/L) = 20/1. Subsequently, any change in the concentration of either bicarbonate or dissolved CO_2 and therefore in the ratio of $cHCO_3^-/cdCO_2$ must be accompanied by a change in pH. Such changes in the ratio can occur through a change either in the numerator (the renal component) or denominator (the respiratory component). Clinical conditions characterized as *metabolic* disturbances of acid-base balance are classified as primary disturbances in HCO_3^- concentration. Those characterized as *respiratory* disturbances are classified as primary disturbances in $cdCO_2$. Various compensatory mechanisms functioning to reestablish the normal ratio of $cHCO_3^-/cdCO_2$ may result in changes in the bicarbonate concentration, dissolved CO_2 concentration, or both. The lever-fulcrum diagram (Figure 35-6) is used to illustrate the application of the Henderson-Hasselbalch equation to human acid-base physiology.

Buffer Systems and their Role in the pH Regulation of Body Fluids

Buffers are defined in Chapter 1. A buffer is a mixture of a weak acid and a salt of its conjugate base that resists changes in pH when a strong acid or base is added to the solution. If the concentrations of the acid and base components of a buffer are equal, the pH equals the pK. Generally, buffers work best at resisting changes in pH in the interval ± 1 pH unit of their pK, where the ratio of acid to base is within the range of 10:1 to 1:10. The buffer value (β) is defined as the amount of base required to cause a change in pH of one unit.

The action of buffers in the regulation of body pH can be explained by use of the bicarbonate buffer system as an example. If a strong acid is added to a solution containing HCO_3^- and H_2CO_3, the H^+ reacts with HCO_3^- to form more H_2CO_3 and subsequently, CO_2 and H_2O. The hydrogen ions thereby are bound, and the increase in the H^+ concentration is minimal, as follows:

$$HCO_3^\ominus + H^\oplus \longrightarrow H_2CO_3 \longrightarrow CO_2 + H_2O$$

The most important physiological buffer systems are those of plasma and erythrocytes.

Bicarbonate/carbonic acid buffer system

The most important buffer of plasma is the bicarbonate/carbonic acid pair; it also is present in erythrocytes, but at a lower concentration. Initially, this buffer may not appear effective because its pK is 6.1, whereas normal plasma pH is 7.4. Furthermore, the ratio of base to acid is approximately 20:1 in plasma, which is outside the general limits for good buffering capacity. However, the effectiveness of the bicarbonate buffer is based on its high concentration and on the fact that the lungs can dispose of readily or retain CO_2. In addition, the renal tubules can increase or decrease the rate of reclamation of bicarbonate from the glomerular filtrate (see Chapter 34). The importance of the high buffer concentration becomes apparent in the consideration that at normal pH, 5 mmol/L of lactate (pK $\sim$4) generates 5 mmol/L of H^+ ion; a normal H^+ ion concentration is only 40 nmol/L. The nonbicarbonate buffers of blood are present at less than 10 mmol/L concentration, whereas the bicarbonate buffer system is present at greater than 20 mmol/L.

Phosphate buffer system

At a plasma pH of 7.4 the ratio $cHPO_4^2/cH_2PO_4^-$ is 4/1 (pK' = 6.8). The total concentration of this buffer in both plasma and erythrocytes is less than that of other major buffer systems, accounting for only about 5% of the nonbicarbonate buffer value of plasma. Organic phosphate, however, in the form of 2,3-diphosphoglycerate (2,3-DPG; present in erythrocytes in a concentration of about 4.5 mmol/L), accounts for about 16% of the nonbicarbonate buffer value of erythrocyte fluid.

Plasma protein and hemoglobin buffer systems

The buffer value of the nonbicarbonate buffers of plasma is about 7.7 mmol/L at pH 7.40 for a normal plasma protein concentration of 72 g/L (7.2 g/dL). Proteins, especially albumin, account for the greatest portion (95%) of the nonbicarbonate buffer value of the plasma. The most important buffer groups of proteins in the physiological pH range are the imidazole groups of histidines (pK $\sim$7.3). Each albumin molecule contains 16 histidines.

The buffer value of the nonbicarbonate buffers of intracellular erythrocyte fluid is about 63 mmol/L at pH 7.20.

Hemoglobin accounts for the major part (53 mmolL), with the remainder primarily in the form of 2,3-DPG. The imidazole groups of hemoglobin are quantitatively the most important buffer groups.

Respiratory Mechanism in the Regulation of Acid-Base Balance

In addition to supplying O_2 to tissue cells for normal metabolism, the respiratory mechanism contributes to the maintenance of normal body pH through elimination or retention of CO_2 in metabolic acidosis and alkalosis, respectively.

Respiration

Exchange of O_2 and CO_2 in the lungs between alveolar air and blood is called **external respiration,** in contrast to **internal respiration** occurring at the tissue level. At inspiration, contraction of the diaphragm and thoracic musculature expands intrathoracic volume and produces a fall in intrapulmonary pressure. Atmospheric air is drawn into the bronchial tree, which terminates at the alveoli. Alveoli are small saclike chambers with very thin walls in close approximation to pulmonary capillaries where the exchange of gases between alveolar air and pulmonary blood occurs. Expiration takes place passively by recoil as the elastic tissues of the lungs and chest wall rebound and the intrathoracic volume is decreased. Loss of elasticity of the lungs and destruction of the alveolar membranes are basic pathological mechanisms underlying many pulmonary diseases.

Peripheral venous blood reaches the pulmonary circulation from the right ventricle of the heart and is "arterialized" in the capillaries of the lungs by uptake of O_2 and loss of CO_2. Pulmonary venous blood then returns to the left ventricle by way of the left atrium and is pumped through the aorta to the peripheral tissues. In the capillaries of peripheral tissues the arterial blood releases O_2 to the tissue cells and takes up CO_2. With return of blood to the lungs the cycle is completed.

In a resting state the respiration rate is normally 12 to 15 respirations per minute. For an average-sized adult with a tidal volume (the amount of air exchanged per breath cycle) of about 0.5 L, 6 to 8 L of air is moved per minute in either direction. Physical activity increases ventilation (respiratory rate $\times$ tidal volume), that is, the amount of air exchanged per minute. Voluntary efforts can increase the rate of ventilation 20 to 30 times over the resting level, but only briefly. Involuntary increases in rate and depth of respiration are regulated by the medullary respiratory center in the brainstem, which in turn is stimulated by central chemoreceptors located on the anterior surface of the medulla oblongata and peripheral chemoreceptors located in the carotid arteries and aorta. Peripheral chemoreceptors are stimulated by a fall in pH due to accumulation of CO_2 or by a decrease in Po_2.

The central chemoreceptors are stimulated only by a decrease in pH of the CSF.

Often an individual's normal response to these chemical receptors that drive respiration is perturbed by a pathological condition in the circulatory or respiratory system. If it is significantly abnormal, the individual requires assisted ventilation with a mechanical device to provide gas mixtures intermittently via an endotracheal tube inserted through the mouth or through a tracheostomy. The selection of conditions for mechanical ventilation carries risks of hyperventilation and excessive loss of CO_2 **(respiratory alkalosis)**or of hypoventilation and excessive retention of CO_2 **(respiratory acidosis)** and reduced uptake of O_2. Gas mixtures containing different fractional compositions of O_2 and CO_2 may be administered in conjunction with assisted ventilation. A physician's adjustments of the conditions of this me-

chanical ventilation depend greatly on the results of blood gas and pH determinations that reflect current acid-base status.

Exchange of gases in the lungs and peripheral tissues

Diffusion of O_2 and CO_2 across alveolar and cell membranes is governed by gradients in the partial pressure of each gas (Figure 35-7). Dry air inspired at a pressure of 1 atm (760 mm Hg) consists of 20.95% O_2 (P_{O_2} ~160 mm Hg), 0.03% CO_2 (P_{CO_2} ~0.25 mm Hg), 78.1% nitrogen, and approximately 0.8% other inert gases. As inspired air passes over the moist mucous membranes of the upper respiratory tract, it is warmed to 37 °C, becomes saturated with water vapor, and mixes with air in the respiratory tree, resulting in partial pressures of approximately 150 mm Hg

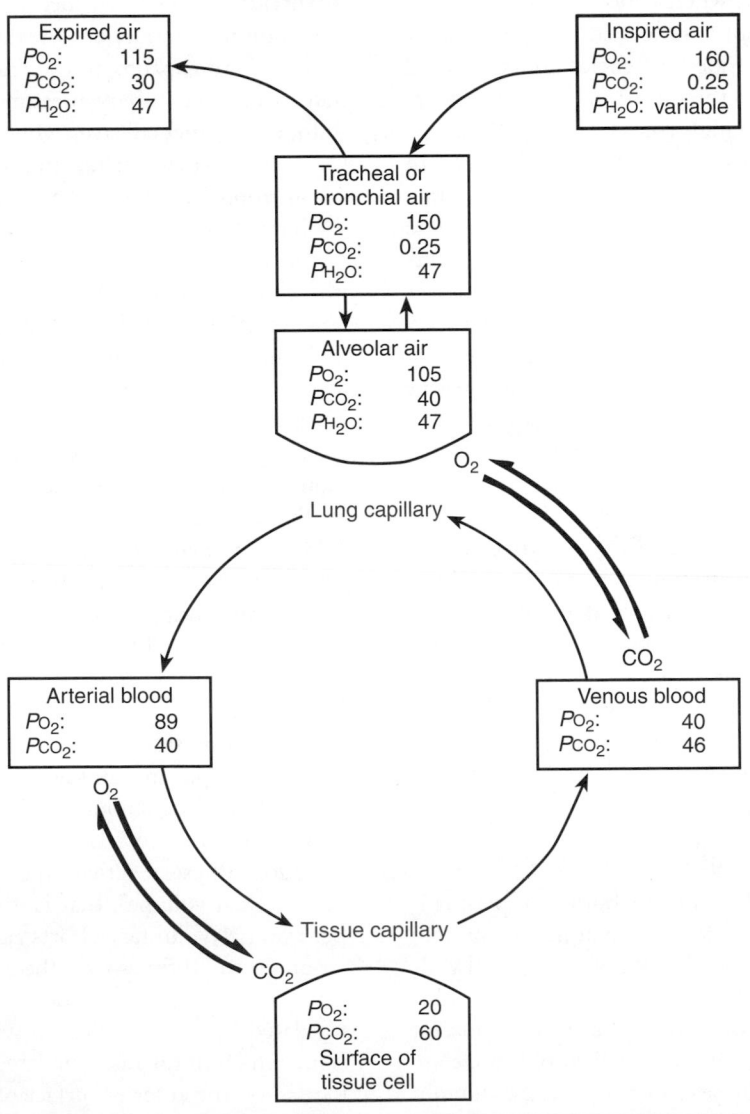

Figure 35-7 Partial pressures of oxygen and carbon dioxide in air, blood, and tissue. Values shown are approximations in mm Hg and calculated under the assumption of a 5% shunt. Note the directions of gradients (*heavy arrows*). P_{O_2}, Partial pressure of oxygen; P_{CO_2}, partial pres-

sure of carbon dioxide; P_{H_2O}, partial pressure of water. (Modified from Tietz NW: Fundamentals of Clinical Chemistry, 3rd edition, Philadelphia, WB Saunders, 1987.)

for O_2, 0.3 mm Hg for CO_2, approximately 47 mm Hg for H_2O, and 563 mm Hg for nitrogen.

Further mixture with alveolar air results in partial pressures at the alveolar membrane of approximately 105 mm Hg for O_2, approximately 40 mm Hg for CO_2, and approximately 47 mm Hg for H_2O. Venous blood on the opposite side of the alveolar membrane contains O_2 at a partial pressure of approximately 40 mm Hg and CO_2 at approximately 46 mm Hg. Thus the gradient for O_2 is inward, toward the blood, and for CO_2, it is outward, toward the alveoli (see Figure 35-7). At the arterial end of capillaries of peripheral tissues, the PO_2 at approximately 90 mm Hg is substantially higher than the average PO_2 at the surface of the tissue cells (20 mm Hg), and the PCO_2 at approximately 40 mm Hg is substantially lower than that in the cells (50 to 70 mm Hg). Thus in the tissue capillary the gradient for O_2 is inward, toward the cell, and for CO_2 it is outward, toward the capillary blood. The arteriovenous difference in partial pressures is approximately 60 mm Hg for O_2 and 6 mm Hg or less for CO_2. This difference in arteriovenous PO_2 is one indicator of the efficiency of O_2 extraction in the passage of blood through the capillaries.

Respiratory response to acid-base perturbations

The respiratory system responds immediately to a change in acid-base status, but 3 to 6 hours are required for the response to become maximal. (Most metabolic acid-base disorders develop slowly, within hours in individuals with diabetic ketoacidosis and months or even years in those with chronic renal disease.) The maximal response is not attained until both the central and peripheral chemoreceptors are stimulated fully. For example, in the early stages of metabolic acidosis, plasma pH decreases, but because ions equilibrate rather slowly across the blood-brain barrier, the CSF pH remains nearly normal. The peripheral chemoreceptors are stimulated by the decrease in plasma pH, hyperventilation occurs, and plasma PCO_2 decreases. The PCO_2 of the ECF of the brain decreases immediately because CO_2 equilibrates rapidly across the blood-brain barrier. Therefore initially the pH of the ECF of the brain tends to rise, and the central chemoreceptors are inhibited; however, as plasma bicarbonate gradually falls, bicarbonate concentration in the ECF of the brain also falls over the subsequent 3 to 6 hours and its pH returns to normal or slightly below normal. At this point, stimulation of respiration becomes maximal. The reverse is true when an individual with metabolic acidosis is treated with HCO_3^-.

Renal Mechanisms in the Regulation of Acid-Base Balance

The average pH of plasma and of the initial glomerular filtrate is approximately 7.4, whereas the average urinary pH is approximately 6.0, reflecting the renal excretion of nonvolatile acids produced by metabolic processes. The various functions of the renal mechanism can respond to specific requirements. In the case of acidosis, excretion of acids is increased and base is conserved; in alkalosis, the opposite occurs. The pH of the urine changes correspondingly and may vary in random specimens from pH 4.5 to 8.2 (reference interval from 4.5 to 8.0). This ability to excrete variable amounts of acid or base makes the kidney the final defense mechanism against changes in body pH.

The various acids produced during metabolic processes are buffered in the ECF at the expense of HCO_3^-. Renal excretion of acid and conservation of HCO^{-3} occur through several mechanisms, as follows:

1. The Na^+-H^+ exchange
2. Production of ammonia and excretion of NH_4^+
3. Reclamation of bicarbonate

Sodium-hydrogen exchange

Nearly all mammalian cells contain a plasma membrane ATP-hydrolyzing protein capable of exchanging sodium ions for protons—the so-called Na^+-H^+ exchanger. In the renal tubules the Na^+-H^+ exchangers extrude H^+ ions into the tubular fluid in exchange for Na^+ ions. Na^+-H^+ exchange is enhanced in states of acidosis and inhibited in alkalotic states. The proximal tubules, however, cannot maintain an H^+-gradient of more than approximately 1 pH unit, whereas the distal tubules cannot maintain one of more than approximately 3 pH units. Thus maximum urine acidity is reached at an approximate pH of 4.4. In some forms of RTA this exchange process is defective and may lead to a decrease in blood pH and an increase in urinary pH.

Potassium ions compete with hydrogen ions in the renal tubular Na^+-H^+ exchanger. If the intracellular K^+ level of renal tubular cells is high, more K^+ and less H^+ are exchanged for Na^+ and the urine becomes less acid, increasing the acidity of body fluids. If K^+ is depleted, more H^+ ions are exchanged for Na^+ and the urine becomes more acid and the body fluids more alkaline. Thus hyperkalemia can contribute to acidosis and hypokalemia to alkalosis.

Renal production of ammonia and excretion of ammonium ions

Renal tubular cells are able to generate ammonia from glutamine and other amino acids derived from muscle and liver cells according to the following reaction:[10]

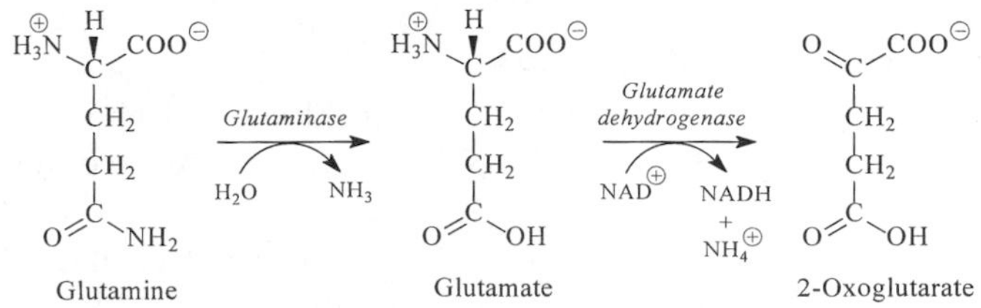

The quantity of ammonium ion produced that dissociates into ammonia and hydrogen ions is dependent on the pH. However, studies[6] indicate that NH_4^+ ions may be transported into the tubular luminal fluid without prior dissociation into NH_3 and H^+. At normal blood pH the ratio of NH_3 to NH_4^+ is about 1 to 100. Ammonia is a gas and diffuses readily across the cell membrane into the tubular lumen, where it combines with hydrogen ions to form ammonium ions. At the acid pH of urine the equilibrium between NH_4^+ and NH_3 shifts markedly to the left ($\sim$10,000 to 1), strongly favoring formation of NH_4^+. The NH_4^+ formed in the tubular lumen cannot cross cell membranes easily and thus is trapped in the tubular urine and excreted with anions, such as phosphate, chloride, or sulfate. In normal individuals, NH_4^+ production in the tubular lumen accounts for the excretion of approximately 60% (30 to 60 mmol) of the H^+ ions associated with nonvolatile acids.

The amount of H^+ excreted bound to NH_3 can be measured as NH_4^+. The H^+ required for NH_4^+ formation may be present in the glomerular filtrate or generated within the tubular cell through the synthesis of carbonic acid from CO_2, catalyzed by carbonic anhydrase (CA). These hydrogen ions are secreted into the tubular lumen through the Na^+-H^+ exchange. In cases of systemic acidosis, NH_4^+ excretion accounts by far for the greatest net excretion of H^+ by the kidneys. However, the maximum rate of glutamine release and therefore of NH_3 production ($\sim$400 mmol/day) is not achieved until acidosis has persisted for 3 days. In individuals with chronic renal insufficiency the kidneys are unable to generate sufficient NH_3 to buffer the nonvolatile acids produced, and this defect contributes significantly to the acidosis in such individuals.

Excretion of H^+ as $H_2PO_4^-$

H^+ secreted into the tubular lumen by the Na^+-H^+ exchanger also may react with HPO_4^{2-} to form $H_2PO_4^-$. This process depends on the amount of phosphate filtered by the glomeruli and the pH of urine. Under normal physiological conditions, approximately 30 mmol of H^+ is excreted per day as $H_2PO_4^-$, and this amount accounts for approximately 90% of the titratable acidity of urine. Acidemia increases phosphate excretion and thus provides additional buffer for reaction with H^+. A decrease in the glomerular filtration rate (GFR), as observed in individuals with renal disease, may result in a decrease of $H_2PO_4^-$ excretion.

Excretion of other acids

Strong acids, such as sulfuric, hydrochloric, and phosphoric, are ionized fully at the pH of urine and excreted only after the H^+ derived from these acids reacts with a buffer base. Excretion of the anions of these acids is accompanied by the simultaneous removal of an equal number of cations, such as Na^+, K^+, or NH_4^+, to provide electrochemical balance. However, some acids, such as acetoacetic acid ($pK = 3.58$) and β-hydroxybutyric acid ($pK = 4.7$), are present in blood almost entirely in ionized form, but at the acid pH frequently prevailing in urine, some are nondissociated and thus may be excreted partially as the nondissociated acid.

Reclamation of filtered bicarbonate

The unmodified glomerular filtrate has the same concentration of HCO_3^- as does plasma; however, with increasing acidification of the proximal tubular urine, the urine $P\text{CO}_2$ increases, and the HCO_3^- concentration decreases. These changes are thought to be initiated by the excretion of H^+ by the Na^+-H^+ exchanger mechanism, which results in a decrease in urinary pH. The H^+ thus excreted reacts with HCO_3^- (catalyzed by CA in the brush border of the proximal tubular cells) to form H_2CO_3 and subsequently, CO_2 and H_2O.

The increase in urinary $P\text{CO}_2$ causes carbon dioxide to diffuse across the tubular wall into the tubular cell, where it reacts with H_2O in the presence of cytoplasmic carbonic anhydrase in the tubular cells to form H_2CO_3 and subsequently, H^+ and HCO_3^-. Thus reclamation of bicarbonate is in fact diffusion of CO_2 into tubular cells and its subsequent conversion to HCO_3^-. Normally, nearly 90% of the filtered HCO_3^- (or about 4500 mmol/day) is reclaimed in the proximal tubule, and the extent of HCO_3^- reclamation parallels Na^+ reabsorption. Thus for each H^+ secreted into the tubular fluid, one Na^+ and one HCO_3^- enter the tubular cell and return to the general circulation.

When plasma HCO_3^- concentration increases above 26 mmol/L, the capacity of the proximal and distal tubules to reclaim HCO_3^- is exceeded, and HCO_3^- is excreted in the urine. The process of bicarbonate reclamation is enhanced in states of acidosis (and decreased in alkalosis), most likely as a result of increased Na^+-H^+ exchange.

■ CONDITIONS ASSOCIATED WITH ABNORMAL ACID-BASE STATUS AND ABNORMAL ELECTROLYTE COMPOSITION OF THE BLOOD

Many pathological conditions are accompanied by disturbances of the acid-base balance and electrolyte composition of the blood.[4,9,15] These changes usually are reflected in the acid-base pattern and anion-cation composition of ECF, as measured in blood. However, results obtained on blood or plasma may not always reflect the acid-base status of the ICF.

Abnormalities of acid-base status of the blood always are accompanied by characteristic changes in electrolyte concentrations in the plasma, especially in metabolic disorders. Hydrogen ions cannot accumulate without concomitant accumulation of anions, such as Cl^- or lactate, or without exchange for cations, such as K^+ or Na^+. For this reason, electrolyte composition of blood serum or plasma often is determined along with measurements of blood gases and

TABLE 35-3   **Classification and Characteristics of Simple Acid-Base Disorders**

Disorder	Primary Change	Compensatory Response	Expected Compensation
Metabolic			
Acidosis	$\downarrow cHCO_3^-$	$\downarrow Pco_2$	$Pco_2 = 1.5\ (cHCO_3^-) + 8 \pm 2$.
			Pco_2 falls by 1 to 1.3 mm Hg for each mmol/L fall in $cHCO_3^-$.
			Last 2 digits of pH = Pco_2 (for example, if Pco_2 = 28, pH = 7.28).
			$cHCO_3^-$ + 15 = last 2 digits of pH ($cHCO_3^-$ = 15; pH = 7.30).
Alkalosis	$\uparrow cHCO_3^-$	$\uparrow Pco_2$	Pco_2 increases 6 mm Hg for each 10 mmol/L rise in $cHCO_3^-$.
			$cHCO_3^-$ + 15 = last 2 digits of pH ($cHCO_3^-$ = 35; pH = 7.50).
Respiratory			
Acidosis			
Acute	$\uparrow Pco_2$	$\uparrow cHCO_3^-$	$cHCO_3^-$ increases by 1 mmol/L for each 10 mm Hg rise in Pco_2.
Chronic	$\uparrow Pco_2$	$\uparrow cHCO_3^-$	$cHCO_3^-$ increases by 3.5 mmol/L for each 10 mm Hg rise in Pco_2.
Alkalosis			
Acute	$\downarrow Pco_2$	$\downarrow cHCO_3^-$	$cHCO_3^-$ falls by 2 mmol/L for each 10 mm Hg fall in Pco_2.
Chronic	$\downarrow Pco_2$	$\downarrow cHCO_3^-$	$cHCO_3^-$ falls by 5 mmol/L for each 10 mm Hg fall in Pco_2.

Modified from Narins RG, Gardner LB: Simple acid-base disturbances. Med Clin North Am 1981; 65:321-346.
Pco_2, Partial pressure of carbon dioxide; $cHCO_3^-$, concentration of bicarbonate; $\uparrow$, increase; $\downarrow$, decrease.

pH and the acid-base parameters derived from them. Acid-base disturbances are classified traditionally in one of the following four groups

1. Metabolic acidosis
2. Metabolic alkalosis
3. Respiratory acidosis
4. Respiratory alkalosis

In simple, straightforward acid-base disorders, the laboratory parameters shown in Table 35-3 are observed. However, interpretation of laboratory values to classify these disorders is rarely straightforward because of compensatory responses by the respiratory and renal systems.

The causes of acid-base disorders, resulting laboratory values, and compensatory responses are discussed in this chapter in the traditional categorization of these disorders. However, remembering which disorders fall into which categories often is difficult, so the use of mnemonic devices or tables to facilitate description of these disorders is common. A useful and more logical approach is to realize that an acidosis can only occur as a result of one (or a combination) of three mechanisms—(1) increased addition of acid, (2) decreased elimination of acid, and (3) increased loss of base. Similarly, alkalosis can occur only by (1) increased addition of base, (2) decreased elimination of base, and (3) increased loss of acid. Dufour has illustrated this simple concept by depicting the body as a two-tank vat—one of acid and one of base—with inputs and outputs for each vat (Figure 35-8).[4] In the normal setting these inputs and outputs are balanced; an acid-base disorder then involves a perturbation in the input or output of these body reservoirs.[1]

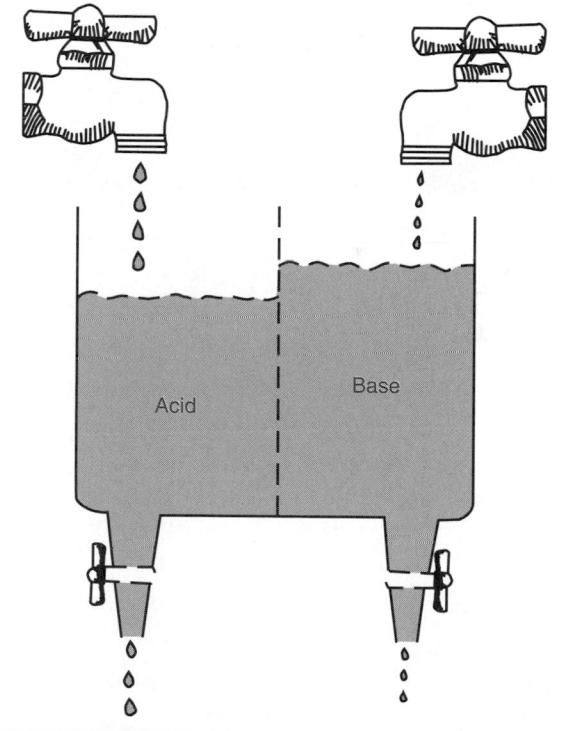

Figure 35-8   Simple depiction of the body as a two-vat system of acid and base. At equilibrium, input and output from each "vat" are equal. (Modified from Dufour DR: Acid-base disorders. In Dufour DR, Christenson RH (eds): Professional Practice in Clinical Chemistry: A Review, pp 604-635, Washington, DC, AACC Press, 1995.

Metabolic Acidosis (Primary Bicarbonate Deficit)

Metabolic acidosis is detected readily by a decreased concentration of plasma bicarbonate, the primary perturbation in this acid-base disorder. Bicarbonate is "lost" in the buffering of excess acid. Causes include the following:

1. Production of organic acids that exceeds the rate of elimination (for example, the production of acetoacetic acid and β-hydroxybutyric acid in states of diabetic acidosis and of lactic acid in those of lactic acid acidosis)
2. Reduced excretion of acids (H^+) as is seen in cases of renal failure and some renal tubular acidoses, resulting in an accumulation of acid that consumes bicarbonate
3. Excessive loss of bicarbonate due to increased renal excretion (decreased tubular reclamation) or excessive loss of duodenal fluid (as with diarrhea). Plasma $cHCO_3^-$ falls; the fall is associated with a rise in the concentration of inorganic anions (mostly chloride) or a concomitant fall in the sodium concentration.

When any of these conditions exists, the ratio of $cHCO_3^-/cdCO_2$ is decreased because of the primary decrease in bicarbonate. The resulting drop in pH stimulates the respiratory compensatory mechanism of hyperventilation, which lowers PCO_2 and thereby raises the pH.

Increased anion gap acidosis (organic acidosis)

Metabolic acidoses can be classified as those associated with either an increased anion gap or a normal anion gap (Table 35-4). The concept of the **anion gap** originally was devised as a quality control rule when the discovery was made that if the sum of Cl^- and HCO_3^- values was subtracted from the Na^+ value ($Na^+ - [Cl^- + HCO_3^-]$), the difference, or "gap," averaged 12 mmol/L in healthy individuals.[2,3] This *apparent* gap is due to unmeasured anions (e.g., proteins, SO_4^{2-}, HPO_4^{2-}) that are present in plasma. Anion gap values outside the interval of 7 to 16 mmol/L suggest the possibility of an error in measurement of one of the electrolytes. However, the anion gap also apparently is increased in many individuals with a metabolic acidosis.[5] For example, a laboratory report that signals an increased anion gap is often the first indication of a metabolic acidosis and should be assessed in the electrolyte profiles of all individuals.[4] The gap can be increased slightly artificially in the absence of acidosis by very low calcium, magnesium, or potassium levels because lower levels of these "unmeasured" cations result in lower levels of anions (Figure 35-9). Conversely, the gap can be narrowed artificially in settings of hypoalbuminemia (negatively charged proteins), hypergammaglobulinemia (positively charged proteins), hypercalcemia, or hypermagnesemia.

TABLE 35-4   **Conditions of Metabolic Acidoses with High and Normal Anion Gaps**

Etiology	Retained Acids	Other Laboratory Findings
High Anion Gap*		
Methanol toxicity	Formate	↑Osmolal gap (>15 mOsm/kg)
Uremia of renal failure	Sulfuric, phosphoric, organic	↑BUN† and serum creatinine
Ketoacidoses		
Diabetes mellitus	Acetoacetate and β-hydroxybutyrate	↑Plasma and urine glucose
Ethyl alcohol toxicity		↑Osmolal gap (>15 mOsm/kg)
Starvation		
Paraldehyde toxicity		
Isoniazid or iron toxicity, also ischemia	Organic, mainly lactate	Isoniazid and iron acting as mitochondrial poisons
Lactic acidosis	Lactate	
Ethylene glycol toxicity	Hippurate, glycolate, oxalate	↑Osmolal gap (>15 mOsm/kg); urine oxalate crystals
Salicylate toxicity	Salicylate, organic	Respiratory alkalosis
Normal Anion Gap		
Gastrointestinal fluid loss	Primary loss of bicarbonate	
Severe diarrhea		Hypokalemia
Pancreatitis		K^+ variable
Intestinal fistula		
RTA	Sulfuric, phosphoric, organic	
Proximal (type II) RTA		Urine pH <5.5, with K^+ normal or low
Distal (type I) RTA		Urine pH >5.5. with hypokalemia (usually)
Type IV RTA		Urine pH <5.5, with hyperkalemia

RTA, Renal tubular acidosis.
*Although considerable variability exists, the anion gap is often greater than 25 mmol/L in these conditions, with the exception of uremic renal failure.
†Blood urea nitrogen (reference interval of 8 to 25 mg/dL, or ~3.0 to 9.0 mmol/L).

All anion gap metabolic acidoses can be explained by one (or a combination) of eight underlying mechanisms listed in the following sections according to the common mnemonic device, MUDPILES (see Table 35-4). The physiological basis for the anion gap in these conditions is the consumption of bicarbonate in buffering excess acid. Cl^- values remain normal when the excess acid is any other than HCl because the lost bicarbonate is replaced by the unmeasured anions.

Methanol

Although nontoxic itself, methanol is metabolized by the liver to formaldehyde and formic acid. Accumulation of this acid leads to metabolic acidosis with a high anion gap and to clinical symptoms of optic papillitis, retinal edema, and ultimately blindness due to optic nerve atrophy and neurological defects that may lead to coma. Methanol and other ingested alcohols, such as ethylene glycol, ethanol, and isopropanol, increase the osmolality of plasma. Thus determination of the osmolal gap (see Chapter 25) can help determine the source of the unmeasured anion and suggest specific toxicological analyses.

Uremia of renal failure

The loss of functional renal tubular mass results in decreased ammonia formation, Na^+-H^+ exchange, and GFR. All result in decreased acid excretion (see Chapter 34). Acidosis usually develops if GFR falls below 20 mL/minute. Serum creatinine and blood urea nitrogen concentrations usually are elevated and used to estimate the degree of renal damage or remaining functional renal capacity.

Diabetes or ketoacidosis

The pathogenesis of ketoacidosis is discussed in detail in Chapter 23. Ketoacids, such as β-hydroxybutyrate and

2-oxoglutarate, accumulate and represent the unmeasured anions. Accumulation of these "ketone bodies" causes a decrease in HCO_3^-, a normal or low serum chloride, and a high anion gap. Ketoacids also can accumulate in states of starvation and alcoholic malnutrition.

Paraldehyde toxicity

Paraldehyde toxicity may develop after chronic paraldehyde ingestion. The pathogenesis is ill defined, but the acidosis actually may be a ketosis (nitroprusside negative), with β-hydroxybutyric acid as the main acidic product. Individuals with paraldehyde toxicity have a pungent, applelike odor to the breath.

Isoniazid, iron, or ischemia

These seemingly unrelated etiologies of high anion gap acidosis share a common feature—the accumulation of organic acids, with a predominance of lactic acid. Thus, the "three I's" actually represent special cases in the general category of lactic acidosis, which is described in the following section. Both isoniazid, an antimycobacterial agent commonly used in the treatment or prophylaxis of tuberculosis, and iron toxicity involve the production of toxic peroxides, which act as mitochondrial poisons and interfere with normal cellular respiration. Tissue ischemia may result from many causes; in general, hypoperfusion leads to hypoxia of cells, which results in anaerobic metabolism with the attendant accumulation of organic (mainly lactic) acids.

Lactic acidosis

Lactic acid, present in blood entirely as lactate ion ($pK = 3.86$), is an intermediate of carbohydrate metabolism and is derived mainly from muscle cells and erythrocytes. It represents the end product of anaerobic metabolism and normally is metabolized by the liver. The blood lactate concentration therefore is affected by the rate of production and rate of metabolism, both of which depend on adequate tissue perfusion. Any increase in the concentration of lactate to greater than 2 mmol/L and the associated increased H^+ leads to a condition called *lactic acidosis*. However, during exercise, lactate levels may increase as high as approximately 12 mmol/L. Under normal conditions the lactate is metabolized rapidly so that the "acidosis" is merely transient.

Lactic acidosis caused by severe tissue hypoxia is seen in cases of severe anemia, shock, cardiac decompensation, and pulmonary insufficiency. Severe oxygen deprivation of tissues blocks aerobic oxidation of pyruvic acid in the tricarboxylic acid cycle and results in the reduction of pyruvate to form lactate. A short-lived lactic acidosis often is observed after epileptic seizures. If the origin of lactate (for example, seizure, hypoxic tissue) can be rectified, lactate is metabolized rapidly to CO_2 and eliminated, provided the respiratory system is intact.

Hyperventilation in lactic acidosis is more intense than in other forms of metabolic acidosis. This intensity is thought

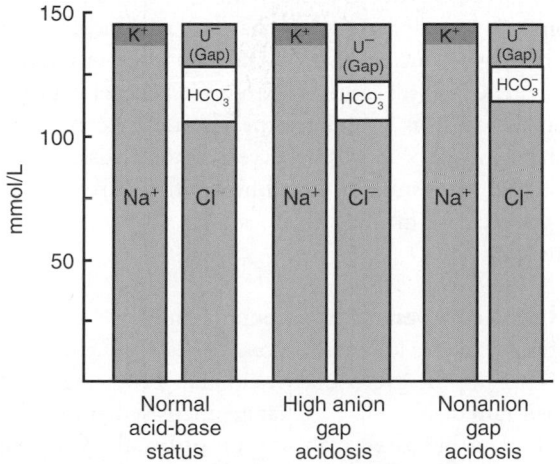

Figure 35-9   Simple "Gambelgram" depiction of normal gap acidosis, anion gap acidosis, and nonanion gap acidosis. Cations, Na^+, and K^+ appear in the left bar for each condition, whereas measured (Cl^- and HCO_3^-) and unmeasured (U^-) anions are in the right bar for each condition. HCO_3^-, Bicarbonate.

to be due to the participation of the respiratory center in lactic acid production and the resulting greater local acidification of the respiratory center.

Lactate in spinal fluid normally parallels blood levels. In case of biochemical alterations in the CNS, however, CSF lactate values change independently of blood values. Increased CSF levels may be seen in individuals with intracranial hemorrhage, bacterial meningitis, epilepsy, and other CNS disorders.[14]

Ethylene glycol

Ethylene glycol, when ingested, is metabolized to glycolic and oxalic acids and other acidic metabolites. Its metabolism leads to an acidosis with high anion and osmolal gaps. Accumulation of toxic metabolites may contribute to lactic acid production and further contribute to the acidosis. Precipitation of calcium oxalate and hippurate crystals in the urinary tract may lead to acute renal failure. Clinically, individuals develop a variety of neurological symptoms that may lead to coma. Some may develop, either singly or in combination, bronchial pneumonia, pulmonary edema, congestive heart failure, hypertension, or cardiopulmonary arrest.

Salicylate intoxication

Salicylate intoxication generally occurs when blood salicylate concentrations increase above 30 mg/dL. Salicylate, itself an unmeasured anion, alters peripheral metabolism, leading to the production of various organic acids. The process eventually results in a metabolic acidosis with a high anion gap. Salicylate also stimulates the respiratory center to increase the rate and depth of respiration, resulting in a low PCO_2, low HCO_3^-, and respiratory alkalosis (see the later discussion on respiratory alkalosis).

Normal anion gap acidosis (inorganic acidosis)

In contrast to high anion gap acidoses in which bicarbonate is consumed in buffering of excess H^+, the cause of acidosis in the presence of a normal anion gap is the loss of bicarbonate-rich fluid from either the kidney or gastrointestinal tract. As bicarbonate is lost, more Cl^- ions are reabsorbed with Na^+ or K^+ to maintain electrical neutrality so that hyperchloremia ensues (see Figure 35-9). Normal anion gap acidosis can be divided into hypokalemic and normokalemic acidoses, which can be helpful in the differential diagnosis of this type of acidosis (see Table 35-4).

Diarrhea

Diarrhea may cause acidosis as a result of loss of Na^+, K^+, and HCO_3^-. One of the primary exocrine functions of the pancreas is the production of HCO_3^- to neutralize gastric contents on their entry into the duodenum. If the water, K^+, and HCO_3^- in the intestine is not reabsorbed, a hypokalemic, normal anion gap metabolic acidosis develops. The resulting hyperchloremia is due to the replacement of lost bicarbonate with Cl^- to maintain electrical balance.

Renal tubular acidosis, types I and II

RTA syndromes are characterized predominantly by a loss of bicarbonate due to decreased tubular secretion of H^+ (distal, or type I, RTA) or decreased reabsorption of HCO_3^- (proximal, or type II, RTA). Recall that the major urine-acidifying power of the kidneys rests in the distal tubules; thus the proximal and distal RTAs may be differentiated by measurement of urine pH. In proximal RTA, urine pH becomes less than 5.5, whereas in distal RTA the distal tubules are compromised and urine pH is greater than 5.5.[8]

Hyperkalemic normal anion gap acidosis (renal tubular acidosis type IV)

Failure of the kidneys to synthesize renin, failure of the adrenal cortex to secrete aldosterone, and renal tubular resistance to aldosterone are the most common causes of hyperkalemic normal anion gap acidosis, often called *type IV RTA*. This condition inhibits Na^+ reabsorption, and both K^+ and H^+ thus are retained abnormally. The result is decreased renal ammonia formation and therefore decreased elimination of H^+. Urine still may be acidified to a pH less than 5.5. Hyperkalemia also usually is present.

Compensatory mechanisms of metabolic acidosis

Table 35-3 depicts the expected **compensation** mechanisms in both acidoses and alkaloses and the corresponding laboratory values.

Respiratory compensatory mechanism

The buffer systems of the blood (mainly the bicarbonate/carbonic acid buffer) minimize changes in pH. In cases of acidoses the bicarbonate concentration is decreased to give a ratio of $cHCO_3^-/cdCO_2$ less than the normal 20/1. The respiratory compensatory mechanism responds to correct the ratio with increased rate and depth of respiration to eliminate CO_2 (see Figure 35-6). The decrease in pH in metabolic acidosis stimulates the respiratory compensatory mechanism and produces hyperventilation (Kussmaul respiration), which results in the elimination of carbonic acid as CO_2, a decrease in PCO_2 (hypocapnia), and consequently, a decrease in $cdCO_2$.

Renal compensatory mechanism

If possible, the kidneys respond to restore the normal pH by increasing the excretion of acid and preserving base (increased rate of Na^+-H^+ exchange, increased ammonia formation, and increased reabsorption of bicarbonate). When the renal compensating mechanisms are functioning, urinary acidity and urinary ammonia are increased. The total amount of H^+ excreted may be as much as 500 mmol/day. As a result, $cHCO_3^-$ increases, for example, to 22/1.1 or 20/1 for a pH of 7.40.

Metabolic Alkalosis (Primary Bicarbonate Excess)

Alkalosis can occur either when excess base is added to the system, base elimination is decreased, or acid-rich fluids are lost (Table 35-5). In **metabolic alkalosis,** any of these occurrences can lead to a primary bicarbonate excess so that the ratio of $HCO_3^-/cdCO_2$ becomes greater than 20/1. For instance, a primary increase in bicarbonate to 48 mmol/L alters the $HCO_3^-/cdCO_2$ to 48/1.5 or 32/1 for a pH of 7.6 (see Figure 35-6). The individual hypoventilates to raise the PCO_2 and therefore lower the pH toward normal. Hypoxia usually prevents the individual from achieving a PCO_2 greater than 55 mm Hg.

If the increase in pH is great enough, increased neuromuscular activity may be noticeable, and above pH 7.55, tetany may develop even in the presence of a normal serum total calcium concentration. The cause of the tetany is a decreased concentration of free ionized calcium due to increased binding of calcium ions by protein and other anions. Measurement of Cl^- status can be helpful because the causes of metabolic alkalosis fall into Cl^- responsive, Cl^-

resistant, and exogenous base categories (see Table 35-5 and Figure 35-3).

Chloride-responsive metabolic alkalosis

Most causes of Cl^- responsive metabolic alkalosis are accompanied by hypovolemia (see Table 35-5). When the ECF is depleted, the acid-base disorder is often referred to as "contraction alkalosis." Renal bicarbonate retention occurs in response to hypovolemia under the action of increased aldosterone. This retention also results in increased reabsorption of Na^+, together with HCO_3^-, and excretion of K^+ and H^+. The resulting hypokalemia contributes to the alkalosis. Urine Cl^- is less than 10 mmolL because both the available Cl^- and HCO_3^- are reabsorbed with Na^+. Common causes of contraction alkalosis include prolonged vomiting or nasogastric suction, pyloric or upper duodenal obstruction, villous adenoma (unregulated secretion of HCl), and the use of certain diuretics that lead to excessive Na^+ and Cl^- excretion. Treatment consists of TBW replacement with water and sodium chloride (NaCl) tablets or saline infusion.

Chloride-resistant metabolic alkalosis

Cl^- resistant metabolic alkalosis is far less common than Cl^- responsive metabolic alkalosis and is associated almost always with either an underlying disease (for example, primary hyperaldosteronism, Cushing's syndrome) or excess addition of exogenous base.

Mineralocorticoid or glucocorticosteroid excess

In states of adrenocortical excess (endogenous or pharmacological, primary or secondary) K^+ and H^+ are "wasted" by the kidneys as a consequence of the increased Na^+ reabsorption stimulated by elevated aldosterone or cortisol. The attendant hypokalemia often further contributes to the alkalosis. The decreased tubular K^+ concentration stimulates NH_3 production and thus renal H^+ excretion as NH_4^+. Diseases in which endogenous mineralocorticoids, glucocorticoids, or both are elevated include primary and secondary hyperaldosteronism, bilateral adrenal hyperplasia, pituitary adrenocorticotropic hormone (ACTH)-producing adenoma (Cushing's disease), and primary adrenal adenomas producing glucocorticoids (Cushing's syndrome) or aldosterone.

Exogenous base

Examples of excess exogenous base include citrate toxicity after massive blood transfusion, aggressive intravenous therapy with bicarbonate solutions, and ingestion of large quantities of milk and antacids in the treatment of gastritis and peptic ulcers ("milk-alkali syndrome"). The latter is seen far less commonly since the introduction and now widespread use of H_2-receptor antagonists and antibiotic treatment for *Helicobacter pylori* infection. Finally, the use of antacids and cationic exchange resins in individuals with renal

---

TABLE 35-5   Conditions Leading to Metabolic Alkalosis

Chloride-Responsive (Urine $Cl^- < 10$ mmol/L)
Contraction alkaloses
  Prolonged vomiting or nasogastric suction
  Pyloric or upper duodenal obstruction
  Prolonged or abusive diuretic therapy (loop diuretics)
  Villous adenoma
Posthypercapnic state
Cystic fibrosis (systemic ineffective reabsorption of Cl^-)

Chloride-Resistant (Urine $Cl^- > 20$ mmol/L)
Mineralocorticoid excess
  Primary hyperaldosteronism (adrenal adenoma or rarely, carcinoma)
  Bilateral adrenal hyperplasia
  Secondary hyperaldosteronism
  Hyperreninemic hyperaldosteronism (hypertension)
  Congenital adrenal hyperplasia (due to adrenal enzyme deficiencies in cortisol production [11β- or 17α-hydroxylase])
Glucocorticoid excess
  Primary adrenal adenoma (Cushing's syndrome)
  Pituitary adenoma secreting ACTH (Cushing's disease)
  Exogenous cortisol therapy
  Excessive licorice ingestion
Bartter's syndrome (defective renal Cl^- reabsorption)

Exogenous Base
Iatrogenic
  Bicarbonate-containing intravenous fluid therapy
  Massive blood transfusion (sodium citrate overload)
  Antacids and cation-exchange resins in dialysis patients
  High-dose carbenicillin or penicillin (associated with hypokalemia)
Milk-alkali syndrome

ACTH, Adrenocorticotropin hormone.

failure (especially those on dialysis) may result in a metabolic alkalosis.

Compensatory mechanisms for metabolic alkalosis

The compensatory mechanisms for metabolic alkalosis include both respiratory compensation and, if physiologically possible, renal compensation.

Respiratory compensatory mechanism

The increase in pH depresses the respiratory center, causing a retention of carbon dioxide (hypercapnia), which in turn causes an increase in cH_2CO_3 and $cdCO_2$. Thus the ratio of $cHCO_3^-/cdCO_2$, which originally was increased, approaches its normal value, although the actual levels of both $cHCO_3^-$ and $cdCO_2$ remain increased. The respiratory response to metabolic alkalosis is erratic, and increases in PCO_2 are variable.

Renal compensatory mechanism

The kidneys respond to the state of alkalosis through a decreased Na^+-H^+ exchange, decreased formation of ammonia, and decreased reclamation of bicarbonate. This response is blunted, however, in the conditions of hypokalemia and hypovolemia.

Respiratory Acidosis

Any condition that decreases elimination of carbon dioxide through the lungs results in an increase in PCO_2 (hypercapnia) and a primary excess of dCO_2, which is seen as an increased PCO_2 (respiratory acidosis). Thus respiratory acidosis can only occur by decreased elimination of CO_2 (or inhalation of excess CO_2). Causes of decreased CO_2 elimination can be classified as acute or chronic (Table 35-6). These conditions may be separated further into those caused by factors that directly depress the respiratory center (such as centrally acting drugs, CNS trauma, and infections) and those that affect the respiratory apparatus or cause mechanical obstruction of the airways. Chronic obstructive pulmonary disease (COPD) is the most common cause. Cardiac disease also may cause respiratory acidosis, although generally it causes a slight respiratory alkalosis because the hypoxemia (caused by increased pulmonary shunting) stimulates hyperventilation. Rebreathing, or breathing air high in CO_2 content, also may produce a high PCO_2. An increase in PCO_2 results in an increase of $cdCO_2$ (and thus H_2CO_3, which dissociates to H^+ and HCO_3^-), which in turn causes a decrease in the $cHCO_3^-/cdCO_2$ ratio (for example, the ratio may be 28/1.7 or 16/1 for a pH of approximately 7.30; see Figure 35-6). A doubling of PCO_2 causes a fall in pH of about 0.23 when extracellular base excess remains constant.

Compensatory mechanisms for respiratory acidosis

Compensation for respiratory acidosis occurs immediately via buffers and with time via the kidneys and, if possible, the lungs.

TABLE 35-6 Conditions Leading to Respiratory Acidosis

Factors that Directly Depress the Respiratory Center
Drugs, such as narcotics and barbiturates
CNS trauma, tumors, and degenerative disorders
Infections of the CNS, such as encephalitis and meningitis
Comatose states, such as cerebrovascular accident due to intracranial hemorrhage
Primary central hypoventilation

Conditions that Affect the Respiratory Apparatus
Chronic obstructive pulmonary disease (most common cause)
Pulmonary fibrosis
Status asthmaticus (severe)
Diseases of the upper airways, such as laryngospasm or tumor
Pulmonary infections (severe)
Impaired lung motion due to pleural effusion or pneumothorax
Adult respiratory distress syndrome
Chest wall diseases and deformities
Neurological disorders affecting the muscles of respiration

Others
Abdominal distention, as in peritonitis and ascites
Extreme obesity (Pickwickian syndrome)
Sleep disorders, such as sleep apnea

CNS, Central nervous system.

TABLE 35-7 Factors Causing Respiratory Alkalosis

Nonpulmonary Stimulation of Respiratory Center
Anxiety, hysteria
Febrile states
Gram-negative septicemia
Metabolic encephalopathy (for example, due to liver disease)
CNS infections, such as meningitis, encephalitis
Cerebrovascular accidents
Intracranial surgery
Hypoxia (for example, severe anemia, high altitudes [acute condition])
Drugs and agents, such as salicylates, catecholamines, and progesterone
Pregnancy, mainly third trimester ($\uparrow$ progesterone?)
Hyperthyroidism

Pulmonary Disorders*
Pneumonia
Asthma
Pulmonary emboli
Interstitial lung disease
Large right to left shunt (PCO_2 <50 mm Hg)
Congestive heart failure
Respiratory compensation after correction of metabolic acidosis

Other
Ventilator-induced hyperventilation

CNS, Central nervous system.
*The severe stages of some of these disorders may be associated with respiratory acidosis if elimination of CO_2 is impaired severely.

Buffer system

Excess carbonic acid present in blood is buffered to a great extent by the hemoglobin and protein buffer systems. The buffering of CO_2 causes a slight rise in $cHCO_3^-$. Thus in the immediate posthypercapnic state this compensation may appear as a metabolic alkalosis (see Table 35-5).

Respiratory mechanism

The increase in P_{CO_2} stimulates the respiratory center and results in increased pulmonary rate and depth of respiration, provided that the primary defect is not in the respiratory center. The elimination of carbon dioxide through the lungs results in a decrease in $cdCO_2$, and thus the ratio of $cHCO_3^-/cdCO_2$ and pH approaches normal.

Renal mechanism

The kidneys respond to respiratory acidosis in the same way that they do to metabolic acidosis—namely, with increased Na^+-H^+ exchange, increased ammonia formation, and increased reclamation of bicarbonate. In an individual with partially compensated chronic respiratory acidosis at steady state, the plasma pH is returned about halfway toward normal, as compared with the acute (uncompensated) situation. Renal compensation is not effective before 6 to 12 hours and is not optimal until 2 to 3 days. In a state of chronic respiratory acidosis, such as occurs in individuals with COPD, full renal compensation may be seen even in those individuals with very high P_{CO_2} (>50 mm Hg). However, these severe COPD patients often present with a superimposed metabolic alkalosis arising from a variety of causes, such as prolonged administration of diuretics.

Respiratory Alkalosis

A decrease in P_{CO_2} (hypocapnia) and the resulting primary deficit in dCO_2 (respiratory alkalosis) are caused by an increased rate or depth of respiration, or both. Therefore the basic cause of respiratory alkalosis is excess elimination of acid via the respiratory route. Excessive elimination of carbon dioxide reduces the P_{CO_2} and causes an increase in the $cHCO_3^-/cdCO_2$ ratio (due to decrease in $cdCO_2$). This increase in the ratio shifts the normal equilibrium of the bicarbonate/carbonic acid buffer system, reducing the hydrogen ion concentration and increasing the pH. This shift also results in a decrease in $cHCO_3^-$, which somewhat ameliorates the change in pH. In a state of respiratory alkalosis the compensation is very efficient and returns the pH almost to the original value.

Analogous to causes of respiratory acidosis, causes of respiratory alkalosis can be classified as those with direct stimulatory effects on the respiratory center and those caused by effects on the pulmonary system. These and some additional conditions underlying respiratory alkalosis are listed in Table 35-7.

Compensatory mechanisms for respiratory alkalosis

The compensatory mechanisms respond to respiratory alkalosis in two stages. In the first stage, erythrocyte and tissue buffers provide H^+ ions that consume a small amount of HCO_3^-. The second stage becomes operational in a state of prolonged respiratory alkalosis and depends on the renal compensation as described for metabolic alkalosis (decreased reclamation of bicarbonate).

References

1. Albert MD, Dell RB, Winters RW: Quantitative displacement of acid-base equilibrium in metabolic acidosis. Ann Intern Med 1967; 66:312-322.
2. Bockelman HW, Cembrowski GS, Kurtycz DFI et al: Quality control of electrolyte analyzers: evaluation of the anion gap average. Am J Clin Pathol 1984; 81:219-223.
3. Cembrowski GS, Westgard JO, Kurtycz DFI: Use of anion gap for the quality control of electrolyte analyzers. Am J Clin Pathol 1983; 79:688-696.
4. Dufour DR: Acid-base disorders. In Dufour DR, Christenson RH (eds): Professional Practice in Clinical Chemistry: A Review, pp 604-635, Washington DC, AACC Press, 1999.
5. Gabow PA, Kaehny WD, Fennessey WD et al: Diagnostic importance of an increased serum anion gap. N Engl J Med 1980; 303:854-858.
6. Halperin ML, Ethier JH, Kamel KS: The excretion of ammonium ions and acid base balance. Clin Biochem 1990; 23:185-188.
7. Haycock GB: The syndrome of inappropriate secretion of antidiuretic hormone (review). Pediatr Nephrol 1995; 9:375-381.
8. Lash JP, Arruda JAL: Laboratory evaluation of renal tubular acidosis. Clin Lab Med 1993; 13:117-129.
9. Lippmann BJ: Fluid and electrolyte management. In Ewald GA, McKenzie CR (eds): Manual of Medical Therapeutics, 28th edition, New York, Little, Brown, 1995.
10. McGilvery RW: Biochemistry, pp 778-782, Philadelphia, WB Saunders, 1983.
11. Robertson GL: Diabetes insipidus (review). Endocrinol Metabol Clin North Am 1995; 24:549-572.
12. Rose AM, Valdes R: Understanding the sodium pump and its relevance to disease. Clin Chem 1994; 40:1674-1685.
13. Thrasher TN: Baroreceptor regulation of vasopressin in renin secretion: low pressure vs. high pressure receptors (review). Front Neuroendocrinol 1994; 15:157-196.

14. Watson MA, Scott MG: Clinical utility of biochemical analysis of cerebrospinal fluid. Clin Chem 1995; 41:343-360.

15. Williamson JC: Acid-base disorders: classification and management strategies. Am Fam Physician 1995; 52:584-590.

Additional Reading

Rose BD, Post T: Clinical Physiology of Acid-Base and Electrolyte Disorders, 5th edition, St Louis, McGraw-Hill, 2000.

Siggaard-Andersen O: The Acid-Base Status of the Blood, 4th edition, Baltimore, Williams & Wilkins, 1974.

CHAPTER 36

Liver Function*

KEITH G. TOLMAN, MD, and ROBERT REJ, PhD

Objectives

1. Describe the microscopic and macroscopic anatomy of the hepatic system.
2. Define the following terms:

   Hepatic lobule   Cirrhosis

   Portal triad   Cholestasis

   Jaundice   Cholecystitis

   Viral and chronic hepatitis
3. List and define the major functions of the liver.
4. List the enzymes synthesized in the liver, as well as their functions and clinical significance, and describe the mechanisms of enzyme release.
5. Describe the three specific patterns of liver cell injury and the causes and symptoms of each pattern.
6. Describe how overdose of certain drugs induces hepatic damage.
7. State the laboratory values obtained with each of the following hepatic diseases: acute hepatitis, chronic alcoholism, cirrhosis, Reye's syndrome, Wilson's disease, and cholestasis.

Key Words

Alcoholic Liver Disease   Irreversible liver disease due to the chronic inflammatory and toxic effects of ethanol on the liver

Apoptosis   Programmed cell death signaled by the nuclei when cells achieve the end of their normal life spans or become damaged

Ascites   Serous fluid that accumulates in the abdominal cavity

Bile   A fluid synthesized by the liver and secreted into the duodenum via the bile ducts, the important constituents of which are conjugated bile salts, cholesterol, phospholipid, bilirubin diglucuronide, and electrolytes

Bile Acids   Any of the steroid carboxylic acids synthesized in the liver from cholesterol; primary bile acids, cholic and chenodeoxycholic acids, being conjugated with glycine or taurine forming bile salts (for example, cholylglycine), which are secreted in the bile and aid in the digestion of fats; secondary bile acids, deoxycholic, lithocholic, and ursodeoxycholic acids, being formed from the primary bile acids by the action of intestinal bacteria

Biliary Cirrhosis   A rare form of liver disease in which small intrahepatic bile ducts are destroyed and replaced with scar tissue, ultimately leading to cirrhosis

Biotransformation   The series of enzyme-mediated alterations of a compound (for example, a drug) that occur within the body and that in general convert foreign compounds from lipophilic to hydrophilic substances

*The authors gratefully acknowledge the original contribution by Dr. William Balistreri, on which portions of this chapter are based.

Cholangitis   Inflammation of the bile duct

Cholangitis, Sclerosing   A chronic, nonbacterial inflammation of the bile ducts, ultimately resulting in narrowing of the bile ducts and cirrhosis; about 50% of the cases being associated with ulcerative colitis

Cholestasis   Decreased bile flow resulting from either intrahepatic or extrahepatic causes

Cirrhosis   Liver disease characterized by diffuse interlacing bands of fibrous tissue dividing the hepatic parenchyma into micronodular or macronodular nodules

Gallstone   A calculus or inorganic mass (concretion), usually of cholesterol, formed in the gallbladder or bile duct

Hemochromatosis   A disorder due to deposition of hemosiderin in the parenchymal cells, causing tissue damage and dysfunction of the liver, pancreas, heart, and pituitary

Hepatic Encephalopathy   A neuropsychiatric syndrome occurring secondary to advanced liver disease and manifested by aberrant behavior, which leads to coma

Hepatitis   Inflammation of the liver, usually caused by a virus or drug

Hepatitis, Alcoholic   An acute or chronic inflammatory lesion of the liver in the alcoholic individual

Hepatitis, Viral   Liver inflammation caused by viruses, the types of which include A, B, C, D, E, G, and TTV

Hepatocyte   An epithelial cell found in the liver

Jaundice   A syndrome characterized by hyperbilirubinemia and deposition of bile pigment in the skin, mucous membranes, and sclera, with resulting yellow appearance of the patient; called also *icterus*

Jaundice, Neonatal   A jaundice seen in newborns; also called *icterus neonatorum*

Necrosis   The sum of the morphological changes that indicate cell death

Portal Hypertension   Any increase in portal vein (in the liver) pressure due to anatomical or functional obstruction (for example, alcoholic cirrhosis) to blood flow in the portal venous system

Reye's Syndrome   A rare, acute, and sometimes fatal disease of childhood, most often occurring as a sequela of varicella or a viral upper respiratory infection; also associated with aspirin ingestion

Varices   Enlarged and tortuous veins, arteries, or lymphatic vessels, usually seen in the esophagus or stomach

Wilson's Disease   An autosomal recessive disorder associated with excessive quantities of copper in the tissues, particularly the liver and central nervous system

Xenobiotics   A chemical substance foreign to the biological system

---

The liver performs many diverse functions essential for life. It receives, processes, and stores amino acids, carbohydrates, lipids, vitamins, and minerals. In addition, many of the proteins in plasma, including albumin, α- and β-globulins, coagulation factors, and transport proteins, are synthesized by the liver. The liver is also the primary site of detoxification of exogenous compounds, such as drugs and toxins.[9] This process, known as **biotransformation,** converts lipophilic substances to hydrophilic ones for subsequent elimination. Another major liver function is the conjugation of birubin with glucuronic acid to produce bilirubin monoglucuronides and diglucuronides, which then are excreted into **bile** (see Chapter 30). The liver also is responsible for the synthesis of bile acids from cholesterol and the secretion of these compounds into the bile, thus regulating cholesterol metabolism and facilitating the absorption of dietary fat. The liver is a major site of catabolism of thyroid, steroid, and other hormones, and thereby helps regulate plasma hormone levels. Many of these specific hepatic functions are assessed by laboratory procedures.

This chapter includes discussions of the anatomy, biochemistry, and pathophysiology of the liver. It concludes with a discussion of relevant laboratory tests and the principles of their measurement.

■ ANATOMY OF THE LIVER

Gross Anatomy

The liver weighs 1.2 to 1.5 kg and is the largest organ in the body. It is located beneath the diaphragm in the right upper quadrant of the abdomen and is protected by the ribs. It is divided into left and right anatomical lobes (Figure 36-1). Two smaller lobes are found on the posterior surface (caudate lobe) and inferior surface (quadrate lobe) of the right lobe. The liver is supplied by the left and right branches of the portal vein and the hepatic artery. The venous drainage is into the hepatic veins, whereas the biliary drainage is into the left and right hepatic ducts. Glisson's capsule, a thin connective tissue, covers the entire liver surface. Connective tissue provides an internal supportive framework for the liver parenchyma, branches to ensheathe vessels and nerves, and subdivides the parenchyma into lobules.

The liver has a dual blood supply—(1) the portal vein that carries nutrient-rich blood from the capillary bed of the alimentary tract and (2) the hepatic artery, which carries well-oxygenated blood from the central circulation to the liver. Venous drainage from the liver is via the right and left hepatic veins, which enter into the inferior vena cava near the right atrium.

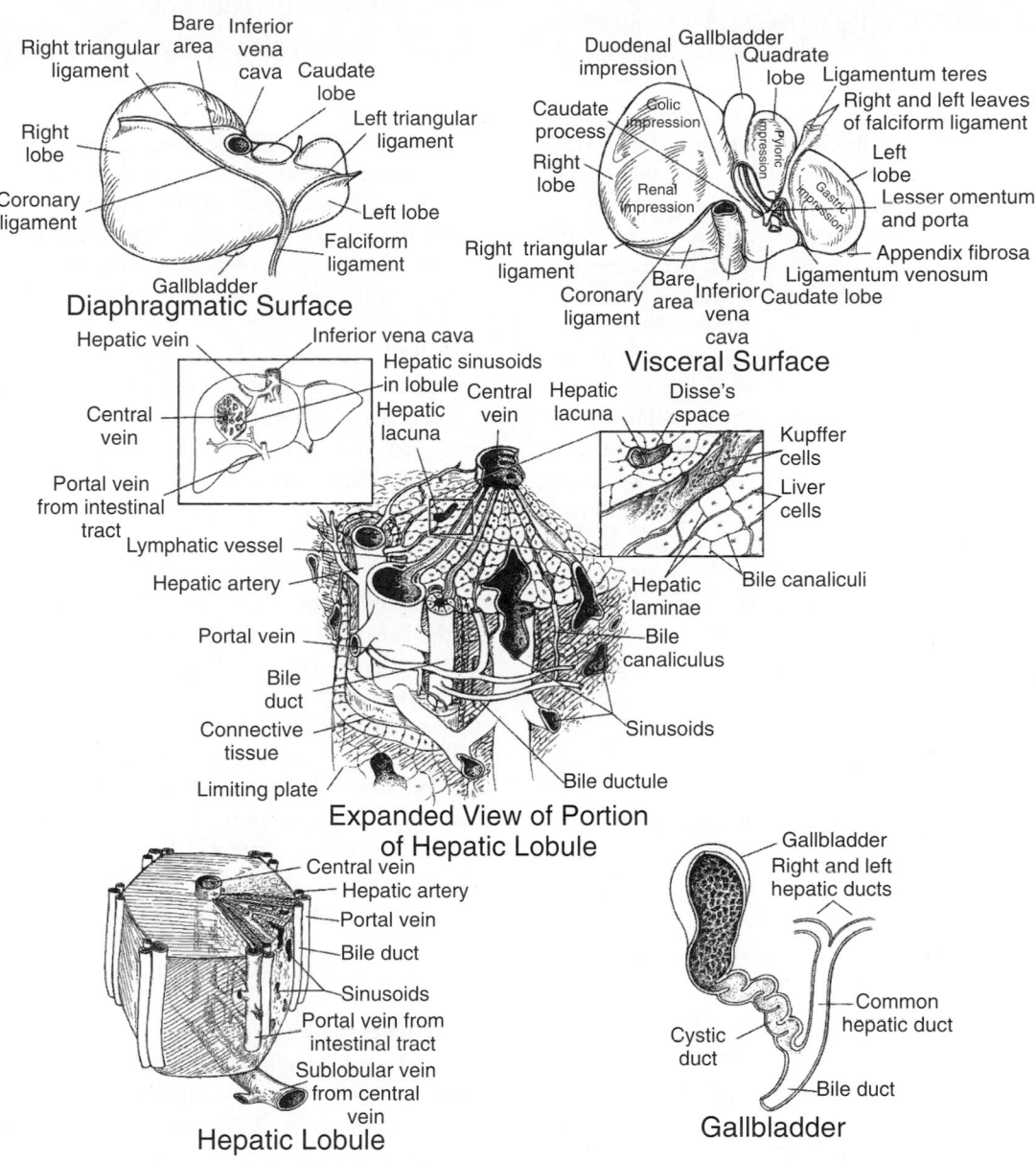

Figure 36-1   Structure of the liver. (Modified from Dorland's Illustrated Medical Dictionary, 28th edition, p 954, Philadelphia, WB Saunders, 1994.)

The portal triad consists of bile ducts that accompany the hepatic artery and portal vein (see Figure 36-1). Bile flows from the hepatocytes into the bile canaliculi and ductules, to the larger intrahepatic bile ducts, and finally to the left and right hepatic bile ducts, which emerge from the liver at the porta hepatis and form the common hepatic duct. The hepatic duct is joined by the cystic duct from the gallbladder to form the common bile duct. The common bile duct and pancreatic duct enter the duodenum at the ampulla of Vater.

The gallbladder is divided into four segments—the neck, infundibulum, body, and fundus. The neck is a transitional zone between the infundibulum and cystic duct. The infundibulum is the transitional area between the body and neck and is attached to the duodenum by a ligament. Hartmann's pouch is an inferior diverticulum of the infundibulum. The body is the largest part of the gallbladder. The fundus is directed forward and may be palpable on abdominal examination if enlarged. The gallbladder itself, in the adult, is 9 to 10 cm long and has a capacity of 50 mL. The gallbladder receives blood from the cystic artery, a large branch of the hepatic artery. The venous drainage is via the cystic vein into the portal venous system.

Microscopic Anatomy

The liver is composed of a large number of functional units or lobules. The classic liver lobule is a polyhedral prism of tissue demarcated by connective tissue septa and the vascular and biliary vessels (see Figure 36-1). The central vein (terminal hepatic vein) is in the center of the lobule. Single cell plates of parenchymal epithelial cells radiate from the central vein. The sinusoids are blood-carrying vascular channels on either side of the liver cell plates; they form a rich, intralobular, vascular network that converges toward the central vein. The sinusoidal lining cells are either endothelial cells or Kupffer cells. The tissue spaces between the endothelial cells and hepatocytes—the space of Disse—contain interstitial fluid, across which the transfer of nutrients and waste products from the blood and liver cells occurs.

Hepatocytes are polygonal cells approximately 30 μm in diameter that constitute about 60% of the liver mass. These cells are the metabolic factory of the liver. The surface of a hepatocyte is specialized into three areas—(1) the sinusoidal surface, which faces the incoming blood (sinusoid and space of Disse); (2) the intercellular surface, contiguous with the sinusoidal surface; and (3) the canalicular surface. The space of Disse is a tissue space between the sinusoids and surrounding hepatocytes. It contains fat-storing cells (Ito cells) that transform into fibroblasts, which synthesize collagen, leading to fibrosis during liver injury. They also regulate portal blood flow.

Ultrastructure of the Hepatocyte

Hepatic parenchymal cells contain the following structures:

1. Numerous mitochondria that participate in energy generation through oxidative phosphorylation and fatty acid oxidation
2. Lysosomes, which contain proteolytic enzymes and have specific degradative functions
3. The endoplasmic reticulum (ER), the site of many functions, including bile acid synthesis and drug metabolism

The smooth ER assumes the form of tubules and vesicles and is the site of bilirubin conjugation, drug detoxification, and cholesterol synthesis. The rough ER forms lamellar profiles lined with ribosomes, which are the site of the specific synthesis of proteins such as albumin, coagulation factors, and various enzymes.

4. The multifunctional Golgi complex, which produces very–low-density lipoproteins and is involved in glycosylation of proteins and albumin secretion
5. Microtubules and microfilaments that maintain cell shape and provide contractile force

■ BIOCHEMICAL FUNCTIONS OF THE LIVER

The liver is a multifunctional organ involved in a number of excretory, synthetic, and metabolic functions. Clinical laboratories perform many tests that are useful in the biochemical assessment of these functions.

Hepatic Excretory Function

Organic anions of both endogenous and exogenous origin are extracted from the sinusoidal blood, biotransformed, and excreted into the bile or urine. Assessment of this excretory function provides valuable clinical information. The most frequently used tests involve the measurement of serum concentrations of endogenously produced compounds, such as bilirubin and bile acids, and determination of the rate of clearance of exogenous compounds, such as indocyanine green or aminopyrine.

Bilirubin

Bilirubin is the yellow pigment derived from senescent red blood cells. It is extracted and biotransformed in the liver and then excreted in bile and urine. The chemistry, biochemistry, and analytical methodology for bilirubin and related compounds are reviewed in Chapter 30.

Bile acids

The regulation of bile acid metabolism is a major function of the liver. Cholesterol homeostasis is maintained in large part by the conversion of cholesterol to bile acids and the subsequent regulation of bile acid metabolism. **Bile acids** themselves provide surface-active detergent molecules that facilitate both hepatic excretion of cholesterol and solubilization of lipids for intestinal absorption. Bile acid homeostasis requires normal terminal ileum function to absorb bile acids for recirculation—the so-called enterohepatic circulation. Alterations in hepatic bile acid synthesis, intracellular metabolism, excretion, intestinal absorption, or plasma extraction are reflected in derangements in bile acid metabolism.

Synthesis of bile acids

Cholesterol is synthesized continually by all tissues but primarily by the liver and small intestine. It is the substrate for many hormones. A portion of cholesterol is converted in the liver to highly polar bile acids, which are secreted subsequently in bile, preventing cholesterol accumulation, which carries the risk of atherosclerosis. This transformation and the ability of bile acids to solubilize additional cholesterol in bile are the major mechanisms of cholesterol elimination from the body.

The products of cholesterol metabolism are cholic acid and chenodeoxycholic acid, which together are termed *primary bile acids* because of their hepatic origin. (The sequence of reactions involved in the synthesis of bile acids from cholesterol is shown in Chapter 24, Figure 24-6.) Before they are secreted into the bile canaliculi, the primary bile acids are conjugated at the carboxylic acid carbon with either glycine or taurine; this action increases their polarity and water solubility (Figure 36-2). Through this mechanism of conjugation, four primary bile acids (cholyltaurine, cholylglycine, chenodeoxycholyltaurine, and chenodeoxycholylglycine) are formed. Conjugation changes the pK_a values of bile acids from approximately 6 to 4 for glycine conjugates and 6 to 2

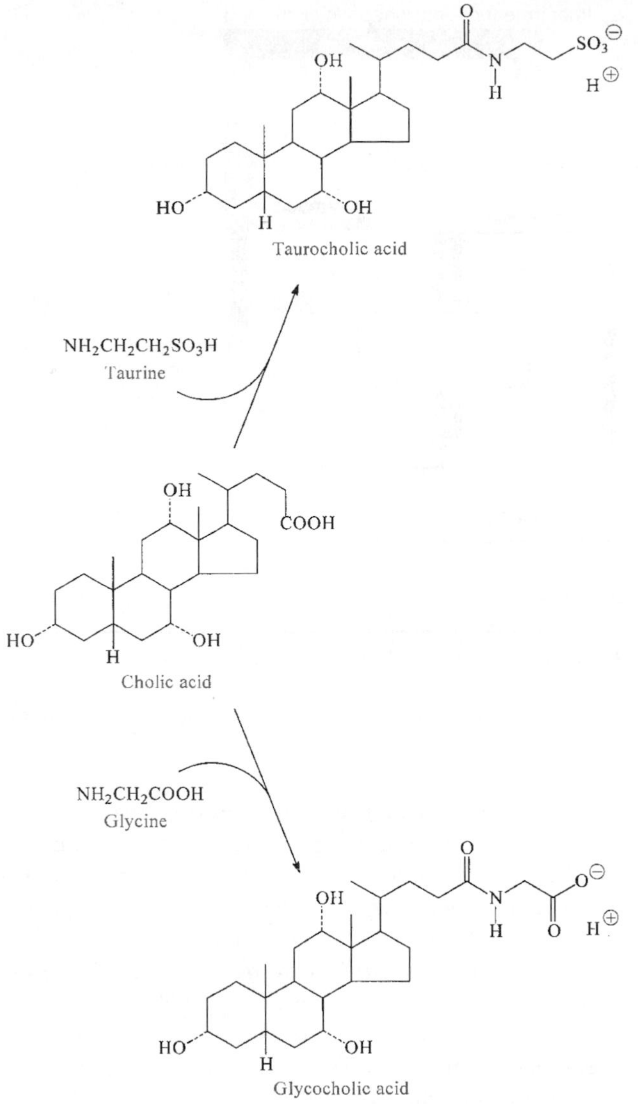

Figure 36-2   Conjugation of cholic acid with either taurine or glycine.

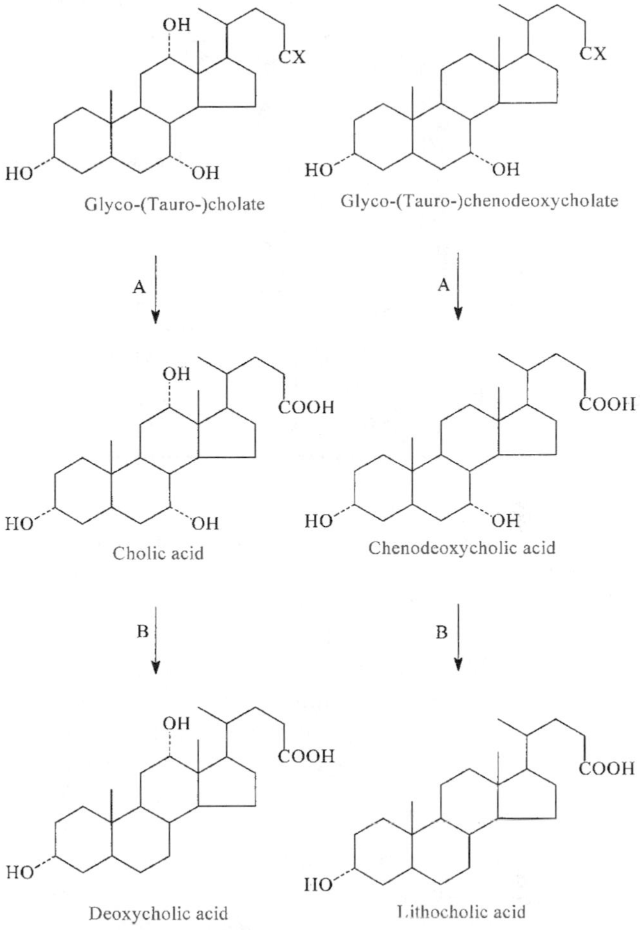

Figure 36-3   Conversion of primary bile acids to secondary bile acids by endogenous microflora. *X*, Glycine or taurine; *A*, bacterial deconjugation; *B*, bacterial transformation (7α-dehydration).

for taurine conjugates. The conjugated bile acids are present in the intestinal lumen in the ionized form because their pK_a values are low, compared with the relatively high pH of the intestinal lumen. In healthy individuals the glycine conjugates predominate in a ratio of approximately 3:1 to 4:1. Unconjugated (free) bile acids are not present in bile.

During passage through the small intestine and colon, bile acid are subject to alterations by enzymes produced by the indigenous bacterial flora, giving rise to the secondary bile acids deoxycholic acid and lithocholic acid (Figure 36-3). Secondary bile acids also are conjugated in the liver with glycine or taurine and join the primary bile acids as components of bile. The average bile acid composition of normal human adult bile is approximately 38% cholate conjugates, 34% chenodeoxycholate conjugates, 28% deoxycholate conjugates, and 1% to 2% lithocholate conjugates.

Hepatic bile formation

Hepatic bile contains 5% to 15% total solids, the major components of which are bile acids. Bile formation occurs in the bile canaliculi, which are specialized modifications of the hepatocyte membrane that ultimately unite to form bile ductules. Transport of bile acids into the bile canaliculi generates osmotic water flow and is a major factor regulating bile formation and secretion. Transport of these organic anions also influences secretion of the remainder of the major components of bile, such as bilirubin, cholesterol, and phospholipids. The latter two compounds do not secrete in the absence of bile acid secretion. The influence of bile acid secretion on biliary lipid excretion is primarily a result of the ability of bile acids to solubilize cholesterol and phospholipids in an aqueous medium in mixed micelles.

Because molecules of bile acids have both polar and nonpolar regions, they can solubilize biliary lipids. Such mol-

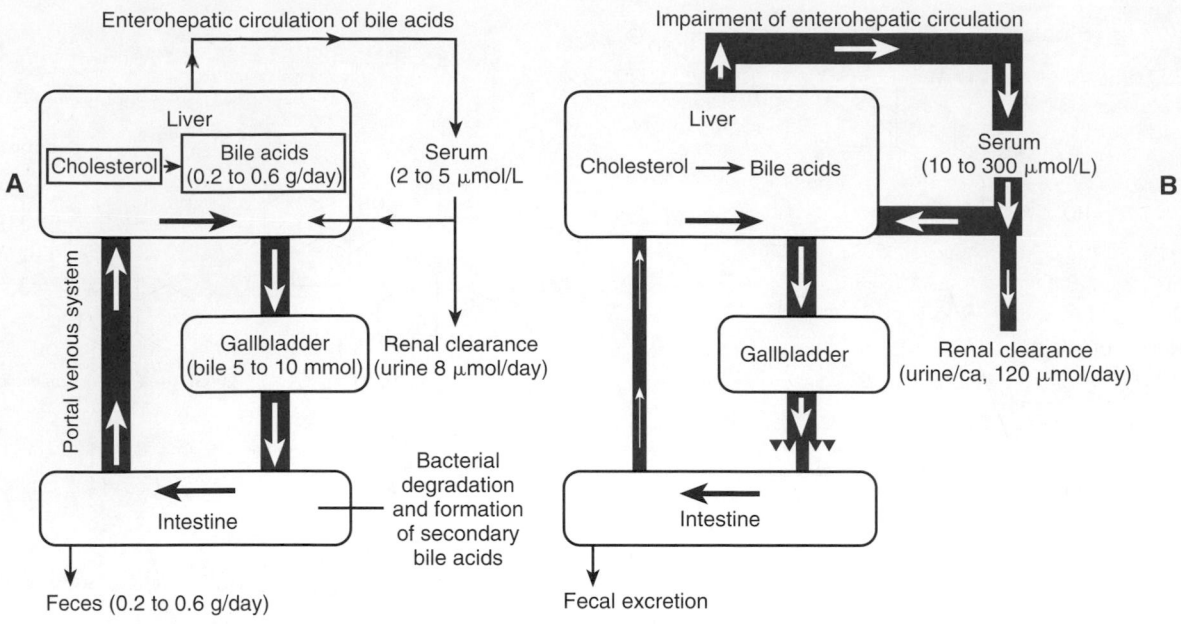

Figure 36-4   Enterohepatic circulation of bile acids. **A,** Normal circulation. **B,** Impaired circulation.

ecules align at water-lipid interfaces and reduce surface tension, thus acting as detergents. In an aqueous solution, bile acids aggregate to form small polymolecular aggregates, approximately 5 nm in diameter, called *micelles;* these aggregates are capable of incorporating cholesterol and phospholipids, and in so doing, maintain cholesterol in solution. Formation of mixed micelles of bile salts and phospholipids enhances the aqueous solubility of cholesterol, a weakly polar compound, and permits cholesterol excretion in bile.

Enterohepatic circulation of bile acids

The body conserves the bile acid pool through a recirculating system known as the *enterohepatic circulation.* The anatomical components of the enterohepatic circulation are the liver, biliary tract, terminal ileum, and portal venous circulation.

During fasting, bile acids are secreted into the bile ducts. They subsequently enter the gallbladder (Figure 36-4), where they undergo a tenfold increase in concentration because of the reabsorption of water and electrolytes by the gallbladder. The bile acids coalesce as micelles, with the lipid-soluble ends directed inward and the water soluble ends directed outward so that the micelles can remain in solution.

In response to food ingestion, cholecystokinin is released, causing the gallbladder to contract and release the micelles into the intestine (see Chapter 37). In the intestinal lumen, dietary cholesterol and the products of triglyceride digestion—predominantly free fatty acids and monoglycerides—are incorporated into the micelles, now known as *mixed micelles.* Micelles facilitate fat absorption in the jejunum by solubilizing the hydrolytic products of fat digestion and delivering those lipolytic products to the mucosal surface. Bile acids are reabsorbed subsequently in the intestine, primarily

in the terminal ileum, and returned via the portal circulation to the liver for recirculation.

Abnormalities of bile acid metabolism

Because of the multiple processes involved in bile acid synthesis, conjugation, and excretion, as well as its hepatic and intestinal uptake, several potential sites exist for primary or secondary disturbances (Table 36-1).

Abnormalities of bile acid delivery to the bowel.
Decreased bile flow from intrahepatic cholestasis or extrahepatic bile duct obstruction due to biliary atresia, stricture, stone, or carcinoma result in bile acid retention and regurgitation from the liver cell into plasma, as well as in a decrease in delivery to the intestine.

Interruption of the enterohepatic circulation of bile acids.   Approximately 95% of the bile acids secreted during a single enterohepatic cycle are recirculating bile acids. Therefore a significant interruption of this cycle leads to a decrease in hepatic bile acid secretion. A negative-feedback increase in bile acid synthesis can compensate only partially for the losses. Resection, inflammation, or bypass of the ileum is associated with specific clinical symptoms and disturbances of bile acid metabolism. The amount of bile acid returned to the liver is reduced, and a loss of feedback inhibition results in accelerated hepatic synthesis of bile acids. The concentration of serum cholesterol is reduced because an increased proportion of this particular compound is used for bile acid synthesis. Levels of serum bile acids decrease and are a reflection of ileal dysfunction because the expected postprandial rise (due to ileal absorption of bile acids) is not present.[2]

Disturbances of bile acid metabolism with hepatocellular disease.   Fasting serum bile acid levels are elevated in

TABLE 36-1   Disturbances in Bile Acid Metabolism

Defective Bile Acid Synthesis
Specific defects in bile acid synthesis
  Cerebrotendinous xanthomatosis
  Intrahepatic cholestasis (familial neonatal hepatitis)
    3β-hydroxysteroid dehydrogenase/isomerase deficiency
    α^4-3-oxosteroid 5β-reductase deficiency
    C_{24} steroid: 7α-hydroxylase deficiency
  Peroxisomal disorders
    Genetic diseases with a general impairment of numerous peroxi-somal functions and reduced or undetectable peroxisome numbers
      Cerebrohepatorenal (Zellweger's) syndrome
      Infantile Refsum's disease
      Neonatal adrenoleukodystrophy
      Rhizomelic chondrodysplasia punctata
      Hyperpipecolic acidemia
    Genetic diseases with generalized impairment of peroxisomal function but normal number of peroxisomes
      Pseudo-Zellweger's syndrome
    Genetic diseases with a single enzyme defect and a normal number of peroxisomes
      X-linked adrenoleukodystrophy
      Adult Refsum's disease
      Acatalasemia
Acquired defects in bile acid synthesis (nonspecific) secondary to parenchymal liver disease (cholestasis, cirrhosis)

Abnormalities of Bile Acid Delivery to the Bowel
Celiac sprue

Extrahepatic Bile Duct Obstruction
Congenital biliary atresia
Stricture
Stone
Carcinoma

Interruption of the Enterohepatic Circulation of Bile Acids
External bile drainage (fistula)
Ileojejunal exclusion for exogenous obesity or hypercholesterolemia
Cystic fibrosis
Contaminated small bowel syndrome (with bile acid precipitation, increased jejunal absorption, and "short circuiting")
Entrapment of bile acids in intestinal lumen by:
  Cholestyramine
  Trivalent cations
  Fiber

Bile Acid Malabsorption
PRIMARY BILE ACID MALABSORPTION (ABSENT OR INEFFICIENT ILEAL ACTIVE TRANSPORT)
Intractable diarrhea (infancy)
Irritable bowel (adults)

SECONDARY BILE ACID MALABSORPTION
Ileal disease or resection
  Crohn's disease
  Ileal resection
  Ileal bypass
  Radiation enteritis
  Postinfectious enteritis
Exogenous bile acid administration (for example, gallstone dissolution)
Cystic fibrosis

TERTIARY BILE ACID MALABSORPTION
Postcholecystectomy
Renal failure
Drugs

Defective Uptake or Altered Intracellular Metabolism
Parenchymal disease (acute hepatitis, cirrhosis) associated with regurgitation from cells or portosystemic shunting
Cholestasis

---

individuals with hepatocellular diseases, such as hepatitis and cirrhosis. The mechanisms responsible are regurgitation of bile acids from cholestatic hepatocytes and portosystemic shunting. These defects allow the serum levels to rise proportionately much higher than normal after meals.

Analytical methodology

Analytical techniques used to quantify either total or individual bile acids in biological fluids include gas-liquid chromatography (GLC), high-performance liquid chromatography (HPLC), enzymatic assay, radioimmunoassay (RIA), and enzyme-linked immunosorbent assay (ELISA).[10]

Clinical significance

Increased serum bile acid concentrations in the fasting state suggest impaired hepatic uptake or secretion or portosystemic shunting. Thus such measurements may be used as sensitive endogenous clearance tests. However, a diagnosis suggested by an increase in serum bile acid concentrations should be confirmed by standard liver function tests. In a similar manner, abnormal standard liver function tests can be confirmed as indicative of hepatic dysfunction by concomitant measurement of serum bile acids. Serum bile acid measurements may be used serially to monitor individuals with suspected or proven hepatic disease. However, these measurements add little to standard tests of liver function and are used rarely in clinical medicine.

Xenobiotic metabolism and excretion

Xenobiotics are foreign substances that are cleared and metabolized by the liver. Most xenobiotics are lipophilic and require biotransformation by the liver to hydrophilic substances for clearance. Others, such as synthetic dyes, are hydrophobic and either are conjugated directly or excreted intact. In practice the excretion of such dyes is measured and used to indicate liver function. Bromsulfophthalein, indocyanine green, aminopyrine, caffeine, lidocaine, and rose bengal are examples of such dyes. However, with the development of more sensitive and specific indicators of liver disease, the dye excretion tests have become almost obsolete. Details of these dye excretion tests are found in an expanded version of this chapter.[10]

Hepatic Synthetic Function

The liver has an extensive synthetic function and plays a major role in the regulation of carbohydrate, lipid, and protein metabolism (see Chapters 19, 23, and 24). A bidirectional flux of precursors and products, such as glucose, amino acids, free fatty acids, and other nutrients, occurs across the hepatocyte membrane. Normal blood glucose concentrations are maintained during short fasts by the breakdown of hepatic glycogen and during prolonged fasts by hepatic glucose synthesis (gluconeogenesis). The primary sources of carbon atoms for gluconeogenesis are amino acids derived from muscle proteins. The main source of energy from metabolic processes, adenosine triphosphate (ATP), arises from hepatic metabolism of glucose by means of the citric acid and Embden-Meyerhof pathways and via fatty acid oxidation. Protein, triglyceride, fatty acid, cholesterol, and bile acid synthesis also occur within the liver.

Hepatic Metabolic Function

Another important function of the liver is the metabolism of drugs (activation and detoxification), as well as the disposal of exogenous and endogenous substances, such as galactose (see Chapter 23) and ammonia (see Chapter 22). In addition, metabolic abnormalities due to specific, inherited enzyme deficiencies affect the liver. A classic example is galactosemia. In this condition the congenital absence of the galactose-1-phosphate uridyltransferase enzyme allows accumulation of the toxic metabolite galactose-1-phosphate, which causes injury to the liver, brain, and kidneys.

■ CLINICAL MANIFESTATIONS OF LIVER DISEASE

Clinical manifestations of liver disease include jaundice, portal hypertension, bleeding esophageal varices, ascites, portosystemic encephalopathy, altered drug metabolism, nutritional and metabolic abnormalities, disordered hemostasis, and release of enzymes into the blood.

Jaundice

Jaundice is a physical sign characterized by a yellow appearance of the skin and sclera, resulting from deposition of bile pigment. It is the most characteristic clinical manifestation of liver disease and is apparent when the serum bilirubin concentration reaches 2 to 3 mg/dL (34 to 51 μmol/L). Other signs of bilirubin retention, such as the passage of tea-colored urine or acholic (tan-colored) stools, also may

be evident. Jaundice is not specific to liver disease and may indicate other disorders, including hemolysis and disorders of bilirubin metabolism. A classification of jaundice, based on the site of altered bilirubin metabolism, is shown in Table 36-2.

Portal Hypertension

The portal circulation includes the venous outflow of the gastrointestinal (GI) tract, spleen, pancreas, and gallbladder. The portal vein is formed by the union of the splenic vein and the superior mesenteric vein. **Portal hypertension** occurs when an obstruction to portal flow exists anywhere along its course. The causes of obstruction leading to portal hypertension are classified as *presinusoidal, sinusoidal,* or *postsinusoidal.* Presinusoidal portal hypertension is caused most commonly by portal vein thrombosis or schistosomiasis. Sinusoidal hypertension is caused most commonly by cirrhosis. Postsinusoidal hypertension is caused most commonly by hepatic vein thrombosis (Budd-Chiari syndrome), veno-occlusive disease (seen after bone marrow transplantation), and constrictive pericarditis.

The major consequences of portal hypertension are (1) bleeding esophageal varices (enlarged tortuous veins), (2) ascites, and (3) hepatic encephalopathy. The condition also compromises many of the metabolic functions of the liver. Because portal shunting decreases effective perfusion of hepatocytes, synthetic functions also are lost, leading to hypoalbuminemia that predisposes the individual to ascites, hypoprothrombinemia that predisposes to bleeding, and loss of thrombolytic factors, such as antithrombin III, which predisposes to venous thrombosis. Paradoxically, coagulation disorders may lead to portal vein thrombosis.

Bleeding Esophageal Varices

Varices (singular: varix) are enlarged and tortuous veins. The most life-threatening consequence of portal hypertension is the development of varices, which are most prominent in the esophagus and the stomach. They are predisposed to bleeding. Bleeding varices are the leading cause of death in individuals with cirrhosis. Patients typically present with hematemesis.

Ascites

Ascites is the effusion and accumulation of serous fluid in the abdominal cavity. It is the most common presenting symptom in patients with cirrhosis (see later discussion under cirrhosis). Although not life-threatening, ascites is uncomfortable and may compromise respiration. It also may predispose an individual to the development of bleeding esophageal varices and spontaneous bacterial peritonitis, both of which are life threatening.

Many causes of ascites exist, and differentiation of ascites secondary to portal hypertension from ascites of other

TABLE 36-2   Physiological Classification of Jaundice

Unconjugated Hyperbilirubinemia (see Chapter 30)

INCREASED PRODUCTION OF UNCONJUGATED BILIRUBIN FROM HEME
Hemolysis
  Hereditary
  Acquired
Ineffective erythropoiesis
Rapid turnover of increased red blood cell mass (in the neonate)

DECREASED DELIVERY OF UNCONJUGATED BILIRUBIN (IN PLASMA) TO HEPATOCYTE
Right-sided congestive heart failure
Portacaval shunt

DECREASED UPTAKE OF UNCONJUGATED BILIBUBIN ACROSS HEPATOCYTE MEMBRANE
Competitive inhibition
  Drugs
  Others?
Gilbert's syndrome
Sepsis, fasting

DECREASED STORAGE OF UNCONJUGATED BILIRUBIN IN CYTOSOL (DECREASED Y AND Z PROTEINS)
Competitive inhibition
Fever

DECREASED BIOTRANSFORMATION (CONJUGATION)
Neonatal jaundice (physiological)
Inhibition (drugs)
Hereditary (Crigler-Najjar)
  Type I (complete enzyme deficiency)
  Type II (partial deficiency)
Hepatocellular dysfunction
Gilbert's syndrome?

Conjugated Hyperbilirubinemia (Cholestasis)

DECREASED SECRETION OF CONJUGATED BILIRUBIN INTO CANALICULI
Hepatocellular disease
  Hepatitis
  Cholestasis (intrahepatic)
Dubin-Johnson and Rotor syndromes
Drugs (estradiol)

DECREASED DRAINAGE
Extrahepatic obstruction
  Stones
  Carcinoma
  Stricture
  Atresia
Sclerosing cholangitis
Intrahepatic obstruction
  Drugs
  Granulomas
  Primary biliary cirrhosis
  Bile duct paucity
  Tumors

causes is essential. This differentiation is done through analysis of ascitic fluid. The feature that distinguishes portal hypertension is an increase in the serum-to-ascitic fluid albumin gradient. A gradient greater than 1.1 g/dL is diagnostic of ascites caused by portal hypertension.

Portosystemic Encephalopathy

Hepatic encephalopathy is a condition used to describe the deleterious effects of liver failure on the central nervous system (CNS). It is characterized by a wide spectrum of neuropsychiatric dysfunction. It may occur as an acute syndrome in individuals with acute hepatic failure from viral or drug-induced hepatitis (fulminant hepatic failure) or as a chronic syndrome associated with liver failure and cirrhosis (portosystemic encephalopathy). Characteristic of all chronic hepatic encephalopathies is an effective decrease in hepatocyte function and some degree of portosystemic shunting, hence the synonym *portosystemic encephalopathy*.

The clinical syndrome follows a reasonably predictable course. Disturbed consciousness always occurs. It usually starts as hypersomnia and progresses to sleep reversal, in which the individual tends to sleep through the day and be awake at night. Personality changes, irritability, and disturbed social behavior may follow. Although difficult to detect in its early stages, intellectual deterioration occurs and generally progresses to overt confusion. This deterioration is followed by decreased spontaneous movement, apathy, and gradually increasing levels of coma. Neurological abnormalities include slurred speech, a characteristic flapping tremor called *asterixis,* increased muscle tone, and abnormal reflexes. The acute encephalopathy of acute hepatic failure, unlike chronic encephalopathy, progresses rapidly (within hours) and is characterized by cerebral edema, which may result in death.[5]

Diagnosis of hepatic encephalopathy is made on clinical grounds. Serum ammonia levels are helpful only rarely, either for diagnosis or for patient monitoring. An exception is a patient who presents with acute encephalopathy of unknown cause. Elevated ammonia levels in that situation suggest acute hepatic failure or Reye's syndrome.

Altered Drug Metabolism

Because of the liver's central role in drug metabolism and disposition, alterations in drug metabolism often occur in individuals with liver disease. In general this alteration is reflected in delayed metabolism, requiring the interval between drug doses to be increased. Only individuals with evidence of liver failure, such as encephalopathy, coagulopathy, or ascites, need alterations in dosing. In general, individuals with liver disease are not more susceptible to drug-induced liver disease. However, those with alcoholic liver disease who continue to consume alcohol are susceptible to liver injury from acetaminophen, even at therapeutic doses.

Nutritional and Metabolic Abnormalities

Chronic liver disease alters the intake and disposition of nutrients, and individuals with this disease are subject to nutritional imbalance. Severe metabolic and nutritional derangements may occur in the cirrhotic individual, such as alterations in glucose metabolism due to insulin resistance and hypokalemia due to excess renal losses of potassium. Hypoalbuminemia is present frequently due to sinusoidal leakage of albumin into the peritoneal space. In the presence of chronic cholestasis, impaired delivery of bile salts to the duodenum results in malabsorption of lipids and fat-soluble vitamins, leading to deficiencies in vitamins A, D, E, and K (see Chapters 28 and 38).

Disordered Hemostasis

The liver manufactures most of the coagulation factors, as well as the bile salts that are essential for absorption of vitamin K. The liver also clears activated clotting factors from the circulation. Thus chronic liver disease is associated with both a hemorrhagic tendency and hypercoagulable state. Disorders that impair the conversion of fibrinogen into stabilized fibrin also occur in the liver. For example, dysfibrinogenemia leads to prolongation of the partial thromboplastin time.

Disseminated intravascular coagulation occurs with severe acute hepatitis, presumably due to release of tissue thromboplastin and defective clearance of inhibitors, such as antithrombin III and protein C. Thrombocytopenia may contribute to ineffective intravascular coagulation. Individuals with chronic or severe liver disease also may be hypercoagulable due to deficiency of fibrinolytic factors, such as antithrombin III and protein C.

Enzymes Released

Serum levels of numerous cytosolic, mitochondrial, and membrane-associated enzymes are increased in individuals with various forms of liver disease. They include aspartate aminotransferase (AST), alanine aminotransferase (ALT), alkaline phosphatase (ALP), and γ-glutamyltransferase (GGT). Details of the measurement of these enzymes are given in Chapter 20.

The detailed mechanisms by which enzymes are released from the cytosol and mitochondria of hepatocytes into the bloodstream are unknown. Clinical observations and experimental studies have shown that subtle membrane changes are sufficient to allow passage of intracellular enzymes to the extracellular space. A very large concentration gradient between the hepatocyte and the sinusoidal space usually exists for enzymes. Cell damage increases membrane permeability, causing cytosolic enzymes to spill into the sinusoids and from there into the peripheral blood. Permeability of mitochondrial membranes also is increased.

The amount of an enzyme in an individual with a diseased hepatocyte is usually significantly different from that in a normal liver cell. For example, GGT was found to be 20% higher than normal in liver specimens from individuals with acute hepatitis, threefold higher in those with **alcoholic hepatitis** and biliary obstruction, and fourfold higher in individuals with metastatic liver disease. In individuals with chronic liver disease the specific activity of ALT in liver tissue decreases to a significantly greater degree than does that of AST. Thus as liver disease progresses, the ratio of serum AST to ALT increases. On the other hand, in cases of acute hepatitis the intracellular specific activities of both aminotransferases decrease significantly, and the increase in ALT is higher than that of AST, except in cases of alcoholic hepatitis. These changes in aminotransferase patterns in tissue are reflected in the pattern of enzyme activities observed in serum. The current belief is that changes in the aminotransferase pattern in tissue account in part for the higher AST levels, compared to ALT levels, in individuals with alcoholic liver disease; in contrast, ALT levels are usually higher than AST levels in individuals with acute hepatitis.

Clearance of liver enzymes from plasma occurs at variable rates. The half-life of ALT is 47 hours, of cytosolic AST is 17 hours, of ALP is 9.7 days, and of GGT is 4.1 days.

■ DISEASES OF THE LIVER

The diseases that occur in the liver are (1) infectious (for example, viral hepatitis), (2) toxic (for example, alcohol-related disease), (3) genetic (for example, hemochromatosis), (4) immune (for example, autoimmune hepatitis and primary biliary cirrhosis), and (5) neoplastic (for example, hepatocellular carcinoma). **Viral hepatitis** is the third or fourth most common reportable infection in the United States, with 500,000 acute cases per year and more than 4 million individuals chronically infected. The death rate from alcoholic liver disease in the United States is 12,000 individuals each year. The gene prevalence of hemochromatosis is 1 in 15 to 20, with a disease prevalence of 1 in 400 individuals. Hepatocellular carcinoma (HCC) accounts for 7500 deaths per year and worldwide is the third or fourth leading cause of cancer death.

Mechanisms and Patterns of Injury

Cell death occurs by **necrosis** or **apoptosis** (programmed cell death), or both. The target cell determines the pattern of injury, with hepatocyte injury leading to hepatitis and biliary cell injury leading to cholestasis. All cellular injury induces fibrosis as a healing response, with the duration of injury and genetic factors determining whether cirrhosis and ultimately carcinoma occur (Figure 36-5).

Cellular necrosis occurs as the result of an injurious environment ("murder").[8] It is characterized by cellular swelling with loss of membrane integrity. Toxic injury from compounds such as carbon tetrachloride, aspirin, and acetaminophen (Figure 36-6) occurs for the most part by necrosis. As the cell dies, it releases its contents, which evoke an inflammatory response that causes further cell injury from cytokines and toxic oxygen species.

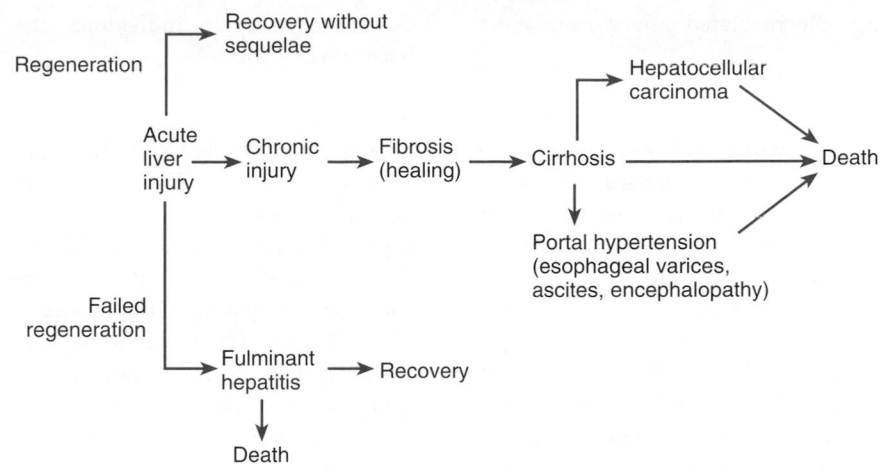

Figure 36-5   Natural history of liver disease.

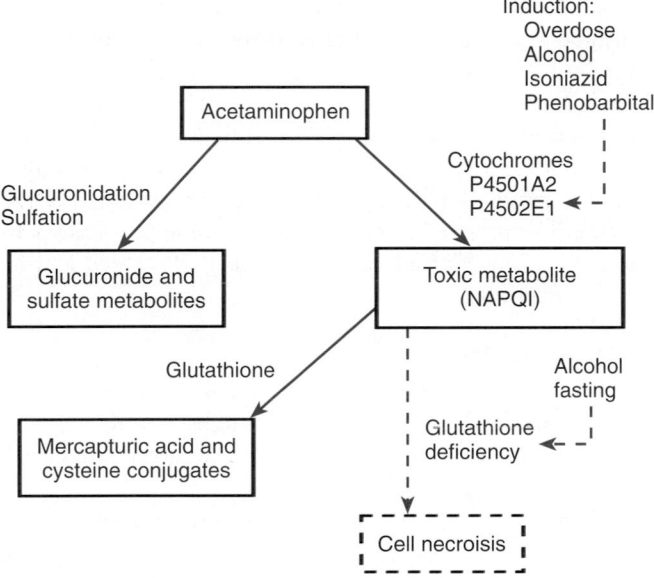

Figure 36-6   Metabolism of acetaminophen by the liver. *NAPQI, N-acetylbenzoquinoneimine.*

Apoptosis occurs as the result of accelerated programmed death, in which the cell participates in its own demise and thus commits "suicide."[6] It is characterized by cell shrinkage, with nuclear chromatin condensation and fragmentation forming apoptotic bodies. The councilman bodies (condensed cosinophilic cytoplasm) found in viral hepatitis and other liver diseases are apoptotic bodies. They are phagocytosed by neighboring epithelial cells and honing mononuclear cells with little if any inflammatory response.

Apoptosis and necrosis may occur together. Whatever the cause of death, but especially with necrosis, intracellular enzymes are released, leading to an increase in the aminotransferase enzymes in serum. The target cell for injury determines the clinical pattern of injury, with hepatocyte injury causing a hepatocellular pattern (with an increase

primarily in aminotransferase enzymes) and vascular and biliary cell injury leading to a cholestatic pattern (with an increase primarily in ALP).

The usual repair response to cell injury is fibrosis. Why this healing process leads to cirrhosis in some individuals but not in others is unknown. For example, only 20% to 25% of heavy consumers of alcohol develop cirrhosis. Genetic factors appear to be involved.

HCC for the most part occurs in the presence of cirrhosis. A wide variation exists in the incidence of HCC in various diseases. For example, hemochromatosis and hepatitis B are associated with a high incidence of HCC, but autoimmune hepatitis and Wilson's disease are associated with a low incidence.

Laboratory tests can help distinguish the pattern of injury (hepatocellular versus cholestatic), the chronicity of injury (acute versus chronic), and severity of injury (mild versus severe). In general the aminotransferase enzymes and ALP are used to distinguish the pattern, serum albumin to determine the chronicity, and the plasma prothrombin time (PT) or factor V concentration to determine the severity. Currently the only way to detect fibrosis is by liver biopsy.

Disorders of Bilirubin Metabolism

Defects in bilirubin metabolism resulting in jaundice occur at each step in the metabolic pathway of bilirubin. Disorders of bilirubin metabolism are discussed in detail in Chapter 30.

Acute Hepatitis

Acute **hepatitis** refers to an acute injury directed against the hepatocytes. The injury may be mediated either directly, as occurs with certain drugs—such as acetaminophen (see Figure 36-6), valproic acid, and isoniazid—or indirectly, as occurs with immunologically mediated injury from most hepatitis viruses.

Toxic hepatitis

Toxins and drugs can cause all patterns of liver disease. The most common drug-induced causes of hepatitis are acetaminophen and nonsteroidal antiinflammatory drugs (NSAIDs). (These causes will be discussed in detail in the section on drug-induced liver diseases.)

Viral hepatitis

Seven viruses have been identified (A, B, C, D, E, G, and TTV) as hepatotropic viruses. In addition, certain other viruses may infect the liver as part of a more generalized infection, among them cytomegalovirus (CMV), Epstein-Barr virus (EBV), and herpes simplex virus (HSV). All forms of acute hepatitis have similar pathological processes (Table 36-3). They are all diagnosed on the basis of marked elevations in aminotransferases, from 4- to 200-fold, with only slight elevations in ALP and little or no decrease in serum albumin levels. More serious disease may manifest in a prolongation of the PT or a decrease in serum albumin. The specific etiological diagnosis is made with serological tests.

Hepatitis A

Hepatitis A virus (HAV) causes a form of viral hepatitis. It is known as *infectious hepatitis* due to its transmission through personal contact with oral secretions or stool. Virus is shed in the stools of an infected individual 2 to 3 weeks before the onset of any symptoms. HAV also may be transmitted sexually. Symptoms are similar to those of influenza, but the skin and eyes may become yellow. Recent travel to a third world country is a risk factor. No specific treatment

exists, but infected individuals should avoid potentially hepatotoxic substances.

HAV accounts for 47% of clinical hepatitis in the United States and 20% to 25% of hepatitis cases worldwide. An immunoglobulin M (IgM) antibody (anti-HAV IgM) appears early in the course of illness and persists for 2 to 6 months. An immunoglobulin G (IgG) antibody (anti-HAV IgG) appears toward the end of the acute illness, persists for several years, and conveys lifelong immunity. HAV occurs in sporadic and epidemic forms, with an incubation period of 15 to 50 days. The incidence of the disease is declining in the developed world as standards of living improve. Most sporadic cases occur from person-to-person contact, such as that in children in day-care centers. Epidemics have been associated with water-borne and food-borne outbreaks. Similar outbreaks have occurred through infected food handlers in restaurants.

The clinical course of acute HAV is usually that of a mild flulike illness that lasts for a few days to a few weeks. It typically goes unrecognized and often is considered to be flu because only 10% of individuals become jaundiced. The disease is more prolonged and serious in individuals over 50 years of age. No chronic form of hepatitis A exists. HAV can be prevented with passive immunization with nonspecific immune serum globulin or active immunization with HAV vaccine. The passive immunization lasts for approximately 6 months. An inactivated vaccine has been developed and is highly effective.

Hepatitis B

Hepatitis B virus (HBV) infects the liver and causes inflammation. HBV is transmitted through body fluids, primarily by parenteral or sexual contact. The carrier rate varies

TABLE 36-3 Types of Viral Hepatitis

Factor	A	B	C	D	E	G
Type	RNA	DNA	RNA	Partial	RNA	RNA
Incubation period (days)	15 to 50	30 to 150	15 to 160	30 to 150	20 to 40	?
Transmission						
Fecal-oral	Yes	No	Min	No	Yes	No
Household	Yes	Min	Min	Yes	Yes	No
Vertical	No	Yes	Min	Yes	No	Yes
Blood	Rare	Yes	Yes	Yes	?	Yes
Sexual	No	Yes	Min	Yes	?	Yes
Diagnosis	Anti-HAV, IgM	HBsAg, PCR, anti-HBc IgM	Anti-HCV, PCR	Anti-HDV	Anti-HEV	Anti-HGV
Carrier state	No	Yes	Yes	Yes	Yes	Yes
Chronic hepatitis	No	10%	80%	Yes	No	No
Liver cancer	No	Yes	Yes	No	No	No
Prevention						
Vaccine	Yes	Yes	No	Yes*	No	No
Immunoglobulin	Yes	Yes	No	Yes*	No	No
Response to interferon	?	50%	20% to 45%	Yes	?	Yes

RNA, Ribonucleic acid; *DNA,* deoxyribonucleic acid; *HAV,* hepatitis A virus; *IgM,* immunoglobulin M; *HBsAg,* hepatic B surface antigen; *PCR,* polymerase chain reaction; *anti-HBc IgM,* hepatitis B core antibody (IgM); *HCV,* hepatitis C virus; *HDV,* hepatitis D virus; *HEV,* hepatitis E virus; *HGV,* hepatitis G virus.
*Vaccination and passive immunization against HBV protects against HDV infection.

from 0.1% to 3% in the developed world to 10% to 15% in sub-Saharan Africa and the Asian subcontinent. An estimated 300 million individuals are infected worldwide. In parts of the world with high carrier rates, most of the transmission is vertical, occurring from mother to newborn child. Male homosexuals have a high infectivity rate. Health-care personnel, especially surgeons and dentists, are at high risk. The residual risk from transfusion is estimated to be 1 in 63,000.

HBV is a 42-nm DNA virus that is a member of the hepadnavirus family. It accounts for 34% of cases of hepatitis in the developed world. The virus consists of a core and a surface envelope. The core is formed in the nucleus of the hepatocyte and contains DNA polymerase, core antigen (HBcAg), and e antigen (HBeAg). The surface particles (HBsAg) are formed in the cytoplasm. The serological course of HBV is illustrated in Figure 36-7.

The development of anti-HBs is associated with recovery and probably lifelong immunity. However, carriers may have persistent HBsAg and anti-HBs, perhaps due to simultaneous infection with different viral subtypes. HBeAg correlates with viral synthesis and implies infectivity. It tends to persist for only a few weeks. Persistence for more than 3 months implies development of chronicity. Anti-HBe is a marker of low or absent infectivity and is strong evidence that recovery will occur. HBV DNA is the most sensitive marker of HBV infection and is detected readily by Southern blot analysis. Polymerase chain reaction (PCR) detection of HBV has been found to correlate with enzyme levels and levels of viremia and is useful in monitoring of patients undergoing treatment.

The clinical course of HBV is similar to that of other types of hepatitis. A characteristic feature of HBV is its propensity to become chronic (see later discussion under chronic hepatitis). Once cirrhosis develops, individuals are susceptible to HCC. On a worldwide basis, HBV is the most common cause of HCC.

HBV may be prevented by either passive (HBV immune globulin [HBIG]) or active (HBV recombinant vaccine) immunization. A universal immunization program in Taiwan has reduced the death rate from HCC.

Hepatitis delta (hepatitis D)

Hepatitis D virus (HDV), also known as the *delta agent*, is a partial virus that requires HBsAg. It is an incomplete, 36-nm RNA particle that cannot replicate on its own. It is coated with HBsAg and depends on HBV for its activation. It is thus a satellite virus similar to those seen in plants. HDV is very infectious and strongly associated with intravenous (IV) drug abuse. It occurs as simultaneous infection with HBV (coinfection) or as superimposed infection in an individual with chronic HBV (superinfection). Coinfection usually runs the same course as the HBV and resolves spontaneously as the HBV resolves. Superinfection often results in a severe course and should be suspected in a chronically infected HBV patient who worsens. It is diagnosed by the finding of anti-HDV IgM, HDVAg, or HDV RNA and anti-HDV IgG in an individual who is HBsAg positive. In individuals with coinfection, anti-HBc IgM may be declining or absent. HBsAg and anti-HBc IgG persist in individuals with superinfection. Treatment is the same as for HBV. HDV reduces the likelihood of HCC development in HCV-infected individuals.

Hepatitis C

Hepatitis C virus (HCV) causes a form of hepatitis, previously referred to as *non-A, non-B hepatitis*. It is the most common form of blood transfusion-acquired hepatitis. Transmission through sexual contact is rare. Risk factors include blood transfusion before 1992, IV drug abuse, or occupational exposure to blood products. A positive test for HCV antibody indicates usually active infection. Unlike HBV, no marker yet can identify those who suffer from chronic HCV.

HCV is highly prevalent in the general population. An estimated 3.9 million individuals in the United States are infected. Worldwide the prevalence is approaching 170 million. Before donor testing was begun, approximately 1.5% of blood donors were infected. Acute HCV accounts for 16% of acute hepatitis cases in the United States but is now on the decline, after peaking in the late 1980s. Because most individuals become chronically infected and the latency period from acquisition of the infection to development of cirrhosis is 20 to 30 years, the disease burden is increasing. In some areas, more than 50% of drug users and hemophiliacs

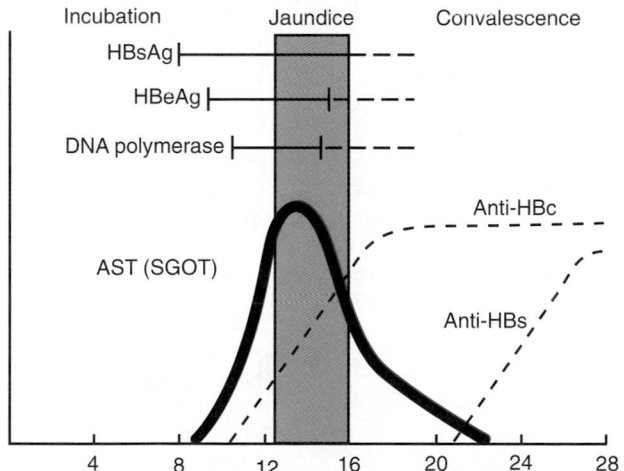

Figure 36-7 Course of acute type B hepatitis with recovery. (1) Onset of hepatitis with jaundice 3 months after exposure; (2) detection of hepatitis B surface antigen (HBsAg) 2 to 8 weeks after exposure, followed by appearance of its antibody (anti-HBs) 2 to 4 weeks after HBsAg is no longer detectable; (3) detection of hepatitis Be antigen (HBeAg) shortly after HBsAg disappears (usually followed by the appearance of antibody to HBeAg [anti-HBe], which persists); (4) detection of hepatitis B core antibody (anti-HBc) at the time of onset of disease 2 to 3 months after exposure. Anti-HBc IgM is detectable in high levels for approximately 5 months. *AST,* Aspartate aminotransferase. (From Balistreri WF: Consultant 1984; 24:131-153.)

are infected. Transmission occurs through blood—primarily in IV drug abusers. Vertical and sexual transmission are relatively inefficient. The risk of infection with a regular sexual partner is 1% to 3% per year. Nevertheless, because of the large number of chronically infected individuals, sexual transmission probably accounts for a large portion of the cases of HCV infection. In community-acquired HCV infection the mode of transmission is unknown. The residual risk from blood transfusion is estimated to be 1 in 103,000.

A number of tests variously referred to as first-, second-, and third-generation ELISA and recombinant immunoblot assay (RIBA) tests have been developed to diagnose HCV infection.[10] These tests, although simple, are compromised by a delay in appearance of the antibody in acutely infected individuals. Qualitative and quantitative PCR tests have proved useful in early detection and subsequent follow-up of infected individuals. Considerable heterogeneity exists in the virus, resulting in distinct subspecies. These subspecies, known as *genotypes,* have different prevalences around the world and some (1a and 1b) may be associated with higher viral loads that are more resistant to therapy. Minor mutations in the virus, known as *quasispecies,* allow the virus to evade immune detection and eradication.

The clinical course of HCV infection is similar to that of other types of viral hepatitis but tends to be mild and unrecognized. Only 25% of individuals are jaundiced, and many are asymptomatic. Fulminant hepatitis is rare. More than 80% of individuals become chronically infected.

Prevention of HCV has proved difficult. Epidemiological approaches have been frustrated by an incomplete knowledge about the mode of transmission. Vaccine development has been compromised because of the many subspecies of virus and its ability to mutate under immune pressure.

Studies have shown that treatment of acute HCV with α-interferon is effective in the prevention of chronic hepatitis in 75% of individuals. Treatment of chronic hepatitis with combination interferon and ribavirin is effective in approximately 50% of individuals.

Hepatitis E

Hepatitis E virus (HEV) causes a form of hepatitis similar to HAV and seen mostly in tropical poor countries. It is a 34-nm, single-stranded, unenveloped RNA virus. Only one species has been identified. It has been detected in stool and serum with a reverse transcription PCR method.[12] HEV accounts for sporadic and epidemic hepatitis in tropical and semitropical countries and in individuals returning from these areas. It has been identified recently in the United States. HEV is transmitted enterically. The virus has been cloned. ELISA IgM and IgG tests have been developed for detection of the virus.

The clinical course of HEV is similar to that of HAV infection in that HEV typically infects young people, has a self-limited course, and is not associated with chronicity. A peculiar feature of this disease is its virulent course in late pregnancy, with mortality rates of 20% to 25%.

Hepatitis G

Hepatitis G virus (HGV), also known as *CBV-C,* is an RNA virus. It has been cloned and is found in 1.5% of the blood supply in the United States. It has a very high infectivity rate in recipients of contaminated blood (>90%) but a very low, if any, disease burden. In fact, little evidence exists to suggest that this virus causes hepatitis. Whether routine testing of donor blood is appropriate has yet to be determined.

Chronic Hepatitis

Chronic hepatitis is defined as a chronic inflammation of the liver that persists for at least 6 months. It is characterized by an ongoing inflammatory assault on the hepatocyte. The causes of chronic hepatitis and the tests used to make a specific etiological diagnosis are listed in Table 36-4.

Chronic hepatitis is a classic immunological disease. Cell-mediated immunity is targeted against the hepatocyte and, for reasons that are unknown, becomes self-perpetuating in some individuals. Other features of autoimmunity or immune complex disease often are present, especially with HCV and autoimmune-type chronic hepatitis.

The clinical features of chronic hepatitis are highly variable. Most individuals are asymptomatic or experience mild fatigue, but crippling exhaustion also occurs. Many patients present with an unexplained abnormality on liver chemistry tests, whereas others may have jaundice. Fatigue is the most common symptom. Moderately elevated aminotransferase activities (twofold to fivefold) are characteristic, and bilirubin levels may be elevated mildly. The ALP concentration is

TABLE 36-4 Causes of Chronic Hepatitis and Diagnostic Strategies

Cause	Diagnosis
Hepatitis B	History, HBsAg, anti-HBs, anti-HBc, HBV DNA
Hepatitis C	Anti-HCV, HCV RNA by PCR
Autoimmune type 1	ANA, ASTHMA
Autoimmune type 2	SLA, anti-LKM₁
Wilson's disease	Ceruloplasmin
Drugs	History
α₁-Antitrypsin deficiency	α₁-AT phenotype
Idiopathic	Liver biopsy, absence of markers

HBV, Hepatitis B virus; *HBsAg,* hepatitis B surface antigen; *anti-HBs,* hepatitis B surface antibodies; *anti-HBc,* hepatitis B core antibody; *HCV,* hepatitis C virus; *anti-HCV,* hepatitis C antibody; *PCR,* polymerase chain reaction; *ANA,* antinuclear antibody; *ASTHMA,* anti-smooth muscle antibody; *SLA,* soluble liver antigen; *LKM₁,* anti-liver-kidney microsomal antibody type 1; *AT,* antitrypsin.

elevated typically less than twofold. Alpha-globulins are increased frequently, and serum albumin levels may be decreased. This type of presentation should lead to an evaluation for chronic hepatitis by use of the tests outlined in Table 36-4. A specific etiological diagnosis is essential because it dictates the treatment. Chronic HBV and HCV are the most common causes of chronic hepatitis.

Chronic hepatitis B

HBV is the most common worldwide cause of chronic hepatitis. Approximately 10% of acutely infected individuals develop chronic hepatitis. The rate is much higher in neonates and younger individuals.

The natural history of chronic HBV is one of slow progression to cirrhosis and, in many individuals, to HCC. Once cirrhosis has developed, the 1- and 5-year survival rates are 84% and 64%, respectively. On a worldwide basis, HBV infection is the most common cause of liver cancer. Most individuals with chronic HBV will be HBsAg positive, anti-HBc positive, HBeAg positive, and anti-HBe negative. AST and ALT levels are elevated moderately, to the 100 to 300 U/L range. Chronic HBsAg carriers with normal aminotransferase levels usually do not have significant disease and have a spontaneous remission rate of approximately 2% to 3% per year. HBV DNA levels are elevated variably. Depending on how advanced the disease is, serum albumin levels may be decreased. The clinical presentation may be complicated by a number of extrahepatic complications, including polyarteritis, glomerulonephritis, polymyalgia rheumatica, cryoglobulinemia, myocarditis, and Guillain-Barré syndrome.

Treatment of chronic HBV consists of subcutaneous injection of 5 million units of α-interferon daily for 6 months. Therapy is monitored by measurement of serum DNA levels.

Chronic hepatitis C

HCV is the most common cause of chronic hepatitis. More than 80% of cases of acute HCV become chronic. For most individuals the infection lasts a lifetime. Approximately 30% of individuals with HCV progress to chronic hepatitis, cirrhosis, and HCC over a period of 15 to 30 years. The remarkable ability of the virus to persist is one of its unique features. The mechanisms involved are understood only partially. Persistence appears to be a feature of the virus's ability to mutate under immune pressure and to exist in lymphocytes, which are privileged cells. These characteristics allow the virus to evade immune detection.

The natural history of liver disease progresses from mild chronic hepatitis to severe chronic hepatitis to cirrhosis to HCC. The rate and frequency with which it does this in part may be a feature of the particular viral genotype and the environment in which the genotype exists. For example, alcohol ingestion, male sex, and genotype 1 all predispose an individual to an accelerated course.

One of the characteristic clinical features of chronic HCV is a wide array of extrahepatic manifestations. For example, approximately 60% of individuals with HCV have autoantibodies, including antinuclear (28%), rheumatoid factor (21%), antithyroid (20%), anti-smooth muscle (11%), and anti-liver-kidney microsomal antibodies. More than 20% of infected individuals have concurrent immune diseases, including autoantigen-driven disease and foreign antigen (immune complex)-driven disease. The autoantigen-driven diseases include Sjögren's syndrome, autoimmune thyroiditis, myasthenia gravis, lichen planus, diabetes mellitus, and Mooren's corneal ulcers.

The diagnosis of chronic HCV may be made with the various ELISA and RIBA antibody tests but is made more reliably by reverse transcription PCR detection of the viral RNA.

Treatment of chronic HCV consists of subcutaneous administration of α-interferon. Treatment can be followed with quantitative PCR assay for HCV RNA levels.

Autoimmune chronic hepatitis

Autoimmune hepatitis is an unresolving predominately periportal hepatitis, usually with hypergammaglobulinemia and serum autoantibodies. It consists of a chronic inflammatory reaction directed against the hepatocytes and in some cases, against the bile ducts. As with most autoimmune diseases, a female predominance exists. Immunological features are prominent in both the clinical and laboratory aspects of the disease. Both liver- and non–liver-related autoantibodies are found in the serum. The diagnosis is based on characteristic histological features and the presence of autoantibodies and hypergammaglobulinemia. The antibodies include antinuclear antibody (ANA), anti-smooth muscle antibody (ASTHMA), anti-liver-kidney microsomal antibody type 1 (LKM_1), and antisoluble liver antigen (cytokeratin) antibody. Autoimmune hepatitis can be subdivided into types 1 (ASTHMA positive) and 2 (anti-LKM_1 positive) based on specific autoantibodies. This classification, although not recommended by the International Association for the Study of Liver Disease, has been accepted widely and has utility based on significant differences in epidemiology, clinical features, prognosis, and response to therapy.

The prognosis for untreated autoimmune chronic hepatitis is poor, with most individuals progressing to cirrhosis. HCC, however, is rare. Prednisone therapy, alone or in combination with azathioprine, induces clinical and histological remission in more than 70% of affected individuals. Cyclosporine has been used in resistant cases. Azathioprine alone, although not effective to induce remission, is effective to sustain remission and is preferred to prednisone because of its fewer side effects. Liver transplantation is successful in individuals who do not respond to therapy. The incidence of recurrence in the graft is very low.

Alcoholic Liver Disease

Ethanol is toxic to the liver. Its excessive consumption is the most common cause of liver disease in the developed world. For most people, the risk dose is about 80 g of alcohol (200 mL of whiskey or equivalent) per day. Daily drinking appears to be riskier than intermittent drinking. Women may be at a greater risk because of reduced alcohol dehydrogenase (ADH) in gastric mucosa, leading to increased blood levels of alcohol.

The average intake of alcohol for individuals with cirrhosis is approximately 160 g/day for approximately 8 years. This quantity is comparable to 1 pint of whiskey or equivalent per day. Both alcoholism and susceptibility to the development of cirrhosis appear to be genetically determined in that only 10% to 15% of heavy consumers of alcohol develop cirrhosis. The predisposition may be related to different rates of alcohol elimination, which are determined by genetic polymorphism of the microsomal ethanol oxidizing system (MEOS) and ADH.

The clinical presentation of **alcoholic liver disease** is nonspecific, ranging from asymptomatic to behavioral changes, to the incidental finding of slightly abnormal serum enzyme activities, to overt signs of liver disease, including jaundice and ascites. The findings of spider telangiectasias, palmar erythema, Dupuytren's contracture, testicular atrophy, and gynecomastia often are associated with alcoholic liver disease and reflect alcohol-inhibited testosterone production.

A large number of biochemical markers have been proposed for the detection of excessive alcohol consumption and associated liver disease.[4] None has proved ideal. Aminotransferase levels rarely exceed 300 U/L. The AST:ALT ratio is usually greater than 2, unlike other liver diseases, in which ALT is typically higher than AST. ALP is elevated typically about twofold but may be fourfold or fivefold elevated in individuals with alcoholic hepatitis. Serum GGT is used commonly as a screening test for alcohol abuse. However, GGT is an inducible enzyme that is elevated by many drugs and many disease states and is not a specific test of chronic alcohol abuse.

PT may be prolonged and serum albumin decreased as the disease becomes more severe. Nonspecific laboratory abnormalities reflecting the diffuse metabolic changes that occur with alcoholism include hyperuricemia, hyperlactic acidemia, hypertriglyceridemia, hypoglycemia, hyperglycemia, hypophosphatemia, hypomagnesemia, and macrocytosis. Liver biopsy is essential for the determination of disease severity and prognosis, as well as to rule out treatable diseases, such as chronic hepatitis and hemochromatosis.

The prognosis of an individual with alcoholic liver disease is better than that for other forms of liver disease, with only 10% to 15% developing cirrhosis and a much smaller fraction developing HCC. Both HBV and HCV appear to accelerate the course of alcoholic liver disease. The 5-year survival rate in individuals with cirrhosis, jaundice, and as-

TABLE 36-5	Causes and Treatment of Cirrhosis	
Cause	Treatment
Viral	
Hepatitis B	Administration of α-interferon
Hepatitis C	Administration of α-interferon
Toxic	
Alcohol	Abstinence, liver transplantation
Methotraxate	Abstinence
Metabolic	
Hemochromatosis	Phlebotomy
Wilson's disease	Penicillamine
α_1-Antitrypsin deficiency	? Gene therapy
Biliary	
Primary biliary cirrhosis	Ursodeoxycholic acid
Primary sclerosing cholangitis	Liver transplantation
Autoimmune hepatitis	Corticosteroids, azathioprine
Idiopathic	Treatment of diabetes, if present
	Liver transplantation

cites is 40% if the individual continues drinking and 60% if the individual abstains.

Successful treatment of alcoholism is very difficult to achieve and maintain. The primary treatment is abstinence from alcohol. Liver transplantation is the treatment of choice for end-stage liver disease.

Cirrhosis

Cirrhosis is defined anatomically as diffuse fibrosis with nodular hepatocyte regeneration. It is the consequence of chronic injury to the liver. The liver's response to injury is hepatocyte regeneration and collagen formation. When the regeneration occurs with distorted architecture in the form of nodules and the collagen synthesis rate exceeds the degradation rate, cirrhosis results. Virtually all cases of chronic liver disease lead to cirrhosis (see Figure 36-5). In most individuals, cirrhosis is the requisite precursor lesion to the development of HCC. Genetic factors may be involved with the balance between regeneration and fibrosis. This response to injury occurs independently of the etiology and thus determination of the cause of cirrhosis based on the histology is not possible in most circumstances. The common causes of cirrhosis and recommended therapies are listed in Table 36-5.

The clinical manifestations of cirrhosis are diverse and include jaundice and portal hypertension. The liver may be enlarged or shrunken in size. An enlarged spleen suggests portal hypertension. Abdominal wall venous dilation also indicates portal hypertension. Evidence of poor nutrition with muscle wasting may be present. Ascites and edema are present in individuals with advanced disease. Gallstones (pigmented type) are common. Spider telangiectasias are common, especially in individuals with alcoholic cirrhosis or women with chronic autoimmune hepatitis as a cause of cirrhosis. Digital clubbing is common in cases of biliary cirrhosis, as is brown skin pigmentation. Dupuytren's contractures and parotid gland enlargement, along with testicular atrophy and gynecomastia, are seen in cases of alcoholic cirrhosis. Infections with enteric organisms, spontaneous bacterial peritonitis, and septicemia also may occur. Bleeding from esophageal and gastric varices may result in hematemesis or melena. Bruising often is prominent due to hypoprothrombinemia and thrombocytopenia. Neurological signs, such as encephalopathy, have a bad prognosis.

The clinical outcome of cirrhosis is variable, depending on the etiology. Regression of fibrosis has been demonstrated after treatment of hemochromatosis, Wilson's disease, and chronic autoimmune hepatitis. The clinical course of cirrhosis may be improved and the onset of HCC delayed by treatment of HBV or HCV. Abstinence from alcohol improves the outcome for individuals with alcoholic cirrhosis. The treatment of complications such as ascites and esophageal varices does not improve survival rates, which depend more on liver function.

Cirrhosis is the usual prerequisite lesion of HCC. Screening for HCC with serial determinations of α-fetoprotein (AFP) and abdominal ultrasound is becoming more common and may improve the prognosis by early recognition of surgically resectable tumors. Up to 70% of adults with HCC have AFP levels above 500 ng/mL. Many false-positive results are obtained due to underlying acute or chronic liver disease—both of which cause AFP elevations, but usually to levels less than 100 ng/mL.

Drug-Induced Liver Diseases

The central role of the liver in drug metabolism predisposes it to toxic injury, not only because of the bioaccumulation of drugs in the liver but also because drug metabolism may go awry, leading to the formation of electrophilic toxic metabolites and immunogenic protein adducts.

Most drugs are lipophilic and are absorbed passively by the GI tract into the portal circulation, where they are delivered to the liver. To eliminate drugs, the body must convert them to hydrophilic compounds so that they can be excreted in urine and bile without being reabsorbed in the GI tract or renal tubules. This process, known as *biotransformation*, occurs in two phases and ordinarily protects the host from accumulation of potentially toxic xenobiotics (Figure 36-8).

Phase I reactions are mediated by cytochrome P_{450}-dependent enzymes and usually consist of oxidation or demethylation. The cytochrome P_{450} enzymes are composed of heme and a unique apoprotein that characterizes the isoenzymes. This reaction results in aliphatic or aromatic hydroxylation. The hydroxyl group participates in the phase II reaction, in which a large polar group is attached to the hydroxyl oxygen by glucuronidation or sulfation. The drug is now water soluble and is eliminated in bile or urine. This biotransformation process is ordinarily protective but may lead to the accumulation of reactive electrophilic molecules that are potentially toxic. These toxic metabolites, however,

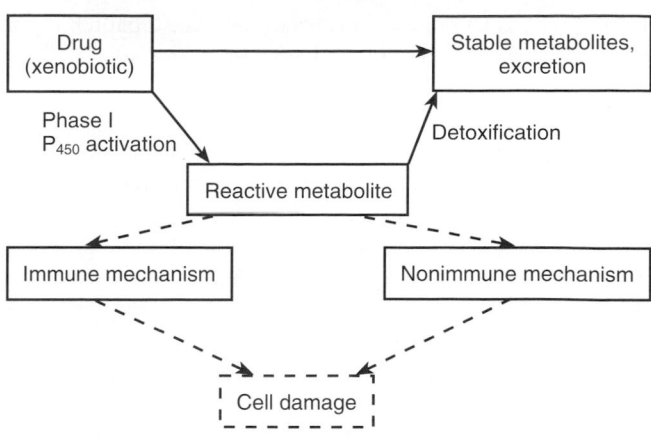

Figure 36-8 Metabolism of xenobiotics by the liver.

also are detoxified by a third phase, in which they react with glutathione. Glutathione is available in limited supply in the body and when it is depleted, toxic metabolites accumulate. Glutathione may be depleted by alcohol ingestion or fasting, both of which predispose an individual to drug-induced injury (for example, acetaminophen hepatotoxicity). Excess drug ingestion or induction of the phase II reaction by other drugs also predisposes an individual to accumulation of toxic electrophiles (for example, alcohol and acetaminophen). These electrophiles interact with cellular proteins to cause direct cellular injury or form protein-drug adducts that become targets for immune-mediated injury.

Metabolic Liver Diseases

Hemochromatosis, Wilson's disease, α_1-antitrypsin deficiency, and the glycogenoses are examples of metabolic liver disease.

Hemochromatosis

Hereditary **hemochromatosis** (HHC) is an autosomal-recessive disorder of iron retention that results in damage to the liver, pancreas, heart, joints, gonads, and skin.[1] The gene for HHC has been identified on chromosome 6 (C 282 Y), and genetic testing is available widely. HHC is the most common inherited liver disorder in Caucasians, with a gene incidence of approximately 1 in 20 and a disease incidence of 1 in 400. The female to male ratio is 1:10. Heightened awareness and gene testing allows for the diagnosis of HHC before symptoms or tissue damage appear.

The typical clinical presentation is a middle-aged man with lethargy, hepatomegaly, grayish skin pigmentation, loss of libido, and sometimes, diabetes. The peak incidence occurs at 40 to 60 years of age but somewhat later in females (because of menstrual iron loss). The skin pigmentation is due to increased deposition of melanin rather than iron.

The diagnosis of hemochromatosis is made on the basis of serum iron, serum ferritin, transferrin saturation, gene testing, and hepatic iron concentrations. (See Chapter 30 for a more detailed discussion of hemochromatosis.)

Wilson's disease

Wilson's disease is an autosomal-recessive disorder of copper metabolism manifested by a neuropsychiatric syndrome or chronic hepatitis. It has a gene frequency of 1 in 200 and a disease frequency of 1 in 30,000. The gene for Wilson's disease is on chromosome 13 and encodes a copper-binding cation transporting ATPase. This enzyme is essential for the addition of copper to ceruloplasmin, a copper-binding protein that contains 95% of serum copper (see Chapters 19 and 29). More than thirty different mutations have been described. These mutations may dictate the variable clinical course of the disease. Wilson's disease usually manifests before the individual reaches 30 years of age. In children, hepatic involvement tends to predominate, whereas in adolescents and adults the neuropsychiatric disease predominates. The hepatic manifestations include fulminant hepatitis, chronic hepatitis, and cirrhosis.

Total body copper is typically 50 to 150 mg, with the highest concentration found in liver as metallothionein and superoxide dismutase. The defective biliary excretion of copper leads to the accumulation of copper in the liver, brain, cornea, kidneys, and joints, resulting in the characteristic clinical features of chronic hepatitis, neuropsychiatric disease, Kayser-Fleischer rings, renal tubular acidosis, and arthritis. The neuropsychiatric changes include behavioral changes, psychosis, extrapyramidal signs, and cerebellar or pseudobulbar signs. Corneal rings known as *Kayser-Fleischer rings* are pathognomonic in the presence of evidence of disturbed copper metabolism but can be seen in individuals with chronic cholestasis. (See Chapter 19 for more information on Wilson's disease and copper metabolism.)

α₁-Antitrypsin deficiency

α_1-Antitrypsin is a glycoprotein that is synthesized and secreted by the liver and is the major protease inhibitor in serum. One of its multiple allelic variants, PiZZ, is characteristic of a homozygous deficiency state, in which serum α_1-antitrypsin concentrations are reduced significantly. Children with the PiZZ genotype are predisposed to liver disease; homozygous and heterozygous (for example, MZ genotype) α_1-antitrypsin-deficient adults are prone to develop chronic obstructive lung disease.

The glycogenoses

The glycogenoses are a group of disorders characterized by excessive and/or aberrant glycogen storage in various tissues. Most such disorders feature deficient glucose production by the liver, leading to hypoglycemia. All are inherited by autosomal-recessive transmission, except for type IV, which is sex linked.

Most glycogenoses are associated with growth retardation and hepatosplenomegaly. Mental development is usually normal. Hypoglycemia is a prominent feature in types I, III, and VI and should be treated with continuous glucose feeding of uncooked cornstarch, a treatment that results in a slow release of glucose.

Diagnosis of the glycogenoses is based on the demonstration of excess glycogen on liver biopsy and tissue identification of the abnormal enzyme or aberrant glycogen. Prognosis and treatment vary with each entity.

Cholestatic Liver Diseases

Cholestasis is defined as a decrease in canalicular bile flow that results in the accumulation of bile in hepatocytes and canaliculi. It implies functional and morphological disturbances in the hepatic excretory process. Intrahepatic cholestasis may be due to functional or structural alterations of the biliary tree. Extrahepatic obstruction can be secondary to a variety of lesions that cause obstruction of the bile ducts, such as choledocholithiasis, biliary strictures, and tumors.

The clinical consequences of prolonged cholestasis of any nature are due to (1) failure of bile to reach the duodenum, with subsequent malabsorption of fat and the fat-soluble vitamins A, D, E, and K, and (2) accumulation in the liver of biliary constituents, such as bile acids, bilirubin, and cholesterol. Vitamin A malabsorption results in night blindness. Vitamin D malabsorption results in calcium malabsorption and secondary osteomalacia with pathological bone fractures. Vitamin K malabsorption results in easy bruising and bleeding. Bile acid retention causes pruritus—the clinical hallmark of cholestasis. Bilirubin retention leads to dark, tea-colored urine and tan-colored stool. The accumulation of cholesterol is associated with the development of hypercholesterolemia and xanthomas. The major cholestatic liver diseases are primary biliary cirrhosis, primary sclerosing cholangitis, post-bone marrow transplant cholangiopathy, post-liver transplant cholangiopathy, and acquired immunodeficiency syndrome (AIDS) cholangiopathy.

Primary biliary cirrhosis

Primary **biliary cirrhosis** (PBC) is a classic autoimmune liver disease and, like most autoimmune diseases, is more common in women. The median age at onset is 50 years. An association exists in some populations with human leukocyte antigen (HLA) class II antigen DR8. Familiality is observed in 1% to 4% of cases.

The pathogenesis of PBC is not understood well, and the target antigens have not been identified. Most individuals have mitochondrial antibodies that react against the pyruvate dehydrogenase complex, part of which is found on the apical surface of biliary epithelial cells.

The clinical presentation of PBC is typically an asymptomatic individual in whom routine screening reveals an elevated ALP value. Aminotransferase activities are elevated only modestly, and bilirubin concentrations are variable. Symptomatic patients present with the insidious onset of pruritus and fatigue. Occasionally, individuals have jaundice or GI bleeding from esophageal varices complicating portal hypertension.

The diagnosis of PBC is established by the combination of cholestatic biochemical tests, the presence of antimitochondrial antibody, and a liver biopsy. Measurement of the M2 antimitochondrial antibody, which is directed against the pyruvate dehydrogenase complex of the inner mitochondrial membrane, has a clinical sensitivity of 98% and a specificity of 96%. It is useful in confirmation of the diagnosis in equivocal cases.

The natural history of PBC is one of slow progression to cirrhosis. PBC is associated frequently with other autoimmune diseases, such as Sicca syndrome (70%), scleroderma (5%), autoimmune hepatitis (20%), pulmonary fibrosis, renal tubular acidosis, and celiac disease. Breast cancer has shown in some studies, but not in others, to be more prevalent in individuals with PBC. Medical management of PBC consists of ursodeoxycholic acid, 13 to 15 mg/kg/day, and can slow the progression of disease and delay liver transplantation—the only definitive treatment.

Primary sclerosing cholangitis

Primary **sclerosing cholangitis** (PSC) is a chronic inflammatory disease of the biliary tree. In contrast to PBC, PSC has a male predominance and a younger median age of onset at 30 years. In 70% of affected individuals, PSC is associated with ulcerative colitis. A markedly increased prevalence of HLA antigens B8 and DR3 also exists.

The clinical presentation of PSC, like that of PBC, is typically an asymptomatic patient with elevated ALP concentrations discovered during routine laboratory screening. Other patients may present with the insidious onset of pruritus. Most patients have ulcerative colitis at the time of presentation. An increased incidence of both cholangiocarcinoma and colon cancer exists when PSC and ulcerative colitis occur simultaneously. The diagnosis of PSC is based on the typical radiographic appearance of beading and irregularity of the bile ducts. Antineutrophil cytoplasmic antibodies (ANCA) are present in approximately 80% of individuals but are not specific for PSC.

The clinical course of PSC is variable. For the most part, it is slowly progressive, but factors such as bile duct strictures, formation of biliary stones, and the development of cholangiocarcinoma can accelerate its course. Liver transplantation is the definitive treatment for PSC.

Post-bone marrow transplant cholangiopathy

The most common cholestatic diseases after bone marrow transplantation are acute and chronic graft-versus-host disease (GVHD), drug injury (especially from cyclosporine), biliary sludge syndrome, and cholangitis lenta.

Acute graft-versus-host disease

Acute GVHD is a consequence of the infusion of allogeneic immune competent T-lymphoid cells into an immunocompromised host who is unable to reject these cells. The periductular epithelial cells and hepatocytes are the target cells that die through accelerated programmed cell death (apoptosis).

The clinical syndrome is characterized by skin rash, intestinal symptoms (nausea, vomiting, diarrhea, and abdominal pain), and cholestatic liver disease. The average time of onset is 15 to 25 days. A progressive rise in bilirubin, aminotransferases (up to tenfold), and ALP with a cholestatic pattern can be detected.

The preferred treatment for acute GVHD is prevention through accurate donor-host matching, depletion of donor T lymphocytes, and pharmacological therapy of the grafted marrow. Once acute disease has occurred, prednisone treatment is 50% to 75% successful.

Chronic graft-versus-host disease

Chronic GVHD is caused by abnormalities of both cellular and humeral immunity in recipients of allogeneic donor marrow up to 2 years after grafting. It is characterized by progressive rises in serum bilirubin and ALP concentrations. It is accompanied often by autoimmune manifestations, such as Sicca syndrome and skin rashes. Chronic GHVD is treated with prednisone and cyclosporine.

Biliary sludge syndrome

The combination of gallbladder stasis (from lack of oral intake), the excretion of precipitable drugs, and exfoliation of mucus-containing epithelial cells from the gallbladder (due to cytoreductive therapy) leads to the accumulation of sludge in the biliary tree. Transient elevations in ALP and rarely, in bilirubin ensue and typically last until the individual starts eating. Most individuals recover uneventfully in a few days, but **cholangitis** may develop when the cystic duct becomes obstructed with the sludge; pancreatitis may develop when the pancreatic duct is obstructed.

Cholangitis lenta

Cholangitis lenta is cholestasis caused by the release of inflammatory mediators in individuals with posttransplantation fever and infections, usually within 30 days of transplantation. It is characterized by an isolated rise in serum bilirubin, although ALP occasionally is elevated mildly.

Post-liver transplant cholangiopathy

The posttransplantation cholangiopathies consist of recurrent PBC and PSC, bile duct leaks, and bile duct strictures. Recurrence of PBC and PSC is rare, but the recurrence has the same clinical presentation and laboratory manifestations as the original disease.

Bile duct leaks occur the site of the anastomosis at the time of transplantation or from the T-tube insertion site.

They often are accompanied by a biloma that causes biliary obstruction and manifests with cholestasis.

Bile duct strictures, probably due to ischemia, manifest 2 to 6 months after transplantation, with asymptomatic rises in ALP. They are diagnosed by cholangiography.

AIDS cholangiopathy

Acquired immunodeficiency syndrome (AIDS) cholangiopathies are infectious and caused by organisms that were not known previously to infect the biliary tree. *Cryptosporidium* is the most common organism. *Microsporidium*, CMV, *Mycobacterium avium* complex, and Cyclospora also have been identified. The clinical presentation usually includes abdominal pain, diarrhea, and cholestatic liver disease manifested by threefold to tenfold elevations in serum ALP and mild elevations in aminotransferase enzymes. Jaundice is uncommon. Papillary stenosis at the ampulla of Vater is present. The bile ducts have features of sclerosing cholangitis; pain is the most characteristic clinical feature. Cholangiography is needed for the diagnosis but is indicated only in patients with pain. Medical therapy (trimethoprim-sulfamethoxazole) has been effective only in individuals with cholangitis caused by Cyclospora. The prognosis is that of the underlying human immunodeficiency virus (HIV) infection.

Nutritional Liver Disease and Fatty Liver

Malnutrition causes fatty liver, hepatic necrosis, and fibrosis. The classic nutritional liver disease is kwashiorkor, but diabetes, obesity, and alcoholic and nonalcoholic fatty liver disease also fall into the broad category of nutritional liver disease. Fatty liver also is caused by urea cycle disorders, fatty acid oxidation disorders, and Reye's syndrome. Steatosis is a common feature of all these diseases.

Fatty liver

The presence of fatty liver is suspected on the basis of hepatomegaly, slight elevations in aminotransferase enzymes, and a computed tomography (CT) scan showing low density with reduced attenuation. Ultimately, the diagnosis requires liver biopsy. The various causes of macrovesicular and microvesicular fatty liver are listed in Tables 36-6 and 36-7, respectively.

Acute fatty liver of pregnancy now is thought to be due to an inherited defect in long-chain 3-hydroxyacyl-coenzyme A dehydrogenase (see Chapter 43). Sodium valproate toxicity has occurred almost exclusively in children receiving polypharmacy for seizure disorders and no longer is being reported. Tetracycline toxicity is seen almost exclusively in pregnant women treated with IV tetracycline for urinary tract infections. The urea cycle disorders and fatty acid oxidation disorders bear a striking resemblance to Reye's syndrome and sodium valproate toxicity, but are very rare.

TABLE 36-6   **Causes of Macrovesicular Fatty Liver**

Nutrition	**Toxic Injury**
Obesity	Alcohol
Intestinal bypass	Corticosteroids
Parenteral nutrition	Amiodarone
Kwashiorkor	
	Miscellaneous
Metabolic Diseases	Febrile illness
Diabetes type 2	Systemic infection
Glycogenoses	Cryptogenic (nonalcoholic
Wilson's disease	steatohepatitis)
Hyperlipidemias	
Acylcoenzyme A deficiency	
Abetalipoproteinemia	

TABLE 36-7   **Causes of Microvesicular Fatty Liver**

Metabolic Diseases	**Miscellaneous**
Urea cycle enzyme defect	Reye's syndrome
Fatty acid oxidation defects	Fatty liver of pregnancy
Cholesterol ester storage disease	
Toxic Injury	
Valproate toxicity	
Salicylate toxicity	
Tetracycline toxicity	

Reye's syndrome

Reye's syndrome is a sudden, sometimes fatal, disease of the brain (encephalopathy), with degeneration of the liver. It occurs in children (primarily 4 to 12 years of age), follows chickenpox (varicella) or an influenza-type illness, and also is associated with the ingestion of medications containing aspirin. The child with Reye's syndrome first tends to be unusually lethargic (stuporous), sleepy, and vomiting. In the second stage the lethargy deepens, and the child becomes confused, combative, and delirious. The child then progresses to decreasing consciousness, coma, seizures, and eventually death. The prognosis depends on early diagnosis and control of the increased intracranial pressure.

Acute encephalopathy in combination with fatty degeneration of the viscera was described initially by Reye and associates in Australia in 1963, with nearly simultaneous case descriptions by Johnson and colleagues in the United States. The etiology of Reye's syndrome is unknown; however, a generalized mitochondrial dysfunction exists, due either to a virus or toxin or to viral potentiation of a chemical toxin.

Laboratory findings indicative of Reye's syndrome are not specific, but a rapid and pronounced elevation of aminotransferases, lactate dehydrogenase (LD), and ALP is seen. The most characteristic feature of the disease is an increase in serum ammonia concentrations, with the degree of increase possibly having prognostic significance. The total bilirubin concentration remains normal or elevated only modestly. Hyperuricemia, hypoglycemia, and hypoprothrombinemia unresponsive to vitamin K are associated with the disease. A PT prolongation greater than 3 seconds and a serum ammonia level greater than 100 μg/dL usually indicate a poor prognosis.

Obesity

Clinically, the degree of steatosis parallels the increase in body weight. Liver function tests reveal trivial elevations in aminotransferase enzymes and occasionally ALP. Weight loss results in improvement in both liver histology and biochemical tests.

Diabetes

Type 2 diabetes causes hepatomegaly. The condition is due to increased deposition of fat (triglyceride). Mild elevations on biochemical tests, such as elevated levels of aminotransferases and ALP, occur. Cirrhosis occurs in approximately 10% of diabetic patients. Type 2 diabetes is the third most common cause of liver disease—surpassed only by alcohol and hepatitis C. Liver disease is caused by the hyperinsulinemia that occurs in the early stages of type 2 diabetes. Treatment with diet, exercise, and insulin-sensitizing drugs, such as metformin, appears to be beneficial.

Nonalcoholic steatohepatitis

In 1981, Ludwig and colleagues described patients who did not have substantial alcohol consumption but had features on liver biopsy that could not be distinguished from alcoholic hepatitis. This condition later was termed *nonalcoholic steatohepatitis (NASH)*. It typically is associated with diabetes, obesity, or hyperlipidemias, as well as with other conditions causing macrovesicular fatty liver. NASH has been reported with increasing frequency and now is considered a distinct entity. The pathogenesis of NASH is unclear. It is more common in women and tends to occur in the fifth and sixth decades of life. Affected individuals are usually asymptomatic, but they may experience vague right upper quadrant discomfort. The liver is usually enlarged. Twofold to threefold increases in aminotransferase enzyme levels are common, as are mild elevations in ALP. Serum bilirubin, albumin, and PT are normal. Progression to cirrhosis occurs in 5% to 10% of individuals, and HCC has been reported. Type 2 diabetes accounts for 50% to 70% of the cases. Some of those who develop fibrosis are heterozygous for hemochromatosis.

The diagnosis is suggested by the appropriate clinical setting and a hyperechoic texture of the liver on ultrasound, along with mild elevations of ALT and AST, but only liver biopsy can prove the diagnosis.

Hepatic Tumors

The liver is host to a wide variety of both benign and malignant primary tumors (Table 36-8). It is also the second

TABLE 36-8   Classification of Hepatic Tumors

Benign	Malignant
Epithelial Tumors	
Adenoma	Hepatocellular carcinoma
Bile duct adenoma	Cholangiocarcinoma
Cyst adenoma	Cystadenocarcinoma
Carcinoid	Squamous carcinoma
Focal nodular hyperplasia	
Diffuse nodular hyperplasia	
Mesenchymal Tumors	
Cavernous hemangioma	Hemangiosarcoma
Fibroma	Fibrosarcoma
Leiomyoma	Leiomyosarcoma
Hematoma	Hepatoblastoma
Metastatic Tumors (Most Common Sources)	
Colon	
Pancreas	
Stomach	
Breast	
Unknown primary	
Bronchogenic	

most common site of metastases. Metastatic tumors account for 90% to 95% of all hepatic malignancies. Primary tumors may arise from any cell line in the liver but most commonly arise from parenchymal and biliary epithelial cells and mesenchymal cells.

Hepatocellular Carcinoma

HCC is a leading cause of cancer death worldwide. Its incidence encompasses wide geographical and ethnic variations, suggesting that both host and environmental factors are involved in its etiology.

Cirrhosis is present in the overwhelming majority of individuals with HCC and is probably a premalignant lesion independent of etiology. The pathogenesis of HCC is unknown. Wide variations exist in the incidence of HCC, with different etiologies of cirrhosis. For example, HCC occurs commonly in individuals with hemochromatosis, α_1-antitrypsin deficiency, type I glycogen storage disease, and porphyria cutanea tarda (see Chapter 30), but the condition is rare in individuals with autoimmune hepatitis, Wilson's disease, and PBC.

The clinical presentation of HCC is variable but is suspected if a cirrhotic individual deteriorates or develops right upper quadrant pain. Fever, malaise, anorexia, and anemia are common; jaundice also may occur. A mass may be palpable on physical examination; the mass often is tender and accompanied by a friction rub or bruit. Ascites is present in approximately half of the affected individuals.

Laboratory findings include markedly elevated levels of serum ALP and mildly elevated aminotransferases. Progressive elevations in α-fetoprotein are usual. Carcinoembryonic antigen levels are elevated usually in individuals with metastatic disease. Serum ferritin concentration is elevated due to increased production by the tumor.

Biliary Tract Diseases

The most common biliary tract diseases are gallstones, cholecystitis, and carcinoma of the gallbladder and bile ducts.

Gallstones

A **gallstone** is a solid concretion in the gallbladder. Although they vary in chemical composition, gallstones generally contain a mixture of cholesterol, bilirubin, calcium, and mucoproteins. In the United States, 70% to 85% of all gallstones are predominantly cholesterol. More than 10% of the adult population is affected.

Three major types of gallstones exist—cholesterol gallstones, pigmented gallstones, and most commonly, mixed gallstones. These stones form whenever bile is supersaturated with cholesterol or unconjugated bilirubin.[7] Most gallstones are mixed cholesterol and pigment stones. For these or cholesterol gallstones to form, bile must be supersaturated with cholesterol. Whenever cholesterol increases or bile acids or lecithin decrease, bile becomes lithogenic (prone to stone formation) as cholesterol precipitates from solution. Factors that predispose to cholesterol hypersecretion are obesity; aging; certain drugs, such as clofibrate; nicotine; and certain hormones, such as estrogen. Factors that decrease bile acid secretion are terminal ileal disease and cholestatic diseases, such as PBC, sclerosing cholangitis, and cystic fibrosis. Genetic factors also appear to be involved. Within racial groups, women are affected more frequently than men. Diet may play a role because individuals who ingest diets high in polyunsaturated fats have a higher incidence, whereas those who follow a diet high in fiber have a decreased incidence.

Pigmented gallstones are associated with conditions in which the bilirubin load is increased, such as hemolytic anemia, or in which bilirubin becomes insoluble (that is, deconjugated), such as occurs with cholestasis or chronic biliary infections.

Cholecystitis

Acute cholecystitis usually is due to gallstones in the gallbladder. Those individuals most susceptible to gallstones are obese women older than 40 years of age. The most common symptom of acute cholecystitis is right upper quadrant abdominal pain that typically is referred to the tip of the right scapula. Nausea, vomiting, and fever often accompany the attacks, which may be initiated by the ingestion of meals but tend to occur late in the evening hours. The pain consists of a persistent, severe ache lasting 1 to 4 hours, during which the individual cannot find a comfortable position. If the stone passes into the common bile duct, dark urine, tan-

colored stool, and jaundice may occur. The individual may experience tenderness in the right upper quadrant.

The diagnosis is made usually by ultrasound. Accompanying laboratory features include leukocytosis and occasionally, mildly fluctuating elevations in bilirubin, ALP, and aminotransferase enzymes.

◼ DIAGNOSTIC STRATEGY

Liver function tests help detect, diagnose, and evaluate liver disease; they also help monitor therapy and assess the prognosis.[3,11] The array of tests useful for these purposes include serum total bilirubin, protein, and albumin levels, as well as the activity of enzymes, such as the aminotransferases (AST and ALT), ALP, LD, and GGT. These tests and their utility are discussed in more detail in earlier sections of this chapter and are listed in Table 36-9. Additional information is found in Chapters 20 and 22. Use of a combination of these tests can help categorize the broad types of liver disease, which then are diagnosed more accurately through disease-specific tests. An algorithm for that process is presented in Figure 36-9.

Serum Enzymes

In practice the serum aminotransferases and ALP are the most useful tests because they allow for the differentiation of hepatocellular disease from cholestatic disease. This differentiation is important because the failure to recognize cholestatic disease caused by extrahepatic biliary obstruction results in liver failure if the obstruction is not corrected rapidly. Recognizing that a gray zone of tests exist that do not distinguish hepatocellular and cholestatic disease also is important. In such unclear instances a wise move is to as-

TABLE 36-9	**Tests of Hepatic Function**
Test	Utility
Bilirubin	Diagnosis of jaundice, modest correlation with severity
Alkaline phosphatase	Diagnosis of cholestasis and space-occupying lesions
Bilirubin fractionation	Diagnosis of disorders of metabolism and of jaundice of the newborn
Aspartate aminotransferase	Sensitive test of hepatocellular disease; AST > ALT in alcoholic disease and chronic severe liver disease
Alanine aminotransferase	Sensitive and more specific test of hepatocellular disease
Albumin	Indicator of chronicity and severity
Prothrombin time	Indicator of severity and of cholestasis

AST, Aspartate aminotransferase; *ALT,* alanine aminotransferase.

sume that the problem is cholestatic and rule out biliary obstruction.

Individuals occasionally are seen with isolated elevations in ALP or aminotransferase enzyme levels. In practice an isolated increase in ALP activity is difficult to interpret. Confirmation that the ALP is of hepatobiliary origin is a necessary first step. This step can be performed by isoenzyme fractionation (see Chapter 20) or measurement of another phosphodiesterase enzyme, such as 5′-nucleotidase (Figure 36-10), or measurement of GGT, which tends to parallel ALP levels. The most important aspect of the workup is to rule out tumors by visualization of the liver with CT and biliary tract obstruction by visualization of the biliary tree with ultrasound or cholangiography.

Elevation of serum levels of AST and ALT is common in individuals with many disorders (see Chapter 20). ALT is more specific to liver. All drugs and alcohol intake (especially if AST is higher than ALT) should be discontinued. More than 50% to 80% of isolated enzyme elevations of liver origin are due to fatty liver, HCV, and HBV. Ultrasound may detect fatty liver, but a liver biopsy is necessary for a more specific diagnosis. The most common cause of fatty liver is insulin resistance—often before the onset of overt type 2 diabetes. A fasting insulin and glucose are needed to make the diagnosis. No reliable test other than liver biopsy exists to detect scarring. Serum procollagen type III peptide has been used, but it correlates better with disease activity than fibrosis.

Serum Albumin

Serum albumin measurements are used to assess of the chronicity and severity of liver disease. For example, the serum albumin concentration is decreased in individuals with chronic liver disease. Its utility for this purpose is limited because the serum albumin concentration also is decreased in cases of severe acute liver and renal disease. Serial measurements of serum albumin also are used to assess the severity of liver disease. Minor elevations of AFP and reversal of the ALT-to-AST ratio are more sensitive tests of severity but one seldom used for that purpose.

Prothrombin Time

PT measurements are used to differentiate between cholestasis and severe hepatocellular disease. If the PT is prolonged, it should be remeasured after vitamin K injection. If the PT corrects after vitamin K replacement (10 mg subcutaneously or intramuscularly, followed by PT measurement 4 hours later), the individual has cholestasis. If the PT does

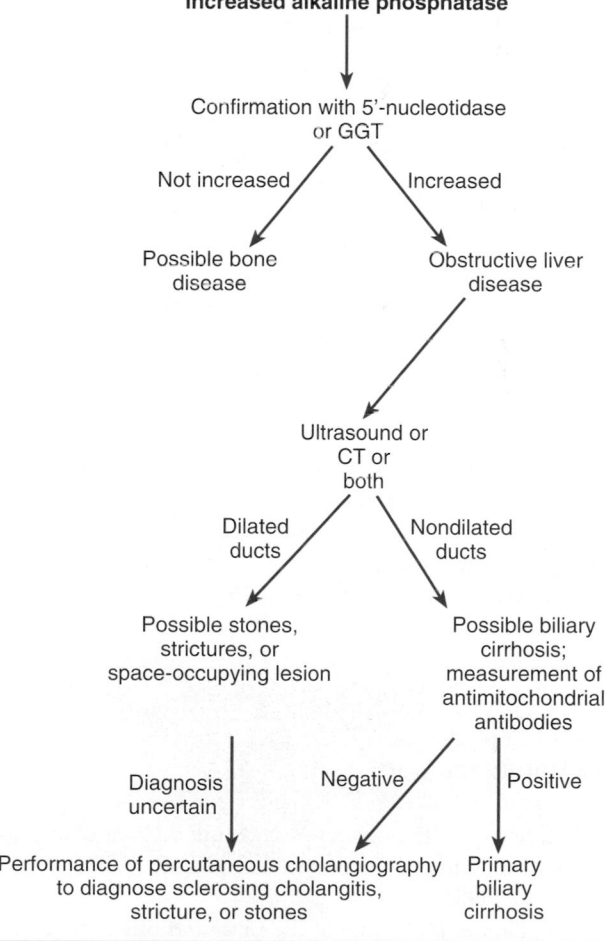

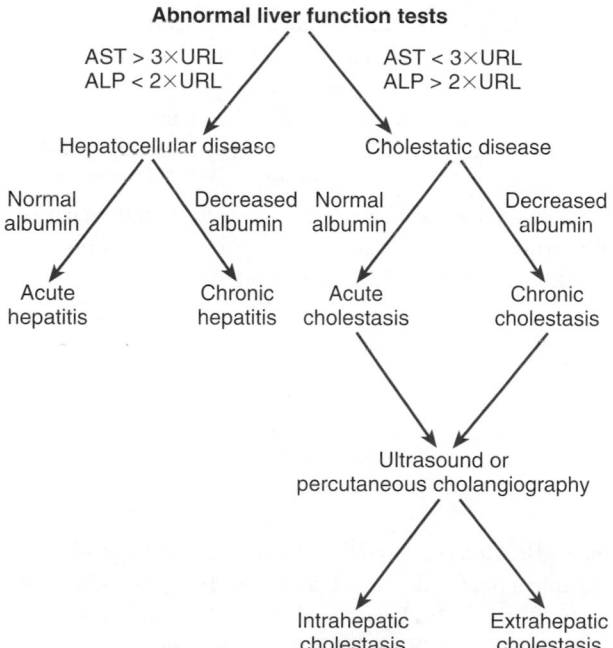

Figure 36-9 Algorithm for the use of abnormal liver function tests to classify and diagnose various types of liver disease. *ALP,* Alkaline phosphatase; *AST,* aspartate aminotransferase; *URL,* upper reference limit.

Figure 36-10 Algorithm for the use of elevated levels of serum alkaline phosphatase in the diagnosis of liver disease in adults. *GGT,* γ-Glutamyltransferase.

not return to normal, the individual has severe hepatocellular disease.

Serum Bilirubin

Serial measurement of bilirubin helps determine the severity of liver disease. Bilirubin fractionation is helpful only in cases of **neonatal jaundice** or isolated elevations of bilirubin in the absence of other liver test abnormalities.

Individuals are seen occasionally with isolated elevations in bilirubin concentration. In most cases this elevation is due to an inherited disorder of bilirubin metabolism, familial hyperbilirubinemia, or hemolysis. Distinguishing hemolysis severe enough to cause hyperbilirubinemia is not difficult because the individual with hemolysis has many other disease manifestations and always is very ill. An algorithm for the differentiation of the familial causes of hyperbilirubinemia is presented in Figure 36-11 (see Chapter 30).

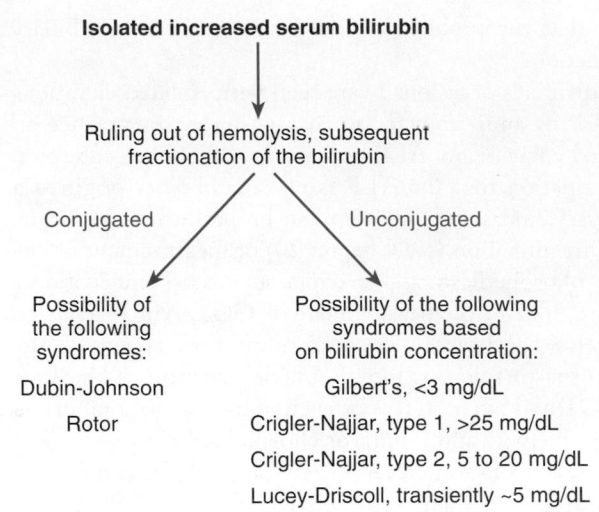

Figure 36-11 Algorithm for the differentiation of the familial causes of hyperbilirubinemia.

References

1. Bacon BR: Diagnosis and management of hemochromatosis. Gastroenterology 1997; 113:995-999.
2. Balistreri WF: Fetal and neonatal bile acid synthesis and clinical implications. J Inherited Metab Dis 1991; 14:459-477.
3. Black ER: Diagnostic strategies and test algorithms in liver disease. Clin Chem 1997; 43:1555-1560.
4. Conigrave KM, Saunders JB, Whitfield JB: Diagnostic tests for alcohol consumption. Alcohol 1995; 30:13-16.
5. Cordoba J, Blei AT: Brain edema and hepatic encephalopathy. Semin Liver Dis 1996; 16:271-280.
6. Patel T, Gores GJ: Apoptosis and hepatobiliary disease. Hepatology 1995; 21:1725-1741.
7. Portincasa P, van de Meeberg P, van Erpecum KJ et al: An update on the pathogenesis and treatment of cholesterol gallstones. Scand J Gastroenterol 1997; 223:60-69.
8. Rosser BO, Gores GJ: Liver cell necrosis: cellular mechanisms and clinical implications. Gastroenterology 1995; 108:252-275.
9. Sturgill MG, Lambert GH: Xenobiotic-induced hepatotoxicity: mechanisms of liver injury and methods of monitoring hepatic function. Clin Chem 1997; 43:1512-1526.
10. Tolman KG, Rej R: Liver Function. In Burtis CA, Ashwood ER (eds): Tietz Textbook of Clinical Chemistry, 3rd edition, pp 1125-1177, Philadelphia, WB Saunders, 1999.
11. Tredger JM, Sherwood RA: The liver: new functional, prognostic, and diagnostic tests. Ann Clin Biochem 1997; 34:121-141.
12. Turkoglu S, Lazizi Y, Meng H et al: Detection of hepatitis E virus RNA in stools and serum by reverse transcription-PCR. Clin Microbiol 1996; 34:1568-1571.

Additional Reading

Schiff ER, Sorrell MF, Maddrey WC: Schiff's Diseases of the Liver, 8th edition, Baltimore, Lippincott Williams & Wilkins, 1998.
Sherlock S, Dooley J: Diseases of the Liver and Biliary System, 10th edition, London, Blackwell Science, 1996.
Worman HJ: Molecular biological methods in diagnosis and treatment of liver diseases. Clin Chem 1997; 43:1476-1486.
Zakim O, Boyer TD: Hepatology: A Textbook of Liver Disease, 4th edition, Philadelphia, WB Saunders, 1998.

Gastric, Pancreatic, and Intestinal Function

A. RALPH HENDERSON, MB, ChB, PhD, FRCPath

Objectives

1. Define the following terms:
    Digestion   Cystic fibrosis
    Absorption   Steatorrhea
    Ulcer
2. List and describe the three phases of digestion.
3. Describe the structure and function of the stomach, intestinal tract, and pancreas.
4. State the function and clinical significance of intrinsic factor.
5. List the hormones and enzymes synthesized in the gastrointestinal tract, as well as their functions and clinical significance.
6. List the procedures and the principles of the procedures used to assess gastrointestinal function.
7. State the laboratory values obtained in the following diseases: ulcer, Zollinger-Ellison syndrome, gastritis, pancreatitis, pancreatic tumor, cystic fibrosis, lactose intolerance, steatorrhea, and diabetes mellitus.

Key Words

Acute Pancreatitis   An acute episode of enzymatic destruction of the pancreatic substance due to the escape of active pancreatic enzymes into the pancreatic tissue

Breath Tests   Tests that detect abnormalities of CO_2 and H_2 elimination in the breath due to abnormalities of digestion, absorption, or bacterial overgrowth

Celiac Disease (Gluten-Sensitive Enteropathy)   A disease caused by the destructive interaction of gluten with the intestinal mucosa, causing malabsorption

Cholecystokinin (CCK)   A polypeptide hormone secreted by the mucosa of the upper intestine and by the hypothalamus; stimulates contraction of the gallbladder (with release of bile) and secretion of pancreatic enzymes

Chronic Pancreatitis   An inflammatory disease characterized by persistent and progressive destruction of the pancreas

Chyme   The semifluid, homogeneous, creamy or gruellike material produced by gastric digestion of food; also called *chymus*

Crohn's Disease   A chronic inflammatory disease affecting any part of the intestine from the mouth to the anus

Cystic Fibrosis (CF)   A genetic disorder affecting many types of exocrine glands, particularly the sweat glands (the sodium and chloride content of sweat being elevated) but also glands in the lung and pancreas

Diarrhea   The passage of liquid stool or the frequent passage of normal stool

Digestion   The process or act by which food is converted into chemical substances that can be absorbed and assimilated

Digestive Process   A three-phase process consisting of neurogenic, gastric, and intestinal phases

Dumping Syndrome   Condition in which after gastric surgery, hyperosmolar chyme is "dumped" into the small intestine, causing rapid hypovolemia and hemoconcentration

Fecal "Occult" Blood (FOB)   The presence of blood in the feces in concentrations in excess of 2 mg/g of stool per day; positive FOB possibly indicating the presence of malignant or premalignant lesions in the colon

Gastric Inhibitory Polypeptide (GIP)   A polypeptide hormone that stimulates insulin release and inhibits the release of gastric acid and pepsin

Gastrin   Polypeptide hormones released from peptidergic fibers in the vagus nerve and from G cells in the pyloric glands in the gastric antrum; stimulates secretion of gastric acid, increases growth of acid-secreting mucosal cells, and weakly stimulates secretion of pancreatic enzymes and gallbladder contraction

Helicobacter Pylori   A bacterium found in the mucous layer of the stomach that has been implicated in the development of duodenal and gastric ulcers

Malabsorption   An abnormality of the small intestine that causes a disorder of the absorptive process

Maldigestion   An abnormality of the digestive process due to dysfunction of the pancreas or small intestine

Peptic Ulcer Disease   The collective name given to duodenal and gastric ulceration

Postgastrectomy Syndrome   A syndrome that occurs after surgery for peptic ulcer disease and includes the dumping syndrome, diarrhea, maldigestion, weight loss, anemia, bone disease, and gastric cancer

Secretin   A polypeptide hormone secreted by the mucosa of the duodenum and upper jejunum when acid chyme enters the intestine; stimulates the pancreatic acinar cells to release bicarbonate and water, which are secreted into the duodenum and change the pH from acid to alkaline, thereby facilitating the action of intestinal digestive enzymes

Steatorrhea   A condition of excessive fat in feces (>7 g/day)

Ulcerative Colitis   A recurrent inflammatory disease of the large bowel that also is known as *inflammatory bowel disease*

Vasoactive Intestinal Polypeptide (VIP)   A polypeptide of the central nervous system that acts as a neuropeptide and is released by specific interneurons

Zollinger-Ellison (Z-E) Syndrome   A condition resulting from a gastrin-secretins tumor (gastrinoma) of the pancreatic islet cells that results in an overproduction of gastric acid, leading to fulminant ulceration of the esophagus, stomach, duodenum, and jejunum

---

Efficient **digestion** and absorption of nutrients are the result of coordinated functions of the stomach, intestinal tract, and pancreas.[2] Coordination and regulation in large measure depend on hormones that stimulate or inhibit secretion of fluids containing hydrochloric acid (HCl), bile acids, bicarbonate, and digestive enzymes.

■ BASIC ANATOMY AND PHYSIOLOGY

The gastrointestinal (GI) tract is a 10-meter tube beginning with the mouth and ending with the anus. The major organs of the GI tract include the stomach, small and large intestines, and pancreas, all of which are involved in the digestive process.

Stomach

The human stomach consists of three major zones—the cardiac zone, the body, and the pyloric zone (Figure 37-1). The upper cardiac zone contains mucus-secreting surface epithe-

lial cells. The body of the stomach contains cells or cell groups of many of the following different types:

1.   The surface epithelial cells, which secrete mucus
2.   The parietal (oxyntic) cells, which secrete HCl and intrinsic factor
3.   The chief, zymogen, or peptic cells, which secrete pepsinogens
4.   The neck chief cells, or mucous cells, which secrete mucus and pepsinogens
5.   Enterochromaffin cells, which secrete serotonin
6.   A number of different types of endocrine-secreting cells

The third portion of the stomach, the pyloric zone, is subdivided into the antrum, pyloric canal, and sphincter. Its cells secrete mucus, some pepsinogens, serotonin, gastrin, and several other hormones, but no HCl.

Small Intestine

In the adult human the small intestine is approximately 7 m long. It consists of the duodenum, jejunum, and ileum and

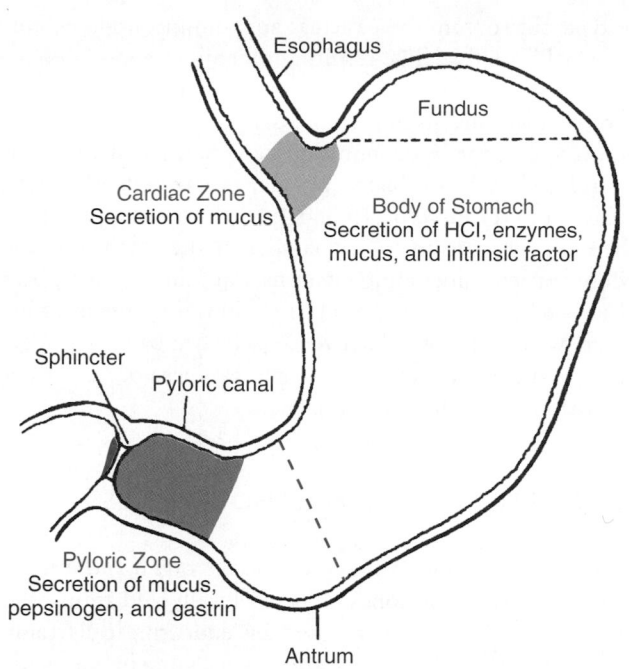

Figure 37-1   Schematic drawing of the stomach, illustrating major zones.

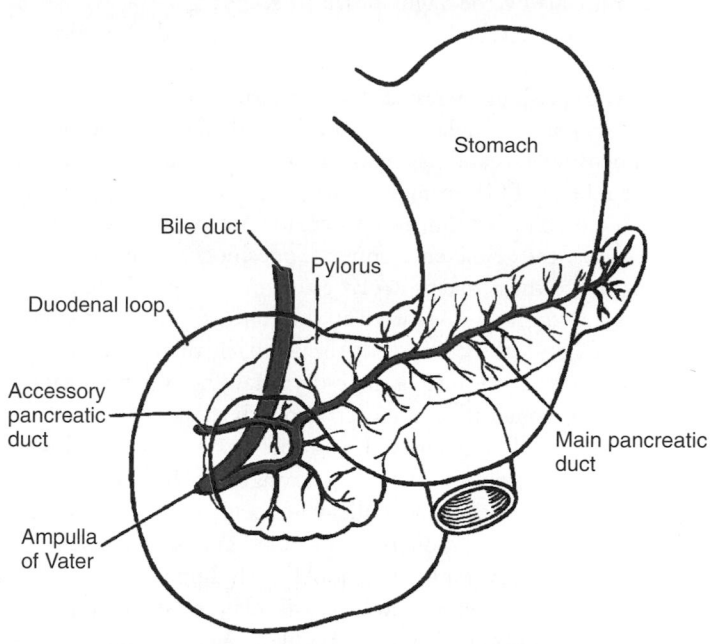

Figure 37-2   Cross-section through the pancreas.

decreases in cross-section as it proceeds from the duodenum to the ileum. The duodenum is the shortest (~25 cm) and widest part of the small intestine. The jejunum and ileum constitute the remainder of the small intestine.

The internal surface of the small intestine contains circular folds and minute villi. The circular folds are valvelike and project 3 to 10 mm into the lumen of the intestine. The villi are very small, fingerlike projections that cover the entire mucosal surface of the small intestine, giving it a "velvety" appearance.

Large Intestine

The large intestine is about 1.5 m long, extending from the ileum to the anus. It is divided into the cecum, appendix, colon, rectum, and anal canal. The cecum is the large blind pouch that begins the large intestine and is approximately 6 to 7 cm long. The appendix is a long, "worm-shaped" tube that connects the cecum and the colon. The colon is divided into the ascending, transverse, descending, and sigmoid sections. The sigmoid section of the colon connects to the rectum, which is approximately 12 cm long. The rectum in turn connects to the anal canal, the terminal end of the large intestine.

Pancreas

The pancreas lies across the posterior wall of the abdomen. Its head is located in the duodenal curve (loop), and the body and tail are directed toward the left, extending to the spleen (Figure 37-2).

Digestive Process

The neurogenic, gastric, and intestinal phases constitute the **digestive process.** The neurogenic (vagal) phase is initiated by the sight, smell, and taste of food, all of which stimulate the cerebral cortex and subsequently the vagal nuclei and result in secretion of pepsinogen, HCl, and gastrin. The process is chemically mediated by acetylcholine from postganglionic parasympathetic nerve endings, which act on gastric parietal cells. The vagus also stimulates gastric chief and parietal (oxyntic) cells to secrete pepsinogen and HCl. Hydrogen ion secretion takes place against a 1 million-fold concentration gradient, an energy-dependent process catalyzed by H^+, K^+-ATPase; it is mediated by acetylcholine, histamine, and gastrin acting through their respective neurocrine, paracrine, and endocrine pathways to stimulate the parietal cells. The important role of histamine in acid secretion also has been confirmed by the findings that histamine H_2-receptor antagonists (cimetidine [Tagamet], ranitidine [Zantac], famotidine [Pepcid], and nizatidine [Axid]) inhibit acid secretion. These drugs block both the morphological transformation of the parietal cell, which precedes H^+ secretion, and H^+ secretion itself. By contrast, the antisecretory drug omeprazole is taken up by the parietal cell and converted to an active metabolite that inactivates the parietal H^+, K^+-ATPase. H^+ secretion is inhibited until new ATPase is synthesized, a process that requires at least 24 hours.

The distention caused by food entry into the stomach initiates the gastric phase of digestion. HCl release is caused by (1) direct stimulation of the parietal cells by the vagus nerve; (2) local distention of the antrum and stimulation of antral cells by the vagus nerve to secrete gastrin, which in turn causes HCl release from parietal cells; and (3) release of gastrin, stimulated by the near neutralization (pH 5 to 7) of gastric HCl by ingested food entering the pyloric zone. Gastrin also stimulates (1) antral motility, (2) the secretion of pepsinogens and pancreatic fluid rich in enzymes, and (3) the release of GI hormones, such as secretin, insulin, acetylcholine, somatostatin, and pancreatic polypeptide (PP). As a result of the acidic environment, pepsinogens are converted rapidly to the active proteolytic enzyme, pepsin. As food enters the stomach, it is mixed by the contractions of the stomach. Chemical secretions of the stomach then partially degrade the food into a mucus-containing mixture called **chyme,** which then is moved through the pylorus into the duodenum. The pylorus plays a role in emptying food into the duodenum by virtue of its strong musculature.

The intestinal phase of digestion begins when the weakly acidic digestive products of proteins and lipids enter the duodenum. Several GI hormones, including gastrin, are released by both neural and local stimulation and act on various regions of the GI tract to regulate digestion and absorption. In addition, the action of gastrin, is potentiated by the secretion of cholecystokinin (CCK). Additional gastrin is released as the upper duodenal mucosa comes in contact with partially digested proteins and lipids and gastric HCl. Cholecystokinin is released in the duodenum in response to the presence of fat, protein, and HCl. Its principal actions are stimulation of gallbladder contraction; secretion of enzymes, bicarbonate, insulin, and glucagon from the pancreas; and stimulation of intestinal motility and stomach contraction.

Secretin is released by gastric acid in the duodenum; it (1) augments the effect of CCK on gallbladder contraction and pancreatic secretions, (2) stimulates pepsinogen secretion by the stomach, (3) inhibits gastrin and gastric acid secretion, and (4) in contrast to CCK, reduces gastric and duodenal motility. Gastric inhibitory polypeptide (GIP) is secreted by the duodenum and jejunum. It inhibits gastric acid, gastrin, and pepsin secretion; reduces intestinal motility; and increases insulin secretion in the presence of hyperglycemia. Vasoactive intestinal polypeptide (VIP), present throughout the gut and in nerve fibers, is a potent vasodilator and aids in the relaxation of smooth muscle. It has a large number of physiological actions, some of which are shared with secretin and GIP. Somatostatin is secreted to inhibit most GI secretory and motor functions, thus preventing excessive reactions.

Pancreatic digestive enzymes, in a bicarbonate-rich juice, enter the duodenum through the ampulla of Vater and sphincter of Oddi (see Figure 37-2) and mix with the food bolus in the duodenum. During passage through the small intestine, carbohydrates are broken down by amylase and saccharidases into monosaccharides, which then are absorbed actively into the bloodstream. Protein is degraded further in the duodenum by trypsin, chymotrypsin, and car-

boxypeptidase from the pancreas and aminopeptidases from the small intestine. The resulting dipeptides and amino acids are absorbed in the jejunum and ileum by specialized absorptive mechanisms in the mucosal surface. Dietary fats are emulsified in the duodenum by the action of bile; they are hydrolyzed by lipase (aided by colipase) to individual fatty acids, monoacylglycerols (monoglycerides), and glycerol and then are absorbed in the remainder of the small intestine. Most nutrients, including vitamins and minerals, have been absorbed by the time the food passes into the large intestine, where water is absorbed actively, electrolyte balance is regulated, and bacterial actions take place. These processes end ultimately in the formation of feces.

◼ GASTROINTESTINAL HORMONES

The GI tract is both a major endocrine organ and a major target for many hormones, released locally and from other sites. GI hormones are released by endocrine cells found throughout the gut mucosa and are so numerous that the gut is recognized as the largest endocrine organ in the body. Collectively the GI hormones influence motility, secretion, digestion, and absorption in the gut. They regulate bile flow and secretion of pancreatic hormones and affect tonicity of vascular walls, blood pressure, and cardiac output. Many of these hormones are present both in the gut and in the central nervous system (CNS), and play an important role in the neuroendocrine control of the gut. In addition, they may have a role as neurotransmitters when they are released from nerve synapses. A listing of the major GI hormones is given in Table 37-1. Other hormones affecting GI function include somatostatin, motilin, and PP.

Gastrin

Biochemistry and physiology

Three molecular forms of **gastrin** are known to exist in blood and tissues—big gastrin, a linear polypeptide of 34 amino acids designated as G-34; little gastrin, or G-17; and mini gastrin, or G-14. All these polypeptides circulate in nonsulfated or sulfated form and have similar biological activities. Derivatives of gastrin, containing the same terminal tetrapeptide residue, are physiologically active, but the potency of each derivative differs. Pentagastrin is a synthetic derivative used for maximal stimulation of HCl secretion in gastric function testing.

Gastrin is produced and stored mainly by special endocrine cells (G cells) of the antral mucosa of the stomach and to a lesser extent by G cells of the proximal duodenum and delta cells of the pancreatic islets. After secretion, gastrin is transported by the blood through the liver to the parietal cells of the fundus of the stomach, where it stimulates the secretion of gastric acid. Gastrin also stimulates secretion of gastric pepsinogens and intrinsic factor by the gastric mu-

TABLE 37-1 **Characteristics of Principal GI Hormones**

Hormone	MW	Number of Amino Acids	Tissues*	Half-Life in Blood (min)	Serum Reference Interval	Principal Actions
Little gastrin	2098 2178	17	Stomach antrum; also vagal fibers, duodenum	~5	<100 ng/L†	Stimulates secretion of gastric acid, pepsinogen, intrinsic factor, secretin, pancreatic enzymes and HCO_3^-, and hepatic bile; increases gastric and intestinal motility and mucosal growth
Big gastrin	3839 3919	34	Duodenum; also stomach antrum	~42	<100 ng/L†	See text for details
Secretin	3056	27	Duodenum	~4	0 to 500 ng/L	Increases pancreatic secretion of HCO_3^-, enzymes, and insulin; promotes pancreatic growth; increases HCO_3^- and water secretion from liver and Brunner's glands; stimulates gallbladder contractions; reduces gastric and duodenal motility; inhibits gastrin release and gastric acid secretion
CCK-PZ	3918	33	Duodenum and jejunum; also CNS	~3	5 to 800 ng/L	Regulates gallbladder contraction; increases motility of small intestine; stimulates secretion of pancreatic enzymes, insulin, glucagon, pancreatic polypeptide, and HCO_3^-; stimulates pancreatic growth and secretion from Brunner's glands; slightly stimulates gastric HCl and pepsinogen
VIP	3326	28	Nervous system; also all areas of GI tract	~1	0 to 100 ng/L; ~tenfold higher in CSF	Causes relaxation of smooth muscles of circulatory system, gut, and genitourinary system; increases water and electrolyte secretion from pancreas and gut; releases hormones from pancreas, gut, and hypothalamus; stimulates lipolysis, glycolysis, and bile flow; inhibits gastrin and gastric acid secretion
GIP	4976	42	Duodenum and jejunum	~15	15 to 100 pmol/L	Stimulates insulin release in hyperglycemia; inhibits gastric acid, pepsin, and gastric secretion; reduces gastric and intestinal motility; increases fluid and electrolyte secretion from small intestine

MW, Molecular weight; *HCO_3^-*, bicarbonate; *CCK-PZ*, cholecystokinin-pancreozymin; *CNS*, central nervous system; *HCl*, hydrochloric acid; *VIP*, vasoactive intestinal polypeptide; *GI*, gastrointestinal; *CSF*, cerebrospinal fluid; *GIP*, gastric inhibitory polypeptide.
*Principal tissue(s) are listed first.
†This value represents gastrin immunoreactivity as measured in "G-17 equivalents" because gastrin assays are standardized by use of synthetic human G-17. Other forms of gastrin (for example, G-34, G-14) have variable cross-reactivities with G-17 antibodies used in these assays.

cosa, release of secretin by the small intestinal mucosa, and secretion of pancreatic bicarbonate ion (HCO_3^-) and enzymes, as well as hepatic bile; it also increases gastric and intestinal motility, mucosal growth, and blood flow to the stomach. Gastrin is secreted in response to (1) antral disten-tion, (2) meals, and (3) the presence of partially digested protein products (peptides and polypeptides) in the stomach. Any free amino acids present also stimulate gastrin secretion; of those, glycine, tryptophan, and phenylalanine are the most potent stimulators. Carbohydrates and fats have little effect on gastrin release. Other stimuli include alcohol, caffeine, insulin-induced hypoglycemia, ingestion or intravenous infusion of calcium, and vagal stimulation initiated by smelling, tasting, chewing, and swallowing of food.

Maximal secretion of gastrin from the fundus occurs at an antral pH of 5 to 7. This secretion is reduced by approximately 80% at pH 2.5, with maximal suppression occurring at a pH of 1.0. Gastrin secretion by antral G cells is inhibited by the direct action of acid on the G cells. This negative-feedback regulation appears to be a safeguard against overacidification by any and all stimulants.

Clinical significance

Zollinger-Ellison syndrome

Knowledge of blood gastrin levels is helpful in the diagnosis of **Zollinger-Ellison (Z-E) syndrome**, which is characterized by the presence of gastrinomas (duodenal or pancreatic endocrine tumors) that produce and secrete large quantities of gastrin. In individuals with Z-E, fasting gastrin levels usually are elevated markedly, ranging from 2 to 2000 times the normal level. Gastrin concentrations greater than 1000 ng/L with gastric acid hypersecretion are virtually diagnostic of gastrinoma. However, substantial overlap in gastrin levels exists among individuals with Z-E syndrome and those with common peptic ulceration and a variety of other diseases.

Because management of the patient with Z-E syndrome requires surgical removal of the tumor, hypergastrinemia caused by gastrinoma should be distinguished from that caused by other conditions. This differential diagnosis is aided by the gastrin response to one of three provocative procedures—secretin infusion, calcium infusion, or a standard meal. Currently the secretin infusion is the most useful provocative test for the diagnosis Z-E syndrome.

Increased fasting serum gastrin concentrations also often are associated with increasing age, especially in individuals older than 60 years who do not demonstrate symptomatic GI diseases. These older individuals may represent cases of unrecognized gastric mucosal atrophy, may have reduced rates of gastric acid secretion, or both. Fasting serum gastrin levels of individuals with duodenal ulcer disease usually do not differ from those of normal subjects, but postprandial serum gastrin responses are usually greater than normal.

Increased basal gastrin concentrations may be classified as "appropriate" or "inappropriate," according to their association with decreased or increased gastric acid secretion. In an individual with very low or absent acid secretion and a functionally intact gastric antrum, an increase in serum gastrin is physiologically appropriate and expected. The increase is due to hyperplasia of antral G cells, as observed in cases of atrophic gastritis, pernicious anemia, previous vagotomy, and renal failure. Inappropriate hypergastrinemia may be caused by gastrinoma, isolated retained antrum after gastric surgery, or primary gastrin cell hyperfunction.

Analytical methodology

Several commercial kit procedures are available for the measurement of gastrin; a sample size of either 100 or 200 μL of serum is required. Most such procedures use a double-antibody separation technique that requires 4 hours for analysis.

Calibrators in most available gastrin assays consist of synthetic human G-17. Because G-34 is the predominant form of gastrin in individuals with gastrinoma but is difficult to obtain in its pure form, measurement of serum gastrin in these individuals should be interpreted in terms of "G-17 equivalents."

Gastrin is unstable in serum, even at refrigerator temperatures. For long-term storage, specimens should be kept at −70 °C in a freezer without a self-defrost cycle. Specimens should be centrifuged promptly and then divided into two aliquots immediately after separation from the clot and kept frozen before they are assayed. If a second analysis is required, the duplicate specimen then is assayed, with minimal loss of immunoreactivity. Specimens must be assayed immediately after thawing; they should not be frozen and thawed repeatedly.

Reference values for serum gastrin in fasting individuals range up to 100 ng/L. Values may be higher in elderly individuals; approximately 15% of those older than 60 years of age have gastrin values between 100 and 800 ng/L. Concentrations may fluctuate throughout the day, according to a circadian rhythm (lowest at 0300 to 0700 hours; highest during daytime), or physiologically, in relation to meals.

Cholecystokinin-Pancreozymin

Biochemistry and physiology

Cholecystokinin (CCK) is an intestinal hormone that activates gallbladder contraction and stimulates secretion of pancreatic enzymes. This dual action was discovered separately; thus two different substances initially were believed to be responsible for these actions. Eventually, CCK and pancreozymin (PZ) were shown to be the same substance. Because gallbladder contraction was the first action described for this hormone, the hormone now usually is called *cholecystokinin*, although *CCK-PZ* also is used.

CCK is found in the I cells of the upper small intestinal mucosa, mainly in the duodenum. Mixtures of polypeptides and amino acids (especially tryptophan and phenylalanine) from partially digested protein stimulate CCK secretion, whereas pure undigested protein does not elicit such a response. Secretion also is stimulated by gastric HCl entering the duodenum and fatty acids with nine-carbon chains or longer, especially in the form of micelles. Although circulating levels of CCK are increased after the ingestion of a mixed meal, CCK is cleared rapidly from plasma, having a half-life of less than 3 minutes. The kidney appears to be the major organ for removal of CCK from the blood. CCK secretion is inhibited completely after somatostatin infusion.

CCK regulates the contraction of the gallbladder and increases the motility of the duodenum and small intestine. Because it possesses the same terminal amino acid pentapeptide as gastrin, CCK has a slight degree of gastrin activity and also competes with gastrin for the receptor sites on the HCl-secreting cells. This action may contribute to the termination of gastric secretion after a meal. The effects of gastrin and CCK activities are cumulative in their stimulation of the pancreas, and both increase the effect of secretin on pancreatic function. In addition, CCK stimulates pancreatic growth, relaxes the sphincter of Oddi, and stimulates secretions from Brunner's (duodenal) glands.

Clinical significance

Little information is available on plasma CCK concentrations for various disorders. However, basal concentrations are increased (up to 8500 ng/L) in individuals with pancreatic exocrine insufficiency and celiac disease. CCK also may be increased in individuals with fatty food intolerance, gastric ulcers, postgastrectomy states, and irritable bowel syndrome. In individuals with diabetes or duodenal ulcers, CCK response to test meals is more rapid than in healthy individuals. The existence of CCK-secreting tumors has not as yet been documented.

Analytical methodology

Currently, no reliable and convenient methods are available for the measurement of CCK. Various radioimmunoassays (RIAs) have been developed, but considerable disagreement exists about circulating CCK values obtained with these different RIAs.

Reference values for fasting serum from healthy individuals have been reported to be less than 80 ng/L, but these types of methods are highly dependent on the method being used.

Secretin

Biochemistry and physiology

Secretin is a linear polypeptide containing 27 amino acids and has structural similarities to glucagon, VIP, GIP, and growth hormone-releasing hormone. The positions of 14 amino acid residues within the molecule are identical with those found in glucagon; 8 are the same as in GIP, and 9 are the same as in VIP. The intact secretin molecule is required for biological activity.

Secretin is secreted by the mucosal granular S cells located in the greatest concentration in the duodenum but present throughout the length of the small intestine. It is released primarily on contact of the S cells with gastric HCl. Alcohol appears to increase secretin release by stimulation of gastric acid secretion, with subsequent lowering of duodenal pH, rather than by a direct stimulatory effect. The half-life of secretin in humans is approximately 4 minutes. The kidney is the major site of its degradation (40%). The

only known physiological inhibitor of secretin release is somatostatin.

The primary physiological role of secretin appears to be the stimulation of the pancreas to secrete an increased amount of juice with a high bicarbonate content. Other actions include (1) stimulation of bicarbonate and water secretion from the liver and from Brunner's glands, (2) augmentation of gallbladder contraction and increased hepatic bile flow, (3) weak stimulation of insulin secretion (a pharmacological effect), (4) stimulation of parathyroid hormone (PTH) release and pancreatic enzymes and of pepsinogen by the chief cells of the stomach, (5) reduction of gastric and duodenal motility, (6) reduction of the lower esophageal sphincter pressure, and (7) promotion of pancreatic growth. Secretin inhibits gastrin release (except in Z-E syndrome) and therefore gastric acid secretion.

Clinical significance

Transient decreases of secretin and prolonged rises after meals constitute the normal diurnal patterns of secretion. Fasting and periods of severe physical stress cause increased secretin levels that are reversed by ingestion of glucose. Currently, little knowledge exists of abnormal secretion of secretin in pathological conditions.

Clinical uses of secretin are limited to diagnostic tests. Secretin infusion in individuals with Z-E syndrome increases serum gastrin and gastric acid output. These responses are not observed in healthy individuals or those with duodenal ulcers. In addition, the secretin-CCK test may be useful for the detection of pancreatic disease.

Analytical methodology

RIAs have been developed that are sufficiently sensitive and specific to measure circulating levels of secretin. However, large variations in results exist among such methods.

Secretin is unstable in plasma or serum because of the presence of proteases. Fasting blood for secretin measurements should be collected into ice-cold, plastic, heparinized tubes; separated immediately; and the plasma stored at −20 °C. Glass containers should not be used because secretin binds to glass surfaces. Serum is also suitable for analysis.

Fasting levels in humans have been reported to be 12 to 75 ng/L. Blood concentrations rise rapidly within 3 minutes after stimulation by duodenal acidification and then decline to basal levels in about 60 minutes.

Vasoactive Intestinal Polypeptide

Biochemistry and physiology

Vasoactive intestinal polypeptide (VIP) is a linear polypeptide consisting of 28 amino acids; it has structural similarities to secretin, GIP, and glucagon. VIP is present throughout the body and is found in highest concentrations in the CNS and gut. VIP-containing nerve fibers are found throughout the GI tract, from the esophagus to the colon, and in all tissue layers of the gut.

Little is known about the conditions that cause VIP secretion into the circulation. For example, no evidence exists that VIP is released during digestion. However, vagal stimulation causes its release. Its plasma half-life is approximately 1 minute, and most of the hormone is inactivated by a single passage through the liver.

VIP has a large number of poorly defined physiological actions, some of which are shared with other similar polypeptide hormones, such as secretin and GIP. It acts as a neurotransmitter in the CNS and autonomic nervous system and causes vasodilation and relaxation of the smooth muscles of the circulatory and genitourinary systems and the gut. Other actions of VIP include increase of water and electrolyte secretion from the pancreas and gut; release of hormones from the pancreas, gut, and hypothalamus; stimulation of lipolysis, glycolysis, and bile flow; and inhibition of gastrin and gastric acid secretion. Most of VIP's actions tend to be short lived because of its rapid degradation.

Clinical significance

Increased plasma concentrations of VIP are found in individuals with Verner-Morrison syndrome (also called *pancreatic cholera*). This syndrome is characterized by watery diarrhea, hypokalemia and achlorhydria, hypotension, and cutaneous flushing (vasodilation); it usually is associated with a pancreatic tumor. Because overproduction of VIP by the tumor is responsible for these symptoms, these tumors are called *VIPomas*. Measurement of VIP concentration is a very useful screening test for the diagnosis of VIP-secreting tumors as a cause of intractable diarrhea and is an effective tumor marker for the detection of occult metastases. Its measurement also has been used to evaluate the effect of surgery or chemotherapy in individuals with VIP-secreting tumors.

Other conditions unassociated with intractable diarrhea also may be associated with increased levels of VIP. For example, individuals with hepatic cirrhosis have markedly elevated VIP concentrations because of failure of the liver to clear VIP from the blood. In addition, increased tissue concentrations and bowel content of VIP have been found in individuals with Crohn's disease.

Analytical methodology

RIAs have been developed to measure circulating plasma concentrations in individuals with pathological conditions in which VIP is elevated; however, many RIA methods are not sensitive enough to measure VIP levels accurately in healthy individuals. Reported reference values for healthy individuals are generally less than 50 ng/L. Concentrations of VIP in cerebrospinal fluid (CSF) are approximately 10 times higher than in plasma. Individuals with VIPomas have plasma VIP concentrations reported to vary from 600 to 9000 ng/L.

Gastric Inhibitory Polypeptide

Biochemistry and physiology

Gastric inhibitory polypeptide (GIP) is a linear peptide consisting of 42 amino acids. Its N-terminal end bears a close resemblance to glucagon and secretin. GIP is synthesized and released by K cells located in the duodenal and jejunal mucosa. Plasma GIP is increased by oral administration of glucose, triacylglycerols, or intraduodenal infusions of solutions containing mixtures of amino acids; however, none of these compounds causes changes in GIP concentrations when administered intravenously. Protein ingestion has not produced any significant elevation of GIP. For food components to stimulate GIP release, they must be absorbed by the intestinal mucosa.

The biological actions of GIP include (1) stimulation of insulin secretion in the presence of hyperglycemia, (2) reduction of intestinal motility, with stimulation of small intestinal fluid and electrolyte secretion, and (3) inhibition of gastric acid, pepsin, and gastrin secretion in supraphysiological concentrations. The insulinotropic action of GIP appears to be the most important of its biological actions, and as a result, this hormone has been called more recently "glucose-dependent insulinotropic peptide" as a more accurate description of its physiological action.

Clinical significance

Fasting baseline levels of GIP are increased in states of starvation, prolonged fasting, type IV hyperlipoproteinemia, and renal failure and in some cases of diabetes, such as untreated ketotic diabetes, in which insulin levels are low. Exaggerated GIP responses to mixed test meals are observed in individuals with severe diabetes and in nondiabetic obese individuals. Individuals with cystic fibrosis (CF) or pancreatitis show increased responses of GIP to glucose and lower-than-normal responses to triglycerides. In individuals with duodenal ulcer disease, GIP shows an increased response to glucose. Surgical procedures and other conditions associated with an accelerated rate of transfer of glucose from the stomach into the small intestine may produce an excessive rise in GIP, glucose, and insulin that leads to hypoglycemia. No documented cases of GI disease resulting from the overproduction of GIP have been observed so far. Lowered basal GIP concentrations and decreased GIP responses to glucose and triglycerides are seen in individuals with untreated celiac disease and malabsorption. Currently the diagnostic or therapeutic value of GIP has yet to be established.

Analytical methodology

Plasma GIP is measured by RIA. Levels of GIP in fasting human plasma have been reported to be less than 100 pmol/L.

Other Hormones of the Gut

Somatostatin is one of the most potent known inhibitors of endocrine secretions. Somatostatin inhibits the release of growth hormone, thyroid-stimulating hormone, insulin, glucagon, gastrin, CCK, secretin, VIP, GIP, motilin, PP, enteroglucagon, neurotensin, substance P, and other hormones. It also inhibits the effect of these hormones on their target tissues.

Motilin is a strong stimulant for contraction of smooth muscles of the upper GI tract, and it increases the motility of the fundus, antrum, and duodenum, as well as the contractions of the lower esophageal sphincter. It is unique in that its actions generally are restricted to the fasting state. Increases in motilin concentrations have been observed in conditions involving acute diarrhea, such as Crohn's disease, acute intestinal infection, irritable bowel syndrome, tropical sprue, and ulcerative colitis.

PP is derived primarily from the pancreas. The exact physiological role of PP is not understood. It has a biphasic effect; it initially increases and then inhibits the secretion of pancreatic enzymes, water, and electrolytes, thus opposing the stimulation effects of secretin and CCK. PP also increases gut motility and gastric emptying, as well as relaxation of the pyloric and ileocecal sphincters, colon, and gallbladder. PP levels are increased in a large percentage of individuals with VIPomas, glucagonomas, gastrinomas, and insulinomas.

■ ENZYMES OF THE GASTROINTESTINAL TRACT

Enzymes are produced both by the GI tract and the pancreas.[7]

Pepsin and Pepsinogen

Pepsin and pepsinogen are general names for several proteinases (pepsin A, B, and C; EC 3.4.23.1, 2, and 3, respectively) and their precursors that are secreted by the chief and mucous neck cells of the oxyntic glands and the mucous cells of the cardiac and pyloric glands (see Figure 37-1; see also Chapter 20).

Biochemistry and physiology

Pepsinogen is a proteolytic enzyme precursor (proenzyme) that, after secretion, is converted by acid to the active enzyme, pepsin. Once pepsin is activated, it is capable of converting more pepsinogen to pepsin (autocatalysis). Pepsins catalyze the hydrolysis of proteins to a mixture of polypeptides and partially digested proteinaceous foods during their passage through the stomach. Pepsinogen I (PG I, also called *pepsinogen A*) is found only in the chief and mucous neck cells of the oxyntic glands. Pepsinogen II (PG II) is found in the chief and mucous neck cells of the oxyntic glands, the cardiac and pyloric glands, and Brunner's glands in the duodenum.

Of the pepsinogen released from the gastric mucosa, about 99% is secreted into the stomach to become part of the gastric fluid. The remaining 1% diffuses into the interstitial fluid surrounding the chief cells and eventually reaches the blood. Any active pepsin that may enter the blood is inactivated rapidly at the near-neutral pH of blood. However, pepsinogen is stable and circulates in blood as such. The portion that reaches the kidneys passes through the glomeruli and is excreted in the urine (PG I only). At the mildly acidic pH of urine, part or all the proenzyme, now called *uropepsinogen,* may be converted (activated) to uropepsin. Daily excretion is fairly constant for any one individual, although a diurnal variation in urine output parallels the diurnal variation in adrenal activity. The quantity excreted is independent of urine pH, volume, and specific gravity. If the pH of the urine specimen is kept between 5.0 and 6.5, the urine enzyme is stable at room temperature for 2 to 3 days and in the refrigerator for 2 weeks. No inhibitor of the enzyme is present in the urine. Pepsinogen secretion, similar to that of gastric lipase, is stimulated by the vagus nerve and by some GI hormones (gastrin, secretin, CCK, and VIP).

Clinical significance

Serum concentrations of PG I reflect the parietal cell mass and correlate well with the maximum acid-secreting capacity. PG I increases with increasing height and is higher in smokers; it decreases as weight increases. Both PG I and PG II increase with increasing age.

Increased PG I and increased pepsin activity have been observed (1) in individuals with diseases associated with increased gastric output and related increased parietal mass; (2) in individuals with gastrinomas, such as Z-E syndrome; (3) in 30% to 50% of individuals with duodenal ulcer; (4) in individuals with acute and chronic superficial gastritis; and (5) after the administration of omeprazole.

Decreased levels of PG I are observed in individuals with diseases associated with decreased chief cell mass, atrophic gastritis, and gastric carcinoma and in those with myxedema (severe hypothyroidism), Addison's disease, and hypopituitarism. Absence of pepsinogen is observed in individuals with achlorhydria, as is seen in cases of pernicious anemia. PG II levels are normal in cases of pernicious anemia, in contrast to the low or undetectable levels of PG I. PG II levels are elevated, like PG I levels, in individuals with acute and chronic superficial gastritis. An elevated serum PG II level is considered a major risk factor for gastric ulcer. However, the location of the ulcer now appears to affect the pepsinogen levels and their ratio. A normal PG I, increased PG II, and decreased PG I/PG II ratio is found in individuals with an ulcer in the gastric body, whereas an elevated PG I, normal PG II, and an increased PG I/PG II ratio occurs in individuals with duodenal ulcers.

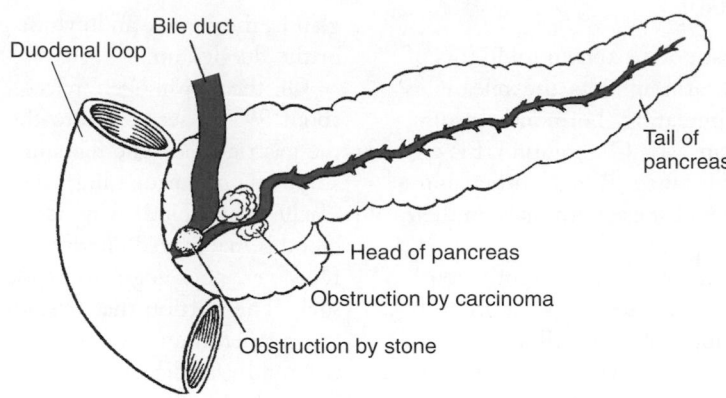

Figure 37-3   Cross-section through the pancreas, showing obstruction of the pancreatic duct by stone and carcinoma.

The most sensitive test for fundic atrophic gastritis is the PG I/PG II ratio in serum. Its clinical sensitivity and specificity are 99% and 94%, respectively. Ratios below about 3.3 are observed in individuals with moderate to severe atrophic gastritis and after total gastrectomy. More slight decreases are seen in individuals with gastric adenocarcinoma and mild atrophic gastritis. The discrimination limit is 5.5.

Analytical methodology

Pepsin, as well as pepsinogen after activation to pepsin, has been measured in mucosal cells, gastric contents, serum, and urine. As noted previously, PG I and PG II are immunologically distinct, thus permitting immunological assays of both proenzymes. These assays are commercially available. Typical reference intervals for serum PG I and PG II are 20 to 107 and 3 to 19 µg/L, respectively. The ratio, PG I/PG II, is about 5 to 6.

Enzymes Derived from the Pancreas

The normal pancreas secretes up to 1500 mL of fluid daily. More than 90% of the protein secretion consists of proenzymes or enzymes[6] that pass almost entirely into the duodenum; only a small fraction of these enzymes reach the blood, where they can be measured. Pancreatic enzymes are synthesized by the acinar cells and stored there in the form of zymogen granules. Enzymes of most clinical interest are amylase, lipase, and proteolytic enzymes. Activities of proteolytic enzymes in pancreatic juice are relatively constant, but they change if the diet is predominantly of one type for long periods of time; for example, proteolytic enzymes are secreted in larger amounts in cases of prolonged high-protein intake. Other enzymes present in pancreatic juice (some in the form of precursors and others, such as ribonucleases, in the active form) include trypsin, chymotrypsin, carboxypeptidases A and B, phospholipase A, ribonucleases, elastase, and collagenase.

On stimulation by CCK and, to a lesser extent, by gastrin and secretin, these enzymes are released from the acinar cells into the acinar lumen in a fluid containing HCO_3^- From the acinar lumen, they pass through the ductules into the main pancreatic duct, which empties into the duodenum through the ampulla of Vater. The bile duct joins the pancreatic duct just proximal to or at the ampulla of Vater (see Figure 37-2). In the duodenum the pancreatic juice mixes with the food material from the stomach. The combination of enzymes secreted by the pancreas, at the proper pH provided by the bicarbonate, digests virtually any food material.

In individuals with some disorders, such as pancreatitis or obstruction of the pancreatic duct due to stones or carcinoma, the flow of enzymes and bicarbonate into the duodenum is impeded (Figure 37-3). This obstruction results in a decreased secretion of pancreatic juice into the duodenum, and in turn an increased amount of pancreatic enzymes reaches the bloodstream (back flooding). The mechanism by which the enzymes enter the circulation is not known exactly, but it is thought to be due to changes in pressure in the pancreatic duct and ductules, changes in permeability of acinar cells, or disruption of the acinar-limiting membrane.

The pancreatic enzymes most commonly measured in serum are amylase, lipase, trypsin, and elastase.

Amylase, lipase, trypsin

The determination of these enzymes and their role in the diagnosis of pancreatic diseases are discussed in more detail in Chapter 20. To summarize their clinical utilities, amylase is measured in serum for the diagnosis of acute pancreatitis, in which case serum amylase activity is increased 2 to 12 hours after an acute attack and reaches a peak 12 to 72 hours after the attack. Determination of salivary (S-) and pancreatic (P-) type isoenzymes increases specificity and aids in the differentiation of hyperamylasemia of pancreatic origin from that due to other causes. Assays for lipase in serum are used chiefly for diagnosis of acute pancreatitis, in which case levels change in a manner similar to those of amylase. Serum trypsin is a highly sensitive and relatively specific indicator of pancreatic disease. Serum levels also are elevated in individuals with renal disease.

Elastase

Elastase (EC 3.4.21.11), unlike trypsin, chymotrypsin, and pepsin, rapidly hydrolyzes elastin, the yellow scleroprotein that is the basic ingredient of yellow elastic connective tissue. Two types of elastase are known—elastase 1, which exists in serum both free and as a complex with α-1-proteinase inhibitor, and elastase 2, which exists in serum mainly in the bound form with α-1-proteinase inhibitor. Elastase 1 is increased in cases of acute and relapsing chronic pancreatitis to a greater degree than is serum amylase activity. Elevations also persist for a longer time and are believed to reflect the clinical course more accurately than amylase activities.

Furthermore, no elevations or only minor elevations in elastase are observed in cases of hyperamylasemia of nonpancreatic origin. Elevations of elastase 1 also have been observed in individuals with carcinoma of the pancreas, especially carcinoma of the head of the pancreas. Its reference interval is about 1 to 4 μg/L, with no difference between men and women. Elastase 2 likewise is increased in individuals with acute pancreatitis, and both amylase activity and trypsin mass decrease in serum at a faster rate than elastase 2, which sometimes remains elevated for as long as 10 days. The reference interval for elastase 2 is 48 to 114 μg/L.

Because elastase is not digested during intestinal passage, concentrations of fecal elastase have been found to reflect accurately the amount of enzyme secreted from the pancreas. Low fecal elastase concentrations are found in individuals with watery diarrhea. In those with chronic pancreatitis but with normal pancreatic function, concentrations are greater than 200 μg/g stool. With moderately impaired pancreatic function, fecal elastase is 100 to 200 μg/g, and with severely impaired pancreatic function, it is less than 100 μg/g stool.

◼ GASTRIC, PANCREATIC, AND INTESTINAL DISEASES

Gastric Diseases

Diseases categorized as "gastric" include various types of ulcers, Z-E syndrome, gastritis, colorectal cancer, gastric cancer, and postgastrectomy syndrome.

Peptic ulcer disease

Peptic ulcer disease is the collective name given to chronic duodenal ulcer and chronic gastric (benign) ulcer. Although both have many features in common, they differ with respect to incidence, pathogenesis, natural history, outcome, and management.

Chronic duodenal ulcer

A duodenal ulcer is a round, sharply punched-out defect in the mucosa of the duodenum or the distal antrum and pyloric channel of the stomach. In time, chronic duodenal ulcers heal by the formation of fibrous scar tissue and the inward growth of the duodenal mucosal epithelium. Apart from the morbidity caused by the ulcer itself, other complications of duodenal ulcer include (1) hemorrhage due to the ulcer's erosion of a blood vessel; (2) perforation through the anterior wall of the duodenal cap, causing peritonitis; (3) penetration of the ulcer into adjacent structures, such as the pancreas, biliary tract, liver, colon, abdominal wall, and even lung; and (4) luminal obstruction (pyloric stenosis), caused by the gradual contraction of the ulcer scar.

Diagnosis of a chronic duodenal ulcer is made primarily by radiological techniques or endoscopy. Serum levels of PGI may be valuable because they reflect the gastric chief cell mass and correlate with the peak acid output (PAO). One third to one half of individuals with duodenal ulcer have PAO about 30 mmol/hour. The most important diseases to exclude during the diagnostic process are gastric ulcer and gastric carcinoma.

Chronic benign gastric ulcer

Gastric ulcers can occur anywhere in the stomach, although most are found along the lesser curvature. Some individuals with gastric ulcer have a coexistent duodenal ulcer. Gastric ulcers heal with the formation of fibrous tissue and the inward growth of the gastric epithelium. As with duodenal ulcers, gastric ulcers may cause hemorrhage or perforate. Chronic benign ulcers must be differentiated from acute gastric erosion and ulceration (see following discussion on gastritis). The PAO of gastric ulcer disease does not differ significantly from that of a healthy individual.

Zollinger-Ellison syndrome

The Z-E syndrome results from a tumor (gastrinoma) of the pancreatic islet cells. Its characteristics include fulminant peptic ulcers, massive gastric hypersecretion, hypergastrinemia, diarrhea, and steatorrhea. About half of all gastrinomas are multiple, and about two-thirds are malignant. One fourth of all gastrinomas are part of the multiple endocrine neoplasia syndrome, type I (MEN I), with associated tumors, or hyperplasia, in pancreatic islets and parathyroid and pituitary glands. In individuals with Z-E syndrome, fasting gastrin levels usually are elevated markedly, ranging from 2 to 2000 times the normal level. Gastrin concentrations greater than 1000 ng/L with gastric acid hypersecretion are virtually diagnostic of gastrinoma. Diarrhea often precedes ulcer symptoms and occurs in about one third of all affected individuals. The hypersecretion of acid causes the diarrhea, but the high blood levels of gastrin also may suppress jejunal absorption of sodium and water. Steatorrhea also occurs because of the lowering of the small intestinal pH, but it is less common than diarrhea. Lipase is inactivated at low pH, bile salts are rendered insoluble, and vitamin B_{12} is not absorbed by the distal ileum; gastric secretion of intrinsic factor is unaffected.

Gastric acid hypersecretion is a common finding of Z-E syndrome. However, a substantial overlap exists in gastric acid production and duodenal ulcer disease. Serum gastrin levels usually are increased markedly in individuals with Z-E syndrome, but sometimes only marginal elevations are found; additional testing, such as by secretin infusion, then is necessary. The 12-hour overnight secretion of HCl and the basal HCl excretion are greater than 100 mmol/L.

Gastritis

Gastritis is the term used to denote mucosal inflammation. Erosive, nonerosive, and specific (very rare) are the classifications of gastritis.

Erosive gastritis

Erosive gastritis (acute gastritis) occurs in individuals after severe trauma or severe burns (Curling's ulcer) and craniotomy or traumatic head injuries. It also is found in individuals with intracranial disease (Cushing's ulcer) and in those who chronically ingest drugs, such as corticosteroids, ethanol, or aspirin or other nonsteroidal antiinflammatory drugs (NSAIDs). Endoscopy is usually the definitive technique to establish the diagnosis.

Nonerosive gastritis

Nonerosive gastritis (chronic gastritis) is associated with peptic ulcer disease or gastric carcinoma, the period after partial gastrectomy, pernicious anemia, *Helicobacter pylori* infection, and healthy elderly individuals. Serum gastrin levels are elevated in achlorhydric individuals because of the absence of negative feedback by HCl.

Colorectal cancer

Colorectal cancer is the second leading cause of cancer deaths in Western Europe and North America. Most malignant colon cancers arise from adenomatous polyps, which are considered premalignant lesions. Most strategies used to detect colorectal cancer at an early, curative, stage are based on the detection of bleeding from the tumor; most individuals with colorectal cancer have fecal hemoglobin concentrations more than 2 mg/g of stool, whereas healthy subjects have less than 2 mg/g/day. The testing of **fecal "occult" blood** (**FOB**; meaning hidden and not apparent on inspection of the stool) is an example of such a strategy. Other techniques used to detect colorectal cancer include sigmoidoscopy and colonoscopy. Unfortunately, about one third of all cancers and polyps are beyond the reach of the rigid or flexible sigmoidoscope examination; this aspect emphasizes the importance of the FOB test.

The fate of intraluminal hemoglobin depends on the bleeding site. Bleeding in the upper gastrointestinal (GI) tract permits complete digestion of the globin and conversion of the heme, which is not absorbed, by bacterial action in the colon to heme-derived porphyrins. Bleeding in the proximal colon allows for the bacterial degradation of globin and for heme's conversion to heme-derived porphyrins, whereas bleeding in the rectosigmoid zone causes minimal

alteration of the hemoglobin molecule. Therefore tests for FOB should detect either heme or heme-derived porphyrins.

The most common FOB test formulation has been heme-based detection of the peroxidase-like activity of heme, of which the guaiac (leuko-dye) test is an example. Unfortunately, guaiac reacts with many nonhemoglobin peroxidases present in stool, such as those found in many vegetables and ingested meat. In addition, many medications, such as salicylates (which may cause bleeding into the gut) or vitamin C supplements (which inhibit the guaiac reaction), may create problems for the interpretation of FOB test results. Thus dietary and other restrictions should be followed before the guaiac test can be used; this aspect often reduces the compliance rate for testing because patients have to collect multiple stool samples over several days. Overall the clinical sensitivity of the guaiac test is about 40%. Thus many tumors are not detected at their earliest, potentially curative stage.

The sensitivity of the guaiac test has been improved by the introduction of a rehydration step (a drop of water on the slide) before testing; this step increases the test sensitivity but decreases its specificity. Thus more cancers are detected after rehydration is performed, but more false positives result, leading to the need for a large number of additional investigations (barium meal or sigmoidoscopy). A more sensitive version has been developed that has a clinical sensitivity and specificity of about 80% and 94%, respectively. A further improvement is the development of an immunochemical assay for human hemoglobin, which removes the need for the burdensome dietary preparations and interferences by several medications.

The major disadvantage to hemoglobin or heme-based testing is that neither type of test detects heme-derived porphyrins that arise from proximal GI bleeding and are less likely to be detected by guaiac or immunochemical testing. A fluorometric assay has been developed specifically to detect these porphyrins and heme. Although it may be affected by ingestion of red meat, the assay does not respond to other dietary peroxidases, medications, or fecal contaminants. With this test, results are reported as milligrams of hemoglobin per gram of stool. Values below 2 mg/g are regarded as normal, and 97% of individuals with colorectal cancers demonstrate values above that level.

Gastric cancer

Gastric cancer (adenocarcinoma) arises from the mucous cells of the gastric mucosa; it is the second most common cancer in the world after lung cancer. It is the third most common GI cancer in the United States. The role of *H. pylori* infection is being recognized increasingly as a significant causative factor.

Diagnosis of gastric cancer is made by biopsy. The majority of individuals have fasting achlorhydria, but less than one quarter of all individuals demonstrate achlorhydria after maximal stimulation. The volume of the gastric residue may be increased, and in some cases, blood may be found in the stomach. Lactate often is present.

Postgastrectomy Syndrome

Despite advances in the development of antiulcer drugs, surgery for peptic ulcer disease by gastric resection (pyloroplasty, gastric resections, gastroduodenostomy, or gastrojejunostomy) or various types of denervation (vagotomy) of the stomach still may be required. A number of these individuals suffer some functional incapacity, to which the name **postgastrectomy syndrome** or dysfunction has been given. This term includes the dumping syndrome, diarrhea, maldigestion, weight loss, anemia, bone disease, and gastric cancer.

The **dumping syndrome** occurs because the stomach, after gastrectomy, empties more rapidly than normal. The individual experiences abdominal pain and diarrhea, together with vagomotor phenomena, such as flushing, light-headedness, and cardiac palpitations 30 to 60 minutes after eating. Because the proximal jejunum contains a hypertonic solution of partially digested food, rapid osmotic equilibrium with blood results in a slight but rapid decrease in the blood volume, with concomitant intestinal distention. Between 90 and 180 minutes after a meal the individual may experience cardiac palpitations, lassitude, mental confusion, or even loss of consciousness; these events may be due to reactive hypoglycemia. Diarrhea may occur usually 1 or 2 hours after food ingestion as a result of rapid filling of the jejunum after meals.

Weight loss and specific nutritional deficiencies are not uncommon after gastric surgery. Anemia develops as a result of decreased absorption of iron, vitamin B_{12}, and folate. Maldigestion may occur due to rapid gastric emptying (resulting in less gastric dispersion of solid food and reduced digestion time), small intestinal "hurry," and reduced pancreatic secretion. In addition, asynchronism exists between the arrival of pancreatic and biliary secretions and the entry of food into the small intestine.

An increased prevalence of metabolic bone disease has been observed in individuals after ulcer surgery. Osteoporosis (loss of bone matrix and bone) occurs more commonly than osteomalacia (deficient calcification). The former is characterized by bone pain, loss of bone, pseudofractures, low serum calcium, and increased serum alkaline phosphatase activity. These manifestations can be reversed by the administration of vitamin D. About one-half the individuals with osteoporosis also have osteomalacia. Metabolic bone disease is estimated to occur in 5% to 15% of individuals who have undergone ulcer surgery.

Pancreatic and Intestinal Diseases

Acute and chronic pancreatitis, pancreatic carcinoma, and CF are classified as pancreatic and intestinal diseases.

Acute pancreatitis

Acute pancreatitis is defined as a discrete, sudden episode of more or less diffuse enzymatic destruction of the pancreatic tissue. It results from the escape of active pancreatic enzymes into the glandular parenchyma. Acute pancreatitis is distinguished from chronic pancreatitis in that in the acute form, normal endocrine and exocrine function are restored on elimination of the causative factor, with no permanent functional damage. Acute pancreatitis is estimated to occur once in about every 500 acute admissions to a general hospital and most frequently in the age group of 50 years and older. It is associated frequently with biliary tract disease, alcoholism, or both. *Relapsing pancreatitis* is a term used to characterize recurrent occasions of either acute or chronic pancreatitis.

Apart from the morbidity resulting from acute pancreatitis itself, four important local complications exist—pseudocyst formation, ascites, pleural effusion, and pancreatic or peripancreatic abscess formation. About one half of all individuals with severe pancreatitis develop pseudocysts (areas of necrosis containing tissue debris, pancreatic juice, blood and fat droplets walled off by fibrous tissue); many of these masses are palpable on physical examination. About one-half all acute pseudocysts resolve spontaneously over several weeks after formation; others may require surgical removal or drainage. Ascites results from a persistent leak of pancreatic juice from a pseudocyst or less frequently, from a disrupted pancreatic duct. The ascites may resolve spontaneously, or it may persist and cause a painless enlargement of the abdomen. Pleural effusion is caused by spread, via the diaphragmatic lymphatics, of the inflammatory exudate into the pleural (usually left-sided) space. The volume may be sufficient to cause impaired ventilation. Abscess formation is rare but very serious. Necrotic pancreatic tissues become infected with coliform bacteria from the colon.

The two leading conditions associated with acute pancreatitis are biliary tract disease, especially cholelithiasis, and excessive alcohol intake. Gallstones are present in about 50% of all cases, and about 5% of individuals with gallstones develop acute pancreatitis. Most alcoholic individuals with pancreatitis progress to chronic pancreatitis (irreversible functional and structural damage). Estimations are that up to 25% of all cases of acute pancreatitis are not associated with a known predisposing factor and therefore are labeled *idiopathic pancreatitis* of unknown etiology or not secondary to any other disease.

Other known causes of acute pancreatitis include (1) drugs (particularly antimetabolites and sulfonamide derivatives), (2) abdominal operations on or near the pancreas, (3) some cases of coronary artery bypass surgery, (4) retrograde injections of radiological media into the pancreatic duct for visualization purposes (endoscopic retrograde cholangiopancreatography), (5) physical trauma, (6) hypercalcemia, (7) obstruction to the outflow of the pancreatic duct, (8) inflammation or spasm caused by a variety of anatomical defects or coexisting diseases, (9) renal transplantation, and (10) the presence of hyperlipidemia. Individuals on estrogen therapy who develop pancreatitis have a type IV or V hyperlipidemia. Up to 20% of alcoholic individuals with pancreatitis have hypertriglyceridemia (type V pattern). A similar association occurs in some individuals with idiopathic pancreatitis. Finally, those individuals with type I, IV, or V hyperlipoproteinemias frequently develop acute pancreatitis that often progresses to chronic pancreatitis. The morphology of the pancreas in cases of acute pancreatitis indicates that proteolysis, lipolysis, and hemorrhage are caused by the pancreatic enzymes.

The diagnosis of acute pancreatitis is principally a diagnosis of exclusion. Abdominal and chest radiographs, upper GI contrast series, ultrasonography, and computed tomography (CT) are clinically useful, particularly for the detection of complications of pancreatitis, such as pseudocyst, abscess, and localized hematoma. Ultrasonography also is useful in the detection of gallstones, which may be a cause of pancreatitis. The clinical laboratory provides a number of chemical and hematological assays (Table 37-2). The enzyme findings in individuals with acute pancreatitis are discussed in Chapter 20. Simultaneous determinations of serum amylase and lipase are recommended, although the severity of the attack does not correlate with the degree of elevation of serum enzyme activity. However, an assessment of the severity and prognosis is made through notation of the clinical features of the patient. One such scoring system is that of Ranson. Three or more positive indices in the following list indicate severe disease:

On admission:

- Age greater than 55 years
- Leukocyte count greater than 16×10^9/L
- Serum glucose greater than 200 mg/dL (>11 mmol/L)
- Lactate dehydrogenase (LD) greater than 350 U/L (normal up to 225 U/L)
- Aspartate transaminase (AST) greater than 250 U/L (normal up to 40 U/L)

During first 48 hours:

- Hematocrit decreased by greater than 10%
- Calcium less than 8 mg/dL (<2 mmol/L)
- Urea nitrogen rise greater than 5 mg/dL (1.8 mmol urea/L)
- P_{O_2} less than 60 mm Hg
- Base deficit greater than 4 mmol/L
- Fluid sequestration greater than 6 L

Chronic pancreatitis

Chronic pancreatitis is defined by the presence of chronic inflammatory lesions characterized by the destruction of exocrine parenchyma and fibrosis. In the condition's late stages the endocrine parenchyma is destroyed. Individuals with chronic pancreatitis may suffer episodes of exacerba-

---

TABLE 37-2 Selected Tests Used to Diagnose Pancreatic and Intestinal Diseases

Pancreatitis, Pseudocyst
Amylase, serum
Amylase, urine
Isoamylase, serum
Lipase, serum
Immunoreactive trypsin, serum
Miscellaneous tests:
   Calcium, serum
   Glucose, serum
   Creatinine, serum
   Albumin, serum
   Hematocrit
Visualization techniques*

Pancreatic Exocrine Insufficiency
Pancreatic juice or duodenal content after stimulation with Lundh meal, secretin, or secretin CCK for volume; concentration of HCO_3^-, trypsin, chymotrypsin, lipase, and amylase
Byz-Tyr-PABA test or FDL test after stimulation with Lundh meal
Stool for trypsin or chymotrypsin, with or without Lundh meal
Breath tests
Stool for fat
Visualization techniques*

Malignant Disease
CA 19-9 antigen, serum
α-Fetoprotein, serum
Special enzyme tests: pancreatic juice or duodenal content
Pancreatic exocrine function tests, with cytological examination
Visualization techniques*

Malabsorption
Breath tests
Disaccharide tolerance tests
Xylose absorption test
Fat, stool
Tests for pancreatic exocrine insufficiency (see previous)
Intestinal biopsy, histochemical study for intestinal enzymes
Iron, folate, vitamin B_{12}, in serum
Visualization techniques*

CCK, Cholecystokinin; HCO_3^-, bicarbonate; *Byz-Tyr-PABA*, N-benzoyl-L-tyrosyl-p-aminobenzoic acid; *FDL*, fluorescein dilaurate; *CA*, carbohydrate antigen.
*Visualization techniques include angiography, computed tomography (CT scan), endoscopic retrograde cholangiopancreatography (ERCP), ultrasound scan, magnetic resonance imaging (MRI), and radiological examination of intestine with contrast media.

---

tion indistinguishable from acute pancreatitis. About one half of all individuals with chronic pancreatitis suffer attacks of acute pancreatitis in the presence of an irreversibly damaged pancreas; one-third of such attacks are continuous or intermittent in nature. Another less common presentation is the sudden appearance of diabetes mellitus, malabsorption, jaundice, or upper GI bleeding. During the course of chronic pancreatitis, 90% of affected individuals suffer "boring," dull, or sharp and steady epigastric or lower abdominal pain that often radiates to the back. The onset of pain may be gradual and usually lasts for several days to weeks.

Etiology and pathogenesis of chronic pancreatitis are unknown largely, but associated factors that may be causative are well recognized. Ethanol abuse is associated clearly with the development of chronic pancreatitis. A substantial proportion of these individuals may also develop hepatic cirrhosis, alcoholic hepatitis, or fatty liver. Other causes of chronic pancreatitis are hyperparathyroidism, other hypercalcemic states, and hyperlipidemia. In the known alcoholic individual a recurring attack of pancreatitis or the presence of pancreatic calcifications suggests the diagnosis. Acute pseudocysts, malabsorption, or diabetes mellitus is a frequent development in these individuals. The diagnostic challenge of chronic pancreatitis occurs in individuals with painless disease or those in whom differentiation between acute relapsing and chronic relapsing pancreatitis is difficult. Serum pancreatic enzyme levels are of limited assistance because the acinar cell mass may be decreased markedly or mild inflammation may not elevate serum enzyme activities. In view of the close association of chronic pancreatitis with alcoholism, checking of liver and biliary function by determination of serum bilirubin and alkaline phosphatase levels is essential.

Tumors of the pancreas

Carcinoma of the pancreas is the major tumor in this organ. Adenocarcinoma of pancreatic ductal epithelium is a common malignancy. It develops insidiously, progresses relentlessly, and is invariably fatal. No characteristic clinical features lead to the diagnosis. About one half of all affected individuals exhibit jaundice because of a tumor in the head of the pancreas obstructing or encircling the distal common bile duct. Radiological tests are used to investigate the possible presence of pancreatic neoplasms.

A wide range of laboratory tests for pancreatic cancer have been proposed, with widely varying sensitivities and specificities. Of these, CA 19-9 appears to be most useful in the clinical setting. Although CA 19-9 is present in several body secretions, very little appears in the blood of healthy individuals or those with benign disorders. However, most individuals with carcinoma of the pancreas have elevated blood levels of CA 19-9. The marker also is useful in the prediction of unresectability because tumors producing blood levels greater than 200 kU/L are unresectable. Blood levels that normalize after surgical removal of the tumor indicate a better postoperative course. Serial assay also may predict also recurrence.

Tumors of the pancreatic islet tissues

Tumors of the pancreatic islet tissues include insulinoma, glucagonoma, gastrinoma (Z-E syndrome), VIPoma (Verner-Morrison syndrome), somatostatinoma, and MEN syndromes.

Insulinoma

These β-cell islet tumors of the pancreas cause variable degrees and symptoms of hypoglycemia, usually after an overnight fast. The diagnosis normally is established by a finding of a low serum glucose value (males <55 mg/dL [<3 mmol/L]; females <35 mg/dL [<2 mmol/L]). The diagnosis can be confirmed by a finding of an inappropriately elevated plasma insulin level of greater than 15 mU/L and a plasma proinsulin level greater than 40 pmol/L. However, these findings may be mimicked by the surreptitious use of oral sulfonylureas.

Glucagonoma

The α-cell islet tumors of the pancreas are mostly malignant and demonstrate progressive metastatic growth. The diagnosis is established by the appearance of clinical symptoms and by the finding of a plasma glucagon level exceeding 500 ng/L.

Somatostatinoma

High circulating levels of somatostatin are found in individuals with somatostatinomas, but somatostatin also may be secreted ectopically by a variety of neoplasms. The pancreatic tumor may secrete adrenocorticotropic hormone and calcitonin. A mild diabetic syndrome usually is present. Gallbladder contraction is inhibited, which, together with inhibition of pancreatic juice secretion, can lead to diarrhea and steatorrhea. Delayed gastric emptying and inhibition of acid secretion produce dyspepsia and achlorhydria.

Multiple endocrine neoplasia syndrome

A number of syndromes are associated with hyperplasia or tumors in two or more endocrine organs. These syndromes have been described as the *MEN syndromes*. One such syndrome (MEN I, or Wermer's syndrome) consists of a highly variable combination of hyperplasia or tumors of the non–β-islet cells of the pancreas, parathyroids, and anterior pituitary, with variable degrees of hyperfunction of these systems. The tumors also may be "nonfunctioning" in the sense that insufficient hormone is secreted to produce symptoms. The most important relationship between pancreatic tumor and MEN I is with gastrinoma, in which case up to one quarter of all individuals with gastrinoma have MEN I.

Cystic fibrosis

Cystic fibrosis (CF) is the most common lethal genetic defect of Caucasian populations.[11] It is inherited in an autosomal-recessive fashion, and its incidence in Caucasian populations ranges from 1:1900 to 1:6500, with an average of 1:2000 live births. These data suggest a heterozygote-carrier incidence of about 1:20. Unfortunately, at present only some alleles have been identified in heterozygotes.

CF is a major cause of malabsorption in infants and children and of chronic pulmonary disease in childhood. All cases of CF eventually develop chronic pulmonary disease and indeed the respiratory disorder is responsible for much of the morbidity and nearly all the mortality associated with this disease. CF is a systemic disease affecting many types of exocrine glands. It is associated with a unique sweat-gland defect, with abnormalities of mucus secretion and the male genital tract. With appropriate long-term treatment, median survival is about 40 years of age for any child born now; previously, more than 80% of individuals with CF survived into their 20s; men survive slightly longer than women.

CF should be suspected in a child with chronic or recurrent respiratory-tract infections. However, many other presentations exist, among them pancreatic exocrine and endocrine dysfunctions, meconium ileus in the newborn, distal intestinal obstruction syndrome, intussusception (invagination of a part of the bowel into the following part of the bowel), rectal prolapse (a protrusion of the rectal mucous membrane through the anus), hepatomegaly, obstructive jaundice, and genital abnormalities in the male. The initial lesion in the lung is bronchial obstruction, which leads to chronic infections and bronchopneumonia, emphysema, atelectasis, and abscesses. Eventually the individual may suffer massive lung destruction. Usually the upper respiratory tract also is infected, and chronic sinus infection is very common. Therefore cough is an early symptom and can become chronic and so frequent that vomiting may occur. By 2 years of age, more than three quarters of children with CF have affected lungs. The individual may have finger clubbing and be cyanotic. Serious complications, such as pneumothorax, hemoptysis, and cor pulmonale, may intervene. Respiratory failure may be—and frequently is—the cause of death.

An estimated 85% of individuals with CF have exocrine pancreatic insufficiency; however, many infants with CF actually have adequate exocrine pancreatic function. The pancreatic lesions are caused by obstruction of the small ducts by secretions that eventually cause necrosis of the acinar and ductal cells. Fibrosis replaces necrosis in the pancreatic lobules. The islets of Langerhans usually are spared until late in the process of the disease. The resulting malabsorption and maldigestion cause bulky and frequent stools, described as light, oily, and foul smelling. Infants may demonstrate diarrhea and failure to gain weight. Another possibility is pancreatic endocrine dysfunction. Approximately 2% of pediatric individuals with CF and 13% of individuals older than 25 years of age have diabetes; many more have glucose intolerance.

Meconium ileus is the presenting symptom in about 10% of infants with CF; meconium (the first material discharged from the bowels of a newborn) is extremely viscous and blocks the distal ileum. The condition presents with signs of intestinal obstruction within 48 hours of birth.

Hepatic abnormalities occur in up to 50% of individuals with CF. Plugging of the biliary tracts with mucus sometimes progresses to periportal inflammation, biliary fibrosis, and, in fewer than 5% of cases, to cirrhosis. Cholestasis therefore is a presentation of CF, and gallstones are an expected complication.

Boys/men with CF experience developmental abnor-malities of the epididymis, vas deferens, and seminal vesicles. An estimated 97% of men are sterile as a result of these abnormalities.

Abnormal electrolyte secretion is a characteristic and constant finding in CF (see Chapter 25). The sodium and chloride and sometimes the potassium content of sweat are elevated. Micropuncture studies of the sweat glands demonstrate that the osmolality and sodium content of the fluid elaborated by the secondary coil are normal. The defect appears to be in the reabsorption of sodium and chloride in the sweat ducts. Abnormal sodium and chloride content also has been noted in submaxillary gland saliva and less often in parotid gland saliva. Duodenal fluid and tears are not affected, but stimulated pancreatic juice exhibits an abnormal electrolyte pattern.

The basic genetic defect in individuals with CF resides on the long arm of chromosome 7 and encodes a protein called the *CF transmembrane conductance regulator (CFTR)*. The allele, which is responsible for about 70% of CF cases, is due to a mutation that deletes a three-base pair sequence coding for phenylalanine at position 508 of the CFTR protein (ΔF508).

CF always must be suspected in cases involving unexplained chronic pulmonary disease, chronic hepatobiliary disease, hypoproteinemia, edema, and failure to thrive. Most children with pancreatic insufficiency or meconium ileus and 30% of those with meconium peritonitis have CF. Using up to 24 mutation probes, estimations are that the detection rate can be as high as 90%.

The diagnosis of CF rests primarily on the findings of the sweat test (see Chapter 25), although these results must be integrated with the clinical findings and family history of the child. An alternative approach for diagnosis is first to measure immunoreactive trypsin in dried blood spots that have been obtained at birth or soon after. If this test is positive, CFTR gene mutation analysis then is performed. This approach has potential as a large-scale screening program. Prenatal screening of all pregnant women, by use of either a blood or mouthwash sample, is a practical alternative to neonatal screening.

Diarrhea

Diarrhea is defined as an abnormal increase in one or more stool characteristics—daily weight, liquidity, and frequency. The normal colon absorbs about 3.8 L of fluid per day (about 2.7 mL/minute); it also absorbs ions against a steep electrochemical gradient. Diarrhea results from (1) prolonged exposure of the colon to fluid volumes exceeding these limits, (2) unusual amounts of poorly absorbable osmotically active solutes, (3) intestinal ion secretion, (4) inhibition of the normal ion absorptive process, (5) deranged intestinal motility, and (6) exudation of mucus, blood, and protein due to inflammatory (infectious) disorders of the bowel.

The ingestion of poorly absorbed, osmotically active solutes, such as some carbohydrates or divalent ions (Mg or

SO_4), causes osmotic diarrhea. If the unabsorbed solute is a carbohydrate, bacterial metabolism in the colon converts this species into many more short-chain fatty acid molecules, thus increasing the number of osmotically active particles in the colon. These species draw water into the gut, and subsequent absorption of sodium and water by the colon leaves a colonic fluid with a low sodium content. Osmotic diarrhea stops when the individual fasts or stops taking the poorly absorbable solute, although the assurance that surreptitious ingestion is not occurring is essential. Determinations of the fecal osmolality and content of sodium, potassium, and magnesium are necessary. An important cause of osmotic diarrhea is the ingestion of magnesium or sulfate salts (for example, magnesium hydroxide [Mylanta, Maalox, or Haley's MO], magnesium trisilicate [Gelusil], magnesium sulfate [Epsom salt], sodium sulfate [Glauber's salt], and other magnesium salts contained in mineral/vitamin supplements). Other causes of osmotic diarrhea include maldigestion and malabsorption of glucose and other sugars present in mucosal disease.

Secretory diarrhea may be due to either inhibition of ion absorption or stimulation of ion secretion. Secretory diarrhea is characterized by the following three features:

1. Stool osmolality is accounted for by normal ionic constituents.
2. The condition usually persists after fasting.
3. Pus, blood, or excess fat are not present.

Some exceptions to these generalizations do exist, such as surreptitious ingestion of laxatives (for example, aloe, senna, oxyphenisatin, phenolphthalein), diarrhea caused by fatty acid malabsorption, and the simultaneous interplay of mechanisms of both secretory and osmotic diarrhea. Causes of secretory diarrhea include, in addition to those listed previously, enterotoxins, such as bacterial exotoxins (for example, *Vibrio cholerae, Escherichia coli, Salmonellae typhimurium, Shigella dysenteriae 1, Staphylococcus aureus*); tumor production of secretagogues, such as VIP, bradykinin, and serotonin; detergents that alter intestinal fluid and electrolyte movement, such as bile acids and some over-the-counter laxatives; inflammatory bowel disease, including parasitic infections; and decreased solute absorption due to loss of mucosal transport function secondary to altered mucosal morphology (celiac disease) or to isolated transport defects (monosaccharide malabsorption).

Deranged motility may be the mechanism for the chronic diarrhea occurring in the individual with irritable bowel syndrome, malignant carcinoid syndrome, medullary carcinoma of the thyroid, postvagotomy and postgastrectomy, and thyrotoxicosis, as well as the acute diarrhea occurring with infections. Inflammatory disorders of the bowel may cause exudative diarrhea when bowel inflammation or ulceration discharges mucus, serum protein, and blood into the lumen.

The loss of diarrhea fluid results in water depletion (hypovolemia), Na^+ and K^+ depletion, and HCO_3^- loss, with the latter resulting in a hyperchloremic metabolic acidosis with a normal anion gap.

Maldigestion, Malabsorption, and Related Disorders

The total quantity of fluid absorbed each day by the gut is estimated to be approximately 9 L, which is composed of 2 L oral intake and 7 L GI secretions. The majority of secretions enter the gut in the upper portion of the tract—from the mouth, stomach, pancreas, and bile duct. More than 90% of the fluid is absorbed in the small intestine. Folds, villi, and microvilli together present an absorptive surface of about 250 m^2, the area of a tennis court!

Several hundred grams of carbohydrates, more than 100 g of fat, and 50 to 100 g of amino acids are absorbed daily in the small gut, but maximal absorptive capacity is believed to be at least 10 times greater. The maximal absorptive capacity for fluid is probably at least 20 L. This considerable reserve capacity may compensate for mild to moderate degrees of dysfunction induced by disease processes.

Different segments of the gut are more or less specialized or adapted to particular stages of digestion and absorption. For convenience these stages are called the *luminal* and *small intestinal stages*. The luminal stage is divided further into the secretory (pancreatic) and biliary stages. The small intestinal stage is divided into the surface (brush border) and cellular (delivery, transport) stages. Defects of digestion or absorption may occur at one or multiple stages and in one or more of the mechanisms of any stage. Defects in digestion and absorption also are related to the nature of the foodstuff that is processed.

Maldigestion is a dysfunction of the digestive process that occurs at a number of sites in the GI tract. For example, hypoacidity in the stomach, hyperacidity of the duodenum, loss of brush border enzymes in the small intestine, and pancreatic insufficiency cause maldigestion of fats and proteins. **Malabsorption** is a dysfunction of the absorptive process by the small gut; it is due to loss of absorptive epithelial cells caused, for example, by gluten, inflammation, infection, surgical resection, and infiltrations. In clinical practice, however, the term *malabsorption* is usually used to encompass all aspects of impaired digestion and absorption.

Carbohydrates

Generalized impairment of carbohydrate absorption occurs as a result of a number of diseases that cause mucosal damage or dysfunction. Examples of such diseases include celiac disease, tropical sprue, and acute gastroenteritis. Absorption defects are caused by a deficiency in a single or all brush border oligosaccharidases. Examples include (1) congenital lactase deficiency, (2) acquired lactase deficiency (hypolactasia), (3) sucrase-isomaltase deficiency, and (4) trehalase deficiency.

If symptoms of flatulence, abdominal discomfort, bloating, or diarrhea occur after consumption of one or two glasses of milk or a large portion of ice cream or yogurt, lactose intolerance should be suspected. Suspicion is increased if the individual belongs to an ethnic group with high prevalence of lactose intolerance—black, Asian, Jewish, Arabic, or other Mediterranean descent or indigenous natives of North, South, or Central America. Lactase intolerance aggravates bowel symptoms of diseases such as ulcerative colitis.

The most direct diagnostic test for an intestinal enzyme deficiency is histochemical examination of the brush border of the intestinal epithelium. A more practical test is to feed the patient one disaccharide (50 g in adults and 2 g/kg in children) at a time, followed by measurement of either breath hydrogen or serum glucose concentrations. If the appropriate disaccharidase is present, the disaccharide is hydrolyzed at the brush border and its component monosaccharide absorbed. A peak rise of breath hydrogen greater than 12 parts per million over the fasting baseline value is considered positive. If this methodology is not available, sequential serum glucose assays may be used. In this latter technique a fasting specimen is drawn, and after consumption of the selected disaccharide, specimens are drawn at 15, 30, 45, 60, and 90 minutes thereafter. An increase of 30 mg/dL (1.7 mmol/L) is considered normal. A rise of 20 to 30 mg/dL (1.1 to 1.7 mmol/L) is inconclusive. An increase of less than 20 mg/dL (1.1 mmol/L) is evidence for a deficiency of the intestinal disaccharidase. Any abnormal test must be followed by a control test, in which 25 g of the each constituent monosaccharide is administered to ensure that the individual has normal tolerance to them. Verification of absorptive ability is made through performance of a glucose tolerance test before the disaccharide challenge test. A normal rise above the fasting glucose level verifies the absence of a transport defect.

Lipids

Conditions associated with maldigestion and malabsorption of lipids include diseases that affect the pancreatic, biliary stage, or cellular and delivery stages, or a combination of these (Table 37-3). Table 37-4 classifies such diseases.

Amino acids and proteins

Pancreatic and small intestinal diseases are major causes of protein maldigestion and malabsorption. Any of the diseases listed under the pancreatic stage in Table 37-3 also results in an impaired assimilation of protein. Note, however, that the reserve capacity of the pancreas is very great, and fecal loss of protein may not become significant in pancreatic insufficiency states until trypsin has fallen to about 20% of its normal value. Mucosal diseases may affect protein assimilation by reduction in the number of mucosal cells, increased turnover of intestinal cells, or increased losses of plasma proteins from the damaged intestinal surface. Surgical resection of the intestine not only reduces the total intestinal absorptive

---

TABLE 37-3　Conditions Associated with Maldigestion and Malabsorption of Lipids

Pancreatic Stage
Isolated pancreatic lipase or colipase deficiency (inherited)
Pancreatic insufficiency
  Cystic fibrosis
  Chronic pancreatitis
  Obstruction of pancreatic duct

Biliary Stage
Decreased synthesis of bile salts in cases of severe hepatic insufficiency
Decreased delivery of bile salts in cases of obstruction in biliary tract or cholestatic biliary disease
Decreased concentration of conjugated bile salts because of increased acidity, drugs affecting micelle formation, intestinal stasis, or bacterial overgrowth
Increased intestinal loss of bile salts because of distal ileal resection, surgical ileal bypass, or diseased terminal ileum

Cellular and Delivery Stages in Small Intestine
Rapid transit, dumping syndrome
Improper emulsification after certain types of gastrectomy
Altered duodenal pH, as in Z-E syndrome
Diseases of small intestinal lymphatics

Defects at Multiple Stages of Digestion and Absorption
Decreased CCK release due to severe mucosal destruction, as in sprue or regional enteritis

Z-E syndrome, Zollinger-Ellison syndrome; *CCK,* cholecystokinin.

---

surface but also may remove a segment of the gut that is specialized for absorption of certain nutrients; an example is resection of the distal ileum, which removes the active transport system for the vitamin B_{12}-intrinsic factor complex. Another cause for reduced protein assimilation is protein-losing enteropathy, a condition in which inflamed or ulcerated mucosa can exude considerable quantities of plasma proteins, which if not digested and reabsorbed subsequently, may represent large fecal losses of nitrogen; these losses cause hypoproteinemia.

Diagnosis of malabsorption and maldigestion

The clinical laboratory plays an important role in the detection or ruling out of malabsorption and the elucidation of its cause.[9] Table 37-2 illustrates the many available diagnostic modalities. The diagnostic process should begin with screening tests, such as one of the simpler tests of fecal lipids. The gold standard test for steatorrhea is the determination of total fecal lipids (because this test provides a measure of the degree of malabsorption), but given the general unpleasantness of the procedure, the xylose absorption test often is used instead. If steatorrhea is not present, hydrogen breath tests and selected disaccharide tolerance tests are used to evaluate bacterial overgrowth or brush border oligosaccharidase deficiencies. Jejunal biopsy for histochemical

TABLE 37-4 Classification of Diseases Causing Maldigestion or Malabsorption

Luminal Phase (Dietary Fats, Proteins, and Carbohydrates Hydrolyzed and Solubilized)

DEFECT AT SECRETORY STAGE
Cystic fibrosis
Chronic pancreatitis
Defective stimulation due to intestinal disease or gastric surgery
Z-E syndrome (low pH inhibiting digestion of fats)
Carcinoma of pancreas
Pancreatectomy
Obstruction of pancreatic duct
Absence of trypsin, lipase, or colipase (inherited)

IMPAIRED MICELLE FORMATION (DUE TO ABSENCE OR DECREASE OF BILE SALTS)
Cholestatic jaundice
Biliary obstruction
Parenchymal liver disease
Drugs (cholestyramine binding and neomycin precipitating bile salts)
Z-E syndrome (low pH precipitating bile salts)
Bacterial overgrowth (deconjugation of bile salts)
Resection or disease of terminal ileum (diminishing enterohepatic circulation of bile salts)

Mucosal Phase (Occurring at the Small Intestinal Mucosa)

DEFECT AT BRUSH BORDER
Disaccharidase deficiencies (inherited and acquired)
Enterokinase deficiency (inherited)

DEFECT AT CELLULAR, DELIVERY, OR REMOVAL STAGE
Amino acid transport defects
Primary vitamin B_{12} malabsorption
Massive small intestinal resection
Radiation enteritis
Intestinal ischemia
Celiac sprue
Tropical sprue
Ulcerative colitis
Regional enteritis
Whipple's disease
Primary intestinal lymphoma
Hypogammaglobulinemia
Food allergy

Multiple-Stage Defects
Postgastrectomy
Diabetes mellitus
Endocrinopathies
Collagen disease

Z-E syndrome, Zollinger-Ellison syndrome.

and morphological examination is helpful to confirm congenital oligosaccharidase deficiencies and is necessary in other conditions to evaluate the nature and degree of damage to the intestinal mucosa. X-rays and other visualization techniques are required to demonstrate abnormal motility or anatomical features of the gut. A wide variety of serum and urine tests (see Table 37-2) are used in specific contexts to refine or confirm possible diagnoses or assign the cause for the presenting malabsorption syndrome.

Related disorders

Tropical sprue, ulcerative colitis, and regional enteritis are types of celiac disease. General symptoms include celiac sprue, idiopathic steatorrhea, nontropical sprue and adult **celiac disease,** also known as **gluten-induced (or sensitive) enteropathy**. Celiac disease is characterized by malabsorption, a specific lesion of the small intestinal mucosa, and an improvement when gluten-containing foods are removed from the diet.

Clinical features of celiac disease include a progressive weight loss, diarrhea, flatulence, and abdominal distention. Stools may be bulky, pale, foul-smelling, and floating; watery diarrhea also may be noticed. In children, an abnormal growth pattern ensues. In both children and adults a range of abnormalities outside the GI tract is present. Iron, folate, and vitamin B_{12}-deficiency anemias occur; calcium and vitamin D deficiencies cause osteomalacia and osteoporosis. Neurological symptoms may be due to multiple vitamin deficiency; secondary hyperparathyroidism due to severely impaired calcium absorption; adrenocortical insufficiency due to electrolyte deficiencies; and panhypopituitarism due to profound malnutrition.

The diagnostic gold standard for detection of celiac disease is biopsy of small intestinal mucosa. However, assays for antigliadin (AGA), antiendomysium (AEA), and antireticulin (ARA) antibodies in serum are useful screening tests because they reduce the need for intestinal biopsy. The AGA antibodies are generated against dietary gliadin (a constitute of wheat flour) and are found in two forms— immunoglobulin A-AGA (IgA-AGA) and immunoglobulin G-AGA (IgG-AGA). IgA-AGA is more specific and IgG-AGA more sensitive for celiac disease. In practice the initial screen for suspected celiac disease should include both tests because the IgA-AGA is a very sensitive marker of gluten-sensitive enteropathy in children and the IgG form is more sensitive in adults. These tests are either based on enzyme-linked immunosorbent assay (ELISA) or the use of an indirect immunofluorescence procedure in which rat kidney tissue is incubated with gliadin before the addition of patient sera. Establishing the reference intervals of both IgA-AGA and IgG-AGA in the local population is essential; at least 100 samples should be used. Values exceeding the median plus two standard deviations are considered abnormal.

The AEA and reticulin antibodies are gluten-inducible, connective tissue reactive autoantibodies that are invoked in individuals with celiac disease and disappear within a few months of a strict gluten-free diet but reappear after a dietary gluten challenge. These tests require the use of tissue sections and the application of fluorescein isothiocyanate-conjugated antihuman IgA, with microscopic detection under indirect ultraviolet illumination. The AEA test (IgA-

AEA) is the best test used to detect celiac disease but requires sections of macaque monkey esophagus, which makes the test very expensive. In addition to the high cost of slides for the monkey esophagus preparation the test requires highly specialized operators and considerable time, thus limiting its use as a screening test. In practice the AEA test is used only when both the IgA-AGA and the IgG-AGA tests are positive.

Tropical sprue

Tropical sprue is a chronic acquired disorder characterized by abnormalities of small bowel structure and function that become progressively more severe and lead to nutritional deficiency. This disorder occurs only among individuals who visit or reside in certain tropical areas and usually is curable by treatment with tetracycline and folic acid. It ordinarily begins as an intestinal infection that resolves itself but then evolves into a stage of milk intolerance as lactase deficiency develops. Eventually, and with a concomitant change in jejunal morphology, a frank syndrome of malabsorption is expressed. Up to 90% of affected individuals have steatorrhea. At the last stage, anorexia, weight loss, megaloblastic anemia, and edema are evident.

Ulcerative colitis

The etiology of the chronic inflammatory disorder of the intestine known as **ulcerative colitis** is unknown. The mucosae of the rectum and left colon are the sites most commonly affected, but any part of the alimentary canal may be involved. Histological changes are not characteristic; the appearance of the inflamed mucosa is similar to that of bacterial infection or other inflammatory conditions. Although the disease process usually is confined to the mucosa, in very serious cases, it may extend into the muscular wall of the colon to become what is called *toxic megacolon*. In ulcerative colitis, intermittent attacks of diarrhea often are associated with rectal bleeding; the diarrhea is often voluminous and may last for several weeks, culminating in water and electrolyte imbalance. The bleeding leads to an iron-deficiency anemia; hypoalbuminemia occurs because of low protein intake resulting from the anorexia or exudative loss of protein from the ulcerated mucosa, or both.

In cases of toxic megacolon, shock and fluid and electrolyte depletion may occur; these symptoms can lead to renal failure and cardiac arrhythmias. Additional complications of ulcerative colitis include perforation or cancer of the colon, massive hemorrhage, liver disease, and renal calculi.

Regional enteritis (Crohn's disease)

Regional enteritis, also known as **Crohn's disease,** is a chronic inflammation of the intestine of unknown etiology. The distal ileum and colon are the sites most often affected, but any part of the gut can be involved. The disease has a variable course, several complications are possible, and it may recur after surgical resection. The inflammatory process affects the entire intestinal wall; it can progress to ulceration, fibrosis leading to contraction and obstruction, and formation of fistulas between loops of the gut or between the gut and other organs. The complications further include development of malignant intestinal neoplasms, arthritis, mild abnormalities of liver function, and renal involvement with increased risk of renal stone formation. The diffuse involvement of the jejunum and ileum affects digestive and absorptive function throughout the gut and leads to numerous problems—disaccharidase deficiency, protein-losing enteropathy, chronic blood loss, lymphatic obstruction, vitamin B_{12}- and folate deficiencies, stasis of intestinal contents, and generalized inadequate caloric and protein malnutrition. Decrease of absorptive surface by fistulas or palliative resection and overgrowth of bacterial flora due to stasis exacerbate the nutritional deficiencies.

■ TESTS OF GASTRIC FUNCTION

The various motor and secretory activities of the stomach are evaluated by a number of clinical laboratory tests, among which are a diagnostic test for infection by *H. pylori* and general tests of gastric function.[5]

Diagnostic Tests for the Detection of *Helicobacter pylori*

About one-third to one-half the world's population harbors the bacterium **Helicobacter pylori.** This organism is a curved, S-shaped, motile organism found in the mucous layer of the stomach. Certain strains of *H. pylori* secrete proteins that cause inflammation of the mucosa, toxins that injure the gastric cells, and urease, the enzyme that breaks down urea to ammonia and CO_2. *H. pylori* infection has been shown to progress to chronic superficial gastritis, which, if untreated, persists for life. A small proportion of those infected may develop peptic ulcer disease, lymphoproliferative diseases, or severe chronic atrophic gastritis leading to stomach cancer. For example, more than 80% of gastric ulcers and 95% of duodenal ulcers are known to be associated with *H. pylori* infection. Such infections have a complex effect on gastric acid secretion. In the early stages of infection, secretion of gastric acid (which permits bacterial growth with consequent inflammation) is reduced. In the latter stages, gastric acid production increases (which causes further mucosal damage).

The laboratory often plays a role in the initial diagnosis and treatment follow-up.[3,8] In symptomatic patients, the gold-standard test is endoscopy (with histological examination), which detects esophageal, gastric, or duodenal lesions that may cause the symptoms; if indicated, a tissue biopsy is performed. A number of other tests also may be performed on this specimen. The initial screening test is often the rapid urease test based on the detection of CO_2 production by the incubated biopsy specimen. However, the sensitivity of this test depends on the number of bacteria in the specimen, so a confirming test may be necessary. Such tests include bacterial culture, smear examination, the application of specific gastric mucosal IgA or IgG, pylori antibodies, or techniques using polymerase chain reaction methodologies. In addition to these invasive tests, several noninvasive and less expensive tests are available, including a rapid whole-blood test providing results in less than 10 minutes, serological examination by several commercially available kits, and the ^{14}C or ^{13}C urea breath tests. The breath test consists of administration, in one formulation, of the isotope in a gelatin capsule and measurement of the production of isotopically labeled CO_2 10 minutes later.

General Tests

A number of general tests are used to assess gastric function. They include detection of compounds not normally seen in gastric contents, analysis of gastric residue (the content of the stomach after fasting), the determinations of the secretion rate in the basal state and after stimulation with appropriate stimuli, and the determination of intrinsic factor and pepsinogens.[4] In the past these tests aided clinicians in diagnosing pernicious anemia, differentiating benign from malignant ulcers, assessing ulcer dyspepsia, and selecting appropriate surgical treatments for duodenal ulcer and recurring postsurgical duodenal ulcer. However, because most of these clinical problems now are addressed by use of different diagnostic strategies, these tests are performed rarely.

■ TESTS MEASURING THE EXOCRINE FUNCTION OF THE PANCREAS

The exocrine function of the pancreas involves the production and secretion of pancreatic juice, which is rich in enzymes and bicarbonate. Normal pancreatic juice is colorless and odorless; it has a pH of 8.0 to 8.3 and a specific gravity of 1.007 to 1.042. The total 24-hour secretion volume may be as high as 3000 mL.

A number of invasive and noninvasive laboratory tests are available to measure exocrine functions in the investigation of pancreatic insufficiency, which is caused most commonly by chronic pancreatitis in adults and CF in children. Invasive tests require GI intubation to collect pancreatic samples. Noninvasive tests were developed to avoid such intubations because they are simpler and cheaper to perform. However, they do not produce results as reproducible, sensitive, or specific as invasive tests.

Invasive Tests of Pancreatic Function

Invasive tests include those that stimulate (1) pancreatic secretion intraluminally (by means of the Lundh test meal or use of a duodenal infusion of essential amino acids) and (2) pancreatic secretion by intravenous hormonal injection with secretin, CCK or a combination of CCK-octapeptide, secretin + CCK.[4] The total volume of pancreatic juice, amount or concentration of bicarbonate, or rates of enzyme secretion are measured either directly on duodenal content or on pancreatic juice obtained by cannulation. The enzyme most commonly measured is trypsin, but amylase and lipase measurements also have been measured. In infants, amylase measurements are unsuitable because this enzyme is synthesized in only small amounts until 1 year of age.

The secretin-CCK stimulation test is regarded as the gold standard for pancreatic function testing. With it, stimulation with secretin followed by stimulation with CCK allows for the assessment of the secretion of enzymes, as well as that of pancreatic juice and bicarbonate. This combination of stimuli is most satisfactory for measurement of pancreatic secretory capacity and thus for separation of individuals with normal from those with impaired pancreatic function.

Noninvasive Tests of Pancreatic Function

Noninvasive tests include (1) measurement of unabsorbed food or fecal pancreatic enzymes (trypsin, chymotrypsin, or elastase); (2) measurement of products of food digestion or synthetic compounds hydrolyzed by intraluminal pancreatic enzymes, absorbed by the gut, and detected in blood, urine, or breath; and (3) measurement of plasma concentrations of hormones, amino acids, or enzymes.

This group of tests is based on the fact that proper pancreatic function is essential for normal intestinal absorption of certain substances. Because the pancreas is the major source of amylase, lipase, and proteolytic enzymes (see Chapter 20), a significant decrease in pancreatic function results in decreased absorption of starch, fats, and protein and a parallel increased excretion of these food materials in the stool. In states of pancreatic deficiency, microscopic examination of stool demonstrates large amounts of undigested cell nuclei and meat fibers (creatorrhea), increased fat **(steatorrhea),** and increased starch (amylorrhea). Demonstration of these conditions suggests impaired absorption. In severe cases the feces are generally pale, bulky, and unusually foul smelling. With steatorrhea of pancreatic origin, fat droplets usually appear on the surface of feces on standing.

Unfortunately, these tests have no diagnostic value in mild cases of pancreatic disease and in cases in which the acute phase has subsided. The greatest value of these tests of pancreatic function seems to be in the exclusion of pancreatic pathology, especially CF.

Measurement of unabsorbed food or fecal pancreatic enzymes

Lipids and trypsin, chymotrypsin, and elastase have been measured in fecal samples to assess pancreatic function.

Fecal lipids

Fecal lipid determinations are performed frequently as part of metabolic or fat-balance studies and in the diagnosis of malabsorption caused by pancreatic or intestinal disorders.[4] The determination of fecal fat is the most definitive test used to determine the presence of steatorrhea, but not for determination of its cause.

Approaches used to measure fecal lipids include (1) gravimetry, (2) near-infrared reflectance, (3) microscopic examination of the stool specimen for fat droplets, (4) fat absorption tests, and (5) the steatocrit.

Gravimetric determination of total fecal lipids.   In the gravimetric method for the determination of total fecal lipids, a preweighed, emulsified stool specimen is acidified to decrease the ionization of fatty acids (present as free acids, or soaps). The lipids, including the less polar nonesterified fatty acids, then are extracted from the stool specimen with an organic solvent, the supernatant is evaporated, and the residue is quantitated by gravimetry. With this method the reference interval for fecal lipids is less than 2 g/day for children up to 6 years of age and 2 to 6 g/day for adults. Values greater than 7 g/day indicate steatorrhea.

Near-infrared reflectance analysis.   Near-infrared reflectance analysis (NIRA) is based on the measurement of radiation in the near-infrared spectrum scattered by the surface of a spot fecal sample. Through variations in wavelength, determinations of dry weight, total nitrogen, total fat, and hydrolyzed fat on a fecal specimen are possible in a matter of minutes. A 72-hour fecal specimen is collected and homogenized. The separate determination of total and hydrolyzed fat permits an indication of the origin of the steatorrhea. In cases of pancreatic insufficiency a decrease in fecal free fatty acids can be detected by the NIRA technique.

Microscopic examination.   Cases of steatorrhea can be determined by the microscopic examination of a stool specimen for fat droplets. The measurement of the diameter of the globules of fatty acid correlates with the measurement of total fecal lipids. On average, individuals with steatorrhea have 10 times as many fat droplets per standard volume of stool as healthy individuals.

Fat absorption test.   In the fat absorption test the individual is administered a fat load (typically, 1 g/kg body weight of butter spread on two slices of toast) after an overnight fast. Then, fasting and 2-hour blood specimens are obtained. The change in light-scattering intensity of the serum indicates the digestion and absorption of the butterfat challenge. More sophisticated versions of this type of test measure the changes in triglyceride and chylomicron concentrations 5 hours after the dietary challenge.

Steatocrit test.   In the steatocrit test a 0.5-g random fecal sample is homogenized with 0.06 g of sand and 2 volumes of water, and 70 μL is placed in a microhematocrit tube, which then is centrifuged for 15 minutes. In individuals with steatorrhea, three distinct layers are visible—a lower layer composed of nonfatty fecal solids, an intermediate liquid layer, and an upper fatty layer. The fatty layer is expressed as a percentage of the total fecal solids, a result termed the "steatocrit." In individuals without steatorrhea, the upper reference value is 2.1%.

Trypsin, chymotrypsin, and elastase in stool

Trypsin and chymotrypsin secreted by the pancreas and present in duodenal contents mix with food material and, except for the fraction digested in the intestinal tract, are excreted in the feces. Measurement of activity of these enzymes in stool (see Chapter 20) has been used for diagnosis of obstruction of the pancreatic duct or of pancreatic insufficiency, as, for example, in cases of CF. In practice, fecal chymotrypsin is considered a better index of pancreatic function. Its output in stool correlates well with chymotrypsin secretion into duodenal contents when both substances are measured after stimulation with secretin-CCK.

With the recommended procedure the stool specimen is extracted with a mixture of salts and a detergent, lauryltrimethylammonium chloride, which fully dissociates the enzyme from particles in stool. The extract is mixed with a synthetic pentapeptide that is covalently tagged with a molecule of 4-nitroaniline (4-NA); the substrate is hydrolyzed by chymotrypsin to produce free 4-NA. Continuous release of 4-NA is measured photometrically at 405 nm. Activity of chymotrypsin in stool remains virtually constant at room temperature for up to 10 days.

The immunoassay of elastase in stool shows promise as an alternative to the more conventional assay of stool chymotrypsin. However, this test does not separate consistently mild to moderate chronic pancreatitis cases from healthy controls.

Measurement of products of food digestion or synthetic substrates

In these tests the products of food digestion or synthetic compounds are measured after they have been hydrolyzed by pancreatic enzymes, absorbed by the gut, and detected in blood, urine, or breath. Examples of such analytes include β-carotene, vitamin A, chymotrypsin, pancreatic arylesterases, and various components of breath.

Serum carotene and vitamin A

Because vitamin A and β-carotene are fat soluble, they are absorbed only if they are hydrolyzed first by pancreatic lipase. Their measurements are discussed in Chapter 28.

Bz-Tyr-PABA test for chymotrypsin

The Bz-Tyr-PABA test for pancreatic chymotrypsin (also known as the *PABA* or *BTP test*) uses the synthetic tripeptide, *N*-benzoyl-L-tyrosyl-p-aminobenzoic acid (BTP). The test is initiated when BTP is administered orally, together with a test meal, to stimulate pancreatic secretion. BTP is hydrolyzed specifically by chymotrypsin in the duodenum to release *p*-aminobenzoic acid (PABA). PABA subsequently is absorbed in the intestinal tract and metabolized in the liver to hippurate, PABA glucuronide, and PABA acetylate. These arylamines then are excreted by the kidney into the urine, where they are measured spectrophotometrically. Low chymotrypsin levels result in less chromogen being excreted into the urine. Such levels are found in cases of pancreatic insufficiency. A high correlation exists between the results of this test and those from the direct test for chymotrypsin in stool.

Test for pancreatic arylesterases

The test for pancreatic arylesterases, also known as the *fluorescein dilaurate (FDL)* or *pancreolauryl test,* is based on the oral administration of FDL in the middle of a standard breakfast (50 g of white bread, 20 g of butter, and one cup of tea). FDL is hydrolyzed specifically by pancreatic arylesterases (EC 3.1.1.2), which require bile acids for its activity. The released fluorescein is water soluble, absorbed readily by the small intestine, conjugated in the liver, and excreted in the urine. Urine is collected for 10 hours. The test is repeated a few days later with free fluorescein to correct for individual variability in intestinal absorption, hepatic conjugation, and urinary excretion. The urinary recovery of fluorescein is measured spectrophotometrically on each day.

The ratio of fluorescein excreted after administration of FDL to that excreted after the free fluorescein dose is greater than 0.30 with normal pancreatic function. Ratios less than 0.20 are obtained in the presence of abnormal function, whereas values between 0.20 and 0.30 are considered inconclusive. The FDL test produces results very similar to those obtained with the PABA test.

Breath tests

Breath tests measure the excretion, by the lung, of either labeled CO_2 (^{14}C or ^{13}C) after the administration of carbon-labeled substrates or of H_2 after the administration of carbohydrate.[10] All CO_2 breath tests are based on the fact that metabolism converts substrates into CO_2, which is excreted by respiration. An example of a CO_2 breath test is the ^{14}C or ^{13}C urea breath test used to diagnose *H. pylori* infection. Breath hydrogen tests are used to investigate carbohydrate malabsorption and as a noninvasive test of intestinal

bacterial overgrowth. The source of H_2 production is due to the fermentation of nonabsorbed carbohydrate in the intestinal lumen or the bacterial metabolism of added fermentable substrates. Hydrogen generated in the gut is absorbed into the circulation and exhaled by the lungs.

■ TESTS OF INTESTINAL FUNCTION

A number of tests are used to determine intestinal function or malfunction.[1] They include the xylose absorption test, sweat test, and hydrogen breath test discussed previously.

D-Xylose absorption test

Xylose is a pentose with a sweet taste that is not present normally in significant amounts in blood. Pancreatic digestive enzymes are not needed for its absorption. When xylose is administered orally, approximately 60% is absorbed passively in the proximal small (duodenojejunal) intestine, and most is excreted subsequently by the kidneys. The amount of xylose recovered in the urine or blood in a specified time interval after administration of a measured dose is used to evaluate mucosal absorption ability.

Low absorption of xylose is observed in individuals with intestinal malabsorption, celiac disease, tropical sprue, Crohn's disease, immunoglobulin deficiency, acquired immunodeficiency syndrome (AIDS), enteropathy, pellagra, ascariasis, blind loop syndrome, radiation enteritis, and surgical bowel resection; low absorption also is present after vomiting or incomplete urine collection, as well as in cases of delayed gastric emptying, inadequate hydration, decreased circulation, intrinsic renal disease, thyroid disease, and sequestration in body fluids, as occurs in states of pregnancy and ascites. In addition, excretory values decrease with age as a reflection of decreased kidney function. In individuals with malabsorption due to pancreatic insufficiency the absorption of xylose is essentially normal, provided that no significant increase exists in intestinal motility; on the other hand, more than 80% of individuals with malabsorption due to jejunal malabsorption demonstrate low values. Therefore the test is of some help to distinguish between these two types of malabsorption and to evaluate the response to therapy.

References

1. Abdelshaheed NN, Goldberg DM: Biochemical tests in diseases of the intestinal tract: their contributions to diagnosis, management, and understanding the pathophysiology of specific disease states. Crit Rev Clin Lab Sci 1997; 34:141-223.

2. Guyton AC, Hall JE: Textbook of Medical Physiology, 9th edition, Philadelphia, WB Saunders, 1995.

3. Hazell SL, Robertson B, Mendz GL: *Helicobacter pylori*—metabolism, physiology and insights from the whole genome [review]. Baillieres Clin Infect Dis 1997; 4:283-317.

4. Henderson AR, Rinker AD: Gastric, pancreatic, and intestinal Function. In Burtis CA, Ashwood ER (eds): Tietz Textbook of Clinical Chemistry, 3rd edition, pp 1271-1327, Philadelphia, WB Saunders, 1999.

5. Henderson AR, Tietz NW, Rinker AD: Gastric, pancreatic, and intestinal function. In Burtis CA, Ashwood ER (eds): Tietz Textbook of Clinical Chemistry, 2nd edition, pp 1576-1644, Philadelphia, WB Saunders, 1994.

6. Moss DW, Henderson AR: Enzymes. In Burtis CA, Ashwood ER (eds): Tietz Textbook of Clinical Chemistry, 3rd edition, pp 617-721, Philadelphia, WB Saunders, 1999.

7. Samloff IM: Peptic ulcer: the many proteinases of aggression. Gastroenterology 1989; 96:586-595.

8. Stone MA: Non-invasive testing for *Helicobacter pylori* [review]. Postgrad Med J 1999; 75:74-77.

9. Toskes PP: Malabsorption. In Bennett JC, Plum F (eds): Cecil Textbook of Medicine, 20th edition, pp 695-707, Philadelphia, WB Saunders, 1996.

10. Vantrappen G, Ghoos Y, Andriulli A: CO_2 and H_2 breath tests in the diagnosis of intestinal malabsorption [review]. Ital J Gastroenterol 1992; 24:212-217.

11. Welsh MJ, Tsui L-C, Boat TF et al: Cystic fibrosis. In Scriver CR, Beaudet AL, Sly WS et al (eds): The Metabolic and Molecular Bases of Inherited Disease, 7th edition, pp 3799-3876, New York, McGraw-Hill, 1995.

Additional Reading

Haubrich WS, Schaffner F, Berk JE: Bockus Gastroenterology, 5th edition, Philadelphia, WB Saunders, 1995.

Weisiger RA, Bilhartz LE: Sleisenger and Fordtran's: Gastrointestinal Disease, 6th edition, Philadelphia, WB Saunders, 1995.

Yamada T, Alpers DH, Laine L et al (eds): Textbook of Gastroenterology, 3rd edition, Philadelphia, Lippincott, Williams & Wilkins, 1999.

CHAPTER 38

Mineral and Bone Metabolism

DAVID B. ENDRES, PhD, and ROBERT K. RUDE, MD

Objectives

1. Describe the structure and function of bone, including matrix and cellular components.
2. State the function and clinical significance of calcium, phosphorus, and magnesium in bone metabolism.
3. State the function and clinical significance of vitamin D, parathyroid hormone, and calcitonin in bone metabolism; describe how these hormones regulate bone metabolism.
4. Describe how the following disease states affect bone: hypercalcemia and hypocalcemia, hyperphosphatemia and hypophosphatemia, hypermagnesemia and hypomagnesemia, hyperparathyroidism and hypoparathyroidism, and decreased vitamin D.
5. List and describe four metabolic bone diseases and state their causes and symptoms.
6. List markers of bone formation and resorption and state how each is affected in normal bone growth and in diseases such as osteoporosis, osteomalacia, and Paget's disease.

Key Words

Calcitonin   A polypeptide hormone produced by the parafollicular cells of the thyroid that causes a reduction of calcium ions in the blood

Collagen   The protein substance of the white fibers (collagenous fibers) of skin, tendon, bone, cartilage, and all other connective tissue

Hypercalcemia   An excess of calcium in the blood, manifestations of which include fatigability, muscle weakness, depression, anorexia, nausea, and constipation

Hypocalcemia   Reduction of the blood calcium below normal; seen in cases of hypoparathyroidism, low vitamin D intake, osteomalacia, and certain kidney diseases

Osteoblasts   Cells that arise from fibroblasts and that, as they mature, are associated with the production of bone

Osteoclasts   Large multinuclear cells associated with the absorption and removal of bone

Osteomalacia   Inadequate or delayed mineralization of osteoid in mature cortical and spongy bone; the adult equivalent of rickets and accompanies that disorder in children

Osteoporosis   A reduction in the amount of bone mass, leading to fractures after minimal trauma

Osteoporosis, Postmenopausal   A metabolic disorder that occurs in women within 3 to 20 years after menopause, affecting trabecular bone more than cortical bone, and manifested mainly by vertebral fractures of the painful crush type, and Colles' fracture of the distal forearem

Paget's Disease   A disease of bone, resulting in the excessive resorption of bone

Parathyroid Hormone (PTH)   A peptide hormone secreted by the parathyroid glands that stimulates osteoclasts to increase blood calcium levels

Parathyroid Hormone-Related Protein (PTHrP)   A protein that mimics most of the actions of PTH; a product of a distinct gene, which is expressed in a variety of normal tissues, including skin, bone marrow, stomach, hypothalamus, thyroid, pituitary, parathyroid, and adrenal gland; overexpressed (by the tumors) in most cases of humoral hypercalcemia of malignancy

Pryridinoline Collagen Cross-Links   Amino acid derivatives of hydroxyl lysine that cross-link type I collagen fibrils in bone and cartilage; two cross-link compounds being pyridinoline and deoxypyridinoline, which add tensile strength and stability to bone

Renal Osteodystrophy   Bone disease resulting from chronic renal failure

Rhabdomyolysis   Disintegration or dissolution of muscle, associated with the excretion of myoglobin in the urine

Rickets   An interruption in the development and mineralization of the growth plate of bone

Telopeptide   Portions of the amino acid sequence of a protein that are removed in maturation of the protein, examples of which are the N and C terminal telopeptides of procollagen that are involved in development of the quaternary structure and then proteolytically removed by procollagen peptidases

---

The main functions of bone are (1) mechanical, for locomotion; (2) protective, for organs; and (3) metabolic, as a reserve for minerals, especially calcium and phosphate. Bones are composed of cortical and trabecular bone. Cortical (compact) bone is 80% to 90% mineralized by volume and constitutes 80% of the skeleton. Its function is primarily mechanical and protective. Trabecular (cancellous or spongy) bone is 15% to 25% mineralized; this particular type of bone constitutes the remaining 20% of the skeleton.

Bone is composed of bone cells and extracellular matrix. **Osteoclasts** and **osteoblasts,** the two main types of bone cells, are responsible for bone resorption and formation, respectively. The extracellular matrix, a mineralized organic matrix, is particularly abundant in bone. The organic matrix is primarily type I collagen (90%). A large number of non-collagenous proteins also are found in bone, including osteocalcin. The organic matrix is mineralized by the deposition of calcium phosphate crystals and lesser amounts of carbonate, magnesium, sodium, potassium and various other ions.

Continuous turnover or remodeling of bone occurs, enabling bone to repair damage and adjust strength. Bone remodeling does not occur at random but instead in discrete packets known as *bone remodeling units.* Bone resorption and formation are coupled. The remodeling cycle can be divided into activation, resorption, reversal, formation and resting phases (Figure 38-1). Circulating osteoclast precursors are recruited, proliferate, and fuse to form osteoclasts. These giant multinucleated cells resorb bone by producing hydrogen ions to mobilize minerals and lysosomal enzymes to digest the organic matrix. Deep foldings of their plasma membrane (ruffled border) are in contact with the bone surface, forming the osteoclastic bone-resorbing compartment. After resorption ceases, a cement line is deposited in the resorption cavity, probably by mononucleated cells. Stromal lining cells differentiate to osteoblasts. Osteoblasts form bone by synthesizing the organic matrix, including type I collagen, and participating in the mineralization process of the newly synthesized matrix. Remodeling is followed by a quiescent phase. An estimated 10% to 30% of the skeleton is remodeled each year.

Bone growth and turnover are influenced and regulated by the metabolism of calcium, phosphate, and magnesium and a number of hormones, the primary ones being parathyroid hormone (PTH) and 1,25-dihydroxyvitamin D (1,25[OH]$_2$D). In addition, a large number of other hormones and factors are involved in regulation of bone formation or resorption, including thyroid hormones, estrogens, androgens, cortisol, insulin, growth hormone, insulin-like growth factors (IGF-I and IGF-II), transforming growth factor β (TGF-β), fibroblast growth factor (FGF) and platelet-derived growth factor (PDGF). A number of cytokines, including interleukin (IL)-1, -4, -6, and -11, macrophage and granulocyte/macrophage colony-stimulating factors, and tumor necrosis factor (TNFα) alter bone remodeling primarily by stimulating resorption.

Significant progress in the study of bone and mineral metabolism has increased the understanding of bone and mineral metabolism and the pathophysiology of associated disorders. Concurrently, improvements in technology have allowed laboratories to expand their role from measuring just total calcium, phosphate and magnesium to measuring other analytes, such as free (ionized) calcium, PTH, vitamin D metabolites, and calcitonin. An aging population is accelerating this trend and increasing the need for the measurement of other analytes, such as biochemical markers of bone formation that include bone alkaline phosphatase and osteocalcin and bone resorption, such as collagen cross-links (deoxypyridinoline and telopeptides) and parathyroid hormone-related protein (PTHrP).

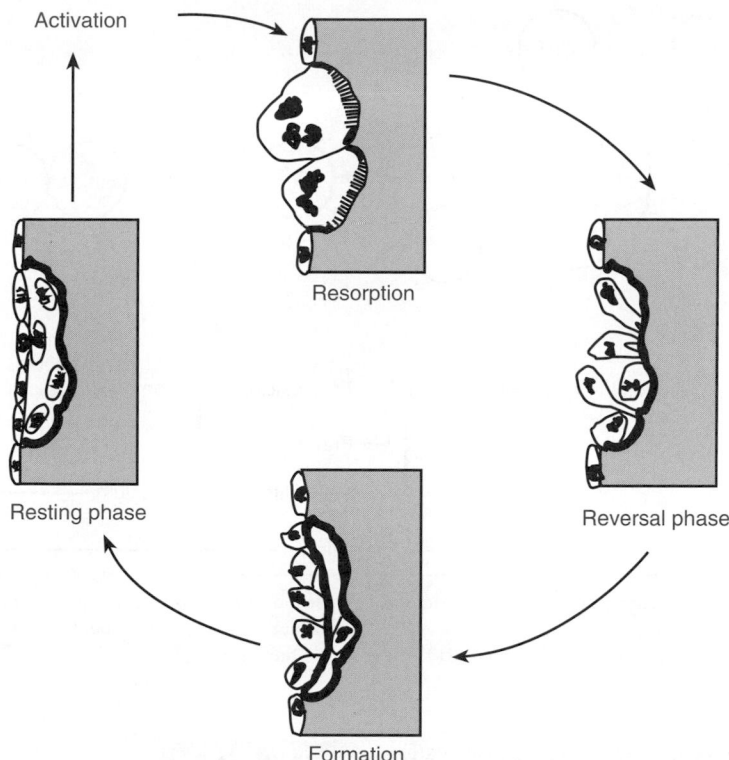

Figure 38-1   Bone remodeling. The bone remodeling sequence—activation, resorption, reversal, formation, and resting phases. (Modified from Baron RE: Anatomy and ultrastructure of bone. In Favus MJ (ed): Primer on the Metabolic Bone Diseases and Disorders of Mineral Metabolism, 3rd edition, p 8, Philadelphia, Lippincott-Raven, 1996.)

TABLE 38-1   Distribution of Calcium, Phosphate, and Magnesium in the Body

| | Relative Distribution (%) | | |
Tissue	Calcium	Phosphate	Magnesium
Skeleton	99	85	55
Soft tissues	1	15	45
Extracellular fluid	<0.2	<0.1	1
Total g (mol)	1000 (25)	600 (19.4)	25 (1.0)

Aurbach GD, Marx SJ, Speigel AM: Parathyroid hormone, calcitonin and the calciferols. In Wilson JD, Foster DW (eds): Williams Textbook of Endocrinology, 8th edition, pp 1397-1476, Philadelphia, WB Saunders, 1992.

TABLE 38-2   Physiochemical States of Calcium, Phosphate, and Magnesium in Normal Plasma

| | Approximate Percent of Total | | |
State	Calcium	Phosphate	Magnesium
Free	50	55	55
Protein bound	40	10	30
Complexed	10	35	15
TOTAL			
(mg/dL)	8.6 to 10.3	2.5 to 4.5	1.7 to 2.4
(mmol/L)	2.15 to 2.57	0.81 to 1.45	0.70 to 0.99

Modified from Marshall RW: Plasma fractions. In Nordin BEC (ed): Calcium Phosphate and Magnesium Metabolism, pp 162-185, London, Churchill Livingstone, 1976.

■ MINERAL METABOLISM

Bone is composed primarily of inorganic minerals (calcium, phosphate, and magnesium) and an organic matrix (type I collagen). Bone contains nearly all the calcium (99%), most of the phosphate (85%), and much of the magnesium (55%) of the body.

Calcium

Calcium is the fifth most common element in the body. It is found mainly in the skeleton, with small amounts in soft tissues and extracellular fluid (Table 38-1).

Biochemistry and physiology

The skeleton contains 99% of the body's calcium, predominantly as extracellular crystals similar to hydroxyapatite $(Ca_{10}[PO_4]_6[OH]_2)$. In blood, approximately 50% of the plasma calcium is free, 40% is protein bound, and 10% is complexed (Table 38-2). About 80% of protein-bound calcium is associated with albumin, with the remaining 20% associated with globulins. Because calcium binds to negatively charged sites on proteins, its binding is pH dependent. Alkalosis leads to an increase in negative charge and bind-

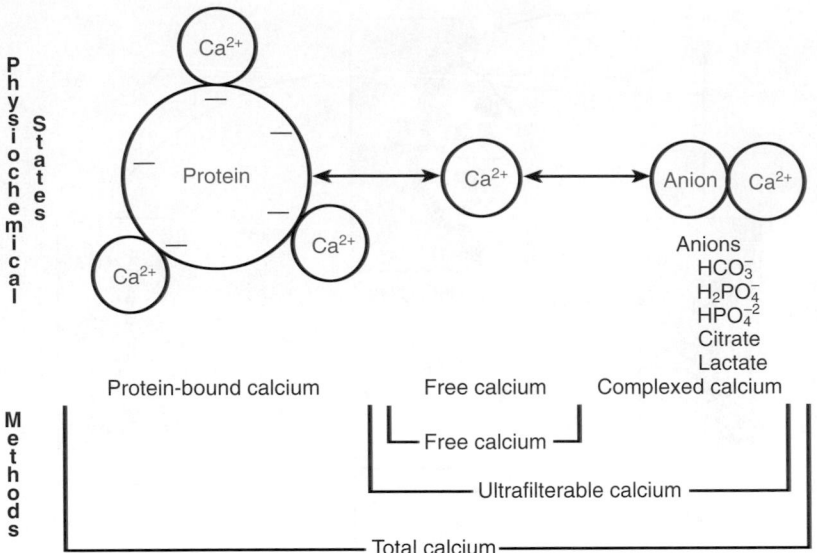

Figure 38-2 Equilibrium between physiochemical states and determination of calcium in serum. Calcium can move among three physiochemical pools—(1) free calcium, (2) protein-bound calcium, and (3) calcium complexed with inorganic and organic anions. Methods for total calcium measure all three pools, whereas methods for free calcium measure only that pool.

ing and a decrease in free calcium; conversely, acidosis leads to a decrease in negative charge and binding and an increase in free calcium. Complexed calcium is complexed with small diffusible anions, including bicarbonate, lactate, phosphate, and citrate. Calcium is redistributed among the three plasma pools by alterations in concentration of protein or small anions, changes in pH, or changes in the quantities of free calcium and total calcium in serum (Figure 38-2).

Physiologically, calcium is classified as either intracellular or extracellular. The skeleton is a major reservoir used to provide calcium for both the extracellular and intracellular pools. Intracellular calcium has many important physiological functions, including muscle contraction, hormone secretion, glycogen metabolism, and cell division.

Extracellular calcium provides calcium ion for the maintenance of intracellular calcium, bone mineralization, blood coagulation, and plasma membrane potential. A decrease in the serum free calcium concentration causes increased neuromuscular excitability and tetany; an increased concentration reduces neuromuscular excitability. Calcium is also important in muscle contraction and as an intracellular second messenger affecting enzyme activity and hormone secretion.

Clinical significance

Certain disorders are characterized by lowered levels of calcium in the blood (hypocalcemia). Other disorders involve elevated levels (hypercalcemia).

Hypocalcemia

Low total serum calcium (**hypocalcemia**) may be due to either a reduction in the albumin-bound or free fraction of calcium (Table 38-3). Hypoalbuminemia is the most

TABLE 38-3	Common Causes of Hypocalcemia

Hypoalbuminemia
Chronic renal failure
Magnesium deficiency
Hypoparathyroidism
Pseudohypoparathyroidism
Osteomalacia and rickets due to vitamin D deficiency or resistance
Acute hemorrhagic and edematous pancreatitis
Healing phase of bone disease of treated hyperparathyroidism, hyperthyroidism, and hematological malignancies (hungry bone syndrome)

common cause of hypocalcemia because 1 gm/dL of albumin binds 0.8 mg/dL of calcium.

Chronic renal failure may result in hypocalcemia because of hypoproteinemia, hyperphosphatemia, low serum $1,25(OH)_2D$, or skeletal resistance to PTH. Magnesium deficiency, as discussed in a later section of this chapter, impairs PTH secretion and causes PTH end-organ resistance.

Other causes of low serum calcium are less common. Hypoparathyroidism is due most commonly to parathyroid gland destruction during neck surgery, whereas pseudohypoparathyroidism is caused by an inherited resistance to PTH. Acute symptomatic hypocalcemia may be associated with rapid remineralization of bone after surgery for primary hyperparathyroidism (hungry bone syndrome) or acute pancreatitis. Vitamin D deficiency also may be associated with hypocalcemia.

Clinically, hypocalcemia most commonly presents with neuromuscular hyperexcitability, such as tetany, paresthesia, and seizures. A rapid fall in the serum calcium also may be associated with hypotension. The initial laboratory evaluation is directed toward the assessment of renal function

TABLE 38-4	Differential Diagnosis of Hypercalcemia

Primary hyperparathyroidism
Malignancy
   Skeletal involvement
   No skeletal involvement (HHM)
   Hematological malignancy
   Coexistent primary hyperparathyroidism
Other endocrine disorders
   Hyperthyroidism
   Hypothyroidism
   Acute adrenal insufficiency
Familial hypocalciuric hypercalcemia
Idiopathic hypercalcemia of infancy
Vitamin D and A overdose
Granulomatous diseases (sarcoidosis and tuberculosis)
Renal failure
Chlorothiazide diuretics
Lithium therapy
Milk-alkali syndrome
Hyperalimentation regimens
Immobilization
Increased serum proteins

and measurement of serum albumin and magnesium concentrations. Serum intact PTH levels are used to diagnose hypoparathyroidism or pseudohypoparathyroidism.

Hypercalcemia

Hypercalcemia is due to an increased flux of calcium into the extracellular fluid compartment from the skeleton, intestine, or kidney. The differential diagnosis of hypercalcemia is shown in Table 38-4; primary hyperparathyroidism is the most common cause in outpatient clinics, whereas malignancy is the most common cause in hospitalized patients. Together, these two disorders account for 90% to 95% of all cases of hypercalcemia.

Hypercalcemia occurs in 10% to 20% of individuals with cancer. Tumors most commonly cause hypercalcemia by production of PTHrP, which is secreted into the circulation and stimulates bone resorption. PTHrP binds to the PTH receptor and is thought to be the principal mediator of humoral hypercalcemia of malignancy (HHM). Tumors that are metastatic to bone also produce factors that stimulate bone resorption. Some lymphomas may produce $1,25(OH)_2D$ and cause hypercalcemia through this mechanism.

Signs and symptoms of hypercalcemia often are evident in patients with hypercalcemia due to malignancy because the serum calcium rises rapidly and often to higher levels than usually are seen in cases of primary hyperparathyroidism. Lethargy, obtundation, nausea, and vomiting are additional symptoms. Laboratory test selection is similar to that of hyperparathyroidism, with the addition of assay for PTHrP in individuals with HHM. In specific instances (for example, lymphoma), determination of $1,25(OH)_2D$ may provide useful information.

Analytical methodology

Various methods are used to quantify either free (ionized) calcium* or total calcium. Free calcium is considered the best indication of calcium status because it is biologically active and tightly regulated by the calcium-regulating hormones PTH and $1,25(OH)_2D$. Although the measurement of free calcium is clinically more useful, it has not yet replaced the measurement of total calcium. However, free calcium determinations have assumed increasing importance because of the availability of improved analyzers and more convenient specimen handling. They are recommended for all requests apart from chemistry panels because of the consequences of delays in treatment and the cost of the working-up of patients with misleading total serum calcium results.

Measurement of total calcium

Both photometric and atomic absorption methods are used to measure total calcium in serum and urine. A serum-based calibrator with calcium levels determined by the definitive method (isotope dilution-mass spectrometry, or ID-MS) is available commercially.

Photometric methods. Total calcium is measured most frequently by photometry or spectrophotometry. Various metallochromic indicators or dyes change color on selectively binding calcium. Although many calcium-binding dyes have been used, only *o*-cresolphthalein complexone (CPC) and arsenazo III are used widely today.

In alkaline solution, CPC forms a red chromophore with calcium, which is measured at 570 to 580 nm. The sample is diluted with acid to release protein-bound and complexed calcium. Interference by magnesium ions is reduced by (1) the addition of 8-hydroxyquinoline; (2) buffering of the reaction mixture to near pH 12; and (3) measurement of the absorbance near 580 nm. Urea may be added to reduce the turbidity of lipemic specimens and enhance complex formation. Ethanol reduces blank formation. Multipoint calibration is recommended, and linearity may be improved with the addition of sodium acetate. The CPC and alkaline reagent are stable as separate reagents but have limited stability when combined.

Arsenazo III has a much higher affinity for calcium than magnesium at mildly acidic pH (approximately 6). Binding of calcium to arsenazo III is influenced by buffer, pH, and sodium concentration. Interference with most biological pigments is reduced by measurement of the calcium-dye complex near 650 nm. Unlike CPC, arsenazo III reagent is stable as a single reagent.

Atomic absorption spectrophotometry. The National Committee for Clinical Laboratory Standards (NCCLS) has approved an atomic absorption spectrophotometry (AAS) reference method to measure total serum calcium. In

---

*Free calcium is the biologically active form of calcium. The term *ionized calcium* was used previously to describe this form of calcium but is a misnomer because all calcium is ionized and associates with protein or small ions.

this method the specimen first is diluted 1 to 50 with a solution of lanthanum-hydrochloric acid ($LaCl_3$, 10 mmol/L; HCl, 50 mmol/L) and then aspirated into an air-acetylene flame, where the ground state calcium atoms absorb incident light from a calcium hollow-cathode lamp (422.7 nm). The amount of light absorbed is measured after the 422.7-nm resonance line is isolated with a monochromator. Absorbance is directly proportional to the number of ground-state calcium atoms in the flame.

Dilution with lanthanum-HCl reduces interference from protein, phosphate, citrate, sulfate, and other anions. Phosphate causes the greatest interference because calcium-phosphate complexes are not dissociated readily by the air-acetylene flame. Lanthanum-HCl dissociates these complexes, ensuring that all fractions of calcium (free, protein bound, and complexed) are measured. Protein also interferes because of its viscosity, which reduces the aspiration rate and atomization of the specimen. Dilution effectively reduces viscosity. Cationic interference, although much less significant than anionic, also can occur. The effect of the three major cations, Na^+, K^+, and Mg^{2+}, generally is offset by their inclusion in calibrators at normal serum concentrations. Strontium may be included in the diluent as an internal standard or calibrator.

Specimen requirements. Serum is the preferred specimen for the measurement of total calcium, although heparinized plasma also is acceptable. Citrate, oxalate, and ethylenediaminetetraacetic acid (EDTA) anticoagulants should not be used because they interfere by forming complexes with calcium. Total calcium is stable in serum for days at 4 °C and for months in a frozen state. Coprecipitation of calcium with fibrin in heparinized plasma or lipids has been reported with storage or freezing.

Urine specimens should be collected in 20 to 30 mL of 6 mol/L HCl per 24-hour specimen (1 to 2 mL for a random specimen) to prevent calcium salt precipitation. Addition of acid after the collection may not dissolve completely precipitated calcium salts.

Care should be taken to handle specimens, calibrators, and solutions to prevent contamination with calcium. Reusable glassware or plasticware should be washed with dilute HCl, followed by distilled water. Corks should not be used because they can contaminate specimens.

Interferences. Hemolysis, icterus, lipemia, paraproteins, and magnesium have been reported to interfere with photometric methods. Many methods use bichromatic or polychromatic analysis or blanking to reduce interference. Lipemic specimens should be clarified by high-speed centrifugation. Although hemolysis causes a negative error because red blood cells contain lower levels of calcium than does serum, more significant errors may be caused by the spectral interference of hemoglobin. Depending on the method, hemoglobin has been reported to cause either negative or positive interference. In photometric methods, if hemolyzed specimens must be analyzed, blanking with ethylene glycol tetraacetic acid (EGTA) is needed.

Serum total calcium and adjusted or corrected total calcium. Various calculations have been used to adjust total calcium determinations to correct for variations in protein concentration. Most of these calculations involve multiplication of the deviation of plasma albumin from its normal concentration by a factor to adjust the measured calcium, as in the following example:

Corrected total calcium (mg/dL) =

Total calcium (mg/dL) + 0.8(4 − albumin [g/dL])

Some factors limiting the usefulness of total and corrected total calcium are pH effects, variations in binding kinetics, amounts of fatty acids, drugs, and other substances that are bound by albumin, heparin, and other anions forming complexes with calcium, and unusual quantities or types of serum proteins (Table 38-5). In addition, calcium binding by proteins varies among individuals and various physiological and pathological states. When possible, mathematical adjustments should be replaced by direct determination of free calcium by an ion-selective electrode (ISE).

Measurement of free calcium

Ion-selective analyzers capable of providing immediate whole-blood determinations of free calcium, electrolytes, and blood gases now are available widely. The free calcium component consists of a system of pumps under microprocessor control that transport calibration solutions, samples, and wash solutions through a measuring cell containing calcium ion-selective, reference, and pH electrodes. Sensitive potentiometers measure the voltage differential between measuring and reference electrodes, while the microprocessor calibrates the system and calculates calcium concentra-

TABLE 38-5 Factors Altering the Distribution among Protein-Bound, Complexed, and Free Calcium and Compounding the Interpretation of Total Calcium

Factors Altering Protein Binding of Calcium	Factors Altering Complex Formation
Altered concentration of albumin or globulins	Citrate
Abnormal proteins	Bicarbonate
Heparin	Lactate
pH	Phosphate
Free fatty acids	Pyruvate and β–hydroxybutyrate
Bilirubin	Sulfate
Drugs	Anion gap
Temperature	

tion and pH. Most instruments simultaneously measure the actual free calcium and pH at 37 °C.

Calcium ISEs contain a calcium-selective membrane, which encloses an internal reference electrode, and an inner reference solution of calcium chloride often containing saturated silver chloride and physiological concentrations of sodium chloride (NaCl) and potassium chloride (KCl). Modern calcium ISEs use liquid membranes containing the ion-selective calcium sensor dissolved in an organic liquid trapped in a polymeric matrix. Neutral carriers (for example, ETH 1001) and ion-exchangers, such as organophosphate sensors (for example, calcium bis[di-*n*-octylphenyl] phosphate dissolved in di-*n*-octylphenyl phosphonate) are commonly used calcium sensors. The electrochemical cell is completed by the external reference electrode in contact with the specimen by a liquid-liquid junction or salt bridge of KCl or sodium formate. The potential difference across the cell is related logarithmically to the activity of free calcium ions in the sample by the Nernst equation.

Interferences. Because ISEs measure ion activity, they are affected by the ionic strength of a specimen. Free calcium analyzers and calibrators are optimized for specimens of serum, plasma, or whole blood. Because the ionic strength of these fluids is primarily a result of Na^+ and Cl^-, calibrators usually are prepared in buffer and NaCl, with a final ionic strength of 160 mmol/kg. Although the range of Na^+ and Cl^- concentrations usually observed in serum or plasma does not cause a clinically significant error, significant errors can occur with other samples unless the matrices and ionic strength of the calibrators and samples are matched closely.

Modern electrodes exhibit high selectivity for calcium over Na^+, K^+, Mg^{2+}, H^+, and Li^+. At normal concentrations these cations have little effect on the accuracy of free calcium measurements. Wide variations in the concentrations of Na^+ and high levels of Mg^{2+} and Li^+ may influence the apparent level of free calcium. Electrodes are quite insensitive to H^+, with insignificant interference between pH 5 and 9.

Whole-blood specimens develop a liquid junction potential different from that of serum or plasma because of the presence of erythrocytes, resulting in a positive bias directly proportional to the hematocrit. Although this effect has been minimized in modern analyzers, if whole blood, plasma and serum are to be analyzed, reference intervals should be established for each of them.

Newer electrodes use a dialysis membrane or neutral carrier to reduce or eliminate the sensitivity to protein concentration. With these electrodes the effect is less than +0.02 mmol/L for 1 g/dL of protein. Regular instrument maintenance and protein removal are reported to minimize this interference.

A number of chemicals may interfere with calcium ISEs or alter free calcium levels. Anionic surfactants and ethanol have been reported to affect the calcium-selective membrane. Physiological anions, including phosphate, citrate, lactate, sulfate, and oxalate, and chemicals such as EDTA and EGTA, form complexes with calcium ions, reducing the concentration of free calcium.

Effect of pH. The binding of calcium by protein and small anions is influenced by pH in vitro and in vivo. Increasing the pH of a specimen in vitro increases the ionization and negative charge on albumin and other proteins, leading to an increase in protein-bound calcium and a decrease in free calcium. Decreasing pH in vitro decreases ionization and negative charge, decreasing protein-bound calcium and increasing free calcium. The concentration of free calcium changes by about 5% for each 0.1-unit change in pH.

Because of this inverse relationship between free calcium and pH, specimens should be analyzed at the patient's in vivo blood pH.

Specimen requirements. Specimens for free calcium should be collected and handled anaerobically, with care taken to prevent an increase in pH because of loss of CO_2. All syringes and tubes should be filled completely and sealed in order to prevent the loss of CO_2.

Specimens also should be treated to prevent a decrease in pH because of production of lactic acid by erythrocytes or white blood cells during anaerobic metabolism. For example, unless the analysis can be completed within minutes of sampling, specimens should be collected, transported, and maintained on ice to prevent anaerobic metabolism.

Free calcium concentration, the actual pH of the specimen, and the patient's pH, should be reported. Such information is useful to verify that the specimen has been properly handled. Aerobic handling of specimens and/or correction of the free calcium to pH 7.4 may be misleading in patients with respiratory or metabolic alkalosis or acidosis and should be avoided.

Free calcium is measured in heparinized whole blood, heparinized plasma, or serum. For laboratories in which specimens are analyzed within a few minutes to an hour, heparinized whole blood may be preferable because it reduces processing time and specimen volume and prevents the alteration in pH associated with centrifugation at temperatures other than 37 °C.

In the measurement of free calcium, heparin is the only acceptable anticoagulant; it does not lower significantly free calcium at levels up to 15 U/mL. However, most heparinized blood gas syringes provide a final heparin concentration of 100 U/mL of blood, which can lower the level of free calcium by 15% to 25%. A number of commercially available syringes are suitable for free calcium determinations— (1) very–low-heparin (2-3 U/mL) syringes, (2) electrolyte-balanced/calcium-titrated heparin (<50 U/mL) syringes, and (3) lithium-zinc heparin (50 U/mL) syringes. Syringes that require liquid heparin to fill the dead space of the syringe should not be used; they can result in errors in measurement of free calcium because of dilution, as well as unacceptably high and variable concentrations of heparin.

If analysis is not completed within an hour or so of collection, serum from specimens collected in evacuated tubes with gel barriers may be the optimal specimens. Once centrifuged, these specimens are stable for hours at 25 °C and for days at 4 °C, provided the tubes are filled completely and remain sealed.

Reference intervals. The reference interval for total calcium in adults by use of a photometric method is 8.6 to 10.3 mg/dL (2.15 to 2.56 mmol/L). The reference interval for free calcium in adults is 4.64 to 5.28, mg/dL (1.16 to 1.32 mmol/L). (The reference intervals for other age groups are listed in Chapter 46.) Total calcium declines in parallel with serum albumin during pregnancy, whereas free calcium remains unchanged.

Interpretation of total and free calcium determinations

Interpretation of total serum calcium is complicated by its association with protein and inorganic and organic ions (see Table 38-5). Calcium status is determined more accurately through measurement of free calcium, especially in hospitalized patients who have received citrated blood or platelets, heparin, bicarbonate, intravenous solutions, or calcium. Alterations in blood pH and temperature further reduce the usefulness of total calcium assay in these patients.

The most common and significant cause of preanalytical error in the measurement of calcium is the increase in total, but not free, calcium concentration associated with venous occlusion (Table 38-6). Errors of 0.5 to 1.0 mg/dL (0.12 to 0.25 mmol/L) in total calcium may result because of the increase in protein-bound calcium caused by the efflux of water from the vascular compartment during stasis. Erect posture also has been reported to result in an increase in total, but not free, calcium of 0.2 to 0.8 mg/dL (0.05 to 0.20 mmol/L) because of fluid shifts. Conversely, mild hypocalcemia is observed commonly in hospitalized patients because of the hemodilution associated with recumbency.

Bone and mineral disorders are common in individuals with renal disease. Therapy and calcium metabolism of these individuals are evaluated best with free calcium assay.

Free calcium is more useful than total calcium in the evaluation of individuals with hypercalcemia caused by primary hyperparathyroidism or malignancy. Paraproteins produced in myeloma may bind calcium, complicating the interpretation of total or adjusted calcium results.

Phosphate

Phosphorus in the form of inorganic or organic phosphate is an important and widely distributed element in the human body (see Table 38-1). In the soft tissues, most phosphate is organic or incorporated into cellular macromolecules. Plasma contains approximately 2.5 to 4.5 mg/dL (0.81 to

TABLE 38-6	Potential Preanalytical Errors in the Measurement of Serum Total or Free Calcium
In Vivo	**In Vitro**
Tourniquet use and venous occlusion	Inappropriate anticoagulants
Changes in posture	Dilution with liquid heparin
Exercise	Interfering levels of heparin
Hyperventilation	Contamination with calcium
Fist clenching	Corks, glassware, tubes
Alimentary status	Specimen handling
Alterations in protein binding (see Table 38-5)	Alterations in pH due to specimen handling
Alterations in complex formation (see Table 38-5)	Adsorption or precipitation of calcium
	Spectrophotometric interference Hemolysis, icterus, lipemia

1.45 mmol/L) of inorganic phosphate, the fraction measured by clinical laboratories.

Biochemistry and physiology

Phosphate in serum exists as both the monovalent ($H_2PO_4^-$) and divalent (HPO_4^{2-}) phosphate anions. The ratio of $H_2PO_4^-/HPO_4^{2-}$ is pH dependent. Approximately 10% of the phosphate in serum is protein bound; 35% forms complexes with sodium, calcium, and magnesium; and the remainder is free (see Table 38-2). Organic phosphate esters are located primarily within the cellular elements of blood.

Inorganic phosphate is a major component of hydroxyapatite in bone, thereby playing an important part in structural support of the body and providing phosphate for the extracellular and intracellular pool.

Phosphate also has many other actions in cells. For example, it has a critical role as a high-energy phosphate bond and a constituent of cyclic adenine and guanine nucleotides, as well as nicotinamide-adenine dinucleotide phosphate (NADP). Phosphate is also an essential element in phospholipid cell membranes, nucleic acids, and phosphoproteins, as well as in gene transcription and cell growth. Phosphate is critical for activity in several important enzyme systems.

Clinical significance
Hypophosphatemia

Hypophosphatemia, defined as a serum inorganic phosphate concentration of less than 2.5 mg/dL (0.81 mmol/L), is relatively common in the hospitalized population (Table 38-7). One major cause of low serum phosphate is carbohydrate-induced stimulation of insulin secretion, which enhances the transport of phosphate into cells. Therefore oral or intravenous carbohydrate or injected insulin results in a fall in serum phosphate. Respiratory alkalosis and refeeding of malnourished individuals also promote an intracellular shift of phosphate, resulting in hypophosphatemia. In some instances, renal phosphate wasting may

TABLE 38-7 Common Causes of Hypophosphatemia and Phosphate Depletion

Intracellular Shift	Decreased Intestinal Phosphate Absorption
Glucose	Increased loss
Oral or intravenous	Vomiting
Hyperalimentation	Diarrhea
Insulin	Phosphate binding antacids
Respiratory alkalosis	Decreased absorption
	Malabsorption syndrome
Lowered Renal Phosphate Threshold	Vitamin D deficiency
Primary or secondary	**Intracellular Phosphate Loss**
hyperparathyroidism	Acidosis
Renal tubular defects	Ketoacidosis
Familial hypophosphatemia	Lactic acidosis
Fanconi's syndrome	

TABLE 38-8 Common Causes of Hyperphosphatemia

Decreased Renal Phosphate Excretion	Increased Extracellular Phosphate Load
Decreased glomerular filtration rate	Transcellular shift
Renal failure, chronic and acute	Lactic acidosis
Increased tubular reabsorption	Respiratory acidosis
Hypoparathyroidism	Untreated diabetic ketoacidosis
Pseudohypoparathyroidism	Cell lysis
Acromegaly	Rhabdomyolysis
Disodium etidronate	Intravascular hemolysis
	Cytotoxic therapy
Increased Phosphate Intake	Leukemia
Oral or intravenous administration	Lymphoma
Phosphate-containing laxatives or enemas	

be the cause of a low serum phosphate, such as occurs in individuals with primary and secondary hyperparathyroidism, Fanconi's syndrome, and X-linked hypophosphatemia. Intestinal phosphate loss is less common but may occur in individuals with malabsorption syndromes and in those ingesting aluminum- and magnesium-containing antacids, which bind to intestinal phosphate and render it nonabsorbable. Acidosis, such as diabetic ketoacidosis, results in catabolism of organic phosphates within the cell. Inorganic phosphate then shifts into the plasma and is excreted into the urine, resulting in intracellular phosphate depletion.

The clinical manifestations of phosphate depletion depend on the length and degree of the deficiency. Because phosphate is an important component of adenosine triphosphate (ATP), cellular function is impaired in individuals with hypophosphatemia. Muscle weakness, respiratory failure, and decreased myocardial output may occur in states of phosphate depletion. At very low serum phosphate levels (<0.5 mg/dL or 0.16 mmol/L), **rhabdomyolysis** may occur. Phosphate depletion also results in decreased erythrocyte 2,3-diphosphoglycerate, which causes tissue hypoxia because of increased affinity of hemoglobin for oxygen. Severe hypophosphatemia may result in hemolysis of red blood cells. Mental confusion to frank coma also may be secondary to the low ATP and tissue hypoxia. If hypophosphatemia is chronic, rickets (in children) or osteomalacia (in adults) may develop.

Hyperphosphatemia

Common causes of hyperphosphatemia are shown in Table 38-8. Hyperphosphatemia usually is related to renal failure. A decrease in glomerular filtration limits the renal excretion of phosphate, and hyperphosphatemia develops. Moderate elevation of serum phosphate occurs in individuals with hypoparathyroidism due to the lack of PTH and in those with acromegaly because growth hormone raises the tubular reabsorption of phosphate. Aggressive phosphate therapy of phosphate-depleted patients may result in a high

serum phosphate. Release of phosphate due to cell breakdown in cases of rhabdomyolysis or chemotherapy of certain malignancies also is associated with hyperphosphatemia. Elevated serum phosphate may cause a decrease in the serum calcium concentration. Therefore tetany and seizures may be presenting symptoms.

Analytical methodology

Photometric measurement

The most common method used to measure phosphate is based on the reaction of phosphate ions with ammonium molybdate to form a phosphomolybdate complex that then is measured photometrically. The colorless phosphomolybdate complex is measured directly by ultraviolet absorption (340 nm), or the colorless complex is reduced to colored molybdenum blue (600 to 700 nm) by various reducing agents. An acid pH is necessary for the formation of complexes but must be controlled because both complex formation and reduction of molybdate depend on pH. Measurement of unreduced complexes has several advantages, including simplicity, speed, and stability. One disadvantage is the greater interference of hemolysis, icterus, and lipemia at 340 nm. Many reducing agents have been used, including aminonaphtholsulfonic acid, stannous chloride, methyl-*p*-aminophenol sulfate, ferrous ammonium sulfate, ascorbic acid, and *N*-phenyl-*p*-phenyldiamine (semidine) HCl.

Specimen requirements

Serum or heparinized plasma is the preferred specimen used for the measurement of phosphate. Anticoagulants, such as citrate, oxalate, and EDTA, should not be used because they interfere with the formation of the phosphomolybdate complex.

Phosphate levels in serum are increased by prolonged storage with cells at room temperature or 37 °C. Hemolyzed specimens are unacceptable because erythrocytes contain high concentrations of organic phosphate esters, which can be hydrolyzed to inorganic phosphate during storage. Phosphate is stable in separated serum for several days at 4 °C and months in its frozen form.

Because a diurnal variation in serum phosphate has been reported, fasting morning specimens are recommended for analysis. Serum phosphate levels are higher in the afternoon and evening and are influenced by dietary intake and meals and increased by exercise.

Interferences

Depending on the specific method used, positive or negative interference has been noted with hemolyzed, icteric, and lipemic specimens. Mannitol and fluoride also have been reported to interfere. Glassware should be cleaned and rinsed properly because phosphate is a common component of many detergents.

Reference intervals

In adults the reference interval for serum phosphate is 2.5 to 4.5 mg/dL (0.81 to 1.45 mmol/L). In children, it is 4.0 to 7.0 mg/dL (1.29 to 2.26 mmol/L). Urinary phosphate varies with age, muscle mass, renal function, PTH, time of day, and other factors. Urinary excretion varies widely with diet and is essentially equivalent to dietary intake. On a nonrestricted diet the reference interval for urinary phosphate is 0.4 to 1.3 g/day (12.9 to 42.0 mmol/day).

Magnesium

Approximately 55% of the total body magnesium is in the skeleton; the remainder is intracellular, where it is the second most prevalent cation (see Table 38-1).

Biochemistry and physiology

Within the cell, magnesium is bound primarily to proteins and negatively charged molecules; 80% of cytosolic magnesium is bound to ATP. Approximately 0.5% to 5.0% of the total cellular magnesium is free, which is the fraction that alters enzyme activity. Extracellular magnesium accounts for about 1% of the total body magnesium content. In serum, about 55% of magnesium is free, 30% is associated with proteins (primarily albumin), and 15% forms complexes with phosphate, citrate, and other anions (see Table 38-2).

Magnesium is a cofactor for more than 300 enzymes in the body. It is required for enzyme substrate formation (for example, MgATP). In addition, magnesium is an allosteric activator of many enzyme systems. Magnesium plays an important role in oxidative phosphorylation, glycolysis, cell replication, nucleotide metabolism, and protein biosynthesis.

Extracellular magnesium provides for the maintenance of intracellular magnesium. Reducing the serum magnesium concentration results in increased neuromuscular excitability

because magnesium competitively inhibits the entry of calcium into neurons.

Clinical significance

Hypomagnesemia/magnesium deficiency

Hypomagnesemia is defined as an abnormally low serum magnesium level resulting from a deficiency of magnesium. Such a deficiency is very common, particularly in large city hospitals and intensive care units. The causes of magnesium deficiency are shown in Table 38-9. Intestinal loss may be due to diarrhea or malabsorption or may result after intestinal surgery. Urinary magnesium loss occurs in cases of alcoholism and diabetes mellitus, with the use of drugs, including loop diuretics, aminoglycoside antibiotics, and with increased renal sodium and calcium excretion.

Neuromuscular hyperirritability with tetany and seizures may be present. Magnesium deficiency induces impaired PTH secretion and PTH end-organ resistance, which may result in hypocalcemia and contribute to neurological symptoms. Cardiac arrhythmias also may be a complication of magnesium deficiency. This effect may be linked to the hypokalemia and intracellular potassium depletion that occurs secondary to magnesium deficiency.

Although extracellular magnesium accounts for only about 1% of total body magnesium, determination of the serum magnesium is the most widely used test to assess magnesium deficiency. A serum magnesium concentration less than 1.7 mg/dL (0.70 mmol/L) indicates deficiency.

Acute symptomatic magnesium deficiency usually is treated with parenteral magnesium; mild depletion may be treated with oral magnesium. Renal function and continuing magnesium losses must be monitored.

TABLE 38-9	Causes of Magnesium Deficiency
Gastrointestinal Disorders	Drugs
Prolonged nasogastric suction	Diuretics (furosemide,
Malabsorption syndromes	ethacrynic acid)
Extensive bowel resection	Aminoglycosides
Acute and chronic diarrhea	Cisplatin
Intestinal and biliary fistulas	Cyclosporin
Protein-calorie malnutrition	Amphotericin B
Acute hemorrhagic pancreatitis	Cardiac glycosides
Primary hypomagnesemia	Pentamidine
(neonatal)	Metabolic acidosis (starvation,
	ketoacidosis, alcoholism)
Renal Loss	Renal diseases
Chronic parenteral fluid therapy	Chronic pyelonephritis, inter-
Osmotic diuresis	stitial nephritis, and glo-
Glucose (diabetes mellitus)	merulonephritis
Mannitol	Diuretic phase of acute
Urea	tubular necrosis
Hypercalcemia	Postobstructive nephropathy
Alcohol	Renal tubular acidosis
	Postrenal transplantation
	Primary hypomagnesemia
	Phosphate depletion

Hypermagnesemia

Hypermagnesemia is caused almost always by excessive intake, resulting from the administration of antacids, enemas, or parenteral therapy or administration of magnesium to an individual with renal failure (Table 38-10).

Depression of the neuromuscular system is the most common manifestation of magnesium intoxication. Deep tendon reflexes disappear at levels between 5 and 9 mg/dL (2.06 to 3.70 mmol/L), whereas depressed respiration may occur at 10 to 12 mg/dL (4.11 to 4.94 mmol/L) and cardiac arrest at even higher concentrations.

Analytical methodology

Various methods are used to quantify total and free magnesium.

Measurement of total magnesium

Both photometric methods and AAS are used to measure total magnesium in serum and urine.

Photometric methods. Magnesium is measured most frequently in clinical laboratories by use of photometric methods. A number of metallochromic indicators or dyes change color on selectively binding magnesium. These include calmagite, formazan dye, methylthymol blue, and magon (xylidyl blue).

Atomic absorption spectrophotometry. As with calcium, AAS methods provide greater accuracy and precision for magnesium measurements than do photometric methods; however, they are not used frequently for routine determination of magnesium. However, the AAS method is used as a reference method for magnesium. Neutron activation with ^{27}Mg is the definitive method for magnesium analysis.

TABLE 38-10 **Causes of Hypermagnesemia**

Excessive intake
  Oral administration (usually in the presence of chronic renal failure)
    Antacids
    Cathartic administration
  Rectal administration
    Purgation
  Parenteral administration
    Treatment of pregnancy-induced hypertension
    Treatment of magnesium deficiency
Renal failure
  Chronic failure (usually with administration of magnesium)
    Antacid
    Magnesium-containing cathartics
    Enema
    Infusion
    Dialysis
  Acute failure
    Rhabdomyolysis
Familial hypocalciuric hypercalcemia
Lithium ingestion

Magnesium is determined by AAS after dilution of the specimen 1 to 50 with a solution of lanthanum-HCl to eliminate interference from anions, including phosphate and protein and metal oxides. The dilution also reduces viscosity, ensuring that the aspiration rates for aqueous calibrators and specimens are comparable. The specimen is aspirated into an air-acetylene flame, in which the ground-state magnesium ions absorb light from a magnesium hollow lamp (285.2 nm). Absorbance at 285.2 nm is directly proportional to the number of ground-state magnesium atoms in the flame.

Measurement of free magnesium

Free magnesium is determined in whole blood, plasma, or serum by use of commercially available ISEs with neutral carrier ionophores. Further improvements in these ISEs and instruments may increase the availability of such determinations.

Specimen requirements

Serum is the preferred specimen for the measurement of magnesium, but heparinized plasma also may be used. Zinc heparin, lithium-zinc heparin, and the new heparins developed for free calcium determinations should not be used because they significantly increase magnesium. Other anticoagulants, such as citrate, oxalate, and EDTA, should not be used because they form complexes with magnesium. Magnesium is stable in serum for days at 4 °C and for months in its frozen state.

Serum or plasma must be separated from red blood cells as soon as possible to avoid increased levels caused by cell leakage. Because erythrocytes contain higher levels of magnesium than do serum or plasma, hemolyzed specimens are unacceptable. Interference by icterus or lipemia depends on the method, use of bichromatic or polychromatic analysis, or blanking. Lipemic specimens should be clarified by high-speed centrifugation. Spectral interference in photometric methods may be overcome with EDTA blanking.

Reference intervals

For adults the reference interval for serum magnesium is 1.7 to 2.4 mg/dL (0.66 to 1.07 mmol/L). Erythrocytes have magnesium levels approximately three times those of serum.

■ HORMONES REGULATING MINERAL METABOLISM

PTH and 1,25(OH)$_2$D are the hormones primarily responsible for regulating bone and mineral metabolism. Calcitonin has pharmacological actions, but a physiological role has not been established in adults. PTHrP is the principal mediator of HHM.

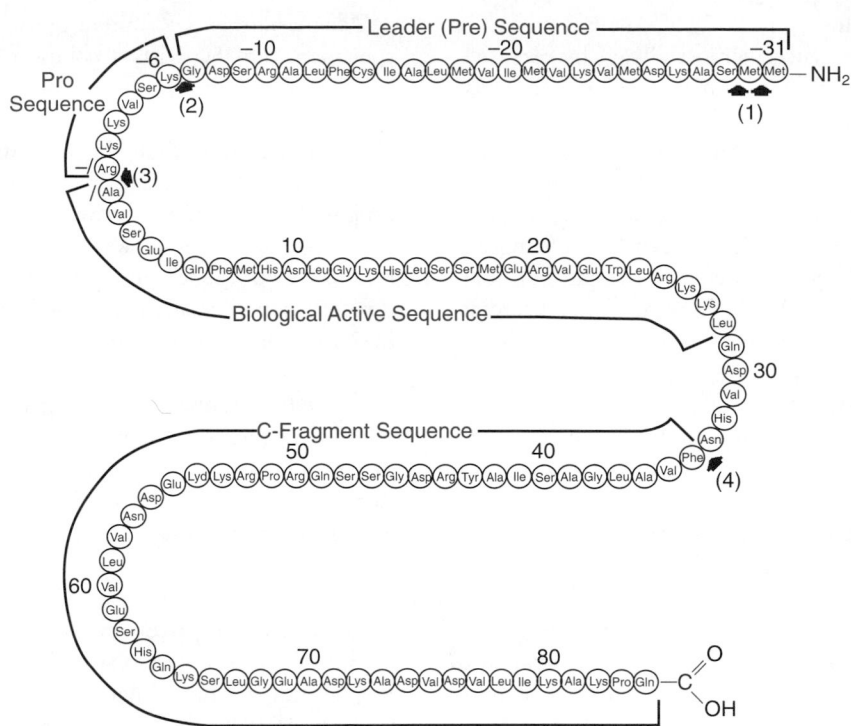

Figure 38-3 Amino acid sequence of preproparathyroid hormone. Note the sites of cleavage by proteases (*arrows*) to remove the N-terminal methionines (*1*), the leader (pre) sequence (*2*), and the pro sequence (*3*), producing intact PTH (1-84). Cleavage at position (*4*) produces inactive carboxyl (C)-terminal fragments. *Met,* Methionine; *Ser,* serine; *Ala,* alanine; *Lys,* lysine; *Asp,* aspartic acid; *Val,* valine; *Ile,* isoleucine; *Leu,* leucine; *Cys,* cysteine; *Phe,* phenylalanine; *Arg,* arginine; *His,* histidine; *Glu,* glutamine; *Asn,* asparagine; *Trp,* tryptophan; *Tyr,* tyrosine; *Gln,* glutamine; *Pro,* proline. (Modified from Habener JF, Rosenblatt M, Potts JT Jr: Parathyroid hormone: biochemical aspects of biosynthesis, secretion, action, and metabolism. Physiol Rev 1984; 64:985-1053.)

Parathyroid Hormone

Parathyroid hormone (PTH) is synthesized and secreted by the four parathyroid glands located bilaterally on or near the thyroid gland capsule. The glands are composed of chief and oxyphil cells; the chief cells synthesize, store, and secrete PTH.

Biochemistry and physiology

Synthesis

PTH is synthesized as a precursor pre-proPTH. Both the "pre" and "pro" segments are cleaved enzymatically during intracellular synthesis and processing. After processing in the Golgi apparatus, PTH is secreted, stored, or degraded intracellularly. Intact PTH contains 84 amino acids and has a molecular weight of 9425 kD (Figure 38-3). Biological activity resides in the amino N-terminal third of the molecule. Synthetic PTH containing the first 34 amino acids generally is considered to have full biological activity.

Secretion

The concentration of free calcium in blood or extracellular fluid is the primary physiological regulator of PTH secretion. Free calcium is sensed by a calcium-sensing receptor in the plasma membrane of the parathyroid cells; this receptor activates intracellular events leading to the release of free calcium from intracellular stores. An increase in extracellular free calcium inhibits PTH synthesis and secretion, whereas a decrease has the reverse effect. An inverse sigmoidal relationship exists between PTH secretion and free calcium (Figure 38-4). Small changes in free calcium cause maximal secretion (decreased calcium) or suppression (increased calcium) of PTH.

Magnesium and $1,25(OH)_2D$ also influence the secretion of PTH. Vitamin D receptors in the parathyroid glands interact with $1,25(OH)_2D$ to suppress chronically PTH synthesis and secretion. Magnesium probably does not play an important physiological role in PTH secretion except at the extremes of magnesium concentration. Chronic severe hypomagnesemia, such as that occurring with alcoholism, has been associated with impaired PTH secretion, whereas acute reduction in serum Mg levels stimulates secretion. Hypermagnesemia suppresses PTH secretion, although not as effectively as calcium.

Biological actions

PTH influences both calcium and phosphate homeostasis directly through its actions on bone and kidney and indirectly on the intestine through $1,25(OH)_2D$. PTH exerts its actions by interacting with PTH receptors, located in the plasma membrane of target cells, such as bone and kidney; stimulating cyclic adenosine monophosphate (cAMP); increasing intracellular calcium, which stimulates phospho-

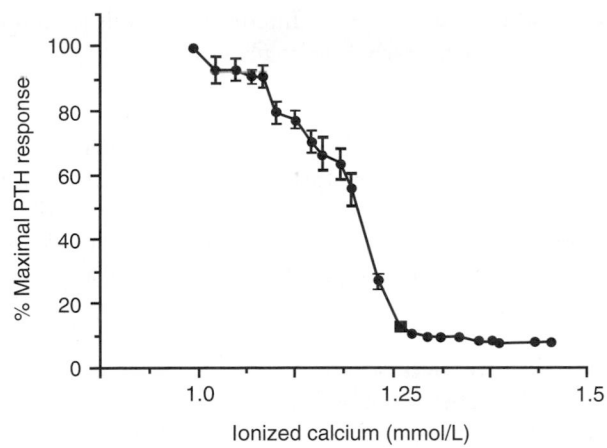

Figure 38-4   Regulation of intact PTH secretion by calcium in normal humans. Calcium and ethylenediaminetetraacetic acid were infused to demonstrate the sigmoidal relationship between PTH secretion and free calcium. *PTH,* Parathyroid hormone. (Modified from Brown EM: Extracellular Ca^{2+} sensing, regulation of parathyroid cell function, and role of Ca^{2+} and other ions as extracellular [first] messengers. Physiol Rev 1991; 71:371-411.)

lipase C and phosphoinositol hydrolysis; and initiating a cascade of intracellular events. In the kidneys, PTH (1) increases calcium reabsorption in the distal tubule of the nephron, (2) decreases reabsorption of phosphate by the proximal tubule, resulting in phosphaturia, and (3) stimulates intestinal absorption of both calcium and phosphate through an increase in $1,25(OH)_2D$ production by inducing 1α-hydroxylase.

The effects of PTH on bone are complex, as evidenced by its stimulation of bone resorption or bone formation, depending on the concentration of PTH and the duration of exposure. Chronic exposure to elevated levels of PTH increases bone resorption. PTH acts directly or indirectly by altering the activity or numbers of osteoblasts (bone-forming cells) and osteoclasts (bone-resorbing cells). Bone resorption, a prompt effect, is important in the maintenance of calcium homeostasis, whereas delayed effects are important for extreme systemic needs and skeletal homeostasis.

Integration of the direct effects of PTH on bone and kidney and the indirect effects on intestine through $1,25(OH)_2D$ results in changes in the calcium and phosphate concentrations in serum and urine. In serum, total and free calcium are increased, but the concentration of phosphate is reduced. In urine, inorganic phosphate and cAMP concentrations are increased. Urinary calcium also is increased because the larger filtered load of calcium overrides the increased tubular reabsorption of calcium. In the absence of disease the increase in serum calcium reduces PTH secretion through a negative-feedback loop, maintaining homeostasis.

Metabolism and circulating heterogeneity

PTH circulates as intact and inactive fragments. Its heterogeneity is a consequence of (1) the secretion of both in-

tact hormone and inactive fragments by the parathyroids, (2) peripheral metabolism of intact hormone by the liver and kidney, and (3) renal clearance of intact hormone and inactive fragments.

The parathyroid glands secrete both biologically active intact hormone and inactive fragments containing the midregion/carboxyl amino acids. In the case of hypercalcemia, secretion of intact hormone is reduced significantly or absent, whereas secretion of inactive fragments persists.

Biologically active intact PTH (half-life <5 minutes) is converted rapidly to inactive fragments by the liver and kidneys. These inactive fragments lack the biologically active amino-terminal region. Although these inactive fragments have not been characterized thoroughly, fragments containing amino acids 34 to 84, 37 to 84 have been reported. Inactive fragments are cleared by glomerular filtration and normally have half-lives of less than 1 hour. Their half-lives and circulating concentrations are increased significantly in individuals with impaired renal function. Generally, 5% to 25% of the total immunoreactive PTH is intact hormone. The remaining 75% to 95% is inactive midregion/carboxyl fragments. The relative concentrations of intact hormone and fragments vary with physiology and pathology.

Clinical significance

Hyperparathyroidism is defined as the overproduction of PTH by the parathyroid glands. Primary hyperparathyroidism is caused by the excessive secretion of PTH by a solitary parathyroid adenoma in 85% of cases. Diffuse hyperplasia of all parathyroid glands accounts for up to 15% of cases, and parathyroid carcinoma is much less common (less than 1%). Parathyroid hyperplasia may be associated with other inherited endocrine disorders (multiple endocrine neoplasia [MEN] types I and IIa).

More than 80% of the individuals with primary hyperparathyroidism are asymptomatic at diagnosis and are discovered by biochemical screening taken for other reasons. Renal stones and bone disease (osteitis fibrosa) are seen in 10% to 20% of affected individuals. Other signs and symptoms of hyperparathyroidism include fatigue, malaise, and weakness. With serum calcium levels more than 12 mg/dL, nausea, vomiting, depression, apathy, and inability to concentrate may be present. Bone pain and joint pain suggest advanced skeletal involvement.

Two-site, labeled antibody methods used to measure intact PTH differentiate individuals with primary hyperparathyroidism from those with nonparathyroid hypercalcemia. PTH levels are elevated in the majority of individuals with primary hyperparathyroidism (Figure 38-5). Levels in the upper end of the normal reference interval are inappropriately high in individuals with significant and stable hypercalcemia. The majority of those with hypercalcemia associated with malignancy have PTH levels below normal or in the lower end of the normal reference interval. Ectopic PTH production is extremely rare. Hypercalcemia in malig-

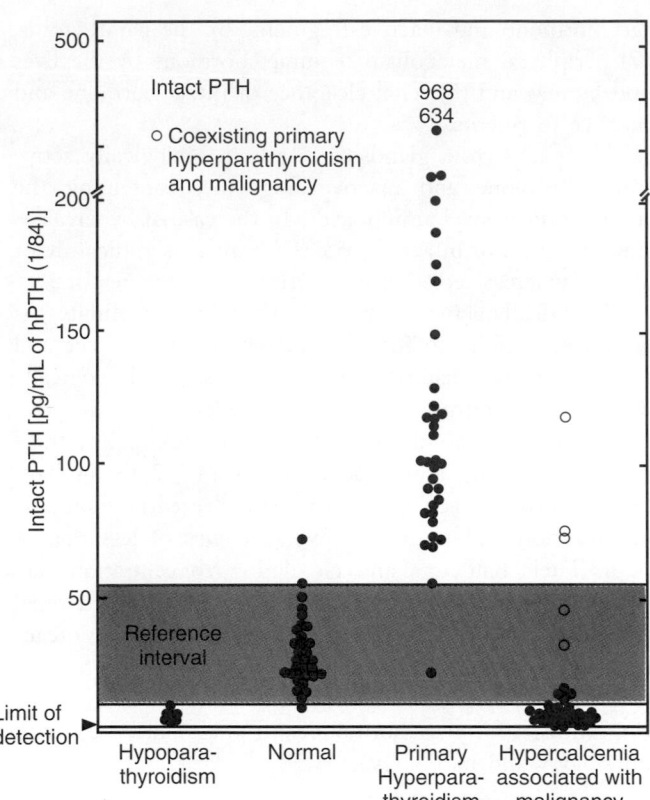

Figure 38-5   Intact PTH in hypoparathyroid patients, normal subjects, patients with primary hypothyroidism, and those with hypercalcemia associated with malignancy. The *open circles* represent patients with coexisting hyperparathyroidism and malignancy. *PTH,* Parathyroid hormone. (Modified from Endres DB, Villanueva R, Sharp CF Jr et al: Measurement of parathyroid hormone. Endocrinol Metab Clin North Am 1989; 18:611-629.)

nancy usually is associated with bone metastases or production of PTHrP, a tumor-product which does not cross-react in PTH immunoassays.

Determination of PTH is useful also in the differential diagnosis of hypercalcemia and hypocalcemia, the assessment of parathyroid function in individuals with renal failure, and the evaluation of parathyroid function in individuals with disorders of bone and mineral metabolism. In practice, both PTH and calcium concentrations should be measured simultaneously because the interpretation of PTH results is difficult without the concomitant calcium results.

Subnormal levels of intact PTH are observed in the majority of individuals with hypoparathyroidism. Apparently detectable levels in many of these individuals may be the result of a matrix effect (nonspecific serum or ligand-free media effect) or the sensitivity of current methods.

In individuals with end-stage renal disease, intact PTH is helpful in the assessment of parathyroid function and the improvement of management. Individuals with advanced osteitis fibrosa caused by secondary hyperparathyroidism have the highest levels of PTH, whereas those with aluminum bone disease, osteomalacia, or low-turnover aplastic

disease have the lowest levels. Intermediate levels are found in individuals with early osteitis fibrosa.

Intact PTH concentrations are correlated inversely with triiodothyronine (T_3) levels in hyperthyroid individuals. PTH levels increase in individuals who become hypothyroid after radioactive iodine treatment and decrease with thyroid replacement therapy. These changes apparently are mediated by serum calcium. Chronic lithium carbonate therapy has been reported to increase parathyroid gland size and circulating intact PTH.

Analytical methodology

Two-site, labeled antibody methods are the method of choice used to measure intact PTH. Older competitive immunoassays or radioimmunoassays (RIAs; C-terminal-, N-terminal-, midregion-PTH, etc.) are inadequate because of their limited specificity and sensitivity and should be discontinued. Because C-terminal and midregion assays measure inactive fragments, they often were elevated falsely in cases of impaired renal function or nonparathyroid hypercalcemia.

The two-site, labeled antibody methods require two different antibodies capable of simultaneously binding PTH—(1) a solid-phase capture antibody often directed against carboxyl-terminal (for example, amino acid sequences 39 to 84, 53 to 84) and (2) a signal or labeled antibody often directed against amino-terminal (for example, amino acids 1-34). Depending on the method, the signal antibody commonly is labeled with a chemiluminescent compound (immunochemiluminometric [ICMA]), radiolabeled with ^{125}I (immunoradiometric [IRMA]), or labeled with the enzyme (alkaline phosphatase) that converts a substrate to a chemiluminescent product. Most methods also have been found to measure unknown circulating species, as well as a synthetic form of PTH missing a few amino terminal amino acids (hPTH [7-84]). However, until more specific methods are available, these methods are considered the most sensitive and specific assessments of parathyroid function.

Specimen requirements

Serum is the specimen of choice for PTH measurements. After collection, serum should be separated and frozen promptly because PTH is unstable at room or refrigerated temperatures. Lower levels of PTH are observed in serum incubated for more than a few hours at room temperature or a day or more at 4 °C. If a specific method permits its use, EDTA plasma has been reported to stabilize PTH, a probable consequence of reduced proteolytic activity.

Reference intervals

The reference interval for intact PTH in adults is 10 to 65 pg/mL (1.05 to 6.84 pmol/L). Levels of intact PTH reportedly are low or normal during pregnancy, lower in fetuses and umbilical cord blood, and increased during the first few days of life in response to early neonatal

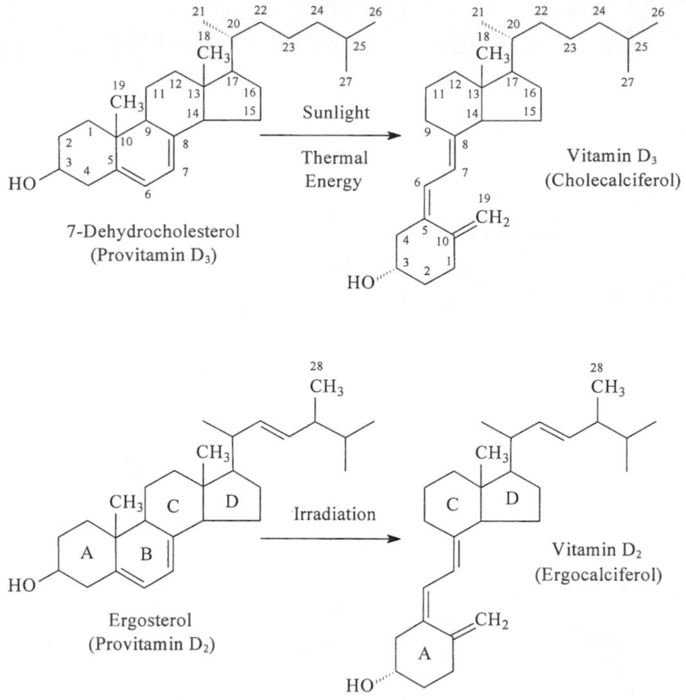

Figure 38-6 Structure of vitamin D_3 (cholecalciferol) and vitamin D_2 (ergocalciferol) and their precursors. Cholecalciferol is produced in the skin from 7-dehydrocholesterol on exposure to sunlight. Ergocalciferol is produced commercially by irradiation of ergosterol. (Modified from Holick MF, Adams JS: Vitamin D metabolism and biological function. In Avioli LV, Krane SM (ed): Metabolic Bone Disease, 2nd edition, pp 155-195, Philadelphia, WB Saunders, 1990.)

hypocalcemia. Levels in children and adolescents are reportedly similar if not identical to those in adults. In healthy adults, circulating concentrations of intact PTH increase with age.

Vitamin D and Its Metabolites

Vitamin D is produced by exposure of human skin to ultraviolet light. It plays an important role in calcium and phosphorus metabolism. Its deficiency is known as *rickets* in children and *osteomalacia* in adults.

Biochemistry and physiology

Vitamin D and its metabolites are categorized as either cholecalciferols or ergocalciferols (Figure 38-6). Cholecalciferol (vitamin D_3) is the parent compound of the naturally occurring family and is produced in skin from 7-dehydrocholesterol on exposure to sunlight. Vitamin D_2 (ergocalciferol) is manufactured by irradiation of ergosterol produced by yeasts. When vitamin D and its metabolites are written without a subscript, both families are included.

Vitamin D may be acquired by exposure of skin to sunlight or ingestion of foods containing vitamin D. Only a few foods, primarily fish liver oils, egg yolks, and liver, naturally contain substantial amounts of vitamin D. A considerable fraction of dietary vitamin D is acquired by ingestion of fortified foods or vitamin D supplements. The recommended daily allowance is 400 IU (10 μg). Groups at risk for developing vitamin D deficiency include breast-fed infants, strict vegetarians who abstain from eggs and milk, and the elderly.

Metabolism, regulation, and transport

Vitamin D is metabolized to 25-hydroxyvitamin D (25[OH]D) in the liver by 25-hydroxylase and to $1,25(OH)_2D$ by 1-hydroxylase in the kidneys and placenta (Figure 38-7). $1,25(OH)_2D$ is the biologically active form of vitamin D. An alternative pathway for the metabolism of 25(OH)D involves the production of inactive 24,25-dihydroxyvitamin D (24,25[OH]$_2$D) by 24-hydroxylase.

Circulating concentrations of $1,25(OH)_2D$ are regulated tightly, primarily by PTH and phosphate. PTH increases the synthesis of $1,25(OH)_2D$. Phosphate restriction and hypophosphatemia also increase $1,25(OH)_2D$, whereas phosphate supplementation and hyperphosphatemia have the opposite effect. Hypocalcemia increases $1,25(OH)_2D$ indirectly by stimulating the secretion of PTH.

Vitamin D, 25(OH)D, and $1,25(OH)_2D$ are bound in the circulation to vitamin D-binding protein (DBP; Table 38-11). The concentration of 25(OH)D, the major circulating form of vitamin D, is approximately 1000 times that of $1,25(OH)_2D$. Only 0.03% of 25(OH)D and 0.4% of $1,25(OH)_2D$ are normally free in plasma.

Biological actions

Serum calcium and phosphate levels are maintained by $1,25(OH)_2D$ stimulation of calcium absorption primarily

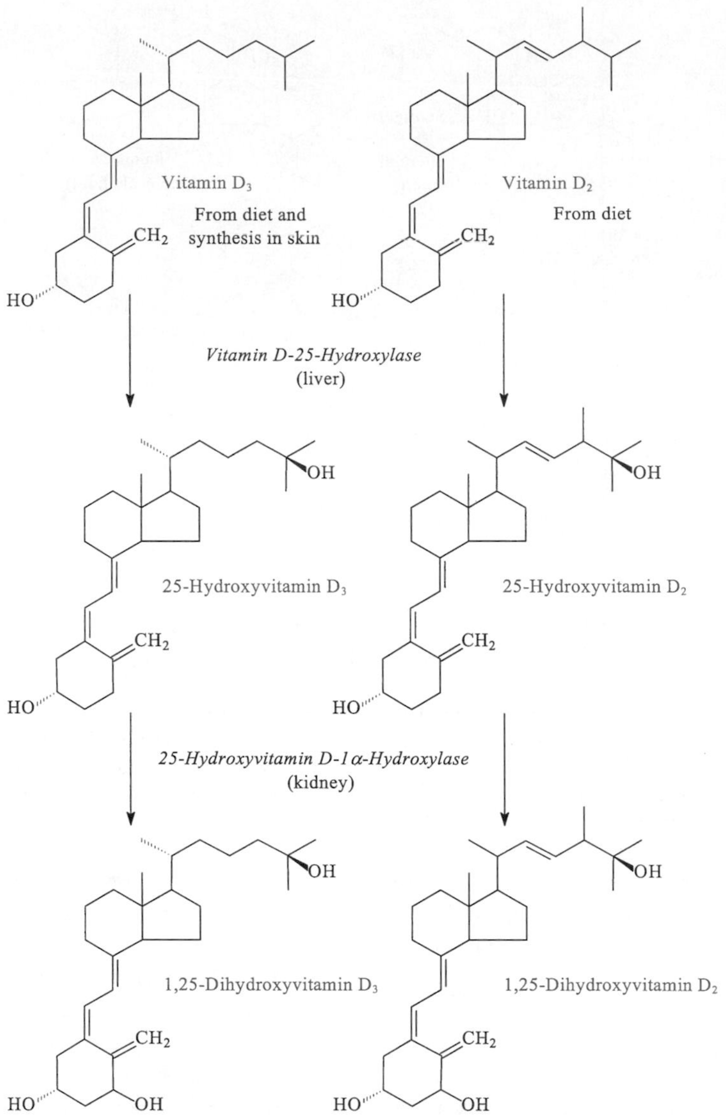

Figure 38-7　Metabolism of vitamin D. Vitamin D_2 and vitamin D_3 are hydroxylated enzymatically to 25-hydroxyvitamin D (25[OH]D) in liver and 1,25-dihydroxyvitamin D (1,25[OH]$_2$D) in the kidneys. 1,25-Dihydroxyvitamin D_2 and 1,25-dihydroxyvitamin D_3 are the biologically active forms of vitamin D.

TABLE 38-11　Vitamin D and Its Metabolites in Plasma

Compound	Concentration	Free (%)	Half-Life
Vitamin D			
(ng/mL)	<0.2 to 20	—	1 to 2 days
(nmol/L)	<0.5 to 52		
25(OH)D			
(ng/mL)	10 to 50	0.03	2 to 3 weeks
(nmol/L)	25 to 125		
1,25(OH)$_2$D			
(pg/mL)	15 to 60	0.4	4 to 6 hours
(pmol/L)	36 to 144		

25(OH)D, 25-Hydroxyvitamin D; 1,25(OH)$_2$D, 1,25-dihydroxyvitamin D.

in the duodenum and phosphate absorption by the jejunum and ileum. 1,25(OH)$_2$D also has a direct effect on the parathyroids, inhibiting the synthesis and secretion of PTH. It exerts its cellular actions by associating with a specific vitamin D receptor. The receptor is found, not only in tissues involved in calcium and phosphate metabolism, but also in a wide variety of normal tissues and tumors. In bone, 1,25(OH)$_2$D and PTH at high concentrations increase bone resorption, mobilizing calcium and phosphate.

Clinical significance

Only the measurement of 25(OH)D and 1,25(OH)$_2$D have proven clinical value. Vitamin D status is determined best by the measurement of 25(OH)D (Table 38-12). Circulat-

TABLE 38-12	Abnormal Circulating Levels of 25(OH)D

Decreased 25(OH)D
Inadequate exposure to sunlight
Inadequate dietary vitamin D
Vitamin D malabsorption
Severe hepatocellular disease
Increased catabolism (for example, drugs such as anticonvulsants)
Increased loss (nephrotic syndrome)

Increased 25(OH)D (Hypercalcemia)
Vitamin D or 25(OH)D intoxication

25(OH)D, 25-Hydroxyvitamin D.

TABLE 38-13	Abnormal Levels of 1,25(OH)$_2$D

Decreased 1,25(OH)$_2$D
Renal failure
Hyperphosphatemia
Hypomagnesemia
Hypoparathyroidism
Pseudohypoparathyroidism
Vitamin D-dependent rickets, type I
Hypercalcemia of malignancy

Increased 1,25(OH)$_2$D
Granulomatous diseases
Primary hyperparathyroidism
Lymphoma
1,25(OH)$_2$D intoxication
Vitamin D-dependent rickets, type II

1,25(OH)$_2$D, 1,25-Dihydroxyvitamin D.

ing levels of 25(OH)D may be decreased by (1) reduced availability of vitamin D, (2) inadequate conversion of vitamin D to 25(OH)D, (3) accelerated metabolism of 25(OH)D, and (4) urinary loss of 25(OH)D with its transport protein. Reduced availability of vitamin D occurs with inadequate exposure to sunlight, dietary deficiency, malabsorption syndrome, or gastric or small-bowel resection. Severe hepatocellular disease has been associated with inadequate conversion of vitamin D to 25(OH)D. Drugs such as phenytoin and phenobarbital induce hepatic enzymes, which accelerate the metabolism of vitamin D and its metabolites. Serum 25(OH)D levels may be reduced in individuals with nephrotic syndrome because of the urinary loss of DBP and 25(OH)D. Levels are increased in vitamin D- or 25(OH)D-intoxicated individuals.

Measurement of 1,25(OH)$_2$D is useful in the detection of certain states of inadequate or excessive production in the evaluation of hypercalcemia, hypercalciuria, hypocalcemia, and bone and mineral disorders (Table 38-13). Increased concentrations have been observed in individuals with sarcoidosis, tuberculosis, other granulomatous diseases, and lymphoma. Levels also are increased in cases of primary hyperparathyroidism, individuals with vitamin D-dependent rickets, type II, and individuals with 1,25(OH)$_2$D intoxication. Reduced levels of 1,25(OH)$_2$D are observed in individuals with renal failure, hypercalcemia of malignancy, hyperphosphatemia, hypoparathyroidism, pseudohypoparathyroidism, type I vitamin D-dependent rickets, hypomagnesemia, nephrotic syndrome, and severe hepatocellular disease.

Analytical methodology

Specific and sensitive assays have been developed for vitamin D, 25(OH)D, and 1,25(OH)$_2$D. The differences in the number of hydroxyl groups cause differences in polarity that have been used to separate chromatographically the metabolites before quantification.

Most assays for vitamin D metabolites require two or three of the following steps:

1. Extraction or deproteinization
2. Purification
3. Quantification

Extraction with organic solvents frees and partially purifies the metabolites that are associated almost completely with DBP and albumin. Chromatographic columns packed with octadecylsilanol (C$_{18}$)-silica or silica are used commonly to separate vitamin D metabolites, lipids, and interfering substances. Partially purified vitamin D metabolites are measured by RIA, competitive protein-binding assay (CPBA), competitive receptor assay, or high-performance liquid chromatography (HPLC) with ultraviolet absorption. For clinical purposes the 25(OH)D and 1,25(OH)$_2$D assays should measure both the D$_2$ and D$_3$ forms.

After deproteinization with acetonitrile, RIA is used most commonly to measure 25(OH)D. RIA also is used to measure 1,25(OH)$_2$D. In addition, a competitive receptor assay using vitamin D receptor from calf thymus has been used to measure 1,25(OH)$_2$D. With both methods, specimens first must be deproteinized and purified by column chromatography.

Specimen requirements

Serum typically is used to measure vitamin D metabolites, although plasma is acceptable for assays using extraction and chromatography. Vitamin D metabolites are relatively stable in serum at both room temperature and 4 °C; however, specimens should be frozen if the analysis is delayed. Vitamin D metabolites in serum do not appear to be sensitive to light and do not require special handling in the laboratory.

Reference intervals

The reference interval for 25(OH)D in serum is 10 to 50 ng/mL (25 to 125 nmol/L). For 1,25(OH)$_2$D the reference interval in serum is 15 to 60 pg/mL (36 to 144 pmol/L). Circulating levels of 25(OH)D are increased by exposure to sunlight. Levels are higher in summer and fall and lower in winter or spring. In addition, levels are influenced by latitude, sunscreen use, and skin pigmentation. 1,25(OH)$_2$D levels are higher in children than in adults, with the highest levels exhibited during periods of the most active growth.

Calcitonin

Biochemistry and physiology

Secretion

Calcitonin is a 32-amino-acid peptide secreted by the parafollicular or C cells of the thyroid gland (Figure 38-8). These cells are included in the amine precursor uptake and decarboxylation (APUD) family. This inclusion explains the association of medullary thyroid carcinoma (MTC), a tumor of the C cells, with other tumors of the APUD family in MEN IIa and MEN IIb. Its secretion is regulated primarily by the level of free calcium in plasma. Increasing serum calcium levels and hypercalcemia stimulate calcitonin secretion. Decreasing calcium levels and hypocalcemia reduce its secretion.

Biological actions

Pharmacological doses of calcitonin reduce serum calcium and phosphate concentrations primarily by inhibiting osteoclastic bone resorption. Pharmacological doses of calcitonin also decrease the renal tubular reabsorption of calcium, phosphate, magnesium, and other ions. Despite these pharmacological effects, the physiological role of calcitonin in adults is uncertain.

Clinical significance

MTC may occur as sporadic disease, familial MEN IIa, familial MEN IIb, or familial MTC. Sporadic MTC is believed to account for about 75% of the cases of the carcinoma. Routine measurement of serum calcitonin in individuals with nodular thyroid diseases assists in the detection of unsuspected sporadic MTC. All MTC accounts for approximately 10% of thyroid cancers. Stimulation of calcitonin with calcium or pentagastrin increases the sensitivity of detection for medullary carcinoma and C-cell hyperplasia. Specificity also is increased with provocative testing, which helps identify false positives. Minimally elevated levels that are not stimulated after provocative testing should be questioned.

More than 90% of individuals with MEN IIa, MEN IIb, and familial MTC now are identified with genetic testing for mutations of the coding sequence of the RET protooncogene transmembrane receptor type tyrosine kinase. Genetic testing provides the most sensitive and specific method for confirmation of MTC in these individuals and, unlike calcitonin, does not require annual testing from 5 to 45 years of age.

Calcitonin levels are increased in individuals with various nonthyroidal cancers. Although calcitonin often is elevated in those with tumors arising from tissues derived from the neural crest, it also may be elevated in individuals with other malignancies. Intestinal, bronchial, and gastric carcinoids; carcinoma of the lung, especially oat- or small-cell carcinoma; melanoma and pheochromocytoma; pancreatic and breast carcinoma; and others have been associated with elevated levels of calcitonin.

Elevated levels of calcitonin or increased responsiveness to stimulation also has been reported in individuals with acute and chronic renal failure, hypercalcemia, hypergastrinemia, other gastrointestinal disorders and pulmonary disease, and severe illness (Table 38-14).

Analytical methodology

Measurement and interpretation of serum calcitonin is complicated by the circulating heterogeneity of calcitonin and wide differences in the sensitivity and specificity of calcitonin immunoassays. Calcitonin circulates as the monomer, a dimeric form, and a number of larger forms. Generally immunoassays recognize multiple forms of calcitonin. Historically, calcitonin was measured primarily by RIA. More recently, several two-site, labeled antibody methods (IRMA, enzyme-linked immunosorbent assay [ELISA]) have been reported for assaying of calcitonin. These methods generally provide improved sensitivity and specificity for the diagnosis of MTC, when compared with earlier competitive immunoassays. Calcitonin levels in healthy individuals are less than 10 to 20 pg/mL (ng/L) with these two-site methods.

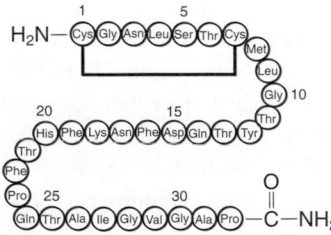

Figure 38-8 Amino acid sequence of calcitonin. *Cys,* Cysteine; *Gly,* glycine; *Asn,* asparagine; *Leu,* leucine; *Ser,* serine; *Thr,* threonine; *Met,* methionine; *Tyr,* tyrosine; *Gln,* glutamine; *Asp,* aspartic acid; *Phe,* phenylalanine; *His,* histidine; *Pro,* Proline; *Val,* valine; *Ala,* alanine.

TABLE 38-14	Increased Circulating Levels of Calcitonin
C-cell hyperplasia	Acute and chronic renal failure
Medullary thyroid carcinoma	Hypercalcemia
Nonthyroidal cancers	Hypergastrinemia and other GI disorders
Oat-, small-cell carcinomas	
Other malignancies	Pulmonary disease

The basal levels of serum calcitonin in men are 25 pg/mL or less; for women the levels are 20 pg/mL or less. Reference intervals for calcitonin vary significantly among different methods. Because calcitonin secretion is stimulated by calcium as well as certain gastrointestinal hormones, calcium and pentagastrin have been used as provocative stimulatory agents to differentiate normal individuals from those with medullary carcinoma.

Parathyroid Hormone-Related Protein

Parathyroid hormone-related protein (PTHrP) was discovered in 1987 through an investigation of the mechanism by which certain cancers cause humoral hypercalcemia of malignancy (HHM).

Biochemistry and physiology

Although the exact circulating forms of PTHrP are unknown, three isoforms of 139, 141, and 173 amino acids in length are produced by alternative messenger RNA (mRNA) splicing (Figure 38-9). The N-terminal end of PTHrP has close homology with PTH (8 of the first 13 amino acids being identical), which may explain the ability of PTHrP to mimic the biological actions of PTH. Like PTH, PTHrP induces hypercalcemia and hypophosphatemia and increases urinary cAMP. In addition to its endocrine role observed in the pathophysiology of malignancy, PTHrP appears to exert its normal physiological actions locally on cells or tissues as an autocrine or paracrine factor. PTHrP may play important roles in fetal life and lactation.

Clinical significance

PTHrP is elevated in 50% to 90% of individuals with hypercalcemia-associated malignancy. In addition to squamous-cell carcinomas of the lung, head and neck, esophagus, cervix, skin, and other sites, levels often are elevated in individuals with a wide variety of malignancies, irrespective of their source or histology.

Increased levels of PTHrP are found in individuals with breast, renal, and ovarian carcinomas. PTHrP levels have been elevated less frequently in individuals with hematological malignancies, including lymphomas, leukemias, and myelomas.

PTHrP level is undetectable or normal in the majority of individuals with malignancy not associated with hypercalcemia, primary hyperparathyroidism, hypoparathyroidism, miscellaneous causes of hypercalcemia, and chronic renal failure (with IRMAs).

Analytical methodology

A number of immunoassays have been used to measure PTHrP in sera from individuals with HHM. Today, PTHrP generally is measured with more sensitive and specific two-site, labeled antibody assays (IRMAs). Currently available assays use antibodies against one end of the molecule as cap-

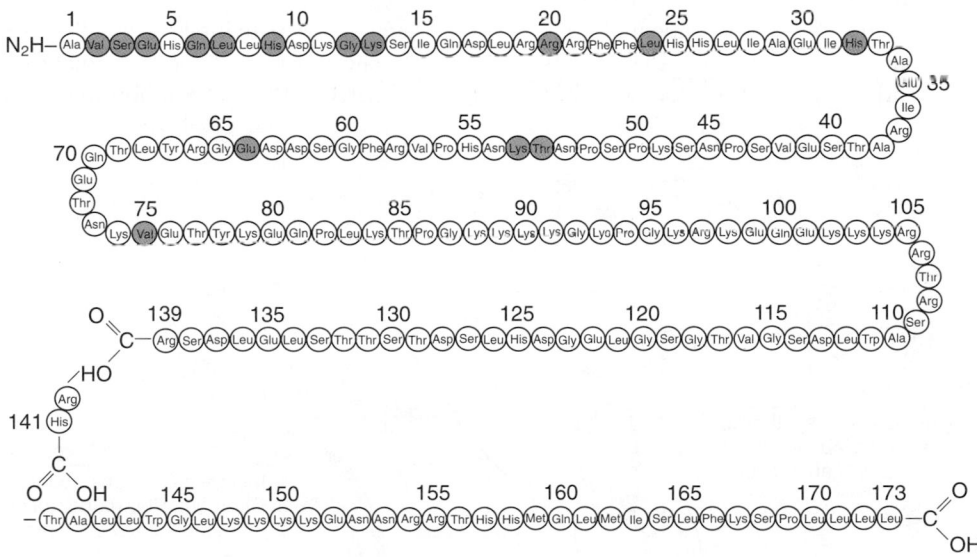

Figure 38-9   Amino acid sequence of parathyroid hormone-related protein (PTHrP). Although the exact length of circulating PTHrP is unknown, proteins of 139, 141, and 173 amino acids have been predicted from alternate splicing events. The *filled circles* show amino acids that are identical for PTH and PTHrP. *Ala,* Alanine; *Val,* valine; *Ser,* serine; *Glu,* glutamic acid; *His,* histidine; *Gln,* glutamine; *Leu,* leucine; *Asp,* aspartic acid; *Lys,* lysine; *Ile,* isoleucine; *Arg,* arginine; *Phe,* phenylalanine; *Thr,* threonine; *Pro,* proline; *Asn,* asparagine; *Tyr,* tyrosine; *Trp,* tryptophan. (Modified from Hendy GN, Goltzman D: Parathyroid hormone-like peptide. In Endocrinology and Metabolism Inservice, vol 9, pp 9-24, Washington, DC, American Association for Clinical Chemistry, 1991.)

ture antibodies and radiolabeled antibodies against the other end of the molecule for the signal.

Specimen requirements

PTHrP is unstable in serum and plasma at 4 °C and at room temperature unless it is collected in the presence of protease inhibitors, such as aprotinin, leupeptin, pepstatin, and EDTA. Serum or plasma should be separated from the cells and frozen promptly.

Reference intervals

Reference intervals are method dependent. With sensitive IRMA, reference intervals up to 1.5 to 2.5 pmol/L have been reported, with detectable levels in 50% to 80% of healthy individuals.

■ INTEGRATED CONTROL OF BONE AND MINERAL METABOLISM

The metabolism of calcium and phosphate is linked intimately (Figure 38-10). The homeostatic mechanisms are directed principally toward the maintenance of normal extracellular calcium and phosphate concentrations, which sustain extracellular and intracellular processes and provide substrate for skeletal mineralization. The parathyroid gland responds to a decrease in free calcium concentration within seconds. During a time of calcium deprivation, the rise in serum PTH rapidly alters both renal and skeletal metabolism. Of the approximately 10 g (250 mmol) of calcium filtered by the kidneys each day, 65% is reabsorbed in the proximal tubule. Calcium reabsorption in the proximal tubule is linked closely to sodium and is independent of PTH. Approximately 20% of calcium is reclaimed in the thick ascending limb of Henle and 5% in the distal convoluted tu-

bule. PTH enhances calcium reabsorption at the distal tubule, presumably through a cAMP mechanism. A small portion of filtered calcium, about 5%, is absorbed in the collecting duct via a PTH-independent mechanism. In contrast to the calcium-conserving effect of PTH on the kidneys, PTH increases renal phosphate excretion at the proximal tubule by directly lowering the tubular maximum for phosphate ($TmPO_4$). Approximately 6.5 g (210 mmol) of phosphate is filtered by the kidneys each day. Normally, 85% to 90% is reabsorbed by the renal tubules (proximal, as well as distal convoluted tubule). PTH is one of the most important factors regulating the $TmPO_4$ and hence the serum phosphate concentration.

PTH also causes an increase of intestinal calcium absorption through its action on the vitamin D endocrine system. PTH is a major trophic factor for the renal 25(OH)D-1-hydroxylase. It increases the conversion of 25(OH)D to the active vitamin D metabolite, 1,25(OH)$_2$D. Calcium is absorbed principally in the duodenum, although it is absorbed also by the distal small bowel and colon. About 30% of the recommended daily calcium intake of 1 g (25 mmol) is absorbed. Approximately 100 mg (2.5 mmol) of calcium is secreted into the gut lumen by intestinal secretion; thus the net calcium absorption is 200 mg (5.0 mmol)/day. Calcium is absorbed by passive diffusion and by an active transport system. Estimations are that passive diffusion accounts for absorption of approximately 10% of ingested calcium per day. Active calcium absorption in the duodenum is under the control of 1,25(OH)$_2$D. This vitamin D metabolite increases the intestinal cell synthesis of a calcium-binding protein (CaBP), which enhances the net absorption of ingested calcium.

Dietary phosphate intake is usually 1.2 to 1.4 g (39 to 45 mmol)/day, nearly twice the recommended intake, of which approximately 60% to 70% is absorbed principally in the je-

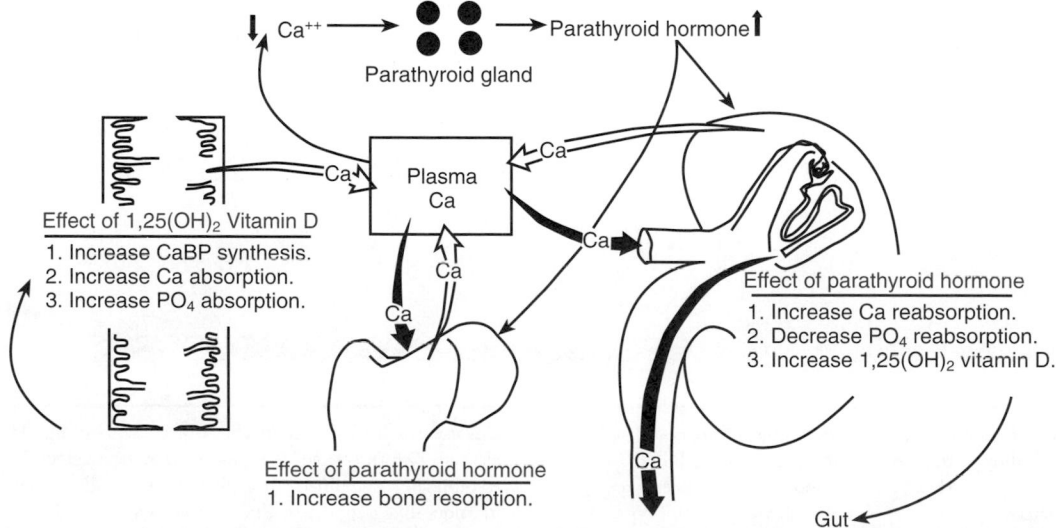

Figure 38-10　Integrated control of mineral metabolism. *CaBP,* Calcium-binding protein.

junum. As with calcium, both passive and active transport systems exist; $1,25(OH)_2D$ is the principal regulator of the active transport of phosphate. PTH-stimulated synthesis of $1,25(OH)_2D$ thus offsets the phosphaturic effect of PTH. The prevailing serum phosphate concentration also modulates renal 25(OH)D-1-hydroxylase. Phosphate deletion, or hypophosphatemia, stimulates formation of $1,25(OH)_2D$ by the kidneys. Calcitonin, in general, has the opposite effect of PTH. Whether calcitonin has any physiological role in mineral homeostasis in adult humans, however, remains unclear.

PTH also has an acute effect on the skeleton because it decreases osteoblastic collagen synthesis and increases osteoclastic bone resorption, with a net increase of mineral (calcium and phosphate) release from bone into the extracellular fluid. Receptors for PTH are found on osteoblasts. The effect of PTH on osteoclasts appears to be indirect, through local mediators produced by the osteoblast or released from the bone matrix. Prolonged calcium deprivation results in enhanced recruitment of osteoclasts and an increased number of mature osteoclasts, which continue to release calcium, phosphate, and peptides, from the bone matrix, such as hydroxyproline and **pyridinoline collagen cross-links.** Prolonged exposure to PTH eventually also increases osteoblast activity, and biochemical markers, such as serum alkaline phosphatase and osteocalcin, rise.

Despite the critical importance of magnesium in physiology, no hormone or factor has been described as regulating magnesium homeostasis. Magnesium is absorbed efficiently from the intestinal tract (most efficiently from the distal small bowel). During a normal dietary magnesium intake, approximately 30% to 40% of magnesium is absorbed. Both active and passive transport systems are present. The kidneys tightly regulate magnesium homeostasis. About 25% to 35% of filtered magnesium is reabsorbed passively in the proximal convoluted tubule, where it is linked closely to sodium and calcium transport. The major site of active reabsorption is the thick ascending limb of Henle, where 60% to 75% of magnesium is reabsorbed. During times of magnesium deprivation, magnesium essentially disappears from the urine (<0.5 mmol/day). The tubular maximum for magnesium is close to the filtered load. When magnesium intake is excessive, any amount greater than this maximum is excreted.

▐ BIOCHEMICAL MARKERS OF BONE TURNOVER

Many methods for markers of bone resorption and formation have been developed. Bone resorption markers (Table 38-15) are produced by osteoclasts during bone resorption. Bone formation markers (Table 38-16) are produced by osteoblasts during bone formation. Markers of bone resorption are measured in urine, whereas formation markers are measured in serum.

Selection and interpretation of biochemical markers of bone resorption and formation for osteoporosis and other metabolic bone diseases are complicated by uncertainties concerning the clinical utility of these new and evolving tests. Measurement of these biochemical markers provides a real-time assessment of bone resorption and/or formation. Although osteoporosis and osteopenia are diagnosed by measurement of bone mass (for example, dual energy x-ray absorptometry), 1 to 3 years are required to identify statistically significant changes in bone mass. Biochemical markers have a number of potential uses including (1) monitoring of therapy, (2) assessment of bone resorption and formation, (3) prediction of future bone loss and fracture risk, and (4) basic and clinical research.

Markers of Bone Resorption

Several analytes are measured as markers of bone resorption (see Table 38-15). The pyridinolines (deoxypyridinoline and pyridinoline) and the N- and C-**telopeptides** of type I collagen are the most frequently measured markers of bone resorption. Other markers include urinary hydroxyproline, galactosyl hydroxylysine, and serum osteoclastic or tartrate-resistant acid phosphatase.

Collagen cross-links

Type I **collagen** (Figure 38-11), a triple helix of two identical α1 (I) chains and an α2 (I) chain, is synthesized as a

TABLE 38-15 Markers of Bone Resorption

Marker	Method
Deoxypyridinoline and/or Pyridinoline	
Total deoxypyridinoline and pyridinoline	HPLC
Free deoxypyridinoline	ELISA
Free deoxypyridinoline and pyridinoline	ELISA
Total or free deoxypyridinoline	RIA
Telopeptides	
N-telopeptide	ELISA
C-telopeptide	ELISA
Other	
Hydroxyproline	Photometric, HPLC
Galactosyl hydroxylysine	HPLC
Osteoclastic acid phosphatase	Photometric, ELISA

HPLC, High-performance liquid chromatography; *ELISA,* enzyme-linked immunosorbent assay; *RIA,* radioimmunoassay.

TABLE 38-16 Markers of Bone Formation

Osteocalcin
Bone alkaline phosphatase
Collagen propeptides

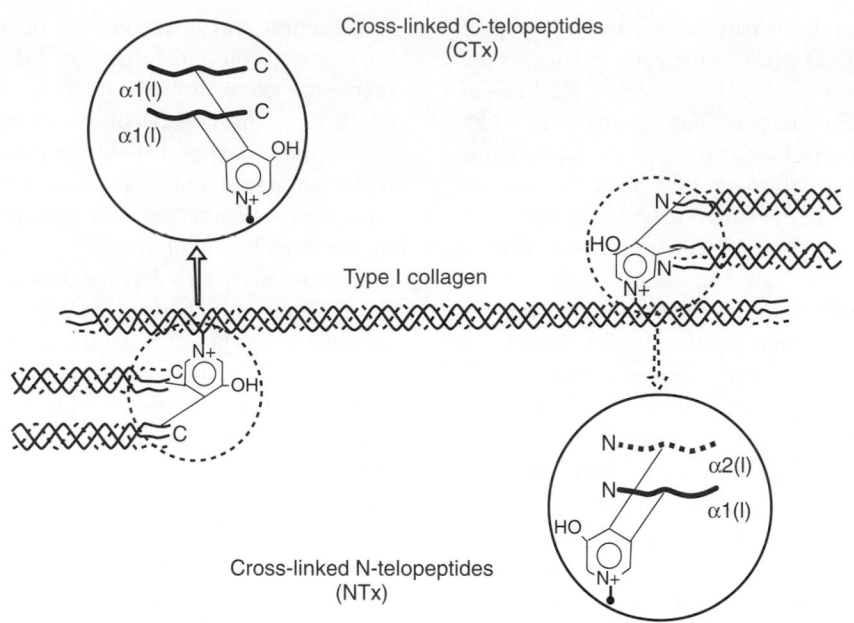

Cross-linked C-telopeptides
(CTx)

Type I collagen

Cross-linked N-telopeptides
(NTx)

Figure 38-11 Collagen pyridinoline cross-links. Cross-links occur at two intermolecular sites in the collagen fibril—(1) two N-telopeptides are linked to a helical site near residue 930 (N-telopeptide) and (2) two C-telopeptides are linked to helical residue 87 (C-telopeptide). (Modified- from Calvo MS, Eyre DR, Gundberg CM: Molecular basis and clinical application of biological markers of bone turnover. Endocr Rev 1996; 17:333-368.)

precursor, type I procollagen, containing both N- and C-terminal extensions. Procollagen undergoes extensive intracellular posttranslational processing, including hydroxylation of proline and lysine residues, glycosylation, and formation of intrachain and interchain disulfide bonds and the triple helix. After it is secreted, procollagen is converted to collagen during extracellular processing by enzymatic removal of N- and C-propeptides.

Type I collagen molecules assemble into immature fibrils with limited tensile strength, then mature by the formation of intramolecular and intermolecular covalent bonds or cross-links. An enzyme, lysyl oxidase, deaminates the side chain ε-amino group of specific lysines or hydroxylysines to produce an active aldehyde. Three amino acid side chains react to form a trivalent amino acid containing a 3-hydroxypyridium ring. The following two nonreducible cross-links have been identified:

1. Deoxypyridinoline formed by reaction of two hydroxylysyl and one lysyl side chain
2. Pyridinoline formed by reaction of three hydroxylysyl chains

Four molecular cross-linking sites have been located for the formation of pyridinolines in type I collagen (see Figure 38-11). Two N-telopeptide sites have been linked to the helical site at amino acid 930 to form the N-telopeptide or two C-telopeptides are linked to the helical site at amino acid 87 to form the C-telopeptide.

Biochemistry and physiology
Pyridinoline (hydroxylysylpyridinoline) and especially

deoxypyridinoline (lysylpyridinoline) (Figure 38-12) have been used to assess bone resorption. Deoxypyridinoline is found in significant quantities in bone, dentine, ligaments, and aorta, whereas pyridinoline is more widespread, occurring in hard connective tissues with high levels in cartilage. Because of the large mass of the skeletal system, bone is usually the major source of both pyridinoline and deoxypyridinoline. Neither substance is present in significant quantities in skin. Deoxypyridinoline is a sensitive and specific marker of bone resorption, for the following reasons:

1. It is formed during collagen maturation, not biosynthesis, and originates only as a breakdown product.
2. It does not appear to be metabolized before it is excreted in urine.
3. Bone is the major source of deoxypyridinoline.
4. It does not appear to be absorbed from the diet.

Clinical significance
Bone resorption markers are reported to be more sensitive than bone formation markers in their assessment of changes in bone turnover in individuals with osteoporosis. Furthermore, because most current therapies are antiresorptive and markers of bone resorption respond more quickly to these therapies, resorption markers have received the greatest attention. Reductions of 30% to 60% usually have been reported with antiresorptive agents. Response to antiresorptive therapies has reportedly been the greatest with telopeptides, intermediate with total pyridinolines, and lowest with free pyridinolines. For N-telopeptide, the therapeutic goal is a decline of 30% or more or levels of 35 nmol bone collagen

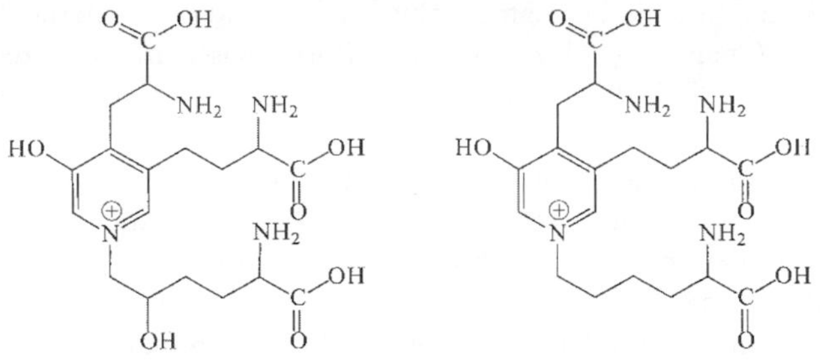

Figure 38-12   Structures of free pyridinoline cross-links, deoxypyridinoline (lysylpyridinoline) and pyridinoline (hydroxylyslpyridinoline).

equivalents (BCE) BCE/nmol of creatinine or less, a level near the premenopausal mean. Current urine assays require either 24 hour collection nor correction for creatinine excretion. More recently, serum assays have been reported for C- and N-telopeptides. These serum assays ultimately may improve substantially both the convenience and reproducibility of resorption markers.

Pyridinolines (deoxypyridinoline and pyridinoline) and telopeptides (N-telopeptide and C-telopeptide) are increased in individuals with metabolic bone diseases with increased bone resorption and formation, including osteoporosis, osteomalacia, primary hyperparathyroidism, hyperthyroidism, and renal osteodystrophy and in those with Paget's disease, glucocorticoid excess, and bony metastases. Levels are decreased in individuals with hypoparathyroidism.

Analytical methodology

Determination of pyridinolines (deoxypyridinoline and pyridinoline).
HPLC has been used to measure deoxypyridinoline and pyridinoline in urine. Because these compounds are present in urine in both free and peptide forms, most HPLC methods use acid hydrolysis to generate free amino acids and measure total deoxypyridinoline and total pyridinoline. After preparative chromatography, deoxypyridinoline and pyridinoline are separated by use of ion-pairing agents on reversed-phase columns and then quantified through measurement of their fluorescence as they elute from the column.

A number of immunoassays have been developed to measure pyridinolines. An older commercially available method measured both free pyridinoline and free deoxypyridinoline. A more useful ELISA method now is available that measures free deoxypyridinoline only. More recently a number of automated methods for free deoxypyridinoline have been introduced that use the same monoclonal antibody as the ELISA.

Recent comparisons of free and total deoxypyridinolines suggest that the ratio of free to total deoxypyridinoline (free and peptide-bound) is not constant in urine and varies with physiology, pathophysiology, and treatment. The ratio of free to total deoxypyridinoline has been reported as lower in individuals with disorders involving increased bone resorption (postmenopausal women, Paget's disease, osteoporosis,

and hyperthyroidism). Furthermore, short-term treatment with bisphosphonates have reduced the total, but not free, deoxypyridinoline, whereas estrogens decreased both.

Determination of N-telopeptides and C-telopeptides.
Immunoassays have been developed for measurement of the NTx and CTx. An ELISA is commercially available for measurement of N-telopeptides by use of a monoclonal antibody against the NTx fraction of adolescent urine. It recognizes a conformational epitope of the cross-linked telopeptide. The assay does not measure the uncross-linked precursor or free pyridinolines. Another ELISA is available for measurement of C-telopeptides by use of a polyclonal antibody against a synthetic fragment of the cross-linking region of the $\alpha2$ (I) chain.

Specimen collection and reference intervals.
Specimen collection should be standardized because pyridinolines and N-telopeptides demonstrate significant diurnal variation. Peak urinary excretion occurs at 0500 to 0800 hours, reflecting a nocturnal peak in bone turnover, with a nadir between 2 and 2300 hours. Although early studies used 24-hour urine specimens, timed and early-morning voids also have been used. A second-morning void, collected by 1000 hours, is recommended. Prolonged exposure to light and exposure to direct sunlight should be avoided, especially with free pyridinolines, which are vulnerable to ultraviolet exposure.

Reference intervals.
For women, reference intervals usually are based on healthy, young premenopausal, not postmenopausal, women. In premenopausal women, reference intervals for the N-telopeptide of 5 to 65 nmol of BCEs per mmol of creatinine and for free deoxypyridinoline of 3.0 to 7.4 nmol per mmol of creatinine have been reported. Levels are markedly higher in children, especially during growth spurts.

Other markers of bone resorption

Other markers of bone resorption include urinary hydroxyproline and galactosyl hydroxylysine and serum osteoclastic or tartrate-resistant acid phosphatase. Hydroxyproline and galactosyl hydroxylysine both are produced during the posttranslational processing of collagen. Hydroxyproline is not a sensitive or specific marker of bone resorption for the following reasons:

1. It is distributed widely in collagens, including those in skin and muscle.
2. Hydroxyproline is absorbed from the diet.
3. Most hydroxyproline is metabolized before it is excreted.
4. It is produced during bone formation.

Galactosyl hydroxylysine is measured by fluorometric detection after dansylation and HPLC. It has not been investigated thoroughly and is not measured widely. Methods for tartrate-resistant acid phosphatase are not specific for the osteoclastic enzyme (see Chapter 20). Ultimately, the development of sensitive and specific immunoassays should facilitate the measurement of this osteoclastic enzyme.

Markers of Bone Formation

Biochemical markers of bone formation (see Table 38-16) include bone alkaline phosphatase, osteocalcin, and collagen propeptides. In practice, bone alkaline phosphatase and osteocalcin are the markers most frequently measured.

Bone alkaline phosphatase

Alkaline phosphatase is found in many tissues, including bone, liver, intestine, kidney, and placenta (see Chapter 20).

Biochemistry and physiology

Four different genes code for the tissue-nonspecific intestinal, placental, and germ-cell (placenta-like) isoenzyme. Alkaline phosphatase from liver, bone, and kidney are isoforms of the same gene product, the tissue-nonspecific gene. These tissue-specific isoforms are produced by tissue-specific posttranslational processing (for example, glycosylation). In bone, osteoblasts are the source of alkaline phosphatase, and serum levels of this isoenzyme reflect osteoblastic activity.

Clinical significance

Bone alkaline phosphatase is increased in metabolic bone diseases with increased bone formation, such as osteoporosis, osteomalacia, primary hyperparathyroidism, hyperthyroidism, and renal osteodystrophy and in individuals with Paget's disease, glucocorticoid excess, and bony metastases.

The measurement of bone alkaline phosphatase has several advantages over osteocalcin measurement. Because of its relatively long half-life (1 to 2 days), it is relatively unaffected by diurnal variation. Bone alkaline phosphatase is measured in serum and does not require special handling. The within-individual biological and analytical variation of total, and presumably, the bone isoform is significantly less than reported for other markers. Bone alkaline phosphatase is more useful in individuals with impaired renal function because it is not cleared by glomerular filtration. The measurement of bone and total alkaline phosphatase are the markers of choice in cases of Paget's disease, with the former being more sensitive and specific.

Measurements of bone alkaline phosphatase may be misleading in individuals with liver disease because of cross-reactivity with liver isoform and in those with severe osteomalacia because of a mineralizing defect. Because $1,25(OH)_2D$ regulates the synthesis of osteocalcin and bone alkaline phosphatase, these markers may be misleading in individuals treated with, or those with abnormal levels of, this hormone. Procollagen peptides may be helpful in the assessment of bone formation in these individuals.

Analytical methodology

Attempts have been made to measure bone alkaline phosphatase specifically by a number of chemical and physical methods or combinations of methods, including heat inactivation, chemical inhibition, electrophoresis, lectin precipitation and chromatography, HPLC, and other methods (see Chapter 20). Despite these efforts, classic methods remain technically complicated, labor intensive, imprecise, and/or inaccurate.

Immunoassays for bone alkaline phosphatase ultimately may provide accurate, reproducible, sensitive, and convenient determinations of bone alkaline phosphatase. Two assays are available commercially, both of which use monoclonal antibodies against bone alkaline phosphatase from SaOS-2, a human osteosarcoma cell line. One assay is an IRMA using two monoclonal antibodies and measuring mass or nanograms per milliliter of enzyme. The other uses a single, solid-phase monoclonal antibody to bind bone alkaline phosphatase. After immunoseparation is performed, the activity of bone alkaline phosphatase is determined with a p-nitrophenyl phosphate substrate. Unfortunately, current immunoassays are not completely specific for the bone isoform and exhibit 5% to 20% cross-reactivity with the liver isoform. They are not reliable in individuals with significant elevations of the liver isoform (for example, liver disease). In spite of these limitations, immunoassays provide improved sensitivity, reproducibility, and convenience in the assessment of bone formation.

The reference intervals for bone alkaline phosphatase are approximately 5 to 20 ng/mL with the IRMA and 7 to 30 U/L with the immunoabsorption assay. However, serum levels are influenced by age and sex. For example, levels are higher in men and increase with age in both men and women, consistent with an age-related increase in bone turnover. Children have much higher levels than adults, especially during growth spurts.

Osteocalcin

Osteocalcin, or bone Gla protein (BGP), is a small protein composed of 49 amino acids (Figure 38-13), with a molecular weight of 5669. It is the major and most thoroughly characterized noncollagenous protein in human bone, accounting for approximately 1% of total protein.

Biochemistry and physiology

Osteocalcin is synthesized by osteoblasts and is considered a marker of bone formation. However, osteocalcin, especially osteocalcin fragments, possibly may be liberated during bone resorption and measured by some methods. Although osteocalcin binds calcium and hydroxyapatite, its physiological role is unknown. Its synthesis is stimulated by $1,25(OH)_2D$. Osteocalcin is cleared rapidly by the kidney, with a short half-life of approximately 5 minutes.

Osteocalcin contains three specific glutamyl residues in amino acid positions 17, 21, and 24 that can be converted to γ-carboxyglutamyl residues by a posttranslational, vitamin K-dependent enzymatic carboxylation. Immunochemical and chromatographic studies have demonstrated considerable heterogeneity in circulating osteocalcin. This heterogeneity may be due at least partially to proteolytic hydrolysis of

Osteocalcin [bone Gla protein (BGP)]

1 Tyr	Leu	Tyr	Gln	5 Trp	Leu	Gly	Ala	Pro	10 Val
11 Pro	Tyr	Pro	Asp	15 Pro	Leu	**Gla**	Pro	Arg	20 Arg
21 **Gla**	Val	Cys	**Gla**	25 Leu	Asn	Pro	Asp	Cys	30 Asp
31 Glu	Leu	Ala	Asp	35 His	Ile	Gly	Phe	Gln	40 Glu
41 Ala	Tyr	Arg	Arg	45 Phe	Tyr	Gly	Pro	49 Val	

Figure 38-13   Amino acid sequence of osteocalcin (bone Gla protein [BGP]). A disulfide bond formed between cysteines in positions 23 and 29 stabilizes two antiparallel α-helical structures representing 40% of the overall structure. Three glutamyl residues at positions 17, 21, and 24 can be carboxylated in a posttranslational, vitamin K-dependent step producing γ-carboxyglutamyl residues (Gla). *Tyr,* Tyrosine; *Leu,* leucine; *Gln,* glutamine; *Trp,* tryptophan; *Ala,* alanine; *Pro,* proline; *Val,* valine; *Asp,* aspartic acid; *Gly,* glycine; *Arg,* arginine; *Cys,* cysteine; *Asn,* asparagine; *His,* histidine; *Ile,* isoleucine; *Phe,* phenylalanine. (Modified from Power MJ, Fottrell P.: Osteocalcin: diagnostic methods and clinical applications. Crit Rev Clin Lab Sci 1991; 28:287-335.)

susceptible peptide bonds, involving arginine residues, at positions 19 and 20 and 43 and 44. Sequence-specific competitive and two-site immunoassays have demonstrated that circulating osteocalcin is composed primarily of an N-terminal/midregion fragment consistent with the predicted 1-43 fragment and intact osteocalcin.

Clinical significance

Osteocalcin is increased in metabolic bone diseases with increased bone formation, such as in osteoporosis, osteomalacia, primary hyperparathyroidism, hyperthyroidism, and renal osteodystrophy and in individuals with Paget's disease, glucocorticoid excess, and bony metastases. Levels are decreased in cases of hypoparathyroidism and glucocorticoid excess.

Analytical methodology

Osteocalcin has been measured by competitive and noncompetitive immunoassays. Both heterologous (bovine and porcine BGP) and homologous (human BGP) assays have been used widely. Competitive immunoassays have used polyclonal and monoclonal antibodies and radioisotopic, enzyme, or chemiluminescent labels. More recently, two-site labeled antibody methods have been developed. Two-site methods measuring intact osteocalcin and especially those measuring both intact osteocalcin plus the N-terminal/midregion (1-43) fragment are of particular interest.

Intact osteocalcin is hydrolyzed rapidly at room temperature and more slowly at 4 °C. Serum osteocalcin levels are more stable when they are measured with methods recognizing both intact and the N-terminal/midregion (1-43) fragment. These fragments may be released by osteoblasts during bone formation or produced in vivo in circulation or in vitro during specimen handling by proteolysis of intact osteocalcin. Protease inhibitors, EDTA tubes, and collection on ice improve stability. Unless proven unnecessary, specimens should be collected on ice, separated within 1 hour, and frozen.

Reference intervals are method dependent but vary between 3 and 27 ng/mL. With one RIA, osteocalcin reference intervals of 3 to 13 ng/mL for men, 0.4 to 8.2 for premenopausal women, and 1.5 to 11.0 ng/mL for postmenopausal women have been reported.

Osteocalcin levels are influenced by age, sex, and diurnal variation. Levels are higher in children than in adults, with the highest levels during periods of rapid growth. Men exhibit somewhat higher levels of osteocalcin. Osteocalcin levels have been reported to increase, decrease, or remain unchanged with age, a probable consequence of the heterogeneity of circulating osteocalcin and differences in immunoassay specificity and sensitivity. Osteocalcin exhibits a diurnal variation, with a nocturnal peak dropping by as much as 30% to a morning nadir. Levels are increased in individuals with renal failure because of impaired clearance by glomerular filtration.

Collagen propeptides

Procollagen peptides are cleaved from type I collagen during collagen maturation. They also have been proposed as a marker of bone formation. Immunoassays have been reported for both C-terminal and N-terminal propeptides. Because type I collagen is widespread, these procollagen peptides are not as sensitive or specific for bone formation as the more widely measured markers.

■ DISEASES OF THE BONE

Metabolic bone diseases result from the uncoupling or imbalance between bone resorption and formation. Osteoporosis is the most common metabolic bone disease. Primary osteoporosis can be separated into **postmenopausal osteoporosis,** the rapid loss of bone occurring in women after menopause, and senile osteoporosis, the slower, age-related loss occurring in both men and women. Bone mass peaks at approximately 30 years of age, remains stable for a few years, and then declines with age.

Osteoporosis

Osteoporosis is the most common metabolic disease of bone in the United States and results in 1.5 million bone fractures each year. One third of women older than 65 years of age suffer vertebral crush fractures, and the lifetime risk of hip fracture is 15%. Exercise and adequate nutrition play important roles in the maintenance of skeletal mass. Aging is a major risk factor because approximately 1% of skeletal mass is lost per year after 35 to 40 years of age. The loss of sex steroids, such as at menopause, accelerates bone loss to 2% per year for approximately a decade. Other risk factors include a positive family history, alcohol abuse, smoking, and chronic disease states. The most common clinical presentation of osteoporosis is crush fracture of the vertebral bodies or fracture of the hip or forearm.

Laboratory evaluation is directed at the ruling out of those diseases associated with osteoporosis (Table 38-17). In postmenopausal women, indicators of high bone turnover, such as a high serum osteocalcin value or increased urinary excretion of collagen cross-links, suggests that therapeutic agents that inhibit osteoclast activity are beneficial. Bone densitometry allows for the accurate assessment of bone mineralization and is useful in the diagnosis of osteoporosis and the monitoring of therapy.

Treatment of osteoporosis is directed toward treatment of any underlying disease present. The prevention of postmenopausal osteoporosis may be achieved by the replacement of estrogen. Alternate forms of therapy include bisphosphonates (alendronate and risidronate), raloxiphene, and calcitonin therapy. Calcium supplements and physiological doses of vitamin D also are indicated. Prevention is of the utmost importance. Adequate nutrition and exercise during growth allow for the achievement of optimal bone mass. Maintenance of high calcium intake during pregnancy and lactation, a regular exercise program during adult life, and early estrogen-replacement therapy after menopause help prevent osteoporotic fractures.

Osteomalacia (Rickets)

Osteomalacia usually is due to either vitamin D deficiency or phosphate depletion. Because many foods in the United States are fortified with vitamin D, nutritional deficiency is uncommon. The most common cause of **rickets** in the United States is hypophosphatemic rickets or osteomalacia (also known as *vitamin D-resistant rickets*), an X-linked dominant disease characterized by renal phosphate wasting. Certain anticonvulsant drugs also have been associated with osteomalacia, presumably by altering hepatic vitamin D metabolism. Phosphate-binding antacids also have been reported to result in osteomalacia.

TABLE 38-17   Causes of Osteoporosis

Failure to develop normal skeletal mass during growth and development due to poor nutrition or inadequate exercise	Immobilization or weightlessness
	Hematological malignancies (multiple myeloma)
Endocrine deficiency or excess	Inherited defects of collagen synthesis (osteogenesis imperfecta)
Estrogen or testosterone deficiency	Systemic mastocytosis
Cushing's syndrome	Heparin therapy
Hyperthyroidism	Rheumatoid arthritis
Hyperparathyroidism	Idiopathic juvenile osteoporosis

Clinical manifestations include muscle weakness and hypotonia. In children, short stature and bowing of extremities (rickets) are common. In adults, bone pain is common, and stress fractures and frank skeletal fractures may occur. X-rays demonstrate rachitic changes and/or pseudofractures.

The major biochemical feature of osteomalacia and rickets is a high serum alkaline phosphatase level due to increased bone turnover. Moderate to severe vitamin D deficiency may cause hypocalcemia so that the resulting elevated serum PTH causes hypophosphatemia. Vitamin nutrition may be assessed by the concentration of serum 25(OH)D, whereas renal phosphate deficiency is assessed best by determination of the renal phosphate threshold.

Treatment of rickets or osteomalacia is dictated by the etiology of the disorder. This treatment includes vitamin D or its metabolites for disorders of vitamin D or phosphate replacement in cases of chronic phosphate depletion.

Paget's Disease

Paget's disease is a localized disease of bone characterized by osteoclastic bone resorption, followed by replacement with bone of chaotic architecture. It may affect one or several bones. The signs and symptoms depend on which skeletal site is affected; the skull, femur, and vertebrae are affected most commonly. In the majority of affected individuals the disease is diagnosed by x-ray or notation of elevated serum alkaline phosphatase in tests performed for another reason. In some cases, bone pain in the affected bone may occur and, if advanced, deformity of the involved bone may develop. Complications of the deformed bone include arthritic symptoms, nerve compression and deafness, and in rare cases, osteogenic sarcoma.

The most common laboratory finding is a markedly elevated serum alkaline phosphatase level (up to tenfold). Increased bone turnover denoted by high urinary collagen cross-links may be found. Characteristic x-ray changes are diagnostic.

Therapy is directed toward a decrease in osteoclastic bone resorption. Bisphosphonates (alendronate, risidronate, pamidronate, etidronate) and calcitonin are effective in decreasing bone pain, serum alkaline phosphatase, and markers of bone resorption.

Renal Osteodystrophy

Renal osteodystrophy comprises various skeletal abnormalities. Renal failure commonly causes hyperphosphatemia and low serum $1,25(OH)_2D$, and secondary hypocalcemia. These conditions result in secondary hyperparathyroidism and the subsequent development of hyperparathyroid bone disease (osteitis fibrosa). Because of decreased renal synthesis of $1,25(OH)_2D$, osteomalacia also may be a complication of chronic renal failure. Aluminum deposition in bone also may result in osteomalacia. Other skeletal abnormalities that may occur in individuals with renal failure include aplastic bone disease and amyloid deposition.

Characteristic biochemical features of renal failure include elevated serum urea nitrogen and creatinine levels. Serum calcium may be low, PTH elevated, and 1,25(OH)$_2$D low. Because magnesium is cleared by the kidney, modest elevations (2 to 4 ng/dl) of the serum magnesium are observed frequently.

Management of renal failure includes dietary phosphate restriction and administration of phosphate-binding agents. Calcium supplements also are added. Administration of 1,25(OH)$_2$D enhances intestinal calcium absorption. 1,25(OH)$_2$D also directly affects the parathyroid gland toward a decrease in PTH biosynthesis. Ultimately, dialysis or renal transplantation may be necessary.

Additional Reading

GENERAL
Favus MJ (ed): Primer on the metabolic bone diseases and disorders of mineral metabolism, 4th edition, Philadelphia, Lippincott-Raven, 1999.

Wilson JD, Foster DW, Kronenberg HM et al (eds): Williams Textbook of Endocrinology, 9th edition, Philadelphia, WB Saunders, 1998.

BIOCHEMICAL MARKERS OF BONE METABOLISM
Endres DB (ed): Biochemical markers of bone metabolism. J Clin Ligand Assay 1998; 21:92-158.

Kallner A, Woloszczuk W, Holzel W (eds): Biochemical Markers for Bone Diseases: Current Status and Future Trends. Proceedings of the 6th Bergmeyer Conference, IFCC Master Discussion, Improving the Clinical Value of Laboratory Data. Scand J Clin Lab Invest 1997; 57(Suppl 227):1-127.

BONE AND METABOLIC BONE DISEASE
Avioli LV, Krane SM (eds): Metabolic bone disease and clinically related disorders, 3rd edition, San Diego, Academic Press, 1998.

Mundy GR (ed): Bone Remodeling and its Disorders, 2nd edition, Malden, Mass, Martin Dunitz, 1999.

CALCITONIN
Chi DD, Moley JF: Medullary thyroid carcinoma: genetic advances, treatment recommendations, and the approach to the patient with persistent hypercalcitoninemia. Surg Oncol Clin N Am 1998; 7:681-706.

VITAMIN D
Feldman D, Glorieux FH, Pike WJ: Vitamin D, San Diego, Academic Press, 1997.

Holick MF (ed): Vitamin D: Physiology, Molecular Biology and Clinical Applications, Totowa, NJ, Humana Press, 1999.

OSTEOPOROSIS
Adams JS, Lukert BP (eds): Osteoporosis: Genetics, Prevention, and Treatment, Boston, Kluwer, 1999.

Watts NB: Postmenopausal osteoporosis. Obstet Gynecol Surv 1999; 54:532-538.

PARATHYROID HORMONE
Bilezikian JP (ed): The Parathyroids: Basic and Clinical Concepts, Philadelphia, Lippincott-Raven, 1994.

Endres DB, Villanueva R, Sharp CF Jr et al: Measurement of parathyroid hormone. Endocrinol Metab Clin North Am 1989; 18: 611-629.

PARATHYROID HORMONE-RELATED PROTEIN
Martin TJ, Moseley JM, Williams ED: Parathyroid hormone-related protein: hormone and cytokine. J Endocrinol 1997; 154:S23-37.

Rankin W, Grill V, Martin TJ: Parathyroid hormone-related protein and hypercalcemia. Cancer 1997; 80:1564-1571.

Horvit PK, Gagel RF: The goitrous patient with an elevated calcitonin—what to do? J Clin Endocrinol Metab 1997; 82:338-341.

CHAPTER 39

Pituitary Function*

LAURENCE M. DEMERS, PhD, DABCC

Objectives

1. Describe the structure and function of the pituitary gland.
2. List the hormones synthesized by the anterior pituitary and those stored in the posterior pituitary gland.
3. State the peripheral effects of normal hormone release for each hormone synthesized or stored in the pituitary gland.
4. State the peripheral effects of increased and decreased hormone release for each hormone synthesized or stored in the pituitary gland.
5. Define *pituitary adenoma* and describe its effect on hormonal activity.
6. List the laboratory tests used to assess pituitary function.

Key Words

Acromegaly   A chronic disease of adults caused by hypersecretion of pituitary growth hormone and characterized by enlargement of many parts of the skeleton

Adrenocorticotropic Hormone (ACTH)   A 39-amino-acid peptide hormone secreted by the anterior pituitary gland that stimulates the adrenal cortex to secrete corticosteroids

Antidiuretic Hormone (ADH)   An octapeptide hormone formed by the neuronal cells of the hypothalamic nuclei and stored in the posterior lobe of the pituitary gland (neurohypophysis) that has antidiuretic and vasopressor activity; also known as *vasopressin*

β-Lipotropin (LPH)   A polypeptide hormone synthesized by the anterior pituitary that is a prohormone of several endogenous opioids and exerts a mild peripheral lipolytic action and promotes darkening of the skin by the stimulation of melanocytes

Corticotropin-Releasing Hormone (CRH)   A neuropeptide released by the hypothalamus that stimulates the release of corticotropin by the anterior pituitary gland

Follicle-Stimulating Hormone (FSH)   A gonadotropic hormone of the anterior pituitary that stimulates the growth and maturation of ovarian follicles, stimulates estrogen secretion, and promotes the endometrial changes characteristic of the first portion (proliferative phase) of the mammalian menstrual cycle; also stimulates spermatogenesis in the male

Growth Hormone (GH)   A polypeptide hormone produced by the anterior pituitary that affects carbohydrate, lipid, and protein metabolism and controls the rate of skeletal and visceral growth

Insulin-Like Growth Factor (IGF)   Serum peptides with insulin-like actions; formerly were known as *somatomedins*

Luteinizing Hormone (LH)   A glycoprotein gonadotropic hormone secreted by the anterior pituitary that acts with FSH to promote ovulation and androgen and progesterone production; referred to in men as *interstitial cell-stimulating hormone*

---

*The author gratefully acknowledges the contributions of Ronald J. Whitley, A. Wayne Meikle, and Nelson B. Watts, on which portions of this chapter are based.

Oxytocin   An octapeptide hormone synthesized in the hypothalamus and stored in the posterior lobe of the pituitary; induces smooth muscle contraction in the uterus and mammary glands

Pituitary Gigantism   Excessive growth that is caused by increased synthesis of hormones of the anterior pituitary

Polydipsia   Chronic excessive intake of water

Polyuria   The passage of a large volume of urine in a given period; a characteristic of diabetes

Prolactin (PRL)   A lactogenic hormone synthesized by the pituitary

Somatomedin   Any of several peptides produced in the liver and released in response to somatotropin; stimulate the growth of bone and muscle and also influence calcium, phosphate, carbohydrate, and lipid metabolism; examples: insulin-like growth factors I and II

Syndrome of Inappropriate Antidiuretic Hormone (SIADH)   A condition in which inappropriate antidiuretic hormone secretion produces hyponatremia, hypovolemia, and elevated urine osmolality

Thyroid-Stimulating Hormone (TSH)   A polypeptide hormone synthesized by the anterior pituitary gland that promotes the growth of, sustains, and stimulates the hormonal secretion of the thyroid gland

Thyrotropin-Releasing Hormone (TRH)   A tripeptide produced in the hypothalamus that stimulates the release of TSH from the anterior pituitary

The pituitary gland (hypophysis) is located at the base of the skull (Figure 39-1) in a bone cavity called the *sella turcica* or *Turkish saddle*. The gland is small—1 cm or less in height and width—and weighs approximately 500 mg. The pituitary consists anatomically of three lobes of differing embryonic origin—the anterior lobe, or adenohypophysis, the posterior lobe, or neurohypophysis, and the intermediate lobe, which is well developed in the human fetus but vestigial in the human adult.

Arterial blood reaches the pituitary gland via the superior hypophyseal artery. Venous blood, carrying neurosecretory hormones from the hypothalamus, reaches the pituitary through the hypothalamo-hypophyseal portal system. These hypothalamic hormones stimulate or inhibit the release of hormones from the adenohypophysis.

The pituitary regulates several endocrine functions by integrating signals from the brain with the feedback effects of peripheral hormones to stimulate intermittent hor-

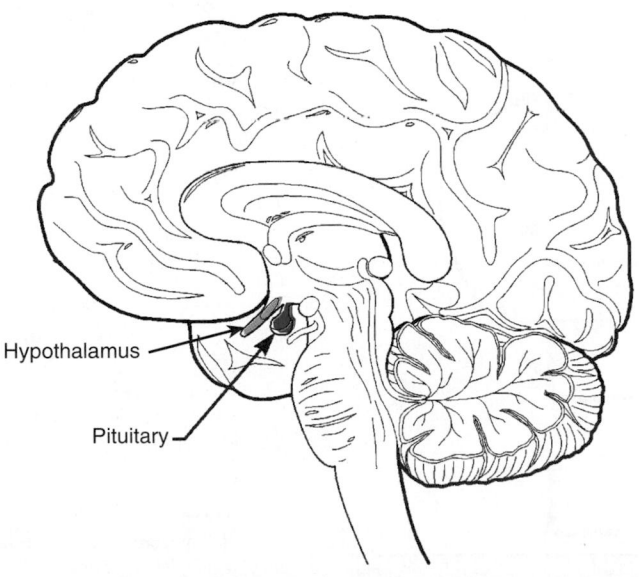

Figure 39-1   Location of pituitary and hypothalamus in the brain.

mone release from target glands (Figure 39-2). It is involved in the regulation of growth and development, thyroid function, adrenal function, reproduction, and water homeostasis.

The adenohypophysis secretes growth hormone (GH), prolactin (PRL), thyrotropin (TSH), adrenocorticotropic hormone (ACTH), follicle-stimulating hormone (FSH), and luteinizing hormone (LH), all of which are proteins or peptides (see Table 26-2). GH and PRL act primarily on diffuse target tissues. TSH, ACTH, and the gonadotropins (LH and FSH) act primarily on the thyroid gland, adrenal cortex, and gonads, respectively. The adenohypophysis also secretes **β-lipotropin (β-LPH)** and a number of smaller peptides of undetermined significance.[8] Antidiuretic hormone (ADH), also known as *Vasopressin*, and oxytocin are synthesized in the hypothalamus and stored in and secreted from the neurohypophysis.

HYPOTHALAMIC REGULATION

Secretion of hormones from the anterior lobe of the pituitary gland is controlled by the hypothalamus, which manufactures small peptides known as *releasing* or *inhibiting factors* (see Figure 39-2). These substances qualify as hormones because they are transported in the portal circulation and produce specific effects on the activities of the pituitary gland. At least six different hypothalamic hormones have been identified—**corticotropin-releasing hormone (CRH), thyrotropin-releasing hormone (TRH),** growth hormone-releasing hormone (GHRH), somatostatin (also called *growth hormone-inhibiting hormone [GHIH]*), gonadotropin-releasing hormone (GnRH; also called *luteinizing hormone-releasing hormone [LHRH]*), and prolactin-inhibiting factor (PIF), which is thought to be dopamine. GnRH stimulates the secretion of FSH and LH; whether a separate releasing factor exists for FSH has not yet been established.

CRH, GnRH, GHRH, and TRH are used to test pituitary reserve. Pulsatile GnRH is used to initiate puberty and to induce ovulation or spermatogenesis. GnRH antagonists are used to treat patients with precocious puberty, endometriosis, uterine fibroids, and prostate carcinoma. GHRH is used to treat patients with GH deficiency resulting from hypothalamic disease.

The neurons that elaborate hypophysiotropic hormones are influenced by the hypothalamic neurotransmitters, such as dopamine, norepinephrine, serotonin, acetylcholine, and endorphins, which also modify the secretory activity of anterior pituitary hormones (Table 39-1). Basal and episodic secretion, diurnal rhythm, and nocturnal release of pituitary hormones all are considered secondary to central nervous system events that are mediated through hypothalamic hormones.

Control of the functional relationship between the pituitary gland and its target glands is based primarily on negative feedback from the target glands to the pituitary gland and hypothalamus (see Figure 39-2). The effect of negative feedback is opposite that of the initial stimulus. Such feedback control maintains an optimal concentration of hormones in the blood under a variety of physiological circumstances.

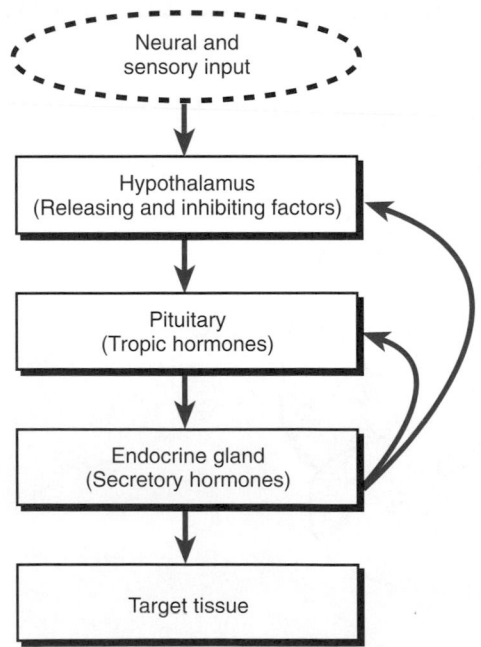

Figure 39-2 Functional interrelationships of the hypothalamus, pituitary, and endocrine glands.

TABLE 39-1	Neurotransmitter Effect on Hormonal Secretions by the Anterior Lobe of the Pituitary Gland	
Hormone	Stimulates Secretion	Inhibits Secretion
ACTH	Serotonin Acetylcholine Endorphins	GABA
TSH	Norepinephrine	Dopamine Serotonin Endorphins
PRL	Norepinephrine Endorphins	Dopamine
GH	Dopamine Norepinephrine Serotonin Endorphins	
Gonadotropins	Norepinephrine Acetylcholine GABA	Serotonin Dopamine Endorphins

ACTH, Adrenocorticotrophic hormone; *GABA,* γ-aminobutyric acid; *TSH,* thyroid-stimulating hormone; *PRL,* prolactin; *GH,* growth hormone.

■ HORMONES OF THE ADENOHYPOPHYSIS

The human anterior pituitary contains the following five types of cell:

1. Somatotrophs, which secrete GH (somatotropin)
2. Mammotrophs, which secrete PRL
3. Thyrotrophs, which secrete TSH (thyrotropin)
4. Gonadotrophs, which secrete both LH and FSH
5. Corticotrophs, which secrete both ACTH and β-LPH

Growth Hormone and Insulin-Like Growth Factors

GH is the most abundant hormone produced by the adenohypophysis.

Biochemistry and physiology

Growth hormone (GH) in humans is a single-chain polypeptide with a molecular mass of 21,500 D that contains 191 amino acids and two intramolecular disulfide bridges. It is structurally similar to PRL and the placental hormone chorionic somatomammotropin, with which it has overlapping biological activities. During most of the day the plasma concentration of GH in normal adults remains stable and relatively low, with several secretory "spikes" occurring approximately 3 hours after meals and after exercise. In addition, adults and children show a significant rise in GH secretion approximately 90 minutes after the onset of sleep; GH concentration reaches a peak value during the period of deepest sleep.

Regulation of secretion

The release of GH is controlled by GHRH, which stimulates GH release, and GHIH, which inhibits GH release. GHIH also is found in the delta cells of the pancreatic islets and in other sites in the digestive tract, where it has important effects on gastrointestinal hormones and inhibits insulin and glucagon release. The hypothalamic influence on GH release seems to be predominantly stimulatory. The release of the two hypothalamic factors is controlled by the higher centers of the brain. Thus stimuli, such as exercise, physical and emotional stress, hypoglycemia, increased amino acid levels, and hormones such as testosterone, estrogens, and thyroxine, all stimulate GH secretion. High levels of glucocorticoids suppress GH secretion. Other hypothalamic hormones, such as TRH and GnRH, may provoke GH release in individuals with acromegaly.

Functions

The overall effect of GH is to promote the growth of soft tissues, cartilage, and bone. The effects of GH on tissues are exerted both directly and by the mediation of insulin-like growth factors (IGFs) produced in the liver and other tissues (for example, bone) under the influence of GH.

GH also produces effects on intermediary metabolism. It stimulates uptake of nonesterified fatty acids by muscle and accelerates the mobilization of fat from adipose tissue. Upon injection, GH causes a decrease in blood glucose levels; however, chronic GH excess stimulates hepatic glycogenolysis and antagonizes the effect of insulin on glucose uptake by peripheral cells (see Chapter 23) so that blood glucose concentrations increase. GH and insulin induce growth in a similar manner because both produce protein anabolic effects and can stimulate the transport of amino acids into peripheral cells. However, their respective effects on glucose homeostasis oppose each other. Most GH effects are delayed rather than immediate.

Relationship of growth hormone to insulin-like growth factors

Insulin-like growth factors (IGFs) I and II, also called somatomedins, are polypeptides with considerable sequence similarity to insulin. They can elicit the same biological responses as insulin, including mitogenesis in cell culture. Of the two, IGF I is the most important. In addition to the growth-promoting effects on cartilage, IGF-I also shows insulin-like activity in other tissues. IGF-I inhibits lipolysis, increases glucose oxidation in adipose tissues, and stimulates glucose and amino acid transport into diaphragmatic and heart muscle. Synthesis of collagen and proteoglycans is enhanced by IGF-I, which also has positive effects on calcium, magnesium, and potassium homeostasis. The insulin-like activity has been attributed in part to the similarity of the structures of insulin and the IGFs. Unlike most other peptide hormones, IGFs circulate in blood in complexes with plasma-binding proteins. Four major IGF-binding proteins have been described in human plasma. IGFBP-3, a glycosylated binding protein, forms complexes with more than 75% of the circulating IGF-I. The concentration of this binding protein is GH dependent and provides for a circulating reserve pool of IGF-I. Dissociation from the binding proteins occurs before passage through capillary membranes and entrance into dense tissues, such as cartilage.

Plasma levels of immunoreactive IGF-I are increased in cases of acromegaly and reduced in GH deficiency states and in individuals with many other forms of growth retardation, hypothyroidism, chronic illness, nutritional deficiency, and liver disease.

Clinical significance

Clinically important states of GH excess or deficiency are rare and often difficult to diagnose.[13,17] GH levels vary widely under normal circumstances, so measurement of GH under random conditions generally is not useful. A single GH measurement cannot be used to distinguish normal fluctuations from the low or high levels that are seen in vari-

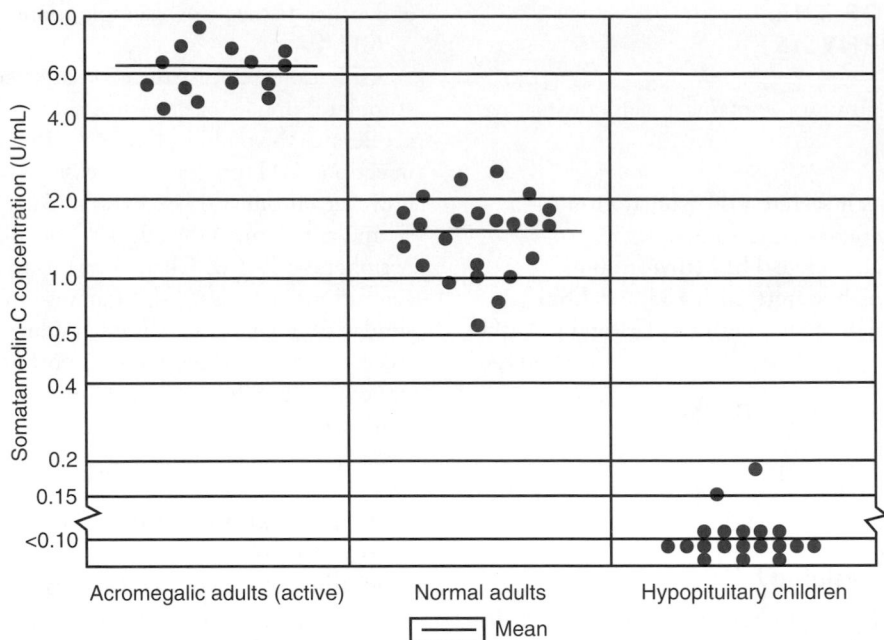

Figure 39-3   Insulin-like growth factor I (IGF-I; somatomedin-C) levels in growth hormone excess and deficiency states. (Modified from Van Wyk JJ, Underwood LE: Growth hormone, somatomedins, and growth failure. Hosp Pract 1978; 13:66.)

ous disease states. GH measurements are most effective as part of dynamic tests with pharmacological or physiological provocative stimuli to stimulate or suppress GH release.

Serum levels of IGF-I are low at birth and rise slowly during the prepubertal period. At puberty, IGF-I levels increase significantly to levels usually found in adults with acromegaly. Serum IGF-I levels remain elevated during the adolescent years of continuous growth, subside in the third decade of life, and remain constant throughout adult life. A single measurement of IGF-I is considered an accurate reflection of IGF-I production. IGF-I concentrations are elevated in conditions of GH excess (for example, acromegaly).[12] Serum levels of IGF-I are low in states of GH deficiency and also in individuals with acute or chronic protein or calorie deprivation.

Growth hormone excess

Excess GH production is associated with adenomas[3] of the pituitary gland; these tumors are large enough to be seen with computed tomography or magnetic resonance imaging in approximately 75% of afficted individuals. Prolonged GH excess causes an overgrowth of the skeleton and soft tissues. This overgrowth occurs most commonly in adults and is known as **acromegaly.** When GH excess is seen before long-bone growth is complete, the condition is called **pituitary gigantism.** With pituitary gigantism, in addition to the overgrowth of bone and soft tissues in the face and extremities, linear growth undergoes a striking acceleration. In severe or advanced cases of GH excess the diagnosis can be made on the basis of physical appearance alone; however, the

changes are often subtle and gradual. In addition to the soft-tissue changes, acromegaly may cause severe disability or death from cardiac or neurological sequelae. The most important requirement for diagnosis is demonstration of inappropriate and excessive GH secretion.

As many as 10% of individuals with active acromegaly have random serum GH levels that fall within the normal reference interval. Essentially, all individuals with acromegaly demonstrate an abnormal response to a glucose load.[7] Individuals with acromegaly typically show either no change in the basal level of GH or a paradoxical increase of GH; normal individuals show suppression of GH levels to less than 2 ng/mL after an oral ingestion of glucose.

Serum IGF-I levels are elevated in individuals with active acromegaly (Figure 39-3). IGF-I levels often correlate better with the clinical severity of acromegaly than with glucose-suppressed or basal GH levels.

Growth hormone deficiency states and growth retardation

Children with insufficient GH production or action do not grow normally. GH deficiency may be (1) congenital or acquired; (2) idiopathic or a result of anatomical damage to the pituitary or hypothalamus; or (3) isolated or associated with deficiencies of other pituitary hormones. About 15% of children with growth retardation have endocrine problems, and approximately half of these (around 8% of all children with short stature) have GH deficiency. However, children with growth retardation or dwarfism with no clear explanation at least should be screened for GH deficiency.

TABLE 39-2	Stimuli for Growth Hormone Release	
Test	Test Conditions and Dosages	Time of Peak GH Release
Exercise	20 min vigorous exercise	20 min after exercise has begun
Sleep	Sample drawn 1 h after the onset of deep sleep (stage III or IV); EEG documentation, if possible	Usually 1 h after onset of deep sleep; coincides with onset of stage III or IV sleep
Arginine*†	Arginine hydrochloride, 0.5 g/kg body weight, given intravenously over a 30-min period	60 to 120 min
Insulin*†‡	Regular insulin, 0.1 to 0.15 U/kg, IV push (Severe hypoglycemia may result, and a physician should be in constant attendance.)	45 to 75 min
Glucagon†	0.03 mg/kg IM or subcutaneously (not to exceed 1 mg)	120 to 180 min
L-Dopa	0.5 g/1.73 m² , usually given with lunch (Responses may be improved by administration of priming doses of L-Dopa, 0.25 g/1.73 m², for one or more days before the test.)	30 to 120 min
Clonidine	0.15 mg/m²	90 min
Diazepam	0.15 mg/kg, orally	60 min
Pentagastrin	IV infusion, 1.5 mg/kg/h	75 min

GH, Growth hormone; *EEG*, electroencephalography; *IV*, intravenous; *IM*, intramuscular.
*Sequential administration of arginine and insulin may reduce the need for additional testing.
†Propranolol, 0.75 mg/kg (20 to 40 mg orally), given 30 to 60 minutes before glucagon, insulin, or arginine, may enhance a normal response.
‡Insulin, thyrotropin-releasing hormone (TRH), and gonadotropin-releasing hormone may be administered as a "cocktail" to evaluate GH, adrenocorticotropic hormone; TSH, prolactin, luteinizing hormone, and follicle-stimulating hormone in a single test period.

With the availability of recombinant GH for therapeutic use, many children with short stature now are being treated selectively with GH to advance their growth pattern closer to normal.

GH deficiency in adults is probably the most common demonstrable abnormality in individuals with large pituitary adenomas[3] or those who have undergone pituitary irradiation; however, GH deficiency in adults is rarely clinically significant.

In normal individuals the basal level of GH is usually low, and the half-life of circulating GH is approximately 20 minutes. Moreover, GH is secreted by the pituitary gland in short pulses or bursts. Thus assays of GH performed on single random or fasting specimens may not distinguish individuals with abnormally low levels from healthy subjects who have GH levels in the lower part of the reference interval. In the evaluation of GH reserve, provocative tests are used commonly. Although a normal GH response to a provocative test is a strong indication that GH deficiency is not present, no single test can be considered diagnostic in this situation; as many as 30% of individuals with normal GH secretion fail to show the expected increase in serum GH in response to a specific provocative stimulus at any given time. For this reason, to diagnose GH deficiency as a cause of growth retardation, demonstration that the serum concentration of GH remains low after the use of at least two different provocative stimuli is necessary. The definition of subnormal responses, however, is arbitrarily defined and assay dependent. In general, a GH response greater than 7 to 10 ng/mL after stimulation is considered normal.

A number of physiological and pharmacological circumstances provoke GH release (Table 39-2). In one simple screening test the patient performs 20 minutes of vigorous exercise, after which a sample is obtained for GH measurement. With the known rise in GH that occurs with deep sleep, a sample may be obtained 60 to 90 minutes after the onset of sleep. A disadvantage of this approach is that the patient must be in the hospital for testing. Insulin infusion and arginine infusion are the standard pharmacological stimuli for GH release; protocols for these are well established and standardized.[7] Other medications that stimulate GH release are L-dopa and glucagon. Intravenous (IV) GHRH administration also has been used to test pituitary GH reserve directly to distinguish between a hypothalamic and pituitary cause for GH deficiency.

IGF-I levels are low in individuals with GH deficiency and growth failure (see Figure 39-2). Individuals with growth failure caused by other endocrine diseases or nonendocrine organic diseases also may exhibit low levels of IGF-I; thus a low level of IGF-I is not a specific indication of GH deficiency. The presence of a normal level of IGF-I, however, does rule out severe GH deficiency.

Analytical methodology

Methods for the determination of growth hormone in blood and urine

Principles.   Bioassays for GH are available, but immunoassays that use specific GH antibodies are preferred for clinical laboratory use. For many years, serum levels were measured by radioimmunoassay (RIA) with reagents from the United States National Hormone and Pituitary Agency. Today a variety of isotopic and nonisotopic assays are available commercially. Many such assays use polyclonal antisera produced in rabbits or guinea pigs against purified pituitary preparations of the unmodified, monomeric hormone. However, many GH assays use mouse monoclonal antibodies, and some of these assays can discriminate GH variants. Most procedures now use recombinant-derived GH (r-hGH) for labeling with a tracer and as a calibration material. The latter usually is prepared gravimetrically and verified by comparison with an international reference preparation (IRP) produced by the World Health Organization (WHO).

Sensitive immunometric assays that use excess labeled antibodies in noncompetitive formats have been developed for GH. Several of these two-site "sandwich" assays are available commercially. Most are immunoradiometric assays (IRMAs) based on the use of two monoclonal antibodies directed at different antigenic sites on the GH molecule; one of the antibodies is labeled with radioactive iodine, whereas the other is anchored to a solid-phase separation system. Procedures using monoclonal antibodies with nonisotopic enzyme or fluorescent labels also have been reported. In addition, chemiluminescence-based GH assays on automated analyzers have been introduced; these tests can make the measurement of GH even easier to perform.[16] The detection limit of immunometric and chemiluminescence assays is approximately 0.1 to 0.5 ng/mL.

Human GH is not a single molecular species but exists in the pituitary gland and circulation as a heterogenous mixture of structural isoforms. Normally the human gene for GH directs the synthesis of a monomeric 22-kD protein; however, approximately 10% of GH from human pituitaries is present in plasma as a 20-kD protein. This smaller form lacks amino acid residues 32 to 46 and is probably a product of posttranslational processing. Fractionation of serum by gel filtration also reveals the presence of aggregates and oligomers of GH. The oligomers are predominately dimers of the monomeric hormone, whereas the large aggregates are mainly complexes formed by GH and its serum-binding protein. All these GH variants are antigenic; in normal plasma, 55% of immunoreactive GH consists of monomeric forms, 27% dimeric, and 18% oligomeric.

Analytically the presence of GH variants in serum often leads to problems with quantification and discrepancies among the results given by different assays.[9] The use of different antibodies, different calibration materials, different labels, and different assay diluents further increases the complexity of GH measurements. For example, immunometric assays using monoclonal antibodies tend to give lower GH estimates than polyclonal RIAs and may not recognize some forms of the hormone. Discordant results also have been noted among immunometric assays.[7]

Specimen requirements. The preferred specimen is serum; plasma with ethylenediaminetetraacetic acid (EDTA) or heparin added to prevent coagulation also may be used, but values are method dependent. Serum specimens should be stored at 2 to 8 °C if they are not to be tested within 8 hours. If they must be stored for long periods, serum samples are frozen at −20 °C. Patients must be fasting and at complete rest 30 minutes before collection. Highly sensitive immunometric assays have been developed that allow direct measurement of GH in untreated urine. Because the concentration of GH in urine is only 0.1% of that in serum, conventional RIAs usually require preliminary extraction and concentration procedures.

Reference intervals. The following intervals are based on a competitive RIA technique that was calibrated against the WHO IRP 80/505 for r-hGH:

	ng/mL
Basal	2 to 5
Insulin tolerance test	>10
Arginine	>7.5
L-DOPA	>7.5

Methods for the determination of insulin-like growth factors

Principles. IGFs are measured in plasma or serum by in vitro bioassay, radioreceptor assay, or immunoassay techniques. Immunoassays for IGF-I (somatomedin C) are based mainly on double-antibody methods (equilibrium or nonequilibrium conditions) and on the use of ^{125}I-labeled tracers. Purified preparations of IGF-I isolated from human serum generally serve as calibrators, although synthetic (recombinant) IGF-I also is available and used in some procedures. To remove interfering IGF-binding proteins, most assays preextract serum specimens by methods such as gel filtration, acid-ethanol precipitation, cryoprecipitation, or reversed-phase chromatography. Direct (no extraction) procedures also are available, but extraction methods help prevent problems associated with the presence of carrier proteins and serum proteases. Commercial RIA and IRMA kits are available for measurement of IGF-I, with little crossreactivity to IGF-II (0% to 3%). Because of the significant differences in adult and pediatric levels, establishment of age-related reference intervals for IGF-I is important.

Specimen collection and storage. Serum or plasma (with heparin or EDTA) can be used, depending on the assay method. Samples are centrifuged within 1 hour of their collection and subsequently stored frozen at −20 °C for up to 30 days.

Reference intervals. Published intervals for IGF-I differ because of variations in methods and calibration. The values in the following table are expressed in nanograms per milliliter of synthetic peptide; dividing by 220 converts IGF-I values to units per milliliter, where one unit is defined arbitrarily as the amount of IGF-I in a pool of normal adult human sera. IGF-I levels are highly dependent on individuals ages.

Age (y)	Men (ng/mL)	Women (ng/mL)
1 to 2	31 to 160	11 to 206
3 to 6	16 to 288	70 to 316
7 to 10	136 to 385	123 to 396
11 to 12	136 to 440	191 to 462
13 to 14	165 to 616	286 to 660
15 to 18	134 to 836	152 to 660
19 to 25	202 to 433	231 to 550
26 to 85	135 to 449	135 to 449

Prolactin

Prolactin (PRL) is a pituitary lactogenic hormone (23 kD) that is synthesized as preprolactin. PRL is formed when an N-terminal signal peptide is cleaved from the preprolactin.

Biochemistry and physiology

PRL is a 198-amino-acid peptide secreted by pituitary lactotropic cells with a structure similar to that of GH. During pregnancy and in the fetal pituitary the relative number and PRL content of lactotropic cells increases as a result of elevated circulating estrogens during pregnancy.

Regulation of secretion

Secretion of PRL is under hypothalamic control and is unique because the main control of its secretion is inhibitory rather than stimulatory. Dopamine is believed to be the principal inhibitory factor that regulates PRL secretion. TRH, the releasing factor that controls TSH release, functions as a PRL-releasing factor (PRF) and stimulates PRL secretion within minutes when injected intravenously into human subjects. TRH, however, is not the only PRF because hypothalamic extracts cause PRL release even when TRH has been inactivated or removed. However, the chemical nature of the other PRFs has not been identified yet.

As with other pituitary hormones the release of PRL is episodic and varies predictably during the day, with the lowest levels at midday and highest values shortly after the onset of deep sleep. The major physiological stimulus for PRL release is suckling; maternal plasma PRL levels increase within minutes after the initiation of breast-feeding. After labor and delivery, PRL levels remain elevated longer when the newborn is breast-fed. Many other stimuli induce PRL release, probably through suppression of dopamine action from the hypothalamus; stress is one important factor. ACTH levels, which also are increased with stress, cause an elevation in plasma PRL levels. Finally, an important influence on PRL regulation appears to be exerted by PRL itself by way of the short feedback loop between the pituitary and hypothalamus.

Function

PRL is the principal hormone controlling the initiation and maintenance of lactation. However, for an appropriate manifestation of PRL action, breast tissue requires priming by estrogens, progestins, corticosteroids, thyroid hormone, and insulin. PRL induces ductal growth, development of the lobular alveolar system, and synthesis of specific milk proteins, including casein and γ-lactalbumin. PRL affects the immune system[18] and is important in the control of osmolality and various metabolic events, including the metabolism of subcutaneous fat, carbohydrate metabolism, calcium and vitamin D metabolism, fetal lung development, and steroidogenesis.

PRL, like other pituitary hormones, binds to specific receptors on the cell membranes of target organs (breast, adrenal, ovaries, testes, prostate, kidneys, and liver). However, the exact intracellular mechanism of PRL action is unknown.

Clinical significance

Hyperprolactinemia is the most common hypothalamic-pituitary disorder encountered in clinical endocrinology.[10] PRL levels also are elevated in women with subtle alterations of fertility, such as (1) anovulation with or without menstrual irregularity, (2) amenorrhea and galactorrhea, or (3) galactorrhea alone. PRL excess in men results in oligospermia, impotence, or both. In addition, men with PRL-secreting pituitary adenomas more often present with macroadenomas and visual field disturbances as a result of a larger tumor pressing on the optic chiasm. Men do not have the subtle reminder of an irregular menstrual period that signals a microadenoma, as do women. As many as 30% of individuals with clinically silent pituitary adenomas have elevated PRL levels. Other causes of PRL elevation are shown in Table 39-3 and should be considered during the evaluation of individuals with elevated PRL levels. As with other pituitary hormones no reliable stimulation or suppression test exists to distinguish tumor from nontumor causes of a PRL elevation.

If a borderline elevation of PRL is found, the measurement should be repeated on at least two other occasions, with care to obtain the specimen in the morning, with minimal excitement to the patient, no trauma, and no breast stimulation; the patient also should not be taking any medication that could stimulate PRL release.

Clinically, medications that provoke PRL release create a biochemical picture of a prolactinoma in an otherwise healthy individual. When an elevation of PRL is confirmed, a careful history must be recorded to rule out the possibility that medications are the cause of the elevated PRL. A significant number of medications elevate PRL levels. In addi-

TABLE 39-3	**Causes of Prolactin Elevation**

Chronic renal failure
Pregnancy
Breast stimulation or chest wall trauma
Primary hypothyroidism
Empty sella syndrome
Pituitary adenoma (microadenoma or macroadenoma)
   "Nonsecretory"
   With galactorrhea and amenorrhea or oligospermia
Idiopathic
Drugs
   Dopaminergic-blocking agents: phenothiazines, butyrophenones, benzamides (metoclopramide, sulpiride)
   Dopamine-depleting agents: α-methyldopa, reserpine
   Noncatecholamine-dependent agents: TRH, estrogens
   H$_2$-receptor blocking agents, such as: cimetidine
   Tricyclic antidepressants
Hypothalamic etiologies

TRH, Thyrotropin-releasing hormone.

tion to estrogens, dopamine antagonists, such as metoclopramide, domperidone, and haloperidol, used to treat gastrointestinal diseases produce significant elevations in PRL release. TSH measurements also should be performed on individuals in whom prolactinoma is suspected to rule out primary hypothyroidism, a thyroid disorder that can elevate PRL levels.

In addition, imaging of the pituitary gland with CT or MRI should be performed. Most individuals with PRL levels greater than 150 ng/mL have PRL-secreting tumors; many large prolactinomas are associated with PRL levels greater than 1000 ng/mL. Most individuals with prolactinomas fail to show a further increase in PRL after TRH stimulation; however, the same is true for most individuals with hyperprolactinemia from other causes. Unless a pituitary tumor can be demonstrated by CT or MRI the diagnosis of a PRL-secreting microadenoma (<10 mm in diameter) is one of exclusion. Because 50% of PRL-secreting microadenomas are too small to be seen with neuroradiological techniques, delineation of the distinction among a small pituitary tumor, PRL-cell hyperplasia, and idiopathic hyperprolactinemia may not be possible without surgical intervention.

Evidence of an elevated PRL level in an individual with a pituitary tumor does not establish a cause-and-effect relationship. Usually a PRL level in excess of 200 ng/mL is sufficient evidence to suspect a PRL-secreting pituitary tumor. "Pseudoprolactinomas" are large nonsecretory tumors that press on the pituitary stalk and disrupt the normal inhibitory flow of dopamine from the hypothalamus, resulting in a modest elevation in PRL levels. Recognizing this distinction is particularly important in the decision regarding treatment because PRL-secreting macroadenomas (>10 mm in diameter) usually decrease in size with medical therapy, whereas "pseudoprolactinomas" do not. (Although PRL levels usually decrease with bromocriptine treatment, pseudoprolactinomas often continue to grow.) In individuals with pituitary macroadenomas a PRL level less than 500 ng/mL usually indicates the presence of a pseudoprolactinoma and a PRL level greater than 1000 ng/mL suggests a true PRL-producing tumor; values between 500 and 1000 ng/mL must be interpreted based on individual circumstances.

Analytical methodology

Principles

Several IRMA and enzyme-linked immunosorbent assay (ELISA) kits used to determine PRL are available. In practice, most routine PRL determinations are performed on automated immunoassay systems with either chemiluminescence or fluorescence-based detection. PRL usually is calibrated against reference materials with WHO reference materials. Without the performance of such calibration, PRL results that are expressed in mass units are not comparable from assay to assay.

Specimen requirements

Serum is the specimen of choice for the PRL assay. No special handling procedures are necessary, and it can be stored at 4 °C for 24 hours. Freezing is preferred for the maintenance of long-term stability. Specimens should be collected 3 to 4 hours after the subject has awakened because PRL levels rise rapidly during sleep and peak in the early-morning hours. Emotional stress, exercise, ambulation, and protein ingestion all can elevate PRL levels; thus specimens should be collected after an overnight fast when the patient is resting. Blood specimens also can be collected by finger puncture, spotted on filter paper, and stored in airtight plastic bags. PRL in blood spots is stable for 1 week at room temperature.

Reference intervals

Reference intervals for PRL by use of an IRMA are as follows:

	μg/L
Cord blood	45 to 539
Children	
Tanner stage	
Stage 1	
Male	<10
Female	3.6 to 12
Stages 2 to 3	
Male	<6.1
Female	2.6 to 18
Stages 4 to 5	
Male	2.8 to 11
Female	3.2 to 20
Adults	
Male	3.0 to 14.7
Female	3.8 to 23.0
Pregnancy, third trimester	95 to 473

Adrenocorticotropic Hormone and Related Peptides

Biochemistry and physiology

Adrenocorticotropic hormone (ACTH) and related peptides originate from a large precursor molecule called *proopiomelanocortin (POMC)*. As shown in Figure 39-4, POMC is processed to smaller peptides in both the anterior and intermediate lobes of the pituitary gland. In the anterior lobe, enzymes hydrolyze POMC to β-LPH and a 22-kD fragment known as *pro-ACTH*. This latter peptide is processed further to ACTH (1-39, a peptide consisting of 39 amino acids) and to a 16-kD peptide, pro-α-melanotropin (pro-MSH). β-LPH in turn is cleaved to two smaller peptides, β-endorphin and γ-LPH. Both β-LPH and β-endorphin are released with ACTH from the anterior lobe of the pituitary gland, but only about one-third the β-LPH is converted to β-endorphin. In contrast, the intermediate lobe fully processes β-LPH to β-endorphin, cleaves pro-MSH to α-melanotropin (α-MSH), and splits ACTH to α-MSH and a corticotropin-like, intermediate-lobe peptide.

Regulation of adrenocorticotropin secretion

Regulation of ACTH secretion is described in Chapter 41.

Clinical significance

With adrenal insufficiency the pituitary release of POMC and ACTH is increased significantly. Individuals with Addison's disease will demonstrate increased circulating levels of ACTH and MSH as a result of the lack of negative feedback to the pituitary from cortisol. The increased levels of MSH can result in hyperpigmentation and darkening of the skin, a characteristic feature of individuals with Addison's disease.

Analytical methodology

Methods used to measure adrenocorticotropic hormone

Principles.   ACTH is measured in the laboratory primarily by immunoassay. Individual immunoassay components (anti-ACTH antisera, ACTH calibrators), as well as complete reagent test kits are available commercially.[14] Older methods used polyclonal antisera directed at a segment of the biologically active N-terminal portion of the molecule. These antisera react with intact ACTH (amino acids 1 to 39) and with ACTH fragments (amino acids 1 to 24) and precursor molecules, such as POMC and pro-ACTH. ACTH has become available more recently on automated immunoassay systems that use chemiluminescence for detection. This method has lowered the detection limit for ACTH measurements and allowed for discrimination of low-normal results from true suppression.

Immunometric assays for ACTH that use labeled monoclonal antibodies in noncompetitive formats also have proven quite reliable. In these assays, two monoclonal antibodies are directed at different sites on the ACTH molecule (for example, the N-terminal and C-terminal regions). In terms of assay detection limit, simplicity, and speed, these two-site "sandwich" immunometric assays easily detect low ACTH levels (1 to 4 pg/mL) and can distinguish true low from low-normal specimens.

Laboratories and manufacturers of commercial kits usually calibrate their assays against ACTH preparations from research centers, such as human-purified ACTH 1-39 (MRC 74/555, 6.2 IU per 25 µg) from the National Institute of Biological Standards and Control (United Kingdom) or synthetic ACTH 1-39 (4.71 IU per 50 µg) supplied by the National Pituitary Agency (Baltimore).

Specimen requirements.   Proper precautions must be taken in the collection, transportation, and storage of specimens for ACTH measurements. ACTH is oxidized easily, strongly adsorbs to glass surfaces, and is degraded rapidly by plasma proteases into immunoreactive fragments during freezing and thawing of the specimen. Factors that influence plasma ACTH, such as prior administration of corticosteroids, time of day at which the specimen is taken (diurnal variation), and stress from a poorly performed venipuncture, also must be considered. To minimize these problems, blood specimens should be collected into prechilled polystyrene (plastic) tubes containing EDTA, immediately placed on ice, and centrifuged at 4 °C. Some laboratories also recommend the use of protease inhibitors, such as aprotinin (Trasylol). The supernatant then is transferred to another plastic tube and stored at −20 °C or colder. To protect the ACTH molecule further, antioxidants such as mercaptoethanol also have been used. Immediately before analysis, frozen

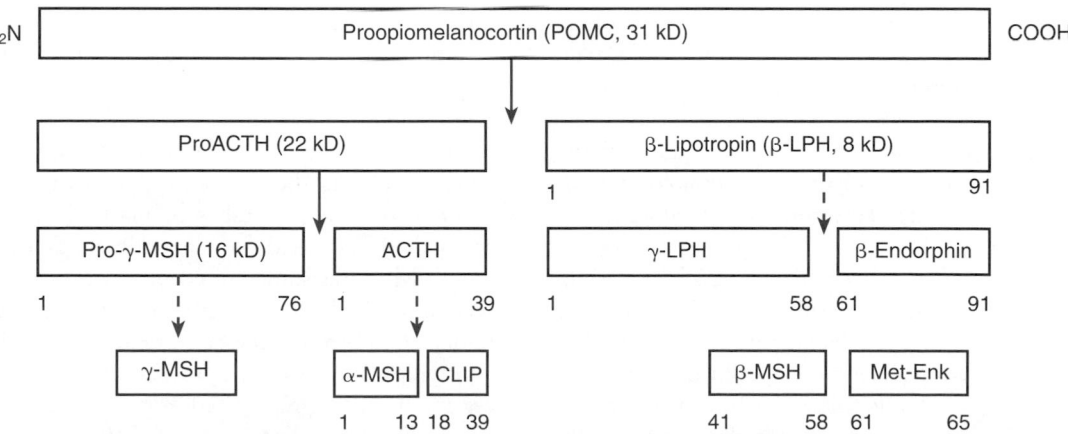

Figure 39-4   Diagrammatic representation of POMC and its precursor relationship to ACTH, β-LPH, α- and β-MSH, and the endorphins. *MSH,* Melanotropin; *CLIP,* corticotropin-like intermediate lobe peptide.

specimens should be thawed and centrifuged to remove any fibrin clots, which interfere with the assay system.

Reference intervals. With an IRMA method, reference intervals for ACTH have been reported as follows:

Adult, 0800 h: unrestricted activity	<120 pg/mL (<26 pmol/L)
Adult, 2400 h: supine	<10 pg/mL (<2.2 pmol/L)

Methods used to measure β-endorphin

Principles. Immunoassay is the method of choice for the analysis of plasma β-endorphin. Both RIAs and direct IRMAs have been developed for this purpose. Commercial reagent kits are available. The level of β-endorphin is usually very low in normal subjects, and samples have to be extracted and concentrated to detect meaningful levels in plasma. The specificity of commercial antibodies for β-endorphin relative to β-LPH varies widely; in some immunoassays, 50% cross-reactivity is seen with β-LPH. With polyclonal antibodies, results may be spuriously high because of cross-reactivity with serum immunoglobulin G (IgG; for example, in individuals with IgG myeloma). The preferred specimen is plasma with EDTA as the anticoagulant. A typical adult reference interval for specimens collected between 0600 and 1000 hours is 16 to 48 pg/mL (5 to 30 pmol/L).

Gonadotropins (Follicle-Stimulating Hormone, Luteinizing Hormone)

Biochemistry and physiology

Luteinizing hormone (LH) and **follicle-stimulating hormone (FSH)** are glycoprotein hormones produced by the pituitary and placenta (see Chapter 43). They are composed of two peptide chains (usually referred to as α and β *subunits*), each with carbohydrate substituent groups attached. The carbohydrate moiety, which accounts for 15% to 31% of the molecular weight (MW), includes mannose, galactose, glucosamine, galactosamine, and sialic acid. The α subunits of these hormones are similar to one another and are interchangeable. The β subunits, which display greater differences in amino acid sequences among the various hormones, confer hormonal and immunological specificity. Isolated α subunits are devoid of biological activity. Isolated β subunits may have slight intrinsic biological activity, but full activity is attained when α and β subunits are recombined.

This combination suggests that the presence of both α and β subunits is important for specific receptor recognition and that the α subunit is responsible for eliciting the specific biological response. The availability of specific antisera for β subunits has led to the development of RIA methods targeted for the specific measurements of these structurally similar glycoprotein hormones (see the discussion of chorionic gonadotropin, Chapter 43).

Secretion

The gonadotropic cells of the anterior lobe of the pituitary gland secrete FSH (MW 30 kD) and LH (MW 32 kD). In men, LH sometimes is referred to as *interstitial cell-stimulating hormone*. Because these two hormones control the functional activity of gonads, they are grouped together under the generic term *gonadotropins*.

Function

In women, FSH stimulates the growth of ovarian follicles and, in the presence of LH, promotes secretion of estrogens by the maturing follicles. LH in females causes release of the ovum from the ovarian follicle, which previously has matured under the influence of FSH, and induces the formation of the corpus luteum from the ruptured follicle. The corpus luteum then secretes progesterone and estradiol under the influence of pulsatile LH release. In men, FSH stimulates spermatogenesis, whereas LH is responsible for the production of testosterone by the Leydig cells of the testes.

Regulation

Regulation of LH and FSH secretion is discussed in Chapter 42.

Clinical significance

The clinical significance of LH and FSH in reproductive endocrinology is discussed in Chapter 42.

Analytical methodology

Methods for the measurement of follicle-stimulating hormone, luteinizing hormone, and free α units

Principles. Methods used to assay gonadotropins have evolved from bioassays to receptor assays to immunoassays that use radioactive and nonisotopic labels. Immunoassays largely have replaced bioassays in the routine clinical laboratory. Many methods have been described for the determination of FSH and LH in blood and urine, and reliable commercial kits are available.

The introduction of two-site immunometric assays has improved significantly gonadotropin measurements. A number of LH and FSH "sandwich" assays are available for manual or automated immunoassay systems. In some commercial kits the first antibody is immobilized on the inner surfaces of test tubes or plastic beads; in others the antibody is attached to magnetic particles or glass-fiber paper. Multiple signal molecules are associated with the second antibody, including radioisotopes, enzymes, fluorophors, and chemiluminescent molecules. With these assays, chorionic gonadotropin (CG) interference in LH assays is essentially negligible (<0.008% cross-reactivity), and detection limits are less than 0.2 IU/L.

In practice, calibration of gonadotropic hormone assays is difficult.[5] The challenge of the use of calibrators that are identical to the analytes found in clinical specimens is confounded by the fact that LH and FSH are not single chemical entities, but rather mixtures of closely related compounds. Partially purified pituitary extracts, such as the first and second WHO IRPs for FSH/LH, have been available for many years but have been replaced by highly purified pituitary preparations that have high biological potency and low potential for contamination with cross-reacting glycoproteins and their subunits. Most manufacturers of immunoassay kits for LH and FSH use one or more pituitary reference materials to standardize their working calibrators. With DNA techniques, recombinant gonadotropin calibrators (rFSH and rLH) have been produced that eliminate many of the problems associated with reference materials isolated from human pituitary glands.[15]

Several immunoassays have been described for the quantification of the free α subunit of pituitary glycoprotein hormones in serum. As expected, monoclonal antibody-based IRMAs of free α subunits are more sensitive and specific than conventional polyclonal RIAs. For example, in one such IRMA used to measure free α subunit, negligible cross-reactivity was observed with intact pituitary glycoprotein hormones (<0.001%). This method was sensitive enough to detect these subunits in healthy, nonpregnant individuals and in those individuals with hormone-secreting tumors (detection limit, ~10 ng/L).

Specimen requirements. Serum is preferred as the specimen of choice for gonadotropins. Hemolyzed, lipemic, or icteric specimens should not be used. Both hormones are stable for 8 days at room temperature and 2 weeks at 4 °C; for longer periods the serum specimen should be stored frozen at or below −20 °C. Because of episodic, circadian, and cyclical variations in the secretion of gonadotropins, a meaningful clinical evaluation of these hormones may require determinations in pooled blood specimens, multiple serial blood specimens, or timed urine specimens. Urine specimens should not contain preservatives; storage at or below −20 °C is recommended.

Reference intervals. Reference intervals for LH and FSH in serum by use of a sensitive ("third-generation") immunochemiluminometric assay are reported as follows:

	LH (IU/L)	FSH (IU/L)
Men	1.2 to 7.8	1.4 to 15.4
Women		
Follicular phase	1.7 to 15.0	1.4 to 9.9
Midcycle peak	21.9 to 56.6	0.2 to 17.2
Luteal phase	0.6 to 16.3	1.1 to 9.2
Postmenopausal	14.2 to 52.3	19.3 to 100.6

Methods for the measurement of urinary gonadotropins

The measurement of FSH and LH in a timed collection specimen of urine allows for integration of the marked pulsatility in gonadotropin secretion. In addition, urine samples can be extracted and concentrated, which results in a fiftyfold decrease in the detection limit of the method. Urine gonadotropin measurements are the preferred method used to assess gonadotropin secretion in prepubertal children and during the prepubertal transition period to adolescence.

Principles. The same methods used to measure gonadotropins in serum are used to measure these analytes in urine.

Specimen requirements. A meaningful clinical evaluation of the levels of FSH and LH in urine may require a timed urine specimen. Urine specimens should not contain preservatives; storage at or below −20 °C is recommended.

Reference intervals. Reference intervals for LH and FSH in urine from a timed 3-hour collection are reported as follows:

	LH (mIU/h)	FSH (mIU/h)
Prepubertal	3 to 97	10 to 160
Pubertal	20 to 1800	18 to 1310
Adult woman	190 to 3350	120 to 1490
Adult man	550 to 2500	190 to 1700

Thyroid-Stimulating Hormone

Like FSH and LH, **thyroid-stimulating hormone (TSH)** is a glycoprotein with an MW of 26.6 kD. It is produced in and released from the anterior lobe of the pituitary gland. It has a specific β subunit and an α subunit chemically similar to the α subunits of LH, FSH, and CG. TSH stimulates growth and vascularity of the thyroid gland and growth of the thyroid follicular cells and promotes most the steps in thyroid hormone synthesis, including iodine uptake, organification of iodine to tyrosine, coupling of tyrosines, and proteolytic release of thyroid hormone from thyroglobulin stores.

The regulation, function, clinical significance, and methodology of TSH are discussed in Chapter 40.

■ HORMONES OF THE NEUROHYPOPHYSIS

The neurohypophyseal system is composed of neurons in the supraoptic and paraventricular nuclei of the hypothalamus. These neurons pass through the median eminence and pituitary stalk, with the nerve endings projecting to the posterior lobe of the pituitary gland. The cell bodies of these neurons synthesize and secrete ADH—also called *arginine vasopressin*—and oxytocin. ADH is a nonapeptide (MW 1.08 kD) consisting of a cyclic hexapeptide and tripeptide side chain. Oxytocin has a structure similar to that of ADH (Figure 39-5) but with isoleucine rather than phenylalanine at position 3 and leucine instead of arginine at position 8.

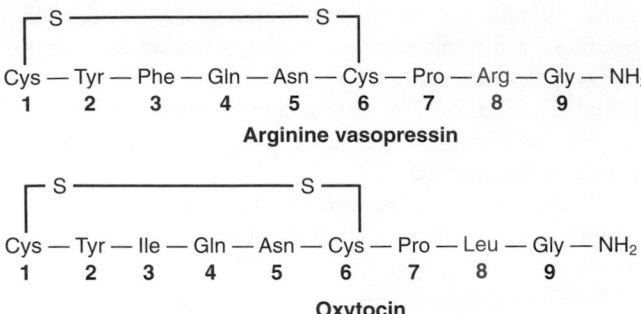

Figure 39-5　The amino acid sequence of arginine vasopressin and oxytocin. *Cys*, Cysteine; *Tyr*, tyrosine; *Phe*, phenylalanine; *Gln*, glutamine; *Asn*, asparagine; *Pro*, proline; *Arg*, arginine; *Gly*, glycine; *Ile*, isoleucine; *Leu*, leucine.

Antidiuretic Hormone

Biochemistry and physiology

Antidiuretic hormone (ADH) is synthesized as part of a large precursor molecule (prepropressophysin) in conjunction with a specific neurophysin-binding protein; the latter serves as a carrier protein for ADH during axonal transport and storage. These molecular complexes are packaged into secretory granules that migrate down the nerve axons for 12 to 14 hours before reaching the posterior pituitary lobe for storage. Release of ADH into the portal circulation occurs via calcium-dependent exocytosis on nerve cell stimulation. ADH exists in plasma mainly in unbound forms.

Regulation of secretion

Osmolality of the blood is the predominant regulator of ADH secretion. Osmoreceptors located in the hypothalamus respond to changes in plasma osmolality; a 2% increase in extracellular fluid osmolality stimulates ADH release (Figure 39-6). A plasma osmolality above 280 mOsm/kg is considered the osmotic threshold for ADH release. The thirst center has a higher set point than the osmoreceptors and responds to osmolalities above 290 mOsm/kg. Responses involving ADH, thirst, and the kidney are coordinated to maintain the plasma osmolality in healthy individuals within a narrow range (284 to 295 mOsm/kg).

Other important stimuli for ADH release include pain, stress, sleep, exercise, and chemical agents, such as catecholamines, angiotensin II, opiates, prostaglandins, anesthetics, nicotine, and barbiturates. An increase in plasma volume, a decrease in plasma osmolality, and agents such as alcohol, phenytoin, and glucocorticoids inhibit ADH release.

Functions

The major physiological function of ADH is its role in maintaining water homeostasis (see Figure 39-6), which allows the kidney to reabsorb water and concentrate urine (see Chapters 34 and 35). When released in sufficient quantity, ADH also induces a generalized vasoconstriction that leads

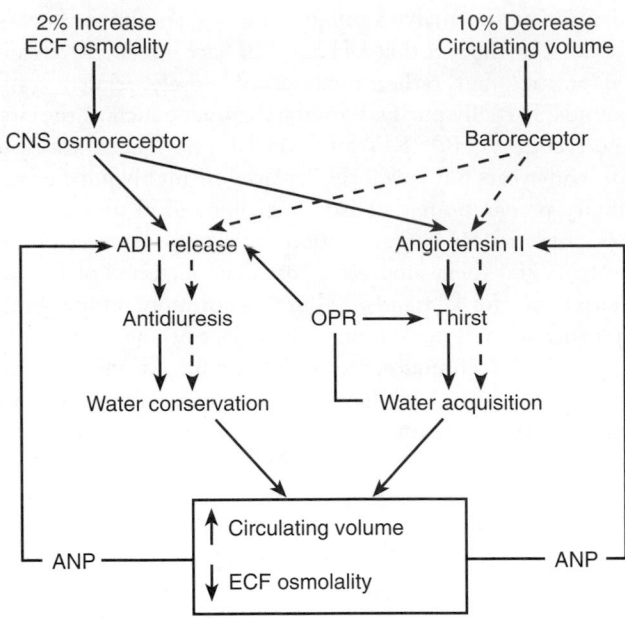

Figure 39-6　Key elements in water homeostasis. Note the osmotically stimulated pathways *(solid lines)*, volume-stimulated pathways *(dashed lines)*, and negative-feedback pathways *(dotted lines)*. *ANP*, Atrial natriuretic peptide; *AVP*, vasopressin; *CNS*, central nervous system; *ECF*, extracellular fluid; *OPR*, oropharyngeal reflex; *ADH*, antidiuretic hormone. (Modified from Reeves W, Andreoli T: The posterior pituitary and water metabolism. In Wilson JD, Foster DW (eds): Williams Textbook of Endocrinology, 8th edition, p 312, Philadelphia, WB Saunders, 1992.)

to a rise in arterial blood pressure. Release of ADH into the pituitary portal system also augments the action of CRH in stimulating the release of ACTH from the neurohypophysis. ADH does not appear to affect the release of other anterior pituitary hormones.

Clinical significance

Disorders of ADH activity are divided into hypofunction (polyuric states) and hyperfunction (syndrome of inappropriate antidiuretic hormone secretion [SIADH]).

Polyuric states

Deficient production or action of ADH results in **polyuria** caused by the failure of the renal tubules to reabsorb solute-free water. When urine output is greater than 2.5 L/day, further investigation usually is required; with complete deficiency of ADH, urine output may approach 1 L/hour. If the thirst response is normal, increased ingestion of fluid **(polydipsia)** follows. If access to water is not restricted, plasma osmolality and serum electrolytes usually remain normal.

Polyuric states are divided further into subcategories of (1) hypothalamic diabetes insipidus (HDI), (2) nephrogenic diabetes insipidus (NDI; deficient ADH action on the kidney), and (3) psychogenic polydipsia. The classic approach to the diagnosis of polyuric disorders is the overnight water-deprivation test.[7]

Hypothalamic diabetes insipidus. Also called *neurogenic, central,* or *cranial diabetes insipidus,* HDI is caused by a failure of the pituitary gland to secrete normal amounts of ADH in response to osmoregulatory factors. Often, HDI occurs without apparent cause or is associated with neoplastic diseases, neurological surgery, head trauma, ischemic or hypoxic disorders, granulomatous diseases, infections, or autoimmune disorders.

Nephrogenic diabetes insipidus. NDI results from a failure of the kidneys to respond to normal or increased concentrations of ADH. A familial form of NDI is inherited as an X-linked trait and mostly affects men. Acquired forms of NDI may be caused by metabolic disorders (hypokalemia, hypercalcemia, amyloidosis), drugs (lithium, demeclocycline, barbiturates), and renal diseases (polycystic disease, chronic renal failure). NDI also may be seen in the absence of these factors (idiopathic).

Psychogenic or primary polydipsia. A chronic, excessive intake of water suppresses ADH secretion and produces hypotonic polyuria. The polyuria and polydipsia are usually not as sustained as in HDI or NDI; nocturnal polyuria also is less frequent. Psychogenic factors are associated most commonly with this disorder, but hypothalamic disease affecting the thirst center may be a cause. Drugs also affect the thirst center and result in primary polydipsia.

Syndrome of inappropriate antidiuretic hormone secretion

Syndrome of inappropriate antidiuretic hormone secretion (SIADH) refers to the autonomous, sustained production of ADH in the absence of known stimuli for its release. Plasma ADH levels are increased "inappropriately" relative to a low plasma osmolality and a normal or increased plasma volume. SIADH may be the result of (1) a malignancy (such as a small-cell carcinoma of the lung), (2) the presence of acute and chronic diseases of the central nervous system, (3) pulmonary disorders, or (4) a side effect of certain drug therapies. In these situations a primary excess of ADH, coupled with unrestricted fluid intake, promotes increased reabsorption of free water by the kidney. The result is a decreased urine volume and an increased urine sodium concentration and osmolality. As a consequence of water retention, these individuals become modestly volume expanded. The increase in intravascular volume causes hemodilution accompanied by dilutional hyponatremia and a low plasma osmolality. Volume expansion also decreases renal sodium reabsorption and thus further increases the urine sodium concentration.

Clinically, SIADH is the most common cause of hyponatremia in hospitalized patients. However, other disorders cause dilutional hyponatremia and must be differentiated from SIADH. These conditions include congestive heart failure, renal insufficiency, nephrotic syndrome, liver cirrhosis, and hypothyroidism. Excessive administration of hypotonic fluids and treatment with drugs that stimulate ADH (for example, chlorpropamide, vincristine, clofibrate, carbamazepine, nicotine, phenothiazines, and cyclophosphamide) also cause dilutional hyponatremia. Hyponatremia also may occur from renal or extrarenal sodium losses (depletional hyponatremia) as a result of vomiting, diarrhea, excessive sweating, diuretic abuse, salt-losing nephropathy, or mineralocorticoid deficiency.

The clinical manifestations of hyponatremia are nonspecific; weakness and apathy occur in mild cases, and central nervous system changes (lethargy, coma, seizures) are present in more severe cases. No signs or symptoms are specific for SIADH. History, physical examination, and routine laboratory test results often suggest that hyponatremia is due to dilution or depletion.

Measurements of sodium and osmolality in blood and urine, combined with a clinical assessment of volume status, usually permit the appropriate differential diagnosis of hyponatremic conditions (Table 39-4). The typical individual with SIADH has a hypo-osmolal plasma (<270 mOsm/kg), a urine osmolality slightly greater than that of plasma, and a urine sodium concentration that is elevated inappropriately ($\sim$40 to 80 mmol/L). Individuals with dilutional hyponatremia resulting from excess water intake have hypotonic plasma, unremarkable urine sodium concentration (<20 mmol/L), and dilute urine (a urine osmolality less than that of plasma). Individuals with depletional hyponatremia caused by extrarenal sodium loss have hypotonic plasma, low urine sodium concentration (usually <20 mmol/L), and urine osmolality greater than that of plasma; individuals with depletional hyponatremia caused by impaired renal conservation of sodium have similar results, except that their urine sodium concentrations are elevated.

TABLE 39-4   **Diagnosis of SIADH**

Document plasma hypo-osmolality ($\leq$275 mOsm/kg) and hyponatremia (sodium level of $\leq$130 mmol/L).

Use history, physical examination, and appropriate laboratory tests to exclude cardiac, hepatic, renal, thyroid, or adrenal failure, as well as the effects of pituitary surgery, diuretic therapy, or medications known to stimulate ADH release. (SIADH cannot be diagnosed unless these factors are corrected.)

Measure urine sodium level and osmolality. Urine osmolality greater than plasma osmolality and without a correspondingly low urine sodium level (usually >60 mmol/L) indicates probable SIADH.

If further tests are indicated:

1. Perform water loading test. Use with caution. Normal results exclude SIADH.

2. Measure plasma ADH and plasma renin levels. SIADH is characterized by high ADH concentration and low renin concentration. If plasma ADH and renin levels are both low, a primary defect in renal water excretion is present.

SIADH, Syndrome of inappropriate antidiuretic hormone; *ADH,* antidiuretic hormone.

If the cause for mild hyponatremia remains unclear after the previously discussed tests are performed, a water loading test may be performed.[7] However, this test is potentially dangerous in individuals with severe hyponatremia and should not be performed if the serum sodium level is less than 130 mmol/L. Individuals with SIADH have impaired excretion of the water load and fail to dilute their urine. Measurements of ADH in plasma usually are not needed to diagnose SIADH, but basal values are expected to be inappropriately high relative to plasma hypo-osmolality. Interpretations of plasma ADH levels sometimes are complicated because values are often within the physiological reference interval or undetectable.

Analytical methodology

Numerous immunoassays used to measure ADH in plasma or urine have been described. However, their routine clinical application has been hampered because of the complexity and poor performance of the methods. With most plasma assays a preliminary extraction procedure is required, not only to concentrate the minute amount of hormone present in the specimen, but also to remove nonspecific interfering substances.

Principles

Procedures used to extract and concentrate ADH from biological fluids often involve the use of solvents, such as acetone, petroleum ether, or ethanol. Alternatively, column chromatography using octadecyl silica (C_{18}) columns is an efficient purification technique. Although a few nonisotopic immunoassays have been developed for ADH, most clinical laboratories use some variant of an RIA; complete test kits or individual components (anti-ADH antisera, ADH tracers) are available commercially.

Specimen requirements

Blood specimens for ADH are collected into prechilled tubes containing EDTA as an anticoagulant. Most procedures recommend that specimens be delivered to the laboratory on ice and centrifuged at 4 °C within 30 minutes of collection. The plasma then is removed and stored frozen at −20 °C until analysis is performed. Random urine specimens are collected without preservatives; alternatively, complete 24-hour urine specimens may be collected in 10 mL of 6 mol/L of hydrochloric acid. Significant deterioration of ADH occurs with prolonged storage.

Reference intervals

The plasma concentration of ADH in healthy adults (24 to 42 years of age) with normal water intake and normal physical activity is 0.35 to 1.94 ng/L (0.32 to 1.80 pmol/L). For the best interpretation of results, plasma ADH values should be correlated with serum or plasma osmolality.

ADH		Osmolality
ng/L	pmol/L	mOsm/kg
<1.5	<1.4	270 to 280
<2.5	<2.3	280 to 285
1 to 5	0.9 to 4.6	285 to 290
2 to 7	1.9 to 6.5	290 to 295
4 to 12	3.7 to 11.1	295 to 300

The reference interval for ADH in a random urine specimen is reportedly 1 to 112 pg/mL.

Oxytocin

Oxytocin is a peptide hormone that induces smooth muscle contraction in the uterus and mammary glands.

Biochemistry and physiology

Oxytocin is synthesized in the hypothalamus as part of a preprohormone, along with a separate neurophysin-binding protein. These molecular complexes are packaged into secretory granules that migrate down the nerve axons for 12 to 14 hours before reaching the posterior pituitary lobe for storage. Release of oxytocin into the portal circulation occurs via calcium-dependent exocytosis on nerve cell stimulation. Oxytocin exists in plasma mainly in unbound forms.

Secretion

The primary stimulus for oxytocin release is suckling. Stimulation of tactile receptors located around the nipples of the breasts initiates an action potential that propagates along afferent nerve fibers through the spinal cord and midbrain to the hypothalamus. The cell bodies in the paraventricular nucleus then are stimulated, resulting in the episodic release of oxytocin. The influence of other parts of the brain on the release of oxytocin has been reported; emotional stress, for instance, inhibits lactation.

Functions

Oxytocin is present in men and women, but its physiological effects are known only for women. Oxytocin stimulates contraction of the estrogen-primed uterus. Oxytocin has been used as a therapeutic agent to induce labor, but the physiological mechanism whereby it induces uterine contractions remains obscure. Oxytocin also stimulates the lactating mammary gland. Progestins are believed to inhibit the action of oxytocin.

Analytical methodology
Principles

Numerous immunoassays used to measure oxytocin in plasma or urine have been described.[7] However, as with ADH, routine clinical application has been hampered because of method complexity. With most plasma assays a preliminary extraction procedure is required, not only to concentrate the minute amount of hormone that is present in the specimen, but also to remove nonspecific interfering substances.

Specimen requirements

Blood specimens for oxytocin are collected into pre-chilled tubes containing EDTA as an anticoagulant. Most procedures recommend that specimens be delivered to the laboratory on ice and centrifuged at 4 °C within 30 minutes of collection. The plasma then is removed and stored frozen at −20 °C until analysis is performed. Random urine specimens are collected without preservatives; alternatively, complete 24-hour urine specimens may be collected in 10 mL of 6 mol/L of hydrochloric acid. Significant deterioration of oxytocin occurs with prolonged storage.

Reference intervals

Oxytocin values are quantified relative to the bioassay potency of a synthetic reference preparation. Plasma results are reported as microunits per milliliter (1 μU is equivalent to 2 pg of synthetic oxytocin).

	Oxytocin μU/mL
Men	1.1 to 1.9
Women	
Nonpregnant	1.0 to 1.8
Second stage of labor	3.1 to 5.3

ASSESSMENT OF PITUITARY FUNCTION

Evaluation of endocrine function is an important part of the management of patients with pituitary tumors.[2,4] Testing of pituitary function[6] in individuals with pituitary tumors has two objectives—(1) detection of hormone deficiencies before and after treatment and (2) recognition of hormone-producing tumors.

Assessment of anterior and posterior pituitary lobe function in individuals with pituitary tumors is important to expose clinically significant hormone-deficiency states. Pituitary hormone secretion failure is due to the tumor itself or is a result of pituitary surgery or irradiation. Testing of pituitary function usually is performed under basal conditions but also under provocative stimuli to bring out mild deficiencies that affect the adrenal, thyroid, or gonads. Evaluation of pituitary reserve for GH or PRL usually is unnecessary in adult patients because deficiencies of these hormones are not clinically important.

Pituitary function assessment should include observation of both clinical signs and symptoms of hormone deficiency and the measurement of hormones secreted by the pertinent endocrine gland, such as T_4, cortisol, testosterone, and the measurement of ACTH, TSH, FSH, and LH. A scheme used to test pituitary reserve is listed in Table 39-5.

TABLE 39-5 **Method of Assessment of Pituitary Reserve**

A. Before Pituitary Surgery
Adrenal glands: measurement of morning serum cortisol level or cosyntropin stimulation test
Thyroid gland: ultrasensitive determination of TSH
Gonads: sex hormone determinations (estradiol in women, testosterone in men) and gonadotropins

B. One Month after Pituitary Surgery
Adrenal glands: cosyntropin stimulation test
Thyroid gland: ultrasensitive determination of TSH level
Gonads: sex hormone determinations (estradiol in women, testosterone in men)

TSH, Thyroid-stimulating hormone.

In practice, different approaches are taken to assess the hypothalamic-pituitary-adrenal, -thyroid, or -gonadal axes.

Hypothalamic-Pituitary-Adrenal Axis

A normal morning serum or plasma cortisol level is usually adequate evidence to document intactness of the hypothalamic-pituitary-adrenal axis. Frequently, however, the cosyntropin stimulation test is used when the morning cortisol results are low or equivocal (<10 μg/dL) or when a strong clinical suspicion of adrenal insufficiency exists. A baseline blood specimen for cortisol is obtained for the performance of provocative testing, followed by the IV administration of 250 μg cosyntropin (a potent analogue of ACTH). Specimens for cortisol then are obtained at 30 or 60 minutes (or both) after the IV injection of cosyntropin. A peak value for plasma cortisol of greater than 20 μg/dL is considered a normal response.

Hypothalamic-Pituitary-Thyroid Axis

When the serum free thyroxine level (FT_4) or ultrasensitive TSH result is normal, the hypothalamic-pituitary-thyroid axis is assumed to be intact. If hypothyroidism is suspected clinically, however, a single measurement of TSH with an ultrasensitive method may be sufficient to confirm the diagnosis.

Hypothalamic-Pituitary-Gonadal Axis

History and physical examination are extremely helpful in the evaluation of the status of the hypothalamic-pituitary-gonadal axis, particularly in women during the reproductive years.[1,11] Normal menstrual cycles usually are indicative of an intact hypothalamic-pituitary-gonadal axis in reproductive-age women. Baseline laboratory assessment for hypothalamic-pituitary-gonadal disregulation should include measurement of serum gonadotropins (LH and FSH) and sex steroids (estradiol in females, testosterone in males). Provocative testing of this axis with GnRH and measurements of FSH and LH may be useful in selected individuals. These tests, however, can be unreliable in the dif-

ferentiation of pituitary disorders from hypothalamic dysfunction; thus the physician usually depends on an accurate determination of gonadotropins and sex steroids, along with good clinical judgment.

References

1. Apter D: Development of the hypothalamic-pituitary-ovarian axis. Ann NY Acad Sci 1997; 816:9-21.

2. Benbow SJ, Foy P, Jones B et al: Pituitary tumours presenting in the elderly: management and outcome. Clin Endocrinol 1997; 46:657-660.

3. Buatti JM, Marcus RB Jr: Pituitary adenomas: current methods of diagnosis and treatment. Oncology 1997; 11:791-796.

4. Bulatov AA, Martynov AV, Grigorian AL et al: Molecular forms of human growth hormone and prolactin, secreted by cultured pituitary tumor cells. Biokhimiia 1995; 60:1637-1646.

5. Canadian Society of Clinical Chemists: Canadian Society of Clinical Chemists position paper: standardization of selected polypeptide hormone measurements. Clin Biochem 1992; 25:415-424.

6. Davies MJ, Howlett TA: A survey of the current methods used in the UK to assess pituitary function. J R Soc Med 1996; 89:159P-164P.

7. Demers LM: Pituitary function. In Burtis CA, Ashwood ER (eds): Tietz Textbook of Clinical Chemistry, 3rd edition, pp 1470-1495, Philadelphia, WB Saunders, 1999.

8. Ghigo E, Arvat E, Muccioli G et al: Growth hormone-releasing peptides. Eur J Endocrinol 1997; 136:445-460.

9. Howanitz J: Review of the influence of polypeptide hormone forms of immunoassay results. Arch Pathol Lab Med 1993; 117:369-372.

10. Kaye TB: Hyperprolactinemia: causes, consequences, and treatment options. Postgrad Med 1996; 99:265-268.

11. Magiakou MA, Mastorakos G, Webster E et al: The hypothalamic-pituitary-adrenal axis and the female reproductive system. Ann N Y Acad Sci 1997; 816:42-56.

12. Melmed S: Unwanted effects of growth hormone excess in the adult. J Pediatr Endocrinol Metab 1996; 9(Suppl 3):369-374.

13. Preece MA: Making a rational diagnosis of growth-hormone deficiency. J Pediatr 1997; 131(1 Part 2):S61-S64.

14. Rosano TG, Demers LM, Hillam R et al: Clinical and analytical evaluation of an immunoradiometric assay for corticotropin. Clin Chem 1995; 41:1022-1027.

15. Rose MP: Follicle-stimulating hormone international standards and reference preparations for the calibration of immunoassays and bioassays. Clin Chim Acta 1998; 273(2):103-117.

16. Veldhuis JD, Liem AY, South S et al: Differential impact of age, sex steroid hormones and obesity on basal versus pulsatile growth hormone secretion in men as assessed in an ultrasensitive chemiluminescence assay. J Clin Endo Metab 1995; 80:3209-3222.

17. Vierhapper H, Nowotny P, Czech T et al: How (not) to diagnose growth hormone deficiency in adults: stimulated serum concentrations of growth hormone in healthy subjects and in patients with pituitary macroadenomas. Metabolism 1997; 46:680-683.

18. Yu-Lee LY: Molecular actions of prolactin in the immune system. Proc Soc Exp Biol Med 1997; 215:35-52.

Additional Reading

DeGroot LJ, Jameson JL (eds): Endocrinology, 4th edition, Philadelphia, WB Saunders, 2000.

Dickson RB, Salomon DS: Hormones and Growth Factors in Development and Neoplasia, New York, John Wiley & Sons, 1998.

Moore WT, Eastman RC: Diagnostic Endocrinology, 2nd edition, St Louis, Mosby, 1996.

Wilson JD, Foster DW, Kronenberg HM (eds): Williams Textbook of Endocrinology, 9th edition, Philadelphia, WB Saunders, 1998.

Thyroid Function

RONALD J. WHITLEY, PhD

Thyroxine (T$_4$) The major hormone synthesized by the thyroid gland that contains four iodine molecules (L-3,5,3′,5′-tetraiodothyronine)

Triiodothyronine (T$_3$) One of the thyroid hormones having three iodine molecules attached to its molecular

structure (L-3,5,3′-triiodothyronine); has several times the activity of T$_4$; reverse T$_3$ also having three iodine molecules attached to its molecular structure (L-3,3′,5′-triiodothyronine) but little biological activity

---

The thyroid gland is composed of two lobes connected by a thin band of tissue, known as the *isthmus,* which gives the gland the appearance of a butterfly (see Figure 26-1, Chapter 26). In the adult the entire thyroid gland weighs approximately 15 to 20 g. Each lobe measures approximately 2.0 to 2.5 cm in thickness and width and 4.0 cm in length.

The **thyroid follicle** is the secretory unit of the thyroid gland and is composed of an outer layer of epithelial cells that encloses an amorphous material known as *colloid.* **Colloid** is composed mainly of **thyroglobulin** (Tg) and small quantities of iodinated thyroalbumin. Important reactions of thyroid hormone synthesis, such as iodination and the initial phase of hormone secretion (colloid resorption), are believed to take place at or near the apical surface of the epithelial cells.

The thyroid gland also contains another type of cell known as *parafollicular* or *C cells.* These cells produce the polypeptide hormone calcitonin (see Chapter 38) and are confined within the follicular basement lamina or exist in clusters in the interfollicular spaces.

▬ THYROID HORMONES

The thyroid gland secretes **thyroxine** (3,5,3′,5′-L-tetraiodothyronine) and **triiodothyronine** (3,5,3′-L-triiodothyronine), hormones commonly known as **T$_4$** and **T$_3$,** respectively (Figure 40-1). In addition, the thyroid gland secretes small amounts of biologically inactive 3,3′,5′-L-triiodothyronine (reverse T$_3$ [rT$_3$]) and minute quantities of monoiodotyrosine (MIT) and diiodotyrosine (DIT), precursors of T$_3$ and T$_4$. At least 85% of normal T$_3$ production and essentially all of rT$_3$ production can be accounted for by peripheral deiodination of T$_4$ rather than by direct secretion by the thyroid gland. T$_3$ is four to five times more potent in biological systems than is T$_4$.

Control of energy expenditure is the primary function of thyroid hormones. In addition, they are indispensable for growth, development, and sexual maturation in mammals. Other actions include stimulation of heart rate and heart contraction, stimulation of protein synthesis and carbohydrate metabolism, increase in the synthesis and degradation of cholesterol and triglycerides, increase in vitamin requirements, and enhancement in sensitivity of β-adrenergic receptors to catecholamines.

Biochemistry and Physiology

Biosynthesis

The biosynthesis of thyroid hormones involves thyroidal trapping of serum iodide (iodide transport), incorporation of iodine into tyrosine, coupling of iodinated tyrosyl residues of Tg, and proteolytic cleavage of follicular Tg to release the iodothyronines (Figure 40-2). Iodine is the key to the synthesis of thyroid hormones and normally is ingested in the form of iodides; iodide transport to the follicles is the first and rate-limiting step in the synthetic process.

Synthesis of T$_3$, T$_4$, DIT, and MIT in Tg molecules occurs mainly at the follicular cell-colloid interface but also within the colloid. Tg, a protein composed of many tyrosine residues, is present in its highest concentrations within the colloid. Lysosomal proteases break the peptide bonds between iodinated residues and Tg, T$_4$ and T$_3$ thus formed diffuse into the systemic circulation, whereas DIT and MIT remain in the follicular cells, where they are deiodinated and the freed iodide reutilized.

Pituitary **thyroid-stimulating hormone (TSH)** regulates the synthesis of thyroid hormones. In addition, TSH

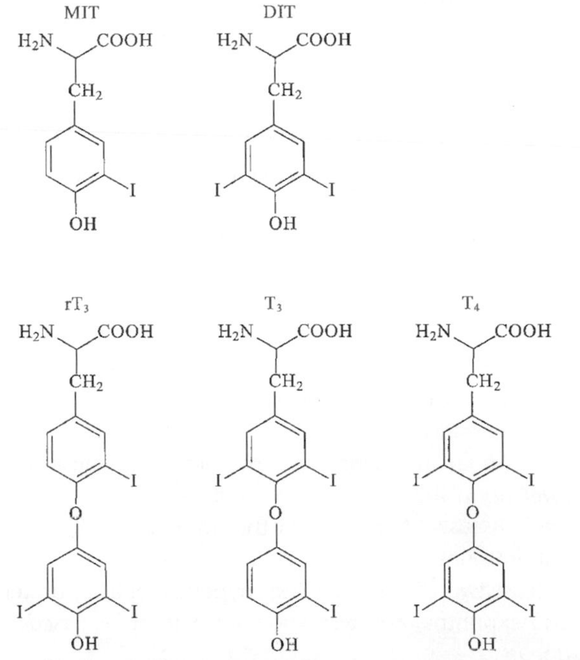

Figure 40-1 Structure of thyroid hormones and their precursors. *MIT,* Monoiodotyrosine; *DIT,* diiodotyrosine; *rT$_3$,* 3,3′,5′-L-triiodothyronine; *T$_3$,* 3,5,3′-L-triiodothyronine; *T$_4$,* 3,5,3′,5′-L-tetraiodothyronine.

induces an increase in the size and number of the thyroidal follicular cells. Prolonged TSH stimulation leads to increased vascularity and eventual **goiter**—hypertrophic enlargement of the thyroid gland.

In the liver, T_3 and T_4 are conjugated to form sulfates and glucuronides. These conjugates enter the bile and pass into the intestine. Thyroid hormone conjugates are hydrolyzed, and some are reabsorbed through the enterohepatic circulation, whereas some are excreted in the stool.[11] For a thorough discussion of thyroid metabolism, secretion, and synthesis, the reader is referred to the endocrinology textbooks listed in the Additional Reading section at the end of this chapter.

Secretion

A tightly coordinated feedback relationship exists among the thyroid gland, hypothalamus, and pituitary gland (Figure 40-3). **Thyrotropin-releasing hormone (TRH),** a tripeptide, is produced in the hypothalamus and acts on the pituitary thyrotropes to stimulate synthesis and release of TSH. A rise in thyroid hormone levels inhibits the pituitary response to TRH (negative feedback). A fall in thyroid hormone levels causes an increase in TRH and TSH secretion.

Metabolism

Free (unbound) T_4 (FT_4) is the primary secretory product of the normal thyroid gland. T_4 undergoes peripheral deiodination of the outer ring at the 5' position to yield T_3. This deiodination occurs in a number of tissues but primarily in the liver. Reverse T_3, produced by removal of one iodine from the inner ring of T_4, is metabolically inactive and an end-product of T_4 metabolism (see Figure 40-1). Peripheral deiodination is a rapidly responsive mechanism of control for thyroid hormone balance. Acute or chronic stress or illness causes a shift in the direction of this deiodination, favoring formation of rT_3 rather than T_3. Various medications also shift peripheral deiodination toward the inactive product rT_3.

T_4 and T_3 in the circulation are bound reversibly and almost completely to carrier proteins. These carrier proteins (thyroxine-binding globulin [TBG], thyroxine-binding prealbumin [TBPA], and albumin) bind 99.97% of T_4 and

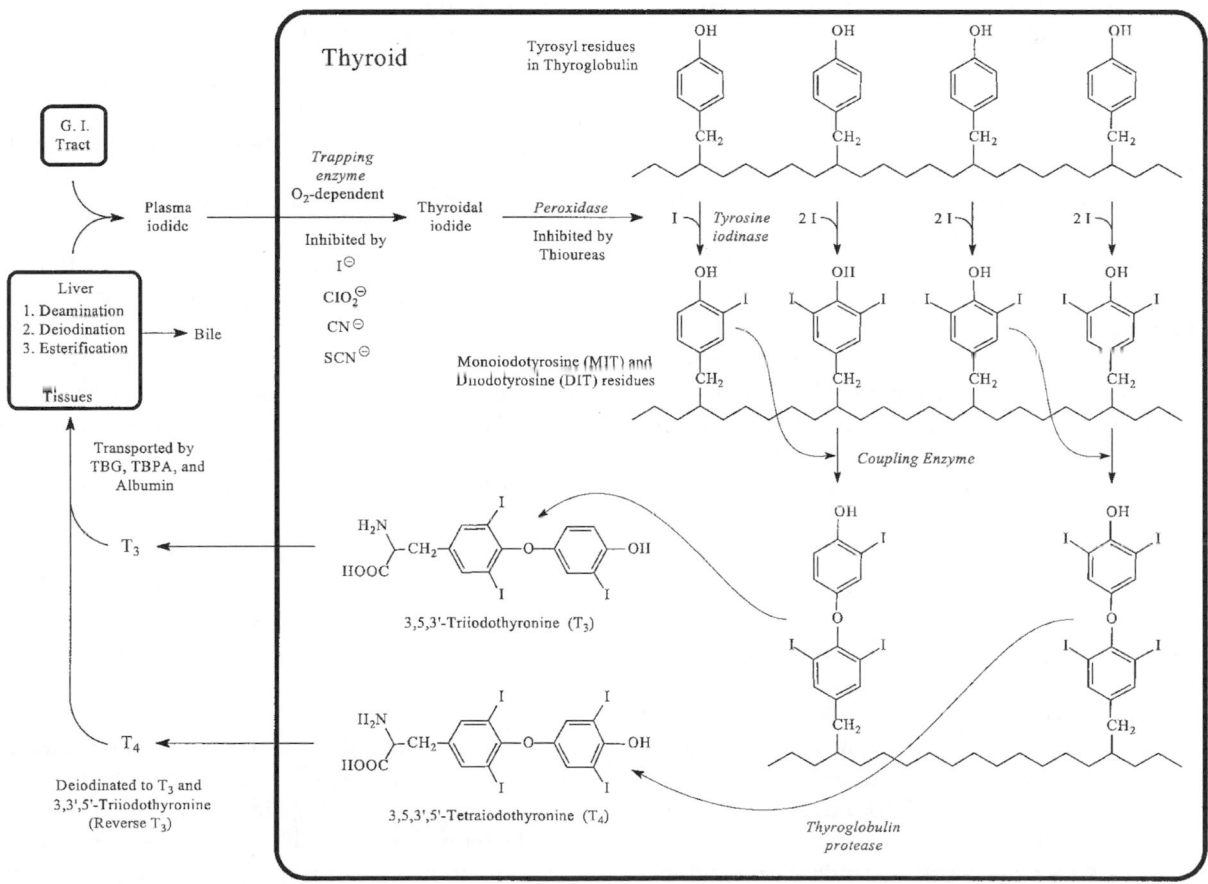

Figure 40-2 The metabolism of iodine, emphasizing formation and secretion of the thyroid hormones. Iodine transport is inhibited by anions such as thiocyanate (SCN^-), perchlorate (ClO^{-4}), and pertechnetate (TcO^{-4}). The oxidation and organic binding of iodide to thyroglobulin is blocked by thiourylenes, sulfonamides, and high concentrations of iodide. *GI,* Gastrointestinal; *TBG,* thyroxine-binding globulin; *TBPA,* thyroxine-binding prealbumin. (Modified from Berger S, Quinn JL: Thyroid function. In Tietz NW (ed): Fundamentals of Clinical Chemistry, 2nd edition, p 585, Philadelphia, WB Saunders, 1976.)

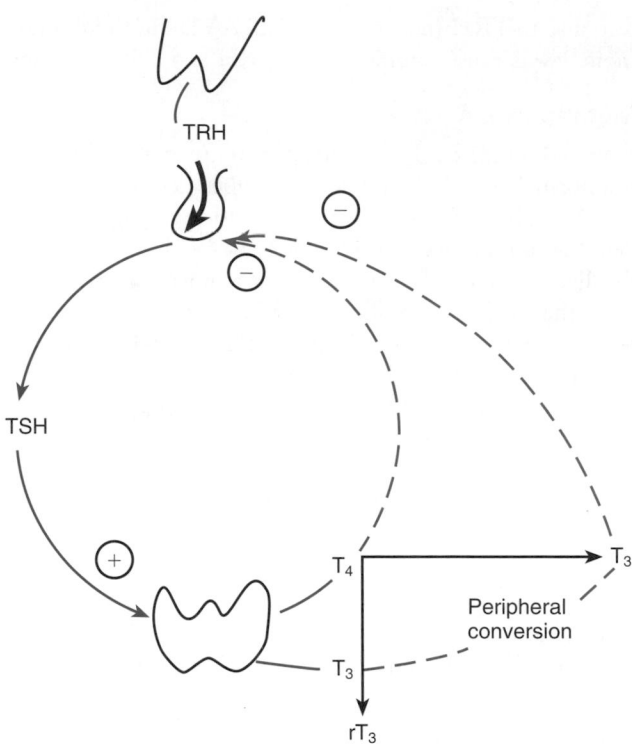

Figure 40-3   Diagram of hypothalamic-pituitary-thyroid interactions. *TRH*, Thyrotropin-releasing hormone; *TSH*, thyroid-stimulating hormone; T_3, triiodothyronine; rT_3, reverse T_3; T_4, thyroxine; +, positive effect; −, negative feedback effect.

TABLE 40-1	Alterations in the Concentration or Affinity of Thyroid Hormone-Binding Proteins

Increases In
  A. TBG concentration (or affinity)
    1. Genetic (inherited) determination
    2. Nonthyroidal illness (HIV infection, infectious and chronic active hepatitis, estrogen-producing tumors, acute intermittent porphyria)
    3. Physiology (pregnancy, newborn)
    4. Drug use (oral contraceptives, estrogens, tamoxifen, methadone)
  B. Prealbumin concentration
  C. Albumin binding (familial dysalbuminemic hyperthyroxinemia)
  D. T_4 binding by antibodies (autoimmune thyroid disease, hepatocellular carcinoma)

Decreases In
  A. TBG concentration
    1. Genetic (inherited) determination
    2. Nonthyroidal illness (major illness or surgical stress, nephrotic syndrome)
    3. Drug use (androgens, anabolic steroids, large doses of glucocorticoids)
  B. TBG binding capacity (drugs bound to TBG such as salicylates and phenytoin)
  C. Prealbumin concentration

TBG, Thyroxine-binding globulin; *HIV*, human immunodeficiency virus; T_4, thyroxine.

99.7% of T_3. Thus only a very small fraction of each of these hormones is unbound and free for biological activity. Because a wide variation exists in the concentration of T_4-binding proteins, even under normal circumstances, a wide variation also exists in total T_4 levels among individuals with normal **(euthyroid)** thyroid function. Total T_3 concentrations also vary with alterations in binding proteins, although usually to a lesser degree than T_4 levels. Circumstances in which thyroid hormone-binding protein levels are increased or decreased are shown in Table 40-1.

ANALYTICAL METHODOLOGY

Laboratory tests most commonly used to evaluate individuals for thyroid hormone dysfunction are listed in Table 40-2. Clinical signs and symptoms of thyroid hormone excess or deficiency are generally nonspecific. When hypothyroidism or hyperthyroidism is suspected, confirmation with laboratory tests generally is necessary. However, normal serum thyroid hormone levels do not exclude thyroid disease, and abnormal thyroid tests do not always indicate thyroid disease. Diffuse or nodular thyroid enlargement may be seen even in euthyroid individuals. Guidelines for the selection of appropriate laboratory determinations have been published by professional organizations, such as the American Thyroid Association[24] and the National Academy of Clinical Biochemistry.[20]

Traditionally, thyroid testing has been performed stepwise, with the initial step being either a serum total T_4 measurement or a free thyroxine estimate (FT₄E). However, these tests are not ideal indicators of thyroid status, in part because (1) of variations in serum binding protein levels, (2) T_3 is the primary active thyroid hormone and (3) the relationships among these hormones (T_4 and T_3) are not always predictable. In individuals with hyperthyroidism, T_3 usually is elevated to a greater degree than T_4 because it is derived from two sources—increased thyroidal secretion of T_3, and increased peripheral conversion of T_4 to T_3. T_3 determination is sometimes a useful adjunctive test in individuals suspected of having hyperthyroidism. However, because T_3 levels fluctuate rapidly in response to stress and other nonthyroidal factors, T_3 levels are low not only in individuals with hypothyroidism, but also in those affected with many other conditions. Thus measurement of T_3 also is not a good general test of thyroid status.

The serum level of TSH reflects the integrative action of thyroid hormone in one of its target tissues—the pituitary cells that secrete TSH. Pituitary TSH secretion is very sensitive to circulating thyroid hormone; in fact a twofold change in FT₄ causes an approximate 100-fold change in serum TSH concentration.[21] Small decreases in thyroid

TABLE 40-2   Nomenclature and Abbreviations for Thyroid Tests

Test	Nomenclature/Abbreviation
Hormone Concentration	
Total thyroxine	T_4
Total triiodothyronine (3,5,3'-triiodothyronine)	T_3
Free thyroxine*	FT_4
Free triiodothyronine*	FT_3
Thyrotropin (thyroid-stimulating hormone)	TSH
Reverse T_3 (3,3',5'-triiodothyronine)	rT_3
Estimates of Free Hormone Fraction	
Free T_4 fraction†	% FT_4
Free T_3 fraction†	% FT_3
Thyroid hormone-binding ratio‡	THBR
Estimates of Free Hormone Concentration	
Free T_4 estimate [$T_4 \times$ % FT_4]	FT_4E
Free T_3 estimate [$T_3 \times$ % FT_3]	FT_3E
Free T_4 index [$T_4 \times$ THBR]	FT_4I
Free T_3 index [$T_3 \times$ THBR]	FT_3I
T_4/TBG ratio	T_4/TBG
Free T_4 estimate (by immunoassay)§	FT_4E
Serum Binding Proteins	
Thyroxine-binding globulin	TBG
Thyroxine-binding prealbumin (transthyretin)	TBPA
Tests for Autoimmune Thyroid Disease	
Antithyroglobulin antibodies	TgAb
Antimicrosomal antibodies	TMAb
Antithyroid peroxidase antibodies	TPO Ab
TSH receptor antibodies	TRAb
Other Hormones and Thyroid-Related Proteins	
Thyrotropin-releasing hormone	TRH
Thyroglobulin	Tg
Calcitonin	CT

TSH, Thyroid-stimulating hormone.
*Measured by "direct" immunoassay of a dialysate (or ultrafiltrate) of undiluted serum.
†Measured by equilibrium dialysis (or ultrafiltration) of diluted serum containing tracer T_4 or T_3.
‡Derived from T_3 or T_4 "uptake" methods (see text for details).
§Measured by two-step or analog (one step) assays.

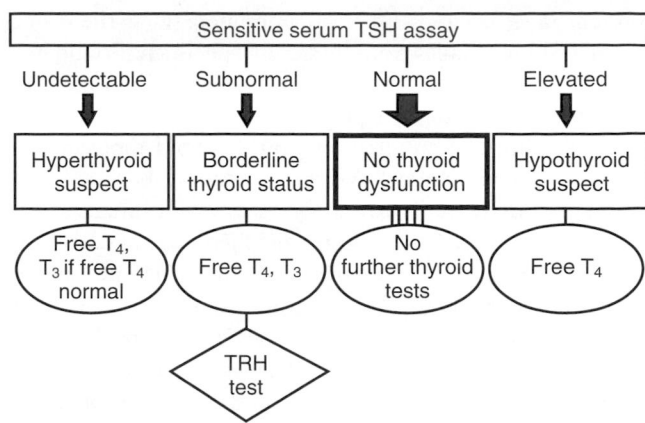

Figure 40-4   Strategies for thyroid diagnosis using a sensitive TSH assay as the initial step. *TSH*, Thyroid-stimulating hormone; T_3, triiodothyronine; T_4, thyroxine; *TRH*, Thyrotropin-releasing hormone. (Modified from Klee GG, Hay ID: Assessment of sensitive thyrotropin assays for an expanded role in thyroid function testing: proposed criteria for analytic performance and clinical utility. J Clin Endocrinol Metab 1987; 64:461-471.)

assay is now the accepted initial screening test of thyroid function in ambulatory individuals with normal pituitary function; TSH levels are high in cases of hypothyroidism and low with hyperthyroidism. FT_4 testing can be ordered when the TSH level is abnormally high or low (Figure 40-4). This TSH-centered strategy for the initial evaluation of thyroid function is both cost effective and efficient.[2,5]

Most laboratory tests for thyroid function are available commercially in kit forms. For detailed descriptions of methods, the reader is referred to the expanded version of this chapter[26] or the documentation accompanying commercial products.

Determination of Thyroid-Stimulating Hormone

Principles

Immunoassay is the standard procedure for the measurement of serum TSH in the clinical laboratory. The older radioimmunoassay (RIA) methods for TSH were based on competition between endogenous and radio-labeled hormone for binding sites on a limited amount of antibody. In such methods the amount of labeled TSH bound to the antibody is inversely related to the amount of unlabeled TSH present in the serum specimen. Most RIAs, however, do not distinguish normal values from subnormal values associated with hyperthyroidism. New immunometric techniques now are capable of measuring TSH at levels that routine clinical laboratories need to detect low levels of serum TSH. These new sensitive methods resulted from the application of the immunometric sandwich configuration, in which a serum TSH molecule forms a bridge between two or more distinct anti-TSH antibodies. The first antibody (of monoclonal origin) often is directed at the specific β-subunit and is anchored to a solid-phase separation system. This antibody is

hormone have resulted in high levels of serum TSH. Similarly, mild degrees of thyroid hormone excess have resulted in very low TSH concentrations. This inverse log-linear relationship explains why some individuals may have normal FT_4 levels and few clinical signs or symptoms of thyroid dysfunction but TSH levels that are abnormally high or low. Not all such "subclinical" thyroid disease warrants treatment, but detection of even mild thyroid function change is important for some individuals.[25]

Improvements in assay technology have altered the approach to thyroid function testing. Instead of thyroid function assessment beginning with a T_4 test, a sensitive TSH present in excess and selectively immunoextracts the majority of TSH molecules from the serum specimen. Bound hormone then is quantitated by use of a second TSH antibody (of either monoclonal or polyclonal origin) that is directed against a different antigenic site on the TSH molecule (for example, the α-subunit). Most procedures label the detection antibody with peroxidase or alkaline phosphatase; sensitive photometric, fluorescent, or chemiluminescent substrates commonly are used to measure enzyme activity. Nonisotopic methods also are available based on direct labeling of antibody with chemiluminescent compounds, such as acridinium esters; fluorescent labels, such as europium chelates; or bioluminescent molecules, such as recombinant aequorin (see Chapter 10). In contrast to RIAs, immunometric assays have positive dose-response curves, with higher levels of signal corresponding to higher concentrations of TSH.

Immunometric assays for TSH are available commercially as manual kit procedures or for use on automated systems. Immunometric assays are more sensitive for TSH measurement and offer rapid turnaround time and a wider linear measurement range, as compared with traditional RIA methods. International Reference Preparation (80/558) and a recombinant TSH (94/674) are available to calibrate TSH assays.[18]

A "generational" classification based on the lowest TSH value detectable with a 20% or less interassay coefficient of variation often is used to describe TSH assays. Each generation of assay represents one log improvement in its detection limit. Thus the first-generation RIAs had a functional detection limit of 1 to 2 mU/L and could distinguish reliably among normal and hypothyroid TSH values. Subsequent immunometric assays had about a tenfold improvement in their functional detection limits (0.1 to 0.2 mU/L) and are considered second-generation TSH assays.

Second-generation assays reliably distinguish normal from both hyperthyroid and hypothyroid TSH values in ambulatory individuals; however, they have limited benefit for distinguishing mildly subnormal values (0.01 to 0.1 mU/L) from the very low values (<0.01 mU/L) that are typical of thyrotoxicosis (severe hyperthyroidism). Third-generation immunometric assays have even lower detection limits; most use chemiluminescent signal detection technologies on automated platforms and have functional detection limits of less than 0.02 mU/L.[22]

Third-generation assays distinguish mildly subnormal TSH values (such as may be seen in euthyroid hospitalized patients with nonthyroidal illness [NTI]) from the very low values of frank hyperthyroidism. In addition, third-generation TSH assays are helpful in classifying hyperthyroid individuals according to their degrees of TSH suppression. They help in the monitoring of thyroid cancer patients who are receiving thyroid medication and who require complete suppression of TSH and monitoring of the adequacy of thyroid hormone replacement in hypothyroid individuals.

Specimen requirements

Serum that is free of hemolysis and lipemia is preferred. Specimens are stable for 5 days at 2 to 8 °C and for at least 1 month when stored frozen. For newborn screening, whole blood is collected by heel puncture 48 to 72 hours after birth.

Reference intervals

TSH is secreted in a circadian fashion. In adults the highest levels prevail at night between 2 and 4 AM, and the lowest levels occur between 1700 and 1800 hours; low-amplitude oscillations also occur throughout the day. TSH measurements are not affected by variations in thyroid hormone-binding proteins. Reference intervals for TSH are listed in the following table:

	mU/L
Prematures, 28 to 36 wk (first week of life)	0.7 to 27.0
Cord blood (>37 wk)	2.3 to 13.2
Children	
Birth to 4 days	1.0 to 39.0
2 to 20 wk	1.7 to 9.1
21 wk to 20 y	0.7 to 64.0
Adults	
21 to 54 y	0.4 to 4.2
55 to 87 y	0.5 to 8.9
Pregnancy	
First trimester	0.3 to 4.5
Second trimester	0.5 to 4.6
Third trimester	0.8 to 5.2

Determination of Thyroxine

Principle

Competitive immunoassays are the methods of choice in the clinical laboratory for the measurement of total T_4; they measure both free and protein-bound T_4.[17] Accurate measurement of total hormone requires dissociation of T_4 from its serum transport proteins. Blocking agents, such as 8-anilino-1-naphthalene-sulfonic (ANS) acid, salicylate, thimerosal (Merthiolate), and phenytoin are used to inhibit binding of T_4 to TBG. Binding of T_4 to TBPA is overcome by the use of barbital buffers. Many T_4 immunoassays use polyclonal antisera produced against an albumin-T_4 conjugate; monoclonal antibodies against T_4 also are available. Both isotopic and nonisotopic methods are available.

Isotopic methods

Radioactive iodine (^{125}I) has been used widely as an immunoassay marker to follow and measure the distribution of T_4 between unbound and antibody-bound fractions. In practice, isotopic methods have been replaced by nonisotopic ones.

Nonisotopic methods

Nonisotopic assays for T_4 are available commercially; many have been developed for use on fully automated immunoassay systems or are compatible with existing chemistry analyzers. A variety of sensitive labels are used to construct these nonisotopic assays. For example, enzymes such as horseradish peroxidase, alkaline phosphatase, and galactosidase are used widely as labels, as are fluorescent and chemiluminescent molecules. Both heterogeneous and homogeneous enzyme immunoassays are available.

Heterogeneous assays require physical separation of free and bound T_4, and a variety of solid-phase supports are used. An assortment of photometric, fluorescent, and luminescent substrates are available for monitoring of the enzyme activity of the antibody-bound fraction. In contrast, homogeneous enzyme immunoassays do not require physical separation of free and bound T_4. These procedures are rapid and simple to use and also have been applied to several major automated instruments. Examples of such assays are the enzyme-multiplied immunoassay technique (EMIT) and the cloned enzyme donor immunoassay (CEDIA).

Fluorescent molecules also are used as labels in both heterogeneous and homogenous fluorescent immunoassays for T_4. Heterogeneous fluorescent immunoassays for T_4 are based on lanthanide rare earth ions (europium chelates) and time-resolved fluorescence. Fluorescence polarization immunoassay is an example of a homogenous technique. In addition, chemiluminescent molecules are used as direct labels for T_4 immunoassays, such as chemiluminescent aryl acridinium ester or electrochemiluminescent ruthenium tris(bipyridyl) ester. Particle-enhanced immunoassays involving turbidimetric measurements also have been developed for measurement of T_4 in serum.

By itself, the total T_4 level does not provide adequate clinical information. In practice an FT_4E (for example, thyroid hormone binding ratio [THBR] and calculated FT_4 index) should be reported with every total T_4 measurement.

Specimen requirements

Serum is the preferred specimen used in the measurement of T_4. Plasma with ethylenediaminetetraacetic acid (EDTA) or heparin as anticoagulant also may be used. T_4 in serum is quite stable; storage of serum specimens at room temperature up to 7 days results in no appreciable loss of T_4. However, storage at 2 to 8 °C or freezing of the specimen is recommended. Frozen specimens are stable for at least 30 days. Repeated freezing and thawing of the specimens should be avoided. Grossly hemolyzed specimens should not be used, and turbid samples should be centrifuged before testing. Individuals undergoing therapy for thyroid disorders should stop treatment 1 month before sampling if a true baseline is to be established. T_4 autoantibodies interfere and have produced artificially low or high results. Specimens are obtained from infants by heel puncture and collected in capillary tubes or on filter paper.

Reference intervals

Reference intervals for T_4 are listed in the following table:

	μg/dL	nmol/L
Cord blood	7.4 to 13.0	95 to 168
Children		
1 to 3 days	11.8 to 22.6	152 to 292
1 to 2 wk	9.8 to 16.6	126 to 214
1 to 4 mo	7.2 to 14.4	93 to 186
4 to 12 mo	7.8 to 16.5	101 to 213
1 to 5 y	7.3 to 15.0	94 to 194
5 to 10 y	6.4 to 13.3	83 to 172
10 to 15 y	5.6 to 11.7	72 to 151
Adults (15 to 60 y)		
Men	4.6 to 10.5	59 to 135
Women	5.5 to 11.0	65 to 138
>60 y	5.0 to 10.7	65 to 138
Newborn screen (whole blood)		
1 to 5 days	>7.5	>97
6 days	>6.5	>84

NOTE: Reference intervals for newborns should be developed by each laboratory that provides screening for neonatal hypothyroidism.

Determination of Triiodothyronine in Serum
Principles

Isotopic and nonisotopic immunoassays are the methods of choice used to measure total T_3 concentrations. Procedures are similar to those described for T_4, except that a ^{125}I-T_3 tracer and T_3-specific antibody are used. Solid-phase systems are preferred to liquid-phase separation systems. As with the T_4 methods, most T_3 methods use ANS to release T_3 from serum binding proteins without disturbing the binding of T_3 to antibody. A typical calibration curve ranges from 25 to 800 ng/dL.

Nonisotopic assays similar to those described for serum T_4 have been applied to the measurement of T_3. Most commercial methods use peroxidase or alkaline phosphatase to label T_3 antigens or T_3 antibodies; enzyme activity is determined commonly by use of a variety of sensitive photometric, fluorescent, or chemiluminescent substrates. Immunoassays for T_3 that use direct fluorescent and chemiluminescent labels also are available.

Typical coefficients of variation for interassay performance are 5% to 7%; the assay detection limit is approximately 10 ng/dL. Most T_3 immunoassays have negligible cross-reactivity with T_4, thus permitting direct measurement of T_3 in serum specimens. T_3 autoantibodies interfere with some assays.

Different T_3 immunoassays may exhibit unexplained discrepancies between values for the same sera. Many factors have been suggested as causes of these discrepancies, including differences in antisera cross-reactivity, protein interferences, and different assay limits of detection. T_3 methods are discussed in more detail in the expanded version of this chapter.[26]

The major clinical roles for total T_3 measurements are in the diagnosis and monitoring of hyperthyroid individuals with suppressed TSH and normal FT_4 concentrations, such as those seen in individuals with T_3-thyrotoxicosis.[8] Serum total T_3 measurements play only a limited role in euthyroid and hypothyroid individuals.

Specimen requirements

Requirements are the same as those previously described for T_4.

Reference intervals

Reference intervals[26] for T_3 may vary from one procedure and reference population to another. Each laboratory should establish its own reference intervals. The following T_3 reference intervals have been obtained through use of an RIA method:[26]

	ng/dL	nmol/L
Cord blood (>37 wk)	5 to 141	0.08 to 2.17
Children		
1 to 3 days	100 to 740	1.54 to 11.40
1 to 11 mo	105 to 245	1.62 to 3.77
1 to 5 y	105 to 269	1.62 to 4.14
6 to 10 y	94 to 241	1.45 to 3.71
11 to 15 y	82 to 213	1.26 to 3.28
Adolescents		
16 to 20 y	80 to 210	1.23 to 3.23
Adults		
20 to 50 y	70 to 204	1.08 to 3.14
50 to 90 y	40 to 181	0.62 to 2.79
Pregnancy		
First trimester	81 to 190	1.25 to 2.93
Second and third trimesters	100 to 260	1.54 to 4.00

Determination of Free Thyroid Hormones

T_4 and T_3 circulate in the blood as equilibrium mixtures of free and protein-bound hormones. Changes in the concentration or affinity of TBG or other transport proteins profoundly affect the total hormone concentration in serum. The steady-state level of the free hormone is independent of these binding protein variations and remains almost constant.

The interaction between free thyroid hormones and their thyroid-binding proteins (TBPs), such as TBG, TBPA, and albumin, conforms to a reversible binding equilibrium that is described by the following mass action relationship:

$$[FT_4] \times [TBP] = K \times [T_4:TBP]$$

where

$[FT_4]$ = Concentration of free T_4 in serum
$[TBP]$ = Concentration of unoccupied binding sites on TBP
K = Association constant

$[T_4:TBP]$ = Concentration of T_4-occupied binding sites on TBP

The relationships among these entities have important diagnostic implications. A primary increase in either $[FT_4]$ or $[TBP]$ drives this reaction to the right, increasing serum $[T_4:TBP]$. The value of $[T_4:TBP]$ is considered equivalent to that of total T_4 because 99.97% of the total T_4 is bound to TBP. Hyperthyroidism produces a primary increase in FT_4, whereas estrogens and idiopathic or genetic conditions may produce a primary increase in TBP. In both cases, $[T_4:TBP]$ increases, but in the former the individual is ill and requires treatment; in the latter the individual is euthyroid. Likewise a low serum $[T_4:TBP]$ may be due to a primary decrease in $[FT_4]$ or to a primary decrease in $[TBP]$. Therefore differentiation between changes in $[T_4:TBP]$ that are due to primary changes in $[FT_4]$ (for example, hyperthyroidism or hypothyroidism) and those that are due to primary changes in $[TBP]$ are clinically important.

Numerous methods have been proposed for the assessment of the concentrations of FT_4 and FT_3 in serum.[3] These include direct assays that currently serve as reference methods, indirect assays for routine use, and uptake methods. Special reports from the Nomenclature Committee of the American Thyroid Association[6] and the National Academy of Clinical Biochemistry[20] discuss some of the issues and concerns regarding free thyroid hormone measurements.

Direct reference methods

Free hormone concentrations are exceedingly low in normal serum (approximately 0.03% of the total serum T_4 and 0.3% of the total serum T_3 concentrations), and a sensitive method with a low limit of detection is required to measure subpicomole amounts. In practice the most reliable methods used to measure FT_4 and FT_3 in serum are equilibrium dialysis and ultrafiltration methods that physically separate free hormone from protein-bound hormone before direct measurement of the free fraction by immunoassay or chromatographic analysis.[17] Only minimal dilution of serum specimens is allowed; dilution alters the binding of drugs, free fatty acids, and other substances to serum proteins, thus disturbing the equilibrium between bound and free hormone.[4] FT_4 assays based on direct equilibrium dialysis or ultrafiltration are unaffected by either variations in serum binding proteins or by thyroid hormone autoantibodies.

Principles

In the simplified equilibrium dialysis method, undiluted serum specimens are dialyzed for 16 to 18 hours at 37 °C in a reusable dialysis chamber. The dialysis buffer provides for minimal changes in the serum matrix. The dialysate then is analyzed directly with a sensitive immunoassay. The reportable range is 2 to 128 ng/L (2.6 to 165 pmol/L), and the interassay coefficient of variation is approximately 7%.

The second method is an ultrafiltration procedure in which the serum specimen is adjusted to pH 7.4, incubated for 20 minutes at 37 °C (to achieve equilibrium of the binding at this temperature), applied to an ultrafiltration device, centrifuged for 30 minutes at 37 °C and 2000 $\times$ g, and the ultrafiltrate analyzed for T_4.

Specimen requirements
Requirements are the same as those previously described for T_4.

Reference intervals
Expected values for FT_4 by use of direct equilibrium dialysis are as follows:

	ng/dL	pmol/L
Newborns (1 to 4 days)	2.2 to 5.3	28.4 to 68.4
Children (2 wk to 20 y)	0.8 to 2.0	10.3 to 25.8
Adults (21 to 87 y)	0.8 to 2.7	10.3 to 34.7
Pregnancy		
First trimester	0.7 to 2.0	9.0 to 25.7
Second and third trimesters	0.5 to 1.6	6.4 to 20.6

Indirect methods for estimation of free thyroid hormones
Most methods used to assess FT_4 and FT_3 concentrations in serum are estimates. These approaches often are more convenient and less expensive than reference methods, and many are available in kit form. Two test strategies currently are used for indirect estimation of the concentrations of free hormones—index methods and immunoextraction assays.

Index methods use two separate tests to estimate the free hormone concentration—a total serum T_4 (or T_3) measurement and an assessment of either the serum TBG level or the free hormone fraction (the latter traditionally derived by use of equilibrium tracer dialysis or uptake methods). Results of these tests then are combined mathematically to provide estimates of the free hormone concentration.

Two-step and one-step immunoassays estimate free hormone concentrations indirectly by use of antibody extraction techniques. Although a frequent claim or implication is that these immunoextraction assays measure FT_4 or FT_4 directly, virtually all methods do so indirectly by relating test results to extracted serum calibrators, the free hormone values of which have been measured independently with reference methods.

Free hormone fraction by indirect equilibrium tracer dialysis
Several isotopic methods are used to estimate the free hormone fraction accurately, including equilibrium tracer dialysis, ultrafiltration, and gel chromatography. Equilibrium tracer dialysis is considered to provide a true measurement of the free hormone fraction. Unfortunately, the free hormone fraction as estimated in normal sera by this technique varies substantially among laboratories. Additional details for this method can by found in an expanded version of this chapter.[26]

Reference values with this method for free T_4 fraction (%FT_4) vary between 0.02% and 0.04% of total hormone concentration. Because T_3 is bound less firmly by TBG than is T_4, the dialyzable fraction of T_3 is appreciably greater (by almost 10 times) than that of T_4. Thus the reference interval for free T_3 fraction (%FT_3) is 0.2% to 0.4%.

Calculation of free hormone estimates
The free hormone fraction, as measured by dialysis or ultrafiltration of diluted serum containing tracer T_4 or T_3, is multiplied by the respective total hormone concentration to obtain indirect estimates of FT_4 or FT_3.

$$FT_4E = total\ T_4 \times \%FT_4$$
$$FT_3E = total\ T_3 \times \%FT_3$$

With equilibrium tracer dialysis the expected reference interval for FT_4 in adults is 0.8 to 2.3 ng/dL (10 to 30 pmol/L) and 260 to 480 pg/dL (4.0-7.4 pmol/L) for FT_3.

Free hormone fraction by uptake methods (thyroid hormone binding ratio)
Principle
Uptake tests are used to estimate the number of unoccupied (unsaturated) thyroid hormone-binding sites on serum proteins. Values obtained by uptake methods are expressed as a THBR that is considered directly proportional to the free hormone fraction. Measurement of THBR, in conjunction with a total hormone concentration, is an accurate and clinically useful indirect method used to calculate the FT_4 (or FT_3) index. Both isotopic and nonisotopic methods are available for estimation of the THBR.

Isotopic methods. Different radioactive tracer methods have been used to estimate the unsaturated thyroid hormone-binding capacity. The simplest is the T_3 uptake test.[26] Traditionally this test is performed by measurement of the distribution of radiolabeled T_3 between serum binding proteins and a solid-phase binding material. In a typical assay a diluted sample of patient serum is allowed to equilibrate with a trace amount of ^{125}I-T_3 and the secondary binder. A portion of the radioactive T_3 binds to empty binding sites on TBG, and the remainder attaches to the solid matrix. At the end of a specific incubation period the reactants are separated, and the proportion of radioactivity bound by the solid matrix (the "uptake") is measured. The amount of T_3 tracer bound to the secondary binder varies inversely with the number of unoccupied TBG binding sites in the serum specimen and directly with the free fraction of T_4 and T_3.

Nonisotopic methods. Several commercial T_4 and T_3 uptake assays use nonisotopic tracers. Most use enzymes to tag T_4 or T_3. A variety of photometric, fluorescent, and luminescent substrates are available for monitoring of the resultant enzyme activity. Assays that utilize direct labeling of T_4 or T_3 antigens with fluorophores or chemiluminescent molecules also are available. These nonisotopic methods are generically named *T uptake* assays, regardless of whether T_4 or T_3 is used as the labeled analog. The competitive binder commonly used in many of these assays is a T_4 antibody. Some methods probe the total binding capacity of all thyroid hormone binding proteins, but most estimate the concentration of unoccupied TBG binding sites.

Specimen requirements

The preferred specimen is serum. Specimens may be stored at 4 °C for 1 week or at −20 °C for 30 days.

Reference intervals

Although centered on a ratio of 1.0, reference values for THBR differ by method and local population. Therefore each laboratory should establish its own reference intervals. The following values are representative:

	THBR
Cord blood	0.75 to 1.05
Infants/children	
1 to 3 days	0.90 to 1.40
1 to 2 wk	0.85 to 1.15
1 to 4 mo	0.75 to 1.05
1 to 15 y	0.88 to 1.12
Adult	
>50 y	0.83 to 1.15
Male	0.87 to 1.11
Female	0.80 to 1.04
Pregnancy (last 5 mo)	0.68 to 0.87

Comments

To improve the understanding of T uptake results from different laboratories, the Committee on Nomenclature of the American Thyroid Association has recommended that uptake results for individuals be normalized to those of a control serum (or reference serum pool) obtained from euthyroid individuals who have normal quantities of TBPs.[10] The quotient of these results is proportional to the free fraction of T_4 or T_3 in serum and is known properly as the *THBR*. A value of 1.0 indicates that the two values are identical. Some laboratories prepare their own normal reference serum pool to analyze in every assay run. This step enables the laboratory to maintain consistency in T uptake values in case of changes in assay procedure or kit components. Other laboratories determine a mean T uptake value for their own local reference populations to use in the calculation of the THBR. Terms such as *T_3-resin uptake* or *T_3 uptake* are a continuing source of confusion and should not be used.

In cases of hyperthyroidism, more binding sites—and with hypothyroidism, fewer binding sites—on TBG are occupied by T_4. As a result the THBR is high in individuals with hyperthyroidism and low in those with hypothyroid-

TABLE 40-3   Diagnostic Utility of THBR and FT₄ Index

Clinical Condition	Total T_4	THBR	FT_4I
Euthyroid	N	N	N
Hyperthyroid	↑	↑	↑
Hypothyroid	↓	↓	↓
Increased TBG	↑	↓	N
Decreased TBG	↓	↑	N

THBR, Thyroid hormone binding ratio; *T_4,* thyroxine; *FT_4I,* free thyroxine index; *N,* normal; ↑, increase; ↓, decrease; *TBG;* thyroxine-binding globulin.

ism. In cases of decreased and increased TBG (see Table 40-1) the THBR is high and low, respectively. Deviations of THBR and total T_4 in the same direction from normal (a condition known as *concordant variance*) suggest an abnormality in thyroid hormone production. Deviations in opposite directions (a discordant variance) suggest a primary change in the concentration or affinity of circulating TBG (Table 40-3).

Calculation of free thyroxine and free triiodothyronine index

The THBR assay is not designed for use as an independent test for thyroid disease. It is useful only when combined mathematically with a total T_4 level to calculate an FT_4 index (FT_4I), as follows:

$$FT_4I = [T_4] \times THBR$$

The FT_3 index is calculated as is the FT_4 index, $[T_3] \times THBR$, and is used in the same way as an estimate of FT_3. In general the FT_3 index offers no advantage over the FT_4 index and is used less frequently in clinical practice.

Reference intervals are numerically close to the reference intervals for total T_4 or T_3. Most automated immunoassay analyzers are capable of performing the THBR and total T_4 tests with online calculation of the FT_4I. Theoretically, because the calculated indices are products of T_4 or T_3 concentrations and a ratio, they have concentration units. However, to avoid confusion with serum T_4 or T_3, the free hormone index units usually are omitted or termed *index units*. Typical values are as follows:

	FT_4 Index	
	μg/dL	nmol/L
Cord blood	6.0 to 13.2	77 to 170
Infants		
1 to 3 days	9.9 to 17.5	128 to 226
1 wk	7.5 to 15.1	97 to 195
1 to 12 mo	5.0 to 13.0	65 to 168
Children		
1 to 10 y	5.4 to 12.8	70 to 165
Pubertal child and adult	4.2 to 13.0	54 to 168

Calculation of T_4/TBG and T_3/TBG ratios

Measurements of serum TBG concentration are used to calculate a T_4/TBG or T_3/TBG ratio. Such indices are derived from mass action expressions and used to approximate FT_4 or FT_3 concentrations. These ratios correlate variably with FT_4 or FT_3 levels and are particularly useful in sera with altered TBG concentrations. The reference interval for T_4/TBG ratios is 3.8 to 4.5 when the reference intervals for total T_4 and TBG are 4.5 to 12.5 µg/dL and 1.2 to 2.8 mg/dL, respectively.

Direct immunoextraction assays used to estimate free thyroid hormones

Immunoassays used in the estimation of free thyroid hormones are categorized as two-step and one-step ("analog") assays. Each procedure involves the direct incubation of serum with a specific anti-T_4 or anti-T_3 antibody. During the incubation period, thyroid hormones reach a new equilibrium, with all the binders present. The amount of immunoextracted T_4 or T_3 closely approximates the undisturbed free hormone concentration that preexists in serum at equilibrium.

Two-step immunoassays

Two-step methods require two processing steps (Figure 40-5). In the first the specimen is incubated briefly with specific antibody; a percentage of the total thyroid hormone proportional to the original FT_4 or FT_3 concentration is extracted and bound by the solid-phase antibody. After washing of the solid phase to remove serum proteins and other interfering substances, a second step estimates the remaining unoccupied (vacant) antibody binding sites by back-titration with labeled T_4 or T_3. Excess label then is washed away, and the quantity of bound tracer is compared with a calibration curve generated from secondary calibrators that have had target values assigned by a reference method. The amount of labeled hormone retained by the antibody is inversely related to the free hormone concentration in the test specimen.

The key feature of a two-step method is that the labeled hormone is prevented physically from interacting with serum binding proteins. This prevention ensures that antibody binding of tracer is governed solely by the free hormone concentration and not by changes in thyroid hormone-binding proteins.

One-step immunoassays

Single-step techniques are available in labeled hormone analog and labeled antibody formats. Both approaches use structurally modified analogs of T_4 or T_3 that theoretically retain the ability to compete with free hormone for binding to specific anti-T_4 or anti-T_3 antibodies but are restricted chemically from interacting with thyroid hormone-binding proteins in the serum specimen. Unlike two-step methods,

1. First incubation step

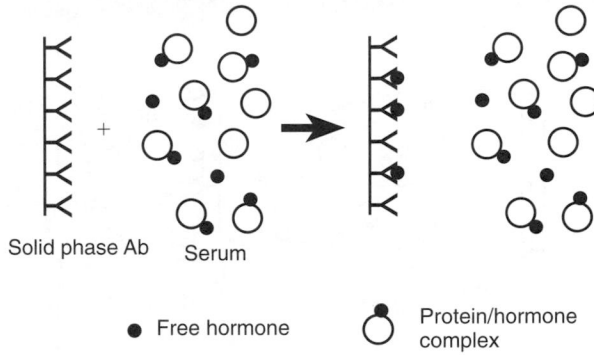

Solid phase Ab   Serum

● Free hormone   ◒ Protein/hormone complex

2. Separation of serum from antibody; washing

3. Second incubation step

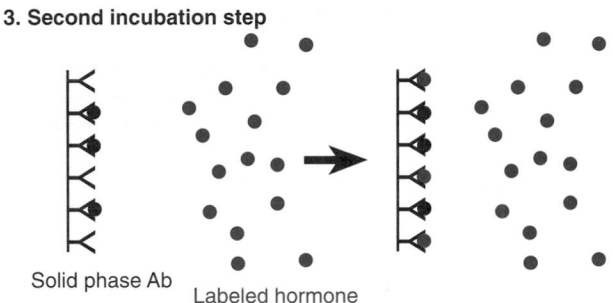

Solid phase Ab   Labeled hormone

4. Separation of labeled hormone from antibody; washing

5. Measurement of antibody-bound activity

Figure 40-5   Summary of a two-step free thyroxine (T_4) immunoassay. After incubation with serum and solid-phase antibody, the serum is removed and the antibody washed, followed by incubation with labeled T_4 to determine empty antibody binding sites. *Ab,* Antibody. (Modified from Ekins R: Free hormone measurement. Part 2. Methods. Endocrinology and Metabolism In-Service Training and Continuing Education Program. AACC Press 1993; 11:181-191.)

analog assays rely on simultaneous rather than sequential back-titration of unoccupied antibody binding sites. For one-step methods to succeed the hormone analog should not displace T_4 (or T_3) from binding proteins; binding of the hormone analog by serum proteins must be either totally absent or essentially insignificant.

Labeled-analog methods. In a typical one-step RIA for FT_4, endogenous free hormone and a ^{125}I-labeled T_4 analog compete for antibody binding sites; the amount of labeled analog bound by the specific antibody is inversely related to the amount of FT_4 in the specimen (Figure 40-6). Test results are expressed relative to secondary serum calibrators that have been calibrated with reference techniques. Abnormal amounts of any substance affecting analog binding, such as endogenous antibody, nonesterified fatty acids, or certain anions, greatly distort assay results.

1. Incubation

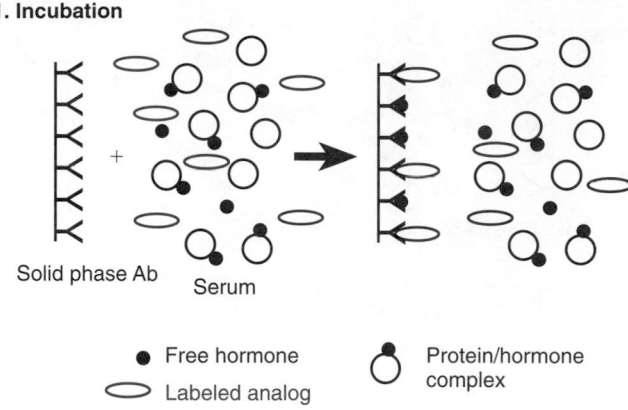

Solid phase Ab   Serum

● Free hormone   ● Protein/hormone
                        ○ complex
○ Labeled analog

2. Separation of serum from antibody; washing

3. Measurement of antibody-bound activity

Figure 40-6   One-step free thyroxine (T_4) immunoassay using labeled analog and solid-phase antibody. *Ab,* Antibody. (Modified from Ekins R: Free hormone measurement. Part 2. Methods. Endocrinology and Metabolism In-Service Training and Continuing Education Program. AACC Press 1993; 11:181-191.)

1. Incubation

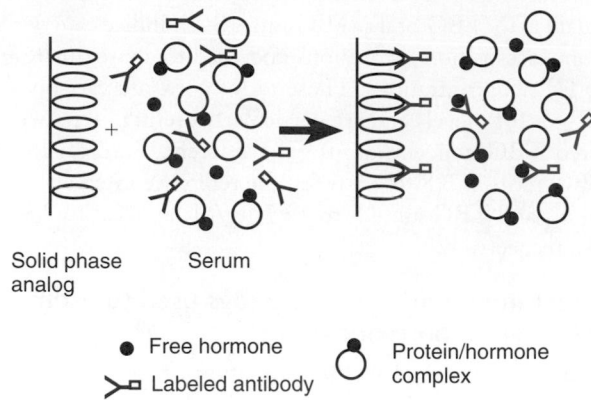

Solid phase   Serum
analog

● Free hormone   ○ Protein/hormone
                        ● complex
⊱▭ Labeled antibody

2. Separation of serum from solid phase analog; washing

3. Measurement of analog-bound activity

Figure 40-7   One-step free hormone immunoassay using labeled antibody and solid-phase analog. (Modified from Ekins R: Free hormone measurement. Part 2. Methods. Endocrinology and Metabolism In-Service Training and Continuing Education Program. AACC Press 1993; 11:181-191.)

Labeled-antibody methods. A number of labeled antibody methods have been developed in which the distribution of a labeled antibody between exogenous solid-phase hormone and free hormone reflects the free hormone concentration (Figure 40-7). This assay design is similar to the labeled-analog principle except that unoccupied antibody-binding sites are identified by their absorption from the reaction mixture onto a hormone analog coupled to a solid support. Linking of T_4 or T_3 to the solid phase creates a macroanalog with a reduced interaction with serum proteins. These labeled-antibody assays are claimed to be less sensitive than labeled-analog methods to protein modifications or progressive serum dilution.

Reference intervals

Expected values by use of a one-step immunochemiluminometric assay are as follows:

- For FT_4, 0.8 to 2.3 ng/dL (10 to 30 pmol/L)
- For FT_3, 230 to 420 pg/dL (3.5 to 6.5 pmol/L)

Selection and use of tests to measure free thyroid hormones

Estimates of FT_4 and FT_3 generally give results that are comparable with those of direct reference methods in healthy individuals, hyperthyroid and hypothyroid individuals, and those individuals with only mild binding protein abnormalities.[13] In these individuals the selection of a specific FT_4 or FT_3 measurement method is based on factors that include technical convenience, turnaround time, com-

mercial availability, and cost. With certain clinical conditions, however, estimated methods may give results that differ from the generally normal values obtained with direct reference methods. These abnormalities, summarized in Table 40-4, are encountered commonly in euthyroid individuals who show significant changes in T_4 or T_3 binding to serum proteins. In these situations the selection of appropriate FT_4 or FT_3 estimate methods should be based more on their analytical and diagnostic reliability than on the ease of performance and cost.

Determination of Thyroxine-Binding Globulin

Of the thyroid hormone binding proteins, TBG has the greatest affinity for T_4 and is the most important in regulating free T_4 concentration. Estrogen-induced TBG excess and congenital TBG deficiency are the most significant TBG abnormalities (see Table 40-1).

Principles

TBG is measured indirectly in terms of its T_4-binding capacity or directly by assessment of the protein concentration of TBG. Direct measurement of the protein concentration of TBG by immunoassay is technically less complex and offers increased precision and immunospecificity. Commercial kits based on both isotopic and nonisotopic formats are available.

TBG tests that use labeled T_4 in a two-site immunoradiometric assay (IRMA) format also have been developed. Individuals with molecular variants of TBG may have

TABLE 40-4   FT$_4$ Measurements in Common Conditions Affecting TBPs

Clinical Condition	Direct Equilibrium Dialysis/RIA*	Other Index Methods	Two-Step Methods	Analog Methods
Near-Normal Concentration of Serum Binding Proteins				
Hypothyroidism	L	L	L	L
Hyperthyroidism	H	H	H	H
Hyperestrogenism	N	N	N	N
Abnormal Concentration of Serum Binding Proteins				
TBG excess	N	H	N	L, N, or H
TBG deficiency	N	L	N	L, N, or H
Dysalbuminemia	N	N to H†	N	H
Hypoalbuminemia	N	N	N	N to L
T$_4$ autoantibody	N	H	N	L
Low T$_4$ NTI	H	L	N to L	L
High T$_4$ NTI	N to H	N to H	N to H	H

From Hay ID, Bayer MF, Kaplan MK et al: American Thyroid Association Assessment of current free thyroid hormone and thyrotropin measurement and guidelines for future clinical assays. Clin Chem 1991; 37:2002-2008.
FT$_4$, Free thyroxine; *TBPs*, thyroid-binding proteins; *RIA*, radioimmunoassay; *TBG*, thyroxine-binding globulin; *L*, low; *H*, high; *N*, normal; *NTI*, nonthyroidal illness; *T$_4$*, thyroxine.
*Methods involving minimal dilution.
†Normal when determined with labeled T$_4$; high when with labeled T$_3$.

discordant results, but the assay is not affected by excess T$_4$ or phenytoin. The specimen and storage criteria that have been discussed previously for T$_4$ also apply to TBG measurements.

Reference intervals

Binding capacity of TBG for T$_4$ in normal serum generally varies from 10 to 25 mg/dL; of prealbumin for T$_4$, from 49 to 70 mg/dL; and of albumin for T$_4$, from 12 to 34 mg/dL.

Determination of Thyroglobulin

Tg is a large glycoprotein (molecular weight [MW] 660 kD) that is stored in the follicular colloid of the thyroid gland. Tg is elevated in individuals with thyroid follicular and papillary carcinoma, thyroid adenoma, subacute thyroiditis, Hashimoto's **thyroiditis,** and **Graves' disease.** Serial measurement of Tg is most useful in the detection of recurrence of differentiated thyroid carcinoma after surgical resection or radioactive iodine ablation.

Principle

Circulating levels of Tg can be measured with double-antibody RIAs and two-site immunometric assays. Commercial kits based on these techniques are available.

A major difficulty in most Tg immunoassays is interference due to endogenous anti-Tg antibodies present in about 15% to 35% of individuals with thyroid cancer. Interference effects can be substantial, causing either an overestimation

or underestimation of the true value.[23] With newer immunometric assays this effect is generally an underestimation. All serum samples must be screened for the presence of anti-Tg with a sensitive immunoassay. When detected, the concentration of such antibodies is reported, and a warning is issued to interpret the serum Tg value with caution.

Specimen requirements

The specimen collection and storage criteria that have been discussed previously for T$_4$ also apply to Tg measurements. Individuals should discontinue thyroid hormone replacement therapy long enough to achieve an elevated TSH level before specimen collection (for example, 6 weeks).

Reference intervals

The reference interval for Tg for a euthyroid individual is 3 to 42 ng/mL (3 to 42 mg/L); 87% of normal adults have serum levels less than 10 ng/mL. For athyroidic individuals not receiving T$_4$ replacement therapy the upper limit of the reference interval is set at less than or equal to 5 ng/mL. Levels are high in the neonate and decrease significantly during the first 2 years of life.

Serum Tg values obtained by different methods are usually not interchangeable, and the same assay should be used to perform serial serum Tg measurements in a patient.

Determination of Antithyroid Antibodies

Antithyroid antibodies are found in a variety of thyroid disorders and in other autoimmune diseases and certain malignancies. These autoantibodies are directed against several thyroid and thyroid hormone antigens, including Tg, thyroidal microsomal antigen, the TSH receptor, a non-Tg colloid antigen, TSH, and T$_4$. Of these antibodies, only antithyroglobulin (anti Tg) and antimicrosomal antibodies are used commonly in the evaluation of thyroid disorders.

Antithyroglobulin antibodies

Principles

In the tanned erythrocyte hemagglutination method used to measure anti-Tg antibodies an aliquot of patient serum is mixed with erythrocytes that have been treated with tannic acid and then coated with purified human Tg. When antibodies in the serum combine with Tg bound to erythrocytes, agglutination of the erythrocytes occurs. The use of Tg-coated erythrocytes makes this agglutination reaction much more sensitive than a simple antigen-antibody reaction. Several commercial kits are available for the measurement of anti-Tg antibodies in serum.

Serial dilutions of the patient serum are used to establish a Tg antibody titer. The reported result is the highest dilution that causes agglutination. Titers usually are considered negative at a dilution ratio less than 1:10. This hemagglutination test is not highly specific, and about 5% to 10% of the normal population may have a low titer of Tg antibodies. Reactivity occurs more frequently in individuals with Hashimoto's thyroiditis (>85%) and Graves' disease (>30%); titers greater than 1:1600 are common.

RIA, enzyme-linked immunosorbent assay (ELISA), and chemiluminescent immunoassays also have been developed for the measurement of anti-Tg antibodies. Several are available as commercial kits. These methods correlate well with agglutination tests but are generally more sensitive and more specific for thyroid autoimmune diseases.

Specimen requirements

The preferred specimen for testing is serum, which should be kept frozen if the test is not performed on the day that the blood is drawn.

Reference intervals

Assessment of a reference interval for anti-Tg antibodies is controversial, mainly because Tg autoantibodies may be found in healthy individuals without apparent thyroid disease. Variable reference intervals have been reported, depending on whether a random population was sampled or a population without present or previous thyroid disease. Tg antibodies follow a logarithmic normal distribution and usually are expressed as units per milliliter. With IRMA and ELISA assays, values less than 5 U/mL are considered nonreactive for Tg autoantibody. With sensitive chemiluminescence assays, values are less than 2 U/mL in normal sera. With the introduction of antithyroid peroxidase (anti-TPO) antibody assays, the measurement of anti-Tg adds little diagnostic information to the definition of autoimmune thyroid disease. However, measurement of anti-Tg is needed to identify sera with autoantibodies that may interfere with serum Tg measurements.

Antimicrosomal/antithyroid peroxidase antibodies

Principles

Antimicrosomal antibodies are directed against a protein component of thyroid cell microsomes. The tanned erythrocyte agglutination method uses cells that have been coated with microsomal antigen isolated from human hyperplastic thyroid glands. The procedure is simple, and commercial kits for it are available. Reactivity occurs in nearly all adults with Hashimoto's thyroiditis and in about 85% of individuals with Graves' disease. Low titers, however, may be seen in 5% to 10% of healthy asymptomatic individuals. Hemagglutination tests for anti-Tg and antimicrosomal antibodies often are performed together. Of the two, the result of the test for microsomal antibody is more frequently positive for thyroid autoimmune disease and usually is in higher titer.

Procedures for the more sensitive ELISA and RIA methods are similar to those previously described for anti-Tg antibodies; a number of quantitative commercial kits are available. The mean antimicrosomal antibody activity, measured with an IRMA kit, is 280 ± 60 U/mL in normal sera.

Thyroid peroxidase (TPO) now is recognized as the main and possibly only autoantigenic component of microsomes. Methods based on TPO itself are preferred for routine clinical use; anti-TPO antibody assays based on RIA or immunometric techniques also are available. These procedures provide greater sensitivity and specificity than passive hemagglutination assays for microsomal antibodies in the detection, confirmation, and monitoring of autoimmune thyroid disorders and are more suitable for screening or high-volume testing.

Reference interval

The normal reference interval for anti-TPO is also controversial. With sensitive assays, values are less than 2 U/mL. Detectable concentrations of anti-TPO antibodies are observed in nearly all individuals with Hashimoto's thyroiditis and idiopathic myxedema, and in the majority of individuals with Graves' disease. Low levels of TPO autoantibodies may be detected in some healthy individuals without thyroid disease, with a prevalence of anti-TPO antibodies in the elderly. The frequency of detectable anti-TPO antibodies observed in nonimmune thyroid disease is similar to that observed in a normal population.

Thyrotropin-receptor antibodies

Thyrotropin-receptor antibodies (TRAbs) are immunoglobulins that bind to thyroid cell membranes at or near the TSH receptor site. These antibodies are found frequently in the sera of patients with Graves' disease or other thyroid autoimmune disorders; some cause thyroid stimulation, whereas others have no effect or decrease thyroid secretion by blocking the action of TSH. At present these abnormal immunoglobulins can be demonstrated with radioreceptor assays or bioassays.[16]

The direct radioreceptor assay for TRAbs assesses the capacity of immunoglobulins to inhibit the binding of labeled TSH to its receptors in thyroid membrane preparations. Such antibodies usually are designated *thyrotropin-binding inhibitory immunoglobulins (TBII)*. This method is available as a commercial kit and requires only 2 to 3 hours to perform. Measurement of TBII is used mainly in pregnant women with present or past Graves' disease to assess the risk of fetal or neonatal hyperthyroidism.

In vitro bioassays assess the capacity of immunoglobulins to stimulate a functional activity of the thyroid gland, such as adenylate cyclase stimulation or cyclic adenosine monophosphate (cAMP) formation. Such antibodies often are referred to as *thyroid-stimulating immunoglobulins (TSIs)*. Measurement of the increase in cAMP level has been accomplished by use of human thyroid slices, frozen human thyroid cells in culture, or a cloned line of thyroid follicular cells (FRTL-5).[26] A sensitive and specific indicator of Graves' disease, TSI measurement sometimes is used to follow the course of therapy and predict relapse and remission.

DISORDERS OF THE THYROID

Disorders of the thyroid include hypothyroidism and hyperthyroidism, nonthyroid illness (NTI), euthyroid sick syndromes, and those resulting from medication.

Hypothyroidism

Hypothyroidism, or underactivity of the thyroid gland, commonly is caused by diseases or treatments that destroy thyroid tissues or interfere with thyroid hormone biosynthesis (primary hypothyroidism) and less often by disorders of the pituitary or hypothalamus (secondary hypothyroidism).[14,19] Thyroid enlargement (goiter) may or may not be present, depending on the underlying cause (Table 40-5). Autoimmune Hashimoto's thyroiditis is the most frequent cause of primary hypothyroidism in developed countries; worldwide, iodine deficiency is the most common cause of thyroid gland failure.

In individuals with primary hypothyroidism, small decreases in T_4 and T_3 concentrations lead to high levels of serum TSH. The latter is a key laboratory finding, particularly in the early detection of thyroid failure. In cases of mild or subclinical hypothyroidism, thyroid hormone levels may remain within the normal reference interval but the TSH concentration is elevated. Primary hypothyroidism is treated easily with oral T_4. Periodic monitoring of serum TSH is recommended to help maintain clinical euthyroidism.

Congenital hypothyroidism may be caused by absence of the thyroid gland (athyreosis) or may occur secondarily to defects of thyroid hormone synthesis. This disorder occurs once in every 3500 to 4000 live births, and early treatment is critical if mental retardation is to be prevented. Neonatal screening programs for congenital hypothyroidism have been established in almost all developed countries of the world.[9] A majority of North American programs use an initial T_4 measurement, followed by TSH determinations on infants with low T_4 values.

Secondary hypothyroidism results from pituitary or hypothalamic diseases that produce a deficiency of TSH, TRH, or both. Isolated TSH deficiency is rare, and most individuals with secondary hypothyroidism also have other pituitary hormone deficiencies. With secondary hypothyroidism, serum thyroid hormone concentrations are low, but TSH levels are either low or within the reference interval. When both T_4 levels and TSH levels are low, a TRH test (see Chapter 39) may be helpful to distinguish pituitary failure from hypothalamic dysfunction.

Hyperthyroidism

Hyperthyroidism is a hypermetabolic disorder caused by excessive amounts of free T_4 and T_3 (Table 40-6).[7,12] These elevated levels may arise from hyperfunction of the thyroid, excessive leakage out of a nonhyperactive gland, or sources outside of the thyroid. Hyperthyroidism generally is easier to diagnose on clinical grounds than is hypothyroidism.

Increases in free T_4 and T_3 suppress circulating TSH to undetectable levels, except in rare cases in which hyperthyroidism is mediated by TSH itself (for example, TSH-secreting pituitary tumor). The pattern of low TSH level and an elevated FT_4 level is usually sufficient to establish the diagnosis of hyperthyroidism. If the TSH level is low but the free T_4 level is normal, a total T_3 measurement should be performed because the serum T_3 concentration often is elevated to a greater degree than is the T_4 concentration in early Graves' disease and in some individuals with Plummer's disease (T_3 thyrotoxicosis). A depressed serum

---

TABLE 40-5   Causes of Hypothyroidism

Primary (Goitrous) Hypothyroidism
Chronic lymphocytic (Hashimoto's) thyroiditis
Subacute thyroiditis
Postpartum thyroiditis
Endemic iodine deficiency
Defects in hormone biosynthesis and action
Drug-induced (lithium, iodine, antithyroid drugs)

Primary (Nongoitrous) Hypothyroidism
Spontaneous thyroid atrophy (atrophic myxedema)
Radioactive iodine therapy
Surgical ablation
External radiation
Sporadic athyreotic cretinism

Secondary Hypothyroidism
Pituitary disease
Hypothalamic disease

Peripheral Resistance to Thyroid Hormones

TABLE 40-6   Causes of Hyperthyroidism

Associated with Thyroid Hyperfunction*	Not Associated with Thyroid Hyperfunction†
Diffuse toxic hyperplasia (Graves' disease)	Subacute thyroiditis
Toxic multinodular goiter (Plummer's disease)	Silent lymphocytic thyroiditis
Solitary toxic adenoma	Thyrotoxicosis factitia
TSH-secreting pituitary tumor	Drug-induced thyrotoxicosis
CG-secreting trophoblastic tumor	Struma ovarii
Iodine-induced hyperthyroidism	Hyperfunctioning metastatic thyroid carcinoma
Hyperemesis gravidarum	

TSH, Thyroid-stimulating hormone; *CG*, chorionic gonadotropin.
*Associated with increased radioactive iodine uptake, except iodine induced.
†Associated with decreased radioactive iodine uptake.

TSH concentration, associated with normal or equivocal concentrations of T_3 and FT_4 may signify a state of subclinical hyperthyroidism when the individual is asymptomatic. Numerous medications, as well as acute and chronic illnesses, may cause a transient lowering of T_3 concentration and a reduction in TSH level. In individuals with nonthyroidal illnesses a definite diagnosis of early hyperthyroidism may not be possible until other illnesses resolve.

Occasionally, increases in serum levels of T_4 and T_3 occur because of the ingestion of large quantities of exogenous thyroid hormones or the release of stored thyroid hormones secondary to subacute thyroiditis or lymphocytic thyroiditis. These increases in T_4 and T_3 may be associated with clinical findings that also are consistent with an overactive thyroid gland. This diagnostic dilemma is solved by the finding of a low radioactive iodine uptake (percent of orally administered radioactive iodine taken up by the gland at 6 or 24 hours) that accompanies the hyperthyroidism of thyroiditis. Most cases of thyroiditis are self-limited conditions that resolve without any residual thyroid function abnormality.

Treatments for hyperthyroidism include antithyroid drugs, radioiodine ablation, and thyroidectomy. Measurements of serum FT_4 usually are performed every few weeks until symptoms abate and serum values normalize; monitoring for recurrence is suggested two or three times a year.[19] Serum TSH is not an accurate measure of effective treatment and remains undetectable for months after the individual becomes clinically euthyroid. Ablation of thyroid tissue or overtreatment with antithyroid drugs may lead to clinical hypothyroidism and an increase in serum TSH.

Nonthyroidal Illness

Many disorders are characterized by thyroid hormone excess or deficiency in the absence of definitive thyroid disease. These abnormalities may result from changes in the concentration of thyroid hormone-binding proteins, actions of certain drugs, effects of acute and chronic NTI, or peripheral resistance to thyroid hormones.

A progressive spectrum of test abnormalities may be seen in NTI in euthyroid individuals (the **"euthyroid sick syndrome"**) (Figure 40-8).[15] The most common changes are a reduction in the serum total and free T_3 and an elevation in the serum level of rT_3 (the "low T_3 state"). Declining levels of total T_4 also may be observed; however, FT_4 concentrations, determined with reference methods, usually remain within the normal reference interval or elevated mildly. Some methods used to estimate FT_4, such as the conventional FT_4I and one-step immunoassays, may provide artifactually low values in euthyroid individuals with increasing severity of chronic illness.

Serum TSH concentrations are usually normal in euthyroid sick individuals but may be depressed mildly during the acute phase of NTI or slightly elevated during recovery from

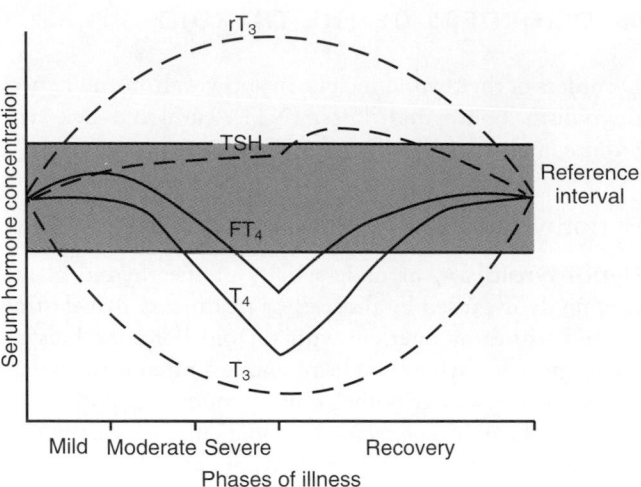

Figure 40-8 The spectrum of thyroid hormone concentrations in ill individuals. rT_3, Reverse triiodothyronine; *TSH*, thyroid-stimulating hormone; FT_4, free thyroxine; T_4, thyroxine; T_3, triiodothyronine. (Modified from Brent GA, Hershman JM: Effects of nonthyroidal illness on thyroid function tests. In Van Middleworth L (ed): The Thyroid Gland: A Practical Clinical Treatise, p 86, Chicago, Year-Book Medical, 1986.)

severe illness. As individuals recover from NTIs, most of these test abnormalities revert to normal. Assessments of thyroid function in ill individuals should be postponed until the illness resolves.

Hypothyroidism Versus Euthyroid Sick Syndrome

The euthyroid sick syndrome is characterized by abnormalities in thyroid hormone and TSH levels, often simulating hypothyroidism, in euthyroid individuals suffering some other illness, such as diabetes mellitus or liver cirrhosis. The most common dilemma presented by the test abnormalities and observed with the euthyroid sick syndrome occurs when hypothyroidism is suspected in an ill individual. Total and free T_3 levels are expected to be low in NTI and should not be measured for this purpose. If the total or free T_4 level is normal, hypothyroidism is most unlikely; however, a low total T_4 and a low FT_4 estimate often are seen in extremely ill euthyroid individuals.

Serum TSH is probably the best single test used to address the differential diagnosis of euthyroid sick and hypothyroidism (in the absence of suspected pituitary or hypothalamic disease). A clear elevation of TSH level (>30 mU/L) indicates moderate to severe hypothyroidism. Lesser TSH elevations may be seen transiently in euthyroid sick individuals during recovery and in those with mild hypothyroidism. If the question of hypothyroidism in acutely ill individuals cannot be resolved with TSH and free T_4 testing, measurement of rT_3 should help (rT_3 being low in individuals with hypothyroidism [either primary or secondary] and normal or high in euthyroid subjects). Documentation of a normal serum cortisol may help distinguish NTI from pituitary or hypothalamic hypothyroidism.

Hyperthyroidism Versus Euthyroid Sick Syndrome

As many as 3% of hospitalized patients, at the time of admission, have subnormal TSH values often associated with the acute phase of illness or glucocorticoid or dopamine therapy. With sensitive TSH assays, separation of hyperthyroid sick individuals with profoundly low TSH values (less than 0.01 mU/L) from critically ill euthyroid individuals with only mild suppression of TSH in the 0.01 to 0.1 mU/L range is possible.

Effect of Drugs

Some medications are known to alter thyroid function and thyroid function tests.[1] For example, glucocorticoids and dopamine reduce TSH levels, whereas amiodarone increases TSH levels. The most commonly encountered variations in thyroid hormone measurements induced by medications are reduced peripheral conversion of T_4 to T_3 and altered binding of T_4 and T_3 to carrier proteins.

References

1. Davies PH, Franklyn JA: The effects of drugs on tests of thyroid function. Eur J Clin Pharmacol 1991; 40:439-451.
2. Demers LM: Thyroid function testing and automation. J Clin Ligand Assay 1999; 22:38-41.
3. Ekins R: Measurement of free hormones in blood. Endocr Rev 1990; 11:5-46.
4. Ekins R: Free hormone measurement (in two parts). Endocrinology and Metabolism In Service Training and Continuing Education Program. AACC Press, 1993; 11:149-157, 181-191.
5. Feldkamp CS, Zafar MS: Thyroid Disease. In Jialal I, Winter WE, Chan DW (eds): Handbook of Diagnostic Endocrinology, pp 23-48, Washington, DC, AACC Press, 1999.
6. Hay ID, Bayer MF, Kaplan MK et al: American Thyroid Association assessment of current free thyroid hormone and thyrotropin measurement and guidelines for future clinical assays. Clin Chem 1991; 37:2002-2008.
7. Kannan CR, Seshadri KG: Thyrotoxicosis. Dis Mon 1997; 43:601-677.
8. Klee GG: Clinical usage recommendations and analytic performance goals for total and free triiodothyronine measurements. Clin Chem 1996; 42:155-159.
9. LaFranchi S: American Academy of Pediatrics. American Thyroid Association. Newborn screening for congenital hypothyroidism. Recommended guidelines. Thyroid 1993; 3:257-263.
10. Larsen PR, Alexander N, Chopra IJ et al: Revised nomenclature for tests of thyroid hormones and thyroid-related proteins in serum. Clin Chem 1987; 33:2114-2117.
11. Larsen PR, Davies TF, Hay ID: The thyroid gland. In Wilson JH, Foster DW, Kronenberg HM et al (eds): Williams Textbook of Endocrinology, 9th edition, pp 389-516, Philadelphia, WB Saunders, 1998.
12. Lazarus JH: Hyperthyroidism. Lancet 1997; 349:339-343.
13. Liewendahl K: Thyroid function tests: performance and limitations of current methodologies. Scand J Clin Lab Invest 1992; 52:435-445.
14. Lindsay RS: Hypothyroidism. Lancet 1997; 349:413-417.
15. McIver B: Euthyroid sick syndrome: an overview. Thyroid 1997; 7:125-132.
16. Morris J, Hay I, Nelson R et al: Clinical utility of thyrotropin-receptor antibody assays: comparison of radioreceptor and bioassay methods. Mayo Clin Proc 1988; 63:707-717.
17. Nelson JC, Wilcox RB: Analytical performance of free and total thyroxine assays. Clin Chem 1996; 42:146-154.
18. Rafferty B, Gaines-Das R: Comparison of pituitary and recombinant human thyroid-stimulating hormone (rhTSH) in a multicenter collaborative study: establishment of the First World Health Organization reference reagent for rhTSH. Clin Chem 1999; 45:2207-2215.
19. Ridgway EC: Modern concepts of primary thyroid gland failure. Clin Chem 1996; 42:179-182.
20. Sawin CT (ed): Laboratory support for the diagnosis and monitoring of thyroid disease. National Academy of Clinical Biochemistry, Standards of Laboratory Practice Monograph, Washington, DC, AACC Press, 1996.
21. Spencer CA: Strategy for use of serum thyrotropin vs. free thyroxin measurement in thyroid testing. Endocrinology and Metabolism In-Service Training and Continuing Education Program. AACC Endo 1991; 10:9-17.
22. Spencer CA, Takeucho M, Kazarosyan M: Current status and performance goals for serum thyrotropin (TSH) assays. Clin Chem 1996; 42:140-145.
23. Spencer CA, Takeucho M, Kazarosyan M: Current status and performance goals for serum Tg assays. Clin Chem 1996; 42:164-173.
24. Surks MI, Chopra IJ, Mariash CN: American Thyroid Association guidelines for use of laboratory tests in thyroid disorders. JAMA 1990; 263:1529-1532.
25. Woeber KA: Subclinical thyroid dysfunction. Arch Intern Med 1997; 157:1065-1068.
26. Whitley RJ: Thyroid Function. In Burtis CA, Ashwood ER (eds): Tietz Textbook of Clinical Chemistry, 3rd edition, pp 1496-1529, Philadelphia, WB Saunders, 1999.

Additional Reading

Braverman LE: Diseases of the Thyroid, Contemporary Endocrinology Series, vol 2, Totowa, NJ, Humana Press, 1996.

Braverman LE, Utiger RD (eds): Werner and Ingbar's The Thyroid: A Fundamental and Clinical Text, 7th edition, Philadelphia, Lippincott Williams & Wilkins, 2000.

DeGroot LJ, Larsen PR, Hennemann G (eds): The Thyroid and Its Diseases, 6th edition, New York, Churchill Livingstone, 1996.

Falk SA: Thyroid Disease: Endocrinology, Surgery, Nuclear Medicine, and Radiotherapy, 2nd edition, Philadelphia, Lippincott-Raven Publishers, 1997.

CHAPTER 41

Adrenocortical Function

LAURENCE M. DEMERS, PhD, DABCC, and RONALD J. WHITLEY, PhD

Objectives

1. Describe the structure and function of the adrenal cortex.
2. Diagram the biosynthesis of adrenocortical hormones from cholesterol.
3. List the hormones synthesized by each specific zone of the adrenal cortex, and state their functions.
4. Describe the following adrenal disorders: Addison's disease, Conn's syndrome, Cushing's syndrome, congenital adrenal hyperplasia.
5. List the laboratory tests used to assess adrenocortical function.

Key Words

Aldosterone   The major mineralocorticoid steroid hormone secreted by the adrenal cortex; controls salt and water balance in the kidney

Androgens   A class of sex hormones that produce masculinization

Androstenedione   An androgenic steroid produced by the testes, adrenal cortex, and ovaries; occurs in nature as Δ^4-androstenedione and Δ^5-delta-androstenedione; is converted metabolically to testosterone and other androgens

Cortisol   The major adrenal glucocorticoid synthesized in the zona fasciculata of the adrenal cortex; affects the metabolism of glucose, proteins, and lipids and has appreciable mineralocorticoid activity

Cushing's Disease   A condition characterized by an increased blood concentration of adrenal glucocorticoid hormone caused by a pituitary adenoma

Dehydroepiandrosterone (DHEA)   A steroid secreted by the adrenal cortex; the major androgen precursor in females

Glucocorticoids   Any of the group of C_{21} steroids produced by the adrenal cortex that regulate carbohydrate, fat, and protein metabolism; also inhibit adrenocorticotropin secretion, act as antiinflammatories, and play a role in various homeostatic processes

Mineralocorticoids   Any of the group of C_{21} corticosteroids (principally aldosterone) that regulate the balance of water and electrolytes in the body

Renin   An enzyme of the hydrolase class that catalyzes cleavage of the leucine-leucine bond in angiotensinogen to create angiotensin I

Zona Fasciculata   The thick middle layer of the adrenal cortex that is the major source of glucocorticoids

Zona Glomerulosa   The thin outer layer of the adrenal cortex that is the source of aldosterone

Zona Reticularis   The inner layer of the adrenal cortex

Humans have an adrenal gland at the upper pole of each kidney (see Figure 26-1). Each adult gland has a pyramidal shape and is approximately 2 to 3 cm wide, 4 to 6 cm long, and 1 cm thick and weighs approximately 4 g, regardless of the person's age, weight, or sex. Each gland consists of a yellow, outer cortex and a gray, inner medulla. The adrenal cortex cells synthesize steroid hormones. The adrenal medulla cells synthesize catecholamines, such as dopamine, norepinephrine, and epinephrine, which have important hormonal functions (see Chapter 27).

The human adrenal cortex secretes three major classes of steroid hormones, including glucocorticoids (such as cortisol), mineralocorticoids (such as aldosterone), and the adrenal androgens (such as dehydroepiandrosterone and androstenedione). These steroids affect a wide range of physiological functions including carbohydrate metabolism, electrolyte balance, and the metabolism of sex steroids.

GENERAL STEROID CHEMISTRY

Chemical Structure

Steroids contain a cyclopentanoperhydrophenanthrene nucleus as their backbone structure (Figure 41-1). The three, six-sided rings *(A, B,* and *C)* constitute the phenanthrene nucleus, which is attached to the cyclopentane ring *(D).* The prefix *perhydro-* refers to the saturation of the compound with hydrogen atoms. This class of compounds includes such natural products as sterols (for example, cholesterol), bile acids (for example, cholanic acid), sex hormones (for example, estrogens and androgens), vitamin D, and the adrenal steroids. Steroid hormones contain up to 21 carbon atoms (C_{21} steroids), which are numbered as shown in Figure 41-1.

Steroids are three-dimensional molecules. Their constituent atoms lie in different planes, which results in the creation of isomers. The direction of the hydrogen atoms, the substituents, and the side chain play a much more important role in the differentiation among various steroid compound isomers than do the relative positions of the carbon atoms in the rings. Thus the isomers resulting from fusion of two rings are identified on the basis of the spatial relationship between the hydrogen atoms or the substituents at common carbon atoms. When rings *A* and *B* are fused, two isomers are possible depending on whether the hydrogen atom at C-5 and the methyl group at C-10 are on the same or the opposite side of the plane of the rings. If the hydrogen atom points in the same direction as that of the angular methyl group at C-10, the compound is in the *cis,* or *normal,* form. However, if they are on opposite sides, the compound is in the *trans,* or *allo,* form. Depending on which side of the molecule the substituents are attached relative to these two methyl groups, they have either an α or β orientation. For example, when the substituents are on the same side as the two methyl groups, they have a β configuration, which is indicated by a solid line (—) joining the substituents to the appropriate carbon atoms in the nucleus. Substituents on the opposite side are attached by a broken line (--) to denote an α configuration.

Individual steroids containing the cyclopentanoperhydrophenanthrene nucleus are differentiated by the presence of double bonds between certain pairs of carbon atoms, the introduction of substituents for the hydrogen atoms, or the addition of a specific type of side chain. On the basis of such structural characteristics, the steroidal compounds are classified as derivatives of certain parent hydrocarbons, namely estrane (for estrogens), androstane (for androgens), and pregnane (for corticosteroids and progestins). Various suffixes and prefixes are used to describe steroids (Table 41-1).

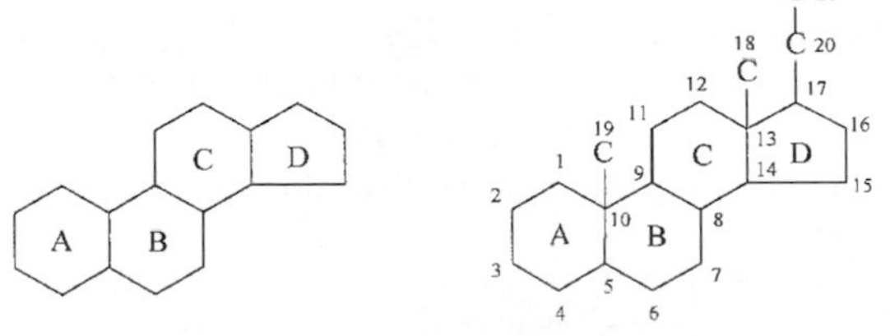

TABLE 41-1	Common Suffixes and Prefixes for Steroids
Suffix or Prefix	**Definition**
Suffix	
-al	Aldehyde group
-ane	Saturated hydrocarbon
-ene	Unsaturated hydrocarbon
-ol	Hydroxyl group
-one	Ketone group
Prefix	
hydroxy- (oxy-)	Hydroxyl group
keto- (oxo-)	Ketone
deoxy- (desoxy-)	Replacement of hydroxyl group by hydrogen
dehydro-	Loss of two hydrogen atoms from adjacent carbon atoms
dihydro-	Addition of two hydrogen atoms
cis-	Spatial arrangement of two substituents on the same side of the molecule
trans-	Spatial arrangement of two substituents on opposite sides of the molecule
α-	Substituent that is *trans* to the methyl group at C-10
β-	Substituent that is *cis* to the methyl group at C-10
epi-	Isomeric in configuration at any carbon atom except at the junction of two rings
Δ^n-	Position of unsaturated bond

Figure 41-1 Common features and numbering system of steroids.

Biochemistry

Synthesis

Normally, steroid hormones are synthesized from cholesterol in the adrenal glands and gonads. In most cases, cholesterol is acquired from circulating low-density lipoproteins; however, all steroidogenic cells are capable of de novo synthesis of cholesterol from acetate. To ensure a continuous supply of free cholesterol for steroid synthesis, lipoprotein cholesterol uptake is linked to intracellular cholesterol synthesis and the mobilization of intracellular cholesteryl ester pools.

The nature and quantity of steroid hormones produced by the adrenal glands and gonads differ. The difference is inherent in the degree of activity of certain enzyme systems. For example, the enzymes 11β-hydroxylase and 21-hydroxylase are present only in the adrenal glands. Similarly, the ovaries and the testes contain enzymes that uniquely synthesize the male and female sex hormones (see Chapter 42).

Transport

Steroid hormones circulate in blood in free and bound forms. In the bound form, they are attached to plasma carrier proteins or albumin. Steroids conjugated to glucuronide or sulfate are excreted by the kidneys or gastrointestinal tract. At physiological concentrations, about 90% to 98% of circulating steroid hormones are bound to some carrier protein and usually have a high affinity for binding of globulin. When a steroid has low affinity for a carrier protein, 60% to 70% of the circulating steroids are bound principally to albumin.

Metabolism

The liver is the major site of steroid metabolism; however, the kidney and gastrointestinal tract also metabolize steroids. In addition to the use of acetate and cholesterol, some steroidogenic tissues produce hormones by conversion of steroid intermediates that originate from other sources. For example, ovarian granulosa cells convert androgens produced in thecal cells to estrogens. Some target cells also convert the circulating form of a steroid to its bioactive form, which then has an effect within the cells. For example, the adrenal androgen precursor **dehydroepiandrosterone (DHEA)** is converted to estrone in fat tissue by the aromatase enzyme.

Important biochemical steps neutralize the potent biological activity of hormones and facilitate their rapid elimination from the systemic circulation; they include (1) the addition of hydroxyl groups (for example, estradiol to estriol), (2) dehydrogenation (for example, testosterone to androstenedione), (3) reduction of double bonds (for example, cortisol to dihydrocortisol), and (4) conjugation of essential hydroxyl groups with a chemical moiety such as glucuronic acid (for example, testosterone to testosterone glucuronide). The conjugation of these hormones and their metabolites with sulfuric or glucuronic acid is the most efficient single metabolic process for their excretion in the urine.

■ ADRENOCORTICAL STEROIDS

The human adrenal cortex secretes steroid hormones from three discrete anatomical zones: the **zona fasciculata, zona reticularis,** and **zona glomerulosa.** Corticosteroids (Figure 41-2), which include the glucocorticoids and mineralocorticoids, and androgens are synthesized within these three adrenal cortex zones. Enzymes that participate in the synthesis of the adrenal steroids include (1) hydroxylases, (2) lyases, (3) dehydrogenases, and (4) isomerases.

The glucocorticoids and mineralocorticoids are physiologically and quantitatively the most important group of

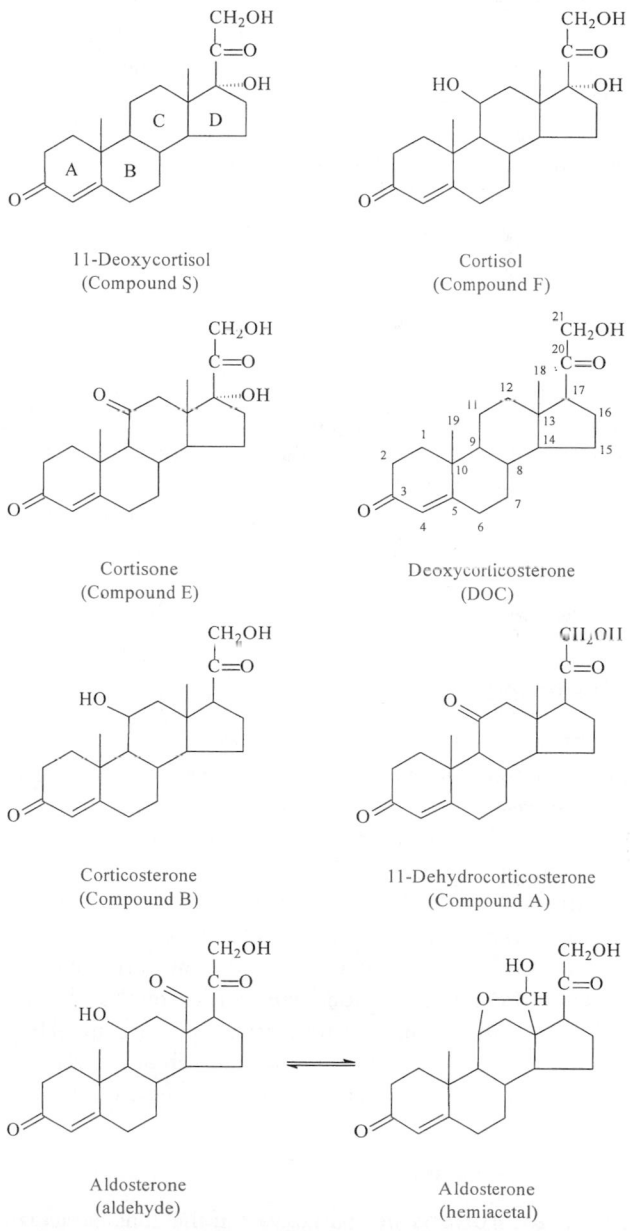

Figure 41-2 Structural formulas and trivial names of some biologically active corticosteroids. Note the alphabetical ring system and numerical system for 21 carbon (C_{21}) atoms.

corticosteroid hormones produced by the adrenal cortex. Cortisol is the major glucocorticosteroid and aldosterone is the major mineralocorticoid (see Figure 41-2) secreted by the adrenal cortex. They are secreted at approximately 25 mg/day and 200 μg/day, respectively. The adrenal androgens include DHEA, **androstenedione,** and testosterone (Figure 41-3). DHEA is the principal adrenal androgen formed by the adrenal cortex and is secreted at a rate of approximately 20 mg/day.[1]

Cortisol

Cortisol is formed from cholesterol in the zona fasciculata and zona reticularis of the adrenal cortex. Several key enzymatic steps are involved in its synthesis, including hydroxylations at carbon atoms 11, 17, and 21, oxidation of the 3-hydroxyl group, and isomerization of a double bond from ring *B* to ring *A* (see Figure 41-3).

When released into the circulation, cortisol is principally bound to corticosteroid-binding globulin (CBG) and transported as such. Cortisol is metabolized and conjugated in the liver to several inactive forms. More than 95% of cortisol and its metabolite cortisone is conjugated to glucuronic acid and excreted into the urine as a conjugate. Less than 2% of cortisol is excreted in the urine unmetabolized as urinary free cortisol.

Glucocorticoids such as cortisol influence carbohydrate metabolism by promoting gluconeogenesis and decreasing glucose utilization. Increased gluconeogenesis results from the catabolism of protein. In addition, glucocorticoids inhibit amino acid uptake and protein synthesis in peripheral tissues (muscle, skin, and bone). Glucocorticoids influence fat metabolism when present in excess and cause a central redistribution of fat to the face, neck, and abdomen.

Aldosterone

Aldosterone is the most potent naturally occurring mineralocorticoid and is synthesized exclusively in the zona glomerulosa region of the adrenal cortex. This zone contains the enzyme 18-hydroxysteroid dehydrogenase, a requisite enzyme for the synthesis of aldosterone.

Mineralocorticoids such as aldosterone regulate sodium conservation, potassium loss, and extracellular fluid volume.[3] Other adrenocortical steroids that have mineralocorticoid properties include deoxycorticosterone (DOC), 18-hydroxy-DOC, and corticosterone (see Figure 41-2). Aldosterone acts directly on the kidney tubules to regulate sodium homeostasis and control arterial pressure.

Adrenal Androgens

Adrenal **androgens** are synthesized in the zona fasciculata and reticularis from pregnenolone and 17OH pregnenolone. They include DHEA, androstenedione, and testosterone (see Figure 41-3). Quantitatively, DHEA and its sulfated derivative (DHEA-S) are the most important adrenal androgens produced by the adrenal. The daily amount of DHEA/DHEA-S released from the adrenal is second in concentration only to cortisol. Approximately 8 to 16 mg of DHEA-S are secreted per day, which accounts for more than 90% of the DHEA-S that circulates in plasma.[1] The major adrenal androgens, DHEA and androstenedione, have no known physiological roles but act as substrates for peripheral conversion to testosterone, estradiol, and estrone. When it is not metabolized to androstenedione, DHEA is converted in the liver to inactive metabolites including etiocholanolone and androsterone.

Hormonal Regulation

As discussed in Chapter 39, the secretion of adrenal glucocorticoids and androgens is regulated by adrenocorticotropic hormone (ACTH) which in turn is under the control of the hypothalamic corticotropin-releasing hormone (CRH). Evidence also suggests that the pituitary gland secretes a separate hormonal factor that regulates adrenal androgen production. The hypothalamic-pituitary-adrenal axis in healthy individuals and in those with various adrenal disorders is shown in Figure 41-4. Aldosterone is controlled by the renin-angiotensin system (see Chapter 34).

CRH/ACTH

Biorhythms and other physiological events in the brain result in episodic and circadian secretion of CRH from the hypothalamus. CRH in turn elicits a similar circadian rhythm in ACTH release from the pituitary. ACTH then stimulates cortisol synthesis in the adrenal gland. Cortisol controls CRH-ACTH secretion through negative feedback. CRH secretion is modulated by neuroendocrine, physical, and emotional factors. In addition to CRH, several other circulating factors influence the secretory dynamics of ACTH release. Antidiuretic hormone (ADH) from the posterior pituitary and other peptides (such as angiotensin II, opiates, somatostatin, and interleukin-1 [IL-1]) and catecholamines modulate the secretion of ACTH from the adenohypophysis.

Cortisol

ACTH has both trophic and steroidogenic effects on the adrenal cortex and is under negative feedback control of non–protein-bound cortisol. Cortisol is secreted within a few minutes of an increase in serum levels of ACTH. Deficiency of ACTH results in atrophy of the zona fasciculata and zona reticularis. Atrophy of the adrenal cortex, which can be caused by various factors, causes plasma ACTH levels to rise. Hypertrophy and hyperplasia occur in response to several hours of ACTH administration. The trophic response to ACTH may be produced by cyclic adenosine monophosphate (cAMP) stimulation of insulin-like growth

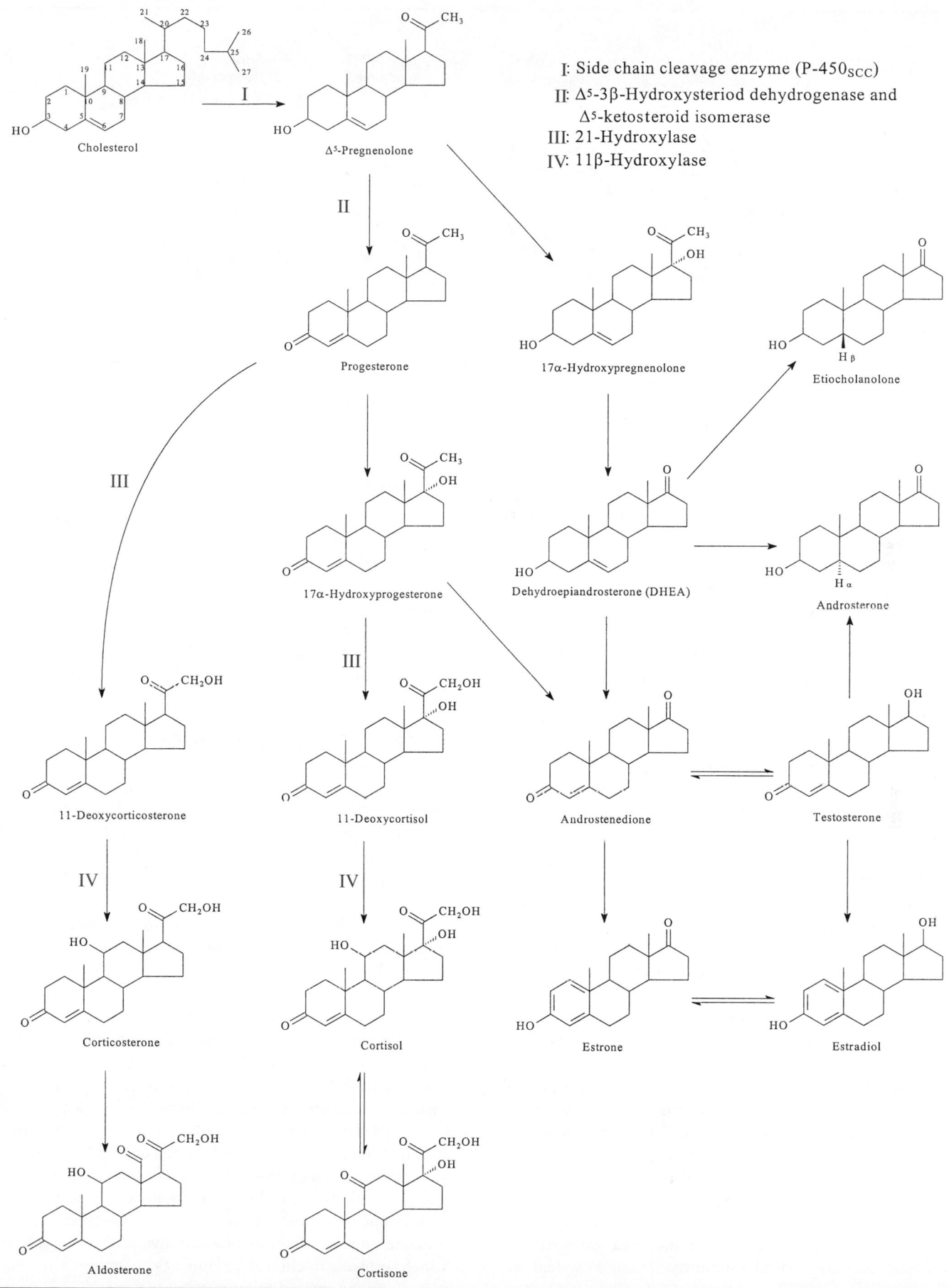

I: Side chain cleavage enzyme (P-450$_{SCC}$)
II: Δ^5-3β-Hydroxysteriod dehydrogenase and
   Δ^5-ketosteroid isomerase
III: 21-Hydroxylase
IV: 11β-Hydroxylase

Cholesterol

Δ^5-Pregnenolone

Progesterone

17α-Hydroxypregnenolone

Etiocholanolone

17α-Hydroxyprogesterone

Dehydroepiandrosterone (DHEA)

Androsterone

11-Deoxycorticosterone

11-Deoxycortisol

Androstenedione

Testosterone

Corticosterone

Cortisol

Estrone

Estradiol

Aldosterone

Cortisone

Figure 41-3   Biosynthesis of corticosteroids. Roman numerals *I* (side-chain cleavage enzyme), *II* (3-β-OH dehydrogenase/Δ4 isomerase), *III* (21-hydroxylase), and *IV* (11β-hydroxylase) indicate sites of major blocks that cause adrenogenital syndromes. (From Netter FH: The CIBA Collection of Medical Illustrations, Basel, Switzerland, CIBA Pharmaceutical Company, 1959.)

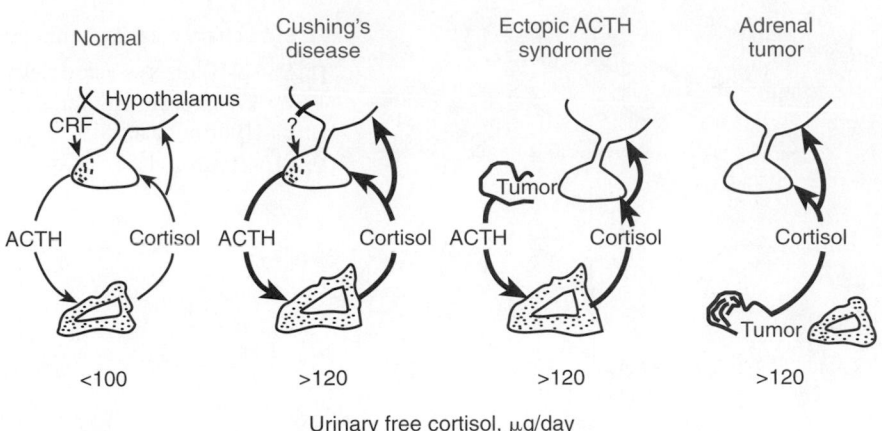

Figure 41-4   Hypothalamic-pituitary-adrenal axis under normal conditions and in individuals with various adrenal disorders. *ACTH,* Adrenocorticotropic hormone; *CRH,* corticotropin-releasing factor. (Modified from Lipsett MB, Odell WD, Rosenberg LE: Humoral syndromes associated with nonendocrine tumors. Ann Intern Med 1964; 61:733; and copyright 1964, American Medical Association.)

factor II (IGF-II) rather than cAMP directly. Prolonged suppression of ACTH by the administration of exogenous glucocorticoids causes adrenocortical atrophy. Recovery of the hypothalamic-pituitary-adrenal axis takes several days to several months after the cessation of exogenous steroid therapy.

During normal wake and sleep cycles, the circadian rhythm of ACTH secretion produces higher cortisol levels in the morning between 0400 and 0900 hours and lower levels in late evening. This pattern is affected by an individual's sleep-wake pattern. Trauma, surgery, hypoglycemia, and systemic illness are physical stressors that elevate plasma cortisol levels and alter the circadian rhythm of secretion. Major depression and severe anxiety are psychological stressors and can also elevate plasma cortisol levels.

Aldosterone

Renin is a proteolytic enzyme synthesized by specialized kidney cells (see Chapter 34). These cells, called *juxtaglomerular cells,* are located along the terminal part of the afferent arterioles of the renal glomeruli. Cells of the juxtaglomerular apparatus are sensitive to sodium concentrations and cause renin to be released when the plasma sodium level decreases to a specific concentration. Renin acts on angiotensinogen, an α-globulin made by the liver, to produce the decapeptide angiotensin I. Angiotensin I is rapidly converted to an octapeptide, angiotensin II, by an angiotensin-converting enzyme (ACE) found in abundance in the lung. Angiotensin II is a potent vasoconstrictor and stimulates the cells of the zona glomerulosa to produce aldosterone. ACTH also increases aldosterone secretion by increasing substrate flow into the zona glomerulosa; however, the steroidogenic activity of the zona glomerulosa is affected primarily by the renin-angiotensin system and potassium.

Androgens

ACTH partially regulates adrenal androgen production in adults because DHEA and androstenedione are secreted simultaneously with cortisol. Adrenal androgen production begins to increase around age 9 or 10; peaks during the 20s, and then gradually decreases, reaching low levels again above age 70. Glucocorticoid therapy also suppresses the secretion of androstenedione and DHEA; if used for several days, it causes a decrease in DHEA-S levels.

◾ ANALYTICAL METHODOLOGY

Numerous methods, including immunoassays and instrumental methods, are used to measure cortisol, aldosterone, and their precursors; renin; and angiotensin I in body fluid.

Cortisol

More than 90% of the circulating cortisol in blood is bound to plasma proteins, primarily to CBG and minimally to albumin. About 2% of cortisol is excreted into the urine as free cortisol.

The principal clinical laboratory method for the quantitative estimation of the cortisol levels in the blood is based on immunoassay techniques.[14] High-performance liquid chromatography (HPLC) has been used as a chromatography method to measure cortisol and other adrenocortical steroids, but it is used primarily for research.[4,6] Fluorescence polarization immunoassay and chemiluminescence-based methods are the procedures of choice for the measurement of cortisol and other adrenocortical steroids in blood and urine.

Immunoassays are the most common methods used to measure cortisol levels in blood, saliva and urine and are widely available in clinical laboratories on various semiautomated and automated immunoassay systems.[13]

Principles

Many immunoassays have been developed to measure cortisol and use different polyclonal and monoclonal antibodies, extraction procedures, labels (isotopic and nonisotopic), and measurement principles, including gamma counting, fluorescence, and chemiluminescence. Most cortisol immunoassays in clinical laboratories today are direct assays and require no initial steroid extraction from the specimen. However, assays used to measure levels of free cortisol in urine still require an extraction step to isolate and concentrate the free cortisol from the many metabolite and conjugate forms found in urine. In direct blood assays, cortisol is quantitatively displaced from endogenous binding proteins by protein-binding agents such as 8-anilino-1-naphthalenesulfonic acid (ANS) or salicylate, low pH, or heat. With the high specificity of the antibodies available today and the use of very sensitive nonisotopic detection methods such as chemiluminescence and fluorescence, the quantitative measurement of cortisol in blood, saliva, and urine is well established.

Specimen requirements

Either serum or plasma (with heparin as an anticoagulant) may be used. No special handling procedures are necessary, and specimens may be refrigerated overnight at 2 to 8 °C. Freezing is preferred for long-term stability. Urinary free cortisol levels are determined by use of a 24-hour urine collection schedule that may include boric acid preservative. If the specimen is collected without preservative, it should be refrigerated between voidings and an aliquot frozen immediately after completion of the 24-hour collection. Salivary samples collected for cortisol measurements should be frozen immediately at −20 °C or colder and remain frozen until the assay is performed. Thawing causes the glycoproteins in the saliva to precipitate, and supernate that remains after centrifugation is processed like serum.

Comments

Blood cortisol levels parallel the episodic and diurnal secretion of ACTH throughout the day. Under normal circumstances the concentration of cortisol at 2000 hours is less than 50% the level obtained at 0800 hours. Increased cortisol secretion occurs in individuals with stress, after exogenous glucocorticoid administration, in individuals who are pregnant, and in individuals with depression, hypoglycemia, and hyperthyroidism. The half-life of cortisol in the circulation is approximately 100 minutes.

Levels of free cortisol in the urine can be used to screen for Cushing's syndrome. After sample extraction with dichloromethane, standard immunoassay methods are used. Care should be taken to ensure a complete 24-hour urine collection (~1 to 1.5 L) for proper interpretation of results.

The measurement of free cortisol in saliva is a practical and convenient approach to assess levels of free cortisol.[5] Salivary cortisol measurements accurately reflect the concentration of non–protein-bound cortisol in blood. Most immunoassay methods for total serum cortisol levels will also measure cortisol in saliva[11]; extraction is not required because saliva contains virtually no cortisol-binding proteins or other cortisol metabolites.

Reference intervals

Representative values of total cortisol (free and bound) in serum assayed by radioimmunoassay (RIA) are as follows:

	µg/dL	nmol/L
Cord blood	5 to 17	138 to 469
Infant (1 to 7 days)	2 to 11	53 to 304
Child (1 to 16 y): 0800 h	3 to 21	83 to 580
Adult		
0800 h	5 to 23	138 to 635
1600 h	3 to 16	83 to 441
2000 h	<50% of 0800 h values	<50% of 0800 h values

Aldosterone

Simple and reliable immunoassay methods used to measure aldosterone in blood and urine are readily available. Methods differ primarily in the specificity of the antialdosterone antibodies used. Most direct RIA methods used to measure aldosterone levels in plasma use antisera generated against an aldosterone-3-mono-oxime-bovine serum albumin (BSA) conjugate, an ^{125}I-labeled ligand, and ANS at pH 3.6 to displace aldosterone from plasma-binding proteins.

Principles

Various commercial immunoassay kits are available for the determination of plasma and urine aldosterone levels. Most assay procedures for total aldosterone levels in urine are similar to those used for plasma except that the urine is acid hydrolyzed before the assay.

Several nonisotopic enzyme immunoassays have been developed to determine serum and urinary aldosterone levels, including chemiluminescence-based immunoassays for direct measurement of aldosterone in serum.[15]

Specimen requirements

Plasma (preserved with heparin, ethylenediaminetetraacetic acid [EDTA], or citrate) or serum samples are used to measure aldosterone. If a blood specimen from a patient in the upright position is needed, the patient should maintain the upright position (standing or seated) for at least 2 hours before the specimen is collected. A complete 24-hour urine collection is needed for urine assays, and boric acid is used as a preservative. Fifty percent acetic acid should also be added to the urine specimen to obtain a pH of between 2 and 4. Specimens should not be acidified with strong mineral acids such as hydrochloric acid. Urine should be refrigerated during collection; aliquots are stored frozen at −20 °C. It is recommended that urine sodium levels also be determined to facilitate interpretation of the aldosterone result.

Reference intervals

The aldosterone level in serum, plasma, and urine are affected by the individual's salt intake and posture at the time of specimen collection. The following serum values are based on a morning specimen collection from individuals on a normal salt diet who have been in an upright position for at least 2 hours:

	ng/dL	nmol/L
Cord blood	40 to 200	1.11 to 5.54
Premature infants	19 to 141	0.53 to 3.91
Full-term infants		
3 days	7 to 184	0.19 to 5.1
1 wk	5 to 175	0.03 to 4.85
1 to 12 mo	5 to 90	0.14 to 2.49
Children		
1 to 2 y	7 to 54	0.19 to 1.50
2 to 10 y	3 to 35	0.08 to 0.97 (supine)
	5 to 80	0.14 to 2.22 (upright)
10 to 15 y	2 to 22	0.06 to 0.61 (supine)
	4 to 48	0.11 to 1.33 (upright)
Adults	3 to 16	0.08 to 0.44 (supine)
	7 to 30	0.19 to 0.83 (upright)

The following aldosterone levels in urine, which were obtained over 24 hours, have been reported:

	µg/day	nmol/day	µg/g Creatinine
Newborns, 1 to 3 days	0.5 to 5	1 to 14	20 to 140
Children, 4 to 10 y	1 to 8	3 to 22	4 to 22
Adults	3 to 19	8 to 51	1.5 to 20

Other Adrenocortical Steroids

When clinical evidence shows an adrenal enzyme block or deficiency, it is customary to measure the steroid just proximal to the suspected enzyme block. For example, the measurement of 11-deoxycortisol confirms an 11β-hydrolyase block. Likewise, the measurement of 17-hydroxyprogesterone verifies a 21α-hydroxylase deficiency. In addition, numerous biosynthetic precursors of cortisol and aldosterone are measured by immunoassay, either directly or after sample extraction or chromatography or both. Other steroids measured include pregnenolone, 17-hydroxypregnenolone, corticosterone, 18-hydroxycorticosterone and DOC. Adrenal androgens measured by immunoassay include DHEA (usually measured as DHEA-S), androstenedione, and testosterone.

11-Deoxycortisol

Estimation of serum or plasma levels of 11-deoxycortisol (compound S) is required for the metyrapone stimulation test. Because metyrapone inhibits 11β-hydroxylase, a large increase in 11-deoxycortisol is expected in individuals with adequate pituitary-adrenal reserves. Consequently, immunoassay methods for 11-deoxycortisol in metyrapone test specimens do not have to be highly sensitive.

Principle

Although methods for direct analysis of plasma levels of 11-deoxycortisol have been reported, very few reliable commercial kits are available. In one commercial kit, plasma specimens are extracted with hexane/ethylacetate and then assayed with antiserum generated against 11-deoxycortisol-3-carboxymethyloxime-BSA. Antibody-bound and free steroid fractions are separated with a double-antibody technique and polyethylene glycol precipitant. The principal interfering steroid in this kit is 17-hydroxyprogesterone (with 29% cross-reactivity). Nonisotopic methods used to measure 11-deoxycortisol in serum exist, but the procedures are not widely used.

Comments

Most immunoassays for 11-deoxycortisol are adequate for monitoring of the metyrapone test but are not sensitive enough to measure the hormone in native serum. A more sensitive assay is recommended for this procedure and for evaluation of adrenocortical hyperplasia caused by 11β-hydroxylase defects.

Reference intervals

Representative values for 11-deoxycortisol in serum are as follows:

	ng/dL	nmol/L
Cord blood	295 to 554	9 to 16
Children and adults	20 to 158	0.6 to 4.6
After metyrapone	4	12

17-Hydroxyprogesterone

Measurement of 17-hydroxyprogesterone in serum or plasma is primarily used to rapidly diagnose congenital adrenal hyperplasia (CAH) and monitor the effectiveness of therapy in newborns. This test is also used to evaluate women with hirsutism or infertility, either of which may be caused by adult-onset 21-hydroxylase deficiency.

Principles

Historically, 17-hydroxyprogesterone has been assayed with competitive protein-binding techniques by use of CBG as the binding reagent. Because of the nonspecificity of CBG, organic solvent extraction of the test sample and chromatographic purification of the extract often preceded the protein-binding assay.

Direct immunoassays assays for 17-hydroxyprogesterone have now replaced the CBG methods. These methods use antisera with sufficient affinity and specificity to permit direct assays of small volumes of serum, saliva, or blood. In addition to high-activity radioiodinated tracers, nonisotopic labels have also been used to develop enzyme, fluorometric, and chemiluminescent immunoassays. These methods usually involve solid-phase coated tube or liquid-phase double-antibody methods to separate free and antibody-bound fractions. Despite the use of highly specific antisera, most direct assays can be affected by cross-reacting substances in neonatal and infant plasma specimens. Thus some form of extraction is needed to analyze these types of specimens. In addition, elevated results obtained by direct methods should be confirmed by another assay that uses an extraction method.

Specimen requirements

The preferred specimen used to measure 17-hydroxyprogesterone is serum; plasma with an EDTA anticoagulant may also be used. Specimens may be stored at 4 °C for up to 4 days or at −20 °C for up to 1 month. Specimens from infants are obtained by heel puncture and collected in capillary tubes or on filter paper. Dried blood specimens are stable and easily transported and thus are ordinarily obtained to screen newborns for CAH.

Reference intervals

The following serum values are representative of expected reference intervals for 17-hydroxyprogesterone:

	ng/dL	nmol/L
Cord blood	900 to 5000	27.3 to 151.5
Premature infant	26 to 568	0.8 to 17
Newborn, 3 days	7 to 77	0.2 to 2.7
Prepubescent child	3 to 90	0.1 to 2.7
Adult		
Male	27 to 199	0.8 to 6.0
Female		
Follicular phase	15 to 70	0.4 to 2.1
Luteal phase	35 to 290	1.0 to 8.7
Pregnancy	200 to 1200	6.0 to 36.0
After ACTH	<320	<9.6
Postmenopause	<70	<2.1

Renin and Angiotensin I

Clinical laboratory assessment of the renin-angiotensin-aldosterone system is usually determined by measurement of plasma renin activity (PRA) levels and aldosterone in plasma. Most clinical laboratories measure PRA with an enzyme kinetic assay in which renin catalyzes the formation of angiotensin I from its substrate, angiotensinogen. The accumulation of angiotensin I during a fixed, timed incubation period is measured by RIA.

Principles

PRA is defined as the rate of angiotensin I produced from angiotensinogen by renin in an individual's plasma. PRA is expressed in nanograms of angiotensin I produced per milliliter of plasma per hour and is determined by assaying of angiotensin I after incubation of plasma at 37 °C for 1 to 1½ hours and then subtraction of the amount of baseline angiotensin I in the unincubated control plasma aliquot stored at 4 °C.

Specimen requirements

Special problems are encountered in the preparation of plasma specimens for RIA of angiotensin I. Angiotensin I and angiotensin II are very labile in plasma and are continuously generated in vitro in untreated plasma, even in the frozen state. Therefore great care must be taken in the collection and storage of specimens for angiotensin assays, with special attention given to the inactivation of angiotensinases.

Specimens for an angiotensin assay are collected in a tube containing EDTA. After centrifugation at room temperature, the plasma is removed and frozen at −20 °C or lower. Plasma for PRA can be stored frozen for up to 1 month. Freeze-thaw cycles should be avoided because of the possibility they can activate prorenin in the sample. At the time of collection, blood should not be chilled or placed on ice because irreversible cryoactivation of prorenin may occur, leading to overestimation of PRA. Factors such as time of day, posture, salt intake, and diuretic or other drug use should be properly documented so that test results can be properly interpreted. The patient should be ambulatory for 2 hours before blood collection. A urine specimen for sodium is collected over 24 hours on the day before the renin test to reference the effect of salt intake. Specimens with high renin activity generate considerable amounts of angiotensin I before and during storage, even at −20 °C. However, this type of storage does not affect the test results because angiotensin I levels are determined before and after the incubation step. An angiotensinase enzyme inhibitor is used in the reaction system to prevent further metabolism of angiotensin I. Buffering plasma samples is also important because any change in pH alters the generation of angiotensin I at 37 °C. Most PRA assays use a pH of 5.7 to 6.3, which is optimal for the renin enzyme.

Reference intervals

Reference intervals for PRA vary depending on salt intake, posture, and certain medications. For adults on a normal sodium diet, a reference interval of 0.3 to 4 ng angiotensin I/mL/hour has been reported.

■ DISORDERS OF THE ADRENAL CORTEX

In general, adrenal cortex diseases are classified as being a disease of hypofunction or hyperfunction.

TABLE 41-2 Hormonal Levels as a Result of Adrenocortical Insufficiency

	Reference Values	Adrenal Insufficiency		
		Primary	Secondary	Tertiary
Screening Tests				
Plasma ACTH (0800 h)	10 to 85 pg/mL	Increased	Normal or decreased	Normal or decreased
Serum cortisol (0800 h)	5-23 μg/dL	Decreased	Normal or decreased	Normal or decreased
Challenge Tests				
Rapid ACTH stimulation, peak cortisol	>20 μg/dL	<20 μg/dL	Any	Any
Overnight metyrapone test				
Plasma 11-deoxycortisol	>7 μg/dL	Not indicated	<7 μg/dL	<7 μg/dL
Plasma ACTH	>150 pg/mL	Not indicated	<150 pg/mL	<150 pg/mL
CRH stimulation test				
Plasma ACTH	Not indicated	Not indicated	Decreased response	Increased response

ACTH, Adrenocorticotropic hormone; *CRH,* corticotropin-releasing hormone.

TABLE 41-3 Causes of Primary Adrenal Insufficiency

Chronic Adrenal Insufficiency
Autoimmune adrenal atrophy
Granulomatous disease: tuberculosis, histoplasmosis, sarcoidosis
Neoplastic infiltration
Metabolic disorders: amyloidosis, hemochromatosis, adrenoleukodystrophy, adrenomyeloneuropathy
Acquired immunodeficiency syndrome
Congenital immunodeficiency syndrome
Abdominal irradiation
After bilateral adrenalectomy

Acute Adrenal Insufficiency
Vascular
Adrenal hemorrhage: infection (caused by organisms such as meningococci and *Pseudomonas*), anticoagulants
Adrenal artery embolism
Adrenal vein thrombosis
After bilateral adrenalectomy

Hypofunction

Adrenal insufficiency

Adrenal insufficiency affects hormone levels (Table 41-2) and is classified as primary, secondary, or tertiary.

Primary adrenal insufficiency, also known as *Addison's disease,* results from progressive destruction or dysfunction of the adrenal glands by a local disease process or systemic disorder (Table 41-3). Because the entire cortex is affected, all classes of adrenal steroids are deficient. The onset of clinical manifestations is usually gradual, and the degree and severity of symptoms depend on the extent of the adrenal failure. In early or mild expressions of primary adrenal insufficiency, hypofunction may not be evident unless the individual is under stress. Complete glucocorticoid deficiency is characterized by chronic fatigue, weakness, weight loss, and postprandial hypoglycemia. Mineralocorticoid deficiency leads to dehydration with hypotension, hyponatre-

mia, and hyperkalemia. Excess release of ACTH and related precursor peptides causes hyperpigmentation and darkening of the skin, a characteristic feature of Addison's disease.

The measurement of basal ACTH and cortisol levels and the use of the ACTH stimulation test* are recommended when primary adrenal insufficiency is suspected.[2] Basal plasma ACTH levels greater than 150 pg/mL with a serum cortisol level of less than 10 μg/dL usually indicates adrenal insufficiency. A suppressed cortisol response to the corsyntropin stimulation test† supports the diagnosis of primary adrenal insufficiency. A normal cortisol rise in response to ACTH stimulation suggests the adrenal cortex is normal. A decreased or delayed response to ACTH stimulation suggests secondary or tertiary adrenal failure.

In individuals with secondary and tertiary adrenal insufficiency, inadequate cortisol production may be caused by destructive processes at the hypothalamic-pituitary level, resulting in a decreased ability to secrete ACTH (secondary adrenal insufficiency) or CRH (tertiary adrenal insufficiency). However, the most common cause of tertiary insufficiency is long-term administration of glucocorticoids that suppress CRH synthesis and therefore ACTH release. Clinical features of secondary and tertiary adrenal insuffi-

---

*Multiple-day ACTH stimulation testing for assessment of adrenal cortex function is required occasionally to evaluate adrenal cortisol responsiveness. For example, it is commonly used in the diagnosis of adrenal insufficiency, which is treated with glucocorticosteroids before establishment of an etiology. Prolonged ACTH stimulation is also used to distinguish primary from secondary or tertiary causes of adrenal insufficiency.
†Administering ACTH to normal patients results in a rapid rise in the serum cortisol level. Patients with adrenal destruction (Addison's disease) show no change in serum cortisol levels after ACTH administration. Patients with atrophy of the adrenal cortex caused by exogenous glucocorticoid treatment or dysfunction of the pituitary gland or hypothalamus may show a slight rise in serum cortisol levels, but the increase is not the normal amount.

TABLE 41-4 Causes of Hypoaldosteronism

Condition	Effects	Comments
Addison's disease	Diffuse destruction of adrenal cortex that includes zona glomerulosa	—
Complication of heparin therapy	Direct effect of heparin therapy	Usually after prolonged treatment
Resection of aldosterone-producing adenoma	Suppression of aldosterone secretion in normal cortical tissue by adenoma with delayed recovery after surgery	Prevention by spironolactone treatment before surgery
Hyperreninemic hypoaldosteronism	Selective injury to the renal zona glomerulosa during hypotensive episodes in critically ill individuals	Normal cortisol secretion; characterized by hyperkalemia in intensive care unit patients
Congenital adrenal hyperplasia with methyloxidase type II defect	Enzymatic block in the conversion of 18-OHβ corticosterone to aldosterone	—
Pseudohypoaldosteronism	Decreased responsiveness to aldosterone caused by mineralocorticoid receptor defect	Higher aldosterone levels
Hyporeninemic hypoaldosteronism	Low renin output causing a decrease in aldosterone secretion	In diabetic and older individuals with mild renal failure

ciency are similar to those of primary insufficiency except that hyperpigmentation is not present and hypotension is less severe. The pituitary ACTH reserve is usually assessed with the metyrapone or insulin-induced hypoglycemia test.[2] A decreased response suggests that the pituitary ACTH reserve is inadequate and supports a diagnosis of secondary or tertiary adrenal insufficiency.

The CRH stimulation test is used to differentiate tertiary from secondary adrenal insufficiency.[2] Individuals with tertiary disease show an elevation in ACTH in response to CRH administration, whereas those with secondary disease show little or no change in ACTH levels.

Hypoaldosteronism

Deficient aldosterone production (Table 41-4) occurs in individuals with Addison's disease and in individuals with (1) inadequate renin production by the kidney, (2) inherited enzyme defects in aldosterone biosynthesis, and (3) acquired forms of primary aldosterone deficiency (such as forms caused by heparin therapy or surgery). The resulting metabolic condition is hyperkalemia and hyponatremia, often with hypochloremic acidosis. Mild or moderate volume depletion, often with postural hypotension, may also develop. Hyporeninemic hypoaldosteronism is diagnosed by demonstration of the failure of PRA and aldosterone to increase in response to furosemide stimulation or an upright posture. Individuals with primary adrenal insufficiency may also have aldosterone deficiency caused by decreased availability of steroid substrate from pregnenolone.

Hyperfunction

Hyperfunction of the adrenal cortex produces the clinical syndromes of glucocorticoid excess, mineralocorticoid excess, and adrenal androgen excess.

TABLE 41-5 Incidence of Clinical Manifestations of Cushing's Syndrome

Clinical Manifestation	Incidence (%)
Obesity	90
Hypertension	>85
Hyperglycemia and decreased glucose tolerance	80
Menstrual and sexual dysfunction	76
Hirsutism, acne, plethora	72
Striae, atrophic skin	67
Weakness, proximal myopathy	65
Osteoporosis	55
Easy bruisability	55
Psychiatric disturbances	50
Edema	46
Polyuria, polyphagia	16
Ocular changes and exophthalmos	8

Corticosteroid excess (Cushing's syndrome)

Cushing's syndrome is the result of autonomous, excessive production of cortisol. Clinical manifestations include truncal obesity, hypertension, hypokalemic metabolic alkalosis, carbohydrate intolerance, and neuropsychiatric symptoms (Table 41-5). Excessive exogenous steroid therapy commonly causes the clinical features of Cushing's syndrome. Endogenous causes for hypersecretion of cortisol are classified as either ACTH dependent or ACTH independent (Table 41-6). In individuals with **Cushing's disease**, increased ACTH secretion caused by a pituitary microadenoma is the primary defect that leads to bilateral adrenal hyperplasia and cortisol overproduction. In the ectopic ACTH syndrome, nonendocrine tumors (for example, lung, gut, ovarian, and carcinoid tumors) secrete ACTH, producing adrenal hyperplasia and excessive cortisol secretion in the face of suppressed pituitary ACTH release. In individuals with Cushing's syndrome that is associated with primary

TABLE 41-6	Causes of Spontaneous Cushing's Syndrome
Underlying Disorder	Incidence (%)
ACTH Dependent	
Cushing's disease	68
Ectopic ACTH-secreting tumor	15
ACTH Independent	
Adenoma	5
Carcinoma	3
Nodular adrenal hyperplasia	9
Adrenocortical rest tumor	<1

ACTH, Adrenocorticotropic hormone.

adrenal disease caused by an adrenal adenoma or carcinoma, increased cortisol secretion suppresses CRH synthesis and ACTH secretion, resulting in atrophy of the nontumorous adrenal tissue.

Screening tests for Cushing's syndrome

The initial diagnosis of Cushing's syndrome, particularly in mild cases or the early stages of the disease, is based on laboratory evidence of excessive and autonomous cortisol production. Two simple screening tests are used to detect Cushing's syndrome (Table 41-7). The first is the measurement of free cortisol in urine over 24 hours. A result of less than 80 μg/day indicates the individual does not have Cushing's syndrome, whereas values greater than 120 μg/day may indicate Cushing's syndrome. Proper specimen collection is important for accurate result interpretation. A complete 24-hour urine collection from a patient who has not used diuretics or consumed excessive amounts of salt reduces the incidence of false-positive results. It is important to note that measurements of free cortisol in urine are used to screen for Cushing's syndrome but do not establish the diagnosis. An abnormal result should be followed up with provocative testing.

A second reliable screening test for Cushing's syndrome is the overnight low-dose dexamethasone suppression test* (1 mg of dexamethasone at midnight). Serum cortisol levels are measured at 0800 hours the next morning; a normal level is less than 5 μg/dL.[2]

Differential diagnosis of Cushing's syndrome

The determination of plasma ACTH and serum cortisol levels in addition to the dexamethasone suppression test is commonly used to establish the differential diagnosis of Cushing's syndrome. ACTH levels are suppressed in indi-

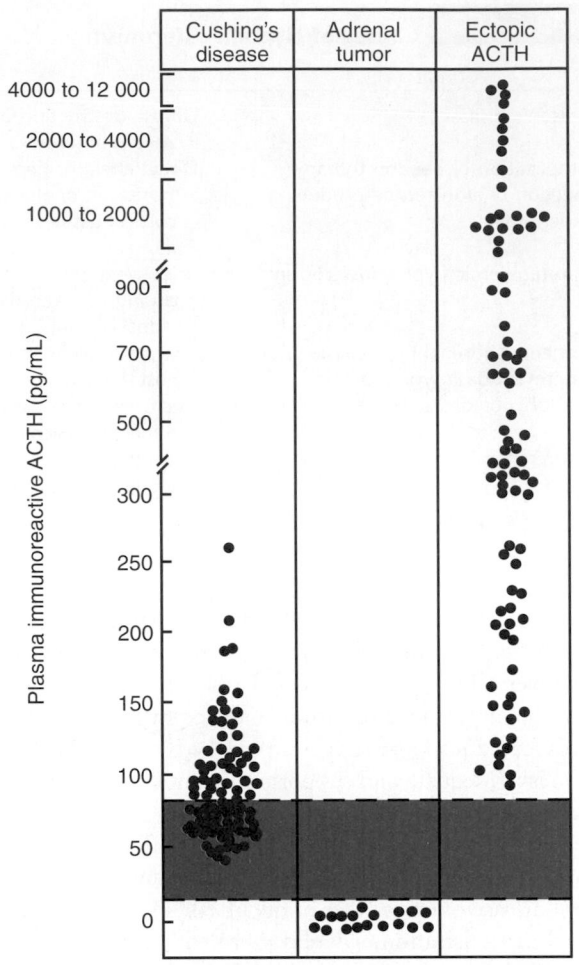

Figure 41-5   Basal plasma adrenocorticotropic hormone (ACTH) concentration in individuals with spontaneous Cushing's syndrome. (Modified from Scott AP et al: Pituitary adrenocorticotrophin and the melanocyte stimulating hormones. In Parsons JA (ed): Peptide Hormones, Baltimore, University Park Press, 1979.)

viduals with primary adrenal tumors and are normal or moderately elevated in individuals with Cushing's disease and macronodular hyperplasia (Figure 41-5). Plasma ACTH levels are usually markedly elevated in individuals with nonendocrine ACTH-secreting tumors. Plasma ACTH levels greater than 300 pg/mL usually support the diagnosis of a nonendocrine ACTH-secreting tumor.

High-dose dexamethasone suppression testing† is used to differentiate among individuals with Cushing's syndrome caused by adrenal tumors or nonendocrine ACTH-secreting

---

*Dexamethasone, a cortisol analogue, suppresses ACTH and cortisol production in healthy patients but not in patients with Cushing's syndrome.

---

†Patients with Cushing's syndrome caused by an ACTH-producing pituitary adenoma usually show suppression of cortisol in response to high doses of dexamethasone. Patients with Cushing's syndrome resulting from other causes (such as adrenocortical adenoma, adrenocortical carcinoma, or ectopic production of ACTH) usually do not demonstrate any changes in cortisol level.

TABLE 41-7	Differential Diagnosis in Cushing's Syndrome			
	Normal	Cushing's Syndrome	Adrenal Tumor	Ectopic ACTH Syndrome
Screening Tests				
Urinary free cortisol	<100 µg/day	>120 µg/day	>120 µg/day	µ120 µg/day
Overnight dexamethasone suppression test				
Serum cortisol (0800 h)	<3 µg/dL	>10 µg/dL	>10 µg/dL	>10 µg/dL
Differential Diagnostic Tests				
Plasma ACTH (0800 h)	10 to 85 pg/mL	40 to 260 pg/mL	<10 pg/mL	Normal to greatly elevated
Serum cortisol (0800 h)	5-23 g/dL	Normal	Normal or elevated	Normal or elevated
High-dose overnight dexamethasone suppression test				
Serum cortisol (0800 h)	50% suppression	Most suppress	Fail to suppress	Fail to suppress
CT or MRI				
Of adrenal glands	−	−	+	−
Of pituitary gland	−	+	−	−
Of other locations	−	−	−	+
CRH stimulation test with IPS venous sampling				
Ratio of ACTH in IPS vein to that in peripheral vein	Not indicated	>3	<3	<3

ACTH, Adrenocorticotropic hormone; *CRH,* corticotropin-releasing hormone; *CT,* computed tomography; *IPS,* inferior petrosal sinus; *MRI,* magnetic resonance imaging.

tumors and individuals with pituitary Cushing's disease. In individuals with adrenal tumors and in most (but not all) individuals with nonendocrine ACTH-secreting tumors, high doses of dexamethasone do not result in ACTH suppression of cortisol. In contrast, most individuals with macronodular hyperplasia show some suppression of cortisol after receiving high doses of dexamethasone, although most show only 50% to 60% suppression.

The CRH stimulation test* produces an exaggerated ACTH or cortisol response in about 90% of individuals with Cushing's disease. Individuals with adrenal tumors and most individuals with nonendocrine ACTH-secreting tumors produce a poor response. If the cause of the individual's Cushing's syndrome is uncertain, measurement of ACTH from the inferior petrosal sinus vein before and after CRH stimulation may be helpful.[9,12]

In addition to suppression and stimulation testing, anatomical localization methods are used to document the diagnosis of Cushing's syndrome. Computed tomography (CT) of the adrenal glands helps to localize adrenal tumors, macronodular hyperplasia, and bilateral hyperplasia of the adrenal glands. CT combined with magnetic resonance imaging (MRI) of the pituitary gland helps detect pituitary microadenomas.

---

*Exogenous CRH stimulates the secretion of ACTH from the anterior pituitary gland in normal patients. The cortisol level is an indicator of the ACTH response.

Congenital adrenal hyperplasia (adrenogenital syndrome)

The biosynthesis of cortisol and aldosterone from cholesterol requires the action of specific enzymes in the adrenal cortex for the chemical modification and introduction of the different functional groups (see Figure 41-3). CAH is characterized by the congenital absence of or deficiency in one or more of the biosynthetic enzymes that participate in cortisol production. If a defect or deficiency in four key enzymes of adrenocorticoid biosynthesis develops, cortisol biosynthesis is impaired, leading to a compensatory increase in ACTH release. ACTH then stimulates steroid biosynthesis excessively and causes an enzyme block. Therefore enzyme defects cause hyperplasia of the adrenal cortex and accumulation of intermediate compounds proximal to the block, with substrate shunting toward the adrenal androgen pathway. Measurements of the specific precursor steroids in blood are useful in the identification of the specific enzyme defect and monitoring of a patient's response to cortisol replacement therapy. A partial enzyme block may cause modest or subtle clinical manifestations, whereas a complete enzyme block is sometimes incompatible with life. The closer the enzyme block is to the final cortisol product, the less life threatening are the symptoms.

The diagnosis of CAH in female individuals, particularly in female newborns, is typically indicated by the presence of ambiguous genitalia. In boys the abnormality may not be suspected until signs of precocious puberty or accelerated growth develop during childhood. Because aldosterone production is also compromised, hypertension and salt wasting also occur. It is not uncommon for the adrenogenital syndrome to be diagnosed in adults. For example, affected adults may have subtle abnormalities that go unrecognized until fertility is desired. In women the clinical symptoms may be indistinguishable from those of polycystic ovary disease or idiopathic hirsutism.

A 21-hydroxylase enzyme deficiency (see Figure 41-3) is the most common form of CAH. An elevated 17α-hydroxyprogesterone level is characteristic of this enzyme defect. In addition, because substrate flow is diverted into the adrenal androgen pathway, DHEA-S levels are also elevated, leading to symptoms caused by excess androgen levels. Late-onset 21-hydroxylase deficiency is associated with mild to moderate hirsutism in women. The ACTH stimulation test and measurement of 17-hydroxyprogesterone is useful in the identification of heterozygotes and individuals with acquired forms of 21-hydroxylase deficiency.[10]

An 11β-hydroxylase deficiency is the second most common form of congenital adrenal hyperplasia and is associated with virilization and hypertension. The mineralocorticoid-induced hypertension is caused by DOC elevations. Levels of 11-deoxycortisol are markedly raised in individuals with an 11β-hydroxylase defect.

A 3β-hydroxysteroid dehydrogenase-isomerase deficiency leads to an increase in the ratio of 17α-hydroxypregnenolone to 17α-hydroxyprogesterone and an increased ratio of DHEA to androstenedione. In severe forms, female infants have pseudohermaphroditism, whereas male infants have incomplete masculinization. A late-onset form has also been reported in women with hirsutism, acne, and menstrual irregularities.

A C-17,20-lyase/17α-hydroxylase enzyme deficiency results in the inability to convert 17-hydroxypregnenolone to DHEA and 17-hydroxyprogesterone to androstenedione. A defect in this enzyme complex in the gonads of genetic females results in pubertal failure (no ovarian maturation or menses), and a defect in genetic males causes pseudoher-

maphroditism. Cortisol, androgen, and estrogen synthesis decrease, and the production of progesterone, corticosterone, and DOC increase. In its complete form, the deficiency causes hypertension and hyperkalemia and prevents sexual development in girls, whereas in boys it causes male pseudohermaphroditism.

The effectiveness of a treatment program for CAH is judged on the basis of the presence or absence of normal linear growth, normal sexual development, and suppression of raised blood and urine steroid levels into the reference interval.

Adrenal tumors

In individuals with virilizing adrenal adenomas and Cushing's syndrome, plasma DHEA-S, androstenedione, and testosterone levels are elevated. Plasma levels of androstenedione and testosterone are also elevated in women with virilizing ovarian tumors. CT scans are useful in the determination of the sites of the tumors.

Adrenal carcinomas are rare, possibly causing only virilization and not the typical features of Cushing's syndrome. Plasma DHEA-S levels are markedly elevated in individuals with adrenocortical carcinoma and frequently exceed 10 μg/mL. High doses of glucocorticoids do not suppress the elevated androgen concentrations.

Feminizing adrenal cortical carcinomas are also rare and result in elevation of plasma adrenal androgen, estrone, and estradiol concentrations. Gynecomastia and sexual dysfunctions develop in boys and men with this disorder, whereas precocious pseudopuberty occurs in girls. Steroid hormone production does not decrease to normal levels after treatment with dexamethasone.

Mineralocorticoid excess (hyperaldosteronism)

Hyperaldosteronism, also referred to as *Conn's syndrome,* is associated with hypersecretion of aldosterone, a major mineralocorticoid (Table 41-8). Types of hyperaldosteronism include primary and secondary hyperaldosteronism.

TABLE 41-8 **Differential Diagnosis of Aldosteronism**

	Plasma Renin	Plasma Aldosterone	Blood Pressure	Serum Potassium
Primary aldosteronism	Low	High	High	Low
Secondary hypertension				
Edematous disorder	High	High	Normal	Low
Malignant hypertension	High	High	High	Low
Renovascular hypertension	Normal or high	Normal or high	High	Normal or low
Renin-secreting tumors	High	High	High	Normal or low
Congenital adrenal hyperplasia (11- and 17-hydroxylase deficiency)	Low	Low	High	Low
Cushing's syndrome	Normal or low	Normal or low	High	Low
Liddle's syndrome	Low	Low	High	Low
Bartter's syndrome	High	High	Normal or low	Low
Licorice ingestion	Low	Low	High	Low
Low-renin essential hypertension	Low	Normal or low	High	Normal
Ingestion of exogenous mineralocorticoids	Low	Low	High	Low

Primary aldosteronism

In individuals with primary hyperaldosteronism, excessive aldosterone production results from an adrenal gland adenoma and is characterized by the presence of hypertension and hypokalemia. Overproduction of aldosterone may be caused by an autonomous aldosterone-secreting adenoma[7] (aldosterone-producing adrenal adenoma [APA] or Conn's syndrome), hyperplasia of aldosterone-producing cells (idiopathic adrenal hyperplasia [IAH]), adrenal carcinoma, or a rare familial condition known as *glucocorticoid-suppressible aldosteronism*. Increased sodium retention caused by the effects of aldosterone on the renal tubular processing of sodium, expansion of extracellular fluid volume, and increased tubular secretion of potassium and hydrogen ions are the key features of primary aldosteronism. Hypokalemia and metabolic alkalosis result as a consequence of a progressive renal depletion of potassium. As a consequence of sodium retention, extracellular fluid volume increases slightly, causing a subsequent increase in arterial blood pressure.

Secondary aldosteronism

In individuals with secondary hyperaldosteronism the stimulus for hypersecretion comes from activation of the renin-angiotensin system. The interaction of renin, angiotensin, and aldosterone is important in the maintenance of extracellular fluid volume, blood pressure, and sodium and potassium balance. An alteration in any one of these variables affects the others. The secondary changes are much more common than the primary abnormalities (see Table 41-8). For example, a decrease in effective plasma volume or mean arterial pressure leads to renin release, resulting in angiotensin I and II production and aldosterone release by the adrenal glands. The end result is (1) retention of sodium and water by the kidneys, (2) an increase in extracellular plasma volume, and (3) a decrease in serum potassium levels. Secondary aldosteronism is common in individuals with congestive heart failure, nephrotic syndrome, cirrhosis of the liver, and other hypoproteinemic states, as well as in individuals with conditions involving chronic plasma volume depletion.

Laboratory diagnosis

Hypokalemia is a major clinical sign that an individual with hypertension may have primary aldosteronism. To establish the diagnosis, it is necessary to demonstrate that (1) hyposecretion of renin is being inappropriately corrected with volume depletion, and (2) hypersecretion of aldosterone cannot be suppressed with an expansion in plasma volume. Figure 41-6 shows a recommended algorithm for the evaluation of patients with suspected mineralocorticoid excess.

Although most individuals with autonomous aldosterone overproduction have hypokalemia, most individuals with hypokalemia do not have primary aldosteronism. In individuals with hyperaldosteronism, urinary potassium excretion is inappropriately high, and a random urine potassium level greater than 30 mmol/L is suggestive of primary aldosteronism or some form of mineralocorticoid excess.

In individuals with primary aldosteronism and a normal salt intake, suppressed renin and high aldosterone levels are expected. It is important to recognize that the individual's posture and salt intake markedly affect renin and aldosterone secretion. Thus it is helpful to compare an ambulatory individual's renin and aldosterone levels with sodium excretion to properly interpret the normality of the renin-aldosterone axis. Provocative testing is also helpful in this regard. A twofold to threefold stimulation of renin release with a potent diuretic, such as furosemide, occurs in individuals with a normal renin-angiotensin-aldosterone system.* A high renin activity level rules out primary hyperaldosteronism and suggests secondary hyperaldosteronism (for example, renovascular hypertension or pheochromocytoma). In contrast, a suppressed rennin level suggests that the individual may have primary aldosteronism or low-renin hypertension.

The measurement of plasma renin responsiveness only is not sufficient to make the diagnosis of primary aldosteronism because suppressed PRA also occurs in about 25% of individuals with essential hypertension. Primary aldosteronism is differentiated from other hypermineralocorticoid states on the basis of inappropriate aldosterone secretion. The demonstration of an elevated aldosterone level in blood or urine in an individual with an unequivocally suppressed PRA level is presumptive evidence of primary aldosteronism. To confirm aldosterone autonomous secretion, the clinician may attempt to suppress aldosterone with rapid volume expansion using a potent mineralocorticoid or with the use of the angiotensin-converting enzyme (ACE) inhibitor, captopril. Failure to suppress aldosterone with these maneuvers confirms the diagnosis of primary aldosteronism.

Once the diagnosis of primary aldosteronism is made, it is necessary to distinguish between an adrenal adenoma and bilateral hyperplasia. This differentiation is important because most individuals with an adenoma respond well to surgical removal of the tumor,[8] whereas individuals with hyperplasia are managed medically. CT scan and ultrasound are commonly used to localize the adenoma. On occasion, select venous catheterization of the right versus left adrenal vein is performed to identify which adrenal is hypersecreting aldosterone.

Other types of hyperaldosteronism

Other unusual conditions that suggest aldosterone excess or deficiency but are not connected to the renin-angiotensin-aldosterone system include *Liddle's syndrome* (pseudohyperaldosteronism), which resembles primary al-

---

*Plasma renin activity varies with the state of hydration and sodium intake. The administration of furosemide, a potent diuretic, provides a stimulus to increase plasma renin secretion.

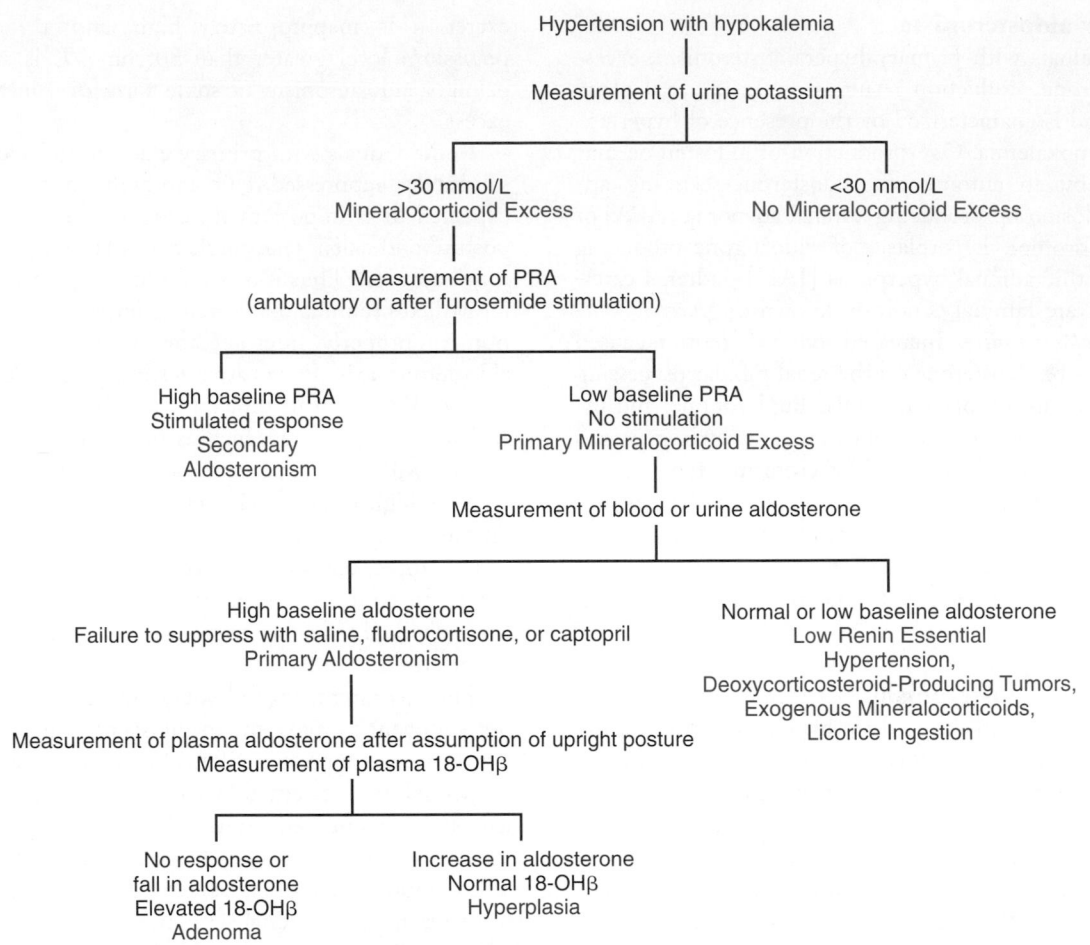

Figure 41-6   Laboratory procedure for individuals with suspected aldosteronism causing hypertension. *PRA,* Plasma renin activity; *18-OHβ,* 18-hydroxycorticosterone.

dosteronism clinically, but aldosterone production is low and hypertension is absent, and *Bartter's syndrome,* which involves prostaglandin-mediated renal potassium wasting and elevated aldosterone and renin levels. Individuals with renal tubular acidosis and pseudohypoaldosteronism have the clinical symptoms of hypoaldosteronism but abnormally high aldosterone levels.

Plasma renin and renovascular hypertension

Used as a screening test, elevated activity of plasma renin after furosemide stimulation or in correlation with urinary sodium excretion suggests renal artery stenosis as the cause of renovascular hypertension. If arteriographic evidence for renal artery stenosis is found, measurements of the activity of renin in plasma specimens obtained from selective renal vein catheterization help predict the response to surgical correction of the renal vascular lesion or nephrectomy. Lateralization of renin in the renal vein to the radiographically involved side, especially after sodium depletion, also predicts a good response to surgery in 90% of cases.

■ TESTING THE FUNCTIONAL STATUS OF THE ADRENAL CORTEX

The functional status of the hypothalamic-pituitary-adrenal axis is assessed by the measurement of ACTH and the adrenocorticosteroids (such as cortisol and aldosterone) in blood under basal and stimulatory conditions. However, relying on basal hormone concentrations to establish the presence of adrenal cortical disorders is problematic because of the episodic and circadian secretory nature of the hormones involved in the hypothalamic-pituitary-adrenal axis. Dynamic testing of this axis helps define abnormalities that are not reflected in basal hormone secretion.

Corticosteroid Function

Basal peptide and steroid hormone levels

Episodic secretion and circadian variation limit the clinical diagnostic accuracy of basal serum cortisol concentrations. Cortisol levels are highest in the early morning and range from 5 to 25 μg/dL between 0400 and 0900 hours. Late afternoon values of cortisol are about half the morning levels. In addition, cortisol concentrations are usually below 5 μg/dL between 2200 and 0200 hours. Serum cortisol levels combined with plasma ACTH determinations improve the diagnostic accuracy of basal values.

Urinary free cortisol levels obtained from a 24-hour urine collection eliminates the circadian influence on cortisol secretion and hence is considered the best screening test for hypercortisolism. The urinary free cortisol excretion rate in normal subjects is between 20 and 80 μg/day.

Mineralocorticoid and adrenal androgen secretion is also circadian and episodic, but the dynamic swing in its levels is not as pronounced as those of cortisol. However, it is usually recommended that blood samples used for testing adrenal steroids be obtained between 0700 and 1000 hours for consistent interpretation of results.

Stimulation tests

Provocative testing is frequently used to verify hyposecretion of the adrenocortical hormones and determine whether the deficiency is primary or secondary. The most common provocative test used to document the functional capacity of the adrenal gland is the cosyntropin (synthetic ACTH) test, or ACTH stimulation test.[2] In healthy individuals the intravenous administration of exogenous ACTH rapidly increases the secretion of cortisol twofold to threefold within 60 minutes. This functional response may be impaired either by adrenal atrophy caused by chronic ACTH deficiency or by destruction of the adrenal cortex itself.

A direct and selective test of pituitary function is the CRH stimulation test.[9] Intravenous administration of ovine CRH stimulates ACTH secretion in normal individuals within 60 to 180 minutes. This test is primarily used in the differential diagnosis of endogenous Cushing's syndrome and to distinguish secondary ACTH deficiency from tertiary ACTH deficiency.

A variation of the CRH stimulation test measures ACTH in blood samples drawn from the inferior petrosal sinus (IPS)* to identify the presence of a pituitary microadenoma and determine on which side of the pituitary the microadenoma is located. Blood samples are collected from the right and left sides of the IPS and from a peripheral vein before and 2, 5, and 10 minutes after the intravenous administration of ovine CRH (1 μg per kilogram of body weight) for 20 to 60 seconds. The ratio of the IPS level to the peripheral venous concentration of plasma ACTH is used to predict the location of excess corticotropin secretion. Some endocrinologists claim that IPS sampling is the best test to distinguish among ACTH-dependent forms of Cushing's syndrome when performed in individuals with prolonged hypercortisolism. ACTH levels are suppressed

in individuals with primary adrenal tumors and raised in cases of Cushing's disease or ectopic ACTH syndrome.

Other indirect tests of ACTH secretion rely on the adrenal glands' response to maneuvers that stimulate endogenous ACTH release. The insulin-induced hypoglycemia stimulation test serves this purpose.[2] Insulin is given to stimulate the release of CRH from the onset of hypoglycemia, and plasma ACTH or cortisol levels are measured and evaluated to determine whether they have increased. This test involves risks and should be performed only with an experienced physician in attendance.

A less risky but indirect test of hypothalamic-pituitary-adrenal axis function involves the administration of metyrapone, an inhibitor of the 11β-hydroxylase enzyme that converts 11-deoxycortisol to cortisol. In healthy individuals, the decrease in the plasma cortisol level that accompanies the metyrapone-induced enzyme block stimulates pituitary ACTH release and increases the concentration of adrenal steroid precursors proximal to the enzyme block. Under normal circumstances, 11-deoxycortisol, the steroid precursor substrate converted to cortisol, increases fortyfold to eightyfold within 3 hours of metyrapone administration. No 11-deoxycortisol increase suggests primary adrenal failure.

Suppression tests

Suppression tests are used to document hypersecretion of adrenocortical hormones. Under normal circumstances an elevation in blood cortisol levels inhibits ACTH release from the adenohypophysis, resulting in decreased production of cortisol and other adrenal steroids from the adrenal cortex. The integrity of this feedback mechanism is tested by administration of a potent glucocorticoid, such as dexamethasone, and judgment of the suppression of ACTH secretion by measurement of serum or urine cortisol levels.

Mineralocorticoid Function
Basal peptide and steroid hormone levels

The measurement of aldosterone and peptides of the renin-angiotensin system is useful to assess sodium homeostasis and normality of the renin-angiotensin-aldosterone axis. Aldosterone and renin secretion are significantly influenced by drugs, posture, and salt intake, so these factors should be considered during the interpretation of test results. In healthy individuals a low-sodium diet, an upright posture, and use of diuretics increase plasma aldosterone levels, whereas a high-sodium diet and a supine position decrease aldosterone secretion. Unlike aldosterone, the plasma renin level is measured in terms of its enzymatic activity. PRA is determined by measurement of the generation of angiotensin I with immunoassay methods. However, the effects of posture, drug ingestion, and diet make it difficult to identify mineralocorticoid secretion disorders on the basis of basal hormone levels

---

*The inferior petrosal sinus arises from the cavernous sinus and runs to the internal jugular vein.

only; thus dynamic testing is used to verify hypersecretion or hyposecretion of aldosterone and renin.

Stimulation tests

The renin-angiotensin-aldosterone system responds to sudden changes in electrolyte balance. Sodium excretion and extracellular fluid volume are inversely associated with PRA and aldosterone concentrations. Protocols for stimulation of the renin-angiotensin system are frequently based on volume-depletion strategies, such as sodium restriction, an upright posture, or administration of diuretics. In the furosemide stimulation test, the patient receives 40 to 80 mg of furosemide orally or intravenously and then maintains an upright posture for 4 hours.[2] A normal patient demonstrates a twofold to threefold rise in PRA in response to the diuretic. Another simple and convenient stimulation test simply restricts sodium intake while the patient maintains an upright posture. Healthy patients placed on a low-salt diet containing less than 20 mmol/day of sodium demonstrate a twofold to threefold increase in PRA.

Suppression tests

Mineralocorticoid suppression tests have been designed to use plasma volume expansion. Saline infusion, oral salt loading, or mineralocorticoid administration is used to suppress aldosterone production by the adrenal gland. In healthy individuals, acute plasma volume expansion caused by the salt intake increases renal perfusion, suppresses renin release,

and decreases aldosterone secretion. In the saline suppression test, isotonic saline is infused intravenously for 4 hours, after which plasma aldosterone levels and renin activity are determined.[2] Aldosterone levels normally decrease to less than 5 ng/dL (<140 pmol/L), and PRA is suppressed. Other suppression tests include the administration of fludrocortisone, a synthetic mineralocorticoid, and the use of an ACE inhibitor to compromise the production of angiotensin II. Healthy individuals suppress plasma aldosterone levels to less than 10 ng/dL (280 pmol/L) during these suppression tests.

Adrenal Androgen Function

Stimulation testing

The responses to ACTH stimulation vary. Plasma DHEA and androstenedione levels increase threefold to fourfold after 90 minutes of stimulation by ACTH (250 μg) administration. In contrast, DHEA-S increases 30% to 50% after ACTH administration. ACTH stimulation studies are useful in the evaluation of hypoandrogenemic disorders.

Suppression tests

Overnight dexamethasone suppression tests produce small changes in adrenal androgen levels compared with those of cortisol. Administered of 0.75 mg of dexamethasone at midnight for several days reliably suppresses adrenal androgen levels in blood. Tissue stores of these androgens may account in part for the delayed response.

References

1. Demers LM : Biochemistry and laboratory measurement of androgens in women. In Redmond GP (ed): Androgenic Disorders, pp 21-34, New York, Raven Press, 1995.
2. Demers LM, Whitley RJ: Function of the adrenal cortex. In Burtis CA, Ashwood ER (eds): Tietz Textbook of Clinical Chemistry, 3rd edition, pp 1530-1569, Philadelphia, WB Saunders, 1999.
3. Funder JW, Krozowski Z, Myles K et al: Mineralocorticoid receptors, salt, and hypertension. Recent Prog Horm Res 1997; 52:247-262.
4. Inoue S: Simultaneous high-performance liquid chromatographic determination of 6 beta-hydroxycortisol and cortisol in urine with fluorescence detection and its application for estimating hepatic drug-metabolizing enzyme induction. J Chromatogr B Biomed Appl 1994; 661:15-23.
5. Kiess W, Meidert A, Dressendorfer RA et al: Salivary cortisol levels throughout childhood and adolescence: relation with age, pubertal stage, and weight. Pediatr Res 1995; 37:502-506.
6. Lensmeyer G, Carlson I, Wiebe D et al: Determination of cortisol (C), cortisone (CN), corticosterone (CC), prednisone (P), and prednisolone (PL) in serum with solid reversed-phase extraction and high-performance liquid chromatography (HPLC). Clin Chem 1992; 38:945.
7. Li JT, Shu SG, Chi CS: Aldosterone-secreting adrenal cortical adenoma in an 11-year-old child and collective review of the literature. Eur J Pediatr 1994; 153:715-717.
8. Lo CY, Tam PC, Kung AW et al: Primary aldosteronism: results of surgical treatment. Ann Surg 1996; 224:125-130.
9. Loriaux DL, Nieman L: Corticotropin-releasing hormone testing in pituitary disease. Endocrinol Metab Clin North Am 1991; 20:363-370.
10. Migeon CJ, Donohoue PA: Congenital adrenal hyperplasia caused by 21-hydroxylase deficiency: its molecular basis and its remaining therapeutic problems. Endocrinol Metab Clin North Am 1991; 20:277-296.
11. Nahoul K, Patricot MC, Bressot N et al: Measurement of salivary cortisol with four commercial kits. Ann Biol Clin (Paris) 1996; 54:75-82.

12. Oldfield EH, Doppman JL, Nieman LK et al: Petrosal sinus sampling with and without corticotropin-releasing hormone for the differential diagnosis of Cushing's syndrome. N Engl J Med 1991; 325:897-905.

13. Price CP, Newman DJ: Principles and Practice of Immunoassay, New York, Stockton Press, 1996.

14. Smith C, Kapsner K: A heterogeneous competitive assay for cortisol using magnetic microparticles and enzyme chemiluminescence. Clin Chem 1992; 38:1085.

15. Stabler T, Siegel A: Chemiluminescence immunoassay of aldosterone in serum. Clin Chem 1991; 37:1987-1989.

Additional Reading

DeGroot LJ, Jameson JL (eds): Endocrinology, 4th edition Philadelphia, WB Saunders, 2000.

Selby C: Interference in immunoassay. Ann Clin Biochem 1999; 36:704-721.

Williams RH, Wilson JD (eds): Williams Textbook of Endocrinology, 9th edition, Philadelphia, WB Saunders, 1998.

Wood PJ, Barth JH, Freedman DB et al: Evidence for the low-dose dexamethasone suppression test to screen for Cushing's syndrome: recommendations for a protocol for biochemistry laboratories. Ann Clin Biochem 1997; 34:222-229.

CHAPTER 42

Reproductive Endocrine Function*

ANN M. GRONOWSKI, PhD, and MARY E. LANDAU-LEVINE, MD

Objectives

1. Define the following terms:

Corpus luteum	Ovum
Gynecomastia	Placenta
Hirsutism	Polycystic ovary syndrome
Leydig cell	Sertoli cell
Menopause	

2. Describe the structure of the female and male reproductive tracts.
3. List the hormones synthesized by the female and male reproductive tracts and their specific sites of synthesis. State the functions of these hormones.
4. State the effects of increased and decreased GnRH, LH, and FSH release.
5. Diagram the female reproductive cycle.
6. List the laboratory tests used to assess reproductive function.

Key Words

Amenorrhea The absence of menstruation

Blastula The usually spherical structure produced by cleavage of a fertilized ovum; consists of a single layer of cells (the blastoderm) surrounding a fluid-filled cavity

Capacitation The process by which a spermatozoon become capable of fertilizing an ovum

Corpus Luteum A yellow glandular mass in the ovary formed by an ovarian follicle that has matured and discharged its ovum; secretes progesterone

Endometritis A condition in which tissue containing typical endometrial elements occurs aberrantly in various locations in the pelvic cavity

Follicle A pouchlike sac that is on the surface of the ovary and contains the maturing ovum (egg)

Gametogenesis The development of the male and female sex cells, or gametes

Gonads A gamete-producing gland (an ovary or a testis)

Gynecomastia Excessive development of the male mammary glands

Hermaphroditism A physical state characterized by the presence of both male and female sex organs

Hirsutism Abnormal hairiness, especially an adult male pattern of hair distribution in women

Infertility A diminished or absent capacity to produce offspring

Kallmann's Syndrome A common form of hypogonadotropic hypogonadism resulting from a deficiency of GnRH in the hypothalamus

Karyotype The full chromosome set of the nucleus of a cell; includes the chromosomal sex of each individual, which is determined by the presence of the XX (female) or the XY (male) genotype in somatic cells

*The authors gratefully acknowledge the original contributions of R.J. Whitley, A.W. Meikle, and N.B. Watts, on which portions of this chapter are based.

Leydig Cells   Cells of the mammalian testis endocrine tissue that produce androgens, primarily testosterone

Menarche   The establishment or beginning of the menstrual function

Menopause   Cessation of menstruation in the woman, which usually occurs around the age 50

Menses   The monthly flow of blood from the genital tract of women

Menstrual Cycle   The reproductive cycle of female humans

Menstruation   The cyclical, physiological discharge of blood and mucosal tissues through the vagina of the uterus of a nonpregnant female

Mullerian Ducts   Two embryonic ducts that in females develop into the vagina, uterus and oviducts but disappear in males, except for the vestigial vagina masculina and the appendix testis

Oophorectomy   Surgery to remove one or both ovaries

Ovum   The female reproductive cell; becomes a zygote after fertilization and develops into a new member of the same species

Placenta   A fetomaternal organ that is characteristic of true mammals during pregnancy

Polycystic Ovary Syndrome (PCOS)   A female condition that is characterized by multiple ovarian cysts and increased androgen production; also known as the *Stein-Leventhal syndrome*

Sertoli Cells   Cells of the mammalian testis to which spermatids become attached; provide support, protection, and nutrition until the spermatids become transformed into mature spermatozoa

Virilization   The induction or development of male secondary sex characteristics; especially the induction of such changes in the female, including enlargement of the clitoris, growth of facial and body hair, development of a typical male hairline, stimulation of secretion and proliferation of the sebaceous glands (often causing acne), and deepening of the voice

Wolffian Duct   An embryonic duct (also known as the *mesonephric duct*) that in males develops into the epididymis, the ductus deferens and its ampulla, the seminal vesicles, and the ejaculatory duct; develops into vestigial structures in females

---

Reproductive function requires the hormones of the hypothalamic-pituitary-gonadal axis, as well as the adrenal glands (see Figure 26-1 and Chapters 39 and 41). These hormones are crucial for proper reproductive function and include gonadotropin-releasing hormone (GnRH), luteinizing hormone (LH), follicle-stimulating hormone (FSH), and numerous sex steroids. The sex steroids are synthesized by the ovaries, testes, and adrenal glands and are responsible for the manifestation of primary and secondary sex characteristics. Steroids that feminize are classified as *estrogens;* those that masculinize are known as *androgens.*

■ MALE REPRODUCTIVE BIOLOGY

Anatomy and Physiology

The male reproductive anatomy includes the penis, two testes (gonads), and a system of exocrine glands (two bulbourethral glands, two seminal vesicles, and the prostate) whose secretions form the seminal fluid. The ducts that connect this system and transport sperm and seminal fluid into and through the urethra are the (1) epididymis, (2) vas deferens, and (3) ejaculatory duct.

Function

The function of the testes is to synthesize sperm and androgens. The mature testis contains a structured network of

tightly packed seminiferous tubules separated by fibrous septa (Figure 42-1). The lumen of the seminiferous tubules are lined by maturing germ cells and **Sertoli cells** (Figure 42-2). Sertoli cells play a crucial role in sperm maturation and secrete inhibin, a glycoprotein that inhibits the pituitary secretion of FSH. The Sertoli cells form a network of

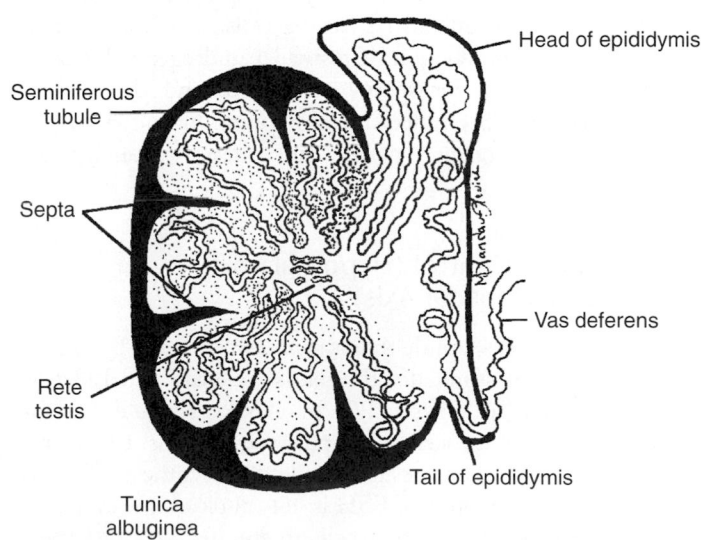

Figure 42-1   Testicular anatomy. (Modified from Ganong WF: Review of Medical Physiology, 11th edition, Los Altos, Calif, Lange Medical Publication, 1983.)

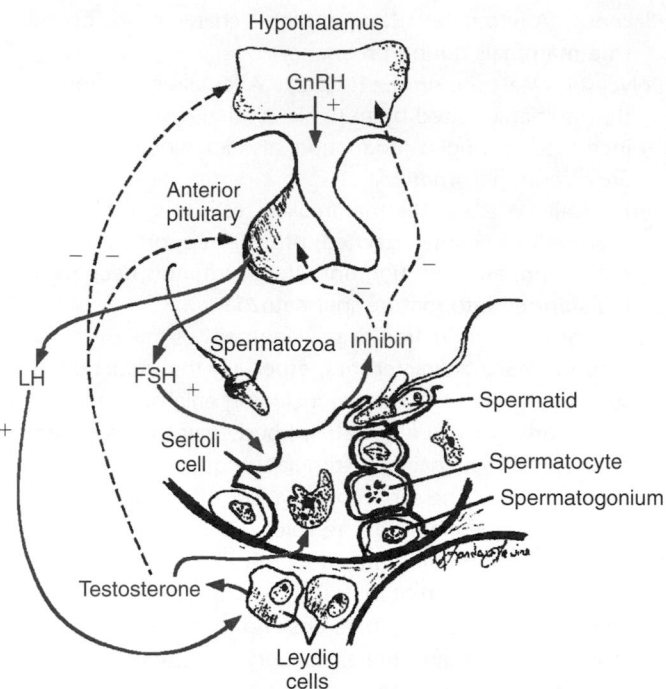

Figure 42-2   Summary of the endocrine control of the testis. Dashed lines indicate inhibitory effects, and solid lines indicate stimulatory effects. *FSH*, Follicle-stimulating hormone; *GnRH*, gonadotropin-releasing hormone; *LH*, luteinizing hormone.

tight junctions that separate the spermatogonia (undifferentiated germ cells) and the more mature primary spermatocytes. Histologically, mature spermatozoa are found at the center of the seminiferous tubules. From this location they are conveyed through the rete testes, the epididymis, and the vas deferens, undergoing minor maturational modifications before ejaculation. Surrounding the tubules are the interstitial Leydig cells, which are responsible for the production of testicular androgens. Testosterone is essential for sperm maturation and the complex endocrine feedback mechanism between Sertoli cells, Leydig cells, maturing sperm, the anterior pituitary, and hypothalamus.

Hormonal Control (Hypothalamic-Pituitary-Gonadal Axis)

GnRH is a decapeptide that is synthesized in the hypothalamus, where it stimulates the release of FSH and LH from the pituitary (see Chapter 39). In men, GnRH and therefore LH and FSH are secreted in pulsatile patterns. LH acts on Leydig cells in the testes to stimulate the synthesis of testosterone. The exact role of FSH is not yet clear; however, FSH is known to act on Sertoli cells to stimulate **gametogenesis** and the synthesis and release of inhibin. The complex feedback mechanism of the hypothalamic-gonadal axis is summarized in Figure 42-2.

Androgens

Androgens are a group of 19-carbon (C_{19}) steroids that cause masculinization of the genital tract and the development and maintenance of male secondary sex characteristics. They also contribute to muscle bulk, bone mass, sex drive, and sexual performance in men. Testosterone is the main androgen secreted by the testes, and its production increases during puberty. Women produce only 5% to 10% as much testosterone as do men.

Biochemistry and Physiology

Biosynthesis

Androgens are synthesized in the testes and adrenal glands. Synthesis begins with the formation of pregnenolone from cholesterol by the action of the cholesterol side-chain cleavage enzyme. The pathway for testosterone formation is shown in Figure 42-3, with the preferred pathway defined by heavy arrows.

Transport in blood

Testosterone and dihydrotestosterone (DHT), a metabolite of testosterone, circulate in plasma either freely (approximately 2% to 3%) or bound to plasma proteins. The binding proteins include the specific sex hormone-binding globulin (SHBG) and nonspecific proteins such as albumin. SHBG has low capacity for steroids but binds with very high affinity for them, whereas albumin has high capacity but low affinity for steroids. Testosterone and SHBG exhibit rhythmic variations in their circulating concentrations.

For many years, the free fraction of testosterone was thought to be the biologically active fraction. Current thought is that dissociation of albumin-bound testosterone occurs within a capillary bed. Therefore the bioavailable testosterone is equal to the free testosterone plus the albumin-bound testosterone. The albumin-bound fraction is referred to as the "non–SHBG-bound" fraction or weakly bound fraction.

Metabolism

Circulating testosterone serves as a precursor for the formation of two types of active metabolites, DHT and estrogen (Figure 42-4). Through the actions of 5α-reductase, testosterone is converted to DHT. Alternatively, testosterone and androstenedione can be converted to estrogens through aromatase. Peripheral aromatization occurs primarily in adipose tissue, and the rate of extraglandular estrogen formation increases with body fat.

Dihydrotestosterone is metabolized to 3α-androstanediol and 3α-androstanediol glucuronide, metabolites that have been used as markers of DHT production in peripheral tissues. The main excretory metabolites of androstenedione, testosterone, and dehydroepiandrosterone (DHEA) are shown in Figure 42-5. Except for epitestosterone, these catabolites constitute a group of steroids known as *17-*

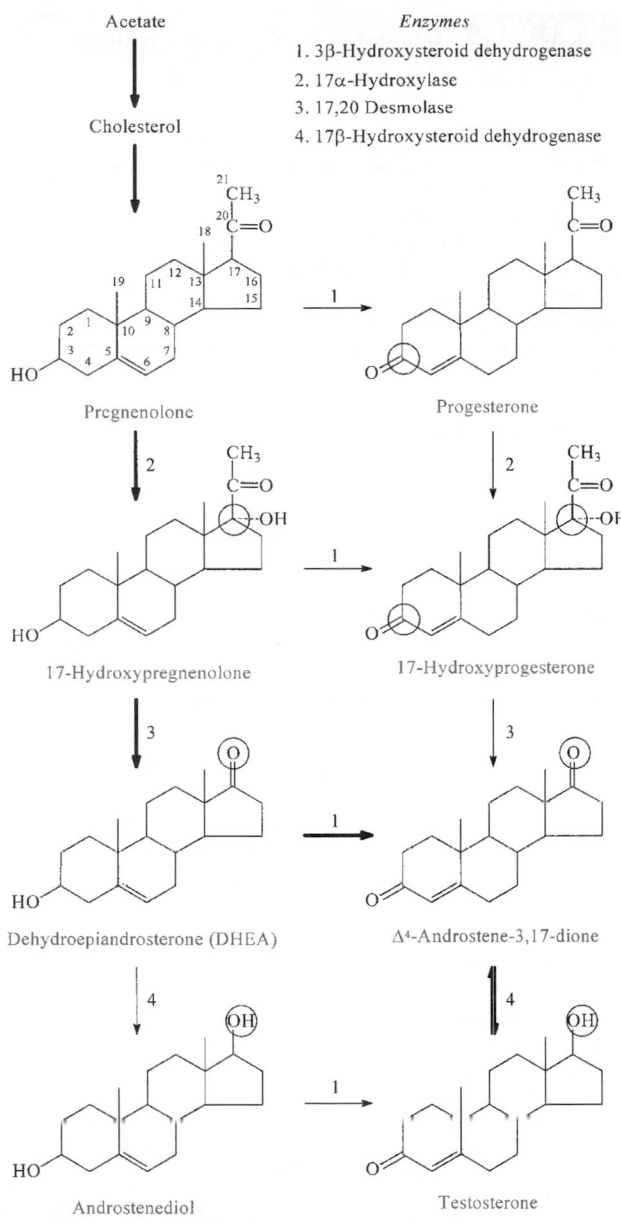

Figure 42-3   Biosynthesis of androgens (in adrenal glands and testes). Heavy arrows indicate the preferred pathways. The circled areas represent the sites of chemical change.

ketosteroids (17-KSs). These metabolites are excreted primarily (>90%) in the urine.

Male Reproductive Development

Fetal

During early embryogenesis, the fetus has **Mullerian ducts** and **Wolffian ducts,** which are the genital ducts for the female and male reproductive tracts, respectively. In male fetuses, testosterone is responsible for maintenance of the Wolffian ducts and virilization of the urogenital sinus and external genitalia. Mullerian inhibiting substance (MIS)

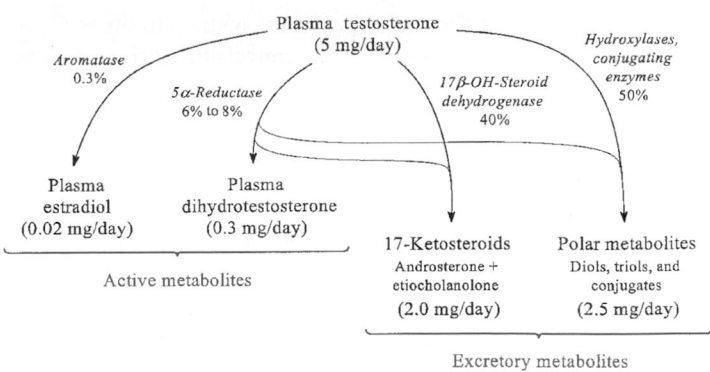

Figure 42-4   Pathways of peripheral metabolism of plasma testosterone. Testosterone can be metabolized into either active metabolites or excretory metabolites. (Modified from Griffin JE, Wilson JD: The testis. In Bondy PK, Rosenberg LE (eds): Metabolic Control and Disease, 8th edition, pp 1535-1578, Philadelphia, WB Saunders, 1980.)

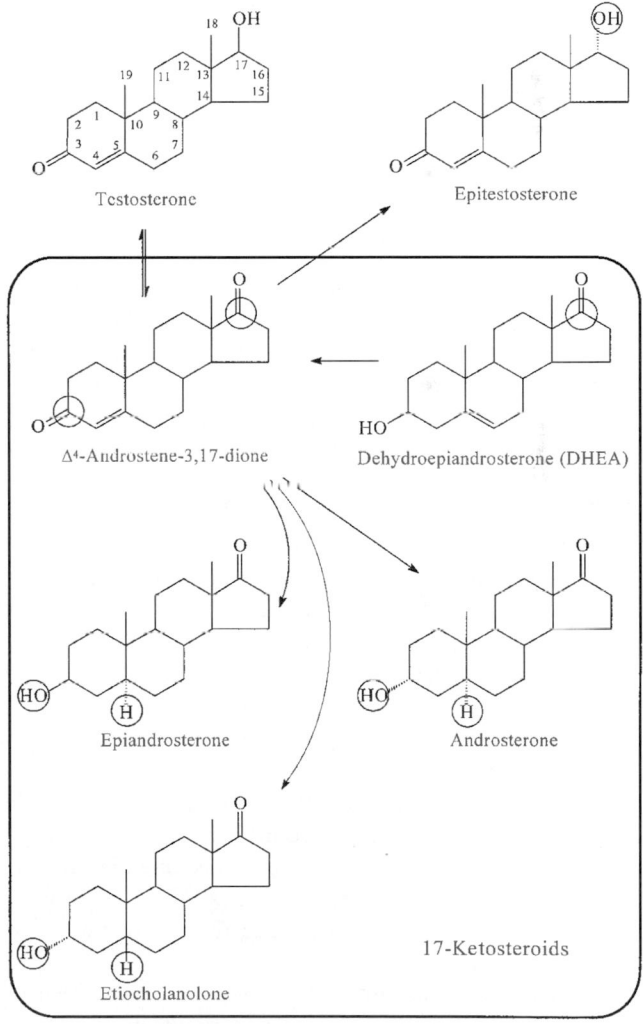

Figure 42-5   Catabolism of $C_{19}O_2$ androgens. The circled areas represent the sites of chemical change.

is responsible for the regression of the Mullerian ducts. Production of MIS and testosterone, conversion of testosterone to DHT, and functioning androgen receptors must occur for normal male sexual development.

Postnatal

At birth the concentration of testosterone is only slightly higher in boys than in girls. Shortly after birth the concentration of testosterone increases, remains elevated for about 3 months, and then falls to baseline (<1 nmol/L) again by 1 year. Although higher in boys than in girls, the concentration of androgens remains low in both until puberty.

Puberty

Concentrations of androstenedione, DHEA, and sulfated dehydroepiandrosterone (DHEA-S) begin to increase as early as 6 to 7 years of age, several years before maturation of the hypothalamic-pituitary-gonadal axis. The onset of puberty is associated with nocturnal surges in LH and to a lesser extent, FSH secretion. The overall changes associated with puberty reflect the theory that the hypothalamic-pituitary system becomes less sensitive to feedback inhibition by circulating androgens, resulting in higher androgen concentrations. On average, puberty is completed between the ages of 16 and 19 years.

Male Reproductive Abnormalities

A wide variety of abnormalities can affect the male reproductive system before birth, in childhood, or in adulthood (Table 42-1). Important abnormalities include (1) hypogonadotropic hypogonadism, (2) hypergonadotropic hypogonadism, (3) Klinefelter's syndrome, (4) prostate cancer, (5) defects in androgen action, (6) impotence, and (7) gynecomastia.

Hypogonadotropic hypogonadism

Male hypogonadism is a condition caused by decreased testes function and leads to slowing of normal sexual development if manifested early in life. The disorder is classified as hypogonadotropic or hypergonadotropic, depending on whether the pituitary gonadotropic hormones (LH and FSH) are decreased or increased, respectively.

Hypogonadotropic hypogonadism occurs when defects in the hypothalamus or pituitary prevent normal gonadotropin production (see Chapter 39). Causative factors include congenital or acquired panhypopituitarism, hypothalamic syndromes, GnRH deficiency, hyperprolactinemia, malnutrition or anorexia, and iatrogenic causes. These abnormalities are all associated with decreased testosterone and gonadotropin concentrations.

Kallmann's syndrome is the most common form of hypogonadotropic hypogonadism and results from a deficiency of GnRH in the hypothalamus. It is characterized by hypogonadism and anosmia (loss of the sense of smell) in males and females; however, it is five times more common in males.[1]

TABLE 42-1	Male Reproductive Abnormalities

Hypogonadotropic Hypogonadism
Panhypopituitarism (congenital or acquired)
Hypothalamic syndrome (acquired or congenital)
   Structural defects (neoplastic, inflammatory, infiltrative)
   Prader-Willi syndrome
   Laurence-Moon syndrome
GnRH deficiency (Kallmann's syndrome)
Hyperprolactinemia (prolactinoma or drugs)
Malnutrition and anorexia nervosa
Drug-induced suppression of LH (androgens, estrogens, tranquilizers, antidepressants, antihypertensives, barbiturates, cimetidine, GnRH analogs, and opiates)

Hypergonadotropic Hypogonadism
Acquired (irradiation, mumps orchitis, castration, and cytotoxic drugs)
Chromosome defects
   Klinefelter's syndrome (47, XXY) and mosaics
   Autosomal and sex chromosomes, polyploidies
   True **hermaphroditism**
Defective androgen biosynthesis
   20α-Hydroxylase (cholesterol 20,22-desmolase) deficiency
   17,20-Lyase deficiency
   3β-Hydroxysteroid dehydrogenase deficiency
   17α-Hydroxylase deficiency
   17β-Hydroxysteroid dehydrogenase deficiency
Testicular agenesis
Selective seminiferous tubular disease
Miscellaneous
   Noonan's syndrome (short stature, pulmonary valve stenosis, hypertelorism, and ptosis)
   Streak gonads
   Myotonia dystrophica
   Acute and chronic diseases

Defects in Androgen Action
Complete androgen insensitivity (testicular feminization)
Incomplete androgen sensitivity
   Androgen receptor defects
   5α-Reductase deficiency

GnRH, Gonadotropin-releasing hormone; *LH,* luteinizing hormone.

Hypergonadotropic hypogonadism

Hypergonadotropic hypogonadism is caused by gonadal dysfunction. Individuals with primary testicular failure have elevated concentrations of LH and FSH and decreased levels of testosterone. Causes for primary hypogonadism are listed in Table 42-1. Aging is also associated with gonadal failure, which occurs in about 20% of men older than 60 years of age who exhibit defects in primary **Leydig cell** function and abnormal gonadotropin secretion in response to GnRH.

Klinefelter's syndrome

Klinefelter's syndrome is a condition characterized by (1) small testes and hyalinization of the seminiferous tubules; (2) varied degrees of masculinization, azoospermia, and **infertility;** and (3) increased gonadotropin excretion in urine.

Individuals tend to be tall with long legs, and about half have gynecomastia. It is associated typically with an XXY chromosome complement, although variants include XXYY, XXXY, XXXXY, and several mosaic patterns (for example, XY/XXY, XXY, XXXY).

Prostate cancer

Prostate cancer is the leading form of cancer in men older than 50. It is a malignant tumor of glandular origin in the prostate, and more than 95% of prostate tumors are adeno-carcinomas. Annual digital rectal examinations and routine prostate-specific antigen (PSA) testing are useful for its early detection (see Chapter 21). When the cancer is detected early and is confined to the gland, some patients can be cured by radical prostatectomy.

Defects in androgen action

The most common and severe defect in androgen action is testicular feminization syndrome. Individuals with this syndrome have female genitalia and develop breast tissue; however, the vagina ends in a blind pouch, and the male testes are internal. The disorder is thought to be caused by a defect in the androgen receptor. Circulating concentrations of testosterone in individuals with this syndrome are the same as or greater than concentrations in healthy men.

Males with 5α-reductase deficiency have ambiguous genitalia. If the deficiency remains undiagnosed until puberty, individuals experience an increase in muscle mass, a voice change, and enlargement of the phallus; however, they lack normal male-pattern hair growth, and their prostate gland remains small.

Impotence

Impotence is the persistent inability to develop or maintain a penile erection that is sufficient for intercourse and ejaculation in 50% or more of attempts. Various organic and psychological abnormalities may cause changes in sexual drive and the ability to have an erection or to ejaculate. Psychogenic impotence is the most common diagnosis. Other causes include vascular disease, diabetes mellitus, hypertension, uremia, neurological disease, hypogonadism, hyperthyroidism or hypothyroidism, neoplasms, and use of certain drugs. If no obvious explanation is found, measurement of morning serum testosterone, LH, and thyroid-stimulating hormone (TSH) concentrations is suggested. Hyperprolactinemia is an uncommon cause but should be considered in unusual situations.

Gynecomastia

Gynecomastia, the benign growth of glandular breast tissue in men, is a common finding in males of various ages.[1] The condition is associated with an increase in the estrogen/androgen ratio, which may be caused by testicular failure or increased body fat, resulting in increased peripheral aromatization of testosterone to estradiol.[1] Gynecomastia may also develop because of various other iatrogenic or sys-temic illnesses. Prolactin plays an important role in galactorrhea (breast discharge) but plays only an indirect role in gynecomastia.

■ FEMALE REPRODUCTIVE BIOLOGY

Anatomy

The female reproductive system consists of a vagina, a uterus, and the bilateral fallopian tubes and ovaries (gonads). The ovaries are located on each side of the uterus close to the fallopian tubes. They produce ova and secrete the sex hormones progesterone and estrogen.

Physiology

Every healthy female infant has approximately 400,000 intraovarian primordial follicles, each containing an immature **ovum.** During the reproductive life span of a woman, 300 to 400 follicles reach maturity and release an egg.[5] One mature **follicle** is produced on approximately the fourteenth day of each normal menstrual cycle. During ovulation the mature follicle ruptures, releasing the oocyte into the space near the fallopian tubes (Figure 42-6). After ovulation, the granulosa and thecal cells of the follicle proliferate to form lipid-rich luteal cells and become the **corpus luteum** (also known as the *yellow body*). The fallopian tubes extend from the uterus toward the ovaries. They transport the sperm upward from the uterine cavity and provide a site for oocyte fertilization. The fertilized egg is transported back by the fallopian tubes to the uterine cavity. The uterine cavity is lined by the endometrium. During the luteal phase of the cycle, the endometrial lining increases in thickness and vascularity and is then shed during **menstruation** (Figure 42-7).

Menstrual cycle

The **menstrual cycle** is the reproductive cycle of the human female. It is characterized by a cyclic, physiological discharge of blood and mucosal tissue through the vagina from the uterus of a nonpregnant female. The cycle is under hormonal control and involves a closely coordinated interaction of feedback effects between the hypothalamus, anterior lobe of the pituitary gland, and ovaries (see Figure 42-7). In nonpregnant females, the cycle occurs at approximately 4-week intervals. During the normal menstrual cycle, the first day of the cycle is the first day of menstrual bleeding. Each cycle consists of a follicular and a luteal phase.

Follicular phase

The follicular phase, the initiation of follicular growth, actually begins during the last few days of the previous luteal phase and ends at ovulation. During the early part of the follicular phase, concentrations of FSH are elevated but decrease until ovulation. One follicle grows, producing increasing amounts of estrogen as it enlarges. LH secretion begins to increase in the middle of the follicular phase. Just before

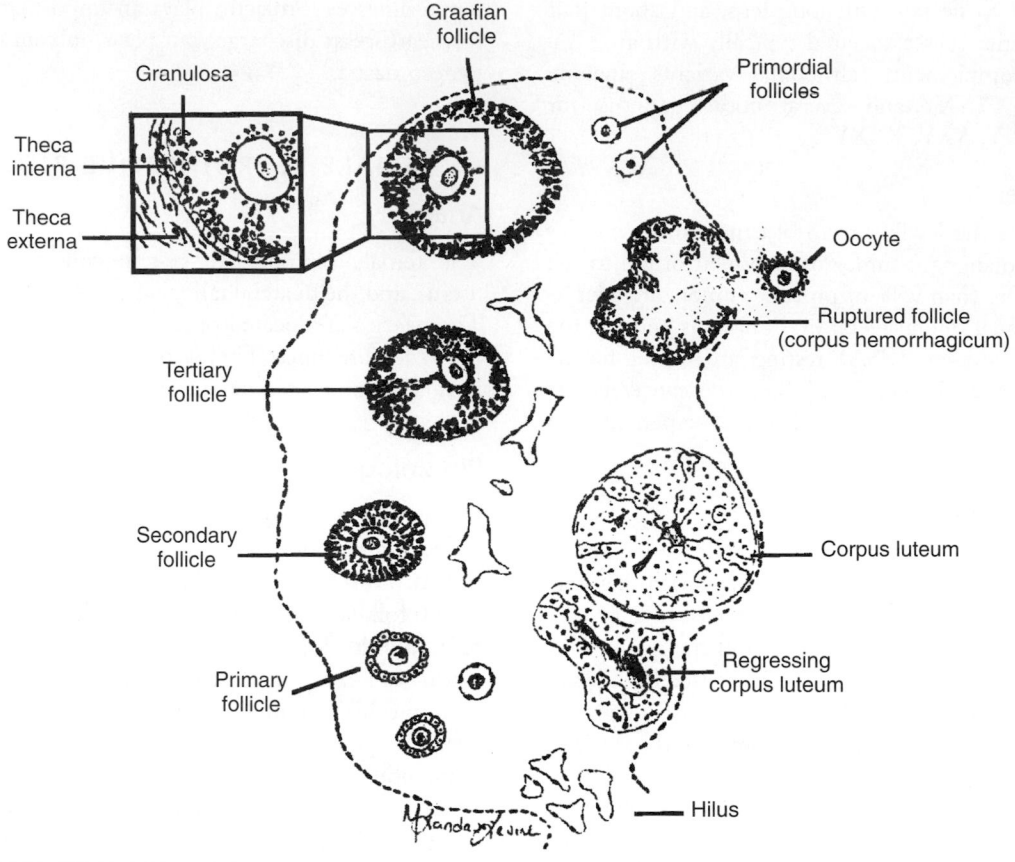

Figure 42-6   Ovarian anatomy.

ovulation, estrogen secretion increases dramatically, which positively stimulates the hypothalamus and triggers an LH surge. The LH surge is a reliable predictor of ovulation, with the onset of the surge occurring 24 to 36 hours before ovulation and the peak occurring 10 to 12 hours before ovulation. Ovulation occurs on approximately the fourteenth day of the menstrual cycle. After ovulation, estradiol levels decline initially, but progesterone secretion continues to increase.

Luteal phase

The luteal phase is the last half of the menstrual cycle and is characterized by increasing production of progesterone and estrogen by the corpus luteum, with consequent gradual lowering of LH and FSH levels. Progesterone reaches a peak of approximately 8 mg/day on approximately the eighth day after ovulation. If ovulation does not occur, the corpus luteum fails to form, and the cyclic rise in progesterone is lower than normal. If the female has not conceived, breakdown of the endometrium begins because the function of the corpus luteum decreases, resulting in a decrease in estrogen and progesterone concentrations. The corpus luteum regresses and is eventually replaced by scar tissue. The endometrium is then sloughed off in 4 to 6 days

as menstrual bleeding. The average menstrual blood loss is 30 mL. The late-cycle FSH peak starts the process again.

If the female becomes pregnant, chorionic gonadotropin (CG), which is produced by the trophoblastic cells of the developing fetus, maintains the corpus luteum, causing progesterone and estrogen concentrations to continue to increase.

Menopause

With advancing age, successive cycles of ovulation and atresia (absence or closure of a normal body orifice or tubular body organ) deplete the ovary of its follicles. The process leads to **menopause,** which is the permanent cessation of menstruation caused by ovarian follicular development in response to gonadotropic stimulation. The ovaries fail to produce adequate amounts of estrogen and inhibin, causing gonadotropin production to increase in a continued attempt to stimulate the ovaries. The mean age of menopause is 51 years but can occur from 45 to 55 years of age. Ovarian failure may occur at any age, but menopause before age 40 is considered premature. Although the ovaries of postmenopausal women do not secrete estrogens, the women have significant blood levels of estrone originating from the peripheral conversion of

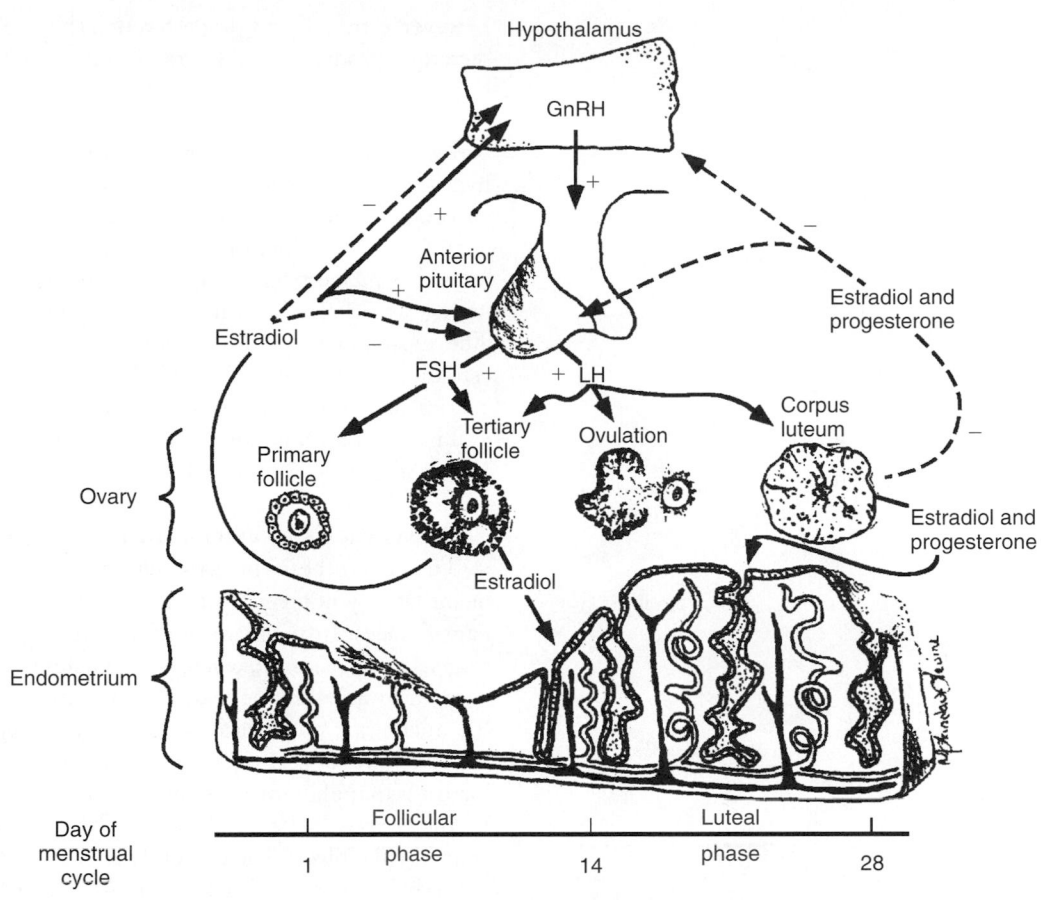

Figure 42-7 Summary of the endocrine control of and changes in ovaries and the endometrium during the menstrual cycle. Dashed lines indicate inhibitory effects, and solid lines indicate stimulatory effects.

FSH, Follicle-stimulating hormone; *GnRH,* gonadotropin-releasing hormone; *LH,* luteinizing hormone.

adrenal androstenedione. Because a major site of this conversion is adipose tissue, estrone increases in obese postmenopausal women, sometimes yielding enough estrogen to produce uterine bleeding.

After menopause the ovary continues to produce androgens, particularly testosterone and androstenedione, as a result of increased LH concentrations. In addition, the adrenal gland continues to secrete androgens. The resulting decrease in the estrogen/androgen ratio is the cause of the hirsutism often seen in postmenopausal women. Prolonged estrogen deficiency results in increased resorption and bone remodeling (see Chapter 38), leading to accelerated bone loss and osteoporosis. Estrogen replacement therapy reduces bone loss and has been reported to reduce fracture risk by half.

Hormonal Control (Hypothalamic-Pituitary-Gonadal Axis)

Women have a tightly coordinated feedback system among the hypothalamus, anterior pituitary, and ovaries that orchestrates menstruation. FSH stimulates follicular growth, and

LH stimulates ovulation and progesterone secretion from the developing corpus luteum (see Figure 42-7).

Estrogens

Estrogens are the sex hormones that are responsible for the development and maintenance of the female sex organs and female secondary sex characteristics. In conjunction with progesterone, they also participate in the regulation of the menstrual cycle and breast and uterine growth, as well as in the maintenance of pregnancy.

Estrogens affect calcium homeostasis and have a beneficial effect on bone mass (see Chapter 38). They decrease bone resorption, and in prepubertal girls estrogens accelerate linear bone growth and result in epiphyseal closure. Long-term estrogen depletion is associated with loss of bone mineral content, an increase in the number of stress fractures, and postmenopausal osteoporosis.

Estrogens also have effects on plasma proteins, which affects endocrine testing. For example, estrogens increase levels of SHBG, corticosteroid-binding globulin (CBG), and thyroxine-binding globulin (TBG). Boys and girls have

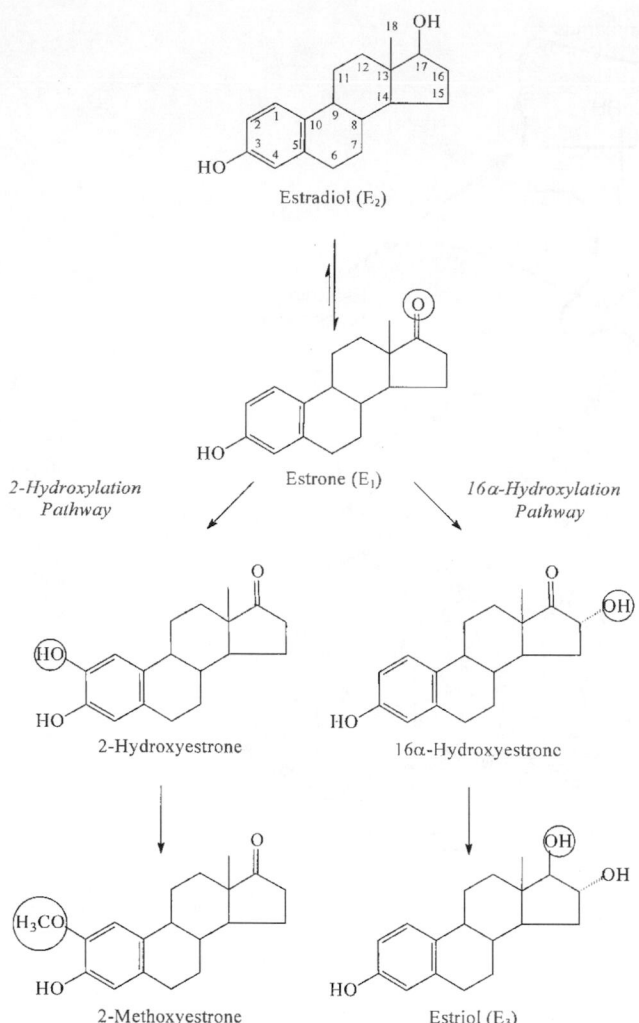

Figure 42-8 Main pathways of estradiol metabolism in humans. The circled areas represent the sites of chemical change.

comparable levels of SHBG, but men have SHBG levels that are about half the levels of SHBG in women.

Chemistry

The names and structural formulas of certain important estrogens are shown in Figure 42-8.

Biochemistry

Biosynthesis

In healthy females, most estrogens are secreted by the ovarian follicles and corpus luteum and by the **placenta** during pregnancy. Adrenal glands and testes are also thought to secrete minute quantities of estrogens. The synthesis of estrogens by the ovaries follows the same steroidogenic pathway as do the other steroid-producing organs. In vivo and in vitro studies indicate that acetate, cholesterol, progesterone, and testosterone can all serve as precursors of estrogens. The normal human ovary produces all three classes of sex steroids, estrogens, progestins, and androgens;

however, estradiol and progesterone are the ovary's primary secretory products. Unlike the testes, the ovaries have a highly active aromatase system that rapidly converts androgens such as testosterone into estrogens. Unlike the adrenal cortex normal ovaries lack the 21-hydroxylase and the 11β-hydroxylase enzymes and therefore cannot produce glucocorticoids and mineralocorticoids. More than 20 estrogens have been identified, but only 17β-estradiol (also known as *E2*), estrone (also known as *E1*), and estriol (also known as *E3*) are known to have any clinical importance. The most potent estrogen secreted by the ovary is 17β-estradiol. Because it is derived almost exclusively from the ovaries, its measurement is often considered sufficient to evaluate ovarian function. The biosynthetic pathway for estradiol is shown in Figure 42-9.

Biosynthesis of estriol during pregnancy

The biosynthesis of estrogens differs qualitatively and quantitatively in pregnant females compared with nonpregnant females. In pregnant females, the major source of estrogens is the placenta, whereas in females who are not pregnant, the ovaries are the main site of synthesis. In contrast to the microgram quantities secreted by nonpregnant females, the amount of estrogen secreted in pregnant women increases to milligram amounts. The major estrogen secreted by the ovaries is estradiol, whereas the major product secreted by the placenta is estriol. Estriol is formed in the placenta by sequential desulfurization and aromatization of plasma DHEA-S. Measurements of estriol have little clinical value (except in pregnant females), because in nonpregnant females, estriol is derived almost exclusively from estradiol (see Chapter 43).

Transport in blood

More than 97% of circulating estradiol is bound to plasma proteins. It is bound specifically and with high affinity to SHBG and nonspecifically to albumin. SHBG concentrations are increased by estrogens and therefore are higher in females than in males. Only 2% to 3% of total estradiol circulates in the free form. Like testosterone, both the free and albumin-bound fractions of estradiol are thought to be biologically available, but measurement of this fraction has not yet been shown to be clinically important.

Metabolism

In the normal course of estrogen metabolism, estradiol is converted to estrone in a reversible reaction (see Figure 42-8). Estrone is then metabolized by one of two alternative pathways. Which pathway is followed depends on the individual's pathophysiological state. For example, obesity and hypothyroidism are associated with an increase in estriol formation, whereas low body weight and hyperthyroidism are associated with the formation of 2-methoxyestrone and 2-hydroxyestrone.

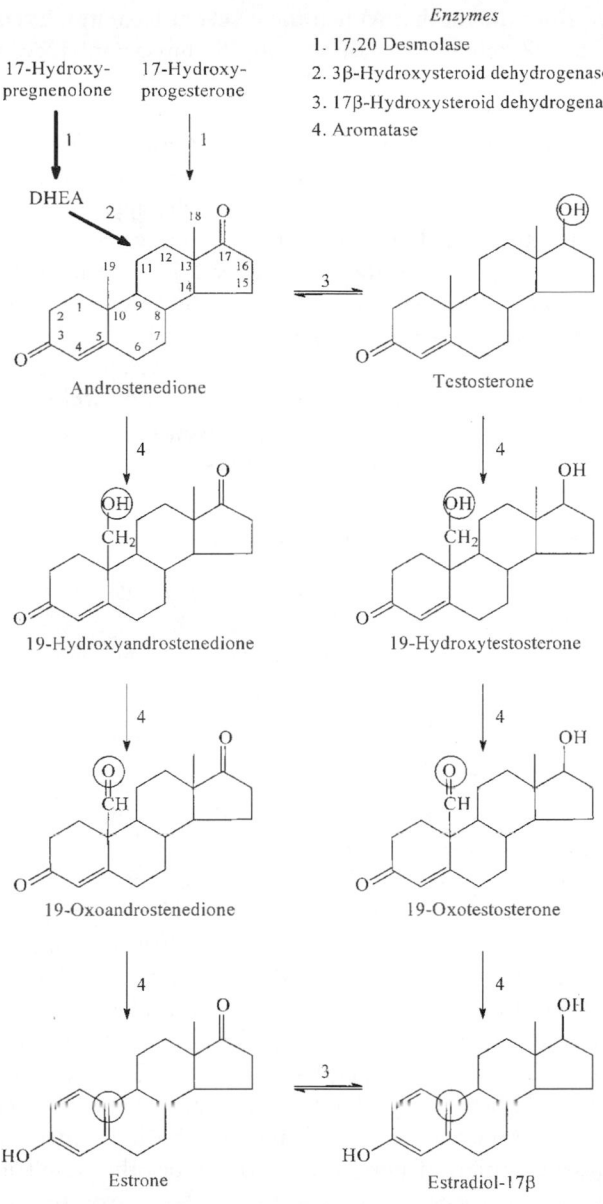

Enzymes
1. 17,20 Desmolase
2. 3β-Hydroxysteroid dehydrogenase
3. 17β-Hydroxysteroid dehydrogenase
4. Aromatase

Figure 42-9 Biosynthesis of estrogens. Heavy arrows indicate the Δ⁵-3β-hydroxy pathway. The circled areas represent the sites of chemical change. (See Figure 42-2 for the early synthetic steps.)

The liver is the primary site for the inactivation of estrogens, as it is for other steroids. The main biochemical reactions are hydroxylation, oxidation, reduction, and methylation. Conjugation with glucuronic or sulfuric acid, which increases the water solubility of these steroids and thus allows them to be eliminated rapidly through the kidney, is the final step in the metabolic process.

Progesterone

Progesterone, like estrogen, is primarily a female sex hormone. In conjunction with estrogens, it helps to regulate the accessory organs during the menstrual cycle. This hormone

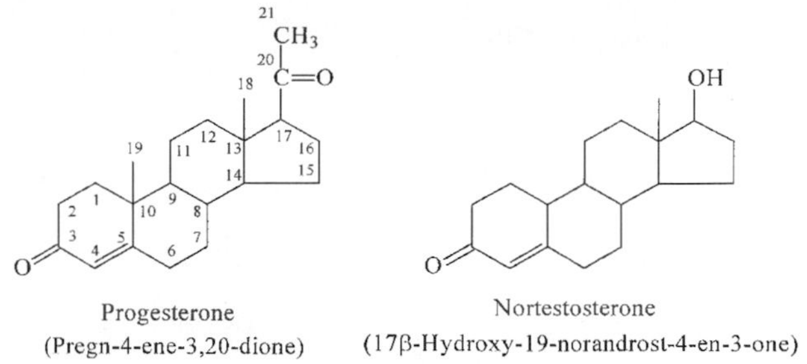

Figure 42-10 Structural formulas of progesterone and 19-nortestosterone.

Progesterone
(Pregn-4-ene-3,20-dione)

Nortestosterone
(17β-Hydroxy-19-norandrost-4-en-3-one)

is especially important in preparing the uterus for the implantation of the **blastula** that is produced by the cleavage of a fertilized ovum. Progesterone continues to be involved in maintaining pregnancy. In nonpregnant females, progesterone is secreted mainly by the corpus luteum. During pregnancy the placenta becomes the major source of the hormone. Minor sources are the adrenal cortex in males and females and the testes in males.

Chemistry

Progesterone is a C_{21} steroid (Figure 42-10). Like the corticosteroids and testosterone, progesterone (pregn-4-ene-3,20-dione) contains a carbonyl group (at C-3) and a double bond between C-4 and C-5 (Δ^4); both structural characteristics are essential for progestational activity. The two-carbon side chain (CH_3CO) on C-17 does not seem have an important physiological action. The synthetic compound 19-nortestosterone (see Figure 42-10) and its derivatives, which are widely used as oral contraceptives, are more potent progestational agents than progesterone itself.

Biochemistry

Biosynthesis

Initiation and control of luteal secretion of progesterone are regulated by LH and FSH (see Chapter 39). Biosynthesis of progesterone in ovarian tissues is believed to follow the same path from acetate to cholesterol through pregnenolone as it does in the adrenal cortex (see Figure 41-3). However, in luteal tissue, low-density lipoprotein (LDL) cholesterol is thought to serve as the preferred precursor.

Transport in blood

Progesterone does not have a specific plasma binding protein but like cortisol is bound to CBG. Reported values for plasma levels of free progesterone vary from 2% to 10% of the total concentrations, and the percentage of unbound progesterone is constant throughout the normal menstrual cycle.

Metabolism

The important metabolic events leading to inactivation of progesterone are reduction and conjugation (Figure

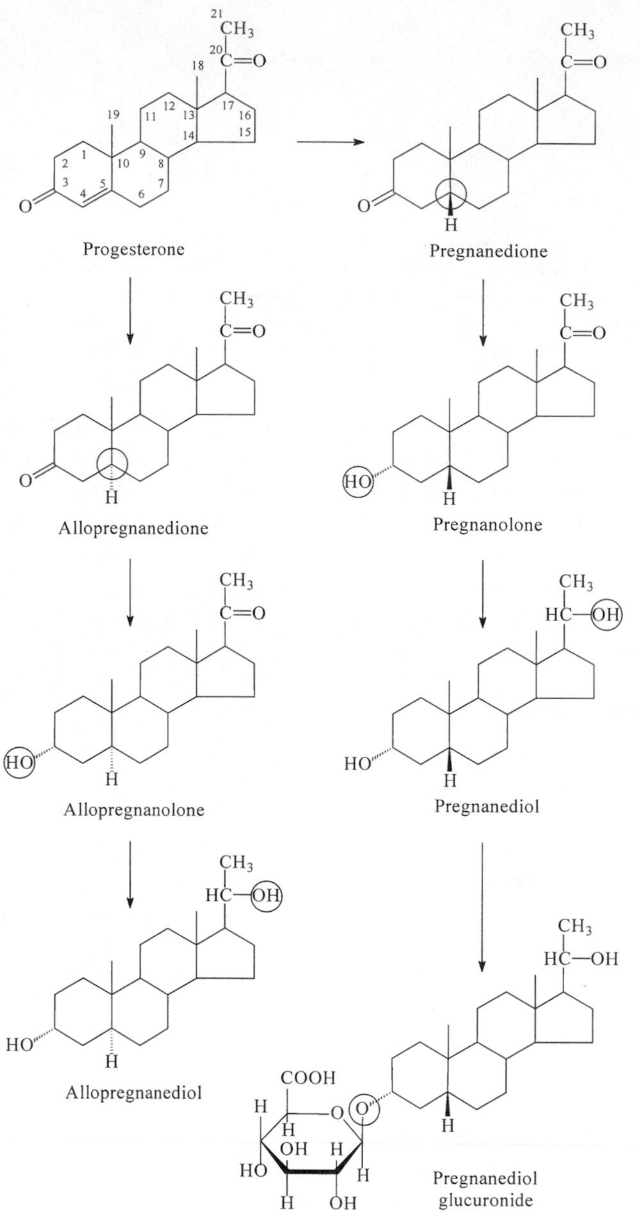

Figure 42-11   Metabolism of progesterone. The circled areas represent the sites of chemical change.

42-11).[6] Metabolites of progesterone are classified into three groups based on the degree of reduction: (1) pregnanediones, (2) pregnanalones, and (3) pregnanediols. Reduced metabolites are eventually conjugated with glucuronic acid and excreted as water-soluble glucuronides.

Female Reproductive Development

In a genotypic female, lack of testosterone and Mullerian inhibiting substance causes the Wolffian ducts to regress and the Mullerian ducts to remain, thus forming the female reproductive tract. Gonadotropin activity in utero is suppressed because of high levels of circulating estrogens de-

rived from the mother. When the placenta separates, levels of fetal sex steroids decrease abruptly. Serum estradiol levels in newborns decrease to basal levels within 5 to 7 days after birth and persist at this level until puberty.

During childhood, circulating concentrations of sex steroids and gonadotropins are low and are similar in both sexes. The transition from sexual immaturity appears to begin with diminished sensitivity of the pituitary gland or hypothalamus or both to the negative feedback effects of the sex steroids. In girls, *precocious puberty* is the onset of pubertal development (secondary sex characteristics) before the age of 8 years, and puberty is considered delayed if no development has occurred by the age of 13 y or **menarche** has not occurred by age 16½ years. The average age of menarche in the United States is 12.8 years.

Female Reproductive Abnormalities

A wide variety of abnormalities affect the female reproductive system, including (1) female pseudohermaphroditism, (2) breast cancer, (3) irregular **menses**, (4) and conditions caused by androgen excess such as polycystic ovary syndrome, hirsutism, and virilization.

Female pseudohermaphroditism

The genotypic sex of an individual with pseudohermaphroditism varies from the phenotypic sex. A female pseudohermaphrodite is genetically female but has phenotypic characteristics that are, to varying degrees, male. Exposure of female fetuses to androgens before the twelfth week of gestation has been known to cause development of ambiguous genitalia; after 13 weeks, it results in clitoral enlargement. In newborns with a 46 XX **karyotype** and ambiguous genitalia, congenital adrenal hyperplasia (CAH) should be considered. CAH is a family of autosomal recessive disorders of adrenal steroidogenesis (see Chapter 41). Each disorder has a specific pattern of hormonal abnormalities that result in androgen deficiency or excess. Only 21-hydroxylase and 11β-hydroxylase deficiencies are predominantly virilizing disorders. A 3β-hydroxysteroid dehydrogenase deficiency is rare, but it may cause virilization in affected girls.

Breast cancer

Estrogen is believed to play a role in the development of breast cancer because (1) the disease predominantly occurs in women who have already gone through puberty (and have higher levels of estrogen), and (2) women who have had their ovaries removed before age 40 have a significantly smaller risk of breast cancer than those who have not. Thus increased exposure to estrogens from early menarche or late menopause are associated with increased risk of breast cancer. Women who have had more completed pregnancies seem to be at lower risk for breast cancer. In addition, pregnancy before age 35 actually also appears to decrease the risk for breast cancer.

TABLE 42-2   Causes of Amenorrhea

Primary Amenorrhea
Lower tract defects
  Vaginal aplasia
  Imperforate hymen
  Congenital vaginal atresia
Uterine disorders
  Congenital absence of the uterus
  Endometritis
  Mullerian agenesis (Mayer-Rokitansky-Küster-Hauser syndrome)
Ovarian disorders
  XO gonadal and X dysgenesis and variants
  XX gonadal dysgenesis
  Turner's syndrome
  Testicular feminization syndrome
  17-Hydroxylase deficiency of the ovaries and adrenal glands
  Autoimmune oophoritis
  Resistant ovary syndrome
  Polycystic ovary syndrome
Adrenal disorders (congenital adrenal hyperplasia)
Thyroid disorders (hypothyroidism)
Pituitary-hypothalamic disorders
  Hypopituitarism
  Constitutional delay in the onset of menses (physiological)
  Nutritional disorders
  Kallmann's syndrome

Secondary Amenorrhea
Pregnancy/lactation
Uterine disorders
  Posttraumatic uterine synechiae (Asherman's syndrome)
  Progestational agents
Ovarian disorders
  Polycystic ovary syndrome (hypothalamic)
  Ovarian tumors
  Premature ovarian failure (idiopathic, autoimmune, injury)
  Antimetabolite therapy

Adrenal disorders
  Late-onset adrenal hyperplasia
  Cushing's syndrome
  Virilizing adrenal tumors
  Adrenocorticoid insufficiency
Thyroid disorders
  Hypothyroidism
  Hyperthyroidism
Pituitary disorders
  Acquired hypopituitarism (trauma, tumors, Sheehan's syndrome, lymphocytic hypophysitis)
  Physiological or pathological hyperprolactinemia
Hypothalamic disorders
  Tumors and infiltrative diseases
  Nutritional disorders
  Hypophysitis
  Excessive exercise
  Stress
Iatrogenic factors
  Antipsychotics (for example, phenothiazines, haloperidol, clozapine, pimozide)
  Antidepressants (for example, tricyclics, monoamine oxidase inhibitors)
  Antihypertensives (for example, calcium-channel blockers, methyldopa, reserpine)
  Drugs with estrogenic activity (for example, digitalis, flavinoids, marijuana, oral contraceptives)
  Drugs with ovarian toxicity (for example, busulfan, chlorambucil, cisplatin, cyclophosphamide, fluorouracil)

The objective of many endocrine therapies for breast cancer is to lower circulating estrogen concentrations. Approximately one third of women with metastatic breast carcinoma are in remission after therapies such as **oophorectomy**, hypophysectomy, and adrenalectomy, as well as administration of antiestrogens and androgens.

The first step in estrogen action is the binding of estrogen to the estrogen receptor, which is found in target tissues such as the uterus, pituitary gland, hypothalamus, and breast. As a prognostic indicator of response to therapy, cytoplasmic estrogen receptors are routinely measured in breast tissue samples after surgical removal of the tumor. Sixty percent of individuals with breast carcinoma have tumors that have increased numbers of estrogen receptors and are termed *estrogen-receptor positive*. Approximately two thirds of individuals with estrogen receptor-positive tumors respond to endocrine therapy, whereas 95% of the individuals with estrogen receptor-negative tumors fail to respond. Thus the greater the estrogen receptor content of the tumor, the higher the response rate to endocrine therapy.

Irregular menses

In a normal ovulatory menstrual cycle, menstruation occurs an average of every 28 days. Healthy females have considerable variation in cycle length, which can last 25 to 30 days. **Amenorrhea,** the absence of menstrual bleeding, is a relatively common disorder, with an estimated prevalence of 5% in the general population and as high as 8.5% in an adolescent postpubescent population. Amenorrhea is traditionally categorized as either primary or secondary (Table 42-2).

Primary amenorrhea

Primary amenorrhea is the failure to establish spontaneous periodic menstruation by the age of 16 years, regardless of whether secondary sex characteristics have developed. About 40% of phenotypic females who have primary amenorrhea (which is nearly always associated with absence of development of secondary sex characteristics) have Turner's syndrome, a rare genetic disorder in females characterized by the absence of an X chromosome (45X) or pure gonadal dysgenesis (either a 46 XX or 46 XY karyotype). When puberty is delayed in a girl, measurement of serum gonadotropins is useful for diagnosis. Low levels may indicate pituitary failure, whereas concentrations that are elevated into the postmenopausal interval indicate gonadal failure. In cases of high concentrations, chromosome studies should be performed. In cases of low concentrations, pituitary function testing and radiography may be helpful.

Secondary amenorrhea

Secondary amenorrhea is an absence of periodic menstruation for at least 6 months in females who have previously experienced menses or for 12 months in females with a history of oligomenorrhea, or infrequent menstruation (less than nine times per year).[13] With a few exceptions the causes of primary and secondary amenorrhea overlap (see Table 42-2). Pregnancy is the most common cause of amenorrhea and should be considered first and ruled out by measurement of CG.[13]

In the evaluation of females with amenorrhea who are otherwise healthy, a careful history and physical examination usually lead to the correct cause. The history should include a complete description of the menstrual patterns as well as documentation of galactorrhea; hot flashes; symptoms of hypothyroidism; hirsutism; previous surgery of the abdomen, pelvis, or uterus; trauma; medications; nutritional history; patterns of exercise; previous contraceptive use; changes in weight; stress; and chronic diseases. Because hypothyroidism and hyperprolactinemia can cause amenorrhea, they can easily be ruled out by measurement of serum TSH and prolactin concentrations.

Often classification of individuals with secondary amenorrhea as those with and without signs of hirsutism and androgen excess is helpful.

Androgen excess

A female with excess androgen levels has symptoms that include, in varying degrees, hair (hirsutism) on the face, chest, abdomen, and thighs; acne; and obesity. Amenorrhea caused by androgen excess may a result of adult-onset CAH, corticotropin-dependent Cushing's syndrome, or polycystic ovary syndrome.

Polycystic ovary syndrome

Polycystic ovary syndrome (PCOS) is a condition characterized by multiple ovarian cysts and increased androgen production. PCOS occurs in about 1% to 2% of women and is thought to be caused by a hypothalamic disorder. The syndrome is defined by symptoms that include hyperandro-

TABLE 42-3	Clinical Features* of the Polycystic Ovary Syndrome
Clinical Feature	**Frequency (%)**
Hirsutism	65
Acne	26
Obesity	37
Infertility	48
Amenorrhea	35
Oligomenorrhea	42
Regular menstrual cycle	20

Modified from Franks S: Polycystic ovary syndrome. N Engl J Med 1995; 333:853.
*Data from three studies. Two used ultrasonography as the primary method of diagnosis, and one used ovarian histology. Total N = 1935.

genism with chronic anovulation without underlying adrenal or pituitary gland disease (Table 42-3).[4] Although the syndrome is associated with polycystic ovaries, they are not essential for the diagnosis.

Individuals with PCOS usually have estradiol concentrations that are greater than 40 pg/mL. The diagnosis of the syndrome can be confirmed with laboratory measurements of serum testosterone, DHEA-S, LH, and FSH. LH concentrations are frequently high, and FSH levels are disproportionately normal or low. It has been suggested that an LH/FSH ratio of greater than 2.5 indicates PCOS.[4] The total testosterone concentration is modestly elevated in 40% to 60% of individuals, with mean values that are 50% to 140% higher than normal. In females with normal testosterone concentrations, free testosterone levels are usually high. Concentrations of DHEA-S are usually normal or slightly elevated.

Hirsutism and virilization

Description. **Hirsutism** is excessive growth of terminal hair on girls, boys, and women in a distribution similar to that occurring in postpubertal men.[11] True hirsutism is responsive to androgens, so women usually either have been exposed to excess androgens or have a heightened sensitivity to normal circulating levels of androgen (Table 42-4). Idiopathic hirsutism, which is characterized by normal physical and laboratory findings in hirsute women, is found in 50% of women evaluated for hirsutism.

Virilization is characterized by clitoral hypertrophy, deepening of the voice, temporal hair recession, baldness, increased libido, decreased body fat, and menstrual irregularities or amenorrhea. Hirsutism is usually associated with normal or slightly elevated serum androgen levels, whereas virilization is associated with marked increases in ovarian or adrenal androgen production.

Laboratory evaluation. The most important screening tests used to evaluate patients for hirsutism and virilization are the measurement of serum levels of total or free tes-

TABLE 42-4	Causes of Hirsutism

Ovarian causes
    Severe insulin resistance
    Hyperthecosis, hilus cell or stromal cell hyperplasia
    Androgen-producing ovarian tumors
    Menopause
Adrenal causes
    Classic congenital hyperplasia
        21-Hydroxylase deficiency
        11-Hydroxylase deficiency
        3β-Hydroxysteroid dehydrogenase deficiency
    Adult or attenuated adrenal hyperplasia
    Androgen-producing adrenal tumors
Familial hirsutism
Endocrine disorders
    Polycystic ovary syndrome
    Hyperprolactinemia
    Acromegaly
    Cushing's syndrome
Idiopathic hirsutism (includes increased skin sensitivity to
    androgens)
Iatrogenic
    Androgens
    Dilantoin
    Diazoxide
    Minoxidil
    Streptomycin
    Cyclosporine
    Danazol
    Metyrapone
    Phenothiazides
    Progestogens (19-norsteroid derivatives)

TABLE 42-5	Male Infertility Factors

Endocrine Disorders	**Abnormal Spermatogenesis**
Hypothalamic dysfunction (Kallmann's syndrome)	Unexplained azoospermia
Pituitary failure (tumor, radiation, surgery)	Chromosomal abnormalities
Hyperprolactinemia (drug, tumor)	Mumps orchitis
	Cryptorchidism
	Chemical or radiation exposure
Exogenous androgens	
Thyroid disorders	**Abnormal Motility**
Adrenal hyperplasia	Absent cilia (Kartagener's syndrome)
Testicular failure	Antibody formation
Anatomical Factors	**Psychosocial Factors**
Congenital absence of vas deferens	Unexplained impotence
Obstructed vas deferens	Decreased libido
Congenital abnormalities of ejaculatory system	
Varicocele	
Retrograde ejaculation	

Modified from Morell V: Basic infertility assessment. Primary Care 1997; 24:195-204.

tosterone and DHEA-S. High DHEA-S concentrations suggest the androgens are adrenal in origin, whereas high testosterone levels suggest either an adrenal or ovarian source. Unless the history suggests possible neoplastic disease, it is unlikely if the serum testosterone concentration is less than 2 ng/mL, the DHEA-S concentration is less than 700 mg/dL, or the 17-KS concentration is less than 30 mg/day. Regardless of the source of the excess androgen production, the androstanediol glucuronide level is elevated in more than 90% of individuals with hirsutism because it is a marker of excessive DHT production in skin.

▩ INFERTILITY

Infertility is the inability to conceive after 1 year of intercourse with no use of contraception.[12] Primary infertility is infertility affecting individuals who have had no previous successful pregnancies. Secondary infertility is infertility affecting individuals who have previously had a successful pregnancy but are currently unable to conceive. Both types

of infertility generally have common causes. Infertility problems are caused by hormonal dysfunction of the hypothalamic-pituitary-gonadal axis. Measurement of peptide and steroid hormones in the serum are therefore essential aspects of the evaluation of infertility.

Male Infertility

Factors

Testosterone is essential for normal sperm development. Therefore any disorder that results in hypogonadism (and hence low testosterone concentrations) results in infertility. Among the causes are hypogonadotropic and hypergonadotropic hypogonadism (Table 42-5). The most common cause of hypothalamic hypogonadism is congenital idiopathic hypogonadotropic hypogonadism or its variant, Kallmann's syndrome (see previous section on male reproductive abnormalities).

Pituitary insufficiency or failure also causes infertility and is caused primarily by adenomas but is also caused by trauma, infiltration, metastases, or hemochromatosis. Hyperprolactinemia is a cause of secondary testicular dysfunction. Prolactin excess likely causes hypogonadism by impairing GnRH release. It also leads to impotence and insufficient androgenization (see previous section on impotence). Pituitary adenomas and drugs such as anxiolytics, antihypertensives, serotonergics, and histamine H_2 receptor antagonists can increase serum prolactin.

Other endocrine causes of male infertility include exogenous androgens, thyroid disorders, adrenal hyperplasia, and testicular failure. Gynecomastia or obesity in the infertile male may signify high concentrations of estrogen and possibly testicular feminization syndrome (see previous section on male reproductive abnormalities).[3] In addition, antibodies to sperm surface antigens also cause of infertility because they decrease motility, cause agglutination, and may be responsible for failure of sperm to penetrate human ova.

Evaluation of male infertility

The laboratory evaluation of male infertility can be separated into three main components: (1) the semen analysis, (2) endocrine parameters, and (3) immunological parameters.

Evaluation of semen

Semen analysis.   The analysis of semen includes the measurement of ejaculate volume and pH, as well as sperm count, motility, and motility direction. Semen should be analyzed within 1 hour of collection. Although the semen analysis is not a test for infertility, it is considered the most important laboratory test in the evaluation of male fertility. Table 42-6 lists characteristics of normal seminal fluid.

Sperm function.   No functional test has yet been established that can unequivocally predict the fertilizing capacity of spermatozoa. However, detailed methods describing the analysis of sperm function exist in the current literature.[3] These methods attempt to measure the functions of sperm necessary for fertilization. For a sperm to be successful, it must be able to reach the ovum through directed motion, undergo **capacitation,** fuse with the oocyte membrane, and be incorporated into the oocyte cytoplasm.[3] The postcoital test (see later section on evaluation of female infertility) is the most widely used measure of sperm adequacy.

Sperm-mucus penetration.   The sperm-mucus penetration test evaluates the ability of sperm to travel through a vaginal mucus sample obtained from either the female partner or a donor. An in vitro test using bovine cervical mucus is available commercially and reduces variables in mucus quality. The mucus is contained in a capillary tube, and migration of sperm into the tube is measured. Factors such as migration distance, penetration density, migration reduction, and duration of progressive movement are measured in this assay.

Evaluation of endocrine parameters

Serum testosterone levels should be measured, especially when the patient history or physical examination suggests deficient development of secondary sex characteristics. Leydig cell function is evaluated in response to a CG stimulation test. An injection of 5000 IU of CG is administered intramuscularly, and the serum testosterone level is measured between 48 and 96 hours later. Males with hypogonadism have a decreased testosterone response to this test.

Hypergonadotropic hypogonadism.   FSH levels should be measured in males with sperm counts of less than 5 to 10 million/mL. Elevated levels of FSH indicate Sertoli cell dysfunction and in males with azoospermia, primary germinal cell failure, Sertoli-cell–only syndrome, or genetic conditions such as Klinefelter's syndrome. Elevated FSH and LH in males with decreased testosterone and oligospermia indicate primary testicular failure, or "andropause."

Hypogonadotropic hypogonadism.   Administering GnRH may help distinguish between gonadal insufficiency caused by pituitary failure and hypothalamic failure. GnRH is injected, and FSH and LH levels are measured before administration and 15, 30, 90, and 120 minutes after administration.[6]

Evaluation of immunological parameters

The method used to measure antisperm antibodies is identical in male and female infertility evaluations. Agglutination; immobilization; and enzyme-linked immunosorbent assays (ELISAs), radioimmunoassays (RIAs), and immunofluorescent assays exist. The immunobead technique, in which polyacrylamide beads are coated with antibodies that recognize human immunoglobulins, is the most widely used method. This technique measures the percentage of sperm bound by immunoglobulin, the immunoglobulin isotype, and the location of the antibody binding (head, midpiece, or tail).

TABLE 42-6   **Normal Seminal Fluid Values**

Parameter	Value
Ejaculate volume	>2 mL*
Sperm density	>20 million/mL*
Total sperm count	>40 million per ejaculate*
Motility	>50% with forward progression or >25% with rapid progression within 60 min of ejaculation*
Morphology	>30% normal*
pH	7.2 to 8*
Color	Gray-white-yellow
Liquefaction	Within 40 min
Fructose	>1200 μg/mL
Acid phosphatase	100 to 300 mg/mL
Citric acid	>3 mg/mL
Inositol	>1 mg/mL
Zinc	>75 μg/mL
Magnesium	>70 μg/mL
Prostaglandins (PGE$_1$ and PGE$_2$)	30-200 μg/mL
Glycerylphosphorylcholine	>650 μg/mL
Carnitine	>250 μg/mL
Glucosidase	>20 mU per ejaculate

From Glezerman M, Bartoov B: Semen analysis. In Insler V, Lunenfeld B (eds): Infertility: Male and Female, 2nd edition, pp 285-515, New York, Churchill Livingstone, 1993.
*Data from World Health Organization: Laboratory Manual for the Examination of Human Semen and Semen-Cervical Mucus Penetration, 3rd edition, Cambridge, Cambridge University Press, 1992.

Female Infertility

Factors

Factors that contribute to female infertility are listed in Table 42-7. Ovulatory disorders (including ovarian and hormonal causes) account for approximately 30%, pelvic factors (including tubal, cervical, and uterine disease) account for approximately 50%, and immunological factors are implicated in approximately 5% of infertility cases.

Ovulatory dysfunction can develop regardless of whether the female has normal menses, making the dysfunction difficult to diagnose. Metabolic diseases of many kinds affect ovulatory function, including diseases that cause androgen levels to increase. PCOS, which results in androgen excess, is the most common cause of anovulation. CAH should be considered as a cause in females with hirsutism. A 21-hydroxylase deficiency or 3-β-hydroxysteroid deficiency may be present in up to 26% of individuals. Ovulatory dysfunction may also be caused by liver or thyroid disorders.

Like male infertility, female infertility can be caused by hypogonadism (hypergonadotropic or hypogonadotropic). Causes of hypergonadotropic hypogonadism include premature ovarian failure (POF), gonadal dysgenesis, resistant ovary syndrome, menopause, and luteal phase deficiency.

TABLE 42-7	Female Infertility Factors

Ovarian or Hormonal Factors	Tubal Factors
METABOLIC DISEASE	Occlusion or scarring
Thyroid	Salpingitis isthmica nodosa
Liver	Infectious salpingitis
Obesity	
Androgen excess	**Cervical Factors**
Polycystic ovary syndrome	Stenosis
	Inflammation or infection
HYPERGONADOTROPIC	Abnormal mucus viscosity
HYPOGONADISM	
Menopause	**Uterine Factors**
Luteal phase deficiency	Leiomyoma
Gonadal dysgenesis	Congenital malformation
Premature ovarian failure (auto-	Adhesions
immune, cytotoxic chemo-	Endometritis or abnormal
therapy, tumor)	endometrium
Resistant ovary syndrome	
	Psychosocial Factors
HYPOGONADOTROPIC	Decreased libido
HYPOGONADISM	Anorgasmia
Hyperprolactinemia (tumor,	
drugs)	**Iatrogenic Factors**
Hypothalamic insufficiency (Kall-	
mann's syndrome)	**Immunological (Antisperm**
Pituitary insufficiency (tumor,	**Antibodies) Factors**
necrosis, thrombosis, stress,	
exercise, anorexia)	

Modified from Morell V: Basic infertility assessment. Primary Care 1997; 24:195-204.

Causes of hypogonadotropic hypogonadism include pituitary or hypothalamic insufficiency and hyperprolactinemia.

Evaluation of female infertility

The initial evaluation of female infertility should include a detailed history and physical examination. After obvious treatable abnormalities have been ruled out, an abnormal menstrual history can indicate further endocrine evaluation and a postcoital test can help determine coital sufficiency (see previous section on irregular menses).

Postcoital test

The postcoital test is a quick assessment of multiple factors affecting fertility. Although widely used, opinions vary regarding its clinical utility. A postcoital sample of endocervical mucus is aspirated from a female who is in the middle of the menstrual cycle; it is placed on a glass slide with two coverslips. Mucus with adequate estrogen stimulation is clear and thin and forms a thread that is 6 cm or greater in length when the coverslip is separated from the slide. When examined under the microscope, air-dried mucus (that has adequate estrogen) forms a fernlike pattern. Before the mucus has dried, more than 20 motile sperm should be seen in the high power field of the microscope. A normal test result suggests coital sufficiency, probable ovulation, "nonlethal" cervical mucus, and a normal male fertility test.[12]

Evaluation of ovulation

Progesterone measurement. Measuring the serum progesterone levels is the primary assay used to evaluate ovulation.[8] Beginning immediately after ovulation, serum progesterone levels rise (Figure 42-12) and peak within 5 to 9 days, during the middle of the luteal phase (on days 21 to 23). If ovulation does not occur, the corpus luteum fails to form, and the expected cyclical rise in progesterone level is lower than normal. Progesterone concentrations of greater than 10 ng/mL indicate normal ovulation; concentrations of less than 10 ng/mL suggest anovulation, inadequate luteal phase progesterone production, or inappropriate timing of the sample collection.

Basal body temperature. Basal body temperature charts have long been accepted as simple and cost-effective indicators of ovulation. Ovulation is associated with a rapid rise in body temperature of 0.5 °F, which persists throughout the luteal phase. However, the rise in body temperature is evident only retrospectively and therefore does not predict imminent ovulation in a way that helps time intercourse.

Measurement of the luteinizing hormone surge. LH appears in the urine just after the physiological LH surge and 24 to 36 hours before ovulation (see Figure 42-12). Measurement of LH cannot confirm ovulation or provide the etiology of anovulation but rather indicates when ovulation should occur and can serve as a guide used to time intercourse.

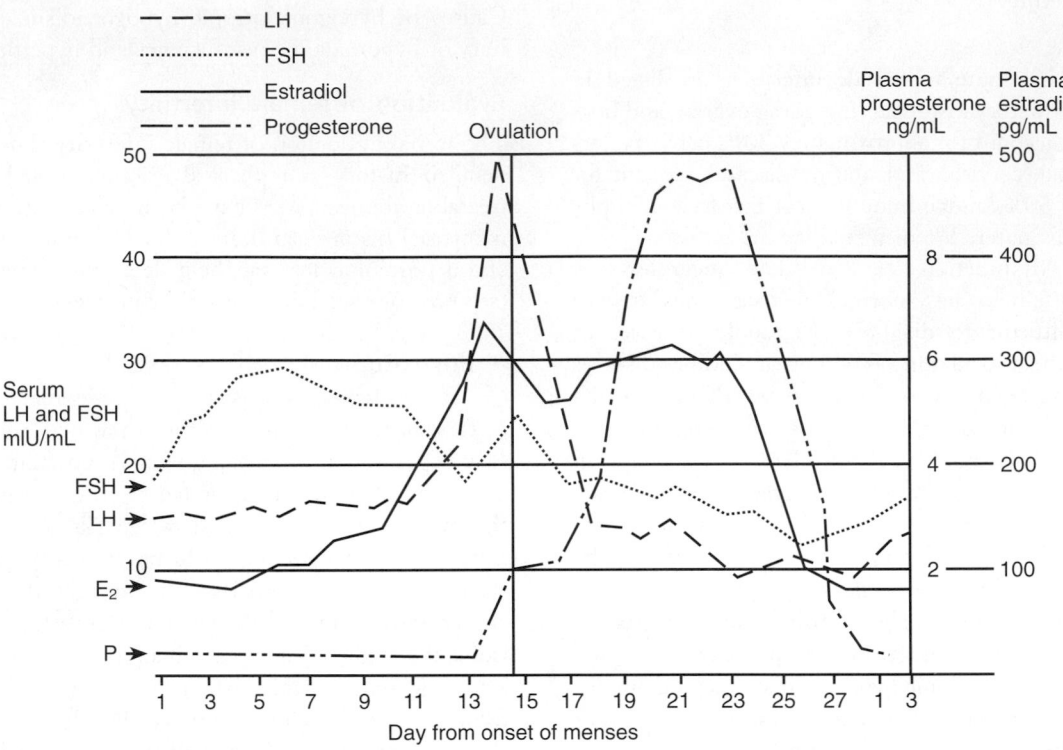

Figure 42-12   Composite of hormone changes during the normal menstrual cycle. *FSH,* Follicle-stimulating hormone; *LH,* luteinizing hormone; *E₂,* estradiol; *P,* progesterone. (Modified from Watts NB, Keffer JH: Practical Endocrine Diagnosis, 3rd edition, Philadelphia, Lea & Febiger, 1982.)

Monoclonal technology has led to the creation of home LH kits. These tests not only provide accurate information about the timing of ovulation but may reduce the stress and cost associated with infertility programs because they are performed at home and are comparatively inexpensive. Most home ovulation kits include a stick that has a two-site, double monoclonal enzyme-linked immunoassay. In one study of 26 healthy females, home LH kits predicted ovulation within 48 hours of a positive urine LH screen with a 92% positive predictive value.[10]

Evaluation of endocrine parameters

Hypergonadotropic hypogonadism.   Primary ovarian failure is indicated by repeatedly elevated basal FSH levels (>30 IU/L) or a single elevation of greater than 40 IU/L. Individuals diagnosed with hypergonadotropic hypogonadism are also hypoestrogenic (with estradiol levels of <20 IU/L).

Hypogonadotropic hypogonadism.   In individuals with hypogonadotropic hypogonadism, serum estradiol levels are less than 40 pg/mL (110 pmol/L). Decreased LH levels (<10 IU/L) and decreased FSH levels (<10 IU/L) are also present. Hyperprolactinemia can cause hypergonadotropic hypogonadal infertility. TSH concentration should be measured to rule out hypothyroidism. Prolactin levels can be high in individuals with PCOS and those taking medications such as antidepressants, cimetidine, and methyldopa. Radiographic imaging of the pituitary gland should be performed to rule out pituitary adenomas or empty sella syndrome.

■ ANALYTICAL METHODOLOGY

Various methods are available for measurement of reproductive hormones in body fluids. (Methods used to measure the reproductive protein hormones are discussed in Chapter 39.)

Determination of Total Testosterone Levels in Blood

Principles

The level of total circulating testosterone (both protein-bound and non–protein-bound forms) once was typically measured by RIA. However, gas chromatography combined with mass spectrometry (GC-MS) is the reference method for testosterone. A high-performance liquid chromatography (HPLC) method that does not require derivatization has also been described for testosterone.

Direct immunoassay methods have been used to determine testosterone levels in serum or plasma. To measure testosterone directly without extraction, the steroid must be displaced from its binding proteins, which is achieved by the addition of 8-anilino-1-naphthalene-sulfonic acid (ANS), danazol, or a competing steroid such as estradiol. Low-pH buffers, surfactants, and protein denaturation with heat treatment have also been used in some methods. Several commercial assay kits for direct assay of testosterone are available.

The use of nonisotopic immunoassays used to measure total testosterone levels is increasing. Enzyme-labeled, fluorescence, and chemiluminescence immunoassays have been used and are commercially available. A direct assay for testosterone has been fully automated and uses antitestosterone-coated magnetic particles and an acridinium ester-chemiluminescent endpoint.

Specimen requirements

Either serum or heparinized plasma are used to measure total or free testosterone. Specimens are stable for 1 week refrigerated and for 2 months frozen at −20 °C.[7] No steroids, thyroid, adrenocorticotropic hormone (ACTH), estradiol, or gonadotropin medications should be given for 48 hours before sample collection. Ethylenediaminetetraacetic acid (EDTA) causes a 10% decrease in total testosterone values when measured by certain RIA assays.

Comments

Estimation of SHBG in serum is sometimes very useful for interpretation of blood levels of testosterone. Two types of assays are generally available: (1) binding assays, in which the quantity of a radiolabeled androgen bound to SHBG is measured, and (2) specific immunoassays for the SHBG protein. Commercial kits used to measure SHBG are available.

Reference intervals

Reference intervals for total testosterone levels in serum are listed in Table 42-8.

Determination of Free and Weakly Bound Testosterone Levels in Blood

Bioavailable testosterone includes circulating free testosterone and albumin-bound (weakly bound) testosterone (see previous section on androgen transport in blood). Various methods[6] are available to determine the concentrations of these different forms of testosterone in serum or plasma: (1) estimation of the free testosterone fraction by equilibrium dialysis or ultrafiltration, (2) estimation of the free hormone by use of a direct (analog tracer) immunoassay, (3) estimation of the combined free and weakly bound (bioavailable) testosterone fractions by selective precipitation of the tightly bound form, (4) calculation of androgen index by use of indexes that reflect ratios of the testosterone pools, and (5) calculation of free and weakly bound testosterone concentrations by mathematical modeling.[14] The last approach uses mass action equations to calculate free and weakly bound testosterone levels from the concentrations of total

testosterone, SHBG, and albumin and from the association constants for the binding of testosterone to the two binding proteins. Reference intervals for free testosterone are listed in Table 42-9.

Determination of DHEA and DHEA-S Levels in Serum and Plasma

Measurements of DHEA or its sulfated conjugate, DHEA-S, in serum and plasma are important during investigations of adrenal androgen production, such as the assessment of hyperplasia, adrenal tumors, adrenarche, delayed puberty, or hirsutism. Circulating DHEA-S originates mostly from the adrenal glands, although in males some may be derived from the testes; none is produced by the ovaries. DHEA is secreted almost entirely by the adrenal glands.

TABLE 42-8	Reference Intervals for Total Testosterone Levels in Serum	
	ng/dL	nmol/L
Prepubertal Levels		
1 To 5 Mo		
Male infant	1 to 177	0.03 to 6.14
Female infant	1 to 5	0.03 to 0.17
6 To 11 Mo		
Male infant	2 to 7	0.07 to 0.24
Female infant	2 to 5	0.07 to 0.17
1 To 5 Y		
Boy	2 to 25	0.07 to 0.87
Girl	2 to 10	0.07 to 0.35
6 To 9 Y		
Boy	3 to 30	0.10 to 1.04
Girl	2 to 20	0.07 to 0.69
Pubertal Levels (Tanner Stage)		
1		
Boy	2 to 23	0.07 to 0.8
Girl	2 to 10	0.07 to 0.35
2		
Boy	5 to 70	0.17 to 2.43
Girl	5 to 30	0.17 to 1.04
3		
Boy	15 to 280	0.52 to 9.72
Girl	10 to 30	0.35 to 1.04
4		
Boy	105 to 545	3.64 to 18.91
Girl	15 to 40	0.52 to 1.39
5		
Boy	265 to 800	9.19 to 27.76
Girl	10 to 40	0.35 to 1.39
Adult Levels		
Man	260 to 1000	9 to 34.72
Woman	15 to 70*	0.52 to 2.43*

*Higher at midcycle peak.

TABLE 42-9	Reference Intervals for Free Testosterone Levels in Serum		
	pg/mL	pmol/L	Free Fraction (% of Total)
Children			
6 To 9 Y			
Boy	0.1 to 3.2	0.3 to 11.1	0.9 to 1.7
Girl	0.1 to 0.9	0.3 to 3.1	0.9 to 1.4
10 To 11 Y			
Boy	0.6 to 5.7	2.1 to 19.8	1
Girl	1 to 5.2	3.5 to 18	1 to 1.9
12 To 14 Y			
Boy	1.4 to 156	4.9 to 541	1.3 to 3
Girl	1 to 5.2	3.5 to 18	1.0 to 1.9
15 To 17 Y			
Boy	80 to 159	278 to 552	1.8 to 2.7
Girl	1 to 5.2	3.5 to 18	1 to 1.9
Adults			
Man	50 to 210	174 to 729	1 to 2.7
Woman	1 to 8.5	3.5 to 29.5	0.5 to 1.8

Principles

Immunoassay is the method of choice for measurements of DHEA and DHEA-S. Analysis of DHEA-S in serum or plasma is routinely performed with direct RIA; neither extraction nor chromatography is required in most methods. Other methods include gas-liquid chromatography, double-isotope derivative methods, and competitive protein-binding assays. The latter actually measures 5-androstenediol derivatives and uses SHBG as a naturally occurring binding protein.

Specimen requirements

Serum or plasma (preserved with EDTA) is suitable for DHEA or DHEA-S immunoassays.[7] No steroid, ACTH, estradiol, or gonadotropin medications should be given for 48 hours before sample collection. Early morning collection, before 1030 hours, is preferred for samples for DHEA testing. Analysis of DHEA by immunoassay usually requires pretreatment of serum samples because the serum concentration of DHEA is 1000-fold lower than that of DHEA-S.

Reference intervals

Reference intervals for DHEA-S and unconjugated DHEA are listed in Table 42-10.

Determination of 17-Ketosteroid Levels in Urine

The 17-KSs are metabolites of precursors secreted by the adrenal glands, the testes, and to some extent the ovaries. In males, approximately one third of the total urinary 17-KSs

TABLE 42-10	Reference Intervals for Dehydroepiandrosterone Sulfate and Unconjugated Dehydroepiandrosterone in Serum		
		μg/mL	μmol/L
Dehydroepiandrosterone Sulfate (DHEA-S)			
CHILDREN			
1 TO 5 DAYS	Male infant	12 to 254	0.3 to 6.9
	Female infant	10 to 248	0.3 to 6.7
1 MO TO 5 Y	Male infant/boy	1 to 41	0.03 to 1.1
	Female infant/girl	5 to 55	0.1 to 1.5
6 TO 9 Y	Boy	2.5 to 145	0.07 to 3.9
	Girl	2.5 to 140	0.07 to 3.8
10 TO 11 Y	Boy	15 to 115	0.4 to 3.1
	Girl	15 to 260	0.4 to 7
12 TO 17 Y	Boy	20 to 555	0.5 to 15
	Girl	20 to 535	0.5 to 14.4
PUBERTAL LEVELS (TANNER STAGE)			
1	Boy	5 to 265	0.1 to 7.2
	Girl	5 to 125	0.1 to 3.4
2	Boy	15 to 380	0.4 to 10.3
	Girl	15 to 150	0.4 to 4
3	Boy	60 to 505	1.6 to 13.6
	Girl	20 to 535	0.5 to 14.4
4	Boy	65 to 560	1.8 to 15.1
	Girl	35 to 485	0.9 to 13.1
5	Boy	165 to 500	4.4 to 13.5
	Girl	75 to 530	2.0 to 14.3
ADULTS			
MAN			
18 to 30 y		125 to 619	3.4 to 16.7
31 to 50 y		59 to 452	1.6 to 12.2
51 to 60 y		20 to 413	0.5 to 11.1
61 to 83 y		10 to 285	0.3 to 7.7
WOMAN			
18 to 30 y		45 to 380	1.2 to 10.3
31 to 50 y		12 to 379	0.8 to 10.2
Postmenopausal		30 to 260	0.8 to 7
		ng/dL	nmol/L
Unconjugated Dehydroepiandrosterone (DHEA)			
CHILDREN			
6 TO 9 Y	Boy	13 to 187	0.45 to 6.49
	Girl	18 to 189	0.62 to 6.55
10 TO 11 Y	Boy	31 to 205	1.07 to 7.11
	Girl	112 to 224	3.88 to 7.77
12 TO 14 Y	Boy	83 to 258	2.88 to 8.95
	Girl	98 to 360	3.4 to 12.5
ADULTS			
Man		180 to 1250	6.25 to 43.4
Woman		130 to 980	4.51 to 34

are metabolites of testosterone secreted by the testes, whereas most of the remaining two thirds are derived from the steroids produced by the adrenal glands. In females, who normally excrete smaller quantities than males, the total

17-KS levels are derived almost exclusively from the adrenal glands. Thus the main purpose in the measurement of these steroid metabolites is to assess adrenal androgen production.

Numerous chemical methods are available to estimate the level of total 17-KSs in urine. Final quantitation in most of these methods is based on the color reaction originally described by Zimmerman. Acid cleavage of glucuronic and sulfuric acid conjugates of 17-KSs is followed by extraction, washing with alkali, and color development. Estrone, which is an acidic 17-KS, is removed by alkali treatment because of its phenolic nature and thus is eliminated before the photometric reaction of the remaining neutral 17-KS fraction. The color formation is based on the reaction of 17-KS with m-dinitrobenzene in alcoholic potassium hydroxide to produce a reddish-purple color with maximum absorption at 520 nm.

Various drugs interfere with the 17-KS assay. Drugs that produce a positive interference include chlorpromazine, ethinamate, meprobamate, nalidixic acid, penicillin, phenaglycodol, and spironolactone. Drugs that produce a negative interference include chlordiazepoxide, progestational agents, propoxyphene, and reserpine. (See Chapter 41 for information on the measurement of 17-ketosteroids in urine.)

The measurement of DHEA-S in blood is a more convenient marker for adrenal androgen production than urinary 17-KS excretion because a 24-hour urine collection is not required, and many drugs interfere with the 17-KS assay. For these reasons, many clinicians now prefer values for plasma DHEA-S to those for urinary 17-KS.

Detection of Anabolic Steroids

The detection of exogenous steroids such as testosterone and DHT, which are used to improve athletic performance, is a challenge for the laboratory. The ratio of testosterone to epitestosterone, its 17α-epimer, has been used for detection of testosterone abuse. A testosterone/epitestosterone ratio of greater than 6 : 1 suggests exogenous testosterone use, so further testing should be performed for confirmation.[2] Others have suggested use of a testosterone/LH ratio in urine as an indication of testosterone abuse. Detailed studies of these ratios are available.[9] GC-MS remains the most widely used method for screening and confirmation.

Determination of Estrogen Levels in Blood

Principles

GC-MS methods coupled with isotope dilution provide the most accurate and reliable measurement of estradiol. The main steps are solvent extraction, chromatographic fractionation, and chemical derivatization before instrumental analysis. In practice these chemical and physical methods have been superseded by immunoassays, which combine the advantages of lowered limit of detection, reliability, and practicality.

Immunoassay is commonly used to measure estradiol. To measure estradiol directly without extraction and chromatography, the steroid must be displaced from its binding proteins. The displacing agents used in commercial methods are often not disclosed, but in some systems effective displacement is achieved by the addition of ANS or an excess of DHT to the sample. Numerous direct RIA kit methods are available commercially to measure serum estradiol. Nonisotopic immunoassays for estradiol have been developed and adapted for use on fully automated immunoassay systems.

Specimen requirements

Either serum or plasma (with EDTA or heparin as anticoagulant) are the specimens of choice for the measurement of estrogen levels in blood. Samples should be centrifuged and separated within 24 hours. Samples may be stored refrigerated for 24 hours or frozen for up to 2 months. Estradiol concentrations are increased in individuals with liver cirrhosis, and oral contraceptives can alter values.[7] No steroid, ACTH, gonadotropin, or estradiol medications should be given within 48 hours of sample collection.

Comments

Measurements of estriol have little clinical value for nonpregnant females because their estriol is derived almost exclusively from estradiol. Estrone measurements can only be used to diagnose causes of postmenopausal bleeding and menstrual dysfunction caused by extraglandular estrone production. Normally, blood estrone levels parallel estradiol levels (but at slightly lower concentrations) throughout the menstrual cycle.

Reference intervals

Reference intervals for serum levels of estradiol and estrone are listed in Table 42-11.

Determination of Progesterone Levels in Blood

Measurement of progesterone in serum or plasma is considered to be the most reliable way to assess its rate of production.

Principles

Double-isotope derivative methods and competitive protein-binding assays have been used to measure serum progesterone levels, but the methods require extensive purification of the steroid and are labor intensive. Gas chromatography procedures using flame ionization, electron capture, or nitrogen detection have been used to improve the accuracy of progesterone analysis. These methods also are time consuming and often require solvent extraction, chro-

TABLE 42-11 Reference Intervals for Estradiol and Estrone Levels in Serum

	pg/mL	pmol/L
Estradiol		
CHILDREN		
1 To 5 Y		
Boy	3 to 10	11 to 37
Girl	5 to 10	18 to 37
6 To 9 Y		
Boy	3 to 10	11 to 37
Girl	5 to 60	18 to 220
10 To 11 Y		
Boy	5 to 10	18 to 37
Girl	5 to 300	18 to 1100
12 To 14 Y		
Boy	5 to 30	18 to 110
Girl	25 to 410	92 to 1505
15 To 17 Y		
Boy	5 to 45	18 to 165
Girl	40 to 410	147 to 1505
ADULTS		
Man	10 to 50	37 to 184
Woman		
Early follicular phase	20 to 150	73 to 550
Late follicular phase	40 to 350	147 to 1285
Midcycle	150 to 750	550 to 2753
Luteal phase	30 to 450	110 to 1652
Postmenopausal	≤20	≤73
PUBERTAL LEVELS (TANNER STAGE)		
1		
Boy	3 to 15	11 to 55
Girl	5 to 10	18 to 37
2		
Boy	3 to 10	11 to 37
Girl	5 to 115	18 to 422
3		
Boy	5 to 15	18 to 55
Girl	5 to 180	18 to 660
4		
Boy	3 to 40	11 to 147
Girl	25 to 345	92 to 1267
5		
Boy	15 to 45	55 to 165
Girl	25 to 410	92 to 1505
Estrone		
Male	15 to 65	55 to 240
Female		
Early follicular phase	15 to 150	55 to 555
Late follicular phase	100 to 250	370 to 925
Luteal phase	15 to 200	55 to 740
Postmenopausal	15 to 55	55 to 204

TABLE 42-12 Reference Intervals for Progesterone Levels in Serum

	ng/dL	nmol/L
Prepubertal child (1 to 10 y)	7 to 52	0.2 to 1.7
Adult man	13 to 97	0.4 to 3.1
Adult woman		
Follicular phase	15 to 70	0.5 to 2.2
Luteal phase	200 to 2500	6.4 to 79.5
Pregnant woman		
First trimester	725 to 4400	23 to 139.9
Second trimester	1950 to 8250	62 to 262.4
Third trimester	6500 to 22 900	206.7 to 728.2

matography, and derivatization before the steroid is quantified. GC-MS has been recommended as a reference method for progesterone determination.

For routine measurement of progesterone in the clinical laboratory, immunoassays using steroid-specific antibodies are preferred. Initial immunoassays for serum progesterone measurement used organic solvents to remove the steroid from endogenous binding proteins such as CBG and albumin. Direct measurement of progesterone in serum or plasma is considered the method of choice for routine applications. Both RIA and nonisotopic immunoassays are available to measure progesterone in body fluids.

Specimen requirements

Either serum or plasma (with heparin or EDTA as anticoagulant) are used as specimens for progesterone analysis and should be separated within 24 hours.[7] The patient does not have to fast, and no special handling procedures are necessary. Samples can be stored refrigerated for up to 25 days at 2 to 8 °C or frozen for up to 7 months at −20 °C. Patients should not receive any corticosteroid, ACTH, estrogen, or gonadotropin medication for at least 48 hours before specimen collection.

Comments

During pregnancy a gradual increase in blood progesterone levels is observed from 5 to 40 weeks of gestation (and may increase tenfold to fortyfold). Previously, measurements of urinary pregnanediol were used as an indirect measure of progesterone. With the advent of specific immunoassays for serum progesterone, assays of urinary pregnanediol are rarely needed.

Reference intervals

Reference intervals for progesterone in serum are listed in Table 42-12.

References

1. Braunstein GD: Gynecomastia. N Engl J Med 1993; 328:490-495.
2. Catlin DH, Hatton CK, Starcevic SH: Issues in detecting abuse of xenobiotic anabolic steroids and testosterone by analysis of athletes' urine. Clin Chem 1997; 43:1280-1288.
3. Fisch H, Lipschultz LI: Diagnosing male factors of infertility. Arch Pathol Lab Med 1992; 116:398-405.
4. Frank S: Polycystic ovary syndrome. N Engl J Med 1995; 333:853.
5. Gougeon A, Ecochard R, Thalavard JC: Age-related changes of the population of human ovarian follicles: increase in the disappearance of non-growing and early growing follicles in aging women. Biol Reprod 1994; 50:653-657.
6. Gronowski AM, Landau-Levine M: Reproductive endocrine function. In Burtis CA, Ashwood, ER (eds): Tietz Textbook of Clinical Chemistry, 3rd edition, Philadelphia, WB Saunders, 1999.
7. Inter Science Institute: Current Unique and Rare Endocrine Assays, Inglewood, Calif, Inter Science Institute, 1997.
8. Jones HW, Toner JP: The infertile couple. N Engl J Med 1993; 329:1710-1715.
9. Kicman AT, Brooks RV, Collyer SC et al: Criteria to indicate testosterone administration. Br J Sports Med 1990; 24:253-264.
10. Miller PB, Soules MR: The usefulness of a urinary LH kit for ovulation prediction during menstrual cycles of normal women. Obstet Gynecol 1996; 87:13-17.
11. Rittmaster RS: Hirsutism. Lancet 1997; 349:191.
12. Viniker DA: Investigations for infertility management. In Rainsbury PA, Viniker DA (eds): Practical Guide to Reproductive Medicine, pp 93-110, New York, Parthenon Publishing Group, 1997.
13. Warren MP: Evaluation of secondary amenorrhea. J Clin Endocrinol Metab 1996; 81:437-442.
14. Wheeler MJ: The determination of bio-available testosterone. Ann Clin Biochem 1995; 32:345-357.

Additional Reading

Lobo, RA, Paulson RJ (eds): Mishell's Textbook of Infertility, Contraception, and Reproductive Endocrinology, 4th edition, Malden, Mass, Blackwell Science, 1997.

Williams RH Wilson JD (eds): Williams Textbook of Endocrinology, 9th edition, Philadelphia, WB Saunders, 1998.

Yen SSC, Jaffe RB, Barbieri RL (eds): Reproductive Endocrinology, 4th edition, Philadelphia, WB Saunders, 1997.

CHAPTER 43

Pregnancy

EDWARD R. ASHWOOD, MD

Objectives

1. Define the following terms:

Amniotic fluid	Embryo	Respiratory Distress Syndrome
Anencephaly	Erythroblastosis fetalis	Spina bifida
Eclampsia	Gestation	Trophoblast
Ectopic pregnancy	Preeclampsia	Zygote

2. List the protein and steroid hormones produced by the placenta and state their functions.
3. Describe the function and composition of amniotic fluid.
4. State the major biochemical changes that take place in a pregnant female during a normal pregnancy.
5. Describe the development of fetal renal, hepatic, pulmonary systems with regard to function and maturity.
6. State the clinical significance of chorionic gonadotropin, placental lactogen, alpha-fetoprotein, and unconjugated estriol analyses in the assessment of maternal and fetal health.
7. List the methods of analysis, principles of the procedures, and laboratory values obtained in the assessment of fetal lung maturity.

Key Words

Amniotic Fluid   Substance that protects the developing fetus; derived mostly from fetal urine

Anencephaly   A birth defect characterized by a brain that does not develop normally

Eclampsia   Convulsions and coma in a pregnant or puerperal woman

Ectopic Pregnancy   A pregnancy in which the embryo develops in the fallopian tube or abdomen instead of in the uterus

Embryo   A developing infant that has not yet finished organ development (less than 10 weeks gestation)

Erythroblastosis Fetalis   A fetal disease caused by maternal antibody-mediated fetal erythrocyte destruction

Fetus   A developing infant that has finished organ development (more than 10 weeks gestation)

Gestation   Length of pregnancy measured in weeks from the first day of the last menstrual period

Preeclampsia   Pregnancy-induced hypertension and increased protein levels in the urine

Respiratory Distress Syndrome   A disease of premature newborns caused by a deficiency of lung surfactant

Spina Bifida   A birth defect characterized by a spinal cord that does not develop normally

Trophoblasts   The cells comprising a layer of extraembryonic ectodermal tissue on the outside of the blastocyst

Zygote   The cell resulting from the union of a male and female gamete

The clinical laboratory has an important role in the management of pregnancy.[2] The health of a mother and her fetus are intertwined; thus pregnancy management must consider both. Laboratory tests are used to detect, evaluate, and monitor pregnancies and include common tests such as chorionic gonadotropin (CG), hematocrit, blood type, and glucose tolerance testing; screening tests, such as the "triple test" (α-fetoprotein [AFP], CG, and unconjugated estriol [uE₃]); and esoteric tests, such as fetal lung maturity tests and amniotic fluid bilirubin examination.

■ HUMAN PREGNANY

Understanding fundamental topics, such as conception, embryo development, fetal growth, the role of the placenta, the importance and composition of amniotic fluid, maternal adaptation to pregnancy, and functional maturation of the fetus, is necessary to appreciate the role of laboratory tests in pregnancy health care.

Conception, Embryo, and Fetus

Normal human pregnancy lasts approximately 40 weeks, as measured from the first day of the last normal menstrual period (LMP or LNMP). An infant's anticipated date of birth is commonly referred to as the *expected date of confinement,* or EDC. When talking with patients, physicians customarily divide **gestation** into three time intervals, or trimesters, each of which is slightly longer than 13 weeks. By convention, the first trimester, 0 to 13 weeks, begins on the first day of the last menses.

Ovulation occurs on approximately the fourteenth day of the regular menstrual cycle (see Chapter 42.) If conception occurs, the ovum is fertilized in the fallopian tube and becomes a **zygote,** which is then carried down the tube into the uterus. The zygote divides and becomes a morula. After 50 to 60 cells are present, the morula develops a cavity, the primitive yolk sac, and becomes a blastocyst, which implants into the uterine wall about 5 days after fertilization. The cells on the exterior wall of the blastocyst become **trophoblasts,** which synergistically invade the uterine endometrium and develop into chorionic villi, creating the placenta.

At this stage the product of conception is referred to as an **embryo.** A cavity called the *amnion* forms within the embryo and enlarges with the accumulation of liquor amnii, commonly referred to as *amniotic fluid.* Nourished by the placenta and protected by the amniotic fluid, the embryo undergoes rapid cell division, differentiation, and growth. From combinations of three primary cell types (ectoderm, mesoderm, and endoderm), organs begin to form, a process termed *organogenesis.* At 10 weeks the embryo has developed most major structures and is referred to as a **fetus.** At 13 weeks, the fetus weighs approximately 13 g and is 8 cm long.

During the second trimester, 13 to 26 weeks, rapid fetal growth occurs. By the end of the second trimester, the fetus weighs approximately 700 g and is 30 cm long, and many fetal organs have begun to mature. The third trimester, 26 to 40 weeks, is the period in which fetal organs complete maturation. During this trimester, the growth rate decelerates; at the end of the third trimester, the fetus weighs approximately 3200 g and is about 50 cm long. *Term* is the interval from 37 to 42 weeks. Normal labor, rhythmic uterine contractions, and birth occur during this period.

Placenta

The placenta's umbilical cord is the primary link between the fetus and mother. The placenta grows throughout pregnancy and is delivered through the birth canal immediately after birth of the infant.

Function

The placenta keeps the maternal and fetal circulations separate, nourishes the fetus, eliminates fetal wastes, and produces hormones vital to pregnancy. It is composed of large collections of fetal vessels called *villi,* which are surrounded by intervillous spaces in which maternal blood flows. For substances to move from the maternal circulation to the fetal circulation, they must cross through the trophoblasts and several membranes. The permeability of any substance depends largely on the concentration gradient between the maternal and fetal circulations, the presence or absence of circulating binding proteins, the lipid solubility of the substance, and the presence of facilitated transport mechanisms such as ion pumps or receptor-mediated endocytosis (Table 43-1). The placenta is an effective barrier to large proteins

TABLE 43-1	Normal Placental Transport
No Transport	**Active Transport Across**
Most proteins	**Cell Membranes**
Thyroid hormones	Glucose
Maternal immunoglobulins M	Many amino acids
and A	Calcium
Maternal and fetal erythrocytes	
	Receptor-Mediated
Limited Passive Transport	**Endocytosis**
Unconjugated steroids	Maternal immunoglobulin G
Steroid sulfates	Insulin
Free fatty acids	Low-density lipoprotein
Passive Transport	
Lipid-soluble molecules up to 5000 D	
Oxygen	
Carbon dioxide	
Sodium and chloride	
Urea	
Ethanol	

and hydrophobic compounds bound to plasma proteins. Maternal immunoglobulin G (IgG) crosses the placenta by receptor-mediated endocytosis. Because of its long half-life, maternally produced IgG protects the newborn for the first 6 months of life.

Placental hormones

The placenta produces several protein and steroid hormones (Figure 43-1). The major protein hormones are CG and placental lactogen (PL). The steroid hormones include progesterone, estradiol, estriol, and estrone. Generally, hormone production by the placenta increases in proportion to the increase in placental mass. Therefore concentrations of hormones derived from the placenta, such as PL and estriol, increase in maternal peripheral blood as the placenta increases in size. CG, which peaks at the end of the first trimester, is an exception.

Chorionic gonadotropin

One of the most important placental hormones is CG. This hormone is commonly called "human chorionic gonadotropin" and is often abbreviated hCG or HCG. This term and its abbreviations should be abandoned because the label "human" is superfluous.

Chemistry. CG is a glycoprotein composed of two different, noncovalently bound glycoprotein subunits, alpha (α) and beta (β). The complete hormone has a molecular weight of approximately 37,900 D and has a higher carbohydrate proportion than any other human hormone. In maternal serum, CG can be in many forms, including unmodified CG dimers with differing carbohydrate side chains, and modified forms with various degrees of degradation. Leukocyte elastase breaks peptide bonds in CGβ at position 47-48 to form nicked CG (CGn). The nicking inactivates the hormone and also reduces ability to bind to some CG antibodies. Other nicking sites are at β44-45, β46-47, and α70-71. Both free CGα (fCGα) and free CGβ (fCGβ) are found in the serum, along with nicked free forms (for example, fCGβn). The C-terminal portion of fCGβ can be cleaved to leave a core fragment of CGβ (CGβcf) with a molecular mass of 13,000 D. Urine contains predominantly CGβcf and some unmodified CG and CGn. The rate of clearance varies for the different forms of CG and has three phases. The rapid, medium, and slow half-lives are, respectively: CG—3.6, 18, and 53 hours; CGβ—1, 23, and 194 hours; and CGα—0.63, 6, and 22 hours.

Biochemistry. CG is synthesized in the syncytiotrophoblast cells of the placenta. A single gene on chromosome 6 codes for the α subunit of all four glycoprotein hormones (thyroid-stimulating hormone [TSH], luteinizing hormone [LH], follicle-stimulating hormone [FSH], and CG). Chromosome 19 contains a family of genes that encodes the CGβ subunit. Separate messenger RNAs (mRNAs) are

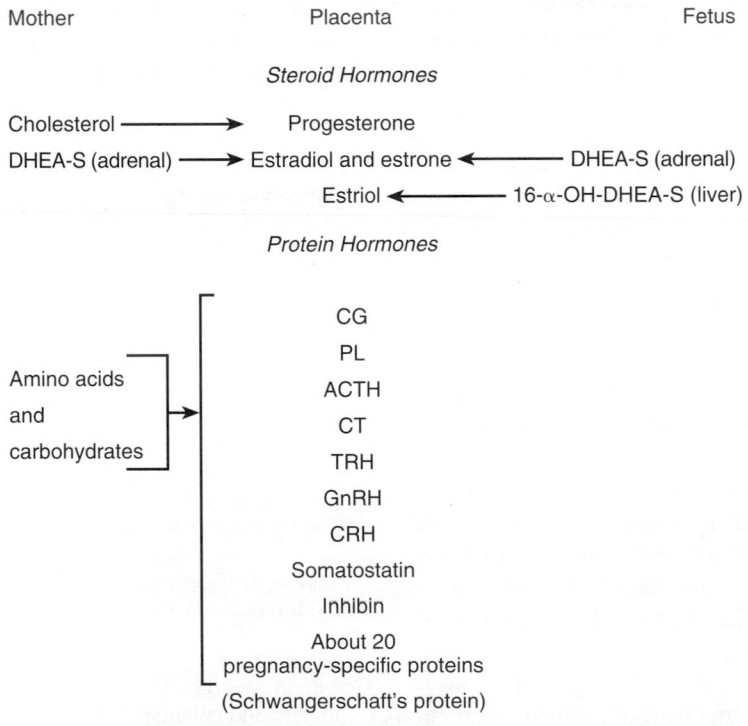

Figure 43-1   Steroid and protein hormone production by the placenta. *DHEA-S,* Dehydroepiandrosterone sulfate; *CG,* chorionic gonadotropin; *PL,* placental lactogen; *ACTH,* adrenocorticotropic hormone; *TRH,* thyroid-stimulating hormone; *CT,* chorionic thyrotropin; *GnRH,* gonadotropin-releasing hormone; *CRH,* corticotropin-releasing hormone.

transcribed from the respective genes, and the α and β subunits are translated from each. The subunits spontaneously combine in the rough endoplasmic reticulum and are then continuously secreted into the maternal circulation. Synthesis of CGβ peaks at about 8 to 10 weeks, but production of the α subunit continues to increase and is thought to be a function of the placental mass.

Extensive homology exists between the peptide portions of CGβ and LHβ subunits. Investigators have proposed that a single deletion in the ancestral LHβ gene lengthened the subunit from 115 amino acids to 145 amino acids; 80% of the first 115 amino acids in both β-subunits are identical, but 30 additional amino acid residues in CGβ are unique. Highly specific monoclonal antibodies have been produced that bind to unique epitopes throughout the CGβ subunit. These antibodies are the most frequently used in assays that measure CG.

Physiology.   CG stimulates the corpus luteum in the ovary to make progesterone during the first weeks of pregnancy. The placenta makes inadequate amounts of progesterone during this time. No specific receptor for CG is known; it binds to and activates the LH receptor in cells of the corpus luteum in the maternal ovary. Receptor activation increases intracellular cyclic adenosine monophosphate (cAMP), which in turn stimulates the production of progesterone, a steroid that prevents menses and thus supports the pregnancy. CG binds weakly to TSH receptors in the maternal thyroid, thus CG concentrations greater than 1,000,000 IU/L are thyrotropic.

Methods used to measure chorionic gonadotropin.   Measurements of CG can be used to diagnose a normal pregnancy, diagnose ectopic pregnancy, screen for Down syndrome, and monitor the course of a patient with certain types of cancer. Because of these diverse uses, many differing assays are used to determine CG, including home test kits, qualitative urine kits, and quantitative serum kits.

- *Home test kits* Assays in home test kits are the most commonly used pregnancy tests. Purchased without a prescription, these tests are simple and can be performed by in the privacy of the home. One third of females who suspect they may be pregnant use home kits.[14] Most kits provide a single test that uses an enzyme immunometric or immunochromatographic strategy. Detection limits are about 50 IU/L, and tests take from 2 to 30 minutes to perform. Although the techniques used are straightforward, consumers do make more mistakes performing these tests than do trained laboratory professionals. An extensive evaluation of home test kits in France revealed that only 11 of 27 home-use tests performed by experienced technologists were as accurate as claimed.[8] When the 11 tests were further evaluated by a group female lay individuals, the clinical specificity ranged from 77% to 100%, and the clinical sensitivity ranged from 31% to 100% even at two times the claimed detection limit of

the test. The high number of false-negative results was attributed to difficulty in understanding of the literature that accompanied the test.

- *Qualitative laboratory test kits* First-morning urine specimens are preferred for qualitative pregnancy tests because they contain abundant CG. False-positive results occur in 1% of tests because of the presence in urine of interfering substances such as proteins, drugs, bacteria, erythrocytes, or leukocytes. False-negative results can occur because the tests usually do not detect CG levels at concentrations of less than 25 to 50 IU/L. Therefore about half of the qualitative tests are positive on the day after the first missed menstrual period. Denaturation of the antiserum to CG caused by high temperature, pH extremes, or old reagents may also yield false results. The use of known positive and negative controls is therefore extremely important in order to obtain reliable results. The simplicity and speed with which the results are obtained make these tests very valuable for pregnancy confirmation. However, these procedures are not quantitative and may not detect an early or abnormal pregnancy.

- *Quantitative laboratory test kits* Immunoassay is a popular technique used to measure CG. Serum samples should be used in quantitative CG assays. Blood specimens are collected into suitable tubes without anticoagulants, allowed to clot at room temperature, and centrifuged to obtain clear serum. All specimens not tested within 48 hours of collection should be stored at −20 °C. As with most biological materials, repeated freezing and thawing should be avoided. Serum specimens showing gross hemolysis, gross lipemia, or turbidity may give false results. Diagnostic companies use five common strategies to measure CG among 10 different CG immunoassay kits: antiCGβ radioimmunoassay (RIA), antiCGβ:antiCGβ sandwich, antiCGβ:antiCGα sandwich, antiCGβ C terminal:antiCGβ sandwich, and antiCG:antiCGβ sandwich. The sandwich techniques used either immunoradiometric assay (IRMA) or (immunoenzymatic assay) IEMA for CG detection. Serum samples from pregnant patients varied by up to 2.2-fold. The differences were attributed to differences in antibody recognition of the various forms of CG (for example, nicked, β subunit, and other fragments) present in serum. The lowest detectable concentration is 1 to 2 IU/L. Typical between-run precision is 10% to 15% at 10 IU/L, 6% to 15% at 30 IU/L, and 7% to 12% at 150 IU/L.

- *Specificity of CG assays* Modern CG immunoassays should have little or no cross-reactivity with LH. To assess the specificity of a CG immunoassay, blood samples with high LH results should be assayed to show that LH does not significantly influence the CG results. Serum from postmenopausal women is a convenient source of specimens with high LH. The assay should be designed so that low concentrations of CG are detected and false-positive values caused by LH interference are minimized.

Placental lactogen

PL, also known as *human placental lactogen (hPL)* and *human chorionic somatomammotropin (hCS)*, is a single-chain polypeptide with a molecular mass of 22,279 D and is composed of 191 amino acids. The structure of PL is exceptionally homologous (96%) with growth hormone (GH) and less with prolactin (67%). Therefore PL, not surprisingly, has potent growth and lactogenic properties. The placental secretion of PL near term is 1 to 2 g/day, more than any other known human hormone. From the physiological point of view, PL has many biological activities, including lactogenic, metabolic, somatotropic, luteotropic, erythropoietic, and aldosterone-stimulating effects. Either directly or in synergism with prolactin, PL has a significant role in preparing mammary glands for lactation. Although PL was used in the past to evaluate fetal well-being, currently no apparent clinical reason exists to measure PL.[6]

Placental steroids

The placenta produces a wide variety of steroid hormones, including phenomenal amounts of progesterone and estrogens at term (see Chapter 42). Estrogen and progesterone induce changes in the endometrium, stimulating uterine growth and uterine blood supply, ensuring adequate fetal nutrition and preparing the uterus for labor. Although measurement of estriol in the third trimester was previously used to assess fetal well-being, many obstetricians consider this practice obsolete.[6] It has been shown that during the second trimester, serum levels of uE_3 are low in cases of fetal Down syndrome.[5]

Chemistry of estriol. Estriol, as its name implies, is an estrogen with three hydroxyl groups (at positions 3, 16, and 17). Its systematic name is 1,3,5(10)-estriene-3,16-α,17-β-triol. Only a minor amount (~9%) of the hormone circulates in plasma unconjugated, and because of its low solubility this form is strongly bound to sex hormone-binding globulin (SHBG). The majority exists as conjugates of glucuronate and sulfate (Figure 43-2). The conjugation occurs in the maternal liver and makes the hormone more soluble, thereby permitting renal clearance.

Biochemistry of estriol. Biosynthesis of estrogens by the placenta differs from that of the ovaries because the placenta has no 17α-hydroxylase. Thus each of the estrogens—estrone (E_1), estradiol (E_2), and estriol (E_3)—must be synthesized from C_{19} intermediates that already have a hydroxyl group at position 17. The fetal adrenal cortex has a unique zone for steroid production. The demand for estrogens is so great that the fetal adrenal gland is massive compared to that of an adult; 80% of the adrenal weight is composed of the fetal zone. The fetal adrenal avidly binds low-density lipoprotein (LDL) particles to take in cholesterol, which is converted into two major steroid intermediates, pregnenolone sulfate and dehydroepiandrosterone sulfate (DHEA-S). The intermediates are secreted into the fetal circulation. The fetal liver converts DHEA-S into 16α-hydroxy-DHEA-S, which is secreted back into the fetal cir-

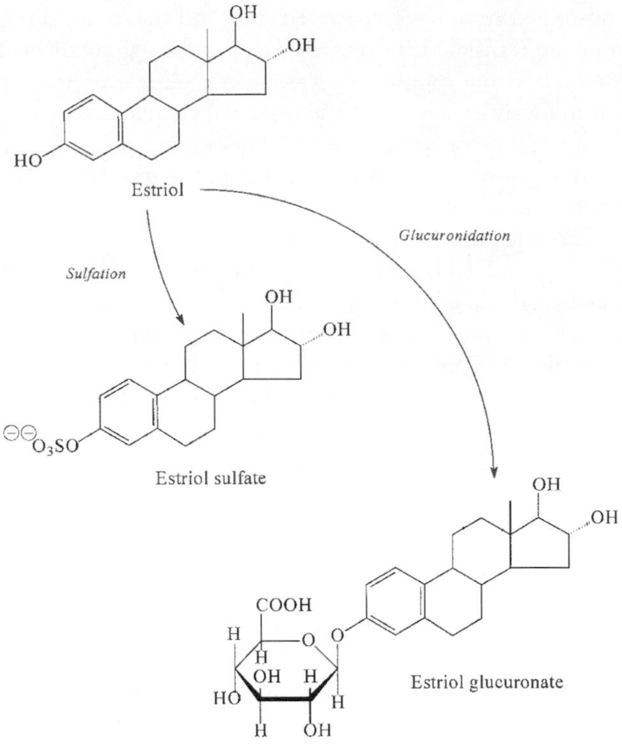

Figure 43-2 Forms of estriol present in maternal serum. Glucuronidation and sulfation also occur at the other hydroxyl positions.

culation. Finally, the placenta synthesizes estriol from 16α-hydroxy-DHEA-S. Approximately 90% of maternal estriol in serum is derived from this pathway. A minor amount is made with precursors from the maternal ovary. The uE_3 concentrations typical for the second trimester of pregnancy, 0.30 to 1.50 μg/L, are shown in Figure 43-3. In nonpregnant women the ovaries secrete 100 to 600 μg/day of estradiol, of which about 10% is metabolized into estriol. During late pregnancy the placenta produces about 250 mg/day of progesterone, 50 to 150 mg/day of estriol, and 15 to 20 mg/day of estradiol and estrone.

Clinical significance of estriol. Down syndrome leads to a modest decrease in uE_3 levels. Any disruption in the biosynthetic pathway leads to very low maternal serum estriol levels. Conditions that cause disruption include fetal **anencephaly,** placental sulfatase deficiency, fetal death, chromosome abnormalities, and molar pregnancy. Placental sulfatase deficiency appears in the infant as X-linked ichthyosis. It is present in approximately 1 in every 2000 males. Because of the lack of uE_3, the mother often has delayed onset of labor. The cesarean section rate is significantly higher in these mothers.

Methods used to measure unconjugated estriol. Most commercial assays were designed to measure estriol in the third trimester and therefore have reportable ranges from 2 to 40 ng/mL. Two ultrasensitive RIA methods are available commercially, and other methods are under development. The most commonly used method uses eight external calibrators from 0.1 to 20 ng/mL in a competitive RIA

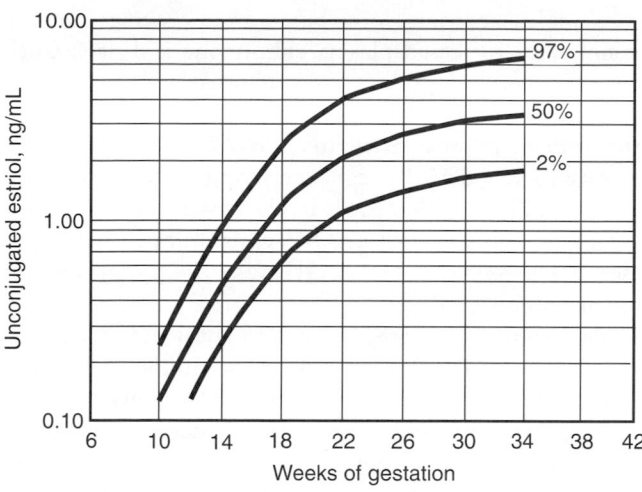

Figure 43-3   Concentration of unconjugated estriol (uE₃) in maternal serum as a function of gestational age.

format; a zero calibrator is also used. The tracer is ^{125}I, which has a shelf life of 12 weeks. Labeled estriol competes with endogenous estriol for binding to rabbit antiestriol. The immune complexes are precipitated with goat-antirabbit γ-globulin and polyethylene glycol. The method uses 50 μL of serum and has a detection limit of 0.03 ng/mL. Precision at 0.70 ng/mL is less than ±7%.

The uE₃ concentration increases in whole blood at room temperature and 4 °C because the conjugated forms can be enzymatically deconjugated to form the parent hormone. Serum collected for uE₃ analysis can be kept at 4 °C for up to 7 days but should be frozen at −20 °C for longer periods. Levels up to 1000 ng/mL of estrone, estriol-3-sulfate, and estriol-3-glucuronide have a cross-reaction rate of less than 0.03%.

Maternal Adaptation

During pregnancy a woman undergoes dramatic physiological and hormonal changes. The large amounts of estrogens, progesterone, PL, and corticosteroids produced during pregnancy affect various metabolic, physiological, and endocrinological systems. An increase in resistance to angiotensin, a predominance of lipid metabolism over glucose utilization, and an increased synthesis by the liver of thyroid- and steroid-binding proteins, fibrinogen, and other proteins are characteristic of pregnancy. As a result of such changes, many of the laboratory reference intervals for nonpregnant patients are not appropriate for pregnant patients. The mean values for selected tests expressed as a percentage of control means are summarized in Table 43-2.[19]

Hematological changes

Maternal blood volume increases during pregnancy by an average of 45%. Plasma volume increases more rapidly than red blood cell mass; therefore despite augmented production, the concentration of hemoglobin, the erythrocyte count, and the

TABLE 43-2	Mean Serum and Plasma Laboratory Values during Normal Pregnancies Expressed as a Percentage of the Nonpregnant Mean*		
	Time of Gestation		
Analyte	12 wk	32 wk	Term
Sodium	97	98	97
Potassium	95	95	100
Bicarbonate	85	85	81
Chloride	98	100	99
Urea nitrogen	77	63	77
Creatinine	71	74	81
Fasting glucose	98	94	94
Bilirubin, unconjugated	56	67	78
Albumin	93	78	78
Protein	92	83	83
Uric acid	68	92	120
Calcium	98	94	97
Free ionized calcium	99	101	102
Parathyroid hormone, intact	—	—	140
Vitamin 1,25-(OH)₂D₃	—	—	400
Phosphate	108	97	96
Magnesium	92	87	87
Alkaline phosphatase	90	203	347
Creatine kinase	87	86	135
α₁-Antitrypsin	129	174	191
Transferrin	105	160	170
Cholesterol	100	144	156
HDL-cholesterol	121	119	130
LDL-cholesterol	80	118	146
Fasting triglycerides	141	300	349
Iron	112	94	94
Iron-binding capacity	95	139	144
Transferrin saturation	136	68	64
Zinc protoporphyrin	107	109	144
Ferritin	81	33	59
Thyroxine	103	107	100
Triiodothyronine	100	121	121
Free thyroxine	98	72	74
Thyroxine-binding globulin	114	155	182
Thyroid-stimulating hormone	111	122	139
Cortisol	111	301	309
Aldosterone	—	—	1500
Prolactin	—	—	800
Hemoglobin	95	90	96
Hematocrit	94	91	97
Leukocyte count	144	167	240
Prothrombin time	99	97	97
Activated partial thromboplastin time	95	91	93
Platelet count	98	96	100
Fibrinogen	119	154	165

Data from Lockitch G (ed): Handbook of Diagnostic Biochemistry and Hematology in Normal Pregnancy, Boca Raton, Fla, CRC Press, 1993.
HDL, High-density lipoprotein; *LDL*, low-density lipoprotein.
*The values are the means in pregnant subjects expressed as a percentage of the means in nonpregnant controls.

hematocrit decrease during normal pregnancy. Hemoglobin concentrations at term average 12.6 g/dL, compared with 13.3 g/dL for nonpregnant individuals.

The concentrations of several blood coagulation factors increase during pregnancy in preparation for birth—a major challenge to hemostasis. Plasma fibrinogen increases approximately 65%, from 275 to 450 mg/dL. The increase contributes to the increase in sedimentation rate. Pregnancy increases the risk of thromboembolism up to five times that of normal.

Chemical changes

During pregnancy the electrolytes show little change, but approximately a 40% increase occurs in serum triglycerides, cholesterol, phospholipids, and free fatty acids. The increase is in response to the maternal switch from carbohydrate metabolism to fat metabolism. Plasma albumin is decreased to an average of 3.4 g/dL in late pregnancy; plasma globulin concentrations increase slightly. Several of the plasma transport proteins increase markedly, including thyroxine-binding globulin (TBG), cortisol-binding globulin (CBG), and SHBG. Serum cholinesterase activity decreases, whereas alkaline phosphatase activity in serum triples, mainly because of an increase in heat-stable alkaline phosphatase from the placenta. Delivery can markedly increase creatine kinase levels.

Renal function

Pregnancy increases the glomerular filtration rate (GFR) to about 170 mL/min/1.73 m^2 by 20 weeks and therefore increases the clearance of urea, creatinine, and uric acid. Up to 1000 mg/day of glucosuria may be present because of the increased GFR, which presents more fluid to the tubules and therefore lowers the renal glucose threshold. Protein loss in the urine can increase to up to 300 mg/day.

Endocrine changes

Progesterone prevents menses and thus allows pregnancy to continue. In early pregnancy, the progesterone is produced by the maternal ovary in response to CG. In later stages the placenta directly produces enough progesterone to maintain the pregnancy.

Throughout pregnancy the plasma level of parathyroid hormone (PTH) is increased by approximately 40%, with almost no change in the plasma levels of free ionized calcium, thus suggesting a new set-point for the secretion of PTH. Calcitonin does not increase predictably during pregnancy, whereas vitamin 1,25-(OH)$_2$D$_3$ increases during pregnancy and promotes increased intestinal calcium absorption. These changes permit the transfer of large amounts of calcium to the developing fetus.

The elevated estrogen levels stimulate increased production of CBG by the liver. For unknown reasons, the metabolic clearance rate of cortisol decreases. Thus the absolute plasma levels of both total and free cortisol are several times higher during pregnancy. The diurnal rhythm of cortisol,

with higher morning levels and lower evening levels, is maintained. Increased plasma aldosterone and deoxycorticosterone concentrations are also observed.

Increasing estrogen levels throughout pregnancy increase the secretion of prolactin up to tenfold. Conversely, the high estrogen levels during pregnancy suppress the secretion of LH and FSH to undetectable levels. Baseline levels of other pituitary hormones such as TSH remain nearly unchanged (see Table 43-2), but the GH response to provocative stimuli is decreased.

Although normal pregnancy is an euthyroid state, many changes occur in thyroid hormone concentrations. The high levels of TBG raise the concentration of total thyroxine (T$_4$) and triiodothyronine (T$_3$), but a slight decrease in free T$_4$ concentration occurs during the second and third trimesters. Very few (less than 0.2%) pregnant individuals develop hyperthyroidism, and hypothyroidism is very rare. However, thyroid dysfunction after birth is common and is frequently unrecognized.

Functional Development of the Fetus

The fetal organs mature during the third trimester but not at the same rate.

Lungs and pulmonary surfactant

In normal air-breathing lungs, a substance called *surfactant* coats the alveolar epithelium and responds to alveolar volume changes by reducing the surface tension in the alveolar wall during expiration. Surfactant is needed because the surface tension is an inverse function of the radius of the airway. Thus small alveoli have a higher collapsing force than larger alveoli. Surfactant opposes the force and keeps the small alveoli from collapsing. Specialized alveolar cells called *type II granular pneumocytes* synthesize pulmonary surfactant and package it into laminated storage granules called *lamellar bodies.* These storage granules are 1 to 5 μm in diameter and contain phospholipids, cholesterol, and protein. Production starts as early as 20 weeks gestation, but adequate amounts do not accumulate until about 36 weeks. The newborn lung contains 100 times more surfactant per cm^3 than the adult lung. The excessive surfactant is needed at birth as the newborn transforms from breathing water to breathing air. The surfactant overcomes the surface tension produced in water-filled alveoli that are admitting air for the first time.

Pulmonary surfactant is a complex mixture of lipids and proteins, and less than 5% is composed of carbohydrates. Most of the lipid is phospholipid, and the majority of that is lecithin (phosphatidylcholine). Unlike lecithin from other organs, pulmonary lecithin has two saturated fatty acids, usually palmitoyl groups. Other lipids present are phosphatidylglycerol (PG), phosphatidylinositol (PI), and phosphatidylethanolamine (see Chapter 24). Sphingomyelin is present in very small amounts (~2%). The protein fraction of lamellar bodies is approximately 4% and is composed of three surfactant-specific proteins, SP-A, SP-B, and SP-C.

Liver

Hematopoiesis occurs in the liver during the first two trimesters and transfers to the fetal bone marrow during the third trimester. The liver is also responsible for producing specific proteins (such as albumin and clotting factors), metabolism and detoxification of many compounds, and secretion of substances such as bilirubin. A clinically useful protein produced by the liver is AFP. Detoxification and bilirubin secretion mechanisms are immature until late in pregnancy and even in the first few months after birth. Thus premature infants often have high serum bilirubin concentrations and metabolize drugs poorly.

Alpha-fetoprotein

Very early in pregnancy, the fetal liver begins to produce the albumin-like protein called *AFP.* Because AFP is produced by only the fetal liver and in some adults with cancer, it is classified as an oncofetal protein. The function of AFP is unknown.

Chemistry.   As its name implies, AFP migrates to the α zone during electrophoresis. It is a glycoprotein with a molecular weight of approximately 70,000 D. The AFP gene, which is located on the long arm (q) of chromosome 4 (q11 to q22), is part of a family of genes that also encode for albumin and vitamin D-binding protein. Although very stable in serum, even at room temperature, for as long as a week, AFP rapidly forms multimers in dilute serum or saline solutions.

Biochemistry.   AFP is produced initially by the fetal yolk sac in small quantities and then in larger quantities by the fetal liver as the yolk sac degenerates. Early in embryonic life, AFP has a high concentration in fetal serum, reaching about one tenth the concentration of albumin. The peak concentration in the fetal serum, approximately 3,000,000 ng/mL, is reached at about 9 weeks gestation. The concentration then declines steadily to about 20,000 ng/mL at term (Figure 43-4). The increase and decrease in concentration of AFP in the amniotic fluid roughly parallels that in the fetal serum but is two to three orders of magnitude lower in concentration (~15,000 ng/mL at 16 weeks gestation). The relationship with respect to maternal serum concentration is slightly more complicated because of fetal-maternal transfer, the rapidly growing fetus, the relatively constant size of the mother, maternal clearance of the protein, and the volume of distribution in the mother, which varies based on maternal weight. Maternal AFP is first detectable (at ~5 ng/mL) in serum at about 10 weeks gestation. The concentration increases about 15% per week to a peak of approximately 180 ng/mL at about 25 weeks. The concentration in maternal serum then subsequently declines slowly until term. After birth the maternal serum AFP level rapidly decreases to less than 2 ng/mL. In an infant, serum AFP levels decline exponentially and reach adult levels by the tenth month of life.

Methods used to measure alpha-fetoprotein.   Although AFP was traditionally measured by RIA, newer

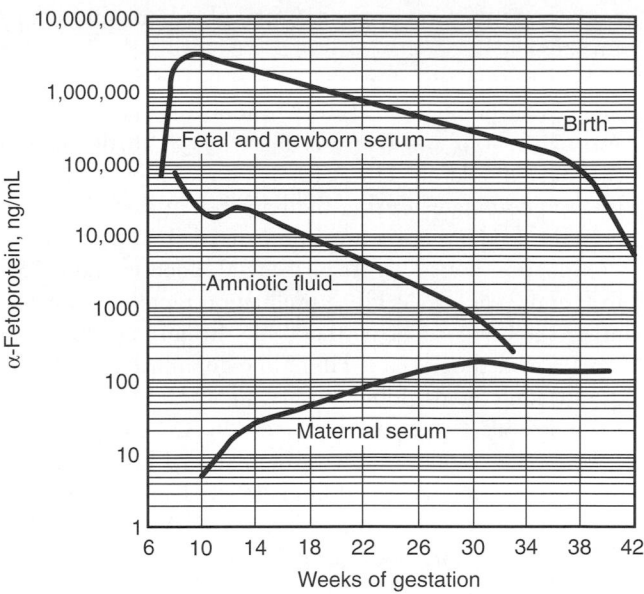

Figure 43-4   Concentrations of α-fetoprotein in fetal and newborn serum, amniotic fluid, and maternal serum.

methods use IEMA because of its lower detection limits, better precision, speed, avoidance of radioactivity, and ease of automation. The Food and Drug Administration (FDA) has licensed three immunoassay AFP kits for use in maternal serum screening for neural tube defects: a monoclonal bead assay, a microparticles immunoassay, and a polyclonal bead assay. Each assay uses a sandwich design: a solid-phase antibody captures the AFP, and after washing, a second enzyme-labeled antibody is added. After a second wash that removes unbound labeled antibody, substrate is added to produce a colored product. Calibration is relative to an international standard, with 1 IU being approximately 1.126 ng. Most laboratories report AFP in units of nanograms per milliliter. Day-to-day precision studies show that the coefficient of variation (CV) is approximately 8% at about 40 ng/mL.

Kidneys

Toward the end of the first trimester the fetal kidneys begin to produce urine, which is the main component of amniotic fluid. The early nephrons cannot produce concentrated urine, and pH regulation is also limited. Complete maturation occurs after birth. Although kidneys are not required for fetal survival, amniotic fluid is required for proper lung development. Thus newborns without kidneys die of pulmonary failure.

Fetal blood development

Fetal blood is produced first by the embryonic yolk sac, then by the liver, and finally by the fetal bone marrow. The yolk sac produces three embryonic hemoglobins: Portland ($\zeta_2\epsilon_2$), Gower-1 ($\zeta_2\epsilon_2$), and Gower-2 ($\alpha_2\epsilon_2$). These normal embryonic hemoglobins are of little importance in clinical chemistry because they are present in fetal blood only in the first trimester.

With the switch of erythropoiesis to the fetal liver and spleen, fetal hemoglobin (Hb F) production begins. Hb F consists of two α and two γ-chains ($\alpha_2\gamma_2$). Small amounts of adult hemoglobin, Hb A ($\alpha_2\beta_2$), are also produced, but Hb F predominates during the remainder of fetal life.

As the fetal bone marrow begins red cell production, Hb A production increases. At birth, fetal blood contains 75% Hb F and 25% Hb A. Hb F production rapidly diminishes during the first year of postnatal life. In normal adults, less than 1% of hemoglobin is Hb F. The difference between fetal and adult hemoglobin is very significant. Hb F has a higher affinity for oxygen than does Hb A. Thus in the placenta, oxygen is released from the maternal Hb A, diffuses into the chorionic villi, and binds to the fetal Hb F. In addition, 2,3-diphosphoglycerate (2,3-DPG) does not bind Hb F and therefore does not affect its affinity for oxygen.

■ MATERNAL AND FETAL HEALTH ASSESSMENT

Individuals who desire optimum health care during pregnancy should consult their physicians before conception. Unfortunately, many conceptions are unexpected—up to 40% of conceptions of married females and higher for unmarried females. The preconception evaluation should include a medical, reproductive, and family history; a physical examination; and laboratory tests. Hematocrit, blood type and Rh factor compatibility, erythrocyte antibody screen, Papanicolaou (Pap) smear, urinalysis, rubella titer, rapid plasma reagin test, gonococcal culture, and hepatitis B surface antigen (HBsAg) tests all are indicated. In addition, patients should be offered a human immunodeficiency virus (HIV) antibody test and an illicit drug screen. Depending on demographic risk factors, genetic testing for disorders such as Tay-Sachs disease, thalassemia, and sickle cell disease may be offered. A careful diet history is warranted. Folic acid supplementation should be recommended to reduce the risk of neural tube defects.[20]

Most individuals consult a physician a few days after a missed menses if they suspect they might be pregnant. Many laboratory tests are useful in the management of normal and abnormal pregnancies. A pregnancy test result is positive (meaning the test can detect a CG concentration of about 25 IU/mL) in about half of pregnant females at the beginning of the missed menses—at about 4 weeks of pregnancy and 2 weeks after conception. Screening for fetal neural tube defects and Down syndrome should be offered to all pregnant patients at 16 to 18 weeks of gestation. Glucose tolerance testing should be performed at 24 to 28 weeks. Some physicians screen patients for preterm labor risk at 24 to 30 weeks. Although PL and estriol measurements were previously used to predict fetal well-being, both tests

are now obsolete for this purpose.[6] Maternal observation and recording of fetal movements, ultrasound examination, and tests that monitor the fetal heart rate during random uterine contractions or fetal movement are the currently accepted methods for monitoring of fetal well-being.

Clinical Specimens

Many different samples are available for clinical laboratory analysis before and during pregnancy. Samples include paternal serum and blood; maternal serum, blood, and urine; amniotic fluid; chorionic villi; and fetal blood and tissue.

Amniotic fluid

Amniotic fluid provides a medium in which a fetus can readily move. It cushions the fetus against possible injury and helps maintain a constant temperature.

Volume and dynamics

The volume of amniotic fluid is 200 to 300 mL at 16 weeks, 400 to 1400 mL at 26 weeks, 300 to 2000 mL at 34 weeks, and 300 to 1400 mL at 40 weeks. Amniotic fluid volume is quickly increased by fetal urination. Slower decreases in volume occur during periods of fetal swallowing, an activity the fetus begins at the end of the first trimester. When the fetus breathes amniotic fluid, the amount "exhaled" is slightly greater than that "inhaled," which moves lung surfactant into the amniotic fluid. Pathological alterations in fluid volume are encountered fairly frequently in clinical practice. Intrauterine growth retardation and anomalies of the fetal urinary tract, such as absence of the kidneys or obstruction of the urine outflow tracts, are associated with *oligohydramnios,* an abnormally low amniotic fluid volume. Increased fluid volume is known as *hydramnios* (or *polyhydramnios*). Conditions associated with hydramnios are maternal diabetes mellitus, severe Rh isoimmune disease, fetal esophageal atresia, multifetal pregnancy, anencephaly, and **spina bifida.**

Composition

Early in gestation the composition of the amniotic fluid resembles a complex dialysate of the maternal serum. As a fetus grows, the amniotic fluid changes in several ways (Table 43-3). Most notably, the sodium concentration and osmolality decrease, and the concentrations of urea, creatinine, and uric acid increase because the fetal kidney begins to be able to produce dilute urine. The major lipids are the phospholipids, whose type and concentrations reflect fetal lung maturity. Numerous steroid and protein hormones are also present in amniotic fluid. Levels of androgens and estrogens have been measured in attempts to predict fetal sex. However, the reference intervals of normal for each group of hormones overlap, and such determinations have not been useful. The rare syndrome congenital adrenal hyperplasia (CAH) has been diagnosed antenatally by measurement of

tional age differs from the pretest estimate by 10 days or more, the screen should be reinterpreted. If the reinterpretation is normal, no further testing is indicated.

Any patient who has had a child with a neural tube defect has a 2% risk of having another. In a subsequent pregnancy, these patients should skip the serum screening, have an ultrasound, and if deemed necessary, obtain a direct prenatal diagnosis with amniotic fluid testing.

Screening with the triple test identifies about 8% of patients at increased risk for neural tube defects (3%) or Down syndrome (5%), whereas it detects approximately 90% of actual cases of neural tube defects and approximately 60% of cases of Down syndrome, as well as many other significant conditions. Thus the screening process concentrates many affected cases into a smaller group of mothers. An abnormal screen is never used for a diagnosis but instead indicates the need for a more extensive medical evaluation. The patients with increased risk can undergo more expensive and definitive testing. When a fetal anomaly is diagnosed, the most significant decision facing a patient is whether to elect abortion. For the mothers who are philosophically opposed to abortion, the knowledge that a birth defect is present can aid in pregnancy and delivery management. For example, some investigators have reported that a cesarean section before labor reduces the residual motor impairment in infants with spina bifida.

Analytes used for maternal serum screening

The triple test for Down syndrome includes measurement of AFP, CG, and uE_3 concentrations in maternal serum. All are measured in a single specimen collected (ideally) between 16 and 18 weeks. The results are analyzed through the assumption that the frequency distribution curves are log-gaussian, the means, standard deviations, and prior probability for each condition is known. During the analysis the result of each test interacts with the others, providing slightly less information than if each was performed independently. One prospective study[12] reported the benefits of using the triple test in the prenatal care of more than 25,000 females. The authors used a risk of 1 in 190 or higher for Down syndrome to define an abnormal screen. Initially, 6.6% of the screens were classified as abnormal, but ultrasound examination reduced the percentage to 3.8%. Twenty-one cases of Down syndrome were found in this final group. From the spectrum of maternal ages of the women in the entire study group, 36 cases of Down syndrome were expected. Thus the detection rate was estimated to be 58%.

Laboratories performing maternal serum screening should enroll in an external proficiency program. Two programs are available in the United States, one from New York and the other conducted jointly by the College of American Pathologists and the Foundation for Blood Research in Scarborough, Maine.

Maternal serum alpha-fetoprotein

Between 16 and 18 weeks gestation the maternal serum AFP concentration rises dramatically. To simplify interpretation of the test results, each patient's AFP result is expressed as a multiple of the median (MoM). A patient's AFP concentration in nanograms per milliliter is divided by the median value appropriate for the patient's gestational age. Adjustments to the AFP MoM are made as needed for maternal weight, maternal race, number of fetuses, and the presence of type 1 diabetes.[1]

Screening programs should determine the AFP medians for each week of pregnancy by use of at least 100 patients at each week. By convention, the number of completed weeks is used; thus a patient who is at 16 weeks 6 days of gestation is included in the 16-weeks group. A method used to determine the medians is described in an expanded version of this chapter (p 1746).[1] Typical medians are shown in Figure 43-4. Screening programs should reevaluate the AFP medians at least annually and whenever the methodology changes.

Although many programs report AFP MoM values to the nearest 0.01, this practice overstates the precision of available AFP assays. Although the medians are quite precise, an individual patient's AFP result has a CV of about ±8%; thus rounding the AFP MoM to 0.1 is more appropriate.

Maternal serum chorionic gonadotropin

The maternal serum CG concentration is an average of 2.04 times higher when fetal Down syndrome is present.[28] Like AFP, maternal serum CG should be reported in conventional units (international units per liter) and in multiples of the median to simplify interpretation. Typically, CG is 20,000 to 40,000 IU/L at this time in pregnancy (see Figure 43-6). The CG MoM is calculated by division of a patient's result by the appropriate median established by the screening program (similar to AFP median programs). Adjustments for maternal weight, multiple fetuses, diabetes, and race should be made.[1] Reporting the CG MoM to the nearest 0.1 is appropriate. As with AFP, the CG medians should be reevaluated annually or whenever the methodology changes.

Maternal serum unconjugated estriol

The maternal serum uE_3 level is an average of 0.72 times lower when fetal Down syndrome is present.[5] Like AFP and CG, maternal serum uE_3 should be reported in conventional units (micrograms per liter) and in multiples of the median to simplify interpretation. Typically, uE_3 is 0.30 to 1.50 μg/L 16 weeks into the pregnancy (see Figure 43-3). Most uE_3 assays are designed to measure from 0 to 20 μg/L. A patient's uE_3 result should be reported to no more than the hundredths place. The uE_3 MoM is calculated by division of a patient's result by the appropriate median established by the screening program (similar to AFP median programs).

Adjustments for maternal weight and multiple fetuses should be made.[1] As with AFP and CG, the uE_3 medians should be reevaluated annually or whenever the methodology changes.

Other markers and combinations of markers

Many other maternal serum markers have been reported to show altered results in association with Down syndrome, including free $CG\beta$, free α subunit, β_1-glycoprotein, dimeric inhibin A, pregnancy-associated protein A (PAP A), and urinary gonadotropin peptide (UGP). Many patients would welcome a first trimester screening test for Down syndrome. A large prospective study[13] started in 1996 reported that CG and PAP A could be feasibly used in the first trimester to screen for Down syndrome; AFP and uE_3 were not useful in early pregnancy. A 1999 report found that urinary hyperglycosylated CG during the second trimester is an excellent predictor of fetal Down syndrome.[16] Both studies used mothers who were primarily more than 35 years of age, thus the results need to be confirmed in a prospective study involving younger mothers.

Risk calculation and results reporting

The maternal serum screening report should contain the following information: the concentration of the measured analytes, an interpretation of "abnormal" or "normal," estimates of risk of disease(s) if the screen is abnormal or if the estimates are requested by the physician, and information provided to the laboratory that affects the interpretation. The physician-provided information should include the first or second specimen, dating by menses or ultrasonography, maternal birth date and age, relevant family history, number of fetuses (if known), and the existence of maternal diabetes requiring insulin therapy. For mothers less than 35 years old, the report should unambiguously state whether the screen is normal and no further evaluation is needed, or the screen is abnormal, requiring a discussion with the mother to determine the extent of further evaluations.

Risk for neural tube defects

The calculation of risk for neural tube defect is based on a patient's a priori risk (before testing), gestational age, and AFP MoM.[27] The distribution of AFP MoM is assumed to be log-gaussian for normal and affected pregnancies. A detailed method used to calculate the risk can be found in an expanded version of this chapter (pp 1748 to 1749).[1]

The risk for neural tube defects is best expressed as a ratio in the laboratory report; for example, a risk of anencephaly of 0.012 should be reported as 1 in 80. The risks are approximate. No more than two significant figures should be used in the laboratory report. In addition to neural tube defects, AFP elevations can be a result of underestimated gestational age (18%), fetal demise (2.5%), and abdominal wall defects (1%).[2] Each screening program should monitor the percentage of high AFP results monthly. Using an AFP MoM cutoff of 2.5 should generate about 3% abnormally high screens.

Down syndrome risk calculation with the triple test

The risk of Down syndrome can be estimated from a patient's a priori risk, which is established from her age, and the results of the maternal serum screening triple test. The results of the tests are expressed in MoM. The distributions of the three markers are assumed to fit a trivariate log-gaussian distribution for normal and affected pregnan-

| TABLE 43-4 | Risk of Down Syndrome and Other Chromosome Disorders in the Second Trimester Based on Maternal Age at Term* |

Maternal Age (y)	Risk of Down Syndrome	Risk of Other Chromosome Disorders
≤15	1 in 720	1 in 680
16	1 in 800	1 in 680
17	1 in 900	1 in 680
18	1 in 1030	1 in 680
19	1 in 1200	1 in 680
20	1 in 1200	1 in 620
21	1 in 1200	1 in 620
22	1 in 1030	1 in 620
23	1 in 1030	1 in 620
24	1 in 900	1 in 570
25	1 in 900	1 in 570
26	1 in 850	1 in 610
27	1 in 800	1 in 610
28	1 in 760	1 in 580
29	1 in 720	1 in 580
30	1 in 690	1 in 580
31	1 in 650	1 in 580
32	1 in 550	1 in 580
33	1 in 440	1 in 370
34	1 in 360	1 in 330
35	1 in 280	1 in 270
36	1 in 210	1 in 230
37	1 in 160	1 in 190
38	1 in 130	1 in 170
39	1 in 100	1 in 140
40	1 in 75	1 in 120
41	1 in 60	1 in 100
42	1 in 45	1 in 80
43	1 in 35	1 in 65
44	1 in 30	1 in 55
45	1 in 21	1 in 45
46	1 in 17	1 in 35
47	1 in 13	1 in 30
48	1 in 10	1 in 24
49	1 in 8	1 in 20

From Hook EB: Rates of chromosome abnormalities at different maternal ages. Obstet Gynecol 1981; 58:282-285; and Hook EB, Cross PK, Schreinemachers DM: Chromosomal abnormality rates at amniocentesis and in live-born infants. JAMA 1983; 249:2034-2038.
*Risks are based on live-birth estimates adjusted for fetal survival. Maternal age is the age of the mother at the expected time of delivery.

TABLE 43-5 Conditions Associated with Abnormal Maternal Serum Screening Results

Condition	AFP	CG	uE₃
Amniocentesis (shortly after)	H	N	N
Anencephaly	H	N	L
Down syndrome	L	H	L
Encephalocele	H	N	N
Esophageal atresia	H	N	N
Fetal blood contamination	H	N	N
Fetal demise	L or H	L	L
Molar pregnancy	U	H	L
Molar pregnancy (partial)	L to N	H	L to N
Normal pregnancy	L, N, or H	L, N, or H	L, N, or H
Open spina bifida	H	N	N
Overestimated gestational age	L	H	L
Preeclampsia	N	H	N
Pseudocyesis (imaginary pregnancy)	U	U	U
Rh isoimmune disease	H	N	N
Spontaneous or impending abortion	H or L	L	L
Sulfatase deficiency (fetal)	N	N	L
Trisomy 18 (Edward syndrome)	L	L	L
Twins and other multiple gestations	H	H	H
Underestimated gestational age	H	L	H

AFP, α-Fetoprotein; CG, chorionic gonadotropin; uE₃, unconjugated estriol; N, not changed (from normal); H, high (>1 MoM); L, low (<1 MoM); U, undetectable.

cies. A detailed method used to calculate the risk can be found in an expanded version of this chapter (pp 1749 to 1752).[1] The age-based midtrimester risks for Down syndrome are listed in Table 43-4.

As is the risk for neural tube defects, the risk for Down syndrome is approximate and should be reported to no more than two significant figures. The definition of normal is a decision each program must address. Although midtrimester risks between 1 in 270 and 1 in 190 are commonly used as cutoffs, programs should use 1 in 190 when the triple test is ordered.[12] The use of 1 in 270 results in an initial positive screening rate of up to 9%. Using 1 in 190 produces a rate of 5% to 6% with a detection rate of approximately 60%. The initial positive rates are typical when women who are less than 35 years of age are screened. The maternal age distribution of the population being screened affects the initial positive rate because maternal age strongly affects the estimated risk.

Causes of an abnormal screen other than Down syndrome are listed in Table 43-5 with the pattern of results typically seen. Besides Down syndrome, high CG levels (>2 MoM) are noted in cases of molar pregnancy (hydatidiform mole), preeclampsia, and multiple fetuses. Very low uE₃ val-

ues (~0.1 MoM) are a result of fetal death, overestimated gestational age, anencephaly, nonpregnancy, chromosome abnormalities, and sulfatase deficiency. If all results are low results, the risk of trisomy 18 is increased.

Additional testing after abnormal screening tests

Patients with abnormal results on the maternal serum screening test should be evaluated by ultrasonography, which usually explains about half of the abnormalities. The most frequent findings are incorrect gestational age, twins, and fetal demise. Often, serious disorders such as anencephaly, moderate to large spina bifida, and gastroschisis are readily apparent. Mothers who have unexplained abnormalities should be offered prenatal diagnosis,[7] including amniocentesis to obtain amniotic fluid. If the serum AFP level is high, the amniotic fluid AFP concentration, acetylcholinesterase (AChE), fetal hemoglobin, and fetal karyotype should be determined. If the patient had an abnormal risk for Down syndrome, testing for just AFP and fetal karyotype is appropriate. The benefits of accurate diagnosis of a neural tube defect or chromosome abnormality early in gestation must be weighed against the potential of harming a normal fetus during amniocentesis. This invasive procedure carries a small but real risk of harming the fetus or causing spontaneous abortion. Even amniocentesis performed by an experienced obstetrician using ultrasonography for guidance has a fetal loss rate of about 1 in 200.[25] One in 100 patients with an unexplained high AFP level has a fetus with a chromosome abnormality; thus fetal karyotyping is reasonable in these cases.

Amniotic fluid alpha-fetoprotein

Testing amniotic fluid for AFP levels can predict open neural tube defects more accurately than maternal serum screening. Patients with unexplained high maternal serum AFP levels and normal ultrasonography findings should be offered amniotic fluid testing.

Amniotic fluid AFP has been measured as early as 8 weeks gestation; the concentration at this gestational age is very high. The concentration rapidly decreases to a lower point at 11 weeks, then increases to reach a second maximum at 13 weeks (see Figure 43-4). The concentration then falls in a log-linear fashion until 25 weeks, when the decline gets steeper. The complex pattern before 14 weeks suggests that amniotic fluid AFP cannot be used in the diagnosis of neural tube defects in early pregnancy.

Laboratories that measure amniotic fluid AFP (AF-AFP) should establish medians for each week between 14 and 25 weeks gestation. Medians from a laboratory are shown in Figure 43-4. AF-AFP concentration is much more powerful for diagnosis of neural tube defects than is maternal serum AFP concentration. The median AF-AFP is approximately 7 MoM for open spina bifida and approximately 20 MoM for anencephaly. A frequent confounding interference is contamination of the fluid with fetal blood.

Elevated AF-AFP levels should be tested for Hb F, a sensitive marker of fetal blood contamination.

Acetylcholinesterase

A useful adjunct in the diagnosis of neural tube defects is the measurement of AChE (EC 3.1.1.7) in amniotic fluid. Some laboratories test both AF-AFP and AChE levels whenever amniotic fluid is collected in the second trimester. The usual technique for identification of AChE is polyacrylamide gel electrophoresis. After separation a specific AChE inhibitor, 1,5-bis(4-allyldimethylammoniumphenyl) pentan-3-one dibromide (BW284C51), is used to distinguish this isoenzyme from other cholinesterases. Amniotic fluid from individuals with normal pregnancies contains a single cholinesterase, which migrates relatively slowly in an electric field. Mothers who have pregnancies in which the fetus has an open neural tube defect and abdominal wall defect have a second cholinesterase, AChE, which migrates more rapidly. AChE appears to be relatively specific for neural tissue but is found in fetal blood, so the presence of fetal erythrocytes in the specimen invalidates the results. Detection of AChE by electrophoresis has a specificity of 99.76% and the following sensitivities: for anencephaly, 97%; for open spina bifida, 99%; and for abdominal wall defects, 94%.

▮ COMPLICATIONS OF PREGNANCY

Although most pregnancies progress without problems, complications are not uncommon. The primary cause of complications can arise in the mother, placenta, or fetus.

Abnormal Pregnancies

Conditions arising primarily in the mother include ectopic pregnancy, hyperemesis gravidarum, preeclampsia, HELLP syndrome, liver diseases, Graves' disease, and isoimmunization disease. The clinician must distinguish abnormal changes in laboratory tests from the normal physiological changes induced by pregnancy (see Table 43-2). Notably, total bilirubin, 5′-nucleotidase, γ-glutamyltransferase (GGT), alanine aminotransferase (ALT), and aspartate aminotransferase (AST) are unchanged in mothers with a normal pregnancy.

Ectopic pregnancy and threatened abortion

When a fertilized egg implants in a location other than the body of the uterus, the condition is called an **ectopic pregnancy.** Most abnormal implantations occur in the fallopian tube, but they can also occur in the abdomen, although it is rare. Tubal rupture and hemorrhage are common serious complications of ectopic pregnancy. About 25% of individuals with an ectopic pregnancy have three classic symptoms: lower abdominal pain, vaginal bleeding, and an adnexal mass. Of all individuals with these symptoms, about 15%

have an ectopic pregnancy and a smaller percentage have had an incomplete or a complete spontaneous abortion. About 2% of all pregnancies are ectopic, and complications from this condition cause approximately 13% of maternal deaths. Management of ectopic pregnancy can be surgical (by laparoscopy) or medical (with intramuscular administration of methotrexate). Early detection and proper management of an ectopic pregnancy are the most effective means to decrease maternal morbidity and mortality.

Ultrasound examination and quantitative measurements of serum CG levels can be useful in identification of patients with ectopic pregnancies or who are at risk for abortion. These conditions frequently produce abnormal CG concentrations and slow rates of increase. In addition, progesterone measurements can be helpful either individually or in combination with CG. Kadar and colleagues reported in 1981 that ultrasonography should detect a gestational sac in the uterus of all patients having CG concentrations greater than 6500 IU/L based on the second internal standard. They called this threshold the "discriminatory zone." The threshold has now decreased because of improvements in ultrasonographic resolution. The current cutoff concentration is 3000 IU/L based on the third internal standard.[15] However, a recent report concludes that the CG concentration should not be used to predict the presence of a gestational sac if the gestational age is known with confidence. The best predictor of the presence of a sac is an accurate gestational age. Failure to detect a gestational sac by sonography 24 days or more after conception is presumptive evidence of an ectopic pregnancy.

Romero and colleagues reported that in 184 patients with ectopic pregnancies, CG levels ranged from 0 to 200,000 IU/L, with a geometric mean of about 1000 IU/L.[22] Concentrations of CG depend on the size and viability of the trophoblastic tissue. In about 1% of patients with an ectopic pregnancy, the CG is undetectable with serum tests capable of measuring concentrations as low as 5 IU/L. To distinguish further between the various possibilities, serial testing of CG may be very helpful. In a normal intrauterine pregnancy a rapid increase in CG occurs. During the second through fifth weeks, the CG concentration doubles in about 1½ days. After 5 weeks of gestation, the doubling time gradually lengthens to 2 to 3 days. Before 7 weeks, calculation of the slope of log(CG) versus time in days is useful in the identification of normal pregnancies. At least two CG determinations should be obtained from specimens collected 1 to 7 days apart. The log-linear slope, $\Delta\log(CG)/\Delta$time (in log[IU/L]/day), is greater than 0.11 in the vast majority of normal pregnancies. In cases of ectopic pregnancies or spontaneous abortions, the slope is usually less than 0.11, and the CG concentrations often decrease.

The serum progesterone concentration is often low in mothers with abnormal pregnancies. In a study of asymptomatic women less than 8 weeks from their last menses, a serum progesterone level of less than 6 ng/mL predicted an abnormal pregnancy outcome with 81% confidence, but the average in nonviable pregnancies was 10 ng/mL. For women with clinical symptoms of an abnormal pregnancy, measurement of both CG and progesterone levels is more predictive of abnormal pregnancy than a single CG measurement. In a large outcome study, 97% of the patients with a CG concentration of less than 3000 IU/L and a progesterone concentration of less than 12.6 ng/mL had an abnormal pregnancy, whereas those with a CG concentration of greater than 3000 IU/L or progesterone concentration of greater than 12.6 ng/mL had a normal pregnancy. Almost all women with progesterone levels greater than 17.5 ng/mL have viable pregnancies and need no additional laboratory tests.

Hyperemesis gravidarum

Nausea and vomiting (morning sickness) complicates up to 70% of pregnancies. Symptoms develop between 4 and 8 weeks gestation and typically lasts 15 weeks. When severe, the condition is called *hyperemesis gravidarum* and can lead to dehydration and malnutrition. Fifty percent of the dehydrated patients have elevated aminotransferase levels up to four times the upper reference limit (URL). Mildly high serum bilirubin levels may develop. However, significant liver disease does not develop, and liver biopsy results are normal. Low–birth-weight babies are common for women who develop hyperemesis gravidarum, especially for women who develop malnutrition.

Preeclampsia

Preeclampsia affects about 5% of pregnancies and is more common among women who are experiencing their first pregnancy. The condition is characterized by hypertension (high blood pressure), proteinuria, and edema, usually late in the second trimester or early in the third trimester. When untreated, preeclampsia can lead to convulsions and is then called **eclampsia,** which is related to abnormal endothelial reactivity that leads to intravascular deposition of fibrin with subsequent organ damage. Most maternal deaths from eclampsia are caused by central nervous system complications, but the liver may also be injured; injury to the liver is ischemic. Modest elevations in ALT and AST occur, typically at 4 to 10 times URL. Hepatic complications including hemorrhage, infarction, and fulminant hepatic failure may occur, necessitating an early delivery.

HELLP syndrome

The HELLP syndrome (*h*emolysis, *e*levated *l*iver enzymes, and *l*ow *p*latelet count in association with preeclampsia) occurs in 0.1% of pregnancies. The most prominent features are thrombocytopenia and disseminated intravascular coagulation (DIC). Most cases occur between the 27th and 36th weeks of pregnancy, but it also may develop after delivery. Women typically have symptoms of epigastric or right upper quadrant pain, malaise, nausea, vomiting, and headache. Jaundice occurs in 5% of patients. Lactate dehy-

drogenase concentrations may be very high, and ALT and AST are usually 2 to 10 times URL. Treatment is delivery of the infant. The postpartum management of the patient may require plasmapheresis or organ transplantation. Recurrence rates are 3% to 27%.

Cholestasis of pregnancy

Cholestasis is a suppression of the flow of bile. It occurs during the third trimester, and although common in Chile (5% of pregnancies) and Sweden (1% of pregnancies), it is less common in the United States. Patients have diffuse itching, and 20% to 60% develop jaundice. The typical signs include pale stools and dark urine. The symptoms last until delivery. Serum bile acid concentrations are markedly increased. Bilirubin levels rarely exceed 5 mg/dL. Alkaline phosphatase levels are typically 2 to 4 times URL. Aminotransferase enzyme concentrations are mildly elevated. The prothrombin time may be slightly increased as a result of vitamin K malabsorption. The condition itself is benign but is associated with an increased risk of prematurity and fetal death. Cholestasis recurs with subsequent pregnancies.

Fatty liver of pregnancy

Fatty liver of pregnancy occurs in 1 in 13,000 pregnancies and is characterized by accumulation of microvesicular fat in the liver. It typically occurs in week 35 or 36 and is manifested clinically by the rapid onset of nausea, vomiting, and right upper quadrant pain. Mild elevations in aminotransferase enzyme concentrations occur, with the AST elevation typically measuring higher than the ALT elevation (but with both less than 6 times URL). The bilirubin concentration is usually greater than 10 mg/dL. Life-threatening hypoglycemia may occur. Hyperuricemia, presumably from tissue destruction and renal failure, is characteristic. Liver histology shows acute fatty infiltration with little necrosis or inflammation. If untreated, fulminant hepatic failure with hepatic encephalopathy ensues. Treatment is immediate termination of the pregnancy, at which time rapid recovery usually occurs. Infant and maternal mortality is approximately 20%. Recurrence in subsequent pregnancies is very rare.

Viral hepatitis infection

Viral hepatitis occurs with the same frequency in pregnancy as would be expected in a comparable age group of nonpregnant women. Women who acquire hepatitis B late in pregnancy or who are chronic carriers are likely to transmit the disease to their babies, especially so if the mother is hepatitis Be antigen (HBeAg) positive (see Chapter 36). The outcome in the infant varies from fulminant hepatitis (rare and usually in infants from antiHBe-positive mothers) to mild hepatitis to chronic hepatitis (the usual outcome in 90% of chronically infected women). All pregnant women should be screened for hepatitis B with HBsAg. If positive, their babies should be immunized with hepatitis B immune globulin (HBIG) and hepatitis B vaccine. Babies born to hepatitis C-positive mothers usually have passively transmitted the antibody for several months, but transmission of active hepatitis is unusual. Because no treatment is known for the newborn, screening for hepatitis C antibody is not recommended.

Neonatal Graves' disease

The fetal thyroid-pituitary axis functions independently from the mother's axis in most cases. However, if the mother has preexisting Graves' disease (see Chapter 40), her autoantibodies can cross the placenta and stimulate the fetal thyroid gland. Thus the fetus can develop hyperthyroidism. Thyroid stimulating immunoglobulin testing is useful for pregnant women with Graves' disease.

Isoimmunization disease

Isoimmunization disease is a fetal hemolytic disorder caused by maternal antibodies directed against antigens on fetal erythrocytes. Commonly used synonyms for this disorder are *Rh isoimmune disease, Rh disease,* or *D isoimmunization.* Any of a large number of erythrocyte surface antigens—Rh C, D, and E; A; B; Kell; Duffy; Kidd; and others—may be responsible for isoimmune hemolysis. When severe, the disorder is called **erythroblastosis fetalis** and is life-threatening to fetuses and newborns. The amount of bilirubin in the amniotic fluid helps determine the severity of the disease. The most common cause of severe disease is sensitization of an RhD-negative woman.

Sensitization, or production of an antibody, may occur in response to any exposure to a foreign antigen. For example, if an RhD-negative woman is inadvertently given a transfusion of D-positive blood, she may respond by producing antibodies. However, with modern transfusion techniques, the source for sensitization in women is more likely to be exposure to D-positive fetal blood during pregnancy. Although the fetal and maternal blood compartments are generally considered separate during normal gestation, small numbers of fetal erythrocytes continuously gain access to the maternal circulation. This antigenic challenge is enough to provoke an antibody response in some women. Substantially larger antigenic exposures may result from the disruptions in the integrity of the fetal compartment that accompany spontaneous or induced abortion, ectopic pregnancy, or delivery of an infant. The larger the fetomaternal hemorrhage, the more likely that the mother will respond to the challenge by developing antibodies.

The central problem is destruction of the fetal erythrocytes, which produces several other problems. Fetal anemia imposes an extra burden on the fetal heart to provide adequate oxygen supply to fetal tissues. Anemia stimulates the fetal marrow and extramedullary erythropoiesis in the liver and spleen to replace the destroyed erythrocytes. Extramedullary erythropoiesis destroys hepatocytes and leads to decreased production of serum albumin and decreased oncotic pressure in the intravascular space. When severe, these changes lead to congestive heart failure and generalized fetal edema, with ascites as well as pleural and pericardial effusions. When the fetal condition has deteriorated to this degree, it is referred to as *hydrops fetalis* and has a grave prognosis. The edema and effusions are readily observable by ultrasonography examination. When these changes are observed and no treatment is given, intrauterine demise occurs in a relatively short time.

Prevention

The best way to manage any disease is to prevent it. Sensitization can be prevented if the potentially stimulating antigens are removed from the circulation before they have the opportunity to reach and stimulate the maternal immune system. A dose of immunoglobulin against RhD (RhoGAM, Ortho-Clinical Diagnostics, Raritan, N.J.) administered intramuscularly to a mother who may have been exposed to D-positive fetal erythrocytes after abortion, fetomaternal hemorrhage, amniocentesis, chorionic villi sampling, or delivery is very effective at preventing sensitization.

To care for sensitized women properly, first they must be identified. Thus a routine step at the first prenatal visit is to determine each patient's blood group and Rh status as well as to screen her serum for erythrocyte antibodies against a standard panel of cells. If an antibody is found, it is identified and titered. If the father possesses the antigen in question and the maternal antibody is of the IgG class and of sufficiently high titer, then a problem may arise for the fetus. Under these circumstances, further prenatal care for this condition is required.

Determination of amniotic fluid bilirubin by ΔA_{450}

The concentration of bilirubin is generally too low (~ 10 to $30\ \mu g/dL$) to be measured by standard photometric techniques, but the determination can be done rapidly, accurately, and directly by absorption spectrophotometry. The sample is centrifuged to remove debris. The absorption is determined from 350 to 550 nm. The maximal absorbance of bilirubin is at 450 nm. In the absence of significant amounts of bilirubin, the absorbance spectrum for the amniotic fluid between 365 and 550 nm is nearly exponential (Figure 43-7). When plotted on a semilog scale, the degree to which the curve deviates from a straight line at 450 nm is linearly proportional to the concentration of bilirubin in the amniotic fluid. This is the change in absorbance at 450 nm (ΔA_{450}), which is still occasionally referred to as ΔOD_{450} in clinical literature. A small amount of bilirubin is normally found in amniotic fluid, and the actual amount changes with gestational age (see Figure 43-7).

Specimen. The amniotic fluid specimen is obtained by amniocentesis, and care should be taken not to contaminate the specimen with blood. Because bilirubin is unstable in light, the specimen should be protected from light during transport to the laboratory and during storage. Most am-

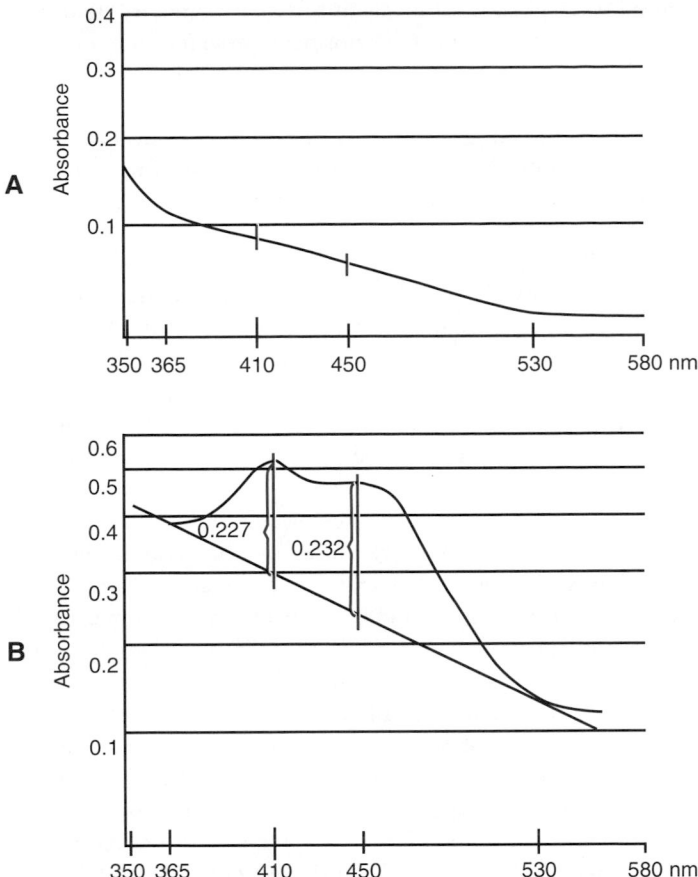

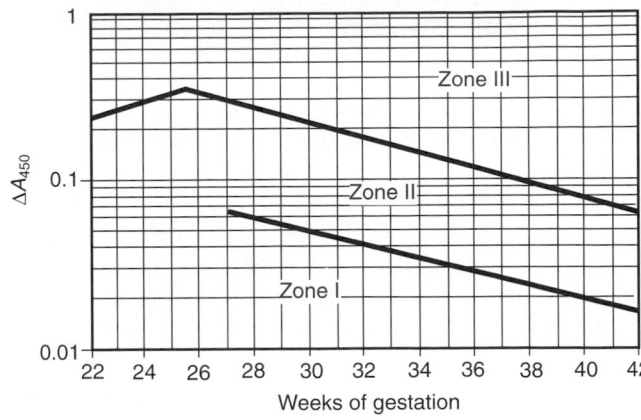

Figure 43-8   Liley's (modified) three-zone chart for interpretation of amniotic fluid change in absorbance at 450 nm (ΔA_{450}). (Modified from Liley AW: Liquor amnii analysis in the management of the pregnancy complicated by rhesus sensitization. Am J Obstet Gynecol 1961; 82:1359-1370.)

Figure 43-7   Absorption spectrophotometry measurement of amniotic fluid. **A,** Normal amniotic fluid. Note that curve is nearly linear when plotted on log-linear graph. **B,** Amniotic fluid showing bilirubin peak at 450 nm and oxyhemoglobin peak at approximately 410 nm. Note baseline drawn between linear parts of curve, from 550 to 365 nm.

niocentesis trays contain a brown plastic tube with a screw top. If a clear tube must be used, it should be wrapped in aluminum foil. Bilirubin's absorbance peak has a half-life of 10 hours in a lighted laboratory and 12 to 18 minutes in winter sunlight. However, bilirubin that is stored in the dark is stable for 30 days at room temperature and for at least 9 months when refrigerated.

Interpretation.   The interpretation of ΔA_{450} depends on knowledge of the gestational age of the pregnancy (Figure 43-8). Values that fall into the bottom zone represent an unaffected or very mildly affected fetus. Values in the middle zone are still representative of a minimally affected fetus, but as values rise within this zone it becomes increasingly likely that the fetus is suffering moderate to marked hemolysis. Depending on the trend and the clinical circumstances, some clinicians recommend intervention when ΔA_{450} has climbed 85% in the middle zone. Values in the top zone (zone III) denote severe disease. Without intervention, a fetus with values in the top zone is likely to die.

Contamination of amniotic fluid with blood should be obvious from the red color and the presence of erythrocytes in the button after centrifugation. When a blood-contaminated specimen is obtained, an important step is to minimize hemolysis of the erythrocytes. Therefore a bloody sample should be refrigerated immediately and processed as soon as possible. Contamination of an amniotic fluid specimen with fetal blood from an affected fetus with a high serum bilirubin level could introduce a substantial error. When a bloody specimen is obtained, a Kleihauer-Betke test should be performed on the erythrocytes to establish their origin. If the erythrocytes are found to be mostly fetal, this should be a factor during interpretation of the fluid results. If the amniotic fluid remaining within the amniotic cavity has been contaminated with blood by traumatic amniocentesis, these erythrocytes lyse and contaminate the fluid with hemoglobin and bilirubinoid pigments. It takes 2 to 3 weeks for these pigments to be cleared and for the fluid to return to the original state.

Occasionally, during monitoring of a sensitized pregnancy, delivery seems imminent and a large dose of glucocorticoids is administered to stimulate fetal lung maturation. If the patient has not delivered and amniocentesis is repeated within 2 to 4 days of the steroid course, the ΔA_{450} is lowered relative to the level found immediately before the steroid administration. Further observation and amniocenteses should show that the ΔA_{450} returns to the previous level or higher within a week. It seems doubtful that this phenomenon represents a decrease in hemolysis; instead, it may be an artifact, possibly from, acute changes in amniotic fluid volume.

Meconium staining of amniotic fluid causes a substantial rise in the ΔA_{450} with a broad and variable peak at 400 to 415 nm. There is no way to compensate quantitatively for meconium contamination. A single episode of meconium passage into the amniotic fluid requires about 3 weeks to clear.

Abnormalities of the Placenta (Trophoblastic Disease)

During some pregnancies the trophoblasts of the placenta proliferate abnormally, leading to molar pregnancy and in rare cases, choriocarcinoma. A molar pregnancy, also called a *hydatidiform mole*, appears grossly as a mass of cysts resembling a bunch of grapes. Microscopically, the epithelial layer of the chorionic villi proliferates, causing the villi to form avascular cysts. If fetal tissue is absent, the mole is called *complete*. The karyotype of the tissue is usually 46 XX, and all chromosomes are from the father. When fetal tissue is present, the mole is *partial*. The molar karyotype is either 69 XXY or 69 XYY, with two of the haploid chromosome sets coming from the father. About 5% of partial moles transform to choriocarcinoma, whereas 20% of complete moles transform. Very high maternal serum CG concentrations can develop in a molar pregnancy. Occasionally the mother becomes hyperthyroid because CG has a slight TSH-like activity. Patients often develop preeclampsia. Molar pregnancies have characteristic ultrasound findings.

Treatment consists of immediate evacuation of the mole by vacuum aspiration. Serum CG measurements are performed every 2 weeks until they are below the level of the assay detection (usually 10 weeks). If the decline is too slow or the CG level starts to rise, additional treatment is needed. The CG level should be less than 20,000 IU/L 1 month after aspiration. Treatments include hysterectomy, repeat aspiration, or chemotherapy using methotrexate.

Fetal Anomalies

Many but not all serious birth defects can be detected with screening tests. The major defects that most screening programs are designed to detect are neural tube defects, Down syndrome, and trisomy 18.

Neural tube defects

Neural tube defects occur early in embryonic development and cause very serious birth defects. By 19 days after fertilization, the area that is to form the central nervous system (brain and spinal cord) has differentiated into a plate of cells. The flat plate then rolls up, and its edges fuse into a hollow neural tube that drops into the embryo to develop just underneath what becomes the skin of the back. Neural tube formation is normally complete 4 weeks after fertilization. Failure of neural tube fusion leads to permanent developmental defects of the brain or spinal cord or both. These defects are called *anencephaly*, *meningomyelocele* (which is commonly called *spina bifida*), and *encephalocele*. Although many heterogeneous causes are known, about 90% fall into the classification of multifactorial inheritance. Folic acid deficiency is clearly related to neural tube closure defects.[20]

The incidence at birth of anencephaly and meningomyelocele is about 1 in 1800 for each. Almost all cases of anencephaly and about 95% of meningomyeloceles have no overlying skin and are therefore called *open neural tube defects*. In these cases, spinal fluid mixes directly with amniotic fluid. Thus the fetal serum proteins normally present in amniotic fluid at low concentrations are present in large quantities. The elevated amniotic fluid AFP concentration leads to increased amounts in the maternal circulation. About 90% of open neural tube defects can be detected by use of maternal serum AFP testing.[27]

Down syndrome

Down syndrome is the most common serious disorder of the autosomal chromosomes, occurring in 1 in 800 live births. An extra copy of the long arm region q22.1 to q22.3 of chromosome 21 results in a phenotype characterized by mental retardation, hypotonia, congenital heart defects, and flat facial profile. Chromosome 21 is the smallest chromosome, making up about 1.7% of the human genome. Usually an affected child has three copies of chromosome 21 (trisomy 21), but 5% of cases are caused by translocations and 1% of cases are mosaics. Older mothers are at dramatically increased risk for having a child with Down syndrome. At 35 years of age the risk at birth is 1 in 385; at age 40 it is 1 in 105. Most obstetricians offer amniocentesis for fetal karyotype determination to all mothers who will be 35 years or older at the time of birth. This strategy detects about 20% of all fetuses with Down syndrome. Using maternal serum AFP screening increases the detection rate to just 33%. Adding maternal serum CG measurements (with a midtrimester risk cutoff of 1 in 270) improves detection to 53%, and the addition of estriol (with a midtrimester risk cutoff of 1 in 190) improves the detection rate to 58%. Approximately 1 in every 50 mothers with abnormal triple test results have a fetus with Down syndrome.[29]

Trisomy 18

The trisomy 18 chromosome disorder is caused by nondisjunction of chromosome 18 during meiosis. The fetus receives an extra copy of chromosome 18. Although it occurs in only 1 in 8000 births, it is probably the most common chromosome defect at the time of conception. The dramatic change in prevalence is caused by the very high fetal loss rate both before 8 weeks (~80%) and during the second and third trimesters (~70%). Approximately 25% of affected fetuses have spina bifida or another serious structural defect. A high cesarean section rate has been noted in undiagnosed cases. After birth, half of the infants die by age 5 days, and 90% die by age 100 days. Maternal serum screening using the triple test often produces a pattern of low results for AFP, CG, and uE_3 levels. Using an algorithm similar to that used for Down syndrome, 60% of cases can be detected with the triple screen, with only a 0.2% false-positive rate. One fetus is affected for every nine fetuses classified as abnormal.

Preterm Delivery

The leading cause of neonatal morbidity and mortality in the United States is preterm delivery. Infants born before 37 weeks gestation often develop respiratory distress syndrome and usually have a low birth weight (<2500 g); some have a very low birth weight (<1500 g). According to the National Center for Health Statistics, 7.2% of all U.S. live-born infants in 1993 had low birth weights, and 1.3% had very low birth weights. Most premature infants spend time in intensive care units at a cost of up to $3500 per day.

Preterm labor

When labor begins before 37 weeks gestation it is called *preterm labor.* Determining the risk of preterm labor would help clinicians manage high-risk patients more aggressively and thereby lower the incidence of preterm delivery. Measuring fetal fibronectin concentration in cervical and vaginal secretions can aid in the prediction of preterm delivery. The symptoms of preterm labor include regular uterine contractions, low back pain, lower abdominal cramping, and vaginal bleeding and increased discharge.

Fetal fibronectin

Fibronectin is a term for a family of ubiquitous adhesive glycoproteins that cross-link to collagen to bind cells together. These proteins are found on cell surfaces and in plasma and amniotic fluid. A unique fetal fibronectin (fFN) can be measured with a specific monoclonal antibody that recognizes the epitope produced by α-N-acetylgalactosamine linked to threonine in the peptide Val-Thr-His-Pro-Gly-Tyr. When labor begins, the disruption of cell adhesion between the placenta and the uterine wall increases the amount of fFN in cervical and vaginal secretions. After these secretions are collected with a swab, the fFN concentration can be determined by immunoassay. Mothers with greater than 50 ng/mL fFN in their secretions are 27 times more likely to deliver in the next 7 days (20 of 150) than those with less than 50 ng/mL (3 of 613). However, the majority of patients with results that are higher than 50 ng/mL repair any placental disruption and successfully continue the pregnancy.[11]

Respiratory distress syndrome

Respiratory distress syndrome (RDS), also called *hyaline membrane disease,* is the most common critical problem encountered in clinical management of preterm newborns. The worldwide incidence of RDS is 1% of live births and 10% to 15% of live preterm births (<37 weeks or <2500 g). In the United States, 300,000 to 500,000 preterm deliveries occur each year. In 1994, RDS killed more than 1500 infants in the United States. Affected infants require supplemental oxygen and mechanical ventilation to remain properly oxygenated. The disorder is caused by a deficiency of pulmonary surfactant (see the previous section on functional development of the fetus). In normal lungs, surfactant coats the alveolar epithelium and responds to alveolar volume changes by reducing the surface tension in the alveolar wall during expiration. When the quantity of surfactant is deficient, many of the alveoli collapse during the expiration and thereby overinflate the remaining airways. Blood flowing through the capillary beds of collapsed alveoli fails to oxygenate properly. During the first few hours of life, affected infants develop tachypnea with or without cyanosis, nasal flaring, expiratory grunting, and intercostal retractions. The disease exacerbates during the next few days and is usually worse on the third or fourth day of life. Infants at risk for development of RDS can be treated with intratracheal administration of exogenous surfactant immediately at birth.

Fetal lung maturity tests help a clinician decide whether the best perinatal survival will be achieved in utero or in the nursery. The most common situation in which a fetal lung maturity test is ordered is before a repeat cesarean delivery when the age of gestation is somewhat uncertain. Another major indication is anticipated early delivery because of some medical or obstetrical factor, such as preterm labor, premature rupture of the membranes, worsening maternal hypertension, severe renal disease, intrauterine growth retardation, or fetal distress. Results indicating immaturity of the fetal lungs might cause postponement of elective delivery or prompt active intervention with tocolytics to suppress preterm labor. Administration of corticosteroids before birth accelerates pulmonary maturation and can prevent RDS. If delivery of an infant is inevitable, transfer to a tertiary health care center is appropriate.

Tests used to evaluate fetal lung maturity

Numerous tests of amniotic fluid have been proposed to measure fetal lung maturity. Some of these, such as creatinine, urea, or the lipid-staining characteristics of cells, correlate with gestational age but do not predict lung maturation. Tests that measure lamellar bodies directly or indirectly, the surfactant contained in lamellar bodies, or the biophysical property of surfactant are the most useful in the evaluation of fetal lung maturity. Surfactant/albumin ratio by fluorescence polarization, PG, lecithin/sphingomyelin (L/S) ratio, foam stability, and lamellar body counts are methods used to measure pulmonary surfactant.

Other surfactant-based tests include those that measure turbidity at either 400 nm or 650 nm. These tests measure the light-scattering effect of lamellar bodies suspended in the amniotic fluid. An absorbance greater than 0.15 at 650 nm is claimed to indicate lung maturity. Unfortunately, the absorbance of amniotic fluid is affected not only by light scattering but also by substances that absorb light.

Hospital laboratories should offer a rapid test, such as fluorescence polarization, lamellar body counts, or PG.[9] The tests should be available daily on a routine and an emergency basis. Requests for an L/S ratio can be sent to a reference laboratory. Analysts should communicate the results of any fetal lung maturity test immediately to the ordering location, because the patient's status may change, and the information might assist with management of labor.

Processing of amniotic fluid before testing

Standards of laboratory practice for fetal lung maturity testing[3] that make several recommendations regarding specimen collection, handling, centrifugation, and mixing have been published. Amniotic fluid is obtained by amniocentesis and although not optimal, from vaginal pools. Whenever possible the fluid should be tested immediately. If a delay of a few hours is unavoidable, the fluid should be refrigerated at 4 °C. The total phospholipid content of amniotic fluid does not change significantly during at least a week of storage. If testing is going to be delayed longer than 1 week (for example, of fluids kept for research studies), fluids should be stored frozen at −20 or −70 °C. Immediately before testing the fluid, it should be gently inverted several times to obtain a uniform suspension. In practice, at least 2 minutes on a test tube rocker is recommended.

Most procedures used to measure fetal lung maturity include a centrifugation step to remove debris from the amniotic fluid. Careful attention to technique is needed to obtain reproducible results. Any centrifugation removes pulmonary surfactant from the specimen. Accidentally prolonged centrifugation can reduce recovery of the phospholipids to less than 50%. For best results, the specimen should be well-mixed, lightly centrifuged for 2 minutes at 400 ×g, decanted, and mixed again. Always note the condition of the specimen: uncontaminated, bloody, meconium stained (green tinged), xanthochromic (yellow tinged), or obviously contaminated with mucus. Keep the specimen on wet ice.

Surfactant/albumin ratio by fluorescence polarization assay

The technique of fluorescence polarization is now the most commonly used quantitative method for fetal lung maturity.[23,26] This rapid test has better precision than the L/S ratio and is equivalent for the prediction of RDS. Initially diphenylhexatriene was used as the fluorescent dye. The technique later was improved with the use of a more stable fluorescent dye, NBD-phosphatidylcholine (NBD-PC), and a commercial polarimeter, the Abbott TDx. A commercial version, (TDX FLM) was developed that used a slightly different dye, PC-16. The results of the two assays have a strong nonlinear, inverse correlation.

Fluorescence polarization is a dimensionless ratio with values from 0.000 to 0.500 (also denoted as 0 to 500 mP) for dilute solutions containing fluorescing compounds (see Chapter 4). Polarization measures the rotational diffusion of the fluorophore relative to its fluorescent half-life. If the half-life is short compared with the rate of rotational diffusion, polarization is high. In contrast, if the molecular rotation is faster than the excited state decay, then polarization is low. PC-16, the commercial dye (or NBD-PC, the non-commercial dye) binds to albumin, which has a high polarization, and to surfactant, which has a low polarization. The resulting polarization is a function of the surfactant/albumin ratio.

The commercial version is calibrated to solutions containing phospholipid and albumin. The units are milligrams of surfactant per gram of albumin. The vast majority of laboratories performing fluorescence polarization testing for fetal lung maturity use the commercial version of the assay. Some laboratories use the NBD-PC method but must prepare the reagents and perform the calculations required for interpretation.

Interpretation. The commercial version of this test, TDx FLM II (Abbott Laboratories, North Chicago, Ill), produces results that vary from 0 to 160 mg/g. Precision is excellent, varying from 4% to 5% CV at 20 and 115 mg/g. Although the manufacturer-sponsored multicenter prospective evaluation[23] recommends a maturity cutoff of greater than 50 mg/g, the kit instructions recommend greater than 70 mg/g. Several studies have confirmed that 50 mg/g has better predictive value for high-risk pregnancies. The more conservative cutoff of 70 mg/g is appropriate for patients who need a cesarean delivery at term, but use of 50 mg/g is better for high-risk pregnancies.

An NBD-PC fluorescence polarization value of less than 260 mP is considered to reflect mature lungs, values between 260 and 290 mP are considered transitional, and values greater than 290 reflect immaturity. Using 260 mP as the cutoff, this test has a clinical sensitivity of 94% and a clinical specificity of 84%. The supplemental use of the L/S ratio for those patients with transitional results is of little benefit. The 260 mP cutoff is appropriate for high-risk pregnancies. For a patient who needs a cesarean section at term and will not be harmed by a delay in delivery, a cutoff of 230 mP is more appropriate.

Fluorescence polarization is unaffected if less than 0.5% blood is in the amniotic fluid. Contamination with more than this tends to increase low results and decrease high results. Clearly mature (>70 mg/g or <230 mP) and immature (<30 mg/g or >290 mP) results from bloody specimens are reliable in the prediction of fetal lung status. Results from bloody specimens between these values cannot be interpreted. Maternal diabetes mellitus does not affect the medical decision limit of the commercial assay and probably does not affect the NBD-PC assay.[18]

Phosphatidylglycerol

Determination of the presence of PG is the most commonly used qualitative method used to assess fetal lung maturity. Measurement of PG was classically performed by thin-layer chromatography. It could be performed alone or in combination with other amniotic fluid phospholipids. The later test was known as a *lung profile* and was invented by Marie Kulovich and Louis Gluck in the early 1970s.[17] Although thin-layer chromatography is still offered by some reference and hospital laboratories, most hospital laboratories use a rapid slide method for the qualitative PG detection. Several enzymatic-based tests for quantitative PG have also been published, but none are widely used.

The exact role of PG in lung surfactant is unclear. Many claim that the appearance of PG in the amniotic fluid indicates the final biochemical maturation of surfactant. However, PG can be found in measurable quantities in amniotic fluid as early as 32 weeks, and its presence in small quantities does not necessarily imply that the fetal lungs are mature. The concentration of PG in amniotic fluid increases with gestational age. Most thin-layer chromatography techniques are positive when PG exceeds about 2 μmol/L. Using this level, results indicating maturity are almost always correct, but results indicating immaturity are frequently wrong.

A qualitative rapid agglutination test (AmnioStat) for PG uses less than 0.5 mL of amniotic fluid. The sample is mixed on a slide with reagents containing particles coated with a substance that binds to PG. Agglutination occurs in the presence of PG. Results are reported as negative, weakly positive, or positive. RDS rarely develops in an infant from a mother with a positive PG determined by AmnioStat. Unfortunately, more than 50% of mothers with a negative AmnioStat PG also have unaffected infants. The major disadvantage to this test is that negative values convey no information. Immature results from quantitative tests are more useful; for example, a surfactant/albumin ratio of 10 mg/g is significantly different from 45 mg/g. The PG test is very useful in low-risk pregnancies that require cesarean section. Determination of PG is also useful for specimens contaminated with blood or meconium. PG is not found in either blood or meconium, and therefore results are not affected by the presence of either of these contaminants.

Lecithin/sphingomyelin ratio

The major surface-active component of the lung surfactant is phosphatidylcholine, which is also called *lecithin*. Nearly all of the sphingomyelin in amniotic fluid is derived from nonlung sources, thus it has no role in the surfactant system in the lungs. However, it is used as a convenient marker against which lecithin is measured. The concentration of lecithin relative to sphingomyelin, the L/S ratio, tends to rise with increasing gestational age. This is not a uniform gradual increase; a rather sudden increase occurs at 34 to 36 weeks of gestation and correlates with the development of fetal lung maturity.[10]

Although most laboratories use a commercially available thin-layer chromatography method for L/S determination, some continue to use methods developed in their own laboratories (so-called "home brew" methods). Because many techniques exist, laboratories should be very careful when establishing medical decision limits. Some methods measure all phosphatidylcholine species, whether saturated or unsaturated. Not all staining methods detect phosphatidylcholine and sphingomyelin equivalently. Because of the need to contain health care costs, many laboratories have stopped performing L/S ratio testing.

Interpretation. The L/S ratio usually indicates lung maturity if it exceeds 2.0. This test predicts fetal lung maturity more reliably than immaturity. About 2% to 3% of babies delivered within 24 hours of the obtaining of an L/S ratio greater than 2.0 can be expected to develop RDS; thus 97% to 98% of babies predicted to have mature lungs do in fact have mature lungs. However, almost half of the infants with L/S ratios between 1.5 and 2.0 do not develop RDS. Thus in contrast to the high degree of reliability of lung maturity prediction, only half of the babies predicted to have immature lungs do in fact have immature lungs.

Numerous investigators have reported that infants of diabetic mothers more frequently develop RDS despite L/S ratios greater than 2.0. For this reason, many laboratories use a different reference interval for lung maturity for an infant of a diabetic mother; the L/S ratio is typically 3.0. Some researchers have proposed a causal relationship between hyperinsulinemia and delayed lung maturity, whereas others have reported no delay in the lung maturity of infants of diabetic mothers.

Serum has a large concentration of lecithin and sphingomyelin. The ratio varies between 1.5 and 2.0, depending on the individual. The values of blood-contaminated specimens therefore tend to be pushed into that range from either higher or lower values. A high L/S ratio in the presence of even substantial blood contamination can safely be interpreted as indicative of mature lungs. Similarly, contaminated samples with very low ratios clearly represent immature lungs. Borderline values of bloody specimens cannot be interpreted because they may represent either very immature values that are falsely elevated or mature values that are falsely depressed. Various effects of meconium contamination have been reported, but the chromatograms of fluids heavily contaminated with meconium are not interpretable.

L/S ratio methods are not very precise. For example, a proficiency testing survey reported the following results (proficiency test sample number, mean, SD, and CV): LM-09, 4.46, 1.18, 26%; and LM-10, 2.31, 0.62, 27%.

Foam stability index

Many laboratories used a commercial version of the foam stability test[24] called *Lumadex, FSI Fetal Lung Maturity Test* (Beckman Instruments, Fullerton, Calif.), which was introduced in 1982. Beckman Instruments discontinued this test in 1997. Laboratories may want to use the "home-brew" procedure described in an expanded version of this chapter as an alternative.[1]

When pulmonary surfactant is present in amniotic fluid in sufficient concentrations, the fluid is able to form a highly stable surface film that can support bubbles. Other substances in the fluid, including proteins, bile salts, and salts of free fatty acids, are also capable of forming stable bubbles, but they can be removed from the film by ethanol, which competes with the other substrates for a position in the surface film. The test makes use of the principle that more surfactant activity is necessary to support a stable foam as the fraction of ethanol in the mixture is increased. Therefore a fixed volume of undiluted amniotic fluid is mixed with increasing volumes of ethanol, and the largest fraction of ethanol in which the amniotic fluid is still capable of supporting a foam is determined. The highest fraction of ethanol at which a positive reading is obtained is the foam stability index (FSI).

Interpretation.   An FSI value of 0.47 or greater is interpreted as mature. In two studies, a combined total of 270 fetuses with an FSI of 0.47 or greater were reported, two of which developed RDS. In 110 fetuses with an FSI of 0.46 or less, 44 (40%) developed RDS. Thus the test is associated with more false predictions of immaturity than the L/S ratio or surfactant/albumin ratio. Tubes and stoppers must be clean and free of detergents to prevent false-positive readings. The final concentration of the ethanol is critical. Ethanol is hygroscopic; therefore careful attention must be paid its preparation and storage. Specimens contaminated with either blood or meconium tend to give a falsely mature result.

Lamellar body counts

Lamellar body particles[4] can be measured directly with the platelet channel of a standard hematology cell counter.

Many of these surfactant particles are from 2 to 20 fL in volume, an interval that is commonly used to enumerate and size platelets in whole blood specimens. Several investigators have proposed that lamellar body counting be used as a rapid fetal lung maturity test. The new method has been shown to be cost effective and reliable in clinical outcome studies.

A typical day-to-day standard deviation is 3500 counts/μL (5%) at 70,500/μL and 7800 counts/μL (4%) at 209 400/μL. Centrifugation slows the procedure, reduces the counts by 8%, and does not improve the precision of the assay, therefore use of uncentrifuged specimens is recommended. Maturity is indicated by a lamellar body count of at least 55,000/μL in a centrifuged specimen or 60,000/μL in an uncentrifuged specimen. A 3-year prospective study[4] found that all 28 cases of RDS were correctly classified by use of these thresholds. Fifty-five percent of infants who did not develop RDS had results greater than the cutoff.

More than 1% v/v blood can decrease lamellar body count by up to 20%. Meconium-stained fluids and vaginal pool fluids containing obvious mucus can have very high and erroneous counts. These contaminated fluids should not be tested with this method.

References

1. Ashwood ER: Clinical chemistry of pregnancy. In Burtis CA, Ashwood ER (eds): Tietz Textbook of Clinical Chemistry, 3rd edition, pp 1736-1775, Philadelphia, WB Saunders, 1999.

2. Ashwood ER: Evaluating health and maturation of the unborn: the role of the clinical laboratory. Clin Chem 1992; 38:1523-1529.

3. Ashwood ER: Standards of laboratory practice: Evaluation of fetal lung maturity. Clin Chem 1997; 43:1-4.

4. Ashwood ER, Palmer SE, Taylor JS et al: Lamellar body counts for rapid fetal lung maturity testing. Obstet Gynecol 1993; 81:619-624.

5. Canick JA, Knight GJ, Palomaki GE et al: Low second trimester maternal serum unconjugated oestriol in pregnancies with Down's syndrome. Br J Obstet Gynaecol 1988; 95:330-333.

6. Cunningham FG, MacDonald PC, Gant NF: The placental hormones, and techniques to evaluate fetal health. In Cunningham FG (ed): Williams Obstetrics, 18th edition, pp 67-85, 277-305, Norwalk, Conn, Appleton & Lange, 1989.

7. D'Alton ME, DeCherney AH: Prenatal diagnosis. N Engl J Med 1993; 328:114-120.

8. Daviaud J, Fournet D, Ballongue C et al: Reliability and feasibility of pregnancy home-use tests: laboratory validation and diagnostic evaluation by 638 volunteers. Clin Chem 1993; 39:53-59.

9. Dubin SB. Assessment of fetal lung maturity. Practice parameter. Am J Clin Pathol 1998; 110:723-732.

10. Gluck L, Kulovich MV: Lecithin/sphingomyelin ratios in amniotic fluid in normal and abnormal pregnancy. Am J Obstet Gynecol 1973; 115:539-546.

11. Goldenberg RL, Mercer BM, Iams JD et al: The preterm prediction study: patterns of cervicovaginal fetal fibronectin as predictors of spontaneous preterm delivery. Am J Obstet Gynecol 1997; 177:8-12.

12. Haddow JE, Palomaki GE, Knight GJ et al: Prenatal screening for Down's syndrome with use of maternal serum markers. N Engl J Med 1992; 327:588-593.

13. Haddow JE, Palomaki GE, Knight GJ et al: Screening of maternal serum for fetal Down syndrome in the first trimester. N Engl J Med 1998; 388:955-961.

14. Jeng LL, Moore RM Jr, Kaczmarek RG et al: How frequently are home pregnancy tests used? Results from the 1988 National Maternal and Infant Health Survey. Birth 1991; 18:11-13.

15. Kadar N, Bohrer M, Kemmann E et al: The discriminatory human chorionic gonadotropin zone for endovaginal sonography: a prospective, randomized study. Fertil Steril 1994; 61:1016 1020.

16. Kole LA, Shahabi S, Oz UA et al: Hyperglycosylated human chorionic gonadotropin (invasive trophoblast antigen) immunoassay: a new basis for gestational Down syndrome screening. Clin Chem 1999; 45:2109-2119.

17. Kulovich MV, Hallman MB, Gluck L: The lung profile: I. Normal pregnancy. Am J Obstet Gynecol 1979; 135:57-63.

18. Livingston EG, Herbert WN, Hage ML et al: Use of the TDx-FLM assay in evaluating fetal lung maturity in an insulin-dependent diabetic population. The Diabetes and Fetal Maturity Study Group. Obstet Gynecol 1995; 86:826-829.

19. Lockitch G (ed): Handbook of Diagnostic Biochemistry and Hematology in Normal Pregnancy, Boca Raton, Fla, CRC Press, 1993.

20. Milunsky A, Jick H, Jick SS et al: Multivitamin/folic acid supplementation in early pregnancy reduces the prevalence of neural tube defects. JAMA 1989; 262:2847-2852.

21. Phillips OP, Elias S, Shulman LP et al: Maternal serum screening for fetal Down syndrome in women less than 35 years of age using α-fetoprotein, hCG, and unconjugated estriol: a prospective 2-year study. Obstet Gynecol 1992; 80:353-358.

22. Romero R, Kadar N, Copel JA et al.: The effect of different human chorionic gonadotropin assay sensitivity on screening for ectopic pregnancy. Am J Obstet Gynecol 1985; 153:72-74.

23. Russell JC, Cooper CM, Ketchum CH et al: Multicenter evaluation of TDx test for assessing fetal lung maturity. Clin Chem 1989; 35:1005-1010.

24. Sher G, Statland BE, Freer DE: Clinical evaluation of the quantitative foam stability index test. Obstet Gynecol 1980; 55:617-620.

25. Simpson JL: Genetic counseling and prenatal diagnosis. In Gabbe SG, Niebyl JR, Simpson JL (eds): Obstetrics: Normal and Problem Pregnancies, 2nd edition, pp 269-298, New York, Churchill Livingstone, 1996.

26. Tait JF, Franklin RW, Simpson JB et al: Improved fluorescence polarization assay for use in evaluating fetal lung maturity: I. Development of the assay procedure. Clin Chem 1986; 32:248-254.

27. UK Collaborative Study: Maternal serum-alpha-fetoprotein measurement in antenatal screening for anencephaly and spina bifida in early pregnancy: report of UK collaborative study on alpha-fetoprotein in relation to neural-tube defects. Lancet 1977; 1:1323-1332.

28. Wald NJ, Cuckle HS, Densem JW et al: Maternal serum screening for Down syndrome in early pregnancy. Br Med J 1988; 297:883-887.

29. Wald NJ, Densem JW, Smith D et al: Four-marker serum screening for Down syndrome. Prenat Diagn 1994; 14:707-716.

Additional Reading

Jauniaux E, Barnea ER, Edwards R (eds): Embryonic Medicine and Therapy, New York, Oxford University Press, 1997.

Johnson TRB, Blakemore K, Callan N: Clinical Fetal Assessment, Philadelphia, WB Saunders, 1996.

Lockitch G (ed): Handbook of Diagnostic Biochemistry and Hematology in Normal Pregnancy, Boca Raton, Fla, CRC Press, 1997.

Quilligan EJ, Zuspan FP: Current Therapy in Obstetrics and Gynecology, vol 5, WB Saunders, 1999.

CHAPTER 44

Inherited Disease

BARBARA G. BORDER, PhD, MT(ASCP), and JOHN F. O'BRIEN, PhD

Objectives

1. Define the following terms:
   - Acquired disease
   - Inherited disease
   - Autosomal dominant
   - Autosomal recessive
   - X-linked inheritance
   - Trinucleotide repeat
   - Inborn error of metabolism
2. Describe and define three types of genetic disorders.
3. List five inherited diseases and the gene mutation involved in each.
4. State the laboratory procedures utilized to assess inherited disease.

Key Words

Acquired Disease   Disease induced by a somatic cell mutation (sometimes referred to as *spontaneous)* that is passed on to daughter cells but not inherited

Alleles   Alternative form of a gene that can occupy a particular chromosomal locus (or position); *homozygous alleles* refers to a pair of identical alleles at a given locus

Autosomal Dominant Inheritance   A Mendelian inheritance pattern in which traits are inherited vertically from parents to offspring; inheritance pattern in which individuals who do not express the trait cannot have offspring that do express the trait, and individuals who express the trait have a parent with the trait; 50% chance that individuals inheriting the trait will pass the trait to their offspring; affects males and females equally; autosomes carry the mutation

Autosomal Dominant Trait   A phenotypic trait that appears because of the presence of a heterozygous allele; *dominant gene mutation*—causes the individual to gain a new protein function

Autosomal Recessive Inheritance   A Mendelian inheritance pattern in which traits appear horizontally in the pedigree; an inheritance pattern in which affected individuals with a homozygous allele have heterozygous parents, and heterozygous parents have a 25% chance of having a homozygous affected offspring; autosomes carry the mutation

Autosomal Recessive Trait   A phenotypic trait that appears because of the presence of a homozygous allele

Genotype   Individual gene sequences on a chromosome; produce specific proteins when translated

Inherited Disease   Disease induced by a mutation (sometimes referred to as a *de novo* or *germline* mutation) that initially develops in a germline cell (sperm or egg) and is then inherited through Mendelian inheritance patterns

Monogenic Disorder   A disorder caused by a single gene or locus mutation

Phenotype   The physical expression of the genotype or the specific proteins produced from transcription and translation of genes

Polygenic Disorder   A disorder caused by several gene mutations and the interaction of environmental and physiological factors

X-Linked Inheritance   A Mendelian inheritance pattern passed on to offspring through the X chromosome in which traits appear primarily in male offspring of carrier females; inheritance pattern in which affected males have normal male offspring but female offspring who are carriers, with a 25% chance that a female carrier will have either an affected son, an unaffected son, a noncarrier daughter, or a carrier daughter

X-Linked Trait   A trait that is differentially displayed depending on the sex of the affected individual; almost always expressed in males who carry the mutated chromosome

The theory of transmission of units of heredity from generation to generation put forth by Gregor Mendel in the 1850s forms the basic principle of inheritance. Genes (the units of heredity referred to by Mendel) are deoxyribonucleic acid (DNA) sequences that code for protein synthesis (see Chapter 11) and are inherited in pairs like chromosomes, with one coming from each parent. An alteration in the nucleotide bases of a gene is called a *mutation.* Heritable gene mutations that lead to a physiological or biochemical abnormality produce diseases referred to as *Mendelian genetic disorders.* These abnormalities can affect a single organ system or have extensive effects on many tissues.

The causes of gene mutation are numerous. Spontaneous mutations in DNA occur as the result of environmental and physiological interactions. Deamination reactions, hydrolysis, or methylation of nucleotides can chemically alter the base pair sequences in DNA. Alterations of infectious viruses that carry oncogenes can affect tumor induction. Alterations of DNA, whether they occur within an intron or exon (a protein-coding sequence) or affect an entire chromosome, increase the chance of altered protein synthesis. If mutations affect the expressed genes of somatic cells and their daughter cells and cause a physiological disorder, the disorder is called an **acquired disease.** However, if the initial mutation affects a germline cell (a sperm or an ovum), the mutation, referred to as a *de novo* or *germline mutation,* is incorporated into the offspring's genotype and becomes heritable. Germline mutations produce **inherited disease** and are inherited through Mendelian inheritance patterns. Disorders caused by autosomal genetic mutations are inherited as either autosomal dominant or autosomal recessive traits, whereas mutated genes on the sex chromosomes (typically the X chromosome) are inherited as X-linked disorders.

Thousands of disorders are caused by mutations of single genes. Most diseases likely have a genetic component, either through inheritance of a susceptibility gene (which occurs in some individuals with neoplastic disease) or through a direct gene mutation that affects essential enzymes (which occurs in some individuals with phenylketonuria [PKU]). Knowledge obtained through the Human Genome Program (HGP) regarding the location of specific gene loci has allowed scientists to examine the genetic alterations and inheritance patterns involved in certain diseases. The HGP, which began in 1990, is an energetic project with the goal to identify all of the 100,000 genes in human DNA and determine the sequences of the three billion bases that make up this DNA.

Data gleaned from the HGP will eventually provide physicians with the ability to diagnose and treat many genetic diseases. The clinical laboratory, as a genetics testing center, has a vital role in determination of whether an individual—an adult, a child, or a fetus—will inherit or has inherited a genetic mutation that is associated with a disease. Some predict that in the future, half of the revenue generated by clinical laboratories will come from gene testing.

■ GENETIC DISORDERS

Genetic disease is categorized into three groups: chromosomal disorders, monogenic disorders, and polygenic (multifactorial) disorders. Although not all of these disorders lead to inherited diseases, a basic background is given for informative purposes.

Chromosomal Disorders

An alteration in the number or arrangement of chromosomes that leads to production of excessive or deficient genetic material is referred to as a *chromosomal disorder.* In chromosomal disorders, large segments of DNA are involved, which include introns and exons. Most (but not all) chromosome abnormalities produce acquired disorders and are not inherited. A common chromosomal disorder is *aneuploidy,* which is characterized by an excess or a loss of one or more chromosomes. *Trisomy,* a type of aneuploidy, is the presence of three copies of a chromosome instead of two (see Chapter 43); the presence of a single copy of a chromosome instead of the typical pair is referred to as *monosomy* (see Chapter 21). When these types of disorders are inherited, they lead to physical birth defects and in some cases, mental retardation. When these types of disorders are acquired, they lead to cancer.

The loss or breakage of a chromosome that results in the loss of the specific genes in the deleted region is referred to as a chromosomal *deletion*. If a particular class of gene such as a protooncogene, which controls cell growth and proliferation, is deleted, alterations in normal cell growth and proliferation occur and usually result in neoplasia. *Amplification* of DNA sequences, which results in an increased number of the affected sequences, causes in increase in synthesis of the proteins coded for by the amplified sequences. *Translocation* of gene segments between chromosomes is the reciprocal exchange of a sequence of DNA between chromosomes. Translocation in which protooncogenes are transposed from one chromosome to another causes uncontrolled cell growth and leads to certain types of lymphoma. Another type of chromosomal abnormality is *isochrome formation*. This abnormality occurs when a chromosome's centromere splits during mitosis, so one set of chromosomal arms is duplicated and the other is lost; a chromosome with four identical arms is produced. The majority of disorders that are caused by these chromosomal abnormalities are acquired diseases and not heritable.

Monogenic Disorders

An aberration of a single gene or a gene locus is referred to as a **monogenic disorder** and is the most likely disorder to result in an inherited disease. Mutations comprise the majority of monogenic disorders and cause the gene sequence to be permanently altered. A mutation that only affects somatic cells only affects daughter cells; the mutation is not inherited. Germline mutations are inherited through autosomal dominant, autosomal recessive, or **X-linked inheritance.** (See Chapter 11 for classifications of the various kinds of mutations.) Point mutations, which involve a single nucleotide substitution, produce a deranged protein product, as do frameshift mutations, which involve the addition or deletion of a single or many nucleotides. Many inherited monogenic disorders are caused by the addition of nucleotides within introns. The clinical significance of a mutation depends on the type of mutation, the location of the mutation in the gene (whether it is in an intron or exon), and the cells or tissues that are affected by the mutation.

Polygenic Disorders

A **polygenic disorder** (or a *multifactorial disorder*) is caused by the interaction of numerous altered genes with chemical and physiological factors. Traits that are the result of the combined effects of multiple genes are *polygenic traits;* the interaction of environmental factors with the trait produces the multifactorial effects. Many of the interactions occur spontaneously and produce greater DNA damage than has initially occurred from a de novo mutation. Multifactorial disorders run in families, but the inheritance pattern is unpredictable and the risk of recurrence is less than the 25% to 50% associated with typical Mendelian genetic disorders. Studies of identical twins with multifactorial disorders who are genetically similar but do not have the same disorders suggest that nongenetic factors are involved in the expression of multifactorial traits. Polygenic, multifactorial inheritance is thought to be involved in such complex disorders as Alzheimer's disease, coronary artery disease, certain cancers, type II diabetes mellitus, and hypertension.

◼ TRADITIONAL INHERITANCE PATTERNS

The human genome is composed of approximately 100,000 genes contained in the 46 chromosomes that are found in each nucleated cell. The chromosomes are grouped into 22 pairs of autosomes and one pair of sex chromosomes (Figure 44-1). Haploid cells (sperm and ova, or *gametes*) contain half of the genetic material necessary for the formation of offspring. During the formation of gametes, the reduction of chromosomes from their diploid number to a haploid number occurs through a process called *meiosis*. The combination of sperm and ova "reunites" the genetic material to produce the 23 pairs of chromosomes found in early embryonic cells. Individual gene sequences within the chromosomes make up an individual's unique **genotype,** and the physical expression of the genotype is referred to as the **phenotype.** Different forms of a gene are called **alleles;** if each allele in the pair of has the same sequence, they are homozygous alleles and if they have different sequences, they are heterozygous alleles. Single gene inheritance patterns are based on traditional Mendelian laws of assortment.

In regard to disease phenotypes, the term *dominance* describes a phenotypic trait that appears because of the presence of heterozygous alleles at a specific locus on a chromosome. Affected individuals have an autosomal dominant disease gene and a normal gene. A *recessive* trait requires homozygosity of alleles at a specific locus on a chromosome before the trait is expressed. If these alleles are located on autosomes, the phenotypes are referred to as either **autosomal dominant traits** or **autosomal recessive traits;** if the alleles are located on the X chromosomes **(X-linked traits),** they are referred to as X-linked dominant or X-linked recessive traits. Mutant alleles are typically the result of single nucleotide mutations. If the altered gene sequence is in an exon, an altered protein product is synthesized. A gene mutation is considered dominant if it produces a protein that is new or has a different function than the normal protein, resulting in a "gain of function." Expression of a dominant mutant allele often increases production of a protein's product or creates a new function, either normal or abnormal, whereas the expression of a recessive allele typically decreases or halts the production of a protein product or creates a nonfunctional protein ("loss of function").

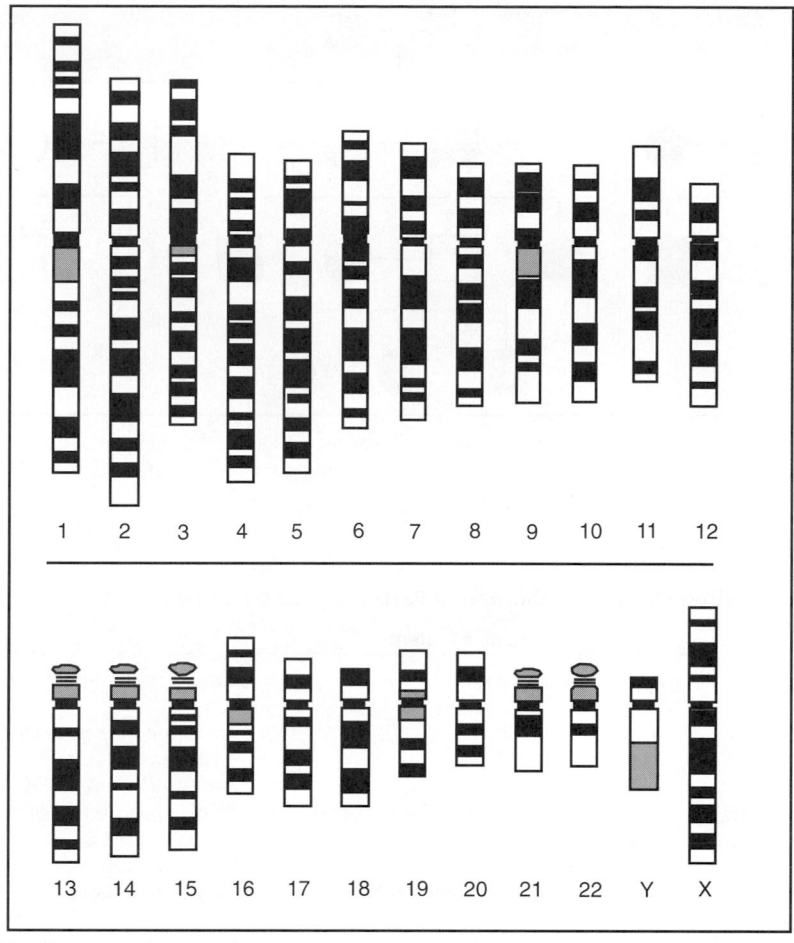

Figure 44-1 An idiogram showing each of the human chromosomes—22 autosomes and the two sex chromosomes, X and Y. The bands shown are typical of those seen when the chromosomes are stained with Giemsa. (From www.pathology.washington.edu/Cytogallery/cytogallery.html)

Autosomal Dominant Inheritance

Pedigrees are diagrams that illustrate inheritance patterns. An example of an **autosomal dominant inheritance** pattern in relation to an inherited disease is shown in Figure 44-2. A pedigree that illustrates an autosomal dominant trait has the following characteristics, as does the individual inheriting the trait:

1. Traits are inherited vertically (from the top to the bottom of the pedigree) from parents to offspring.
2. Females and males have an equal chance of expressing the trait.
3. Individuals who inherit the trait have a 50% chance of passing the trait on to offspring.
4. Individuals who do not express the trait cannot have offspring that do express the trait.
5. Individuals who express the trait have a parent who expressed the trait.

Approximately four times more autosomal dominant traits than recessive traits exist. Examples of diseases that are inherited through autosomal dominant inheritance include familial hypercholesterolemia, Huntington disease, factor V Leiden thrombophilia, early onset familial Alzheimer disease, and multiple endocrine neoplasia (Table 44-1). Autosomal dominant traits are typically *pleiotropic*, meaning the inherited mutation has diverse and multiple effects on various tissues and organs.

Variations in Autosomal Dominant Inheritance

Occasionally, the pedigree of a family who has a member with an autosomal dominant disorder does not follow the five traits listed previously. In rare situations, a parent has a normal phenotype but has an autosomal dominant mutation in the germline cells; the remaining cells are normal. This phenomenon is known as *germline mosaicism*. Approximately half of the parent's children will be affected.

Another situation in which an affected offspring can be born to phenotypically normal parents is in cases of *incomplete penetrance*. *Penetrance* refers to the number of individu-

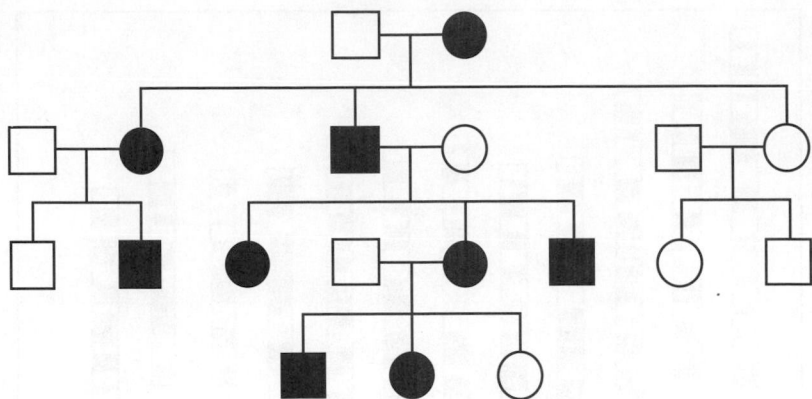

Figure 44-2 Pedigree of an autosomal dominant inheritance pattern. The squares represent males and the circles represent females. White symbols represent unaffected individuals; black symbols represent affected individuals. Examples of autosomal dominant disorders include Huntington disease and familial hypercholesterolemia.

TABLE 44-1	Selected Inherited Diseases, Inheritance Patterns, and Gene Loci

Disease	Inheritance Pattern	Gene Map Locus and Mutation Type
Achondroplasia	Autosomal dominant	Various mutations at the FGFR3 gene located at 4p16.3
Adenomatous polyposis coli	Autosomal dominant	Nonsense or frameshift mutations in APC gene at 5q21
Familial Alzheimer disease, type 3	Autosomal dominant	Point mutations in PSEN1 gene at 14q24.3
Familial amyotrophic lateral sclerosis, type 1	Autosomal dominant and a recessive juvenile form	Point, or missense, mutations at SOD1 gene at 21q22.1-22.2
Ataxia telangiectasia	Autosomal recessive	Various mutations in ATM gene at 11q22.3
Breast cancer, type 1 (BRCA1)	Autosomal dominant and multifactorial	Various mutations in susceptibility gene, BRCA1 at 17q21
Breast cancer, type 2 (BRCA2)	Autosomal dominant and multifactorial	Various mutations in susceptibility gene, BRCA2 at 13q12.3
Congenital adrenal hyperplasia	Autosomal recessive	De novo point mutations in CYP21A2 gene at 6p21.3
Cystic fibrosis	Autosomal recessive	Various mutations in CFTR gene at 7q31.2
Duchenne's muscular dystrophy	X linked	Frameshift mutation in DMD gene at Xp21.2
Factor V Leiden thrombophilia	Autosomal dominant Autosomal recessive	Point mutations in F5 gene at 1q23
Familial hypercholesterolemia	Autosomal dominant and multifactorial	Various mutations in LDLR gene at 19p13.3
Fanconi anemia A	Autosomal recessive	Various mutations in FANCA gene 16q24.3
Fragile X syndrome	X linked	CGG repeat expansion in FMR1 gene at Xq27.3
Hemochromatosis	Autosomal recessive	Various mutations in HFE gene at 6p21.3
Huntington disease	Autosomal dominant	CAG repeat expansion in HD gene at 4p16.3
Multiple endocrine neoplasia, type 1	Autosomal dominant	Various mutations in MEN1 gene at 11q13
Obesity caused by leptin deficiency	Autosomal recessive and multifactorial	Various mutations in LEP gene at 7q31.3
Prader-Willi syndrome	Uniparental disomy	Deletion of paternally derived PWCR region of 15q11 to 15q12 containing the SNRPN and NDN genes
Wilson's disease	Autosomal recessive	Frameshift mutation in ATP7B gene at 13q14.2-q21

---

als who have inherited a mutant gene and who actually exhibit the disease phenotype. Penetrance is calculated through mathematical division of the number of mutant gene carriers who have the disease by the total number of mutant gene carriers (who have the disease and do not have the disease). Anything less than 100% is incomplete penetrance. For example, if 65 out of 100 mutant gene carriers have the associated disease, the gene is said to have a 65% penetrance. Incomplete penetrance involves multiple factors. For example, if a single mutated gene that normally codes for tumor suppression is inherited, its paired normal gene must also be mutated for neoplastic growth to actually occur. This second mutation usually occurs spontaneously through some environmental factor. Thus not everyone who inherits a mutated tumor suppressor develops tumors. As mentioned previously, multifactorial disorders include the heritable forms of some cancers (such as breast and colon cancer) and certain complex diseases.

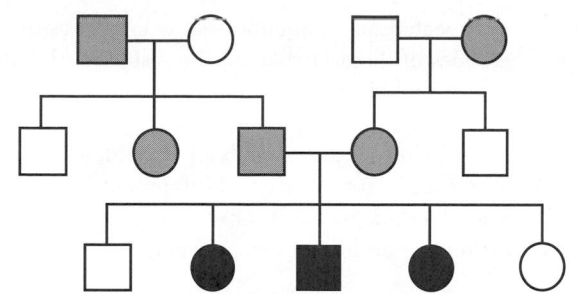

Figure 44-3   Pedigree of an autosomal recessive inheritance pattern. The squares represent males, and the circles represent females. White symbols represent unaffected, noncarriers; gray symbols represent carriers; black symbols represent affected individuals. Examples of autosomal recessive disorders include cystic fibrosis, phenylketonuria, and Tay-Sachs disease.

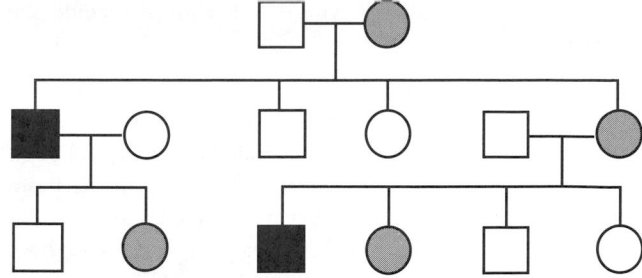

Figure 44-4   Pedigree of an X-linked recessive inheritance pattern. The squares represent males, and the circles represent females. White symbols represent unaffected noncarriers; gray circles represent female carriers; black squares represent affected males. Examples of X-linked recessive disorders include Duchenne's muscular dystrophy and factor VIII hemophilia.

The appearance of mild, moderate, or severe disease symptoms in individuals who inherit the same mutation is referred to as *variable expressivity.* Variable expressivity is common in individuals with autosomal dominant traits and is related to penetrance. If a phenotype is exhibited by an individual, it can have variable degrees of clinical involvement. Numerous factors cause variable expressivity, including environmental factors, the multiple effects of a gene on different tissues, and the presence of genes that can modify the abnormal gene.

Autosomal Recessive Inheritance

Families with autosomal recessive traits have pedigrees that differ in appearance and in characteristics from those families with autosomal dominant traits. The pedigree illustrated in Figure 44-3 shows an **autosomal recessive inheritance** pattern. The characteristics of this type of inheritance include the following:

1. Horizontal appearance of the trait on the pedigree.
2. Affected individuals with a homozygous allele have unaffected heterozygous parents.
3. Heterozygous parents have a 25% chance of having a homozygous, affected offspring.

Examples of diseases that demonstrate an autosomal recessive inheritance pattern include cystic fibrosis, sickle cell anemia, PKU, and Tay-Sachs disease (see Table 44-1). The majority of enzyme abnormalities (such as inborn metabolic errors) are autosomal recessive. Some disorders (such as PKU) exhibit *locus heterogeneity*—are caused by mutations in different genes at different loci. In individuals with PKU, a deficiency of phenylalanine hydroxylase caused by a mutation in the gene that codes for the enzyme is typically the cause of the disease. However, in some individuals, a mutation in the gene responsible for the synthesis of tetrahydrobiopterin (a cofactor of phenylalanine hydroxylase) leads to PKU symptoms, and the gene responsible for phenylalanine hydroxylase synthesis is normal. Many other disorders exhibit *allelic heterogeneity.* These diseases can be caused by different mutations within a single gene at one locus. An example is cystic fibrosis; the large 250-kilobase cystic fibrosis gene has approximately thirty exons (and introns). Hundreds of mutations within the expressed regions have been discovered, and each one individually leads to the symptoms of cystic fibrosis. The allelic heterogeneity leads affects the severity of cystic fibrosis in affected individuals.

X-Linked Patterns of Inheritance

Inheritance patterns of X-linked phenotypes have pedigrees that exhibit differential genotype inheritance that depends on whether the offspring are male or female. Genes responsible for X-linked disorders are located on the X chromosome. Males have only one X chromosome; therefore the presence of an abnormal gene on the X chromosome is almost always expressed, and the male develops signs of the disease. Because no normal gene exists to compensate for the X-linked diseases such as muscular dystrophy or certain mental retardation syndromes, the conditions are transmitted by unaffected carrier mothers and expressed in their male offspring. In females an X chromosome is randomly and irreversibly inactivated early in embryogenesis (a process called *lyonization*).[16] Approximately half of the females cells contain the paternally derived active X chromosome; the others contain the maternally derived active X chromosome. The genes on the inactivated X chromosome do not produce any protein products.

The concept of dominance and recessiveness in X-linked disorders has little significance. In a female the expression of a mutant allele is dependent on whether it is located on an active or inactive X chromosome. A recessive gene in a carrier female is occasionally expressed because of the inactivation of a significant number of the X chromosomes containing the normal gene, whereas a dominant gene's expression can be masked if it is located on a preponderance of inactivated X chromosomes. However, in males the mutant allele is always expressed because they have only one X chromosome. A typical pedigree is shown in Figure 44-4.

The characteristics of this type of inheritance include the following:

1. A carrier female has a 50% chance of donating a normal X chromosome to her male or female offspring.
2. Affected males have normal male offspring, although all female offspring are carriers. A carrier female has a 25% chance of having either an affected son, an unaffected son, a noncarrier daughter, or a carrier daughter.

Examples of X-linked disorders include hemophilia, Duchenne's muscular dystrophy (DMD), and fragile X syndrome (see Table 44-1).

■ NONTRADITIONAL PATTERNS OF INHERITANCE

Exceptions to the patterns of inheritance previously described include uniparental disomy, imprinting, mosaicism, and anticipation.

Uniparental disomy occurs when an individual inherits two copies of a chromosome from one parent and none from the other parent.

Imprinting refers to the differential expression of a gene in an offspring, which is determined by whether the gene was inherited from the mother or father. Several human genes exhibit differential parental expression. Prader-Willi syndrome is an example of a disorder caused by inheritance of a deleted chromosome segment from the father. If the same deletion is inherited from the mother, a different clinical syndrome is observed.[2]

Another nontraditional pattern of inheritance is called *mosaicism*, which is the presence of two or more distinct cell types, one with a normal genetic makeup and the other with an abnormal genetic makeup. Mosaicism was first observed in the chromosomal disorder Turner syndrome. About half of women with Turner syndrome have 45,X in all their cells. The remaining affected females have mosaicism with chromosomally normal and abnormal cells in differing proportions. Mosaicism for a gene abnormality involves cells from certain parts of the body that have genes coding for a specific mutated protein, whereas cells from other regions of the same body have normal gen If the abnormal cells affect the gonads, the abnormal gene is passed on to offspring, who are then fully affected even though the parent may be only partially affected.[14]

Many disorders are associated with expansions of *triplet repeats*. A triplet repeat consists of three DNA base pairs repeated sequentially various times in introns. In the human genome, triplet repeats are common and normal; however, in a diseased individual, the number of triplet repeats is much higher than normal. As the repeated sequences are passed on to offspring, they can increase in number as a result of meiotic recombination. In some cases the meiotic expansion increases with each generation. Thus the disease onset is earlier than expected, phenomenon that is known as *anticipation*. Examples of diseases that are the result of triplet repeat expansions include Huntington disease, fragile X syndrome, and myotonic dystrophy. Myotonic dystrophy is an autosomal dominant condition with an expanded CTG repeat. An interesting note is that development of prostate cancer is related to a *decreased* number of a certain triplet repeat (CAG) on the androgen receptor gene.[15]

■ MITOCHONDRIAL INHERITANCE

Mitochondria are cellular organelles that provide essential energy for cellular metabolism. A unique DNA genome referred to as *mitochondrial DNA* (mtDNA), is found within each mitochondria and is separate from nuclear DNA. The replication and transcription of mtDNA is under regulatory control that is separate from nuclear DNA. mtDNA codes for approximately 15 of the proteins used by mitochondria, and the remainder are encoded by DNA in the cell's nucleus. mtDNA is inherited exclusively from the cytoplasm of the ovum, and the mode of inheritance is vertical. The approximately 50 harmful mtDNA disorders affect male and female offspring.[5] Examples of mitochondrial diseases include mitochondrial myopathy and Leber optic neuropathy.

■ SPECIFIC INHERITED DISEASES

As the genetic components of more diseases are being discerned, the number of known inherited diseases grows. The following section includes only diseases that are commonly encountered in the clinical laboratory. Table 44-1 includes certain other inherited diseases, inheritance patterns, and the mutations that cause each disease. For complete information, see the additional reading list at the end of this chapter.

Neoplastic Disease

Cancer involves neoplastic cell changes that are caused by somatic and inherited mutations. The initiation of these changes is called *carcinogenesis,* a multistep process interpreted through a progression of morphological changes in benign or premalignant cells that lead to formation of malignant cells or a tumor (see Chapter 21). In cases of familial or inherited cancers, identification of specific mutations in affected individuals aids in screening of other family members who are at risk for inheriting the cancer. Numerous criteria must be met for a gene mutation to be considered a heritable factor in familial cancer (Table 44-2). Linkage analysis and segregation analysis are typically performed if enough family members are available for testing.

Cancer susceptibility is likely an inherited component and when the germline genes are altered, family members

TABLE 44-2   Criteria Used to Classify a Cancer Gene as Familial

1. The cellular DNA of affected individuals must contain the specific gene mutation.
2. The tumor cell DNA of affected individuals must contain the specific gene mutation.
3. An assessment of the family pedigree must demonstrate germline transmission of the specific gene mutation to offspring.
4. The inheritance pattern should demonstrate autosomal dominance.
5. Segregation analysis of the specific mutated gene must demonstrate linkage to cancer susceptibility in family members.
6. The specific gene mutation should be demonstrated in multiple family pedigrees and must not be observed in healthy control populations.

TABLE 44-3   Selected Familial Cancer Susceptibility Genes

Gene*	Locus	Cancer Type
APC	5q21	Colon, malignant polyps
NPAT	11q22.3	Various malignancies
BRCA1	17q21	Breast, uterine
BRCA2	13q12.3	Breast, uterine
MEN1	11q13	Parathyroid, thyroid

*Most of the listed genes are considered tumor suppressor genes.

become susceptible to any neoplastic disease. Numerous tumor suppressor genes have been identified as familial cancer susceptibility genes (Table 44-3). Mutations associated with familial cancers comprise gene amplification, gene deletion, point mutations, and gene rearrangement, and the mutations are typically inherited through autosomal dominant inheritance. The affected genes are typically protooncogenes and tumor suppressor genes, in which one (the protooncogene) is activated to form an oncogene and the other (the tumor suppressor gene) is inactivated, resulting in loss of the proliferative control of cell growth. Other genes possibly affected in individuals with cancer include genes coding for proteins involved in DNA repair and genes coding for kinases that govern cell cycle progression.

Several heritable cancers have a particularly high incidence. Genetic susceptibility to colorectal cancer is associated with familial adenomatous polyposis coli, a disorder that involves the formation of malignant colonic polyps. The mutation involves a gene on chromosome 5q21 referred to as the *adematous polyposis coli* (APC) gene, which becomes inactivated after a frameshift or nonsense mutation.[1] Familial breast and ovarian cancers comprise approximately 5% of all breast and ovarian cancer cases. Heritable genes involved in breast cancer genesis include the susceptibility genes BRCA1 (17q21) and BRCA2 (13q12.3). Germline mutations that occur in the BRCA1 gene confer a 90% risk of developing either breast or ovarian cancer by age 70.[13]

Although many cancers occur sporadically and involve acquired somatic mutations, several malignancies are considered inherited diseases because of familial clustering. The early age of onset and hereditary patterns indicate that these cancers are inheritable in familial groups.

Cardiovascular Disease

Most cardiac disorders have a genetic component, and external factors (such as diet, age, and the environment) probably interact with the genetic components to affect risk. Heart disease is a polygenic, multifactorial disease, and cer-

tain genetic alterations are inherited. In some cases of familial hypertriglyceridemia, the primary defect is either overproduction of certain apoproteins or defective lipoprotein lipase. Inherited alterations in the genes that code for these proteins initiate the elevation in blood triglyceride levels, and secondary factors such as excess weight or diabetes exacerbate the disorder. Familial hypercholesterolemia is induced either by a mutation in the gene that codes for apoprotein B (chromosome 2p) or the low-density lipoprotein (LDL) receptor gene (chromosome 19p).[6] Many mutations have been noted on the LDL receptor gene locus, and individuals heterozygous for these mutations typically develop coronary artery disease between ages 40 and 50 years. Individuals who are homozygotic for the disease are rare and suffer acute myocardial infarctions by the age of 20 years.

Factor V mutation

Thrombosis plays a major role in cardiovascular disease, and inherited defects that affect coagulation or anticoagulation lead to an increased risk of forming thrombotic plaques in coronary arteries. Although many genetic defects lead to imbalances in hemostasis, such as mutations in the fibrinogen gene locus, defects in the genes coding for factor V are the most common cause of venous thromboembolism.

Factor V Leiden thrombophilia is characterized by an increased risk of venous thromboembolism. A point mutation in the factor V gene (F5 on 1q23) causes resistance to cleavage by activated protein C.[7,18] Thus factor V is inactivated for longer than usual, resulting in an increase in thrombin generation and a hypercoagulable state. About 5% of the Caucasian population is heterozygous for this mutation. Although factor V thrombophilia is an autosomal dominant disorder—with the presence of one mutated gene increasing the risk of thromboembolism about fivefold—being homozygous for factor V Leiden increases the risk about thirtyfold.

Neuromuscular Disease

Inherited muscular diseases include many childhood- and adult-onset disorders. Duchenne's muscular dystrophy (DMD) is characterized by generalized weakness and muscle wasting with an onset of about 2 to 6 years of age. All voluntary muscles are affected, and survival beyond the age of 25 is rare. DMD is inherited as an X-linked recessive disorder. The mutation involves a large frameshift on the short arm of the X chromosome at locus 21.2.[18] Individuals with myotonic dystrophy (MD), also known as *Steinert's disease,* have similar symptoms, although prolonged muscular contraction is a characteristic of MD. Age of onset of the disease ranges from childhood to middle age. The congenital form is the most severe and includes delayed muscle development and mental retardation. MD is an expanded triplet repeat (CTG) disorder inherited by autosomal dominant inheritance. Progression of this disease is slow, spanning 50 years.

Other heritable disorders of the neuromuscular system include familial amyotrophic lateral sclerosis[8] (FALS), spinal muscular atrophy (SMA), and various ataxias. ALS is the most common form of progressive motor neuron disease caused by the degeneration of lower motor neurons in the spinal cord and upper motor neurons in the cerebral cortex. Some of these disorders are inherited through autosomal dominant inheritance (such as ALS), and others are inherited through autosomal or X-linked recessive inheritance (such as SMA). SMA and certain ataxias are other examples of trinucleotide repeat disorders.

Neurological Disease

The number of neurological disorders that can be traced to a DNA mutation has increased significantly since 1990. The use of DNA probes, linkage analysis, and pedigree assessment has revealed the loci of the mutant genes involved in Huntington disease, familial Alzheimer disease, certain neuroblastomas, fragile-X syndrome, Tourette's syndrome, and many other neuropathies. Presymptomatic testing of individuals who may inherit a mutant gene that affects neurological function has had a major effect on the practice of neurology.

Huntington disease

Huntington disease is inherited as an autosomal dominant trait characterized by writhing movements of the upper extremities and progressive dementia. The age of onset is typically in middle age, and survival after onset of symptoms is between 15 to 20 years. Because of the incapacitating symptoms of Huntington disease, as well as its inheritance pattern, presymptomatic screening for Huntington disease is one of the most requested genetic tests. The disorder is caused by an expansion of a trinucleotide repeat (CAG) in the Huntington disease gene on chromosome 4p16.3.[17,18] Diagnosis of Huntington disease depends on a positive family history of the disease, clinical findings, and demonstration of the expanded CAG repeat in the Huntington disease gene.

Fragile X syndrome

Disturbance of brain function, or mental retardation, is primarily traced to a neural development disorder. Many medical conditions can be associated with mental retardation, including disorders involving lysosomal enzyme function, aminoacidopathies, and intrauterine infection. In individuals with fragile X syndrome, mental retardation and dysmorphic physical characteristics become more obvious with increased age, particularly during puberty. The disorder is caused by an expanded trinucleotide repeat (CGG) at the X chromosome locus Xq27.3 in the *FMR1* gene.[12] Fragile X syndrome is an X-linked genetic disorder.

Familial early-onset Alzheimer disease

Alzheimer disease is a devastating neurological disorder that begins with progressive dementia during late adulthood and can only be definitively diagnosed after death. Examination of an individual with Alzheimer reveals a brain that is riddled with unusual formations, notably amyloid plaques and neurofibrillary tangles, and a significantly atrophied cerebral cortex. Families who have more than one member with Alzheimer disease who had symptoms that appeared before the age of 55 to 60 years old, have early-onset familial Alzheimer disease (EOFAD). Several different genes are implicated in EOFAD; a point mutation in the *PSEN1* gene at locus 14q24.3[11,18] is the most common mutation (referred to as AD3, or FAD type 3). EOFAD is inherited through autosomal dominant inheritance in families with several affected generations.

Inborn Errors of Metabolism

Inborn error of metabolism is a general term that is applied to numerous genetic disorders with pathological symptoms that are usually attributable to excessive tissue stores or circulating concentrations of a specific undegraded metabolite. One type of inborn error is associated with the amino acid metabolic disorders (see Chapter 18). In individuals with these disorders, such as PKU or maple syrup urine disease, a certain mutated enzyme can no longer act on its substrate, resulting in the accumulation of substrate in the urine. The lysosomal storage diseases, some of which are summarized in Table 44-4, are another subset of inborn errors.

The lysosomal storage diseases result from accumulation in lysosomes of metabolites that would normally be degraded by one of the many hydrolytic enzymes residing in these subcellular organelles. The lysosomal enzymes are unique because they are functional at an acid pH. The specific enzyme deficiencies of the lysosomal storage diseases have been elucidated through identification of products stored in tissues or eventually excreted in urine. The nomenclature of enzymes, substrates, storage products, and metabolites is not always systematic. The lysosomal storage disorders are referred to simply as *storage disorders*

TABLE 44-4 Selected Lysosomal Storage Disorders

Storage Disorder	Clinical Features*	Enzyme Deficiency	Current Diagnostic Approach†
Sphingolipidoses			
Niemann-Pick disease (sphingomyelin lipidosis)	*Type IA (acute):* neuropathic; foamy histiocytes in bone marrow; acute neuropathic progressive loss of motor and intellectual capacity early in life; hepatosplenomegaly; cherry red macula; usually fatal in infancy	Sphingomyelinase	*Quantitative enzyme assay.* Three mutations account for 92% of Ashkenazi Jewish cases. Mutation analysis is necessary for carrier detection.
	Type IS (subacute): similar to IA but nonneuropathic and slightly older age at onset	Sphingomyelinase	*Quantitative enzyme assay*
Gaucher's disease (glucosylceramide lipidosis)	*Type 1 (chronic nonneuropathic):* hepatosplenomegaly; Gaucher's cells; anemia; elevated phosphatase levels; bone pain and lytic lesions; striking elevation of angiotensin-converting enzyme (most frequently seen storage disease, with highest incidence in Ashkenazi Jews)	β-Glucosidase	*Quantitative enzyme and DNA analysis.* Carriers are best diagnosed by DNA analysis of the four most common mutations in the Ashkenazi Jewish population, in which the carrier frequency is 1 in 14.
	Type 2 (infantile acute neuropathic): rapidly degenerative central nervous system manifestations; peripheral symptoms similar to type 1 but greatly exaggerated, with death usually occurring by 1 y of age	β-Glucosidase	*Quantitative enzyme and molecular analysis.* Carriers are best diagnosed by DNA analysis of the four most common mutations.
	Type 3 (subacute neuronopathic): similar to type 2 except later onset and a milder course, eventually causing death in early childhood	β-Glucosidase	*Quantitative enzyme and molecular analysis.* Carriers are best diagnosed by DNA analysis of the four most common mutations.
Krabbe's disease (galactosylceramide lipidosis, globoid cell leukodystrophy)	Numerous recognized forms, differing significantly in age at onset and severity of symptoms: progressive psychomotor retardation; globoid cells in central nervous system; spastic quadriparesis; hypertonicity; hyperthermia; elevated cerebrospinal fluid protein levels	Galactosylceramide β-galactosidase	*Quantitative enzyme assay with radiolabeled substrate.* DNA structure and mutations currently are being discovered.
Metachromatic leukodystrophy (MLD) (sulfatide lipidosis)	Several closely related disorders with differing ages of onset, from 1 y into adulthood: peripheral neuropathy; intermittent pain in arms and legs and eventual difficulty in sitting; gait disturbance; absence of deep tendon reflexes; plantar flexion of feet. *Adult form:* slowly progressive dementia (often confused with nonorganic psychoses)	Arylsulfatase A	*Quantitative enzyme assay: urinary sulfatide, fibroblast loading with labeled sulfatide.* DNA analysis is currently impractical except in special circumstances because of the frequent occurrence of a pseudodeficient allele and multiple MLD-causing mutations.
Fabry's disease (angiokeratoma corporis diffusum universale)	Severe pain in extremities; angiokeratoma on buttocks and around navel; tortuous, dilated conjunctival and retinal venules; neuropathy; hypertension; myocardial ischemia (may manifest in female carriers in later life)	α-Galactosidase (X-linked)	*Quantitative enzyme assay for affected males; high-performance thin-layer or column chromatography identification of ceramide trihexoside for carriers.* Molecular testing is possible.
G$_{M2}$-gangliosidosis (Tay-Sachs disease) (β-N-acetylhexosaminidase isoenzyme A-deficient variant, infantile onset); also allelic defects in juvenile and adult onset forms	Early motor weakness; psychomotor deterioration after 1 y of age; progressive deafness; blindness; startle response; red macula	β-N-Acetyl-glucosaminidase A	Molecular testing available for most common mutations, but because of efficiency of enzyme testing molecular testing is not the current standard of practice.
Mucopolysaccharidoses (MPS)			
Hurlers' syndrome (MPS I)	Progressive mental and physical debilitation beginning at age 1; corneal opacities; coarse facies; gingival hyperplasia; dysostosis multiple; stiff joints (claw hands); dwarfing; organomegaly	α-L-Iduronidase	*Quantitative enzyme assay; demonstration of excess urinary mucopolysaccharide consisting of dermatan and heparan sulfates*

*Because biochemical and more recently, molecular genetic, approaches have been refined and developed, the presence of allelic variants of specific enzyme deficiencies have become apparent. For example, Tay-Sachs variants in which affected individuals live well into adulthood have been described. This general phenomenon is common in other lysosomal storage disorders. Some nonallelic variants that result from deficiency of activator proteins (saposins) have also been described.

†Testing for the molecular defect in most of the lysosomal storage disorders is not routine because of the heterogeneity of the mutations. However, automation of sequence-based testing will likely cause molecular methods to be used more frequently.

lipidoses, mucopolysaccharidoses, or *mucolipidoses.* Synonymous with lipidoses are the sphingolipidoses. Although the nomenclature regarding mucopolysaccharides has been changed to more accurately reflect the structure of the polysaccharide—the new name is *glycosaminoglycans*—the medical genetic literature still refers to these diseases as *mucopolysaccharidoses.* The original grouping of lipidoses and mucopolysaccharidoses was largely based on phenotypic symptoms and observation of abnormal cells in marrow or tissues caused by lipid or complex carbohydrate storage.

Tay-Sachs disease and other lysosomal storage diseases

Among the lysosomal storage diseases, Tay-Sachs disease has been the most thoroughly studied. The biochemical defect responsible for Tay-Sachs disease is a near total deficiency of the enzyme *N*-acetyl-β-hexosaminidase A (β-NAG A; hex A). This enzyme is responsible for the hydrolysis of the β (1→4)-glycosidic bond between *N*-acetylgalactosamine and galactose in the G_{M2} ganglioside (Figure 44-5). The absence of enzyme activity results in the neuronal storage of the G_{M2} ganglioside and the clinical symptoms described in Table 44-2. Because of the G_{M2} ganglioside storage, Tay-Sachs disease and at least three of its variants are classified as G_{M2} gangliosidoses.[10]

In the recessive inherited disorders (except for X-linked Fabry's disease), clinical symptoms are apparent only in homozygotes. However, unaffected heterozygotes can often be detected by enzyme assays. In laboratories where such assays are performed, detection of heterozygotes of recessive inherited disorders has become an important function. The activities of lysosomal enzymes in heterozygotes are usually below the reference interval but higher than those obtained in specimens from affected homozygotes. A frequently cited example is the identification of heterozygotes for Tay-Sachs disease. Tay-Sachs disease is rare in the general population, but the increased incidence of carriers in Ashkenazi Jews—1 in 28—makes screening for carriers in the subpopulation practical and desirable. Genetic counseling of mates who have both been identified as carriers clarifies the risk of an infant. Identifying carriers of Tay-Sachs disease has become the most frequently requested function of laboratories engaged in enzymatic diagnosis of lysosomal storage diseases.

Identification of heterozygotes of X-linked disorders is more difficult than identification of disorders caused by autosomal mutations. Because of the random inactivation of one X chromosome in each cell, assays of lysosomal enzyme activity may not identify certain women who are carriers of X–chromosome-linked disorders.

Other Common Inherited Disorders

Two additional diseases, hemochromatosis and cystic fibrosis, are significant because of their high gene frequency. Hemochromatosis is an iron metabolism disorder, and cystic fibrosis is a chloride transport disorder.

Hereditary hemochromatosis

Hereditary hemochromatosis is a common inherited iron metabolism disorder. Symptoms include elevated circulating serum iron levels caused by increased iron absorption, increased transferrin saturation, and increased iron storage, particularly in the liver; cirrhosis eventually develops. In many cases the cause of death is hepatocellular carcinoma. Reducing the amount of circulating iron is accomplished by simple weekly phlebotomy procedures in which a specified

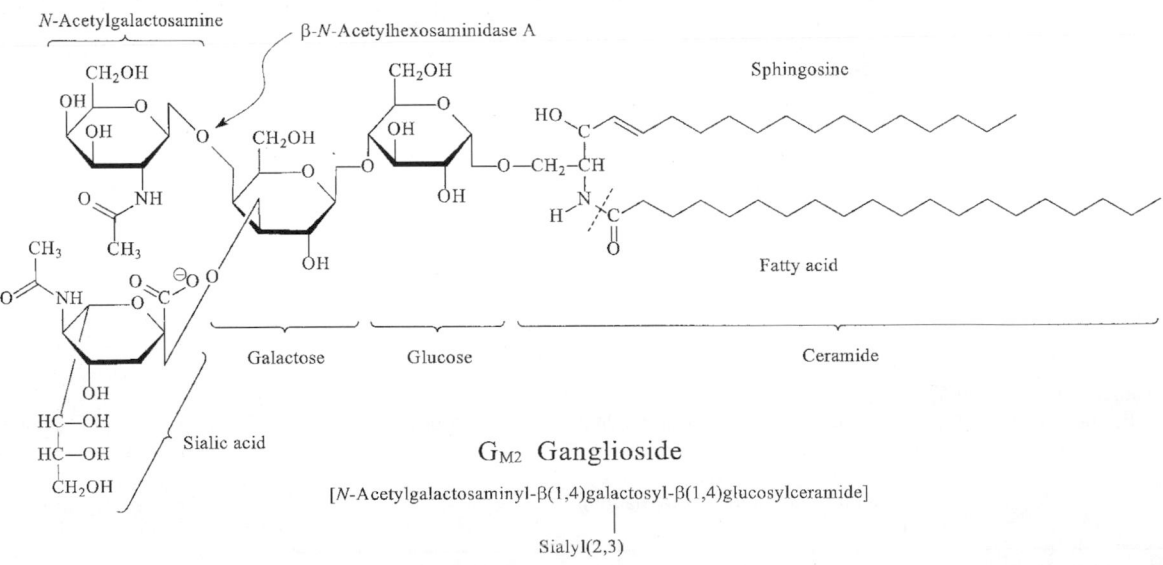

Figure 44-5   The structure of the G_{M2} ganglioside that accumulates in neurons of the central nervous system in individuals with Tay-Sachs disease.

mount of blood is removed from the affected patient. Hereditary hemochromatosis is inherited through autosomal recessive inheritance, and the mutated gene *(HFE)* is on the short arm of chromosome 6 at locus 21.3.[3,18,19] (See Chapter 30 for more detailed information regarding hemochromatosis.)

Cystic fibrosis

Disruption of endocrine gland function is a typical symptom of cystic fibrosis (see Chapters 35 and 37). Cystic fibrosis is an autosomal recessive disorder with various mutations leading to similar symptoms. Chromosome 7q at locus 31.2 contains the *CFTR* gene of the mutation and its variants.[9,18]

■ CLINICAL LABORATORY ASSESSMENT OF INHERITED DISEASES

In the past, laboratory testing for genetic diseases focused on assessment of metabolite accumulation, the absence of enzyme activity, the lack of an enzyme-substrate reaction product, or the increased concentration of precursor proteins. However, the HGP has recently identified the gene sequences and mutations involved numerous inherited diseases, and genetics testing has become an appropriate diagnostic tool in many situations.

Techniques for DNA Testing

DNA analysis is accomplished by extraction of DNA from cells, in some cases fragmentation of the DNA with restriction enzymes, amplification of the fragments or segments, and separation of normal DNA from mutated DNA (often by electrophoresis and hybridization). As with all laboratory procedures, calibrators and controls are needed (see Chapter 11). DNA analysis procedures are typically used for presymptomatic testing of individuals who may develop the disease, prenatal screening, and carrier screening. Use of DNA tests to confirm a clinical disorder, such as factor V Leiden thrombophilia, in a patient who has abnormal phenotypic tests is becoming more common.

In some cases, routine laboratory phenotype testing provides better diagnostic information than genetic tests; reasons include (1) lack of chromosome and gene sequence information related to a particular disease, (2) allelic heterogeneity of a mutation, (3) locus heterogeneity of a mutation, (4) the presence of susceptibility genes in individuals with polygenic disorders, (5) the analytical requirements of the genetic testing procedure, and (6) ethical considerations. For example, genetic testing is not recommended for assessment of hereditary hemochromatosis because of the uncertainty of the mutation's penetrance. To diagnose an individual who has symptoms, often a simple laboratory test is less expensive than a complex genetic analysis. Assessing coronary artery disease by examination of serum cholesterol concentrations, LDL and high-density lipoprotein (HDL) ratios and concentrations, and lipoprotein (a) [LP(a)] values is more financially feasible than by performance of a series of genetic tests.

Recent developments in the testing of lysosomal storage diseases involve more complete genotyping of mutations of specific enzymes. DNA-based assays are now available to help distinguish many of the mutations responsible for Tay-Sachs variants.[4] The assays use a polymerase chain reaction (PCR) technique to amplify specific segments in the α-subunit gene. Although the three most prevalent mutations causing Tay-Sachs disease have been found, the current standard of practice is to use enzyme screening to identify carriers and affected individuals; except in very special circumstances, the enzyme assay is not allele specific and therefore is a better general screening technique.

Numerous new techniques are being developed for genetics testing, including DNA chip technology, microfluidics, and hand-held DNA sensors. Chip-based microfluidic systems will be able to amplify DNA, digest the product with restriction enzymes, and perform electrophoresis. A hand-held sensor might be able to detect an electrical signal generated by DNA as it hybridizes to a target probe. These rapid screening methods may one day allow clinicians to diagnose genetic disease at a patient's bedside.

Genetic diagnosis and gene therapy likely will become effective partners with environmentally- and nutritionally-based medicine and treatment. The costs of genetic services will decrease as the services are incorporated into mainstream health care.

Ethics of DNA Testing

Many questions, ethical and investigative, surround genetics testing. According to the HPG, "Genetic information is personal, powerful, potentially predictive, pedigree-sensitive, permanent, and prejudicial." Genetic counseling, before and after a gene test, should be part of every genetics-related laboratory procedure. An important consideration is the proper use of gene testing and its results. Should molecular testing be used only to confirm specific disorders or to identify possible disease carriers? Should genetic disorders be diagnosed before the appearance of symptoms? Should children be genetically tested? What should be done with the results of genetics tests? Do all patients want to know their results?

To guarantee that pretest genetic counseling has taken place, laboratories should insist on getting a copy of the signed informed consent form. Patients must be made aware of the implications of the information obtained through genetics testing. The language used in obtaining informed consent from a patient must be clear and

concise, and the informed consent document must contain appropriate confidentiality protection. (This issue applies to other situations, such as HIV testing.) Confidentiality is particularly important in regards to health insurability, because certain tests, such as presymptomatic tests, are only predictive, not descriptive, as are many pathology laboratory analyses.

Applying basic DNA science to clinica serious ethical issues. The information obtai tests has enormous psychological, economi implications. Pretest and posttest education and are essential. One of the HGP's goals is to ad ethical, legal, and social issues that might result fr project.

References

1. Beroud C, Soussi T: APC gene: database of germline and somatic mutations in human tumors and cell lines. Nucleic Acids Res 1996; 24:121-124.

2. Buiting K: Sporadic imprinting defects in Prader-Willi Syndrome and Angelman Syndrome: implications for imprint-switch models, genetic counseling, and prenatal diagnosis. Am J Hum Genet 1998; 63:170-180.

3. Burke W, Thomson E, Muin JK, et al: Hereditary hemochromatosis: gene discovery and its implications for population-based screening. JAMA, 1998; 280:172-178.

4. Chong GL, Thibodeau SN, O'Brien JF: DNA-based assays for detecting carriers of Tay-Sachs disease: a comparison with enzymatic assays. Clin Chem 1991; 36:1018.

5. Clark KM: Reversal of a mitochondrial DNA defect in human skeletal muscle. Nature Genetics 1997; 16:222-224.

6. Coleman WB, Tsongalis GJ, (eds): Molecular Diagnostics for the Clinical Laboratorian, p 277, Totowa, New Jersey, Humana Press, 1997.

7. Coleman WB, Tsongalis GJ, (eds): Molecular Diagnostics for the Clinical Laboratorian, pp 286-289, Totowa, New Jersey, Humana Press, 1997.

8. de Belleroche J, Orrel R, King A: Familial amyotrophic lateral sclerosis/motor neuron disease (FALS): a review of current developments. J Med Genet 1995; 32:841-847.

9. Fanen P, Ghanem N, Vidaud M, et al: Molecular characterization of cystic fibrosis: 16 novel mutations identified by analysis of the whole cystic fibrosis conductance transmembrane regulator (CFTR) coding regions and splice site junctions. Genomics 1992; 13:770-776.

10. Gravel RA, Clarke JTR, Kaback MM, et al: The G_{M2} gangliosidoses. In Scriver CR, Beaudet AL, Sly WS, et al (eds): The Metabolic and Molecular Bases of Inherited Disease, 7th edition, pp 2839-2882, New York, McGraw-Hill, 1995.

11. Gustafson L, Brun A, Englunc E, et al: A 50-year perspective of a family with chromosome-14-linked Alzheimer's disease. Hum Genet 1998; 102:253-257.

12. Hammond LS, Macias MM, Tarleton JC: Fragile X syndrome and deletions in FMR1: new case and review of the literature. Am J Med Genet 1997; 72:430-434.

13. Hauser AR, Lerner IJ, King RA: Familial breast cancer. Am J Med Genet 1992: 44:839-840.

14. Johnson VP, Christianson C: Clinical genetics: a self study for health care providers: lesson 1. Virtual Hospital 1999, http://www.vh.org/Providers/Textbooks/Clinical Genetics.

15. Kantoff P, Giovannucci E, Brown M: The androgen receptor CAG repeat polymorphism and its relationship to prostate cancer. Biochim Biophys Acta 1998; 1378(3):C1-5.

16. Lyon MF: X-chromosome inactivation spreads itself: effects in autosomes. Am J Hum Genet 1998; 63:17-19.

17. MacMillan JC, Davies P, Harper PS: Molecular diagnostic analysis for Huntington's disease: a prospective evaluation. J Neurol Neurosurg Psych 1995; 58:496-498.

18. Online Mendelian Inheritance in Man, OMIM: Center for Medical Genetics, Johns Hopkins University, Baltimore, Md; and National Center for Biotechnology Information, National Library of Medicine, Bethesda, Md, 1999. http://www.ncbi.nlm.nih.gov/omim.

19. Totaro A, Rommens JM, Grifa A, et al: Hereditary hemochromatosis: generation of a transcription map within a refined and extended map of the HLA class I region. Genomics 1996; 31:319-326.

Additional Reading

Coleman WB, Tsongalis GJ (eds): Molecular Diagnostics for the Clinical Laboratorian, New Jersey, Humana Press, 1997.

Ethical, Legal, and Social Issues (ELSI) of the Human Genome Program: US Department of Energy and the National Institutes of Health. www.ornl.gov/hgmis/resource/elsi.html#issues.

Farkas DH: DNA Simplified II, Washington, DC, AACC Press, 1999.

Heim RA, Silverman LM: Molecular Pathology: Approaches to Diagnosing Human Disease in the Clinical Laboratory, Durham, North Carolina, Carolina Academic Press, 1994.

Human Genome Program. US Department of Energy and the National Institutes of Health. www.ornl.gov/TechResources/Human_Genome/home.html

Motulsky AG: Screening for genetic diseases. N Engl J Med 1997; 336:1314-1316.

Lewin B: Genes VI, Parts 1 and 7, Oxford, Oxford University Press, 1997.

Scriver CR, Sly WS, Beaudet AL, et al (eds): The Metabolic and Molecular Bases of Inherited Disease, 7th edition, New York, McGraw-Hill, 19

Shaw DJ, (ed): Molecular Genetics of Human Inherited Disease, New York, John Wiley & Sons, 1995.

CHAPTER 45

Nutritional Assessment, Therapy, and Monitoring

MEGAN S. VELDEE, MS, RD

Objectives

1. Define the following terms:
   Nutrition
   Total parenteral nutrition
   Body mass
   Macronutrients
   Micronutrients
   Conditionally essential nutrients
2. List the essential nutrients required for metabolism, and state their role in energy production.
3. List the chemical components of body mass and their percent contribution to total body mass.
4. Describe the anthropometric and biochemical tests used to assess nutritional status.

Key Words

Basal Metabolic Rate (BMR)   An expression of the rate at which oxygen is utilized by the body cells, or the calculated equivalent heat production by the body (in a fasting person at complete rest)

Body Mass Index (BMI)   The weight in kilograms divided by the square of the height in meters; alternatively, 703.1 times the weight in pounds divided by the square of the height in inches

Enteral Nutrition   A means to provide food through a tube that has been placed in the nose, stomach, or small intestine; also called *tube feeding*

Kwashiorkor   A syndrome produced by severe protein deficiency; characterized by retarded growth, changes in hair and skin pigment, edema, and pathological changes in the liver including fatty infiltration, necrosis, and fibrosis

Malnutrition   Any disorder caused by an unbalanced or insufficient diet or defective assimilation or utilization of foods

Marasmus   A form of protein-calorie malnutrition that primarily occurs during the first year of life; characterized by growth retardation and progressive wasting of subcutaneous fat and muscle, although the person usually retains an appetite and mental alertness

Nutrient   Any item of food, whether essential or nonessential, that nourishes or promotes growth and metabolism; conventionally, refers to the macronutrients (water, protein, fats, and carbohydrates) and the micronutrients (vitamins, minerals, and trace elements) that are essential for energy and growth

Nutrition   The sum of the processes involved in the taking in of nutrients and the assimilation and use of them

Obesity   A body weight that is beyond the limitation of skeletal and physical requirements resulting from an excessive accumulation of body fat

Protein-Energy Malnutrition (PEM)   The lack of sufficient energy or protein to meet the body's metabolic demands, resulting either from an inadequate dietary intake of protein, intake of poor quality dietary protein, increased demands for proteins caused by disease, or increased nutrient losses

Total Parenteral Nutrition (TPN)   The administration of nutrient by intravenous infusion; supplies all the necessary calories, water, amino acids, electrolytes, vitamins, minerals, and trace metals

---

Nutrition is the life-sustaining process by which elements of nature are assimilated and used (1) for growth and development, (2) for maintenance of healthy tissue, and (3) as mediators of physiological and metabolic processes. When good nutrition is lacking, impairments occur in immune function, wound healing, muscle and bone strength, and mental processes. The costs of medical care for a malnourished patient are directly related to length and frequency of hospitalization and pharmaceutical and medical supply costs.

Advances in feedings that are supplied directly to the gastrointestinal tract (**enteral nutrition** therapies) and the introduction of intravenous nutrition (**total parenteral nutrition [TPN]**) have revolutionized the field of clinical nutrition. Under most conditions, medical treatments now include therapies that are designed to prevent or correct nutritional deficiencies. However, because both excessive **nutrient** intakes and deficiencies negatively affect patient outcome, administration of nutrients in the proper proportions and at the proper time to ensure optimal nutritional status is still difficult. Therefore accurate and specific nutritional assessments and effective monitoring of nutritional therapies are of utmost importance. Biochemical and direct physical measurements are the most objective and quantitative measures of nutritional status.

Reliable nutrition tests and measurements are available that detect nutrient deficiencies, such as **protein-energy malnutrition (PEM),** before they have had a prolonged effect on biological function and before they are detected by physical examination. Consequently, laboratory tests are a component of nutrition assessments, identifying patients who can benefit from nutrition risk screening and planned interventions (monitoring) that satisfy the 1995 standards of the Joint Commission on Accreditation of Healthcare Organizations (JCAHO) standards.[4] (See Chapters 28 and 29 for detailed discussions of vitamins and trace elements, respectively.)

■ NUTRIENTS AND NUTRIENT REQUIREMENTS

In addition to energy, there are 40 dietary components recognized as essential for human metabolism (Table 45-1). Essential nutrients are categorized as *macronutrients* (needed in amounts of a gram or more per day); *micronutrients*

(needed in quantities of a milligram or less per day); and *conditionally essential nutrients* (may be macro or micro). Macronutrients are used primarily for energy metabolism and as sources of essential amino acids and fatty acids. Macronutrients serve as the backbone of all physiological processes involving proteins, sugars, eicosanoids, phospholipids, or steroids, including muscle contraction, enzyme catalysis, intracellular and intercellular communication, and vascular transport. Excessive intakes of macronutrients are associated with adverse consequences and the development of chronic disease states. Micronutrients generally function as gene activators, free-radical scavengers, or coenzymes or cofactors in metabolic reactions. Excessive intakes of micronutrients can result in toxicity. Nutrients classified as *conditionally essential* are compounds or elements needed by individuals who have lost the ability to absorb, retain, or synthesize such nutrients at an adequate rate because of factors such as immaturity, states of metabolic disorder, or during severe stress.

Recommended Dietary Allowances

Recommended dietary allowances (RDAs) are the essential nutrient intake levels that are adequate to meet the known nutrient needs of most healthy people.[10] The 1989 dietary

---

TABLE 45-1   Essential Nutrients in Human Metabolism

Water
Carbohydrates
Amino acids
  Threonine, tryptophan, valine, isoleucine, leucine, lysine, methionine, phenylalanine
Fatty acids
  Linoleic, linolenic
Vitamins
  Fat soluble: retinol (A), 25-hydroxycholecalciferol (D), α-tocopherol (E), phylloquinone (K)
  Water soluble: thiamine (B_1), riboflavin (B_2), pyridoxine (B_6), niacin (B_3), folic acid (M), cobalamin (B_{12}), biotin, pantothenic acid (B_5), ascorbic acid (C)
Minerals
  Sodium, potassium, calcium, magnesium, phosphorus, chloride
Trace elements
  Copper, chromium, iodine, iron, manganese, selenium, zinc, fluoride, molybdenum

TABLE 45-2 1989 Recommended Dietary Allowances

Nutrient	Men (25 to 50 Years)	Women (25 to 50 Years)
Vitamin A (μg RE)*	1000	800
Vitamin D (μg)†	5	5
Vitamin E (mg α-TE)‡	10	8
Vitamin K (μg)	80	65
Ascorbic acid (mg)	60	60
Thiamine (mg)	1.5	1.1
Riboflavin (mg)	1.7	1.3
Niacin (mg NE)§	19	15
Vitamin B_6 (mg)	2.0	1.6
Folate (μg)	200	180
Cobalamin (μg)	2.0	2.0
Calcium (mg)	800	800
Phosphorus (mg)	800	800
Magnesium (mg)	350	280
Iron (mg)	10	15
Zinc (mg)	15	12
Iodine (μg)	150	150
Selenium (μg)	70	55

Modified from National Academy of Sciences: Recommended Dietary Allowances, 10th edition, National Academy Press, Washington, DC, 1989.
RDAs are expressed as quantities of a nutrient recommended for a reference individual per day, where per day is intended to be the average intake during at least 3 days for nutrients with short biological half-lives, and for others (such as vitamins A and B_{12}), they are the average intakes during several months. Only a time-averaged intake needs to approximate the RDA in healthy individuals. RDAs also differ based on age and gender. The values given in this table are for individuals 25 to 50 years of age. (NOTE: RDAs are recommended levels of intake; they are set to exceed the requirements of most individuals.)
*Retinol equivalents: 1 RE = 1 μg retinol or 6 μg β-carotene.
†As cholecalciferol: 10 μg cholecalciferol = 400 IU of vitamin D.
‡α-Tocopherol equivalents: 1 mg d-α-tocopherol = 1 α-TE.
§Niacin equivalent: 1 NE = 1 mg of niacin or 60 mg of dietary tryptophan.

recommendations for adults 25 to 50 years of age are summarized in Table 45-2. In general the requirements of infants and children are equated with the levels that maintain a satisfactory rate of growth and development. RDAs for biotin, pantothenic acid, copper, and manganese also are available (see Chapters 28 and 29).

RDAs now are called *dietary reference intakes (DRIs)*, which is appropriate because the information has such broad applications. Three guidelines have been established, including *estimated average requirements (EARs)*, which are determined from the mean nutrient requirement for a specific age-sex category; *RDAs for an individual*, which will likely be calculated as the EAR plus two standard deviations needed to meet the biological need of 97.5% of the reference population; and the *maximum upper level* of intake known or predicted to be associated with a low risk for adverse effects. The DRIs will take into consideration the relationship between nutrient intake and the development of chronic diseases, creating recommendations for optimal intakes. The DRI approach focuses on health maintenance, which differs markedly from the RDA approach used previously, which focused on avoiding nutrient deficiencies. The DRIs will

also address nonessential but valuable components of food such as dietary fiber, carotenoids, phytoestrogens, and carnitine.

Micronutrient Needs of Patients

The micronutrient requirements of a person with an acute or a chronic illness are poorly understood. However, nutrients are required for wound healing or to fight infection, such as protein, ascorbic acid, or zinc, are needed in higher amounts. In addition, higher levels of ascorbic acid (500 to 1000 mg/day), thiamine (200 mg/day), and pyridoxine (20 mg/day) and higher levels of potassium, magnesium, zinc, and phosphate have been recommended for patients with sepsis.[14] Two to five times the RDA for most vitamins and minerals have been recommended for burn patients.[1]

Energy

Carbohydrates, lipids, proteins, and alcohol are dietary sources of energy. Proteins and carbohydrates yield 4 kcal/g (17 kJ/g), lipids yield 9 kcal/g (38 kJ/g), and alcohol yields 7 kcal/g (29 kJ/g). Foods typically contain varying proportions of carbohydrates, lipids, and proteins.

Carbohydrates are the primary source of energy for the body. Major food sources include breads, cereals, fruits, root crops, and sugars. At least 60 g of carbohydrate is needed daily by adults to provide exogenous glucose substrate for brain and red blood cell energy metabolism. An insufficient carbohydrate intake causes ketosis and accompanying malaise.

Energy needs are the sum of the energy required for basal needs (postabsorptive, resting conditions), activity, healing, and specific dynamic action (diet-induced thermogenesis). The metabolic rate measured under basal conditions is known as the *basal energy expenditure (BEE)* or **basal metabolic rate (BMR)**. The BEE is affected by body composition, sex, age, muscle tone, thyroid function, growth, and pregnancy. Metabolic adaptation to starvation also affects the BEE, often lowering energy needs to 50% of normal.

Various methods have been used to measure energy expenditure in healthy people and acutely ill patients (Table 45-3). In clinical practice the BEE (kilocalories per 24 hours) is most commonly estimated by use of the following regression equations:

$$BEE \text{ for a woman (kcal/24 hours)} = 655.096 \\ + 9.563 \text{ (W)} \\ + 1.85 \text{ (H)} \\ - 4.676 \text{ (A)} \quad (1)$$

$$BEE \text{ for a man (kcal/24 hours)} = 66.473 \\ + 13.752 \text{ (W)} \\ + 5.003 \text{ (H)} \\ - 6.755 \text{ (A)} \quad (2)$$

TABLE 45-3   Measurement of Energy Expenditure

Method	Parameter Measured	Principle
Direct calorimetry	Heat	The amount of heat produced by metabolism is a direct measure of energy expenditure.
Respiratory indirect calorimetry	Oxygen, carbon dioxide, and nitrogen	The metabolic rate determined by oxygen consumption, carbon dioxide production, and urinary nitrogen excretion corresponds with energy expenditure per m² per hour
Circulatory indirect calorimetry (Fick equation)	Cardiac output (liters per minute), arterial and mixed venous oxygen, and hemoglobin concentration	The resting energy expenditure is calculated from oxygen consumption and the known caloric value of oxygen.
Balance studies	Caloric intake, fecal losses, and body composition indexes	Changes in body energy stores (usually assessed as net weight change) occur with inadequate or excessive energy intake adjusted for the energy content of feces.
Double-labeled water	Oxygen and hydrogen stable isotope excretion in water and carbon dioxide	Orally administered $^2H_2{}^{18}O$ equilibrates with total body water within 3 hours. Deuterium (^2H) leaves as water, whereas oxygen-18 leaves as both water and exhaled carbon dioxide. The difference in total body water deuterium and oxygen-18 measured at two time intervals is therefore proportional to carbon dioxide production, from which energy expenditure can be calculated if the respiratory quotient is known.
Heart rate	Heart beats per minute	A portable heart monitor integrates beats per minute throughout the measurement period, creating a frequency histogram. The energy expenditure at each heart rate is determined by regression analysis and summed.

where

W = Weight in kilograms
H = Height in centimeters
A = Age in years

This formula estimates the BEE in individuals who have a normal body weight with an accuracy of ±10% to 15%. The formula grossly overestimates the energy requirements of obese people because of the low metabolic activity of adipose tissue. To estimate total energy needs, the BEE is multiplied by a factor between 1.1 and 2, depending on the person's activity level, extent of healing, and hypermetabolism after surgery or trauma. Administration of excessive calories has caused hepatic dysfunction, carbon dioxide retention, acidosis, and an inability to be weaned from mechanical ventilation.

Energy Deficiency

Chronically inadequate food intake or malabsorption leads to energy deficiency and weight loss. Intake of protein, vitamins, and minerals is often concomitantly inadequate, leading to multiple deficiencies. PEM describes the spectrum of clinical disorders caused by protein and energy deficiency. **Marasmus** and nonedematous PEM refer to the condition caused by a primary lack of dietary energy, a condition characterized by growth retardation, anemia, and fat and muscle wasting. In individuals with marasmus, starvation adaptations cause serum protein and electrolyte concentrations to remain within their normal reference intervals. **Kwashiorkor** and edematous PEM refer to the condition caused by severe protein deficiency in individuals with an adequate or

a marginally inadequate energy intake. The clinical symptoms of kwashiorkor include severe edema associated with a low serum albumin level, dermatosis, and mild wasting of fat and muscle. *Marasmic kwashiorkor* is a term that is used to describe two conditions, one that is characterized by a combination of chronic energy deficiency and chronic or acute protein deficits and one that develops when a chronically starved person undergoes additional stress (such as trauma, surgery, or infection). Marasmic kwashiorkor is characterized by severe depletion of muscle and adipose tissue, edema, and a low serum albumin level. Individuals with marasmic kwashiorkor have a poor prognosis because of the resulting immunoincompetence and poor wound healing.

Protein

Dietary amino acids (see Chapter 18) are needed to synthesize structural proteins, enzymes, antibodies, some hormones, and other metabolically active compounds. The protein requirement for healthy individuals is currently based on the sum of the requirements for the essential amino acids multiplied by a factor of 1.25 to account for inefficient utilization of mixed protein in the diet. Protein or amino acids are constantly lost in feces, sweat, and shedding of skin, hair, and nails. Excess amino acids are deaminated, and their carbon skeletons are used directly as a fuel source or in gluconeogenesis. In the absence of adequate carbohydrates, a larger percentage of dietary protein is used for gluconeogenesis.

Depletion of skeletal muscle and catabolism of visceral and plasma proteins occur during starvation. Complete starvation in an adult initially results in catabolism of approximately 75 g/day of body protein (12 to 15 g of nitrogen per day), which is equivalent to a daily 300-g loss of the body cell mass. In individuals experiencing starvation (with no other complications), protein is removed from skeletal and visceral tissues (including the heart, liver, kidneys, and diaphragm) in amounts proportional to their contribution to the total body mass and metabolic rate. Biochemically, a nonstressed person adapts to starvation by having a lower metabolic rate and using more of the stored lipids as an energy source, thereby reducing the rate of protein catabolism. A reduction in blood volume and an increase in biological half-life restore plasma protein concentrations to normal. However, starvation is fatal when body protein losses approach 30% to 40%.

Starvation accompanied by stress such as sepsis, trauma, or surgery accelerates the loss of skeletal proteins, with relative sparing of organ protein. Hypermetabolic individuals do not adapt to starvation. During an acute illness, endogenous amino acids are used for gluconeogenesis and the synthesis of acute-phase proteins, immune proteins, and proteins for wound repair. Prolonged insufficient nutrition in individuals who are metabolically stressed eventually compromises skeletal muscle and viscera size and function. Muscle depletion is attenuated by the provision of exogenous energy substrates to support protein synthetic needs. Recommendations for protein or amino acid intake in patients with hypermetabolism are 1.2 to 3 g/kg/day.

In clinical practice, whole-body protein levels are difficult to restore. For example, nutrition support has been unable to significantly increase whole-body protein levels of hospitalized critically ill patients and patients with malignant disease. In these situations, weight gain is primarily a result of water and fat accumulation. Anabolic stimuli, such as growth hormone and its mediator insulin-like growth factor 1 (IGF-1) or insulin, have been administered as adjunctive therapy with nutrition support to increase whole-body protein levels.

Alanine and glutamine are essential for hepatic gluconeogenesis and protein synthesis. These amino acids are synthesized de novo in skeletal muscle from branched-chain amino acids (BCAAs). However, increased catabolism of BCAAs occurs in muscle during states of hypermetabolism, such as sepsis and trauma, because of insulin resistance and reduced intracellular glucose levels.

The subsequent imbalance of hepatic amino acids impairs hepatic protein synthesis and increases amino acid oxidation for the release of energy. BCAA-enriched enteral feedings have been advocated for use in patients with hepatic encephalopathy as a means to normalize the plasma amino acid pattern (by reducing muscle breakdown and increasing protein synthesis) and competitively inhibiting false neurotransmitters (such as aromatic amino acids) across the blood-brain barrier.

Glutamine, the most abundant amino acid in the body, plays a central role in metabolic adaptation during severe illness, functioning as the principal carrier of nitrogen from skeletal muscle to visceral organs. Glutamine is also a preferred fuel for enterocytes, endothelial cells, renal tubular cells, and rapidly proliferating immune cells and a precursor in nucleotide and neurotransmitter synthesis. Increased glutamine utilization without supplementation results in an efflux of glutamine from skeletal muscle, subsequently impairing skeletal muscle protein synthesis, increasing skeletal muscle protein catabolism, and increasing urinary nitrogen loss. Glutamine supplementation is limited by its instability in aqueous solutions. This problem has been circumvented by supplementation with glutamine dipeptides or 2-oxoglutarate.

Evidence indicates that arginine becomes an indispensable amino acid under conditions of severe stress resulting from sepsis or trauma or under conditions caused by nitrogen overload. Arginine is integral to urea synthesis and is a precursor for the synthesis of polyamines, nucleic acids, and nitric oxide. Arginine supplementation in humans stimulates immune responses, enhances wound healing, and improves nitrogen balance. Combined administration of arginine, omega-3 (ω-3) fatty acids, and ribonucleic acids has been associated with a significant reduction in infectious and wound complications and a significant decrease in hospital stay duration.

Carnitine is an amino acid required for transport of long-chain fatty acids into mitochondria for β-oxidation and adenosine triphosphate (ATP) production. One third of the daily carnitine requirement of adult humans is met by endogenous synthesis, whereas two thirds is met by diet. Carnitine is synthesized in liver, kidney, and brain tissue and travels to other tissues through the blood. An increased rate of endogenous carnitine synthesis compensates for carnitine-deficient diets only if hepatic and renal functions are adequate. Carnitine deficiencies have been found in individuals with cirrhosis, renal failure, and long-term TPN or enteral nutritional therapy, as well as in premature infants. Foods with high carnitine contents include red meat, eggs, and dairy products. Enteral and parenteral nutrition formulas designed for adults do not contain carnitine. Symptoms of carnitine deficiency include weakness, hypotonia, growth failure, liver dysfunction and steatosis, and episodic hypoglycemia. Carnitine supplementation has been shown to restore plasma carnitine to normal levels.

Lipids and Essential Fatty Acids

Energy-releasing lipids include free fatty acids, neutral fats (monoglycerides, diglycerides, and triglycerides), phospholipids, and carbohydrate-containing glycolipids. Fat is considerably more energy dense than carbohydrate or protein, containing 9 kcal/g rather than 4 kcal/g. Dietary fat sources include vegetable oils; margarine; butter; nuts; seeds; and some dairy, meat, bakery, and snack food products. More than 95% of ingested fat is in the form of triglycerides. A high-fat diet has been associated with an increased incidence of atherosclerosis, **obesity,** and certain types of cancer (including colon, breast, and prostate). The average American consumes 34% of dietary calories as fat, which is 13% more than the amount that was consumed in 1910 and 75% more than the amount consumed in the early 1800s. However, today's fat consumption levels indicate a downward trend in fat intake that is partly attributable to the success of nutrition education programs and published dietary guidelines. A downward trend in both plasma cholesterol levels and coronary heart disease mortality has also occurred. The current recommendation of several major health organizations is for Americans to reduce their fat intake to 20% to 30% of their total calories. (See Chapter 24 for a discussion on the metabolism and pathogenesis of dietary fats.)

Fatty acids, the basic component of most complex lipids, are unbranched monocarboxylic acids with the chemical formula $CH_3(CH_2)_nCOOH$, where n is any number from 2 to 22 (see Table 24-2). Fatty acids differ in the number of double bonds present—fatty acids with no double bonds are saturated fatty acids; fatty acids with only one double bond are monounsaturated fatty acids; and fatty acids with two or more double bonds are polyunsaturated fatty acids. The position of the first double bond within the molecule also varies; fatty acids are categorized as being in either the ω-3 or n-3, ω-6 or n-6, ω-7 or n -7, ω-9 or n-9, or ω- or n-11 family. Fatty acids also differ in their physical and metabolic properties. Vegetable oils contain numerous long-chain (16 carbons or more) monounsaturated and polyunsaturated fatty acids, as well as shorter-chain fatty acids, and are liquid at room temperature. Lard contains relatively more highly saturated long-chain fatty acids and is solid at room temperature. Palmitic acid (16 carbon atoms: 0 double bonds, 16:0), stearic acid (18:0), oleic acid (18:1n-9), and linoleic acid (18:2n-6) together account for more than 90% of the fatty acids in the U.S. diet.

Humans are unable to incorporate a double bond between the third and fourth or sixth and seventh carbon atoms of a fatty acid and require dietary sources (about 2% to 4% of total calories) of linoleic and linolenic acids (the essential fatty acids). Linoleic acid is found in a variety of vegetable oils; corn and safflower oils are particularly good sources of linoleic acid. Rapeseed oil and leafy vegetables are good dietary sources of linolenic acid. Elongated and desaturated linoleic and linoleic acids form arachidonic acid (20:4n-6) and eicosapentaenoic acid (EPA, 20:5n-3), respectively. EPA can be further elongated and desaturated to form docosahexaenoic acid (DHA, 22:6n-3). Arachidonic acid, EPA, and DHA are readily incorporated into phospholipids. Arachidonic acid and EPA are the precursors of 2- and 3-series prostaglandins and thromboxanes, respectively and the 4- and 5-series leukotrienes, respectively. Humans are limited in their capacity to convert linolenic acid to EPA, therefore a dietary source of EPA is sometimes necessary to promote 3- and 5-series metabolites. Oils from marine food sources are the primary dietary source of EPA and DHA. A high dietary intake of fish and marine oils has been associated with a reduced risk of cardiovascular disease and chronic inflammatory diseases such as rheumatoid arthritis, psoriasis, and ulcerative colitis. The positive effects are thought to be attributable to the increased proportion of 3- and 5-series metabolites produced from EPAs that are less inflammatory and prone to promote platelet aggregation compared with the 2- and 4-series metabolites of arachidonic acid.

Essential fatty acid deficiency (EFAD) is characterized by dermatitis; immunoincompetence; anemia; thrombocytopenia; peripheral neuropathy; growth retardation; infertility; and cardiac, hepatic, and pulmonary dysfunctions. The most commonly used biochemical index of EFAD is a plasma phospholipid/eicosatrienoic acid (20:3n-9)/20:4n-6 ratio greater than 0.2. In the general population, EFAD is rare but in the early 1970s, linoleic acid deficiency occurred frequently in patients receiving TPN therapy. Few cases of EFAD in patients receiving TPN have been reported since the 1975 Food and Drug Administration (FDA) approval of inclusion of intravenous fat emulsions in TPN.

Some triglycerides have properties that make them preferred supplemental energy sources for hospitalized patients. Medium-chain triglycerides (triglycerides comprising 10 to 14 carbon fatty acids) are absorbed by passive diffusion across the wall of the small intestine without the aid of pancreatic enzyme hydrolysis. In addition, medium-chain triglycerides enter the mitochondria without carnitine as a carrier. Structured lipids (triglycerides synthesized with specific fatty acids esterified to specific carbons of the glycerol backbone) manipulate fatty acid balance and metabolic pathways. Enteral formulas containing medium-chain triglycerides and structured lipids are now available for patient use.

Diet Therapy

Because of the wealth of information produced during the past 50 years on the relationship between diet and the incidence of chronic disease, the U.S. government and other groups have proposed dietary guidelines aimed at reducing the risk of chronic disease in Americans. The 1995 Dietary Guidelines published by the U.S. Department of Agriculture and U.S. Department of Health and Human Services urge Americans to (1) eat a variety of foods; (2) balance the food eaten with physical activity for maintenance or improvement of body weight; (3) choose a diet with plenty of grain products, vegetables, and fruits; (4) choose a diet low in overall fat, saturated fat, and cholesterol; (5) choose a diet moderate in sugar; (6) choose a diet moderate in salt and sodium; and (7) moderate the consumption of alcoholic beverages. Official recommendations are for Americans to consume at least five servings of fruits and vegetables each day. Data from the 1989 to 1991 U.S. Department of Agriculture's Continuing Survey of Food Intakes by Individuals indicate that the mean numbers of servings of fruits and vegetables consumed by Americans are much less than recommended levels.

Many chronic diseases and risk factors are managed or controlled through manipulation of dietary factors on an individual basis. Examples include renal insufficiency (which can be managed through protein intake), renal failure (which can be managed through fluid and electrolyte intake), cirrhosis (which can be managed through fluid and sodium intake), diabetes (which can be managed through carbohydrate intake, meal timing, and weight control), hyperlipidemia (which can be managed through fat and cholesterol, carbohydrate, and fiber intake), hypertension (which can be managed through electrolyte intake and weight control), cholecystitis (which can be managed through fat intake), cystic fibrosis (which can be managed through fat, protein, and carbohydrate intake), inborn errors of metabolism such as phenylketonuria (which can be man-

aged through phenylalanine intake) and maple syrup urine disease (which can be managed through leucine, isoleucine, and valine intake), and celiac sprue (which can be managed through gluten intake). A patient's physician prescribes dietary change as part of the medical treatment of diet-responsive diseases. Dietary compliance is greatly enhanced through diet instruction and follow-up sessions with a registered dietitian.

■ NUTRITION SUPPORT

Individuals who are at risk for development of PEM or have preexisting protein-energy deficits and poor likelihood of recovery without deliberate interventions are candidates for nutrition support therapies. Nutrition support options include oral supplements, tube feedings, and parenteral nutrition. Figure 45-1 summarizes the decision-making process used to select the appropriate nutrition support modality.

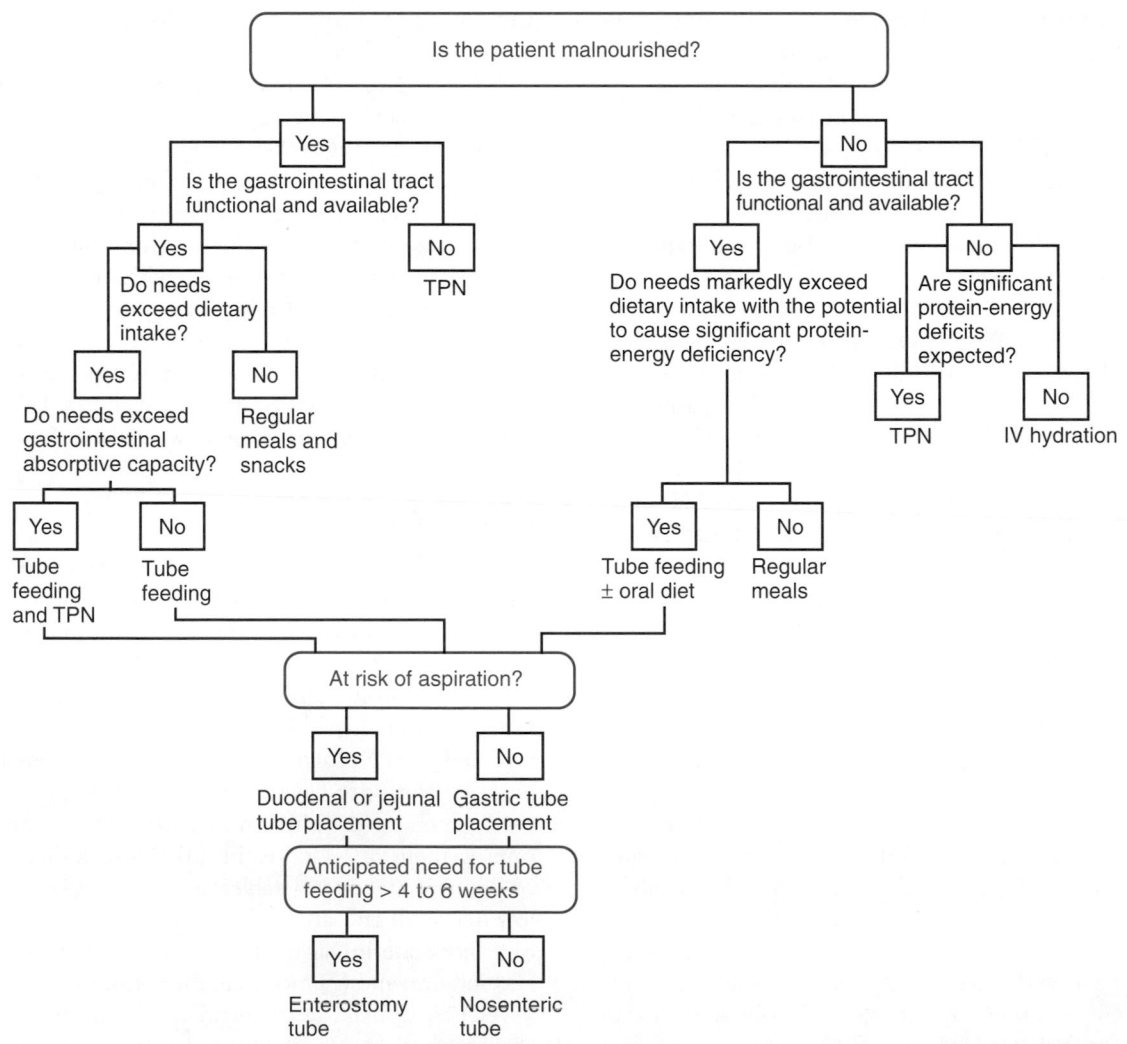

Figure 45-1   Decision tree used to select an appropriate nutrition support modality. *TPN,* Total parenteral nutrition.

Oral Supplementation

Patients who meet 50% to 75% of their estimated energy needs by consuming a normal diet are often able to achieve 100% of their needs by emphasizing intake of energy- and protein-dense foods. Common practice is to encourage the consumption of food items such as milk shakes, puddings, gravies, and sauces. Success with this approach depends on the patient's ability to digest large amounts of fat and lactose. Pharmaceutical companies make a variety of nutrient-dense, lactose-free products with various fat contents for oral supplementation. These products are used extensively in the hospital setting and usually are well tolerated by most patients.

Tube Feedings

Individuals who are unable to meet their maintenance or repletion protein-energy needs by oral supplementation and have a functional gastrointestinal tract can be nourished by administration of a liquid formula diet through a tube placed into the stomach or small intestine. Formula is pumped in at a constant rate (75 to 150 mL/hour for adults) for 8 to 24 hours or administered as a bolus into the stomach in 250- to 500-mL increments as needed. In general, continuous feedings are better tolerated by hospitalized patients. Bolus feedings are reserved for ambulatory, alert patients.

Formula selection depends on volume tolerance, nutrient and fluid needs, digestive capability, diameter of the feeding tube, and preferences of the patient or clinician. Whole foods may be homogenized in a blender, but commercially prepared products have largely replaced blended formulas. Many prepared formulas are available commercially that meet nearly all patient needs. Formulas range from 1 to 2 kcal/mL and have kilocalorie/gram nitrogen ratios of 75:1 to 200:1. Formulas are commonly lactose free because lactase deficiencies are prevalent in nonwhite patients and frequently develop transiently in patients of all races after abdominal surgery or trauma. Formulas composed of "predigested" nutrients such as amino acids, dipeptides, glucose oligosaccharides, and medium-chain triglycerides are available for patients with inadequate digestion or absorption, such as patients with pancreatic insufficiency or short bowel syndrome.

Feeding tubes may be orally, nasally, or surgically placed so that the tip (where formula is discharged) is in the stomach, duodenum, or jejunum. Nasogastric feeding tubes are used frequently for short-term nutrition support in noncomatose patients. Nasoduodenal feeding tubes are preferred for short-term use when the patient is at risk for gastroesophageal reflux, which can lead to pulmonary aspiration of formula and development of pneumonia. Unfortunately, placing and maintaining the tip of the feeding tube in the duodenum is difficult because of gastric motility. Gastrostomies or jejunostomies (using larger-diameter tubes) are preferred for long-term nutritional support.

Diarrhea is one of the most frequent complications of enteral nutrition, with an incidence ranging from 2% to 60%. Clinically defined, diarrhea is an increase in stool weight of more than 150 g in 24 hours or an increase in stool water of more than 1500 mL in 24 hours;[12] it may be osmotic or secretory in origin. Hypertonic formulas draw water into the gastrointestinal tract and cause an osmotic diarrhea in some patients.

Osmotic diarrhea may also be attributed to the administration of hyperosmolar drug solutions through the feeding tube. Secretory diarrhea may be caused by malabsorptive syndromes, gastrointestinal infections, metastatic carcinoid tumors, vasoactive intestinal peptide-secreting adenomas, and intestinal motility disorders. Fiber-containing formulas are available that have been associated with increased gastrointestinal transit time and reduced risk for diarrhea. Osmotic and secretory diarrhea are differentiated by use of the following formula to calculate the osmotic gap between the concentration of ions in the colonic fluid and the stool osmolality:

$$\text{Stool osmotic gap} = \text{stool osmolality} - 2\left([\text{stool Na}^+] + [\text{stool K}^+]\right) \quad (3)$$

Patients with osmotic diarrhea have a stool osmotic gap of greater than 160 mOsm/L, whereas those with secretory diarrhea have a stool osmotic gap of less than 160 mOsm/L (including negative values).

Other complications of enteral nutrition include nausea, vomiting, constipation, dehydration, and potential nutrient deficiencies. Long-term administration of elemental formulas has been associated with the development of copper and selenium deficiencies.

Laboratory monitoring of enteral nutrition support should include at least (1) measurement of baseline and daily serum electrolytes, glucose, blood urea nitrogen, and creatinine levels until stable (with weekly monitoring thereafter); (2) measurement of baseline and daily serum PO_4 and Mg levels until stable in patients at risk for refeeding syndrome or every-other-day monitoring until stable (with weekly monitoring of all patients thereafter); (3) measurement of baseline and weekly monitoring of serum albumin concentrations for evaluation of hydration status and as an index of patient prognosis; (4) measurement of baseline and every-other-day monitoring of serum transthyretin (TTR) concentrations until stable or until a trend has been positively established that ensures the adequacy of the nutrition support; and (5) measurement of baseline and every-other-day monitoring of C-reactive protein (CRP) levels in patients undergoing hypermetabolic stress responses for assistance in the interpretation of changes in TTR. Assessment of nitrogen balance and specific nutrients, such as ascorbic acid and zinc, is also recommended as needed.

Enteral nutrition support is preferred to parenteral nutrition for the patient who has at least a partially functional gastrointestinal tract. Intestinal integrity and function appear to be better maintained or enhanced through early initiation (within 12 to 24 hours of the injury or surgery) of enteral feeding and by the use of specialty formulas that include glutamine, arginine, nucleotides, and fish oil. Compared with TPN, enteral nutrition is associated with a more rapid return in hepatic transport protein synthesis (and normalization of plasma protein concentrations) after injury or surgery.

Parenteral Nutrition

Intravenous nutrient solutions became available for clinical use in humans in the early 1970s. The terms *hyperalimentation, TPN, parenteral nutrition support,* and *parenteral feeding* have all been used to describe this type of therapy.

Parenteral nutrition bypasses gastrointestinal digestion and absorption by delivering predigested energy and protein sources as well as essential fatty acids, vitamins, and minerals directly to the venous system. This approach to nutrition support is valuable in the management of gastrointestinal disorders in patients who need bowel rest, such as those with gastrointestinal obstructions or fistulas. Supplemental use of TPN is helpful for patients with compromised or inadequate intestinal function, such as patients with Crohn's disease or short bowel syndrome. TPN has also been used in the postoperative period in patients with prolonged paralytic ileus; however, these patients usually can be fed enterally if a feeding tube is placed in the small bowel during the surgical procedure. Poor nutritional status prolongs ileus, causing further nutritional decline and an increased risk of postoperative complications if nutritional needs are not met by either enteral or parenteral nutrition.

Dextrose (glucose) is the major energy source for TPN solutions. Most patients tolerate 1 L of 50% dextrose every 24 hours without complications. Lipid emulsion is an alternative energy source in patients with glucose intolerance or poor carbon dioxide clearance. When used as a source of energy for critically ill patients, 15% to 50% of total energy may be supplied as fat. Under extenuating circumstances such as respiratory failure, extreme glucose intolerance, and hypervolemia, up to 60% of the total energy intake can be supplied as fat. However, to prevent the fat overload syndrome, the maximum intravenous fat intake should not exceed 2.5 g/kg/day. The fat overload syndrome is potentially lethal, causing lipemic serum, massive fat deposition in the lungs and liver, spleen and reticuloendothelial blockaded, sepsis, and thrombocytopenia. To prevent fatty acid deficiencies, linoleic acid must be provided as 2% to 4% of the total energy intake. Because of potential intolerance, the plasma triglyceride level should be checked before the initial infusion and repeated 6 hours after the lipid infusion is complete.

Protein is supplied in TPN as 5.5%, 8.5%, 10%, or 15% solutions of crystalline amino acids. The caloric density of crystalline amino acids is 4 kcal/g. The nitrogen content of crystalline amino acids is 5% higher than that in a typical diet because of the select mixture of amino acids.

Vitamins and trace minerals are routinely added to daily TPN formulations; however, the amounts may not be adequate for all patients. Chromium deficiency occurs in parenterally fed patients, partly because of the suboptimal chromium status of the general population. In addition, the suboptimal chromium status is exacerbated in TPN patients because of elevated urinary losses associated with high glucose infusions and stress conditions and the variable chromium content of parenteral products. Similarly, the amount of selenium routinely added may be inadequate for patients receiving long-term TPN because of increased urinary selenium excretion. Copper deficiency that presents as pancytopenia has been seen after 15 months of TPN. Vitamin K is not included in the standard vitamin preparations manufactured for TPN because of frequent contraindications in patients receiving warfarin. Patients with gastrointestinal fluid losses may have increased zinc requirements and should receive additional zinc in their TPN. Zinc and chromium are eliminated by renal excretion and should be administered cautiously to patients with renal dysfunction to avoid toxicity.

Laboratory monitoring of parenteral nutrition support is similar to that described previously for enteral nutrition, with the following additional recommendations. Serum glucose levels are more closely monitored in TPN patients, commonly every 6 hours until tolerance is established. A baseline and every-other-day ionized calcium levels in serum are recommended in critically ill patients until they are stable because of the inherent calcium-phosphorus imbalance in TPN solutions resulting from the tendency of calcium-phosphorus salts to precipitate. Liver enzymes (alkaline phosphatase, aspartate aminotransferase, and total bilirubin) are monitored weekly to detect TPN-induced hepatic damage or symptomatic cholestasis. Serum triglyceride levels are monitored before and 6 hours after an initial infusion of parenteral lipids to ensure clearance; they are monitored periodically thereafter. Prothrombin time should be monitored weekly to ensure adequacy of vitamin K supplementation.

Refeeding Syndrome

Starved or severely malnourished patients can experience life-threatening fluid and electrolyte shifts after the initiation of aggressive nutrition support therapies. This phenomenon is known as the *refeeding syndrome* and has developed in patients receiving either enteral or parenteral nutrition support. Patients at risk for development of refeeding syndrome include those with classic kwashiorkor, marasmus, or anorexia nervosa, or a history of chronic undernutrition, chronic alcoholism, or massive weight loss. To prevent the development of the syndrome, nutrition support for patients at risk should be increased slowly but should still provide adequate amounts of vitamins and minerals. Organ function, fluid balance, and serum electrolyte levels (especially of phosphorus, potassium, and magnesium) need to be monitored daily during the first week of enteral tube feeding or TPN and less often thereafter.

CLINICAL NUTRITION ASSESSMENT

The objectives of a clinical nutrition assessment are to (1) identify patients who will benefit from nutrition interventions, (2) determine baseline values by which to measure the effectiveness of nutrition therapies, and (3) detect and treat macronutrient and micronutrient deficiencies.

Nutrition assessment in the hospital setting begins with screening to identify newly admitted patients with existing **malnutrition** or at risk for development of malnutrition and its associated complications.[5] Patients identified as malnourished (Table 45-4) or at risk subsequently receive a comprehensive nutrition assessment by a registered dietitian, beginning with a thorough history and physical examination. The history should include specific questions concerning usual body weight, recent weight changes, dietary habits (including frequency and amount of alcohol consumption), appetite, gastrointestinal function, the use of vitamin and mineral supplements, and the use of drugs that could interfere with nutrient absorption or utilization.[6] A complete history alerts the dietitian to potential underlying energy, protein, vitamin, or mineral deficiencies. The physi-

TABLE 45-4	Physical Signs Suggestive of Malnutrition	
Organ	Signs Associated with Malnutrition	Deficiency
Hair	Lack of luster, thinness, sparseness, easy pluckability, abnormal pigmentation, alternating bands of light and dark	Energy, protein
Face	Nasolabial seborrhea, diffuse depigmentation	Riboflavin
	Paleness	Iron
Eyes	Pale conjunctiva	Iron
	Poor dark adaptation, Bitot's spots, corneal or conjunctival xerosis, papilledema	Retinol
	Angular blepharitis	Riboflavin, niacin
	Intraocular hemorrhage	Ascorbic acid
Lips	Bilateral angular stomatitis	Riboflavin
	Cheilosis	Niacin or riboflavin
Tongue	Scarlet and raw tongue	Niacin
	Magenta tongue	Riboflavin
	Glossitis (beefy, red tongue)	Folic acid, niacin, riboflavin, cobalamin, iron
	Atrophic filiform papilla (slick tongue)	Niacin, folate, riboflavin, iron, cobalamin
Teeth	Mottled enamel, caries	Fluoride
Gums	Paleness	Iron
	Sponginess, bleeding	Ascorbic acid
Endocrine system	Thyroid enlargement	Iodine
	Parotid enlargement	Protein
Skin	Purpura	Vitamin K
	Hyperpigmentation	Energy, cobalamin, folic acid, niacin
	Desquamatory dermatitis	Biotin, essential fatty acids, zinc, pyridoxine
	Follicular hyperkeratosis, xerosis, mosaic dermatosis	Retinol, essential fatty acids
	Petechial hemorrhages	Ascorbic acid
	Thickening and pigmentation of pressure points and areas exposed to sunlight	Niacin
	Scrotal and vulval dermatosis	Riboflavin
Nails	Koilonychia (spoon nail), paleness	Iron
Subcutaneous tissue	Decreases or increases in fat	Energy (deficit or surfeit)
	Edema	Protein, thiamine
Musculoskeletal system	Wasting	Energy, protein
	Craniotabes, frontal bossing, knock knees, beading of ribs, bow legs	Vitamin D
	Musculoskeletal hemorrhage	Ascorbic acid
Cardiovascular system	Cardiomegaly, tachycardia, congestive heart failure, wet beriberi	Thiamine
Nervous system	Mental confusion, encephalopathy	Thiamine, protein
	Calf tenderness, sensory loss, motor weakness, dry beriberi	Thiamine
	Bilateral loss of ankle and knee jerks	Thiamine, cobalamin
Gastrointestinal system	Hepatomegaly	Protein

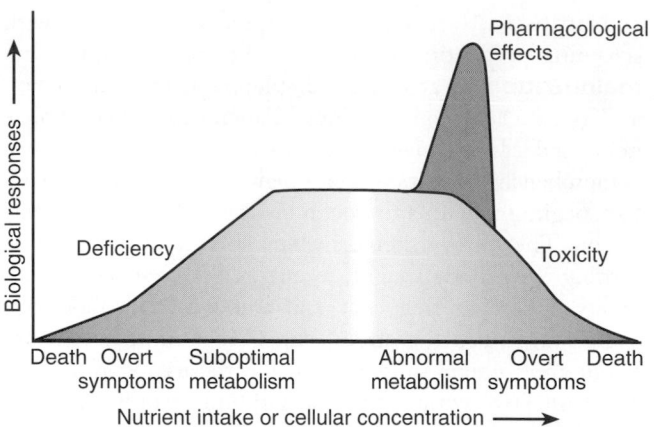

Figure 45-2 Physiological continuum of an essential nutrient. High intakes of some nutrients (such as niacin) cause pharmacological effects; the resulting biological response may not be related to the physiological function of the nutrient at normal intake levels.

cal examination reveals overt symptoms of nutrient deficiencies. Although frank deficiencies are seen today, they are rare in developed nations. More common is a patient with a general appearance of poor health and subcutaneous fat and muscle wasting. However, suboptimal nutrient stores have adverse biochemical effects before any overt clinical symptoms develop. Therefore a nutritional assessment should take into account the physiological continuum from frank deficiency to toxicity, with optimal status being somewhere between these extremes (Figure 45-2). Suspected micronutrient deficiencies are often confirmed by laboratory testing.

Numerous methods are available for the evaluation of PEM, including measurements of body composition, muscle function, and biochemical tests. (See Chapters 28 and 29 for a discussion of laboratory tests used to evaluate micronutrient status.)

Measurements of Body Composition

Measuring body composition has proven to be useful in monitoring of nutritional status because of the marked changes in body composition that occur in individuals with malnutrition.[3,15] Body composition methods differ in ease of determination, accuracy, total cost, and applicability to the hospital setting. Methods used to determine body composition have been used extensively to assess the response to exercise and weight-reducing therapy and to assess various disease states.

Body composition is described at the atomic, molecular, cellular, tissue-system, and whole-body levels.[15] At the atomic level, approximately 50 elements are found in the human body, with oxygen, carbon, hydrogen, calcium, nitrogen, and phosphorus accounting for more than 98% of body weight. Oxygen itself constitutes more than 60% of the total body mass. The 11 principal elements found in the human body (oxygen, carbon, hydrogen, nitrogen, calcium, phosphorus, potassium, sulfur, sodium, chlorine, and magnesium) form more than 100,000 chemical compounds, which have been grouped at the molecular level into the following categories: water, lipid, protein, mineral, and glycogen. Lipids are further classified as functionally essential (such as sphingomyelin and phospholipids in cell membranes) and nonessential (such as stored triglycerides). *Lean body mass (LBM)* is the body weight minus the nonessential lipid weight. Body composition described at the cellular level is divided into three main categories: (1) cells (connective, epithelial, nervous, and muscular), (2) extracellular fluid (plasma and interstitial), and (3) extracellular solids (primarily collagen, elastin, and calcium hydroxyapatite). *Body cell mass* is a term frequently used to describe the metabolically active portion of the body that is responsible for essentially all oxygen consumption and carbon dioxide production. Therefore, body cell mass does not include stored triglycerides that occupy 85% to 90% of adipocyte weight and the extracellular mass (solids and fluids).

Components of the cellular level are organized into tissues, organs, and systems in the fourth level of body composition, the tissue-system level. Tissues are grouped into four categories: muscular, connective, epithelial, and nervous. Organs consist of two or more tissues combined to form large functional units such as skin, kidneys, and blood vessels. Systems comprise several organs whose functions are interrelated (for example, the digestive system, which includes the esophagus, stomach, intestine, liver, and pancreas).

Nine main systems are found in the human body: the musculoskeletal, skin, nervous, circulatory, respiratory, digestive, urinary, endocrine, and reproductive systems. Body composition at the whole-body level involves body size, shape, and exterior and physical characteristics. Frequently used dimensional measurements of the body include stature, segment lengths (such as of the thigh length or elbow-wrist length), body breadths (such as of the elbow or ankle), circumferences (such as of the upper arm, waist, or thigh), skinfold thickness (such as of the triceps), body surface area, body volume, body weight, **body mass index (BMI),** and body density. Methods used to quantify body composition are described in Table 45-5. Methods of body composition measurement are categorized as direct, indirect, or doubly indirect.[3] Indirect methods rely on data obtained by direct chemical cadaver analysis. Doubly indirect methods are generally based on a statistical relationship between easily measurable body parameters and data obtained by direct or indirect methods.[16]

Anthropometric Measurements

Anthropometric methods used in nutritional assessments include measurements of body weight and skinfold thick-

TABLE 45-5   **Body Composition Measurement Methods**

Level	Component Measured	Method Category	Method	Principle
Atomic	Individual elements	Direct	Whole-body or tissue ash analysis	This method is the traditional approach to elemental analysis using human cadavers.
	Potassium	Direct	Whole-body potassium-40 counting	γ-Rays (1.46 MeV) emitted by potassium-40, a naturally occurring isotope that exists in the body at a known natural abundance (0.012%) are counted.
	Hydrogen, carbon, sodium, phosphorus, and potassium	Direct	MRI	Atomic nuclei, attempting to align with an external magnetic field, are simultaneously activated by a radiofrequency wave. When the radio wave is turned off, the activated nuclei emit the signal absorbed, which is used to produce an image by computer.
	Sodium, chlorine, calcium, phosphorus, magnesium, and nitrogen	Direct	Neutron activation analysis	The body is bombarded with fast neutrons of a known energy level, which are captured by specific elements forming unstable isotopes such as calcium-40 and nitrogen-15. The isotopes naturally revert to a stable condition by emitting one or more γ-rays of characteristic energy. The energy level identifies the element, and the level of activity indicates its abundance.
Molecular	Total body water	Indirect	Isotope dilution	Water is not present in stored fat and occupies about 73% of the fat-free mass; therefore the plasma equilibrium concentration of injected or ingested isotopically labeled water (deuterium oxide [D_2O], tritiated water [^3H_2O] and water [H_2O^{18}]) represents the total body water after correction for urinary loss of the tracer.
	Osseous mineral and LBM	Indirect	Whole-body dual-photon absorptiometry	The body's entire length is scanned by radiation from ^{153}Gd, which emits two γ-rays of different energies (44 and 100 keV). Measurement of γ-ray attenuation allows for quantitation of bone mineral and soft tissue. The ratio of attenuation at 44 to 100 keV indicates the fat content of the soft tissue, from which the percent body fat and LBM are derived.
	Protein	Indirect	Neutron-activation analysis for nitrogen	See previous entry; protein is estimated assuming that 16% of protein is nitrogen.
	Bone mineral; fat; bone mineral-, fat-free lean	Indirect	Dual-energy x-ray absorptiometry	Photons at two energy levels (40 and 70 KeV) are passed through tissue. X-ray attenuation is related to elemental composition.
Cellular	BCM (LBM)	Indirect	Whole-body potassium-40 counting	Potassium is essentially an intracellular cation that is not present in stored triglycerides with an estimated concentration of 2.28 to 2.66 g K/kg LBM.
	BCM	Indirect	Potassium isotope dilution	98% of potassium is found intracellularly. The plasma equilibrium concentration of an administered isotope therefore reflects the BCM.
	Extracellular fluid	Indirect	Sodium radioisotope dilution	Sodium is the principal extracellular cation. The plasma equilibrium concentration of injected or ingested sodium-22 represents the extracellular fluid after correction for urinary loss of the tracer.

BCM, Body cell mass; *CT,* computed tomography; *LBM,* lean body mass; *3-MH,* 3-methylhistidine; *MRI,* magnetic resonance imaging.   *Continued*

TABLE 45-5   Body Composition Measurement Methods—cont'd

Level	Component Measured	Method Category	Method	Principle
Tissue system	Subcutaneous and visceral adipose, skeletal muscle mass, organ size	Indirect	CT	High-resolution cross-sectional images are produced by attenuation in x-rays related to differences in tissue density. Integration of sequential images is used to quantify fat, lean tissue, and bone.
		Indirect	MRI	See previous entry; integration of sequential cross-sectional images is used to quantify fat, lean tissue, and bone based on characteristic chemical composition.
	Adipose tissue mass	Doubly indirect	Infrared	An infrared light beam is used to penetrate tissue to a depth of about 1 cm. The absorptive, reflective, and transmissive properties of the tissue depend on the tissue's composition.
	Skeletal muscle mass	Indirect	Whole-body postassium-40 counting and neutron activation nitrogen analysis	Total-body potassium and nitrogen data are used together to calculate skeletal muscle mass based on the known and constant potassium/nitrogen ratios in skeletal muscle and nonskeletal muscle lean mass of 3.03 mmol/g and 1.33 mmol/g, respectively.
		Doubly indirect	24-h urinary creatinine excretion	Creatinine is produced during the dephosphorylation of creatine phosphate, which is primarily located in skeletal muscle. Creatinine is excreted in the urine at a daily rate of about 1 g per 20 kg skeletal muscle.
		Doubly indirect	24-h urinary 3-MH excretion	3-MH is a modified amino acid produced posttranslationally on actin and myosin. It is released from skeletal muscle during normal myofibrillar protein turnover and excreted in urine.
Whole body	Growth, LBM, percent of adipose tissue, metabolic rate	Doubly indirect	Dimensional body measurements	Mathematical relationships between dimensional measurements and body composition have been described and validated.
	Skeletal muscle and adipose mass	Doubly indirect	Ultrasound	High-frequency ultrasonic energy is transmitted into the body in short pulses. Part of the energy is reflected as it intercepts tissues that differ in acoustical properties. Depth readings of changes in tissue density allow measurement of skinfold thicknesses.
	Total body water (LBM)	Doubly indirect	Bioelectrical impedance analysis	A 50-kHz alternating electrical current is applied to the extremities, and the tissue-induced impedance (or resistance) change is recorded by a detector. Only water and dissolved electrolytes conduct the current. Impedance is directly related to the proportion of fat mass and body water distribution. LBM is calculated under the assumption that LBM is about 73% water.
	Percent body fat	Indirect	Whole-body densitometry	Archimedes' principle; the difference between mass in air and mass in water corrected for water temperature and lung volume is used to calculate body volume and density. Percent body fat is calculated from the known density of adipose (0.9 g/cm^3) and LBM (1.1 g/cm^3).

BCM, Body cell mass; *CT,* computed tomography; *LBM,* lean body mass; *3-MH,* 3-methylhistidine; *MRI,* magnetic resonance imaging.

ness. Details of these physical methods are found in Table 45-5 and in an expanded version of this chapter.[14]

Biochemical Measurements

After protein-energy reserves are assessed, protein-energy requirements estimated, and nutrition support therapies initiated, determination of the adequacy of prescribed therapy is necessary. Biochemical markers identify when anabolism has been induced before measurable improvements in body composition occur. The ideal biochemical protein-energy markers should have (1) a short biological half-life, (2) exist primarily within an accessible body fluid, (3) have limited homeostatic regulation and a constant catabolic rate, and (4) be unaffected by vitamin or mineral status or pathophysiological states. Because an ideal marker does not exist, analytes that are affected by several factors that include protein-energy balance are often used to monitor protein-energy status. The following are common biochemical protein-energy balance markers.

Urinary creatinine and creatinine/height index

Creatinine is a normal waste product of muscle energy metabolism formed by the nonenzymatic hydrolysis of free creatine liberated during the dephosphorylation of creatine phosphate. The 24-hour urinary creatinine excretion level correlates well with total body muscle mass in people with normal renal function, sufficient food intake, and a diet of constant composition. Creatinine excretion declines with age and is increased by acute infection, injury, severe emotional stress, rigorous exercise, and diets high in protein, creatine, and creatinine.

The CHI is used to determine the size of muscle mass. With this parameter, an individual's 24-hour urinary creatinine content subsequently is compared with standard values for a given height, sex, and age, as shown in the following CHI equation:

$$CHI = \frac{mg\ creatinine/24\ hours\ (patient)}{mg\ creatinine/24\ hours\ (control)} \times 100 \qquad (4)$$

A decrease in muscle mass is reflected in a proportionate decrease in the CHI. Index values of 80% to 90% are indicative of mild muscle mass depletion; values of 70% to 80% indicate moderate depletion; values less than 70% are evidence of severe depletion.

Endogenous 3-methylhistidine excretion

The measurement of 3-MH formation and excretion has been used as a simple test to estimate skeletal muscle mass. Posttranslational methylation of specific histidine residues in muscle fiber actin and in white muscle fiber myosin produces 3-MH. As a consequence of normal myofibrillar protein turnover, 3-MH is released and subsequently excreted

in the urine in amounts proportional to total body skeletal muscle mass as determined by densitometry and indirect measurements of total body nitrogen and potassium levels. The 3-MH excretion test has been shown to predict the LBM with an error of approximately ±4 kg in the range of 50 to 82 kg, versus the approximately ±5-kg error associated with creatinine excretion tests.

Use of the 3-MH excretion test to predict skeletal muscle mass in the acute care setting is limited by several factors. Sepsis, trauma, steroid administration, or starvation accelerates protein degradation and thereby disproportionately increase 3-MH excretion. Therefore 3-MH excretion should be normalized for creatinine excretion and body weight before it is used as a marker of skeletal muscle catabolism and thus adequacy of nutrition therapy. The excretion of 3-MH also is significantly higher in individuals who eat meat, and individuals who are tested must follow a relatively controlled, meat-free diet. This requirement is easily met in patients receiving tube feeding or parenteral nutrition. Some concern exists over the contribution of nonskeletal muscle 3-MH efflux (gastrointestinal and dermal), especially in surgical or trauma cases. Finally, reference intervals are inadequate for the evaluation of individual 3-MH excretion levels.

Methods used to measure 3-MH include ion exchange chromatography with either a ninhydrin or ninhydrin orthophthalaldehyde postcolumn reactor or by high performance liquid chromatography (HPLC) with precolumn derivatization with fluorescamine.

Plasma proteins

Several plasma proteins of hepatic origin have been used as markers of nutritional status.[9] During relatively short periods of inadequate dietary protein or energy intake (as opposed to chronic starvation), a reduction in hepatic synthesis and secretion of these proteins causes plasma levels to fall. Reinstitution of an adequate diet induces protein synthesis, returning plasma concentrations to normal. In individuals with chronic starvation, the opposite effects occur; a reduced rate of protein catabolism and a reduction in blood volume tend to keep plasma protein concentrations within the normal reference interval. The rate of change in a protein's plasma concentration in response to nutritional inadequacy depends in part on the protein's biological half-life.

Plasma protein concentrations are also influenced by nonnutritional factors, including (1) normal biological variation, (2) physiological function, (3) physiological and pathological consumption; (4) hydration status; (5) patient posture at the time of phlebotomy; (6) hepatic and renal function (which can alter synthetic and catabolic rates); (7) drug or hormone therapy; and (8) inflammatory disease. Consequently, the effects of these factors must be considered in the nutritional interpretation of protein levels.

Acute-phase proteins

Several acute-phase proteins, such as ceruloplasmin, fibrinogen, α_1-antitrypsin, CRP, and α_1-acid glycoprotein (AAP) have been evaluated as indicators of protein-energy status. Like the transport proteins, plasma levels of acute-phase proteins decrease when an individual becomes protein-energy deprived and rise in response to adequate support. However, because synthesis of these proteins is greatly increased by inflammatory disease, their use as nutritional markers is limited and has no advantage over TTR.

Albumin

Albumin is the most commonly measured plasma protein for evaluation of PEM.[9] It is present in the highest concentration of all plasma proteins, usually representing more than 50% of total plasma protein (see Chapter 19). Albumin is vital for regulating osmotic pressure and water balance and stabilizing blood volume. Any sizable loss of albumin reduces blood osmolality, leading to edema. Albumin also serves as a transport protein for bilirubin, fatty acids, cortisol, thyroxin, and many drugs. Protein deficiencies (when no other complications are present) causes albumin concentrations to decrease. The values for mild, moderate, and severe depletion are usually 28 to 35, 21 to 27, and less than 21 g/L, respectively. Surveys have found hypoalbuminemia to be a sensitive prognostic indicator of morbidity, mortality, and increased length of stay among hospitalized patients. Albumin's predictive ability as a nutritional marker is compromised because it decreases in concentration during inflammatory disease, with levels corresponding to the severity of insult and degree of hypermetabolism. In addition, albumin is a poor indicator of the adequacy of recent nutritional intake because of its long half-life (18 to 20 days) and the multiple nonnutritional factors that alter or maintain its plasma concentration. Albumin has a large extravascular pool ($1\frac{1}{2}$ to 2 times the amount in blood) that tends to cause its plasma levels to remain steady during periods of reduced synthesis. Administration of exogenous human albumin, used to help mobilize extravascular fluids, raises serum albumin levels and thus negates its value as a marker of nutritional progress. Other factors result in a decrease in serum albumin levels; for example, albumin is lost from the intravascular compartment during conditions involving increased capillary permeability, such as hepatic cirrhosis (ascites) or inflammation, and it is lost from the extravascular compartment in burn or wound exudates. Various methods are used to quantify serum albumin (see Chapter 19).

Insulin-like growth factor 1

IGF-1 may be a superior protein-energy balance marker because of its sensitivity to nutritional adequacy and independence from the effects of inflammatory disease.[11] Serum IGF-1 levels have been shown to correlate positively with nitrogen balance during an inflammatory disease, whereas a relationship between TTR and nitrogen balance is abolished. IGF-1 is synthesized by various cell types, but most circulating IGF-1 is of hepatic origin. IGF-1 is not subject to diurnal variation or affected by changes in sleep, exercise, or circulating levels of nutrients. However, IGF-1's clinical application is currently limited because of the few available analytical methods and associated costs.

Retinol-binding protein

Serum retinol-binding protein (RBP) levels correlate with protein-energy status in uncomplicated PEM.[8] However, the circulating level of RBP is strongly influenced by its glomerular filtration rate and by the metabolic response to injury and infection (MRII). Hepatic secretion of RBP depends on adequate retinol status. Retinol deficiency is considered rare in the general U.S. population; however, the retinol status of hospitalized patients has not been adequately studied and feasibly could influence serum RBP levels. High serum RBP levels are associated with renal impairment and acute or early liver damage caused by release of hepatic RBP stores. Both TTR and RBP are measured by radial immunodiffusion, rocket electroimmunoassay, turbidimetry, and nephelometric immunoassay (see Chapter 10).

Transferrin

Several studies have shown transferrin, which has a half-life of 8 days, to be a sensitive protein-energy balance marker and a prognostic indicator. Transferrin has a small extravascular pool, making its plasma concentrations more sensitive than albumin to decreases in hepatic synthetic rates. However, the use of transferrin as a nutritional marker is complicated by the opposing effects of iron deficiency. In response to iron deficiency (the most common nutrient deficiency in affluent countries), the liver increases transferrin synthesis and secretion. When a patient is iron and protein deficient, transferrin levels may remain within the normal reference interval. Transferrin can be measured by several methods, including radial immunodiffusion, turbidimetry, and nephelometric immunoassay (see Chapter 10). Transferrin is also estimated from total iron-binding capacity.

Transthyretin

TTR (formerly known as "prealbumin" and "thyroxine-binding prealbumin") has a relatively short half-life of 1 to 2 days, enabling it to respond rapidly to nutritional adequacy. Consequently, TTR has become a frequently assayed protein for the assessment of PEM.[9] The high tryptophan content and high ratio of essential to nonessential amino acids of TTR make its plasma concentration sensitive to the quality of protein provided. TTR transports thyroxin and also complexes in plasma with the low–molecular-weight RBP, helping to prevent glomerular filtration and subsequent loss of RBP and retinol. TTR synthesis and secretion require adequate zinc. The circulating level of TTR is affected by the availability of its transport ligand, thyroxine (mainly triiodothyronine [T_3]). Consequently, in conditions in which the circulating level of T_3 is decreased (such as hypothyroidism), the use of TTR as a nutritional marker may be compromised. After abatement of the inflammatory disease, plasma TTR can be used for nutritional monitoring. TTR concentrations have been shown to increase more than 4 mg/dL/wk in patients given optimal nutrition support.[13] However, persistent sepsis, adult respiratory distress syndrome, and purulent abscesses preclude the return to normal concentrations. Elevated TTR concentrations are associated with renal insufficiency (reduced catabolism) and steroid administration.

Combined assay

A combined assay of acute-phase proteins, albumin, and TTR has been used as a means to discriminate between nutritional deprivation and metabolic stress.[7] Their prognostic inflammatory and nutrition index (PINI) is calculated according to the following formula:

$$PINI = \frac{\alpha_1\text{-AGP (g/L)} \times \text{CPR (g/L)}}{\text{albumin (g/L)} \times \text{TTR (g/L)}} \quad (5)$$

Infection-free, well-nourished individuals have PINI values of less than 1. Low-, medium-, and high-risk patients have values of 1 to 10, 11 to 20, and 21 to 30, respectively. This index has been validated in children, adults, and older patients, but further evaluation is needed before it is recommended for general usage.

Monitoring protein-energy balance

Monitoring changes in protein-energy balance by use of plasma protein concentrations requires an appreciation of the expected biological and analytical variations for the chosen analytes. A statistically significant difference, or critical difference (CD), between two successive values is calculated from the analytical coefficient of variation (CV_a) and the intraindividual coefficient of variation (CV_i) according to the following formula:

$$CD\ (\%) = 2^{1/2} \times Z \times (CV_i^2 + CV_a^2)^{1/2} \quad (6)$$

where Z is the *Z-score*, or the number of standard deviations appropriate for a chosen level of probability (P; P usually equal to 0.05). The CD for the plasma proteins albumin and TTR have been determined to be 8% and 32% respectively.[2] Thus plasma albumin must change by at least 8% or TTR by at least 32% to confirm that the change is attributable to improvements in nutritional health rather than expected daily variations. The absolute amount of change required is reduced by serial monitoring (three or more sequential observations). Three or four observations of TTR reduce the absolute change required (with P equal to 0.05) between each observation to 12% or 6%, respectively; 24% and 18% changes are required for the entire observational period. Similarly, use of two or more proteins simultaneously reduces the CDs required by each protein. Unfortunately, albumin's long biological half-life makes it unsuitable for this application.

Nitrogen balance studies

Nitrogen balance is the difference between dietary nitrogen intake and excretion (or losses) and is widely used as an index of protein requirements. In clinical practice, nitrogen intake is considered to be 16% of dietary protein or 16.8% of crystalline amino acids (which is used in parenteral nutrition therapy). Nitrogen excretion occurs mainly in urine, but appreciable amounts of nitrogen may be lost in feces, skin, exudates, or drainage. An accurate and precise nitrogen balance must account for all routes and types of nitrogen loss.

In the absence of diarrhea or abnormal routes of nitrogen loss, nitrogen balance (NB) is calculated as follows:

NB = 24-hour nitrogen intake (g) −
        [24-hour total urine nitrogen (g) + 2 g]   (7)

NOTE: The 2 g of nitrogen is added to the measured 24-hour total urinary nitrogen level to account for average skin sloughing and fecal losses.) Because complete 24-hour urine collections are difficult to obtain, clinicians have sought to validate 4-, 8-, and 12-hour extrapolations. Unfortunately, because of normal diurnal variations and the effects of injury, random short-interval collections do not accurately predict 24-hour totals. For greater accuracy in highly stressed patients, the recommendation is to take sequential 24-hour urine collections and average total urinary nitrogen level measurements from several days. A positive 3 g/day to 5 g/day nitrogen balance is desired to promote anabolism and wound healing.

Because clinical laboratories once found impractical the measurement of total urine nitrogen levels, urine urea nitrogen levels were measured, and the results were used to estimate the total urinary nitrogen level. On average, 80% of the total urinary nitrogen level is in the form of urea; however, this value varies significantly in hospitalized patients.

Several factors must be considered in the evaluation of nitrogen balance in hospitalized patients. Most important, nitrogen loss measurements in patients with chronic renal failure, renal insufficiency, or changing renal function need to be adjusted for accumulation of blood urea nitrogen, which involves the determination of urea generation and protein catabolic rates. It also is important to recognize that nitrogen excretion affects the metabolic response to injury, immobilization, and total caloric support. Finally, inadequate caloric support causes additional protein catabolism and thus excretion of nitrogen as urea. Therefore increasing caloric input in a patient with a constant nitrogen input usually leads to an improved nitrogen balance.

Urinary nitrogen can be used as an indicator of the catabolic stress level. As the severity of stress increases and catabolism becomes pronounced, the total urinary nitrogen and urine urea nitrogen excretion levels increase. For example, increasing levels of metabolic stress cause total urinary nitrogen level values to increase from less than 5 μmol/L (level 0) to 5 to 10 μmol/L (level 1); 10 to 15 μmol/L (level 2); and greater than 15 μmol/L (level 3), respectively.

Other protein-energy status markers or tests

Other markers or tests of nutritional status include (1) plasma free amino acid levels in plasma, (2) indicators of immunocompetence, (3) urine hydroxyproline levels, and (4) biochemical analysis of skeletal muscle.

Free amino acids in plasma

Various diseases and stress conditions are characterized by an altered protein metabolism that is detected through evaluation of plasma or urinary amino acid profiles. The clinical management of such conditions often includes a nutrition component. For example, amino acid analysis is routinely used to diagnose inborn errors of metabolism (see Chapter 18) and as a prognostic index in multiple organ failure syndrome. Cirrhosis and encephalopathy are associated with an increase in aromatic and sulfur-containing amino acids that are normalized by the administration of formulas enriched with BCAAs. The metabolic response to injury is associated with tissue-specific requirements for certain amino acids. Under these circumstances, plasma amino acid profiles may be used to indicate the need for specialized formulas. Starvation without concomitant disease is characterized by a reduction in the plasma ratio of essential to nonessential amino acid concentrations. However, plasma amino acid levels are a poor indicator of developing PEM, because homeostatic mechanisms tend to keep concentrations constant until depletion is severe (and readily apparent during a clinical examination).

Indicators of immunocompetence

Malnutrition is associated with a progressive decline in immune function that is measured either quantitatively or qualitatively. Total lymphocyte count, T-lymphocyte count, immunoglobulin levels, and complement levels are useful quantitative measures. Degrees of malnutrition are commonly defined by total lymphocyte counts of 1200 to 1500 cells/mL (mild), 800 to 1200 cells/mL (moderate), and less than 800 cells/mL (severe). A delayed or absent cutaneous hypersensitivity response to common skin test antigens (such as those for mumps, *Candida* organisms, streptokinase-streptodornase, *Trichophyton* organisms, and tuberculin) is a qualitative measure of impaired immune function. An induration of at least 5 mm in diameter 24 or 48 hours after testing is considered a positive response. The delayed cutaneous hypersensitivity response correlates well with serum protein levels, morbidity, and mortality and is restored to normal by nutritional intervention. Many nonnutritional factors such as cancer, human immunodeficiency virus (HIV) infection, immunosuppressive drugs,

and recent use of anesthetics also alter immunocompetence and must be considered before attributing dysfunction to malnutrition.

Urine hydroxyproline

Proline is hydroxylated by an ascorbic acid-dependent reaction during collagen synthesis. Because the resulting hydroxyproline is not recycled and is released during collagen breakdown, urinary excretion of hydroxyproline reflects the rate of collagen turnover and has been used to indicate the adequacy of protein-energy intake. Hydroxyproline excretion decreases when a low-protein diet is consumed and increases during anabolism. Excretion is age dependent and varies throughout the day, so 24-hour urine collections are necessary. Consumption of meat and gelatin-containing foods and fever also increase hydroxyproline excretion.

Biochemical analysis of skeletal muscle

Direct tissue analysis has been used as a safe, simple, and accurate means to assess protein-energy status in hospitalized patients. Human muscle samples are obtained by a needle biopsy. Suggested analytes include water, electrolytes, glycogen, energy-rich organic phosphates, enzymes, and amino acids.

Combined Testing for Improved Diagnostic and Prognostic Value

Because of the multiple factors that must be considered in the evaluation of a patient's nutritional state, no single measurement or test consistently reflects protein-energy status. Consequently, several multiparameter nutritional indexes have been developed to increase diagnostic and prognostic test sensitivity, specificity, and accuracy. Table 45-6 summarizes the clinical sensitivity, specificity, and ability to predict mortality of single parameter and multiparameter nutritional assessment tests. In general, multiparameter tests have improved diagnostic and predictive abilities.

One of the simplest prognostic multiparameter nutritional tests is the instant nutritional assessment that requires the simultaneous measurement of both albumin and total lymphocyte count. When both analytes were measured, low values for either test in intensive care patients were associated with a twentyfold increased risk of death and a fourfold increased risk of complications. In comparison, when the analytes were assayed and interpreted individually, increases in risk for complications were sixfold and fourfold higher for albumin only and fourfold and eightfold for total lymphocyte count only. Combinations of serum levels of albumin and cholesterol, serum levels of transferrin, or body weight have similarly been evaluated.

The prognostic nutritional index (PNI) is a multiparameter nutritional test that was developed to provide a quantitative estimate of surgical risk and selection criteria for pre-

TABLE 45-6 Single-Parameter and Multiparameter Nutritional Assessment Tests as Predictors of Mortality

Single-Parameter Tests

Parameter	Sensitivity	Specificity	Diagnostic Accuracy
Weight loss	0.86	0.69	0.72
Albumin	0.69	0.82	0.81
Transferrin	0.77	0.39	0.48
DHR	0.52	0.86	0.82
TLC	0.76	0.62	0.63
CHI	0.65	0.58	0.6

Multiparameter Tests

INA	0.71	0.7	0.71
PNI >50	0.79 to 0.86	0.58 to 0.69	0.63 to 0.72
PNI >40	0.93	0.44	0.51
HPI	0.74	0.66	0.72
MRI	0.9	0.9	0.9

Modified from Dempsey DT, Mullen JL: Prognostic value of nutritional indices. JPEN 1987; 11:1095-1145; and Pinchofsky-Devin GD, Kaminski MV, Pfeifer E: Mortality risk index for predicting futility of nutritional support. Nutr Support Serv 1986; 6:14.
DHR, Delayed cutaneous hypersensitivity response; *TLC,* total lymphocyte count; *CHI,* creatinine/height index; *INA,* instant nutritional assessment; *PNI,* prognostic nutrition index; *HPI,* hospital prognostic index; *MRI,* mortality risk index.

operative nutrition support. This index uses serum albumin, transferrin, triceps skinfold thickness, and delayed cutaneous hypersensitivity reactivity in the following equation:

$$PNI\ (\%) = 158 - 16.6(ALB) - 0.2(TFN) - 0.7(TSF) - 5.8(DHR) \quad (8)$$

where

ALB = Albumin (g/dL)
TFN = Transferrin (mg/dL)
TSF = Triceps skinfold thickness (mm)
DHR = Delayed cutaneous hypersensitivity reactivity (0 = nonreactive, 1 = <5 mm induration, 2 = >5 mm induration)

Patients with PNI values less than 40% are considered low risk, 40% to 49% are intermediate risk, and higher than 50% are high risk. Patients identified as high risk have been shown to have a sixfold increase in complications, a tenfold increase in major sepsis, and a twelvefold increase in mortality compared with low-risk patients. Application of the PNI has been limited by the relative inconvenience and morbidity of delayed cutaneous hypersensitivity reactivity.

A likelihood of malnutrition (LOM) score was developed in the mid-1970s based on a combination of serum chemistries (folate, ascorbate, and albumin), hematocrit, total lymphocyte count, and anthropometric measurements. With this test a graded score (5, 10, or 25 points) is given for each abnormal measurement depending on the severity of the abnormality and the total points. Patients with total scores higher than 25 points are considered to have a high LOM. A high LOM score predicts subsequent morbidity and mortality during the hospital stay.

Other multiparameter indexes include clinical or disease factors as well as nutritional markers. The hospital prognostic index uses serum albumin, delayed cutaneous hypersensitivity reactivity, the presence of sepsis, and diagnosis (cancer or noncancer). The mortality risk index (MRI) uses serum albumin, serum transferrin, delayed cutaneous hypersensitivity reactivity, triceps skinfold, a diagnosis severity score, and a treatability score. As indicated in Table 45-6, the MRI has achieved very high clinical sensitivity levels, specificity, and accuracy in the prediction of death.

References

1. Alexander JW, Gottschlich MM: Nutritional immunomodulation in burn patients. Crit Care Med 1990; 18:S149-S153.
2. Clark GH, Fraser CG: Biological variation of acute phase proteins. Ann Clin Biochem 1993; 30:373-376.
3. Deurenberg P, Schutz Y: Body composition: Overview of methods and future directions of research. Ann Nutr Metab 1995; 39:325-333.
4. Dougherty D, Bankhead R, Kushner R et al: Nutrition care given new importance in JCAHO standards. Nutr Clin Pract 1995; 10:26-31.
5. Gallagher-Allred CR, Voss AC, Finn SC et al: Malnutrition and clinical outcomes: the case for medical nutrition therapy. J Am Diet Assoc 1996; 96:361-366.
6. Hark L, Deen D Jr: Taking a nutrition history: a practical approach for family physicians. Am Fam Physician 1999; 59:1521-1528, 1531-1532.
7. Ingenbleek Y, Carpentier YA: Prognostic inflammatory and nutritional index scoring critically ill patients. Int J Vit Nutr Res 1985; 55:91-101.
8. Inoue Y, Okada A, Nezu R et al: Rapid turnover proteins as index of nutritional status in benign diseases. Nutrition 1991; 7:45-49.

9. Johnson AM: Low levels of plasma proteins: malnutrition or inflammation? Clin Chem Lab Med 1999; 37:91-96.

10. National Research Council: Recommended Dietary Allowances, 10th edition, Washington, DC, National Academy Press, 1989.

11. Rabkin R: Nutrient regulation of insulin-like growth factor-1. Miner Electrolyte Metab 1997; 23:157-160.

12. Rombeau JL, Kripke SA: Enteral nutrition. In Fischer J (ed): Total Parenteral Nutrition, 2nd edition, pp 423-445, Boston, Little, Brown, 1991.

13. Spiekerman AM: Nutritional assessment (protein nutriture). Anal Chem 1995; 67:429R-436R.

14. Veldee MS: Nutritional Assessment, Therapy, and Monitoring. In Burtis CA, Ashwood ER (eds): Tietz Textbook of Clinical Chemistry, 3rd edition, pp 1359-1394, Philadelphia, WB Saunders, 1999.

15. Wang ZM, Pierson RN, Heymsfield SB: The five-level model: a new approach to organizing body-composition research. Am J Clin Nutr 1992; 56:19.

16. Wang ZM, Heshka S, Pierson RN et al: Systematic organization of body-composition methodology: an overview with emphasis on component-based methods. Am J Clin Nutr 1995; 61:457-465.

Additional Reading

Dietary Reference Intakes for Calcium, Phosphorus, Magnesium, Vitamin D, and Fluoride, Washington DC, National Academy Press, 1997.

Dietary Reference Intakes for Vitamin C, Vitamin E, Selenium, and Beta-Carotene, and Other Carotenoids, Washington DC, National Academy Press, 2000.

Dietary Reference Intakes for Thiamine, Riboflavin, Niacin, Vitamin B6, Folate, Vitamin B12, Pantothenic Acid, Biotin, and Choline, Washington DC, National Academy Press, 1999.

Krummel DA, Kris-Etherton PM: Nutrition in Women's Health, Gaithersburg, Md, Aspen, 1996.

Marshall JR, Chen Z: Diet and health risk: risk patterns and disease-specific associations. Am J Clin Nutr 1999; 69:1351S-1356S.

Peckenpaugh NJ, Poleman CM: Nutrition: Essentials and Diet Therapy, 8th edition, Philadelphia, WB Saunders, 1999.

Seiler O, Stahelin HB (eds): Malnutrition in the Elderly: A National Crisis, New York, Springer-Verlag, 1999.

CHAPTER 46

Reference Information for the Clinical Laboratory

PENNELL C. PAINTER, PhD, JUNE Y. COPE, MT(ASCP)SC, and JANE L. SMITH, MS, MT(ASCP)SI, DLM

■ CONTENTS

Reference Intervals and Values

The results of laboratory tests have little practical utility until clinical studies have ascribed various states of health and disease to intervals of values. Reference intervals are useful because they attempt to describe the typical results found in a defined population of apparently healthy individuals. Different methods may yield different values, depending on calibration and other technical considerations. Therefore different reference intervals and results may be obtained in different laboratories. Variability among methods is particularly characteristic of methods that use antibodies to detect the material of interest and when results are reported as relative units of activity. Values from apparently healthy and diseased individuals may overlap significantly. Therefore reference intervals, although useful for clinicians, should not be used as absolute indicators of health or disease (see Chapter 14).

The reference intervals presented in this chapter are for general informational purposes only. Guidelines for defining and determining reference intervals have been discussed in Chapter 14 and published in the 1995 National Committee for Clinical Laboratory Standards (NCCLS) C28-A guideline.

The values given in this chapter are for adults who are fasting unless otherwise stated. When included, values for other age groups are clearly identified. Specific methods or instrumental systems are given for some intervals. Most values given were taken from *Tietz Clinical Guide to Laboratory Tests* and *Tietz Textbook of Clinical Chemistry*. For several proteins, reference intervals—obtained after calibration of the analytical system with the international protein reference, RPPHS/CRM 470—are listed in Chapter 19.

All reference intervals are given in conventional and international units. In general, the international units given conform to the SI system (Système International d'Unités). However, in some cases the recommendations of the International Union of Pure and Applied Chemistry (IUPAC) and the Commission on World Standards (COWS) of the World Association of Societies of Pathology (WASP) are used, because these are more widely accepted in clinical laboratories and offer advantages over the units recommended in the SI system. If the exact molecular weight of a

TABLE 46-1 Metric Prefixes of SI Units*

Factor	Prefix	Symbol	Factor	Prefix	Symbol
10^{24}	yotta	Y	10^{-1}	deci	d
10^{21}	zetta	Z	10^{-2}	centi	c
10^{18}	exa	E	10^{-3}	milli	m
10^{15}	peta	P	10^{-6}	micro	μ
10^{12}	tera	T	10^{-9}	nano	n
10^{9}	giga	G	10^{-12}	pico	p
10^{6}	mega	M	10^{-15}	femto	f
10^{3}	kilo	k	10^{-18}	atto	a
10^{2}	hecto	h	10^{-21}	zepto	z
10^{1}	deka†	da	10^{-24}	yocto	y

From The International System of Units [SI]. Washington, DC, National Institute of Standards and Technology, 1991.
*The Eleventh Conférence Générale des Poids et Mésures (CGPM) (1960, Resolution 12) adopted a first series of prefixes and symbols of prefixes to form the names and symbols of the decimal multiples and submultiples of SI units. Prefixes for 10^{-15} and 10^{-18} were added by the twelfth CGPM (1964, Resolution 8), those for 10^{15} and 10^{18} by the fifteenth CGPM (1975, Resolution 10), and those for 10^{21}, 10^{24}, and 10^{-24} were proposed by the CIPM (1990) for approval by the nineteenth CGPM (1991).
†Outside the United States, the spelling "deca" is used extensively.

Conversion Charts

TABLE 46-2 Units of Length

Kilometer (km)	Meter (m)	Decimeter (dm)	Centimeter (cm)	Millimeter (mm)	Micrometer (μm)	Nanometer (nm)	Angstrom (Å)	Picometer (pm)	Inch (in)
1	10^3	10^4	10^5	10^6	10^9	10^{12}	10^{13}	10^{15}	39.37×10^3
10^{-3}	1	10	10^2	10^3	10^6	10^9	10^{10}	10^{12}	39.37
10^{-4}	10^{-1}	1	10	10^2	10^5	10^8	10^9	10^{11}	39.37×10^{-1}
10^{-5}	10^{-2}	10^{-1}	1	10	10^4	10^7	10^8	10^{10}	39.37×10^{-2}
10^{-6}	10^{-3}	10^{-2}	10^{-1}	1	10^3	10^6	10^7	10^9	39.37×10^{-3}
10^{-9}	10^{-6}	10^{-5}	10^{-4}	10^{-3}	1	10^3	10^4	10^6	39.37×10^{-6}
10^{-12}	10^{-9}	10^{-8}	10^{-7}	10^{-6}	10^{-3}	1	10	10^3	39.37×10^{-9}
10^{-13}	10^{-10}	10^{-9}	10^{-8}	10^{-7}	10^{-4}	10^{-1}	1	10^2	39.37×10^{-10}
10^{-15}	10^{-12}	10^{-11}	10^{-10}	10^{-9}	10^{-6}	10^{-3}	10^{-2}	1	39.37×10^{-12}

TABLE 46-3 Units of Mass*

Kilometer (kg)	Gram (g)	Decigram (dg)	Centigram (cg)	Milligram (mg)	Microgram (μg)	Nanogram (ng)	Picogram (pg)	Ounce (Av.) (oz)	Pound (Av.) (lb)
1	10^3	10^4	10^5	10^6	10^9	10^{12}	10^{15}	35.27	2.2
10^{-3}	1	10	10^2	10^3	10^6	10^9	10^{12}	35.27×10^{-3}	2.2×10^{-3}
10^{-4}	10^{-1}	1	10	10^2	10^5	10^8	10^{11}	35.27×10^{-4}	2.2×10^{-4}
10^{-5}	10^{-2}	10^{-1}	1	10	10^4	10^7	10^{10}	35.27×10^{-5}	2.2×10^{-5}
10^{-6}	10^{-3}	10^{-2}	10^{-1}	1	10^3	10^6	10^9	35.27×10^{-6}	2.2×10^{-6}
10^{-9}	10^{-6}	10^{-5}	10^{-4}	10^{-3}	1	10^3	10^6	35.27×10^{-9}	2.2×10^{-9}
10^{-12}	10^{-9}	10^{-8}	10^{-7}	10^{-6}	10^{-3}	1	10^3	35.27×10^{-12}	2.2×10^{-12}
10^{-15}	10^{-12}	10^{-11}	10^{-10}	10^{-9}	10^{-6}	10^{-3}	1	35.27×10^{-15}	2.2×10^{-15}

*According to the SI system, *mass* is the preferred term; the term *weight* is more commonly used in the United States.

compound has not been established (for example, for a protein), values in the conventional unit are converted to values expressed in mass per liter (mass/L).

Throughout this chapter, the prefixes for units used are those approved by the Conférence Générale des Poids et Mésures (CPGM), 1964, and IUPAC and International Federation of Clinical Chemistry (IFCC) (Clin Chim Acta 1979; 96:157F-183F [see Chapter 1]).

For convenience and to preserve space, the standard abbreviations common in laboratory medicine are used. Less-

TABLE 46-4   Units of Capacity

Kiloliter (kL)	Liter (L)	Deciliter (dL)	Centiliter (cL)	Milliliter (mL)	Microliter (μL)	Nanoliter (nL)	Picoliter (pL)	Ounce (oz)	Quart (qt)
1	10^3	10^4	10^5	10^6	10^9	10^{12}	10^{15}	33.81×10^3	1.06×10^3
10^{-3}	1	10	10^2	10^3	10^6	10^9	10^{12}	33.81	1.06
10^{-4}	10^{-1}	1	10	10^2	10^5	10^8	10^{11}	33.81×10^{-1}	1.06×10^{-1}
10^{-5}	10^{-2}	10^{-1}	1	10	10^4	10^7	10^{10}	33.81×10^{-2}	1.06×10^{-2}
10^{-6}	10^{-3}	10^{-2}	10^{-1}	1	10^3	10^6	10^9	33.81×10^{-3}	1.06×10^{-3}
10^{-9}	10^{-6}	10^{-5}	10^{-4}	10^{-3}	1	10^3	10^6	33.81×10^{-6}	1.06×10^{-6}
10^{-12}	10^{-9}	10^{-8}	10^{-7}	10^{-6}	10^{-3}	1	10^3	33.81×10^{-9}	1.06×10^{-9}
10^{-15}	10^{-12}	10^{-11}	10^{-10}	10^{-9}	10^{-6}	10^{-3}	1	33.81×10^{-12}	1.06×10^{-12}

common abbreviations and some nonstandard abbreviations are given below.

Abbreviations

ACD	Acid-citrate-dextrose
Amf	Amniotic fluid
Ascf	Ascitic fluid
BPH	Benign prostatic hypertrophy
Br	Breath
Cit	Citrate
CN⁻	Cyanate ion
CSF	Cerebrospinal fluid
EDTA	Ethylenediaminetetraacetic acid
F	Feces
F⁻	Fluoride
F⁻/Ox	Fluoride and oxalate
Gast Cont	Gastric contents
Gastf	Gastric fluid
Gast Res	Gastric residue
H	Hair
Hep	Heparin
Occup. exp.	Occupational exposure
Ox	Oxalate
Pericf	Pericardial fluid
Placent	Placental
Plf	Pleural fluid
Plt	Platelets
post-stim	Post-stimulation
pp	Postprandial
RBC	Red blood cells
S	Serum
Sal	Saliva
SCN⁻	Thiocyanate ion
Semf	Seminal fluid
Serf	Serous fluid
Swt	Sweat
Synf	Synovial fluid
T	Tissue
U	Urine
WB	Whole blood

Drugs

Therapeutic drug monitoring and detection of drug overdose have become increasingly important aspects of the laboratory's role in patient care. The information given for the drugs in this table has been gathered from published sources. Because knowledge and drug measurement methodologies are continuously improving, it may be necessary to supplement the information given here with information obtained from other sources as it becomes available. Reliable drug analysis information depends on a well-coordinated sample collection, assay methodology characteristics, and patient-associated considerations such as age, disease state, concomitant drug administration, and clinical procedures that the patient may have undergone.

Many tests for therapeutic drugs require careful timing between administration and sample collection if the measured drug level is to be of optimal use clinically. Therapeutic or toxic ranges for which definitive limits do not exist have been omitted from the table. Drugs are listed by their chemical or generic name and a commercial brand of the drug (as appropriate).

For convenience and to preserve space, standard abbreviations common in laboratory medicine are used. Less common abbreviations and some nonstandard abbreviations are given below.

Abbreviations

EDTA	Ethylenediaminetetraacetic acid
Hep	Heparin
Occup. exp.	Occupational exposure
P	Plasma
prem.	Premature
S	Serum
Therap.	Therapeutic
U	Urine
WB	Whole blood

Critical values

Critical values, also known as *panic values,* are laboratory results that indicate a life-threatening situation for the patient. Because of their critical nature, urgent notification of a critical value to the appropriate health-care professional is necessary. Table 46-10 has been adapted from an extensive national survey conducted by Kost (Kost GJ: Critical limits for urgent clinician notification at US medical centers. JAMA 1990; 263:704-707; Kost GJ: Using critical limits to improve patient outcome. Med Lab Observ 1993; 25:22-27). The limits listed were obtained from 92 U.S. medical centers. In practice, each situation should have its own set of critical limits and physician notification policy.

Text continued on p. 1028

Nomograms

TABLE 46-5   **Nomogram for the Determination of Body Surface Area of Children***

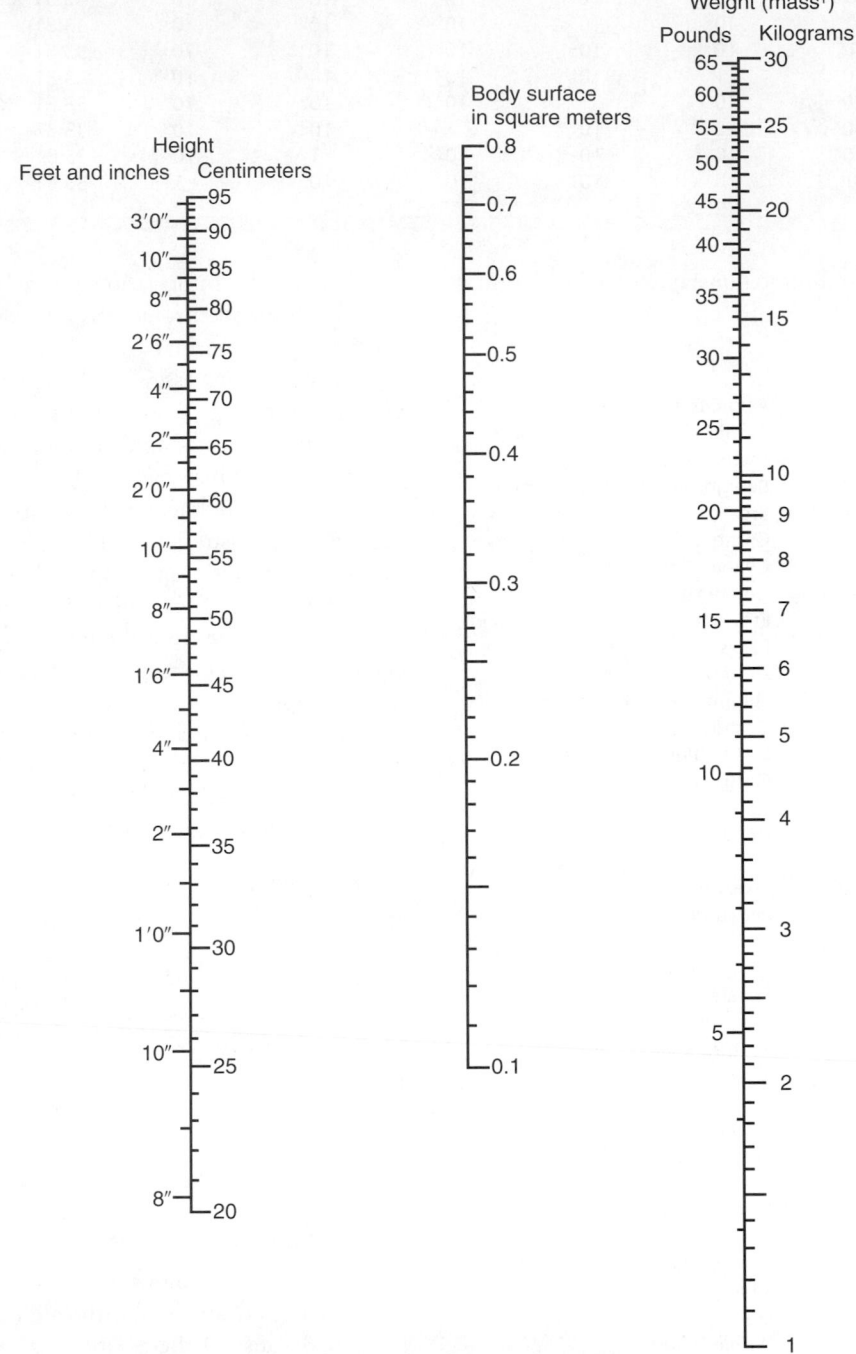

*From DuBois EF: Basal Metabolism in Health and Disease, Philadelphia, Lea & Febiger, 1936.
†According to the SI system, *mass* is the preferred term; the term *weight* is more commonly used in the United States.

TABLE 46-6   Nomogram for the Determination of Body Surface Area of Children and Adults*

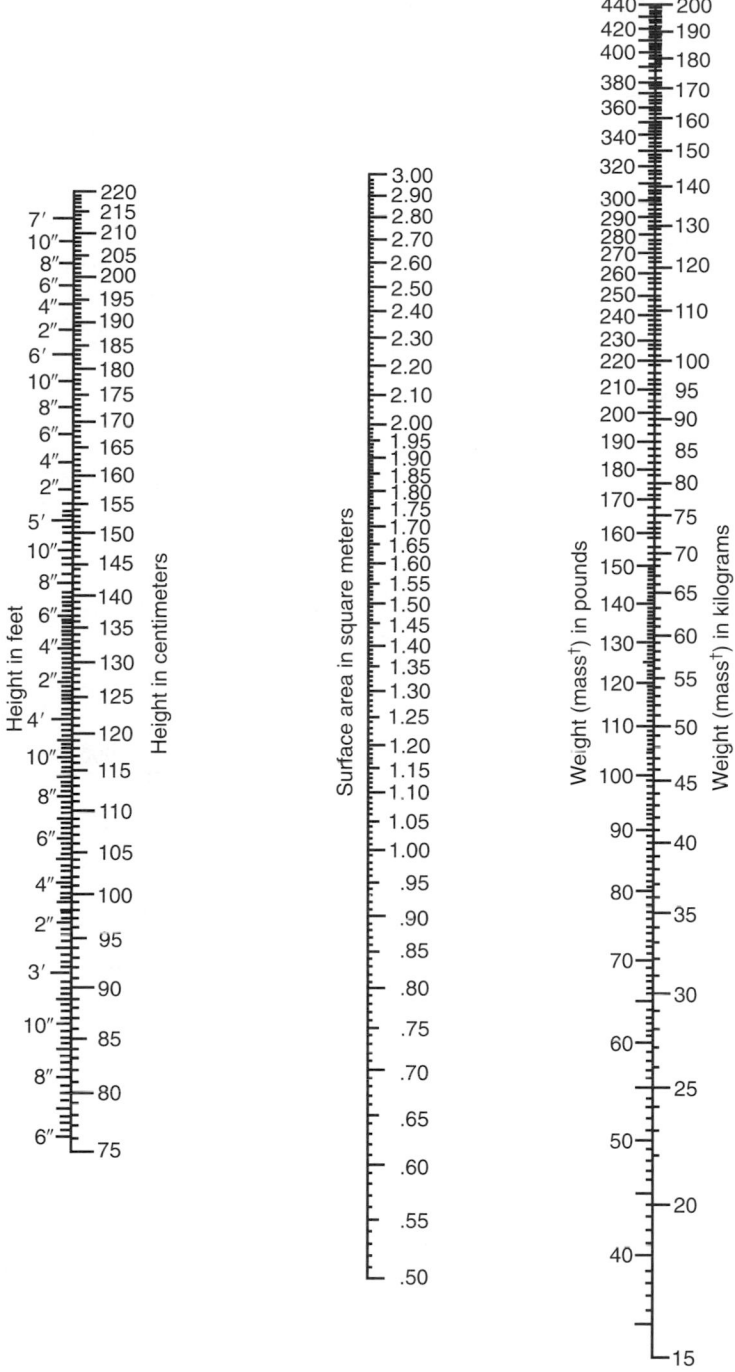

*From Boothby WM, Sandiford RB: Nomographic charts for the calculation of the metabolic rate by the gasometer method. Boston Med Surg J 1921; 185:337.
†According to the SI system, *mass* is the preferred term; the term *weight* is more commonly used in the United States.

TABLE 46-7 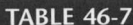 Nomogram for Calculating Relative Centrifugal Force*

Scale A

Scale B

Scale C

Rotating radius—inches

Rotating radius—centimeters

Relative centrifugal force—gravities

Speed—revolutions per minute

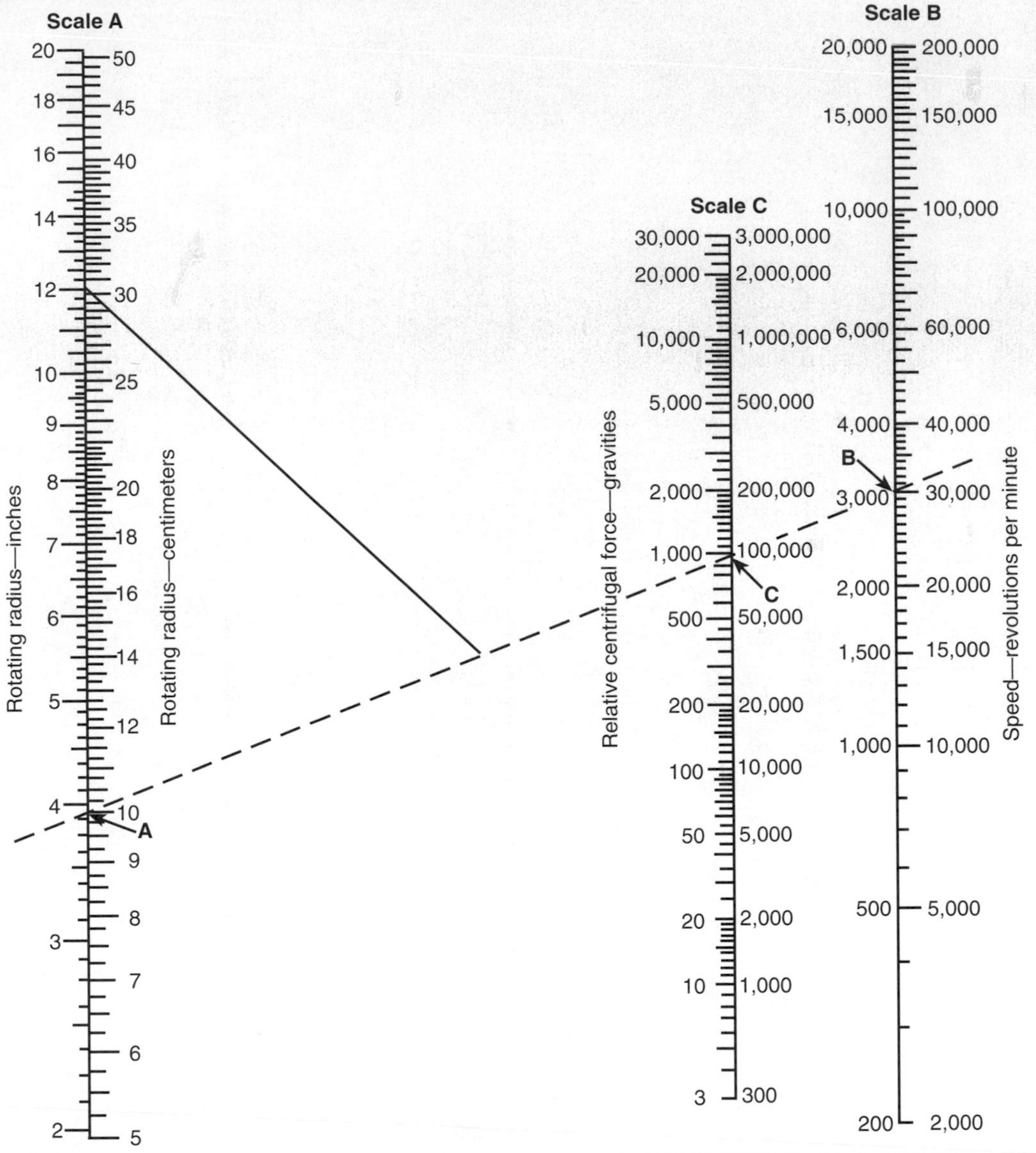

*Modified from the International Equipment Company (IEC) Relative Centrifugal Force Nomograph.

Instructions: To find, for example, the relative centrifugal force (RCF) at a radial distance of 10 cm from the center of rotation when the centrifuge is operated at a speed of 3000 rpm, place a straightedge on the chart, and connect the 10 cm point on scale A (rotating radius) with the 3000 rpm point on scale B (speed). Read the point at which the straightedge intersects scale C (relative centrifugal force); in this example, that point is 1000 × *g*. Use the right side of scales B and C for high-speed and ultracentrifuges.

If the desired RCF is known, the necessary speed for a particular rotating radius may be determined by connecting appropriate points on scales A and C and reading speed from scale B.

Equation for calculating RCF:

$$RCF = 1.118 \times 10^{-5} \times r \times n^2$$

where

RCF is obtained in gravities (× *g*),

r is rotating radius in centimeters, and

n is rotating speed in revolutions per minute

TABLE 46-8   **Chemistry and Toxicology**

Test	Specimen		Reference Interval	Conversion Factor	Reference Interval (International Units)
Acetaldehyde	WB (F⁻/Ox)		**mg/L**		**μmol/L**
			<0.2	× 22.7	<4.5
		Occup. exp.:	<0.5		<11.4
		Toxic:	1 to 2		22.7 to 45.4
Acetoacetate					
Semiquant.	S or P (F⁻/Ox)		Negative (<1 mg/dL)	× 0.098	Negative (<0.1 mmol/L)
	U		Negative (<50 mg/dL)		Negative (<4.9 mmol/L)
Acetone					
Semiquant.	S or P (F⁻/Ox)		Negative (<1 mg/dL)	× 0.172	Negative (<0.17 mmol/L)
			mg/dL		**mmol/L**
Quant.	S or P (F⁻/Ox)		0.3 to 2.0	× 0.172	0.05 to 0.34
		Ketoacidosis:	10 to 70		1.72 to 12.04
		Occup. exp.:	<10		<1.72
		Toxic:	>20		>3.44
Semiquant.	U	Negative	0.3	× 0.172	0.05
Quant.		Occup. exp.:	>27		>4.64
			mg/L		**μmol/L**
	Br	Negative	0.003	× 17.2	0.52
		Occup. exp.:	0.006		1.03
Acetonitrile	WB (F⁻/Ox)		**mg/L**		**μmol/L**
		CN⁻:	<0.04	× 38.4	<1.5
		SCN⁻:	<12	× 17.2	<206
		Occup. exp., CN⁻:	<0.1	× 38.4	<3.8
		Toxic,			
		CN⁻:	>3	× 38.4	115
		SCN⁻:	>160	× 17.2	>2752
	U	SCN⁻:	<17		<292
		Occup. exp., SCN⁻:	<20		<344
Acetylcholinesterase in Erythrocytes	WB (ACD, EDTA, or Hep)	Adult:	36.9 ± 3.83 U/g Hb (SD)	× 0.0645	2.38 ± 0.23 MU/mol Hb
			1070 ± 111 U/10¹² RBC	× 10⁻³	1.07 ± 0.11 nU/RBC
			12.5 ± 1.30 U/mL RBC	× 1	12.5 ± 1.30 kU/L RBC
			Lower in newborns		
α₁-Acid-Glycoprotein (Orosomucoid)	S (Neph)	Adult:	25 to 135 mg/dL	× 0.2439	6.1 to 32.9 μmol/L
	S	Adult:	55 to 140 mg/dL	× 0.2439	13.4 to 34.1 μmol/L
	U		0.29 to 0.68 mg/day	× 24.39	7.1 to 16.6 nmol/day
	CSF		0.28 to 0.54	× 0.2439	0.07 to 0.13 μmol/L
Acrylonitrile	WB (F⁻/Ox)		**mg/L**		**μmol/L**
		CN⁻:	<0.04	× 38.4	<1.5
		SCN⁻:	<0.12	× 17.2	<2.1
		Toxic (SCN⁻):	>160	× 17.2	>2752
		Toxic (CN⁻):	>3	× 38.4	>115
	U	Toxic (SCN⁻):	>20	× 17.2	>344
Adrenocorticotropic Hormone (ACTH)	P (EDTA)		**pg/mL**		**pmol/L**
		Cord:	50 to 570	× 0.22	11 to 125
		Newborn:	10 to 185		2.2 to 41
		Adult:			
		0800 h: unrestricted activity	<120	× 0.22	<26
		2400 h: supine	<10		<2.2
	Amf	10 to 18 wk:	209 (mean)	× 0.22	46 (mean)
		26 to 30 wk:	430		95
		35 to 36 wk:	162 and maintained thereafter		36 and maintained thereafter

Continued

TABLE 46-8   Chemistry and Toxicology—cont'd

Test	Specimen		Reference Interval	Conversion Factor	Reference Interval (International Units)
Adrenocorticotropic Hormone-Insulin Stimulation Test Dose: 0.05 to 0.15 U insulin/kg, IV, after overnight fast	S: fasting, 30, 60, and 90 min post-stim	Cortisol:	>10 μg/dL rise ½ h after max. fall in blood glucose, >20 μg/dL	× 27.6	>276 μmol/L rise ½ h after max. fall in blood glucose, >552 nmol/L
		Peak response:	>20 μg/dL	× 27.6	552 nmol/L
		Glucose:	≤40 mg/dL or signs of hypoglycemia	× 0.0555	<2.2 nmol/L or signs of hypoglycemia
Adrenocorticotropic Hormone Stimulation Test (Prolonged Infusion) Dose: 50 units ACTH or 500 μg Cortrosyn/day × 3	U, 24-h	17-KGS: 17-KS: 17-OHCS:	Twofold to fourfold rise Twofold rise Twofold to fivefold rise		Same
	S	Cortisol:	25 to 50 μg/dL	× 27.6	Cortisol: 690 to 1380 nmol/L
Adrenocorticotropic Hormone Stimulation Test (Rapid Test) Dose: 250 μg Cortrosyn, IM	S: baseline, 30 and 60 min post-stim	Cortisol: Baseline After Cortrosyn: Rise above baseline Peak response	>5.0 μg/dL >7 >20	× 27.6	Baseline: >138 nmol/L >193 nmol/L >552 nmol/L
Alanine	S		**mg/dL**		**μmol/L**
		Premature, 1 day:	3.34 ± 0.45 (SD)	× 112.2	375 ± 50 (SD)
		Newborn, 1 day:	2.10 to 3.65		236 to 410
		1 to 3 mo:	2.45 ± 0.63 (SD)		275 ± 71 (SD)
		2 to 6 mo:	1.58 to 3.68		177 to 413
		9 mo to 2 y:	0.88 to 2.79		99 to 313
		3 to 10 y:	1.22 to 2.71		137 to 305
		6 to 18 y:	1.72 to 4.85		193 to 545
		Adult:	1.87 to 5.88		210 to 661
	U, 24-h		**mg/day**		**μmol/day**
		10 days to 7 wk:	4.1 to 9.3	× 11.2	46 to 104
		3 to 12 y:	9.1 to 39.2		102 to 439
		Adult:	7.9 to 48.3		88 to 541
Alanine Aminotransferase (ALT, SGPT) Henry, optimized, 37 °C	S		**U/L**		**μkat/L**
		Newborn/infant:	13 to 45	× 0.017	0.22 to 0.77
		Adult:			
		Man:	10 to 40		0.17 to 0.68
		Woman:	7 to 35		0.12 to 0.06
IFCC, with P-5'-P, 37 °C		Adult:			
		Man:	13 to 40		0.22 to 0.68
		Woman:	10 to 28		0.17 to 0.48
Albumin Nephelometric, photometric	S	0 to 4 days:	2.8 to 4.4 g/dL	× 10	28 to 44 g/L
		4 days to 14 y:	3.8 to 5.4 g/dL		38 to 54 g/L
		Adult:	3.5 to 5.2 g/dL		35 to 52 g/L
		>60 y:	3.2 to 4.6 g/dL		32 to 46 g/L
		Average ~0.3 g/dL higher in ambulatory individuals			Average ~3 g/L higher in ambulatory individuals
Nephelometric, rate	CSF	3 mo to 4 y:	0 to 45 mg/dL	× 10	0 to 450 mg/L
		>4 y:	10 to 30 mg/dL	× 10	100 to 300 mg/L
	U	At rest:	<45 mg/days	× 10	Same
		Ambulatory:	20 to 30 mg/days		
		Adult:	0.0 to 2.0 mg/dL	× 10	0.0 to 20 mg/L

TABLE 46-8 Chemistry and Toxicology—cont'd

Test	Specimen	Reference Interval		Conversion Factor	Reference Interval (International Units)	
Alcohol Dehydrogenase 340 nm, 30 °C	S	≤2.8 U/L		× 0.017	≤0.05 μkat/L	
Aldolase Spectrophotom. 340 nm, 37 °C	S	Adult:	1.0 to 7.5 U/L (30 °C) 0.3 to 3.0 U/L at bed rest	× 0.017	0.02 to 0.13 μkat/L 0.01 to 0.05 μkat/L	
		Child: 10 to 24 mo: 25 mo to 16 y:	3.4 to 11.8 1.2 to 8.8		0.06 to 0.20 μkat/L 0.02 to 0.15 μkat/L	
Aldosterone	S or P (Hep, EDTA)		**ng/dL**		**nmol/L**	
		Cord blood:	40 to 200	× 0.0277	1.11 to 5.54	
		Premature infant:	19 to 141		0.53 to 3.91	
		Full-term infant: 3 days:	7 to 184		0.19 to 5.10	
		1 wk:	5 to 175		0.03 to 4.85	
		1 to 12 mo:	5 to 90		0.14 to 2.49	
		Child: 1 to 2 y:	7 to 54		0.19 to 1.50	
		2 to 10 y: Supine:	3 to 35		0.08 to 0.97	
		Upright:	5 to 80		0.14 to 2.22	
		10 to 15 y: Supine:	2 to 22		0.06 to 0.61	
		Upright:	4 to 48		0.11 to 1.33	
		Adult: Supine:	3 to 16		0.08 to 0.44	
		Upright:	7 to 30		0.19 to 0.83	
	U, 24-h		**μg/day**		**nmol/d μg/g creatinine**	
		Newborn, 1 to 3 days:	0.5 to 5	× 2.77	1 to 14 20 to 140	
		Prepubertal child: 4 to 10 y:	1 to 8		3 to 22 4 to 22	
		Adult:	3 to 19		8 to 51 1.5 to 20	
Aluminum (Al)			**μg/L**		**μmol/L**	
	S		<5.41	× 0.0371	<0.2	
	P	Patients on hemodialysis Al medication	20 to 550 <30	× 0.0371	0.74 to 20.4 <1.11	
	U, random		5 to 30	× 0.0371	0.19 to 1.11	
α-Amino Acid Nitrogen (AAN) Ninhydrin Naphthoquinone and FDNB	P (EDTA) U, 24 h		3.2 to 5.5 mg/dL 50 to 200 mg/day	× 0.714 × 0.0714	2.28 to 3.93 mmol/L 3.57 to 14.28 mmol/day	
5-Aminolevulinate Dehydratase Photometric, 38 °C	RBC (Hep)		108 to 299 U/mL erythrocytes	× 1	108 to 299 kU/L	
5-Aminolevulinic Acid (5-ALA)	S		15 to 23 μg/dL; lower in children	× 0.076	1.14 to 1.75 μmol/L	
	U		1.3 to 7.0 mg/day	× 7.262	9.9 to 53.4 μmol/day	

Continued

TABLE 46-8 Chemistry and Toxicology—cont'd

Test	Specimen		Reference Interval	Conversion Factor	Reference Interval (International Units)
Ammonia Nitrogen Resin or enzymatic	S or P (NaHep)		**µg N/dL**		**µmol N/L**
		Newborn:	90 to 150	× 0.714	64 to 107
		0 to 2 wk:	79 to 129		56 to 92
		>1 mo:	29 to 70		21 to 50
		Adult:	15 to 45		11 to 32
		Values for arterial plasma are lower than for venous plasma.			
	U, 24-h		**mg N/d**		**mmol N/d**
		Infant:	560 to 2900	× 0.0714	40 to 207
		Adult:	140 to 1500	× 0.0714	10 to 107
Ammonia Chloride Loading Test Dose: 0.1 g ammonium chloride/kg orally at 0800 h after complete midnight fast	U, hourly between 1000 and 1600 h		pH should fall to ≤5.2 between 2 and 8 h after the dose.		H⁺ concentration should increase to >6 µmol/L between 2 and 8 h after the dose.
Amniotic Fluid Analysis ΔA_{450}	Amf				Same
		28 wk:	0 to 0.048 ΔA		
		40 wk:	0 to 0.02 ΔA		
Amylase UV-method, Beckman	S				
		Newborn:	5 to 65 U/L	× 0.017	0.09 to 1.11 µkat/L
		Adult:	27 to 131 U/L		0.46 to 2.23 µkat/L
		>70 y:	24 to 151 U/L		0.41 to 2.57 µkat/L
	U, timed		1 to 17 U/h		1 to 17 U/h
Amylase/Creatinine Clearance Ratio	S and U, random		1% to 4%	× 0.01	Clearance fraction: 0.01 to 0.04
Amyloid-Associated Protein (Amyloid A Protein, AA Protein)	S	0 to 5 y:	<0.4 mg/dL	× 10	<200 mg/L
		Adult:	<40 mg/dL		
			Levels may increase up to 3 orders of magnitude with inflammation		
Androstenedione	S		**ng/dL**		**nmol/L (mean ± SE)**
		Cord:	30 to 150	× 0.0349	1.0 to 5.2
		Premature:	80 to 446		2.8 to 15.6
		1 to 12 mo:	6 to 68		0.2 to 2.4
		1 to 7 days:	20 to 290		0.7 to 10.1
		Prepubertal (1 to 10 y):	8 to 50	× 0.0349	0.3 to 1.7
		Puberty (10 to 17 y): (varies with Tanner stage and sex)	8 to 240		0.3 to 8.4
		Adult:			
		Man:	75 to 205	× 0.0349	2.6 to 7.2
		Woman:	85 to 275		3.0 to 9.6
	Amf	Midpregnancy	**ng/mL**		**nmol/L**
		Male fetus:	1.0	× 3.49	3.49
		Female fetus:	0.7		2.44
		Term:	0.7 to 3.5		2.44 to 12.22

TABLE 46-8   Chemistry and Toxicology—cont'd

Test	Specimen		Reference Interval	Conversion Factor	Reference Interval (International Units)
Angiotensin I	P (KEDTA), periphvein		<25 pg/mL	× 1	<25 ng/L
Angiotensin II	P (KEDTA)		10 to 60 pg/mL	× 1	10 to 60 ng/L
Anion Gap	P (Hep)	$[Na - (Cl^- + HCO_3^-)]$	7 to 16 mmol/L	× 1	7 to 16 mmol/L
		$[(Na + K) - (Cl^- + HCO_3^-)]$	10 to 20 mmol/L	× 1	10 to 20 mmol/L
α_1-Antichymotrypsin (α_1AC)	S	Newborn:	~1 mg/dL	× 10	~10 mg/L
		Adult:	30 to 60 mg/dL		300 to 600 mg/L
Antidiuretic Hormone (ADH, Vasopressin)	P (EDTA)	**Plasma mOsmol/kg**	**Plasma ADH pg/ml**		**Plasma ADH ng/L**
		270 to 280:	<1.5	× 0.926	<1.4
		280 to 285:	<2.5		<2.3
		285 to 290:	1 to 5		0.9 to 4.6
		290 to 295:	2 to 7		1.9 to 6.5
		295 to 300:	4 to 12		3.7 to 11.1
Antimony NAA, AAS	P (Hep)		0.052 ± 0.019 µg/dL	× 82.1	4.27 ± 1.56 nmol/L (SD)
	U		<10 µg/L	× 8.21	<82.1 nmol/L
		Toxic:	>1 mg/L	× 8.21	>8.21 µmol/L
Antithrombin III RID	P (citrate)		85% to 115% of normal human plasma	× 0.01	0.85 to 1.15
α_1-Antitrypsin Nephelometric	S		**mg/dL**		**g/L**
		Newborn:	145 to 270	× 0.1	1.45 to 2.70
		Adult:	78 to 200		0.78 to 2.0
		>60 y:	115 to 200		1.15 to 2.0
Apolipoprotein A-I (Apo A-I) Nephelometric (Beckman)	S		**mg/dL**		**g/L**
		Male: APA:	94 to 178	× 0.01	0.94 to 1.78
		APA/APB:	0.80 to 2.33		Same
		APB/APA:	0.43 to 1.25		Same
		Female: APA:	101 to 199	× 0.01	1.01 to 1.99
		APA/APB:	0.94 to 2.63		Same
		APB/APA:	0.38 to 1.07		Same
Apolipoprotein B (Apo B100) Nephelometric (Beckman)	S		**mg/dL**		**g/L**
		Male: APB:	63 to 133	× 0.01	0.63 to 1.33
		APA/APB:	0.80 to 2.33		Same
		APB/APA:	0.43 to 1.25		Same
		Female: APB:	60 to 126	× 0.01	0.60 to 1.26
		APA/APB:	0.94 to 2.63		Same
		APB/APA:	0.38 to 1.07		Same
Arsenic	WB (Hep)		**µg/L**		**µmol/L**
			2 to 23	× 0.0133	0.03 to 0.31
		Chronic poisoning:	100 to 500		1.33 to 6.65
		Acute poisoning:	600 to 9300		7.98 to 124
	U, 24-h		5 to 50 µg/day	× 0.0133	0.07 to 0.67 µmol/day

Continued

TABLE 46-8   Chemistry and Toxicology—cont'd

Test	Specimen		Reference Interval		Conversion Factor	Reference Interval (International Units)
Ascorbic Acid (*see Vitamin C*)						
Aspartate Aminotransferase (AST, SGOT), (30 °C)	S		**U/L**			**μkat/L**
		Newborn:	25 to 75		× 0.017	0.43 to 1.28
		Infant:	15 to 60			0.26 to 1.02
		Adult:	8 to 20			0.14 to 0.34
		With P-5′-P	10 to 30			0.17 to 0.51
Base Excess	WB (Hep)		**mmol/L**			Same
		Newborn:	(−10) to (−2)			
		Infant:	(−7) to (−1)			
		Child:	(−4) to (+2)			
		Adult:	(−2) to (+3)			
Benzene	S	Negative:	None detected			None detected
			mg/L			**μmol/L**
		Toxic:	>1.0		× 12.8	>13
	U	As phenol:	<20.0		× 10.6	<213
		Toxic, as phenol:	>30.0			>319
Beryllium Fluorometric, AAS	U, 24-h	Negative:	None detected			None detected
		Toxic:	>20 μg/L		× 0.111	>2.22 μmol/L
Bicarbonate (HCO$_3^-$)	S	Arterial:	21 to 28 mmol/L		× 1	21 to 28 mmol/L
		Venous:	22 to 29 mmol/L			22 to 29 mmol/L
			mEq/L			**mmol/L**
	WB, arterial (Hep; anaerobic)	Cord blood:				
		Arterial:	22.3 ± 2.5 (SD)		× 1	22.3 ± 2.5 (SD)
		Venous:	20.4 ± 4.1 (SD)		× 1	20.4 ± 4.1 (SD)
		Newborn:	17 to 24		× 1	17 to 24
		Infant:	19 to 24			19 to 24
		2 mo to 2 y:	16 to 24			16 to 24
		Adult:	22 to 26			22 to 26
			μg/mL			**μmol/L**
Bile Acids, Total GLC	S	Deoxycholic	0.09 to 0.35		× 2.547	0.23 to 0.89
		Chenodeoxycholic	0 to 0.63		× 2.547	0 to 1.61
		Cholic	0.03 to 0.37		× 2.448	0.08 to 0.91

Bilirubin Total	S		**Premature mg/dL**	**Full term mg/dL**		**Premature μmol/L**	**Full term μmol/L**
		Cord:	<2.0	<2.0	× 17.1	<34.2	<34.2
		0 to 1 day:	<8.0	1.4 to 8.7		<137	24 to 149
		1 to 2 day:	<12.0	3.4 to 11.5		<205	58 to 197
		3 to 5 day:	<16.0	1.5 to 12.0		<274	26 to 205
		Adult:		0.3 to 1.2			5 to 21
	U		Negative			Negative	
	Amf	28 wk:	<0.075 mg/dL (or ΔA_{450} < 0.048)		× 17.1	<1.28 μmol/L	
		40 wk:	<0.025 mg/dL (or ΔA_{450} < 0.02)			<0.43 μmol/L	
Conjugated (direct)	S		0 to 0.2 mg/dL		× 17.1	0 to 3.4 μmol/L	

TABLE 46-8 Chemistry and Toxicology—cont'd

Test	Specimen		Reference Interval	Conversion Factor	Reference Interval (International Units)
Bismuth	P (Hep)		<0.1 to 3.5 µg/L	× 4.785	<0.5 to 16.7 nmol/L
	U, 24-h		<0.3 to 4.6 µg/L	× 4.785	<1.4 to 22.0 nmol/L
Blood Volume	WB (Hep)	Male:	52 to 83 mL/kg	× 0.001	0.052 to 0.083 L/kg
		Female:	50 to 75 mL/kg		0.050 to 0.075 L/kg
Borate	S		**mg/L**		**µmol/L**
		Child:	<7	× 16.4	<115
		Adult, man:	<2		<33
		Toxic:	>20		>329
Bromosulfophthalein (BSP) Test (5mg/kg)	S		<6% retention at 45 min	× 0.01	Fraction dye retained: <0.06
Cadmium	WB (Hep)	Nonsmokers:	0.3 to 1.2 µg/L	× 8.897	2.7 to 10.7 nmol/L
		Smokers:	0.6 to 3.9 µg/L		5.3 to 34.7 nmol/L
	U, 24-h	Toxic:	100 to 3000 µg/L	× 0.0089	0.9 to 26.7 µmol/L
Calcitonin (CT)	S or P (Hep or EDTA)		**pg/mL**		**ng/L**
		Newborn:	70 to 348	× 1	70 to 348
		Term, cord:	25 to 150		25 to 150
		48 h:	91 to 580		91 to 580
		7 days:	77 to 293		77 to 293
		Premature, cord:	30 to 265		30 to 265
		48 h:	108 to 670		108 to 670
		7 days:	79 to 570		79 to 570
		Adult:			
		Man:	≤100		≤100
		Woman:	≤30		<30
			Increases in pregnancy		
			Concentrations decrease with age.		
Calcitonin-Calcium Infusion Stimulation Test Dose: 15 mg Ca (as gluconate)/kg, IV infusion/4h	S or P (Hep or EDTA): baseline, 3 and 4 h	Peak hCT level, Male: Female:	≤190 pg/mL ≤130 pg/mL	× 1	<190 ng/L <130 ng/L
Calcium, Free ISE			**mg/dL**		**mmol/L**
	WB (Hep)	>18 y:	4.6 to 5.1	× 0.25	1.15 to 1.27
	P (Hep)	>18 y:	4.12 to 4.92		1.03 to 1.23
	S	1 to 18 y:	4.80 to 5.52		1.20 to 1.38
		>18 y:	4.64 to 5.28		1.16 to 1.32
	WB, capillary	Newborn, full-term:			
		1 day (6 to 36 h):	4.20 to 5.48		1.05 to 1.37
		2 days (60 to 84 h):	4.40 to 5.68		1.10 to 1.42
		5 days (108 to 132 h):	4.80 to 5.92		1.20 to 1.48

Continued

TABLE 46-8　Chemistry and Toxicology—cont'd

Test	Specimen		Reference Interval	Conversion Factor	Reference Interval (International Units)
Calcium, Total	S		**mg/dL**		**mmol/L**
		Cord:	8.2 to 11.2	× 0.25	2.05 to 2.80
		Premature:	6.2 to 11.0		1.55 to 2.75
		0 to 10 days:	7.6 to 10.4		1.90 to 2.60
		10 days to 24 mo:	9.0 to 11.0		2.25 to 2.75
		Child, 2 to 12 y:	8.8 to 10.8		2.2 to 2.70
		Adult:	8.6 to 10.3		2.15 to 2.50
		Man, >60 y:	8.8 to 10.2		2.20 to 2.55
	CSF		4.2 to 5.4	× 0.25	1.05 to 1.35
	U, 24-h	**Ca in diet**	**mg/day**		**mmol/day**
		Ca-free:	5 to 40	× 0.025	0.13 to 1.00
		Low to average:	50 to 150		1.25 to 3.75
		Average (800 mg/day):	100 to 300		2.50 to 7.50
	F	Average:	420 to 560	× 0.025	10.5 to 14
Cancer Antigen 125 (CA125)	S		<35 U/mL	× 1.0	<35 kU/L
Cancer Antigen 15-3 (CA 15-3)	S		<30 U/mL	× 1.0	<30 kU/mL
Carbohydrate Antigen 19-9 (CA 19-9)	S		<37 U/mL	× 1.0	<37 kU/L
Cancer Antigen 27-29 (CA 27-29)	S		0 to 40 *U/mL*	× 1000	0 to 40,000 *U/L*
Carnitine (Free and Total) Enzymatic	S		**μmol/L**		
		Total:	2.6 to 8.1	× 1	Same
		Free:	2.3 to 7.0		
		Esterified (acyl):	0.0 to 1.9		
Cannabinoids	P (Hep or EDTA)		Negative		Negative
		THC after smoking 10 mg:	0.019 to 0.026 mg/L	× 3.18	0.060 to 0.083 μmol/L
	U	Negative			Negative
Carbon Dioxide, Partial Pressure (*PCO_2*)	WB, arterial (Hep)		**mm Hg**		**kPa**
		Newborn:	27 to 40	× 0.133	3.59 to 5.32
		Infant:	27 to 41		3.59 to 5.45
		Adult,			
		Man:	35 to 48		4.66 to 6.38
		Woman:	32 to 45	× 0.133	4.26 to 5.99
		Cord blood:			
		Arterial:	49 ± 8.4 (SD)		6.54 ± 1.12
		Venous:	38 ± 5.6 (SD)		5.08 ± 0.74
Carbon Dioxide, Total (*tCO_2*)	S or P (Hep)		**mmol/L**		Same
		Cord:	14 to 22		
		Newborn:	13 to 22		
		Premature, 1 wk:	14 to 27		
		Infant:	20 to 28		
		Child:	20 to 28		
		Adult:	22 to 28		
		>60 y:	23 to 31		

TABLE 46-8   Chemistry and Toxicology—cont'd

Test	Specimen	Reference Interval		Conversion Factor	Reference Interval (International Units)
Carbon Disulfide GLC, color (metabolites)	WB (F⁻/Ox) U	Negative: Occup. exp.: Toxic: Exposure index:	None detected <0.3 mg/L >0.5 mg/L 6 to 10 mg · L⁻¹ · s	× 13.1	None detected <3.9 μmol/L >6.6 μmol/L 6 to 10 mg · L⁻¹ · s
Carbon Monoxide	WB (EDTA)	Nonsmokers: Smokers, 1 to 2 pack/day: >2 packs/day: Toxic: Lethal:	**% HbCO** 0.5 to 1.5 4 to 5 8 to 9 >20 >50	× 0.01	**HbCO fraction** 0.005 to 0.015 0.04 to 0.05 0.08 to 0.09 >0.20 >0.5
Carboxyhemoglobin, *see Carbon Monoxide*					
Carcinoembryonic Antigen (CEA)	S	Nonsmokers: 99% of healthy Smokers: 95% 4%	<5.0 ng/mL <5.0 ng/mL 5.1 to 10.0 ng/mL	× 1	<5.0 μg/L <5.0 μg/L 5.1 to 10.0 μg/L
β-Carotene HPLC	S		**μg/dL** 10 to 85	× 0.0186	**μmol/L** 0.19 to 1.58
β-Carotene Absorption Test Dose: 15,000 U carotene orally, 3 × daily with meals for 3 days	S	Increase by ≥35 μg/dL after loading.		× 0.0186	Increase by ≥0.65 μmol/L after loading
Catecholamines, Total Fluorometric	U, 24-h	Adult: Infant: 2 to 3 mo: 4 to 11 mo: 12 to 19 mo: Adult:	**μg/m²/day** <100 5 to 34 8 to 51 19 to 48 <100 μg/day	× 5.91	**nmol/m²/day** <100 30 to 201 47 to 301 112 to 284 <591 nmol/day Conversion factor based on norepinephrine, MW 169.18)
Catecholamines, Fractionated HPLC	U, 24-h	Norepinephrine: 1 to 4 y: 4 to 10 y: 10 to 15 y: Adult: Epinephrine: 1 to 4 y: 4 to 10 y: 10 to 15 y: Adult: Dopamine: 1 to 4 y: >4 y:	**μg/day** 0 to 29 8 to 65 15 to 80 15 to 80 **μg/day** 0 to 6.0 0 to 10.0 0.5 to 20 0 to 20 **μg/day** 10 to 260 65 to 400	× 5.91 × 5.46 × 6.53	**nmol/day** 0 to 171 47 to 384 89 to 473 89 to 473 **nmol/day** 0 to 32.8 0 to 54.6 2.7 to 109 0 to 109 **nmol/day** 65 to 1698 425 to 2610

Continued

TABLE 46-8 | Chemistry and Toxicology—cont'd

Test	Specimen	Reference Interval		Conversion Factor	Reference Interval (International Units)
Catecholamines HPLC	P (EDTA and Na met-abisulfite)		**pg/mL**		**pmol/L**
		Epinephrine, random:	<140	× 5.46	<764
		Norepinephrine, random:	<1700	× 5.91	<10,047
		Dopamine, random:	<30	× 6.53	<196
		Lower values with patient supine			
Cerebrospinal Fluid Volume	CSF	Child:	60 to 100 mL	× 0.001	0.06 to 0.10 L
		Adult:	100 to 160 mL		0.10 to 0.16 L
Ceruloplasmin RID	S		**mg/dL**		**mg/L**
		1 day to 3 mo:	5 to 18	× 10	50 to 180
		6 mo to 1 y:	33 to 43		330 to 430
		1 to 7 y:	24 to 56		240 to 560
		Thereafter:	18 to 45		180 to 450
		Levels rise during pregnancy and may peak at levels 3 times normal.			
Chenodeoxycholic Acid, Total	S		0.31 ± 0.32 µg/mL	× 2.55	0.79 ± 0.82 µmol/L
Chenodeoxycholyl-glycine, Conjugated	S		0.09 ± 0.01 µg/mL	× 2.22	0.2 ± 0.03 µmol/L
Chloride	S or P (Hep)		**mmol/L**		Same
		Cord:	96 to 104		
		Newborn, 0 to 30 days:	98 to 113		
		Thereafter:	98 to 107		
	CSF	Infant:	110 to 130		
		Adult:	118 to 132		
	U, 24-h		**mmol/day**		Same
		Infant:	2 to 10		
		Child:	15 to 40		
		Thereafter:	110 to 250		
		Varies greatly with Cl intake.			
	Swt		**mmol/L**		Same
		Normal:	5 to 35		
		Marginal:	30 to 70		
		Cystic fibrosis:	60 to 200		
	RBC, lysed		49 to 54		
			mmol/L		Same
	Sal	Without stimulation:	5 to 20		
		After stimulation:	44		
	WB		77 to 87		

TABLE 46-8 Chemistry and Toxicology—cont'd

Test	Specimen	Reference Interval		Conversion Factor	Reference Interval (International Units)
Cholesterol, Total	S, P (EDTA or Hep)		**mg/dL** **Fifth to ninety-fifth percentile**		**mmol/L** **Fifth to ninety-fifth percentile**
		Cord blood:			
Liebermann-Burchard, Zlatkis-Zak (ferric chloride–sulfuric acid), color, enzymatic		Male:	44 to 103	× 0.0259	1.14 to 2.66
		Female:	50 to 108		1.29 to 2.79
		0 to 4 y, Boy:	114 to 203		2.95 to 5.25
		Girl:	112 to 200		2.90 to 5.18
		5 to 9 y, Boy:	121 to 203		3.13 to 5.25
		Girl:	126 to 205		3.26 to 5.30
		10 to 14 y, Boy:	119 to 202		3.08 to 5.23
		Girl:	124 to 201		3.21 to 5.20
		15 to 19 y, Boy:	113 to 197		2.93 to 5.10
		Girl:	119 to 200		3.08 to 5.18
		20 to 24 y, Man:	124 to 218		3.21 to 5.64
		Woman:	122 to 216		3.16 to 5.59
		25 to 29 y, Man:	133 to 244		3.44 to 6.32
		Woman:	128 to 222		3.32 to 5.75
		30 to 34 y, Man:	138 to 254		3.57 to 6.58
		Woman:	130 to 230		3.37 to 5.96
		35 to 39 y, Man:	146 to 270		3.78 to 6.99
		Woman:	140 to 242		3.63 to 6.27
		40 to 44 y, Man:	151 to 268		3.91 to 6.94
		Woman:	147 to 252		3.81 to 6.53
		45 to 49 y, Man:	158 to 276		4.09 to 7.15
		Woman:	152 to 265		3.94 to 6.86
		50 to 54 y, Man:	158 to 277		4.09 to 7.17
		Woman:	162 to 285		4.20 to 7.38
		55 to 59 y, Man:	156 to 276		4.04 to 7.15
		Woman:	172 to 300		4.45 to 7.77
		60 to 64 y, Man:	159 to 276		4.12 to 7.15
		Woman:	172 to 297		4.45 to 7.69
		65 to 69 y, Man:	158 to 274		4.09 to 7.10
		Woman:	171 to 303		4.43 to 7.85
		>70 y, Man:	144 to 265		3.73 to 6.86
		Woman:	173 to 280		4.48 to 7.25
		In North America, a reference interval, based on an "apparently healthy population," is relatively high, primarily because of diet. Values for blacks are approximately 10 mg/dL (0.26 mmol/L) higher than for whites after age 10 y. Adult levels in terms of risk for coronary heart disease:			
		Recommended (desirable):	<200 mg/dL [<5.18 mmol/L]		
		Moderate risk:	200 to 239 mg/dL [5.18 to 6.19 mmol/L]		
		High risk:	≥240 mg/dL [≥6.22 mmol/L]		
Cholic Acid, Total	S		0.20 ± 0.17 µg/mL	× 2.45	0.49 ± 0.42 µmol/L

Continued

TABLE 46-8   Chemistry and Toxicology—cont'd

Test	Specimen		Reference Interval	Conversion Factor	Reference Interval (International Units)
Cholinesterase II (S-Pseudocholines- erase)					
Photometric			4.9 to 11.9 U/mL	× 1.0	4.9 to 11.9 kU/L
Dade aca			7 to 19 U/mL		7 to 19 kU/L
Inhibition:	S	Dibucaine:	79% to 84% inhibition	× 0.01	0.79 to 0.84
		Fluoride:	58% to 64% inhibition		0.58 to 0.64 Fraction of activity inhibited
Cholylglycine, Conjugated	S		0.13 ± 0.01 μg/mL	× 2.15	0.27 ± 0.03 μmol/L
Chorionic Gonadotropin, Intact Molecule	S		**mIU/mL**		**IU/L**

Male and nonpregnant female: <5.0   × 1   <50

Female:

After fertilization	After last menstrual period				
2 wk:	4 wk:	5 to 100			5 to 100
3 wk:	5 wk:	200 to 3000			200 to 300
4 wk:	6 wk:	10,000 to 80,000			10,000 to 80,000
5 to 12 wk:	7 to 14 wk:	90,000 to 500,000			90,000 to 500,000
13 to 24 wk:	15 to 26 wk:	5000 to 80,000			5000 to 80,000
26 to 38 wk:	27 to 40 wk:	3000 to 15,000			3000 to 15,000
Trophoblastic disease:		>100,000			>100,000

Values based on the Second International Standard for CG.

Test	Specimen	Reference Interval	Conversion Factor	Reference Interval (International Units)
Chromium	WB (Hep)	0.7 to 28.0 μg/L	× 19.23	14 to 538 nmol/L
AAS	S	<0.05 to 0.5 μg/L		1 to 10 nmol/L
	U, 24-h	0.1 to 2.0 μg/day		1.9 to 38.4 nmol/day
	RBC	20 to 36 μm/L		384 to 692 nmol/L
Chymotrypsin	S or P (EDTA and poly-brene)	~10 μg/L	× 1.0	~10 μg/L
	F	120 to 1265 μg/g stool (mean: 290)	× 1.0	120 to 1265 mg/kg stool (mean: 290)
Cobalt	S	0.11 to 0.45 μg/L	× 16.97	1.9 to 7.6 nmol/L
	U	1 to 2 μg/L		17.0 to 34.0 nmol/L
	RBC	16 to 46 μg/kg		272 to 781 nmol/kg
Complement Components				
Total hemolytic complement activity	S, P (EDTA)	75 to 160 U/mL	× 1000	75 to 160 kU/mL
Classic pathway components (RID)		**mg/dL**		**mg/L**
C1q	S, P (EDTA)	14.9 to 22.1	× 10	149 to 221
C1r	S, P	2.5 to 10.0		25 to 100
C1s (C1 esterase)	S, P	5 to 10.0		50 to 100
C2	S, P	1.6 to 3.6		16 to 36
C3 (β₁ C-globulin) Neph	S, P	83 to 177		830 to 1770

TABLE 46-8 Chemistry and Toxicology—cont'd

Test	Specimen	Reference Interval		Conversion Factor	Reference Interval (International Units)
Complement Components—cont'd		**mg/dL**			**mg/L**
Classic pathway components (RID)					
C4 (β_1 E-globulin) Neph	S, P	29 to 68			290 to 680
C5 (β_1 F-globulin)	S, P	5.5 to 11.3			55 to 113
C6	S, P	17.9 to 23.9			179 to 239
C7	S, P	2.7 to 7.4			27 to 74
C8	S, P	4.9 to 10.6			49 to 106
C9	S, P	3.3 to 9.5			33 to 95
Alternative pathway components					
Factor D RIA, ELISA	S, P (EDTA, EGTA, citrate)	1 to 5 µg/mL		× 1.0	1 to 5 mg/L
Properdin RID, ELISA	S, P (EDTA, EGTA, citrate)	**µg/mL**			**mg/L**
		Cord serum:	8.1 to 23.4	× 1.0	8.1 to 23.4
		Adults:	10 to 30		10 to 30
			10.5 to 36.5		10.5 to 36.5
Factor B (Properdin factor B, Bf, C3-proactivator, C3PA) RID, nephelom		**µg/mL**			**mg/L**
		Adults:	127 to 278	× 1.0	127 to 278
		mg/dL			**mg/L**
		Cord serum:	7.8 to 15.8	× 10	78 to 158
		Adults:	14.7 to 33.5		147 to 335
Regulatory components					
C1-INH (C1 esterase inhibitor, C1-inactivator, C1-INH) RID, FIA, nephelom	S, P (EDTA, EGTA, citrate)	**mg/dL**			**mg/L**
		8 to 19.5		× 10	80 to 195
		12.4 to 24.0			124 to 240
		12.6 to 14.8			126 to 148
C1-INH Functional assays RID, ELISA		RID results are reported as "normal" or "abnormal" ELISA results: >68% of mean normal function			
C4-binding Protein (C4bp) RID	S, P (EDTA, EGTA, citrate)	18 to 32 mg/dL		× 10	180 to 320 mg/L
		250 µg/mL		× 1.0	250 mg/L
		470 µg/L		× 1.0	470 µg/L
Factor H RID		40.5 ± 71.7 mg/dL		× 10	405 ± 717 mg/L
		0.025 to 0.05 mg/mL		× 1000	25 to 50 mg/L
Factor I RID		35 µg/mL		× 1.0	35 mg/L
		25 µg/mL		× 1.0	25 mg/L
Copper AAS	S	**µg/dL**			**µmol/L**
		Birth to 6 mo:	20 to 70	× 0.157	3.14 to 10.99
		6 y:	90 to 190		14.13 to 29.83
		12 y:	80 to 160		12.56 to 25.12
		Adult:			
		Man:	70 to 140		10.99 to 21.98
		Woman:	80 to 155		12.56 to 24.34
		Pregnancy at term:	118 to 302		18.53 to 47.41
		Values for blacks ~8% to 12% higher			Blacks ~8% to 12% higher
	RBC (Hep)	90 to 150 µg/dL		× 0.157	14.13 to 23.55 µmol/L
	U, 24-h	3 to 35 µg/day		× 0.0157	0.047 to 0.55 µmol/day
		2 to 80 µg/L		× 0.0157	0.03 to 1.26 µmol/L

Continued

TABLE 46-8　Chemistry and Toxicology—cont'd

Test	Specimen		Reference Interval	Conversion Factor	Reference Interval (International Units)
Coproporphyrin	U, 24-h		19 to 34 μmol/mol creatinine	× 10.3	195 to 320 nmol/day
	F, 24-h		<30 μg/g dry wt	× 1.53	<46 nmol/g dry wt
			400 to 1200 μg/day		612 to 1836 nmol/day
Corticobinding Globulin (CBG) *(see Transcortin)*					
Corticosterone	S or P (Hep, EDTA, or Ox)	Adult,			
		0800 h:	130 to 820 ng/dL	× 0.0289	4 to 24 nmol/L
		1600 h:	60 to 220 ng/dL		2 to 6 nmol/L
Cortisol	S or P (Hep)	0800 h:	5 to 23 μg/dL	× 27.6	138 to 635 nmol/L
		1600 h:	3 to 16 μg/dL		83 to 441 nmol/L
		2000 h:	≤50% of 0800 h	× 0.01	Fraction of 0800 h: ≤0.50
Cortisol, Free HPLC	U, 24-h		**μg/day**		**nmol/day**
		Child:	1 to 21	× 2.76	3 to 58
		Adolescent:	2 to 38		6 to 105
		Adult:	≤50		≤138
C-Peptide RIA	S	Adult:	0.78 to 1.89 ng/mL	× 0.33	0.26 to 0.62 nmol/L
	U		44.1 to 85.1 ng/mL		14.5 to 28.2 nmol/L
C-Reactive Protein (CRP)	S		<1 mg/dL	× 10	<10 mg/L
RIA		Lower 95th percentile:	20 to 610 μg/dL	× 0.01	0.20 to 6.10 mg/L
Neph	S		**μg/dL**		**μg/L**
		Cord:	1 to 35	× 10	10 to 350
		Adult:	6.8 to 820		68 to 8200
Creatine	S or P	Male:	0.17 to 0.70 mg/dL	× 76.3	13 to 53 μmol/L
		Female:	0.35 to 0.93 mg/dL		27 to 71 μmol/L
	U, 24-h	Male:	0 to 40 mg/day	× 7.63	0 to 305 μmol/L
		Female:	0 to 80 mg/day		0 to 609 μmol/day
Creatine Kinase (CK) Total, 30 °C	S		**U/L**		**μkat/L**
		Newborn:	10 to 200	× 0.017	0.17 to 3.40
		Adult,			
		Male:	15 to 105		0.26 to 1.79
		Female:	10 to 80		0.17 to 1.36
		>60 y,			
		Male:	20 to 110		0.34 to 1.87
		Female:	16 to 18		0.27 to 0.31
		>70 y,			
		Man:	22 to 90		0.37 to 1.53
		Woman:	19 to 76		0.32 to 1.29
		Ambulatory:			
		Male:	25 to 90		0.43 to 1.53
		Female:	10 to 70		0.17 to 1.19
			Higher after exercise		
Total, CK-NAC, 30 °C		Newborn:	68 to 580		1.16 to 9.86
		Adult,			
		Man:	25 to 130		0.43 to 2.21
		Woman:	10 to 115		0.17 to 1.96

TABLE 46-8 Chemistry and Toxicology—cont'd

Test	Specimen		Reference Interval	Conversion Factor	Reference Interval (International Units)
Creatine Kinase (CK)—cont'd			**U/L**		**μkat/L**
Isoenzymes		Fraction 2 (MB):	<4% to 6% of total (method dependent)	× 0.01	Fraction of total: <0.04 to 0.06
Immunoenzymetric, CK-2 (Hybritech Tandem-E)	S	CK-2:	0 to 9 μg/L		

$$\text{CK-2 relative index (\%)} = \frac{\text{CK-2 μg/L}}{\text{Total CK (U/L)}} \times 100 = <3.9\% \times 0.01 \; [<0.039, \text{fractional activity}]$$

Test	Specimen		Reference Interval	Conversion Factor	Reference Interval (International Units)
Creatine Kinase Isoforms (CK Isoforms) EP	S		**% of Total Activity**		**Fraction of Total Activity**
		CK-3_1:	42 to 75	× 0.01	0.42 to 0.75
		CK-3_2:	18 to 51		0.18 to 0.51
		CK-3_3:	2 to 14		0.02 to 0.14
Creatinine	S or P		**mg/dL**		**μmol/L**
Jaffe, kinetic, or enzymatic		Cord:	0.6 to 1.2	× 88.4	53 to 106
		Newborn, 1 to 4 days:	0.3 to 1.0		27 to 88
		Infant:	0.2 to 0.4		18 to 35
		Child:	0.3 to 0.7		27 to 62
		Adolescent:	0.5 to 1.0		44 to 88
		Adult:			
		Man:	0.7 to 1.3		62 to 115
		Woman:	0.6 to 1.1		53 to 97
Jaffe, manual	S or P		0.8 to 1.5 mg/dL	× 88.4	71 to 133 μmol/L
	Amf	After 37 wk gestation:	>2.0 mg/dL	× 88.4	>177 μmol/L
	U, 24-h		**mg/kg/day**		**μmol/kg/day**
		Infant:	8 to 20	× 8.84	71 to 177
		Child:	8 to 22		71 to 194
		Adolescent:	8 to 30		71 to 265
		Adult:			
		Man:	14 to 26		124 to 230
		Woman:	11 to 20		97 to 177
		Declines with age to (10 mg/kg)/d at age 90 y			
Creatinine Clearance (Endogenous)	S or P, and U	20 to 29 y:	**mL/min/1.73 m²**		**mL/s/m²**
		Man:	94 to 140	× 0.00963	0.91 to 1.35
		Woman:	72 to 110		0.69 to 1.06
			Decreases ~6.5 per decade		Decreases (~0.06) per decade
		Impairment			
		Borderline:	62.5 to 80	× 0.00963	0.60
		Slight:	52 to 63		0.50 to 0.60
		Mild:	42 to 52		0.41 to 0.50
		Moderate:	28 to 42		0.27 to 0.40
		Marked:	<28		<0.27
Cyanide	S		**mg/L**		**μmol/L**
		Nonsmokers:	0.004	× 38.4	0.15
		Smokers:	0.006		0.23
		Nitroprusside therapy:	0.01 to 0.06		0.38 to 2.30
		Toxic:	>0.1		>3.84

Continued

TABLE 46-8　Chemistry and Toxicology—cont'd

Test	Specimen		Reference Interval	Conversion Factor	Reference Interval (International Units)
Cyanide—cont'd			**mg/L**		**μmol/L**
	WB (Ox)	Nonsmokers:	0.016		0.61
		Smokers:	0.041		1.57
		Nitroprusside therapy:	0.05 to 0.5		1.92 to 19.20
		Toxic:	>1		>38.40
Cyclic AMP	P (EDTA)	Male:	4.6 to 8.6 ng/mL	× 3.04	14 to 26 nmol/L
		Female:	4.3 to 7.6 ng/mL		13 to 23 nmol/L
	U, 24-h		0.3 to 3.6 mg/day	× 3.04	1 to 10.9 μmol/day
			0.29 to 2.1 mg/g creatinine	× 344	100 to 723 μmol/mol creatinine
Cystine	P (hep)	Adult:	0.40 to 1.40	× 83.3	33 to 117 μmol/L
Qual.	U, random		Negative		Negative
Quant.	U, 24-h		<38.1 mg/day	× 8.32	<317 μmol/day Conversion based on cysteine (MW 121.16)
			2 to 14 mg/g creatinine	× 0.94	1.9 to 13.1 mmol/mol creatinine
Dehydroepiandrosterone (DHEA)					
Total unconjugated	S		**ng/dL**		**nmol/L**
		Cord:	200 to 1590	× 0.0347	6.9 to 55.1
		1 to 10 y:	<20 to 345		<0.7 to 12.0
		Adult:			
		Man:	180 to 1250		6.2 to 43.3
		Woman:	130 to 980		4.5 to 34.0
Unconjugated	U, 24-h	Child:	**mg/day**		**μmol/day**
		0 to 5 y:	<0.1	× 3.47	<0.3
		6 to 9 y:	<0.2		<0.7
		10 to 15 y:	<0.4		<1.4
		Adult:			
		Man:	<3.1		<10.8
		Woman:	<1.5		<5.2
Dehydroepiandrosterone Sulfate (DHEA-SO$_4$)	S or P (Hep or EDTA)		**μg/mL**		**μmol/L**
		Newborn:	88 to 356	× 0.027	2.4 to 9.6
		1 to 5 y:	<30		<0.8
		6 to 11 y:	<150		<4.1
		12 to 17 y:	30 to 550		0.8 to 14.9
		Adult:			
		Male, 31 to 50 y:	59 to 452		1.6 to 12.2
		Female, premenopausal, 31 to 50 y:	12 to 379		0.8 to 10.2
		Postmenopausal:	30 to 260		0.8 to 7.1
	Amf		10 to 50 ng/mL	× 2.7	27 to 136 nmol/L
Deoxycholic Acid, Total	S		0.22 ± 0.13 μg/mL (SD)	× 2.55	0.56 ± 0.33 μmol/L (SD)
11-Deoxycorticosterone (DOC)	S or P (Hep, EDTA, or Ox)	Ad lib diet, 0800 h:	2 to 19 ng/dL	× 30.3	61 to 576 nmol/L
11-Deoxycortisol (Compound S)	P (Hep, EDTA, or Ox)		**μg/dL**		**μmol/L**
		1 to 10 y, 0800 h	20 to 155	× 0.029	0.6 to 4.5
		Adult, 0800 h	12 to 158		0.3 to 4.6

TABLE 46-8   Chemistry and Toxicology—cont'd

Test	Specimen	Reference Interval			Conversion Factor	Reference Interval (International Units)
Dexamethasone Single Dose Overnight Suppression Test Dose: 1 mg orally at 2300 or 2400 h	S, 0800 h	Cortisol: Suppression to <3 µg/dL			× 0.0276	Cortisol: Suppression to <0.08 µmol/L
Dexamethasone Suppression Test (Standard)	S, 0800 h Control, day 2 and 3	Cortisol: Suppression on day 4 to <50% of baseline or to <5 µg/dL			× 0.01 × 27.59	Cortisol: Suppression on day 4; fraction of baseline: <0.50 or <138 nmol/L
Low dose, adult: 0.5 mg q 6 h × 8	U, 24-h Control, day 1, 2, and 3	17-KGS: Suppression on day 4 to <7.5 mg/day			× 3.467	17-KGS: Suppression on day 4 to <26 µmol/day
		17-OHCS: Suppression on day 4 to <4.5 mg/day			× 2.76	17-OHCS: Suppression on day 4 to <12.4 µmol/d
		Free cortisol: <50% of baseline			× 0.01	Free cortisol: Fraction of baseline <0.50
High dose, adult: 2 mg q 6 h × 8		Free cortisol, 17-KGS, 17-OHCS: Suppression on day 6 to <50% of baseline			×0.01	Free cortisol, 17-KGS, 17-OHCS: Suppression on day 6; fraction of baseline: <0.50
Dihydrotestosterone (DHT)	S	**ng/dL** Pubertal Tanner stage 1: 2: 3: 4-5: Adult:	Boy <3 3 to 17 8 to 33 22 to 65 30 to 85	Girl <3 5 to 12 7 to 19 3 to 18 4 to 22	× 0.0344	**nmol/L** Male Female <0.10 <0.10 0.10 to 0.58 0.17 to 0.41 0.27 to 1.14 0.24 to 0.65 0.76 to 2.24 0.10 to 0.62 1.03 to 2.92 0.14 to 0.76
Disaccharide Absorption Test	S	**mg/dL** Change in glucose from fasting value: Inconclusive: Abnormal:	>30 20 to 30 <20		× 0.055	**mmol/L** Change in glucose from fasting >1.67 1.11 to 1.67 <1.11
Estradiol (E$_2$), Unconjugated	S	**pg/mL** Boy, pubertal stage I: II: III: Adult: Man: Woman, pubertal stage I: II: III: IV:	3 to 15 3 to 10 5 to 15 10 to 50 5 to 10 5 to 155 5 to 180 25 to 410		× 3.67	**pmol/L** 11 to 55 11 to 37 18 to 55 37 to 184 18 to 37 18 to 422 18 to 661 19 to 1266
	U, 24-h	**µg/day** Adult: Man: Woman, follicular: Ovulatory peak: Luteal: Postmeno-pausal:	1 to 4 1 to 13 4 to 20 1 to 17 0 to 4		× 3.67	**nmol/day** 0.4 to 1.7 0.4 to 5.4 1.7 to 8.3 0.4 to 7.1 0 to 15

Continued

TABLE 46-8 Chemistry and Toxicology—cont'd

Test	Specimen	Reference Interval		Conversion Factor	Reference Interval (International Units)
Estriol (E₃), Free	S	Pregnancy (wk):	**ng/mL**		**nmol/L**
		22:	2.6 to 8.0	× 3.47	9.0 to 27.8
		26:	2.5 to 13.5		8.7 to 46.8
		30:	3.5 to 19.0		12.1 to 65.9
		34:	5.8 to 18.3		18.4 to 63.5
		38:	8.6 to 38.0		29.8 to 131.9
		40:	9.6 to 28.9		33.3 to 100.3
	Amf	Pregnancy (wk):	**ng/mL (95% range)**		**nmol/L (95% range)**
		16 to 20:	1.0 to 3.2	× 3.47	3.5 to 11.1
		20 to 24:	2.1 to 7.8		7.3 to 27.1
		24 to 28:	2.1 to 7.8		7.3 to 27.1
		28 to 32:	4.0 to 13.6		13.9 to 47.2
		32 to 36:	3.6 to 15.5		12.5 to 53.8
		36 to 38:	4.6 to 18.0		16.0 to 62.5
		38 to 40:	5.4 to 19.8		18.7 to 68.7
Estriol (E₃), Total	S	Pregnancy (wk):	**ng/mL**		**nmol/L**
		28 to 30:	38 to 140	× 3.47	132 to 486
		32:	35 to 330		121 to 1145
		36:	48 to 350		167 to 1215
		40:	95 to 460		330 to 1596
	U, 24-h	Pregnancy (wk):	**μg/day**		**nmol/day**
		First trimester:	0 to 800	× 3.47	0 to 2776
		Second trimester:	800 to 12,000		2776 to 41,640
		Third trimester:	5000 to 50,000		17,350 to 173,500
					Fraction of previous value of <0.60 suggests fetus at risk.
	Amf	Pregnancy (wk):	**ng/mL**		**nmol/L**
		21 to 32:	5 to 50	× 3.47	17 to 174
		33 to 35:	9 to 240		31 to 833
		36 to 41:	150 to 213		521 to 739
Estrogen Receptor Assay (ERA)	T		**fmol/mg protein**		**nmol/kg protein**
		Negative:	<6	× 1	<6
		Borderline positive:	6 to 10		6 to 10
		Positive:	>10		>10
Estrogens, Total	S		**pg/mL**		**ng/L**
		Child (1 to 10 y):	<25	× 1	<25
		Adult:			
		Man:	20 to 80		20 to 80
		Woman:			
		Follicular:	60 to 200		60 to 200
		Luteal:	160 to 400		160 to 400
		Postmeno-pausal:	<130		<130
	U, 24-h		**μg/day**		
		Child:	<10		Same
		Boy, pubertal stage I:	2.5 (mean)		
		II:	5.9 (mean)		
		III:	6.2 (mean)		
		Adult,			
		Man:	15 to 40		
		Woman:			
		Postmeno-pausal:	<20		
		Premenopausal:	15 to 80		

TABLE 46-8   Chemistry and Toxicology—cont'd

Test	Specimen	Reference Interval		Conversion Factor	Reference Interval (International Units)
Estrone (E₁)					
Unconjugated	S		**ng/mL**		**pmol/L**
		Boy, pubertal stage			
		I:	0.50 to 1.7	× 37	18 to 63
		II:	1.0 to 2.5		37 to 92
		III:	1.5 to 2.5		55 to 92
		Adult:			
		Woman, pubertal	1.5 to 6.5		55 to 240
		stage I:	0.4 to 2.9		15 to 107
		II:	7.0		37 to 122
		III:	1.5 to 4.3		55 to 159
		IV:	1.6 to 7.7		59 to 285
		Follicular:	1.5 to 25		55 to 925
	U, 24-h		**μg/day**		**nmol/day**
		Adult:			
		Man:	3 to 8	× 3.70	11 to 30
		Woman:			
		Ovulatory peak:	11 to 31		41 to 115
		Luteal:	10 to 23		37 to 85
		Postmeno-pausal:	1 to 7		4 to 26
	Amf	38 to 40 wk:	2.3 to 4.0	× 3.70	9 to 15 nmol/L
Ethanol	WB (Ox) or S		**mg/dL**		**mmol/L**
		Impairment:	50 to 100	× 0.217	11 to 22
		Depression of CNS:	>100		>21.7
		Fatalities reported:	>400		>86.8
		Serum levels 10% to 35% greater than whole blood levels			
Ethylene Glycol	P (EDTA)		0 mg/L	× 16.1	0 μmol/L
	U		0 mg/L		0 μmol/L
		Toxic	>200 mg/L		3200
Fat, Fecal	F, 72-h		**g/day**	× 1	Same
		Infant, breast fed:	<1		
		0 to 6 y:	<2		
		Adult:	<7		
		Adult (fat-free diet):	<4		
Fatty Acid Profile	S or P (Hep)		**Percent of total non-esterified fatty acids**		**Fraction of total non-esterified fatty acids**
		Oleic:	26 to 45	× 0.01	0.26 to 0.45
		Palmitic:	23 to 25		0.23 to 0.25
		Stearic:	10 to 14		0.10 to 0.14
		Linoleic:	8 to 16		0.08 to 0.16
		Linoleate:	≥25		0.25
		Arachidonate:	≥6		0.06
Fatty Acids, Nonesterified Free	S or P (Hep)		**mg/dL**		**mmol/L**
		Adult:	8 to 25	× 0.0354	0.28 to 0.89
		Child and obese adult:	<31		<1.10 Conversion factor based on oleic acid, MW 282.47
Ferric Chloride Test	U, random		Negative		Negative

Continued

TABLE 46-8   Chemistry and Toxicology—cont'd

Test	Specimen		Reference Interval	Conversion Factor	Reference Interval (International Units)
Ferritin	S		**ng/mL**		**µg/L**
		Newborn:	25 to 200	× 1	25 to 200
		1 mo:	200 to 600		200 to 600
		2 to 5 mo:	50 to 200		50 to 200
		6 mo to 15 y:	7 to 140		7 to 140
		Adult:			
		Man:	20 to 250		20 to 250
		Woman:	10 to 120		10 to 120
α₁-Fetoprotein (AFP)	S	Adult:	<15 ng/mL	× 1	<15 µg/L
		Fetus:	Peak of 200 to 400 mg/dL in 1st trimester, falls to 1% of peak (<5 mg/dL) in cord blood	× 0.01	Peak of 2 to 4 g/L in first trimester; falls to 1% of peak (<0.05 g/L) in cord blood.
		1 y:	<30 ng/mL	× 1	<30 µg/L
	S, maternal	Pregnancy (week)	**ng/mL (median)**		**µg/L (median)**
		14	25.6		25.6
		15	29.9		29.9
		16	34.8		34.8
		17	40.6		40.6
		18	47.3		47.3
		19	55.1		55.1
		20	64.3		64.3
		21	74.9		74.9
	Amf	Pregnancy (week)	**µg/mL (median)**	× 1	**mg/L (median)**
		15	16.3		16.3
		16	14.5		14.5
		17	13.4		13.4
		18	12.0		12.0
		19	10.7		10.7
		20	8.1		8.1
		21	6.2		
		22	5.5		
Fibrinogen	P (NaCit)	Adult:	200 to 400 mg/dL	× 0.01	2.00 to 4.00 g/L
		Newborn:	125 to 300 mg/dL	× 0.01	1.23 to 3.00 g/L
FIGLU (Formiminoglutamic Acid) Dose: 5 g histidine q 4 h × 3	U, 24-h, after initial dose	Normal: Folate deficiency:	<35 mg/day >35 mg/day	× 5.74	<201 µmol/day >201 µmol/day
Fluoride			**µg/mL**		**µmol/L**
	P (Hep)		0.01 to 0.2	× 52.6	0.5 to 10.5
	U		0.2 to 3.2		10.5 to 168
		Occup. exp.:	<8.0		<421
Folate	S	2 to 16 y:	5 to 21 ng/mL	× 2.265	11 to 48 nmol/L
		>16 y:	3 to 20 ng/mL		7 to 45 nmol/L
	RBC (EDTA)	2 to 16 y:	>160 ng/mL		>362 nmol/L
		>16 y:	140 to 628 ng/mL		>317 to 1422 nmol/L
Folate Absorption Test	U, 24-h		45 ± 7% of dose	× 0.01	Fraction of dose: 0.45 ± 0.07

TABLE 46-8   Chemistry and Toxicology—cont'd

Test	Specimen	Reference Interval		Conversion Factor	Reference Interval (International Units)
Follicle-Stimulating Hormone (FSH, follitropin) Numerical values based on WHO 2nd IRP 78/549 reference materials	S or P (Hep)		**mIU/mL**		**IU/L**
		2 to 11 mo:			
		Male:	0.19 to 11.3	× 1.0	0.19 to 11.3
		Female:	0.1 to 11.3		0.1 to 11.3
		Adult:			
		Man:	1.4 to 15.4		1.4 to 15.4
		Woman:			
		Follicular:	1 to 10		1 to 10
		Ovulatory peak:	6 to 17		6 to 17
		Luteal:	1 to 9		1 to 9
		Postmenopausal:	19 to 100		90 to 100
	U, 24-h		**IU/day***		**IU/L**
		Prepubertal child:	<1.0 to 3.4		Same
		Puberty, Tanner stage:			
		1: Boy, girl:	<1.3		
		2: Boy:	1 to 7		
		Girl:	2 to 6		
		3: Boy:	2 to 9		
		Girl:	3 to 8		
		4: Boy:	2 to 10		
		Girl:	3 to 9		
		5: Boy:	3 to 12		
		Girl:	2 to 11		
		Adult:			
		Man:	3 to 11		
		Woman: nonmidcycle:	2 to 15		
Formaldehyde			**mg/L**		**μmol/L**
	WB (F$^-$/Ox)	Occup. exp.:	0.6 to 4.0	× 33.3	20 to 133
	U	Formic acid:	<17	× 21.7	<369
Free Thyroxine Index (FT$_4$I) Calculation	S		**FT$_4$ index**		Same
		Cord blood:	6.0 to 13.2		
		1 to 3 days:	9.9 to 17.5		
		1 wk:	7.5 to 15.1		
		1 to 12 mo:	5.0 to 13.0		
		1 to 3 y:	5.4 to 12.5		
		3 to 10 y:	5.7 to 12.8		
		>10 and adult:	4.2 to 13.0		
		Borderline low:	4.8		
		Borderline high:	14.0		
Free Thyroxine (see Thyroxine, Free)					
Free Triiodothyronine, (see Triiodothyronine, Free)					
Fructose	S		1 to 6 mg/dL	× 55.5	55.5 to 333 μmol/L
	U		<30 to 65 mg/day	× 5.55	<130 to 360 μmol/day
	Semf		>150 mg/dL	× 0.0555	>8.33 mmol/L

*WHO, First International Reference Preparation of FSH/LH 69/104.

Continued

TABLE 46-8   Chemistry and Toxicology—cont'd

Test	Specimen		Reference Interval	Conversion Factor	Reference Interval (International Units)
Fructosamine	S	Child:	5% less than adult levels		Same
		Adult:	1.61 to 2.68 mmol/L		
Galactose	S	Newborn:	0 to 20 mg/dL	× 0.0555	0 to 1.11 mmol/L
		Thereafter:	<5 mg/dL		<0.28 mmol/L
	U	Newborn:	≤60 mg/dL	× 0.0555	≤3.33 mmol/L
		Thereafter:	<14 mg/d	× 0.00555	<0.08 mmol/day
Galactose Tolerance Test Dose: 40 g in 250 mL H_2O, orally	WB (Hep with NaF)	60 min:	40 to 60 mg/dL	× 0.0555	2.22 to 3.33 mmol/L
		Sum of 30-, 60-, 90-, 120-min specimens:	<110 mg/dL		<6.11 mmol/L
	U, 5-h		≤3 g/5 h	× 5.55	<16.7 mmol/5 h
Galactose-1-Phosphate Uridyl Transferase Enzymatic	P (EDTA)		**U/g hemoglobin** 14.7 to 25.4	0.0645	**MU/mol hemoglobin** 0.9 to 1.6
Gastric Acid	Gast Res		**Without stimulation mmol/L**		Same
		Free:	0 to 40		
		Total:	10 to 50		
Gastric Content	Gast Res	Volume:	20 to 100 mL	× 0.001	0.02 to 0.1 L H^+ concentration
		pH:	1.5 to 3.5		32 to 316 µmol/L
Gastric Secretion Rate	Gast Cont, total; six 15-min spec.	BAO: M	0 to 10.5 mmol/h		Same
		PAO: M	12 to 60 mmol/h (after Pentagastrin)		
		BAO/PAO:	0.20% or 20%		
Gastrin	S		**pg/mL**		**ng/L**
		Cord, venous:	20 to 290	× 1	20 to 290
		0 to 4 days:	120 to 183		120 to 183
		Child:	<10 to 125		<10 to 125
	S		**pg/mL**		**ng/L**
		Adult:			
		16 to 60 y:	25 to 90		25 to 90
		>60 y:	<100		<100
Gastrin-Calcium Infusion Stimulation Test	S	Gastrin:	Slight or no increase		Same
Gastrin-Secretin Stimulation Test	S	Gastrin:	No response or slight suppression		Same
Glucagon	P (Hep or EDTA)		**pg/mL**		**ng/L**
		Adult:	20 to 100	× 1	20 to 100
	Amf	Midgestation:	43 ± 10 (SE)		43 ± 20 (SE)
		Term:	117 ± 38		117 ± 38

TABLE 46-8   Chemistry and Toxicology—cont'd

Test	Specimen		Reference Interval	Conversion Factor	Reference Interval (International Units)
Glucose	S, fasting		**mg/dL**		**mmol/L**
		Cord:	45 to 96	× 0.0555	2.5 to 5.3
		Premature:	20 to 60		1.1 to 3.3
		Neonate:	30 to 60		1.7 to 3.3
		Newborn:			
		1 day:	40 to 60		2.2 to 3.3
		>1 day:	50 to 80		2.8 to 4.5
		Child:	60 to 100		3.3 to 5.6
		Adult:	74 to 106		4.1 to 5.9
		Adult (Normal)	<110 with 8-h fast		<6.1 with 8-h fast
		>60 y:	82 to 115		4.6 to 6.4
		>90 y:	75 to 121		4.2 to 6.7
	WB (Hep)	Adult:	65 to 95		3.5 to 5.3
	CSF	Infant, child:	60 to 80		3.3 to 4.5
		Adult:	40 to 70		2.2 to 3.9
	U		<0.5 g/day	× 5.55	<2.8 mmol/day
	U		1 to 15 mg/dL	× 0.0555	0.1 to 0.8
Glucose-6-Phosphate Dehydrogenase (G-6-PD) in Erythrocytes WHO and ICSH	WB (ACD, EDTA, or Hep)		12.1 ± 2.09 U/g Hb (SD)	× 0.0645	0.78 ± 0.13 MU/mol Hb
			351 ± 60.6 U/10^{12} RBC	× 10^{-3}	0.35 ± 0.06 nU/RBC
			4.11 ± 0.71 U/mL RBC	× 1	4.11 ± 0.71 kU/L RBC
Glucose, 2-h Postprandial	S		<120 mg/dL	× 0.0555	<6.7 mmol/L
			Diabetes (See glucose tolerance test, oral)		
Glucose Tolerance Test (GTT) Oral	S	Normal fasting:	**mg/dL glucose** 110 or below with 8-h fast	× 0.0555	**mmol/L** 6.1
75-g Dose, nonpregnant 100-g Dose, pregnant Child, 1.75 g/kg up to 75 g max IV		Second h:	140 or below with 75 g dose		7.8
		Impaired glucose tolerance Fasting:	110 to 126 with 8-h fast		6.1 to 7.0
		Second hr:	140 to 200 with 75-g dose		7.8 to 11.1
	S	Diabetic fasting:	126 or higher on 2 days		7.0
		Second h:	200 or higher with 75 g dose		11.1
Glutamine (Gln)	S, P (heparin)		**mg/dL**		**μmol/L**
		3 mo to 6 y:	6.93 to 10.89	× 68.5	475 to 746
		6 to 18 y:	5.26 to 10.80		360 to 740
		Adult:	5.78 to 10.38		396 to 711
	U, 24-h		**mg/day**		**μmol/day**
		10 days to 7 wk:	12.4 to 25.8	× 6.85	85 to 177
		3 to 12 y:	20.4 to 113.7		140 to 779
		Adult:	43.8 to 151.8		300 to 1040
			mg/g creatinine		**mmol/mol creatinine**
		or	40 ± 19 (SD)	× 0.77	30.8 ± 14.6

Continued

TABLE 46-8   Chemistry and Toxicology—cont'd

Test	Specimen		Reference Interval	Conversion Factor	Reference Interval (International Units)
Glutamine (Gln)—cont'd	CSF		**mg/dL**		**μmol/L**
		Neonate:	10.34 ± 3.60 (SEM)	× 68.5	708 ± 246
		3 mo to 2 y:	7.27 ± 1.30 (SD)		498 ± 89
		2 to 10 y:	6.76 ± 1.20		463 ± 82
		Adult:	8.61 ± 0.50		590 ± 34
		Adult:	6 to 15 mg/dL	× 68.5	411 to 1028 μmol/L
γ-Glutamyltransferase (GGT) 37 °C	S	Male:	2 to 30 U/L	× 0.017	0.03 to 0.51 μkat/L
		Female:	1 to 24 U/L		0.02 to 0.41 μkat/L
Glutathione, Reduced (GSH)	WB (ACD, EDTA or Hep)		6.57 ± 1.04 μmol/g RBC	× 0.0645	0.42 ± 0.07 mol/mol Hb
			190 ± 30.16 μmol/10^{12} RBC	× 1	190 ± 30 amol/RBC
			2.23 ± 0.35 μmol/mL RBC	× 1	2.23 ± 0.35 mmol/L RBC Conversion factor based on hemoglobin, MW 64,500
Glutathione Reductase in Erythrocytes ICSH, 37 °C	WB (ACD, EDTA, or Hep)	Adult (reaction without FAD):	7.18 ± 1.0 U/g Hb (SD)	× 0.0645	0.46 ± 0.07 MU/mol Hb
			208 ± 31.6 U/10^{12} RBC	× 10^{-3}	0.21 ± 0.03 nU/RBC
			2.44 ± 0.37 U/mL RBC	× 1	2.44 ± 0.37 kU/L RBC
		Adult (reaction with FAD):	10.4 ± 1.5 U/g Hb (SD)	× 0.0645	0.67 ± 0.10 MU/mol Hb
			302 ± 43.5 U/10^{12} RBC	× 10^{-3}	0.30 ± 0.04 nU/RBC
			3.54 ± 0.51 U/mL RBC	× 1	3.54 ± 0.51 kU/L RBC
Glycated Hemoglobin(s)	WB (EDTA, Hep, or Ox)		**% total Hb**		**Hb fraction**
Agar gel (EP)			5.0 to 7.5	× 0.01	0.05 to 0.075
Hb A$_{1c}$ (HPLC)			4.5 to 5.7		0.045 to 0.057
HbA$_{1c}$			**% Total Hb**		**Hb fraction**
(Column chromatography, cation exchange)			4.5 to 8.5	× 0.01	0.045 to 0.085
Total glycated Hb (Column or affinity chromatography)			5.3 to 7.5		0.053 to 0.075
Glycerol, Free	P (EDTA)	3 to 10 y:	0.56 to 2.14 mg/dL	× 0.1086	0.061 to 0.232 mmol/L
		11 to 80 y:	0.29 to 1.72 mg/dL		0.032 to 0.187 mmol/L
Glycine	U, 24-h		**mg/day**		**mmol/day**
		10 days to 7 wk:	15 to 59	× 0.01332	0.20 to 0.79
		3 to 12 y:	12 to 107		0.16 to 1.43
		Adult:	59 to 294		0.79 to 3.92
			or 60 ± 24 mg/g creatinine (SD)	× 1.51	or 90.6 ± 36.2 mmol/mol creatinine (SD)
Glycolic Acid	U, 24-h	Adult:	15 to 60 mg/day	× 0.0131	0.20 to 0.79 mmol/day
Gold	S		<10 μg/dL	× 0.0508	<0.51 μmol/L
		Therap.:	100 to 200 μg/dL		5.1 to 10.2 μmol/L
	U, 24-h		<1 μg/day	× 5.08	<5.08 nmol/day
Gonadotropins (see Pregnancy Tests and Chorionic Gonadotropin Intact Molecule)					

TABLE 46-8   Chemistry and Toxicology—cont'd

Test	Specimen	Reference Interval		Conversion Factor	Reference Interval (International Units)
Growth Hormone (hGH, Somatotropin)	S		**ng/mL**		**µg/L**
		Cord:	8 to 41	× 1	8 to 41
		Newborn, 1 day:	5 to 53		5 to 53
		Child, 1 to 12 mo:	2 to 10		2 to 10
		Adult,			
		Man:	<0 to 4		<0 to 4
		Woman:	<0 to 18		<0 to 18
		>60 y:			
		Man:	1 to 9		1 to 9
		Woman:	1 to 16		1 to 16
	Amf	20 wk:	10		10
		Term:	30		30
Haptoglobin Nephelometry	S		**mg/dL**		**mg/L**
		Newborn:	5 to 48	× 10	50 to 480
		Adult:	26 to 185		260 to 1850
		>60 y:			
		Man:	35 to 164		350 to 1640
		Woman:	40 to 175		400 to 1750
Hematocrit	WB (EDTA)	**% Packed red cell volume (V red cells/V whole blood × 100)**			**Volume fraction (V red cells/V whole blood)**
		Fetal:			
		18 to 20 wk:	35.86 ± 3.29 (SD)	× 0.01	0.36 ± 0.03
		21 to 22 wk:	38.53 ± 3.21		0.39 ± 0.03
		23 to 25 wk:	38.59 ± 2.41		0.39 ± 0.02
		26 to 30 wk:	41.54 ± 3.31		0.42 ± 0.03
		Cord blood:	42 to 60		0.42 to 0.60
		0.5 mo:	41 to 65		0.41 to 0.65
		1 mo:	33 to 55		0.33 to 0.55
		2 mo:	28 to 42		0.28 to 0.42
		4 mo:	32 to 44		0.32 to 0.44
		6 mo:	31 to 41		0.31 to 0.41
		9 mo:	32 to 40		0.32 to 0.40
		12 mo:	33 to 41		0.33 to 0.41
		1 to 2 y:	32 to 40 (95% range)		0.32 to 0.40
		3 to 5 y:	32 to 42		0.32 to 0.42
		6 to 8 y:	33 to 41		0.33 to 0.41
		9 to 11 y:	34 to 43		0.34 to 0.43
		12 to 14y:			
		Boy:	35 to 45		0.35 to 0.45
		Girl:	34 to 44		0.34 to 0.44
		15 to 17 y:			
		Boy:	37 to 48		0.37 to 0.48
		Girl:	34 to 44		0.34 to 0.44
		18 to 44 y:			
		Man:	39 to 49		0.39 to 0.49
		Woman:	35 to 45		0.35 to 0.45
		45 to 64 y:			
		Man:	39 to 50		0.39 to 0.50
		Woman:	35 to 47		0.35 to 0.47
		65 to 74 y:			
		Man:	37 to 51		0.37 to 0.51
		Woman:	35 to 47		0.35 to 0.47

Continued

TABLE 46-8   Chemistry and Toxicology—cont'd

Test	Specimen	Reference Interval		Conversion Factor	Reference Interval (International Units)
Hemoglobin, Total Cyanmethemoglobin	WB (EDTA)		**g/dL**		**g/L**
		Fetal:			
		18 to 20 wk:	11.47 ± 0.78 (SD)	× 10	115 ± 7.8
		21 to 22 wk:	12.28 ± 0.89		123 ± 8.9
		23 to 25 wk:	12.40 ± 0.77		124 ± 7.7
		26 to 30 wk:	13.35 ± 1.17		134 ± 11.7
		Cord blood:	13.5 to 20.5 (2 SD)		135 to 205
		0.5 mo:	13.4 to 19.8		134 to 198
		1 mo:	10.7 to 17.1		107 to 171
		2 mo:	9.4 to 13.0		94 to 130
		4 mo:	10.3 to 14.1		103 to 141
		6 mo:	11.1 to 14.1		111 to 141
		9 mo:	11.4 to 14.0		114 to 140
		12 mo:	11.3 to 14.1		113 to 141
		0.5 to 2 y:	11.0 to 14.0		110 to 140
		2 to 5 y:	11.0 to 14.0		110 to 140
		5 to 9 y:	11.5 to 14.5		115 to 145
		9 to 12 y:	12.0 to 15.0		120 to 150
		12 to 14 y:			
		Boy:	12.0 to 16.0		120 to 160
		Girl:	11.5 to 15		115 to 150
		15 to 17 y:			
		Boy:	11.7 to 16.6		117 to 166
		Girl:	11.7 to 15.3		117 to 153
		18 to 44 y:			
		Man:	13.2 to 17.3		132 to 173
		Woman:	11.7 to 15.5		117 to 155
		45 to 64 y:			
		Man:	13.1 to 17.2		131 to 172
		Woman:	11.7 to 16.0		117 to 160
		65 to 74 y:			
		Man:	12.6 to 17.4		126 to 174
		Woman:	11.7 to 16.1		117 to 161
	P (EDTA, ACD, or Hep)		<3 mg/dL	× 0.155	<0.47 μmol/L
	U, fresh, random	Negative	<0.03 mg free Hb/dL	× 10	<0.03 mg free Hb/L
Hemoglobin A₁c *(see Glycated Hemoglobin(s))*					
Hemoglobin A₂ (HbA₂)	WB (EDTA or Ox)	Adult: Lower in infants <1 y	1.5% to 3.5%	× 0.01	0.015 to 0.035
		β-Thalassemia trait:	3.75% to 6.5%		0.038 to 0.065
Hemoglobin (Hb) Electrophoresis	WB (EDTA, Cit, or Hep)		**% of total Hb**		**Hb fraction**
		HbA:	>95%	× 0.01	>0.95
		HbA₂:	1.5 to 3.7%		0.015 to 0.037
		HbF:	<2%		<0.02
Hemoglobin F Alkali denaturation (White)	WB (EDTA)		**% HbF**		**Mass fraction HbF**
		1 day:	77.0 ± 7.3	× 0.01	0.77 ± 0.073
		5 days:	76.8 ± 5.8		0.768 ± 0.058
		3 wk:	70.0 ± 7.3		0.70 ± 0.073
		6 to 9 wk:	52.9 ± 11.0		0.529 ± 0.11
		3 to 4 mo:	23.2 ± 16.0		0.232 ± 0.16
		6 mo:	4.7 ± 2.2		0.047 ± 0.022
		8 to 11 mo:	1.6 ± 1.0		0.016 ± 0.010
		Adult:	<2.0		<0.020

TABLE 46-8 Chemistry and Toxicology—cont'd

Test	Specimen		Reference Interval	Conversion Factor	Reference Interval (International Units)
Hemoglobin H (HbH) Isopropanol precipitation	WB (ACD, EDTA, or Hep)		No precipitation at 40 min HbH: slight opacity at 10 min		No precipitation at 40 min
Hemopexin	S	Fetus, term:	>30% of mean adult conc. or 18% of maternal conc.	× 0.01	Fraction of adult conc.: >0.30 Fraction of maternal conc.: 0.18
		Maternal:	>1.5 times that of non-pregnant adults		Same
		Adult:	50 to 115 mg/dL	× 1	0.50 to 1.15 g/L
	U	Mean:	0.2 mg/day		0.2 mg/d
HER 2/neu (c-erbB-2)	S		**U/mL** <20: negative 20 to 30: intermediate >30: positive (poor prognosis)	× 1000	**U/L** <20,000: negative 20,000 to 30,000: intermediate >30,000: positive (poor prognosis)
Hexachlorophene	WB		**mg/L**		**μmol/L**
		Infant:	<0.182	× 2.46	<0.448
		Adult:	<0.089		<0.219
		After use:	0.1 to 0.655		0.246 to 1.611
	Milk		<0.009 mg/L		<0.022
	Fat		<0.05 mg/kg		<0.123 μmol/kg
High-Density Lipoprotein Cholesterol (HDL-C) Lipoprotein precipitation	S, P (EDTA)		**mg/dL** **Fifth to ninety-fifth percentile**		**mmol/L** **Fifth to ninety-fifth percentile**
		Cord blood:			
		Male:	6 to 53	× 0.0259	0.16 to 1.37
		Female:	13 to 56		0.34 to 1.45
		5 to 9 y:			
		Boy:	38 to 75		0.98 to 1.94
		Girl:	36 to 73		0.93 to 1.89
		10 to 14 y:			
		Boy:	37 to 74		0.96 to 1.91
		Girl:	37 to 70		0.96 to 1.81
		15 to 19 y:			
		Boy:	30 to 63		0.78 to 1.63
		Girl:	35 to 74		0.91 to 1.91
		20 to 24 y:			
		Man:	30 to 63		0.78 to 1.63
		Woman:	33 to 79		0.85 to 2.04
		25 to 29 y:			
		Man:	31 to 63		0.80 to 1.63
		Woman:	37 to 83		0.96 to 2.15
		30 to 34 y:			
		Man:	28 to 63		0.72 to 1.63
		Woman:	36 to 77		0.93 to 1.99
		35 to 39 y:			
		Man:	29 to 62		0.75 to 1.60
		Woman:	34 to 82		0.88 to 2.12
		40 to 44 y:			
		Man:	27 to 67		0.70 to 1.73
		Woman:	34 to 88		0.88 to 2.28

Continued

TABLE 46-8 Chemistry and Toxicology—cont'd

Test	Specimen	Reference Interval	Conversion Factor	Reference Interval (International Units)
High-Density Lipoprotein Cholesterol (HDL-C)—cont'd	S, P (EDTA)	**mg/dL** **Fifth to ninety-fifth percentile**		**mmol/L** **Fifth to ninety-fifth percentile**
Lipoprotein precipitation—cont'd		45 to 49 y:		
		Man: 30 to 64	× 0.0259	0.78 to 1.66
		Woman: 34 to 87		0.88 to 2.25
		50 to 54 y:		
		Man: 28 to 63		0.72 to 1.63
		Woman: 37 to 92		0.96 to 2.38
		55 to 59 y:		
		Man: 28 to 71		0.72 to 1.84
		Woman: 37 to 91		0.96 to 2.35
		60 to 64 y:		
		Man: 30 to 74		0.78 to 1.91
		Woman: 38 to 92		0.98 to 2.38
		65 to 69 y:		
		Man: 30 to 75		0.78 to 1.94
		Woman: 35 to 96		0.91 to 2.48
		>70 y:		
		Man: 31 to 75		0.80 to 1.94
		Woman: 33 to 92		0.85 to 2.38

Values for blacks are approximately 10 mg/dL [0.26 mmol/L] higher than for whites after age 10 y.

		HDL-C, percent of total cholesterol			**Fraction HDL-C of cholesterol**	
		CHD risk				
			Male	*Female*	*Male*	*Female*
		Dangerous:	<7	<12	× 0.01	<0.07	<0.12
		High:	7 to 15	12 to 18		0.07 to 0.15	0.12 to 0.18
		Average:	15 to 25	18 to 27		0.15 to 0.25	0.18 to 0.27
		Below average:	25 to 37	27 to 40		0.25 to 0.37	0.27 to 0.40
		Protection probable:	>37	>40		>0.37	>0.40

Test	Specimen	Reference Interval	Conversion Factor	Reference Interval (International Units)
Homocyst(e)ine	P (EDTA)	**μmol/L** Male 4.0 to 12.0 Female 4.0 to 12.0	× 1	Same
	U, random	Negative		Negative
Homogentisic Acid	U, random	Negative		Negative
Homovanillic Acid (HVA) HPLC	U, 24-h	**μg/mg creatinine**		**mmol/mol creatinine**
		Child:		
		3 to 6 y: 5.4 to 15.5	× 0.621	3.4 to 9.6
		6 to 10 y: 4.4 to 11.5		2.7 to 7.1
		10 to 16 y: 3.3 to 10.3		2.0 to 6.4
Hydrogen Sulfide	WB (F⁻/Ox)	<0.05 mg/L	× 29.3	<1.5 μmol/L
	Toxic:	>0.90 mg/L		>26.4 μmol/L
β-Hydroxybutyric Acid	S or P	0.21 to 2.81 mg/dL	× 96.05	20 to 270 μmol/L

TABLE 46-8 Chemistry and Toxicology—cont'd

Test	Specimen	Reference Interval		Conversion Factor	Reference Interval (International Units)
17-Hydroxycortico-steroids (17-OHCS)	U, 24-h		**mg/day**		**μmol/day**
		0 to 1 y:	0.5 to 1.0	× 2.76	1.4 to 2.8
		Child:	1.0 to 5.6		2.8 to 15.5
		Adult:			
		Man:	3.0 to 10.0		8.2 to 27.6
		Woman:	2.0 to 8.0		5.5 to 22
					Conversion based on hydrocortisone, MW 362
			or 2 to 6.5 mg/g creatinine	× 0.312	or 0.62 to 2.03 mmol/mol creatinine
	Amf	Pregnancy:	Increases fourfold to sixfold throughout		Same
5-Hydroxyindoleacetic Acid (5-HIAA)					
Qual.	U, random		Negative (<25mg/day)	× 5.2	Negative (<130 μmol/day)
Quant.	U, 24-h		2 to 7 mg/day	× 5.2	10.4 to 36.6 μmol/day
17-Hydroxyproges-terone (17-OHP)	S		**ng/dL**		**nmol/L**
		Male, pubertal			
		stage I:	3 to 90	× 0.03	0.1 to 2.7
		Adult:	27 to 199		0.8 to 6
		Female, pubertal	3 to 82		0.1 to 2.5
		stage I:	15 to 70		0.4 to 2.1
		Follicular:	35 to 290		1 to 8.7
		Luteal:	<70		<2.1
		Postmenopausal:	Values are highest at birth but decrease rapidly during first week of life.		
Hydroxyproline, Free	S		**mg/dL**		**μmol/L**
		Premature, 1 day:	0.52 ± 0.52	× 76.3	40 ± 40
		6 to 18 y:			
		Boy:	0 to 0.66		0 to 50
		Girl:	0 to 0.58		0 to 44
		Adult:			
		Man:	0 to 0.55		0 to 42
		Woman:	0 to 0.46		0 to 34
	U, 24-h		**mg/day**		**μmol/L**
		Adult	0 to 1.3	× 7.63	0 to 10
Immunoglobulin A (IgA)					
Nephelometric	S		**mg/dL**		**mg/L**
		Cord:	1 to 4	× 10	10 to 40
		Newborn, 1 mo:	2 to 50		20 to 500
		2 to 9 mo:	4 to 80		40 to 800
		10 to 12 mo:	15 to 90		150 to 900
		1 to 5 y:	15 to 160		150 to 1600
		6 to 12 y:	35 to 250		360 to 2500
		12 to 60 y:	40 to 350		400 to 3500
RIA	CSF		**mg/dL ± SD**		**mg/L ± SD**
		15 to 20 y:	0.07 ± 0.04	× 10	0.7 ± 0.4
		21 to 40 y:	0.07 ± 0.03		0.7 ± 0.3
		41 to 60 y:	0.10 ± 0.03		1.0 ± 0.3
		61 to 87 y:	0.11 ± 0.06		1.1 ± 0.6

Continued

TABLE 46-8 Chemistry and Toxicology—cont'd

Test	Specimen		Reference Interval	Conversion Factor	Reference Interval (International Units)
Immunoglobulin D (IgD)	S	Newborn:	0 to 1.0 mg/dL	× 10	0 to 10 mg/L
		Adult:	0 to 8 mg/dL		0 to 80 mg/L
Immunoglobulin E (IgE)	S		**IU/mL**		**kIU/L**
		Adult:	3 to 423	× 1	3 to 423
Immunoglobulin G (IgG)	S		**mg/dL**		**g/L**
			565 to 1765	× 0.01	5.65 to 17.65
			mg/dL		**g/L**
Nephelometric	S	Cord:	650 to 1600	× 0.01	6.5 to 16.0
		1 mo:	250 to 900		2.5 to 9.0
		2 to 5 mo:	200 to 700		2.0 to 7.0
		6 to 9 mo:	220 to 900		2.2 to 9.0
		10 to 12 mo:	290 to 1070		2.9 to 10.7
		1 y:	340 to 1200		3.4 to 12.0
		2 to 3 y:	420 to 1200		4.2 to 12.0
		4 to 6 y:	460 to 1240		4.6 to 12.4
		>6 y:	650 to 1600		6.5 to 16.0
		Subclass	**mg/dL**		**g/L**
		IgG_1	500 to 1200	× 0.01	5 to 12
		IgG_2	200 to 600		2 to 6
		IgG_3	50 to 100		0.5 to 1
		IgG_4	50 to 100		0.5 to 1
RIA	CSF		**mg/dL ± SD**		**mg/L ± SD**
		15 to 20 y:	3.5 ± 2.0	× 10	35 ± 20
		21 to 40 y:	4.2 ± 1.4		42 ± 14
		41 to 60 y:	4.7 ± 1.0		47 ± 10
		61 to 87 y:	5.8 ± 1.6		58 ± 16
Immunoglobulin G/Albumin Ratio (IgG index) Calculation	CSF and S		0.3 to 0.6		0.3 to 0.6
Immunoglobulin G Synthesis Rate Calculation	CSF and S		−9.9 to +3.3 mg/day		−9.9 to +3.3 mg/d
Immunoglobulin M (IgM)	S				
			mg/dL		**mg/L**
Nephelometric; Calib.; Beckman; Atlantic Antibodies; WHO		Cord:	<25	× 10	<250
		Newborn (1 mo):	20 to 80		200 to 800
		2 to 5 mo:	25 to 100		250 to 1000
		6 to 12 mo:	35 to 150		350 to 1500
		1 to 8 y:	45 to 200		450 to 2000
		9 to 12 y:	50 to 250		500 to 2500
		>12 y:	50 to 300		500 to 3000
		Results vary with ref. preparation.			
	CSF		**mg/dL ± SD**		**mg/L ± SD**
RIA		15 to 20 y:	0.020 ± 0.009	× 10	0.20 ± 0.09
		21 to 40 y:	0.016 ± 0.003		0.16 ± 0.03
		41 to 60 y:	0.017 ± 0.004		0.17 ± 0.04
		61 to 87 y:	0.017 ± 0.005		0.17 ± 0.05
Insulin Free	S		**µU/mL**		**pmol/L**
		Infant:	0 to 13	× 6.945	0 to 90
		Adult:	0 to 17		0 to 118
Insulin Antibodies	S		Undetectable		Undetectable

TABLE 46-8   Chemistry and Toxicology—cont'd

Test	Specimen	Reference Interval		Conversion Factor	Reference Interval (International Units)
Insulin and Glucose Suppression Test	S, every 6 to 12 h	>40 mg glucose/dL during a 72-h period of fasting, with values slightly lower in females		× 0.0555	>2.2 mmol glucose/L during a 48-h period of fasting, with values slightly lower in females
		Insulin: <4 µU/mL or undetectable		× 6.945	Insulin: <28 pmol/L or undetectable
		Normal fasting insulin/glucose ratio: <0.3			Normal fasting insulin-glucose ratio: <5.4

Insulin-Like Growth Factor I

RIA extracted

S or P (EDTA)   × 1   Same

	ng/mL	
	Male	Female
0 to 5 y	17 to 248	17 to 248
6 to 8 y	88 to 474	88 to 474
9 to 11 y	110 to 565	117 to 771
12 to 15 y	202 to 957	261 to 1096
16 to 25 y	182 to 780	182 to 780
>25 y	123 to 463	123 to 463

Insulin with Oral Glucose Tolerance Test
75 g glucose dose

S   × 6.945

Min	Insulin, µIU/mL	pmol/L
0:	3 to 28	21 to 194
30:	20 to 112	139 to 778
60:	29 to 88	201 to 611
120:	22 to 79	153 to 549
180:	4 to 62	28 to 431

Test	Specimen	Reference Interval	Conversion Factor	Reference Interval (International Units)
Insulin Tolerance Test Dose: 0.1 to 0.15 U/kg, IV	S	*Glucose:* Decrease ~50% of the fasting level by 30 min and return to normal fasting limits by 90 to 120 min.	× 0.01	Fractional decrease in glucose ~0.50 of the fasting level by 30 min and return to normal fasting limits by 90 to 120 min
		GH: Increase of >5 ng/mL within 60 min of hypoglycemia.	× 1	*GH:* Increase of >5 µg/L within 60 min of hypoglycemia
		Cortisol: Increase of >7 µg/dL with peak of >20 µg/dL.	× 27.59	*Cortisol:* Increase of >193 nmol/L with peak of >552 nmol/L

Intrinsic Factor *(see Vitamin B₁₂ Intrinsic Factor)*

Inulin Clearance Test   S and U

	(mL/min)/1.73 m²			(mL/s)/m²	
	Man	Woman		Man	Woman
20 to 29 y:	90 to 174	84 to 156	× 0.00963	0.87 to 1.68	0.81 to 1.50
30 to 39 y:	88 to 168	82 to 150		0.85 to 1.62	0.79 to 1.44
40 to 49 y:	78 to 162	82 to 146		0.75 to 1.56	0.79 to 1.41
50 to 59 y:	68 to 152	66 to 142		0.65 to 1.46	0.63 to 1.37
60 to 69 y:	57 to 137	58 to 130		0.55 to 1.32	0.56 to 1.25
70 to 79 y:	42 to 122	45 to 121		0.40 to 1.17	0.43 to 1.17
80 to 89 y:	39 to 105	39 to 105		0.38 to 1.01	0.38 to 1.01

Continued

TABLE 46-8   Chemistry and Toxicology—cont'd

Test	Specimen	Reference Interval		Conversion Factor	Reference Interval (International Units)
Iron ICSH	S		**μg/dL**	× 0.179	**μmol/L**
		Newborn:	100 to 250		17.9 to 44.8
		Infant:	40 to 100		7.2 to 17.9
		Child:	50 to 120		9.0 to 21.5
		Adult:			
		Man:	65 to 175		11.6 to 31.3
		Woman:	50 to 170		9.0 to 30.4
			Strongly method dependent		
Iron-Binding Capacity, Total (TIBC)	S	Infant:	100 to 400 μg/dL	× 0.179	17.9 to 71.6 μmol/L
		Adult:	250 to 425 μg/dL		44.8 to 71.6 μmol/L
Iron Saturation	S				**Fraction saturation**
		Male:	20% to 50%	× 0.01	0.20 to 0.50
		Female:	15% to 50%		0.15 to 0.50
Isocitrate Dehydrogenase (ICD), 37 °C	S	Adult:	1.2 to 7.0 U/L	× 0.017	0.02 to 0.12 μkat/L
Isoleucine	S		**mg/dL**	× 76.3	**μmol/L**
		Premature, 1 day:	0.26 to 0.78		20 to 60
		Newborn, 1 day:	0.35 to 0.69		27 to 53
		1 to 3 mo:	0.59 to 0.95		45 to 73
		2 to 6 mo:	0.50 to 1.61		38 to 123
		9 mo to 2 y:	0.34 to 1.23		26 to 94
		3 to 10 y:	0.37 to 1.10		28 to 84
		6 to 18 y:	0.50 to 1.24		38 to 95
		Adult:	0.48 to 1.28		37 to 98
	U, 24-h		**mg/day**	× 7.62	**μmol/day**
		10 day to 7 wk:	trace to 0.4		trace to 3
		3 to 12 y:	2 to 7		15 to 53
		Adult:	5 to 24		38 to 183
			or 3 ± 1 mg/g creatinine	× 0.86	2.6 ± 0.9 mmol/mol creatinine
Kappa Light Chain	S		574 to 1276 mg/dL	× 0.001	5.74 to 12.76 g/L
17-Ketogenic Steroids (17-KGS)	U, 24-h		**mg/day**	× 3.467	**μmol/day**
		0 to 1 y:	<1.0		<3.5
		1 to 10 y:	<5		<17
		11 to 14 y:	<12		<42
		Adult:			
		Man:	5 to 23		17 to 80
		Woman:	3 to 15		10 to 52
		>70 y:			
		Man:	3 to 12		10 to 42
		Woman:	3 to 13		10 to 45 (Conversion based on dehydroepiandrosterone, MW 288)
Ketone Bodies Qual.	S		Negative		Negative
	U, random		Negative		Negative
Quant.	S		0.5 to 3.0 mg/dL	× 10	5 to 30 mg/L

TABLE 46-8   Chemistry and Toxicology—cont'd

Test	Specimen		Reference Interval	Conversion Factor	Reference Interval (International Units)
17-Ketosteroids (17 KS), Total	U, 24-h		**mg/day**		**μmol/day**
Zimmermann reaction		1 to 4 y:	<2	× 3.467	<7
		5 to 9 y:	<3		<10
		10 to 12 y:	1 to 5		3 to 17
		12 to 14 y:	1 to 6		3 to 21
		14 to 16 y:	2 to 13		8 to 45
		Adult:			
		Man:	10 to 25		38 to 87
		Woman:	6 to 14		21 to 49
			Decreases with age		Decreases with age
GLC		Adult:			
		Man:	5 to 12		17 to 42
		Woman:	3 to 10		10 to 35
					Conversion based on de-hydroepiandrosterone, MW 288
L-Lactate			**mg/dL**		**mmol/L**
	P (NaF)	Venous:	4.5 to 19.8	× 0.111	0.5 to 2.2
		Arterial:	4.5 to 14.4		0.5 to 1.6
	WB (Hep)	on bed rest,			
		Venous:	8.1 to 15.3		0.9 to 1.7
		Arterial:	<11.3		<1.3
	U, 24-h		496 to 1982 mg/day	× 0.0111	5.5 to 22 mmol/day
	CSF	Adult:	10 to 22 mg/dL	× 0.111	1.1 to 2.4 mmol/L
Qual.	Gastf		Negative		Negative
Lactate/Pyruvate Ratio	WB (Hep)		10/1		10/1
Lactate Dehydrogenase (LD)	S				
Total (L → P), 37 °C			**U/L**		**μkat/L**
		0 to 4 days:	290 to 775	× 0.017	4.9 to 13.2
		4 to 10 days:	545 to 2000		9.3 to 34.0
		10 days to 24 mo:	180 to 430		3.1 to 7.3
		24 mo to 12 y:	110 to 295		1.9 to 5.0
		12 to 60 y:	100 to 190		1.7 to 3.2
		>60 y:	110 to 210		1.9 to 3.6
	CSF		~10% of serum value	× 0.01	~0.10 fraction of serum value
	S		**Percent of total**		**Fraction of total**
Isoenzymes, Agarose		Fraction 1:	14 to 26	× 0.01	0.14 to 0.26
		Fraction 2:	29 to 39		0.29 to 0.39
		Fraction 3:	20 to 26		0.20 to 0.26
		Fraction 4:	8 to 16		0.08 to 0.16
		Fraction 5:	6 to 16		0.06 to 0.16
Lambda Light Chain	S		269 to 638 mg/dL	× 0.01	2.69 to 6.38 g/L
Lactose	S		<0.5 mg/dL	× 29.21	<14.6 μmol/L
	U		12 to 40 mg/dL	× 29.21	350 to 1168 μmol/L

Continued

TABLE 46-8   Chemistry and Toxicology—cont'd

Test	Specimen	Reference Interval	Conversion Factor	Reference Interval (International Units)
LDL-Cholesterol (LDL-C) Calculated	S or P (EDTA)	**mg/dL** **Fifth to ninety-fifth percentile**		**mmol/L** **Fifth to ninety-fifth percentile**
		Cord blood,		
		Male: 20 to 56	× 0.0259	0.52 to 1.45
		Female: 21 to 58		0.54 to 1.50
		5 to 9 y:		
		Boy: 63 to 129		1.63 to 3.34
		Girl: 68 to 140		1.76 to 3.63
		10 to 14 y:		
		Boy: 64 to 133		1.66 to 3.44
		Girl: 68 to 136		1.76 to 3.52
		15 to 19 y:		
		Boy: 62 to 130		1.61 to 3.37
		Girl: 59 to 137		1.53 to 3.55
		20 to 24 y:		
		Man: 66 to 147		1.71 to 3.81
		Woman: 57 to 159		1.48 to 4.12
		25 to 29 y:		
		Man: 70 to 165		1.81 to 4.27
		Woman: 71 to 164		1.84 to 4.25
		30 to 34 y:		
		Man: 78 to 185		2.02 to 4.79
		Woman: 70 to 156		1.81 to 4.04
		35 to 39 y:		
		Man: 81 to 189		2.10 to 4.90
		Woman: 75 to 172		1.94 to 4.45
		40 to 44 y:		
		Man: 87 to 186		2.25 to 4.82
		Woman: 74 to 174		1.92 to 4.51
		45 to 49 y:		
		Man: 97 to 202		2.51 to 5.23
		Woman: 79 to 186		2.05 to 4.82
		50 to 54 y:		
		Man: 89 to 197		2.31 to 5.10
		Woman: 88 to 201		2.28 to 5.21
		55 to 59 y:		
		Man: 88 to 203		2.28 to 5.26
		Woman: 89 to 210		2.31 to 5.44
		60 to 64 y:		
		Man: 83 to 210		2.15 to 5.44
		Woman: 100 to 224		2.59 to 5.80
		65 to 69 y:		
		Man: 98 to 210		2.54 to 5.44
		Woman: 92 to 221		2.38 to 5.72
		>70 y:		
		Man: 88 to 186		2.28 to 4.82
		Woman: 96 to 206		2.49 to 5.34
		Adult levels in terms of risk for coronary heart disease:		
		Recommended (desirable): <130 mg/dL [<3.37 mmol/L]		
		Moderate risk: 130 to 159 mg/dL [3.37 to 4.12 mmol/L]		
		High risk: ≥160 mg/dL [≥4.14 mmol/L]		

TABLE 46-8 Chemistry and Toxicology—cont'd

Test	Specimen		Reference Interval	Conversion Factor	Reference Interval (International Units)
Lead	WB (Hep)		**μg/dL**		**μmol/L**
		Child:	<25	× 0.0483	<1.21
		Adult:	<25		<1.21
		Toxic:	≥100		≥4.83
	U, 24-h		<80	× 0.00483	<0.39
Lecithin-Cholesterol Acyltransferase 37 °C	P (Hep, EDTA, or Cit) or S		(92 ± 14.2 μmol/h)/L	× 0.0167	154 ± 0.24 U/L plasma
Lecithin/ Sphingomyelin (L/S) Ratio	Amf	Immature:	<1.5		Same
		Intermediate:	1.5 to 1.9		
		Mature:	≥2.0		
		Diabetic:	≥3.5		
Lecithin Phosphorus	Amf		>0.10 mg/dL indicates probable adequate fetal lung maturity	× 0.3229	>0.33 mmol/L indicates probable adequate fetal lung maturity
Leucine			**mg/dL (SD)**		**μmol/L (SD)**
		Premature, 1 day:	0.92 ± 0.33	× 76.3	70 ± 25
		Newborn, 1 day:	0.62 to 1.43		47 to 109
		1 to 3 mo:	1.36 ± 0.39		104 ± 30
		9 mo to 2 y:	0.59 to 2.03		45 to 155
		3 to 10 y:	0.73 to 2.33		56 to 178
		6 to 18 y:	1.03 to 2.28		79 to 174
		Adult:	0.98 to 2.29		75 to 175
	U, 24-h		**mg/day**		**μmol/day**
		10 days to 7 wk:	0.9 to 2.0	× 7.624	7 to 15
		3 to 12 y:	3 to 11		23 to 84
		Adult:	2.6 to 8.1		20 to 62
			or 4 ± 2 mg/g creatinine	× 0.86	or 3.4 ± 1.7 mmol/mol creatinine
Leukocyte Count (WBC Count)	WB (EDTA)		**Cells × 10³/μL**		**Cells × 10⁹/L**
		18 to 20 wk:	4.20 ± 0.83	× 10⁶	4.20 ± 0.83
		23 to 25 wk:	3.95 ± 0.69		3.95 ± 0.69
		26 to 30 wk:	4.44 ± 0.85		4.44 ± 0.85
		1 to 3 y:	6.0 to 17.5		6.0 to 17.5
		4 to 7 y:	5.5 to 15.5		5.5 to 15.5
		8 to 13 y:	4.5 to 13.5		4.5 to 13.5
		Adult:	4.5 to 11.0		4.5 to 11.0
	CSF		0 to 5 mononuclear cells/μL		0 to 5 × 10⁶/cells/L
Lipase Turbidimetric 30 °C	S	Adult:	31 to 186 U/L	× 0.017	0.5 to 3.2 μkat/L
		>90 y:	0 to 302 U/L		0.5 to 4.5
Lipoprotein (LDL, Low-Density Lipoprotein)	S, 12- to 14-h fasting		28% to 53% of total lipoproteins	× 0.01	Mass fraction of total; 0.28 to 0.53
Lipoprotein Electrophoresis	S		Distinct β-band; negligible chylomicron and pre–β-bands		Same

Continued

TABLE 46-8   Chemistry and Toxicology—cont'd

Test	Specimen		Reference Interval	Conversion Factor	Reference Interval (International Units)
Lutropin (Luteinizing Hormone, LH) RIA	S or P (Hep); avoid EDTA		**mU/mL (WHO 1st IRP 68/40)**		**U/L**
		Cord blood:	0.04 to 2.6	× 1	0.04 to 2.6
		Prepubertal child:			
		2 to 11 mo:	0.02 to 8.0	× 1	0.02 to 8.0
		1 to 10 y:	0.08 to 3.9		0.08 to 3.9
		Puberty, Tanner stage			
		1, Boy:	0.04 to 3.6		0.04 to 3.6
		Girl:	0.03 to 3.0		0.03 to 3.0
		2, Boy:	0.26 to 4.8		0.26 to 4.8
		Girl:	0.10 to 4.1		0.10 to 4.1
		3, Boy:	0.56 to 6.3		0.56 to 6.3
		Girl:	0.20 to 9.1		0.20 to 9.1
		4 to 5, Boy:	0.56 to 7.8		0.56 to 7.8
		Girl:	0.50 to 15.0		0.5 to 15.0
	S or P (Hep); avoid EDTA		**mU/mL (WHO 1st IRP 68/40)**		**U/L**
		Adult:			
		Man:	1.24 to 7.8		1.24 to 7.8
		Woman:			
		Follicular phase:	1.68 to 15.0		1.68 to 15.0
		Ovulatory peak:	21.9 to 56.6		21.9 to 56.6
		Luteal phase:	0.61 to 16.3		0.61 to 16.3
		Postmeno-pausal:	14.2 to 52.5		14.2 to 52.3
Lysozyme (Muramidase)	S or P (EDTA)		0.4 to 1.3 mg/dL	× 10	4.0 to 13.0 mg/L
Macroamylase	S		Present in ~1% of healthy subjects with normal serum amylase activity and in 2.5% of patients with abnormal activity		Same
Magnesium	S		**mg/dL**		**mmol/L**
		Newborn, 2 to 4 days:	1.5 to 2.2	× 0.4114	0.62 to 0.91
		5 mo to 6 y:	1.7 to 2.3		0.70 to 0.95
		6 to 12 y:	1.7 to 2.1		0.70 to 0.86
		12 to 20 y:	1.7 to 2.2		0.70 to 0.91
		Adult:	1.6 to 2.6		0.66 to 1.07
		Higher in females during menses			
	U, 24-h		6.0 to 10.0 mEq/day	× 0.5	3.00 to 5.00 mmol/day
Melanin	U, random		Negative		Negative
Mercury	WB (EDTA)		0.6 to 59 µg/L	× 4.99	3.0 to 294.4 nmol/L
	U, 24-h		<20 µg/L	× 4.99	<99.8 nmol/L
		Toxic:	>150 µg/L		>748.5 nmol/L
		Lethal:	>800 µg/L		3992 nmol/L

TABLE 46-8   Chemistry and Toxicology—cont'd

Test	Specimen		Reference Interval	Conversion Factor	Reference Interval (International Units)
Metanephrine, Total	U, 24-h		**µg/mg Creatinine**		**mmol/mol Creatinine**
		<1 y:	0.001 to 4.60	× 0.574	0.0006 to 2.64
		1 to 2 y:	0.27 to 5.38		0.15 to 3.09
		2 to 5 y:	0.35 to 2.99		0.20 to 1.72
		5 to 10 y:	0.43 to 2.70		0.25 to 1.55
		10 to 15 y:	0.001 to 1.87		0.0006 to 1.07
		15 to 18 y:	0.001 to 0.67		0.0006 to 0.38
		Adult:	0.05 to 1.20		0.03 to 0.69
Methanol	WB (F⁻/Ox)		**mg/L**		**mmol/L**
			<1.5	× 0.0312	<0.05
		Toxic:	>200		>6.24
	U	Occup. exp.:	<50		<1.56
	Br		0.8 ppm	× 0.0312	0.03
		Occup. exp.:	2.5 ppm		0.08
Methemoglobin (MetHb, Hemiglobin)	WB (EDTA, Hep, or ACD)		0.06 to 0.24 g/dL or	× 155	9.3 to 37.2 µmol/L Conv. factor based on hemoglobin, MW 64,500;
			0.78% ± 0.37% of total Hb	× 0.01	Mass fraction of total Hb: 0.008 ± 0.0037
Methionine	S		**mg/dL**	× 67.1	**µmol/L**
		Premature, 1 day:	0.52 ± 0.07 (SD)		35 ± 5 (SD)
		Newborn, 1 day:	0.13 to 0.61		9 to 41
		1 to 3 mo:	0.31 ± 0.13 (SD)		21 ± 9
		2 to 6 mo:	0.24 to 0.73		16 to 49
		9 mo to 2 y:	0.04 to 0.43		3 to 29
		3 to 10 y:	0.16 to 0.24		11 to 16
		6 to 18 y:	0.24 to 0.55		16 to 37
		Adult:	0.09 to 0.60		6 to 40
	U, 24-h		**mg/day**		**µmol/day**
		10 days to 7 wk:	0.1 to 1.9	×6.70	0.7 to 13
		3 to 12 y:	3 to 14		20 to 95
		Adult:	Trace to 9.0		Trace to 62
			or 4.5 ± 2.5 mg/g creatinine (SD)	× 0.76	or 3.4 ± 1.9 mmol/mol creatinine (SD)
Metyrapone (Metopirone) Stimulation Test	S	11-Deoxycortisol:	>7.0 µg/dL	× 28.86	11-Deoxycortisol: >200 nmol/L
		Cortisol:	<3 µg/dL	× 27.59	Cortisol: <83 nmol/L
Dose, adult: 750 mg every 4 h × 6; child: 300 mg/m²	U, 24-h	17-KGS:	Twofold to fourfold rise, but at least 10 mg/day	× 3.467	17-KGS: 2 to 4-fold rise but at least 35 µmol/day Conv. factor based on DHEA, MW 288
		17-KS:	>2 × base level		Same
		17-OHCS:	3 to 5 × base level		Same
Single-dose metyrapone test	S, 0800 h	11-Deoxycortisol:	>7 µg/dL	× 28.86	>200 nmol/dL
Dose: 30 mg/kg orally with milk or snack at midnight		Cortisol:	<3 µg/dL	× 27.6	<83 nmol/L
		ACTH:	>150 pg/mL	× 0.22	>33 pmol/L

Continued

TABLE 46-8　　**Chemistry and Toxicology—cont'd**

Test	Specimen		Reference Interval	Conversion Factor	Reference Interval (International Units)
Microalbumin (*see Urine Albumin*)					
β₂-Microglobulin (β₂M) RIA	S		**mg/dL (x̄)**		**mg/L (x̄)**
		Newborn:	0.30	× 10	3.0
		0 to 59 y:	0.19		1.9
		60 to 69 y:	0.21		2.1
		>70 y:	0.24		2.4
Microsomal Antibodies, Thyroid, (*see Thyroid Microsomal Antibodies*)					
Molybdenum	S		0.1 to 3.0 µg/L	× 10.42	1.0 to 31.3 nmol/L
Mucopolysaccharide Screen (MPS)	U, random		Negative		Negative
Myelin Basic Protein	CSF		<2.5 ng/mL	× 1	<2.5 µg/L
Myoglobin RIA	S	Male:	19 to 92 µg/L	× 1	Same
		Female:	12 to 76 µg/L Increases slightly with age		
	U, random		Negative		Negative
N-Telopeptide, Cross Linked (NTx) ELISA	U	Adult: Woman: Man:	**nmol/mmol creatinine** 5 to 65 3 to 51	×1	Same
Niacin	U, 24-h		2.4 to 6.4 mg/day	× 7.30	17.5 to 46.7 µmol/day
Nickel			**µg/L**		**nmol/L**
	S or P (Hep)		0.14 to 1.0	× 17	2.4 to 17.0
	WB		1.0 to 28.0		17 to 476
	U, 24-h		0.1 to 10 µg/day	× 17	2 to 170 nmol/day
	F		260 ± 120 µg/day	× 0.017	4.4 ± 2.1 µmol/day
	H		0.01 to 1.8 µg/g dry wt.	× 17	0.2 to 30.6 nmol/g dry wt.
Nitrites	U		Negative		Same
		Toxic:	Methemoglobin, 5% of total Hg		Same
Nitrogen, Total	F	Infant:	0.11 to 0.52 g N/day	× 71.4	7.9 to 37 mmol N/day
		Adult:	<2 g N/day		<143 mmol N/day
Nonprotein Nitrogen (NPN)	WB (Ox)		<50 mg/dL	× 0.714	<35.7 mmol/L
	S		<35 mg/dL		<25.0 mmol/L
Normetanephrine, Total	P (EDTA and Na met-abisulfite)	Normotensive:	1.2 ± 0.1 ng/mL (SEM)	× 5.46	6.55 ± 0.55 nmol/L
		Primary hypertensive:	2.5 ± 0.2 ng/mL (SEM)		13.65 ± 1.09 nmol/L

TABLE 46-8   Chemistry and Toxicology—cont'd

Test	Specimen	Reference Interval		Conversion Factor	Reference Interval (International Units)
Occult Blood	F, random		Negative (<2 mL blood/150 g stool per day)	× 6.67	Negative (<13.3 ml blood/kg stool per day)
Qual.	U, random		Negative		Negative
Orosomucoid (see α_1-Acid Glycoprotein)					
Osmolality	S	Newborn:	May be as low as 266 mOsmol/kg		Same
		Child, adult:	275 to 295 mOsmol/kg		
		>60 y:	280 to 301 mOsmol/kg		
	U, random		50 to 1200 mOsmol/kg, depending on fluid intake		Same
	U, random		After 12 h fluid restriction >850 mOsmol/kg		
	U, 24-h		~300 to 900 mOsmol/kg		
Osmolality Ratio, Urine/Serum	U and S		1.0 to 3.0 3.0 to 4.7 after 12 h fluid restriction		Same
Osteocalcin (Bone G1a Protein) Immunoradiometric Assay	S		Method Dependent **ng/mL**		**µg/mL**
		1 to 10 y:	10 to 50	× 1	10 to 50
		11 to 15 y:	10 to 100		10 to 100
		16 to 22 y:	10 to 50		10 to 50
		Adult:			Adult:
		Man:	5.8 to 14		Man: 5.8 to 14
		Woman:	3.1 to 14.4		Woman: 3.1 to 14.4
Oxalate	S		1.0 to 2.4 mg/L	× 11.4	11 to 27 µmol/L
		Ethylene glycol poisoning:	>20 mg/L		>228 µmol/L
	U, 24-h	Adult:			
		Man:	20 to 60 mg/day	× 11.4	228 to 684 µmol/day
		Woman:	20 to 55 mg/day		228 to 627 µmol/day
		Ethylene glycol poisoning:	>150 mg/L		>1710 µmol/L
Oxygen, P$_{50}$	WB (Hep)	Newborn:	18 to 24 mm Hg	× 0.133	2.39 to 3.19 kPa
		Adult, adjusted to pH (P) 7.4:	25 to 29 mm Hg		3.33 to 3.86 kPa
Oxygen, Partial Pressure (P_{O_2})	WB, arterial (Hep)	Cord:	**mm Hg**		**kPa**
		Arterial:	5 to 30	× 0.133	0.6 to 4.0
		Venous:	17 to 41		2.2 to 5.5
		Birth:	8 to 24	× 0.133	1.1 to 3.2
		5 to 10 min:	33 to 75		4.4 to 10.0
		30 min:	31 to 85		4.1 to 11.3
		>1 h:	55 to 80		7.3 to 10.6
		1 day:	54 to 95		7.2 to 12.6
		Thereafter:	83 to 108		11.1 to 14.4
		Decreases with age and high altitude $P_{O_2} = (-0.27 \times age) + 104$			

Continued

TABLE 46-8   Chemistry and Toxicology—cont'd

Test	Specimen	Reference Interval		Conversion Factor	Reference Interval (International Units)
Oxygen Saturation	WB, arterial (Hep)	Newborn:	40% to 90%	× 0.01	Fraction saturated: 0.40 to 0.90
		Thereafter:	95% to 98%		0.95 to 0.98
			Values decrease with age		
Oxytocin	P (EDTA)		**μU/mL**		**mU/L**
		Male:	1.5 ± 0.2	× 1	1.5 ± 0.2
		Female:			
		Nonpregnant:	1.4 ± 0.2		1.4 ± 0.2
		Second trimester:	4.2 ± 1.1		4.2 ± 1.1
Po$_2$ (see Oxygen, Partial Pressure)					
Pancreatic Polypeptide	S	**Age**	**pg/mL**		**ng/L**
		20 to 29:	26 to 158	× 1	26 to 158
		30 to 39:	55 to 284		55 to 284
		40 to 49:	64 to 243		64 to 243
		>50:	51 to 326		51 to 326
Pantothenic Acid (Vitamin B$_3$)	WB (NaCit) or S	Total:	0.2 to 1.8 μg/mL	× 4.56	0.9 to 8.2 μmol/L
Parathyroid Hormone (PTH)	S			× 0.1053	
RIA		N-terminal:	8 to 24 pg/mL		0.84 to 2.52 pmol/L
		C-terminal:	50 to 330 pg/mL		5.26 to 34.74 pmol/L
		Intact molecule:	10 to 65 pg/mL		1.05 to 6.84 pmol/L
		Varies with laboratory			
Pentachlorophenol (PCP)	P (EDTA)		**mg/L**		**μmol/L**
			<1	× 3.75	<3.8
		Occup. exp.:	<20		<75
		Toxic:	>30		>113
	U		<0.6		<2.3
		Occup. exp.:	<4		<15
		Toxic:	>4		>15
Pentoses	U, 24-h	**Total pentoses**			
		Fruit-free diet:	2 to 5 mg/kg/day or	× 6.66	13.3 to 33.3 μmol/kg/day
			225 mg/day	× 0.00666	or 1.50 mmol/day
		Slightly higher in children			
	U, 24-h				
		L-Xylulose:	<60 mg/day	× 6.66	<400 μmol/day
		D-Ribose:	<15 mg/day	× 6.66	<100 μmol/day
		D-Ribulose:	Trace		
	S	L-Xylulose:	<2 mg/dL	× 66.6	<133.2 μmol/L
Pepsinogen (PG I)	S		**ng/mL ± SEM**		**μg/L ± SEM**
		Premature:	22 ± 2	× 1	22 ± 2
		Cord:	26 ± 2		26 ± 2
		<1 y:	77 ± 5		77 ± 5
		1 to 2 y:	98 ± 8		98 ± 8
		3 to 6 y:	92 ± 12		92 ± 12
		7 to 10 y:	95 ± 8		95 ± 8
		11 to 14 y:	107 ± 11		107 ± 11
		Adult:	133 ± 9		133 ± 9
		Woman at delivery:	127 ± 11		127 ± 11

TABLE 46-8   Chemistry and Toxicology—cont'd

Test	Specimen		Reference Interval	Conversion Factor	Reference Interval (International Units)
pH (37 °C)	WB, arterial (Hep)	Premature, 48 h:	7.35 to 7.50		Same
		Birth, full term:	7.11 to 7.36		
		5 to 10 min:	7.09 to 7.30		
		30 min:	7.21 to 7.38		
		>1 h:	7.26 to 7.49		
		1 day:	7.29 to 7.45		
		Thereafter:	7.35 to 7.45		
		or H^+ conc.:	36 to 44 nmol/L	× 1	36 to 44 nmol/L
			pH in plasma is 0.001 to 0.003 higher		
	U, random	Newborn:	5 to 7		Same
		Thereafter:	4.5 to 8		
		Average:	5 to 6		
	Serf (Plf, Pericf, Ascf)		6.8 to 7.6		
	Synf		Parallels serum		
	CSF		7.35 to 7.40		
	Semf		7.2 to 8.00 (average: 7.8)		
	F		7.0 to 7.5		
			May be acid with high lactose intake		
Phenols	U		**mg/L**		**μmol/L**
		Phenol:	<10	× 10.6	<106
		p-Cresol:	20 to 200	× 9.25	185 to 1850
		Toxic:			
		Phenol:	>10	× 10.6	>106
		o-Cresol:	>2	× 9.25	>19
		m-Cresol:	>2	× 9.25	>19
		p-Cresol:	>200	× 9.25	>1850
Phenolsulfonphthalein Test (PSP Test) Dose: 1 mL (6 mg), IV, 30 min after patient has voided and drunk 600 mL water	U, timed		**% dose excreted**		**Fraction of dose excreted**
		15 min:	28 to 51	× 0.01	0.28 to 0.51
		30 min:	13 to 24		0.13 to 0.24
		60 min:	9 to 17		0.09 to 0.17
		120 min:	3 to 10		0.03 to 0.10
		Total 2 h:	63 to 84		0.63 to 0.84
Phenylalanine	Whole blood on filter paper		≤2mg/dL	× 60.5	≤121 μmol/L
			mg/dL		**μmol/L**
	S	Premature:	2.0 to 7.5	× 60.5	121 to 454
		Newborn:	1.2 to 3.4		73 to 206
		Adult:	0.8 to 1.8		48 to 109
			mg/day		**μmol/day**
	U, 24-h	10 days to 7 wk:	1.2 to 1.7	× 6.05	7 to 10
		3 to 12 y:	4.0 to 17.5		24 to 106
		Adult:	<16.5		<100
			or 6 ± 2 mg/g creatinine (SD)	× 0.68	or 4.1 ± 1.4 mmol/mol creatinine (SD)

Continued

TABLE 46-8   Chemistry and Toxicology—cont'd

Test	Specimen	Reference Interval		Conversion Factor	Reference Interval (International Units)	
Phosphatase, Acid Prostatic (RIA)	S		<2.5 ng/mL	× 1	<2.5 μg/L	
		U/L			**μkat/L**	
4-Nitrophenyl-phosphate, 37 °C		Total, Male:	2.5 to 11.7	× 17	42 to 199	
		Female:	0.3 to 9.2		5 to 153	
		Tartrate-inhibited fraction,				
		Male:	0.2 to 3.5		3 to 60	
		Female:	0 to 0.8		0 to 14	
Thymolphthalein mono-phosphate, 37 °C	S		<0.8		<14	
4-Nitrophenyl-phosphate (with tar-trate inhibition), 37 °C	Semen or seminal plasma. Treat like serum.		~50,000 U/L	× 0.017	850 μkat/L	
	Vaginal swab		<2 U/L	× 17	<34 μkat/L	
Immunoassay for Prostate-Specific Acid Phosphatase	Male, with benign hypertrophy		<0.3 μg/L	× 1	<0.3 μg/L	

Phosphatase, Alkaline AACC, IFCC reference method (4-NPP, AMP), 30 and 37 °C	S	**U/L (central ninety-fifth percentile)**		× 0.017	**μkat/L**		
		30 °C	**37 °C**		**30 °C**	**37 °C**	
	20 to 50 y, Man:	38 to 94	53 to 128		0.65 to 1.60	0.9 to 2.18	
	Woman:	28 to 78	42 to 98		0.50 to 1.33	0.71 to 1.67	
	≥60 y, Man:	43 to 88	56 to 119		0.73 to 1.50	0.95 to 2.02	
	Woman:	40 to 111	53 to 141		0.68 to 1.89	0.90 to 2.40	

IEF

Percentage of total activity

Isoenzyme	<1 y	1 to 15 y	Adult	Pregnant woman	Postmenopausal woman
Biliary:	3 to 6	2 to 5	1 to 3	1 to 3	0 to 12
Liver:	20 to 34	22 to 34	17 to 35	5 to 17	17 to 48
Bone:	20 to 30	21 to 30	13 to 19	8 to 14	8 to 21
Placental:	8 to 19	5 to 17	13 to 21	53 to 69	7 to 15
Renal:	1 to 3	0 to 1	0 to 2	3 to 6	0 to 2
Intestinal:	0 to 2	0 to 1	0 to 1	0 to 1	0 to 1

Fraction activity

	<1 y	1 to 15 y	Adult	Pregnant woman	Postmenopausal woman
Biliary:	0.03 to 0.06	0.02 to 0.05	0.01 to 0.03	0.01 to 0.03	0.0 to 0.12
Liver:	0.20 to 0.34	0.22 to 0.34	0.17 to 0.35	0.05 to 0.17	0.17 to 0.48
Bone:	0.20 to 0.30	0.21 to 0.30	0.13 to 0.19	0.08 to 0.14	0.08 to 0.21
Placental:	0.08 to 0.19	0.05 to 0.17	0.13 to 0.21	0.53 to 0.69	0.07 to 0.15
Renal:	0.01 to 0.03	0.0 to 0.01	0.0 to 0.02	0.03 to 0.06	0.0 to 0.02
Intestinal:	0.0 to 0.02	0.0 to 0.01	0.0 to 0.01	0.0 to 0.01	0.0 to 0.01

TABLE 46-8   Chemistry and Toxicology—cont'd

Test	Specimen		Reference Interval	Conversion Factor	Reference Interval (International Units)
Phosphatidylglycerol (PG)	Slide Agglutination (Amino-stat-FLM)	High positive: Low positive: Negative:	**mg/L** >2.0 >0.5 <0.5		None found
	Amf	Absent:	Fetal immaturity (method-dependent)		Same
	(TLC)	Present:	Fetal maturity (method-dependent)		
Phosphofructokinase (PFK) in Erythrocyles, IFCC, 30 °C	WB (ACD, EDTA, or Hep)		9.05 ± 1.89 U/g Hb (SD) 262 ± 55 U/10^{12} RBC 3.08 ± 0.64 U/mL RBC lower in newborns	× 0.0645 × 10^{-3} × 1	0.58 ± 0.12 MU/mol Hb 0.26 ± 0.05 nU/RBC 3.08 ± 0.64 kU/L RBC
Phospholipids, Total	S or P (EDTA)	Newborn: Infant: Child: Adult: >65 y:	**mg/dL** 75 to 170 100 to 275 180 to 295 125 to 275 196 to 366	× 0.01	**g/L** 0.75 to 1.70 1.00 to 2.75 1.80 to 2.95 1.25 to 2.75 1.96 to 3.66
Phosphorus, Inorganic	S	Cord: 0 to 10 day: 10 days to 24 mo: 24 mo to 12 y: Thereafter: >60 y: Man: Woman:	**mg/dL** 3.7 to 8.1 4.5 to 9.0 4.5 to 6.7 4.5 to 5.5 2.7 to 4.5 2.3 to 3.7 2.8 to 4.1	× 0.323	**mmol/L** 1.20 to 2.62 1.45 to 2.91 1.45 to 2.16 1.45 to 1.78 0.87 to 1.45 0.74 to 1.20 0.90 to 1.32
	U, 24-h	Adults on diet containing 0.9 to 1.5 g P and 10 mg Ca/kg:	<1.0 g/day	× 32.3	Adults on diet containing 29 to 48 mmol P and 0.25 mmol Ca/kg: <32.3 mmol/day
		On nonrestricted diet:	0.4 to 1.3 g/day	× 32.3	On nonrestricted diet: 12.9 to 42.0 mmol/day
Placental Lactogen (PL)	S	Male and nonpregnant female:	**μg/mL** Not detected		Not detected
		Pregnancy, 5 to 38 wk:	0.5 to 11	× 46.30	23 to 509 nmol/L
	Amf	Rises slowly during pregnancy, <20 wk: 30 to 40 wk:	0.3 to 0.4 μg/mL 0.4 to 0.6 μg/mL		14 to 18 nmol/L 18 to 28 nmol/L
Plasma Volume ^{125}I-albumin	P (Hep)		45 to 50 mL/kg	× 0.001	0.04 to 0.05 L/kg
Plasminogen	P or S		10 to 30 mg/dL	× 10	100 to 300 mg/L
Porphyrins HPLC	U	Uroporphyrin: Heptacarboxylate: Coproporphyrin:	**μmol/mol creatinine** 0 to 4 0 to 2 0 to 22	× 1	Same
	Fecal	Coproporphyrin: Protoporphyrin:	**nmol/g dry wt** 0 to 45 0 to 150	× 1	Same

Continued

TABLE 46-8　Chemistry and Toxicology—cont'd

Test	Specimen		Reference Interval	Conversion Factor	Reference Interval (International Units)
Porphobilinogen (PBG)					
Quant.	U, 24-h		0 to 2.0 mg/day	× 4.42	0 to 8.8 μmol/day
Qual.	U, random		Negative		Negative
Potassium	S		**mmol/L**		**mmol/L**
		Premature cord:	5.0 to 10.2	× 1	5.0 to 10.2
		48 h:	3.0 to 6.0		3.0 to 6.0
		Cord blood:	5.6 to 12.0	× 1	5.6 to 12
		Newborn:	3.7 to 5.9		3.7 to 5.9
		Infant:	4.1 to 5.3		4.1 to 5.3
		Child:	3.4 to 4.7		3.4 to 4.7
		Thereafter:	3.5 to 5.1		3.5 to 5.1
	P (Hep)	Male:	3.5 to 4.5		3.5 to 4.5
		Female:	3.4 to 4.4		3.4 to 4.4
	U, 24-h	Adult:	25 to 125 mmol/day; varies with diet		25 to 125 mmol/day; varies with diet
	CSF		70% of plasma level; 2.5 to 3.2 mmol/L, rises with plasma hyperos-molality	× 0.01 × 1	0.70 plasma level fraction; 2.5 to 3.2 mmol/L, rises with plasma hyperos-molality
	F, 24-h		~5 mmol/day	× 1	~ 5mmol/day
	Gastf		~10 mmol/L; parietal and nonparietal juice have the same conc.	× 1	10 mmol/L, parietal and nonparietal juice have the same conc.
	RBC		96 to 109 mmol/L	× 1	96 to 109 mmol/L
	Sal	Without stimulation:	19 to 23 mmol/L	× 1	19 to 23 mmol/L
		With stimulation:	18 to 19 mmol/L		18 to 19 mmol/L
	Swt	Male:	4.4 to 9.7 mmol/L		
		Female:	7.6 to 15.6 mmol/L		
		Cystic fibrosis:	14 to 30 mmol/L		14 to 30
Prealbumin, *see* **Transthyretin**					
Pregnancy Tests Chorionic Gonadotropin (CG) Tube Test Qual.	S or U		Negative Positive by fourth to eighth day after ex-pected menstrual period		Same
Quant.	S or U, 24-h		Peak values up to 120,000 mIU/mL	× 1	Peak values up to 120,000 IU/L
Chorionic Gonadotropin (β-CG), *see* Chorionic Gonadotropin					
Pregnanediol	U, 24-h		**mg/day**		**μmol/day**
		<2 y:	<0.1	× 3.12	<0.3
		3 to 5 y:	<0.3		<0.9
		6 to 9 y:	<0.5		<1.6
		Boy, 10 to 15 y:	0.1 to 0.7		0.3 to 2.2
		Girl, 10 to 15 y:	0.1 to 1.2		0.3 to 3.7
		Adult, Man:	0 to 1.9		0 to 5.9
		Adult, Woman:			
		Follicular:	<2.6		<8
		Luteal:	2.6 to 10.6		8 to 33
		Pregnancy (wk),			
		First trimester:	10 to 35		31 to 109
		Second trimester:	35 to 70		109 to 218
		Third trimester:	70 to 100		218 to 312
		Term:	145 ng/dL		452 nmol/L

TABLE 46-8 Chemistry and Toxicology—cont'd

Test	Specimen	Reference Interval		Conversion Factor	Reference Interval (International Units)
Pregnanetriol	U, 24-h		**mg/day**		**μmol/day**
		0 to 5 y:	<0.1	× 2.97	<0.3
		6 to 9 y:	<0.3		<0.9
		Adult:			
		Man:	0.4 to 2.5		1.2 to 7.5
		Woman:			
		Follicular:	0.1 to 1.8		0.3 to 5.3
		Luteal:	0.9 to 2.2		2.7 to 6.5
Pregnenolone	S	Adult:	46 to 225 ng/dL	× 0.0316	1.5 to 7.1 nmol/L
Progesterone (P₄)			**ng/dL**		**nmol/L**
		Cord blood:	8000 to 56,000	× 0.0318	254 to 1780
		Premature:	84 to 1360		2.7 to 43.2
RIA	S	Prepubertal child (1 to 10 y):	7 to 52		0.2 to 1.7
		Puberty:			
		Tanner stage			
		1, Boy:	<10 to 33		<0.3 to 1.0
		Girl:	<10 to 33		<0.3 to 1.0
		2, Boy:	<10 to 33		<0.3 to 1.0
		Girl:	<10 to 55		<0.3 to 1.7
		3, Boy:	<10 to 48		<0.3 to 1.5
		Girl:	<10 to 450		<0.3 to 14.3
		4, Boy:	<10 to 108		<0.3 to 3.4
		Girl:	<10 to 1300		<0.3 to 41.3
		5, Boy:	21 to 82		0.7 to 2.6
		Girl:	10 to 950		0.3 to 30.2
		Adult:			
		Man:	13 to 97		0.4 to 3.1
		Woman:			
		Follicular:	15 to 70		0.5 to 2.2
		Luteal:	200 to 2500		6.4 to 79.5
		Pregnancy:			
		7 to 13 wk:	1025 to 4400		32.6 to 139.9
		14 to 37 wk:	1950 to 8250		62.0 to 262.4
		30 to 42 wk:	6500 to 22,900		206.7 to 728.2
Progesterone Receptor Protein (PRP)	T, tumor		**fmol/mg of protein**		**nmol/kg of protein**
		Normal, or benign and nonresponsive tumor:	<6	× 1	<6
		Indeterminate:	6 to 10		6 to 10
		Positive:	>10		>10
Proinsulin	S		2.0 to 26 pmol/L	× 1	Same
Prolactin (PRL)	S		**ng/mL**		**μg/L**
Immunometric Assay		Cord blood:	45 to 539	× 1.0	45 to 539
		Newborn, 1 to 7 days:	30 to 495		30 to 495
		Children:			
		Tanner stage			
		1, Boy:	<10		<10
		Girl:	3.6 to 12		3.6 to 12
		2 to 3, Boy:	<6.1		<6.1
		Girl:	2.6 to 18		2.6 to 18
		4 to 5, Boy:	2.8 to 11.0		2.8 to 11.0
		Girl:	3.2 to 20		3.2 to 20

Continued

TABLE 46-8 Chemistry and Toxicology—cont'd

Test	Specimen		Reference Interval	Conversion Factor	Reference Interval (International Units)
Prolactin (PRL)—cont'd					
Immunometric assay—cont'd					
		Adult:	**ng/mL**		**µg/L**
		Man:	3.0 to 14.7		3.0 to 14.7
		Woman:	3.8 to 23.2		3.8 to 23.2
		Pregnancy:			
		Third trimester:	95 to 473		95 to 473
	Amf		Low before 12 wk; increases rapidly to peak levels of 2000 to 3000 ng/mL [2 to 3 mg/L] between 15 to 20 wk and declines gradually in the last trimester		
Properdin	S		**mg/dL ± SD**		**mg/L ± SD**
		Cord:	1.5 ± 0.1	× 10	15 ± 1
		1 mo:	1.4 ± 0.4		14 ± 4
		6 mo:	1.9 ± 0.3		19 ± 3
		Adult:	2.8 ± 0.4		28 ± 4
Prostaglandins, E	P (Hep)		25 to 200 pg/mL	× 2.82	71 to 564 pmol/L
F			25 to 150 pg/mL		71 to 423 pmol/L
Prostate-specific Antigen (PSA)	S	Healthy males >40 y (percent of population):		× 1.0	
			ng/mL		**µg/L**
RIA, IRMA, IEMA		96	<4.0		<4.0
		3.5	4.1 to 10.0		4.1 to 10.0
		0.5	10.1 to 30		10.1 to 30
		0	>30		>30
			Values vary with method.		
Protein	S		**g/dL**		**g/L**
Total		Cord:	4.8 to 8.0	× 10	48 to 80
		Premature:	3.6 to 6.0		36 to 60
		Newborn:	4.6 to 7.0		46 to 70
		1 wk:	4.4 to 7.6		44 to 76
		7 mo to 1 y:	5.1 to 7.3		51 to 73
		1 to 2 y:	5.6 to 7.5		56 to 75
		≥3 y:	6.0 to 8.0		60 to 80
		Adult:			
		Ambulatory:	6.4 to 8.3		64 to 83
		Recumbent:	6.0 to 7.8		60 to 78
		>60 y:	Lower by ~0.2		~2
Electrophoresis (agarose)		Albumin:	**g/dL**		**g/L**
		Adult:	3.9 to 5.1		39 to 51
		α_1-Globulin:			
		Adult:	0.2 to 0.4		2 to 4
		α_2-Globulin:			
		Adult:	0.4 to 0.8		4 to 8
		β-Globulin:			
		Adult:	0.5 to 1.0		5 to 10
		γ-Globulin:			
		Adult:	0.6 to 1.3		6 to 13
Total	U, 24-h		1 to 14 mg/dL	× 10	10 to 140 mg/L
			50 to 80 mg/d (at rest)		Same
			<250 mg/d after intense exercise		

TABLE 46-8   Chemistry and Toxicology—cont'd

Test	Specimen	Reference Interval		Conversion Factor	Reference Interval (International Units)
Protein—cont'd					
Electrophoresis		**Average % of total protein**			**Fraction of total**
		Albumin:	37.9	× 0.01	0.379
		α_1-Globulin:	27.3		0.273
		α_2-Globulin:	19.5		0.195
		β-Globulin:	8.8		0.088
		γ-Globulin:	3.3		0.033
Total		**mg/dL**			**mg/L**
Column Turbidimetry	CSF, lumbar:		8 to 32	× 10	80 to 320
		Premature:	15 to 130		150 to 1300
		Full-term newborn:	40 to 120		400 to 1200
		<1 mo:	20 to 80		200 to 800
		Thereafter:	8 to 32		80 to 320
Electrophoresis		**% of Total**			**Fraction of total**
		Prealbumin:	2 to 7	× 0.01	0.02 to 0.07
		Albumin:	56 to 76		0.56 to 0.76
		α_1-Globulin:	2 to 7		0.02 to 0.07
		α_2-Globulin:	4 to 12		0.04 to 0.12
		β-Globulin:	8 to 18		0.08 to 0.18
		γ-Globulin:	3 to 12		0.03 to 0.12
Electrophoresis	Synf	Albumin:	63		0.63
		α_1-Globulin:	7		0.07
		α_2-Globulin:	7		0.07
		β-Globulin:	9		0.09
		γ-Globulin:	14		0.14
		Fibrinogen:	0		0
Protein C and S	P (citrate)	%			
EI		Protein C total:	69 to 125	× 1	Same
		Protein S total:	58 to 146		
Clotting					
		Protein functional:	52 to 131		
		Protein S functional Male:	82 to 177		
		Protein S functional Female:	67 to 146		
Prothrombin Time	WB (NaCit)	In general:	11 to 15 s (varies with type of thromboplastin)		Same
One-stage (Quick)		Newborn:	Prolonged by 2 to 3 s		
		Premature:	Prolonged by 3 to 5 s, reaches adult level by day 3 or 4		
Two-stage modified (Ware and Seegers)			18 to 22 s		
Protoporphyrin	WB (Hep or EDTA)	Total:	<60 μg/dL	× 10	<600 μg/dL
	F, 24-h		<200 nmol/g dry wt.	× 1	<200 nmol/g dry wt.
Pseudocholinesterase (PChE), *see* *Cholinesterase II*					

Continued

TABLE 46-8   Chemistry and Toxicology—cont'd

Test	Specimen		Reference Interval	Conversion Factor	Reference Interval (International Units)
Pyridinium Collagen Crosslinks (Pyridinoline)	Urine, 24h		**nmol/mmol creatinine**	1.0	Same
		Child,			
		2 to 10 y:	160 to 440		
		11 to 14 y:	105 to 400		
		15 to 17 y:	42 to 200		
		Man:	20 to 61		
		Woman: pre-menopausal:	28 to 89		
(Deoxypyridinoline)	Urine, 24h		**nmol/mmol creatinine**	1.0	Same
		Child,			
		2 to 10 y:	31 to 110		
		11 to 14 y:	17 to 100		
		15 to 17 y:	<60		
		Man:	4 to 19		
		Woman: pre-menopausal:	4 to 21		
Pyruvic Acid	WB, arterial:		0.02 to 0.08 mg/dL	× 114	2 to 9 μmol/L
	WB, venous (Hep):		0.3 to 0.9 mg/dL	× 114	34 to 103 μmol/L
	U		88.1 mg/day	× 0.0114	1 mmol/day
	CSF		0.5 to 1.7 mg/dL	× 11.4	6 to 19 μmol/L
Renal Plasma Flow (RPF)	P and U	Male:	560 to 830 mL/min	× 0.01667	9.34 to 13.84 mL/s
		Female:	490 to 700 mL/min or (390 mL/min)/m^2 body surface		8.17 to 11.67 mL/s or (6.50 mL/s)m^2 body surface
		>40 y:	Decreases ~75 mL/decade		
Renin	P (EDTA)	**Normal sodium diet:**	**ng/mL/h**		**μg/L/h**
		Supine:	0.2 to 1.6	× 1	0.2 to 1.6
		Standing (4h):	0.7 to 3.3		0.7 to 3.3
		Low sodium:			
		Supine:	1.0 to 5.4		1.0 to 5.4
		Standing (4h):	0 to 19		0 to 19
Reverse Triiodothyronine (rT$_3$)	S		**ng/dL**		**nmol/L**
		Cord:	130 to 300	× 0.0154	2.00 to 4.62
		1 day:	83 to 194		1.28 to 2.99
		2 days:	107 to 209		1.65 to 3.22
		3 days:	102 to 166		1.57 to 2.56
		1 mo to 20 y:	10 to 35		0.15 to 0.54
		Adult:	10 to 28		0.15 to 0.43
		Material serum,			
		15 to 40 wk:	11 to 33		0.17 to 0.51
		Amf, <17 wk:	130 to 599		2.00 to 9.22
		17 to 22 wk:	163 to 599		2.51 to 9.22
		35 to 42 wk:	15 to 98		0.23 to 1.57
Rheumatoid Factor (*Nephelom.*)	S		<30 U/mL	× 1	<30 kU/L
Riboflavin (Vitamin B$_2$)	S		4 to 24 μg/dL	× 26.6	106 to 638 nmol/L
	Erythrocytes		10 to 50 μg/dL	× 26.6	266 to 1330 nmol/L
	U, random		>80 μg/g creatinine	× 0.3	>24 μmol/mol creatinine
	U, 24-h		>100 μg/day	× 2.66	>266 nmol/day

TABLE 46-8   Chemistry and Toxicology—cont'd

Test	Specimen		Reference Interval	Conversion Factor	Reference Interval (International Units)
Schilling Test (Intrinsic Factor Test) Dose: 0.5 to 1.0 μCi ^{58}Co-Vitamin B$_{12}$	U, 24-h		>7.5% of dose	× 0.01	Fraction of dose: 0.075
Secretin	S or P (Hep or EDTA)		12 to 75 pg/mL	× 1	12 to 75 ng/L
Selenium	WB (Hep) S U, 24-h Toxic conc.:		58 to 234 μg/dL 46 to 143 μg/dL 7 to 160 μg/L >400 μg/L	× 0.0127	0.74 to 2.97 μmol/L 0.58 to 1.82 μmol/L 0.09 to 2.03 μmol/L >5.08 μmol/L
Serotonin	WB (EDTA) Plt		50 to 200 ng/mL 125 to 500 ng/10^9 platelets	× 0.00568	0.28 to 1.14 μmol/L ~0.7 to 2.8 amol/platelet
Sex Hormone Binding Globulin RIA	S	Male: Female: Third trimester pregnancy: Hirsuitism:	**nmol/L** 10 to 55 30 to 95 220 to 450 20 to 40	× 1	Same
Sodium	S or P (Hep)	Premature, Cord: 48-h: Newborn, Cord: Newborn: Infant: Child: Thereafter:	**mmol/L** 116 to 140 128 to 148 126 to 166 133 to 146 139 to 146 138 to 145 136 to 145	× 1	**mmol/L** 116 to 140 128 to 148 126 to 166 133 to 146 139 to 146 138 to 145 136 to 145
	U, 24-h	6 to 10 y: Boy: Girl: 10 to 14 y: Boy: Girl: Adult:	**mmol/day** 41 to 115 20 to 69 63 to 177 49 to 168 40 to 220	× 1.0	**mmol/day** 41 to 115 20 to 69 63 to 177 48 to 168 40 to 220
		Full-term, 7- to 14-day-old newborns have sodium clearance of about 20% of adult values.			
Iontophoresis, photometric, coulometric, ISE	Swt	Child and adult: Child, $\bar{x}$: Adult, $\bar{x}$: Cystic fibrosis:	**mmol/L** 10 to 40 27 33 70 to 190	× 1.0	**mmol/L** 10 to 40 27 33 70 to 190
Soluble Transferrin Receptor EI	S	Normal: Elevated:	**nmol/L** Less than 28.1 More than 28.1	× 1	Same
Somatomedin C (see Insulin Growth Factor 1)					
Somatostatin	P (EDTA)		<25 pg/mL	× 1	<25 ng/mL

Continued

TABLE 46-8 **Chemistry and Toxicology—cont'd**

Test	Specimen	Reference Interval			Conversion Factor	Reference Interval (International Units)
Specific Gravity	U, random	Newborn:	1.012			Same
		Infant:	1.002 to 1.006			
		Adult:	1.002 to 1.030			
		After 12-h fluid restriction:	>1.025			
		U, 24-h	1.015 to 1.025			
Sucrose	S or P		0.06 mg/dL		× 29.21	1.75 μmol/L
	U		2.2 mg/dL			64.26 μmol/L
Sulfhemoglobin	WB (EDTA, Hep or ACD)		≤1.0% of total Hb		× 0.01	≤0.010 of total Hb (mass fraction)

Testosterone, Free S			pg/mL	pmol/L	Percent of total		Fraction of total
RIA (equilibrium dialysis)	Cord:					× 0.01	
		Male:	5 to 22	× 3.47 17.4 to 76.3	2.0 to 4.4		0.02 to 0.04
		Female:	4 to 16	13.9 to 55.5	2.0 to 3.9		0.02 to 0.04
	Newborn (1 to 15 days):						
		Male:	1.5 to 31.0	5.2 to 107.5	0.9 to 1.7		0.1 to 0.017
		Female:	0.5 to 2.5	1.7 to 8.7	0.8 to 1.5		0.008 to 0.015
	1 to 3 mo:						
		Male:	3.3 to 18.0	11.5 to 62.5	0.4 to 0.8		0.004 to 0.008
		Female:	0.1 to 1.3	0.3 to 4.5	0.4 to 1.1		0.004 to 0.011
	3 to 5 mo:						
		Male:	0.7 to 14.0	2.4 to 48.6	0.4 to 1.1		0.004 to 0.011
		Female:	0.3 to 1.1	1.0 to 3.8	0.5 to 1.0		0.005 to 0.01
	5 to 7 mo:						
		Male:	0.4 to 4.8	1.4 to 16.6	0.4 to 1.0		0.004 to 0.01
		Female:	0.2 to 0.6	0.7 to 2.1	0.5 to 0.8		0.005 to 0.008
	Prepubertal child (6 to 9 y):						
		Boy:	0.1 to 3.2	0.3 to 11.1	0.9 to 1.7		0.009 to 0.017
		Girl:	0.1 to 0.9	0.3 to 3.1	0.9 to 1.4		0.009 to 0.014
	Adult:						
		Man:	50 to 210	174 to 729	1.0 to 2.7		0.010 to 0.027
		Woman:	1.0 to 8.5	3.5 to 29.5	0.5 to 1.8		0.005 to 0.018

Testosterone, Total S			ng/dL		nmol/L
RIA	Cord:				
		Male:	13 to 55	× 0.0347	0.45 to 1.91
		Female:	5 to 45		0.17 to 1.56
	Premature:				
		Male:	37 to 198		1.28 to 6.87
		Female:	5 to 22		0.17 to 0.76
	Newborn:				
		Male:	75 to 400		2.6 to 13.9
		Female:	20 to 64		0.69 to 2.22
	Prepubertal child (1 to 10 y):				
		Boy:	2 to 30		0.07 to 1.04
		Girl:	1 to 20		0.03 to 0.69

TABLE 46-8   Chemistry and Toxicology—cont'd

Test	Specimen	Reference Interval		Conversion Factor	Reference Interval (International Units)	
Testosterone, Total—cont'd		**ng/dL**			**nmol/L**	
RIA—cont'd		Puberty:				
		Tanner stage				
		1, Boy:	2 to 23		0.07 to 0.8	
		Girl:	2 to 10		0.07 to 0.35	
		2, Boy:	5 to 70		0.17 to 2.43	
		Girl:	5 to 30		0.17 to 1.04	
		3, Boy:	15 to 280		0.52 to 9.72	
		Girl:	10 to 30		0.35 to 1.04	
		4, Boy:	105 to 545		3.64 to 18.91	
		Girl:	15 to 40		0.52 to 1.39	
		5, Boy:	265 to 800		9.19 to 27.76	
		Girl:	10 to 40		0.35 to 1.39	
		Adult:				
		Man:	280 to 1100		0.52 to 38.17	
		Woman:	15 to 70 (higher at midcycle peak)		0.52 to 2.43	
		Pregnancy:	3 to 4 × the adult level			
		Postmenopause:	8 to 35		0.28 to 1.22	
	U, 24-h	**µg/kg of body weight**			**nmol/kg of body weight**	
		Pubertal stage I:				
		Boy:	0.25	× 3.47	0.87	
		Girl:	0.16		0.56	
		Pubertal stage II,				
		Boy:	0.34		1.18	
		Girl:	0.16		0.56	
		Pubertal stage III,				
		Boy:	0.37		1.28	
		Girl:	0.16		0.56	
		µg/day			**nmol/day**	
		20 to 50 y:				
		Man:	50 to 135	× 3.47	173 to 470	
		Woman:	2 to 12		7 to 42	
		>50 y:				
		Man:	40 to 60		139 to 210	
		Woman:	2 to 8		7 to 28	

	Amf	**ng/dL**				**nmol/L**		
		Fetal age (wk)	**Median**	**Interval**		**Median**	**Interval**	
		9 to 12:						
		Male:	5.0	2.0 to 72.6	× 0.0347	0.17	0.07 to 2.52	
		Female:	2.7	1.3 to 4.0		0.09	0.05 to 0.14	
		12 to 16:						
		Male:	25.0	7.0 to 72.4		0.87	0.24 to 2.51	
		Female:	2.6	1.3 to 10.0		0.09	0.05 to 0.35	
		16 to 19:						
		Male:	19.3	8.4 to 29		0.67	0.29 to 1.0	
		Female:	2.9	1.0 to 9.0		0.10	0.03 to 0.31	
		28 to 34:						
		Male:	12.3	8.4 to 26.4		0.43	0.29 to 0.92	
		38 to 40:						
		Male:	18.0	2.0 to 16.0		0.62	0.07 to 0.56	
		Female:	3.4	2.2 to 10.2		0.12	0.08 to 0.35	

Test	Specimen	Reference Interval	Conversion Factor	Reference Interval (International Units)
Tetrahydrocortisol (THF)	U, 24-h	Adult: 0.5 to 1.5 mg/day	× 2.72	1.4 to 4.1 µmol/day

Continued

TABLE 46-8 Chemistry and Toxicology—cont'd

Test	Specimen		Reference Interval	Conversion Factor	Reference Interval (International Units)
Tetrahydrodeoxy-cortisol	U, 24-h		20 to 130 µg/day <25% of total 17-hydroxycorticosteroids	× 0.0029	0.1 to 0.4 µmol/day
Thallium	WB (NaHep)		<0.5 µg/L	× 48.9	<24.5 nmol/L
	Toxic		10 to 800 µg/dL	× 0.0489	0.5 to 39.1 µmol/L
	U, 24-h		<2.0 µg/L	× 4.89	<9.78 nmol/L
	Toxic		1.0 to 20.0 mg/L	× 4.89	4.9 to 97.8 µmol/L
Thiocyanate Spectrometric	S, P (EDTA)		**mg/ml**	× 17.2	
		Nonsmoker:	1 to 4		17 to 69
		Smoker:	3 to 12		52 to 207
		Toxic:	>50		> 860
		Nitroprusside therapy:	6 to 29		>103 to 499
	U, 24 h		**mg/day**		
		Nonsmoker:	1 to 4		17 to 69
		Smoker:	7 to 17		121 to 292
Thyroglobulin (Tg)	S	Adult:	3 to 42 ng/mL	× 1	3 to 42 µg/L
Thyroid Peroxidase Antibodies	S	Adult:	Negative (≤1:10 dilution)		Same
Thyroid Microsomal Antibodies	S		Nondetectable (hemag-glutination) and <1:100		Same
Thyroid-Stimulating Hormone (TSH) (Thyrotropin)	S or P	Adult:	**µU/mL** 0.4 to 4.2	× 1	**mU/L** 0.4 to 4.2
Thyrotropin-Releasing Hormone (TRH)	P	Newborn, 30 min after delivery:	78 pg/mL (mean), falling to normal at 24 h	× 1	78 ng/L (mean)
		Adult:	5 to 60 pg/mL		5 to 60 ng/L
	U, 24-h	Adult:			
		Man:	195 ng/d (mean)		Same
		Woman:	119 ng/d (mean)		
Thyroxine-Binding Globulin (TBG)	S		**mg/dL**		**mg/L**
		Cord:	3.6 to 9.6	× 10	36 to 96
		1 to 3 days:	5.0 ($\bar{x}$)		50 ($\bar{x}$)
		1 to 12 mo:	3.1 to 5.6		31 to 56
		1 to 5 y:	2.9 to 5.4		29 to 54
		5 to 10 y:	2.5 to 5.0		25 to 50
		10 to 15 y:	2.1 to 4.6		21 to 46
		Adult:	1.2 to 3.0		12 to 30
		Pregnancy, third trimester:	4.1 to 6.5		41 to 65
		As T_4 binding capacity, Adult:	16 to 24 µg/dL	× 12.9	206 to 309 µg/L

Thyroxine Index, Free
(see Free Thyroxine Index)

TABLE 46-8   Chemistry and Toxicology—cont'd

Test	Specimen		Reference Interval	Conversion Factor	Reference Interval (International Units)
Thyroxine Ratio, Effective (ETR)			0.86 to 1.13	× 1	0.86 to 1.13
Thyroxine/TBG Ratio	S		3 to 5	× 0.065	0.19 to 0.32 (mole ratio)
Tyroxine, Free (FT₄)	S		**ng/dL**		**pmol/L**
		Cord:	1.7 to 4.0	× 12.9	21.9 to 51.6
		Newborn:	2.6 to 6.3		33.5 to 81.3
		Adult:	0.8 to 2.7		10.3 to 35.0
Thyroxine (T₄), Total	S		**μg/dL**		**nmol/L**
		Cord:	7.4 to 13.0	× 12.9	95 to 168
		1 to 3 day:	11.8 to 22.6		152 to 292
		1 to 2 wk:	9.8 to 16.6		126 to 214
		1 to 4 mo:	7.2 to 14.4		93 to 186
		4 to 12 mo:	7.8 to 16.5		101 to 213
		1 to 5 y:	7.3 to 15.0		94 to 194
		5 to 10 y:	6.4 to 13.3		83 to 172
		Adult:	5 to 12		65 to 155
		Man:	4.6 to 10.5		59 to 135
		Woman:	5.5 to 11.0		71 to 142
		Pregnancy, 15 to 40 wk:	9.1 to 14.0		117 to 181
T-uptake (Thyroxine uptake, T-U) Abbott IM$_x$	S		3 to 5	× 0.065	0.19 to 0.32 mole ratio
Transcortin	S		**mg/L**		**nmol/L**
		Male:	18.8 to 25.2	× 17.18	323 to 433
		Female:	14.9 to 22.9		256 to 393
		Pregnancy:	31.5 to 60.0		541 to 1031
		Oral contraceptives:	20.2 to 52.3		347 to 899
		Child:			
		Boy:	18.3 to 28.3		314 to 486
		Girl:	14.3 to 26.7		246 to 458
Transferrin Nephelometric	S		**mg/dL**		**g/L**
		0 to 4 days:	130 to 275	× 0.01	1.30 to 2.75
		3 mo to 10 y:	203 to 360		2.03 to 3.6
		Adult:	215 to 380		2.15 to 3.8
		>60 y:	190 to 375		1.90 to 3.75
		Maternal (at term):	305		3.05
		Adult levels reached by 9 mo.			
	U		0.04 to 0.45 mg/day	× 1	0.04 to 0.45 mg/day
Transketolase Ribose/sedoheptulose, 37 °C	WB (Hep)		(9 to 12 μmol/h)/mL whole blood	× 16.67	150 to 200 U/L whole blood

Continued

TABLE 46-8   Chemistry and Toxicology—cont'd

Test	Specimen	Reference Interval			Conversion Factor	Reference Interval (International Units)	
Transthyretin		**mg/dL**				**mg/L**	
(Prealbumin, PA,	Cord:	13			× 10	130	
Tryptophan-Rich	1 y:	10				100	
Prealbumin,	Maternal:	23				230	
Thyroxine-	Adult:	10 to 40				100 to 400	
Binding	Male, $\bar{x}$:	21.5				215	
Prealbumin,	Female, $\bar{x}$:	18.2				182	
TBPA)	2 to 36 mo:	16 to 28.1				160 to 281	
TRH (Thyrotropin-Releasing Hormone) Stimulation Test	S before and 30 and 60 min after TRH	TSH:	The minimum normal response is an increase of 1 to 2 μU/mL (1 to 2 mU/L) above baseline. The typical normal response is an increase of fivefold to tenfold above baseline.				

Triglycerides (TG)   S, ≥12-h fast
Fluorometric, photometric

		mg/dL			**mmol/L**	
		Male	**Female**		**Male**	**Female**
	Cord blood:	13 to 95	11 to 76	× 0.0113	0.15 to 1.07	0.12 to 0.86
	0 to 9 y:	30 to 100	35 to 110		0.34 to 1.13	0.40 to 1.24
	10 to 14 y:	32 to 125	37 to 131		0.36 to 1.41	0.42 to 1.48
	15 to 19 y:	37 to 148	39 to 124		0.42 to 1.67	0.44 to 1.40
	20 to 29 y:	44 to 201	37 to 144		0.50 to 2.27	0.41 to 1.63
	30 to 39 y:	51 to 321	39 to 176		0.56 to 3.62	0.44 to 1.99
	40 to 49 y:	55 to 327	45 to 214		0.62 to 3.70	0.51 to 2.42
	50 to 59 y:	58 to 286	52 to 262		0.62 to 3.23	0.59 to 2.62

Values decrease slightly after age 60.
Levels for blacks are 10 to 20 mg/dL lower.
Values for women on oral contraceptives 20 to 40 mg/dL higher than those not taking such drugs.

Levels for blacks are 0.11 to 0.23 mmol/L lower

Recommended: (desirable) levels for adults:
Normal: <250 mg/dL   × 0.013   <2.83 mmol/L
Borderline high: 250 to 500 mg/dL   2.83 to 5.67 mmol/L
Hypertriglyceridemic: >500 mg/dL   >5.65 mmol/L

Triiodothyronine, Free   S
Equilibrium Dialysis

RIA (direct analog)

		pg/dL		**pmol/L**
	Cord:	15 to 391	× 0.0154	0.2 to 6.0
	Child and adult:	260 to 480		4.0 to 7.4
	Pregnancy:			
	First trimester:	211 to 383		3.2 to 5.9
	Second and third trimesters:	196 to 338		3.0 to 5.2

Triiodothyronine Resin Uptake Test (T$_3$RU)   S

		% of total		**Fraction of total**
	Newborn:	25 to 37	× 0.01	0.25 to 0.37
	Adult:	24 to 34		0.24 to 0.34
	>60 y,			
	Man:	24 to 32		0.24 to 0.32
	Woman:	22 to 32		0.22 to 0.32

TABLE 46-8　Chemistry and Toxicology—cont'd

Test	Specimen		Reference Interval	Conversion Factor	Reference Interval (International Units)
Triiodothyronine, Total T$_3$ (RIA)	S		**ng/dL**		**nmol/L**
		Cord:	5 to 141	× 0.0154	0.08 to 2.17
		1 to 3 days:	100 to 740		1.54 to 11.40
		1 to 5 y:	105 to 269		1.62 to 4.14
		5 to 10 y:	94 to 241		1.45 to 3.71
		10 to 15 y:	83 to 213		1.28 to 3.28
		Adult:	70 to 204		1.08 to 3.14
Troponin-I	S		<10 µg/L	× 1	<10 µg/L
Troponin-T	S		0 to 0.1 µg/L		0 to 0.1 µg/L
Tubular Reabsorption of Phosphate (TRP)	U, 4-h (0800 to 1200 h) and S		82% to 95%	× 0.01	Fraction: 0.82 to 0.95
Tumor Necrosis Factor ELISA	S,P (EDTA or Heparin)		**ng/mL**		**µg/L**
		Serum:	0.2 to 7.1	× 1	Same
		Plasma (EDTA):	0.5 to 5.5		
		Plasma (Heparin):	0.3 to 7.2		
Tyrosine Fluorometric	S		**mg/dL**		**mmol/L**
		Premature:	7.0 to 24.0	× 55.2	386 to 1325
		Newborn:	1.6 to 3.7		88 to 204
		Adult:	0.8 to 1.3		44 to 72
Urea, *see Urea Nitrogen*					
Urea Nitrogen	S		**mg/dL**		**mmol Urea/L**
		Cord:	21 to 40	× 0.357	7.5 to 14.3
		Premature (1 wk):	3 to 25		1.1 to 8.9
		Newborn:	4 to 12		1.4 to 4.3
		Infant/child:	5 to 18		1.8 to 6.4
		Adult:	6 to 20		2.1 to 7.1
		>60 y:	8 to 23		2.9 to 8.2
		Higher after protein intake			
	U		12 to 20 g/day	× 0.0357	0.43 to 0.71 mol/day
Urea Nitrogen/ Creatinine Ratio	S		12/1 to 20/1	× 4.04	48 to 80 (urea/creatinine mole ratio)
Uric Acid Phosphotungstate	S		**mg/dL**		**mmol/L**
		Adult:			
		Male:	4.4 to 7.6	× 0.059	0.26 to 0.45
		Female:	2.3 to 6.6		0.13 to 0.39
		>60 y:			
		Male:	4.2 to 8.0		0.25 to 0.47
		Female:	3.5 to 7.3		0.20 to 0.43
Uricase		Child:	2.0 to 5.5		0.12 to 0.32
		Adult:			
		Male:	3.5 to 7.2		0.21 to 0.42
		Female:	2.6 to 6.0		0.15 to 0.35

Continued

TABLE 46-8 Chemistry and Toxicology—cont'd

Test	Specimen	Reference Interval		Conversion Factor	Reference Interval (International Units)
Uric Acid—cont'd Uricase—cont'd	U, 24-h		**mg/day**		**mmol/day**
		Free-purine diet:			
		Male:	<420	× 0.0059	<2.48
		Female:	slightly lower		Slightly lower
		Low-purine diet:			
		Male:	<480		<2.83
		Female:	<400		<2.36
		High-purine diet:	<1000		<5.90
		Average diet:	250 to 750		1.48 to 4.43
Urine Volume	U, 24-h		**mL/day**		Same
		Newborn (1 to 2 days):	30 to 60		
		Infant, 3 to 10 days:	100 to 300		
		10 to 60 days:	250 to 450		
		60 to 365 days:	400 to 500		
		Child, 1 to 3 y:	500 to 600		
		3 to 5 y:	600 to 700		
		5 to 8 y:	650 to 1000		
		8 to 14 y:	800 to 1400		
		Adult:			
		Man:	800 to 1800		
		Woman:	600 to 1600		
		Older adult: (varies with water intake and other factors)	250 to 2400		
Urobilinogen	U, 2-h		0.1 to 0.8 EU*/2 h		Same
	U, 24-h		0.5 to 4.0 EU/day		
	F		75 to 275 EU/100 g	× 10	750 to 2750 EU*/kg
			75 to 400 EU/day		75 to 400 EU/day
			40 to 280 mg/day	× 1.69	67 to 473 μmol/day
Uroporphyrin	U, 24-h		32 to 63 nmol/d		Same
			3.5 to 5.7 μmol/mol creatinine		
Valine	S		**mg/dL**	× 85.5	**μmol/L**
		Premature, 1 day:	1.52 ± 0.59 (SD)		130 ± 50 (SD)
		Newborn, 1 day:	0.94 to 2.88		80 to 246
		1 to 3 mo:	2.27 ± 0.57 (SD)		194 ± 49 (SD)
		9 mo to 2 y:	0.67 to 3.07		57 to 262
		3 to 10 y:	1.50 to 3.31		128 to 283
		6 to 18 y:	1.83 to 3.37		156 to 288
		Adult:	1.65 to 3.71		141 to 317
	U, 24-h		**mg/day**		**μmol/day**
		10 d to 7 wk:	1.4 to 3.2	× 8.55	12 to 27
		3 to 12 y:	1.8 to 6.0		15 to 51
		Adult:	2.5 to 11.9		21 to 102
			or 4 ± 1 mg/g creatinine (SD)	× 0.97	or 3.9 ± 1.0 mmol/mol creatinine (SD)
Vanillylmandelic Acid (Vanilmandelic Acid) HPLC	U, 24-h		**mg/day**	× 5.05	**μmol/day**
		3 to 6 y:	1.0 to 2.6		5 to 13
		6 to 10 y:	2.0 to 3.2		10 to 16
		10 to 16 y:	2.3 to 5.2		12 to 26
		16 to 83 y:	1.4 to 6.5		7 to 33

*Ehrlich units.

TABLE 46-8   Chemistry and Toxicology—cont'd

Test	Specimen	Reference Interval		Conversion Factor	Reference Interval (International Units)
Vasoactive Intestinal Polypeptide (VIP)	P (Hep)	Child and adult:	<50 pg/mL	× 1	<50 ng/L
Viscosity	S		1.00 to 1.24 cP (relative to water at 37 °C)		Same
Vitamin A	S		**µg/dL**	× 0.0349	**µmol/L**
		1 to 6 y:	20 to 43		0.70 to 1.50
		7 to 12 y:	26 to 49		0.91 to 1.71
		13 to 19 y:	26 to 72		0.91 to 2.51
		Adult:	30 to 80		1.05 to 2.80
Vitamin B1 (Thiamine) HPLC for Thiochrome	P (EDTA or Heparin)		**µg/dL** 0.2 to 2.0	× 29.6	5.9 to 59.2
	WB (EDTA or Heparin)		1.6 to 4.0		47.3 to 118.4
	U		Adult >100 µ/day Adult deficient <40 µg/s		> 2960 nmol/day <1184 nmol/day
Vitamin B₂, see Riboflavin					
Vitamin B₆	P (EDTA)		5 to 30 ng/mL Deficiency: <5 ng/mL	× 4.046	20.2 to 121.8 nmol/L <20.2 nmol/L
Vitamin B₁₂, True	S		**pg/mL**	× 0.738	**pmol/L**
		Newborn:	160 to 1300		118 to 959
		Adult:	200 to 835		148 to 616
		>60 y:	110 to 800		81 to 590
Vitamin B₁₂ Intrinsic Factor	Gastf	50% to 400% enhancement of ^{57}Co-B$_{12}$ uptake by guinea pig intestinal mucosal homogenate		× 0.01	Fractional increase in ^{57}Co-B$_{12}$ uptake by GPIMH: 0.50 to 4.00
Vitamin C Dinitrophenylhydrazine, photometric	P (Ox, Hep, or EDTA)		0.4 to 1.5 mg/dL Deficiency: <0.2 mg/dL	× 56.78	23 to 85 µmol/L <11 µmol/L
	Buffy coat (Hep)		20 to 53 µg/10⁸ WBC	× 0.0568	1.14 to 3.01 fmol/cell
Vitamin C Saturation Test Dose: 0.5 to 2.0 g ascorbate orally over a period of 4 days	U, 24-h		60% to 80% of test dose excreted	× 0.01	Fraction test dose excreted: 0.60 to 0.80
Vitamin D₃, 1,25-dihydroxy	S		16 to 65 pg/mL	× 2.4	42 to 169 pmol/L
Vitamin D₃, 25-hydroxy	P (Hep)		14 to 60 ng/mL	× 2.496	35 to 150 nmol/L
Vitamin E (α-Tocopherol)	S	Adult:	0.5 to 1.8 mg/dL	× 2.32	12 to 42 µmol/L

Continued

TABLE 46-8		Chemistry and Toxicology—cont'd			
Test	Specimen		Reference Interval	Conversion Factor	Reference Interval (International Units)
Vitamin K (Phylloquinone)	S		0.13 to 1.19 ng/mL	× 2.22	0.29 to 2.64 nmol/L
Xylene	WB (F/Ox)		Negative		Negative
		Occup. exp.:	<1 mg/L	× 9.42	<9.4 μmol/L
		Toxic:	>3 mg/L		>28.3 μmol/L
Xylose Absorption Test	WB (NaF)		**mg/dL**		**mmol/L**
		Child, 1-h (5-g dose):	>30	× 0.0666	>2
		Adult, 2-h (25-g dose):	>25		>1.67
	U, 5-h	Child:	16% to 33% of ingested dose	× 0.01	Fraction ingested dose: 0.16 to 0.33
		Adult:	**g/5 h**		**mmol/5 h**
		5-g dose:	>1.2	× 6.66	>8.00
		25-g dose:	>4.0		>26.64
		>65 y:	>3.5		>23.31
Zinc	S		70 to 120 μg/dL	× 0.153	10.7 to 18.4 μmol/L
Zinc Protoporphyrin (ZPP)	WB (Hep, EDTA)		17 to 77 μg/dL	× 0.0160	0.27 to 1.23 μmol/L
			30 to 80 μmol ZPP/mol heme	×1	Same

TABLE 46-9   **Reference Values for Therapeutic and Toxic Drugs**

Drug	Specimen	Reference Interval		Conversion Factor	Reference Interval (International Units)
Acetaminophen (Tylenol)	S or P (Hep or EDTA)	Therap: Toxic:	10 to 30 μg/mL >200 μg/mL	× 6.62	66 to 199 μmol/L >1324 μmol/L
Amikacin (Amikin)	S or P (EDTA)		**μg/mL**		**μmol/L**
		Therap.: Peak: Trough:	25 to 35	× 1.71	43 to 60
		Less severe infection:	1 to 4		1.7 to 6.8
		Life-threatening infection:	4 to 8		6.8 to 13.7
		Toxic: Peak: Trough:	>35 to 40 >10 to 15		>60 to 68 >17 to 26
ε-Aminocaproic acid (Amicar)	S or P (Hep or EDTA); trough	Therap.: Toxic:	100 to 400 μg/mL Not defined	× 0.00762	0.76 to 3.05 mmol/L
Amitriptyline (Elavil)	S or P (Hep or EDTA); trough (>12 h after dose)	Therap.: Toxic:	80 to 250 ng/mL >500 ng/mL	× 3.61	289 to 903 nmol/L >1805 nmol/L
Amobarbital, quant. (Amytal)	S	Therap.: Toxic:	1 to 5 μg/mL >10 μg/mL	× 4.42	4 to 22 μmol/L >44 μmol/L
Amphetamine	S or P (Hep or EDTA)	Therap.: Toxic:	20 to 30 ng/mL >200 ng/mL	× 7.40	148 to 222 nmol/L >1480 nmol/L
Bromide	S	Therap.: Toxic:	750 to 1500 μg/mL >1250 μg/mL	× 0.0125	9.4 to 18.7 mmol/L >15.6 mmol/L
Caffeine	S or P (Hep or EDTA)	Therap.: Infant: Toxic:	3 to 15 μg/mL 8 to 20 μg/mL >50 μg/mL	× 5.15	15 to 77 μmol/L 41 to 103 μmol/L >258 μmol/L
Carbamazepine (Tegretol)	S or P (Hep or EDTA); trough	Therap.: Toxic:	4 to 12 μg/mL >15 μg/mL	× 4.23	17 to 51 μmol/L >63 μmol/L
Carbenicillin (Geopen)	S or P (Hep or EDTA)	Therap.: Toxic:	Dependent on minimum inhibition conc. of specific organism >250 μg/mL (neurotoxicity)	 × 2.64	Same >660 μmol/L
Chloral hydrate (Noctec)	S	As trichloroethanol: Therap.: Toxic:	 2 to 12 μg/mL >20 μg/mL	 × 6.69	 13 to 80 μmol/L >134 μmol/L
Chloramphenicol (Chloromycetin)	S or P (Hep or EDTA); trough	Therap.: Toxic: Gray baby syndrome:	10 to 25 μg/mL >25 μg/mL 40 to 100 μg/mL	× 3.09	31 to 77 μmol/L >77 μmol/L 124 to 309 μmol/L
Chlordiazepoxide (Librium)	S or P (Hep or EDTA); trough	Therap.: Toxic:	700 to 1000 ng/mL >5000 ng/mL	× 0.0033	2.34 to 3.34 μmol/L >16.7 μmol/L

Continued

TABLE 46-9   Reference Values for Therapeutic and Toxic Drugs—cont'd

Drug	Specimen	Reference Interval		Conversion Factor	Reference Interval (International Units)
Chlorpromazine (Thorazine)	S or P (Hep or EDTA); trough	Therap.: Adult: Child: Toxic:	50 to 300 40 to 80 >750 ng/mL	× 3.14	157 to 942 126 to 251 >2355 nmol/L
Cimetidine (Tagamet)	S or P (Hep or EDTA)	Therap.: Toxic:	0.5 to 1.2 μg/mL (trough) >1.3	× 3.96	2.0 to 5.0 μmol/L (trough) >5.1 μmol/L
Clonazepam (Klonopin)	S or P (Hep or EDTA); trough	Therap.: Toxic:	15 to 60 ng/mL >80 ng/mL	× 3.17	48 to 190 nmol/L >254 nmol/L
Clonidine (Catapres)	S or P (Hep or EDTA)	Therap.: Toxic:	1.0 to 2.0 ng/mL Not defined	× 4.35	4.4 to 8.7 nmol/L
Clorazepate (Tranxene)	S or P (Hep or EDTA)	As desmethyldiaz-epam: Therap.:	0.12 to 1.0 μg/mL	× 3.01	0.36 to 3.01 μmol/L
Cocaine	S or P (Hep or EDTA); on ice U	Toxic: Toxic:	>1000 ng/mL 1 to 215 mg/L	× 3.3	>3300 nmol/L
Codeine GLC, GC-MS, RIA, EIA, HPLC	S	Therap. conc.: Toxic conc.:	**ng/mL** 10 to 100 >200	× 3.34	**nmol/L** 33 to 334 >668
Cyclosporine (Sandimmune) RIA	S	**Renal transplant** Therap. conc.: 12 h after dose: 24 h after dose: **Cardiac transplant** Therap. conc.: 12 h after dose: 24 h after dose: **Bone marrow transplant** Therap. conc.: 12 h after dose: Toxic conc.:	**ng/mL** 100 to 400 100 to 200 100 to 300 100 to 200 100 to 300 >400	× 0.832	**nmol/L** 83 to 333 83 to 166 83 to 250 83 to 166 83 to 250 >333
HPLC	WB (EDTA)	**Renal transplant** Therap. conc.: 24 h after dose: **Cardiac transplant** Therap. conc., 12 h after dose: **Hepatic transplant** Therap. conc., 12 h after dose:	**ng/mL** 100 to 200 150 to 250 100 to 400	× 0.832	**nmol/L** 83 to 166 125 to 208 83 to 333
Desipramine (Norpramin)	S or P (Hep or EDTA); trough (≥12 h after dose)	Therap.: Toxic:	**ng/mL** 75 to 300 >400	× 3.75	**nmol/L** 281 to 1125 >1500

TABLE 46-9   **Reference Values for Therapeutic and Toxic Drugs—cont'd**

Drug	Specimen		Reference Interval	Conversion Factor	Reference Interval (International Units)
Diazepam (Valium)	S or P (Hep or EDTA); trough	Therap.: Toxic:	100 to 1000 ng/mL >5000 ng/mL	× 0.0035	0.35 to 3.51 μmol/L >17.55 μmol/L
Digitoxin	S or P (Hep or EDTA); ≥8 h after dose	Therap.: Toxic:	20 to 35 ng/mL >45 ng/mL	× 1.31	26 to 46 nmol/L >59 nmol/L
Digoxin (Lanoxin)	S or P (Hep or EDTA); ≥12 h after dose	Therap.: CHF: Arrhythmias: Toxic: Adult: Child:	**ng/mL** 0.8 to 1.5 1.5 to 2.0 >2.5 >3.0	× 1.28	**nmol/L** 1.0 to 1.9 1.9 to 2.6 >3.2 >3.8
Diphenylhydantoin (*see Phenytoin*)					
Disopyramid (Norpace)	S or P (Hep or EDTA); trough	Therap.: Arrhythmias Atrial: Ventricular: Toxic:	**μg/mL** 2.8 to 3.2 3.3 to 7.5 >7	× 2.95	**μmol/L** 8.2 to 9.4 9.7 to 22.1 >20.6
Doxepin (Sinequan, Adapin)	S or P (Hep or EDTA); trough (≥12 h after dose)	Therap.: Toxic:	150 to 250 ng/mL >500 ng/mL	× 3.58	537 to 895 nmol/L >1790 nmol/L
Ephedrine (Ectasule)	S	Therap.: Toxic:	0.05 to 0.10 μg/mL >2	× 6.05	0.30 to 0.61 μmol/L >12.1
Ethchlorvynol (Placidyl)	S or P (Hep or EDTA)	Therap.: Toxic:	2 to 8 μg/mL >20 μg/mL	× 6.92	14 to 55 μmol/L >138 μmol/L
Ethosuximide (Zarontin)	S or P (Hep or EDTA); trough	Therap.: Toxic:	40 to 100 μg/mL >150 μg/mL	× 7.08	283 to 708 μmol/L >1062 μmol/L
Fenoprofen (Nalfon)	P (EDTA)	Therap.:	20 to 65 μg/mL	× 4.12	82 to 268 μmol/L
Flecainide (Tambocor)	S (Hep, EDTA)	Therap. conc.: Toxic conc.:	**μg/mL** 0.2 to 1.0 >1.0	× 2.41	**μmol/L** 0.5 to 2.4 >2.4
Flurazepam (Dalmane)	S or P (EDTA)	Therap. conc.: Toxic conc.:	Not well defined >0.2 μg/mL	× 2.58	>0.5 μmol/L

Continued

TABLE 46-9   Reference Values for Therapeutic and Toxic Drugs—cont'd

Drug	Specimen	Reference Interval		Conversion Factor	Reference Interval (International Units)
Gentamicin (Garamycin)	S or P (EDTA)		**μg/mL**		**μmol/L**
		Therap.:			
		Peak (less severe infection):			
		(severe	5 to 8	× 2.09	10.5 to 16.7
		infection):	8 to 10		16.7 to 20.9
		Trough (less severe			
		infection):	<1		<2.1
		(moderate			
		infection):	<2		<4.2
		(severe infection):	<2 to 4		<4.2 to 8.4
		Toxic:			
		Peak:	>10 to 12		>21 to 25
		Trough:	>2 to 4		>4.2 to 8.4
Glutethimide (Doriden)	S	Therap.:	2 to 6 μg/mL	× 4.60	9 to 28 μmol/L
		Toxic:	>5 μg/mL		>23 μmol/L
Haloperidol (Haldol)	S, P (Hep, EDTA)	Therap. conc.:	6 to 245 ng/mL, tentative	× 2.66	16 to 652 nmol/L
		Toxic conc.:	Not defined		
Hydromorphone (Dilaudid)	S		**ng/mL**		**nmol/L**
		Therap. conc.:	1 to 3	× 3.50	4 to 105
		Toxic conc.:	>100		>350
Ibuprofen (Motrin)	S, P (EDTA)		**μg/mL**		**μmol/L**
		Therap. conc.:	10 to 50	× 4.85	49 to 243
		Toxic conc:	100 to 700		485 to 3395
Imipramine (Tofranil)	S or P (Hep or EDTA); trough (≥12 h after dose)	Therap.:	150 to 250 ng/mL	× 3.57	536 to 893 nmol/L
		Toxic:	>500 ng/mL		>1785 nmol/L
Isoniazid (Hyzyd, Nydrazid)	S or P (Hep or EDTA)	Therap.:	1 to 7 μg/mL	× 7.29	7 to 51 μmol/L
		Toxic:	20 to 710 μg/mL		146 to 5176 μmol/L
Kanamycin (Kantrex)	S or P (EDTA)		**μg/mL**		**μmol/L**
		Therap.:			
		Peak:	25 to 35	× 2.06	52 to 72
		Trough (less severe			
		infection):	1 to 4		2 to 8
		(life threatening			
		infection):	4 to 8		8 to 17
		Toxic:			
		Peak:	>35 to 40		>72 to 82
		Trough:	>10 to 15		>21 to 31
Lidocaine (Xylocaine)	S or P (Hep or EDTA); ≥45 min following bolus dose		**μg/mL**		**μmol/L**
		Therap.:	1.5 to 6.0	× 4.27	6.4 to 26
		Toxic:			
		CNS, cardiovascular depression:	6 to 8		26 to 34.2
		Seizures, obtundation, decreased cardiac output:	>8		>34.2

TABLE 46-9   **Reference Values for Therapeutic and Toxic Drugs—cont'd**

Drug	Specimen		Reference Interval	Conversion Factor	Reference Interval (International Units)
Lithium (Eskalith)	S or P (Hep or EDTA); ≥12 h after last dose	Therap.: Toxic:	0.6 to 1.2 mmol/L >2 mmol/L	× 1	0.6 to 1.2 mmol/L >2 mmol/L
Lorazepam (Ativan)	S or P (Hep or EDTA)	Therap.: Toxic:	50 to 240 ng/mL Not defined	× 3.11	156 to 746 nmol/L
Lysergic Acid Diethylamide (LSD)	P (EDTA) U	After hallucinogenic dose:	5 to 9 ng/mL 1 to 50 ng/mL	× 3.09	15 to 28 nmol/L 3 to 155 nmol/L
Meperidine (Demerol)	S or P (Hep or EDTA)	Therap.: Toxic:	0.4 to 0.7 μg/mL >1 μg/mL	× 4.04	1.62 to 2.83 μmol/L >4.04
Meprobamate (Equanil)	S	Therap.: Toxic:	6 to 12 μg/mL >60 μg/mL	× 4.58	28 to 55 μmol/L >275 μmol/L
Methadone (Dolophine)	S or P (Hep or EDTA)	Therap.: Toxic:	100 to 400 ng/mL >2000 ng/mL	× 0.00323	0.32 to 1.29 μmol/L >6.46 μmol/L
Methamphetamine (Desoxyn)	S	Therap.: Toxic:	0.01 to 0.05 μg/mL >0.5 μg/mL	× 6.70	0.07 to 0.34 μmol/L >3.35 μmol/L
Methaqualone (Quaalude)	S or P (Hep or EDTA)	Therap.: Toxic:	2 to 3 μg/mL >10 μg/mL	× 4.00	8 to 12 μmol/L >40 μmol/L
Methotrexate	S or P (Hep or EDTA)	Therap.:	Variable **μmol/L**		Variable
		Toxic conc.: 1 to 2 wk after low-dose therapy:	>0.02		Same
		24 h after high-dose therapy:	≥5		Same
		48 h after high-dose therapy:	≥0.5		Same
		72 h after high-dose therapy:	≥0.05		Same
Methsuximide (**N-desmethyl methsuximide**) (**Celontin**)	S	Therap. Toxic:	10 to 40 μg/mL >40 μg/mL	× 5.29	53 to 212 μmol/L >212 μmol/L
Methyldopa (Aldomet)	P (EDTA)	Therap.: Toxic: (not well defined)	1 to 5 μg/mL >7 μg/mL	× 4.73	4.7 to 23.7 μmol/L >33 μmol/L
Methyprylon (Noludar)	S	Therap.: Toxic:	8 to 10 μg/mL >50 μg/mL	× 5.46	43 to 55 μmol/L >273 μmol/L
Morphine	S or P (Hep or EDTA)	Therap.: Toxic:	10 to 80 ng/mL >200 ng/mL	× 3.50	35 to 280 nmol/L >700 nmol/L
N-acetylprocainamide	S or P (Hep or EDTA); trough	Therap.: Toxic:	5 to 30 μg/mL >40 μg/mL	× 3.61	18 to 108 μmol/L >144 μmol/L

Continued

TABLE 46-9 Reference Values for Therapeutic and Toxic Drugs—cont'd

Drug	Specimen		Reference Interval	Conversion Factor	Reference Interval (International Units)
Netilmicin (Netromycin)	S or P (EDTA)	Therap. conc.: Peak:	**μg/mL**		**μmol/L**
		Less severe infections:	5 to 8	× 2.10	10 to 17
		Severe infections:	8 to 10		17 to 21
		Trough:			
		Less severe infections:	<1		<2
		Moderate infections:	<2		<4
		Severe infections:	<2 to 4		<4 to 8
		Toxic conc.:			
		Peak:	>10 to 12		>21 to 25
		Trough:	>2 to 4		>4 to 8
Nortriptyline (Aventyl)	S or P (Hep or EDTA); trough (≥12 h after dose)	Therap.: Toxic:	50 to 150 ng/mL >500 ng/mL	× 3.80	190 to 570 nmol/L >1900 nmol/L
Oxazepam (Serax)	S or P (Hep or EDTA)	Therap.: Toxic:	0.2 to 1.4 μg/mL Not defined	× 3.49	0.70 to 4.9 μmol/L
Oxycodone (Percodan)	S	Therap.: Toxic:	10 to 100 ng/mL >200	× 3.17	32 to 317 nmol/L >634
Paraldehyde	S or P (Hep or EDTA)	Therap.:	**μg/mL**		**μmol/L**
		Sedation:	10 to 100	× 7.57	76 to 757
		Anesthesia:	>200		>1514
		Toxic:	200 to 400		1514 to 3028
		Lethal:	>500		>3785
Paraquat	WB (EDTA)	Toxic:	0.1 to 1.6	× 3.89	0.39 to 6.2
	U	Occup. exp.:	0.3		1.17
		Toxic:	0.9 to 64		3.50 to 2.49
Pentazocine (Talwin)	S or P (Hep or EDTA)	Therap. conc.:	**μg/mL** 0.05 to 0.2	× 3.50	**μmol/L** 0.2 to 0.7
		Toxic conc.:	>1.0		>3.5
	U	Toxic conc.:	>3.0		>10.5
Pentobarbital (Nembutal)	S or P (Hep or EDTA); trough	Therap.:	**μg/mL**		**μmol/L**
		Hypnotic:	1 to 5	× 4.42	4 to 22
		Therap. coma:	20 to 50		88 to 221
		Toxic:	>10		>44
Phenacetin	P (EDTA)	Therap.: Toxic:	1 to 30 μg/mL 50 to 250 μg/mL	× 5.58	6 to 167 μmol/L 279 to 1395 μmol/L
Phencyclidine (Sernylan)	S or P (Hep or EDTA)	Toxic: Fatal:	90 to 800 ng/mL 500 to 4000 ng/mL	× 4.11	370 to 3288 nmol/L 2055 to 16,440 nmol/L

TABLE 46-9 Reference Values for Therapeutic and Toxic Drugs—cont'd

Drug	Specimen	Reference Interval		Conversion Factor	Reference Interval (International Units)

Pentobarbital (Luminal)	S or P (Hep or EDTA); trough	Therap.:
		Toxic:
		  Slowness, ataxia
		    nystagmus:
		  Coma with re-
		    flexes:
		  Coma without
		    reflexes:
			µg/mL
			15 to 40
			
			35 to 80
			
			65 to 117
			
			>100
				× 4.31	**µmol/L**
					65 to 172
					
					151 to 345
					
					280 to 504
					
					>431

Phensuximide (both parent and *N*-desmethyl metabolites) (Milontin)	S or P (Hep or EDTA)	Therap.:	40 to 60 µg/mL	× 5.71	228 to 324 µmol/L
Phenylbutazone (Butazolidin)	P (EDTA)	Therap.: (not well-defined) Toxic:	50 to 100 µg/mL >100 µg/mL	× 3.08	162 to 324 µmol/L >324 µmol/L
Phenytoin (Dilantin)	S or P (Hep or EDTA); trough	Therap.: Toxic:	10 to 20 µg/mL >20 µg/mL	× 3.96	40 to 79 µmol/L >79 µmol/L
Primidone (Mysoline)	S or P (Hep or EDTA); trough	Therap.: Toxic:	5 to 12 µg/mL >15 µg/mL	× 4.58	23 to 55 µmol/L >69 µmol/L
Procainamide (Pronestyl)	S or P (Hep or EDTA); trough	Therap.: Toxic: Also consider effect of metabolite (NAPA)	4 to 10 µg/mL >10 to 12 µg/mL	× 4.23	17 to 42 µmol/L >42 to 51 µmol/L
Propoxyphene (Darvon)	P (EDTA)	Therap.: Toxic:	0.1 to 0.4 µg/mL >0.5 µg/mL	× 2.95	0.3 to 1.2 µmol/L 1.5 µmol/L
Propanolol (Inderal)	S or P (Hep or EDTA); trough	Therap.: Toxic:	50 to 100 ng/mL Not defined	× 3.86	193 to 386 nmol/L
Protriptyline (Vivactil)	S or P (Hep or EDTA); collect at trough (≥12 h after dose)	Therap.: Toxic:	70 to 260 ng/mL >500 ng/mL	× 3.80	266 to 988 nmol/L >1900 nmol/L
Quinidine	S or P (Hep or EDTA); trough	Therap.: Toxic:	2 to 5 µg/mL >6 µg/mL	× 3.08	6.2 to 15.4 µmol/L >18.5 µmol/L

Continued

TABLE 46-9   Reference Values for Therapeutic and Toxic Drugs—cont'd

Drug	Specimen	Reference Interval		Conversion Factor	Reference Interval (International Units)
Salicylates	S or P (Hep or EDTA); trough		**μg/mL**		**μmol/L**
		Therap. conc.: Analgesia, anti-pyresis:	<100	× 0.00724	<0.72
		Anti-inflammatory:	150 to 300		1.09 to 2.17
		Toxic conc.: Gastric intolerance, impaired hemostasis:	>100		>0.72
		Deafness, headache, vertigo, tinnitus:	150 to 300		1.09 to 2.17
		Nausea, vomiting, hyperventilation:	250 to 400		1.81 to 2.9
		Intoxication:	>500		>3.62
Secobarbital (Seconal)	S	Therap.:	1 to 2 μg/mL	× 4.20	4.2 to 8.4 μmol/L
		Toxic:	>5 μg/mL		>21.0 μmol/L
Theophylline	S or P (Hep or EDTA)		**μg/mL**		**μmol/L**
		Therap.: Bronchodilator:	8 to 20	× 5.55	44 to 111
		Prem. apnea:	6 to 13		33 to 72
		Toxic:	>20		>110
Thiopental (Pentothal)	S or P (Hep or EDTA); trough		**μg/mL**		**μmol/L**
		Hypnotic:	1 to 5	× 4.13	4 to 21
		Coma:	30 to 100		124 to 413
		Anesthesia:	7 to 130		29 to 536
		Toxic conc.:	>10		>41
Thioridazine (Mellaril)	S or P (Hep or EDTA)	Therap.:	1.0 to 1.5 μg/mL	× 2.70	2.7 to 4.1 μmol/L
		Toxic:	>10 μg/mL		>27 μmol/L
Tobramycin (Nebcin)	S or P (Hep or EDTA); trough		**μg/mL**		**μmol/L**
		Therap.: Peak (less severe infection):	5 to 8	× 2.14	11 to 17
		(severe infection):	8 to 10		17 to 21
		Trough (less severe infection):	<1		<2
		(moderate infection):	<2		<4
		(severe infection):	<2 to 4		<4 to 9
		Toxic: Peak:	>10 to 12		>21 to 26
		Trough:	>2 to 4		>4 to 9
Tolbutamide (Orinase)	S	Therap. conc.:	80 to 240 μg/mL, tentative	× 3.70	299 to 888 μm/L
		Toxic conc.:	>640 μg/mL		>2368 μmol/L
Valproic Acid (Depakene)	S or P (Hep or EDTA); trough	Therap.:	50 to 100 μg/mL	× 6.93	346 to 693 μmol/L
		Toxic:	>100 μg/mL		>693 μmol/L
Vancomycin (Vancocin)	S or P (Hep or EDTA); trough	Therap.: Peak:	20 to 40 μg/mL	× 0.690	14 to 28 μmol/L
		Trough:	5 to 10 μg/mL		3 to 7 μmol/L
		Toxic:	>80 to 100 μg/mL		>55 to 69 μmol/L
Warfarin (Coumadin)	S or P (Hep or EDTA)	Therap.:	1 to 10 μg/mL	× 3.24	3 to 32 μmol/L
		Toxic:	>10		>32 μmol/L

TABLE 46-10 Critical Values

Test	Units	Lower Limit	Upper Limit	Comments
Blood Gases				
pH		7.2	7.6	Arterial, capillary
PCO_2	mm Hg	20	70	Arterial, capillary
PO_2	mm Hg	45		Arterial
PO_2	mm Hg	20		Capillary
HCO_3	mmol/L	10	40	Arterial, capillary
Chemistry				
Bilirubin (newborn)	mg/dL	—	15	Serum
Calcium	mg/dL	6	13	Serum
Glucose	mg/dL	40	450	Serum
Glucose (<1 y old)	mg/dL	40	400	Serum
Glucose (newborn)	mg/dL	30	200	Serum
Potassium	mmol/L	2.8	6.2	Serum
Potassium (newborn)	mmol/L	2.8	6.5	Serum
Sodium	mmol/L	120	160	Serum
Sodium (<1 y old)	mmol/L	125	150	Serum
Magnesium	mg/dL	1.0	4.7	Serum
Microalbumin	mg/g creatinine	—	<30	Urine
Hematology				
Hematocrit				
Adult	%	18	60	First report only
0 to 1 wk	%	30	65	
1 mo	%	25	65	
3 mo to 12 y	%	25	65	
Hemoglobin				
Adult	g/dL	6	20	First report only
0 to 1 wk	g/dL	10	21	
1 mo	g/dL	8	21	
3 mo to 12 y	g/dL	9	21	
WBC (adult)	$\times 10^3$	1.5	30	First report only
ER, L&D, and prenatal				
screen	$\times 10^3$	1.5	20	
12 h to 1 day	$\times 10^3$	1.5	30	
1 wk	$\times 10^3$	1.5	25	
1 wk to 12 y	$\times 10^3$	1.5	20	
Platelets	$\times 10^3$	40	1000	
Bands	%	—	23	First report only
Myelocytes	%	—	6	First report only
Blast	Leukemia patients >100,000; other patients—any seen (first report)			
Coagulation				
Fibrinogen	mg/dL	100	—	
PT	s	—	25	All patients
PTT	s	—	Method-dependent	All patients
Urinalysis				
Microscopic			RBC casts	
Cerebrospinal Fluid				
WBC (newborns)	Cells per μL	—	>30	
(>3 mo)	Cells per μL	—	>5	
Malignant cells		Any		

Selected References

Emancipator K: Critical values: ASCP practice parameter. American Society of Clinical Pathologists. Am J Clin Pathol 1997; 108:247-253.

Hortin GL, Csako G: Critical values, panic values, or alert values? Am J Clin Pathol 1998; 109:496-498.

Kost GJ: Critical limits for urgent clinician notification at US medical centers. JAMA 1990; 263:704-707.

McPherson RA (ed): Tietz Clinical Guide to Laboratory Tests, 4th edition, Philadelphia, WB Saunders, 2000.

Painter PC, Cope JY, Smith JL: Appendix. In Burtis CA, Ashwood ER (eds): Tietz Textbook of Clinical Chemistry, 3rd edition, Philadelphia, WB Saunders, 1999.

Sasse EA: How to Define, Determine, and Utilize Reference Intervals in the Clinical Laboratory. NCCLS Guideline C28-A. Wayne, Pa, National Committee for Clinical Laboratory Standards, 1995.

Tietz NW (ed): Clinical Guide to Laboratory Tests, 3rd edition, Philadelphia, WB Saunders, 1990.

Tietz NW, (ed): Clinical Guide to Laboratory Tests, 4th edition, Philadelphia, WB Saunders, 1995.

INDEX

A

AA amyloidosis, 342-343
Abdomen, peritoneal fluid
    specimen and, 39, 41
Abortion, threatened, 912
Absorbance
    of acidic potassium dichromate
      solution, 70t
    definition of, 59, 59t
    in fluorescence, 75
    of porphyrins, 587
    in spectrophotometry, *58*, 58-59
Absorbed dose of radiation, 100,
    101t
Absorption
    biotin, 563
    cholesterol, 464-465
    drug, 611-612, *612*
    flameless atomic, 56
    folic acid, 562
    iron, 597
    niacin, 557
    pantothenic acid, 563
    radioactive material, 102
    riboflavin, 553
    thiamine, 551
    vitamin A, 546
    vitamin B_6, 555
    vitamin B_{12}, 558-559
    vitamin D, 548
    vitamin K, 550
Absorption cell in
    spectrophotometry, 65
Absorption spectrophotometry,
    atomic; *see* Atomic
    absorption
    spectrophotometry
Absorption spectrum, 56, 66, *66*
Absorption test
    D-zylose, 793
    for fecal lipids, 792

Page numbers in italics indicate illustrations; *t* indicates tables; *n* indicates notes.

Absorptivity, 56
    molar, 56, 59, 59t
Abuse, drug, 659-675; *see also*
    Drug abuse
ACAT, 466
Accounting, test-cost, 277-278
ACCR, 374
Accreditation, 296
Accuracy, statistical, 234, 239, *239*
    in evaluation experiment,
      246-247
Acetaminophen
    analytical techniques for, 675
    liver disease and, 756, *757*, 763
    toxicology of, 643-645, *645*
Acetest for ketones, 449-450
Acetic acid, added to buffer, 20
Acetone, 42t
Acetylcholinesterase in pregnancy,
    912
Acetyl-CoA, 470
Acetylsalicylic acid, 645-647, *646,*
    647
Acid
    acetylsalicylic, 645-647, *646,*
      647
    amino; *see* Amino acid
    ascorbic, 544t, 564-566, *565*
    bile; *see* Bile acid
    fatty; *see* Fatty acid
    folic, 544t, *560,* 560-563, *561,*
      561t, *562*
    homogentisic
      reduction test for, 323
      as urine preservative, 40t
    homovanillic, 529, 537-538
      as urine preservative, 40t
    hydrocyanic, 638-639
    5-hydroxyindolacetic, 538-541
      smoking affecting, 48
    keto, 323
    lactic, 450
    nicotinic, 544t
      toxicity of, 557

Acid—cont'd
    nucleic; *see* Nucleic acid
    pantothenic, 544t, 563-564, *564*
    perchloric, handling of, 26
    phenylpyruvic, 323
    splattering of, 26
    uric, 422-426; *see also* Uric acid
    valproic, 624
    vanillylmandelic, 530, 537
      as urine preservative, 40t
    weak, dissociation constant for,
      19
Acid phosphatase, 352, 383-385
    blood specimen handling and,
      42t
    circadian variation in, 45t
    distribution of, 354t
    specimen preservation and, 41
Acid-base balance
    buffer systems and, 734-735
    definition of, 723
    disorders of, 738-745
      classification of, 739t
      metabolic acidosis, 740-742,
        740t
    Henderson-Hasselbalch
      equation and, 734
    mixed disorder of, 724
    parameters for, 733-734
    physiology of, 732-734, *733,*
      734
    renal mechanisms in, 737-738
    respiratory mechanism in
      regulation of, 735-737,
      736
    status of, 732-733
Acid-base measurement, 494
Acid-base property of amino acid,
    301
Acid-base titration, 116
Acidemia, 723
    methylmalonic, 309t
Acidic potassium dichromate
    solution, 70t